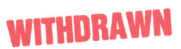

Handbook of
Nonprescription Drugs
An Interactive Approach to Self-Care

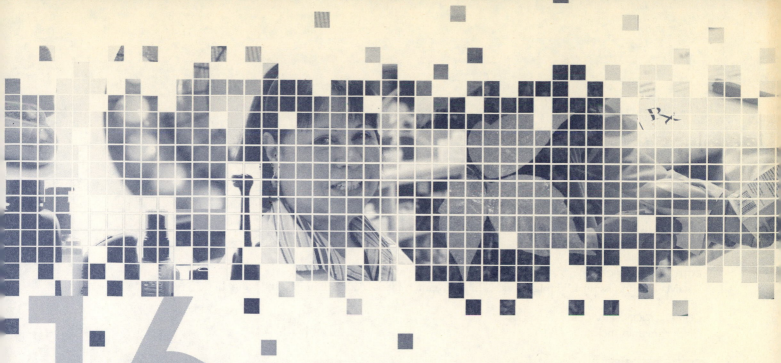

16

SIXTEENTH EDITION

Handbook of
Nonprescription Drugs

An Interactive Approach to Self-Care

Rosemary R. Berardi

Stefanie P. Ferreri

Anne L. Hume

Lisa A. Kroon

Gail D. Newton

Nicholas G. Popovich

Tami L. Remington

Carol J. Rollins

Leslie A. Shimp

Karen J. Tietze

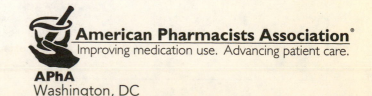

American Pharmacists Association®
Improving medication use. Advancing patient care.

APhA
Washington, DC

MANAGING EDITOR
Linda L. Young

EDITORIAL SERVICES
DataMasters Professional Editing Services, Eileen Kramer, Linda Young, Potomac Indexing, LLC

COMPOSITION SERVICES
Circle Graphics Inc.

COVER DESIGNER
Scott Neitzke, APhA Creative Services

ANATOMIC DRAWINGS
Aaron Hilmers, Gray Matter Studio, Walter Hilmers, Jr.

Published by the American Pharmacists Association
1100 15th Street, NW, Suite 400
Washington, DC 20005-1707
www.pharmacist.com

To comment on this book via e-mail, send your message to the publisher at aphabooks@aphanet.org.

Library of Congress Cataloging-in-Publication Data
Main entry under the title: Handbook of Nonprescription Drugs

ISSN 0889-7816
ISBN-13 978-1-58212-122-2

How to Order This Book
Online: www.pharmacist.com
By phone: 800-878-0729 (770-280-0085 from outside the United States and Canada)
VISA®, MasterCard®, and American Express® cards accepted.

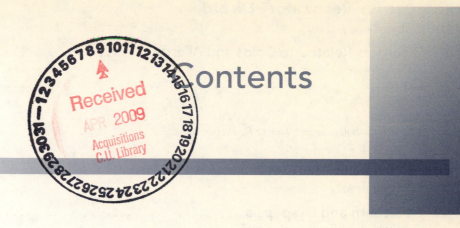

Contents

SECTION I: The Practitioner's Role in Self-Care
Editor: Nicholas G. Popovich

SECTION II: Pain and Fever Disorders
Editor: Tami L. Remington

SECTION III: Reproductive and Genital Disorders
Editor: Leslie A. Shimp

SECTION VIII: Dermatologic Disorders

Editor: Gail D. Newton

SECTION IX: Other Medical Disorders

Editor: Lisa A. Kroon

SECTION X: Home Medical Equipment

Editor: Leslie A. Shimp

SECTION XI: Complementary and Alternative Medicine
Editor: Anne Lamont Hume

Foreword

The publication of the sixteenth edition of the American Pharmacists Association's *Handbook of Nonprescription Drugs: An Interactive Approach to Self-Care* could not be more timely. The Consumer Healthcare Products Association indicates that "retail sales of nonprescription medications in the United States in 2007 exceeded $16.1 billion (excluding sales at Wal-Mart), reflecting an increase from $3.1 billion in 1972 (http://www.chpa-info.org/OTC_Retail_Sales_1964_2007_.aspx?pid=77&cc=6; last accessed November 20, 2008). Other similar surveys confirm the increased use of nonprescription medications. Sales may also be boosted by the Internal Revenue Service Ruling 2003-102, which went into effect October 1, 2003. This ruling allows employers to reimburse properly substantiated nonprescription medication expenses, but not dietary supplements, from flexible health care spending accounts. (http://www.irs.gov/pub/irs-drop/rr-03-102.pdf; last accessed November 20, 2008). The anticipated increase in the number of prescription medications that will be reclassified as nonprescription will further confound the patient's dilemma in selecting appropriate self-treatment.

The use of complementary and alternative therapies, dietary supplements, nondrug measures, diagnostic tests, and medical devices is also an integral part of self-care. The paucity of clinical evidence as to their safety and effectiveness and the potential for serious adverse events when these products are combined with nonprescription or prescription medications demand that health care practitioners be knowledgeable about alternatives to traditional medications and be able to provide therapeutic information and guidance to the consumer. Unlike nonprescription medications, no federal regulatory agency evaluates the safety and effectiveness of complementary and alternative therapies.

Numerous other factors have contributed to the growing self-care movement in the United States, including an increase in direct-to-consumer advertising of prescription and nonprescription medications. Information obtained from television commercials, newspaper and magazine advertisements, the Internet, and health-related articles serves to empower the consumer to make decisions about their own health care. However, individuals who wish to self-treat minor health disorders are faced with a staggering number of single-entity and combination nonprescription products and may not have adequate information to determine if their medical condition is amenable to self-treatment and if the self-selected treatment is appropriate for the condition.

All health care practitioners should be able to assist individuals in the management of their own self-care. However, pharmacists, because of their accessibility and expertise with respect to nonprescription and prescription medications, are in a unique position to fulfill the self-care needs of most individuals with minor health ailments. Thus, designing a self-care curriculum for pharmacy students with learning outcomes that ensure appropriate knowledge and skills is now more important than ever. The importance of this objective is reflected in the most recent Accreditation Council for Pharmacy Education's Accreditation Guidelines (http://www.acpe-accredit.org/deans/standards.asp; last accessed November 20, 2008) and the Competency Statements of the North American Pharmacist Licensure Examination (NAPLEX) taken by all United States pharmacy graduates prior to licensure (http://www.nabp.net/ftpfiles/NABP01/updatednaplexblueprint.pdf; last accessed November 20, 2008).

The sixteenth edition of the American Pharmacists Association's *Handbook of Nonprescription Drugs: An Interactive Approach to Self-Care* is an excellent and up-to-date resource for all health care educators, students, and practitioners engaged in self-care.

JOHN A. GANS, PHARMD
Executive Vice President & CEO
American Pharmacists Association

Preface

The newly revised and updated sixteenth edition of the *Handbook of Nonprescription Drugs: An Interactive Approach to Self-Care* is a comprehensive and authoritative textbook on self-care and nonprescription medications. The goal for this edition was to produce an up-to-date reference that is not only helpful to all health care professionals and students—but is also user-friendly. This edition remains true to the sprit of previous editions, namely to assist practitioners and students in developing knowledge and problem-solving skills needed to:

■ Assess a patient's health status, medical problems, and current practice of self-treatment including nonprescription and prescription mediations, dietary supplements, and other self-care measures.

■ Determine whether self-care and/or self-testing and monitoring are appropriate

■ If appropriate, recommend safe and effective self-care measures, taking into account the patient's treatment preferences.

Written and reviewed by experts, this edition of the *Handbook* continues to serve as an authoritative source for students and practitioners who guide and care for individuals undertaking self-treatment.

Highlights of New Features and Revisions

Considerable time and effort have been invested in improving this edition. We are hopeful that the following changes continue to improve the quality and usability of the book, and to provide increased clarity and convenience for students and practitioners.

■ Complementary and Alternative Medicine (CAM) Chapters: The CAM section consists of three chapters that have been significantly revised and reorganized. A new introductory chapter provides a foundation for understanding current issues with regard to natural products. This chapter also addresses quackery and provides tips to educate consumers on how to spot fraudulent claims. The botanical and nonbotanical CAM chapters in the previous edition have been combined into a single chapter and organized according to an organ system approach. In previous editions, the third CAM chapter focused solely on homeopathy. Although the homeopathy chapter possessed valuable information, it has been revised to address key points related to six different types of CAM health systems/healing practices, including naturopathy and massage. The intent of these changes was to provide the reader with a broad overview of the different health systems/healing practices that a consumer may be using.

■ Standardization of CAM Discussions in Disease-Specific Chapters: In addition to revising the CAM section, the discussions of natural products in the individual disease-specific chapters have been carefully evaluated and standardized to ensure greater consistency in the assessment of the evidence supporting or refuting the use of natural products.

■ Prevention of Pregnancy and Sexually Transmitted Infections Chapter: This chapter has been updated to include new and expanded information on the emergency contraceptive Plan B that is now available as a nonprescription product for women 18 years of age and older.

■ Primary Drug/Therapy Chapters: Selected chapters have been designated as the primary chapter to discuss the basic information about a drug or other therapy (such as fiber, nutrition, dietary supplements) when these agents are used to treat multiple disorders. Other chapters that discuss the use of these drugs or therapies will focus on information relevant to the specific disorder and will cross-reference the primary chapter for basic information.

■ Case Assessment Model: New cases were developed for each disease-related chapter.

Chapter Content

All disease-oriented chapters in this edition include the following features and information:

■ Up-to-date information on nonprescription medications including indications, dosages, interactions, supportive evidence for efficacy and safety, medical conditions or symptoms amenable to self-treatment, prescription-to-nonprescription reclassifications, and nonprescription drug withdrawals from the market.

■ Treatment algorithms that outline triage and treatment.

■ Controversies in self-care therapeutics.

■ Self-care treatment or prevention guidelines.

■ Product tables with examples of specific nonprescription products.

- New nonprescription medications and dietary supplements. Nutrition-related dietary supplements, such as vitamins and minerals, continue to be discussed in the nutrition section of the book.

Chapter Features

Most chapter features remain unchanged and are intended to promote an interactive approach to self-care. Students and practitioners can use these features to develop or improve problem-solving and critical thinking skills.

- Disease-oriented chapters are grouped primarily according to body systems. These chapters begin with a discussion of the epidemiologic, etiologic, and pathophysiologic characteristics and the clinical manifestations of the disorder. These discussions are followed by a comprehensive discussion of self-care options. The inclusion of dietary supplements, as well as nonpharmacologic and preventive measures, completes the discussion of self-care options.
- Case studies, treatment algorithms, comparisons of self-treatments, patient education boxes, and product selection guidelines foster an interactive therapeutic approach to learning.
- Sections on the evaluation of patient outcomes reinforce follow-up of patients who are self-treating. This section defines the parameters for confirming successful self-treatment and those that indicate the need for medical referral.
- Chapters include tables that list interactions (drug–drug, drug–supplement, drug–nutrient), as well as dosage and administration guidelines.
- Authors provide comparisons of agents based on clinical studies of safety and efficacy, as well as product selection guidelines based on patient factors and preferences.
- Authors discuss the role of nonprescription therapies among the available treatment options for a specific disorder and describe other options in the event that nonprescription therapy fails or is not appropriate.
- The book's organization and content allow students and practitioners to quickly identify the information needed to make a treatment recommendation and to counsel patients.

Acknowledgments

We would like to acknowledge the many individuals who contributed to the new edition of this textbook. We are grateful to the 77 authors and coauthors and 131 reviewers who contributed to this comprehensive and authoritative textbook. These individuals were selected from many practice settings and health professions throughout the country. Their scholarship and clinical experience reflect a broad perspective and interdisciplinary approach to patient care. The dedication of the authors and reviewers in ensuring that chapters were accurate, comprehensive, balanced, and relevant to practice and of the highest quality is deeply appreciated.

The editors acknowledge the work of Celtina K. Reinert, PharmD, in standardizing the discussion of natural products in the disease chapters in this edition. At that time, she was a Natural Product Information and Research Fellow, University of Missouri-Kansas City School of Pharmacy Drug Information Center.

The authors of Chapter 55 also respectfully acknowledge the work of members of the Natural Standard Research Collaboration for their support in the development of the chapter, especially the efforts of Dr. Wendy Chao, Dawn Costa, Wendy Weissner, and Jen Woods.

We would like to convey a special thanks to Linda Young, our managing editor. Ms. Young provided invaluable guidance and support to the editors and authors in all aspects related to the publication of this edition of the textbook. She contributed to the copyediting of chapters, and managed the design, editorial, and composition stages of the book. Without her experience and attention to detail, the improvements in this edition would not have been possible.

We are confident that the combined efforts of these individuals will ensure that the *Handbook of Nonprescription Drugs: An Interactive Approach to Self-Care* continues to serve as the worldwide practice and teaching resource on self-care and nonprescription products.

ROSEMARY R. BERARDI
STEFANIE P. FERRERI
ANNE L. HUME
LISA A. KROON
GAIL D. NEWTON
NICHOLAS G. POPOVICH
TAMI REMINGTON
CAROL J. ROLLINS
LESLIE A. SHIMP
KAREN J. TIETZE

February 2009

Editors

Editor in Chief and Section Editor

Rosemary R. Berardi, PharmD, FCCP, FASHP
Professor of Pharmacy, Department of Clinical Sciences,
The University of Michigan College of Pharmacy, Ann Arbor

Section Editors

Stefanie P. Ferreri, PharmD, CDE
Clinical Assistant Professor and Director, Community
Pharmacy Residency Program, University of North Carolina
Eshelman School of Pharmacy, Chapel Hill

Anne Lamont Hume, PharmD, FCCP, BCPS
Professor of Pharmacy, Department of Pharmacy Practice,
University of Rhode Island College of Pharmacy, Kingston;
Adjunct Professor of Family Medicine, Brown
University/Memorial Hospital of Rhode Island, Providence

Lisa A. Kroon, PharmD, CDE
Associate Professor of Clinical Pharmacy, Department of
Clinical Pharmacy, University of California at San Francisco
School of Pharmacy

Gail D. Newton, PhD, RPh
Associate Professor, Department of Pharmacy Practice,
Purdue University School of Pharmacy and Pharmaceutical
Sciences, West Lafayette, Indiana

Nicholas G. Popovich, PhD
Professor and Head, Department of Pharmacy Administration,
University of Illinois at Chicago College of Pharmacy

Tami L. Remington, PharmD
Clinical Pharmacist, Department of Pharmacy, The
University of Michigan Hospitals and Health System; Clinical
Associate Professor, Department of Clinical Sciences, The
University of Michigan College of Pharmacy, Ann Arbor

Carol J. Rollins, MS, RD, PharmD, BCNSP
Coordinator, Nutrition Support Pharmacy, University
Medical Center, Tucson; Associate Clinical Professor,
Department of Pharmacy Practice and Science, University of
Arizona College of Pharmacy, Tucson

Leslie A. Shimp, PharmD, MS
Professor of Pharmacy, The University of Michigan College
of Pharmacy, Ann Arbor

Karen J. Tietze, PharmD
Professor of Clinical Pharmacy, Department of Pharmacy
Practice and Pharmacy Administration, Philadelphia College
of Pharmacy, University of the Sciences in Philadelphia,
Philadelphia, Pennsylvania

Contributors

Authors

Note: Numbers in parentheses denote the chapter(s) authored or co-authored.

Mitra Assemi, PharmD (47)
Director, UCSF Fresno Pharmacy Education Program, Fresno, California; Associate Professor of Clinical Pharmacy, Department of Clinical Pharmacy, University of California at San Francisco School of Pharmacy

Cathy L. Bartels, PharmD, FAAIM (27)
Associate Professor, Department of Pharmacy Practice, Creighton University School of Pharmacy and Health Professions, Omaha, Nebraska

Rosemary R. Berardi, PharmD, FCCP, FASHP (14, 18)
Professor of Pharmacy, Department of Clinical Sciences, The University of Michigan College of Pharmacy, Ann Arbor

Daphne B. Bernard, PharmD, CACP (42)
Associate Professor, Department of Pharmacy Practice, Howard University College of Pharmacy, Nursing, and Allied Health Sciences, Washington, DC

Ilisa B. G. Bernstein, PharmD, JD (4)
Senior Advisor for Regulatory Policy, Office of Policy, Food and Drug Administration, Rockville, Maryland

Suzanne G. Bollmeier, PharmD, BCPS, AE-C (13)
Associate Professor of Pharmacy Practice, St. Louis College of Pharmacy, St. Louis, Missouri

Geneva Clark Briggs, PharmD, BCPS (51)
Clinical Associate, MedOutcomes, Inc., Richmond, Virginia

Lawrence M. Brown, PharmD, PhD (2)
Assistant Professor, Department of Pharmaceutical Sciences, College of Pharmacy; Assistant Professor, Department of Preventive Medicine, College of Medicine, University of Tennessee Health Sciences Center, Memphis

Wayne Buff, PharmD (37)
Associate Dean and Clinical Associate Professor, Department of Pharmacy Practice and Outcomes Sciences, South Carolina College of Pharmacy, Univeristy of South Carolina Campus, Columbia

Demetris M. Butler, PharmD (16)
Director of Clinical Pharmacy Programs, Clinical Pharmacy Associates, Inc., Laurel, Maryland

Juliana Chan, PharmD (18)
Clinical Assistant Professor, Department of Pharmacy Practice, College of Pharmacy; Department of Medicine, Sections of Digestive Diseases & Nutrition & Section of Hepatology, University of Illinois at Chicago

Katherine H. Chessman, PharmD, FCCP, BCNSP, BCPS (26)
Associate Professor, Department of Pharmacy Practice and Clinical Sciences, Clinical Pharmacy Specialist, Pediatrics/Pediatric Surgery, and Residency Program Director, Pediatric Pharmacy Practice, South Carolina College of Pharmacy, Medical University of South Carolina Campus, Charleston

Cynthia W. Coffey, PharmD (45)
Clinical Pharmacist, Pride Medical Pharmacy, Atlanta, Georgia

Robin L. Corelli, PharmD (50)
Professor of Clinical Pharmacy, Department of of Clinical Pharmacy, University of California at San Francisco School of Pharmacy

Kimberly M. Crosby, PharmD, BCPS (39, 40)
Clinical Assistant Professor, Department of Clinical and Administrative Sciences, The University of Oklahoma College of Pharmacy–Tulsa; Clinical Pharmacist, USA Drug, Tulsa

Barbara Insley Crouch, PharmD, MSPH (21)
Director, Utah Poison Control Center and Professor (Clinical) and Vice Chair, Department of Pharmacotherapy, University of Utah College of Pharmacy, Salt Lake City

Clarence E. Curry, Jr., PharmD (16)
Associate Professor of Pharmacy Practice, Department of Clinical and Administrative Pharmacy Sciences, Howard University College of Pharmacy, Nursing and Allied Health Sciences, Washington, DC

Patricia L. Darbishire, PharmD (35)
Clinical Assistant Professor, Department of Pharmacy Practice, Purdue University School of Pharmacy and Pharmaceutical Sciences, West Lafayette, Indiana

Lawrence W. Davidow, PhD (1)
Director, Pharmacy Skills Laboratory, Clinical Assistant Professor, Department of Pharmacy Practice, and Director, Integrated Laboratory, Kansas University School of Pharmacy, Lawrence

Cathi Dennehy, PharmD (53)
Department of Clinical Pharmacy, University of California at San Francisco School of Pharmacy

Janet P. Engle, PharmD, RPh, FAPhA (29)
Associate Dean for Academic Affairs and Clinical Professor of Pharmacy Practice, University of Illinois at Chicago College of Pharmacy

Brett Feret, PharmD (6)
Clinical Associate Professor, University of Rhode Island College of Pharmacy, Kingston

Richard G. Fiscella, RPh, MPH (28)
Clinical Professor, Department of Pharmacy Practice, College of Pharmacy; Adjunctive Assistant Professor, Department of Ophthalmology, University of Illinois at Chicago

Karla T. Foster, PharmD (38, 45)
Clinical Assistant Professor, Department of Clinical and Administrative Sciences, Mercer University Southern School of Pharmacy, Atlanta, Georgia

Cliff Fuhrman, PhD (37)
Clinical Associate Professor, Department of Pharmaceutics and Biomedical Sciences, South Carolina College of Pharmacy, University of South Carolina Campus, Columbia

Jeffery A. Goad, PharmD, MPH (19)
Associate Professor of Clinical Pharmacy, Coordinator, Community Pharmacy Program, and Director, Community Pharmacy Practice Residence, University of Southern California School of Pharmacy; Travel Health Consultant, University of Southern California Pharmacy, Student Health and Family Medicine, Los Angeles

Nicholas E. Hagemeier, PharmD, MS (36)
Pharmacist, Cowan Drugs, Inc., Lebanon, Indiana

Jennifer L. Hardman, PharmD (10)
Clinical Pharmacist and Clinical Assistant Professor, Department of Pharmacy Practice, University of Illinois at Chicago College of Pharmacy (1999–2007)

Michael D. Hogue, PharmD (46)
Assistant Professor, Department of Pharmacy Practice, Samford University McWhorter School of Pharmacy, Birmingham, Alabama

Yvonne Huckleberry, RD, PharmD (23)
Clinical Staff Pharmacist, Department of Pharmacy, University Medical Center, Tucson; Clinical Assistant Professor, College of Pharmacy, University of Arizona, Tucson

Karen Suchanek Hudmon, DrPH, MS, RPh (50)
Associate Professor, Department of Pharmacy Practice, Purdue University School of Pharmacy and Pharmaceutical Sciences, Indianapolis, Indiana

Holly Hurley, PharmD (51)
Assistant Professor of Pharmacy Practice, University of Appalachia College of Pharmacy, Grundy, Virginia

Brian J. Isetts, PhD, BCPS, FAPhA (2)
Associate Professor, Peters Institute of Pharmaceutical Care, Department of Pharmaceutical Care and Health Systems, University of Minnesota College of Pharmacy, Minneapolis

Michael Kirk Jensen, RPh, MS (28)
Clinical Associate Professor of Pharmacy Practice, University of Utah College of Pharmacy; Clinical Ophthalmic Pharmacy Specialist, John A. Moran Eye Center, Salt Lake City, Utah

Cynthia K. Kirkwood, PharmD, BCPP (48)
Vice Chair for Education and Associate Professor of Pharmacy, Virginia Commonwealth University, Richmond

Wendy Klein-Schwartz, PharmD, MPH (21)
Coordinator of Research and Education, Maryland Poison Center and Associate Professor, Department of Pharmacy Practice and Science, University of Maryland School of Pharmacy, Baltimore

Lisa A. Kroon, PharmD, CDE (50)
Associate Professor of Clinical Pharmacy, Department of Clinical Pharmacy, University of California at San Francisco School of Pharmacy

Linda Krypel, PharmD, FAPhA (30)
Professor of Pharmacy Practice, Department of Pharmacy Practice, Drake University College of Pharmacy and Health Sciences, Des Moines, Iowa

Nicole M. Lodise, PharmD (8)
Assistant Professor of Pharmacy Practice-Women's Health/Tobacco Cessation, Union University Albany College of Pharmacy; Clinical Pharmacy Specialist, Albany Medical Center, Albany, New York

Joycelyn Mallari, PharmD (19)
Assistant Professor, Department of Pharmacotherapy and Outcome Sciences, Loma Linda University School of Pharmacy, Loma Linda, California

Macary Weck Marciniak, PharmD, BCPS (32)
Clinical Associate Professor, University of North Carolina Eshelman School of Pharmacy, Chapel Hill

Cydney E. McQueen, PharmD (54)
Assistant Director, Natural Product Information and Assistant Clinical Professor, Pharmacy Practice, University of Missouri-Kansas City Drug Information Center

Patrick D. Meek, PharmD, MS (15)
Assistant Professor, Department of Pharmacy Practice, Union University Albany College of Pharmacy, Albany, New York

Sarah T. Melton, PharmD, BCPP, CGP (48)
Associate Professor of Pharmacy Practice, University of Appalachia College of Pharmacy, Oakwood, Virginia

Sarah J. Miller, PharmD (27)
Professor of Clinical Pharmacy, Department of Pharmacy Practice, University of Montana Skaggs School of Pharmacy, Missoula

Candis M. Morello, PharmD, CDE (47)
Assistant Professor of Clinical Pharmacy, Skaggs School of Pharmacy and Pharmaceutical Sciences, University of California San Diego; Clinical Pharmacist, Veterans Affairs San Diego Healthcare System, La Jolla, California

Mark Newnham, PharmD, BCPS, BCNSP (25)
Clinical Affiliate Assistant Professor, College of Pharmacy, NOVA Southeastern University, Fort Lauderdale, Florida; Clinical Coordinator, Lawnwood Regional Medical Center, Fort Pierce, Florida

Gail D. Newton, PhD, RPh (43, 44)
Associate Professor, Department of Pharmacy Practice, Purdue University School of Pharmacy and Pharmaceutical Sciences, West Lafayette, Indiana

Gloria J. Nichols-English, BSP, MED, PhD (3)
Associate Professor and Senior Fellow, Center for Minority Health Services Research, Department of Clinical and Administrative Pharmacy Sciences, Howard University College of Pharmacy, Nursing, and Allied Health Sciences, Washington, DC

Lynda Oderda, PharmD (20)
Clinical Assistant Professor, Department of Pharmacy Practice, University of Utah College of Pharmacy, Salt Lake City

Christine K. O'Neil, PharmD, BCPS, FCCP, CGP (52)
Professor of Clinical Pharmacy, Department of Pharmacy Practice, Duquesne University Mylan School of Pharmacy, Pittsburgh, Pennsylvania

Katherine Kelly Orr, PharmD (54)
Clinical Assistant Professor, University of Rhode Island College of Pharmacy, Kingston

Louise Parent-Stevens, PharmD, BCPS (10)
Clinical Assistant Professor, Department of Pharmacy Practice and Clinical Pharmacist, Family Medicine Center; University of Illinois at Chicago College of Pharmacy

Kimberly S. Plake, PhD (35)
Assistant Professor, Department of Pharmacy Practice, Purdue University School of Pharmacy and Pharmaceutical Sciences, West Lafayette, Indiana

Nicholas G. Popovich, PhD (43, 44)
Professor and Head, Department of Pharmacy Administration, University of Illinois at Chicago College of Pharmacy, University of Illinois at Chicago

Valerie T. Prince, PharmD, FAPhA, BCPS (41)
Assistant Professor of Pharmacy Practice, Samford University McWhorter School of Pharmacy; Family Practice Pharmacist, Medical Center East Family Practice Residency Program, Birmingham, Alabama

Theresa R. Prosser, PharmD, FCCP, BCPS, AE-C (13)
Professor of Pharmacy Practice, St. Louis College of Pharmacy, St. Louis, Missouri

Kristi Quairoli, PharmD (38)
Primary Care Clinical Pharmacist, Grady Health System, Atlanta, Georgia; At the time of writing: Clinical Assistant Professor and Director, Community Practice Residency, Department of Pharmacy Practice, Mercer University College of Pharmacy and Health Sciences, Atlanta, Georgia

Tami L. Remington, PharmD (5)
Clinical Pharmacist, Department of Pharmacy, The University of Michigan Hospitals and Health System; Clinical Associate Professor, Department of Clinical Sciences, The University of Michigan College of Pharmacy, Ann Arbor

Edward D. Rickert, JD, RPh (4)
Partner, Smith, Rickert, and Smith, Downers Grove, Illinois; Instructor, Adjunct Professor, Pharmacy Law, Department of Pharmacy Administration, University of Illinois at Chicago College of Pharmacy

Magaly Rodriguez de Bittner, PharmD, BCPS, CDE (3)
Chair and Professor, Department of Pharmacy Practice and Science, University of Maryland School of Pharmacy, Baltimore

Carol J. Rollins, MS, RD, PharmD, BCNSP (23, 24)
Coordinator, Nutrition Support Pharmacy, University Medical Center, Tucson; Associate Clinical Professor, Department of Pharmacy Practice and Science, University of Arizona College of Pharmacy, Tucson

Erica Rusie-Seamon, PharmD (55)
Clinical Research Associate, Natural Standard, Washington, DC

Kelly L. Scolaro, PharmD (11)
Clinical Assistant Professor and Director of Pharmaceutical Care Laboratory, Division of Pharmacy Practice and Experiential Education, The University of North Carolina Eshelman School of Pharmacy, Chapel Hill

Steven A. Scott, PharmD (33, 34)
Associate Professor of Clinical Pharmacy and Associate Head, Department of Pharmacy Practice, Purdue University School of Pharmacy and Pharmaceutical Sciences, West Lafayette, Indiana

Joan Lerner Selekof, BSN, RN, CWOCN (22)
Certified Wound Ostomy Continence Nurse, University of Maryland Medical Center, Baltimore

Laura Shane-McWhorter, PharmD, BCPS, FASCP, CDE, BC-ADM (20)
Professor (Clinical), Department of Pharmacotherapy, University of Utah College of Pharmacy, Salt Lake City

Leslie A. Shimp, PharmD, MS (8, 9)
Professor of Pharmacy, The University of Michigan College of Pharmacy, Ann Arbor

Karen J. Tietze, PharmD (12)
Professor of Clinical Pharmacy, Department of Pharmacy Practice and Pharmacy Administration, Philadelphia College of Pharmacy, University of the Sciences in Philadelphia, Philadelphia, Pennsylvania

Candy Tsourounis, PharmD (53)
Associate Professor of Clinical Pharmacy, Department of of Clinical Pharmacy, University of California at San Francisco School of Pharmacy

Catherine Ulbricht, PharmD, MBA [c] (55)
Founder, Natural Standard, Editor-in-Chief, *Journal of Herbal Pharmacotherapy*, and Senior Attending Pharmacist, Massachussetts General Hospital, Cambridge

Paul C. Walker, PharmD (17)
Clinical Associate Professor, College of Pharmacy, Department of Clinical Sciences, The University of Michigan College of Pharmacy; Manager of Clinical Services, Department of Pharmacy, The University of Michigan Health System, Ann Arbor

Amy L. Whitaker, PharmD (31)
Assistant Professor, Department of Pharmacy, Virginia Commonwealth University School of Pharmacy, Richmond

Sharon Wilson, PharmD (22)
Clinical Specialist-Surgery/Transplantation, University of Maryland Medical Center; Clinical Assistant Professor, Department of Pharmacy Services, University of Maryland School of Pharmacy, Baltimore

Michael Z. Wincor, PharmD, BCPP (49)
Director of External Programs and Associate Professor of Clinical Pharmacy, Psychiatry, and the Behavioral Sciences, Schools of Pharmacy and Medicine, University of Southern California, Los Angeles

Eric Wright, PharmD, BCPS (7)
Associate Professor, Department of Pharmacy Practice, Wilkes University Nesbitt School of Pharmacy, Wilkes-Barre, Pennsylvania

Ann Zweber, B. Pharm (14)
Senior Instructor, Department of Pharmacy Practice, Oregon State University College of Pharmacy, Corvallis

Reviewers

Note: Numbers in parentheses denote the chapter(s) reviewed.

Stephen R. Abel, PharmD (28, 29)
Assistant Dean for Clinical Programs, and Bucke Professor and Head, Department of Pharmacy Practice, Purdue University School of Pharmacy and Pharmaceutical Sciences, Indianapolis, Indiana

Renee Ahrens, PharmD, MBA (12, 18)
Associate Professor, Shenandoah University Bernard J. Dunn School of Pharmacy, Winchester, Virginia

Nicole Paolini Albanese, PharmD (31, 32)
Clinical Assistant Professor, Department of Pharmacy Practice, The State University of New York at Buffalo School of Pharmacy and Pharmaceutical Sciences; Director, Buffalo Medical Group–PGY1: Primary Care; Director, Lifetime Health - PGY1: Managed Care, Buffalo

Emily M. Ambizas, PharmD (30)
Assistant Clinical Professor, St. John's University College of Pharmacy and Allied Health Professions, Jamaica, New York; Clinical Specialist, Brooks Eckerd Pharmacy, Whitestone, New York

Kenneth A. Bachmann, PhD, FCP (49)
Distinguished University Professor (Emeritus), Department of Pharmacology, The University of Toledo College of Pharmacy; Interim Chief Executive Officer, CeutiCare, LLC, Toledo, Ohio

Becky K. Baer, BS, PharmD (40)
Associate Professor, South Dakota State University College of Pharmacy, Brookings

Danial E. Baker, PharmD, FASHP, FASCP (2)
Associate Dean for Clincial Programs, Professor of Pharmacotherapy, Department of Pharmacotherapy, Washington State University Spokane College of Pharmacy

Erin Ballard, PharmD, BCNSP (27)
University of Arizona College of Pharmacy, Tucson

Veronica T. Bandy, PharmD (30)
Clinical Assistant Professor, Pharmacy Practice Department, University of the Pacific Thomas J. Long School of Pharmacy and Health Sciences, Stockton, California

Jeffrey L. Barnett, MD (18)
Private Practitioner, Huron Gastroenterology Associates, Ypsilanti, Michigan

Cathy L. Bartels, PharmD, FAAIM (53)
Associate Professor of Pharmacy Practice, Creighton University School of Pharmacy and Health Professions, Omaha, Nebraska

Hildegarde J. Berdine, BS, PharmD, BCPS (7)
Assistant Professor of Pharmacy Practice, Department of Clinical, Social, and Administrative Sciences, Duquesne University Mylan School of Pharmacy, Pittsburgh, Pennsylvania

Tricia M. Berry, PharmD, BCPS (43, 46)
Associate Professor, Division of Pharmacy Practice, St. Louis College of Pharmacy, St. Louis, Missouri

Elizabeth Ewing Betchick, PharmD, BCPS, BCNSP (23)
Assistant Professor, Department of Pharmacy, University of Tennessee College of Pharmacy, Memphis; Clinical Pharmacy Specialist, Methodist LeBonheur Healthcare–Germantown, Germantown, Tennessee

Missy L. Blue, RPh, JD (4)
Staff Pharmacist, Walgreens, Lebanon, Indiana

Karen Beth Bohan, PharmD, BCPS (45)
Assistant Professor, Wilkes University Nesbitt College of Pharmacy and Nursing, Wilkes-Barre, Pennsylvania

Donald J. Brideau Jr., MD, MMM (50)
Family Physician, Springfield Family Medicine, Alexandria, Virginia; Assistant Clinical Professor, Georgetown Unviersity and George Washington University Schools of Medicine, Washington, DC

Tina Penick Brock, RPh, MS, EdD (50)
Management Sciences for Health, Arlington, Virginia

Wayne Buff, PharmD (1)
Associate Dean, and Clinical Associate Professor, Department of Pharmacy Practice and Outcomes Sciences, South Carolina College of Pharmacy, University of South Carolina Campus, Columbia

Stephen M. Caiola, MS, FRSH (15, 51)
Associate Professor and Director, Postgraduate/Continuing Education Program, University of North Carolina Eshelman School of Pharmacy, Chapel Hill

Lingtak-Neander Chan, PharmD, BCNSP (24)
Associate Professor, School of Pharmacy and Graduate Program in Nutritional Sciences, University of Washington, Seattle

Hae Mi Choe, PharmD, CDE (12)
Clinical Assistant Professor, Department of Pharmacy Practice, The University of Michigan College of Pharmacy, Ann Arbor

Peter A. Chyka, PharmD (21)
Professor and Associate Dean, University of Tennessee College of Pharmacy, Knoxville Campus

Martha D. Cobb, MS, MEd, CWOCN (22)
Clinical Associate Professor (Emeritus), University of Arizona College of Nursing, Tucson

Mary Petrea Cober, PharmD (6)
Clinical Pharmacist–Pediatric Surgery/Intestinal Failure Program, University of Michigan CS Mott Children's Hospital; Clinical Adjunct Assistant Professor, University of Michigan College of Pharmacy, Ann Arbor

Andrea D. Collaro, PharmD, CDM, RPh (47)
Category Manager-Diagnostics, Walgreens Company, Deerfield, Illlinois; Adjunctive Faculty, Clinical Assistant Professor, Department of Pharmacy Practice, University of Illinois at Chicago

Janice C. Colwell, MS, RN, CWOCN (22)
University of Chicago Medical Center, Chicago, Illinois

Susan Cornell, PharmD, CDE, CDM (47)
Assistant Director of Experiential Education and Assistant Professor of Pharmacy Practice, Midwestern University Chicago College of Pharmacy, Downers Grove, Illinois

Catherine M. Crill, PharmD, BCPS, BCNSP (26)
Associate Professor, Department of Clinical Pharmacy, The University of Tennessee Health Science Center, Memphis

Lourdes M. Cuellar, MS, RPH, FASHP (3)
Director, Pharmacy Department and Patient Safety Officer, Memorial Hermann–TIRR, Houston, Texas

Jeffrey C. Delafuente, MS, FCCP, FASCP (11)
Associate Dean for Professional Education, Professor of Pharmacy and Director of Geriatric Programs, Virginia Commonwealth University School of Pharmacy, Richmond

Thomas Scott Devetski, OD (29)
Associate Optometrist, Alamance Eye Center, Burlington/Chapel Hill; Clinical Assistant Professor, Department of Ophthalmology, University of North Carolina, Chapel Hill

Joseph T. DiPiro, PharmD (17)
Executive Dean, South Carolina College of Pharmacy, The Medical University of South Carolina Campus, Charleston, and The University of South Carolina Campus, Columbia

Michael B. Doherty, PharmD (47)
Director of Experiential Training and Assistant Professor of Clinical Pharmacy Practice, University of Cincinnati College of Pharmacy, Cincinnati, Ohio

Janell Norris Downing, PharmD (32)
Community Pharmacist and Medication Therapy Management Coordinator, Bear Drug, Kitty Hawk, North Carolina; Pharmacy Student Preceptor, University of North Carolina Eshelman School of Pharmacy, Chapel Hill

Jeremiah Duby, PharmD, BCPS (25)
Critical Care Clinical Pharmacist, Department of Pharmacy, U.C. Davis Medical Center, Sacramento, California; Clinical Associate Professor, College of Pharmacy, Touro University, Mare Island, Vallejo, California

B. DeeAnn Dugan, PharmD (6)
Assistant Professor of Community Pharmacy Practice, Lloyd L. Gregory School of Pharmacy, Palm Beach Atlantic University, West Palm Beach, Florida

Kaelen C. Dunican, PharmD, RPh (43)
Assistant Professor, Pharmacy Practice, Massachusetts College of Pharmacy and Health Sciences School of Pharmacy, Worcester, Massachusetts

Herbert L. DuPont, MD (17)
Chief, Internal Medicine Service, St. Luke's Episcopal Hospital; Director, Center for Infectious Diseases, University of Texas School of Public Health; Clinical Professor and Vice-Chairman of the Department of Medicine, Baylor College of Medicine, Houston, Texas

Marilyn S. Edwards, PhD, RD (25)
Professor, Department of Internal Medicine, Division of Gastroenterology, Hepatology, and Nutrition, The University of Texas Medical School at Houston

Patricia M. Elsner, PharmD (42, 43)
Staff Pharmacist, Walgreens 10974, Lafayette, Indiana

Carl F. Emswiller Jr, BS Pharmacy, FACA (30)
Pharmacist (Retired), Leesburg, Virginia

Linda M. Farho, PharmD (16)
Assistant Professor, Pharmacy Practice, University of Nebraska Medical Center College of Pharmacy, Omaha

Stefanie P. Ferreri, PharmD, CDE (16)
Clinical Assistant Professor and Director, Community Pharmacy Residency Program, University of North Carolina Eshelman School of Pharmacy, Chapel Hill

Richard Finkel, PharmD (48)
Assistant Professor, Department of Pharmaceutical and Administrative Sciences, College of Pharmacy, Nova Southeastern University, Fort Lauderdale, Florida

Daniel Forrister, PharmD (31)
Clinical Assistant Professor, Department of Clinical and Administrative Pharmacy, The University of Georgia College of Pharmacy, Athens

Karla T. Foster, PharmD (20, 33)
Clinical Assistant Professor, Department of Clinical and Administrative Sciences, Mercer University Southern School of Pharmacy, Atlanta, Georgia

Andrea R. Franks, PharmD, BCPS (18)
Associate Professor, Departments of Clinical Pharmacy and Family Medicine, University of Tennessee Health Science Center Colleges of Pharmacy and Medicine, Knoxville Campus

Conchetta White Fulton, PharmD (7)
Clinical Associate Professor, Department of Pharmacy Practice, Xavier University of Louisiana College of Pharmacy, New Orleans

Candice Garwood, PharmD, BCPS (53)
Clinical Assistant Professor, Department of Pharmaceutics/Pharmacy, Wayne State University Eugene Applebaum College of Pharmacy and Health Sciences; Clinical Pharmacy Specialist, Ambulatory Care, Harper University Hospital, Detroit Medical Center, Detroit, Michigan

Diane B. Ginsburg, MS, RPh, FASHP (3)
Clinical Professor, Division of Pharmacy Practice, Assistant Dean for Student Affairs, and Regional Director, Internship Program, The University of Texas at Austin College of Pharmacy

Jeffery A. Goad, PharmD, MPH (17)
Associate Professor of Clinical Pharmacy, Coordinator, Community Pharmacy Program, and Director, Community Pharmacy Practice Residence, University of Southern California School of Pharmacy, Los Angeles; Travel Health Consultant, University of Southern California Pharmacy, Student Health and Family Medicine, Los Angeles

William C. Gong, PharmD, FASHP, FCSHP (2)
Associate Professor of Clinical Pharmacy, and Director, Residency and Fellowship Training, University of Southern California School of Pharmacy, Los Angeles

Philip Gregory, PharmD (54)
Assistant Professor, Department of Pharmacy Practice, Creighton University, Omaha

Nicholas E. Hagemeier, PharmD, MS (39, 41)
Pharmacist, Cowan Drugs, Inc., Lebanon, Indiana

Judy Sommers Hanson, PharmD, CDM (30)
Manager, Clinical Education and Shared Faculty, Walgreens Health Initiatives, Deerfield, Illinois

Ila M. Harris, PharmD, FCCP, BCPS (55)
Associate Professor, Department of Pharmaceutical Care and Health Systems, College of Pharmacy; Adjunct Associate Professor, Medical School, Department of Family Medicine and Community Health, University of Minnesota, Minneapolis

Jan K. Hastings, PharmD (3)
Associate Professor, Department of Pharmacy Practice, University of Arkansas for Medical Services College of Pharmacy, Little Rock

Katherine Heller, PharmD (7)
Assistant Professor of Pharmacy Practice, Lloyd L. Gregory School of Pharmacy, Palm Beach Atlantic University, West Palm Beach, Florida

Metta Lou Henderson, RPh, PhD (1)
Professor Emerita of Pharmacy, Raabe College of Pharmacy, Ohio Northern University, Ada, Ohio

Karl Hess, PharmD (19)
Assistant Professor of Pharmacy Practice, Western University of Health Sciences College of Pharmacy, Pomona, California

Michelle L. Hilaire, PharmD, CDE (28)
Clinical Assistant Professor, Department of Pharmacy Practice, University of Wyoming School of Pharmacy, Laramie; Clinical Pharmacist, Fort Collins Family Medicine Residency Program, Fort Collins, Colorado

Thomas J. Holmes Jr, PhD (44)
Associate Dean and Professor, Medicinal/Pharmaceutical Chemistry/Pharmacognosy, Campbell University School of Pharmacy, Buies Creek, North Carolina

James P. Hoover, DPM (44)
Private Practitioner, Lafayette, Indiana

Daniel A. Hussar, BS Pharmacy, MS, PhD (2)
Remington Professor of Pharmacy, Philadelphia College of Pharmacy, University of the Sciences in Philadelphia, Philadelphia, Pennsylvania

Eric Jackson, PharmD, BCPS (54, 55)
Associate Professor of Family Medicine, Family Medicine Center at Asylum Hill, University of Connecticut School of Medicine and Saint Francis Hospital and Medical Center, Hartford

Pramodini B. Kale-Pradhan, PharmD (12, 20)
Associate Clinical Professor, Department of Pharmacy Practice, Eugene Applebaum College of Pharmacy and Health Sciences, Wayne State University; Clinical Specialist–Surgery, Department of Pharmacy Services, St. John Hospital and Medical Center, Detroit, Michigan

William D. King, RPh, MPH, DrPH (20)
Division Director and Professor of Pediatrics, Department of Pediatarics, The University of Alabama at Birmingham

Erika Kleppinger, PharmD, BCPS, CDE (29)
Assistant Clinical Professor, Department of Pharmacy Practice, Auburn University Harrison School of Pharmacy, Auburn, Alabama

Teresa B. Klepser, PharmD, BCPS (35)
Associate Professor, Department of Pharmacy Practice, Ferris State University College of Pharmacy, Kalamazoo, Michigan; Clinical Pharmacist, Borgess at Woodbridge Hills, ProMed Family Practice, Portage, Michigan

Erin Koopman, PharmD, BCNSP (23)
Clinical Pharmacy Specialist in Nutrition Support, Saint Marys Hospital, Mayo Clinic, Rochester, Minnesota

Jeffrey Kreitman, PharmD (6)
Regional Clinical Pharmacist, AmeriHealth Mercy Health Plan, Harrisburg, Pennsylvania

Thomas E. Lackner, PharmD (52)
Professor, Experimental and Clinical Pharmacology and Institute for the Study of Geriatric Pharmacotherapy, University of Minnesota College of Pharmacy, Minneapolis

J. Kyle Lawson, PharmD (35, 37, 38)
Pharmacist, Kroger Pharmacy J-81, Crawfordsville, Indiana

Cherokee Layson-Wolf, PharmD, CGP (28)
Assistant Professor, Department of Pharmacy Practice and Science, and Director, Community Residency Program, University of Maryland School of Pharmacy; Patient Care Program Coordinator, NeighborCare Professional Pharmacies. Baltimore, Maryland

Karen W. Lee, PharmD, CDM (11)
Associate Director of Professional Development, Clinical Pharmacy Services of Commonwealth Medicine and University of Massachusetts Medical School, Shrewsbury

Howard Madsen, RD, PharmD, CNSD (23)
Nutrition Support/Clinical Pharmacist, Samaritan Health Services, Lebanon, Oregon

Patricia Marshik, PharmD (13)
Director, Pediatric Asthma Outreach Clinics and Associate Professor of Pharmacy, University of New Mexico Health Sciences Center School of Pharmacy, Albuquerque

Beth A. Martin, PhD, RPh (50)
Assistant Professor (CHS), University of Wisconsin–Madison School of Pharmacy

Linda Gore Martin, PharmD, MBA, BCPS (8, 9)
Associate Professor, Department of Social and Administrative Pharmacy, University of Wyoming School of Pharmacy, Laramie

Marsha McFalls-Stringert, RPh, PharmD (41)
Assistant Professor of Pharmacy Practice, and Director, Academic Center for Pharmacy Practice, Department of Clinical, Social, and Administrative Sciences, Duquesne University Mylan School of Pharmacy, Pittsburgh, Pennsylvania

Emily K. Meuleman, RN, C, MS (8, 9)
Family Nurse Practitioner, Department of Family Medicine, University of Michigan, Chelsea

Susan M. Meyer, BS Pharmacy, MS, PhD (51)
Associate Dean for Education and Professor, University of Pittsburgh School of Pharmacy, Pittsburgh, Pennsylvania

Jill E. Michels, PharmD (21)
Managing Director, Palmetto Poison Center and Clinical Assistant Professor, South Carolina College of Pharmacy, University of South Carolina Campus, Columbia

Janis Miller, RN, PhD (52)
Assistant Professor of Nursing and Associate Research Scientist, Nursing, The University of Michigan School of Nursing; Research Assistant Professor of Obstetrics and Gynecology, The University of Michigan Medical School, Ann Arbor

Brad A. Miller, PharmD (5)
Clinical Specialist-Emergency Medicine, Pharmacy Department, Spectrum Health System, Grand Rapids, Michigan

Jane R. Mort, PharmD (16)
Professor of Pharmacy Practice, South Dakota State University College of Pharmacy, Brookings

David Paquette, DMD, MPH, DMSc (31, 32)
Associate Professor and Graduate Program Director, Department of Periodontology, University of North Carolina School of Dentistry, Chapel Hill

Jeegisha Patel, PharmD (28)
Clinical Assistant Professor, Department of Pharmacy Practice, Oregon State University College of Pharmacy, Oregon Health & Science University, Portland

Karen Steinmetz Pater, PharmD, BCPS, CDE (5)
Assistant Professor, University of Pittsburgh School of Pharmacy, Pittsburgh, Pennsylvania

Roy Alton Pleasants II, PharmD, BCPS (13)
Associate Professor, Campbell University School of Pharmacy, Buies Creek, North Carolina; Clinical Pharmacist in Pulmonary Medicine, Division of Pulmonary, Allergy, and Critical Care Medicine, Department of Medicine, Duke University, Durham, North Carolina

Charles D. Ponte, PharmD, BC-ADM, BCPS, CDE, FAPhA, FASHP, FCCP (10, 38)
Professor of Clinical Pharmacy and Family Medicine, Departments of Clinical Pharmacy and Family Medicine, West Virginia University Robert C. Byrd Health Sciences Center Schools of Pharmacy and Medicine, Morgantown

David R. Potts, MD (42)
Private Practitioner, Unity Healthcare, Lafayette, Indiana

Pamela Ringor, MBA, RPh (37, 39)
Staff Pharmacist, PayLess Pharmacy, Lafayette, Indiana

Ronald J. Ruggiero, PharmD (9, 10)
Clinical Professor (Emeritus), Departments of Clinical Pharmacy and Obstetrics, Gynecology, and Reproductive Sciences, Schools of Pharmacy and Medicine, The UCSF National Center of Excellence in Women's Health, The Medical Center at University of California, San Francisco

Gina J. Ryan, PharmD, BCPS, CDE (3)
Clinical Assistant Professor of Pharmacy Practice, Mercer University College of Pharmacy and Health Sciences, Atlanta, Georgia

Jasmine K. Sahni, PharmD (26)
Assistant Professor, Department of Clinical Pharmacy, University of Tennessee College of Pharmacy, Memphis

Elizabeth J. Scharman, PharmD, ABAT, BCPS, FAACT (21)
Director, West Virginia Poison Center; Professor, Department of Clinical Pharmacy, West Virginia University School of Pharmacy, Charleston

Philip Schneider, PharmD (16, 20)
Director of Pharmacy, Olathe Medical Center, Olathe, Kansas; Adjunct Clinical Assistant Professor, Department of Pharmacy Practice, University of Kansas School of Pharmacy, Lawrence

Kelly L. Scolaro, PharmD (51)
Clinical Assistant Professor and Director of Pharmaceutical Care Laboratory, Division of Pharmacy Practice and Experiential Education, The University of North Carolina Eshelman School of Pharmacy, Chapel Hill

Steven A. Scott, PharmD (45)
Associate Professor of Clinical Pharmacy and Associate Head, Department of Pharmacy Practice, Purdue University School of Pharmacy and Pharmaceutical Sciences, West Lafayette, Indiana

Chad Shedron, PharmD (33, 34)
Owner, Family Pharmacare, Lafayette, Indiana

Debra Sibbald, BSc Phm, ACPR, MA, PhD [candidate] (36)
Coordinator, Pharmaceutical Care I, University of Toronto Faculty of Pharmacy, Mississauga, Ontario, Canada

John K. Siepler, PharmD, BCNSP, FCCP (14)
Research Specialist, Nutrishare, Inc., Elk Grove, California; Clinical Professor, University of California at San Francisco School of Pharmacy

Heather Skillman, MS, RD, CSP, CNSD (26)
Pediatric Critical Care Dietitian, The Children's Hospital, Denver, Colorado

Susan Claire Smolinske, PharmD (21)
Poison Control Center, Children's Hospital of Michigan, Detroit

Jenelle L. Sobotka, PharmD (1)
Manager, Professional Relations, The Procter and Gamble Company, Cincinatti, Ohio

Vanessa A. Stanford, MS, RD, CSCS (25)
Research Specialist, Sr., Department of Nutritional Sciences, University of Arizona College of Agriculture and Life Sciences, Tucson

Scott K. Stolte, PharmD (17)
Chair, Department of Pharmacy Practice, Shenandoah University Bernard J. Dunn School of Pharmacy, Winchester, Virginia

Donald L. Sullivan, PhD (51)
Associate Professor of Pharmacy Practice, Department of Pharmacy Practice, Ohio Norhtern University College of Pharmacy, Ada

Keith A. Swanson, PharmD (48)
Associate Professor, Department of Pharmacy Practice, University of Oklahoma College of Pharmacy, Oklahoma City

Larry N. Swanson, PharmD, FASHP (34)
Professor and Chairman, Department of Pharmacy Practice, Campbell University School of Pharmacy, Buies Creek, North Carolina

Sahar Swidan, PharmD (5)
Clinical Associate Professor, Department of Clinical Sciences, The University of Michigan College of Pharmacy; President and CEO, Pharmacy Solutions, Ann Arbor, Michigan

Jane Takagi, PharmD, FCSHP, FASHP (27)
Adjunct Associate Professor of Pharmacy Practice, University of Southern California School of Pharmacy, Los Angeles; Assistant Clinical Professor, Department of Clinical Pharmacy, University of California at San Francisco School of Pharmacy; Kaiser Permanente Drug Information Services, Downey, California

Jeff G. Taylor, PhD (11)
Associate Professor of Pharmacy, University of Saskatchewan College of Pharmacy and Nutrition, Saskatoon

Jeremy Lynn Thomas, PharmD (15)
Assistant Professor, Department of Clinical Pharmacy, University of Tennessee Health Science Center College of Pharmacy, Memphis

Cynthia Thomson, RD, PhD (24)
Associate Professor, Department of Nutritional Sciences, University of Arizona, Tucson

Michael S. Torre, MS, RPh, CDE (47)
Clinical Professor of Pharmacy, Department of Clinical Pharmacy Practice, College of Pharmacy and Allied Health Professions, St. John's University, Jamaica, New York

Dominic P. Trombetta, PharmD, BCPS, CGP (46)
Associate Professor of Pharmacy Practice, Wilkes University Nesbitt School of Pharmacy, Wilkes-Barre, Pennsylvania; Allied Services Rehabilitation Hosptial & Outpatient Centers, Scranton, Pennsylvania

Candy Tsourounis, PharmD (48, 49)
Associate Professor of Clinical Pharmacy, Department of of Clinical Pharmacy, University of California at San Francisco School of Pharmacy

Angela R. Vinti, PharmD, BCPS (30)
Assistant Clinical Professor, Department of Pharmacy Practice, Auburn University Harrison School of Pharmacy, Mobile Satellite Campus; Adjunct Assistant Professor, Department of Family Medicine, University of South Alabama College of Medicine, Mobile

Paul C. Walker, PharmD (19, 36)
Clinical Associate Professor, College of Pharmacy, Department of Clinical Sciences, The University of Michigan; Manager of Clinical Services, Department of Pharmacy, The University of Michigan Health Systems, Ann Arbor

Geoffrey C. Wall, RPh, PharmD, BCPS, CGP (14)
Associate Professor of Pharmacy Practice, College of Pharmacy and Health Sciences, Drake University; Internal Medicine Clinical Pharmacist and Director, Pharmacy Practice Residency Program, Iowa Methodist Medical Center; Clinical Assistant Professor of Pharmacology/Physiology, Des Moines University College of Osteopoathic Medicine, Des Moines, Iowa

C. Wayne Weart, PharmD (14)
Professor, Department of Pharmacy and Clinical Sciences, South Carolina College of Pharmacy, Medical University of South Carolina Campus; Associate Professor of Family Medicine, Medical University of South Carolina, Charleston

Kristin Weitzl, PharmD (19)
Assistant Editor, *Pharmacist's Letter* and *Prescriber's Letter*, Stockton, California; Clinical Associate Professor (Adjunct), Department of Pharmacy Practice, University of Florida College of Pharmacy, Gainesville, Florida

Amy L. Whitaker, PharmD (40)
Assistant Professor, Department of Pharmacy, Virginia Commonwealth University School of Pharmacy, Richmond

G. Thomas Wilson, BS Pharm, JD (4)
Associate Professor of Pharmacy Practice and Law, Department of Pharmacy Practice, Purdue University School of Pharmacy and Pharmaceutical Sciences, West Lafayette, Indiana

Kenneth W. Witte, PharmD (24)
Adjunct Clinical Associate Professor, University of Illinois at Chicago College of Pharmacy; President, Clinical Pharmacy Consultants, Inc., LaGrange, Illinois

Supakit Wongwiwatthananukit, PharmD, PhD (50)
Assistant Professor, Department of Pharmacy Practice, College of Pharmacy, University of Hawaii, Hilo

John R. Yuen, PharmD, BCNP (28, 29)
Board Certified Nuclear Pharmacist, Oncology Pharmacist Specialist (Hospital and Ambulatory Care), Kaiser Permanente Los Angeles Medical Center; Adjunct Assistant Professor of Pharmacy Practice, University of Southern California School of Pharmacy, Los Angeles

Ann Zweber, B. Pharm (15)
Senior Instructor, Department of Pharmacy Practice, Oregon State University College of Pharmacy, Corvallis

How to Use the Case Problem-Solving Model

Rationale for Case Format

Use of a problem-solving model is one mechanism for developing problem-solving skills. Repeated exposure to the model in a variety of contexts aids students in learning the model and applying it in various circumstances. Use of the model in each diseases-related chapter in this text provides repeated exposure and reinforces learning.

Case Format Description

The case format is based on the guided-design instructional format that models the steps of decision making. This format facilitates student development of a framework for the organization and application of acquired information to the solution of novel problems. The basic steps used in the guided-design decision-making format are as follows.

- Gather information pertinent to the problem and its solution.
- Identify the problem.
- Identify exclusions for self-treatment.
- Perform patient assessment and triage.
- Identify alternative solutions.
- Select an optimal solution.
- Prepare and implement a plan to solve the problem.
- Provide patient education.
- Evaluate patient outcome.
- When outcomes do not achieve the self-treatment goal, start the process again from the beginning.

Steps 1 and 2: Gather Information

When a patient presents to a practitioner and is in need of self-care advice, the practitioner must collect information about the patient that may be pertinent to solving the patient's problem. This information falls into two general categories: (1) information about the symptoms that prompted the patient to seek assistance and (2) information about the patient's background characteristics (history). The first two steps in the case format direct the student to elicit this type of information.

It may be argued that it is unnecessary to collect all the patient's background characteristics to solve every patient problem. However, it should be remembered that novice problem solvers do not yet have the expertise to selectively elicit the most pertinent information to a specific situation. Thus, the model prompts them to ask about all of the listed characteristics to avoid overlooking information that is critical to the solution of the problem.

Step 3: Identify the Problem

The third step involves the evaluation of information gathered in the previous steps to identify the patient's problem, its severity, and its most probable cause. Clear articulation of the problem is critical to (1) assist with differentiation among conditions with similar symptoms and (2) determine the goals of self-treatment. A comparison of the patient's symptoms to the usual or typical presentation of symptoms for a particular disease will help to differentiate and determine the most likely primary problem. For example, it is inadequate to conclude that a patient's problem is a common cold. In this instance, the therapeutic goal—to relieve the cold—is too vague to be useful, because there are dozens of symptoms that may or may not be associated with the common cold and there are even more alternatives for symptomatic relief. On the other hand, if the patient's problem is nasal congestion, the goal would be to relieve the congestion: This goal is a much more useful criterion against which to evaluate a more limited set of potential therapeutic options.

Step 4: Identify Exclusions for Self-Treatment

There are several reasons why it may be inappropriate for an individual to self-treat the symptoms or problems they are experiencing, which include (1) symptoms should not be self-treated because medical referral is necessary (e.g., eye pain); (2) patient is not an appropriate candidate for self-care (e.g., a woman with diabetes who develops a vaginal candidal infection); (3) symptoms are too severe or long-lasting for self-treatment; or (4) effective nonprescription therapy is not available, or nonprescription dosages or duration of treatment is inadequate to treat the disorder.

Assessing the severity and determining the most likely primary problem that a patient is experiencing are essential in making appropriate recommendations for treatment or referral. For example, a patient who complains of a cough associated with a cold is often a candidate for self-care. However, if the cough is significantly hampering the patient's ability to sleep or carry out routine activities, or if the cough produces pain in the chest area, referral to a primary care provider may be appropriate. In another instance, a patient who complains of a mild cough may not be a candidate for self-care if other information about the condition (e.g., history of tobacco use and emphysema) suggests an etiology that is not amenable to self-management.

Step 5: Identify Alternative Solutions

The fifth step involves formulation of a list of possible approaches to the patient's problem. At this point, no alternative is prejudged or omitted. Four general options are available to practitioners who are advising patients about self-care: (1) recommend self-care with drug, nondrug, and/or alternative/complementary therapies; (2) refer patient to an appropriate primary care provider for treatment; (3) recommend self-care until an appropriate primary care provider can be consulted; and (4) take no action. In the context of self-treatment, all potentially plausible product categories, dosage forms, and nondrug products and measures should be included in the list. In the context of self-treatment, all potentially plausible product categories, dosage forms, and nondrug products and measures should be included in the list. Similarly, all potentially useful sources of primary care (e.g., urgent care clinic, dentist, or emergency department) should be considered.

Critics of this approach have sometimes indicated that including no action as an option is unconscionable or not in the best interest of patients. In fact, there are situations in which this option may be preferred. For example, consider a situation involving a patient on a limited income who suffers from an asymptomatic, common wart that is in a location where it is neither noticeable nor likely to be spread easily to others. Because most common warts resolve spontaneously without treatment and the patient has limited income to pay for a nonprescription product, taking no action may indeed be an optimal solution in this instance. Furthermore, the crucial point often overlooked by critics is that, at this point in the decision-making process, all ideas are listed and none are prejudged. Thus, it is entirely appropriate to consider no action, even if it turns out to be an inappropriate alternative. Again, this format is targeted at novice problem solvers who have little experience in identifying alternative therapeutic options. Thus, the model prompts them to formulate a list of all possible alternatives to prevent them from prematurely ruling out appropriate options.

Step 6: Select an Optimal Solution

During the sixth step, each of the plausible solutions is evaluated to determine whether and to what extent each achieves the intended goal and is concordant with the patient's preferences in terms of goals of therapy, cost of therapy, and overall approach (e.g., personal philosophy, health beliefs) to self-care. Next, one of the alternatives that may adequately achieve the goal is selected on the basis of a variety of patient-specific and therapy-specific variables. Therapy-specific variables include dosage forms, ingredients, side effects, adverse reactions, relative effectiveness, and price. Patient-specific variables may include age, sex, medication history, concurrent medical conditions, patient preferences, and economic status.

Steps 7 and 8: Prepare and Implement a Plan

These steps involve the communication of a therapeutic plan to the patient. The plan should include a summary of the condition and the reasons for treatment. The patient should be made aware of the available treatment options and their relative merits should also be included in the plan. When the recommended solution involves drug therapy, the plan should include monitoring parameters.

Steps 9-11: Educate Patient

Patient education is designed to provide a clear and concise description of administration of the treatment, side effects and precautions, expected outcome, and guidelines for appropriate use. When appropriate, the plan should also include nondrug measures, lifestyle changes, and additional information resources.

The practitioner should ensure that the patient understands the plan by having the patient repeat it and by correcting any misunderstandings. Finally, after answering any remaining questions from the patient, the practitioner should encourage the patient to call or return if the symptoms fail to resolve. If symptoms are not resolved, the entire decision-making procedure begins anew.

SECTION

1

The Practitioner's Role in Self-Care

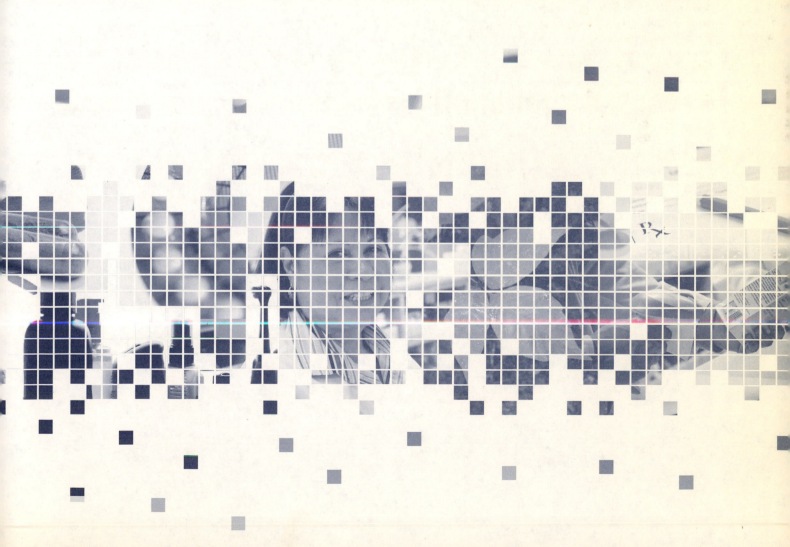

Self-Care and Nonprescription Pharmacotherapy

Lawrence W. Davidow

Self-Care

Self-care is the independent act of preventing, diagnosing, and treating one's own illnesses without seeking professional advice. Preventive self-care involves maintaining well-being and appearance through exercise and a healthy lifestyle. For many individuals, a healthy lifestyle includes controlling their diet; taking vitamins, minerals, and herbal supplements; and maintaining their appearance by using dental, skin, and hair-care products. However, sickness self-care for individuals involves diagnosing their conditions, and obtaining products for the goal of mitigating illness and relieving symptoms. Examples of sickness self-care include dietary options (e.g., feeding warm soup for a cold), using devices for both disease assessment (e.g., home blood glucose meters and pregnancy tests) and treatment (e.g., ice packs, first-aid bandages, vaporizers, and nasal strips), as well as taking nonprescription medications. The use of sickness self-care products is limited to mild illness or short-term management of illness, and most products warn users to contact a health care provider if conditions do not improve within a short period of time.

For the provision of sickness self-care, a single individual from each household usually plays a leading role in adopting a course of action. This individual must determine whether to consult a health care provider or whether the use of home remedies and self-care will suffice. Furthermore, the number of individuals involved in choosing the most appropriate self-care option is increasing, owing to the growth of the U.S. geriatric population and the decreasing number of persons per household.[1]

Individuals responsible for providing self-care to themselves or family members rely on knowledge and experience to guide their decisions. For better or worse, there is no shortage of information, given the wealth of health-related self-help books, newspaper feature articles, television advertisements, magazine and radio programs, instructional audio- and videotapes, and Internet sites, all of which provide self-care advice. The abundance of health-related information available, especially from the Internet, helps consumers become more "self-empowered" to address their own health care issues and leads to an aggressive use of self-care alternatives. Nevertheless, although it is more accepted today for people to attempt to manage their own health-related issues rather than to consult a health care provider, the concern is whether they are making appropriate and informed judgments. Furthermore, all this health information can become overwhelming, driving some individuals to seek advice from family and friends. This well-intentioned advice can be prob-

lematic, because it is often biased, and most people are not sufficiently informed to consider another's health conditions or medications before making a recommendation. They simply state what has worked best for them and fail to consider how their approach might apply to someone else.

Commercial products used for preventive or sickness self-care are often classified together as health and beauty care (HBC) products. Staggering numbers of HBC products are available. For example, Figure 1-1 illustrates the number of commercial products available in 2006 for various categories of preventive and sickness self-care.[2] Although access to quality HBC products is crucial to the goal of self-care, the vast number of similar, competing products makes appropriate selection difficult. Yet, in one consumer poll in which 66% of adults believed that the wide range of competing products made selection difficult, less than half (43%) said they consulted a pharmacist before making a purchase.[3] The pharmacist plays a crucial role in assisting patients who are seeking both types of self-care products. The practicing pharmacist has the expertise to screen patient health information and apply his or her knowledge and training to select products according to individual health care needs. Therefore, for pharmacies to provide pharmacist-assisted self-care, only quality HBC products should be stocked, and access to a pharmacist for assistance should be readily available for patients who request it.

Self-Medication

Self-medication is often the most sought-after first level of self-care. As self-care has increased, so has the practice of self-medication with vitamins (i.e., nutritional dietary supplements), natural products (i.e., herbal/botanical and nonherbal dietary supplements [e.g., glucosamine]), and nonprescription medications. Factors that help drive reliance on self-medication include (1) the increase in size of the aging population, (2) restricted access to prescribers through health management organizations, (3) the increasing costs of health care, and (4) the high proportion of underinsured or uninsured people in the U.S. population. It is the easy access and cost-effectiveness of self-medication products that ensure their essential role in the U.S. health care system.

The results of a survey conducted for the National Council on Patient Information and Education (NCPIE)[4] illustrate how ubiquitous the use of nonprescription medications has become. According to the survey, 59% of Americans had taken at least

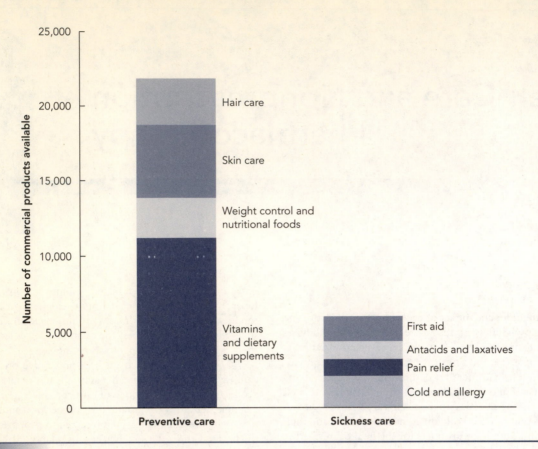

FIGURE 1-1 Number of HBC products for selected departments in 2006. (*Source:* Reference 2.)

one nonprescription medication in the last 6 months. Conditions commonly treated with nonprescription medications included:

- Pain (78%)
- Cough/cold/flu/sore throat (52%)
- Allergy/sinus problems (45%)
- Heartburn, indigestion (37%)
- Constipation/diarrhea/gas (21%)
- Minor infections (12%)
- Skin problems (10%)

Approximately 20% of Americans believe that they are consuming more nonprescription medications and taking them more frequently than they did 5 years ago.[4] This increase in nonprescription drug use may reflect a consumer belief that self-medication can be accomplished safely. A survey published by Roper Starch Worldwide "Self-Care in the New Millennium" supports the view that American consumers are confident in their use of nonprescription medications.[5] Survey results show that:

- 73% would rather try and treat their own condition than go to a physician.
- More than 80% stated that they were satisfied with the nonprescription medications they used to treat their most recent health problems.
- 87% believe that nonprescription medications are safe when used as directed.
- 90% or more stated that the first time they took a nonprescription medication, they took time to read package labels regarding the correct choice, directions for use, and side effects and drug interactions.

In addition, self-medication plays an increasing role as adjunctive therapy for chronic diseases that are managed by physicians with prescription medications. Examples include low-dose aspirin for reducing heart attack risk, fish oil (omega-3 fatty acids) to help treat certain dyslipidemias, and glucosamine with chondroitin to help reverse osteoarthritis. However, the benefits of using nonprescription products as adjunctive therapy come with a risk of harm resulting from incorrect selection of products. For example, many patients who require daily low-dose aspirin do not fully understand the difference between the many different aspirin products. There are different strengths (low-dose, regular, and extra-strength) and products (chewable, buffered, and enteric-coated). Selection of the wrong product by a patient could result in adverse reactions (e.g., gastritis or ulcer) or drug–drug interactions (e.g., warfarin, blood pressure medications). The pharmacist plays an important role in helping these patients select the correct products for their condition.

Options for Self-Medication

Three general categories of products are available to consumers for self-medication: (1) nonprescription medications, (2) nutritional dietary supplements, and (3) natural products and homeopathic remedies.

Nonprescription Medications

Nonprescription medications are regulated by the Center for Drug Evaluation and Research, a division of the U.S. Food and Drug Administration (FDA)—the same agency that regulates prescription drug products. As such, nonprescription medications are held to the same standards of drug product formulation (e.g., purity and stability), labeling, and safety (benefits outweigh risks) as those for prescription medications. It is worth noting that, although nonprescription medications are regulated in a manner equivalent to that of prescription medications, the sales of nonprescription medications are not limited to pharmacies; they are commonly sold at discount stores and supermarkets.

The provisions of the 1951 Durham-Humphrey Amendment to the Food, Drug, and Cosmetic Act (FDC Act) of 1938 gives FDA the final authority to categorize a medication as prescription or nonprescription. Nonprescription medications are judged by FDA as safe and effective when used without a prescriber's directive and oversight. In 2000, more than 100,000 FDA-approved nonprescription drug products, including more than 800 active ingredients that covered more than 100 therapeutic categories, were available.[6] Table 1-1 illustrates some of the conditions that are self-treatable with nonprescription medications.

Sales of nonprescription medications were estimated in 2003 at $17.5 billion dollars. Sales of the top 15 therapeutic categories of nonprescription medications for the years 2003–2006 are shown in Figure 1-2.[7] Not surprisingly, the dollars spent, as shown in Figure 1-2, correspond to what consumer surveys have reported as the most common conditions. For example, in a survey in which consumers were asked what health problems they had experienced in the preceding 6 months, the most frequent response was muscle/back/joint pain and cough/cold/flu/sore throat, both categories at 48%, with headache and heartburn/indigestion trailing at 43% and 32%, respectively.[5] The correlation between common types of illnesses and dollars spent implies that most Americans provide self-care for these conditions using nonprescription medications.

Dietary Supplements

The Dietary Supplement Health and Education Act of 1994 amended the 1983 FDC Act to establish standards with respect to dietary supplements. This new act defined dietary supplements as products that are intended to supplement the diet and bear or contain one or more of the following dietary ingredients: (1) a vitamin, (2) a mineral, (3) an herb, or (4) an amino acid. A 1999–2000 survey indicated that 52% of consumers had taken a dietary supplement in the previous month.[8] The most common supplements taken in this survey were multivitamin/multimineral formulations (35%), vitamin E (13%), vitamin C (12%), and calcium (10%). High demand has created a huge dietary supplement industry, with yearly sales in 2003 totaling nearly $18.8 billion dollars.[8]

CAM and Homeopathic Remedies

Because of factors such as high health care costs and restricted access to conventional practitioners, many consumers seek treatment from providers of complementary and alternative medicine (CAM). The National Center for Complementary and Alternative Medicine and the National Center for Health Statistics reported survey results on the use of CAM by Americans.[9] Between 36% and 74% of the people surveyed reported having used some form of CAM therapy. Some of the most common forms of CAM therapy were prayer, natural and vitamin products, deep breathing, chiropractic care, and yoga.[9]

Self-medication is a component of many CAM therapies. In 2005, total estimated sales of natural products were $4.41 billion, the top-selling supplements being garlic, echinacea, saw palmetto, and *Ginkgo biloba*.[10] A 2002 National Health Survey indicated that

TABLE 1-1 Selected Medical Disorders Amenable to Nonprescription Drug Therapy[a]			
Abrasions	Colds (viral upper respiratory infection)	Gastritis	Ostomy care
Aches and pains (general, mild-to-moderate)	Congestion (chest, nasal)	Gingivitis	Ovulation prediction
Acidity	Constipation	Hair loss	Periodontal disease
Acne	Contact lens care	Halitosis	Pharyngitis
Albumin testing	Contraception	Morning hangover relief	Pinworm infestation
Allergic reactions	Corns	Head lice	Pregnancy (diagnostic)
Allergic rhinitis	Cough	Headache	Premenstrual syndrome
Anemia	Cuts (superficial)	Heartburn	Prickly heat
Arthralgia	Dandruff	Hemorrhoids	Psoriasis
Asthma	Decongestant, nasal	Herpes	Ringworm
Athlete's foot	Dental care	Impetigo	Seborrhea
Bacterial infection	Dermatitis (contact)	Indigestion	Sinusitis
Blisters	Diabetes mellitus (insulin, monitoring equipment, supplies)	Ingrown toenails	Smoking cessation
Blood pressure monitoring		Insect bites and stings	Sprains
Boils		Insomnia	Strains
Bowel preparation (diagnostic)	Diaper rash	Jet lag	Stye (hordeolum)
Burns (minor, thermal)	Diarrhea	Jock itch	Sunburn
Calluses	Dry skin	Migraine	Teething
Candidal vaginitis	Dyslipidemia	Motion sickness	Thrush
Canker sores	Dysmenorrhea	Myalgia	Toothache
Carbuncles	Dyspepsia	Nausea	Vomiting
Chapped skin	Fever	Nutrition (infant)	Warts (common and plantar)
Cold sores	Flatulence	Obesity	Xerostomia
		Occult blood, fecal (detection)	Wound care

[a] The pertinent nonprescription medication(s) for a particular disorder may serve as primary or major adjunctive therapy.
Source: Rulemaking History for Nonprescription Products: Drug Category List. Available at: http://www.fda.gov/cder/otcmonographs/rulemaking_index.htm. Last accessed July 28, 2008.

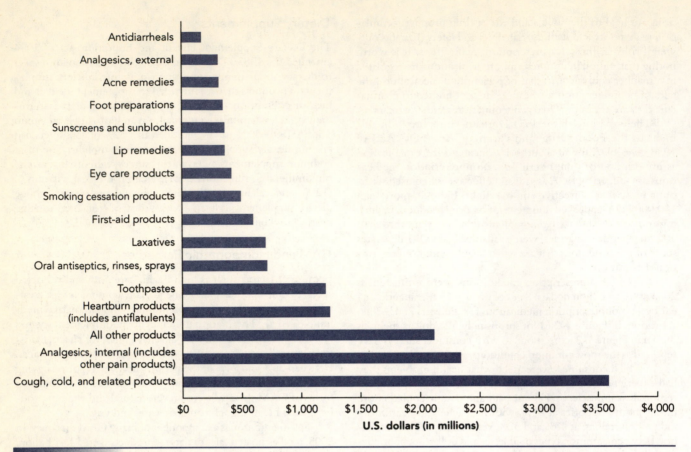

FIGURE 1-2 2006 sales of U.S. nonprescription drugs. (*Source:* Reference 7.)

about 13% of elderly patients had used an herbal supplement during the preceding year.[11] The use of combined herbal and conventional therapy raises safety concerns, because 51% of patients failed to inform their health care provider about their herbal therapy.[11] These safety concerns include the potential for herbal supplement–drug interactions. *Facts & Comparisons: Drug Interaction Facts* (St. Louis: Wolters Kluwer Health; 2007) lists approximately 150 herb–drug interactions, with St. John's wort and *Ginkgo biloba* having 59 and 20 interactions, respectively. Therefore, individuals who take prescription or nonprescription medications should consult with a pharmacist or other health care provider before self-medicating with herbal supplements.

Influences on Self-Medication

Costs

Individuals can save money by purchasing nonprescription medications using money from a flexible spending account (FSA). These accounts were established when the Internal Revenue Service began allowing reimbursement of medically substantiated nonprescription medications with pretax dollars.[12] Reimbursable expenses include "nonprescription drugs" defined in the 1938 FDC Act as "alleviating or treating" personal injuries/illness, but only those that make such therapeutic claims on their labels are eligible. Also qualified for pretax reimbursements of health care dollars are dietary supplements if the patient's physician has suggested their use for the treatment/mitigation of an illness, such as iron for iron-deficiency anemia. Dietary supplements such as vita-

mins, minerals, and natural products, which are "merely beneficial to the general health," are not eligible as pretax expenses.

In 2006, approximately 10% of Americans used FSAs to pay for health care expenses.[13] The disadvantage of using FSAs is that the money must be allocated in advance and is either used within a plan year or lost. This "use-it-or-lose-it" feature encourages people to limit their FSA contributions.[14] Furthermore, consumers are confused about what purchases are FSA-eligible. For example, it has been reported that less than half of the money spent from FSA accounts is for eligible purchases.[13] Pharmacists play a role in educating patients about what purchases are FSA-eligible and in encouraging FSA use by reminding patients to use their FSA debit card when purchasing nonprescription medications.

In 2003, the Medicare Modernization Act established Health Savings Accounts (HSAs), whereby individuals who are enrolled in a High Deductible Health Plan may contribute pretax dollars that can be used to pay for health-related expenses. These accounts function as normal savings accounts with accruable and interest-bearing balances that grow over time. However, with HSAs, both contributions and disbursements are tax-free as long as they are spent on health care.[14] Unlike FSAs, purchases for nonprescription medications from HSAs have no time limit; the HSA balance will roll over to the next tax year.

Whether from FSA or HSA accounts, the medical expense "pretax" deduction is becoming increasingly popular as Americans pay more for "out-of-pocket" health care costs. In 2004, 5.02% of taxpayers claimed medical expense deductions, up from 4.3% in 1997.[15] Consumers have an economic incentive to use low-cost nonprescription medications rather than expensive prescription medications (with high insurance copayments), which in turn gives pharmacists greater opportunity for therapeutic counseling.

The Medicare Modernization Act of 2003 also established Medicare Part D prescription coverage. When the plan was first introduced, it did not pay for nonprescription medications, even when their use was directed by a physician.[16] However, beginning in 2007, the Centers for Medicare & Medicaid Services began loosening restrictions on coverage of nonprescription medications that are less expensive than prescription alternatives in a Medicare Part D plan's formulary. It is expected that many Medicare drug plans will likely pay for nonprescription medications to drive utilization and reduce costs for medications such as proton pump inhibitors, nonsteroidal anti-inflammatory drugs, and antihistamines, which all have low-cost nonprescription alternatives.[16]

Aging Population

New projections illustrate the magnitude of the still-to-come elderly boom. The average life expectancy for Americans has increased, with individuals reaching age 65 expected to live an additional 12.4 years.[17] The percentage of older Americans started to increase sharply as the baby boom generation approached the 65 and older age group.[18] By 2030, an estimated 20% (70 million) of the U.S. population will be 65 years or older, up from 12.6% (35 million) in 2000.[19] The fastest-growing segment of the elderly are those older than 85 years.[18] Because these patients tend to be in poorer health and require more services than patients between 65 and 85 years, they will have a bigger impact on the future of the U.S. health care system.

Elderly patients consume a disproportionately larger share of nonprescription medications; patients older than 65 years purchase 40% of all nonprescription medications, although they represent only 12% of the population.[20] One study in elderly nursing home patients showed that use of nonprescription medications (93.9%) was only slightly less than that of prescription medications (98.2%).[21] This study noted that, on average, nursing home residents used 8.8 unique medications per month, one-third (2.8) of which were nonprescription medications. Increased use

of nonprescription medications in the elderly can be attributed to the following:

- Conditions for which nonprescription medications are used, such as arthritis pain, insomnia, and constipation, become more prevalent with advancing age.
- Nonprescription medications provide low-cost alternatives to more expensive primary care visits and prescription medications.
- Accessibility to pharmacists in the community setting makes nonprescription medications an acceptable alternative to scheduling visits with primary care providers.

There are heightened safety concerns for elderly patients who use nonprescription medications because of the likelihood for multiple disease states and concurrent use of prescription medications. For example, one study documented the use of nonprescription medications and dietary supplements in 45 elderly patients (average age: 85 years) residing in assisted-living facilities.[22] The results showed that elderly residents used an average of 3.4 nonprescription products, the most common being nutritional dietary supplements (32%), gastrointestinal products (17%), pain relievers (16.3%), and herbal products (14.4%). Potential safety concerns of drug duplication (70%) and potential drug/disease/food interactions (20.8%) were identified in more than one-half of these patients.

Gender Differences

As is true worldwide, there are more women than men in the United States. The gender gap widens dramatically with age. For example, in 2000, comparison of the number of all males to females, regardless of age, showed a ratio of 95.5 males/100 females.[19] This ratio decreased to 68.9 males/100 females at age 65 years or older and plummeted to 40.5 males/100 females in the 85 years or older age group.

The preponderance of elderly women has a considerable influence on self-medication. In the "Self-Care in the New Millennium" survey, women consistently reported having a variety of health problems more frequently than men.[5] Figure 1-3 shows

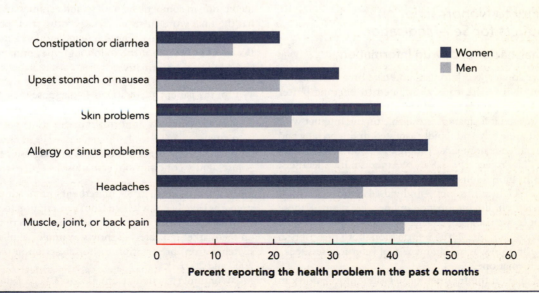

FIGURE 1-3 Selected ailments self-treated by men and women. (*Source:* Reference 5.)

that, across the board, more women than men (in the range of 31%–65%) report having each of six ailments. Women in this survey were also more likely to report using nonprescription medications (82%) than were men (71%). This gender difference was also observed in dietary supplement use, which was reported by 30% of women but only 23% of men.[5] Therefore, the increasing population of older women will increase demand for nonprescription products in the future.

There are also gender-specific self-medication concerns such as the use of nonprescription medications during pregnancy. More than 80% of pregnant women reported taking at least one medication, with about 30% using more than four.[23] This same study reported that 6 of the top 10 medications used were nonprescription medications. However, the ability of pregnant women to self-medicate safely is limited by the fact that most products state "if pregnant or breast-feeding, ask a health care professional before use." Pharmacists are trained to assess whether a nonprescription medication is safe for use during pregnancy.

Breast-feeding mothers are also faced with difficult choices when selecting nonprescription medications. All three main active ingredients in nonprescription pain relievers (i.e., aspirin, acetaminophen, and ibuprofen) have the potential to enter breast milk. The following are recommendations a pharmacist can make to help avoid problems in women who are breast-feeding[24]:

■ Use nonpharmacologic therapy if possible.
■ Take medications immediately after nursing or before the infant's longest sleep period.
■ Avoid recommending any medications that are extra-strength, maximum-strength, or long-acting.
■ Avoid recommending combination products.
■ Counsel about potential side effects that could occur in the child.

Nonprescription status of an emergency contraception (Plan B) is another example for which female patients will need direct access to the pharmacist. The pharmacist plays an important role in screening the patient's age and ensuring timely access to the medication. In some states pharmacists need to become certified and trained to provide Plan B directly to patients.

Accessibility to Nonprescription Drug Products for Self-Medication

Internet Pharmacies and Drug Information

As people live longer, work longer, and take on a more active role in their own health care, they need to become better informed about self-care options and how to safely self-medicate. Health care–related information is available on the Internet with resources that are easily and rapidly accessed in the privacy and comfort of a patient's home. According to a 2006 Pew Internet & American Life Project report, 80% of American Internet users, or some 113 million adults, have searched for information on at least one of 17 health topics.[25] Individuals who were most likely to search for health information online were women, those younger than 65 years of age, college graduates, and those with broadband access at home. Drug information (both prescription and nonprescription) was sought by 37% of Internet users seeking health information.[25]

Dependence on the Internet for self-care information can be problematic, given the lack of quality control, which in many instances compromises patients' welfare.[26] No single organiza-

tion is accountable for the quality or accuracy of health-related information available on Web sites.[27] The sheer number and diversity of Internet sources increase the likelihood that patients unknowingly view biased or outdated information. The Pew report concluded that "most internet users start at a search engine when looking for health information online and very few check the source and date of the information they find."[25] Because many sites contain inadequate, outdated, or incomplete information, it is not safe to simply "surf" and self-medicate.[28] For example, one study that evaluated the suitability of written supplemental materials available on the Internet for nonprescription medications determined that most manufacturer-sponsored Web sites intended for consumers had information that scored poorly in the areas of reading level and use of uncommon words.[29]

In response to public-safety concerns, the National Association of Boards of Pharmacy (NABP) has started to evaluate the credentials of online pharmacies (also known as e-pharmacies) through the Verified Internet Pharmacy Practice Sites (VIPPS) program.[30] The VIPPS program is voluntary, and an e-pharmacy must agree to strict conditions including NABP inspections to be certified under its auspices. Use of the VIPPS logo on Web pages confers credibility to each e-pharmacy that meets the NABP standards. As of December 2007, there were 15 VIPPS-approved Web site addresses in the United States.[31] Although prescription medications are dispensed at all of these sites, some also sell nonprescription medications, nutritional dietary supplements, herbal products, and medical devices, in addition to providing "on site" medical/pharmaceutical information for patients.

Rx-to-OTC Switch

An Rx-to-OTC switch is defined as over-the-counter (OTC) marketing of a drug product that was once a prescription (Rx) drug for the same indication, with the same strength, dose, duration of use, dosage form, and route of administration.[32] Pharmaceutical companies can benefit financially by requesting that FDA switch from prescription to nonprescription status a medication that is about to lose market share because of patent expiration and subsequent generic drug competition. The much longer period of sales generated as a nonprescription medication can offset the decreased revenue associated with the agent being a prescription medication in competition with generic entities. However, FDA has the final word in reclassifying a drug from prescription to nonprescription status. The Agency considers a medication for Rx-to-OTC switch if the following types of questions can be answered in the affirmative:

1. Can the patient adequately self-diagnose the clinical abnormality?
2. Can the clinically abnormal condition be successfully self-treated?
3. Is the self-treatment product safe and effective for consumer use, under conditions of actual use?

Since 1976 more than 80 ingredients, indications, or dosage strengths have been switched from prescription to nonprescription status, resulting in more than 700 nonprescription products on the market.[33] Table 1–2 shows examples of pharmaceuticals switched from prescription to nonprescription status between 2000 and 2007.[34]

Consumers benefit from Rx-to-OTC switches because they broaden access to important medications. In addition, the nonprescription versions are more cost-effective for consumers

TABLE 1-2 Examples of Prescription-to-Nonprescription Switches, 2000–2007

Year of Approval	Ingredient	Brand Name	Use
2000	Ibuprofen	Motrin Migraine Pain	Migraine
2000	Ibuprofen	Advil Migraine Liqui-Gels	Migraine
2000	Famotidine, calcium carbonate, magnesium hydroxide	Pepcid Complete	Heartburn, acid indigestion
2001	Butenafine hydrochloride	Lotrimin Ultra	Athlete's foot, jock itch, ringworm
2002	Ibuprofen, pseudoephedrine	Children's Advil Cold	Cold symptoms
2002	Guaifenesin extended-release tablet	Mucinex	Loosens mucus
2002	Nicotine polacrilex	Commit	Smoking cessation
2002	Loratadine	Claritin	Allergy symptoms
2002	Loratadine, pseudoephedrine	Claritin-D	Allergy symptoms
2003	Omeprazole	Prilosec OTC	Acid reducer, heartburn
2003	Loratadine	Claritin	Hives relief
2005	Diphenhydramine, ibuprofen	Advil PM	Pain relief, sleep aid
2006	Ecamsule (combined with avobenzone and octocrylene)	Anthelios SX	Sunscreen
2006	Levonorgestrel	Plan B	Contraception
2006	Polyethylene glycol 3350	MiraLAX	Constipation
2006	Ketotifen	Zaditor	Itchy eyes
2007	Orlistat	alli	Weight loss aid
2007	Cetirizine	Zyrtec	Allergy symptoms
2007	Cetirizine, pseudoephedrine	Zyrtec-D	Allergy symptoms

Source: Reference 34.

and third-party insurers. One study estimated Rx-to-OTC switches have saved consumers $13 billion and managed care organizations $20 million.[35] Additional examples of the cost benefits of Rx-to-OTC switches include the following:

■ A female patient can save as much as $80 by using switched nonprescription vaginal antifungal products for recurring yeast infections, according to the American Pharmacists Association. A nonprescription drug can be obtained for less than $20; however, a physician's visit and prescription–only vaginal anti-fungal drug can cost almost $100. Savings can be even greater when indirect (e.g., travel, lost time from work) costs are considered.[36]

■ A survey found that consumers save up to $750 million a year as a result of using nonprescription cough/cold medications that once were available only by prescription. The same study demonstrated that physician visits for the common cold dropped by 110,000 a year between 1976 and 1989.[36]

The pharmacist is ideally situated to advise patients on appropriate choices of recently switched nonprescription medications. For example, in 1996 an entirely new nonprescription drug category called "smoking cessation aids" was created when Nicorette chewing gum, NicoDerm CQ transdermal patch, and Nicotrol transdermal patch were switched from prescription to nonprescription status. A 10-year review of the effect of nonprescription

nicotine replacement therapy (NRT) concluded "Studies over the decade of OTC nicotine replacement therapy (NRT) availability demonstrate that OTC availability increased access and utilization of treatment, while also demonstrating that the projected adverse effects of OTC switch have not materialized: OTC NRT is being used safely and effectively, without substantial misuse or abuse. . . ."[37]

Behind-the-Counter (BTC) Medications

FDA is exploring whether to expand the use of a third drug class, which would be kept behind the pharmacy counter and require a pharmacist to dispense but without the need of a prescription. These behind-the-counter (BTC) medications are also sometimes referred to as "pharmacist only" or "Schedule 3" medications. This class of medications could provide patients greater access to medications that require safeguards for their use. Pharmacists could ensure appropriate drug selection while screening for potential drug–disease or drug–drug interactions. Examples of BTC medications already used in countries such as Canada and the United Kingdom include emergency contraception and simvastatin, a "statin" used to lower cholesterol.

One current example of a BTC medication in the United States is pseudoephedrine (PSE). Nonprescription pseudoephedrine is used to manufacture methamphetamine illicitly and has become a major public health concern. PSE-containing products were moved behind the counter on the recommendation of the Drug Enforcement Administration to combat shoplifting and the sale of bulk quantities needed to manufacture methamphetamine. Consumers must show pharmacy staff photograph identification and sign a logbook when purchasing PSE-containing products. Quantities of PSE-containing products available for purchase are also limited. One report suggests that the BTC status of PSE-containing products is reducing their sales.[38] However, the report noted that it is unclear whether the decreased sales are related to the burden of having to request the BTC drug or to the reformulation of many products with phenylephrine, a decongestant that does not require BTC status.[38]

Another example of making a nonprescription medication BTC is Plan B, an emergency contraceptive. In this instance, FDA wanted to ensure that Plan B was dispensed only to women 18 years or older so they placed it BTC. A pharmacist must verify the patient's age before this product can be sold. However, this requirement also places the pharmacist in the perfect situation to be able to counsel a patient about the proper use and potential side effects of the drug.

Despite the potential advantages, several strong lobbying groups oppose the expansion of BTC medications. Manufacturers of nonprescription medications oppose the creation of BTC medications, because it would reduce the number of retail outlets for their products and thereby reduce sales. Some grocery stores and other mass retailers without pharmacies that have traditionally sold nonprescription medications would be unable to sell BTC medications. The pharmaceutical manufacturers have stated that they can work with FDA and design the appropriate tools to address any challenges to a particular nonprescription medication without having to make it BTC.[33]

Other groups opposed to BTC medications cite a 1995 U.S. Government Accounting Office (GAO) report "Nonprescription Drugs, Value of a Pharmacist-Controlled Class Has Yet to Be Demonstrated."[39] The GAO report gave several observations to support its conclusion, including: (1) while a pharmacy or pharmacist class is assumed by some to improve safeguards against drug misuse and abuse, in the 10 countries studied these safeguards were easily circumvented, and studies showed that pharmacist counseling was infrequent and incomplete; and (2) experience in Florida with a class of drugs similar to a BTC class had not been successful, because pharmacists did not regularly prescribe the drugs and record-keeping requirements were frequently not followed.

Self-Medication and the Safe Use of Nonprescription Drug Products

Informed, appropriate, and responsible use of nonprescription medications is crucial for effective self-medication. Casual or inappropriate use of nonprescription medications can lead to serious adverse effects (e.g., liver toxicity with prolonged intake of high doses of acetaminophen), drug–drug interactions, and indirect effects (e.g., from delay in seeking appropriate medical attention). Pharmacists can combat misuse of nonprescription medications through the following measures:

- Ensure that patients are able to read and understand product labeling.
- Help patients avoid drug interactions.
- Warn about potential allergic reactions and side effects.
- Discuss appropriate drug storage and handling.

Nonprescription Drug Labeling

The Omnibus Budget Reconciliation Act of 1990 mandates pharmacists to "offer to counsel" on the prescription medications they dispense. However, nonprescription medications are exempted from this provision. Therefore, it is also up to the consumer to seek information from the pharmacist when they have a question. In the absence of this verbal consultation, the consumer must understand what is written on the product label to ensure proper use.

To assist consumers with reading of product labels, FDA has mandated use of a standard label format for each of the product categories, namely, herbals, dietary supplements, and nonprescription medications.[40] The standard product label for nonprescription medications, titled "Drug Facts," has specific sections for active ingredients, uses, warnings, when to use the product, directions, and inactive ingredients (see Chapter 4). The new label was designed to be easy to read, with all relevant information about taking the drug appearing in the same sequence on all package labels. This consistency in labeling enables patients to find information in a familiar spot on the label regardless of the use for the product (e.g., pain, cough/cold, and diarrhea). Initiated in 2002, the "Drug Facts" label has been on all nonprescription medications since May 15, 2005.

NCPIE commissioned a survey to determine if the "Drug Facts" label has helped to promote the message that nonprescription medications must be taken with care.[3] Results of this survey include the following:

- As for reading the label: 44% looked for the active ingredient, 20% read about possible side effects, and 8% read nothing on the label.
- As for following the dosing recommendations: 48% of respondents confided that, if needed to increase product effectiveness, they would take more than the recommended dose by either taking the next dose sooner than directed (35%), taking more than the recommended amount at a single time (32%), or taking the medication more times during the day than recommended (18%).
- Practitioners cited nonprescription medications being used incorrectly in the following ways: combining nonprescription and prescription medications (51%), chronic use of a nonprescription medication (44%), using a nonprescription drug for a prescription indication (32%), and taking more than one nonprescription product with the same active ingredient (27%).

The likelihood of inappropriate nonprescription drug use resulting from misreading of product labels increases when patients have limited reading skills or language barriers. The National Adult Literacy Survey found that nearly 44 million Americans cannot read and write, and 90 million adults have difficulty understanding information related to health care.[41] Effects of health illiteracy are particularly profound for Medicaid recipients, 90% of whom have reading skills at the fifth-grade level. Such a low level of literacy could be expected to adversely affect health care in patients using nonprescription medications, because a ninth-grade reading level is required to comprehend most nonprescription drug labels.[42] Other factors that can impair a consumer's ability to read nonprescription drug labeling include the size of type and price or antitheft tags improperly placed over critical information.[43,44]

Despite literacy concerns many studies have concluded that nonprescription medications are being used safely. For example, appropriate use of nonprescription medications such as topical steroids (hydrocortisone),[45] proton pump inhibitors (omeprazole),[46] and NRT[37] has been documented. Nevertheless, in January 2008 FDA began warning consumers to avoid treating children younger than 2 years with nonprescription cough and cold products because of an increased risk of overdose requiring emergency medical treatment. FDA cited studies that estimated that during a 2-year period, 1519 children younger than 2 years were admitted to emergency departments (EDs) for evaluation after known or possible exposure to cough/cold products. Of these incidents, it was noted that a large percentage of ED visits were related to inappropriate dosing and inappropriate use of the drug based on its labeling. Pharmacists can take a prominent role in ensuring the safe use of cough/cold medications in children by counseling parents to (1) carefully determine their child's dose according to weight not age, (2) avoid mistakenly duplicating ingredients if giving multi-ingredient products (e.g., adding a dose of Tylenol after administering a cough/cold medication that contains acetaminophen), and (3) use the provided dosing device correctly to measure the amount needed.

Nonprescription Drug Product Reformulation

Reformulation of nonprescription drug products is sometimes initiated by FDA because of safety or efficacy concerns. For example, Kaopectate is a brand-name antidiarrheal product that has been on the market for many years and has strong name recognition. The name "Kaopectate" was originally derived from its active ingredients kaolin and pectin. However, in 1992 it was reformulated with attapulgite, because FDA banned the use of pectin in nonprescription products because of insufficient data about its safety and efficacy. The product was reformulated again in 2003 to contain bismuth subsalicylate given that all attapulgite-containing medications were discontinued.

Confusion and misuse can occur when a nonprescription drug product is reformulated to contain different active ingredient(s) but does not change its brand name. Although reformulated products may be labeled as being "new and improved," there may be no indication that the active ingredient in a product is entirely different. Again using Kaopectate as an example, the product prior to its reformulation in 2003 could be used in children and had pediatric dosing instructions on the label. However, in 2004, the FDA ruled that antidiarrheals containing bismuth subsalicylate could be labeled for use by only adults and children 12 years and older. Therefore, the most recent version of the Kaopectate label does not include pediatric dosing information. As a result of all these formulation changes, there was a time in 2004 when consumers were faced with three different bottles labeled "Kaopectate": one containing attapulgite, one with bismuth subsalicylate and pediatric dosing information, and a third with bismuth subsalicylate and no pediatric dosing information. In addition, patients with aspirin or salicylate allergies who may have previously taken the old formulation of Kaopectate should not take the new version because it contains bismuth subsalicylate. A potentially serious adverse reaction could occur in a patient who does not carefully recheck the label of a "new and improved" product that they have used safely in the past.

It is also important to note that drug manufacturers can reformulate products for their own reasons. Changes to PSE-containing products are an example of a drug manufacturer–driven product reformulation. When the government restricted the sale of PSE-containing products to BTC status, many large pharmaceutical companies rushed to reformulate their brand-name products to contain a different decongestant, phenylephrine, which was not restricted. In most cases the brand names of these products did not change. This therapeutic switch was not because of safety or efficacy concerns but because of fears that BTC restrictions would decrease sales. In fact, phenylephrine prior to the reformulation was not used widely because of its limited effectiveness. Moreover, there have been recent reports questioning phenylephrine's efficacy at its FDA-approved adult dose of 10 mg, including a letter published in the *Journal of Allergy and Clinical Immunology,* which concluded that there is "virtually no evidence to show that phenylephrine oral nasal decongestants at the FDA-sanctioned dose of 10 mg are effective."[47] FDA has been subsequently petitioned to review dosing guidelines toward establishing a more effective 25 mg dose (FDA Docket #2007P-0047; www.fda.gov/ohrms/dockets).

Drug Interactions

The risk for drug interactions increases as consumers use more nonprescription medications, many of which have active ingredients that interact with the human body in different ways in a few individuals. In addition, diet and lifestyle can have a considerable effect on a medication's ability to work in the body. Certain foods, beverages (e.g., grapefruit juice), alcohol, caffeine, and even cigarette smoking can interact with medications. These interactions may make the medications less effective or may cause dangerous side effects or other therapeutic problems. For example, one study concluded that older adults were unaware of the adverse risks associated with concurrent use of nonprescription pain medications, alcohol, high blood pressure medications, and regular caffeine use, and that health care practitioners need to increase their educational efforts.[48] To avoid drug interactions, patients should consult pharmacists when first selecting herbal products, nutritional dietary supplements, or nonprescription medications. Table 1-3 lists some commonly used nonprescription medications and their interactions with food, alcohol, certain disease conditions, and other nonprescription medications.

Allergies to Active or Inactive/Inert Ingredients

Although the likelihood is low, any medicine can cause an allergic reaction. For example, allergic reactions have occurred in patients taking common nonprescription pain relievers such as aspirin, ibuprofen, naproxen, and ketoprofen. Patients should always be counseled about the signs and symptoms of an allergic reaction (itching, hives, and trouble breathing) and instructed to seek medical care immediately. Allergic reactions and side effects are caused by active ingredients and can also involve inactive ingredients. Inactive ingredients in nonprescription medications—such as binders, disintegrants, fillers, and preservatives—can cause reactions in a few individuals. Therefore, for safety reasons, FDA requires inactive ingredients to also be listed on the label. Table 1-4 lists some of the common inactive ingredients used in drug formulations and their known adverse effects.

TABLE 1-3 Potential Interactions with Selected Nonprescription Drugs

Drug–Drug Interactions

Drug	Drug	Potential Adverse Effect
Aluminum-containing antacids	Ascorbic acid	Decreased aluminum absorption
Aspirin	Products containing aluminum, calcium, or magnesium	Decreased blood aspirin concentration by increasing aspirin elimination
Iron	Products containing aluminum, calcium, or magnesium	Decreased iron absorption
Mineral oil	Docusate	Increased mineral oil absorption
Psyllium	Antidiabetic agents (metformin)	Decreased metformin absorption

Drug–Food/Beverage Interaction

OTC Drug	Food/Beverage	Potential Adverse Effect
Acetaminophen	Garlic	Delayed acetaminophen absorption
Aspirin	Garlic	Increased risk of bleeding
Calcium	Oxalic acid foods (spinach, rhubarb); phytic acid foods (bran/whole-grain cereal)	Altered calcium absorption
Zinc	Caffeine; dairy products (milk)	Decreased zinc absorption

Drug–Disease Interactions

OTC Drug	Condition	Mechanism
Aspirin	Hyperuricemia	Decreased renal excretion of uric acid
Doxylamine succinate, phenylephrine HCl	Glaucoma	Obstructed aqueous outflow
Naproxen, ketoprofen	Peptic ulcer disease	Altered gastric mucosal barrier
Pheniramine maleate, naphazoline HCl, nicotine	Hypertension	Increased vascular resistance

Drug–Alcohol Interactions

OTC Drug	Potential Adverse Effect	Mechanism
Aspirin	Increased gastrointestinal blood loss	Prolongs bleeding time
Diphenhydramine HCl	Increased sedation	Depresses central nervous system
Insulin	Increased hypoglycemia	Decreases hepatic gluconeogenesis
Ketoconazole (topical)	Vomiting, tachycardia	Causes disulfiram-like reaction
Yohimbine	Increased blood pressure	Increases norepinephrine level

Source: Wolters Kluwer Health. *Facts & Comparisons 4.0.* Available at: http://online.factsandcomparisons.com/login.aspx?url=/index .aspx&qs=. Last accessed July 28, 2008.

Handling and Storage of Nonprescription Medications

For a consumer to benefit from using a nonprescription medication, it must have the potency stated on its label. Consumers reasonably assume that, because nonprescription drug products are under the aegis of the FDA, they are pure and have their stated potency. Although this is usually the case, recalls of nonprescription medications because of impurity, contamination, or incorrect potency can occur. Some "out of the ordinary" clues that should arouse suspicion before one uses a nonprescription prod-

uct include abnormal odors, color changes, texture differences, and abnormal shape of a solid dosage form. Consumers should avoid taking any drug product they suspect is bad. Pharmacists should also actively remove any recalled drug product from their shelves and post notices informing patients of the recall and what action they should take.

Before any product is used, consumers should check the expiration date that appears on the product label. However, health care providers should be aware that there is a lot of conflicting information for consumers about the real meaning of a drug prod-

TABLE 1-4 Adverse Effects of Some Inactive Ingredients Used in Drug Preparations

Inactive Ingredient	Use	Where Found	Adverse Events
Aspartame	Sweetener	Liquid sucrose-free preparations	Headaches, hallucinations, panic attacks
Benzalkonium chloride	Preservative	Anti-asthmatic drugs, nasal decongestants	Airway constriction
Benzyl alcohol	Preservative	Liquid preparations	Neonatal deaths, severe respiratory and metabolic complications
Lactose	Filler	Capsules and tablets	Diarrhea, dehydration, cramping
Propylene glycol	Solubilizes drugs	Liquid preparations	Respiratory problems, irregular heartbeat, low blood pressure, seizure, skin rashes
Saccharin	Sweetener	Liquid preparations	Cross-sensitivity with sulfonamides, dermatologic reactions, pruritus
Sulfites	Antioxidant	Anti-asthmatic drugs; anti-inflammatories	Wheezing, breathing difficulties
Yellow tartrazine	Coloring agent	Solid/liquid preparations	Allergic reaction similar to that of aspirin

Source: Wolters Kluwer Health. *Facts & Comparisons 4.0.* Available at: http://online.factsandcomparisons.com/login.aspx?url=/index.aspx&qs=. Last accessed July 28, 2008.

uct expiration date. Many publications including *Consumer Reports* and the *Wall Street Journal* have published articles stating that many drug products are still potent for a long time after their expiration date.[49] These articles suggest that expiration dates may be shortened by drug manufacturers for the purpose of increasing sales. Pharmacists should help patients understand that after the expiration date, the product is no longer under the manufacturer's "warranty" and that the product "may" no longer work.

To retain its potency, a drug must be stored properly. Prescription and nonprescription medications are often mistakenly stored in bathroom cabinets, usually above the sink. Humidity and heat from the shower and sink are easily trapped in the cabinet, accelerating the degradation of the medications, even if they are in a prescription vial or bottle. Consumers need to be aware that all medications should be stored away from high humidity in a cool, dark place to ensure that they retain their potency and effectiveness. Furthermore, all medications should be stored a sufficient distance from the ground to ensure that they are kept out of a child's reach. This precaution is especially important for the many nonprescription medications that are not packaged in child-resistant containers. Examples of nonprescription product packaging that is not childproof include blister packs, lozenges, topical creams or ointments, spray canisters, and bulk powder containers (e.g., laxatives). Table 1-5 lists some nonprescription medications and health care products, with storage recommendations, generally kept on hand to treat minor ailments or injuries. It is a good practice to encourage patients to check product expiration dates and purge medicine cabinets at least once every 6 months.

Pharmacists' Role in Nonprescription Drug Therapy

The public's ability to discern critical information about the condition being treated and the clinical risk–benefit of a nonprescription drug is highly variable. The array of product choices; line extensions; and overstated, vague, or misleading marketing messages lead to consumer confusion. Generally package labeling is limited in the breadth and depth of the message it communicates;

it can never address the informational needs of all patients. Therefore, the pharmacist–patient interaction is vital for ensuring optimal nonprescription drug therapy. In 2007, *U.S. Pharmacist* published survey results of pharmacists (41.4% chain store, 34.4% independent retail) about their roles in counseling on nonprescription medications.[50] More than 90% of pharmacists surveyed stated that they have an active role in counseling patients on nonprescription medications, with more than 40% recommending 6 to 10 products per day. Table 1-6 shows how pharmacists ranked the importance of various counseling topics. Pharmacists clearly feel

TABLE 1-5 Recommended Storage Places of Selected Nonprescription Health Care Products

Closet/Kitchen Cabinet or Shelf	Bathroom Medicine Cabinet
Analgesics (relieve pain)	Adhesive bandages
Antacids (relieve upset stomach)	Adhesive tape
Antibiotic ointments (reduce risk of infection)	Alcohol wipes
Antihistamines (relieve allergy symptoms)	Calibrated measuring spoon
Antipyretics (reduce fever; adult and child formulations)	Dental floss
Antiseptics (help prevent infection)	Disinfectant
Decongestants (relieve stuffy nose and cold)	Gauze pads
Hydrocortisone (relieves itching and inflammation)	Thermometer

Source: Adapted from Lewis C. Your medicine cabinet needs an annual checkup, too. *FDA Consum.* 2000;34(2):25–8.

TABLE 1-6 Pharmacist Ranking of Nonprescription Drug Counseling Topics

Survey Question

"Which of the following counseling topics are most important when discussing OTC-related products with patients?"	Average Rank (1 = highest importance; 5 = lowest importance)
Selection of right product	1.5
Rx-to-OTC drug interactions	2.5
Side effects/adverse reactions	3.0
Directions/instructions	3.0
Cost	4.4

Source: Reference 50.

that their main service is to help patients select the most appropriate drug for their condition while avoiding drug interactions.

The underlying goal of pharmacists' counseling is to ensure that the patient gets correct, practical information and understands it in the context of the ailment being treated. Validation of the patient's understanding is also critically important. The pharmacist should always encourage the patient to ask questions and learn more. In the initial encounter with a patient who is seeking assistance with nonprescription medications, the pharmacist should:

■ Assess, by interview and observation, the patient's physical complaint/symptoms and medical condition (see Chapter 2).
■ Differentiate self-treatable conditions from those requiring a primary care provider's intervention.
■ Advise and counsel the patient on the proper course of action (i.e., no drug treatment, self-treatment with nonprescription medications, or referral to a primary care provider or other health care provider).
■ Advise the patient on the outcome of the selected course of action.
■ Assure the patient that the desired therapeutic outcome can be achieved if nonprescription medications are taken as directed on the label and/or recommended by the physician/pharmacist.
■ Reinforce the concept that the pharmacist and physician are qualified to perform follow-up assessment of the treatment.

If self-care with nonprescription medications is in the best interest of the patient, then pharmacists can help in the following ways:

■ Assist in product selection.
■ Assess patient risk factors (e.g., contraindications, warnings, precautions, comorbidities, age, and organ function).
■ Counsel the patient about proper drug use (e.g., dosage, administration technique, monitoring parameters, and duration of self-therapy).
■ Maintain an accurate patient drug profile that includes prescription, nonprescription, and herbal/dietary supplement products.

■ Assess the potential of nonprescription medications to mask symptoms of a more serious condition.
■ Prevent delays in seeking appropriate medical attention.

Key Points for Self-Care and Nonprescription Pharmacotherapy

➤ Self-care will play an increasingly important role in health care, and self-medication represents a significant element in the self-care process.
➤ Nonprescription medications are used by millions of Americans each year, because they offer safe and effective relief for a variety of common health care ailments.
➤ Health care professionals and FDA agree that nonprescription medications, although safe and effective, bear some risks associated with patients not reading and closely following the label instructions when taking the medications.
➤ Patients, manufacturers, governmental agencies, and, particularly, pharmacists should become even more intent on recognizing that each group fulfills essential functions in ensuring the safe, appropriate, effective, and economical use of nonprescription medications.

REFERENCES

1. U.S. Department of Commerce, Bureau of the Census. Statistical Abstracts of the United States. Historical Statistics of U.S. Colonial Times to 1990. Washington, DC: US Government Printing Office; 1995.
2. New OTC/HBC Stars of 2006. *Drug Top.* 2007;151(7):34.
3. Uses and Attitudes about Taking Over-the-Counter Medications: Findings of a 2003 National Opinion Survey Conducted for The National Council on Patient Information and Education. Harris Interactive, Inc; Bethesda, Md: National Council on Patient Information and Education; 2003. Available at: http://www.bemedwise.org/survey/summary_survey_findings.pdf. Last accessed July 28, 2008.
4. The Attitudes and Beliefs about the Use of Over-the-Counter Medicines: A Dose of Reality: A National Survey of Consumers and Health Professionals. Harris Interactive, Inc; Bethesda, Md: National Council on Patient Information and Education; 2002. Available at: http://www.bemedwise.org/survey/summary_survey.pdf. Last accessed July 28, 2008.
5. Self-Care in the New Millennium: American Attitudes toward Maintaining Personal Health and Treatment. New York: Roper Starch World Wide; 2001. Available at: http://www.chpa-info.org/ChpaPortal/Press Room/Statistics/ConsumerSurveyonSelfMedication.htm. Last accessed August 4, 2008.
6. CDER, Over-the-counter drug products; public hearing. *Fed Regist.* April 27, 2000;65:24704–6.
7. Consumer HealthCare Products Association: OTC Sales by Category: 2003–2006. Available at: http://www.chpa-info.org/ChpaPortal/Press Room/Statistics/OTCSalesbyCategory.htm. Last accessed July 28, 2008.
8. Radimer K, Bindewald B, Hughes J, et al. Dietary supplement use by US adults: data from the National Health and Nutrition Examination Survey, 1999–2000. *Am J Epidemiol.* 2004;160:339–9.
9. National Center for Complementary and Alternative Medicine. The Use of Complementary and Alternative Medicine in the United States. Available at: http://nccam.nih.gov/news/camsurvey_fs1.htm. Last accessed July 28, 2008.
10. Blumenthal M, Ferrier GKL, Cavaliere C. Total sales of herbal supplements in United States show steady growth. *HerbalGram* (American Botanical Council). 2006;71:64–6.
11. Bruno JJ, Ellis JJ. Herbal use among US elderly: 2002 National Health Interview Survey. *Ann Pharmacother.* 2005;39:643–8.
12. Department of Treasury, Internal Revenue Service. Over-the-Counter Drugs to be Covered by Health Care Flexible Spending Accounts. Available at: http://www.irs.gov/newsroom/article/0,,id=112623,00.html. Last accessed July 28, 2008.

13. Koutnik-Fotopoulos E. Finpago to the rescue for mass merchants. *Pharm Times*. 2006;72:92.

14. Blacker K, Dow HW, Wolfson J. Health savings accounts: implications for health spending. *Natl Tax J*. 2006;59:463–75.

15. Consumer HealthCare Products Association. FAQs about the OTC Medicine Tax Fairness Act and making OTCs tax deductible. Available at: http://www.chpa-info.org/ChpaPortal/Issues/CongressionalIssues/OTCTaxFairness. Last accessed August 4, 2008.

16. Piper Report. Over-the-Counter Drugs in Medicare Part D: Impact of OTCs on Medicare Drug Plans, Medicaid Programs, Pharmacies, and Drug Manufacturers. Available at: http://www.piperreport.com/archives/2006/06/overthecounter_1.html. Last accessed July 28, 2008.

17. Centers for Disease Control and Prevention. United States life tables, 2003. *Natl Vital Stat Rep*. 2006;54:1–40.

18. US Census Bureau. Statistical Abstract of the United States:2004–2005: Decennial Census and Projections. Available at: http://www.census.gov/prod/2004pubs/04statab/pop.pdf. Last accessed July 28, 2008.

19. US Department of Health and Human Services, Administration on Aging. Aging into the 21st Century. Available at: http://www.aoa.gov/prof/statistics/future_growth/aging21/demography.aspx. Last accessed July 28, 2008.

20. WebMD Health: Medications and Older Adults. Available at: http://www.webmd.com/healthy-aging/medications-older-adults. Last accessed July 28, 2008.

21. Simoni-Wastila L, Stuart BC, Shaffer T. Over-the-counter drug use by medicare beneficiaries in nursing homes: implications for practice and policy. *J Am Geriatr Soc*. 2006;54:1543–9.

22. Lam A, Bradley G. Use of self-prescribed nonprescription medications and dietary supplements among assisted living facility residents. *J Am Pharm Assoc*. 2006;46:574–81.

23. Mitchell AA, Hernández-Díaz S, Louik C, et al. Medication use in pregnancy: 1976–2000. *Pharmacoepidemiol Drug Saf*. 2001;10:S146.

24. Nice FJ, Snyder JL, Kotansky BC Review: breastfeeding and over-the-counter medications *J Hum Lact*. 2000;16:319–31.

25. Pew Internet & American Life Project. Online Health Search 2006: Most internet users start at a search engine when looking for health information online. Very few check the source and date of the information they find. October 29, 2006. Available at: http://www.pewinternet.org/pdfs/PIP_Online_Health_2006.pdf. Last accessed July 28, 2008.

26. Henkel J. Buying drugs online: it's convenient and private, but beware of "rogue sites." *FDA Consum*. 2000;34(1):5–9.

27. Anderson C. A call for Internet pharmacies to comply with quality standards. *Qual Saf Health Care*. 2003;12:86.

28. Bessell TL, Anderson JN, Silagy CA, et al. Surfing, self-medicating and safety: buying non-prescription and complementary medicines via the Internet. *Qual Saf Health Care*. 2002;11:88–92.

29. Wallace, LS, Rogers, ES, Turner, LW, et al. Suitability of written supplemental materials available on the Internet for nonprescription medications. *Am J Health-Syst Pharm*. 2006;63:71–8.

30. National Association of Boards of Pharmacy. VIPPS Accreditation Fact Sheet. Available at: http://www.nabp.net/ftpfiles/NABP01/PSsummaries/VIPPS.pdf. Last accessed July 28, 2008.

31. National Association of Boards of Pharmacy. Verified Internet Pharmacy Practice Sites™ (VIPPS®): List of Pharmacies. Available at: http://www.nabp.net/vipps/consumer/listall.asp. Last accessed July 28, 2008.

32. Mahecha LA. Rx-to-OTC switches: trends and factors underlying success [serial online]. *Nature Rev Drug Discov*. April 7, 2006; doi:10.1038/nrd2028.

33. Consumer Healthcare Products Association. FAQs About Rx-to-OTC Switch. Available at: http://www.chpa-info.org/ChpaPortal/Science/Switch/Switch.htm. Last accessed August 4, 2008.

34. Consumer Healthcare Products Association. Rx-to-OTC Switch List. Available at: http://www.chpa-info.org/ChpaPortal/Science/Switch/Press_SwitchList.htm. Last accessed August 4, 2008.

35. Pawaskar MD, Balkrishnan R. Switching from prescription to over-the-counter medications: a consumer and managed care perspective. *Manag Care Interface*. 2007;20(1):42–7.

36. Consumer Healthcare Products Association. The Switch Process. Available at: http://www.chpa-info.org/ChpaPortal/Science/Switch/SwitchProcess.htm. Last accessed August 4, 2008.

37. Shiffman S, Sweeney CT. Ten years after the Rx-to-OTC switch of nicotine replacement therapy: what have we learned about the benefits and risks of non-prescription availability [serial online]? *Health Policy*. 2008;86:17–26. doi:10.1016/j.healthpol.2007.08.006.

38. Bodine, WK. A third category? Medicines go behind the counter. *Pharm Times*. 2007;73(1):96–7.

39. United States General Accounting Office. Nonprescription Drugs: Value of a Pharmacist-Controlled Class Has Yet to Be Demonstrated. 1995. Available at: http://www.gao.gov/archive/1995/pe95012.pdf. Accessed December 5, 2007.

40. US Food and Drug Administration. New OTC drug facts label. *FDA Consum*. July–August 2002; Available at: http://www.fda.gov/FDAC/features/2002/402_otc.html. Last accessed August 4, 2008.

41. Kirsch I, Jungeblut A, Jenkins L, et al. *Adult Literacy in America: A First Look at the Findings of the National Adult Literacy Survey*. Washington, DC: US Department of Education, National Center for Education Statistics; 1993.

42. Sangsiry SS, Cady PS, Patil S. Readability of over-the-counter medication labels *J Am Pharm Assoc*. 1997;NS37:522–8.

43. Sangsiry SS, Pawaskar MD. Obstruction of critical information on over-the-counter medication packages by external tags. *Ann Pharmacother*. 2005;39:249–54.

44. Wogalter MS, Vigilante WJ Jr. Effects of label format on knowledge acquisition and perceived readability by younger and older adults. *Ergonomics*. 2003;46:327–44.

45. Ellis CN, Pillitteri JL, Kyle TK, et al. Consumers appropriately self-treat based on labeling for over-the-counter hydrocortisone. *J Am Acad Dermatol*. 2005;53:41–51.

46. Fendrick AM, Shaw M, Schachtel B, et al. Self-selection and use patterns of over-the-counter omeprazole for frequent heartburn. *Clin Gastroenterol Hepatol*. 2004;2:17–21.

47. Hendeles L, Hatton RC. Oral phenylephrine: an ineffective replacement for pseudoephedrine? *J Allergy Clin Immunol*. 2006;118:279–80.

48. Amoako EP, Richardson-Campbell L, Kennedy-Malone L. Self-medication with over-the-counter drugs among elderly adults. *J Gerontol Nurs*. 2003;29(8):10–5.

49. Cohen, LP. Safe and effective: many medicines prove potent for years past their expiration dates. *Wall Street Journal*. March 28, 2000;sect A:1.

50. Pharmacists take center stage in OTC counseling. *U.S. Pharm* 2007; 32(7):4–6.

Patient Assessment and Consultation

Lawrence M. Brown and Brian J. Isetts

The development of viable pharmaceutical care business models is helping pharmacists to respond more effectively to the drug-related needs of patients. One important development relates to the use of a clearly defined patient care process to fulfill a patient's self-care needs. In addition, decisions made by pharmacists, who function to identify, resolve, and prevent drug therapy problems, are valid, or clinically credible, as judged by panels of physicians and pharmaceutical care practitioners. This chapter describes the consistent and systematic process used to meet the drug-related needs of patients with self-care concerns.

The patient care process pertaining to medication therapy management includes assessment, care planning, and evaluation and follow-up. Assessment represents the first set of clinical judgments made by a practitioner when caring for a patient. The purpose of assessment is to determine, describe, and define the patient's drug-related needs, including the goals of therapy and identification of drug therapy problems that the patient may be experiencing. Assessment provides the practitioner with a basis for consulting with a patient to decide which of the patient's drug therapy problems the practitioner will help resolve. A care plan is a detailed schedule of responsibilities for achieving treatment goals and for resolving and preventing drug therapy problems, whereas follow-up evaluation represents an accounting of actual patient outcomes.

Patients expect pharmacists to assist them with many health care concerns and to help them interpret treatment options within the health care delivery system. This chapter is divided into six sections:

1. A brief review of the demands for self-care.
2. An introduction to the consistent and systematic patient care process used by practitioners when assuming responsibility for a patient's drug-related needs.
3. A description of the rational and ordered process for conducting an assessment, developing a care plan, and completing a follow-up evaluation of a patient's drug-related needs.
4. A discussion of the skills required by pharmacists to care for patients with self-care needs.
5. A summary of special considerations when caring for selected high-risk and special patient populations (infants and children, persons of advanced age, and pregnant and breast-feeding women).
6. Key points for integrating these principles into pharmacy practice.

Because the federal government and the medical profession have helped to clarify the relationship of "medication therapy management services" (MTMS) provided within the practice of pharmaceutical care, there is commonality in the use of these terms in this chapter. The term MTMS first appeared in federal legislation introduced, but not passed, in the late 1990s, proposing to compensate pharmacists for pharmaceutical care services. Throughout this chapter a case-based format is used to demonstrate how a pharmacist can apply this information to the care of patients with self-care needs.

Demand for Self-Care

The U.S. health care system is dynamic and marked by rapid change. Access, cost, and quality of health care are debated extensively at a public policy level. Our complicated, diverse, and fractionated health care system can leave consumers frustrated when confronted with personal health care concerns. Fortunately, patients have come to trust and depend on their pharmacists when faced with their own personal health care needs.

Pharmacists, who are often on the front line of the health care delivery system, are called on to help patients evaluate therapeutic options. In most cases, the pharmacist can help patients by (1) recommending no treatment at all, (2) recommending self-care therapy, or (3) referring patients to other health care providers. Several chapters in this book contain information and tables on exclusions for self-care treatment that pharmacists may find helpful in deciding when to refer patients to other health care providers. In addition, issues relating to special populations such as infants and young children, persons of advanced age, and pregnant or breast-feeding women are also addressed in this text.

Self-care, self-diagnosis, and self-medication are important components of the health care system in the United States. Instead of seeking the advice of a medical care provider, many people self-diagnose and treat their symptoms using a vast array of self-care options, ranging from nonprescription medications, herbal products, and home remedies to yoga, meditation, and spiritual healing, among others. Survey data show that about 80% of Americans who have conditions that can be treated with nonprescription medications use self-care for those conditions.[1] Nonprescription medications allow individuals to manage their many medical problems rapidly, economically, and conveniently, and may prevent unnecessary visits to a primary care provider or specialist. Patients often believe that products that move from prescription to nonprescription status are more effective than other nonprescription medications, and 87% of Americans believe that nonprescription medications are safe when used as directed.[2] The demand for and shift toward self-medication are further described and documented in Chapter 1.

The appropriate use of a nonprescription product, like the use of any other medication, requires attention to the intended use, effectiveness, safety, and convenience of administration. Although warnings are required on the labels of such products, labeling alone may be inadequate, and the patient may need assistance in selecting and properly using nonprescription medications. Inappropriate use and misuse of nonprescription medications can increase the risk of drug misadventures,[3] resulting in increased health care costs and more serious illness. Therefore, the pharmacist's role is crucial in assessing a patient's need for nonprescription medications.

The magnitude of drug misadventures, or drug therapy problems, has been described in terms of drug-related morbidity and mortality.[4,5] In addition, one category of drug therapy problems, referred to as medication safety, has received extensive national attention in reports such as those issued through the Institute of Medicine and the work of organizations such as the Institute for Safe Medication Practices. From 1995 to 2000, the cost of drug therapy problems more than doubled.[5] Drug therapy problems are defined as any aspect of a patient's drug therapy that is interfering with a desired, positive therapeutic outcome.[6] A patient who requires a nonprescription medication pursuant to a self-care consultation with a pharmacist is experiencing a drug therapy problem, because he or she has an untreated medical condition and requires the intervention of a pharmacist. A pharmacist's interpretation that use of a nonprescription product can help the patient achieve a desired therapeutic outcome is an intervention intended to resolve the patient's drug therapy problem (i.e., the patient needs additional drug therapy). In addition, it is noted that 23% of all drug therapy problems involve one or more nonprescription drug products, either as the cause of the drug therapy problem or in its resolution.[6]

Many patients do not appreciate, or are not aware of, the need for professional assistance in selecting nonprescription medications. The presence of a pharmacist differentiates the nonprescription drug department in a pharmacy from a similar department in a nonpharmacy outlet. To better serve patients, pharmacists need to maximize the personal service they offer. Patient inquiries should be referred to pharmacists, who must actively promote the value of their guidance in selecting and monitoring treatment with a nonprescription medication. It is essential to increase a patient's awareness of the importance of consulting a pharmacist, not only when considering a medication for the first time but also when making subsequent purchases.

A patient's primary patronage motive, or choice of pharmacy, is convenience, followed by price and service.[7] A random-sample telephone interview survey of 1009 adults found that 80% of Americans purchase specific OTC products on the basis of what their pharmacist recommends. Nevertheless, only 43% of those interviewed seek information from a pharmacist about treatment before they buy an OTC product.[1]

The principles of pharmaceutical care are available to help practitioners more effectively address the self-care needs of patients. A consistent and systematic patient care process helps practitioners to be complete and concise when assuming responsibility for a patient's self-care needs. In addition, the use of the systematic patient care process is important in obtaining compensation for the pharmacist's care.

Introduction to MTMS Provided within the Practice of Pharmaceutical Care

The profession of pharmacy has recently achieved two important goals: recognition of pharmacists as health care practitioners, and inclusion of pharmacists' services within the authoritative health care reporting and billing system. The two federal laws significantly affecting pharmacist practitioner classification are HIPAA[8] and the Medicare Modernization Act.[9] These two laws helped the profession of pharmacy work with the American Medical Association (AMA) and the Centers for Medicare & Medicaid Services (CMS) to establish pharmacists' professional service billing codes described in *Current Procedural Terminology* (i.e., CPT codes) and to include pharmacies as a "Place of Service" in the *CPT Manual*.[10] The significance of these new developments to the care delivered by pharmacists is highlighted throughout this chapter.

Evidence of the effectiveness and safety of MTMS contained in the original CPT code proposal was derived from literature on the practice of pharmaceutical care. The detailed CPT reference guide description of MTMS reflects this literature by describing the service as face-to-face patient assessment and intervention to identify and resolve drug therapy problems; formulating a medication treatment plan to optimize the response to medications and achieve patients' goals of therapy, and monitoring and evaluating patient outcomes of therapy.[11] The relationship of MTMS as a distinct procedure provided within the practice of pharmaceutical care was included in this body of evidence.[12,13]

The practice of pharmaceutical care has fulfilled an unmet need in the health care delivery system by providing a systematic approach for consistently achieving intended drug therapy treatment goals while avoiding adverse, unintended, and ineffective medication consequences. In addition, pharmaceutical care has clarified the responsibilities of pharmacists as health care practitioners, and defined the relationship between the profession and society.[14] Now that pharmacists are officially classified as health care practitioners eligible for patient care compensation, the principles of pharmaceutical care will be important to the growing number of pharmacists who are building and expanding patient care practices.

The established characteristics of a pharmaceutical care practice were based on the rules governing the conduct of other professional practices. A practice may be viewed as the application of knowledge—guided by a commonly held social purpose—to the resolution of specific problems in a standard manner accepted and recognized by society. The definition of a pharmaceutical care practice, developed through analysis of other professional practices, is "a practice in which the practitioner takes responsibility for all of a patient's drug-related needs and is held accountable for this commitment."[6] The clinical and economic outcomes of MTMS provided within the practice of pharmaceutical care have been summarized previously.[15]

The goal when assuming responsibility for a patient's drug-related needs is to help the patient achieve the intended therapeutic goals and ensure a positive outcome. A standard problem-solving process, originally termed the "Pharmacist's Workup of Drug Therapy" and now referred to as the "Pharmacotherapy Workup," was developed to help pharmacists systematically address all of a patient's drug-related needs.[6] This standard problem-solving process is designed to move the pharmacist through an ordered sequence of decisions related to the intended use, effectiveness, safety, and convenience of use of the patient's drug therapies. The purpose of defining a common patient care process is to accomplish positive patient care objectives, not to constrain the freedoms or decisions of individual practitioners.[16]

Pharmacists must use a systematic, comprehensive, and efficient process to take responsibility for a patient's drug-related needs. To meet this objective, the patient care process involves the following three major steps[6]:

1. Assess, or systematically review, the patient's drug-related needs, including identifying any and all drug therapy problems.
2. Create a care plan or detailed schedule that outlines both the practitioner's and the patient's activities and responsibilities, and that is designed to resolve any drug therapy problems and achieve treatment goals, and to prevent any potential drug therapy problems.
3. Evaluate the patient's outcome and current status at planned follow-up intervals.

The care plan and evaluation provide the accountability and results that are often lacking in the health care delivery system. The following section focuses on conducting an assessment of a patient's drug-related needs, with an emphasis on assessing the drug-related needs of patients who present with self-care concerns.

Assessment of a Patient's Drug-Related Needs

Identifying drug therapy problems is a primary clinical decision made by the practitioner. From a consumer perspective, pharmaceutical care is a new and emerging concept. Patients are now seeking the personal attention of a trusted professional to help them achieve drug therapy treatment goals, while avoiding or minimizing the adverse consequences of taking medications. The rational and ordered process for conducting an assessment helps the pharmacist—functioning as a health care practitioner—maintain a disciplined approach when confronted with this changing societal demand. Assessing all of a patient's drug-related needs comprises a variety of actions including taking a history, obtaining information, and collecting data.

Before presenting specific examples of how to use the information presented in this chapter, it is important to discuss the realities of providing self-care consultations during the course of a typical day for a pharmacist working in the dispensing business of a pharmacy, compared with consulting with a patient in a practice that receives reimbursement through the patient care business of a pharmacy. Obviously, pharmacists who are asked to conduct a self-care consultation while fulfilling prescription dispensing responsibilities will have less time to devote to working with the patient than pharmacists who are working in the patient care business. For those pharmacists who have not yet worked in the patient care business of a pharmacy, it is important to point out that there are a number of proven strategies and approaches for starting a patient care business in relationship to a pharmacy's traditional prescription-dispensing business. Payment for the provision of MTMS provided within the practice of pharmaceutical care is a reality, and pharmacists who desire a future focused on working in a pharmacy's patient care business can now seek out these employment opportunities.

Skills Necessary to Care for Patients with Self-Care Needs

Advising patients on self-treatment is an important part of a pharmacist's professional responsibilities. When pharmacists use a standard care process to address a patient's self-care needs, they serve in the role of a primary care practitioner. Often the pharmacist is a patient's first contact with the health care system, and the pharmacist can evaluate the situation and recommend a course of action. This role may include recommending a nonprescription medication, dissuading patients from buying a medication when drug therapy is not indicated, recommending a nondrug treatment, or referring patients to another health care practitioner. If the pharmacist deters healthy people from using more costly health care services or products and refers more seriously ill patients to other primary care providers, health care delivery in the United States can be improved and health care resources can be conserved.

The following case study, presented in five parts, illustrates a few important pharmacotherapy assessment skills necessary to care for patients with self-care needs.

PATIENT–PHARMACIST CONSULTATION

General Patient Presentation

Mrs. E.J. is a 66-year-old female patient in good medical condition taking three prescription medications (lisinopril, atenolol, and lovastatin) to manage two chronic medical conditions (hypertension and dyslipidemia). Mrs. E.J.'s primary concern relates to the fact that she has been finding it a little more difficult to initiate a bowel movement.

Regardless of whether a pharmacist is working in a busy dispensing pharmacy or caring for patients during scheduled appointments, working with patients to identify their drug-related needs is at the center of the pharmacist's communication process during interaction with patients. Drug-related needs are defined as those health care needs of a patient that have some relationship to drug therapy and for which the practitioner is able to offer professional assistance.[6] Patients will tell their story or present a picture (e.g., "When I urinate, I feel as though I am going to pass out") in a random fashion. It is the pharmacist's job to interpret a patient's explicit and implicit drug-related needs. This skill is somewhat analogous to throwing a deck of cards into the air and reassembling the deck according to suits.

In the case of Mrs. E.J., the pharmacist will listen to the patient's concerns to ascertain the nature and extent of her problem. The pharmacist will also want to know the patient's current medications to determine whether the condition may be caused by a medication and to select a product appropriate for the patient. The pharmacist will then move forward to assess all of the patient's current medications, supplements, and remedies for indication, effectiveness, safety, and convenience of use. Proceeding systematically in this order is critical to avoid missing an important piece of information or jumping to an erroneous conclusion. Patients express their drug-related needs as understanding (or sometimes as a lack of understanding), expectations, concerns, and behavior (nonadherence). The pharmacist translates a patient's expression of drug-related needs into an assessment of drug therapy problems.

A final determination of drug therapy problems is conducted in consultation and agreement with the patient. Pharmacists cannot force their will on patients. A therapeutic relationship is a partnership between the practitioner and the patient, formed for the purpose of identifying the patient's drug-related needs.[6] When pharmacists care for patients using this systematic process, physicians and pharmaceutical care practitioners have been found to agree with 94.2% of all the pharmacists' clinical decisions made to identify, resolve, and prevent drug therapy problems, and to achieve intended drug therapy treatment goals.[12]

Communication

Interactions by pharmacists through consultation and effective assessment strategies can enhance patient outcomes. Patients' expression of their drug-related needs is one of the most important sources of information pharmacists need to provide pharmaceutical care services related to nonprescription medications. Each step of the patient care process involves communicating with the patient, gathering information from the patient, and transmitting information back to the patient. This process is particularly important during the assessment step, because these data form the basis for the care plan and subsequent follow-up evaluation.

Interaction between the pharmacist and the patient establishes a therapeutic relationship, or an alliance, needed to identify the patient's drug-related needs. It is characterized by trust, empathy, respect, authenticity, and responsiveness. This relationship allows the pharmacist to gather detailed, sometimes intimate, information from patients. In return, patients rely on the pharmacist to use knowledge, skills, and experience to ensure safe and effective drug therapy. Scheduled patient follow-up and reassessment are vital components of this therapeutic relationship and are used to determine actual patient outcomes and progress toward meeting therapeutic objectives. These components allow a pharmacist to reassess whether a patient is experiencing drug therapy problems. In the case of Mrs. E.J., the goal of therapy is a return to the patient's normal bowel movement pattern within 1 week.

The patient–pharmacist relationship is dynamically affected by numerous variables. A positive interaction one day could be followed by a negative interaction a few days later for reasons unrelated to the pharmacist's care. The pharmacist must become adept at interpreting nonverbal cues (e.g., facial expression or body position), as well as at responding to voice tones, inflection, and mood.[17] If a patient has a drug-related need but does not have the time or inclination to discuss it during a particular encounter, the pharmacist should schedule an alternative time to gather additional information to assess the patient's drug-related needs and determine an appropriate intervention. The potential severity of a drug therapy problem will dictate the timetable for these actions.

General Principles of Communication

To establish an effective therapeutic relationship with the patient, the pharmacist must be capable of demonstrating empathy to objectively identify with the patient's affective state.[18] Because the pharmacist's underlying attitude toward the patient will influence the quality of communication, the pharmacist must eliminate barriers by avoiding biases toward a patient's level of education, socioeconomic or cultural background, interests, or attitudes. In addition, the pharmacist must assure patients that any information they discuss will be kept in strict confidence.

A first step in a patient encounter is to assess what the patient already knows and determine where gaps in knowledge exist. This step is important because patients may resent being told what they already know and may be confused if the pharmacist wrongly assumes that they understand more than they do. When interacting with patients, the pharmacist should use words that a layperson can understand.

Effective communication occurs when the receiver of a message hears and understands exactly what the sender wants to communicate. One way to ensure understanding is through active listening, a process in which the receiver repeats the information to the sender. As information is exchanged, the participants change roles as receivers and senders of information. The message received is influenced by its content and context, as well as by how it is sent. Communications can be improved by paying attention to the interaction between sender and receiver.

Effective Questioning

Skillful questioning is a mark of a good communicator. Patients should feel that the pharmacist's questions convey a genuine interest in them and a desire to help. Because a patient may be uncooperative if the questions suggest only superficial curiosity, the pharmacist should explain the reason for asking personal questions (e.g., "I want to obtain additional information so I can determine if a nonprescription medication will help treat your specific problem"). It is important to avoid interrupting, or cutting off the patient in the middle of a response, which can occur when thinking ahead to the next question without adequately processing the current response.

When the pharmacist is unfamiliar with the patient, he or she should start the patient encounter by stating, "My name is ____, and I'm the pharmacist." The pharmacist should begin the exchange with an open-ended query such as, "How may I help you?" or "Would you please tell me more about the symptoms/problems you have?" Such valuable open-ended queries allow for increased flexibility and provide greater information than will questions that can be answered with only a yes or no response. Such open-ended queries enable a good practitioner to collect information efficiently and to establish better communications. If a patient's response wanders, however, the pharmacist must keep the interaction focused. To be sure that a patient understands dosage instructions, the pharmacist could ask, "So I know that I haven't forgotten to tell you anything, would you please tell me how you plan to take this medicine?"

Summarizing the important points or redirecting the interaction with a closed-ended question is useful. A question such as "How long have you had this pain?" may help the pharmacist gather specific information or clarify information obtained through earlier open-ended questions. It is important to ask one question at a time; asking two questions in rapid succession or multiple-choice questions will cause confusion and restrict communication. It is also important to avoid leading questions or judgmental questions such as "You don't smoke, do you?"

Effective Listening

Effective listening is a vital component of communication. When the pharmacist really listens, patients are free to state their problem completely and are assured of receiving the pharmacist's undivided attention. The pharmacist must focus on the patient and exclude distractions such as a telephone or a computer screen. The pharmacist may need to clarify the details of a patient's problem and should be receptive to a patient's response to questions. The pharmacist should respond with empathy, perhaps by paraphrasing a patient's words or by reflecting on what was said in terms of the patient's own experience. For instance, after listening to a complaint of pain, the pharmacist could say, "You have a sharp, stabbing pain in your wrist; is that right?" and end with a statement such as "That must be very uncomfortable." Interrupting or demonstrating lack of interest or disapproval may inhibit a patient's discussion of problems and concerns. Encouraging a patient to talk, exploring a patient's comments, and expressing understanding all facilitate communication. The pharmacist should reinforce wise decisions that a patient has made while reserving judgment about potentially unhealthy behaviors.

Nonverbal Communication

Nonverbal communication skills are important when conducting an assessment. A pharmacist's body language, such as posture and facial expression, communicates strong, direct messages.[17] Pharmacists should be aware of their own nonverbal behavior as well as that of the patient. An open body posture—facing the patient with arms and legs uncrossed—indicates openness, honesty, and a willingness to communicate and listen. Maintaining an appropriate distance from a patient will facilitate confidential communication without making patients uncomfortable. If a patient backs away or moves closer, the pharmacist should maintain the new distance the patient has established. Pharmacists should maintain eye contact with a patient and control their facial expressions to avoid showing negative emotions such as disapproval or shock.

The patient's nonverbal communication is equally important. If a patient has a closed body posture—arms crossed, legs crossed, body turned away—the pharmacist may need to find out why the patient is uncomfortable and then try to allay any concerns. The pharmacist should watch a patient's facial expressions for signs of anxiety, nervousness, and physical symptoms such as pain.

Physical Barriers to Communication

High counters, glass separators, cluttered aisles, and elevated platforms inhibit communication and provide physical barriers. Pharmacists should try to be at eye level with the patient. A tall pharmacist may need to sit on a stool or lower his or her body position to avoid "hovering over" the patient. Discussions between patient and pharmacist should be as private and uninterrupted as possible. If the pharmacist expects or perceives that a patient is uncomfortable discussing the problem, a quiet semiprivate or private consultation area should be sought and used. Ideally, a specific, private area should be designated for patient consultations.

Communication Techniques for Special Populations

Special communication techniques may be required with some patients.[19] Writing or printing out the information to provide a quality copy may be necessary if the patient is deaf or hearing-impaired. If a patient who is hearing-impaired reads lips, the pharmacist should be physically close to, and directly in front of, the patient and maintain eye contact while speaking. The pharmacist should speak slowly and distinctly in a low-pitched, moderate tone, because yelling further distorts the sound and might embarrass the patient. A quiet, well-lit environment is essential, because background noise and dimness can markedly diminish a hearing-impaired individual's ability to communicate. Using written or printed information alone can create misunderstandings with language that confuses the patient and requires further explanation. However, using printed information in conjunction with patient discussions has been found to be more effective than using written information alone.[19]

When interacting with a patient who is blind or visually impaired, the pharmacist should first state, "I am the pharmacist." Because a blind patient cannot perceive most nonverbal communication, the pharmacist should depend on tone of voice and verbal feedback to convey empathy and interest in the patient's problem. If the pharmacist needs to touch the patient to obtain additional information about the patient's condition, such as might be the case with a sprained ankle or to obtain a fingerstick blood glucose measurement, permission should first be obtained.

An estimated 13% to 40% of Americans are illiterate, and another 20% are considered marginally literate.[19] For these patients, written information or directions on a label are barriers, and the pharmacist cannot rely on them to reinforce information provided orally. Patients with reading impairments may be less inclined to ask questions or express their concerns. Although some common characteristics of illiteracy are related to age, education, and employment status,[19] an understanding of the patient's literacy status may take time to determine through the development of a therapeutic relationship.

The pharmacist must build a caring relationship to provide effective communication and consultation. The pharmacist can facilitate communication by using simple language and pictorial labels. Language and cultural barriers to communication may occur when interacting with patients of unfamiliar ethnic backgrounds.[20] Interpreters are also available as a resource in some communities and medical care facilities, and pharmacists may ask questions related to cultural beliefs to assess how these beliefs influence the patient's use of medications (see Chapter 3). Similarly, cultural behaviors may result in failure to make eye contact and should not be interpreted as a lack of interest or understanding.

Patient Consultation

Interacting with a patient regarding self-treatment is a primary care activity that carries a great professional responsibility. Patients with self-care needs present differently from those who have already received a treatment decision from a health care provider. To ensure that a particular drug product is appropriate for a patient, the pharmacist needs to perform an assessment by eliciting information from the patient, integrating these data to determine if any drug therapy problems exist, and then develop a patient care plan. As mentioned previously, pharmacists functioning in the dispensing business of a pharmacy, as well as pharmacists being reimbursed for providing pharmaceutical care, both start from the same point in interacting with a patient with self-care concerns (i.e., nature and extent of the patient's problem, current medications, and other medical conditions).

The self-care encounter in a pharmacy can be initiated by either the patient or the pharmacist (Figure 2-1). Although patients often initiate the consultation, an increasing number of pharmacists greet patients who are entering the self-care section of the premises and initiate an assessment of the patient's self-care concerns and drug-related needs.

Information-Gathering Process

Before formulating a plan for self-treatment or medical referral, the pharmacist must obtain enough information to identify and assess the patient's medical condition and drug therapy problem(s). Important data include the patient's perceived needs and concerns, demographics (i.e., patient-related variables), diseases, and medications. With experience, the pharmacist will be able to gather the necessary information to assess a particular condition within a relatively short period of time.

In a pharmaceutical care practice, the pharmacist will also conduct a general review of systems. A verbal review of the patient's physiologic systems, from head to toe, can help account for all of a patient's drug-related needs. The Pharmacotherapy Workup provides pharmacists with a complete listing of all body organ systems needed to conduct this review of systems: neurologic, psychological, eye-ear-nose-throat, endocrine, vital signs, cardiovascular, hematologic, pulmonary, musculoskeletal, gastrointestinal (GI), fluid/electrolyte status, renal, hepatic, genitourinary/reproductive, and skin.

Other important information gathering is an accurate accounting of each medication a patient is using to treat all medical conditions. This list includes prescription, nonprescription, and herbal products, and vitamins and dietary supplements. Thorough questioning is important given that patients tend to underreport use of nonprescription medications and dietary supplements.[21] If possible, the pharmacist may find it helpful to have the patient's medication history available at the start of the patient consultation.

The pharmacist can explain the need to review all medications by saying, "I would like to review each of the medications you are currently taking so that the drug product we might select for you fits with your current therapy. Here is a list of medications you have received at our pharmacy. Let's take a minute to see which ones you are currently taking, as well as what other medications you may be using." It may also be helpful for the pharmacist to have patients describe their daily activities and medication schedule in case they have difficulty recalling the names of all the medications they are taking.

When an accurate picture of the patient's active medication list has been obtained, the pharmacist in a pharmaceutical care practice will tie all active medications to each of the patient's medical conditions. A patient's drug allergies and medical history may be obtained at this point. The assessment process is dictated by the patient's knowledge level, as well as by the amount of time available to continue the interaction. Therefore, to obtain the needed information quickly and efficiently, the pharmacist should approach the problem logically and keep the questioning direct and to the point.

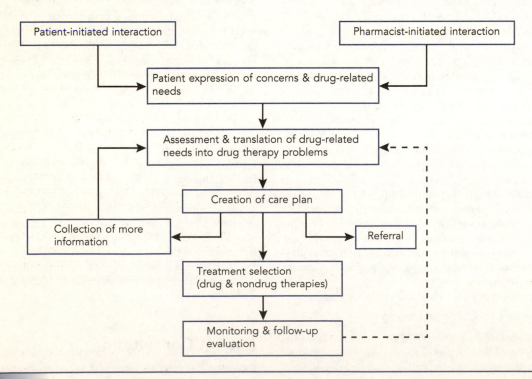

FIGURE 2-1 Patient–pharmacist consultation process.

Fortunately, within the context of providing MTMS within the practice of pharmaceutical care, the pharmacist need not try to obtain all relevant information in one encounter. The planned follow-up evaluation extends the initial assessment process and allows the pharmacist to obtain additional information. With continual practice, the pharmacist will learn to use every patient encounter to gather important additional information. The pharmacist will develop a sense, based on the patient's expression of needs, as to when to bring the initial assessment to a close and, in a pharmaceutical care practice, how to establish appropriate follow-up.

Patient History

After the pharmacist has accounted for the patient's other medications and drug-related needs, it is time to return to the patient's initial presentation of his or her self-care concerns. If the patient is not using any medications, supplements, or other remedies, the pharmacist commences the self-care encounter with a broad overview of the patient's health to determine the nature and extent of the problem. This overview of the patient's health enables the pharmacist to understand the patient's condition and make the most appropriate recommendation, regardless of whether a medication is included. Pharmacists should start by determining a patient's needs with an open-ended question such as "How may I help you?" Patients may initially present incomplete and vague information. To determine the specific symptoms and whether they are amenable to self-treatment, the pharmacist can pose the following open-ended queries or requests:

- Describe your problem.
- Describe to me how your problem has changed over time.
- How does the problem limit your daily activities (e.g., sleeping, eating, working, or walking)?
- Tell me about any foods, medications, and/or physical activities that make the problem worse.
- What have you done to relieve this problem in the past?
- What have you been doing so far to treat the problem?

The next step is to gather patient-specific data, including demographic information and medical history. The pharmacist should selectively elicit the following information:

- Who is the patient? Is the patient the person in the pharmacy or someone else?
- How old is the patient?
- Is the patient male or female? If the patient is female, is she pregnant or breast-feeding?
- Does the patient have any other medical problems that may alter the expected effects of a nonprescription medication or be aggravated by the medication's effects? Is the complaint related to a chronic illness?
- Does the patient have any allergies?
- Is the patient using any prescription, nonprescription, or social drugs (e.g., vitamins or food supplements, caffeine, nicotine, alcohol, or marijuana)?
- Has the patient experienced adverse drug reactions in the past?

Throughout the encounter, the pharmacist is formulating a clinical decision-making hypothesis based on identifying drug therapy problems. The pharmacist should determine whether the patient has misinterpreted the condition, done any harm by waiting to seek advice, or caused the condition to worsen by previous attempts at self-treatment.

Observed Physical Data

In addition to the historical data, physical data are helpful in determining the patient's self-care needs. Physical data include pulse rate, heart sounds, respiration rate, age, and weight. Depending on training and skills, the pharmacist can collect physical data by all or some of the following techniques: observation or inspection, palpation or manipulation, percussion, and auscultation. The importance of each technique in the process of data collection depends on the body system involved. For example, the skin is easily assessed by inspection and palpation, the lungs require percussion and auscultation, and all four skills are essential in examining the abdomen. However, most pharmacists obtain physical data primarily through observation.

Many clues to a patient's general health and the seriousness of a condition can come from simple observation. The degree of discomfort caused by pain may be judged from a patient's facial expressions or lack of use of a limb. Manifestations of an infection may include lethargy and pallor. The practitioner needs to inspect the patient's skin before offering advice about a skin rash, which may result from a simple contact phenomenon or be suggestive of systemic disease. It is recommended that nonlatex examination gloves be available for use when physical contact with the patient is required.

Patient Assessment

Assessment of a patient's drug-related needs during a self-care consultation involves evaluating data collected from the patient to determine the etiology and severity of the medical condition. This assessment is essential for reaching appropriate conclusions about treatment or the need for referral. Methods of assessing severity will vary, depending on the problem. Pharmacists and students of pharmacy who are learning how to conduct an assessment have found it useful to view the initial patient interaction as having a flow consisting of three broad, general phases: (1) establishing a therapeutic relationship, including determining the patient's primary concerns about his or her health; (2) reviewing all of the patient's active medications to assess indication, effectiveness, safety, and convenience of use; and (3) conducting a verbal review of systems to ensure that no drug-related needs have been overlooked.[22]

Assessing the severity of the patient's condition is an important component of deciding on treatment or referral. Many times, however, the etiology and severity of a condition cannot be conclusively determined because data are not accessible. Referral may be required when available information suggests that a certain etiology is responsible or a condition may be particularly severe. In general, the more severe the problem, the greater is the potential for referral.

Patients of advanced age, infants, children, patients with multiple chronic diseases, recently hospitalized patients, and patients who are receiving treatment from several health care providers are at greater risk for complications and require more careful evaluation.

Care Plan Development

After collecting all available information, evaluating the patient's condition, and assessing the patient's drug-related needs, the pharmacist formulates a care plan. A care plan is simply an understanding of the intended goals of therapy with an accompanying time frame for achieving these goals. The patient and pharmacist work together to establish realistic and observable goals. A care plan is a detailed schedule outlining the activities and responsibilities of the pharmacist and patient.[6] A care plan is constructed to:

1. Resolve any drug therapy problems identified during the assessment.
2. Meet the goals for each of the patient's medical conditions.
3. Prevent future drug therapy problems.

A pharmacist may create a care plan without having all desired information. Areas of uncertainty may exist, but a well-designed plan can help the patient properly manage his or her medical conditions. For a more detailed description of documentation systems and principles pertinent to recording a patient's care plan, the reader is referred to texts that review these subjects in detail.[6,12] The importance of documenting care delivered to a patient cannot be overstated. Developing a sound care plan for a patient with self-care needs will most likely include the following five steps:

1. Collect additional information.
2. Refer the patient to a primary care provider, if warranted.
3. Select self-treatment, if appropriate.
4. Advise the patient about self-treatment.
5. Evaluate progress toward achieving treatment goals.

COLLECT ADDITIONAL INFORMATION

The pharmacist may need more information to assess the patient's condition, which may require specific action such as either talking to a parent/caregiver or calling a health care provider. Communication between the pharmacist and health care provider is often desirable to avoid conflict in managing the patient and to overcome problems of overlapping responsibilities. When such communication becomes necessary, the pharmacist should do the following:

- Obtain data on preexisting medical conditions to determine whether self-treatment is appropriate.
- Determine whether the health care provider wants to address the patient's problem over the telephone.
- Determine whether the health care provider wants to see the patient or whether the patient should be referred to an urgent care center or a hospital emergency department.
- Provide information on the reason for referral.

PATIENT–PHARMACIST CONSULTATION

Collecting Additional Information and Referring Patient

One month after accepting your decision to start a stool softener, Mrs. E.J. returns to your pharmacy to inquire which iron product is best to "help give her more red blood cells." During the course of the assessment, the patient reveals that she has felt a little run-down, because she has been losing a little blood in her stools. As you collect additional information, the patient reports that this condition started about a week ago and that she has had three instances in which she noted blood in the stool. Without alarming the patient, you recommend that she consult her health care provider and offer to help her set up the appointment.

REFER PATIENT

When enough information is available to evaluate the condition, the pharmacist must decide whether to refer the patient to a health care provider or to advise on self-treatment. If the plan involves a medical referral, the pharmacist must consider both the type of treatment center to which the patient will be referred (clinic or emergency care facility) and the urgency for treatment. Some conditions do not require the immediate attention or extensive evaluation by emergency care personnel.

When advising a patient to see a health care provider, the pharmacist should discuss with the patient why the referral is being made. The pharmacist must use tact and firmness so the patient is not unnecessarily frightened but is convinced of the need for concern. Medical referral is indicated in the following situations:

- The symptoms are too severe to be endured by the patient without definitive diagnosis and treatment.
- The symptoms are minor but persistent and do not appear to be the result of some easily identifiable cause.
- The symptoms have repeatedly returned with no readily recognizable cause.
- The pharmacist is in doubt about the patient's medical condition.

In the case of Mrs. E.J., the pharmacist collected additional information from the patient to address her concerns about fecal blood loss. However, her condition is persistent (lasting 1 week), there is no readily recognizable cause, and the pharmacist is in doubt about the patient's condition without a definitive medical diagnosis. Therefore, a referral for medical evaluation is warranted.

SELECT SELF-TREATMENT

Selecting self-treatment in collaboration with a patient requires the pharmacist to consider several factors. First, the pharmacist must identify a measurable and achievable therapeutic objective, based on the patient's condition and clinical status. A therapeutic modality—either drug or nondrug—may then be recommended. Choosing a specific treatment requires reviewing drug variables (e.g., dosage forms, ingredients, adverse reactions, relative effectiveness, and price) and matching them with patient variables (e.g., age, gender, drug history, other physiologic problems, and ability to pay).

If self-treatment without the use of a medication is indicated, selection of the nondrug modality would similarly be modified using patient variables. For example, the pharmacist may suggest that a patient with vomiting and diarrhea consider drinking only fluids for a brief period. However, if the patient has insulin-dependent diabetes, the pharmacist must modify this possible course of action, because patients with diabetes have specific caloric requirements. Communicating with the patient, and possibly another health care provider, about modifying the dose of insulin to compensate for changes in caloric intake would be prudent in this situation.

To measure the success of treatment, the pharmacist should set goals and measurement parameters based on the therapeutic objective, the toxic or adverse effects of treatment, the nature and severity of the condition, the patient's ability to understand the condition and its treatment, and the anticipated time to symptom resolution. Toxicity includes those symptoms associated with an excess dose or an untoward reaction. The pharmacist should identify toxicities that suggest the problem may be worsening and require special attention. Finally, queries related to the patient's understanding of the condition and its treatment can include determining the appropriateness of the patient's questions to the pharmacist as well as the patient's response to those questions.

ADVISE PATIENT ON SELF-TREATMENT

The fourth step in the care plan is to advise the patient about self-treatment. The primary purposes are to develop a plan of action with the patient and obtain the consent necessary to enact the plan. Specifically, the pharmacist should provide advice in the following areas:

- Reasons for self-treatment
- Description of the medication and/or treatment
- Administration of the medication and/or treatment
- Adverse reactions and precautions
- General treatment guidelines

In advising the patient about a suggested treatment plan, the pharmacist should summarize the patient's condition, explain the significance of the symptoms, and outline the reasons for treatment. The pharmacist should clearly explain the therapeutic objectives and provide a realistic time frame for achieving the objectives. If the patient desires information on alternative treatments, the pharmacist should be prepared to present such information about their relative merits and drawbacks without biasing the information and jeopardizing the patient–health care provider relationship. The pharmacist should then discuss the nonprescription medications selected, describing in lay terms both the therapeutic action of the ingredients (e.g., decongestants, antihistamines, and laxatives) and the effect the products will have on the patient's symptoms and condition.

The pharmacist should explain administration guidelines clearly and concisely. Because many patients may remember only part of the information, some thought should be given to deciding what is most important for the patient to remember. Covering a few of the most important points is better than overwhelming a patient with a lot of information. In addition, patients will remember dosage instructions better if administration is linked to specific times of the day, rather than just "three times daily." Having a patient review normal daily activities will help establish the best times to take the medication. It is also important to include information about the duration of treatment.

The patient should be told about the most common adverse reactions associated with a medication and be instructed on how to manage them. The pharmacist should describe activities, other medications, foods, or beverages that should be avoided, as well as discuss which of the patient's medical conditions may be complicated by use of the medication. Information should be written down if it is extensive or complex.

The pharmacist should offer the patient some general treatment guidelines that may be helpful in managing the condition. These guidelines might include lifestyle changes, additional products or services, informational sources, and a list of signs and symptoms that indicate whether the medication is working, whether it is causing adverse effects, and when a health care provider's advice is needed. The patient should be informed about the expected response time to the treatment, the time required for the condition to resolve, and what to do if response is delayed.

PATIENT–PHARMACIST CONSULTATION

Advising Patient on Treatment and Care Plan Development

Mrs. E.J. visits her primary care provider for assessment of blood loss and returns to your pharmacy 1 week later with a copy of her laboratory results. She presents a note from the physician asking you to help the patient select an iron product for her to take twice a day that is easy on the stomach. On questioning, the patient indicates that her physician did a full medical workup and she is happy to report that she does not have any type of serious anemia. In collaboration with the patient, you determine that the patient will begin taking ferrous gluconate 324 mg twice daily. Mrs. E.J. then reports that she is scheduled for follow-up blood work in the clinic in 3 weeks.

EVALUATE PROGRESS TOWARD ACHIEVING TREATMENT GOALS

The final area in the patient care process is follow-up evaluation. Evaluation is defined as the practitioner's determination—at planned intervals of follow-up—of the patient's outcome and current status.[6] The purpose of the evaluation is to determine whether previous drug therapy problems have been resolved, to evaluate the patient's progress toward achieving therapeutic goals, and to assess whether new problems have developed from the drug therapy.

PATIENT–PHARMACIST CONSULTATION

Evaluation of Patients' Outcomes

You determined that the use of ferrous gluconate, rather than ferrous sulfate, might cause Mrs. E.J. less gastric irritation. The pharmacist would advise the patient on the proper use of ferrous gluconate and encourage her to return to the clinic in 3 weeks to see how the medication is working. In a pharmaceutical care practice, the pharmacist would review the patient's copy of her laboratory results to set goals of therapy and the anticipated time frame for achieving those goals. A follow-up appointment would then be made with Mrs. E.J. after her clinic appointment to account for progress toward achieving goals of therapy and to reassess for additional drug-related needs.

Documentation systems used by pharmacists in a pharmaceutical care practice typically have a way of tracking the safety and effectiveness of drug therapies that may include an evaluation of outcomes for each of the patient's medical conditions and a resolution status of drug therapy problems. Pharmacists may also include a brief progress note in a patient's pharmaceutical care chart after each patient encounter. Evaluation notes help pharmacists convey important aspects of the patient's care in a clear and concise manner to fellow practitioners.

Aspects of care that pharmacists convey, in written format, may include the patient's expression of drug-related needs, goals of therapy, monitoring parameters, assessment of drug therapy problems, and a plan for resolving and preventing drug therapy problems and achieving treatment goals. An evaluation note can take on an appearance similar to the SOAP (subjective data, objective data, assessment, plan) format used in the field of medicine for the problem-oriented medical record system. When the pharmacist assumes responsibility for all the patient's drug-related needs within each of the patient's medical conditions, the evaluation note may reflect this holistic approach to care.

Follow-up allows the pharmacist to determine whether self-treatment has resulted in an appropriate therapeutic response and whether the patient has used medications appropriately or experienced any drug therapy problems, including drug-related toxicity.

Follow-up provides feedback that allows pharmacists to determine whether their communication skills require modification and whether useful information has been provided. At the same time, the patient will sense that the pharmacist cares. The pharmacist's concern for the correct use of nonprescription medications will also reinforce the notion that these products are medications and must be used carefully.

Pharmaceutical Care for High-Risk and Special Groups

Pharmaceutical care should be an important part of health care for all of our patients, but it is especially important for vulnerable populations. Certain groups of patients—infants and children, persons of advanced age, and pregnant and breast-feeding women—may experience a higher incidence of drug therapy problems than other patients. Because such problems can have dire consequences, these high-risk patients require special attention. Awareness of the physiologic state, possible pathologic conditions, and social context of these patients is necessary to properly assess their medical conditions and recommend appropriate treatment.

In many respects, persons of advanced age, infants, and children require surprisingly similar considerations. They all have a need for drug dosages that differ from those for other age groups because of the following features:

- They have altered pharmacokinetic parameters.
- Their ability to cope with illness or adverse drug events is decreased because of physiologic changes associated with either normal aging or child development.
- Their patterns of judgment are impaired because of either altered sensory function or immaturity.
- They have drug effects and potential adverse reactions that are unique to their age groups.
- They have a need for special consideration in administering medications.

Yet, because each of these groups of patients is heterogeneous, it is important to consider these features for each individual patient.

Special Considerations in Infants and Children

A study of the prevalence of nonprescription medication use in 3-year-old children found that 53.7% had been given a nonprescription medication within the preceding 3 months. The most commonly used medications were acetaminophen and cough or cold products.[23] An analysis of vitamin supplement use found that 54.4% of 3-year-olds in the United States were given vitamin and mineral supplements within the preceding 3 months. Providing pharmaceutical care to pediatric patients is challenging because of differences in physiology and pharmacokinetics,

lack of clinical data, insufficient drug labeling, and problems associated with drug dosing and administration.[24] In considering nonprescription medications for infants and children, the pharmacist should note that the pediatric population might vary substantially among age groups. It is appropriate to differentiate among relatively distinctive pediatric ages as follows[25,26]:

- *Premature:* gestation of less than 36 weeks
- *Neonate:* first postnatal month of life
- *Infant (baby):* ages 1 to 12 months
- *Toddler:* ages 1 to 3 years
- *Preschool or early childhood:* ages 3 to 6 years
- *Middle childhood:* ages 6 to 12 years
- *Adolescence:* ages 13 to 18 years

For most products, the Food and Drug Administration (FDA) recommends against self-medication in children younger than 2 years, especially using cough and cold products. Pharmacists can provide recommendations regarding medications with which they are familiar and for which dosage guidelines are readily available (e.g., pediatric acetaminophen products), but they should recommend evaluation by a primary care provider for medical conditions or medications for which they do not have pediatric experience. Some package labeling provides dosage guidelines by age group rather than by weight.

Physiologic and Pharmacokinetic Differences

Pediatric patients are at risk for drug therapy problems given that their body and organ functions are in a continuous state of development. Not only do the pharmacokinetic properties of medications differ in children compared with adults, but these properties can undergo rapid change as children grow and mature.[26] Furthermore, illness in children is potentially more serious than in adults, because the physiologic state of children is less tolerant of changes. Fever, vomiting, and diarrhea represent greater potential risks to children, because they are more susceptible to the effects of fluid loss. Therefore, the pharmacist should consider referral to a health care provider sooner for a condition in a child than for an adult with the same condition.

Other Potential Drug Therapy Problems

The pharmacist should be sensitive to the potential for drug therapy problems among children. In some illnesses such as diarrhea, nondrug therapy is often more appropriate than therapy with nonprescription antidiarrheal medications. In some situations, specific medications are contraindicated; for example, aspirin should not be administered to young children with certain viral illnesses (especially influenza and varicella) because of its association with Reye's syndrome (see Chapter 5). After warnings against using aspirin in children with viral illnesses were issued, the number of cases of Reye's syndrome dropped dramatically.[27] Pharmacists should counsel parents of children and adolescents with febrile viral illnesses against using aspirin. For younger children, solid dosage forms are inappropriate, and the pharmacist will need to guide parents to liquid medications or chewable tablets.

INACCURATE DOSING

Labeling for nonprescription medications generally uses age-based guidelines to determine dosages; however, many products do not provide dosage information for children younger than

6 years. Following the nonprescription medication's label, instructions for dosing a child older than 6 years can result in too high a dose and potential toxicity for the younger child. Inaccurate dosing by parents can result from determining an incorrect dose from the label instructions, by measuring out an incorrect amount, or both. A study of 200 children, 10 years of age and younger, who had been given a dose of acetaminophen or ibuprofen in the preceding 24 hours, found that 51% of them had been given an incorrect dose by their caregiver.[28] Pharmacists must better educate parents about dosing and administering nonprescription medications by helping parents interpret labels and demonstrating the appropriate use of measuring devices.

IMPROPER ADMINISTRATION/DOSAGE FORMS

Selecting the proper medication and dosage is not beneficial unless a medication is actually administered. Proper administration of medications to pediatric patients requires an appreciation of dosage forms, delivery methodology, routes of administration, palatability, and other factors. The discussion that follows focuses on oral medications.

Liquids are relatively easy to administer, and the dose can be titrated to the patient's weight; therefore, liquid medications are often used in pediatric populations. Because elixirs and syrups can have high alcohol and sugar content, respectively, these liquid forms may be less desirable than suspensions and solutions. A suspension may also mask the disagreeable taste of a medication.

Problems with drug administration can result in the child receiving the wrong dose. In a mock dosing scenario in which caregivers had the choice of using teaspoons, tablespoons, syringes, droppers, measuring cups, and measuring tubes, only 67% of the caregivers accurately measured the dose they intended to administer.[28] The volume delivered by household teaspoons ranges from 2.5 to 7.8 mL and may also vary greatly when the same spoon is used by different individuals. The American Academy of Pediatrics Committee on Drugs highly recommends the use of appropriate devices for liquid administration, such as a medication cup, cylindrical dosing spoon, oral dropper, or oral syringe. Ease of administration and accuracy should be considered when choosing a dosing device. Plastic medication cups are fairly accu-

rate for volumes of exact multiples of 5 mL (i.e., 5 mL, 10 mL, 15 mL). An oral syringe is preferable to the other oral dosing devices for higher viscosity liquids, because the syringe completely expels the total measured dose. Potent liquid medications should be administered with an oral syringe to ensure that the correct dose is given; the pharmacist should briefly explain to caregivers how to use and read an oral syringe. However, drawing up the dose in the syringe requires dexterity.

The use of precision devices for oral dosing helps ensure adequate therapeutic response by reducing the incidence of underdoses and eliminating adverse drug effects from potential overdoses. These devices may also enhance acceptance of medication by infants and children. Parents or caregivers may need instructions on using these devices to measure doses accurately, as well as advice on giving medications to reluctant or struggling children. The pharmacist may need to demonstrate to parents and older children how to take the medication.

A child older than 4 years can usually swallow tablets or capsules. Tablets that are not sustained-release or enteric-coated formulations may be crushed. Most capsules may be opened and the contents sprinkled on small amounts of food (applesauce, jelly, or pudding) to ensure that all the medication is taken. If the child does not eat the full portion, underdosing can occur. If multiple medications are prescribed, the child may be more cooperative if allowed to choose what flavored drink to use and which medication to take first. Table 2-1 presents selected guidelines for administering oral medications to pediatric patients.

ADVERSE DRUG EFFECTS

Adverse reactions are another potential drug therapy problem in children. Adverse drug events in children may differ from those in adults. For example, as in the older population, antihistamines and central nervous system (CNS) depressants may cause excitation in children. Except for Claritin (loratadine) syrup, FDA recommends not administering antihistamines to children younger than 6 years.[29] In contrast, sympathomimetics such as pseudoephedrine may cause drowsiness in children. In the United States, drug-induced acute liver failure is most commonly caused by acetaminophen, and about 18% of those cases were a result of accidental overdose. In addition, administration

---

TABLE 2-1 Selected Medication Administration Guidelines for Oral Medications

Infants
- Use a calibrated dropper or oral syringe.
- Support the infant's head while holding the infant in the lap.
- Give small amounts of medication to prevent choking.
- If desired, crush non–enteric-coated or non–sustained-release tablets into a powder and sprinkle them on small amounts of food.
- Provide physical comfort while administering medications to help calm the infant.

Toddlers
- Allow the toddler to choose a position in which to take the medication.
- If necessary, disguise the taste of the medication with a small volume of flavored drink or small amounts of food. A rinse with a flavored drink or water will help remove an unpleasant aftertaste.
- Use simple commands in the toddler's jargon to obtain cooperation.

- Allow the toddler to choose which of the medications (if multiple) to take first.
- Provide verbal and tactile responses to promote cooperative taking of medication.
- Allow the toddler to become familiar with the oral dosing device.

Preschool Children
- If possible, place a tablet or capsule near the back of the tongue; then provide water or a flavored liquid to aid the swallowing of the medication.
- If the child's teeth are loose, do not use chewable tablets.
- Use a straw to administer medications that could stain teeth.
- Use a follow-up rinse with a flavored drink to help minimize any unpleasant medication aftertaste.
- Allow the child to help make decisions about dosage formulation, place of administration, medication to take first, and type of flavored drink to use.

of acetaminophen at doses above the recommended daily dose over a period of 2 to 4 days can result in hepatotoxicity in children.[30]

NONADHERENCE

Nonadherence may occur when children refuse to take medication or when caregivers give up before the child receives the entire dose. Adherence may be improved by recommending a sweetly flavored product, because children may be more willing to take a medication if they like the flavor, consistency, or texture.[31] Nonadherence can also occur when caregivers do not understand instructions or do not pass them on to daycare providers, teachers, or school nurses. A 2003 survey study of 82 child daycare centers found that 52% of centers reported missing a dose during the preceding year, and 49% reported that the child's medication was not available.[32]

Assessment and Consultation

Assessment and consultation for pediatric patients usually involve the parents or caregivers. A 2003 article by Sleath and coworkers,[33] list six overall steps for communicating with children and improving their medication use process (Table 2-2). One should remember that it is important to include the child and parent during the patient counseling process, and that the child's and parents' concerns or fears about the medication should be considered.

Special Considerations in Persons of Advanced Age

Social, economic, physiologic, and age-related health factors place persons of advanced age at high risk for medical problems, and prompt them to be large consumers of nonprescription medications. Indeed, this population as a group consumes more medications than any other age segment of our society. Although individuals aged 65 years or older take on average 1.8 nonprescription medications daily, geographic area, race/ethnicity, and gender affect this number.[34] Nonprescription drug use in this population is highest in the midwestern United States, in Caucasians, and in women. Analgesics, laxatives, and nutritional supplements are the most common nonprescription

---

TABLE 2-2 Six Steps for Improving Medication Use in Children

Pharmacists should use a patient-centered style that focuses on the following steps:

1. Educating both the child and parents about the medication.
2. Investigating any concerns or fears that the child or parents may have about the medication.
3. Asking the child and parents about priorities for improved quality of life.
4. Following up with the child and parents to learn if they consider the child's treatment effective.
5. Offering to follow up with the pediatrician to improve the child's therapy (if needed).
6. Encouraging the child or parents to ask questions about the medication.

Source: Reference 33.

---

medications used by persons of advanced age. A study in 86 women who were 65 years of age or older reported an average use of 3.8 nonprescription medications per person.[35] In the 45% of women who used herbal products, the average number of herbal products was 2.5. The response to drug therapy by older patients is more scattered and unpredictable than that of other populations. Pharmacokinetic, pharmacodynamic, and various nonpharmacologic factors predispose these patients to potential problems with nonprescription medications. Preexisting medical conditions in older persons may affect the use of some nonprescription medications. For example, antihistamines should be avoided in patients with emphysema, bronchitis, glaucoma, and urinary retention from prostatic hypertrophy. Although nasal and oral decongestants can be used without adverse effect in many older persons, caution may be necessary in some patients with heart disease, hypertension, thyroid disease, and diabetes because of potential adverse effects of sympathomimetics on blood pressure, heart rate, and blood glucose.

Physiologic and Pharmacokinetic Differences

Persons of advanced age often have impaired vision (e.g., difficulty reading and differentiating colors) and hearing loss. The pharmacist should be aware of patient behaviors that indicate visual or hearing loss and should consider these impairments when communicating with older patients. Additional instructions for nonprescription medications may need to be provided in larger, high-contrast, dark print. Asking the patient to repeat counseling instructions can ensure that the directions were heard correctly and understood.

Subtle changes in mental status, such as confusion, may be anticipated in older patients who are anxious about their state of health. Older patients with cognitive impairments may have difficulty comprehending directions. Patients may not remember the names of all their medications or may not be able to remember instructions. Because of memory lapses, some older patients may require special drug delivery systems (e.g., transdermal patches or sustained-release preparations) to help them adhere to their dosage regimen. Older patients with cognitive impairments are less likely to read and interpret labels correctly,[36] which further emphasizes their need for special dosage form considerations.

Older patients are believed to confuse at least one-third of their problems with age-associated problems and, therefore, misreport their symptoms. Accurate perception and reporting of symptoms is vital to the successful use of any medication. In addition, older patients are often reluctant to share health information with others.

The aging process, as well as many chronic diseases, can alter a patient's nutritional status. Older patients who are most at risk for undernourishment or malnutrition are homebound patients and nursing home residents. Poverty, multiple chronic diseases, multiple drug therapy, or a combination of these factors may cause malnutrition in these patients. The patient's nutritional status and weight are important, because these factors can alter the pharmacokinetics and pharmacodynamics of medications.

Aging alters the absorption, distribution, metabolism, and elimination of certain medications, increasing the susceptibility of older patients to drug therapy problems. Pharmacokinetic changes, which have been well described in the literature, are caused not only by advancing age but also by the effects of disease states, and often by multiple drug use.

Older persons appear to have a greater sensitivity to some medications, particularly to anticholinergic medications, which may relate in part to alterations in cholinergic transmission.[37] Nonprescription medications with anticholinergic effects, such as certain antihistamines, may worsen preexisting medical conditions such as angina, congestive heart failure, constipation, diabetes mellitus, glaucoma, urinary dysfunction, sleep disturbance, and dementia.[37] The risk of accidents such as falls may also increase as a result of pupillary dilatation induced by anticholinergic medications and the inability to accommodate the effect.

Both subjective and objective evidence indicates that older patients have an enhanced CNS sensitivity to medications, especially CNS depressants such as sedatives and antidepressants. Increased brain sensitivity and other changes (e.g., decreased coordination, prolongation of reaction time, and impairment of short-term memory) manifest as increased frequency of confusion, urinary incontinence, and number of falls, especially among older women. Drug therapy may exaggerate all these changes, particularly if medications are taken in the "usual" dose or if multiple medications are used.

Control of bowel and bladder function lessens with advancing age. A further decrease in efficiency is likely with laxative use. Anticholinergic and CNS medications may reduce neurologic control. Antihistamines have sedative properties that may reduce bladder control in older persons.[37] Adverse effects of nonprescription medications often increase when such medications are added to an existing medication regimen.

Nonsteroidal anti-inflammatory drugs (NSAIDs) are widely used, especially by patients with osteoarthritis and rheumatoid arthritis. The absolute number of events of NSAID-related toxicity is greater for older patients because of their frequent use of NSAIDs and the increased prevalence of comorbid conditions coupled with concomitant drug therapies.[38] These patients may be especially susceptible to NSAID-associated peptic ulcer disease as well as congestive heart failure in susceptible individuals.[39] There is also some evidence that the chronic use of NSAIDs may elevate blood pressure in women ages 31 to 50.[40] Many patients were switched from NSAIDs to a cyclooxygenase-2 (COX-2) inhibitor; the latter was thought to be safer because of fewer serious GI-related adverse events. However, recent evidence suggests that the risk of cardiac events from taking rofecoxib, such as thrombotic stroke and myocardial infarction, far outweigh the beneficial GI profile. Rofecoxib has already been withdrawn from the market because of the increased risk of cardiac events.[41]

Other Potential Drug Therapy Problems

DUPLICATE THERAPY

Patients of advanced age can receive unnecessary drug therapy when medications are added to their therapeutic regimen without a reevaluation of the entire regimen to determine whether certain medications should be deleted. Duplicate therapy may occur if these patients are seeing multiple health care providers for their various medical problems or using multiple pharmacies. Use of a single pharmacy can significantly lower the risk of inappropriate drug combinations. Nonprescription medications commonly involved in drug interactions in older persons include aspirin, other NSAIDs, antacids, cimetidine, and antihistamines.[42] Many older patients have serious and multiple diseases such as coronary artery disease, chronic renal failure, or congestive heart failure, which can be aggravated by concurrent therapy for other acute problems. Concomitant illnesses or certain medications may contraindicate the use of other medica-

tions. It is important to consider whether an older patient is requesting a nonprescription medication to treat an adverse reaction from another medication.

INACCURATE DOSING/DOSAGE FORMS

Normal drug doses of analgesics and sedating antihistamines may be too high for patients of advanced age because of their impaired hepatic and renal function. These situations would necessitate either lowering the dose or increasing the dosing interval. Furthermore, older patients may experience difficulty with some dosage forms (e.g., swallowing large calcium or vitamin tablets, or using inhalers) because of physical impairments. Arthritis or tremors may make it difficult for older patients to open and close containers. Child-resistant containers may be especially difficult for older patients to open if they have deficits in physical dexterity. A pharmacist should direct older patients to products without child-resistant containers but also warn them of the potential poisoning hazard for visiting grandchildren or other young visitors.

NONADHERENCE

The prevalence of nonadherence with medications is high in the advanced-age population and is often the result of inadequate understanding of their medication regimen. Poor adherence may result from difficulty in swallowing or administering the medication. It may also result from an inability to afford the medication because of a limited or fixed income. Older patients may lack a social support network to supply the aid required by an illness. Pharmacists may need to involve caregivers in administering medications to these patients.

Special Considerations in Pregnant Patients

Drug therapy during pregnancy may be necessary to treat medical conditions or to manage common complaints of pregnancy such as vomiting or constipation. However, because most medications cross the placenta to some extent, a mother who takes a medication might expose her fetus to it. Therefore, the desire to ease the mother's discomfort must be balanced with concern for the developing fetus.

A 2001 study found that 13% of pregnant women from an academic setting birthing center used dietary supplements.[43] Of these women, 25% reported using supplements to relieve nausea and vomiting, and 25% reported stopping the use of these products because of concern for their fetus. The authors concluded that, although the use of dietary supplements was low among these women, the lack of safety data for these products is of concern. In another study, women attending an antenatal clinic reported using an average of 2.3 to 2.6 nonprescription medications in the three pregnancy trimesters, which was slightly higher than nonprescription drug use in the 3 months before pregnancy.[44] The most frequently taken medications were analgesics, vitamin and mineral supplements, and GI medications. Approximately 10% of pregnant women used herbal products.

Potential Drug Therapy Problems

Pregnant women should never presume that a nonprescription medication is safe to use during pregnancy. They should first consult with a pharmacist or primary care provider to determine whether a medication is teratogenic (i.e., causes abnormal embryonic development). Nausea and vomiting can cause another medication-related problem: difficulty in taking oral dosage forms of medications.

TERATOGENIC EFFECTS

Several factors are important in determining whether a medication taken by a pregnant woman will adversely affect the fetus. Two such factors are the stage of pregnancy and the ability of the medication to pass from maternal to fetal circulation through the placenta. The first trimester, when organogenesis occurs, is the period of greatest risk for inducing major anatomic malformations. However, exposure at other periods of gestation may be no less important, because the exact critical period depends on the specific medication in question.

Drug therapy problems are also important considerations for pregnant patients. Although dosage guidelines for some prescription medications (e.g., phenytoin) differ for pregnant patients, no information on dosage adjustments exists for nonprescription medications. Unnecessary drug therapy should be avoided. Nondrug therapy is often more appropriate than drug therapy for pregnant women. Use of cigarettes and ingestion of alcohol should be avoided or limited, because they have been associated with increased risk to the fetus.[45] Consumption of moderate doses of caffeine appears to be safe.[46]

In pregnant patients, the primary concern is related to drug safety. All pharmacists should be familiar with the A-B-C-D-X system for evaluating the safety of medications in pregnancy that were first introduced in 1979.[46] However, the FDA has recently announced a plan to strengthen drug labels to give patients and health care providers more precise information about how medications affect women during pregnancy and breast-feeding. The Agency has stated that consumers and health care providers have expressed concerns that these categories are overly simplistic, confusing, and inaccurate. Under the proposed rule, there will not be any letter categories. Instead, information will be provided in three sections:

1. *Fetal Risk Summary:* What is the risk of the medication to the fetus and the basis for the information, that is, animal or human studies?
2. *Clinical Consideration:* Explains the risks to the woman who took the medication before learning she was pregnant.
3. *Data:* Available about the drug in human and animal studies.

Often the issue is not whether a more effective medication is available but whether a safer medication is available. For example, evidence exists that aspirin is associated with congenital defects, incidence of stillbirths, neonatal deaths, and reduced birth weight.[43,46] Use of aspirin late in pregnancy has been associated with increases in length of gestation and duration of labor. These effects are related to aspirin's inhibition of prostaglandin synthesis. In addition, because aspirin affects platelet function, perinatal aspirin ingestion has been found to increase the incidence of hemorrhage in both the pregnant woman and the newborn during and after delivery. Therefore, a woman should avoid using aspirin during pregnancy, especially during the last trimester. Instead, because acetaminophen is generally considered safe for use during pregnancy, it is the nonprescription medication of choice for antipyresis and analgesia when taken in standard therapeutic doses.[43] NSAIDs such as ibuprofen and naproxen can be taken early in pregnancy.[46] However, they should not be used late in pregnancy given that they are potent prostaglandin synthetase inhibitors. Not only can they cause problems in the

newborn, but they can also affect the duration of gestation and labor. Chronic use of large doses of antitussive products that contain codeine may cause withdrawal in the newborn after delivery.[46] Severe CNS depression and hypoventilation at birth have been reported following maternal use of diphenhydramine, which was taken for several weeks prior to delivery for severe itching.[47]

NONADHERENCE

Nausea and vomiting associated with pregnancy may make it difficult for the pregnant woman to adhere to instructions for taking oral medications. Pharmacists can recommend eating small meals, frequent snacks, and crackers to alleviate or minimize nausea and vomiting. The patient should avoid foods, smells, or situations that cause vomiting. If necessary, an effervescent glucose or buffered carbohydrate solution, or the use of ginger may be effective. Only if those measures are ineffective should an antihistamine or antiemetic be considered. Consultation with a primary care provider may be indicated at this point.

Management of the Pregnant Patient

The pharmacist can aid the self-treating pregnant woman in deciding which drug or nondrug treatments she should consider and when self-treatment may be harmful to her or her unborn child. The decision to suggest a medication must be based on both an up-to-date knowledge of the literature and a critical risk–benefit evaluation of the mother and the fetus. Pharmacists should consult a reference such as the *Drugs in Pregnancy and Lactation* by Briggs and others[46] to check for the safety of medications in this population.

When the pharmacist has a choice between two medications, the preferred medication will be the one that has been in use for a longer period. Ascertaining the trimester of pregnancy is important, because it is a factor in determining whether some nonprescription medications can be used safely. The pharmacist should discourage pregnant women from self-medicating with nonprescription medications without receiving counseling from a primary care provider or pharmacist. The assessment and management of the pregnant patient require observation of the following principles:

1. The pharmacist must be alert to the possibility of pregnancy in any woman of childbearing age who has certain key symptoms of early pregnancy, such as nausea, vomiting, and frequent urination. Any woman who fits this description should be warned not to take a medication that might be of questionable safety if she is pregnant.
2. The pharmacist should advise the pregnant patient to avoid using medications, in general, at any stage of pregnancy unless the patient's health care provider deems such use essential. In addition, because the safety and effectiveness of homeopathic and herbal remedies in pregnancy have not been established, their use should be discouraged.
3. The pharmacist should advise the pregnant patient to increase her reliance on nondrug modalities as treatment alternatives (see Nonadherence).
4. The pharmacist should refer the patient to a primary care provider for certain problems that carry increased risk of poor outcomes in pregnancy (e.g., high blood pressure, vaginal bleeding, urinary tract infections, rapid weight gain, and edema).

Special Considerations in the Nursing Mother

A mother's drug use while breast-feeding can have an adverse effect on the infant. The concentration of a medication in the mother's milk depends on a number of factors, including the medication's concentration in the mother's blood; the medication's molecular weight, lipid solubility, degree of ionization, degree of binding to plasma and milk protein; and the medication's active secretion into the milk. Other important considerations include the relationship between the time of taking a medication and the time of breast-feeding, as well as the medication's potential for causing toxicity in infants. In addition, some medications (e.g., decongestants) may decrease milk supply.

When advising a nursing mother on self-care, the pharmacist should first decide whether a medication is really necessary, then recommend the safest one (e.g., acetaminophen instead of aspirin), and advise the mother to take the medication just after breast-feeding or just before the infant's lengthy sleep periods.[48,49] It is preferable to select a medication that has been in use for a long time and that has shown no apparent harm to nursing infants. If appropriate, topical or local therapy may be preferred to oral systemic therapy. In general, advise against medications that are extra-strength, maximum-strength, or long-acting, or products that contain a variety of active ingredients.[49]

When taken in therapeutic doses, most medications are not present in breast milk in sufficient concentrations to cause significant harm to the infant. However, several medications are contraindicated for use while breast-feeding, and others should be used with caution by nursing mothers. The amount of caffeine in caffeine-containing beverages is not harmful, but higher doses (i.e., more than 1 gram daily) have been reported to cause irritability and poor sleep patterns in infants.[49] Many nonprescription medications exist for which there are no data on their transfer into breast milk and their possible clinical effects.

Nonprescription medications that are usually considered compatible with breast-feeding include the following[46,50]:

- *Analgesics:* acetaminophen, ibuprofen, naproxen, and ketoprofen
- *Antacids*
- *Antidiarrheals:* kaolin-pectin, attapulgite, and loperamide
- *Antihistamines:* brompheniramine, chlorpheniramine, diphenhydramine, and triprolidine
- *Antisecretory agents:* cimetidine, famotidine, ranitidine, and nizatidine
- *Cough preparations:* dextromethorphan
- *Cromolyn sodium*
- *Decongestants:* phenylephrine and pseudoephedrine
- *Fluoride*
- *Laxatives:* bran type, bulk-forming type, docusate, glycerin suppositories, magnesium hydroxide, and senna
- *Vitamins*

CAM Use in Special Populations

Special consideration should be given to the assessment of complementary and alternative medicine (CAM) use in children, pregnant and nursing women, and the elderly, because the level of use is high in these populations. The use of herbals in a study population of children ages 3 weeks to 18 years was 45% during the year before they were surveyed.[51] In the adult population, the use of these products is estimated to be about 57%. Of these, only 33% of patients told their health care provider about their use of these products.[52]

During a typical patient medication interview, the emphasis is usually on prescription and nonprescription medications. However, specific questions need to be asked to assess the current use of herbal and home remedies, because the use of these products may also cause drug therapy problems and patients may not even consider them to be drug products. There is a tendency for patients to view herbal products as safe for use given that they are natural products and not drugs. In the previously mentioned study of herbal use, "77% of patients or caregivers did not believe or were uncertain if herbal products had any side effects and only 27% could name a potential side effect. Sixty-six percent were unsure or thought that herbal products did not interact with other medications."[51]

Therefore, it is imperative that a specific assessment of herbal use be made. To improve the process, it is best to ask about herbal use but also include examples. You might say, "Okay, now I am going to ask you about any herbal or natural products you are taking. This would be things like St. John's wort, echinacea, cod liver oil, or even home remedies that you might use. We know that many patients use products like these, because they feel they are safer, which is fine, but they might not realize that some of them interact with the other medications they are taking." Phrased this way, the question leaves little doubt as to the type of products to which the pharmacist is referring. Furthermore, it takes patients off the defensive, while still expressing the possible danger of using these products. Case 2-1 illustrates the assessment of a patient using an herbal product.

Key Points for Patient Assessment and Consultation

The use of nonprescription medications represents an important component of the health care system. Under ideal conditions, consumers can diagnose their own symptoms, select a nonprescription drug product, and monitor their own therapeutic response. If properly used, nonprescription medications can relieve patients' minor physical complaints and permit primary care providers to concentrate on more serious illnesses. If used improperly, however, nonprescription products can create a multitude of drug therapy problems. The key points discussed in this chapter include the following:

➤ Twenty-three percent of all drug therapy problems experienced by patients have a cause or resolution associated with the use of nonprescription medications.

➤ Interacting with patients to address self-care needs requires attention to the principles of communication discussed in this chapter.

➤ A systematic patient care process has been established to effectively address a patient's self-care needs.

➤ The consistent and systematic patient care process helps practitioners be complete and concise when assuming responsibility for a patient's self-care needs.

➤ A pharmacist working in a busy dispensing pharmacy can establish a relationship with the patient, determine the patient's self-care needs, and ascertain a list of the patient's current medications and medical conditions before recommending an appropriate course of action.

➤ The extent to which pharmaceutical care is implemented and documented, regarding patients with self-care needs, ultimately depends on compensation for services.

Relevant Evaluation Criteria	Scenario/Model Outcome
Information Gathering	
1. Gather essential information about the patient's symptoms, including:	
a. description of symptom(s) (i.e., nature, onset, duration, severity, associated symptoms)	Patient complains of muscle weakness and pain for last 2 weeks.
b. description of any factors that seem to precipitate, exacerbate, and/or relieve the patient's symptom(s)	None
c. description of the patient's efforts to relieve the symptoms	Patient took some acetaminophen, which helps a little bit with the pain, but the weakness is still there.
2. Gather essential patient history information:	
a. patient's identity	Mrs. Lisa Miller
b. patient's age, sex, height, and weight	65-year-old female, 50 inches tall, 100 lb
c. patient's occupation	N/A
d. patient's dietary habits	Balanced and appropriate diet
e. patient's sleep habits	Averages 5–7 hours per night
f. concurrent medical conditions, prescription and nonprescription medications, and dietary supplements	High cholesterol; lovastatin 20 mg each day (started a year ago), One-A-Day vitamin, red yeast rice 1200 mg twice daily; coenzyme Q10 (CoQ10) 200 mg daily
g. allergies	NKA
h. history of other adverse reactions to medications	None
i. other (describe) _____	Except for high cholesterol, Mrs. Miller is in good health. A friend of hers recommended taking red yeast rice to reduce her cholesterol further, and the Red Yeast company recommended she take the CoQ10. She has been taking both for about 3 weeks. She doesn't think these products could be causing her problem, because they are natural products.
Assessment and Triage	
3. Differentiate patient's signs/symptoms and correctly identify the patient's primary problem(s).	Muscle weakness and pain possibly resulting from addition of red yeast rice. Patient states she has not been involved in any strenuous exercise or walking or gardening.
4. Identify exclusions for self-treatment.	Possible adverse effect of rhabdomyolysis; requires referral to provider
5. Formulate a comprehensive list of therapeutic alternatives for the primary problem to determine if triage to a health care provider is required, and share this information with the patient.	Options include: (1) Refer Mrs. Miller to her provider for care. (2) Recommend discontinuing red yeast rice and CoQ10. (3) Recommend discontinuing red yeast rice and CoQ10, and refer Mrs. Miller to her provider for care. (4) Take no action.
Plan	
6. Select an optimal therapeutic alternative to address the patient's problem, taking into account patient preferences.	Recommend discontinuing red yeast rice and CoQ10, and refer Mrs. Miller to her provider for care.
7. Describe the recommended therapeutic approach to the patient.	Discontinue red yeast rice and CoQ10.
8. Explain to the patient the rationale for selecting the recommended therapeutic approach from the considered therapeutic alternatives.	Discontinuing red yeast rice and CoQ10 is needed, because red yeast rice contains lovastatin, which you are currently taking. Referral to your provider is necessary so that the provider is aware of the muscle weakness and pain, and can make further therapeutic changes if necessary.

> **CASE 2-1** (continued)

Relevant Evaluation Criteria	Scenario/Model Outcome
Patient Education	
9. When recommending self-care with nonprescription medications and/or nondrug therapy, convey accurate information to the patient.	Criterion does not apply in this case.
10. Solicit follow-up questions from patient.	Will the muscle weakness and pain go away?
11. Answer patient's questions.	Normally the weakness and pain go away within a couple of weeks after stopping the medication.

Key: NKA, no known allergy.

➤ Compensation for the provision of medication therapy management services provided within pharmaceutical care practices is a reality.

➤ In a pharmaceutical care practice, the pharmacist devotes attention to assessing patients' drug-related needs in which the identification of drug therapy problems and establishment of treatment goals take place.

➤ Addressing the special drug-related needs of selected high-risk groups such as infants and children, people of advanced age, and pregnant and breast-feeding women has been highlighted in this chapter.

To be of greatest service to patients, pharmacists must continually expand their therapeutic knowledge and must improve their interpersonal communication skills. As pharmacists strive to fulfill their responsibilities as health care practitioners and continue to expand their patient care services, people will learn of those services and seek their pharmacist's assistance whenever they are in doubt about self-treatment. The result will be better-informed patients who will not only use the professional services of pharmacists but who will also recognize pharmacists' contributions to health care.

REFERENCES

1. National Council on Patient Information and Education (NCPIE). 2003 National Opinion Survey Conducted for The National Council on Patient Information and Education. Available at: http://www.bemedwise.org/survey/survey.htm. Last accessed August 6, 2008.
2. Consumer Healthcare Products Association. OTC Facts and Figures. Available at: http://www.chpa-info.org/ChpaPortal/PressRoom/Statistics/OTCFactsandFigures.htm. Last accessed August 4, 2008.
3. Manasse HR Jr. Medication use in an imperfect world: drug misadventuring as an issue of public policy: parts 1 and 2. *Am J Hosp Pharm*. 1989; 46:929–44, 1141–52.
4. Johnson JA, Bootman JL. Drug-related morbidity and mortality: a cost of illness model. *Arch Intern Med*. 1995;155:949–56.
5. Ernst FR, Grizzle AJ. Drug-related morbidity and mortality: updating the cost-of-illness model. *J Am Pharm Assoc*. 2001;41:192–9.
6. Cipolle RJ, Strand LM, Morley PC. *Pharmaceutical Care Practice: A Clinician's Guide*. 2nd ed. New York: McGraw Hill Inc; 2004.
7. Stergachis A, Maine LL, Brown LM. The 2001 national pharmacy consumer survey. *J Am Pharm Assoc*. 2002;42:568–76.
8. Public Law No. 104-191: Health Insurance Portability and Accountability Act of 1996.
9. Public Law No. 108-173: Medicare Prescription Drug, Improvement, and Modernization Act of 2003.
10. Beebe M, Dalton, JA, Duffy C, et. al., eds. *Current Procedural Terminology—CPT® 2008*. Chicago: American Medical Association; 2008.
11. Beebe M, Rozell D, JA, Hayden D, et. al., eds. *CPT Changes 2006: An Insider's View*. Chicago: American Medical Association; 2005:309–12.
12. Isetts BJ, Brown LM, Schondelmeyer SW, et al. Quality assessment of a collaborative approach for decreasing drug-related morbidity and achieving therapeutic goals. *Arch Intern Med*. 2003;163:1813–20.
13. Isetts BJ, Buffington DE. CPT code-change proposal: National data on pharmacists' medication therapy management services. *J Am Pharm Assoc*. 2007;47:491–5.
14. Hepler CD, Strand LM. Opportunities and responsibilities in pharmaceutical care. *Am J Hosp Pharm*. 1990;47:533–43.
15. Isetts BJ, Schondelmeyer SW, Artz MB, et al. Clinical and economic outcomes of medication therapy management services: the Minnesota experience. *J Am Pharm Assoc*. 2008;48:203–11.
16. Willink DP, Isetts B. J. Becoming 'indispensible': developing innovative community pharmacy practices. *J Am Pharm Assoc*. 2005;45;376–89.
17. Purtillo RB, Haddad A. *Health Professional and Patient Interaction*. Philadelphia: WB Saunders; 1996.
18. Berger BA. *Communication Skills for Pharmacists: Building Relationships Improving Patient Care*. Washington, DC: American Pharmacists Association; 2002.
19. Rantucci MJ. *Pharmacists Talking with Patients: A Guide to Patient Counseling*. Baltimore: Williams & Wilkins; 1997.
20. Siganga WW, Huynh TC. Barriers to the use of pharmacy services: the case of ethnic populations. *J Am Pharm Assoc*. 1997;37:335–40.
21. Hensrud DD, Engle DD, Scheitel SM. Underreporting the use of dietary supplements and nonprescription medications among patients undergoing periodic health examination. *Mayo Clin Proc*. 1999;74:443–7.
22. Isetts BJ, Sorensen TD. Use of a student-driven, university-based pharmaceutical care clinic to define the highest standards of patient care. *Am J Pharm Educ*. 1999;63:443–9.
23. Kogan MD, Pappas G, Yu SM, et al. Over-the-counter medication use among U.S. preschool-age children. *JAMA*. 1994;272:1025–30.
24. Zenk KE. Challenges in providing pharmaceutical care to pediatric patients. *Am J Hosp Pharm*. 1994;51:688–94.
25. Wong DL. Developmental influences on child health promotion. In: Wong DL, ed. *Essentials of Pediatric Nursing*. 5th ed. St. Louis: Mosby; 1997:83–103.
26. Skaer TL. Dosing considerations in the pediatric patient. *Clin Ther*. 1991;13:526–44.
27. Belay ED, Bresee JS, Holman RC, et al. Reye's syndrome in the United States from 1981 through 1997. *N Engl J Med*. 1999;340:1377–82.
28. Li SF, Lacher B, Crain EF. Acetaminophen and ibuprofen dosing by parents. *Pediatr Emerg Care*. 2000;16:394–7.
29. Pray WS. The pharmacist as self-care advisor. *J Am Pharm Assoc*. 1996; 36:329–41.

30. Larsen OM, Ostapowicz G, Fontana RJ, et al. Outcome of acetaminophen-induced liver failure in the USA in suicidal vs accidental overdose: preliminary results of a prospective multicenter trial. *Hepatology.* 2000;32:396A.

31. Compounding for the pediatric patient. *Pharm Compound.* 1997;1:84–6.

32. Sinkovits HS, Kelly MW, Ernst ME. Medication administration in day care centers for children. *J Am Pharm Assoc.* 2003;43:379–82.

33. Sleath B, Bush PJ, Pradel FG. Communicating with children about medicines: a pharmacist's perspective. *Am J Health Syst Pharm.* 2003;60:604–7.

34. Hanlon JT, Fillenbaum GG, Ruby CM, et al. Epidemiology of over-the-counter drug use in community dwelling elderly: United States perspective. *Drugs Aging.* 2001;18:123–31.

35. Yoon SJ, Horne CH. Herbal products and conventional medicine used by community-residing older women. *J Adv Nurs.* 2001;33:51–9.

36. Meyer ME, Schuna HH. Assessment of geriatric patients' functional ability to take medication. *Drug Intell Clin Pharm.* 1989;23:171–4.

37. Mintzer J, Burns A. Anticholinergic side-effects of drugs in elderly patients. *J R Soc Med.* 2000;93:457–62.

38. Solomon DH, Gurwitz JH. Toxicity of nonsteroidal anti-inflammatory drugs in the elderly: is advanced age a risk factor? *Am J Med.* 1997;1:208–15.

39. Page J, Henry D. Consumption of NSAIDs and the development of congestive heart failure in elderly patients: an underrecognized public health problem. *Arch Intern Med.* 2000;160:777–84.

40. Curhan GC, Willett WC, Rosner B, et al. Frequency of analgesic use and risk of hypertension in younger women. *Arch Intern Med.* 2002;162:2204–8.

41. FitzGerald GA. Coxibs and cardiovascular disease. *N Engl J Med.* 2004; 351:1709–11.

42. Seymour RM, Routledge PA. Important drug-drug interactions in the elderly. *Drugs Aging.* 1998;12:485–94.

43. Tsui B, Dennehy CE, Tsourounis C. A survey of dietary supplement use during pregnancy at an academic medical center. *Am J Obstet Gynecol.* 2001;185:433–7.

44. Henry A, Crowther C. Patterns of medication use during and prior to pregnancy: the M A P study. *Aust N Z J Obstet Gynaecol.* 2000;40:165–72.

45. Wagner CL, Katikaneni LD, Cox TH, et al. The impact of prenatal drug exposure on the neonate. *Obstet Gynecol Clin North Am.* 1998;25: 169–94.

46. Briggs GG, Freeman RK, Yaffe SJ. *Drugs in Pregnancy and Lactation: A Reference Guide to Fetal and Neonatal Risk.* 5th ed. Baltimore: Williams & Wilkins; 1998:73a–81a, 125c–31c, 254c–5c, 524i–6i, 757n–8n.

47. Miller AA. Diphenhydramine toxicity in a newborn: a case report. *J Perinatol.* 2000;20:390–1.

48. American Academy of Pediatrics Committee on Drugs. Transfer of drugs and other chemicals into human milk. *Pediatrics.* 2001;108:776–89.

49. Dillon AE, Wagner CL, Wiest D, et al. Drug therapy in the nursing mother. *Obstet Gynecol Clin North Am.* 1997;24:675–96.

50. Nice FJ, Snyder JL, Kotansky BC. Breastfeeding and over-the-counter medications. *J Hum Lact.* 2000;16:319–31.

51. Lanski SL, Greenwald M, Perkins A, et al. Herbal use in a pediatric emergency department population: expect the unexpected. *Pediatrics.* 2003; 111:981–5.

52. Kennedy J. Herb and supplement use in the U.S. adult population. *Clin Ther.* 2005;27:1847–58.

Multicultural Aspects of Self-Care

Magaly Rodriguez de Bittner and Gloria J. Nichols-English

Culture influences beliefs about the health care system and may impact patients' decisions regarding self-care. This chapter addresses important aspects of patients' health beliefs and use of nonprescription products to help guide pharmacists in the delivery of pharmaceutical care and in counseling patients from diverse backgrounds and cultures.

The ability of pharmacists to gather information, assess patient complaints, guide a patient's product selection, and/or advise patients to seek care from another health care provider is an important component of pharmaceutical care. Through data collection and proper assessment of the patient's symptoms, important health issues can be identified and solved. However, if cultural issues are not considered during the patient interview, it may be difficult for a health care provider to assess and/or counsel a patient effectively. Practitioners can choose a more appropriate self-care plan for the health issue presented if they understand the patient's cultural framework and incorporate the patient's health care beliefs into the formulation of the care plan.

This chapter highlights common issues and challenges faced by individuals of diverse backgrounds in self-care management of health conditions involving the use of nonprescription products. Barriers to participating in medical decision making are also discussed, and approaches to promoting the exchange of ideas about alternative care strategies and recommendations for optimizing patient outcomes and quality of care are delineated. In addition, practical approaches to providing care and counseling of patients of diverse cultural backgrounds are presented.

Major shifts in the composition of the U.S. population are reviewed to illustrate the relevance of cultural issues in health and the overall delivery of health care. Emphasis is placed on defining and listing important cultural terms and theoretical frameworks for cross-cultural pharmaceutical care so that pharmacists are able to better understand the cultural framework of patients. Characteristics of the four major ethnic/minority groups in the United States are discussed, as well as differences in cultural approaches to seeking care, particularly self-care. Emphasis is placed on cultural assessment techniques and communication strategies to assist pharmacists in communicating effectively with patients of diverse cultures and in developing a culturally competent self-care plan.

In this chapter the terms *Western, American,* or *conventional medicine* are used synonymously to mean therapies regulated by the Food and Drug Administration (FDA), including prescription and nonprescription products. The terms *complementary, alternative,* and *traditional* are referred to as complementary and alternative medicine (CAM). These alternative health systems encompass a large array of health practices from all over the world, consisting of essentially natural botanical and non-botanical therapies, and products ranging from relatively new modalities to ancient skills and traditions such as magnet therapy, acupuncture, herbs, mind/body techniques, homeopathy, and massage therapy. The concept of CAM is introduced in this chapter to denote the need for health care providers to evaluate the specific variation in the use of CAM modalities among ethnically diverse patient population groups. This evaluation is particularly important for tailored medication consultations. Researchers have found that patterns of CAM use vary by each ethnic group. Minority populations and foreign immigrants self-treat with unconventional preparations according to their traditional values, health beliefs, and normative patterns of health-seeking behaviors. Furthermore, predictor characteristics for differences in CAM use include ethnicity, age, gender, educational attainment, number of health conditions, and geographical regions. Because the patient's self-management and decision-making process in selecting CAM modalities may impact the patient's health outcome, it is important to develop appropriate fact-gathering skills that include ethnically specific surveys to capture specific patient information needs.[1] Readers are referred to Chapters 53 through 55 for an in-depth discussion of selected alternative health systems and commonly used therapies.

Demographic Changes in the U.S. Population

For statistical purposes, the U.S. Census Bureau classifies ethnic minorities as Hispanics or Latino, Black or African American, Asian, Native Hawaiian and other Pacific Islanders, and American Indian and Alaska Natives.[2] Because ethnic groups can be racially diverse, further classifications were made during the 2000 census to estimate more accurately the composition of the U.S. population. For the first time in the history of the United States, population estimates were published by race and Hispanic origin categories. Race and Hispanic origin are considered two separate categories; Hispanics may be of any race or races. People can also be classified racially as non-Hispanic White, Hispanic White, non-Hispanic Black, Hispanic Black, American Indian and Alaska Natives, Asian, and Native Hawaiian and Pacific Islander. In addition, people were allowed to define themselves as belonging to more than one racial group in the 2000 census.

It is important to keep in mind the heterogeneity of these classifications. For example, the groups included in the classification of Asian American and Pacific Islanders have great variability among them. The same holds true for the Hispanic American classification, which includes four diverse groups: Mexican Americans, Puerto Ricans, Cubans, and others (e.g., Central Americans, South Americans, and Spaniards). Many people in the United States may belong to two or more ethnic groups, making the issue of race and ethnic background very complex.[2]

Shift in the Composition and Geographic Distribution of the U.S. Population

In the past decade, the rapid growth of the racial and ethnic minorities in the United States has resulted in a significant shift in the composition of the U.S. population. The latest U.S. census estimates concur with projections that members of minorities will constitute a majority of the nation's population by 2050.[2] In 2006, the number of foreign-born inhabitants was 37.5 million,[2] with Mexico the leading country of origin. The nation's minority population rose from 98.3 million in 2006 to 100.7 million in 2007, according to a U.S. Census Bureau report based on the national and state estimates by race, Hispanic origin, gender, and age. In perspective, "One in three U.S. residents is a minority."[2] During the July 1, 2005, to July 1, 2006, period, the U.S. Census Bureau reported the Hispanic group as the fastest growing minority. Having increased by 3.4%, this group totaled 44.3 million or 14.8% of the total population, making this group the largest minority in the United States. African Americans were the second largest minority group, having increased by 1.3% and totaled 40.2 million or 12.6% of the population. The third largest minority group was Asian American (14.9 million) or 4.5% of the population. Their 2.9% growth rate was second to that of Hispanics. American Indian and Alaska Native (4.5 million) were 0.8 percent of the total population and had risen by 1%. Native Hawaiian and Other Pacific Islander (1 million) had risen by 1.7% and were 0.1% of the population. From 2005–2006 non-Hispanic White Americans represented 73.9% of the total population (221 million) and grew by only 0.3% during this same time period. This population makes up the largest percentage of aging baby boomers. People older than 65 years make up 12.4% of the population.[2]

In terms of geographical distribution, larger percentages of the nation's population are moving south and west.[3] Minorities are the greatest contributors to this migration trend. Nearly one-third of people classified as minorities live in California and Texas. Four states and the District of Columbia have populations in which minority populations are the majority. In 2006, Hawaii led the nation with a population that was 75% minority, followed by the District of Columbia (68%), New Mexico (57%), California (57%), and Texas (52%).[3]

Although all geographical areas of America are aging, selective areas are becoming younger owing to the lower median childbearing age of minorities and foreign immigrants. By 2006 in two of the nation's fastest growing states, Florida and Nevada, followed by Maryland and New York, members of racial and ethnic minorities comprised the majority of children younger than 15 years.[3]

The Challenges of Cultural Competency and Diversity in the Pharmacy Profession

Current trends in diverging migration patterns have created unevenly distributed racial and ethnic diversity across America's regions. Therefore, transformation in ethnic consumer markets will be more pronounced in certain locales across the nation. In addition to racial/ethnic characteristics, the U.S. population is diverse according to gender, age, physical disabilities, religious preference, and sexual orientation. These demographic changes have penetrated most areas in the United States that were considered homogeneous in culture, making the importance of cultural competence a national issue. Pharmacists in every practice setting are likely to interact with patients from diverse cultures and backgrounds. Other stimulating sweeping changes in health service delivery demands include aging of the baby boomer generation, which parallels growth in prescription medication usage and the expanding need for pharmacists to perform more clinical activities.[4] Minority health disparities for certain diseases and the need for accessible care will continue to fuel the increasing demand for cultural and linguistic competence in pharmacy clinical services, as well as preventive activities.

One difficult challenge related to minorities is worsening shortages of pharmacy manpower in regions where there is an increasing minority population. The Aggregate Demand Index (ADI), a monthly national survey of the unmet demand for pharmacists conducted by the Man Power Project, has consistently shown that the regional workforce outlook for pharmacists in Western states (e.g., California, Hawaii, and New Mexico) have the highest level of unmet pharmacist demand compared with other regions.[5] Rural and Southern areas are also facing similar shortages. Patients in these regions have disproportionately higher rates of chronic disease, lower income, and lower insurance coverage.[5] The negative implications of the pharmacist manpower shortage and the increasing pharmacist workload are the counterbalance of time that could be devoted to providing patient-centered services such as advising patients on drug therapies, evaluating the safety of drug therapy, administering vaccines, and counseling patients on services such as chronic disease management and self-care management.

Another important aspect of the changes in population demographics is that the current racial/ethnic composition of health care professionals in the United States does not reflect the changes observed in the general population. The pharmacy profession must address the under-representation of minority pharmacists in the workforce. Statistics indicate White health care providers are caring for the majority of the patients from minority groups.[6] This issue highlights the need for pharmacists of all races to understand the influences of culture in health care and for schools of pharmacy to institute curricular content that incorporates cultural competency. White Americans received 63% of the first professional doctor of pharmacy degrees conferred in 2007. Under-represented minorities received 11.4%, with African Americans earning 7.0%, Hispanics 3.9%, and American Indian 0.5%. Asian Americans are the only minority group over-represented in the pharmacy profession compared with their racial/ethnic composition in the U.S. population: Asian Americans earned 20.1% of professional pharmacy degrees.[6]

A review of the evidence for a more diverse professional workforce indicates that health care professionals who are from the same racial ethnic minority and socially disadvantaged backgrounds as the patients they serve are more likely than others to (1) serve racially and socioeconomically disadvantaged populations; (2) provide concordance that improves the quality of communication when it is possible for the patient to consult a practitioner from their own racial or ethnic group or, for patients with limited English proficiency, to consult a practitioner who speaks their own primary language; (3) improve trust and comfort for follow-up and partnership; and (4) provide advocacy and leadership for policies and programs aimed at improvements for vulnerable populations. These qualities ultimately improve access to care and outcomes for those patient populations served by these providers.[7]

The Accreditation Council for Pharmacy Education 2007 accreditation standards and guidelines require a commitment to cultural competence training in the doctor of pharmacy curriculum to prepare candidates to practice in currently diverse environments.[8] During the accreditation visits to schools of pharmacy, the accrediting team must confirm that the curriculum provides opportunities to students didactically and experientially in the area of cultural competence. Many schools of pharmacy are completing curricular revision to meet this standard.

Definition of Culture

First, it is important to define what is considered culture in the context of this chapter. Cultural identity is developed on the basis of characteristics such as ethnicity, gender, age, race, country of origin, language, sexual orientation, and religious and spiritual beliefs. An official definition of *culture* is provided by the National Center for Cultural Competence (NCCC) as an "... integrated pattern of human behavior that includes thoughts, communications, languages, practices, beliefs, values, customs, courtesies, rituals, manners of interacting and roles, relationships and expected behaviors of a racial, ethnic, religious or social group; and the ability to transmit the above to succeeding generations." The NCCC embraces the philosophy that culture influences all aspects of human behavior. Of particular importance is the role of culture in help-seeking and health maintenance behaviors, and how these health beliefs and practices are passed from generation to generation. The NCCC home page can be accessed at www11.georgetown.edu/research/gucchd/nccc/index.html.

For the purpose of this chapter, another definition of *culture* is the sum total of socially inherited characteristics of a human group; this definition comprises socially transmitted assumptions about the nature of the physical, social, and supernatural world, as well as the goals of life and the permissible means that one can take to achieve them.[9] Culture is a learned set of values, beliefs, and meanings that guide decisions, attitudes, and action. It is important to remember that unique individuals with slightly different characteristics or beliefs may belong to the same cultural group. Individual differences must be considered when dealing with patients from specific ethnic or cultural groups. There is a great risk in making generalizations or assumptions that a person within a group will always behave in the same manner. This is known as stereotyping.

Variations in behaviors among members of a group become more important when people belonging to a specific cultural group migrate and live in places that have a different, but dominant, culture. In this case, the effect of acculturation or assimilation can be observed. *Acculturation* is a process by which members of a specific cultural group adopt the beliefs and behaviors of a dominant group, but may still value and practice their own traditional beliefs and behaviors when in the presence of their own group members.[9] On the other hand, *assimilation* of one cultural group into another may be evidenced by complete changes in language preference, adoption of common attitudes and values, membership in common social groups and institutions, and loss of separate political or ethnic identification.[9] Subsequently, in the acculturation process, people influenced by the dominant culture may behave differently from their own culture group's norm. Although acculturation is usually in the direction of a minority group adopting habits and language patterns of the dominant group, the outcomes of acculturation can be reciprocal, and the dominant group may also adopt patterns typical of the minority group. For instance, the adoption of ethnic "slang words," the enjoyment of ethnic foods and dances, and dressing in a manner that represents a particular ethnic group are examples of reciprocal acculturation practices. In the United States, reciprocal acculturation is evident by the practice of eating a larger proportion of nachos than the traditional potato chips at many holiday celebrations or major sporting events.

When persons lose or modify their cultural identity to acquire a new identity that differs from their original cultural group, an underlying assumption is that these behaviors and adaptations may cause internal conflicts among members of the cultural group. For example, conflicts can arise when younger members of a cultural group (second- or third-generation immigrants) do not follow traditions of the older generation, and exhibit differences in behaviors and beliefs more consistent with the dominant culture. In many instances, the children of immigrants do not even speak their parents' native language.

Culture can influence an individual's beliefs and attitudes toward health, illness, and treatment, which will influence the person's decisions regarding health issues. The inability of a pharmacist or any health care professional to understand an individual's culture may impede the effective delivery of targeted and patient-centered care and, consequently, the achievement of optimal health outcomes. Incongruent beliefs and expectations between the practitioner and the patient may lead to misunderstandings, confusion, and, ultimately, undesirable therapeutic outcomes.

Sociocultural Framework for Self-Care Practices

Interpretations of illnesses are usually influenced by religious beliefs, family and social contacts, cultural expectations, educational training, and personal experiences; these interpretations are within the foundations of an ethnomedical model of care.[10] According to Kleinman,[10] the patient's understanding of a disease is based on a consensus of beliefs, information, and expectations pertaining to the illness that are shared with a social network. This consensus constitutes the criteria for interpreting conditions for sickness and healing. Normative beliefs are generated by social interaction and personal experiences, which may differ completely from a scientific research approach to evidence-based medicine and the use of technology to diagnose and treat patients, which are within the biomedical model of care.[10] For example, the group may view "hypertension" as caused by "bad nerves" or "high excitement," but may not understand that the disease is the chronic elevation of arterial blood pressure. The group may not perceive the risk factors of obesity, family history, and/or dietary sodium intake as precursors to the development of coronary artery disease and stroke.

Practitioners who give little or no consideration to the beliefs and expectations of their patients will likely encounter resistance to their professional advice. Expecting patients to respond to the practitioner's advice solely on the basis of biomedical principles is naive and could evoke considerable frustration for the patient and the practitioner. Each patient may have different social support needs and concerns related to making decisions about self-care behaviors and medication use. Providers must remember the significance of "groupness" in minority population's self-care behaviors. One classic example includes patients who are neither able to nor willing to modify their dietary intake of certain foods (high-fat, salty, low-fiber) in an effort not to impose these restrictions on the whole family. They are willing to sacrifice their own health not to inconvenience their family.

The group's cultural beliefs and normative patterns of behavior provide the criteria by which the individual judges whether or not he/she is sick or should assume sick role behaviors. The need to include family members and/or designated caregivers in awareness and informational counseling sessions about the diagnosis and severity of an illness is illustrated by the remarks of an African American widow after the death of her husband from a myocardial infarction: "I knew that he was taking those pills for his high blood pressure and sugar. But I did not know that he was so sick. He still continued to work his two jobs and was always looking out for us. He ate as he always did, pretty much anything he wanted. Had I known that he was sick, I would have insisted that he change what he was doing, and I would have changed how I was cooking."

Normative beliefs based on the group's experiences also may assist the individual in making the decision whether to seek care from the health system, or whether it is more appropriate to use complementary or alternative therapies.[11] Self-care practices of many cultural groups involve use of home remedies, herbs, or other alternative treatments that are passed down from generation to generation. Communicating within the framework of the patient's culture helps break down barriers, and facilitates trust and understanding between the patient and health care professional. Through this knowledge, the provider is able to lead a patient successfully away from harmful practices and provide safe culturally sensitive alternatives. Subsequently, the practitioner can develop interventions (even biomedical ones) within the context of the patient's belief system. If the folk practices are not harmful or even found to be beneficial to the patient, the practitioner is encouraged to accept them as aspects of the treatment plan so the effects can be monitored and considered when evaluating patient outcomes. For example, a patient who is being monitored and treated through Western or conventional medicine might also use a folk healer. Some common healing methods include prayers, massage, and aromatherapy. Because these practices may be harmless and potentially additive to Western medicine, the practitioner may want to accept and even encourage their use.

It may be helpful if the pharmacist maintains consistent communication with the patient, folk healer, and other health care practitioners throughout the treatment to keep the channels of communication open for new information concerning alternative treatments. This issue is especially true in the case of many "curanderos" who may be advising the use of medications such as "Mexican aspirin" (dipyrone, an antipyretic drug that has been associated with agranulocytosis). It is banned in the United States but is available in Mexico under the name Neo-melubrina. In a recent study by Taylor et al.,[12] of the 200 patients in the study, 76 (38.0%) reported a lifetime use of Neo-melubrina for pain and fever. Most health care providers surveyed in the study were unable to identify correctly why Neo-melubrina might be used or its adverse effects. Many health care providers taking care of Hispanic patients are not aware of this fact and therefore unable to counsel the patient about therapeutic alternatives.

We know that patients are responsible for taking care of the day-to-day management of their illness. Consequently, better methods need to be developed to determine the patient's health-seeking behaviors, informational needs, preferences, and expectations about treatment management approaches. As stated earlier, the pharmacist is encouraged to use the ethnomedical model of care, as a framework for understanding how patients interpret their illness experiences. This framework according to Kleinman[10] goes beyond discrete medical episodes of "controlling the biological malfunctionings of disease" to include the psychosocial dynamics of family-based care, healer–client transactions, spiritualism, shamanic cures, and other important holistic approaches based on the patient's world view as mentioned above. Using this approach reduces the adverse impact of miscommunication, misinformed decisions, and harmful health behaviors.

General Description of Beliefs by Different Population Groups

Table 3-1 lists some of the characteristics shared by people in the major ethnic/minority groups in the United States (i.e., Hispanic Americans, Asian Americans, American Indians, and African Americans). It is imperative to clarify that these characterizations are generalizations. It is not safe to assume that every member of an ethnic or cultural group will conform to these attitudes and beliefs. This chapter uses examples of these beliefs and attitudes in an attempt to help sensitize practitioners to aspects of health behavior they may encounter with some patients. Health beliefs and behaviors, as well as the interplay of biological and societal influences, are documented in the literature.[9,11,13] Awareness of these differences in beliefs and expectations allows the pharmacist to provide pharmaceutical care in a more effective and culturally competent manner.

Religious beliefs are also important in patients' acceptance of the diagnosis and treatment. The set of beliefs, attitudes, and expectations of illness and treatment based on religion may cause friction with the health care system and the health care team. A typical example of how religion affects the acceptance of a treatment modality is the case of the Jehovah's Witnesses. Members of this religious group oppose the use of blood transfusions as a means of medical treatment. In some instances, attending physicians and/or health care institutions have initiated legal action to force a patient or his/her parents to allow the administration of a life-saving blood transfusion. This example illustrates the complexity of the issue and incongruity between Western medicine and some religious beliefs.

Individuals from different cultures may choose to treat illnesses using different rituals and religious items that are outside the realm of Western medicine. For example, Hispanic patients may use home remedies or other artifacts recommended by the *curanderos/curanderas,* who are spiritual healers and members of the community. On many occasions, these healers may use a combination of herbal remedies and religious rituals. Practitioners

TABLE 3-1 Examples of Cultural Behaviors Observed among Selected Ethnic Groups

Group	General Characteristics
Hispanic Americans	■ Family is very important (family members are deeply involved in the care of the patient) ■ Use *curanderos/curanderas* (healers) ■ Use home remedies (mostly tea or herbal remedies) that contain one ingredient ■ Use religious medals for good luck ■ Believe that health is a matter of "luck" ■ Have pessimistic attitude toward recovery ("fatalism") ■ Believe illnesses are classified as hot and cold (treatment is chosen depending on the classification of the disease)
Asian Americans	■ Family is important ■ Balance between forces defines health ("ying" and "yang") ■ Believe illnesses are caused by an imbalance of cold and hot forces ■ Use alternative medicine ■ Use Chinese herbal products (mostly a blend of a variety of herbs) ■ May have a distrust of Western medicine
African Americans	■ Use home remedies and folk medicine ■ Distrust the health care system because of previous experiences with the system ■ Religion is important in achieving cure ■ Family is also very important
American Indians	■ Use sweat lodges as a method of cure ■ Use herbal medicine/natural roots ■ Use prayer for cure of illnesses ■ Believe that health is a harmony with "Mother Earth" ■ Use healers (medicine man)

Source: Seidl HM, Ball JW, Dains JE, et al. Cultural awareness. In: *Mosby's Guide to Physical Examination.* 6th ed. St Louis: Mosby; 2006.

can better tailor therapy to the patient's needs if they understand these rituals and the belief systems. When practitioners appear nonjudgmental about different approaches, they can better understand how and when the patient plans to use drug therapy or another alternative treatment method. Knowing this information can help the pharmacist determine what prior treatments the patient used or is going to use, or whether there are major interactions between the nonprescription product to be recommended and the patient's alternative treatment.

Use of Nonprescription Medications by Culturally Diverse Patients

Limited data in the literature assess the use of nonprescription products among patients of diverse cultural groups or patients with diverse sexual, gender, or religious preferences. It is known that, for many cultural groups, especially those without drug cov-

erage, nonprescription products represent the most frequently used treatments prior to consulting a primary care provider.[14] Because of monetary constraints, fear of the health care system, and cultural beliefs, some immigrants will use the pharmacist as the first source of care. In many countries, the pharmacist plays a very important and significant role in assessing patient symptoms and triaging the patient to appropriate medical care.

Because of the limited access to health care facilities in many countries, pharmacists have served as primary care providers. It is important for pharmacists to understand that a large number of patients from other countries may seek this same level of pharmacist involvement in their care. There has been consistent evidence of a link between health-seeking behaviors and inappropriate antibiotic use in underserved Hispanic patients.[15] Patients' expectations may include that the pharmacist will provide them with prescription medications such as antibiotics as nonprescription products. Failure to do so may negatively influence the patients' expectations of the pharmacist. Understanding these expectations will allow the pharmacist to be prepared for the encounter and communicate to the patient the rationale for the therapeutic recommendations. Effective interventions for this population could include targeted messages to stakeholders, such as community organizations and other Hispanic community members, to address knowledge deficits and awareness of the harmful affects of antibiotic misuse.[15]

It is also important for pharmacists and other health practitioners to document the use of nonprescription products and CAM therapies in the patient's medical records. In a study conducted by the Mayo Clinic,[16] half of the patients who took nonprescription medication or dietary supplements did not report them to their health care provider, even when a written questionnaire was provided. However, most patients revealed their use during a structured interview.

Suboptimal Responses to Nonprescription Drug Therapy

The improper use of nonprescription products places vulnerable populations at an increased risk for adverse drug reactions, drug–drug interactions, and toxicities from long-term exposure. Therefore, the misuse and abuse of drugs that are available for self-treatment may outweigh the benefit–risk ratio in some high-risk patients. Increased use of nonprescription products by minority groups may create another challenge in self-care management. Self-care is important for patients with multifaceted chronic illnesses (e.g., human immunodeficiency virus/acquired immunodeficiency syndrome).[17] The need for quick relief may prompt more frequent use of nonprescription medicines, thus raising the risk of overmedication and a tendency for people to self-medicate for nonpathologic conditions. Lowered tolerance for discomfort can also lead people to rely on medications, especially nonprescription pain relievers, instead of seeking longer-term behaviorally oriented prevention strategies.

Another example of this behavior is the use of vitamins, laxatives, and antacids to counteract poor eating habits. It is more important to realize that these poor self-management practices can mask more serious symptoms and complicate the diagnosis of serious diseases.

Several other factors contribute to the increased vulnerability of low-income minority patients to the harmful effects of overuse of nonprescription products. First, patients with poor health status, low education, and low income are most likely to reduce consumption of prescription drugs when their costs increase.[18] Second, many uninsured patients use nonprescription products as alternatives to prescription drugs simply because of cost factors.[19] Third, these same patients may seek medical care only for the most recognizable and urgent symptoms, delaying regular, routine visits to their primary care provider's office. Practitioners who counsel patients on the use of nonprescription products can help prevent delays in seeking needed medical care. In addition, many "silent" medical conditions, such as hypertension and hyperlipidemia, are most likely not recognized.[20] Nonprescription products may be used by patients to treat minor symptoms associated with these conditions such as headache, nosebleeds, or chest discomfort. The key problem with a suboptimal response to a nonprescription medication is that more serious conditions may not be diagnosed until the patient experiences a negative consequence or complication.

Pharmacogenetics and Drug Response

Culturally diverse populations have been underrepresented in clinical research trials. This problem has been addressed in part by the NIH Revitalization Act of 1993, amended October 2001. This act requires ethnic minorities and women to be included in clinical research studies funded by the National Institutes of Health (NIH).[21] More research is needed on the pharmacokinetics and pharmacodynamic differences in drug metabolism among different ethnic/racial groups. In addition, very little data exist concerning differences in response to nonprescription drugs among patients of diverse cultural groups.

To date, researchers are discovering that variability in drug responses can be determined by racial or ethnic background, but the data are limited in scope.[22] The field of pharmacogenetics or pharmacogenomics uses genome-wide approaches to study the inherited basis of differences between persons in the response to drugs.[22] The genetic makeup of a race or ethnic group may be such that many people within that group are simply unable to produce certain enzymes needed to adequately metabolize certain pharmacologic classes of drug. Genetics is estimated to account for 20% to 95% of variability of drug disposition and effects.[22] The inherited variability in drug response has been associated with variants in the genes encoding drug-metabolizing enzymes, drug transporters, or drug targets. These differences in drug response do not change over time; instead they remain stable throughout the patient's life. Drug safety and efficacy are compromised when genetic variability in drug response is coupled with other nongenetic factors such as age, organ function, gender, concomitant therapy, drug interactions, and environmental factors.[22]

Armed with specific education and skill development, pharmacists can assist in the detection and reporting of unexpected adverse drug reactions, atypical drug responses from nonprescription and prescription drug interactions, and adverse affects in ethnic minorities. Therefore, it is important for pharmacy educators and institutions to provide this education and skill development in the pharmacy curricula and continuing professional education programs. In addition, practitioners can inform their ethnic minority patients of the need for their participation in pharmacodynamic and pharmacokinetic studies to gather more data in this area.

Providing Care to Culturally Diverse Groups

Barriers to care presented by differences in language, health literacy, and culture are challenges that health care providers confront every day in their practice. Providing services in cross-cultural situations can be extremely challenging and rewarding. In some cases, small differences in the interpretation of language, gesture, or eye contact may lead to misunderstandings between people of different cultures and their health care providers. In many cases, the health care provider's lack of cultural competency may impede the delivery of appropriate care and triage.

In addition, major health disparities among members of minority groups have been identified.[23] It is well-known that people of some minority groups do not equally experience long life spans, good health, and access to health services. Current data from the U.S. census and the Department of Health and Human Services (DHHS) indicate that index measures of the health status of the U.S. population show marked disparities in the health of different racial and ethnic groups. In many cases, these health disparities cannot be explained solely on the basis of current information about the biological and genetic characteristics of African Americans, Hispanic Americans, American Indians, Alaska Natives, Asians, Native Hawaiians, and Pacific Islanders. They may be the result of the complex interactions among genetic variations, environmental factors, socioeconomic factors, and specific health beliefs and behaviors.[23]

Many aspects of the health of the United States have improved, but the health of some racial and ethnic groups has improved less than others. The gap in life expectancy between the Black and White populations has narrowed but persists. Disparities in risk factors, access to health care, and morbidity also remain. In 2002, DHHS selected six focus areas as the corner stone for the 2010 Healthy People goal of reducing health disparities. The six health areas reflect serious disparities in disease burden and known risk factors affecting multiple racial and ethnic minority groups at all life stages in health access and outcomes. The priority health disparity focus areas established were (1) infant mortality, (2) deficits in breast and cervical cancer screening and management, (3) cardiovascular diseases, (4) diabetes, (5) HIV infections/AIDS, and (6) child and adult immunizations.[24]

The Healthy People 2010 Midcourse Review on the six focus areas show that infant mortality rates have not declined significantly since 2000. African American women had the highest infant mortality rates in 2004, which was more than twice that of White women. American Indian and Puerto Rican infants also have higher infant mortality rates than White infants. The death rate for all cancers is 30% higher for African Americans than for Whites; for prostrate cancer, the African American death rate is more than double that of Whites. African American women are two times more likely than White women to die of cervical cancer, and more likely than women of any other racial group to die of breast cancer. Heart disease and stroke are the leading causes of death for all U.S. racial and ethnic groups. The rate of death from heart disease and stroke is 29% and 40% higher, respectively, among African American adults than among White adults. Compared with non-Hispanic White Americans, American Indians and Alaskan Natives are 2.6 times and African Americans are 2.0 times as likely to have diabetes. African Americans and Hispanic Americans represent 66% of adult AIDS cases. African Americans 65 years of age and older are less likely than non-Hispanic Whites to report having received influenza and pneumococcal vaccines.[25]

Other diseases and conditions are glaring examples of racial disparity in health status. Obesity, a major risk factor for many chronic diseases, varies by race and ethnicity—39% of Black non-Hispanic women 20 years of age and older had the highest obesity prevalence in 2007, followed by non-Hispanic Black men (32.1%).[26] Mental health is disproportionately burdensome in American Indians and Alaskan Natives who have higher death rates from unintentional injuries and suicide.[27] Access to mental health care among this population is lacking in terms of quality. Many receive poor-quality care because of insensitivity in provider–patient interactions and program offerings. The incidence of hepatitis C infection is higher in African Americans, and African American teenagers and young adults become infected with hepatitis B three or four times more often than those who are White.[28]

Ethnic minorities bear a disproportionate burden of the tuberculosis cases in the United States, a continuing trend that may be due to factors of immigration and health care accessibility. In 2007, foreign-born persons accounted for a majority of tuberculosis cases among Hispanics (77.2%) and Asians (96.1%). Overall, the rate of tuberculosis cases in foreign-born persons was 9.7 times higher than in native-born persons. However, the majority of cases in African American populations were native-born (71.2%). Within native-born populations, African Americans were nearly eight times more likely than White Americans to have tuberculosis.[29]

Although the rate of primary and secondary (P&S) syphilis in the United States declined 89.7% between 1990 and 2000, the rate of P&S syphilis increased between 2001 and 2006. Syphilis remains an important problem in the South and in urban areas in other regions of the country. From 2005 to 2006, the rate of P&S syphilis increased in all racial and ethnic groups. The Centers for Disease Control and Prevention (CDC) STD Surveillance 2006 reports show that the rates per 100,000 population by race/ethnicity increased 5.6% among non-Hispanic White Americans (from 1.8 to 1.9), 16.5% among African Americans (from 9.7 to 11.3), 12.5% among Hispanics (from 3.2 to 3.6), 18.2% among Asian/Pacific Islanders (from 1.1 to 1.3), and 37.5% among American Indian/Alaska Natives (from 2.4 to 3.3).[28] The rise in sexually transmitted diseases in adults has been characterized by high rates of HIV coinfection.[30]

Factors linked to disparities in health status include race, socioeconomic status, health practices, psychosocial stressors, lack of resources, environmental exposures, discrimination, and access to health care.[29] These factors will likely continue to influence future patterns of disease, disability, and health care utilization unless they are addressed appropriately. For instance, Hispanics and American Indians under 65 years are more likely to be uninsured than those in other racial and ethnic groups. Persons living in poverty are considerably more likely to be in fair or poor health and to have disabling conditions. Adults 45 to 64 years of age living below the federal poverty line were two to three times as likely as those with incomes of 200% or higher of the poverty line to have three or more chronic conditions, and are less likely to have used the most advanced treatment technologies.[31]

The federal government has implemented a public policy to address the health needs of minority groups and to reduce racial and ethnic health disparities. These efforts are well summarized in the publication *Healthy People 2010,* which established goals aimed at decreasing disparities in health care and outcomes of therapy for all Americans, with a special focus on decreasing health disparities among minority groups.[30] *Healthy People 2010* offers a simple but powerful idea: provide health objectives in a format that enables diverse groups to combine their efforts and work as a team. It is a road map to better health for all and can be used by many different people, states, communities, professional organizations, and groups to improve health. The initiative has partners from all sectors.

Table 3-2 summarizes the major goals to decrease health disparities among minority groups. In addition, the Center for Minority Health and Health Disparities (www.ncmhd.nih.gov)

TABLE 3-2 Overarching Goals for *Healthy People 2010*

1. Increase quality and years of healthy life, including:
   —Improving access to comprehensive, high-quality health care services.
   —Improving patient's healthier self-behaviors.
2. Eliminate health disparities among segments of the population, including:
   —Differences that occur by gender, race, ethnicity, education, income, disability, geographic location, or sexual orientation.

Source: US Department of Health and Human Services, Office of Disease Prevention and Health Promotion. *Healthy People 2010.* Available at: http://www.healthypeople.gov. Last accessed August 27, 2008.

---

is a part of the NIH. These national initiatives have created an interest among the health care system, health care providers, and government agencies in identifying those factors that contribute to health disparities, and in developing strategies to decrease the gap that currently exists.[31]

One of the factors identified by many government agencies and health care groups as a cause of health disparities is the lack of awareness of cultural issues and health disparities among health care providers. This lack of awareness may be attributed to lack of formalized training on cultural issues in health care at higher education institutions. Cultural issues are not often an integral part of the curricula or textbooks used in many institutions. In addition, there are few opportunities for practitioners to receive skill development as part of continuing professional education because of the limited number of courses devoted to this topic.

To ensure effective delivery of culturally and linguistically appropriate care in cross-cultural settings, practitioners need to understand cultural issues related to health and illness, health disparities among different groups, and communication strategies to deal with culturally diverse patients.[32] The Institute of Medicine highlighted the need to train culturally competent health care providers to decrease the racial and ethnic health disparities observed among different minority groups.[33] In 1997, the Office of Minority Health also developed the National Standards for Culturally and Linguistically Appropriate Services in Health Care.[32] These standards are based on an in-depth review of the literature, regulations, laws, and standards currently used in federal and state agencies. One intended purpose of the national standards is to provide criteria that credentialing and accreditation agencies can use to ensure the level and quality of culturally competent care that providers and institutions provide. Some of these agencies include the Joint Commission, the National Committee for Quality Assurance, professional organizations such as the American Medical Association and American Nurses Association, and quality review organizations such as peer review organizations.

Communication with Culturally Diverse Groups

Data Gathering

When preparing to interact with patients from different cultures, practitioners must use specific communication skills aimed at elucidating the patient's cultural beliefs. Some of the required communication skills include (1) an openness to alternative viewpoints and approaches; (2) a clear understanding of one's own prejudices and biases (self-awareness); (3) engagement to identify the patient's beliefs, expectations, and barriers to treatment; (4) understanding of the influences of the patient's beliefs and attitudes in the treatment plan; and (5) an ability to negotiate treatment that is acceptable to the patient and the practitioner. Preestablished trust and effective communication are essential for this process to succeed. Trust is essential to gaining awareness of the issues involved in the interaction, and appropriate language is crucial to effective communication.[33]

Many techniques have been suggested to improve communication and care in cross-cultural settings. The organization Diversity R_x hosts a Web site that provides a link to the classic model proposed and developed by Berlin in 1983 for cross-cultural training.[34] This model has been proposed and described for individual and institutional cultural development. This technique, described with the acronym "LEARN," may be used in all clinical encounters to assist the health care provider. The primary steps in the LEARN technique are:

- *L*isten with sympathy and understanding to the patient's perception of the problem.
- *E*xplain your perceptions of the problem.
- *A*cknowledge and discuss the differences and similarities.
- *R*ecommend treatment.
- *N*egotiate agreement.

Tables 3-3 and 3-4 provide guidelines to help the practitioner communicate better with culturally diverse patients. In many instances, the communication barrier may include the patient's inability to speak English. Table 3-5 lists some approaches that the practitioner can use with patients who speak another language. On many occasions, practitioners may need to work with an interpreter. An interpreter provides a means of dealing with a language barrier, but this approach has limitations. On many occasions, problems may arise when family members are used as interpreters. The patient and family members may be put in

an uncomfortable position. This situation becomes more critical when a younger family member, sometimes a child, is asked to interpret for his/her parents or grandparents in a clinical encounter. This position of responsibility is unacceptable and leads to family conflicts by altering the hierarchy within the family. It also places an undue burden on the child, so this situation should be avoided.

The use of family members or untrained personnel to interpret may lead to receiving or transmitting inaccurate information because of the lack of training or failure to translate in a proper manner. The health care provider may fail to detect relevant, critical information or the information provided by the clinician may be mistranslated between clinician, interpreter, and patient. These problems may be avoided when the health care provider uses trained translators who are prepared in medical language and in interpretation, and are familiar with the provider and his or her practice.

Assessment of Cultural Issues on Patient Adherence

Practitioners can assess the role that culture may play in a patient's acceptance of the diagnosis and treatment of an illness by following the recommendations listed in Table 3-6, and by

---

TABLE 3-3 Recommended Actions to Develop Effective Cross-Cultural Communication

- Acknowledge diversity exists.
- Understand culture is part of what makes individuals unique.
- Respect people or cultures that may be unfamiliar or different from one's own.
- Conduct a self-assessment to identify one's own cultural beliefs and biases.
- Recognize there are differences in the way people define and value health and illness.
- Be patient, flexible, and willing to modify health care delivery to meet the cultural needs of the patient.
- Allow for differences among members of the same cultural group (do not expect all individuals from a cultural group to behave identically at all times).
- Appreciate the richness of culture.
- Embrace diversity.
- Understand that cultural beliefs and values are difficult to change and in many instances are learned from birth.

Source: Adapted with permission from Schrefer S. *Quick Reference to Cultural Assessment.* St Louis: Mosby; 1994:IV.

TABLE 3-4 Guidelines for Communicating with Culturally Diverse Patients

- Assess your personal beliefs surrounding persons from different cultures.
- Assess your own biases and prejudices.
- Assess communication variables from a cultural perspective (language barriers, nonverbal communication, and use of interpreters, beliefs, and feelings).
- Plan care based on communicated needs and cultural background. Adapt care to meet the cultural needs of the patient.
- Modify communication approaches to meet cultural needs (use more than one method to communicate the stated plan).

Source: Adapted with permission from Schrefer S. *Quick Reference to Cultural Assessment.* St Louis: Mosby; 1994:33.

TABLE 3-5 Communication Strategies for Non–English-Speaking Patients

- Use a caring tone of voice and facial expression to demonstrate your interest in the patient.
- Speak slowly and clearly, not loudly. Do not yell.
- Use gestures, pictures, and other role-playing techniques to help the patient understand.
- Repeat the message in many ways, using different communication approaches.
- Avoid using medical terms, slang terms or jargon, and/or abbreviations.
- Keep the message simple, and repeat it in several ways.

Source: Adapted with permission from Schrefer S. *Quick Reference to Cultural Assessment.* St Louis: Mosby; 1994:34.

TABLE 3-6 Cultural Assessment of Diagnosis and Treatment of Illness

Diagnosis	Treatment
What is the patient's understanding of the diagnosis?	What motivates the patient to recover?
What does this diagnosis mean to the patient?	Why does the patient want to recover?
How does the patient interpret the illness?	For whom does the patient want to recover?
Does the patient believe that the diagnosis is terminal?	What are the patient's feelings and beliefs about the treatment?
	How will the treatment affect the patient's relationship with his/her family?
	What are the expectations of the family regarding the treatment?
How is the patient accepting the diagnosis?	What is the role of the family in the treatment?
Is the patient in denial?	Is the family involved in administration of the medications or treatment?
How does the patient think others view/feel about the illness?	What effect does the treatment have in the patient's religious and/or cultural beliefs?
How will the diagnosis affect the patient's social status or social acceptance within their culture?	Is there a concordance between the patient's beliefs and the treatment plan?

Source: Adapted with permission from Schrefer S. *Quick Reference to Cultural Assessment.* St Louis: Mosby; 1994:35–36.

paying attention to verbal and nonverbal cues given or displayed by the patient. These recommendations will help the health care provider conduct a better assessment of the impact that cultural health beliefs and perceptions may have on the patient's acceptance of a diagnosis or treatment. For example, many Hispanic patients may have the perception that injectable dosage forms are more effective than oral tablets. This belief is probably based on the practice, in many Hispanic countries, particularly Central America, of primary care providers using injectable drugs with repository drug delivery forms to provide more sustained drug delivery. This technique is used to deal with the geographic distances many patients have to travel to receive care and helps achieve a more predictable duration of treatment. Furthermore, this form of drug delivery ensures adherence with treatment. Because a cure is most likely achieved with this repository of products, the patient most likely associates the effectiveness of care with this method of drug administration.

In the United States, however, injectable dosage forms are not commonly and routinely used. Therefore, Hispanic patients may leave a health facility with a prescription for an oral product believing that the treatment is not going to be effective. This lack of trust in the therapy may affect adherence with the regimen and impair achievement of a cure. If health care providers are aware of this particular cultural belief and take the time to assess the patient's preferences or beliefs to a variety of treatments, they can modify the treatment plan or educate the patient about the benefit of the oral dosage form. Even though this approach seems simplistic, it is a very complex process that requires time and individual assessment of the patient's beliefs and preferences.

Development of a Self-Care Plan

Self-care refers to strategies that individuals can use to manage their health problems, or to improve their health. Activities of self-care can include a range of individual health behaviors such as health maintenance, use of preventive health services, symptom evaluation, self-treatment, interaction with health care professionals, and the seeking of advice through lay and alternative care networks.[35] Generally, health care professionals encourage and support their patients' participation in self-care behaviors. The derived benefits are empowerment of patients to follow through on a health care plan and to actively participate in their own care, which is broader than just following a doctor's advice. Unfortunately, some health care professionals do not encourage self-care behaviors, because they are not aware of appropriately targeted techniques, strategies, and support systems that patients can use.

Current changes in the health care environment signal the increasing importance of self-care and self-medication. As primary care providers, pharmacists can be of great benefit to the public health agenda for health disparities. As a response to the demands and trends of modern-day pharmacy practice, the North American Pharmacist Licensure Examination has included competencies in nonprescription and self-care medication as a component of the licensing examination for pharmacists.[36] As pharmacists become more involved in self-care, they assume increased responsibility toward their patients. In the provision of pharmacy care skills for facilitating self-care behavior and self-medication, pharmacists serve primarily as communicators to initiate dialogue with the patient for informed decision making. They provide and interpret patient information, make referrals, and collaborate with other providers. Pharmacists can also serve in health and wellness promotion as they participate in health screening to identify health risks in the community and lead health awareness and prevention campaigns.[37]

The information gathered in the interview and physical assessment processes needs to be incorporated into the development of a self-care plan. The self-care plan must consider the cultural differences and beliefs identified by the patient. These beliefs, as well as the role of the family in the patient's care, will help dictate the most appropriate treatment recommendation for the patient. The pharmacist will be able to design pharmacy care plans that incorporate strategies to maximize the patient's goals and expectations of therapy. These strategies can achieve better adherence to drug therapy and treatment recommendations.[37]

Assessment of the problem must consider the patient's beliefs, values, and expectations of treatment. The practitioner must then use this information to delineate and develop his or her self-care recommendations and patient education strategies. In addition, there should be communication with other health care providers, particularly with the physician, about the patient's cultural beliefs and preferences. A collaborative approach ensures that all health care providers involved in the care of this particular patient are aware of his or her cultural preferences. For example, when developing a plan of care for the treatment of a self-limiting illness that requires nonprescription drug therapy, the practitioner must:

1. Consider the patient's beliefs and perceptions of the problem.
2. Find out if the patient has treated the problem with any non-prescription or herbal products/alternative treatments.
3. Identify any communication issues that cast doubt on whether the patient understood the questions being asked and/or whether the data gathered are accurate.
4. Identify any cultural/religious beliefs that may influence the patient's acceptance or willingness to use a specific product.
5. Identify the patient's perceptions/acceptance of the recommended treatment.
6. Identify other methods/resources to help the patient better understand the appropriate use of the product. For example, is a family member present who can understand the instructions and explain them to the patient? Is an interpreter available? Are materials written in the patient's language available? Can diagrams or pictograms be used to communicate the information?
7. Ensure that the patient knows what to do if the product/treatment does not solve the problem.
8. Ensure that the patient knows when to contact the practitioner again or to seek the care of a primary care provider.

Decision Making and Nonprescription Products

The market for nonprescription drugs is expanding, and patient autonomy concerning health care extends to taking part in the decision making for the need for treatment; monitoring treatment progress; and using nonprescription medications, home monitoring devices, and diagnostic kits at intervals during the treatment process. Because there are higher rates of chronic conditions and diseases within minority populations, drugs (even nonprescription drugs) to treat these conditions and symptoms will be more widely used.[16]

Pharmacists can help the patient in the decision to use non-prescription products by conducting thorough assessments to determine whether the patient has the proper skills and motivation to follow through on a recommended self-care plan. Pharmacists should plan to interact with the patient at regular, usually brief, intervals during prescription refills to reinforce nonprescription product selection decisions, make adjustments to the self-care plan, and detect possible adverse effects. Pharmacists may be the health care providers best suited to orient patients toward appropriate referral and self-care behavior.[35]

Barriers to Self-Care Management
Fear and Mistrust of Health Care Providers

Mistrust of providers creates a barrier to self-care management, because it reduces the tendency of patients to seek preventive care and to avoid following the practitioner's advice for follow-up care. Patients may feel practitioners did not consider their concerns; therefore, their expectations are not met. The disparities for minorities, especially African Americans and Native Americans, have been associated historically with discriminatory treatment and systemic racism in America. Although measures have been taken to correct many historical aspects of the health care environment, many negative institutionalized health care policies and social aspects of provider–patient relationships remain as barriers to effective patient care. Racism is insidious, cumulative, and chronic. Persistency in patient mistrust and perceptions of cultural racism directly impact patient satisfaction and health outcomes.[38]

The NIH mandates for inclusion of racial/ethnic minorities have succeeded in encouraging accountability in research design, institutional review board approval, and federal research funding.[39] However, there has not been as much success in sustained recruitment and retention of minority populations into research studies. Persistently poor participation of minorities in research studies is also linked to barriers to the optimal utilization of medical health care facilities, willingness to seek care, and follow-up on treatment recommendations. These factors are linked to the problems of recruitment of minority patients and the need for the patients to continue a path of therapy that requires long-term follow-up. Although minority population groups share such characteristics as low socioeconomic status, poorer access to health care, poorer quality of care, and health disparities, minority cultural subgroups differ in their perception about health care and health care utilization. Minority groups are also likely to differ in their perceptions about research and research participation and how they align themselves to health care.

African Americans and Native Americans are uniquely impacted by structural aspects of the American society that allowed institutionalized domination by White individuals who have repeatedly mistreated them through one social system or another. Health care is one such system with a legacy of poor treatment and abuse. Today there are long-lasting effects of the United States Public Health Service Syphilis Study at Tuskegee (1932–1972) on the Black community. Because of the abuses of that study, many African Americans are unwilling to participate in clinical trials and other aspects of the medical system; they fear unfair treatment and further abuses will occur.[39]

Native Americans have survived a past that includes an onslaught of government policies and wars dedicated to destroying them as a people along with their culture. They have sustained their traditions through traditional family and clan relationships, kinships with their homelands, religious ceremonies, and ancient rituals and shared traditions that maintained their tribal traditions.[39]

The long history of Native Americans and African Americans with the public health services reflects mistrust in multiple aspects: (1) the sentiment that providers are prejudiced against them; (2) the fear that providers do not have their best interest in mind and treat them differently from other patients; (3) the concern that providers have different opinions about time and space, and spend less time listening to the patients about their concerns and problems; (4) the concern that providers do not recognize their traditional medical practices/beliefs and think of them as primitive; and (5) a lack of confidence in the health care providers' skills based on the quality of the historical resources and referrals provided by the U.S. Public Health Service or through the Indian Health Services.[40]

Other minorities such as Hispanic or Asian Americans can also have perceptions of mistrust, but the mistrust is usually derived from sources in their past history outside the United States. Many immigrants have experienced political oppression or government policies that fostered mistrust or unfair practices. Their fears are centered on deportation if they entered the country illegally, or there may be mistrust because of problems of language misconceptions.

Reducing medical mistrust takes repeated encounters over a continuum of interactions. Some key practices that health care providers can do to foster trusting relationships include one-on-one outreach, as well as frequent involvement of the provider with the targeted community through volunteerism and partnering with community leaders (e.g., tribal leaders for Native Americans or pastors for African Americans) to form networks and program approval at the earliest stage of the program-planning process.[41]

Training of community health workers can be effective for garnering trust in the community, especially when there is a dearth of time and resources. Frequent training of these community liaisons provides methods for diffusing health messages; integrating culturally and linguistically diverse prevention programs; and providing information about new health technologies and screening in the language and the context that the group understands. Health care providers should embrace cultural competency training with the intent of making local culture and folklore the central focus of the training. Specifically, pharmacists equipped with cultural competence will be able to develop more targeted and tailored self-care plans and better marketing approaches for social marketing of health messages.

Language Barriers and Unfamiliarity with Medical Terms

Inability to speak or read English makes it difficult for many patients to communicate with their health care providers or to read instructions on a nonprescription product label. Low English proficiency creates a significant barrier to seeking self-care or the advice of a health care provider such as the pharmacist. Because of language barriers, many patients rely on television advertisements (on channels in their language of origin) or on the recommendations of family members or relatives. Problems in interpreting professional jargon are important factors that may impede effective self-care management.

In many cultures, patients may express their symptoms in a different manner than what is typically encountered in a Western medical system. It is not uncommon to observe that patients of different cultural groups express pain or symptoms of mental illnesses differently from the typical White patient. One example of this difference is when a practitioner asks Hispanic patients whether they are depressed. The patient most likely will answer "no" and may get upset with the inference that she or he may be depressed. On further questioning, the patient may say, "I have little or no energy" or other statements that may lead the practitioner to realize that the patient may be depressed. If the practitioner asks whether the patient is "feeling down or blue" or uses jargon, the patient may not understand these expressions. In such cases, the use of validated questionnaires to determine diagnosis may not be useful in capturing the patient's feelings because of cultural differences in the meaning of the words. In this example, the term "feeling blue" has no cultural meaning to the Hispanic patient and probably

will be interpreted as a very confusing and silly question. The practitioner should seek out and use questionnaires that have been validated for use in the languages of the populations being served. These validations can be conducted by testing educational materials or surveys with a group of patients prior to broad dissemination of the instrument.

Another example is the interpretation and expressions of pain by patients of Asian descent. Many Asian American patients do not request pain relief medications even when they are in extreme pain. It has been reported that Asian Americans exhibit a higher tolerance of pain, which may lead to undertreatment of pain in many of these patients.

Health Illiteracy

The lack of health literacy is an important barrier to self-management and decision making about nonprescription products. The prerequisite requirements of the FDA Durham-Humphrey (1951) and Kefauver-Harris (1962) amendments, used in evaluating new drug applications for proposed nonprescription drugs, demonstrate the need for improved health literacy. The required criteria for nonprescription approval include demonstrated evidence that (1) patients can recognize and diagnose themselves for the condition specified in the proposed indication, (2) patients can read the product label and extract the key information necessary to use the drug properly, (3) the drug is effective when used as recommended, and (4) the drug is safe when used as instructed. The consumer must be able to read and understand the information on the label to know the proper dose, recognize warnings and contraindications, and determine whether contraindications apply. New FDA labeling requirements implemented in 2002 were intended to make it easier for patients to read and understand nonprescription drug labels. The standard product label for nonprescription drugs, titled "Drug Facts," has specific sections for active ingredients, uses, warnings, when to use the product, directions, and inactive ingredients (see Chapters 1 and 4). Manufacturers are required to use large print, simple language, and an easy-to-read format on the nonprescription drug labels to help patients with product selection and dosage instruction. In addition to these requirements, pharmacists and other health care providers should be on the alert to meet the educational needs of all patients, particularly those with poor reading skills.

Illiteracy is a pervasive, but often unrecognized, problem that affects all population groups and threatens the health of millions of Americans. Health illiteracy is more prevalent in minority groups because of high poverty and school dropout rates. Many immigrants including Hispanic patients from Central America have completed only a third- or fourth-grade education, in many cases because of the prolonged military conflicts and poverty rates in their country of origin. Lack of education impairs patients' ability to read Spanish, making it difficult for pharmacists to rely on drug information pamphlets or prescription labels produced by the pharmacy computer systems. Through verbal communication with the patient, interpreter, or an adult family member, pharmacists must confirm that the patient understands the instructions and/or prescription label directions. People with low literacy skills are less likely to adhere to medication regimens and appointments or to present for care in the course of treatment of a disease. In a study of hospitalized patients, 49% of patients with hypertension and 44% of those with diabetes were found to have inadequate health literacy for managing their self-care treatment plans.[42]

Studies have documented a relationship between poor reading skills and poor health.[41] Twenty-five percent of U.S. adults (approximately 90 million) read with only marginal literacy skills. It is estimated that 40 million are functionally illiterate, making it difficult or impossible for them to understand routine written information such as dosage instructions on medication bottles, poisoning warnings, appointment slip reminders, or consent forms.[43]

Low literacy has been called "a quiet disability" because many patients do not acknowledge the problem.[44] People who cannot read often hide their illiteracy because of shame, embarrassment, low self-esteem, and fear. As a result of this behavior, many pharmacists and other health care providers often overlook this potential source of nonadherence to prescription drugs and misinformation concerning nonprescription products.

To detect literacy problems, the practitioner should be sensitive to cues that indicate patient difficulty with reading. For example, patients may say they "forgot their glasses" when asked to read something, or ask the practitioner "to fill out a form for me." Poor readers do not like to be exposed and may never join a group education or support group session. Instead, such patients may prefer one-on-one consultations with their health care providers. To ensure that patients understand aspects of their condition and their responsibility for self-care, integrating the following tips may improve clinical outcomes. First, the provider should never take for granted that the patient can comprehend fully all medical instructions whether written or spoken. Providers should be aware of shame and treat the patient with respect. Patient education specialists suggest using the teach-back method to ensure the clarity of the message. This method involves using phrases such as, "Can you tell me in your own words, how are you going to do XYZ?" Gaps in the patient's interpretation will provide additional opportunities to explain the process again or to correct gaps using different methods to deliver the message. Counseling should always be followed up with supplemental materials such as pictorials or demonstration products.[45]

A series of nine health literacy fact sheets are available from the Center for Health Care Strategies, Inc. (CHCS). The fact sheets are created for those who are designing patient education materials for consumers with low health literacy skills. These sheets define health literacy and describe its impact on health. They also provide targeted educational strategies and additional health literacy resources and information. The Health Literacy Fact Sheets can be downloaded from the CHCS Web site (www.chcs.org/publications3960/publications_show.htm?doc_id=291711).

Practitioners are encouraged to assess the health literacy of their self-care plans by using the Test of Functional Health Literacy in Adults (TOFHLA), which is available in English and Spanish,[46] or the Rapid Estimate of Adult Literacy in Medicine (REALM).[47] The TOFHLA tests include items that assess the patient's ability to understand labeled prescription vials, blood glucose test results, clinic appointment slips, and financial information forms. REALM tests a person's ability to read through a list of medical words, moving from short and easy words to difficult and multiple-syllable words. This test correlates well with reading tests and offers a good marker for literacy levels. The National Work Group on Literacy recommends that educational materials be developed at a fifth-grade level, and that a variety of media be used to convey a message.[48]

Ensuring Cultural Competence in Health Care and Elements of Cultural Competence

Cultural competence has been defined as a set of congruent behaviors and attitudes among professionals that enables them to work effectively in cross-cultural situations.[49] Cultural competence is a continuous process undertaken to ensure that care is delivered in an effective manner among diverse populations of patients and practitioners while avoiding cultural generalizations.[49] Development of cultural competence in pharmaceutical care has the potential to increase effectiveness and favorably affect health outcomes, and it helps the practitioner understand the treatment of choice and the monitoring parameters to follow. This competency is very important in the area of self-care, when the patient has the opportunity to select the therapy of choice. By having knowledge in the area of cultural competence and possessing the skills to assess patient's cultural beliefs, the practitioner can help the patient choose treatment options that are congruent with the patient's cultural beliefs. It is believed that this action will lead to better adherence with the treatment and optimal outcomes. Some important elements related to cultural competence are listed in Table 3-7.

At Georgetown University, researchers have described a series of stages that define the continuum of cross-cultural process toward achieving cultural proficiency.[50] The six stages are as follows:

1. *Cultural destructiveness*. This stage is the beginning of the continuum and represents the most negative stage, in which there is bigotry, racism, discrimination, and exploitation that can harm other cultures and the patients within them. Cultural destructiveness could be an intentional or unintentional behavior. Many health care systems are in this stage but simply do not realize it. They have policies that can harm patients from different cultures.

2. *Cultural incapacity*. In this stage, an organization or health care practitioner does not have any programs or services available to respond to the needs of patients from other

---

TABLE 3-7 Concepts of Cultural Competence

- Demonstrate understanding of and respect for the values, beliefs, and expectations of patients.
- Modify communication approaches, allowing for incorporation of a variety of communication techniques to meet the patient's cultural needs.
- Apply new knowledge and skills to each patient encounter to improve outcomes.
- Apply new knowledge of cultural preferences and drug response variability among patients of different cultures/races to the selection of the best therapy for the patient.
- Adapt and modify the treatment plan on the basis of negotiated agreements.

cultures. There is a sense of ethnocentrism in which the dominant culture assumes a paternalistic stance toward other cultures.

3. *Cultural blindness.* In this stage, organizations or individuals try to remain unbiased. They believe that culture or race makes no difference and they treat everyone the same. This is probably the stage that prevails in many health care organizations. In this stage the organization does not have any programs or policies addressing cultural needs of different groups.

4. *Cultural pre-competence.* This stage is the first on the positive end of the continuum. Organizations or individuals start to reach out to other cultures by hiring a diverse workforce, hiring translators, or translating materials into different languages. Organizations at this stage of the continuum limit their efforts to one or two initiatives and, at times, they become frustrated with the lack of progress.

5. *Cultural competence.* In this stage, there is an ongoing acceptance and respect for the differences among cultural groups. Practitioners and organizations are continually increasing their knowledge and skills in the area of cultural competence. Models to deliver culturally appropriate care are implemented, and there is true commitment to cultural competence and to improving the outcomes of patients from diverse cultures.

6. *Cultural proficiency.* This stage is the highest level in the continuum. The organizations and practitioners in this stage have a true commitment to culturally competent practices by engaging in research, evaluating new therapies and approaches to care, publishing their findings, conducting training, and disseminating their findings. They have a true commitment to achieving cultural proficiency and value the positive impact that culture has in health care.

To achieve cultural competence, health care professionals and the health care systems in which they work will increasingly be expected to undertake major initiatives aimed at achieving changes in awareness, attitude, skills, and behaviors that will enable them to provide effective culturally competent care. This competency can be achieved only by having a true commitment to change, a real conviction of the significance of the task, and an in-depth assessment of the beliefs and attitudes of the personnel and the institution. The first step in this effort is to conduct a self-assessment of the level of cultural competence in the institution and the care being provided by practitioners. The literature describes many self-assessment instruments. One of these instruments, created by the Georgetown Center on Cultural Competence, is a survey containing a series of questions and statements aimed at having the institution and the practitioner assess current activities in the area of cultural competence. This survey can be found at www.aafp.org/fpm/20001000/58cult.html.

Important elements of a culturally competent practice include dissemination of cultural knowledge and skills as well as advocacy. The dissemination of cultural knowledge and skills should be targeted at decreasing racism or other forms of bias and increasing awareness among practitioners of the influence of culture in health. Advocacy efforts should involve recognition of racism in the health care provider and actions taken by the health care provider to reverse racism. Only by incorporating these two final elements can a practitioner deliver culturally competent care. Unfortunately, cultural competence often requires on-the-job training because of a lack of formalized training in many health care professional schools. An increased level of cultural competence training in the health professions' schools and continuing professional education programming is needed.

To develop targeted health service programs that are culturally competent, the practitioner may want to follow the recommendations and guidelines made available by the Georgetown University National Center for Cultural Competence (NCCC). The NCCC Web site offers a plethora of resource materials including planning guides, policy briefs, monographs, and multimedia products. The resource materials are designed to assist meeting and conference planners in infusing principles, content, and themes related to cultural and linguistic competence into their service delivery systems. The NCCC activities are funded through a collaborative agreement between the Department of Health and Human Services Administration (DHHS), the Bureau of Primary Health Care and the Maternal and Child Health Bureau, and the Department of Health Resources and Services Administration. Resource materials are available at: www11.georgetown.edu/research/gucchd/nccc/index.html. A practical guide to the development of culturally competent health promotion materials can be found at www11.georgetown.edu/research/gucchd/nccc/features/voices.html.

The case scenarios on the following pages illustrate important aspects of cultural competence care in the area of self-care. These cases are examples of issues that are commonly observed in community practice.

Key Points for Multicultural Aspects of Self-Care

➤ Major shifts in the demographics of the U.S. population are affecting the delivery of care to patients.

➤ Currently, minority populations are experiencing a broad range of health disparities compared with their White counterparts. A disproportionately high number of minority patients are experiencing increased rates of complications with chronic diseases compared with other populations.

➤ Cultural issues affect patients' attitudes and behaviors toward health and illness, as well as their acceptance and adherence to treatment plans.

➤ The inability of health care providers, including pharmacists, to deliver effective culturally competent care can affect the health outcomes of diverse patient populations.

➤ To become culturally competent, health care providers need to evaluate their biases and prejudices, and acquire the knowledge and skills to become culturally competent. Cultural competence implies that the health care provider has the knowledge and skills to deal effectively with diverse patient populations and is able to apply these to the care of patients.

➤ Delivering culturally competent pharmaceutical care should be a goal of every health care provider, particularly in the area of self-care. Self-care lends itself very well to the practice of culturally competent pharmaceutical care. Many minority groups seek nonprescription products, herbal medicines, and other complementary and alternative therapies as their main source of care. The reader is referred to the Chapters 53 through 55 for an in-depth discussion of complementary and alternative therapies.

48   SECTION I   *The Practitioner's Role in Self-Care*

CASE 3-1
CULTURAL COMPETENCE IN SELF-CARE

Patient Complaint/History

Mr. Truong is a 44-year-old Vietnamese man who comes to the pharmacy complaining of weight loss and a decreased appetite. The patient enters the pharmacy and looks confused as he wanders in the nonprescription drug aisles. He speaks limited English and is not comfortable asking for help. After approximately 20 minutes of waiting, a clerk offers to assist the patient. The patient proceeds to tell the clerk that he would like to talk to the pharmacist. The pharmacist approaches the patient and proceeds to ask the patient about his condition. The patient states that he does not speak English well and answers with "yes" and "no" responses. The pharmacist elicits the following information:

■ The patient has lost a lot of weight (15 pounds in 2 months) because of his inability to eat.
■ He has had epigastric pain for the last 3 months.
■ He says that he has been drinking every night to relieve his "nerves."
■ He moved to this country 5 years ago.
■ Currently, he is worried and in a lot of pain, but says everything is "OK."

The patient wants the pharmacist to give him something for "his problem," because he cannot afford to miss days at work.

What would be an appropriate action at this time?
What do you think of Mr. Truong's reaction to his condition?
Is this reaction what you would expect in a situation like this?
How would you communicate with Mr. Truong?

Clinical/Cultural Considerations

Mr. Truong is reacting to his symptoms and condition in a manner that differs from what you would expect from someone with significant alarming symptoms such as weight loss. He does not seem to realize the severity of his symptoms. This reaction could be based on his approach to health issues, which could be routed in his cultural upbringing. It is important to assess what his beliefs are and what other treatment (alternative treatments or herbals) he has tried previously. This patient is of Asian descent, which puts him at a high risk for stomach cancer based on incidence and prevalence data from the U.S. DHHS. It is important to assess the patient's symptoms and other medical conditions the patient may have. Pain perception is also influenced to a very large extent by our cultural definition of pain. How pain and discomfort are perceived varies among cultures. The fact he is seeking help from the pharmacist may indicate the pain is severe. He has probably tried familiar home remedies, which have failed.

All of these factors indicate that this patient needs to be referred for further evaluation. The clinical scenario in this case does not indicate the use of nonprescription products. The pharmacist must speak clearly and assess the patient's level of health literacy and his command of the English language. It is important to explain to the patient that he must seek medical care. It may be appropriate to ask whether the patient wants the pharmacist to speak with a relative of the patient to explain his/her recommendation of seeking care. If the patient does not have a health care provider, the pharmacist may want to recommend appropriate resources for the patient (i.e., community centers, local physicians). If the patient has difficulty understanding the pharmacist or does not want the pharmacist to call relatives, the use of an interpreter who is aware of the Vietnamese culture is a good alternative. Interpreters could be located at community centers, health systems (hospitals, clinics), or AT&T translation services. A follow-up telephone call may be needed to ensure that the patient did seek medical evaluation.

CASE 3-2
CULTURAL COMPETENCE IN SELF-CARE

Patient Complaint/History

Mrs. Perez is a 38-year-old Hispanic woman with diabetes type 2 and hypertension. She comes to your pharmacy on a regular basis to get her prescription medications, but you have not seen her in the last 2 months. She is looking in the nonprescription aisle for a product. You proceed to greet Mrs. Perez and offer your assistance. When you ask Mrs. Perez why she has not come to get her medications, she states that the medications were too expensive and because she lost her job she cannot buy them anymore. She is looking for cinnamon tablets that she was told are good for her diabetes. She also asks for a medication to treat her "vaginal itching"; a friend told Mrs. Perez the itching should be treated with an antibiotic.

What would be an appropriate action at this time?
What do you think is going on with Mrs. Perez?

Clinical/Cultural Considerations

Mrs. Perez is confronting financial issues that prevent her from obtaining her medications. Her symptom of "vaginal itching" may be consistent with a complication of an uncontrolled diabetes-vaginal infection. It is important to ask whether the patient has any other acute symptoms at this time such as fever, increased thirst, hunger, or urination. It is important that the pharmacist not criticize the patient for not getting her diabetes medications on time. The pharmacist should offer help in referring the patient to resources where she may be able to get her medication. These resources include community centers, free health clinics, manufacturer's indigent programs, and government programs. The patient must feel there is *respeto* (respect) and *confianza* (trust) in her relationship with the pharmacist. Most Hispanic patients value these two components of their relationships with health care providers. It is important to educate the patient about the complications of diabetes and that the cinnamon tablets are not enough to treat her condition. Referral to community resources is important to find assistance in getting her medications. After careful evaluation of the vaginal itching symptoms, the pharmacist must determine whether an appropriate nonprescription product is available at this time. The use of antibiotics or the sharing of medications currently being used by the patient's family members should be discouraged. These are common practices observed in many Hispanic communities.

REFERENCES

1. Hsiao Af, Wong MD, Goldstein MS, et al. Variation in complementary medicine (CAM) use across racial/ethnic groups and the development of ethnic-specific measures of CAM use. *J Altern Complement Med*. 2006;12: 281–90.
2. US Department of Commerce, US Census Bureau News. Population Estimates. Available at: http://www.census.gov/popest/estimates.php. Last accessed August 27, 2008.
3. US Department of Commerce, US Census Bureau. American Community Survey. Available at: http://factfinder.census.gov. Last accessed August 27, 2008.
4. Mahrous S, Maziarz D. Community pharmacist shortage: fact or fiction? *Pharm Times*. Available at: http://www.pharmacytimes.com/issues/articles/2008-02_016.asp. Last accessed August 27, 2008.
5. Western Interstate Commission for Higher Education. A Closer Look at Healthcare Workforce Needs in the West. Available at: http://www.

CASE 3-3
CULTURAL COMPETENCE IN SELF-CARE

Patient Complaint/History

Mr. James is a 50-year-old African American man with a history of hypertension (HTN) and cardiovascular disease (CVD). He comes to the pharmacy and asks the pharmacist for a remedy for his "stomach acid." He has been using "Alka-Seltzer" and "soda water" with little relief. He uses "garlic tablets" to treat his hypertension and currently is taking a "water pill" to treat his high blood pressure and amlodipine for his "heart."

What would be an appropriate action at this time?
What do you think is going on with Mr. James?

Clinical/Cultural Considerations

Mr. James has HTN and CVD; these conditions must be considered when recommending a nonprescription product. In African American patients, HTN is known to be more sensitive to changes in plasma volume including sodium changes. The use of Alka-Seltzer is not recommended owing to its high sodium bicarbonate content. The pharmacist must ask further questions to assess the patient's complaint of stomach acid, including its duration and frequency. The pharmacist may be able to recommend an antacid, a histamine$_2$-blocker, or a proton pump inhibitor, or refer the patient for further assessment by a health care provider. The patient should be educated about the need to determine the sodium content in food and nonprescription products. The ability of the patient to read the nonprescription labels or his level of health literacy must be evaluated to ensure that he can make appropriate self-care decisions concerning the effect of many nonprescription products on blood pressure control. In many cases, it is important to provide patient education materials appropriate for low literacy to educate the patient concerning products to avoid because of his HTN and CVD.

wiche.edu/sep/psep/workforcePharmacy.pdf. Last accessed September 5, 2008.

6. American Association of Colleges of Pharmacy. *2007–08 Profile of Pharmacy Students*. Alexandria, Va: American Association of Colleges of Pharmacy; 2008:1–4.

7. US Department of Health and Human Services, Health Resource and Service Administration. Executive Summary. The Rationale for Diversity in the Health Professions: A Review of the Evidence. October 2006. Available at: http://bhpr.hrsa.gov/healthworkforce/reports/diversity/default.htm. Last accessed August 27, 2008.

8. *Accreditation Standards and Guidelines for the Professional Program in Pharmacy Leading to the Doctor of Pharmacy Degree. Accreditation Council for Pharmacy Education*. Chicago: Accreditation Council for Pharmacy Education. Adopted January 15, 2006; released February 17, 2006; effective July 2007.

9. Specter RE. *Cultural Diversity in Health and Illness*. 6th ed. Upper Saddle River, NJ: Pearson Prentice Hall; 2004.

10. Kleinman A. *Patients and Healers in the Context of Culture*. Berkeley: University of California Press; 1980.

11. Brashers DE, Goldsmith DJ, Hsieh E. Information seeking and avoiding in health contexts. *Hum Commun Res*. 2002;28;258–71.

12. Taylor L, Abarca S, Henry B, et al. Use of Neo-melubrina, a banned antipyretic drug, in San Diego, California: a survey of patients and providers in San Diego. *West J Med*. 2001;175:159–63.

13. Institute of Medicine. *Health and Behavior: The Interplay of Biological, Behavioral, and Societal Influence*. Washington, DC: National Academy Press; 2001.

14. The Commonwealth Fund. *2001 Health Quality Survey*. New York: The Commonwealth Fund; 2002. Publication No. 523.

15. Larson EL, Dilone J, Garcia M, et al. Factors which influence Latino community members to self-prescribe antibiotics. *Nurs Res*. 2006;55:94–102.

16. Hensrud DD, Engle DD, Sheitel SM. Underreporting the use of dietary supplements and nonprescription medications among patients undergoing a periodic health examination. *Mayo Clin Proc*. 1999;74:443–7.

17. Chou FY. Testing the predictive model of the use of HIV/AIDS symptom self-care strategies. *AIDS Patient Care STDS*. 2004;18:109–17.

18. Brass EP. Drug therapy: changing the status of drugs from prescription to over-the-counter availability. *N Engl J Med*. 2001;345:810–6.

19. Lundberg L, Johannesson M, Isacson D. The effects of user charges on the use of prescription medicines in different socio-economic groups. *Health Pol*. 1998;44:123–34.

20. Oborne CA, Luzac ML. Over-the-counter medicine use prior to and during hospitalization. *Ann Pharmacother*. 2005;39:268–73.

21. National Institutes of Health, US Department of Health and Human Services. NIH Guidelines on the Inclusion of Women and Minorities as Subject in Clinical Research—Amended October 2001. Available at: http://grants.nih.gov/grants/funding/women_min/guidelines_amended_10_2001.htm. Last accessed August 27, 2008.

22. Evans WE, McLeod HL. Pharmacogenomics: drug disposition, drug targets, and side effects. *N Engl J Med*. 2003;348:538–49.

23. Centers for Disease Control and Prevention, Office of Minority Health and Health Disparities. Disease Burden and Risk Factors (OMHD). Last modified 2007. Available at: http://www.cdc.gov/omhd/AMH/dbrf.htm. Last accessed August 27, 2008.

24. Centers for Disease Control and Prevention, Office of Minority Health and Health Disparities. Racial and Ethnic Populations. Last modified 2007. Available at: http://www.cdc.gov/omhd/Populations/populations.htm. Last accessed August 27, 2008.

25. Centers for Disease Control and Prevention, Office of Minority Health and Health Disparities. Eliminating Racial and Ethnic Health Disparities. Last modified 2007. Available at: http://www.cdc.gov/omhd/About/disparities.htm. Last accessed August 27, 2008.

26. Centers for Disease Control and Prevention. State specific prevalence of obesity among adults—United States, 2007. *MMWR Morb Mortal Wkly Rep*. 2008;15:765–8. Available at: http://www.cdc.gov/mmwr/preview/mmwrhtml/mm5728a1.htm. Last accessed August 27, 2008.

27. Centers for Disease Control and Prevention, Office of Minority Health and Health Disparities. American Indian and Alaskan Native Population. Available at: http://www.cdc.gov/omhd/Populations/AIAN/AIAN.htm#high. Last Accessed. August 27, 2008.

28. Centers for Disease Control and Prevention, Division of STD Prevention, National Center for HIV, STD, and TB Prevention. Health Disparities in HIV/AIDS, Viral Hepatitis, STDs, and TB. Updated January 2008. Available at: http://www.cdc.gov/nchhstp/healthdisparities. Last accessed August 16, 2008.

29. Collins KS, Hughes DI, Doty MM, et al. Diverse communities, common concerns; assessing health care quality for minority Americans. Findings from the Commonwealth Fund 2001 Health Quality Survey. New York: The Commonwealth Fund; 2002. Publication No. 523.

30. US Department of Health and Human Services, Office of Disease Prevention and Health Promotion. *Healthy People 2010*. Available at: http://www.healthypeople.gov. Last accessed August 27, 2008.

31. Smedley BD, Stith AY, Nelson AR, eds. *Committee on Understanding and Eliminating Racial and Ethnic Disparities in Health Care, Board on Health Sciences Policy. Unequal Treatment: Confronting Racial and Ethnic Disparities in Health Care*. Washington, DC: National Academy Press; 2002.

32. Carrillo EJ, Green AR, Batancourt JR. Cross-cultural primary care: a patient-based approach. *Ann Intern Med*. 1999;130:830–4.

33. US Department of Health and Human Services, Office of Minority Health. *National Standards for Culturally and Linguistically Appropriate Services in Health Care: Final Report*. Washington, DC: US Department of Health and Human Services, Office of Minority Health; March 20, 2001. Available at: http://www.omhrc.gov/assets/pdf/checked/finalreport.pdf. Last accessed August 27, 2008.

34. Diversity R$_x$. L-E-A-R-N Model of Cross Cultural Encounter Guidelines for Health Practitioners. Available at: http://www.diversityrx.org/HTML/MOCPT2.htm. Last accessed September 5, 2008.

35. Answers.com. Encyclopedia of Public Health: Self-Care Behavior. Available at: htpp://www.answers.com/topic/self-care. Last accessed August 27, 2008.

36. Matthew, LA. Nonprescription medicines and the North American pharmacist licensure examination. *Am J Pharm Educ.* 2006:70(6):Article 138.

37. Nichols-English G, Poirier S. Optimizing adherence to pharmaceutical care plans. *JAPhA.* 2000;40:475–85.

38. Shoor S, Lorig KR. Self-care and the doctor-patient relationship. *Med Care.* 2002;40(4 suppl):II40–4.

39. Benkert R, Peters R, Clark R, et al. Effects of perceived racism, cultural mistrust and trust in providers on satisfaction with care. *J Natl Med Assoc.* 2006;98:1532–40.

40. Shavers VL, Lynch CF, Burmeister LF. Factors that influence African-Americans' willingness to participate in medical research studies. *Cancer.* 2001;91(1 suppl):233–6.

41. Calderon L, Baker RS, Fabrega H. An ethno-medical perspective on research participation: a qualitative pilot study. *MedGenMed.* 2006;8(2):23. Available at: http://www.medscape.com/viewarticle/525132. Last accessed August 27, 2008.

42. Williams MV, Baker DW, Parker RM, et al. Relationship of functional health literacy to patient's knowledge of their chronic disease: a study of patients with hypertension and diabetes. *Arch Intern Med.* 1998;158: 166–72.

43. Baker DS, Parker RM, Williams MV, et al. The relationship of patient reading ability to self-reported health and use of health services. *Am J Public Health.* 1997;87:1027–30.

44. Parikh NS, Parker RM, Nurss JR, et al. Shame and health literacy: the unspoken connection. *Patient Educ Couns.* 1996;27:33–9.

45. Villaire M, Mayer G. Low health literacy. *Prof Case Manag.* 2007;12:213–6.

46. Parker RM, Baker DW, Williams MV, et al. The test of functional health literacy in adults: a new instrument for measuring patients' literacy skills. *J Gen Intern Med.* 1995;10:537–41.

47. Davis TC, Crouch MA, Long SW, et al. Rapid assessment of literacy levels of adult primary care patients. *J Fam Med.* 1991;23:433–5.

48. Weiss BD. Communicating with patients who have limited literacy skills: report of the National Work Group on Literacy and Health. *J Fam Pract.* 1998;46:168–76.

49. Cohen E, Goode TD. *Policy Brief 1: Rationale for Cultural Competence in Primary Health Care.* Washington, DC: National Center for Cultural Competence; 1999.

50. Kim-Godwin YS, Clarke PN, Burton L. A model for the delivery of culturally competent community care. *J Adv Nurs.* 2001;35:918–25.

Legal and Regulatory Issues in Self-Care Pharmacy Practice

Ilisa B. G. Bernstein and Edward D. Rickert

This chapter analyzes the federal laws and regulations that govern the manufacturing, distribution, labeling, and marketing of the products that patients commonly use for self-care. Nonprescription drugs are regulated differently than prescription-only drugs and other consumer health care products, such as dietary supplements and homeopathic medicines. It is important that health care providers have a basic understanding of these regulations so they can respond to their patients' questions and concerns about the self-care products they use.

Regulation of Nonprescription Drugs

The first major federal legislation enacted in the United States to regulate drugs was the Pure Food and Drugs Act of 1906.[1] "Unsafe" and "nonefficacious" drug products were not actually prohibited by the statute; drugs were required to meet only the standards of strength, quality, and purity claimed by the manufacturers. Laws did not mandate drug safety until passage of the 1938 Federal Food, Drug, and Cosmetic Act (FDC Act). In 1951, an amendment to the FDC Act in essence established two classes of drugs: prescription-only and nonprescription (also referred to as over-the-counter, or OTC). Before that time, manufacturers were free to determine to which category their drug product belonged. Drugs that could be used safely without medical supervision and had labeling that included adequate directions for use could be marketed without a prescription. In 1962, a major amendment to the FDC Act was enacted, requiring that all new drugs be shown to be effective, as well as safe, for their intended uses. As a result of this amendment, the Food and Drug Administration (FDA) undertook a review of the effectiveness of 4500 new drug products, including 512 nonprescription drugs that had been approved for only safety since 1938.

In 1972, FDA initiated a massive scientific review of the 700 active ingredients in 300,000 nonprescription drug formulations to ensure that they were safe and effective, and bore fully informative labeling. This review process, which is still underway, is often referred to as the "OTC Drug Review."

The FDA is also responsible for the labeling of nonprescription drugs and reclassifying (i.e., switching) drugs from prescription to nonprescription status. Consequently, nonprescription drugs that are on the market today fall into one of the three following categories (from a legal and regulatory perspective):

1. Approved through the drug approval process and either
   (1) reclassified (i.e., switched) from prescription to non-

prescription status or (2) approved directly as a nonprescription drug.
2. Marketed in accordance with the OTC monograph for that ingredient (see the section OTC Monograph Process).
3. On the market pending a determination under the OTC Drug Review monograph process of the drug's disposition.

Drug Approval Process

The FDC Act of 1938, as amended in 1962, requires that all new drugs introduced for marketing be cleared in advance through a new drug application (NDA), which requires that the drugs be proven safe and effective for human use before being marketed. Products marketed before 1938 were exempted from the NDA requirement under a grandfather clause. However, FDA's Office of Nonprescription Products has evaluated, or is in the process of evaluating, all nonprescription drugs for safety, effectiveness, and labeling, regardless of the date of marketing entry.[2]

A new chemical entity never before marketed in the United States would be classified as a new drug and, in most cases, would be approved initially for prescription use only. An NDA for a nonprescription drug product can also be approved directly (without reclassification), as occurred with ibuprofen 200 mg (a dose that was never available by prescription). When a new drug is used for many years by many patients (referred to in the FDC Act as "used for a material time and material extent"), it may be considered generally recognized as safe and effective and qualifies for marketing as a nonprescription drug. In addition, under new regulations, certain data regarding the safety, efficacy, and use of the product in a foreign country can be used to determine whether a drug can be marketed as a nonprescription product in the United States.[3]

Some drugs are available as prescription-only and nonprescription in the same strength, but they are marketed for different uses. For example, nonprescription meclizine is available for motion sickness, which is easy to diagnose, and by prescription for vertigo, which is a complex condition that is not easy to diagnose and treat.

New Drug Application

An NDA is the vehicle through which sponsors apply to FDA to seek approval of a new pharmaceutical for sale and marketing in the United States. The data gathered during the animal studies and human clinical trials of an Investigational New Drug (IND) become part of the NDA. The goals of the NDA are to provide FDA with enough information to determine, among other things, whether (1) the drug is safe and effective for its proposed use(s), (2) the benefits of the drug outweigh the risks, (3) and the methods and controls used in manufacturing the drug are adequate to preserve the drug's identity, strength, and quality, and purity.[4] The approved NDA is manufacturer-specific and allows only the sponsor (applicant) to market the product. Any other manufacturer interested in marketing a similar product would first need to seek FDA approval through its own NDA. In some cases, a full NDA is not necessary for the second manufacturer; an abbreviated NDA (ANDA) may be submitted instead, eliminating the need for duplicative testing. All NDAs must contain, among other things, complete labeling information; the final printed labeling is usually the last step before approval (see the section Drug Facts Labeling for Nonprescription Drugs).

OTC Monograph Process

An OTC monograph is developed for therapeutic classes of ingredients that are generally recognized as safe and effective (also referred to as "GRAS/E"). A manufacturer desiring to market a product that contains an ingredient covered under an OTC monograph need not seek FDA's prior approval. In this case, marketing is not exclusive; any manufacturer may market a similar product without specific approval. Under the monograph approach, all data and information supporting safety and efficacy of the product and its nonprescription status are publicly available. The FDA Office of Nonprescription Products has established the monographs through a complex administrative process called "rulemaking," which allows the general public, manufacturers, and other interested parties to comment on proposed rules. Each individual rulemaking has resulted in an extensive administrative record. Figure 4-1 illustrates the process by which the OTC drug monographs are reviewed.

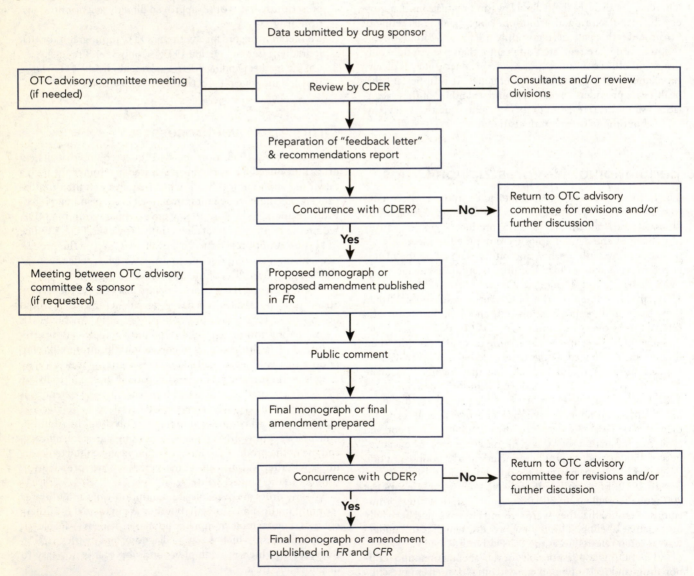

FIGURE 4-1 OTC drug monograph review process, showing how CDER determines the safety and effectiveness of OTC drug products. Key: CDER, Center for Drug Evaluation and Research; *CFR, Code of Federal Regulations; FR, Federal Register;* OTC, over-the-counter. (*Source:* http://www.fda.gov/cder/handbook/otc.htm. Last accessed August 11, 2008.)

Under a final OTC monograph, the manufacturer has considerable flexibility in labeling. All the required monograph labeling must be included; for example, antacids must include terms such as *heartburn, acid indigestion,* and *sour stomach.* In addition, certain language not included in the monograph may be used in specific places on the label without prior approval. For example, *hospital-tested* or *pleasant-tasting antacid* are terms considered outside the scope of the monograph but are permissible in antacid labeling. However, even though these permissible terms are not preapproved, they are subject to the general labeling provision of the FDC Act and may not be false or misleading.

Monographs primarily address active ingredient(s) in the product and, in most cases, final formulations are not subject to monograph specifications. Manufacturers are free to include any inactive ingredients that serve a pharmaceutical purpose, provided those ingredients are safe and do not interfere with either product effectiveness or any required final product testing. In a few instances, even though the product contains generally recognized safe and effective ingredients, it may need to meet a monograph-testing procedure; for example, antacids must pass an acid-neutralizing test.

Laws and regulations require the manufacturer, packer, or distributor whose name appears on the label of an OTC drug to report certain adverse events associated with such drug.[5,6] FDA's MedWatch program is a safety information and adverse event reporting system for medical products, including nonprescription drugs. Health care professionals and consumers are encouraged by FDA to report serious adverse events that they suspect are associated with the drugs they dispense, prescribe, or use. Reporting can be done online (www.fda.gov/medwatch) or by telephone, fax, or mail.[7] FDA uses this information to examine adverse trends and, if necessary, take appropriate action (see the section Adverse Event Reporting).

Labeling and Packaging Issues

"Drug Facts" Labeling for Nonprescription Drugs

It is essential that the labeling of nonprescription drug products clearly communicate to the patient the important information on how to use the product safely and effectively. In recent years, FDA and consumers have been concerned about the adequacy of labeling for nonprescription drugs.[8] This concern is heightened because an increasing number of prescription drugs are being reclassified from prescription to nonprescription status. Many of these "switch" drugs require the patient to perform more sophisticated self-diagnostic and self-monitoring evaluations. Therefore, to provide adequate directions and safety information, a greater number of sophisticated messages must be communicated through the nonprescription label.

Recognizing these concerns, FDA has changed nonprescription drug labeling requirements. FDA regulations now require a standardized content and format for the labels on the estimated 100,000 nonprescription drugs on the market.[9] Nonprescription drug labels have an area on the package designated as the "Drug Facts" box, which contains the information required by FDA to be on the label.[10] A nonprescription product that lacks this new labeling feature may be considered misbranded and subject to the same enforcement approach that FDA can take with other misbranded drugs, including issuance of a warning letter, product seizures, and injunctions.

The nonprescription labeling regulations make it easier for consumers to read and understand information about the product's benefits and risks, and how it should be taken. It also helps consumers select the right product to meet their needs. The format enables consumers to determine readily and easily whether a product contains ingredients they need, do not need, or should not take. It also makes it easy for consumers to compare similar products to determine which has the appropriate ingredients for their symptoms or personal health situation.

The Drug Facts labeling format, with standardized headings and subheadings, also uses terms that are familiar to consumers, for example, *uses* instead of *indications.* Lay terms are also used instead of medical jargon (e.g., *lung* instead of *pulmonary*).

The population of persons 65 years of age or older is increasing. Older people are significant users of nonprescription products, and they may have greater difficulty reading product labels because of decreasing visual functioning. The labeling requirements set a minimal type size that labels must use, and labels cannot use any type smaller than the minimal standard. An easy-to-read font style is also required, as are other graphic features that enhance the ability to read the information on the label clearly.

Pharmacists should be familiar with the Drug Facts format. It is an essential counseling tool for nonprescription drugs. This format allows pharmacists to readily find information on the label and point it out to the patient. Figure 4–2 illustrates the basic Drug Facts format and the standardized headings and order of information. Figures 4–3 and 4–4 show examples of product labels in the Drug Facts format.

Dietary supplements are not regulated as "drugs" under the FDC Act. Consequently, they do not follow the Drug Facts format (Figure 4–5). Dietary supplements must be labeled in accordance with the regulations discussed in Chapter 53.

Expiration Date Labeling

Most nonprescription drug products are required to include an expiration date on the labeling.[11] This is the date beyond which the product should not be used, because the stability, potency, strength, or quality may have been affected over time. FDA regulations govern how this date is determined and tested. Most nonprescription drug product labels must also include any special storage conditions or requirements for the product. Nonprescription drug products that do not have a dosage limit and are stable for at least 3 years are exempt from the requirement to include the expiration date on the label. Such products include certain topical drugs, skin protectants, lotions, and astringents.

Health care providers should remind patients to check their nonprescription product labels periodically to ensure that the expiration date has not passed. Patients often ask whether a nonprescription drug product they have at home is still good if the expiration date has passed. Safety issues rarely arise from using a drug that is modestly past its expiration date; however, the patient should be advised that the product might have lost some of its ability to work as effectively as possible for the particular symptom or medical problem and that the product should be discarded.

Tamper-Evident Packaging

In the wake of several high-profile tampering incidents involving nonprescription drug products, FDA instituted several packaging, labeling, and manufacturing requirements to protect consumers. Historically, the term *tamper-resistant* was used to

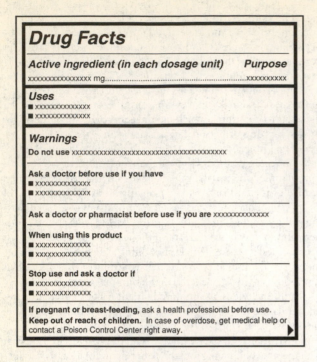

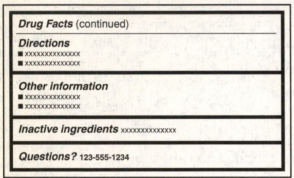

FIGURE 4-2 Drug facts labeling outline. (*Source:* 21 CFR § 201.66.)

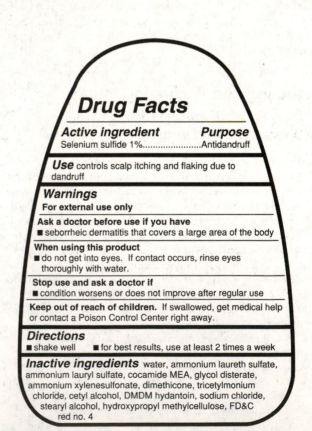

FIGURE 4-3 Drug facts labeling sample 1. (*Source:* 21 CFR § 201.66.)

FIGURE 4-4 Drug facts labeling sample 2. (*Source:* 64 *Federal Register* 13301 (1999).)

describe methods used to prevent tampering. The focus has shifted to "tamper-evident," to heighten consumer awareness of any evidence of tampering, rather than attempt to make products difficult to breach or tamper-proof.

With few exceptions (dermatologics, dentifrice, insulin, and lozenge products), nonprescription drug products must have one or more barriers to entry that, if breached or missing from the package, provide consumers with evidence that tampering may have occurred.[12] Packages must contain unique designs or other characteristics that typically cannot be duplicated. In addition, to alert the consumer to the specific tamper-evident features, the retail package must contain a statement that identifies the feature; the statement must be prominently placed on the package in a way that it will be unaffected if the tamper-evident feature is missing or breached. For example, the statement on a bottle with a shrink band might say, "For your protection, this bottle has an imprinted seal around the neck."

Patients should be educated to check for the tamper-evident features on every nonprescription product they purchase and, if the features are missing or look suspicious, to return the product as soon as possible to the pharmacy or store where it was purchased.

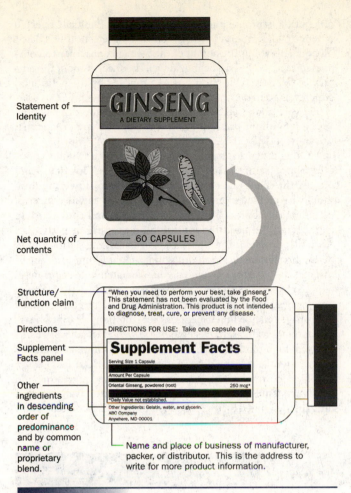

Statement of Identity

Net quantity of contents

Structure/function claim

Directions

Supplement Facts panel

Other ingredients in descending order of predominance and by common name or proprietary blend.

Name and place of business of manufacturer, packer, or distributor. This is the address to write for more product information.

FIGURE 4-5 Statutory labeling format for certain dietary supplements. (*Source:* US Food and Drug Administration. Anatomy of the New Requirements for Dietary Supplement Labels. Available at: http://www.cfsan.fda.gov/~acrobat/fdsuppla.pdf. Last accessed August 11, 2008.)

Drug Reclassification: Prescription-to-OTC Switch

Traditionally, a prescription-to-OTC switch occurs in one of three ways:

1. The drug is switched through the nonprescription drug review process.
2. The manufacturer requests the switch by submitting a supplemental application to its approved NDA.
3. The manufacturer or other party petitions FDA.

Through the OTC drug review process, panels of nongovernment experts are reviewing the prescription drug products that were on the market before 1962 to determine whether some are appropriate for nonprescription marketing. This ongoing process has produced more than 40 reclassifications from prescription-only to nonprescription status since the 1970s.

Another common way that a prescription drug is switched to nonprescription status is for the manufacturer to submit data

to FDA, in the form of a supplemental NDA, demonstrating that the drug is appropriate for self-administration. Typically, these applications include studies showing that the product's labeling can be read, understood, and followed by a consumer without the guidance of a health care provider.[13] FDA reviews this information, along with any information known about the drug from its prescription use history. All of this information is usually presented to FDA's Nonprescription Drug Advisory Committee, which is composed of nongovernment experts. This committee serves as a forum for the exchange of ideas and recommends to FDA whether the drug in question should be switched to nonprescription status. The FDA is not bound by the committee's recommendation, but the agency usually follows the committee's advice.

Overall, more than 700 nonprescription drug products on the market today use ingredients or dosages once available only by prescription.[14] The categories of drug products that have seen the most activity in this area are analgesics, H_1 and H_2 histamine-receptor antagonists, antifungal medications, smoking deterrents, and topical medications used to treat minor skin conditions. Drug products in these categories are good candidates for prescription-to-nonprescription reclassification, because they are used to treat self-limiting conditions that are easily identified by laypersons, with or without the assistance of a health care provider.

A company, usually the manufacturer, can also petition FDA to switch a drug or class of drugs to nonprescription status. In recent years, however, FDA has received petitions that originated not from the drug's manufacturer, but from third-party payers.[15] Citing FDA's statutory authority under Section 503(b) of the FDC Act to remove the prescription requirement for a drug when doing so will not create a threat to public health, third-party payers have petitioned FDA, seeking to have certain drugs switched from prescription to nonprescription status. Three recent examples include the nonsedating antihistamines loratadine, fexofenadine, and cetirizine. In 2002, loratadine was switched to nonprescription status after the manufacturer dropped its original opposition to the switch, and cetirizine was switched to nonprescription status in 2007. However, fexofenadine has retained its prescription-only status.

It is easy to understand why third-party payers, employers, and state and federal health care programs have taken a strong interest in increasing the number of prescription-to-OTC switches. The availability of nonprescription products for self-treatment may save consumers millions of dollars in health care costs by reducing the number of physician visits, preventing unnecessary sick days from work, and decreasing costs associated with the advancement of disease states that could have been limited by treatment with a nonprescription product. In one study, it was estimated that Americans saved approximately $1 billion in health care costs in the first 3 years after topical hydrocortisone acetate was switched from prescription to nonprescription status.[16] That said, out-of-pocket expenditures may increase for many consumers, if employers, insurers, and other third-party payers no longer cover the cost of the medications as the result of a prescription-to-OTC switch. It will, nevertheless, be important for health care providers to stress to their patients the importance of continuing needed drug therapy, even if the cost of the medication is no longer covered by insurance.

Exact standards or switch criteria are very difficult to set, because many factors must be carefully considered. The information that must be gathered from the expert opinions of advisers and consultants regarding a drug's classification as nonprescription includes, but is not limited to, the following:

- Is the condition self-diagnosable?
- Is the condition self-treatable?
- Does the product possess misuse and/or abuse potential?
- Is the product habit forming?
- Do methods of use preclude nonprescription availability?
- Do the benefits of availability outweigh the risks?
- Can adequate directions for use be written?

Further scientific scrutiny typically addresses the following questions as well:

- Does the reclassification candidate have an adequate margin of safety?
- Has the reclassification candidate been used for a sufficiently long time (e.g., 3–5 years) on the prescription market to yield a full characterization of its safety profile?
- Has a vigorous risk analysis been performed? If so, what are the results?
- Has the efficacy literature been reviewed in a way that supports the expected use and labeling of the reclassification candidate?
- Have potential drug interactions for the reclassification candidate been characterized?

Table 4-1 lists some of the prescription drugs reclassified as nonprescription since 1975. A recent addition to this list is omeprazole, a proton pump inhibitor. FDA had initially rejected omeprazole for nonprescription status. The rejection was based on concerns about the ability of the average consumer to comprehend the proposed labeling, as well as concerns about the efficacy of the nonprescription dosage proposed by the petitioner, which was 10 mg, or half of the prescription dose.[17] FDA's concerns were addressed by the petitioner, and the drug is now available without prescription in the same 20 mg dosage that was previously available only by prescription.[18]

Other drugs that have been considered for a switch to nonprescription status include two of the "statins," lovastatin and pravastatin. The issue of whether a cholesterol-lowering drug should be granted nonprescription status has raised concerns, including the ability of the public to understand cholesterol in general and the need for routine blood testing in particular. Also, if approved for nonprescription status, the statins would be the first nonprescription drugs indicated for long-term use to manage and control a potentially life-threatening condition, as opposed to short-term use to control symptoms, such as a runny nose or heartburn. The manufacturers of these recently rejected drugs have renewed their petitions seeking nonprescription status for their products. In December 2007, an FDA advisory panel rejected, for a third time, one manufacturer's efforts to reclassify its cholesterol-lowering drug to nonprescription status.[19]

FDA currently is exploring the benefits and regulatory and legislative issues related to behind-the-counter availability of drugs in the United States.[20] Products in this class would be avail-

---

TABLE 4-1   Selected List of Reclassified Drugs

Ingredient	Indication(s)	Ingredient	Indication(s)
Acidulated phosphate fluoride	Dental rinse	Loperamide HCl	Antidiarrheal
Brompheniramine maleate	Antihistamine	Miconazole nitrate	Antifungal
Butoconazole nitrate	Antifungal	Minoxidil	Baldness
Cetirizine	Antihistamine	Naproxen	Analgesic
Chlorpheniramine maleate	Antihistamine	Nicotine	Smoking cessation
Cimetidine	Heartburn	Nicotine polacrilex	Smoking cessation
Clemastine fumarate	Antihistamine	Nizatidine	Heartburn
Clotrimazole	Antifungal	Omeprazole	Heartburn (proton pump inhibitor)
Cromolyn sodium	Allergy prevention/treatment	Orlistat	Weight-loss aid
Dexbrompheniramine maleate	Antihistamine	Oxymetazoline HCl	Decongestant
Diphenhydramine HCl	Antihistamine	Phenylephrine HCl	Decongestant
Docosanol	Cold sore/fever blister	Polyethylene glycol 3350	Laxative
Doxylamine succinate	Sleep aid	Pseudoephedrine HCl	Decongestant
Dyclonine HCl	Oral anesthetic	Pyrantel pamoate	Pinworm treatment
Ephedrine sulfate	Bronchodilator, vasoconstrictor	Ranitidine	Heartburn
Famotidine	Heartburn	Sodium fluoride	Dental rinse
Guaifenesin	Expectorant	Stannous fluoride	Dental rinse or gel
Haloprogin	Antifungal	Terbinafine HCl	Antifungal
Hydrocortisone	Antipruritic, anti-inflammatory	Tioconazole	Antifungal
Ibuprofen	Analgesic	Tolnaftate	Antifungal
Ketoconazole	Antifungal (shampoo only)	Triclosan	Antigingivitis
Ketoprofen	Analgesic	Triprolidine HCl	Antihistamine
Ketotifen	Antihistamine	Xylometazoline HCl	Decongestant
Levonorgestrel	Contraception		
Loratadine	Nonsedating antihistamine		

able without a prescription, but they would be stored behind the pharmacy counter and sold only by a pharmacist. Such a class of drugs may address concerns surrounding the desire for increased availability of certain drug products, while also ensuring oversight of a health care provider, particularly pharmacists, to ensure that these medications are used appropriately. A de facto third class of drugs has been created and currently exists, however. For example, the sale of certain Schedule V controlled substances is permitted without a prescription, but only from a pharmacist. Also, many states have passed laws permitting pharmacists to prescribe in certain circumstances, often through a collaborative practice arrangement with a physician. Evidence that consumers have benefited and pharmacists have successfully managed risks in these areas could be used as support for a broader, federally sanctioned third class of drugs.

Activity in the area of prescription-to-OTC switches seems certain to increase in the coming years. Health care providers can reasonably expect that more prescription drugs will be subjected to review, as payers, the pharmaceutical industry, and FDA continue to grapple with the difficult task of balancing economic pressures with safety concerns. As more drugs are switched to nonprescription status, health care providers will be called on to play a greater role in assessing the need for treatment and monitoring the use of these drugs.

Regulation of Methamphetamine Precursors

Over the past several years, state and federal regulators have taken steps for increasingly stringent regulation of sale of nonprescription products containing pseudoephedrine. Federal law requires sellers of these products to monitor and report sales above a certain threshold amount, and to prohibit sales in quantities that exceed certain thresholds. State lawmakers have enacted laws restricting the sale of cough and cold products containing pseudoephedrine, in some cases requiring that such products be purchased only from the pharmacy. These laws were enacted to combat the growing problem of illicit methamphetamine laboratories, operated by "garage chemists" who use pseudoephedrine as the precursor in the manufacturing process.

Under federal law, the Comprehensive Methamphetamine Control Act of 1996 and the Combat Methamphetamine Epidemic Act of 2005 regulate the sale of pseudoephedrine-containing products by limiting the quantities that can be purchased in a single transaction and by imposing certain record-keeping and reporting requirements on sellers, including pharmacies.[21] Pseudoephedrine, along with other substances that can be used in manufacturing illegal drugs, are regulated as List I chemicals, and sellers of these substances are required to register with the Drug Enforcement Administration (DEA). Pharmacies that possess a valid DEA registration for dispensing controlled substances are not required to obtain a separate List I registration, but they are required to comply with the record-keeping and other requirements under the act. Threshold quantities have been set for sales of listed chemicals contained in drug products. If the pharmacy engages in any above-threshold retail transactions of pseudoephedrine (3.6 grams), phenylpropanolamine (PPA) (3.6 grams),[22] combination ephedrine (24 grams) and single-entity ephedrine drug products, it must maintain a record of these transactions for 2 years. Pharmacies must also check the identity of the purchasers and maintain a log of each sale that includes the purchaser's name, address, and signature; name and quantity of the product sold; and date and time of sale. Furthermore, suspicious

above-threshold retail transactions must be reported to DEA. The regulations exempt single transactions of regulated products packaged in blister packs from being treated as "regulated transactions,"[23] but caution that such sales of pseudoephedrine and PPA products, regardless of packaging, should be below the 3.6-gram threshold. Nonliquid forms of scheduled listed chemical products (including gel capsules) must be sold in only blister packs, with no more than two dosage units per blister, unless blister packs are technically infeasible. In that case, the dosage units must be in unit dose packages or pouches. For individuals, purchases in a 30-day period should not exceed 9 grams. If a pseudoephedrine-containing product is purchased through mail order, the seller has to confirm the identity of the purchaser before shipping the product; sales are limited to 7.5 grams per customer during a 30-day period. The DEA Drug Diversion Web site (www.deadiversion.usdoj.gov) has additional information regarding the federal laws that regulate the sale of methamphetamine precursors, including a chart showing what quantity of pseudoephedrine-, ephedrine-, and PPA-containing products would exceed the threshold.

In addition to federal law, many states have enacted their own laws to regulate the sale of methamphetamine precursors. As of June 2007, at least 43 states have passed their own laws restricting the sale of methamphetamine precursors.[24] The approaches taken by the states vary from state to state; sales and age restrictions are similar among the states but are more stringent than federal law in many states. Some states have classified pseudoephedrine and ephedrine as Schedule V controlled substances. Practitioners are required to comply with the most stringent law. It is, therefore, essential that all practitioners be familiar with the methamphetamine precursor laws in their states.

Marketing Issues
Product Line Extensions

Increasingly, product line extensions are becoming more commonplace in the nonprescription market. Product line extensions include new strengths, formulations, combinations of ingredients, and even a totally different therapeutic entity (e.g., a device) of a brand-name product that was originally marketed as a single-ingredient product at a specific dose to treat a specific symptom. In developing product line extensions, manufacturers hope to capitalize on the loyalty created by consumer recognition and trust of a brand name.

Product line extensions can create consumer confusion and inappropriate drug selection and use. Pharmacists must be familiar with the range of products within a brand name to recommend them safely and correctly, and to counsel patients on these products. Particular care must be taken with respect to the active ingredients, because these often differ within a product line. Some product line extensions that carry the original brand name as the prefix also retain the active ingredient of the original product, but strengths may vary. Some manufacturers with many product line extensions continue to use the original brand name as the prefix, but they use none of the active ingredients of the original products and attach a suffix for differentiation (e.g., PM, EX, DM, AF, Cold and Flu, Non-Drowsy, Extra, Allergy-Sinus-Headache, Advanced Formula, PH, Day/Night, and Plus).

Nonprescription Drug Advertising

The Federal Trade Commission (FTC) is responsible for matters involving claims made in advertisements for nonprescription drug products. FDA handles most matters involving the labeling, as opposed to the advertisement, of nonprescription drugs. In the 1970s, the Federal Trade Commission Act (FTC Act) was amended to prohibit advertisers from using language to describe the therapeutic benefits of a nonprescription drug product that differs from language approved by FDA for use in the product labeling.

The FTC Act requires that advertising be truthful and nondeceptive. Depending on the claim, advertisers may be required to back up their representations with competent and reliable scientific evidence, including tests, studies, or other objective data.

In 1973, the National Association of Broadcasters and the Consumer Healthcare Products Association developed a code of guidelines for manufacturers to follow in creating television advertisements for nonprescription drugs.[25] The guidelines, which are updated periodically, set standards for truthfulness and honesty, and suggest that an advertisement should, among other things, do the following:

- Comply with all relevant applicable laws and regulation.
- Urge the consumer to read and follow label directions.
- Contain no claims of product effectiveness that are unsupported by clinical or other scientific evidence, responsible medical opinion, or experience through use.
- Present no information in a manner that suggests the product prevents or cures a serious condition that must be treated by a licensed practitioner.
- Emphasize the uses, results, and advantages of the particular product.
- Reference no doctors, hospitals, or nurses, unless such representations can be supported by independent evidence.
- Present no negative or unfair reflections about competing nonprescription drug products, unless those reflections can be supported scientifically and presented in a manner that consumers can perceive differences in the uses.

Consumers should be analytical when listening to or reading marketing messages, particularly because some can be subjective, superficial, vague, or potentially misleading. Health care professionals, particularly the pharmacist and the primary care provider, are well positioned to assist patients in separating fact from ambiguity with regard to nonprescription drug use and to serve the public interest as an objective, informed source of nonprescription drug information.

Vitamins, Minerals, Botanical Medicines, and Other Dietary Supplements

Dietary supplements are regulated under the federal Dietary Supplement Health and Education Act of 1994 (DSHEA). DSHEA became law in recognition that many consumers believe dietary supplements have health benefits. The law represents a balancing between consumer access to dietary supplements and the authority of the FDA to withdraw dangerous products, and address false and misleading claims. FDA's authority to regulate dietary supplements is significantly less than that for prescription and nonprescription products. A thorough discussion of dietary supplements, including regulatory issues, clinical issues, and patient assessment issues, can be found in Chapter 53.

Homeopathy

Homeopathic drugs are recognized as drugs under the FDC Act, which defines the term *drug* as "articles recognized in the official United States Pharmacopoeia, official Homeopathic Pharmacopoeia of the United States ("HPUS"), or official National Formulary, (i) or any supplement to any of them. . . ."[26] Furthermore, the act provides that whenever a drug is recognized in both the *United States Pharmacopoeia* and the *HPUS,* it is subject to the requirements of the *United States Pharmacopoeia,* unless it is labeled and offered for sale as a homeopathic drug, in which case it is subject to the provisions of the *HPUS.* A thorough discussion of homeopathic products can be found in Chapter 55.

Drug–Cosmetic Products

Some nonprescription drug products are also considered cosmetic products.[27] The claim(s) made for the product determine whether it is a drug, a cosmetic, or a drug–cosmetic. Labeling and marketing requirements differ depending on how a product is classified. Often this distinction is not apparent to consumers, but they may wonder why a product they considered to be a cosmetic contains Drug Facts labeling. If a product has a "drug"-intended use and a "cosmetic"-intended use, it is considered a drug–cosmetic. For example, a shampoo is a cosmetic because its intended use is to clean the hair, which is a cosmetic claim. An antidandruff shampoo is a drug because its intended use is to treat dandruff, which is considered a drug claim. Therefore, an antidandruff shampoo that claims to clean the hair and treat dandruff would be a drug–cosmetic and have OTC Drug Facts labeling. Other drug–cosmetic products include toothpastes that contain fluoride, deodorants that are also antiperspirants, moisturizers, and some makeups that are marketed with sun-protection claims.

Identifying and Removing Potentially Dangerous Products from the Market
Adverse Event Reporting

The pharmacist stands out as the one health care provider who has the most frequent and ready access to consumers of prescription and nonprescription drugs. Through counseling of patients in the pharmacy or assisting a customer in selecting the appropriate nonprescription treatment for some health-related condition, pharmacists often obtain information that suggests a drug or other FDA-related product, including dietary supplements, may be causing unintended and unexpected adverse health consequences. Pharmacists play a critical role in helping FDA, consumers, and the pharmaceutical industry manage the risks associated with regulated products. To fulfill this responsibility, it is important for the pharmacist to understand FDA's adverse event reporting system.

The FDA MedWatch program is a voluntary adverse event reporting system that allows health care providers and consumers to report serious adverse drug reactions directly to the agency.[28] FDA analyzes trends and correlations between drug use and adverse reports from information submitted to MedWatch. There is no cost to either the health care professional or the consumer for filing a report. Although the program is voluntary, it is ineffective unless properly used. Health care providers should take their role in patient safety seriously and, as part of that responsibility, make sure that serious adverse drug reactions suspected to be associated with drugs are reported to FDA. Official reporting forms are available from FDA by calling 1-800-FDA-1088. Reports can also be submitted online by accessing the MedWatch Web site (http://www.fda.gov/medwatch/index.html). FDA safety alerts and product recall information are also accessible at this site.

It is important to understand that submitting a report to FDA does not constitute a legal claim, nor does it in any way constitute an acknowledgment that there has even been an adverse drug reaction associated with use of the product. The identities of the practitioners and the patients are confidential. Health care providers are encouraged to report all suspected adverse reactions and to ensure effective review of the reports. FDA asks that practitioners describe the reaction, the exposure to the regulated product, the time between exposure and reaction, and the underlying disease.

Product Recalls

When a product regulated by FDA is identified as a potential risk to the public, removal of the product from the market may be necessary. Products may pose a risk for a variety of reasons, including adulteration, misbranding, or discovery of an unacceptable risk of adverse effects through postmarket surveillance.

FDA has two methods available to force the removal of a product from the market. First, if the drug is misbranded, adulterated, or an unapproved new drug, the FDC Act allows FDA to seize the product and order that it be held pending a review by the court.[29] Second, FDA can also seek a court injunction, preventing further distribution or sale of the product. Both of these remedies are potentially expensive and time-consuming and, more importantly, do not address the issue of retrieving drugs that have already been purchased.

A third avenue that FDA may pursue is to request the manufacturer to recall the product from the market. FDA has no statutory authority to order a recall, but when potentially serious health risks are associated with the use of a drug product, manufacturers typically are more than willing to institute a recall. If a recall is instituted, FDA does have the authority to prescribe the procedures to which the recall must conform. This cooperation between FDA and its regulated industries has proven over the years to be the quickest and most reliable method for removing potentially dangerous products from the market. This method has been successful, because it is in the interest of both FDA and the industry to remove unsafe and defective products from consumer hands as soon as possible. FDA guidelines governing product recalls make clear that FDA expects manufacturers to take full responsibility for product recalls, including follow-up checks to ensure that recalls are successful. Under the guidelines, companies are expected to notify FDA when recalls are started, to make reports to FDA on their progress, and to undertake recalls when asked to do so.[30]

The guidelines categorize all recalls into one of three classes according to the level of hazard associated with the product at issue:

■ *Class I* recalls are for dangerous or defective products that predictably could cause serious health problems or death.
■ *Class II* recalls are for products that might cause a temporary health problem or pose only a slight threat of a serious nature.

■ *Class III* recalls are for products that are unlikely to cause any adverse health reaction but violate FDA labeling or manufacturing regulations.

The manufacturer is responsible for notifying sellers of the recall. The sellers, including pharmacists, are responsible for contacting customers, if necessary. A pharmacist is also responsible for knowing what drugs or other regulated products have been recalled. Failing to remove a recalled product from the shelf—and subsequently providing the product to a consumer—may violate the FDC Act and also exposes the pharmacist to civil liability in the event that someone is injured by use of the product.

FDA issues general information about new recalls that it is monitoring through FDA Enforcement Reports, a weekly publication available on FDA's Internet page (www.fda.gov).

Nonprescription Products and Civil Liability

Nonprescription drug products are, by nature, deemed to be safe and effective for use by the general public for self-care, without the oversight of a health care practitioner. However, no drug, whether prescription or nonprescription, is completely safe. As with any product, injuries can result from the use of a nonprescription product. For example, a patient can have an allergic reaction to an ingredient in a nonprescription product, can become injured as a result of an interaction between a nonprescription product and another drug, or suffer injury resulting from a side effect associated with the use of the drug. The fact that these types of injuries can and do occur, however, does not mean that the drugs causing the problem are inherently dangerous or unsafe, or that they should not be available without a prescription.

Whether a health care practitioner can be held liable for money damages for recommending or selling a nonprescription drug that causes an injury is an issue that is decided under state law, and legislation varies from state to state. A complete analysis of the nuances of the various theories of liability is beyond the scope of this chapter. There are, however, some general principles that practitioners may find useful to understand and guard against potential civil liability.

Initially, it is important to note that regardless of what a court may decide in any given case, the primary obligation of a health care provider is to provide health care. This obligation may include recommending or selling appropriate nonprescription products for patient self-care. A health care provider who refuses to recommend or sell a product for fear of incurring civil liability is not providing health care, and is doing a disservice to himself or herself, the profession, and the patient.

Theories of Civil Liability

The body of law concerning civil liability is guided by the general principle that, in a civilized society, people are responsible for their actions. If one's actions cause an injury to another person, the law may require that the injured person be compensated or made whole. In the U.S. justice system, an injured person who seeks compensation for the injuries that he or she has sustained as a result of another's actions has the right to bring a civil lawsuit against the person who caused the injury. Typically, the injured party (the "plaintiff") will ask the court to award money damages to be paid by the party causing the injury (the "defendant"). For example, a plaintiff who sustains an injury after taking a nonprescription medication recommended by a pharmacist can file a lawsuit against the pharmacist, seeking monetary compensation for the injuries. The plaintiff may seek compensation for the past, present, and future medical bills that he or she has incurred or will incur as a result of the injury, for income lost from missing work, for the pain and suffering endured, and for any permanent injury or damage.

The mere fact that an injury occurred does not, however, entitle the plaintiff to damages. The plaintiff has the burden of proving that he or she has satisfied each of the elements required to be proved under the theory of liability alleged in the complaint. The theories of liability that can be alleged against a health care provider in connection with an injury caused by a nonprescription drug include negligence, breach of warranty, and strict product liability.

Negligence

The mere fact that an injury has occurred does not mean that a party can be found liable for negligence. Similarly, even if a health care provider makes a mistake, that action alone does not necessarily entitle the injured party to compensation. To prevail in a case alleging negligence of a health care provider, the plaintiff must prove four elements: (1) that the defendant owed the plaintiff a duty of care, (2) that the defendant by his or her conduct breached that duty, (3) that the breach caused the injury complained of, and (4) that, in fact, the plaintiff sustained some cognizable injury or damage. If the plaintiff cannot prove all of these elements, there can be no liability.

The first element, duty, is decided by the court. The relevant inquiry is whether the health care provider failed to exercise the degree of care that a reasonable and prudent person would have used under similar circumstances. Courts will examine the relationship between the parties; the foreseeability that the defendant's actions, or failure to act, could cause an injury; and the gravity of harm that resulted from the act or failure to act. After the court defines the duty, the jury will decide whether the duty has been breached by the health care provider.

In one very old case that addressed liability for injuries resulting from a pharmacist's recommendation of a nonprescription product, the court defined the duty as requiring the pharmacist to exercise a high degree of care in advising the purchaser of the injurious effects of the recommended nonprescription product.[31] In that case, the patient presented the pharmacist with a prescription for a product to treat poison ivy. The pharmacist advised the patient to use a nonprescription product instead of the product prescribed by the doctor. A reaction between the nonprescription ointment and a residue present on the patient's skin caused the skin to turn black. The court stated:

> In the discharge of their functions, druggists, apothecaries, and other persons dealing in drugs, poisons, and medicines, are required, not only to be skillful, but also exceedingly cautious and prudent, in view of the terrific consequences which may attend the least inattention on their part. The highest degree of care known among practical men must be used by them to prevent injury from the use of their compounds, and they are held to a special degree of responsibility corresponding with their superior knowledge and are generally held liable for the slightest negligence.

The court sustained a jury verdict awarding money damages to the plaintiff, finding that the recommendation of the nonprescription product and the recommendation that the plaintiff continue to use the product even after she began to notice that her skin was turning black constituted a breach of the standard of care owed to the patient.

Although each state's law differs, and the ruling in any case is dependent on the facts presented, it is likely that courts will hold pharmacists and other health care providers to a high standard of care in connection with the recommendation of nonprescription products. A reasonable pharmacist likely would not, for example, recommend that a patient discontinue all antidepressant medications and take St. John's wort to treat clinical depression. Nor would a reasonable health care provider recommend that a patient take aspirin if it is known that the patient is also on warfarin therapy. The health care provider must act reasonably and make recommendations that are in the patient's best interest. If, despite the exercise of due care, an injury results, a provider likely would not be held liable for negligence.

Of course, even if a duty and a breach were found, the provider would not be liable for injuries that were not caused by the negligent conduct. If, for example, the evidence in the poison ivy case described above showed that the patient's skin turned black not because of any reaction between the product recommended by the pharmacist, but because of some inherent condition the patient suffered from, which coincidentally manifested itself at the same time as the patient began using the nonprescription ointment, the pharmacist would not be held liable. Again, the plaintiff must prove all four elements—duty, breach, causation, and injury—to prevail.

Breach of Warranty

Liability for breach of warranty is based on the theory that the defendant violated either an express or implied agreement concerning the quality of the product in connection with its sale. Express warranties arise out of specific statements made by the seller, whereas implied warranties are created by and imposed by law. Keep in mind that warranty liability can arise only if the health care provider sold the product that fails to perform. Therefore, a recommendation by a health care provider that the patient buy a certain cough and cold preparation that causes injury will not result in warranty liability if the provider merely recommended but did not sell the product.

The Uniform Commercial Code (UCC), which has been adopted by nearly every state, defines an express warranty as "an affirmation of fact or promise made to the buyer, that relates to the goods and becomes a basis of the bargain."[32,33] In one of the few published cases addressing the breach of an express warranty made by a pharmacist in connection with the sale of a drug product, the court found the representation that the product sold "was the same as what the plaintiff's prescription called for" created an express warranty, and when the product sold was in fact different—and caused an injury—the pharmacist was held liable.[34] Using the poison ivy case again as an example, the pharmacist advised the plaintiff that the blackened skin that resulted after the first use of the nonprescription product would clear up with continued use of the ointment. Instead, it worsened. On those facts, the plaintiff likely could have stated a claim for breach of express warranty.

Express warranties should not be confused with "sales talk," or puffery, which are statements made to induce a sale that do not specifically relate to the ability of the product. For example, a statement such as "this is the best ointment you will ever buy" would likely be viewed as sales talk—not an express warranty.

Implied warranties are created by law. Two implied warranties included in the UCC should most concern health care providers who sell goods—the implied warranty of fitness for a particular purpose and the implied warranty of merchantability. When a seller recommends a particular product to meet the buyer's specific needs, it is implied that the product recommended is fit for that purpose. Therefore, for example, if a health care provider recommends and sells a product to treat a specific condition, and it turns out that the product should not have been used for that purpose, the plaintiff could claim the provider breached the warranty of fitness for a particular purpose.

The implied warranty of merchantability states that the product sold is fit for all general purposes for which the product typically is sold. Included within this warranty is the understanding that the products sold and their containers meet certain minimum quality standards. If a pharmacist sells a product that is outdated, contaminated, or subpotent, he or she has breached the implied warranty of merchantability.

Warranty claims often are brought against not just the immediate seller of the product but also against the product's manufacturer. However, if the condition that has rendered the product unfit for ordinary purposes was caused by the manufacturer, and not the seller, that would not necessarily relieve the seller of responsibility. State laws vary in this area, with some states having laws that limit the liability of the seller in those circumstances. In general, to avoid warranty liability, the provider must be mindful of the source and origin of the products it sells.

Strict Product Liability

The last type of liability that will be discussed is strict product liability. Unlike a negligence or warranty theory, strict liability is imposed when a product causes an injury to the user, even if the seller was not negligent and made no express or implied representations regarding the product. Although this type of case is typically brought against the manufacturer, it remains a viable theory of recovery against retail sellers of products in many states. The theory is based on the idea that a seller of a product that has profited from the sale should also be required to compensate victims who are injured by the product, even if the seller was not in any way negligent in causing the injury. The mere sale of a product that is found to be defective, even if the defect is unknown or even unknowable to the seller, can form the basis for imposing strict liability.

When the product involved is a prescription product, courts have almost universally held that pharmacists cannot be held strictly liable for injuries caused by products they dispense. However, when a pharmacist acts as a retailer and sells goods that cause injuries, the theory may remain viable. Again, many states have laws that will automatically pass liability up the chain, past the retailer to the manufacturer.

Again, the most important rule that a pharmacist or any health care provider can follow to avoid civil liability is to simply practice health care as it should be practiced. Caring for the patient and acting in the patient's best interest to improve the patient's health and well-being should be the primary concern of all health care providers. More often than not, adherence to that general principle will provide a defense in the event that a patient claims that the provider's conduct in connection with the recommendation or sale of a product caused an injury.

Key Points for Legal and Regulatory Issues in Self-Care Pharmacy Practice

➤ Although nonprescription drug products are readily available, they are subject to regulatory and legal requirements to ensure their safety and efficacy.

➤ The Drug Facts labeling panel is a useful consumer counseling tool for pharmacists.

➤ Homeopathic products are not subject to all the regulations that govern prescription and nonprescription drugs.

➤ Pharmacists play a critical role in helping FDA, consumers, and industry manage risks associated with nonprescription drugs and should voluntarily report adverse events to FDA's MedWatch program or the manufacturer.

➤ With increasing frequency, FDA is approving product switches from prescription to nonprescription status. Health care providers play a crucial role in educating their patients as to the safe and proper use of recently switched products.

➤ Although liability risks may be associated with the sale of a nonprescription product, health care providers must remember their primary role is to provide health care, and that the best way to protect themselves is to act reasonably and in the best interest of their patient when recommending a nonprescription product.

REFERENCES

1. The Pure Food and Drugs Act of 1906, PL 59-386, 34 Stat 768 (1906) (Repealed in 1938 by 21 USC Sec 329(a)).
2. US Food and Drug Administration, Center for Drug Evaluation and Research. Rulemaking History for OTC Drug Products: Drug Category List. Available at: http://www.fda.gov/cder/otcmonographs/rulemaking_index.htm. Last accessed August 18, 2008.
3. 67 *Federal Register* 3060 (2002) (codified at 21 CFR §330.14).
4. US Food and Drug Administration, Center for Drug Evaluation and Research. Drug Applications. Available at: http://www.fda.gov/cder/regulatory/applications/nda.htm#Introduction. Last accessed July 29, 2008.
5. Public Law 109-462.
6. 21 CFR § 314.80 and 314.98.
7. US Food and Drug Administration. Reporting Adverse Experiences to FDA. Available at: http://www.fda.gov/medwatch/how.htm. Last accessed August 11, 2008.
8. 62 *Federal Register* 9024 (1997).
9. 62 *Federal Register* 13254 (1999). Available at: http://www.fda.gov/cder/consumerinfo/OTClabel.htm. Last accessed August 18, 2008.
10. 21 CFR §201.66.
11. 21 CFR §211.137.
12. 21 CFR §211.132.
13. Nordenberg, T. Now available without a prescription. *FDA Consum.* November 1996.
14. US Food and Drug Administration. Over-the-counter medicines: What's right for you? Available at: http://www.fda.gov/cder/consumerinfo/WhatsRightForYou.pdf. Last accessed August 18, 2008.
15. Newton GD, Benninghoff AJ, Popovich NG. New OTC drugs and devices: a selective review. *J Am Pharm Assoc.* 2002;42:267–77.
16. Shih YT, Prasad M, Luce BR. The effect on social welfare of a switch of second-generation antihistamines from prescription to over-the-counter status: a microeconomic analysis. *Clin Ther.* 2002;24:701–16.
17. Erickson A. RX-to-OTC switches offer golden opportunity. *Pharm Today.* 2002;8:1, 5, 35.
18. FDA approves Prilosec OTC to treat frequent heartburn [press release]. Available at: http://www.fda.gov/bbs/topics/news/2003/NEW00916.html. Last accessed August 18, 2008.
19. FDA advisory panel rejects OTC status for Merck's Mevacor. *Drug Top Daily News Articles.* Available at http://drugtopics.modernmedicine.com/drugtopics/Drug+Topics+Daily+News/FDA-advisory-panel-rejects-OTC-status-for-Mercks-M/ArticleStandard/Article/detail/479448. Last accessed August 11, 2008.

20. US Food and Drug Administration. Behind the Counter Availability of Certain Drugs. Available at: http://www.fda.gov/oc/op/btc. Last accessed August 11, 2008.

21. Drug Enforcement Administration, Office of Diversion Control. Combat Methamphetamine Epidemic Act 2005 (Title VII of Public Law 109-177). Available at: http://www.deadiversion.usdoj.gov/meth/index.html. Last accessed August 11, 2008.

22. 70 *Federal Register* 75988 (2005).

23. 21 CFR §1300.02(b)(28).

24. National Association of Chain Drug Stores. Federal & State Laws Restricting the Sales of OTC Meth Precursor Products. Available at: http://www.nacds.org/user-assets/PDF_files/Meth_Law_Chart.pdf. Last accessed August 18, 2008.

25. Consumer Healthcare Products Association. Voluntary codes and guidelines of the self-care industry: code of advertising practices for nonprescription medicines. Available at: http://www.chpa-info.org/content.aspx?id=82&pid=3&cc=2. Last accessed August 18, 2008.

26. 21 USC §321(g)(1).

27. US Food and Drug Administration. Is it a cosmetic, a drug, or both? July 8, 2002. Available at: http://www.cfsan.fda.gov/~dms/ cos-218.html. Last accessed August 18, 2008.

28. USCA § 379aa-1, *et seq.* [The Dietary Supplement and Nonprescription Drug Consumer Protection Act, was enacted on December 22, 2006. Public Law 109-462 amends the Federal Food, Drug, and Cosmetic Act (the Act) to add safety reporting requirements for OTC drug products that are marketed without an approved application under section 505 of the Act (21 U.S.C. 355).]

29. 21 USC § 334.

30. 21 CFR § 7.40.

31. *Fuhs v. Barber,* 36 P.2d 962 (Kan 1934).

32. Uniform Commercial Code. Article 2 § 2313.

33. Fink J, Vivian J, Bernstein I. *Pharm Law Dig.* 40th ed. St. Louis: Facts and Comparisons; 2006:287–8.

34. Jacobs Pharmacy Co. v. Gibson, 159 S.E.2d 171 (Ga 1967).

SECTION

11

Pain and Fever Disorders

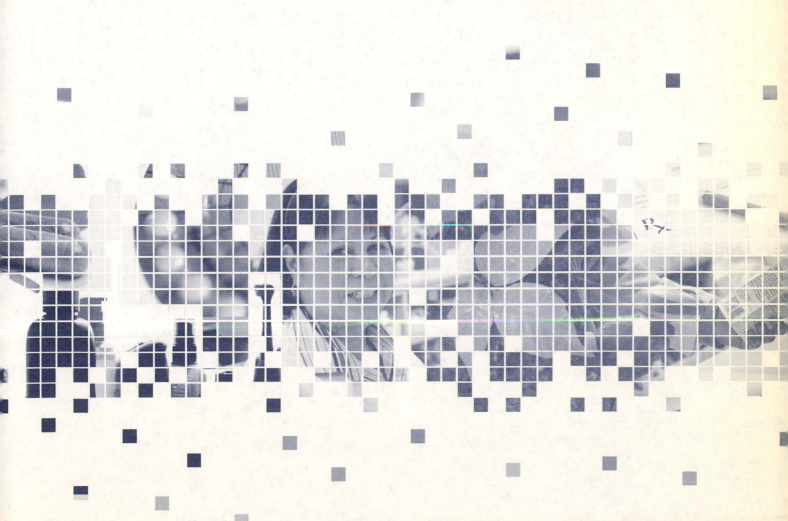

Headache

Tami L. Remington

More than 90% of people experience headache at some time during their lives.[1] In an international survey of people seeking primary care, 22% reported experiencing pain for at least 6 months during the preceding year, with 45% reporting headache.[2] Many headache sufferers self-treat with nonprescription remedies rather than seek medical attention. It is estimated that one-third of nonprescription analgesic use is for headache.[3] Migraine headache is a significant cause of absenteeism and lost productivity in the workplace, and affects relationships with family and friends.[3,4]

Nearly half of patients using nonprescription pain relievers do not read the labeling on the container, and 43% of people surveyed were unaware of the risks associated with taking these agents with prescription medications.[5] Clearly, an opportunity to improve medication use exists among patients self-treating for various pain syndromes.

Headaches are generally classified as primary or secondary.[6] Primary headaches (approximately 90% of headaches) are not associated with an underlying illness. Examples include episodic and chronic tension-type headaches, migraine headache with and without aura, cluster headaches, and medication-overuse headaches. Secondary headaches are symptoms of an underlying condition such as head trauma, stroke, substance abuse or withdrawal, bacterial and viral diseases, and disorders of craniofacial structures.

This chapter focuses on the most common headaches that are amenable to self-treatment: tension-type, diagnosed migraine, and sinus headaches. Nonprescription analgesics are useful in treating headache, either as monotherapy or as adjuncts to non-pharmacologic or prescription therapy. Throughout this chapter, the abbreviation *NSAID* will be used to denote the class of nonsalicylate nonsteroidal anti-inflammatory agents (ibuprofen and naproxen).

Tension-type headaches, also called stress headaches, can be episodic or chronic. More than 75% of the U.S. population will experience tension-type headaches at some time, with the 1-year prevalence being 38%.[1,4] Almost half of patients with tension-type headache report reduced effectiveness at work caused by headache, with about 10% to 12% reporting absenteeism because of head pain. Patients with chronic tension-type headaches have more absenteeism, missing about 18 more days per year than people with episodic headache.[1]

The prevalence of migraine headache in the United States is about 18% for women and 6% for men.[3] Onset usually begins in the first three decades of life, with greatest prevalence at around age 40 years. Among children, boys and girls are affected equally, but attacks usually disappear in boys after puberty.[4] Migraine without aura occurs almost twice as frequently as migraine with aura, and many individuals may have both types of headaches. Up to 70% of patients with migraine have family histories of migraine, suggesting that this disease is influenced by heredity.

The impact of migraine headache is substantial. Direct costs for medical services, taken from 1994 utilization data, were estimated at $1 billion in the United States. A greater burden comes in the form of lost productivity and wages, with migraine costing $13 billion for American employers. Migraine headaches affect health-related quality of life in a manner similar to that of depression, despite the episodic nature of the headaches.[3]

Headache is a frequently reported symptom in patients with acute sinusitis. These patients will also experience other sinus symptoms such as toothache in the upper teeth, facial pain, nasal stuffiness, and nasal discharge. The actual frequency of occurrence of sinus headache is low, and up to 90% of patients who believe they have sinus headache may actually be experiencing migraine headache.[7]

Pathophysiology of Headache

Tension-type headaches often manifest in response to stress, anxiety, depression, emotional conflicts, and other stimuli. It is likely that tension-type and migraine headache share pathophysiologic features, making them more similar than distinct.[8,9]

Migraine headaches probably arise from a complex interaction of neuronal and vascular factors. Stress, fatigue, oversleeping, fasting or missing a meal, vasoactive substances in food, caffeine, alcohol, menses, and changes in barometric pressure and altitude may trigger migraine. Medications (reserpine, nitrates, oral contraceptives, and postmenopausal hormones) can also trigger migraine. Although still debated, personality features of migraine sufferers include perfectionism, rigidity, and compulsiveness. Menstrual migraines appear at the menstrual stage of the ovarian cycle and occur in less than 10% of women. Most women with migraines experience attacks in the premenstrual period and, for some women, migraine headaches recur at specific times before, after, or during the menstrual cycle.

Most investigation into the pathophysiology of headache has centered on migraine headache. The best evidence suggests that migraine occurs through dysfunction of the trigeminovascular system. Neuronal depolarization that spreads slowly across the cerebral cortex is observed during the aura phase. Magnesium deficiency may contribute to this state. Stimulation (by an axon reflex) of trigeminal sensory fibers in the large cerebral and dural vessels causes neuropeptide release with concomitant neurogenic inflammation, vasodilation, and platelet and mast cell activation during the headache phase.

Sinus headache occurs when infection or blockage of the paranasal sinuses causes inflammation or distention of the sensitive sinus walls (see Chapter 11). Most patients who believe they have sinus headache may actually have migraine headache.[7] Pathophysiologic mechanisms at work during migraine headache can produce prominent sinus congestion.

Although a number of medications can cause headache as a side effect, issues discussed here relate to overuse (rebound) and withdrawal of agents used for analgesia. Medication-overuse headaches are a challenging area for clinicians. Agents associated with these headaches are acetaminophen, aspirin, caffeine, triptans, opioids, butalbital, and ergotamine formulations.[8] Medication-overuse headaches are usually associated with frequent use (more than twice weekly) for 3 months or longer, and occur within hours of stopping the agent; re-administration provides relief. Symptomatology shifts from the baseline headache type to a nearly continuous headache, particularly noticeable on awakening. This continuous headache may be punctuated by periodic headaches of the baseline type; some patients note an increased frequency of their baseline headache type. When medication-overuse headache is suspected, use of offending agent(s) should be tapered and subsequently eliminated. Most often, this should be done with medical supervision, because use of prescription therapies may be needed to combat the increased headaches that temporarily ensue during the days to weeks of the withdrawal period.[10,11]

Clinical Presentation of Headache

Headaches can be differentiated by their signs and symptoms (Table 5-1). Shivering or cold temperatures may increase pain from tension-type headaches. Chronic tension-type headaches occurring at least 15 days per month for at least 6 months, may be a manifestation of psychologic conflict, depression, or anxiety, and may be associated with sleep disturbances, shortness of breath, constipation, weight loss, fatigue, decreased sexual drive, palpitations, and menstrual changes. The severity of pain associated with tension-type headaches is variable; some headaches are so mild as

to not require treatment, whereas others are sufficiently severe to be disabling.[1]

Migraine headaches are classified as migraine with or without aura. Aura manifests as a series of neurologic symptoms: shimmering or flashing areas or blind spots in the visual field, difficulty speaking, visual and auditory hallucinations, and (usually) one-sided muscle weakness. These symptoms may last for up to 30 minutes, and the throbbing headache pain that follows may last from several hours to 2 days. Migraines without aura begin immediately with the throbbing headache pain. Both forms of migraine are often associated with nausea, vomiting, photophobia, phonophobia, sinus symptoms, tinnitus, light-headedness, vertigo, and irritability, and are aggravated by routine physical activity. A migraine attack may have a prodrome of a burst of energy or fatigue, extreme hunger, and nervousness. Migraine pain tends to be much more severe than that associated with tension-type headaches, with 80% of migraineurs reporting their pain as severe.[1]

Sinus headache is usually localized to facial areas over the sinuses and is difficult to differentiate from migraine without aura. The pain quality is typically dull and pressure-like. Stooping or blowing the nose often intensifies the pain, but sinus headache is not accompanied by nausea, vomiting, or visual disturbances. Persistent sinus pain and/or discharge suggests possible infection and requires referral for medical evaluation.

Treatment of Headache
Treatment Goals

The goals of treating headache are to (1) alleviate acute pain, (2) restore normal functioning, (3) prevent relapse, and (4) minimize side effects. For chronic headache, an additional goal is to reduce the frequency of headaches.

General Treatment Approach

Most patients with episodic headaches respond adequately to self-treatment with nonpharmacologic interventions, nonprescription medications, or both. Some patients with episodic headaches and most with chronic headaches are candidates for prescription treatments. However, these patients will often use nonprescription therapies adjunctively.

TABLE 5-1 Characteristics of Tension-Type, Migraine, and Sinus Headaches

	Tension-Type Headache	Migraine Headache	Sinus Headache
Location	Bilateral Over the top of head, extending to base of skull	Usually unilateral	Face, forehead, or periorbital area
Nature	Varies from diffuse ache to tight, pressing, constricting pain	Throbbing May be preceded by an aura	Pressure behind eyes or face Dull, bilateral pain Worse in the morning
Onset	Gradual	Sudden	Simultaneous with sinus symptoms, including purulent nasal discharge
Duration	Minutes to days	Hours to 2 days	Days (resolves with sinus symptoms)

Source: References 6 and 7.

Episodic tension-type headaches often respond well to nonprescription analgesics, including acetaminophen, NSAIDs, and salicylates, especially when taken as soon as the headache starts. If nonprescription analgesics are used to treat chronic headache, frequency of use should be limited to prevent medication-overuse headache. Chronic tension-type headaches usually benefit from physical therapy and relaxation exercises in addition to nonprescription or prescription medication. Figure 5-1 outlines the self-treatment of headaches and lists exclusions for self-treatment.

A medical diagnosis of migraine headache is required before self-treatment can be recommended. Taking an NSAID or salicylate at the onset of symptoms can abort mild or moderate migraine headache. Once a migraine has evolved, analgesics are less effective. Patients with migraines who can predict the occurrence of the headache (e.g., during menstruation) should take an analgesic (usually an NSAID) before the event known to trigger the headache, as well as throughout the duration of the event.

For patients with coexisting tension and migraine headaches, treatment of the initiating headache type can abort the mixed headache problem. It is not always necessary to treat both types.

For patients with sinus headache, decongestants (e.g., pseudoephedrine) are often useful in facilitating drainage of the sinuses (see Chapter 11). Concomitant use of decongestants and nonprescription analgesics can relieve the pain of sinus headache.

Nonpharmacologic Therapy

Chronic tension-type headaches often respond to relaxation exercises and physical therapy that emphasizes stretching and strengthening of head and neck muscles. General treatment measures for migraine include maintaining a regular sleeping and eating schedule, and practicing methods for coping with stress. Some patients with migraines benefit from use of ice (ice bags or cold packs) combined with pressure applied to the forehead or temple areas to reduce pain associated with acute migraine attacks.

Nutritional strategies are intended to prevent migraine and are based on (1) dietary restriction of foods that contain triggers, (2) avoidance of hunger and low blood glucose (a trigger of migraine), and (3) magnesium supplementation. Advocates of nutritional therapy recommend avoiding foods with vasoactive substances such as nitrites, tyramine (found in red wine and aged cheese), phenylalanine (found in the artificial sweetener aspartame), monosodium glutamate (often found in Asian food), caffeine (in coffee, tea, cola beverages, and chocolate),

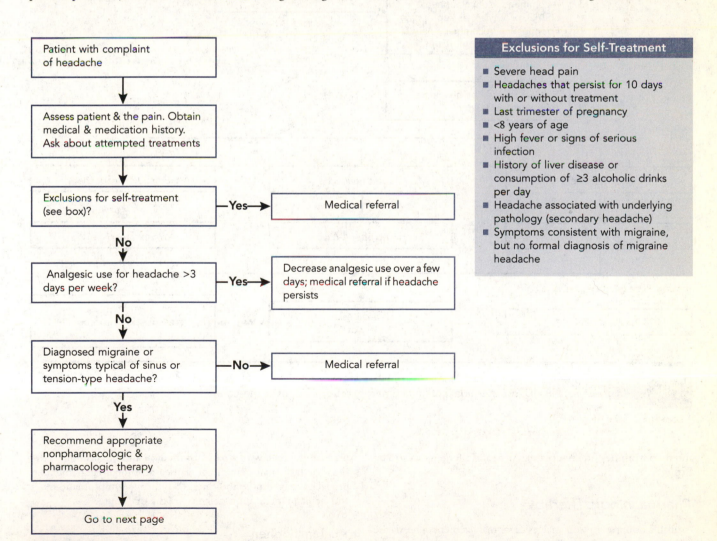

Exclusions for Self-Treatment

- Severe head pain
- Headaches that persist for 10 days with or without treatment
- Last trimester of pregnancy
- <8 years of age
- High fever or signs of serious infection
- History of liver disease or consumption of ≥3 alcoholic drinks per day
- Headache associated with underlying pathology (secondary headache)
- Symptoms consistent with migraine, but no formal diagnosis of migraine headache

FIGURE 5–1 Self-care of headache. Key: CHF, congestive heart failure; GI, gastrointestinal; HBP, high blood pressure; NSAID, nonsteroidal anti-inflammatory drug; OTC, over-the-counter. *(continued on next page)*

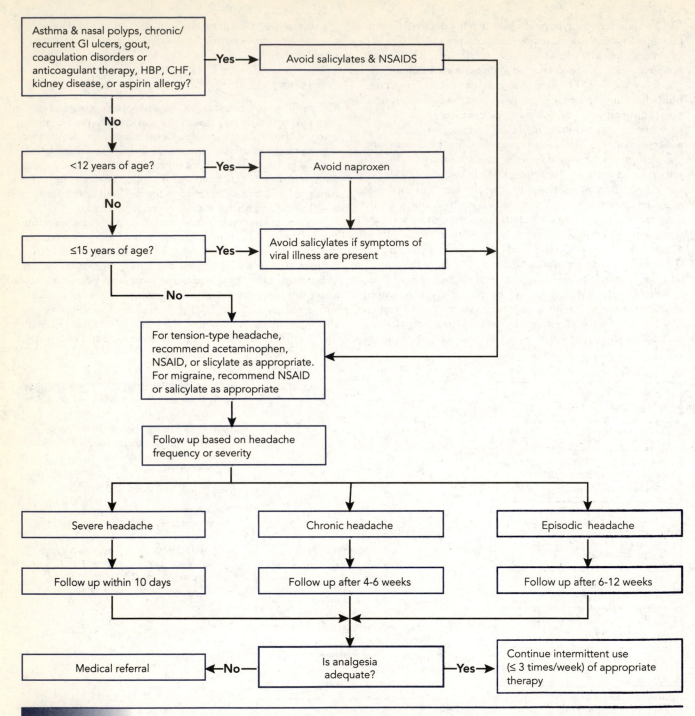

FIGURE 5-1 *(Continued)* Self-care of headache. Key: CHF, congestive heart failure; GI, gastrointestinal; HBP, high blood pressure; NSAID, nonsteroidal anti-inflammatory drug; OTC, over-the-counter.

and theobromines (in chocolate). Any food allergen can also be a trigger.[12]

Pharmacologic Therapy

Available nonprescription analgesics for management of headache include acetaminophen, NSAIDs (ibuprofen and naproxen), and salicylates (aspirin, magnesium salicylate, and sodium salicylate). Although these agents are available without a prescription, they are not benign; selection of an analgesic should be based

on a careful review of a patient's medical and medication histories. Medical management of nausea accompanying migraine headache may also be indicated to improve symptomatic relief and facilitate medication delivery by the oral route.

Acetaminophen

Acetaminophen is an effective analgesic and antipyretic, but it does not possess anti–inflammatory activity. Acetaminophen produces analgesia through a central inhibition of prostaglandin synthesis.

Acetaminophen is rapidly absorbed from the gastrointestinal (GI) tract and extensively metabolized in the liver to inactive glucuronic and sulfuric acid conjugates. In addition, acetaminophen is metabolized to a hepatotoxic intermediate metabolite by the cytochrome P450 enzyme system. This intermediate metabolite is detoxified by glutathione. Rectal bioavailability of acetaminophen is approximately 50% to 60% of that achieved with oral administration. Onset of analgesic activity of acetaminophen is about 30 minutes after oral administration. Duration of activity is about 4 hours and is extended to 6 to 8 hours by using an extended-release formulation.

Acetaminophen is effective in relieving mild-to-moderate pain of nonvisceral origin. Randomized, double-blind, placebo-controlled studies have documented superiority of acetaminophen 1000 mg over placebo in patients with migraine and tension-type headache.[13,14]

Recommended pediatric and adult dosages of acetaminophen are provided in Tables 5-2 and 5-3. Table 5-4 lists select trade-name products.

Acetaminophen is available for administration in various oral and rectal dosage forms. Acetaminophen oral capsules contain tasteless granules that can be emptied onto a spoon containing a small amount of drink or soft food. Patients and parents should not add contents of the capsules to a glass of liquid, because large numbers of granules may adhere to the side of the glass. Mixing with a hot beverage can result in a bitter taste.

Acetaminophen is potentially hepatotoxic in doses exceeding 4 g/day, especially with chronic use. Patients should be cautioned against exceeding this dose limit. More conservative dosing (i.e., 2 g/day or less) or avoidance may be warranted in patients at increased risk for acetaminophen-induced hepatotoxicity, including those with concurrent use of other potentially hepatotoxic drugs, poor nutritional intake, or ingestion of three or more alcoholic drinks per day.[15,16]

Acetaminophen poisoning is a major reason for contacting poison control centers and the leading cause of acute liver failure in the United States.[17–19] Hepatotoxicity from acetaminophen is probably dose-related and is uncommon at recommended doses.[20,21] In a prospective study, 83% of patients presenting with acetaminophen hepatotoxicity had taken more than 4 g/day.[18] Unintended chronic overdose comprises about half of the cases of acetaminophen-induced acute liver failure. Contributing factors include repeated dosing in excess of package labeling, use of more than one product containing acetaminophen, and alcohol ingestion.[19] In an attempt to reduce the occurrence of accidental overdose, the Food and Drug Administration (FDA) recommended labeling changes for prescription and nonprescription products to make acetaminophen content more evident.[22] In the United Kingdom, limiting package size to 16 tablets has reduced deaths attributable to acetaminophen overdose.[23]

It has been proposed that malnutrition and alcohol intake are risk factors for acetaminophen-induced hepatic injury, but this proposal is refuted owing to the paucity of clinical evidence supporting the relationships.[15,24–28] Of interest to note, nearly two-thirds of subjects in one study who reported daily alcohol consumption also reported daily use or abuse of acetaminophen. Despite these usage patterns, none of them developed hepatotoxicity.[26]

Early symptoms of acetaminophen intoxication can include nausea, vomiting, drowsiness, confusion, and abdominal pain, but these symptoms may be absent, belying the potential gravity of the exposure. Serious clinical manifestations of hepatotoxicity

TABLE 5-2 Recommended Pediatric Dosages for Nonprescription Analgesics

Agent	Dose by Body Weight (mg/kg)	Weight or Age	Single Dose (mg)
Acetaminophen[a]	10–15	6–11 lb	40[c]
		12–17 lb	80[c]
		18–23 lb	120[c]
		24–35 lb	160
		36–47 lb	240
		48–59 lb	320
		60–71 lb	400
		72–95 lb	480
		≥96 lb	650
Ibuprofen[b]	7.5	12–17 lb	50[c]
		18–23 lb	75[c]
		24–35 lb	100
		35–47 lb	150
		48–59 lb	200
		60–71 lb	250
		72–95 lb	300
		>95 lb	200–400 mg (maximum 1200 mg/day)
Naproxen sodium		<12 years	Not recommended
		>12 years	220–440 mg, then 220 mg every 8–12 hours (maximum 660 mg/day)
Aspirin[a]	10–15	<24 lb	As directed by health care provider
		24–35 lb	162[c]
		36–47 lb	243[c]
		48–59 lb	324
		60–71 lb	405
		72–95 lb	486
		≥96 lb	648

[a] Individual doses may be repeated every 4–6 hours as needed, not to exceed five doses in 24 hours.

[b] Individual doses may be repeated every 6–8 hours as needed, not to exceed four doses in 24 hours.

[c] Data from *The Harriet Lane Handbook: A Manual for Pediatric House Officers*. 17th ed. Philadelphia: Elsevier Mosby; 2005.

begin 2 to 4 days after acute ingestion of acetaminophen and include increased plasma aspartate aminotransferase and alanine aminotransferase (ALT), increased plasma bilirubin with jaundice, prolonged prothrombin time, and obtundation. In the majority of cases, hepatic damage is reversible over a period of weeks or months,[18] but fatal hepatic necrosis can occur.

TABLE 5-3 Recommended Adult Dosages of Nonprescription Analgesics

Agent	Dosage Forms	Usual Adult Dosage (Maximum Daily Dosage)
Acetaminophen	Immediate-release, extended-release, effervescent, disintegrating, rapid-release, and chewable tablets; capsules; liquid drops; elixir; suspension; suppositories	325–1000 mg every 4–6 hours (4000 mg)
Ibuprofen	Immediate-release and chewable tablets; capsules; suspension; liquid drops	200–400 mg every 4–6 hours (1200 mg)
Naproxen sodium	Tablets	220 mg every 8–12 hours (660 mg)
Aspirin	Immediate-release, buffered, enteric-coated, film-coated, effervescent, and chewable tablets; suppositories; chewing gum	650–1000 mg every 4–6 hours (4000 mg)
Magnesium salicylate	Tablets	650 mg every 4 hours or 1000 mg every 6 hours (4000 mg)

Because of the potential seriousness of acetaminophen overdose, all cases should be referred to a poison control center or emergency department. In addition to supportive care, activated charcoal (or other method of gut decontamination) is used to reduce the absorption of acetaminophen in patients who present shortly after acute overdose. When acetaminophen serum levels (related to time since ingestion) exceed those known to cause hepatic injury, administration of acetylcysteine is warranted. Prompt administration is important given that acetylcysteine's effectiveness is reduced when administration is delayed beyond 8 hours after acute ingestion. For patients with chronic ingestions of greater than 4 g/day, administration of acetylcysteine is indicated until liver toxicity is ruled out by assessing liver enzymes and liver function.

TABLE 5-4 Selected Single-Entity Acetaminophen Products

Trade Name	Acetaminophen Content
Pediatric Formulations	
Children's Tylenol Meltaway Tablets	80 mg
FeverAll Infants' Suppositories	80 mg
FeverAll Children's Suppositories	160 mg
FeverAll Junior Strength Suppositories	325 mg
Jr Tylenol Meltaway Tablets	160 mg
ElixSure Children's Oral Solution	160 mg/5 mL
Infants' Tylenol Drops	80 mg/0.8 mL
Adult Formulations	
Tylenol Arthritis Pain Caplets	650 mg
Tylenol Extra Strength Caplets/Cool Caplets/Rapid Release Gelcaps/ Go Tabs/EZ Tabs	500 mg
Tylenol Rapid Blast Liquid	500 mg/15 mL
Tylenol Regular Strength Tablets	325 mg

Asymptomatic elevations in serum ALT have been reported in otherwise healthy individuals taking acetaminophen 4 g/day. In a prospective study, 39% of patients experienced ALT elevations greater than three times the upper limit of normal. These elevations generally appeared in the first week of use, with some resolution despite continued dosing. The clinical significance of this observation is uncertain.[29]

Patients with glucose-6-phosphate dehydrogenase deficiency should also use caution when medicating with acetaminophen. Use of acetaminophen is contraindicated in patients who are hypersensitive to the medication.

Clinically important drug interactions of acetaminophen are listed in Table 5-5. For patients taking warfarin, acetaminophen is considered the analgesic of choice; however, it has been associated with increases in international normalized ratio (INR). Regular acetaminophen use should be discouraged in patients on warfarin. Patients who require higher scheduled doses (e.g., those with osteoarthritis) should have their INR monitored and warfarin adjusted as acetaminophen doses are titrated.

Nonsteroidal Anti-Inflammatory Drugs

NSAIDs relieve pain through peripheral inhibition of cyclo-oxygenase (COX) and subsequent inhibition of prostaglandin synthesis.

All nonprescription NSAIDs are rapidly absorbed from the GI tract with consistently high bioavailability. They are extensively metabolized to inactive compounds in the liver, mainly by glucuronidation. Elimination occurs primarily through the kidneys. Naproxen sodium and ibuprofen have onsets of activity of about 30 minutes. Analgesia from naproxen sodium lasts up to 12 hours, whereas ibuprofen lasts about 6 to 8 hours.

The FDA-approved uses for nonprescription NSAIDs include reducing fever and relieving minor pain associated with headache, the common cold, toothache, muscle ache, backache, arthritis, and menstrual cramps. NSAIDs have analgesic, antipyretic, and anti-inflammatory activity, and are useful in managing mild-to-moderate pain of nonvisceral origin. Two agents (propionic acid derivatives) are available for nonprescription use: ibuprofen (1984) and naproxen sodium (1994).

Tables 5-2, 5-3, and 5-6 list pediatric and adult doses and selected trade-name products of nonprescription NSAIDs. A

TABLE 5-5   Clinically Important Drug–Drug Interactions with Nonprescription Analgesic Agents

Analgesic/ Antipyretic	Drug	Potential Interaction	Management/Preventive Measures
Acetaminophen	Alcohol	Increased risk of hepatotoxicity	Avoid concurrent use if possible; minimize alcohol intake when using acetaminophen.
Acetaminophen	Warfarin	Increased risk of bleeding (elevations in INR)	Limit acetaminophen to occasional use; monitor INR for several weeks when acetaminophen 2–4 g daily is added or discontinued in patients on warfarin.
Aspirin	Valproic acid	Displacement from protein-binding sites and inhibition of valproic acid metabolism	Avoid concurrent use; use naproxen instead of aspirin (no interaction).
Aspirin	NSAIDs, including COX-2 inhibitors	Increased risk of gastroduodenal ulcers and bleeding	Avoid concurrent use if possible; consider use of gastroprotective agents (e.g., PPIs).
Ibuprofen	Aspirin	Decreased antiplatelet effect of aspirin	Aspirin should be taken at least 30 minutes before or 8 hours after ibuprofen. Use acetaminophen (or other analgesic) instead of ibuprofen.
Ibuprofen	Phenytoin	Displacement from protein-binding sites	Monitor free phenytoin levels; adjust dose as indicated.
NSAIDs (several)	Bisphosphonates	Increased risk of GI or esophageal ulceration	Use caution with concomitant use.
NSAIDs (several)	Digoxin	Inhibit renal clearance of digoxin	Monitor digoxin levels; adjust dose as indicated.
Salicylates and NSAIDs (several)	Antihypertensive agents, beta-blockers, ACE inhibitors, vasodilators, diuretics	Antihypertensive effect inhibited; possible hyperkalemia with potassium-sparing diuretics and ACE inhibitors	Monitor blood pressure, cardiac function, and potassium levels.
Salicylates and NSAIDs	Anticoagulants	Increased risk of bleeding, especially GI	Avoid concurrent use, if possible; lowest risk with salsalate and choline magnesium trisalicylate.
Salicylates and NSAIDs	Alcohol	Increased risk of GI bleeding	Avoid concurrent use, if possible; minimize alcohol intake when using salicylates and NSAIDs.
Salicylates and NSAIDs (several)	Methotrexate	Decreased methotrexate clearance	Avoid salicylates and NSAIDs with high-dose methotrexate therapy; monitor levels with concurrent treatment.
Salicylates (moderate-to-high doses)	Sulfonylureas	Increased risk of hypoglycemia	Avoid concurrent use, if possible; monitor blood glucose levels when changing salicylate dose.

Key: ACE, angiotensin-converting enzyme; COX, cyclooxygenase; GI, gastrointestinal; INR, international normalized ratio; NSAID, nonsteroidal anti-inflammatory drug; PPI, protein pump inhibitor.

dose–effect relationship has been demonstrated for ibuprofen analgesia in the range of 100 to 400 mg.

Overdoses of NSAIDs usually produce minimal symptoms of toxicity and are rarely fatal. In a prospective study of 329 cases of ibuprofen overdose, 43% of ibuprofen-overdose patients were asymptomatic. Among patients with symptoms, GI and central nervous system (CNS) symptoms were most common (in 42% and 30% of patients, respectively) and included nausea, vomiting, abdominal pain, lethargy, stupor, coma, nystagmus, dizziness, and light-headedness. Hypotension, bradycardia, tachycardia, dyspnea, and painful breathing were also reported.[30]

The most frequent adverse effects of NSAIDs involve the GI tract and include dyspepsia, heartburn, nausea, anorexia, and epigastric pain, even among children using pediatric formulations. These agents produce less GI upset and bleeding than aspirin.[31] NSAIDs may be taken with food, milk, or antacids if they upset the stomach. Tablets should be taken with a full glass of water, suspensions should be shaken thoroughly, and enteric-coated

TABLE 5-6	Selected Single-Entity Nonsteroidal Anti-Inflammatory Drugs

Trade Name	Primary Ingredients
Pediatric Formulations of Ibuprofen Products	
Children's Advil Suspension	Ibuprofen 100 mg/5 mL
Children's Advil Chewable Tablets	Ibuprofen 50 mg
Junior Strength Advil Chewable and Swallow Tablets	Ibuprofen 100 mg
Children's Motrin Suspension	Ibuprofen 100 mg/5 mL
Infants' Motrin Concentrated Drops	Ibuprofen 50 mg/1.25 mL
Junior Strength Motrin Tablets/Caplets	Ibuprofen 100 mg
Adult Formulations of Ibuprofen Products	
Advil Migraine Capsules	Ibuprofen 200 mg
Advil Tablets/Caplets/Gel Caplets	Ibuprofen 200 mg
Midol Cramps & Body Aches Tablets	Ibuprofen 200 mg
Motrin IB Tablets/Caplets	Ibuprofen 200 mg
Naproxen Products	
Aleve Tablets/Caplets/Liquid Gels/Smooth Gels	Naproxen sodium 220 mg
Midol Extended Relief Caplets	Naproxen sodium 220 mg

or sustained-release preparations should be neither crushed nor chewed. Other adverse effects include dizziness, fatigue, headache, or nervousness. Rashes or itching may occur in some patients, and some cases of photosensitivity have been reported. Fluid retention can occur and, in some cases, edema develops. At normal nonprescription doses, these effects are usually rare.

GI ulceration, perforation, and bleeding are uncommon but serious complications of NSAID use. Risk factors include age older than 60 years, prior ulcer disease or GI bleeding, concurrent use of anticoagulants (including aspirin), higher dose or longer duration of treatment, and moderate use of alcohol. Package labeling for NSAIDs include warnings about stomach bleeding.[22]

NSAIDs are associated with increased risk for myocardial infarction, heart failure, hypertension, and stroke. The mechanism by which they confer this risk is not clear, but may be related to increased thromboxane A2 activity and suppressed vascular prostacyclin synthesis, resulting in vasoconstriction and platelet aggregation. On the basis of the results from meta-analyses of randomized trials, it appears that the cardiovascular risk of nonselective NSAIDs is dose- and duration-dependent. In addition, there are differences in risk between individual nonselective NSAIDs: ibuprofen has been associated with a significant increase in cardiovascular risk, whereas naproxen has not.

The American Heart Association recommends that patients with or at high risk for cardiovascular disease (hyperlipidemia, hypertension, diabetes, or other macrovascular disease) should avoid NSAIDs. Even patients at low risk should use these agents cautiously, at the lowest dose and shortest duration needed to control symptoms. Naproxen was identified as a preferred drug because it appears to be safer than ibuprofen.[32] FDA has emphasized that patients using NSAIDs for longer than 10 days should do so only with medical supervision.[33]

Clinically important drug–drug interactions of NSAIDs are listed in Table 5-5. Ibuprofen increases bleeding time by reversibly inhibiting platelet aggregation. Patients taking aspirin for cardiovascular prophylaxis should take it at least an hour before or 8 hours after ibuprofen to avoid a pharmacodynamic interaction that inhibits the antiplatelet effect of aspirin. In doses of 1200 to 2400 mg/day, ibuprofen does not appear to affect the INR in patients taking warfarin. However, ibuprofen should not be recommended for self-treatment in patients who are concurrently taking anticoagulants because its antiplatelet activity could increase GI bleeding.

As with other nonprescription analgesics, patients who have three or more alcoholic drinks per day should be cautioned about the increased risk of adverse GI events, including stomach bleeding, and be referred to their primary care provider regarding use.

NSAIDs may decrease renal blood flow and glomerular filtration rate as a result of inhibition of renal prostaglandin synthesis. Consequently, increased blood urea nitrogen and serum creatinine values can occur, often with concomitant sodium and water retention. Advanced age, hypertension, diabetes, atherosclerotic cardiovascular disease, and use of diuretics appear to increase the risk of renal toxicity with ibuprofen use. As a result, patients with a history of impaired renal function, congestive heart failure, or diseases that compromise renal hemodynamics should not self-medicate with NSAIDs.

Salicylates

Salicylates inhibit prostaglandin synthesis from arachidonic acid by inhibiting both isoforms of the enzyme cyclooxygenase (COX-1 and COX-2). The resulting decrease in prostaglandins reduces the sensitivity of pain receptors to the initiation of pain impulses at sites of inflammation and trauma. Although some evidence suggests that aspirin also produces analgesia through a central mechanism, its site of action is primarily peripheral.

Salicylates are absorbed by passive diffusion of the nonionized drug in the stomach and small intestine. Factors affecting absorption include dosage form, gastric pH, gastric-emptying time, dissolution rate, and the presence of antacids or food. Absorption from immediate-release aspirin products is complete. Rectal absorption of salicylate is slow and unreliable, as well as proportional to rectal retention time.

Once absorbed, aspirin is hydrolyzed in the plasma to salicylic acid in 1 to 2 hours. Salicylic acid is widely distributed to all tissues and fluids in the body including the CNS, breast milk, and fetal tissue. Protein binding is concentration-dependent. At concentrations lower than 100 mg/mL, approximately 90% of salicylic acid is bound to albumin, whereas at concentrations greater than 400 mg/mL approximately 75% is bound. Salicylic acid is largely eliminated through the kidney. The pH of the urine determines the amount of unchanged drug eliminated, with urinary concentrations increasing substantially in more alkaline urine (pH ~8).

Dosage-form alterations include enteric coating, buffering, and sustained release. Such formulations were developed to change the rate of absorption and/or reduce the potential for GI toxicity. Enteric-coated aspirin is absorbed only from the small intestine; its absorption is markedly slowed by food, attributed to prolonged gastric-emptying time. Hypochlorhydria from acid-suppressing agents (especially proton pump inhibitors) may result in dissolution of enteric-coated products in the stomach, negating any potential benefit on local gastric toxicity. For patients requiring rapid pain relief, enteric-coated aspirin is inappropriate because of the delay in absorption and the time to analgesic effect.

Buffered aspirin products are available in both tablet and effervescent forms. Although they are absorbed more rapidly than nonbuffered products, time to onset of effect is not improved appreciably. Common buffers include aluminum hydroxide; magnesium carbonate, hydroxide or oxide; calcium carbonate; and sodium bicarbonate (in effervescent formulations). Some effervescent aspirin solutions contain large amounts of sodium and must be avoided by patients who require restricted sodium intake (e.g., patients with hypertension, heart failure, or renal failure). Sustained-release aspirin is formulated to prolong the product's duration of action by slowing dissolution and absorption.

The salicylate content of 377 mg of magnesium salicylate tetrahydrate is equivalent to 325 mg of sodium salicylate.

Salicylates are approved for treatment of symptoms of osteoarthritis, rheumatoid arthritis, and other rheumatologic diseases, and for temporary relief of minor aches and pains associated with backache or muscle aches. They are also effective in treating mild-to-moderate pain from musculoskeletal conditions and fever. Aspirin possesses other important uses for indications unrelated to pain syndromes. It is indicated for prevention of thromboembolic events, such as myocardial infarction and stroke, in high-risk patients, owing to its inhibitory effects on platelet function.

Tables 5-2 and 5-3 list pediatric and adult dosages of nonprescription salicylates. Table 5-7 provides select salicylate products. Aspirin dosages in the range of 4 to 6 g/day are often needed to produce anti-inflammatory effects. The maximum analgesic dosage for self-medication with aspirin is 4 g/day; therefore, anti-inflammatory activity often will not occur unless the drug is used at the high end of the acceptable dosage range.

Mild salicylate intoxication (salicylism) occurs with chronic therapy that produces toxic salicylate plasma concentrations. Chronic intoxication in adults generally requires taking salicylate 90 to 100 mg/kg/day for at least 2 days. Conditions that predispose patients to salicylate toxicity include (1) marked renal or hepatic impairment (i.e., uremia, cirrhosis, or hepatitis); (2) metabolic disorders (i.e., hypoxia or hypothyroidism); (3) unstable disease (i.e., cardiac arrhythmias, intractable epilepsy, or brittle diabetes); (4) status asthmaticus; and (5) multiple comorbidities. Symptoms include headache, dizziness, tinnitus, difficulty hearing, dimness of vision, mental confusion, lassitude, drowsiness, sweating, thirst, hyperventilation, nausea, vomiting, and occasional diarrhea. These symptoms are all reversible in response to lowering the plasma concentration to a therapeutic range. Tinnitus, typically one of the early signs of toxicity, should not be used as a sole indicator of salicylate toxicity.

Acute salicylate intoxication is categorized as mild (ingestion of <150 mg/kg), moderate (ingestion of 150–300 mg/kg), or severe (ingestion of >300 mg/kg). Symptoms are concentration-dependent and include lethargy, nausea, vomiting, dehydration, tinnitus, hemorrhage, tachypnea and pulmonary edema, convulsions, and coma. Acid–base disturbances are prominent and range from respiratory alkalosis to metabolic acidosis. Initially, salicylate affects the respiratory center in the medulla, producing hyperventilation and respiratory alkalosis. In severely intoxicated adults and in most salicylate-poisoned children younger than 5 years, respiratory alkalosis progresses rapidly to metabolic acidosis. Children are more prone than adults to develop high fever in salicylate poisoning. Hypoglycemia resulting from increased glucose utilization may be especially serious in children. Bleeding may occur from the GI tract or mucosal surfaces, and petechiae are a prominent feature at autopsy.

Emergency management of acute salicylate intoxication is directed toward preventing absorption of salicylate from the GI tract and toward supportive care. Activated charcoal should be used at home only if recommended by poison control or emergency department personnel. In an emergency department setting, gut decontamination with gastric lavage or activated charcoal may be undertaken. Enhancing renal elimination can be accomplished through alkalinization of the urine. Dosing recommendations for the use of activated charcoal are included in Chapter 21.

Upper GI symptoms occur in about half of people who take aspirin. Dyspepsia, epigastric discomfort, nausea, and vomiting have all been reported, and may be lessened by taking aspirin with food. These symptoms are not necessarily related to more serious GI adverse events from aspirin.

Aspirin is associated with gastritis and ulceration of the upper GI tract. It produces GI mucosal damage by penetrating the protective mucous and bicarbonate layers of the gastric mucosa and permitting back-diffusion of acid, thereby causing cellular and vascular erosion. Two distinct mechanisms cause this problem: (1) a local irritant effect resulting from the medication contacting the gastric mucosa and (2) a systemic effect from prostaglandin inhibition.

Endoscopy studies reveal upper GI mucosal damage from episodic and chronic aspirin ingestion. Gastric petechiae and erosions occur within 1 to 2 hours after a single 600 mg dose. Lower doses of 300 mg/day for 14 days also show gastric and duodenal petechiae, erosions, and endoscopic ulcers. Other data have shown that 10% of patients taking daily doses of 300 mg or less for 12 weeks have documented gastric ulcers.[35] However, the clinical importance of these findings is uncertain because they do not necessarily correlate with symptoms or adverse clinical outcomes.[36]

GI blood loss with aspirin is dose-dependent and has been demonstrated in patients taking only 75 mg/day. Normal subjects with no aspirin exposure lose approximately 0.5 mL of blood per

TABLE 5-7 Selected Adult Formulations of Single-Entity Salicylate Products	
Trade Name	**Primary Ingredient**
Alka-Seltzer Original Effervescent Tablets	Aspirin 325 mg
Bayer Low-Dose Chewable Aspirin Tablets	Aspirin 81 mg
St. Joseph 81 mg Chewable Aspirin	Aspirin 81 mg
Ecotrin Adult Low Strength Tablets	Aspirin 81 mg
Ecotrin Regular Strength Safety-Coated Tablets	Aspirin 325 mg
Extra Strength Bayer Aspirin Coated Caplets and Gelcaps	Aspirin 500 mg
Genuine Bayer Aspirin Tablets	Aspirin 325 mg
Doan's Pills	Magnesium salicylate 377 mg
Momentum Maximum Strength Backache Relief Coated Caplets	Magnesium salicylate tetrahydrate 580 mg

day in the stool. Moderate aspirin intake increases this amount to 2 to 6 mL per day, and up to 15% of patients will lose in excess of 10 mL per day. Chronic GI bleeding of this magnitude can deplete total body iron and produce iron deficiency anemia.

Patients with risk factors for upper GI bleeding should avoid self-treatment with aspirin. These risk factors include (1) history of uncomplicated or bleeding peptic ulcer; (2) age older than 60 years; (3) concomitant use of other NSAIDs, anticoagulants, antiplatelet agents, bisphosphonates, selective serotonin reuptake inhibitors, or systemic corticosteroids; (4) higher dose of aspirin; (5) infection with *Helicobacter pylori;* (6) rheumatoid arthritis; (7) NSAID-related dyspepsia; and (8) concomitant use of alcohol.[36,37]

Various aspirin formulations may have different rates of GI side effects. Enteric coating may reduce occurrence of mucosal lesions identified by endoscopy, as well as decrease local gastric irritation.[38] Therefore, enteric-coated aspirin is a preferred dosage form for patients requiring chronic therapy with medium-to-high doses.[38] However, no difference among plain, enteric-coated, and buffered products has been identified for risk of major upper GI bleeding that results in hematemesis or melena.[35] Endoscopic evaluation comparing buffered and nonbuffered aspirin products suggests similar rates of gastric damage.[35]

Serious aspirin intolerance is uncommon and consists of two types: urticaria-angioedema type and bronchospastic type. These adverse effects usually occur within 3 hours of aspirin ingestion and present with urticaria, angioedema, difficulty with breathing, bronchospasm, profuse rhinorrhea, and shock. The mechanism is not immunologically mediated and does not preclude use of nonacetylated salicylates.

Risk factors for serious aspirin intolerance include chronic urticaria (for urticaria-angioedema type) and asthma with nasal polyps (for bronchospastic type). In patients with one of these conditions, the incidence of serious aspirin intolerance has been reported to range from 10% to 30%. Severity of the intolerance is variable, ranging from minor to severe.

Nonprescription salicylates interact with several other important drugs and drug classes. Table 5-5 lists clinically important drug interactions reported for salicylates. Clinicians should review current drug interaction references for newly identified interactions when monitoring therapy in patients who are taking high-dose salicylates.

Aspirin ingestion may produce positive results on fecal occult blood testing; therefore, its use should be discontinued for at least 3 days before testing. Similarly, aspirin should be discontinued 2 to 7 days before surgery and should not be used to relieve pain after tonsillectomy, dental extraction, or other surgical procedures, except under the close supervision of a health care provider or dentist. Aspirin can potentiate bleeding from capillary sites such as those found in the GI tract (with ulcers), tonsillar beds (after tonsillectomy), and tooth sockets (after dental extractions). A single 650 mg dose of aspirin can double bleeding time, and low doses also increase bleeding time.

Because of the effect on hemostasis, aspirin is contraindicated in patients with hypoprothrombinemia, vitamin K deficiency, hemophilia, history of any bleeding disorder, or history of peptic ulcer disease. Sodium salicylate does not affect platelets, but it does increase prothrombin time.

The maximum 4 gram dose of sodium salicylate contains 560 mg (25 mEq) of sodium. Consequently, patients on strict sodium restriction should avoid using sodium salicylate; they may take magnesium salicylate instead. Patients with compromised renal function have the potential for decreased renal excretion of

magnesium, allowing accumulation of toxic levels when taking magnesium salicylate. The maximum 24-hour dose of magnesium salicylate contains 264 mg (11 mEq) of magnesium.

All salicylates should be avoided in patients with a history of gout or hyperuricemia because of their dose-related effects on renal uric acid handling. Dosages of 1 to 2 g/day inhibit tubular uric acid secretion without affecting reabsorption and may increase plasma uric acid levels, which can precipitate or worsen a gout attack. Moderate dosages of 2 to 3 g/day have little effect on uric acid secretion. More than 5 g/day may decrease plasma uric acid by increasing its renal excretion, but because these are toxic salicylate doses, they should not be used in the clinical management of gout or hyperuricemia.

Reye's syndrome is an acute illness occurring almost exclusively in children 15 years of age or younger. The cause is unknown, but viral and toxic agents, especially salicylates, have been associated with the syndrome. The onset usually follows a viral infection with influenza (type A or B) or varicella zoster (i.e., chickenpox). Reye's syndrome is characterized by progressive neurologic damage, fatty liver with encephalopathy, and hypoglycemia. The mortality rate may be as high as 50%.

The American Academy of Pediatrics, FDA, the Centers for Disease Control and Prevention, and the Surgeon General have issued warnings that aspirin and other salicylates (including bismuth subsalicylate and nonaspirin salicylates) should be avoided in children and young adults who have influenza or chickenpox. The following contraindication is listed on labels of nonprescription aspirin and aspirin-containing products:

> Aspirin should not be used in children and teenagers for viral infections, with or without fever, because of the risk of Reye's syndrome with concomitant use of aspirin in certain viral illnesses.

Although a simple viral upper respiratory infection (e.g., a common cold) is not a contraindication to aspirin use, it can be difficult to differentiate symptoms of this type of infection from those of influenza and chickenpox. Many clinicians, therefore, recommend a conservative approach of avoiding aspirin whenever symptoms resembling those of influenza are present. The use of aspirin as a pediatric antipyretic has all but ceased in the United States, as have reports of Reye's syndrome.

Since 1999, FDA has required a warning label regarding alcohol use on all nonprescription analgesic/antipyretic products for adult use. Concurrent use of aspirin with alcohol increases the risk of adverse GI events, including stomach bleeding. Patients who consume three or more alcoholic drinks daily should be counseled about the risks and referred to their primary care provider before using aspirin.

Combination Products

Many nonprescription analgesics are available in combination products (Table 5-8).

The efficacy of caffeine/analgesic combinations has been demonstrated for a variety of conditions, including tension-type and migraine headaches.[34] However, these products have the potential to cause medication-overuse headache with frequent use. Combination dosage forms containing a decongestant and either acetaminophen or an NSAID are also available. Such combinations appear logical for use in sinus headaches or other indications for which both analgesia and decongestion are needed.

In addition, enhanced analgesia has been reported for various antihistamine/analgesic combinations, including orphenadrine/acetaminophen and phenyltoloxamine/acetaminophen. Although

TABLE 5-8 Selected Combination Analgesic Products

Trade Name	Primary Ingredients
Advil Cold & Sinus Caplets and Liqui-Gels	Ibuprofen 200 mg; pseudoephedrine 30 mg
Aleve-D	Naproxen sodium 220 mg; pseudoephedrine 120 mg
Alka-Seltzer Plus Sinus Formula Effervescent Tablets	Acetaminophen 250 mg; phenylephrine 5 mg
Anacin Advanced Headache Formula Coated Tablets	Acetaminophen 250 mg; aspirin 250 mg; caffeine 65 mg
Excedrin Migraine tablets	Acetaminophen 250 mg; aspirin 250 mg; caffeine 65 mg
Extra Strength Bayer Back and Body Pain Coated Caplets	Aspirin 500 mg; caffeine 32.5 mg
Excedrin Tension Headache Geltabs	Acetaminophen 500 mg; caffeine 65 mg
Goody's Extra Strength Powder	Acetaminophen 260 mg; aspirin 520 mg; caffeine 32.5 mg

these combinations have demonstrated superior efficacy in acute pain, compared with acetaminophen alone, their use is limited by the sedating effects of the antihistamines.

Pharmacotherapeutic Comparison

ASPIRIN VERSUS NONACETYLATED SALICYLATES
Although definitive clinical data are lacking, aspirin and non-acetylated salicylates are believed to be equal in anti-inflammatory potency; however, aspirin is thought to be a superior analgesic and antipyretic.[39]

ASPIRIN VERSUS ACETAMINOPHEN
Numerous controlled studies have demonstrated the equivalent analgesic efficacy of aspirin and acetaminophen on a milligram-for-milligram basis in various pain models, including postoperative pain, cancer pain, episiotomy pain, and oral surgery pain. In a placebo-controlled trial involving 542 patients, single doses of acetaminophen 500 mg and 1000 mg were compared with single doses of aspirin 500 mg and 1000 mg for the treatment of tension-type headache. Two hours after taking the study medication, both aspirin groups and the acetaminophen 1000 mg group produced superior pain relief compared with placebo. Although the study was not powered to detect differences between active treatment arms, the percentage of patients reporting adequate or total relief was similar among these three groups.[14]

ASPIRIN VERSUS IBUPROFEN
Ibuprofen has been shown to be at least as effective as aspirin in treating various types of pain, including dental extraction pain, dysmenorrhea, and episiotomy pain. Because aspirin must be dosed near the self-care maximum to achieve anti-inflammatory effects, NSAIDs may be preferred for self-treatment of inflammatory disorders such as rheumatoid arthritis or acute muscle injury.

NSAID VERSUS ACETAMINOPHEN
For episodic tension-type headache, acetaminophen 1000 mg appears to provide relief that is equivalent to naproxen 375 mg.[40] For moderate-to-severe (dental or sore throat) pain in children, single doses of acetaminophen 7 to 15 mg/kg produced similar pain relief, compared with ibuprofen 5 to 10 mg/kg. Both drugs were well tolerated.[41]

NAPROXEN VERSUS IBUPROFEN
Naproxen sodium 220 mg appears to be similar in efficacy to ibuprofen 200 mg. The onset of activity is similar between the two NSAIDs. Naproxen's duration of action is somewhat longer than that of ibuprofen, but the clinical significance of that difference is not clear. Nonetheless, some patients report better response to one NSAID than to another for reasons that are unclear.

Product Selection Guidelines

SPECIAL POPULATION CONSIDERATIONS
Age is an important consideration in the selection of an appropriate nonprescription medication for self-treatment of headache. Parents of children younger than 8 years should seek the advice of their pediatrician before embarking on self-treatment. Children 2 years and older may use acetaminophen or ibuprofen, and naproxen has been approved for use in patients at least 12 years of age. Parents should not use aspirin or aspirin-containing products in children ages 15 years or younger, unless directed to do so by a primary care provider, because of the risk for Reye's syndrome.

Persons of advanced age are at increased risk for many adverse effects of salicylates and NSAIDs. Comorbidities, impaired renal function, and use of other medications may contribute to the increased risk. In particular, older adults are more vulnerable to serious GI toxicity,[42] as well as to the hypertensive and renal effects of these agents. For this reason, acetaminophen is generally recognized as the treatment of choice for management of mild-to-moderate pain in older adults.[43]

When peripheral anti-inflammatory activity is not needed and aspirin's effect on hemostasis is a concern, acetaminophen is an appropriate analgesic for self-medication. Prescription salicylate compounds salsalate and choline magnesium trisalicylate do not have appreciable effects on platelet aggregation and are reasonable alternatives when a peripheral anti-inflammatory agent is indicated.

Acetaminophen crosses the placenta, but it is considered safe for use during pregnancy.[44] It appears in breast milk, producing a milk-to-maternal plasma ratio of 0.5:1.0. On the basis of a 1 gram maternal dose, the estimated maximum infant dose is 1.85% of the maternal dose. The only adverse effect reported in nursing infants exposed to acetaminophen through breast milk is a rarely occurring maculopapular rash, which subsides when drug exposure is discontinued. Acetaminophen use is considered compatible with breast-feeding.[45]

No evidence exists that NSAIDs are teratogenic in either humans or animals. However, use of these agents is contraindicated during the third trimester of pregnancy, because all potent prostaglandin synthesis inhibitors can cause delayed parturition, prolonged labor, and increased postpartum bleeding. These agents can also have adverse fetal cardiovascular effects (e.g., premature closure of the ductus arteriosus). Lactating women taking up to 2.4 grams of ibuprofen per day showed no measurable excretion of ibuprofen into breast milk, and ibuprofen is considered compatible with breast-feeding. Naproxen is also considered compatible with breast-feeding.[45]

Women should be advised to avoid aspirin during pregnancy, especially during the last trimester, and when breast-feeding. Aspirin consumption during pregnancy may produce adverse maternal effects, including anemia, antepartum or postpartum hemorrhage, and prolonged gestation and labor. Aspirin ingestion on a regular basis during pregnancy may increase the risk for complicated deliveries, including césarean sections, as well as breech and forceps deliveries. However, definitive data supporting this concern are lacking. In 1990, FDA required oral and rectal nonprescription drug products that contain aspirin to carry labels that warn against using the drugs during the last 3 months of pregnancy unless the patient is directed to do so by a medical provider.

Aspirin readily crosses the placenta and can be found in higher concentrations in the neonate than in the mother. Salicylate elimination is slow in the neonate because of the liver's immaturity and underdeveloped capacity to form glycine and glucuronic acid conjugates, and because of reduced urinary excretion resulting from low glomerular filtration rates.

Fetal effects of in utero aspirin exposure include intrauterine growth retardation, congenital salicylate intoxication, decreased albumin-binding capacity, and increased perinatal mortality. In utero mortality results, in part, from antepartum hemorrhage or premature closure of the ductus arteriosus. In utero aspirin exposure within 1 week of delivery can produce hemorrhagic episodes and/or pruritic rash in the neonate. Reported neonatal bleeding complications include petechiae, hematuria, cephalhematoma, subconjunctival hemorrhage, and bleeding after circumcision. An increased incidence of intracranial hemorrhage in premature or low-birth-weight infants has also been reported after maternal aspirin use near birth.[45] The relationship between maternal aspirin ingestion and congenital malformation is unresolved. An association between maternal aspirin ingestion, oral clefts, and congenital heart disease has been reported. However, other studies have failed to confirm increased risk for fetal malformation resulting from maternal aspirin exposure.

Aspirin and other salicylates are excreted into breast milk in low concentrations. After single-dose oral salicylate ingestion, peak milk levels occur at about 3 hours, producing a milk-to-maternal plasma ratio of 3:8. Although no adverse effects on platelet function in the nursing infant exposed to aspirin through the mother's milk have been reported, these agents still must be considered a potential risk.[45]

Patients with renal impairment should exercise caution when using salicylates. Clinically important alterations in renal blood flow resulting in acute reduction in renal function can result from use of even short courses of salicylates. These patients should be referred for medical evaluation for assistance in selecting an analgesic.

PATIENT FACTORS

Nonprescription analgesics are available in a number of dosage forms. During the patient assessment, clinicians should determine which dosage form will provide the patient with an optimum outcome. If rapid response is desired, then immediate-release oral dosage forms would be preferred over coated or extended-release forms. For patients experiencing migraine headache with severe nausea, rectal dosage forms may be preferred. Analgesic/decongestant combination products should be discouraged in patients with frequent migraine, because nasal congestion may be a consequence of trigeminal nerve activity during the headache and because of the potential for rebound congestion with frequent use.

Use of acetaminophen in the pediatric population is complicated by the various available strengths and formulations. Unintended over- or underdosing can occur when parents switch between infant drops (80 mg/0.8 mL) and elixir (160 mg/5 mL), incorrectly assuming that they are the same concentration. In addition, rapidly growing infants quickly outgrow previous dose requirements. Therefore, recalculation of the pediatric dose according to present age and body weight is appropriate at the time of each treatment course.

Patients with significant alcohol ingestion (more than two drinks per day) should avoid self-treatment with nonprescription analgesics.

Patients intolerant to aspirin may also cross-react with other chemicals or drugs. Up to 15% of patients who are intolerant to aspirin may cross-react when exposed to tartrazine (Food Drug and Cosmetic Yellow Dye No. 5), which can be found in many drugs and foods. Cross-reaction rates for acetaminophen, ibuprofen, and naproxen in documented aspirin-intolerant patients are 7%, 98%, and 100%, respectively.[44] High cross-reaction rates are also reported with some prescription NSAIDs. The proposed mechanism of cross-sensitivity between aspirin and NSAID involves shunting arachidonic metabolism down the lipoxygenase pathway (because of inhibition of the COX pathway), resulting in accumulation of leukotrienes that can cause bronchospasm and anaphylaxis. Therefore, patients with a history of aspirin intolerance should be advised to avoid all aspirin- and NSAID-containing products, and to use acetaminophen preferentially for analgesic self-medication.

PATIENT PREFERENCES

One area in which the clinician can be instrumental in affecting outcomes is in determining which dosing frequency will be needed for an individual patient. Naproxen can be taken two to three times daily and may improve patient adherence. Conversely, acetaminophen, ibuprofen, and salicylates may require dosing as frequently as every 4 hours. Because of the delayed absorption of sustained-release aspirin, such products are not useful for rapid pain relief but may be useful as bedtime medication.

Complementary Therapies

Feverfew, butterbur, and topical peppermint oil are the most commonly used natural products for headache (Table 5-9). (See Chapter 54 for further discussion of these products.)

Acupuncture has been used to prevent migraine and tension-type headache. Evaluation of acupuncture is complicated by difficulties in blinding and differences in identifying acupuncture points. Overall, results have been variable, but several randomized, placebo-controlled trials found acupuncture effective in reducing frequency and severity of headache.[46]

Assessment of Headache: A Case-Based Approach

Before self-treatment of headache can be recommended, the clinician must assess the patient's headache—the type, severity, location, frequency, intensity over time, and age at onset—and obtain a medical and psychosocial history. All current medications should be inventoried, and all past and present headache treatments should be reviewed, with emphasis on determining which treatments, if any, were successful or preferred.

TABLE 5-9 Selected Complementary and Alternative Medicines Used to Treat Headache

Agent	Risks	Use/Effectiveness
Botanical Medicines (Scientific Name)		
Butterbur (*Petasites hybridus*)	Belching; avoid during pregnancy and lactation; avoid products with UPA constituents; UPA-free products seem safe for use ≤16 weeks	Prevention of migraine headache; PC RT demonstrated ≥50 mg/day may reduce frequency by ~50%.
Feverfew (*Tanacetum parthenium*)	Possible rebound headache with chronic use; mouth ulceration with direct contact with leaves; possible anticoagulant effect	Treatment and prevention of migraine headache; mixed results from clinical trials, possibly because of differences in formulations.
Peppermint oil (*Mentha piperita*)	Skin irritation at application site; avoid during pregnancy and lactation	Topical treatment of tension headache; preliminary evidence suggests peppermint oil applied to forehead and temples may relieve tension headaches.
Nonbotanical Natural Medicines		
Coenzyme Q10	Avoid during pregnancy and lactation; minor GI disturbances most common side effects	Prevention of migraine headache; small, open label trial demonstrated 150 mg/day reduced frequency by ~33%.
Nutritional Supplements		
Magnesium	Diarrhea; GI upset	Treatment and prevention of migraine headache; PC, blinded RTs of 20–24 mmol/day yielded mixed results for prevention; patients with hypomagnesemia may respond to IV magnesium administered during acute attack.
Riboflavin	Diarrhea; polyuria	Prevention of migraine headache; small RT of 400 mg/day showed reduced frequency of migraine headaches.

Key: GI, gastrointestinal; IV, intravenous; PC, placebo-controlled; RT, randomized trial; UPA, unsaturated pyrrolizidine alkaloid.

Secondary headaches other than minor sinus headache are excluded from self-treatment. Headache associated with seizures, confusion, drowsiness, or cognitive impairment may be a sign of brain tumor, ischemic stroke, subdural hematoma, or subarachnoid hemorrhage. Headache accompanied by nausea, vomiting, fever, and stiff neck may indicate brain abscess or meningitis.

Headache with night sweats, aching joints, fever, weight loss, and visual symptoms (such as blurring) in patients with rheumatoid arthritis may indicate cranial arteritis. Headache associated with localized facial pain, muscle tenderness, and limited motion of the jaw may indicate temporomandibular joint disorder.

Case 5-1 illustrates assessment of a patient with headache.

C A S E   5 - 1

Relevant Evaluation Criteria	Scenario/Model Outcome
Information Gathering	
1. Gather essential information about the patient's symptoms, including:	
a. description of symptom(s) (i.e., nature, onset, duration, severity, associated symptoms)	Patient describes occasional headaches that tend to occur during work, which are characterized by throbbing pain that comes on suddenly toward the end of her shift. Although she is able to continue working, she feels nauseated and is not as productive.
b. description of any factors that seem to precipitate, exacerbate, and/or relieve the patient's symptom(s)	Her work schedule consists of four midnight shifts per week, and she has noticed that her headaches tend to occur on the first one or two nights. Bright sunlight on her drive home worsens the pain. Going to sleep after she comes home helps resolve the pain.
c. description of the patient's efforts to relieve the symptoms	A trial of acetaminophen 650 mg during two separate headaches did not improve her symptoms.

Relevant Evaluation Criteria	Scenario/Model Outcome
2. Gather essential patient history information:	
a. patient's identity	Heather Moran
b. patient's age, sex, height, and weight	26-year-old female, 5 ft 5 in, 140 lb
c. patient's occupation	Respiratory therapist in an intensive care unit
d. patient's dietary habits	Combination of healthy and processed foods; drinks about 4 cups of coffee per night at work
e. patient's sleep habits	Sleeps about 7 hours during the morning and early afternoon after each work shift, but the sleep is restless and often fragmented. She sleeps about 10 hours per night on nights she is not working and feels this sleep is much more restorative.
f. concurrent medical conditions, prescription and nonprescription medications, and dietary supplements	She was diagnosed with migraine headache 6 months ago and has prescription abortive therapy (sumatriptan). Although she has used it and experienced relief from her headache, she prefers not to take it because of concerns about side effects and high cost. She has seasonal allergies and uses nonprescription loratadine as needed. She uses oral contraception; her last menstrual period was 2 weeks ago.
g. allergies	NKA
h. history of other adverse reactions to medications	Sumatriptan worsens nausea. Diphenhydramine causes excessive drowsiness.
i. other (describe) _____	

Assessment and Triage

3. Differentiate the patient's signs/symptoms and correctly identify the patient's primary problem(s) (see Table 5-1).	Ms. Moran is experiencing episodic migraine headache possibly related to shifting sleep patterns.
4. Identify exclusions for self-treatment (see Figure 5-1).	Ms. Moran has no exclusions for self-treatment.
5. Formulate a comprehensive list of therapeutic alternatives for the primary problem to determine if triage to a medical practitioner is required, and share this information with the patient.	Options include: (1) Refer for medical evaluation. (2) Recommend a nonprescription analgesic. (3) Suggest nondrug measures, alone or in combination with drug therapy. (4) Take no action.

Plan

6. Select an optimal therapeutic alternative to address the patient's problem, taking into account patient preferences.	Normalizing her sleep schedule might help Ms. Moran reduce the frequency of her migraine headaches. Specifically, sleeping during the same hours each day, regardless of whether she is working, might help. Because her pain is not severe (she is able to continue working), nonprescription analgesics can be used. Acetaminophen should be avoided because it is generally not recommended for migraine headache, and because she has already tried it and found no relief.
7. Describe the recommended therapeutic approach to the patient.	Your headaches seem to be caused by your irregular sleeping habits. Try to adjust your sleep times so that they are the same each day, rather than sleeping at night some days and in the morning/afternoon other days. When headaches occur, take ibuprofen, naproxen, or aspirin early in the course of the headache.
8. Explain to the patient the rationale for selecting the recommended therapeutic approach from the considered therapeutic alternatives.	Most mild or moderate migraine headaches respond to self-treatment. Although any nonprescription product containing an NSAID or salicylate could be helpful, avoid using combination products containing caffeine, because you already consume liberal amounts of caffeine during your work shift.

Patient Education

9. When recommending self-care with nonprescription medications and/or nondrug therapy, convey accurate information to the patient:	
a. appropriate dose and frequency of administration	Naproxen 220 mg 1 tablet at the first sign of headache, and every 8 hours if you need it. Do not take more than 3 tablets in 24 hours.

CASE 5-1 *(continued)*

Relevant Evaluation Criteria	Scenario/Model Outcome
b. maximum number of days the therapy should be employed	Use nonprescription analgesics up to 3 days per week.
c. product administration procedures	Take it as soon as possible after the start of a headache.
d. expected time to onset of relief	Pain relief is expected to begin in 30–60 minutes.
e. degree of relief that can be reasonably expected	Many people report a noticeable lessening of the pain. Complete resolution of headache is possible.
f. most common side effects	Watch for stomach upset, stomach pain, and worsening of your nausea with naproxen. Taking it with some food can help if your nausea does not prevent you from doing that.
g. side effects that warrant medical intervention should they occur	Stop using naproxen and seek medical attention if you have severe stomach pain, throw up blood, or have black stools; if you have rash or hives, or red, peeling skin, or swelling in the face or around the eyes; if you develop wheezing or trouble breathing; or if you have unexplained bruising and bleeding.
h. patient options in the event that condition worsens or persists	If naproxen is not helpful for your headaches, then try ibuprofen or aspirin. If you need medicine for your headaches more than 3 days per week, then see your medical provider.
i. product storage requirements	Keep your nonprescription medicines in a tightly closed container and away from children.
j. specific nondrug measures	See comments in step 6 regarding improving your sleep habits.
10. Solicit follow-up questions from patient.	Why can't I take medicines more than 3 days per week?
11. Answer patient's questions.	Using headache medicines more than 3 days per week can cause rebound headaches. Also, frequent headaches may be better treated with preventive medicines that are available by prescription only.

Key: NKA, no known allergies.

Patient Counseling for Headache

To optimize outcomes from therapy, the practitioner should instruct patients to take an appropriate dose of analgesic early in the course of the headache. The use of nonprescription analgesics to preempt or abort migraine headaches should also be explained to patients with migraines whose headaches are predictable. Patients who have headaches with some frequency should be encouraged to keep a log of their headaches to document triggers; frequency, intensity, and duration of episodes; and response to treatment. This record may also be helpful in identifying factors that can improve headache prevention and treatment. Patients should be advised that continuing or escalating pain can be a sign of a more serious problem and that prompt medical attention is warranted. The box Patient Education for Headache lists specific information to provide patients. The clinician should explain appropriate drug and nondrug measures for treating headaches. Frequent use of nonprescription analgesics is not appropriate because of the risk for medication-overuse headache. It should be conveyed that nonprescription analgesics are potent medications with accompanying potential adverse effects, interactions, and precautions/warnings.

PATIENT EDUCATION FOR **Headache**

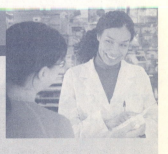

The objectives of self-treatment are to (1) relieve headache pain, (2) prevent headaches when possible, and (3) prevent medication-overuse headaches by avoiding chronic use of nonprescription analgesics. Carefully following product instructions and the self-care measures listed here will help ensure the best results.

Tension-Type Headaches

■ Nonprescription pain relievers (analgesics) are usually effective for episodic tension-type headaches. However, consult a medical provider before using them for chronic tension-type headache.

■ If nonprescription pain relievers are used for chronic headaches, keep records of how often they are used, and share this information with your medical provider.

■ Do not use products containing caffeine because of the risk of caffeine-withdrawal headaches.

Migraine Headache

- Avoid substances (food, caffeine, alcohol, medications) or situations (stress, fatigue, oversleeping, fasting, or missing meals) that you know can trigger a migraine.
- Use the following nutritional strategies to prevent migraine:
  —Avoid foods or food additives known to trigger migraines, including red wine, aged cheese, aspartame, monosodium glutamate, coffee, tea, cola beverages, and chocolate.
  —Avoid foods to which you are allergic.
  —Eat regularly to avoid hunger and low blood glucose.
  —Consider taking magnesium supplements.
- If onset of migraines is predictable (e.g., headache occurs during menstruation), take aspirin, ibuprofen, or naproxen to prevent the headache. Start taking the analgesic 2 days before you expect the headache and continue regular use during the time the headache might start.
- Try to abort a migraine by taking aspirin or an NSAID at the onset of headache pain.
- If desired, use an ice bag or cold pack applied with pressure to the forehead or temples to reduce the pain associated with acute migraine attacks.

Other Headaches

- Consider using a combination of a decongestant and non-prescription analgesics to relieve the pain of sinus headache.

Precautions for Nonprescription Analgesics

- If you are pregnant or breast-feeding, consult a primary care provider before taking any nonprescription medications.
- Obtain medical advice before taking any of these medications if you have a medical condition or are taking prescription medications. Nonprescription analgesics are known to interact with several medications.
- Do not take these medications for longer than 10 days unless a medical provider has recommended prolonged use.
- Do not take these medications if you consume three or more alcoholic beverages daily.
- Do not exceed recommended dosages.
- Products containing aspartame and/or phenylalanine (usually chewable tablets) should not be given to individuals with phenylketonuria.

Salicylates and NSAIDs

- Do not take aspirin during the last 3 months of pregnancy unless a primary care provider is supervising such use. Unsupervised use of this medication could harm the unborn child or cause complications during delivery.
- Do not give aspirin or other salicylates to children 15 years of age or younger who are recovering from chickenpox or influenza. To avoid the risk of Reye's syndrome, a rare but potentially fatal condition, use acetaminophen for pain relief.

- Do not take aspirin or NSAIDs if you are allergic to aspirin or have asthma and nasal polyps. Take acetaminophen instead.
- Do not take aspirin or NSAIDs if you have stomach problems or ulcers, liver disease, kidney disease, or heart failure.
- Do not take NSAIDs if you have or are at high risk for heart disease or stroke unless such use is supervised by a medical provider.
- Do not take aspirin if you have gout, diabetes mellitus, or arthritis, unless such use is supervised by a medical provider.
- Do not take salicylates or NSAIDs if you are taking anticoagulants.
- Do not take magnesium salicylate if you have kidney disease.
- Do not take sodium salicylate if you are on a sodium-restricted diet.
- Do not give naproxen to a child younger than 12 years.

 Stop taking salicylates or NSAIDs and seek medical attention if any of the following symptoms occur:
  —Headache, dizziness, ringing in the ears, difficulty in hearing, dimness of vision, mental confusion, lassitude, drowsiness, sweating, thirst, hyperventilation, nausea, vomiting, or occasional diarrhea. These symptoms indicate mild salicylate toxicity.
  —Dizziness, nausea and mild stomach pain, constipation, ringing in the ears, or swelling in the feet or legs. These symptoms are common side effects of salicylates and NSAIDs.
  —Rash or hives, or red, peeling skin; swelling in the face or around the eyes; wheezing or trouble breathing; bloody or black tarry stools; severe stomach pain or bloody vomit; bloody or cloudy urine; or unexplained bruising and bleeding. These symptoms require immediate medical attention.

Acetaminophen

- To avoid possible damage to the liver, do not take more than 4 grams of acetaminophen a day from all over-the-counter and prescription single-ingredient or combination products containing acetaminophen.
- Do not drink alcohol while taking this medication.
- Follow dosage instructions for acetaminophen carefully if you have glucose-6-phosphate dehydrogenase deficiency.

 Stop taking acetaminophen and seek medical attention if you develop nausea, vomiting, drowsiness, confusion, or abdominal pain.

Evaluation of Patient Outcomes for Headache

Appropriate follow-up will depend on headache frequency and severity, and patient factors. For patients with episodic headaches, a trial of 6 to 12 weeks may be needed to assess efficacy of treatment. For chronic headache, follow-up after 4 to 6 weeks should be adequate to assess treatment efficacy. For severe headaches, clinicians should communicate with patients within 10 days of initiation of self-treatment to assess efficacy and tolerability. In all cases, the patient should seek medical attention if headaches persist longer than 10 days or become worse despite self-treatment.

It is notable that more than half of patients with migraine headache use only nonprescription medications, despite the severity of pain.[4] Patients with migraine headaches that are not adequately self-treated should be referred for a medical evaluation because effective prescription therapies are available that can substantially limit pain and disability.

Key Points for Headache

➤ Most tension-type, migraine, and sinus headaches are amenable to treatment with nonprescription medications.

➤ Patients with symptoms suggestive of secondary or undiagnosed migraine headaches should be referred for medical attention.

➤ Many patients with frequent headaches may improve by identifying and modifying environmental, behavioral, nutritional, or other triggers for their headaches.

➤ The choice of nonprescription analgesic for an individual patient depends on patient preferences, presence of precautionary or contraindicating conditions, concomitant medications, cost, and other factors.

➤ Pharmacists have been identified as key sources of information for nonprescription analgesic users to reduce risk for acetaminophen-induced hepatotoxicity and NSAID-induced GI bleeding, cardiovascular events, and nephrotoxicity.

➤ Use of nonprescription analgesics for headache should be limited to 3 days per week to prevent medication-overuse headache.

REFERENCES

1. Smith TR. Epidemiology and impact of headache: an overview. *Prim Care Clin Office Pract*. 2004;31:237–41.
2. Gureje O, Von Korff M, Simon GE, et al. Persistent pain and well-being: a World Health Organization study in primary care. *JAMA*. 1998;280:147–51.
3. Lipton RB. Migraine: epidemiology, impact, and risk factors for progression. *Headache*. 2005;45(suppl 1):S3–13.
4. Mannix LK. Headache: epidemiology and impact of primary headache disorders. *Med Clin North Am*. 2001;85:887–95.
5. Consumers uninformed about nonprescription pain relievers. *Am J Health-Syst Pharm*. 1998;55:2597.
6. Headache Classification Subcommittee of the International Headache Society. The international classification of headache disorders, 2nd edition. *Cephalalgia*. 2004;24(suppl 1):1–160.
7. Cady RK, Dodick DW, Levine HL, et al. Sinus headache: a neurology, otolaryngology, allergy, and primary care consensus on diagnosis and treatment. *Mayo Clin Proc*. 2005;80:908–16.
8. Krusz JC. Tension-type headaches: what they are and how to treat them. *Prim Care Clin Office Pract*. 2004;31:293–311.
9. Schreiber CP. The pathophysiology of primary headache. *Prim Care Clin Office Pract*. 2004;31:261–76.
10. Diener H-C, Limmroth V. Medication-overuse headache: a worldwide problem. *Lancet Neurol*. 2004;3:475–83.
11. Ward TN. Medication overuse headache. *Prim Care Clin Office Pract*. 2004;31:369–80.
12. Loder E. Migraine diagnosis and treatment. *Prim Care Clin Office Pract*. 2004;31:277–92.
13. Lipton RB, Baggish JS, Stewart WF, et al. Efficacy and safety of acetaminophen in the treatment of migraine. *Arch Intern Med*. 2000;160:3486–92.
14. Steiner TJ, Lange R, Voelker M. Aspirin in episodic tension-type headache: placebo-controlled dose-ranging comparison with paracetamol. *Cephalalgia*. 2003;23:59–66.
15. Krahenbuhl S, Brauchli Y, Kummer O, et al. Acute liver failure in two patients with regular alcohol consumption ingesting paracetamol at therapeutic dosage. *Digestion*. 2007;75:232–7.
16. Farrell GC. Liver disease caused by drugs, anesthetics, and toxins. In: Feldman M, Friedman LS, Sleisenger MH, eds. *Sleisenger & Fordtran's Gastrointestinal and Liver Disease*. 7th ed. Philadephia: Saunders; 2002:1403–47.
17. Bronstein AC, Spyker DA, Cantilena LR Jr, et al. 2006 Annual Report of the American Association of Poison Control Centers' National Poison Data System (NPDS). *Clin Toxicol* (Phila). 2007;458:815–917.
18. Ostapowicz G, Fontana RJ, Schiodt RV, et al. for the US Acute Liver Failure Study Group. Results of a prospective study of acute liver failure at 17 tertiary care centers in the United States. *Ann Intern Med*. 2002;137:947–54.
19. Larson AM, Polson J, Fontana RJ, et al. Acetaminophen-induced acute liver failure: results of a United States multicenter, prospective study. *Hepatology*. 2005;42:1364–72.
20. Bolesta S, Haber SL. Hepatotoxicity associated with chronic acetaminophen administration in patients without risk factors. *Ann Pharmacother*. 2002;36:331–3.
21. Dart RC, Bailey E. Does therapeutic use of acetaminophen cause acute liver failure? *Pharmacotherapy* 2007;27:1219–30.
22. US Food and Drug Administration. FDA proposes labeling changes to over-the-counter pain relievers. *FDA News*. December 19, 2006.
23. Hawton K, Simkin S, Deeks J, et al. UK legislation on analgesic packs: before and after study of long term effect on poisonings. *BMJ*. 2004;329:1076–80.
24. Rumack BH. Acetaminophen misconceptions. *Hepatology*. 2004;40:10–15.
25. Prescott LF. Paracetamol, alcohol and the liver. *Br J Clin Pharmacol*. 2000;49:291–301.
26. Seifert CF, Anderson DC. Acetaminophen usage patterns and concentrations of glutathione and gamma-glutamyl transferase in alcoholic subjects. *Pharmacotherapy*. 2007;27:1473–82.
27. Heard K, Green JL, Bailey JE, et al. A randomized trial to determine the change in alanine aminotransferase during 10 days of paracetamol (acetaminophen) administration in subjects who consume moderate amounts of alcohol. *Aliment Pharmacol Ther*. 2007;26:283–90.
28. Moling O, Cairon E, Rimenti G, et al. Severe hepatotoxicity after therapeutic doses of acetaminophen. *Clin Ther*. 2006;28:755–60.
29. Watkins PB, Kaplowitz N, Slattery JT, et al. Aminotransferase elevations in healthy adults receiving 4 grams of acetaminophen daily. *JAMA*. 2006;296:87–93.
30. McElwee N, Veltri JC, Bradford DC, et al. A prospective, population-based study of acute ibuprofen overdose: complications are rare and routine serum levels not warranted. *Ann Emerg Med*. 1990;19:657–62.
31. Hersh EV, Moore PA, Ross GI. Over-the-counter analgesics and antipyretics: a critical assessment. *Clin Ther*. 2000;22:500–48.
32. Antman EM, Bennett JS, Daugherty A, et al. Use of nonsteroidal anti-inflammatory drugs: an update for clinicians. *Circulation*. 2007;115:1634–42.
33. US Food and Drug Administration. Public health advisory: non-steroidal anti-inflammatory drug products (NSAIDs). Rockville, Md: Center for Drug Evaluation and Research; December 23, 2004.
34. Lipton R, Steward W, Saper J, et al. Efficacy and safety of acetaminophen, aspirin, and caffeine in alleviating migraine headache pain: three double-blind, randomized, placebo-controlled trials. *Arch Neurol*. 1998;55:210–7.
35. Lanas AI. Current approaches to reducing gastrointestinal toxicity of low-dose aspirin. *Am J Med*. 2001;110(1A):70S–3S.
36. Lanas A, Hunt R. Prevention of anti-inflammatory drug-induced gastrointestinal damage: benefits and risks of therapeutic strategies. *Ann Med*. 2006;38:415–28.
37. Berardi RR, Welage LS. Peptic ulcer disease. In: DiPiro JT, Talbert RL, Yee GC, et al., eds. *Pharmacoterhapy: A Pathophysiologic Approach*. 7th ed. New York: McGraw-Hill, Inc, 2008. 571.
38. Dammann HG, Burkhardt F, Wolf N. Enteric coating of aspirin significantly decreases gastroduodenal mucosal lesions. *Aliment Pharmacol Ther*. 1999;13:1109–14.
39. Altman RD. Salicylates in the treatment of arthritic disease: how safe and effective? *Postgrad Med*. 1988;84:206–10.
40. Prior MJ, Cooper KM, May LG, et al. Efficacy and safety of acetaminophen and naproxen in the treatment of tension-type headache: a randomized, double-blind, placebo-controlled trial. *Cephalalgia*. 2002;22:740–8.
41. Perrott DA, Piira T, Goodenough B, et al. Efficacy and safety of acetaminophen vs ibuprofen for treating children's pain or fever. *Arch Pediatr Adolesc Med*. 2004;158:521–6.
42. Wolfe MM, Lichtenstein DR, Singh G. Gastrointestinal toxicity of nonsteroidal anti-inflammatory drugs. *N Engl J Med*. 1999;340:1888–99.
43. AGS Panel on Persistent Pain in Older Persons. The management of persistent pain in older persons. *J Am Geriatr Soc*. 2002;6:S205–24.

44. Jenkins C, Costello J, Hodge L. Systematic review of prevalence of aspirin induced asthma and its implications for clinical practice. *BMJ*. 2004;328: 434–40.

45. Briggs G, Freeman R, Yaffe S, eds. *Drugs in Pregnancy and Lactation*. 6th ed. Baltimore: Williams & Wilkins; 2002.

46. Melchart D, Linde K, Berman B, et al. Acupuncture for idiopathic headache. *Cochrane Database System Rev* 2001;1:CD001218.

Additional Information Resources

http://www.ahrq.gov/ (Agency for Healthcare Research and Quality)

http://www.ampainsoc.org (American Pain Society)

http://www.fda.gov/cder/consumerinfo/otc_all_resources.htm (US Food and Drug Administration consumer education on nonprescription medicine)

Fever

Brett Feret

Fever is the 16th most common reason patients seek medical care.[1] In 2002, patients complaining primarily of fever made approximately 12,250,000 medical office visits, with men making a slightly greater number of visits.[2] Fever is also one of the most common reasons that parents seek medical care for their children. One of every five emergency room visits for children is related to fever, and 19% to 30% of children presenting to their pediatrician's office have fever as a complaint.[2] Overall, 69.6% of all fevers in children younger than 5 years are referred to a health care provider for medical evaluation; however, only 57.2% of patients with fever in the total population seek medical care.[1] Children have fevers more often than adults do. The rate of reported fevers in children younger than 5 years is 10 in 100 persons versus the rate of 0.5 in 100 adults. Nonetheless, the rate of fever does not seem to differ significantly when distinguishing among gender, race, or geographic area of residence in the United States.[2] Of all the therapeutic classifications of drugs on the market, antipyretics are the seventh most commonly mentioned medications at medical office visits.[3]

Most fevers are self-limited and nonthreatening; however, fever can cause a great deal of discomfort and, in some cases, may indicate serious underlying pathology (e.g., acute infectious process) for which prompt medical evaluation is indicated. The principal reason for treating fever is to alleviate discomfort; however, the underlying cause should be identified before treatment.

Fever is defined as a body temperature higher than the normal core temperature of 100°F (37.8°C). It is important to distinguish "fever" from "hyperthermia" and "hyperpyrexia." Fever is a regulated rise in body temperature maintained by the hypothalamus in response to a pyrogen; it is a sign of an increase in the body's thermoregulatory set point. In contrast, hyperthermia represents a malfunctioning of the normal thermoregulatory process at the hypothalamic level.[4] Because of their different mechanisms, treatment of fever versus hyperthermia also varies. Hyperpyrexia is a body temperature greater than 106°F (41.1°C) that typically results in mental and physical consequences.

Pathophysiology of Fever

Core temperature refers to the temperature of the blood that surrounds the hypothalamus, which may differ from that of the surrounding body or skin temperature. Core temperature is regulated by a feedback system that involves information transmitted between the thermoregulatory center located in the anterior hypothalamus and the thermosensitive neurons located in the skin and central nervous system (CNS). Physiologic and behavioral mechanisms regulate body temperature within the normal range. Behavioral adaptations to temperature changes include wearing additional clothing, rubbing the hands together, adjusting air conditioning, and seeking shade for relief from the hot sun. Compensatory physiologic mechanisms such as heat dissipation (e.g., sweating, vasodilation, and hyperventilation) in response to heat, as well as heat production or conservation (e.g., shivering, goose bumps, and vasoconstriction) in response to cold, are mediated by alterations in the secretion of various hormones, such as thyroxine, aldosterone, serotonin, and catecholamines.[5] Therefore, although skin temperature may fluctuate greatly in response to environmental conditions, the core temperature is regulated within a narrow range.

Normal thermoregulation prevents wide fluctuations in body temperature; the average temperature is usually maintained between 97.5°F and 98.9°F (36.4°C and 37.2°C). Temperature maintained in this range is considered to be the "set point," or the point at which the physiologic or behavioral mechanisms are not activated. In addition, normal body temperature varies throughout the day, peaking daily between 4 pm and 6 pm and reaching its lowest point at approximately 6 am.[6] This consistent rhythm occurs at ages older than 2 years and is more pronounced in children than in adults. Body temperature can vary by as much as 1.8°F (1°C) in adults and as much as 2.58°F (1.48°C) in children each day, depending on normal circadian rhythm and activity level, such as vigorous activity or exercise. Because circadian variation continues during febrile illness, patients may be described incorrectly as afebrile when they have a relatively normal temperature in the early morning, and a moderately high evening temperature may be misinterpreted as fever. Therefore, body temperature and fever may be better defined as a range versus a single number.

An increase in body temperature may be idiopathic or can be caused by a variety of mechanisms, including an infectious process, pathologic processes, a response to certain drugs, or vigorous activity.

Most febrile episodes are caused by microbial infections (i.e., viruses, bacteria, fungi, yeasts, or protozoa). Elevated temperatures associated with bacterial infections generally are higher than those associated with viral infections, but there is no absolute temperature at which these infections can be differentiated. In addition, there is no basis for differentiating viral from bacterial infections according to the magnitude of temperature reduction from antipyretic drug therapy. Fever is often less pronounced in patients of advanced age than in younger individuals. Consequently, infection may not be recognized easily in older patients if fever is the primary assessment criterion.[7]

Noninfectious pathologic causes of increases in temperature include malignancies, tissue damage (e.g., myocardial infarction or surgery), antigen–antibody reactions, dehydration, heat stroke, CNS inflammation, and metabolic disorders such as hyperthyroidism or gout. Many of these processes actually may cause hyperthermia rather than fever, because they interfere with the hypothalamic regulation of temperature.

Drug-induced fever, more appropriately termed *drug-induced hyperthermia,* occurs via a variety of mechanisms. Its incidence is unknown, but this type of fever may account for more than 3% to 5% of all adverse drug reactions and occurs in up to 10% of all hospitalized patients (Table 6-1). Drug-induced fevers usually range from 102°F (38.8°C) to 104°F (40°C), but occasional elevations may be as high as 108°F (42.2°C).[8–10] Failure to discontinue the offending drug can result in substantial morbidity, and even mortality. However, drug-induced hyperthermia often goes unrecognized because of inconsistent signs and symptoms.[10]

Drug-induced hyperthermia occurs independent of atopy, gender, age, or existing medical conditions. It has been attributed to one of the following mechanisms: (1) altered thermoregulation, (2) pharmacologic action, (3) drug administration, (4) hypersensitivity, or (5) an idiosyncrasy, all of which lead to the body's inability to maintain core temperature.[10]

The most common mechanism is hypersensitivity, wherein rash, urticaria, and eosinophilia may accompany the fever. Some drugs or their metabolites, as well as some biologic preparations such as infliximab, streptokinase, or vaccine products, have antigenic properties that produce a hypersensitivity reaction from the formation of antibody–antigen complexes. Fever usually develops after 7 to 10 days of treatment; however, symptoms may occur shortly after initiation of therapy, especially if there was previous

exposure to the medication.[10] However, vaccine-associated drug fever usually occurs within 48 hours of administration. Antibiotics, phenytoin, methyldopa, isoniazid, and quinidine are frequently administered drugs that cause fever attributable to a hypersensitivity reaction.[9]

Some medications elevate body temperature by altering normal thermoregulatory mechanisms, thereby causing hyperthermia. Large doses of phenothiazines, tricyclic antidepressants, or drugs with anticholinergic properties decrease sweating and thus reduce heat dissipation. Sympathomimetics such as amphetamines, cocaine, and epinephrine also decrease heat dissipation by inducing vasoconstriction. Thyroid hormones may increase the metabolic rate and thus increase heat generation.

Fever may be a direct result of the pharmacologic effect of a medication. The release of endotoxin from bacteria after the initiation of parenteral antibiotic therapy or the release of endogenous pyrogens associated with cellular injury or death after cancer chemotherapy can result in high fever.

Increased temperature secondary to idiosyncratic reactions such as malignant hyperthermia and neuroleptic malignant syndrome (NMS) is rare, but potentially life-threatening.[11,12] Malignant hyperthermia is characterized by temperature greater than 104°F (40°C), muscle rigidity, and metabolic acidosis. NMS typically presents with high temperature, muscle rigidity, abnormal body movements, sweating, tachycardia, high or low blood pressure, incontinence, and altered consciousness including delirium, stupor, or coma.[9] NMS occurs most commonly in young male patients or dehydrated patients taking neuroleptic medications (e.g., phenothiazines, butyrophenones, and thioxanthenes).

Drug-induced hyperthermia may be differentiated from other causes by establishing a temporal relationship between the fever and the administration of a medication, observing a temperature elevation despite improvement of the underlying disorders, and identifying possible "allergic" symptoms. Symptoms associated with drug fever vary. One study of drug-induced

TABLE 6-1 Selected Medications That Induce Hyperthermia

Anti-Infectives	Antineoplastics	Cardiovascular	CNS Agents	Other Agents
Aminoglycosides	Bleomycin	Epinephrine	Amphetamines	Allopurinol
Amphotericin B	Chlorambucil	Hydralazine	Barbiturates	Atropine
Cephalosporins	Cytarabine	Methyldopa	Benztropine	Azathioprine
Clindamycin	Daunorubicin	Nifedipine	Carbamazepine	Cimetidine
Chloramphenicol	Hydroxyurea	Procainamide	Haloperidol	Corticosteroids
Imipenem	l-Asparaginase	Quinidine	Lithium	Folate
Isoniazid	6-Mercaptopurine	Streptokinase	MAOIs	Inhaled anesthetics
Macrolides	Procarbazine		Nomifensine	Interferon
Mebendazole	Streptozocin		Phenytoin	Iodides
Nitrofurantoin			Phenothiazines	Metoclopramide
Para-aminosalicylic acid			SSRIs	Propylthiouracil
Penicillins			Trifluoperazine	Prostaglandin E$_2$
Rifampin			Thioridazine	Salicylates
Streptomycin			TCAs	Tolmetin
Sulfonamides				
Tetracyclines				
Vancomycin				

Key: CNS, central nervous system; MAOIs, monoamine oxidase inhibitors; SSRIs, selective serotonin reuptake inhibitors; TCAs, tricyclic antidepressants.
Source: References 4, 9, and 10.

fever identified skin rash in only 18% of patients, with less than half experiencing urticaria (hives); mild eosinophilia was present in only 22% of the patients.[10] The presence of high temperature and shaking chills may make differentiation of drug fever from infection difficult. Drug-induced hyperthermia may also be associated with a shift to the left in the white blood cell differential.[10] Diurnal temperature variation in drug fever is often minimal.

The management of drug-induced hyperthermia involves discontinuing the suspected medication whenever possible. If feasible, all medications should be temporarily discontinued. If the hyperthermia is drug-induced, the patient's temperature will generally decrease within 24 to 72 hours after the offending agent is withdrawn. After patient safety and the identification of the offending medication have been considered, each medication may be restarted, one at a time, while monitoring for fever recurrence.

Pyrogens are fever-producing substances that activate the body's host defenses, resulting in an increase in the hypothalamic heat regulatory set point. Pyrogens can be exogenous, originating outside the body (e.g., microbes or toxins), or they can be endogenous, originating within the body (e.g., immune cytokines). Exogenous pyrogens do not independently increase the hypothalamic temperature set point. They stimulate the release of endogenous pyrogens and thereby increase the core temperature.[5,13,14] Endogenous pyrogens are products released in response to or from damaged tissue such as interleukins, interferons, and tumor necrosis factor.

Prostaglandins of the E_2 series (PGE_2) are produced in response to circulating pyrogens and elevate the thermoregulatory set point in the hypothalamus.[5] Within hours, body temperature reaches this new set point and fever occurs. During the period of upward temperature readjustment, the patient experiences chills caused by peripheral vasoconstriction and muscle rigidity to maintain homeostasis. Because the new set point is regulated by negative feedback, body temperature rarely exceeds 106°F (41.1°C).[5]

Clinical Presentation

Because the symptoms of fever are nonspecific and do not occur in all patients, the etiology of the fever is difficult to determine from the symptomatology. The most important sign of fever is an elevated temperature; therefore, accurate temperature measurement is paramount. Fever is a symptom of a larger underlying process, whether it is an infection, abnormal metabolism, or drug induced. Once the symptom of fever is established, investigation into the underlying cause is important. Signs and symptoms that typically accompany fever and cause a great deal of discomfort include headache, diaphoresis, generalized malaise, chills, tachycardia, arthralgia, myalgia, irritability, and anorexia. Symptoms such as sweating, tachycardia, and chills are related directly to the adjustment in temperature set point during fever, whereas symptoms such as myalgias and arthralgias are related more to the release of endogenous pyrogens. Most children will tolerate a fever well, so if they continue to be alert, play normally, and stay hydrated, there is not a great concern. However, high body temperature dulls intellectual function and causes disorientation and delirium, especially in individuals with preexisting dementia, cerebral arteriosclerosis, or alcoholism.

Detection of Fever

Subjective assessment of fever typically involves feeling a part of the body, such as the forehead, for warmth. Although this method may identify an increase in skin temperature, it does not accurately detect a rise in core temperature. The most accurate method of detecting fever is measuring body temperature with a thermometer using proper technique. The patient's age and level of physical and emotional stress, environmental temperature, time of day, and anatomic site at which the temperature is measured are important considerations, because these factors can affect the results of temperature measurement.

Core temperature is estimated with various types of thermometers used at the rectal, axillary, oral, temporal, or ear canal sites. Body temperature should be measured with the same thermometer at the same site over the course of an illness, because the readings from different thermometers or sites may vary (Table 6-2). The rectal method is considered the gold standard measurement, because it most consistently estimates core body temperature. However, most patients prefer other methods of temperature measurement because of comfort and ease of use. A rectal temperature greater than 100.4°F (38.0°C), an oral temperature greater than 99.7°F (37.6°C), or an axillary temperature greater than 99.3°F (37.4°C) is considered elevated.[15] Rectal temperatures are 0.8° to 1.8°F (0.4°C–1.0°C) higher than oral readings, and oral temperature readings may be up to 1.6°F (0.9°C) higher than tympanic readings.[16] Axillary temperatures range from 0.7°F to 3.6°F (0.4°C–2°C) lower than rectal temperatures. The discrepancy between the various sites of temperature measurement is normal and should not be ascribed to improper measurement technique. As noted previously, normal body temperature may range 1.8°F to 2.5°F (1°C–1.4°C) from these norms, and diurnal rhythm causes variances in body temperature during the day.

Over the last several years, there have been many advances in the types of thermometers available for use. Because the Food and Drug Administration (FDA) regulates thermometers as medical devices, all approved types of thermometers are accurate and reliable, if used appropriately. Although most people are familiar with the mercury-in-glass thermometers, more recent innovations include electronic, infrared, and color-change thermometers. Many of these innovations may have stemmed

TABLE 6-2 Body Temperature Range Depending on Site of Measurement

Conversion formulas: Celsius = 5/9 (°F − 32); Fahrenheit = (9/5 × °C) + 32.

Site of Measurement	Normal Range	Fever
Rectal	97.9°F–100.4°F (36.6°C–38°C)	>100.4°F (38.0°C)
Oral	95.9°F–99.5°F (35.5°C–37.5°C)	>99.7°F (37.6°C)
Axillary	94.5°F–99.2°F (34.7°C–37.3°C)	>99.3°F (37.4°C)
Tympanic	96.3°F–99.9°F (35.7°C–37.7°C)	>100°F (37.8°C)

Source: References 15 and 19.

from the Environmental Protection Agency's (EPA's) position on reducing the number of mercury-based products in the United States.[17] Many states have banned the sale of mercury-in-glass thermometers, and many retail pharmacies have voluntarily phased out the sale of these thermometers. Along with EPA, the American Academy of Pediatrics also supports the elimination of these thermometers.[18] Practitioners should not recommend mercury-in-glass thermometers for use at this point. To properly dispose of these thermometers, patients and clinicians should contact their local municipality.

Electronic probe thermometers are available for oral, rectal, and axillary temperature measurements. The probes have an electronic transducer that provides a temperature reading in about 10 to 60 seconds. The oral electronic probes are available in both pen and pacifier shapes. The pacifier-shaped electronic thermometer is for oral use only and takes about 2 minutes to provide a reading, but it is useful in infants who are unable to hold probes under their tongue. The pen-shaped probe may be used in the oral, rectal, or axillary area. Advantages of the electronic thermometers include quick readings and the elimination of glass breakage, mercury toxicity, and risk of cuts. The use of disposable probe covers with these thermometers also eliminates the need for disinfection after their use. In addition, the electronic digital temperature display makes these thermometers easier to read than the traditional glass thermometers. Most electronic thermometers require batteries and may need to be calibrated periodically. Because calibration is difficult to do accurately with home use, it may be preferable for patients to purchase a new thermometer or call the manufacturer's customer service.

Infrared thermometers are available for tympanic and temporal temperature measurements. These thermometers use infrared technology to detect heat from the arterial blood supply. Therefore, they must be placed directly in the line of a blood supply, whether near the temporal artery or the tympanic membrane. Infrared thermometers measure body temperature in less than 5 seconds and are considered very accurate, if used appropriately. The major problem with these thermometers is that they are not always placed appropriately and consequently may give inaccurate readings. The tympanic and temporal thermometers are relatively expensive and require batteries, but many families with young children prefer them because of their convenience and noninvasive nature.

Color-change thermometers are easy to use; however, they are not sufficiently accurate or reliable. The thermometer is an adhesive strip containing heat-sensitive material that changes color in response to different temperature gradients. The strip may be placed anywhere on the skin, but the forehead is used most often; skin has less variation in temperature than other parts of the body. Although this method may detect changes in skin temperature, it does not reliably detect changes in core temperature. Skin temperature is influenced by many factors, including temperature of the environment and skin perfusion. Color-change thermometers may be useful in noting temperature trends but not absolute temperature.

Different types of thermometers may be used through different routes to detect temperature. Each thermometer should be used correctly to obtain an accurate reading. Patient-related factors may preclude the use of a particular type of thermometer through a given route. Although there are a variety of routes of temperature measurement, rectal temperature measurement still remains the gold standard because of its reliability and accuracy. Oral, tympanic, and temporal routes are all appropriate for temperature measurements, given that the proper procedure is followed.

Table 6-3 describes the proper methods of taking oral measurements with electronic thermometers.[19] Oral temperature should not be obtained when an individual is mouth breathing or hyperventilating; has recently had oral surgery; is not fully alert; or is uncooperative, lethargic, or confused. Oral digital probe thermometers may not be appropriate for use in most children younger than 3 years. Children this young may find it difficult to maintain a tight seal around the thermometer and keep the thermometer under the tongue, in which case pacifier thermometers may be recommended. Pacifier thermometers provide reliable temperature readings with a sensitivity of approximately 72% and specificity of 98%, compared with rectal measurements; however, in children younger than 3 months, pacifier thermometers are less accurate.[20,21] Sensitivity is defined as the ability of the test to correctly identify individuals who have a fever, whereas specificity is defined as the ability of the test to accurately identify those who do not have a fever. To ensure reliable measurement, the patient should neither engage in vigorous physical activity nor heat nor cool the oral cavity artificially by smoking or drinking hot or cold beverages for a minimum of 20 minutes before temperature is measured.

Table 6-4 describes the proper methods of taking rectal temperatures in children and adults. Rectal temperature measurement is the standard because of its predictable rise and high sensitivity and specificity, compared with the body's core temperature. Although the rectal route is the closest estimate of the core temperature, its intrusive nature can be very frightening to young children. In children younger than 6 months, however, rectal temperature is the preferred method of estimating fever and should be recommended if feasible. Risks associated with

---

TABLE 6-3 Guidelines for Oral Temperature Measurements Using Electronic Thermometers

Digital Probe

1. Wait 20–30 minutes after drinking or eating.
2. Place a clean disposable probe cover over tip.
3. Turn on the thermometer and wait until it is ready for use.
4. Place tip of thermometer under tongue.
5. Close mouth and breath through nose.
6. Hold thermometer in place until it beeps and temperature has been recorded (usually after 5–30 seconds).
7. Record the displayed temperature.
8. Remove and dispose of probe cover.

Digital Pacifier Thermometer

1. Wait 30 minutes after drinking or eating.
2. Inspect the pacifier for any tears or cracks. Do not use if worn.
3. Press the button to turn on thermometer.
4. Place the pacifier in child's mouth.
5. Have the child hold pacifier in mouth without moving if possible for specified time on packaging of thermometer (2–6 minutes).
6. Record temperature when thermometer beeps.

Source: Reference 19.

TABLE 6-4 Guidelines for Rectal Temperature Measurements Using Electronic Thermometers

1. Cover the tip of thermometer with a probe cover.
2. Turn on the thermometer and wait until it is ready for use.
3. Apply a water-soluble lubricant to tip of thermometer to allow for easy passage through the anal sphincter and to reduce the risk of trauma.
4. For infants or young children, place child face down over your lap, separate the buttocks with the thumb and forefinger of one hand, and insert the thermometer gently in the direction of the child's umbilicus with the other hand. For infants, insert the thermometer to the length of the tip. For young children, insert it about 1 inch into the rectum.
5. For adults, have the patient lie on one side with the legs flexed to about a 45° angle from the abdomen. Insert the tip 0.5–2 inches into the rectum by holding the thermometer 0.5–2 inches away from the tip and inserting it until the finger touches the anus. Have the patient take a deep breath during this process to facilitate proper positioning of the thermometer.
6. Hold the thermometer in place until it beeps and a temperature is displayed.
7. Remove the thermometer. Clean by wiping away from the stem toward tip.
8. Dispose of probe cover and clean and disinfect the tip with an antiseptic such as alcohol or a povidone/iodine solution and rinse with cool water.
9. Wipe away any remaining lubricant from the anus.

TABLE 6-5 Guidelines for Tympanic Temperature Measurements

1. Place a clean disposable lens cover over ear probe.
2. Turn on thermometer and wait until it is ready for use.
3. For children younger than 1 year, pull ear backward to straighten ear canal. Place ear probe into canal, and aim the tip of the probe toward patient's eye.
4. For patients older than 1 year, pull ear backward and up to straighten ear canal. Place the ear probe into canal, and aim the tip of probe toward patient's eye.
5. Press the button for temperature measurement (usually for only 1–5 seconds).
6. Read and record temperature.
7. Discard lens cover.

Source: Reference 19.

taking a rectal temperature include retention of the thermometer, rectal or intestinal perforation, and peritonitis. The patient should never be left unattended while the rectal thermometer remains in place, because a positional change may cause the thermometer to be expelled or broken. Rectal temperature measurement is relatively contraindicated in patients who are neutropenic, have had recent rectal surgery or injury, or have rectal pathology (e.g., obstructive hemorrhoids or diarrhea). Rectal temperature measurement is slow to measure changes in body temperature because of the large muscle mass and poor blood flow to the area; therefore, the thermometer must be left in place longer compared with the oral and axillary route.[15,19,22,23] The most common sources of error in rectal temperature measurement include stool impaction and poor technique in taking the temperature.[24]

Table 6-5 describes the proper method of using tympanic thermometers, which varies slightly, depending on the age of the patient.[19] Tympanic thermometers have digital readouts, and many can be set to provide either a rectal or an oral temperature equivalent. The tip of the tympanic thermometer, which is placed in the ear canal, measures body temperature by sensing infrared heat from the blood vessels in the eardrum. The tympanic membrane is close to the hypothalamus, and the blood supply to these two anatomic areas is at the same temperature, providing an accurate reading of the body core temperature. The thermometer must be positioned in the ear canal properly to ensure that the measured infrared radiation is from the tympanic membrane and not from the ear canal or adjacent areas.

In clinical trials, accuracy of tympanic thermometers has varied, compared with the rectal and oral routes.[25–27] Variations in temperature assessment have been attributed to cerumen impaction, inflammation in the ear canal (otitis media), age of patient (size of ear canal), and inappropriate technique.[16] Comparisons of tympanic and rectal measurements showed tympanic measurement to be 94.8% to 100% specific but only 58% to 68.3% sensitive for fever detection.[25,28] Tympanic thermometers are not recommended in infants younger than 6 months, because their ear canals are not developed fully, leading to inappropriate technique and inaccurate readings. However, if used correctly, tympanic thermometry is found to be more reliable than axillary or oral thermometry in measuring core temperature in adults.[22]

Temporal thermometers are placed on the side of the forehead directly over the temporal artery and moved across the forehead (Table 6-6). The temporal artery is one of the few arteries close enough to the skin surface to detect heat changes. The thermometer is capable of providing a temperature reading in a few seconds. Its rapid, noninvasive nature makes it a preferable route of temperature measurement, and the temporal

TABLE 6-6 Guidelines for Temporal Temperature Measurements

1. Disinfect thermometer by drawing it through a swab moistened with an antiseptic such as alcohol or povidone/iodine solution.
2. Place probe on one side of forehead (near temporal area).
3. Turn on thermometer and wait until it is ready for use.
4. Sweep thermometer across hairline to other side of forehead. Ensure that probe remains in contact with skin at all times.
5. Lift thermometer from forehead, and read and record temperature.
6. Turn off thermometer.

Source: Reference 29.

thermometer is significantly more sensitive than the tympanic thermometer for detecting fever.[29] However, compared with rectal temperature measurement, temporal measurement is close to 100% sensitive but has variable specificity (40%–86%), which indicates that rectal temperature measurement is still the most accurate. Temporal temperature measurement may differ from rectal temperature measurement by ±1.3°C (2.3°F).[21,30] The presence of hair near the temporal area may confound the temperature reading, so hair must be pushed away before a reading is obtained.

Axillary temperature measurement performed with electronic thermometers (Table 6-7) is not recommended routinely because, compared with the oral and rectal routes, it is not as reliable for detecting fever. In clinical studies, axillary temperature measurement was found to be only 63.5% to 75% sensitive and 64% to 92.6% specific in detecting fever, compared with rectal measurement.[25,28] Large variations in temperatures have been reported with axillary measurements attributable to inappropriate placement of the thermometer, movement of arms during measurement leading to a poor seal around the thermometer, and measurements taken for a shorter period.[24] Axillary temperature should not be taken directly after vigorous activity or bathing, because both can affect body temperature. If a fever is detected using the axillary method, a confirmation reading using another method is recommended.

The presence of fever is a cause of great concern, although in most cases fever may be self-limiting and serious complications are rare. In one study, 56% of caregivers were "very worried" about the potential complications of fever, and 34% were "somewhat worried." There is less concern about complications of fever now than 20 years ago; however, 67% of interviewed caregivers still list seizures, brain damage, and death as the main complications of fever.[31] Overall, the major risks of fever are rare but may include acute complications such as seizures, dehydration, and change in mental status.

Febrile seizures are defined as a seizure accompanied by fever in the absence of another cause such as an acute metabolic disorder or CNS inflammation. These seizures occur in 2% to 5% of all children from the ages of 6 months to 5 years.[32] The most common seizures associated with fever are simple febrile seizures, which are characterized by nonfocal movements, generally of less than 15 minutes in duration. Significant neurologic sequelae (e.g., impaired intellectual development or epilepsy) are unlikely after a single pediatric febrile seizure. High, rapidly increasing temperatures have been associated with febrile seizures. Although both the magnitude and rate of temperature increase appear to be critical determinants in precipitating febrile seizures, the temper-

ature at which a particular child will seize is unpredictable. Most initial febrile seizures occur in children younger than 3 years. Seizures occurring after that age are usually unrelated to fever. The risk of recurrence is increased in children who have experienced a previous febrile seizure (especially if it occurred before 1 year of age or was a complex febrile seizure), in children who have documented seizure or other CNS disorder, or in those whose family history includes febrile seizures.[32,33] Prophylaxis against simple febrile seizures with antiepileptic or antipyretic drugs is not recommended by the American Academy of Pediatrics.[33]

Serious detrimental effects (e.g., dehydration, delirium, seizures, coma, irreversible neurologic, or muscle damage) occur more often in patients with hyperpyrexia [temperatures greater than 106°F (41.1°C)], which is usually associated with hyperthermia and not fever. It is rare that a febrile person will have temperatures exceeding 106°F (41.1°C) owing to the homeostatic mechanisms of the hypothalamus. However, even lower body temperature elevations may be life-threatening in patients with heart disease and pulmonary dysfunction. Increased risk of complications exists in infants and patients with brain tumors or hemorrhage, CNS infections, preexisting neurologic damage, and decreased ability to dissipate heat attributed to lower tolerance of elevated body temperature. Patients of advanced age are at a higher risk for fever-related complications because of their decreased thirst perception and perspiration ability.[6,34]

Treatment of Fever

Fever is a sign of an underlying process. Treatment of fever should focus on the primary cause rather than on the temperature reading. No correlation exists between the magnitude and pattern of temperature elevation (i.e., persistent, intermittent, recurrent, or prolonged) and the principal etiology or severity of the disease. Therefore, it is difficult to determine the cause of the fever on the sole basis of the temperature reading. Patient discomfort associated with fever is the main indication for antipyretic therapy, but arguments against such treatment include the generally benign and self-limited course of fever, the possible elimination of a diagnostic or prognostic sign, the attenuation of enhanced host defenses (i.e., possible therapeutic effect of fever), and the untoward effects of antipyretic medications.

The decision to treat fever is based on a patient-specific risk–benefit ratio. Fever increases oxygen consumption, production of carbon dioxide, and cardiac output. However, fever is not associated with many harmful effects unless the temperature exceeds 106°F (41.1°C), and there is evidence that fever is an adaptive response and that elevated body temperature may be beneficial. Certain microbes are thermolabile; therefore, their growth is impaired by higher than normal temperatures. Clinical reports suggest that treating chickenpox with acetaminophen and rhinovirus with aspirin may increase the duration of the symptoms, compared with no treatment.[35] Therefore, overtreatment of fever may also be detrimental. Furthermore, low-grade fever may have beneficial effects on host-defense mechanisms (e.g., antigen recognition, T-helper lymphocyte function, and leukocyte motility), but these effects have not been shown to favorably alter the course of infectious diseases.[5] Because there is no overwhelming amount of data to support either the beneficial or the harmful effects of fever, it is important to consider other patient-specific factors when recommending treatment.

TABLE 6-7 Guidelines for Axillary Temperature Measurements Using Electronic Thermometer

1. Place a clean disposable probe cover over tip.
2. Turn on thermometer and wait until it is ready for use.
3. Place tip of thermometer in armpit. Ensure that armpit is clean and dry. Thermometer must be touching skin, not clothes.
4. Hold child close to secure the thermometer under armpit, if necessary.
5. Read and record temperature when thermometer beeps.

Treatment Goals

The major goal of self-treatment is to alleviate the discomfort of fever by reducing the body temperature to a normal level.

General Treatment Approach

Treatment for fever using antipyretics (see Chapter 5, Tables 5–2 and 5–3) is most often indicated for patients with elevated temperatures, accompanied by discomfort. Fever exceeding 101°F (38.3°C) orally may be treated with antipyretic agents, as well as nonpharmacologic measures. Treatment with antipyretics may also be indicated at lower temperatures if the patient is experiencing discomfort or is of advanced age. Studies sug-

gest that for each decade increase in age, average temperature is decreased by 1.4°F (0.8°C); temperatures less than 101°F (38.3°C) may indicate fever in older populations.[34] The discomfort associated with a fever of less than 101°F (38.3°C) may be the primary indication for any of the nonprescription antipyretic medications, given that all of these agents are also analgesics.

Self-care measures, including antipyretics, are appropriate initial therapy, unless there is an exclusion for self-treatment (Figure 6–1). In addition, parents of children should be urged to call their pediatrician immediately or seek urgent medical care if their child has a history of seizure; refuses to stay hydrated; develops a rash; has a rectal temperature greater than 104°F (40.0°C); or is very sleepy, irritable, or difficult to wake. In all

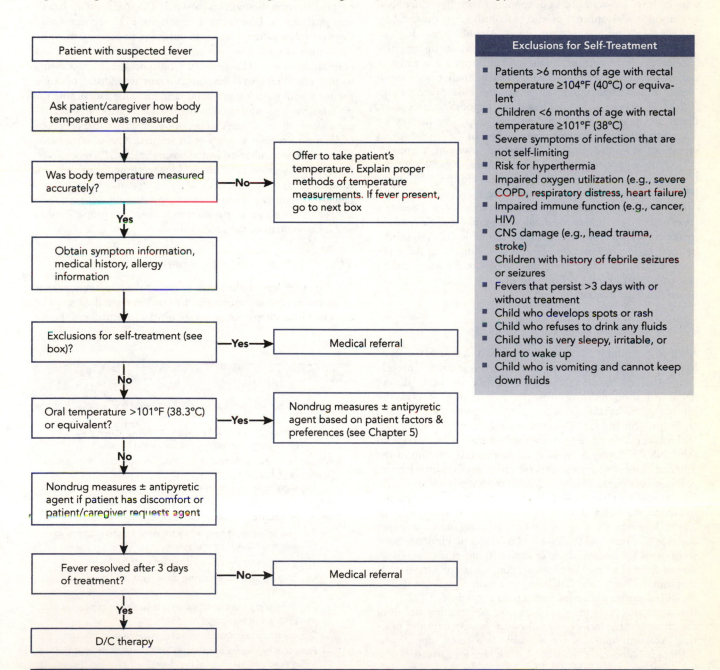

Exclusions for Self-Treatment

- Patients >6 months of age with rectal temperature ≥104°F (40°C) or equivalent
- Children <6 months of age with rectal temperature ≥101°F (38°C)
- Severe symptoms of infection that are not self-limiting
- Risk for hyperthermia
- Impaired oxygen utilization (e.g., severe COPD, respiratory distress, heart failure)
- Impaired immune function (e.g., cancer, HIV)
- CNS damage (e.g., head trauma, stroke)
- Children with history of febrile seizures or seizures
- Fevers that persist >3 days with or without treatment
- Child who develops spots or rash
- Child who refuses to drink any fluids
- Child who is very sleepy, irritable, or hard to wake up
- Child who is vomiting and cannot keep down fluids

FIGURE 6-1 Self-care of fever. Key: CNS, central nervous system; COPD, chronic obstructive pulmonary disease; D/C, discontinue; HIV, human immunodeficiency virus.

cases, self-care measures may be started while medical evaluation is being sought.

Nonpharmacologic Therapy

Nonpharmacologic therapy consists mainly of adequate fluid intake to prevent dehydration. Sponging or baths have limited utility in the management of fever. Body sponging with tepid water may facilitate heat dissipation, because only a small temperature gradient between the body and the sponging medium is necessary to achieve an effective antipyretic response. However, sponging is not routinely recommended for those with a temperature less than 104°F (40°C); sponging is usually uncomfortable and often induces shivering, which could further raise the temperature. Ice-water baths or sponging with hydroalcoholic solutions (e.g., isopropyl or ethyl alcohol) is uncomfortable, unnecessary, and not recommended. Alcohol poisoning can result from cutaneous absorption or inhalation of topically applied alcohol solutions. Infants and children are at a higher risk of alcohol poisoning because of their smaller body mass. Unlike acetaminophen and nonsteroidal anti-inflammatory drugs (NSAIDs), sponging does not reduce the hypothalamic set point; therefore, sponging should follow oral antipyretic therapy by 1 hour to permit the appropriate reduction of the hypothalamic set point and a more sustained temperature-lowering response.[36]

Other nonpharmacologic interventions, regardless of the temperature, include wearing lightweight clothing, removing blankets, maintaining a room temperature at 78°F (25.6°C), and drinking sufficient fluid to replenish insensible losses. Because a fever will cause a child to lose fluids more rapidly, sufficient fluid intake is recommended. Fluid intake in febrile children should be increased by at least 30 to 60 mL (1–2 ounces) of fluids per hour (e.g., sports drinks, fruit juice, water, or ice pops) and by at least 60 to 120 mL (3–4 ounces) of fluids per hour in adults, unless fluids are contraindicated.

Pharmacologic Therapy

Antipyretics inhibit PGE_2 synthesis, which decreases the feedback between the thermoregulatory neurons and the hypothalamus, thereby reducing the hypothalamic set point during fever. All antipyretics decrease the production of PGE_2 by inhibiting the cyclooxygenase (COX) enzyme. NSAIDs and aspirin inhibit the COX enzyme in the periphery and CNS, whereas acetaminophen mainly inhibits the COX enzyme in the CNS.[37] Chapter 5 provides an in-depth discussion of the pharmacokinetics, dosing, adverse effect profile, interactions, contraindications, and precautions of the antipyretic agents.

Acetaminophen typically reaches a maximum temperature reduction at 2 hours at the usual recommended dosing of 10 to 15 mg/kg every 4 to 6 hours with a maximum of five doses per day (see Chapter 5, Table 5-2 and 5-3). Some clinicians have recommended loading doses of acetaminophen for the reduction of fever at 30 mg/kg per dose, consequent to a small study that found a faster (one-half hour) and more significant (0.5°C [0.9°F]) decrease compared with a traditional dose.[38] This practice is not recommended, owing to the size and limitations of this study and the lack of any follow-up evidence for this practice. Acetaminophen is also available as a rectal suppository. Although a suppository may be an advantage for caregivers who have problems giving their children oral medications or for children who are vomiting or having a febrile seizure, its absorption is erratic and the dosing often does not reach levels sufficient to produce antipyretic activity.

Ibuprofen is the most common NSAID used as an antipyretic and typically reaches a maximum temperature reduction at 2 hours at the recommended dosing of 5 to 10 mg/kg per dose every 6 to 8 hours with a maximum of four doses per day (see Chapter 5, Tables 5-2 and 5-3). Some studies have shown that ibuprofen may be more effective at higher doses (10 mg/kg), especially when temperatures exceed 102.5°F (39.2°C).[39] It is important to note that ibuprofen is approved in only patients older than 6 months for the reduction of fever.

Although NSAIDs and acetaminophen are safe and effective when used at low doses for a short duration, they should not be used more than 3 days to treat fever without referral for further evaluation to determine the underlying cause. In addition, recent reports of medication errors and increased adverse events involving these agents have led FDA to encourage health care providers to take preventive actions. FDA recommendations include a patient education campaign to decrease medication errors as well as to increase awareness of side effects and contraindications[40] (Table 6-8). Common medication errors include overdosing or duplicating therapy when using multiple products with similar ingredients, and inappropriate dosing for pediatric patients attributed to mathematical errors in calculating a weight-based dose. A recent study has shown that only 30% of parents were able to measure an accurate dose of acetaminophen, whereas another study demonstrated that 51% received an inaccurate dose of medication (62% for acetaminophen and 26% for ibuprofen).[41] Because of these alarming statistics, it is important for pharmacists to provide an appropriate measuring device and/or demonstrate to patients and caregivers proper dosing and measurement of the medications.

Pharmacotherapeutic Comparison

To date, very few clinical trials compare the antipyretic effects of ibuprofen and acetaminophen in recommend dosages. The trials that have been completed are usually in a small number of

---

TABLE 6-8 FDA Recommendations for Improving Safety of Antipyretic Agents

Health care providers should educate patients actively about antipyretic agents, including the following measures:

- A wide variety of different strengths, formulations, and combinations of acetaminophen- and NSAID-containing products are available over the counter or by prescription.
- Any nonprescription analgesic is a drug, and should be taken and stored appropriately. Specific precautions include:
  - The correct dosing frequency for each of the acetaminophen or the NSAID formulations.
  - The correct weight-based dose for each child.
  - Use of the correct measuring device for the liquid formulations.
  - Risks of taking nonprescription analgesics with prescription or other nonprescription medications.
  - Signs and symptoms of self-recognizable side effects.
  - Potential problems associated with simultaneous use of more than one pain-relief product.

Key: NSAID, nonsteroidal anti-inflammatory drug.
Source: Reference 40.

patients with various dosages, making conclusions on superiority of one agent difficult. A recent review of 14 clinical trials comparing ibuprofen and acetaminophen in febrile children did find that ibuprofen was slightly more effective than acetaminophen in reducing fever after a single dose and furthermore was found to be more effective after 6 hours, thus showing a longer duration of action for ibuprofen.[42] The same review found that multiple-dose studies failed to show any statistically significant clinical difference between acetaminophen and ibuprofen. The risk of serious adverse effects did not differ between the medications. The authors concluded that the efficacy and safety between acetaminophen and ibuprofen are similar in recommended dosages, with slightly more benefit shown with ibuprofen in terms of onset of action and fever reduction; however, more conclusive findings are needed. Although ibuprofen has been studied most frequently, other NSAIDS such as naproxen and aspirin may also be appropriate as an antipyretic in adults.

Alternating different antipyretics for fever reduction has now become a widespread practice. A survey of 256 caregivers showed that 67% alternated acetaminophen and/or ibuprofen, and 81% of those stated that their health care provider/pediatrician advised them to do so. Although this approach was recommended, only 61% received any type of written instructions on how to dose the medications, and the dosing intervals varied from 2 to 6 hours.[41] Despite these practices and a recent clinical trial to show its efficacy over monotherapy in children aged 6 to 36 months,[43] the American Academy of Pediatrics at this time does not recommend alternation of antipyretics because of the risk of overdose, medication errors resulting from the complexity of the regimens, and increased side effects.[39,41,44]

Complementary and Alternative Therapies

There is currently insufficient evidence to recommend any dietary supplement or other complementary and alternative therapy modality for the treatment of fever.

Assessment of Fever: A Case-Based Approach

The first step in assessing a patient with a complaint of fever is to obtain an objective temperature measurement to determine whether fever is actually present. Subjective or inaccurate temperature measurement must be ruled out. If fever is present, assessment of its severity, the seriousness of the underlying cause, and other associated symptoms is indicated. Children who are capable of providing and understanding information should be included in any dialogue concerning their care.

CASE 6-1

Relevant Evaluation Criteria	Scenario/Model Outcome
Information Gathering	
1. Gather essential information about the patient's symptoms, including:	
a. description of symptom(s) (i.e., nature, onset, duration, severity, associated symptoms)	Child daycare provider reported to parents that their daughter has felt warm and is not eating well, although she continues to play with the other children. They took an oral temperature, which was 101.4°F. They did not notice any other symptoms other than a slight runny nose.
b. description of any factors that seem to precipitate, exacerbate, and/or relieve the patient's symptom(s)	The parents have not tried anything up to this point.
c. description of the patient's efforts to relieve the symptoms	None reported by Julianna or her parents
2. Gather essential patient history information:	
a. patient's identity	Julianna Smith
b. patient's age, sex, height, and weight	3-year-old female, 3 ft 0 in, 28 lb
c. patient's occupation	None
d. patient's dietary habits	Normal healthy toddler diet. She has not eaten much today, but she is drinking.
e. patient's sleep habits	Normal sleep pattern
f. concurrent medical conditions, prescription and nonprescription medications, and dietary supplements	Flintstone's vitamins
g. allergies	Penicillin
h. history of other adverse reactions to medications	None
i. other (describe) _____	Julianna seems slightly cranky and tired. She was not herself in daycare today, and she has a runny nose. The oral temperature remeasured in the pharmacy is 101.6°F.

Relevant Evaluation Criteria	Scenario/Model Outcome
Assessment and Triage	
3. Differentiate the patient's signs/symptoms and correctly identify the patient's primary problem(s).	Julianna has a low-grade fever that is causing her some discomfort. It is most likely related to a virus being transmitted through the daycare.
4. Identify exclusions for self-treatment (see Figure 6-1).	None
5. Formulate a comprehensive list of therapeutic alternatives for the primary problem to determine if triage to a health care provider is required, and share this information with the caregivers.	Options include: (1) Refer Julianna for medical attention. (2) Monitor her symptoms and fever and recommend nondrug measures only. (3) Recommend a medication alone or combined with nondrug measures. (4) Make no recommendations.
Plan	
6. Select an optimal therapeutic alternative to address the patient's problem, taking into account patient preferences.	Julianna has no symptoms of a bacterial infection and she has no exclusions for self-care (see Figure 6-1); therefore, therapy with either acetaminophen or ibuprofen is appropriate combined with nondrug measures. Julianna's parents would also like a chewable tablet, if possible, to ease administration. She should not receive any aspirin-containing products.
7. Describe the recommended therapeutic approach to the caregivers.	See Table 5-2 in Chapter 5 for recommended doses. If fever persists for 72 hours, take Julianna to her clinician for follow-up.
8. Explain to the patient the rationale for selecting the recommended therapeutic approach from the considered therapeutic alternatives.	Julianna has a low-grade fever that is causing her discomfort, so minimizing the fever with the medications and nondrug measures should help her. She does not need to see her clinician, because she is otherwise healthy and does not exhibit any signs of a bacterial infection for which she might need an antibiotic.
Patient Education	
9. When recommending self-care with nonprescription medications and/or nondrug therapy, convey accurate information to the caregivers:	
a. appropriate dose and frequency of administration	Acetaminophen 160 mg (two 80 mg chewable tablets) orally every 4–6 hours. Do not exceed 5 doses per 24 hours.
b. maximum number of days the therapy should be employed	3 days
c. product administration procedures	Chew tablets and swallow.
d. expected time to onset of relief	1–2 hours
e. degree of relief that can be reasonably expected	Complete resolution of symptoms may take anywhere from 2 days to 3 weeks, depending on the underlying cause of the fever.
f. most common side effects	Rare; possible gastrointestinal effects or rash
g. side effects that warrant medical intervention should they occur	Can take with food if gastrointestinal effects occur
h. patient's options in the event that condition worsens or persists	Contact health care provider if symptoms worsen or persist after 72 hours of pharmacologic therapy.
i. product storage requirements	Keep medication in a tightly secured container away from any extreme temperatures.
j. specific nondrug measures	Maintain room temperature at 78°F. Maintain fluid intake and wear lightweight clothing.
10. Solicit follow-up questions from caregivers.	May I give Julianna ibuprofen as well?
11. Answer caregivers' questions.	You should not. The American Academy of Pediatrics does not recommend alternating ibuprofen and acetaminophen because of the increased risk of medication errors and side effects.

Patient Counseling for Fever

Although fever is a common symptom, it often is misunderstood and poorly treated. Studies suggest that fever is incorrectly considered a disease associated with detrimental consequences rather than a symptom, is frequently treated inappropriately; and is evaluated improperly.[45,46] Many parents and caregivers have "fever phobia" that results in heightened anxiety and inappropriate treatment of fever.[30,47] Health care providers can improve patient outcomes by educating patients and caregivers about fever, and by teaching patients self-assessment skills and the proper methods for measuring body temperature and interpretation of the results with the variety of thermometers available. If patients continue to use mercury-in-glass thermometers they should be urged to dispose of them according to their local environmental standards. Health care providers should also explain the appropriate nonpharmacologic and pharmacologic treatments for fever and when to seek further medical care. Discussions of pharmacologic treatments should highlight methods for safe use of antipyretics and the avoidance of complementary therapies (Table 6–8).

Evaluation of Patient Outcomes for Fever

The primary monitoring parameters for febrile patients include temperature and discomfort. In one study, 52% of caregivers said that they would check a patient's temperature at least every hour in a febrile patient.[31] Overaggressive monitoring may result from fever phobia. Although most patients demonstrate a reduction in temperature after each individual dose of an antipyretic, pharmacologic therapy for fever may take up to 1 day to result in a decrease in temperature; therefore, body temperature should be monitored only two to three times a day. Associated symptoms including headache, diaphoresis, generalized malaise, chills, tachycardia, arthralgia, myalgia, irritability, and anorexia should also be monitored daily. If symptoms are not improving or are worsening over the course of 3 days with self-treatment, regardless of a drop in temperature, a health care provider should be consulted either by phone or appointment for further evaluation. Timeliness of patient follow-up with medical care is important in determining the presence of a non–self-limiting underlying cause.

PATIENT EDUCATION FOR Fever

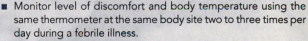

The primary objectives of treating fever are to (1) relieve the discomfort of fever by returning the body temperature to the normal level and (2) prevent complications associated with fever. For most patients, carefully following product instructions and the self-care measures listed here will help to ensure optimal therapeutic outcomes.

Temperature Measurement

- Do not rely on feeling the body for fever. Take a temperature reading with an appropriate thermometer.
- For children up to 6 months of age, the rectal method of temperature measurement is preferred (see Table 6-5). Use of a tympanic thermometer is not recommended in children younger than 6 months because of the size and shape of the infant's ear canal.
- For children ages 6 months to 5 years, the rectal method is still preferred; however, the tympanic, temporal, or oral method may be used if proper technique is followed (see Tables 6-3 through 6-6).
- For individuals older than 5 years, the oral, temporal, or tympanic method is appropriate (see Tables 6-3, 6-5, and 6-6).

Nondrug Measures

- Do not use isopropyl or ethyl alcohol for body sponging. Alcohol poisoning can result from skin absorption or inhalation of topically applied alcohol solutions.
- For all levels of fever, wear lightweight clothing, remove blankets, and maintain room temperature at 78°F.
- Unless advised otherwise, drink or provide sufficient fluids to replenish body fluid losses. For children, increase fluids by at least 1–2 ounces per hour. Sports drinks, fruit juice, or water is acceptable.

Nonprescription Medications

- Nonprescription analgesics/antipyretics (see Chapter 5, Tables 5-2 and 5-3) help in alleviating discomfort associated with fever and reducing the temperature.
- Nonprescription analgesics/antipyretics typically take one-half to 1 hour to begin to decrease temperature and discomfort.
- Monitor level of discomfort and body temperature using the same thermometer at the same body site two to three times per day during a febrile illness.
- Use single-entity nonprescription analgesics/antipyretics at low doses for up to 3 days for treatment of fever (see Chapter 5, Tables 5-2 and 5-3 for dosages), unless you have an exclusion to self-care (see Figure 6-1).
- Avoid alternating antipyretics because of the complexity of the dosing regimens, increased risk of medication errors, and adverse effects.
- Dosing of either ibuprofen or acetaminophen in children should be based on body weight and not age.
- Use a measuring device such as a syringe, dosing spoon, or medicine cup when administering liquid medication to avoid incorrect dosing.
- If you are pregnant or have uncontrolled high blood pressure, congestive heart failure, renal failure, or an allergy to aspirin, avoid use of nonsteroidal anti-inflammatory drugs (ibuprofen and naproxen sodium) or aspirin-containing products.
- Avoid using aspirin and aspirin-containing products for fever in children younger than 15 years because of the possible risk of Reye's syndrome.

 Seek medical attention if fever or discomfort persists or worsens after 3 days of drug treatment.

Key Points for Fever

➤ Fever is self-limiting and rarely poses severe consequences unless the oral temperature is greater than 106°F (41.1°C).

➤ The main treatment goal of fever is to eliminate the underlying cause as well as to alleviate the associated discomfort.

➤ Fever should be confirmed only by using a thermometer and appropriate measurement techniques.

➤ Rectal temperature measurement is the most accurate method; however, oral, tympanic, and temporal measurements are also accurate if taken appropriately.

➤ Patients should be referred for further evaluation if their rectal temperature or its equivalent is greater than 104°F (40°C), they have a history of febrile seizures, they have comorbid conditions compromising their health, or they are younger than 6 months with a temperature exceeding 101°F (38.3°C).

➤ Sponge baths using topical isopropyl or ethyl alcohol to reduce fever should be discouraged.

➤ Referral for further medical evaluation is appropriate to detect an underlying cause if 3 days of self-treatment are not successful.

➤ Clinicians should counsel patients on the proper use of nonprescription antipyretic agents to limit medication errors and side effects.

REFERENCES

1. *National Ambulatory Medical Care Survey; 2002 Summary. Advance data from vital and health statistics*. Washington, DC: US Department of Health and Human Services. ADR No. 346. Available at: http://www.cdc.gov/nchs/data/ad/ad346.pdf. Last accessed August 3, 2008.
2. Rehm KP. Fever in infants and children. *Curr Opin Pediatr*. 2001;13:83–8.
3. Cherry DK, Woodwell DA, Rechsteiner EA. *National Ambulatory Medical Care Survey: 2005 Summary. Advance data from vital and health statistics*. Hyattsville, Md: National Center for Health Statistics. 2007. ADR No. 387. Available at: http://www.cdc.gov/nchs/data/ad/ad387.pdf. Last accessed August 3, 2008.
4. Halloran LL, Bernard DW. Management of drug-induced hyperthermia. *Curr Opin Pediatr*. 2004;16:211–5.
5. Mackowiak PA. Concepts of fever. *Arch Intern Med*. 1998;158:1870–81.
6. Dinarello CA, Gelfand JA. Fever and hyperthermia. In: Kasper DL, Braunwald E, Fauci AS, et al., eds. *Harrison's Principles of Internal Medicine*. 16th ed. New York: McGraw Hill, Inc; 2005:104.
7. Norman DC. Fever in the elderly. *Clin Infect Dis*. 2000;31:148–51.
8. DiPiro JT, Ownby DR, Schlesselman LS. Allergic and pseudoallergic drug reactions. In: DiPiro JT, Talbert RL, Yee GC, et al., eds. *Pharmacotherapy: A Pathophysiologic Approach*. 6th ed. New York: McGraw-Hill, Inc; 2005:1599.
9. Kumar KL, Reuler JB. Drug fever. *West J Med*. 1986;144:753–5.
10. Johnson DH, Cunha BA. Drug fever. *Infect Dis Clin North Am*. 1996;10:85–91.
11. Chan T, Evans S, Clark R. Drug-induced hyperthermia. *Crit Care Clin*. 1997;13:785–809.
12. Velammor V. Neuroleptic malignant syndrome: recognition, prevention, and management. *Drug Saf*. 1998;19:73–82.
13. Dinarello CA, Bunn PA. Fever. *Semin Oncol*. 1997;24:288–98.
14. Netea MG, Kullberg BJ, Van der Meer JW. Circulating cytokines as mediators of fever. *Clin Infect Dis*. 2000;31:S178–84.
15. El-Radhi AS, Barry W. Thermometry in paediatric practice. *Arch Dis Child*. 2006;91:351–6.
16. Rabinowitz RP, Cookson ST, Wasserman SS, et al. Effects of anatomic site, oral stimulation, and body position on estimates of body temperature. *Arch Intern Med*. 1996;156:777–80.
17. US Environmental Protection Agency. State and Local Mercury Collection/Recycling/Exchange Programs. Available at: http://www.epa.gov/epaoswer/hazwaste/mercury/collect.htm. Last accessed August 3, 2008.
18. Goldman LR, Shannon MW; Committee on Environmental Health. Technical Report: mercury in the environment: implications for pediatricians. *Pediatrics*. 2001;108(1):197–205.
19. Thermometer comparison. *Pharmacist's Letter/Prescriber's Letter*. 2007;23(10):231006.
20. Press S. Quinn BJ. The pacifier thermometer: comparison of supralingual with rectal temperatures in infants and young children. *Arch Pediatr Adolesc Med*. 1997;151:551–4.
21. Callanan D. Detecting fever in young infants: reliability of perceived, pacifier, and temporal artery temperatures in infants younger than 3 months of age. *Pediatr Emerg Care*. 2003;19:240–3.
22. Robinson JL, Seal RF, Spady DW, et al. Comparison of esophageal, rectal, axillary, bladder, tympanic, and pulmonary artery temperatures in children. *J Pediatr*. 1998;133:553–6.
23. Greenes DS. Fleisher GR. When body temperature changes, does rectal temperature lag? *J Pediatr*. 2004;144:824–6.
24. Bernardo LM, Henker R, O'Connor J. Temperature measurement in pediatric trauma patients: a comparison of thermometry and measurement routes. *J Emerg Nurs*. 1999;25:327–9.
25. Wilshaw R, Beckstrand R, Waid D, et al. A comparison of the use of tympanic, axillary, and rectal thermometers in infants. *J Ped Nurs*. 1999;14:88–93.
26. Craig JV, Lancaster GA, Taylor S, et al. Infrared ear thermometry compared with rectal thermometry in children: a systematic review. *Lancet*. 2002;360:603–9.
27. Varney SM, Manthey DE, Culpepper VE, et al. A comparison of oral, tympanic, and rectal temperature measurement in the elderly. *J Emerg Med*. 2002:22:153–7.
28. Jean-Mary MB, Dicanzio J, Shaw J, et al. Limited accuracy and reliability of infrared axillary and aural thermometers in a pediatric outpatient population. *J Pediatr*. 2002;141:671–6.
29. Greenes DS, Fleisher GR. Accuracy of a noninvasive temporal artery thermometer for use in infants. *Arch Pediatr Adolesc Med*. 2001;155:376–81.
30. Siberry GK, Diener-West M, Schappell E, et al. Comparison of temple temperatures with rectal temperatures in children under two years of age. *Clin Pediatr*. 2002;41:405–14.
31. Crocetti M, Moghbeli N, Serwint J. Fever phobia revisited: have parental misconceptions about fever changed in 20 years? *Pediatrics*. 2001;107:1241–6.
32. Baumann RJ, D'Angelo SL. The neurodiagnostic evaluation of the child with a first simple febrile seizure. *Pediatrics*. 1996;97:773–5.
33. Practice parameter: long-term treatment of the child with simple febrile seizures. *Pediatrics*. 1999;103:1307–9.
34. Roghmann MC, Warner J, Mackowiak PA. The relationship between age and fever magnitude. *Am J Med Sci*. 2001;322:68–70.
35. Plaisance KI, Mackowiak PA. Antipyretic therapy: physiologic rationale, diagnostic implications, and clinical consequences. *Arch Intern Med*. 1996;160:449–56.
36. Axelrod P. External cooling in the management of fever. *Clin Infect Dis*. 2000;31(suppl 5):S224–9.
37. Aronoff DM, Neilson EG. Antipyretics: mechanisms of action and clinical use in fever suppression. *Am J Med*. 2001;111:304–15.
38. Treluyer JM, Tonnelier S, d'Athis P, et al. Antipyretic efficacy of an initial 30-mg/kg loading dose of acetaminophen versus a 15-mg/kg maintenance dose. *Pediatrics*. 2001;108:e73.
39. Bahal O'Mara, Neeta. Antipyretics and fever in children. *Pharmacist's Letter/Prescriber's Letter*. 2006;22(4):220409.
40. Safety Concerns Associated with Over-the-Counter Drug Products Containing Analgesic/Antipyretic Active Ingredients for Internal Use. 2004. Food and Drug Administration Science Background. Available at: http://www.fda.gov/cder/drug/analgesics/SciencePaper.htm. Last accessed August 4, 2008.
41. Wright AD, Liebelt EL. Alternating antipyretics for fever reduction in children: an unfounded practice passed down to parents from pediatricians. *Clin Pediatr*. 2007;46:146–5.
42. Goldman RD, KO K, Linett, LJ, et al. Antipyretic efficacy and safety of ibuprofen and acetaminophen in children. *Ann Pharmacother*. 2004;38:146–50.
43. Sarrell EM, Wielunsky E, Cohen HA. Antipyretic treatment in young children with fever. *Arch Pediatr Adolesc Med*. 2006;160:197–202.
44. Mayoral CE, Marino RV, Rosenfeld W, et al. Alternating antipyretics: is this an alternative? *Pediatrics*. 2000;105:1009–12.
45. Ey JL. Fever commentary. *Clin Pediatr*. 2002;41:14–6.
46. Lagerlov P, Helseth S. Holager T. Childhood illnesses and the use of paracetamol: a qualitative study of parent' management of common childhood illnesses. *Fam Practice*. 2003;20:717–23.
47. Parkinson GW, Gordon KE, Camfield CS, et al. Anxiety in parents of young febrile children in a pediatric emergency department: why is it elevated? *Clin Pediatr*. 1999;38:219–26.

Musculoskeletal Injuries and Disorders

Eric Wright

Pain is one of the most common symptoms that prompts a visit to a health care provider.[1] Because pain is a common symptom of disease, patients often seek medical attention, although many seek to relieve the pain without notifying their health care provider. Much of the pain for which people attempt self-treatment arises from the musculoskeletal system. Musculoskeletal pain may be felt in the affected tissue itself or referred from another anatomic source (e.g., hip pain referred from its primary source in the low back).[2]

Musculoskeletal pain arises from the muscles, bones, joints, and connective tissue. Similar to other types of pain phenomena, musculoskeletal pain can be idiopathic, iatrogenic, or related to injury. The development of musculoskeletal pain can be acute such as acute sport injuries (e.g., tendonitis, sprains, and strains) or chronic such as pain from stable degenerative joint disease or osteoarthritis. Unfortunately, musculoskeletal pain is also used to describe regional discomfort arising from any soft tissue source (including the skin), which leads to confusion among clinicians and in the medical literature. Table 7-1 describes these and other types of musculoskeletal complaints/disorders.

Use of nonprescription analgesics and external counter-irritants remains high, with more than $2 billion spent per year in the United States on these nonprescription remedies.[3] In addition, nearly 80% of adults admit to taking a pain reliever at least once a week, with many taking these products inappropriately. This high medication use and misuse present significant challenges for providers. Ideally, a patient experiencing pain will ask a health care provider to assist in selecting a nonprescription or prescription product. Health care providers need to understand the types of pain for which patients are seeking treatment and to communicate effectively with patients to better understand the nature of a specific patient's pain complaint. They must also be ready to provide reasonable recommendations for either treatment or further evaluation.

Musculoskeletal complaints result in a significant amount of lost work days, work limitations, and loss of employment, and are believed to be the greatest contributors to the economic burden of chronic pain; musculoskeletal complaints are estimated to cost the U.S. economy more than $60 billion annually.[4] Backache and osteoarthritis are highly prevalent pain complaints with approximately one-half of the U.S. population older than 70 years having osteoarthritis.[5] Approximately one-tenth of the working population is being treated for arthritis with prescription medications, whereas many choose to self-treat and go unreported.[6] Hence, the incidence and prevalence of reported skeletal muscle injuries may be underestimated.

Pathophysiology of Musculoskeletal Injuries and Disorders

The musculoskeletal system includes the muscles, tendons, ligaments, cartilage, and bones (Figure 7-1). Muscles are attached to bones by tendons, and ligaments connect bone to bone. Under normal conditions, tendons and ligaments have limited ability to stretch and twist. Because of their tensile strength, tendons and ligaments rarely rupture unless subjected to intense forces, but they may become damaged when hyperextended or overused. Synovial bursae are fluid-filled sacs located between joint spaces to provide lubrication and cushioning.

Cartilage functions as protective pads between bones in joints and in the vertebral column. Skeletal, or striated muscle, is composed of cells (myocytes) in which two constituents (actin and myosin) are primarily responsible for contraction. Muscle contraction also involves several electrolytes within the muscle tissue, including calcium and potassium. Pain receptors are located in skeletal muscle and the overlying fascia, and can be stimulated as a result of overuse or injury to the muscle or surrounding structures.

Somatic pain occurs when pain impulses are transmitted from peripheral nociceptors to the central nervous system (CNS) by nerve fibers. Common sites of origin of somatic pain are muscles, fascia, bones, and nerves. Somatic pain is most commonly myofascial, as in a muscle strain, or musculoskeletal, as in arthritis. Trigger points, which can occur following injury or immobility of the affected tissues, cause a reproducible, referred pain pattern when pressure is applied. (See Chapter 5 for discussion of transduction, transmission, perception, and modulation of pain.)

Mechanoreceptors and chemoreceptors mediate muscle pain. These nerve endings are heterogeneous in that only a single chemical can stimulate some endings, whereas a variety of chemical, mechanical, and thermal triggers can stimulate others. Ischemic muscle pain is caused by intramuscular pressure during activity that reduces blood supply to the muscle. Normally this effect disappears within seconds of muscle relaxation. Ischemic muscle pain lasting for longer periods is believed to be mediated by the actions of histamine, acetylcholine, serotonin, bradykinin, adenosine, and potassium.

Erythema (redness), edema, and tenderness (hyperalgesia) at the affected site characterize the inflammatory response, which develops through participation of multiple mediators, including histamine, bradykinin, serotonin, leukotrienes, and prostaglandins of the E series. Opioid receptors in peripheral tissues may play a

TABLE 7-1 Common Musculoskeletal Complaints and Disorders

Myofascial pain: pain originating in the fascia

Musculoskeletal pain: pain originating in the muscle

Myalgia: generalized muscle pain

Fibromyalgia: chronic pain syndrome characterized by diffuse muscle and joint pain, joint stiffness, fatigue, and sleep disturbances

Strain: injury to a muscle or tendon caused by overextension

Sprain: injury to a ligament caused by joint overextension

Muscle spasm: involuntary contraction of muscle

Muscle cramp: prolonged muscle spasm that produces painful sensations

role in the inflammatory response and may exert antihyperalgesic activity.[7] Because pain and inflammation increase prostaglandin production, drugs that inhibit peripheral prostaglandin production (e.g., nonsteroidal anti-inflammatory drugs [NSAIDs]) reduce the transmission of pain impulses from the periphery to the CNS.

Muscle injuries can be categorized as strains (see subsequent text), contusions caused by blunt trauma, and delayed onset muscle soreness (e.g., overexertion).

Overexertion or *repeated unaccustomed eccentric muscle contraction* is associated with delayed-onset (8 hours or more) muscle soreness, which can last for days, usually peaking at 24 to 48 hours. This pain reflects muscle damage that was presumably initiated by force generated in the muscle fibers, and is thought to be induced by inflammation, acidosis, muscle spasms, and/or microlesions. Prolonged tonic contraction produced by exercise, tension, or poor posture, and by body mechanics can also produce muscle pain.

Myalgia can also result from systemic infections (e.g., influenza, coxsackievirus, measles, and other illnesses), chronic disorders (e.g., fibromyalgia and polymyalgia rheumatica), and medications (e.g., some cholesterol-lowering agents such as statins).[8] Abuse of alcohol may precipitate acute alcoholic myopathy. Bone and muscle pain (from osteomalacia) may also occur, resulting from a diet deficient in vitamin D.

Tendonitis is the inflammation of a tendon, which results from acute injury or from chronic overuse of a body part (Figure 7-1). An example of an overuse injury is carpal tunnel syndrome, a condition characterized by tingling or numbness of the first digits of the hand caused by repetitive use of the hands and wrists. Tendon sheaths become inflamed and constrict the median nerve as it passes through a narrow channel between the wrist bones. In industry, factors such as poorly designed equipment, awkward working positions, lack of job variation, long work hours, and inadequate rest breaks contribute to its development. In sports-related overuse injuries, contributing factors for tendonitis can include increased age, poor technique, improper conditioning, exercise of prolonged intensity or duration, and poorly designed equipment for specific activities (e.g., poor cushioning of athletic shoes). Tendons can become strained when their stretch capacity is exceeded, such as in a hyperextension injury of an arm or leg. Eccentric contraction of the muscle while the muscle is lengthening causes the injury. Lastly, fluoroquinolone antimicrobials have been suspected in the development of tendonitis and tendon rupture, and these medications carry a boxed warning. Patients older than 60 years who are taking steroids, or have had heart, lung, or kidney transplantation are at greater risk.[9]

Bursitis is a common cause of localized pain, tenderness, and swelling, which is worsened by any movement of the structure adjacent to the bursa (Figure 7-1). Bursitis generally results from either an acute injury to the joint or over-repetitive joint action. When pain is accompanied by presence of a puncture site (possibly from intra-articular injection), an adjacent source of infection, or severe inflammation, an infectious cause should be suspected and ruled out before recommending self-treatment.

Sprains are the most common problem with ligaments. Sprains are characterized by grade, with grade I sprains resulting from excessive stretching, grade II sprains from a partial tear, and grade III sprains involving a complete tear of the tissue. The tear or rupture of a ligament is more common than that of a tendon. Examples of ligament sprains include inversion of the ankle (turning inward at an extreme angle) and tearing of the anterior cruciate ligament of the knee during rotation or twisting motions. Anterior cruciate ligament tears are relatively common injuries in sports such as basketball, volleyball, football, tennis, and skiing, in which knees are involved in both propelling and pivoting the body.

Low back pain is the fifth most likely reason for a physician visit; the lifetime prevalence of developing low back pain approaches 80%.[10] Main risk factors for the development of low back pain include sedentary lifestyle (particularly one disrupted by bursts of activity), as well as poor posture, improper shoes, excessive body weight, poor mattresses and sleeping posture, and improper technique in lifting heavy objects. Although most patients recover within a few days to a few weeks with conservative treatment, low back pain is likely to recur if the initial episode of pain is severe, and if the patient has had multiple prior episodes.[11]

Other causes of low back pain include congenital anomalies, osteoarthritis, vertebral fractures and compressions, spinal tuberculosis, and referred pain from diseased kidneys, pancreas, liver, or prostate.

Pain from arthritis has been attributed to a number of different sources including joint instability, increased pressure in the

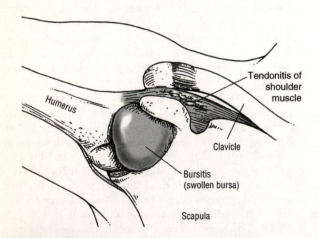

FIGURE 7-1 Bursitis and tendonitis. These two painful injuries, which often result from overuse of a joint or tendon, can cause inflammation, swelling, and tenderness in the injured area. (*Source:* Reprinted with permission from *US Pharm.* January 1995;20(1).)

spaces between bones, inflammatory synovitis, periarticular involvement (e.g., bursitis), muscle atrophy, periosteal elevation, fibromyalgia, pain amplification, and central pain mechanisms. Even in the same individual, the pain may arise from different sources at any given time.

Osteoarthritis is characterized by a gradual softening and destruction of the cartilage between bones. Cartilage and bone are destroyed in the joint spaces and regenerated, causing a rearrangement of the synovial architecture. Often referred to as "degenerative joint disease," osteoarthritis is caused by genetic, metabolic, and environmental factors. Heavy physical activity, repetitive movement, and lifting of heavy weights may aggravate this condition, whereas light-to-moderate activity does not and is generally helpful.[12]

Clinical Presentation of Musculoskeletal Injuries and Disorders

Table 7-2 lists many of the presenting signs and symptoms of musculoskeletal disorders and also differentiates other factors. Pain is a common symptom among all the musculoskeletal disorders.

In addition to the pain induced by a sprain, patients have variable degrees of joint function. With functional limitations, the injury is most likely to be a grade II or grade III sprain and needs proper workup to rule out a fracture or tear. If visibly deformed, a joint is probably ruptured or fractured and requires emergency assistance.

Patients with carpal tunnel syndrome often experience a sense of heat or cold, a sense that their hands are swollen when they are not, weakness, and a tendency to drop things. Symptoms persist during sleep and even when the hand is not being used, a characteristic that can be used to distinguish this disorder from others.

The pain of osteoarthritis does not correlate directly with the degree of joint damage. Pain is often referred, and proximal muscles could be involved if a person with osteoarthritis guards the affected joint by changing the gait to reduce discomfort. The pain caused by chronic osteoarthritis often limits the patient's activities of daily living (ADLs) (e.g., unable to grip containers or walk more than a short distance). It is unclear which joint structures are responsible for the pain and discomfort, but the pain has variably been ascribed to derangements of bone, cartilage, muscle, connective tissue, and nerves supplying the affected joint(s).

Pain and tightness in the low back are also often caused by posture, muscle support, and degenerative changes, and often limit a patient's ability to bend, move, sit, or walk. Low back pain can be neuropathic in nature and involve the sciatic nerve, causing sharp referred pain into one or both of the patient's legs.

Signs and symptoms that preclude self-treatment of these disorders are listed in Figure 7-2.

Complications of untreated pain-inducing injuries include further tissue damage and, in advanced arthritis, bone and cartilage remodeling. The most serious complication of poorly managed pain is disability and loss of function. Pain is associated with significant limitations including a reduction in ADLs, loss of work time, and physical impairments such as insomnia. Complications may also arise if the etiology of the pain is misdiagnosed or misjudged. It is important to look for warning signs (see exclusions for self-treatment in Figure 7-2) that indicate the pain cannot be managed with nonprescription analgesics.

Treatment of Musculoskeletal Injuries and Disorders

Acute pain is the body's alarm system; it signals injury by trauma, disease, muscle spasms, or inflammation. Chronic pain, conversely, may or may not be indicative of injury and requires a primary care provider's assessment before treatment is initiated.

Treatment Goals

Treatment of the patient with musculoskeletal complaints encompasses many different goals, including (1) decreasing the subjective intensity (severity) and duration of the pain; (2) restoring function of the affected area; (3) preventing reinjury and disability (i.e., improve ADLs); and (4) preventing acute pain from becoming chronic persistent pain.

General Treatment Approach

Patients with musculoskeletal injuries present with similar symptoms, especially pain and swelling of the affected area. These conditions have similar self-treatment approaches. Nonpharmacologic therapy consisting of rest, ice, compression, and elevation (RICE) along with nonprescription analgesics (i.e., NSAIDs or acetaminophen) and/or external analgesics during the first 1 to 3 days following injury are helpful. Before treatment can be recommended, however, the patient should be carefully screened to ensure appropriateness of self-treatment. The algorithm in Figure 7-2 presents a stepwise approach to self-management of pain associated with these complaints for patients who do not meet the criteria for exclusion for self-care.

Patients with acute low back pain are candidates for self-treatment. Chronic low back pain (i.e., lasting more than 6–7 weeks) requires medical evaluation before initiating therapy. Management of acute back pain includes rest and ice, nonprescription oral analgesics, and nonprescription topical analgesics. Approaches to chronic low back pain also include therapeutic interventions such as heat therapy, massage with traction (contraindicated for pregnant women and people with osteoporosis, tumor, or spine infection) and, most importantly, mobilization with exercise (a program of techniques and exercises to restore back mechanics and movement). Chiropractic manipulation and acupuncture (often with electrical stimulation) are also commonly used for the treatment of back pain, with mixed results.[13,14]

Rheumatoid arthritis, gouty arthritis, Lyme arthritis, and osteoarthritis all cause arthritic pain, but only the pain of osteoarthritis is approved for self-treatment after an initial medical diagnosis. The general treatment approach includes appropriate lifestyle changes (including physical therapy and weight loss) and systemic therapy with standard doses of acetaminophen or lower-dose NSAIDs, with or without topical therapy.[15]

Nonpharmacologic Therapy

Injury from playing sports or exercising is preventable by warming up and stretching muscles before physical activity, ensuring proper hydration, and not exercising to the point of exhaustion. Stretching must be done cautiously, without bouncing, to avoid muscle strain. For muscle cramps, stretching and massaging the affected area immediately followed by rest, or at least reduced activity, will loosen the muscle. For electrolyte depletion, appropriate oral supplementation of wasted electrolytes can be

TABLE 7-2 Comparison of Musculoskeletal Disorders

	Myalgia	Tendonitis	Bursitis	Sprain	Strain	Osteoarthritis
Location	Muscles of the body	Tendon locations around joint areas	Inflammation of the bursae within joints; common locations include knee, shoulder, big toe	Stretching or tearing of a ligament within a joint	Hyperextension of a muscle or tendon	Weight-bearing joints, knees, hip, low back, hands
Signs	Possible swelling (rare)	Warmth, swelling, erythema	Warmth, edema, erythema, and possible crepitus	Swelling, bruising	Swelling, bruising	Noninflammatory joints, narrowing of joint space, restructuring of bone and cartilage (resulting in joint deformities), possible joint swelling
Symptoms	Dull, constant ache (sharp pain relatively rare); weakness and fatigue of muscles also common	Mild-to-severe pain generally occuring after use; loss of range of motion	Constant pain that worsens with movement or application of external pressure over the joint	Initial severe pain followed by pain, particularly with joint use; tenderness; reduction in joint stability and function	Initial severe pain with continued pain upon movement and at rest, muscle weakness, loss of some function	Dull joint pain relieved by rest, joint stiffness <20–30 minutes, localized symptoms to joint
Onset	Depending on cause (i.e., trauma = acute, but drug-induced = insidious)	Often gradual, but can develop suddenly	Acute with injury; recurs with precipitant use of joint	Acute with injury	Acute with injury	Insidious development over years
Etiology	Trauma, overuse, infection, drug- and alcohol-induced	Trauma, overuse, drug-induced, inflammatory diseases	Trauma and excessive wear/use; septic bursitis (most frequently preceded by trauma and caused by *Staphylococcus aureus*) presenting with fever and acute painful swelling	Hyperextension of joint ligament	Excessive stretch of muscle or tendon	Degeneration of joint space from genetic, metabolic, and environmental factors
Exacerbating Factors	Contraction of muscle	Movement of affected joint	Movement of affected joints	Movement of affected joint	Use of affected muscle or tendon	Obesity, lack of activity, heavy physical activity, repetitive movement, trauma

TABLE 7-2 Comparison of Musculoskeletal Disorders *(continued)*

Myalgia	Tendonitis	Bursitis	Sprain	Strain	Osteoarthritis
Modifying Factors					
Eliminate cause; use stretching, rest, heat, topical analgesics, systemic analgesics	Eliminate cause; use of stretching, rest, ice, heat, topical analgesics, systemic analgesics	Joint rest, immobilization, topical analgesics, systemic analgesics	RICE; stretching; use of protective wraps (e.g., ankle tape, knee brace, cane), topical counterirritants, systemic analgesics	RICE; stretching; use of protective wraps, topical counterirritants, systemic analgesics	Continuous exercise (light-to-moderate activity), weight loss, analgesic medication, topical pain relievers

Key: RICE, rest, ice, compression, elevation (see Table 7-3).

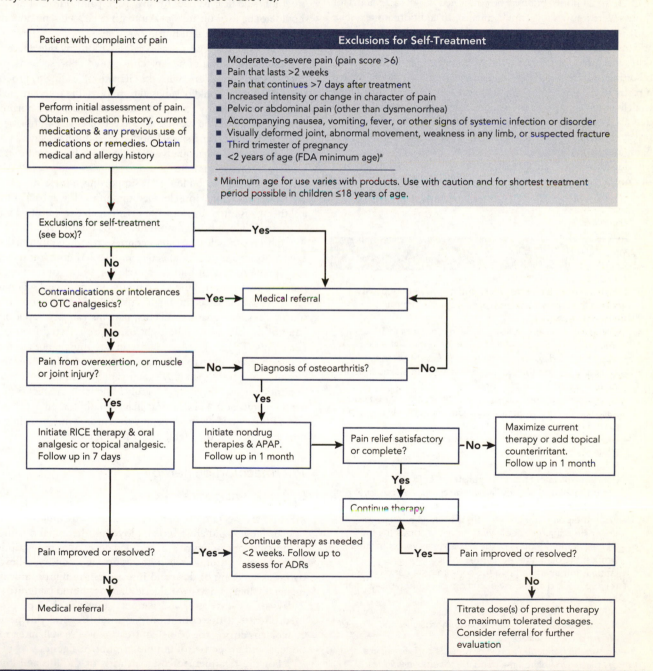

FIGURE 7-2 Self-care of musculoskeletal injuries and disorders. Key: ADR, adverse drug reaction; APAP, acetaminophen; OTC, over-the-counter; RICE, rest, ice, compression, elevation. (Adapted from Self-care of self-limited pain. In: Albrant DH, ed. *The American Pharmaceutical Association Drug Treatment Protocols.* 2nd ed. Washington, DC: American Pharmaceutical Association; 2001:424–5.)

used, with the selection of fluids containing potassium, sodium, and magnesium.

Posture and the use of ergonomic controls (such as a chair with back support or ergonomic keyboard) improve function and reduce pain. Heel lifts and better-fitting shoes are recommended for patients with Achilles tendonitis. RICE therapy promotes healing, and helps reduce swelling and inflammation associated with muscle and joint injuries (Table 7-3). Ice should not be applied for more than 15 minutes, because excessive icing causes considerable vasoconstriction and reduces vascular clearance of inflammatory mediators from the damaged area. Ice therapy should be used as close as possible to the time of injury and applied three to four times a day until the swelling decreases, generally 12 to 24 hours, but may be continued for 48 to 72 hours for more severe injuries (e.g., ankle sprains). In addition, postexercise icing is often appropriate to reduce the likelihood of inflammation and to reduce pain. Ice, as well as heat, at temperatures outside the skin's threshold for tolerance can be damaging and can result in blistering or burning; therefore, neither therapy should be applied directly to the skin. Although the purchase of a product designed to deliver ice therapy is not needed for effective use, many products are available for purchase, which ease the application. Compression and elevation also assist in reducing the swelling and pain, and should be instituted whenever possible.

Heat therapy is an alternative for patients who develop pain of a noninflammatory nature. It has been studied in the treatment of acute low back pain (<4 weeks' duration) with favorable effects.[14] Although its mechanism of action is not fully understood, heat may help to reduce pain by increasing blood flow. Heat is applied for 15 to 20 minutes, three to four times a day. Heat should not be applied to recently injured (<48 hours) or inflamed areas, because it will intensify vasodilation and exacerbate vascular leakage and tissue damage. Furthermore, heat should not be used with other topical agents or over broken skin. Heat should be applied to the affected area in the form of a warm wet compress, heating pad, or hot-water bottle. Ease of use favors newer heat-generating adhesive products (e.g., ThermaCare), which can be worn on the affected area up to 8 hours. Product formulations are now widely available for the area affected (i.e., adhesive heat patches for low back pain). Heating devices should not be used on areas of skin with decreased sensation; this practice can lead to a skin burn.

Although not generally associated with many side effects, at least one formulation of heat patches caused first-, second-, and third-degree burns along with skin irritation, leading to product recall.[16] Patients should be advised to remove the patch immediately if they have any pain or discomfort, itching, or burning. Heat wraps should be worn over a layer of clothing in patients older than 55 years and should not be used during sleep.

Physical and rehabilitative therapies have been used to treat acute pain from sports injuries and to treat chronic pain. Physical therapy can assist in building up supporting muscle structures, such as the abdominal muscles that support the lower back. Physical therapy is often supplemented with deep tissue heating with ultrasound, which has demonstrated some positive results.[13,14]

Chronic muscle pain often requires structured physical therapy to isolate and stretch affected muscles. Although it may be appropriate to rest an injured muscle for a few days, failure to mobilize the area once the acute injury begins to heal will often result in the muscle becoming tight, weak, and overly contracted (guarded). Once guarding occurs, patients can develop a tight band of muscle tissue. The tight bands are referred to as trigger points. Trigger points can arise in any muscle but are most commonly seen in large muscle groups. If muscle pain becomes chronic, the painful area may require application of ice or vapocoolant sprays, or injections, typically using local anesthetics (trigger point injections [TPIs]) to facilitate remobilization. Analgesics and TPIs facilitate physical therapy for chronic muscle pain syndromes; however, the medications are not curative.

Pharmacologic Therapy

Systemic Analgesics

NSAIDs and acetaminophen are commonly used nonprescription analgesics, and are often employed in the initial treatment of musculoskeletal injuries. Scheduled doses of nonprescription strengths are instituted early in the course of an injury, followed by quick tapering of dose and interval as the injury improves (generally in 1–3 days). Analgesic therapy should be limited to 7 days of self-care use, and patients should seek appropriate medical care if the condition continues beyond this period or worsens during the course of treatment. (See Chapter 5 for dosages and properties of nonprescription analgesics.)

For the treatment of osteoarthritis of the hip and knee, acetaminophen is the recommended first-line therapy versus NSAIDs, despite data suggesting that NSAIDs provide slightly improved pain relief.[17–19] Responses to analgesics vary from patient to patient, and initial treatment recommendations are

---

TABLE 7-3 Guidelines for RICE Therapy

- Rest the injured area after injury and continue until pain is reduced (generally 1–2 days). Slings, splints, or crutches can be used if necessary.
- Apply ice as soon as possible to the injured area in 10- to 15-minute increments, 3–4 times a day. Continue the ice-pack therapy for 1–3 days, depending on the severity of injury.
- Apply compression to the injured area with an elastic support or an elasticized bandage as follows:
  —Choose the appropriate size bandage for the injured body part. If preferred, purchase a product specifically designed for the injured body part.
  —Unwind about 12–18 inches of bandage at a time and allow the bandage to relax.
  —If ice is also being applied to the injured area, soak the bandage in water to aid the transfer of cold.
  —Wrap the injured area by overlapping the previous layer of bandage by about one-third to one-half its width.
  —Wrap the point most distal from the injury. For example, if the ankle is injured, begin wrapping just above the toes.
  —Decrease the tightness of the bandage as you continue to wrap. If the bandage feels tight or uncomfortable or circulation is impaired, remove the compression bandage and rewrap it. Cold toes or swollen fingers would indicate that the bandage is too tight.
  —After using the bandage, wash it in lukewarm, soapy water; do not scrub it. Rinse the bandage thoroughly and allow to air dry on a flat surface.
  —Roll up the bandage to prevent wrinkles and store it in a cool, dry place. Do not iron the bandage to remove wrinkles.
- Elevate the injured area at or above the level of the heart 2–3 hours a day to decrease swelling and to relieve pain.

Key: RICE, rest, ice, compression, elevation.

made on the basis of drug safety rather than efficacy, while adjusting drug therapy according to patient response.[15,20] Chronic use of NSAIDs leads to more severe and prevalent side effects such as nephropathy, gastrointestinal ulcerations and bleeding, and the potential for cardiac events.[21] Acetaminophen has a proven safety record if given in the recommended dosage. Chapter 5 describes the safety of acetaminophen and NSAIDs in greater detail.

Topical Products

Topical analgesics may have local analgesic, anesthetic, antipruritic, and/or counterirritant effects. Counterirritants are approved specifically for the topical treatment of minor aches and pains of muscles and joints (simple backache, arthritis pain, strains, bruises, and sprains).[22] They are recommended as adjuncts to pharmacologic and nonpharmacologic therapy of musculoskeletal injuries and disorders.

COUNTERIRRITANTS

Topical counterirritants are topically applied to relieve pain. The difference between counterirritants and other external analgesics (anesthetics, analgesics, and antipruritics) is that the pain relief results more from nerve stimulation than depression.[22] Counterirritation is the paradoxical pain-relieving effect achieved by producing a less severe pain to counter a more intense one. On the basis of their topical effects, counterirritants are classified into four types (Table 7-4). Table 7-5 lists examples of commercially available products.

Undoubtedly, the action of counterirritants in relieving pain has a psychological component. These agents may exert a placebo effect through pleasant odors, or by the sensation of warmth or coolness they produce on the skin. Other factors, which influence the intensity of response to the counterirritation, include the irritant used, its concentration, the solvent in which it is dissolved, and the duration of its contact with the skin.

All regulations and labeling for topical counterirritants are based on the detailed previous proposed rulemaking documents published in the *Federal Register* in 1979 and 1983.[22,23] The U.S. Food and Drug Administration (FDA) has recognized the ingredients in Table 7-4 as safe and effective (Category I) counterirritants for use in adults and in children ages 2 years and older.[23]

Labels for counterirritants indicate that the product is to be used for "the temporary relief of minor aches and sprains of muscles and joints." In addition, the labeling recommended by most of FDA's review panels includes claims for "simple backache, arthritis pain, strains, bruises, and sprains."[22] Product labels may contain descriptors such as "external analgesic" or "topical" or "pain-relieving" cream, lotion, or ointment. However, these terms are not necessarily similar to the manufacturer's advertising claims.[23] The following sections describe the commonly used counterirritants currently available in the United States.

Methyl Salicylate   Methyl salicylate occurs naturally as wintergreen oil or sweet birch oil; gaultheria oil and teaberry oil are other names for the natural compound. In some areas of the United States, it is still referred to as "mountain tea." Synthetic methyl salicylate is prepared by the esterification of salicylic acid with methyl alcohol. Methyl salicylate is usually combined with other ingredients with antipruritic or analgesic properties, such as menthol and/or camphor.

When applied to the skin at pain sites, methyl salicylate and other counterirritants produce a mild, local, inflammatory reaction, which provides relief at another site that is usually adjacent to, or underlying, the skin surface being treated. These induced sensations distract from the deep-seated pain in muscles, joints, and tendons. Pain is only as intense as it is perceived to be, and the perception of other sensations caused by the counterirritant or its application (e.g., massage, warmth, or redness) causes the sufferer to disregard the sensation of pain. The result is that the patient's attention is diverted from the injured structure by the application of the counterirritant medication.

Methyl salicylate, as a rubefacient, causes vasodilation of cutaneous vasculature, thereby producing reactive hyperemia; it is hypothesized that this increase in blood pooling and/or flow is accompanied by an increase in localized skin temperature, which then may exert a counterirritant effect. Because of this rubefacient action, methyl salicylate is responsible for the "hot" action in many topical counterirritant products (Table 7-5).

TABLE 7-4   Classification and Dosage Guidelines[a] for Nonprescription Counterirritant External Analgesics

Group	Mechanism of Action	Ingredients	Concentration (%)	Frequency and Duration of Use
A	Rubefacients	Allyl isothiocyanate Ammonia water Methyl salicylate Turpentine oil	0.5–5.0 1.0–2.5 10–60 6–50	For all counterirritants: Apply no more often than 3–4 times/day for up to 7 days
B	Produce cooling sensation	Camphor Menthol	3–11 1.25–16.0	As above in group A
C	Cause vasodilation	Histamine dihydrochloride Methyl nicotinate	0.025–0.1 0.25–1.0	As above in group A
D	Incite irritation without rubefaction; are as potent as group A ingredients	Capsicum Capsicum oleoresin Capsaicin	0.025–0.25 0.025–0.25 0.025–0.25	Acute pain: As above in group A Chronic pain: Apply 3–4 times/day for duration of pain (often long-term use with medical supervision)

[a] Dosages approved for adults and for children 2 years and older.

Source: Reference 22.

TABLE 7-5 Selected External Analgesic Products

Trade Name	Primary Ingredients
Menthol-Containing Products	
Aspercreme Heat Pain Relieving Gel	Menthol 10%
Icy Hot Pain Relieving Gel	Menthol 2.5%
Icy Hot Patch	Menthol 5%
Camphor-Containing Products	
JointFlex Pain Relieving Cream	Camphor 3.1%
Capsaicin-Containing Products	
Capzasin Arthritis Pain Relief No-Mess Applicator	Capsaicin 0.15%
Capzasin-HP Lotion/Cream	Capsaicin 0.075%
Zostrix Arthritis Pain Relief Cream	Capsaicin 0.025%
Zostrix-HP Cream	Capsaicin 0.075%
Histamine Dihydrochloride–Containing Products	
Australian Dream Pain Relieving Arthritis Cream	Histamine dihydrochloride 0.025%
Trolamine Salicylate–Containing Products	
Aspercreme Cream/Lotion	Trolamine salicylate 10%
Sportscreme Deep Penetrating Pain Relieving Rub Cream/Lotion	Trolamine salicylate 10%
Combination Products	
ActivOn Topical Analgesic Ultra Strength Arthritis	Histamine dihydrochloride 0.025%, menthol 4.127%
ActivOn Topical Analgesic Ultra Strength Joint and Muscle	Histamine dihydrochloride 0.025%, menthol 4.127%, camphor 3.15%
Arthritis Hot Cream	Methyl salicylate 15%; menthol 10%
Bengay Ultra Strength Pain Relieving Cream	Methyl salicylate 30%; menthol 10%; camphor 4%
Flexall Plus Maximum Strength Pain Relieving Gel	Menthol 16%; methyl salicylate 10%; camphor 3.1%
Icy Hot Chill Stick	Methyl salicylate 30%; menthol 10%
Mentholatum Ointment	Camphor 9%; natural menthol 1.3%
Mentholatum Deep Heating Extra-Strength Pain Relieving Rub Cream	Methyl salicylate 30%; menthol 8%
Sloan's Liniment	Turpentine oil 47%; capsaicin 0.025% (from capsicum oleoresin)
Tiger Balm Arthritis Rub Cream	Camphor 11%, menthol 11%

The exact mechanism by which methyl salicylate produces its analgesic effect is not known, but in addition to the mechanisms described previously, it is generally accepted that both central and peripheral inhibition of prostaglandin synthesis occurs. Studies on the rate and extent of percutaneous absorption of various commercially available methyl salicylate preparations show direct tissue penetration, rather than redistribution by the systemic blood supply, indicating a localized effect of the topical product.[24] However, systemic bioavailability increases with occlusive dressings, multiple applications, and application of the agents to different areas of the body in this order: plantar, heel, instep, forearm, and abdomen.[25]

At very low concentrations (0.04%), methyl salicylate is used in oral preparations for its pleasant flavor and aroma.

The longer methyl salicylate or any counterirritant remains in contact with the skin, the longer is its duration of action. Little agreement exists on how long the counterirritants should remain in contact with the skin for optimal results; however, a practical guideline is that preparations should be applied no more than four times a day. Table 7-4 provides dosing information.

Localized reactions (i.e., skin irritation or rash) and systemic reactions (i.e., salicylate toxicity) may occur with the use of methyl salicylate. Strong irritation may cause local reactions such as erythema, blistering, neurotoxicity, or thermal hyperalgesia. There is no evidence that the risk of adverse reactions to counterirritants increases when the application site is lightly bandaged; however, an increased risk of irritation, redness, or blistering does exist with tight bandaging or occlusive dressing.[23,26] Heating pads used in conjunction with counterirritants containing methyl salicylate have produced the elevated temperature, vasodilation, and occlusion necessary to greatly enhance percutaneous absorption of menthol and methyl salicylate, causing full-thickness skin and muscle necrosis as well as persistent interstitial nephritis.[27] In addition, heat exposure and exercise after applying methyl salicylate have shown a threefold increase in systemic absorption of salicylate, which can lead to increases in adverse systemic reactions.[28] Therefore, patients should avoid using heating pads or other heating devices in conjunction with any external analgesics. Because percutaneous absorption can occur, methyl salicylate should be avoided in children, as well as used with caution in individuals who are sensitive to aspirin or have severe asthma or nasal polyps.

Although an FDA survey found that oral ingestion of methyl salicylate formulated as ointments caused no deaths and that few cases manifested severe symptoms,[22] regulations require the use of child-resistant containers for liquid preparations containing concentrations greater than 5%.[29]

Concomitant use of salicylate–containing external analgesics and maintenance warfarin therapy has been implicated in prolonging prothrombin time.[30] Both methyl salicylate and trolamine salicylate were implicated. A later study showed that 11 patients had an abnormally elevated international normalized ratio after significant use of topical methyl salicylate ointment.[31] Chapter 5 describes other potential drug interactions related to systemically absorbed salicylates.

Camphor   Although camphor occurs naturally and is obtained from the camphor tree, approximately three-fourths of the camphor used is prepared synthetically.

In concentrations of 0.1% to 3.0%, camphor depresses cutaneous receptors and is used as a topical analgesic, anesthetic, and antipruritic. In concentrations exceeding 3%, particularly when combined with other counterirritant ingredients, camphor stimulates the nerve endings in the skin and induces relief of pain and discomfort by masking moderate-to-severe deeper visceral pain with a milder pain arising from the skin at the level of innervation. When applied vigorously, it produces a rubefacient reaction.

Camphor has the same indications as those for methyl salicylate. Table 7-4 provides dosing information.

Concentrations higher than those recommended are not more effective and can cause more serious adverse reactions if accidentally ingested.[23] The risk of toxicity relates to both the concentration of camphor in the ingested product and the extent of absorption of camphor into the body. CNS toxicity, expressed primarily as tonic–clonic seizures, is the major toxicity and begins to occur as early as 10 minutes following ingestion. In children, 5 mL of a 20% camphor liniment is a potentially lethal dose, and death resulting from respiratory depression or complications of status epilepticus can occur.[32] Accordingly, preparations with camphor concentrations exceeding 11%, such as camphorated oil (camphor liniment), which is a solution of 20% camphor in cottonseed oil, are not considered safe for nonprescription use and have been removed from the market. However, even products considered safe and effective (e.g., vapo-rubs) have been associated with reports of serve adverse reactions with ingestion.[33] Gastric lavage and activated charcoal administered shortly after ingestion have been used to avoid continued toxicity.[34] Emesis will increase the risk of gastrointestinal toxicity and is generally avoided.

High doses of camphor can cause nausea, vomiting, colic, headache, dizziness, delirium, convulsion, coma, and death.

Placing camphor into the nostrils of an infant may cause immediate respiratory collapse. In 1994, the American Academy of Pediatrics Committee on Drugs noted that, although nonprescription camphor-containing preparations cannot exceed concentrations of 11%, camphor toxicity continues. The academy advised parents to be aware of this potential danger and recommended use of modalities that do not contain camphor.[35]

Menthol   Menthol is either prepared synthetically or extracted from peppermint oil (which contains a 30%–50% concentration of menthol). Menthol may be used safely in small quantities as a flavoring agent and has found wide acceptance in candy, chewing gum, cigarettes, cough drops, toothpaste, nasal sprays, and liqueurs.

At concentrations less than 1%, menthol depresses cutaneous receptor response (i.e., acts as an anesthetic), whereas it stimulates response in concentrations greater than 1.25% (i.e., acts as a counterirritant).

Recent studies have led to the identification of heat- and cold-sensitive receptors within sensory neurons called transient receptor potential (TRP) cation channels. There are five other TRP receptors, the most notable of which is the vanilloid receptor, TRPV1; capsaicin activates this receptor, providing a hot sensation. Topically applied menthol activates the TRPM8 menthol receptor (discovered in 2002), triggering the sensation of cold.[36] The initial feeling of coolness is soon followed by a sensation of warmth. The resultant cold sensation travels along pathways similar to the somatic pain sensations from the affected muscle or joint, which distracts from the sensation of pain.

Menthol, which has the same self-treatment indications as methyl salicylate, is also used as a permeability enhancer to increase absorption of other topically administered medications.[36] In smaller concentrations, menthol is commonly used for upper respiratory congestion and rhinitis (in cough drops and vapo-rubs). Menthol may also provide symptomatic relief of dyspnea.[37]

Table 7-4 provides dosing information for menthol. The fatal dose in humans is approximately 2 grams. In acute studies, however, menthol appears to be a substance of very low toxicity.[36]

Although of low occurrence, menthol use results in sensitization in certain individuals, causing symptoms such as urticaria, erythema, and other cutaneous lesions.[36]

Menthol is contraindicated in patients with hypersensitivity to the agent. Treatment should be discontinued if the patient develops irritation, rash, burning, stinging, swelling, or infection.

Methyl Nicotinate   Although nicotinic acid is inactive topically, methyl nicotinate readily penetrates the cutaneous barrier. Vasodilation and elevation of skin temperature result from very low concentrations, with higher penetration rates seen with hydrophilic mediums (i.e., gels). Studies have shown that indomethacin, ibuprofen, and aspirin significantly depress the skin's vascular response to methyl nicotinate. Because these three drugs suppress prostaglandin biosynthesis, it was concluded that the vasodilator response to methyl nicotinate is mediated, at least in part, by prostaglandin biosynthesis.[38]

Methyl nicotinate has the same indications as methyl salicylate. Table 7-4 provides dosing information.

Generalized vascular dilation can occur when methyl nicotinate passes through the skin into the circulatory system.

Susceptible persons who apply methyl nicotinate over large areas may experience a drop in blood pressure, a decrease in pulse rate, and syncope caused by generalized vascular dilation.

Capsicum Preparations   Capsicum preparations (capsaicin, capsicum, and capsicum oleoresin) are derived from the fruit of various species of plants of the nightshade family. Capsicum contains about 1.5% of an irritating oleoresin, the major component of which is capsaicin (0.02%). Capsaicin is the major pungent ingredient of hot (chili) pepper.

When applied to normal skin, capsaicin elicits a transient feeling of warmth through stimulation of the TRPV1 receptor.[39] More-concentrated solutions produce a sensation of burning pain. However, as a result of tachyphylaxis, this local effect diminishes with repeated applications. Capsicum preparations do not cause blistering or reddening of the skin, even in high concentrations, because they do not act on capillaries or other blood vessels.

The mechanism of action is thought to be directly related to capsaicin's effects on the depletion of substance P. This substance is found in slow-conducting, unmyelinated type C neurons that innervate the dermis and epidermis. It is released in the skin in response to endogenous (stress) and exogenous (trauma or injury) factors. It appears that pruritic stimuli along with pain impulses are conveyed to central processing centers by type C fibers in the skin, for which capsaicin has selective activity. Local application of capsaicin to the peripheral axon appears to deplete substance P from sensory neurons. The depletion occurs both peripherally and centrally, presumably as the result of impulse initiation. When substance P is released, burning pain occurs but abates with repeated applications. This initial burning sensation or the diminishing burn experienced with repeated applications can lead to adherence-related failures, and health care providers should inform their patient's about these effects and the importance of continuing therapy.

Capsaicin has the same indications as those of methyl salicylate. Capsaicin is used to reduce the pain, but not the inflammation, of rheumatoid arthritis and osteoarthritis, and is used in a wide variety of other pain disorders (e.g., postherpetic neuralgia, psoriasis, and diabetic neuropathy). The efficacy of capsaicin is difficult to assess when compared with placebo, owing to the difficulty in blinding patients because of the recognition of burning and stinging. For the treatment of musculoskeletal pain, capsaicin 0.025% used for 4 weeks would improve pain by at least 50% in one of every eight patients treated. Improved efficacy is seen with 0.075% used in the treatment of neuropathic pain, suggesting dose-related effects.[40]

Like menthol, capsaicin has been identified as a penetration enhancer. Concomitant administration with capsaicin enhances the penetration of naproxen through human skin, suggesting efficacy with combined therapy that is improved over that produced by either agent alone.[41] However, this combination is only speculative, given that it has not been clinically studied.

Table 7-4 lists dosing information for capsaicin. The optimal dose of this agent varies among patients. It appears that efficacy decreases and local discomfort increases when capsaicin is applied less often, because the drug's duration of action is 4 to 6 hours. Pain relief is usually noted within 14 days after therapy has begun, but relief will occasionally be delayed by as much as 4 to 6 weeks. Notably, because capsicum lots vary, the concentration range for capsaicin cannot be expressed as a percentage and must be calculated for each lot.

Once capsaicin has begun to relieve pain, its use must continue regularly three or four times a day to keep the pain from returning. If capsaicin treatment is stopped and the pain returns, treatment can be resumed. To reduce the likelihood of capsaicin reaching topically sensitive areas, such as mucous membranes, patients should be instructed to use a glove or plastic bag for application and wash their hands following use.

Overdose with use of capsaicin has not been reported, but use of topical preparations with concentrations greater than 1% have been associated with neurotoxicity and hyperalgesia.

Burning and stinging occur with the application of capsaicin in 40% to 70% of patients. However, this effect generally diminishes in intensity with continued use. If capsaicin gets into the eyes or on other sensitive areas of the body, it will cause a burning sensation. Concentrations greater than 0.025% have also been associated with a cough.[40]

Use in patients with hypersensitivity to capsaicin is contraindicated. The agent should be discontinued temporarily if skin breaks down (weeping, red, and presence of small ulcers), and the agent should not be applied to wounds or damaged skin.

Other Counterirritants   Allyl isothiocyanate, ammonia water, turpentine oil, and histamine dihydrochloride are also classified as Category I counterirritants by the FDA, but fewer commercially available preparations contain these ingredients. Most products that contain these ingredients also contain other topical analgesics, making any beneficial action or side effects of these products indistinguishable from other ingredients. In addition, very little evidence supports the efficaciousness of these compounds. Allyl isothiocyanate, ammonia water, and turpentine oil are rubefacients, and should be expected to have effects similar to those of methyl salicylate, whereas histamine dihydrochloride causes vasodilation, similar in action to methyl nicotinate.

Category III ingredients (insufficient data are available to establish safety and efficacy) include eucalyptus oil, trolamine salicylate, and topical NSAIDs. Despite this designation, several nonprescription products contain trolamine salicylate as the primary ingredient (Table 7-5).

Eucalyptus oil may produce some minor counterirritant effects, but it is not recommended for use as a counterirritant because of inconclusive efficacy data. Eucalyptus is often noted as an inactive ingredient in some products because of its characteristic odor.

Trolamine salicylate, although a salicylate salt, is not a counterirritant analgesic. Trolamine salicylate is absorbed through the skin and results in synovial fluid salicylate concentrations slightly below those of oral aspirin. The recommended topical dosage of trolamine salicylate for adults and for children 2 years and older is a 10% to 15% concentration applied to the affected area not more than three or four times a day.

Several studies led FDA to conclude that topical trolamine salicylate does not show any significant benefit over placebo in the treatment of musculoskeletal pain. Reports published after the review have shown limited effectiveness in alleviating neuralgia caused by unaccustomed strenuous exercise[42] and muscle soreness induced by a reproducible program of weight training.[43] Trolamine salicylate has also demonstrated improved playing time in musicians with localized pain in the arms, wrists, hands, and fingers, and improved pain and stiffness in patients with osteoarthritis of the hands.[44,45] Trolamine salicylate is still available over the counter and may be most useful to those patients who do not favor the localized irritation or the scent of Category I counterirritants.

Trolamine salicylate has the same drug interactions as other salicylates (see Chapter 5). Use is contraindicated in people with renal insufficiency or with hypersensitivity to trolamine or salicylates. People who have liver disease, hypoprothrombinemia (a deficiency of thrombin in the blood), or vitamin K deficiency, or who are scheduled for surgery or are chronic alcohol users should not use this agent. During use, the agent should not contact the eyes or mucous membranes.

TOPICAL NSAIDS

Topical NSAIDs are not currently available for nonprescription use in the United States, but FDA approved them for prescription use in 2007 (Flector, 1.3% diclofenac epolamine patch) for the treatment of acute pain caused by strains, sprains, or contusions. Topical NSAIDs have been used for years in Europe for the treatment of musculoskeletal pain. They are not counterirritants and presumably act locally in a manner analogous to their systemic mechanism of action. Their application on acute soft tissue strains and sprains, where the target tissue is situated closer to the skin surface, are reported to provide the benefits of oral NSAIDs with minimal systemic side effects.

Systematic reviews have concluded that topical NSAIDs are more effective than placebo in the treatment of musculoskeletal pain for short-term use, but they lose effectiveness beyond 2 weeks.[46,47] A well-designed trial of 1.5% topical diclofenac solution applied four times a day demonstrated symptomatic improvement in osteoarthritis of the knee following 12 weeks of treatment.[48] Dimethyl sulfoxide was used to help improve diclofenac penetration and also was present in the placebo. No significant gastrointestinal side effects were noted in the trial, but localized dryness and rash were more prevalent in the treatment group. Evidence to date suggests that topical NSAIDs provide effects on chronic knee pain comparable to those of systemic NSAIDs, with fewer systemic side effects.[49]

Combination Products

General guidelines for nonprescription drug combination products state that Category I active ingredients from the same therapeutic category should not ordinarily be combined, unless the combination is deemed safer or more effective and has enhanced patient acceptance or quality of formulation.[23] Four separate chemical and/or pharmacologic groups of counterirritants provide four qualitatively different types of irritation. Many marketed preparations aim for at least two such effects when greater potency is desired. Table 7-4 lists the individual ingredients and classifies them according to their relative potency and acceptable concentration ranges. Manufacturers may combine active ingredients from one group of counterirritants with one, two, or three other active ingredients, provided that each active ingredient is from a different group.

It is irrational to combine counterirritants with local anesthetics, topical antipruritics, or topical analgesics. Because these agents depress sensory cutaneous receptors, their effects oppose the counterirritant stimulation of cutaneous sensory receptors. It is also irrational to combine counterirritants with skin protectants, because the protectants oppose and may nullify counterirritant effects.

Preparation labels must list the active ingredients, including their concentrations, and must identify them by their officially recognized, established names. In addition, manufacturers voluntarily list ingredients on the label. Many manufacturers of combination products list only some of the active ingredients under the "active" heading, and many of the other pharmacologically viable products in the inactive ingredient section (e.g., BenGay Vanishing Scent Gel lists camphor, and Aspercreme Heat Pain Relieving Gel lists capsaicin under inactive ingredients). Although the concentrations of inactive ingredients are not listed, they are generally below therapeutically determined amounts and are added for reasons other than pain-relieving effects. The manner of use and the frequency of applications should also be indicated.[22]

Product Selection Guidelines

SPECIAL POPULATIONS

No significant variability in response has been noted among patients of different ages or racial backgrounds.

Variability related to the minimum age of patients, however, does exist in product labeling. According to the tentative final monograph published in the *Federal Register* in 1983, use of external analgesics, as labeled within the confines of the statement, is to be avoided in children younger than 2 years.[19] However, most available products elect to label the minimum age as older than 12 years, and some products (particularly capsaicin products) list 18 years and younger. This more restricted labeling is prudent considering the indications for the products and the potential for systemic absorption, but at this time this labeling is not mandated by law. Practitioners should follow labeling instructions for the products used. If a product is to be used in a child 18 years of age or younger, it should be used with caution and for the least amount of time necessary.

PATIENT FACTORS

The choice of treatment for acute pain syndromes and chronic conditions such as osteoarthritis is patient-dependent. In addition to nonpharmacologic treatment, oral therapy is often employed. One should consider a patient's history, taking note of exclusions for self-treatment, other medications the patient is taking, and any known allergies to medications. Topical therapy is used as an adjunct or substitute to oral therapy. If a counterirritant is selected, one with Category I ingredients should be recommended. Patients with precautions for the use of individual counterirritants should also be cautioned about the use of certain products, particularly combination products. Product concentrations are variable and, in general, the lowest effective dose should be recommended for the shortest duration needed.

PATIENT PREFERENCES

Factors that impact product selection include dosage form, ease of use, cost, and even odor of the preparation. Dosage forms available include solutions, liniments, gels, lotions, ointments, creams, and patches. Oleaginous preparations (ointments and oil-based liniments) have increased absorption compared with solutions, gels, lotions, and creams, but they are greasy and generally less acceptable to patients. The use of patches is becoming more popular, owing to their simple application and duration of action, but use of a patch eliminates any benefit of a therapeutic rubbing action.[3] With the exception of patches and solutions, topical products should be rubbed into the skin. Alcoholic liniments and gels may produce a response more intense than that of equal quantities in other preparations, and excessive rubbing should be avoided to reduce the risk of unpleasant burning sensations with these preparations. Additional information about formulation characteristics is described elsewhere.[50,51]

Complementary Therapies

A variety of complementary therapies containing many different compounds and ingredients are marketed for the management of pain. It is difficult to find well-designed controlled clinical trials for many of these agents in humans. The most commonly used products are glucosamine, chondroitin, methyl-sulfonyl-methane, and S-adenosyl-L-methionine. Additional products are summarized in Table 7-6.[52-61] Additional information on these products and other complementary therapies such as massage, chiropractic care, and acupuncture have been described elsewhere and are discussed in greater detail in Chapters 54 and 55, respectively.[52,53,62]

TABLE 7-6 Selected Complementary and Alternative Medicines Used for Treatment of Pain

Agent	Uses	Risks	Effectiveness
Botanical Medicines (*Scientific Name*)			
Cat's claw (*Uncaria tomentosa*)	OA, rheumatoid arthritis Other: HIV, GI ulcers, skin disorders, cancer	Bleeding risk with anti-coagulants	Trials mainly in animals and in vitro Anecdotal improvements[55]
Devil's claw (*Harpagophytum procumbens*)	OA, tendonitis, appetite stimulant	GI (higher doses), headache, tinnitus	Short-term improvement in low back pain similar to 12.5 mg rofecoxib[56]
Peppermint (*Mentha piperita*)	Myalgias (topical) Other (oral): irritable bowel syndrome, dyspepsia	Allergic reactions, respiratory collapse	Topical efficacy similar to menthol (*Note:* Herb contains menthol.)
Willow bark (*Salix* sp.)	Anti-inflammatory, pain	Gastric ulceration, hyper-sensitivity, bleeding, tinnitus, nausea and vomiting, skin rashes	Short-term improvement in low back pain similar to 12.5 mg of rofecoxib[56]
Nonbotanical Natural Medicines			
Chondroitin sulfate	OA	Mild GI pain and nausea	Improvement in pain and reduction in disease progression in patients with knee OA[53,57,58]
Glucosamine sulfate	OA	Mild GI complaints	Probable pain improvement and reduced disease progression in patients with knee OA[59] No benefit in patients with hip OA[60]
Methyl-sulfonyl-methane (MSM)	Acute and chronic pain (arthritis, bursitis, tendonitis)	Nausea, diarrhea, headache, pruritus, allergy symptoms	Pain improvement similar to glu-cosamine[54]
S-Adenosyl-L-methionine (SAMe)	OA	Multiple dose-dependent GI complaints	Improvement in functional limitation similar to NSAIDs, but delayed response and less pain improvement[61,62]

Key: GI, gastrointestinal; HIV, human immunodeficiency disorder; NSAID, nonsteroidal anti-inflammatory drug; OA, osteoarthritis.
Source: References 53–62.

Assessment of Musculoskeletal Injuries and Disorders: A Case-Based Approach

Routinely, the health care provider should inventory all past and present medications, including pain medications, and should note the patient's satisfaction with or preference for past treatments. In addition, the health care provider should ask about aspects of the patient's medical history that relate directly to the origin or treatment of pain.

Before an attempt is made to treat a pain complaint, the health care provider should qualify and quantify the pain. Inquiry about the cause, duration, location, and severity of pain, as well as factors that relieve and exacerbate the pain, will help assess the pain. Chapter 2 outlines effective strategies for obtaining information from patients about specific complaints. When a complaint of pain is expressed by a patient, the health care provider should use effective communication to gather the needed information including symptoms, characteristics, history, onset, location, and aggravating and remitting factors.

Using a pain scale helps to quantify the intensity of a patient's pain. With the numerical pain scale, the health care provider asks patients to rank the present pain on a scale of 0 to 10, with 0 being no pain and 10 being the worst pain the patient can imagine. Scores greater than 3 indicate the need for an intervention, as do any scores that increase 2 or more points on the 10-point scale. Initially, pain scores establish a baseline for pain

before treatment. In addition, a high pain score can be used to screen for patients who would be better served by seeking an appropriate medical evaluation. Pain scores also serve as a measuring device for therapeutic outcomes. In general, nonprescription medications are appropriate for numerical rating scale scores of 1 to 3. These medications may also be appropriate for scores of 4 or 5. Scores of 6 or higher indicate pain that requires medical referral. Other scales are available for pain rating in children (Faces Pain Scale), adolescents, people who do not speak English, and other special populations.

A chronic painful condition presents a different set of challenges. An observant health care provider should intervene with a patient who frequently or regularly purchases aspirin, other NSAID products, or acetaminophen. If additional interviewing indicates an inadequately treated pain problem, additional workup by an appropriate provider should be made. The workup will prevent unwanted long-term adverse consequences of drug therapy (e.g., renal impairment) as well as assist the patient in receiving the appropriate care for the pain problem. Education should be offered regarding the risks of inadequate treatment as well as the overuse of medications.

On the basis of the information collected, the health care provider can appropriately determine whether the patient may self-treat or should be referred for further evaluation. (Figure 7-2).

Cases 7-1 and 7-2 are examples of the assessment of patients with musculoskeletal injuries and disorders.

CASE 7-1

Relevant Evaluation Criteria	Scenario/Model Outcome
Information Gathering	
1. Gather essential information about the patient's symptoms, including:	
a. description of symptom(s) (i.e., nature, onset, duration, severity, associated symptoms)	Patient notes improved pain in knees following the addition of acetaminophen to her osteoarthritic regimen, but still has some pain (1 month ago, rated walking pain as 5/10; now it is 3/10).
b. description of any factors that seem to precipitate, exacerbate, and/or relieve the patient's symptom(s)	Walking long distances is difficult. Needs to rest at regular intervals. Patient notes that the acetaminophen she began taking seems to help, but it wears off midway through the day.
c. description of the patent's efforts to relieve the symptoms	Patient started Tylenol arthritis 1300 mg 1 month earlier and takes it 1–2 times a day (usually in the morning, sometimes at night).
2. Gather essential patient history information:	
a. patient's identity	Margaret Butler
b. age, sex, height, and weight	67-year-old female, 5 ft 2 in, 176 lb
c. patient's occupation	School bus driver
d. patient's dietary habits	Patient eats out 3–4 times a week at a buffet-style restaurant, snacks while driving bus, and does not use tobacco or drink alcohol.
e. patient's sleep habits	Sleeps 6–8 hours a night with no complaints
f. concurrent medical conditions, prescription and nonprescription medications, and dietary supplements	Osteoarthritis of bilateral knees was diagnosed within the preceding year; medical management suggested by provider at this time; initiated acetaminophen 1 month earlier. Calcium carbonate 600 mg (elemental) twice daily, multivitamin, and ranitidine occasionally for heartburn
g. allergies	NKA
h. history of other adverse reactions to medications	None
i. other (describe) _____	
Assessment and Triage	
3. Differentiate patient's signs/symptoms and correctly identify the patient's primary problem(s) (see Table 7-2).	Patient has osteoarthritis of the knee with improved symptoms on oral therapy.
4. Identify exclusions for self-treatment (see Figure 7-2).	PCP is aware of patient's status, which has improved recently with no alarming symptoms; self-treatment could be recommended. If, however, this patient's pain is worsening or does not improve with recommended treatment, the patient should discuss her care with her PCP.
5. Formulate a comprehensive list of therapeutic alternatives for the primary problem to determine if triage to a medical practitioner is required and share this information with the patient.	Options include: (1) Recommend nondrug measures (e.g., exercise, weight loss, use of cane). (2) Recommend adjustment of oral OTC analgesic to appropriate analgesic doses (i.e., acetaminophen 1300 mg [arthritis formula] every 8 hours). (3) Recommend adjunctive use of a topical counterirritant. (4) Recommend alternative therapy (e.g., glucosamine). (5) Refer patient to PCP for further assessment and treatment. (6) Take no action.
Plan	
6. Select an optimal therapeutic alternative to address the patient's problem, taking into account patient preferences.	The recommended therapy is exercise, rest, and weight loss, along with acetaminophen 1300 mg (arthritis formula) every 8 hours and a topical counterirritant applied 3–4 times a day to the knees.

C A S E   7 - 1 *(continued)*

Relevant Evaluation Criteria	Scenario/Model Outcome
7. Describe the recommended therapeutic approach to the patient.	Exercise 3–5 times/week by walking, biking, and/or stretching as tolerated. Exercise will improve circulation; weight loss will reduce pressure on the joint. Continue acetaminophen. Do not take any other product (prescription or non-prescription) that contains acetaminophen, because you risk taking too much acetaminophen. Capsaicin or other topical counterirritant is an appropriate agent to use in conjunction with oral therapy at this time.
8. Explain to the patient the rationale for selecting the recommended therapeutic approach from the considered therapeutic alternatives.	Because you are experiencing some benefit with acetaminophen, you should continue this therapy, but take it before the drug loses effectiveness to avoid recurrence of pain. Despite the improvement with acetaminophen, you may continue to have pain even when taking it. A topical counterirritant is a useful adjunct to effective oral therapy in osteoarthritis.

Patient Education

9. When recommending self-care with nonprescription medications, convey accurate information to the patient:	
a. appropriate dose and frequency of administration	(1) You should take the acetaminophen 1300 mg (arthritis formula) every 8 hours. You can skip the nighttime dose of acetaminophen if the pain does not disrupt your sleep. (2) Apply small amount of capsaicin 0.025% gel to knees 3 times daily.
b. maximum number of days the therapy should be employed	Chronically administered acetaminophen (as initially prescribed by the primary care provider), as well as topical capsaicin The response should be evaluated in 4 weeks. If helpful, continue; if not helpful, discontinue.
c. product administration procedures	Apply three times a day; you can apply the gel at the same time you take acetaminophen. Be sure to wash hands before and after application, and do not use an occlusive bandage. (See the box Patient Education for Musculoskeletal Injuries and Disorders.)
d. expected time to onset of relief	Some improvement will occur shortly after application, but maximal benefits will take up to 6 weeks.
e. degree of relief that can be reasonably expected	Osteoarthritis is a chronic condition for which acetaminophen and capsaicin assist with the perceived pain by the patient. You will continue to suffer from the condition, but you should expect a noticeable reduction in pain along with improved activities of daily living.
f. most common side effects	Capsaicin is expected to produce a localized burning-like sensation; however, this sensation is reduced within a few days with consistent application 3 times daily. Contamination of mucous membranes will produce significant discomfort because of the intense burning sensation.
g. side effects that warrant medical intervention should they occur	Localized rash. See the box Patient Education for Musculoskeletal Disorders and Injuries.
h. patient options in the event that condition worsens or persists	As noted, osteoarthritis is expected to persist. Pain improvement indicates continued therapy. No improvement or worsening of pain warrants further evaluation by medical provider.
i. product storage requirements	Keep out of the reach of children.
j. specific nondrug measures	Reduced signs and symptoms, as well as a slowed progression of the disease, can be obtained with exercise and weight loss, and should be undertaken as tolerated.
10. Solicit follow-up questions from patient.	Should I use the cream only when the pain happens or all the time?
11. Answer patient's questions.	This cream works better when it is applied 3–4 times a day consistently, rather than only once a day or as needed. You likely will not receive the full benefits of the therapy if you do not use the medication 3–4 times every day. Therefore, once it starts working, you should continue applying it.

Key: NKA, no known allergies; OTC, over-the-counter; PCP, primary care provider.

Relevant Evaluation Criteria	Scenario/Model Outcome
Information Gathering	
1. Gather essential information about the patient's symptoms, including:	
a. description of symptom(s) (i.e., nature, onset, duration, severity, associated symptoms)	Patient presents with a slight gait disturbance and wants to purchase some regular-strength aspirin and a heating patch. Patient notes that he was playing racquetball at the health club earlier in the day and twisted his ankle. He says that he had twisted it before, but this one "really hurt." When he had his ankle sprains in the past, he was always able to walk shortly afterward without much difficulty.
	Upon inspection, the patient has a swollen right ankle that is tender to the touch, but otherwise not visibly deformed. The patient has a diminished range of motion of his ankle with tenderness upon manipulation.
b. description of any factors that seem to precipitate, exacerbate, and/or relieve the patient's symptom(s)	The patient can still walk, but it is difficult and causes sharp pain in his ankle on a scale of 7/10.
c. description of the patent's efforts to relieve the symptoms	He applied an ice pack for 10 minutes at the gym after the sprain. He also elevated and rested the ankle at home for about an hour after the twist, which helped only a little.
2. Gather essential patient history information:	
a. patient's identity	Jack Mouser
b. age, sex, height, and weight	39-year-old male, 5 ft 11 in, 214 lb
c. patient's occupation	Information technologist
d. patient's dietary habits	Eats a balanced diet during the week, but eats "whatever" on the weekends
e. patient's sleep habits	No problems sleeping; sleeps about 7 hours a night
f. concurrent medical conditions, prescription and nonprescription medications, and dietary supplements	Mega-man multivitamin daily, occasional loratadine 10 mg daily for allergic rhinitis (not taking currently)
g. allergies	NKA
h. history of other adverse reactions to medications	None
i. other (describe) _____	Last ankle sprain occurred 2 weeks earlier. He intended to purchase ankle braces for his activities but has yet to do so.
Assessment and Triage	
3. Differentiate patient's signs/symptoms and correctly identify the patient's primary problem(s) (see Table 7-2).	Patient's presentation is consistent with an ankle sprain.
4. Identify exclusions for self-treatment (see Figure 7-2).	Patient does have limitations for self-treatment, because his mobility is lessened with the sprain, and he develops severe pain with movement.
5. Formulate a comprehensive list of therapeutic alternatives for the primary problem to determine if triage to a medical practitioner is required, and share this information with the patient.	Options include: (1) Refer patient to PCP for further assessment. (2) Recommend nonpharmacologic treatment (e.g., RICE therapy). (3) Recommend oral nonprescription analgesic (e.g., acetaminophen, nonsalicylate NSAIDs, or salicylate). (4) Recommend topical counterirritant. (5) Fit patient with crutches or cane. (6) Take no action.
Plan	
6. Select an optimal therapeutic alternative to address the patient's problem, taking into account patient preferences.	Refer patient to his primary care provider immediately to rule out severe injury or fracture and to determine degree of sprain. Recommend RICE therapy (see Table 7-3). Advise against aspirin or heat therapy at this time.

CASE 7-2 *(continued)*

Relevant Evaluation Criteria	Scenario/Model Outcome
7. Describe the recommended therapeutic approach to the patient.	Patients with gait disturbances and severe pain upon movement indicate a potentially severe sprain and should not be advised to self-treat.
8. Explain to the patient the rationale for selecting the recommended therapeutic approach from the considered therapeutic alternatives.	Your symptoms are consistent with an ankle sprain, but unlike your previous sprains, this sprain is more severe and should be evaluated by your health care provider before self-treatment. You should call your health care provider to be seen as soon as possible.

Patient Education

9. When recommending self-care with nonprescription medications and/or nondrug therapy, convey accurate information to the patient.	In the meantime, you should rest your ankle by elevating it on some pillows or in a recliner; then place ice over the ankle for 10- to 15-minute intervals about 4 times a day, and wrap the ankle in a bandage. You may take some nonprescription medication while waiting to be seen by your provider. You may choose from any of the nonprescription agents, but aspirin is not recommended because of its higher side effect profile. Also, heat should be avoided until after the swelling subsides.
a. appropriate dose and frequency of administration	Ibuprofen 400 mg every 8 hours as needed for pain
b. maximum number of days the therapy should be employed	Patient should be seen by provider as soon as possible and should self-treat only until evaluated.
c. product administration procedures	Take two 200 mg tablets every 8 hours as needed for pain relief. Take product with a little food to reduce gastrointestinal irritation.
d. expected time to onset of relief	Improvement in pain is expected within 30–60 minutes after taking the medication.
e. degree of relief that can be reasonably expected	Your pain will not go away completely, but you should be able to walk with a little less pain. Rest, ice application, and elevation are also helpful in this process of reducing the pain. Consider crutches or a cane to help with walking while the ankle heals and gait returns to normal.
f. most common side effects	Minimal with short-term use, but some gastrointestinal complaints may present.
g. side effects that warrant medical intervention should they occur	See the box Patient Education for Headache in Chapter 5.
h. patient options in the event that condition worsens or persists	At this time, this condition should be evaluated by the medical provider.
i. product storage requirements	Keep medication in container and away from children.
j. specific nondrug measures	See Table 7-3.
10. Solicit follow-up questions from patient.	Should I purchase ankle braces to help prevent these injuries in the future?
11. Answer patient's questions.	Certainly the best situation would be not to have any more ankle sprains. Unfortunately, certain sports and activities place patients at higher risk for these injuries. Properly designed footwear for a given sport is advisable. Because of the side-to-side movements in racquetball, a higher ankle shoe could be helpful in sprain prevention. Ankle braces are also available, and many are self-adjustable for a better fit. In addition, proper preparation for exercise, like stretching, could help lower the risk of injuries.

Key: NKA, no known allergies; NSAID, nonsteroidal anti-inflammatory drug; PCP, primary care provider; RICE, rest, ice, compression, elevation.

Patient Counseling for Musculoskeletal Injuries and Disorders

Consultation with the patient should include explanation of the expected benefit of any recommended medication, the appropriate dose and drug administration schedule, potential adverse reactions, potential drug–drug or drug–disease interactions, and self-monitoring techniques for assessing response to therapy. The consequences of nonadherence should be emphasized.

Printed materials reinforce verbal information. Many such pamphlets or single-page handouts are available from national professional societies (e.g., www.arthritis.org), including those that educate on various chronic pain syndromes such as osteoarthritis. These materials offer advice on exercise, diet, and sleep habits, and the advantages as well as disadvantages of pharmacologic therapy. Generally, these materials can be obtained for free or for a nominal delivery fee. Health care providers may wish to design their own supplementary materials.

Patients taking NSAIDs should be warned about possible drug–drug interactions, including antihypertensive medications, warfarin, aspirin, and phenytoin, and drug–disease interactions such as heart failure and renal insufficiency. Patients should be cautioned not to take more than the recommended nonprescription dose or to exceed the recommended duration of treatment. Duplication of acetaminophen and NSAIDs is probably more common than recognized, because patients often do not realize that nonprescription products contain the same or similar drugs found in their prescription drug. Failure to recognize this duplication can significantly increase the risk of serious adverse events and patients should be warned of the risk. In acute pain management, early administration of nonprescription analgesics should be employed to prevent escalating pain, with downward tapering of the analgesic doses as pain severity allows, generally 1 to 2 days after the precipitating event.

Patients should be instructed to notify their primary care provider whenever the pain changes in character or severity, or if new acute pain develops. Other sudden uncharacteristic pains may be harbingers of new tissue damage. Patients should be advised to obtain their prescriptions from as few prescribers as possible and to get their prescriptions drugs, nonprescription drugs, and complementary remedies at the same pharmacy to minimize the potential for drug interactions.

The box Patient Education for Musculoskeletal Injuries and Disorders lists specific information to provide patients about topical analgesics and preventive and nondrug measures.

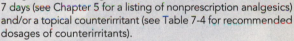

PATIENT EDUCATION FOR
Musculoskeletal Injuries and Disorders

The objectives of self-treatment are to (1) reduce the severity and duration of pain, (2) restore function of the affected area, (3) prevent reinjury and disability, and (4) prevent acute pain from becoming chronic persistent pain. Certain nondrug measures and nonprescription counterirritants can relieve the symptoms of pain from a sudden and recent muscle, tendon, or ligament injury; an overuse injury (tendonitis, bursitis, or repetitive stress injury); low back pain; or arthritis. For most patients, carefully following product instructions and the self-care measures listed here will help ensure optimal therapeutic outcomes.

Nondrug Measures

- For pain related to muscle or joint injuries, begin treatment with RICE therapy (see Table 7-3).
- For periodic muscle cramps, stretch and massage the affected area immediately; then rest or reduce activity of the muscle to allow it to loosen.
- For persistent cramps, apply heat to the affected area in the form of a warm wet compress, a heating pad, or a hot-water bottle.
- For osteoarthritis, try a combination of nondrug measures, including applying heat or cold to the affected area, supporting the area with splints, and doing range-of-motion and strength-maintenance exercises.

Preventive Measures

- To prevent muscle or joint strains and sprains, do warm-up and stretching exercises before playing sports or exercising, and wrap injured muscle or joint with protective bandage or tape.
- To prevent repetitive strain, exercise the muscles that are vulnerable to the injury, and use ergonomic controls to adjust posture, stresses, motions, and other damaging physical factors.
- To prevent tendonitis and cramps, warm up and stretch muscles before physical activity, drink sufficient fluids, and do not exercise to the point of exhaustion. To help prevent nocturnal leg cramps, raise the foot of the bed. If you have Achilles tendonitis, try wearing better-fitting shoes with heel lifts to reduce the symptoms.
- To prevent or reduce the occurrence of low back pain, do exercises to strengthen the muscles of the lower back and abdomen, and use assistive devices (i.e., cane or walker) if needed.
- To prevent or reduce the occurrence of osteoarthritis, avoid a sedentary lifestyle, keep the joints active, lose weight if overweight, and use assistive devices if needed.

Nonprescription Medications

- For mild-to-moderate muscle pain, take a nonprescription analgesic for no longer than 7 days (see Chapter 5 for a listing of nonprescription analgesics) and/or a topical counterirritant (see Table 7-4 for recommended dosages of counterirritants).
- Do not use counterirritants if your skin is abraded, sunburned, or otherwise damaged.
- When using counterirritants, wash your hands after application and before touching your eyes and mucous membranes, or before handling contact lenses.
- Gently rub a thin layer of counterirritant product into affected muscles or joints until you cannot see the product. Thick application of the product does not make the product work better.
- Do not put a tight bandage or dressing over an area treated with a counterirritant. Do not use warming devices with counterirritants.
- Do not treat a child 2 years of age or younger with counterirritants unless a primary care provider supervises the use.
- If you have arthritis, consult your doctor before attempting to treat your pain with counterirritants or with topical or internal analgesics.
- If you have asthma, and symptoms of wheezing and shortness of breath worsen while you are using a mentholated formulation, stop using it.
- Do not use any product containing salicylates (including aspirin, methyl salicylate, and trolamine salicylate) if you are receiving anticoagulation therapy (especially warfarin).
- If a counterirritant causes excessive redness and blistering or hives and vomiting, stop using it.

 If you experience nausea, vomiting, colic, and other unusual symptoms while using a product containing camphor, seek medical care immediately.

 If the pain was present for more than 2 weeks before you sought treatment or has worsened, consult a primary care provider.

 If the symptoms persist after more than 7 days of treatment or if the pain is constant and felt in any position, consult a primary care provider.

Evaluation of Patient Outcomes for Musculoskeletal Injuries and Disorders

The primary indicator of treatment effectiveness is the patient's perception of pain relief. If a patient reports the pain is still present or has worsened after 7 days of using nonprescription analgesics, the health care provider should refer the patient for further evaluation. In many instances, the lack of a return visit indicates a successful treatment regimen. Patients with minor sprains or strains will not require a second visit as the tissues heal and they return to normal function. If the health care provider has a good relationship with the patient, he or she may call the patient in a few days to determine whether the complaint has resolved. However, a patient who does return with signs of continued swelling, pain, or inflammation should be referred for medical evaluation. The continued pain may indicate an ongoing process that could lead to long-term disability or decreased mobility.

Key Points for Musculoskeletal Injuries and Disorders

➤ Self-treatment of patients presenting with pain secondary to an injury or a disorder of the musculoskeletal system should be limited to those with mild-to-moderate pain who have no exclusions for self-treatment such as a visibly deformed joint or systemic symptoms (Figure 7-2).

➤ Self-treatment of acute musculoskeletal injuries should include nondrug therapy, such as rest, ice, compression, and elevation (RICE). Heat therapy may also provide benefit after swelling abates.

➤ Patients self-treating the chronic pain of osteoarthritis should be advised to employ nondrug therapy such as weight loss, exercise and stretching, and use of assistive devices (i.e., cane).

➤ Clinicians should advise patients on the proper selection of a product for their musculoskeletal injury or disorder, taking into account the patient's preferences.

➤ Systemic analgesics are valid first-line treatments for the majority of musculoskeletal injuries and disorders. Acetaminophen is preferred in noninflammatory diseases, whereas NSAIDs are preferred if inflammation is present. Side effects and drug interactions should be considered before therapy is chosen (see Chapter 5).

➤ Topical counterirritants are useful for treatment of acute musculoskeletal injuries and as an adjunct in the treatment of chronic musculoskeletal disorders. They are to be used only topically and on skin that is intact. Patients should be advised not to use heating devices with topical counterirritants or to cover the counterirritant with a tight bandage.

➤ Complementary therapy with glucosamine may provide benefit in patients with mild-to-moderate osteoarthritis of the knee.

➤ Health care providers should monitor the outcome of self-treatments and advise patients who self-treat their acute musculoskeletal injury to seek medical attention if their symptoms do not improve after 7 days.

➤ Health care providers can assist patients through direct support and education by counseling in a nonjudgmental way and providing other resources to help manage their pain.

REFERENCES

1. Loeser JD, Melzack R. Pain: an overview [review]. *Lancet.* 1999;353: 1607–9.
2. Mense S, Simons DG, Russell IJ. *Muscle Pain: Understanding Its Nature, Diagnosis and Treatment.* Baltimore: Lippincott William & Wilkins; 2001: 1–20.
3. Hacher Research Group. Analgesics: the relentless search for relief. *Drug Top.* December 13, 2004.
4. Stewart WF, Ricci JA, Chee E, et al. Lost productive time and cost due to common pain conditions in the US workforce [see comment]. *JAMA.* 2003;290:2443–54.
5. Pendleton A, Arden N, Dougados M, et al. EULAR recommendations for the management of knee osteoarthritis: report of a task force of the Standing Committee for International Clinical Studies Including Therapeutic Trials (ESCISIT) [see comment]. *Ann Rheum Dis.* 2000;59:936–44.
6. Burt VL, Harris T. The third National Health and Nutrition Examination Survey: contributing data on aging and health. *Gerontologist.* 1994; 34:486–90.
7. Yaksh TL. Pharmacology and mechanisms of opioid analgesic activity [review]. *Acta Anaesthesiol Scand.* 1997;41(1 pt 2):94–111.
8. *Meyler's Side Effects of Drugs.* 14th ed. Oxford: Elsevier Science; 2000.
9. FDA Alert: Fluoroquinolone Antimicrobial Drugs and Tendinitis and Tendon Rupture. Available at: http://www.fda.gov/cder/drug/InfoSheets/HCP/fluoroquinolonesHCP.htm. Last accessed: August 12, 2008.
10. Wilson JF. In the clinic. Low back pain [review]. *Ann Intern Med.* 2008; 148(9):ITC5-1–16.
11. Chou R, Qaseem A, Snow V, et al. Diagnosis and treatment of low back pain: a joint clinical practice guideline from the American College of Physicians and the American Pain Society. *Ann Intern Med.* 2007; 147:478–91.
12. McAlindon TE, Wilson PW, Aliabadi P, et al. Level of physical activity and the risk of radiographic and symptomatic knee osteoarthritis in the elderly: the Framingham study. *Am J Med.* 1999;106:151–7.
13. Wright A, Sluka KA. Nonpharmacological treatments for musculoskeletal pain [review; see comment]. *Clin J Pain* 2001;17:33–46.
14. Chou R, Huffman LH. Nonpharmacologic therapies for acute and chronic low back pain: a review of the evidence for an American Pain Society/American College of Physicians Clinical Practice Guideline. *Ann Intern Med.* 2007;147:492–504.
15. Recommendations for the medical management of osteoarthritis of the hip and knee: 2000 update. American College of Rheumatology Subcommittee on Osteoarthritis Guidelines [see comment]. *Arthritis Rheum.* 2000;43:1905–15.
16. Chattem Issues URGENT Voluntary Nationwide Recall of Icy Hot® Heat Therapy™ Products. Available at: http://www.fda.gov/oc/po/firmrecalls/chattem02_08.html. Last accessed: August 12, 2008.
17. Zhang W, Doherty M, Arden N, et al. EULAR evidence based recommendations for the management of hip osteoarthritis: report of a task force of the EULAR Standing Committee for International Clinical Studies Including Therapeutics (ESCISIT) [review; see comment]. *Ann Rheum Dis.* 2005;64:669–81.
18. Wegman A, van der Windt D, van Tulder M, Stalman W, de Vries T. Nonsteroidal antiinflammatory drugs or acetaminophen for osteoarthritis of the hip or knee? A systematic review of evidence and guidelines [review; see comment]. *J Rheumatol.* 2004;31:344–54.
19. Lee C, Straus WL, Balshaw R, et al. A comparison of the efficacy and safety of nonsteroidal antiinflammatory agents versus acetaminophen in the treatment of osteoarthritis: a meta-analysis. *Arthritis Rheum.* 2004;51: 746–54.
20. Nikles CJ, Yelland M, Del MC, et al. The role of paracetamol in chronic pain: an evidence-based approach [review]. *Am J Ther.* 2005;12:80–91.
21. Hippisley-Cox J, Coupland C. Risk of myocardial infarction in patients taking cyclo-oxygenase-2 inhibitors or conventional non-steroidal antiinflammatory drugs: population based nested case-control analysis. *BMJ.* 2005;330:1366.
22. Department of Health and Human Services. External analgesic products for over-the-counter human use; establishment of a monograph and notice of proposed rulemaking. *Fed Regist.* 1979;44:69768–874.

23. Department of Health and Human Services. External analgesic drug products for over-the-counter human use: tentative final monograph. *Fed Regist*. 1983;48:5852–69.

24. Cross SE, Anderson C, Roberts MS. Topical penetration of commercial salicylate esters and salts using human isolated skin and clinical microdialysis studies. *Br J Clin Pharmacol* 1998;46:29–35.

25. Roberts MS, Favretto WA, Meyer A, et al. Topical bioavailability of methyl salicylate. *Austral N Z J Med*. 1982;12:303–5.

26. Bell AJ, Duggin G. Acute methyl salicylate toxicity complicating herbal skin treatment for psoriasis. *Emerg Med*. 2002;14:188–90.

27. Heng MC. Local necrosis and interstitial nephritis due to topical methyl salicylate and menthol. *Cutis*. 1987;39:442–4.

28. Danon A, Ben-Shimon S, Ben-Zvi Z. Effect of exercise and heat exposure on percutaneous absorption of methyl salicylate. *Eur J Clin Pharmacol*. 1986;31:49–52.

29. Methyl salicylate. In: Reynolds JEF, ed. *Martindale—The Extra Pharmacopoeia*. 33rd ed. London: The Royal Pharmaceutical Society; 2002:1090–1.

30. Littleton F Jr. Warfarin and topical salicylates. *JAMA*. 1990;263:2888.

31. Yip AS, Chow WH, Tai YT, et al. Adverse effect of topical methylsalicylate ointment on warfarin anticoagulation: an unrecognized potential hazard. *Postgrad Med J*. 1990;66:367–9.

32. Siegel E, Wason S. Camphor toxicity [review]. *Pediatr Clin North Am*. 1986;33:375–9.

33. Gouin S, Patel H. Unusual cause of seizure [review]. *Pediatr Emerg Care* 1996;12:298–300.

34. Lahoud CA, March JA, Proctor DD. Campho-Phenique ingestion: an intentional overdose [review]. *South Med J*. 1997;90:647–8.

35. Camphor revisited: focus on toxicity. Committee on Drugs. American Academy of Pediatrics. *Pediatrics*. 1994;94:127–8.

36. Patel T, Ishiuji Y, Yosipovitch G. Menthol: a refreshing look at this ancient compound [review]. *J Am Acad Dermatol*. 2007;57:873–8.

37. Eccles R. Menthol: effects on nasal sensation of airflow and the drive to breathe [review]. *Curr Allergy Asthma Rep*. 2003;3:210–4.

38. Wilkin JK, Fortner G, Reinhardt LA, et al. Prostaglandins and nicotinate-provoked increase in cutaneous blood flow. *Clin Pharmacol Ther*. 1985;38:273–7.

39. Pingle SC, Matta JA, Ahern GP. Capsaicin receptor: TRPV1 a promiscuous TRP channel [review]. *Handb Exp Pharmacol*. 2007;179: 155–71.

40. Mason L, Moore RA, Derry S, et al. Systematic review of topical capsaicin for the treatment of chronic pain [review; see comment]. *BMJ*. 2004;328:991.

41. Degim IT, Uslu A, Hadgraft J, et al. The effects of Azone and capsaicin on the permeation of naproxen through human skin. *Int J Pharm*. 1999; 179:21–5.

42. Politino V, Smith SL, Waggoner WC. A clinical study of topical 10% trolamine salicylate for relief of delayed-onset exercise-induced arthralgia/myalgia. *Curr Ther Res*. 1985;38:321–7.

43. Hill DW, Richardson JD. Effectiveness of 10% trolamine salicylate cream on muscular soreness induced by a reproducible program of weight training. *J Orthop Sports Phys Ther*. 1989;11:19–23.

44. Hochberg FH, Lavin P, Portney R, et al. Topical therapy of localized inflammation in musicians: a clinical evaluation of Aspercreme versus placebo. *Med Probl Perform Arts*. 1988;3:9–14.

45. Rothacker DQ, Lee I, Littlejohn TW. Effectiveness of a single topical application of 10% trolamine salicylate cream in the symptomatic treatment of osteoarthritis. *J Clin Rheumatol*. 1998;4:12.

46. Moore RA, Tramer MR, Carroll D, et al. Quantitative systematic review of topically applied non-steroidal anti-inflammatory drugs [see comment] [erratum appears in BMJ 1998;316:1059]. *BMJ*. 1998;316:333–8.

47. Lin J, Zhang W, Jones A, et al. Efficacy of topical non-steroidal anti-inflammatory drugs in the treatment of osteoarthritis: meta-analysis of randomised controlled trials [see comment]. *BMJ*. 2004;329:324.

48. Roth SH, Shainhouse JZ. Efficacy and safety of a topical diclofenac solution (Pennsaid) in the treatment of primary osteoarthritis of the knee: a randomized, double-blind, vehicle-controlled clinical trial. *Arch Intern Med*. 2004;164:2017–23.

49. Underwood M, Ashby D, Cross P, et al. Advice to use topical or oral ibuprofen for chronic knee pain in older people: randomised controlled trial and patient preference study. *BMJ*. 2008;336:138–42.

50. Block LH. Medicated topicals. In: Hoover JE, ed. *Remington: The Science and Practice of Pharmacy*. 20th ed. Easton, Pa: Mack Publishing; 2000:836–57.

51. Nairn JG. Solutions, emulsions, suspensions, and extracts. In: Hoover JE, ed. *Remington*. 20th ed. Easton, Pa: Mack Publishing; 2000:721–52.

52. Soeken KL. Selected CAM therapies for arthritis-related pain: the evidence from systematic reviews [review]. *Clin J Pain*. 2004;13–8.

53. Usha PR, Naidu MU. Randomised, double-blind, parallel, placebo-controlled study of oral glucosamine, methylsulfonylmethane and their combination in osteoarthritis. *Clin Drug Investig*. 2004;24:353–63.

54. Hardin SR. Cat's claw: an Amazonian vine decreases inflammation in osteoarthritis [review]. *Complement Ther Clin Pract*. 2007;13(1):25–8.

55. Gagnier JJ, van Tulder MW, Berman B, et al. Herbal medicine for low back pain: a Cochrane review [review] [erratum appears in *Spine*. 2007; 32:1931]. *Spine* 2007;32(1):82–92.

56. Richy F, Bruyere O, Ethgen O, et al. Structural and symptomatic efficacy of glucosamine and chondroitin in knee osteoarthritis: a comprehensive meta-analysis [see comment]. *Arch Intern Med*. 2003;163:1514–22.

57. Michel BA, Stucki G, Frey D, et al. Chondroitins 4 and 6 sulfate in osteoarthritis of the knee: a randomized, controlled trial. *Arthritis Rheum*. 2005;52:779–86.

58. Reginster JY, Bruyere O, Neuprez A. Current role of glucosamine in the treatment of osteoarthritis [review]. *Rheumatology*. 2007;46:731–5.

59. Rozendaal RM, Koes BW, van Osch GJVM, et al. Effect of glucosamine sulfate on hip osteoarthritis: a randomized trial. *Ann Intern Med*. 2008; 148:268–77.

60. Najm WI, Reinsch S, Hoehler F, et al. S-Adenosyl methionine (SAMe) versus celecoxib for the treatment of osteoarthritis symptoms: a double-blind cross-over trial. [ISRCTN36233495]. *BMC Musculoskelet Disord*. 2004;5(1):6.

61. Soeken KL, Lee WL, Bausell RB, et al. Safety and efficacy of S-adenosylmethionine (SAMe) for osteoarthritis [review; see comment]. *J Fam Pract* 2002;51:425–30.

62. Little CV, Parsons T. Herbal therapy for treating osteoarthritis [review]. *Cochrane Database Syst Rev*. 2001;1:CD002947.

Reproductive and Genital Disorders

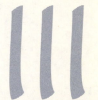

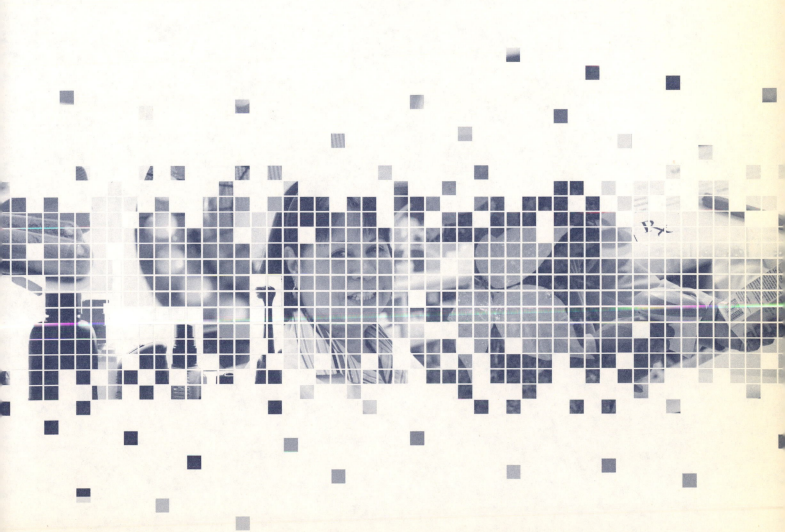

Vaginal and Vulvovaginal Disorders

Nicole M. Lodise and Leslie A. Shimp

Vaginal symptoms are among the most common health concerns of women of reproductive age and older women. Vaginal symptoms may be experienced by women from all walks of life: married or single, sexually active or sexually abstinent, homosexual or heterosexual, and premenopausal or postmenopausal.[1] Vaginal discharge is among the top 25 reasons that women seek medical care and accounts for more than 10 million office visits annually.[2] It is estimated that about 65% of women who experience vaginal symptoms have a vaginal infection caused by one of the three most common vaginal infections: bacterial vaginosis (BV), vulvovaginal candidiasis (VVC), and trichomoniasis.[1] Infections may also be mixed, with more than one causative organism.

Vaginal infections are generally perceived as minor health problems. However, bacterial vaginosis and trichomoniasis have been linked to significant health problems.[3,4] In view of the large number of women seeking diagnosis and treatment for vaginal infections, and the approval of nonprescription vaginal antifungal compounds for the treatment of VVC, it is imperative that practitioners understand the therapeutic management of these three vaginal infections and the appropriate patient education for VVC.

Women may also self-treat noninfectious vaginal symptoms such as vaginal dryness, atrophic vaginitis, and allergic or chemical dermatologic reactions.[1,4] Many women use douches for routine vaginal hygiene. Unfortunately, women are not always knowledgeable about normal vaginal health and the consequences of improper douching methods. Therefore, consumers and health care providers need to understand vaginal health to make informed and appropriate decisions about self-care for vaginal symptoms and vaginal hygiene.

The vagina is an elastic fibromuscular tube that extends 8 to 10 cm from the vulva to the uterus. The upper end of the vagina is closed except for the cervical os, the opening to the cervix. Anatomically, the vagina lies between the urinary bladder and the rectum. At the lower (vulvar) end of the vagina are the Bartholin's glands, which produce secretions in response to sexual stimulation. At puberty, under the influence of estrogen, the vaginal lining changes to stratified squamous epithelium, which contains glycogen. The glycogen is acted on by *Lactobacillus* bacteria to form lactic acid, which creates an acidic pH of about 4 to 4.5. This acidic pH and the production of hydrogen peroxide by these bacteria help protect the vagina from infection with other bacteria. After menopause, thinning of the vaginal lining occurs, the lactobacilli decline, and the pH rises.[5]

The mature vagina is colonized by a variety of organisms. *Lactobacillus* species predominate, accounting for 90% to 95% of the vaginal flora. Another 5 to 10 species of bacteria (e.g., *Corynebacteria, Streptococcus, Staphylococcus epidermidis, Gardnerella vaginalis, Peptostreptococcus,* and *Bacteroides*) are present in small quantities, with anaerobes being more common than aerobes.[4,6] *Candida albicans* and *Escherichia coli* may also be isolated in the absence of active infection in about 20% of women.[6,7]

Various factors influence the vaginal ecosystem (i.e., the number and type of endogenous organisms, vaginal pH, and glycogen concentration), including hormonal fluctuations of the menstrual cycle; aging; certain diseases (e.g., diabetes mellitus); use of various medications (e.g., contraceptive preparations, hormones, and antibiotics); douching; and number of sex partners (increasing exposure to additional organisms).

The healthy vagina is cleansed daily by secretions that lubricate the vaginal tract. Normal vaginal discharge (leukorrhea) consists of about 1.5 grams of vaginal fluid daily, which is odorless, clear or white, and viscous or sticky.[7] This physiologic discharge consists of endocervical mucus, serum transudate from vaginal capillary beds, endogenous vaginal flora, and epithelial cells.[6,7] An increase in vaginal secretions is normal during ovulation, during pregnancy, following menses, and with sexual excitement or emotional flares. An alteration in vaginal secretions may also occur in response to vaginal irritants (e.g., feminine hygiene deodorant products, vaginal douches, and other cleansing products); contraceptive products and devices; or use of tampons.

DIFFERENTIATION OF COMMON VAGINAL INFECTIONS

The signs and symptoms for various vaginal infections may be similar, and the characteristic symptoms that often help distinguish infections may be absent (Table 8-1). Both patients and clinicians may have difficulty accurately determining the type of infection on the sole basis of symptoms.[8,9]

Accurately distinguishing VVC from BV and trichomoniasis is especially important because of the availability of nonprescription antifungal therapy. In addition, BV and trichomoniasis

TABLE 8-1 Differentiation of Common Vaginal Infections

Classic Symptoms[1]	Differentiating Signs and Symptoms	Etiology and Epidemiology[1]
Bacterial Vaginosis		
Thin (watery), off-white or discolored (green, gray, tan), sometimes foamy discharge; unpleasant "fishy" odor that increases after sexual intercourse or with elevated vaginal pH (e.g., menses)	Vaginal irritation, dysuria, and itching less frequent with BV than with VVC or trichomoniasis[19] Malodor strongly associated with BV; absence of malodor virtually rules out BV Increased vaginal discharge ("wetness") more common with BV than with VVC or trichomoniasis	Polymicrobial infection resulting from imbalance in normal vaginal flora with increase in *G. vaginalis* and anaerobes (*Peptostreptococcus, Mobiluncus, Prevotella,* and *Mycoplasma hominis*) and decrease in lactobacilli Risk factors: new sexual partner, African American race, use of IUD, douching, receptive oral sex, tobacco use (smoking alters vaginal flora), and prior pregnancy Possible protective factors: use of female hormones, including OC, and condoms Responsible for 33% of vaginal symptoms Predominately affects young sexually active women but can arise spontaneously regardless of sexual activity; found in 12% of virginal adolescents; lower prevalence in postmenopausal women, even with use of postmenopausal hormones
Trichomoniasis		
Copious, malodorous, yellow-green (or discolored), frothy discharge; pruritus; vaginal irritation; dysuria No symptoms initially in ~50% of affected women Most men are asymptomatic and serve as reservoirs of the disease	Erythema and vulvar edema can occur with this infection[9] Yellow discharge: increased likelihood of trichomoniasis	STI caused by *Trichomonas vaginalis,* a protozoan Risk factors: multiple sex partners, new sexual partner, nonuse of barrier contraceptives, and presence of other STIs Responsible for 15%–20% of vaginal infections
Vulvovaginal Candidiasis		
Thick, white ("cottage cheese") discharge with no odor; normal pH (see text for detailed information; also referred to as "yeast infection" or "moniliasis")	Presence of erythema, itching, and/or vulvar edema, and absence of malodor: increased likelihood of VVC; thick, "cheesy" discharge: strongly predictive of VVC[9,18]	Organisms: *C. albicans, Candida glabrata, Candida tropicalis,* and *Saccharomyces* Some medications: antibiotics, immunosuppressants No identifiable cause for most infections Responsible for 20%–25% of vaginal infections

Key: BV, bacterial vaginosis; HIV, human immunodeficiency virus; IUD, intrauterine device; OC, oral contraceptive; PID, pelvic inflammatory disease; STI, sexually transmitted infection; UTI, urinary tract infection; VVC, vulvovaginal candidiasis.

are associated with potential complications such as pelvic inflammatory disease (PID), urinary tract infections, cervicitis, endometriosis, preterm labor, and tubal infertility, in addition to the facilitation of transmission of human immunodeficiency virus (HIV).[3,10,11]

Given the availability of nonprescription topical vaginal antifungal preparations and the cost and inconvenience of an office evaluation, many patients prefer to self-treat empirically for presumed VVC. In a study by Foxman et al.,[12] women with at least one physician–diagnosed episode and a reported presumed episode of VVC within the preceding 2 months were as likely to self-diagnose VVC as to contact a prescriber by phone or through an office visit. Women who reported having four or more episodes of VVC were the most likely to self-diagnose.

Sales of nonprescription vaginal antifungals are greater than the predicted number of VVC cases, illustrating the difficulty with accurate self-diagnosis.[13] Recent studies indicate that many women have trouble identifying VVC on the basis of their symptoms.[9,14] One study found that when women who had previously

been diagnosed with VVC read a description of the classic symptoms of the infection, only 35% could accurately recognize it.[15] Similarly, among a group of women who purchased a nonprescription vaginal antifungal to self-treat for vaginal symptoms only about half had a candidal infection when they were evaluated by a primary care provider.[14] Ferris and coworkers[14] found that women with a greater number of lifetime vaginal candidal infections were more likely to make an error in self-diagnosis.

The symptom most apt to differentiate a candidal vaginal infection from that of bacterial vaginosis and trichomoniasis is the absence of an offensive odor of the vaginal discharge.[16]

Noninfectious conditions that may be confused with vaginal infections are vulvovaginal irritation or pruritus caused by allergic or hypersensitivity reactions. These reactions may be a result of allergy to latex; spermicides; vaginal lubricants containing potential irritants (e.g., propylene glycol); or anesthetics (used by males to delay ejaculation).[4] Irritation secondary to douches, feminine hygiene products, soaps/detergents, or frequent use of panty liners or sanitary napkins may also cause these reactions.[4] In

Complications[2,3,10,11]	Treatment
PID, UTI, cervicitis, endometriosis, and infections after gynecologic surgical procedures Risks for pregnant patients: preterm labor and low-birth-weight infants May facilitate transmission of HIV	Topical 2% clindamycin inserted vaginally for 7 days or metronidazole 0.75% gel 5 g inserted vaginally twice daily for 5 days Oral metronidazole single 2 g dose 7-day oral course of metronidazole 500 mg twice daily or clindamycin 300 mg twice daily Povidine/iodine 5 g vaginal suppositories inserted twice daily for 14–28 days Oral/vaginal *L. acidophilus* or yogurt Routine treatment of sexual partners not warranted
Increased risk for low-birth-weight infants and tubal infertility May facilitate transmission of HIV	Metronidazole 2 g as single dose or 500 mg twice daily for 7 days Tinidazole 2 g as single dose (new option for metronidazole-resistant infections) Successful treatment requires concurrent treatment of sexual partner(s) and avoidance of sexual intercourse until patient and partner(s) have completed therapy and are asymptomatic
Increased risk of other infections	Typically does not include male partners (Table 8-2)

addition, urethral irritation and dysuria resulting from vulvovaginitis may be mistaken for a urinary tract infection.

Inappropriate use of vaginal antifungal products does have some risks, including (1) unnecessary use of the antifungal agent and (2) delay in effective treatment and possible delay in treatment of a serious condition. The risks of exposure to the vaginal antifungals in the absence of VVC are minor—primarily local irritation and the cost of therapy.[13] Labeling instructions advise patients to seek help for persistent symptoms and, if these guidelines are followed, the delay in treatment from misdiagnosis will likely present few serious consequences for most women. However, repeated use of nonprescription agents for persistent or recurrent symptoms can delay appropriate therapy with potentially significant health implications and may allow transmission of infections. A study evaluated the use of pH devices in symptomatic women. Nearly 57% of women who believed they had a yeast infection did not, which was confirmed by self-testing with the pH device and an examination by a health care provider.[17] The use of pH self-testing devices may be beneficial in reducing inappropriate

self-treatment with antifungals. Two products to test vaginal pH have recently been marketed: Fem-V Vaginal Infection Test and Vagisil Screening Kit for Vaginal infections.

Table 8-1 describes the classic symptoms of the three common vaginal infections as well as the symptoms that women typically experience.[1–3,9–11,18,19]

VULVOVAGINAL CANDIDIASIS

Vulvovaginal candidiasis (also referred to as "yeast infection" and "moniliasis") is second only to BV as the most common vaginal infection, accounting for approximately 20% to 25% of cases of vaginitis. VVC is uncommon prior to menarche, but by age 25 about 50% of women will have had one or more episodes of VVC.[6] A study of 2000 women found that 6.5% of women 18 years of age and older reported experiencing an episode of

VVC within the previous 2 months.[12] Black women reported three times the number of VVC episodes (17.4% of women) compared with white women (5.8%) or women of other races or ethnic groups (4.8%).[12] Recurrent infections (defined as four or more infections within a 1-year period) occur in fewer than 5% of women.[3] About 20% of women may be colonized with *Candida albicans* without experiencing vaginal symptoms.[9]

Pathophysiology of Vulvovaginal Candidiasis

Candida fungi are the causative organisms of this vaginal infection, with about 80% to 92% of cases caused by *C. albicans*.[3] The incidence of non–*C. albicans* infections has increased in the past two decades; *Candida glabrata, Candida tropicalis,* and *Saccharomyces cerevisiae* now account for a significant minority of candidal vaginal infections.[3,7] This increase may be a result of the widespread use of nonprescription antifungals, short courses of azole therapy, and long-term suppressive therapy with azole antifungals.[3]

No precipitating factor is identified for most episodes of VVC. However, a number of physiologic and behavioral factors have been studied as possible risk factors for VVC. The risk factors discussed below are not consistently associated with symptomatic candidal vaginitis, and their presence does not clearly establish an increased likelihood of VVC in a patient with vaginal symptoms. Most women with sporadic and infrequent candidal vaginitis do not have a readily apparent "cause" for the infection.[3] Modification of factors linked to VVC is not warranted for most patients.[1]

Pregnancy, high-dose estrogen oral contraceptives, and estrogen replacement therapy (ERT) may increase vaginal susceptibility to candidal infections by increasing the glycogen content of the vagina. However, studies do not support an increased risk for candidal infections with low-dose estrogen oral contraceptives, and studies on risk during pregnancy or use of postmenopausal ERT are inconsistent.[20,21] Vaginal pH increases during menstruation, which may predispose menstruating women to cyclic fungal vaginal infections. During the reproductive years, the vaginal epithelium cells are thick and contain an abundant amount of glycogen.[22] These cells exfoliate and continually provide the lactobacilli with the glycogen to produce lactic acid.[22] At menopause, there is a decline in glycogen caused by a decrease in epithelial cells, leading to a decrease in lactic acid production and an increase in vaginal pH, which can alter vaginal ecology and may also predispose to vaginal infections. Women with diabetes mellitus are known to be at greater risk for skin and vaginal candidal infections, particularly if glycemic control is poor.

A number of patients (25%–70% in several studies) report developing candidal vaginal infections during or just after treatment with broad-spectrum antibiotics such as tetracycline, ampicillin/amoxicillin, and cephalosporins.[23,24] The proposed mechanism is a decrease in normal vaginal flora, especially lactobacilli, allowing an overgrowth of *Candida* organisms. However, neither an increase in vaginal *Candida* organisms nor a decrease in lactobacilli occurs in all women who have taken antibiotics.

Patients who are taking systemic corticosteroid, antineoplastic, or immunosuppressant drugs may be at increased risk for developing candidal infections. This risk is well-known for certain patient populations such as recipients of an organ transplant and patients with HIV infection.

An increased frequency of VVC is associated with the onset of regular sexual activity. However, neither the number of sexual partners nor the frequency of sexual intercourse is related to the occurrence of VVC episodes.[3] There is some evidence suggesting an increase in risk associated with receptive oral sex.[1] In addition, use of an intrauterine or vaginal sponge contraceptive has been shown to increase the risk for VVC.[3]

Studies do not demonstrate a consistent association between tight-fitting, nonabsorbent clothing or pantyhose and vaginal candidal infections. However, clothing of this type may increase risk by creating a warm and moist environment. Some studies have suggested that foods that may increase urinary sugar (e.g., dietary sugars, refined carbohydrates, milk, and artificial sweeteners) may increase risk for candidal vaginal infections.[1,2] It has been suggested that consumption of yogurt may have a potential prophylactic benefit against VVC.[25] More studies are needed to determine the influence of diet as a preventive or risk factor for candidal vaginal infections.

The treatment of candidal vaginal infections does not typically include treatment of the male partner. If treatment is necessary, topical imidazoles may be applied to the affected area twice a day for 2 to 4 weeks. No controlled studies have shown that treatment of male partners prevents recurrence of candidal vaginal infections in women. However, in cases of recurrent infections, male partners may be treated with a topical imidazole.

Clinical Presentation of Vulvovaginal Candidiasis

The characteristic signs, symptoms, and complications of VVC are described in Table 8-1. Fungal vaginal infections typically do not affect vaginal pH, whereas a pH greater than 4.5 indicates a bacterial or trichomonal vaginal infection. Vaginal pH testing devices use pH to assist consumers in distinguishing candidal vaginal infections that can be self-treated from infections requiring medical evaluation and prescription drug therapy. The Fem-V Vaginal Infection Test (panty liner) and the Vagisil Screening Kit for Vaginal Infections (vaginal swab) both use a color test to determine vaginal pH; Fem-V also measures the wateriness of the vaginal discharge. Both products have a number of limitations to use; testing cannot occur until (1) 72 hours after use of any vaginal preparation such as a contraceptive spermicide or antifungal product, (2) 48 hours after sexual intercourse or douching, and (3) 5 days after a menstrual period. These products are easy to use and are inexpensive (approximately $ 5.00 per test).

Treatment of Vulvovaginal Candidiasis

The treatment of VVC is determined by the severity of symptoms and the frequency of episodes. VVC can be categorized as uncomplicated or complicated; recurrent VVC is a type of complicated infection.[16] Complicated infections occur in only about 5% of women. These more severe infections may occur because of host factors—an inability of normal factors to prevent candidal colonization—or the presence of fungal organisms that are more resistant to azole antifungal therapy.

Treatment Goals

The goals of therapy for vaginal fungal infections are (1) relief of symptoms, (2) eradication of the infection, and (3) reestablishment of normal vaginal flora.

A single course of drug therapy is effective in achieving these goals for virtually all patients. However, a small percentage of patients will experience persistent or recurrent infections and will require prolonged therapy or higher doses of medication.

General Treatment Approach

Self-treatment of VVC with nonprescription antifungal therapy can be appropriate for patients with uncomplicated disease (infrequent episodes, mild-to-moderate symptoms), whereas women with complicated (more severe symptoms, or concurrent predisposing illness or medications) or recurrent infections should be referred for assessment and treatment by a primary care provider. (See Figure 8-1 for a list of exclusions for self-care.)

By definition, recurrent VVC occurs when a woman experiences at least four (documented) infections within a 12-month period.[3] Patients with such symptoms should be evaluated for the possibility of a mixed infection or a strain of candidal infection other than *C. albicans,* which may be resistant to standard therapy. Recurrent candidal infections often require long-term suppressive prophylactic therapy. About two-thirds of surveyed physicians report seeing patients who had delayed treatment because of inappropriate use of nonprescription products.[24] In addition, frequent or recurrent episodes of VVC may be an early sign of HIV infection or diabetes. The Food and Drug Administration (FDA) now requires labels of nonprescription products to include a warning similar to the following:

Symptoms that return within 2 months or infections that do not clear up easily with proper treatment require medical evaluation. Possible causes of the infection include pregnancy or a serious underlying medical disorder, such as diabetes or a damaged immune system (including damage from infection with HIV, the virus that causes acquired immunodeficiency syndrome).

Preventive measures are not a standard part of therapy for vaginal fungal infections. However, women with infections that are more frequent or are not responsive to antifungal therapy may try dietary changes; nondrug measures (e.g., avoidance of nonabsorbent clothing); or alteration in other drug therapy known to be a risk factor for VVC. A 3- to 4-month trial of these approaches will reveal whether they are useful for individual patients.[1] Figure 8-1 outlines the appropriate approach to treating the patient with vaginal symptoms.

Nonpharmacologic Therapy

Decreased consumption of sucrose and refined carbohydrates, as well as consumption of yogurt containing live cultures (see Complementary Therapies), have been suggested as measures to decrease VVC, particularly for women who experience recurrent infections.[1,2,25]

Discontinuing a drug known to increase susceptibility to vaginal fungal infections might be effective in decreasing the incidence of this disorder. Low-dose oral contraceptives are unlikely to contribute to the occurrence of VVC, but they might be discontinued to see whether the frequency of infection is altered. Patients taking broad-spectrum antibiotics or immunosuppressants should consult their primary care provider before discontinuing these medications.

Pharmacologic Therapy

Vaginal Antifungals

Currently, a nonprescription, FDA-approved imidazole (butoconazole, clotrimazole, miconazole, or tioconazole) product is the recommended initial therapy for uncomplicated VVC, and relief of external vulvar itching and irritation associated with the infection. These products are available as vaginal creams, suppositories, and tablets. Tables 8-2 and 8-3 provide proper dosing and administration guidelines, respectively.

The major antifungal effect of the imidazole compounds is accomplished by altering the membrane permeability of the fungi. These agents inhibit cytochrome P450 enzymes in the fungal cell membrane, thereby decreasing synthesis of the essential fungal sterol ergosterol. The reduced membrane ergosterol content is accompanied by a corresponding increase in lanosterol-like methylated sterols. These lanosterol-like sterols cause structural damage to fungal membranes, resulting in the loss of normal membrane function.

Topical vaginal imidazole preparations are not appreciably absorbed. Systemic absorption of butoconazole, clotrimazole, miconazole, and tioconazole is about 1.7%, between 3% and 10%, 1.4% and negligible amounts of a vaginal dose, respectively.[26] Fungicidal clotrimazole concentrations are detectable in the vaginal fluid for up to 3 days after a single 500 mg dose.

Side effects from topical imidazoles are minimal and include vulvovaginal burning, itching, and irritation in 3% to 7% of patients.[20] These side effects are more likely to occur with the initial application of the vaginal preparation and are similar to symptoms of the vaginal infection. Abdominal cramps (3%), penile irritation, and allergic reactions (3%–7%) are uncommon, and headache may occur in up to 9% of women.[1]

Because of the limited absorption of topical antifungals, drug interactions are unlikely. However, a case report documented an interaction between miconazole vaginal suppositories (100–200 mg) and warfarin.[27] In this patient, international normalized ratio (INR) levels were significantly increased on two occasions when vaginal miconazole was used. Miconazole and warfarin are both metabolized by cytochrome P4502C9; concurrent use may decrease the clearance of warfarin and increase unbound drug. The prescriber should be contacted to consider reducing the dose of warfarin during concurrent therapy to avoid an increase in INR. Nonprescription vaginal antifungal product information warns women using warfarin in combination with these products that bleeding or bruising might occur. Aside from an allergy to the imidazoles, there are no contraindications to use of the vaginal imidazoles.

Pharmacotherapeutic Comparison

Studies have shown the imidazoles to be equally effective, with effectiveness rates of approximately 80% to 90%.[3,6] Different treatment durations have been studied. Miconazole single-dose and 7-day treatments were compared, resulting in similar overall cure rates with significantly faster rates of symptom relief by day 3 in the 3-day group compared with the 7-day treatment groups.[28] Butoconazole nitrate 2% single-dose cream has also been compared with miconazole 7-day treatment, resulting in nonsignificant differences in cure rates.[29] Seven-day regimens of clotrimazole and miconazole, 3-day regimens of butoconazole,

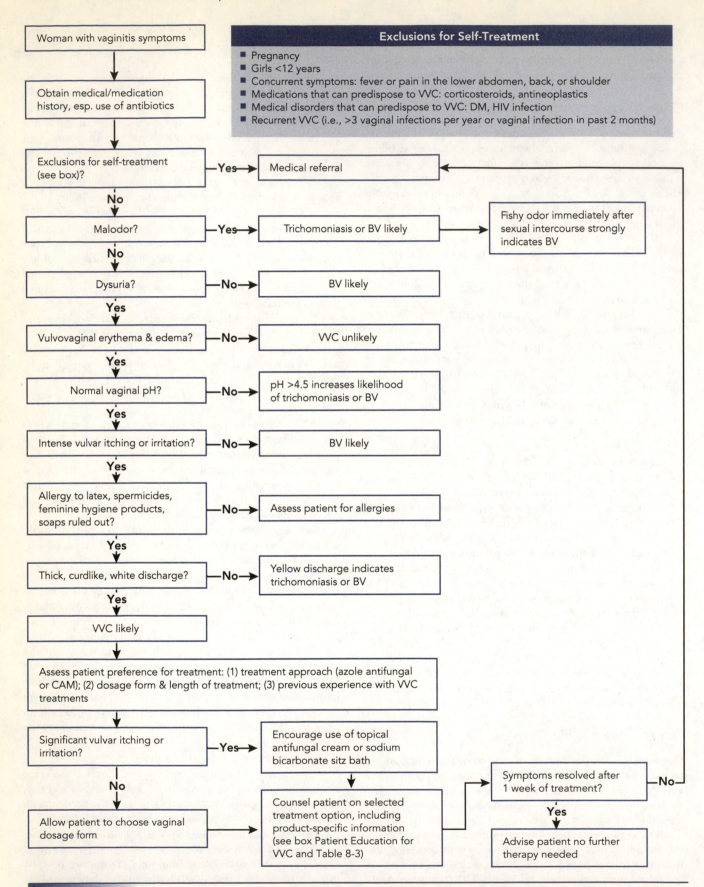

TABLE 8-2 Selected Vaginal Antifungal Products and Their Dosages

Primary Ingredient	Trade Name	Dosage
Butoconazole Nitrate Products		
Butoconazole nitrate 2%	Mycelex-3 Cream	Insert cream into vagina daily for 3 days; apply to vulva twice daily as needed for itching.
Clotrimazole Products		
Clotrimazole 1%	Gyne-Lotrimin 7 Cream Mycelex-7 Cream	Insert cream into vagina daily for 7 days; apply to vulva twice daily as needed for itching.
Tablet: clotrimazole 100 mg	Mycelex-7 Combination Pack	Insert tablet into vagina daily for 7 days; apply cream to vulva twice daily for itching.
Cream: clotrimazole 1% Clotrimazole 2%	Gyne-Lotrimin 3 Cream	Insert cream into vagina daily for 3 days; apply to vulva twice daily for itching.
Miconazole Nitrate Products		
Cream: miconazole nitrate 2% Suppository: miconazole nitrate 1200 mg	Monistat 1 Combination Pack Monistat 1 Daytime Ovule	Apply cream to vulva twice daily as needed for itching; insert suppository into vagina daily (morning or at bedtime) for 1 day.
Cream: miconazole nitrate 2% Suppository: miconazole nitrate 200 mg	Monistat 3 Combination Pack[a] M-zole 3 Combination Pack	Apply cream to vulva twice daily as needed for itching; insert suppository into vagina daily for 3 days.
Miconazole nitrate 4%	Monistat 3 Cream[a]	Insert cream into vagina daily for 3 days; apply to vulva twice daily as needed for itching.
Miconazole nitrate 100 mg	Monistat 7 Suppository	Insert suppository into vagina daily for 7 days.
Miconazole nitrate 2%	Monistat 7 Cream Femizole-M Cream	Insert cream into vagina daily for 7 days; apply to vulva twice daily as needed for itching.
Cream: miconazole nitrate 2% Suppository: miconazole nitrate 100 mg	Monistat 7 Combination Pack M-zole 7 Combination Pack	Apply cream to vulva twice daily as needed for itching; insert suppository into vagina daily for 7 days.
Tioconazole Products		
Tioconazole 6.5%	Vagistat-1 Ointment 1-Day Ointment	Insert ointment into vagina daily for 1 day.

[a] Prefilled applicators are available for this product.

clotrimazole, and miconazole, and 1-day regimens of clotrimazole, miconazole, and tioconazole are available without a prescription. Monistat 1 has also been approved for insertion in the morning or at bedtime. A similar cure rate exists for the daytime and bedtime treatments.[30] Table 8-2 lists the recommended nonprescription dosage regimens for products containing these ingredients. Information on currently available prescription and nonprescription products and regimens for acute infections, recurrent infections, and prophylactic therapy is presented in several reviews.[1–3,16]

Several nonspecific, nonprescription vaginal preparations, including Vagisil and Yeast-Gard (benzocaine and resorcinol) and Vaginex (tripelennamine), are also available. These agents are used for the relief of itching; however, they do not address the cause of the itching in the case of VVC. The use of these agents for VVC is rarely, if ever, appropriate given the obvious advantages of the azole antifungals, including superior efficacy, improved patient compliance associated with ease of use, less frequent local reactions, and shorter treatment durations. The nonspecific products and medicated douches are more appropriate for vaginal and vulvar irritation and itching. They should be used for a limited time or on the advice of a primary care provider. (See Table 8-4 for additional examples of these products.)

Product Selection Guidelines

SPECIAL POPULATIONS

Self-treatment of VVC is not appropriate for girls younger than 12 years. This condition is rare in premenarchal girls, and any vaginal symptoms in this age group warrant a medical referral to determine the cause. Vaginal infections in prepubertal children may indicate potential sexual abuse.[31]

Treatment of VVC in pregnancy should consist of one of the imidazoles (butoconazole, clotrimazole, or miconazole); however, when possible, withholding treatment during the first trimester may be preferable.[32] Self-treatment during pregnancy is not appropriate. Prescriber assessment is important to evaluate for complications (e.g., elevated blood sugar) and to assess for other vaginal organisms, because bacterial vaginosis and trichomoniasis have the potential for adverse pregnancy outcomes. Breast-feeding women can use any of the nonprescription vaginal antifungals.[20]

No special considerations are necessary to treat geriatric patients presenting with a VVC infection.

TABLE 8-3 Guidelines for Applying Vaginal Antifungal Products

1. Start treatment at night before going to bed. Lying down will reduce leakage of the product from the vagina.
2. Wash the entire vaginal area with mild soap and water, and dry completely before applying the product.
3. *Vaginal cream:* (If prefilled applicators are being used, skip to step 4.) Unscrew the cap; place the cap upside down on the end of the tube. Push down firmly until the seal is broken. Attach the applicator to the tube by turning the applicator clockwise. Squeeze the tube from the bottom to force the cream into the applicator. Squeeze until the inside piece of the applicator is pushed out as far as possible and the applicator is completely filled with cream. Remove the applicator from the tube. *Vaginal tablets/suppositories:* Remove the wrapper and place the product into the end of the applicator barrel.
4. While standing with your feet slightly apart and your knees bent, as shown in drawing A, or while lying on your back with your knees bent, as shown in drawing B, gently insert the applicator into the vagina as far as it will go comfortably.
5. Push the inside piece of the applicator in and place the cream as far back in the vagina as possible. To deposit vaginal tablets/suppositories, insert the applicator into the vagina and press the plunger until it stops.
6. Remove the applicator from the vagina.
7. After use, recap the tube (if using cream). Then clean the applicator by pulling the two pieces apart and washing them with soap and warm water.
8. If desired, wear a sanitary pad to absorb leakage of the vaginal antifungal. Do not use a tampon to absorb leakage.
9. Continue using the product for the length of time specified in the product instructions. Use the product every day without skipping any days, even during menstrual flow.

A

B

PATIENT PREFERENCES

Selection of cream, tablet, or suppository formulations can be left to patient preference; some patients may prefer the convenience of prefilled applicators. Studies have found that women who have previously experienced VVC prefer shorter courses of therapy than do women who have not had a prior infection; physicians tend to prefer longer courses of therapy.[1] If vulvar symptoms are significant, a cream preparation, or the combination of a cream with vaginal suppositories or tablets is preferred.

Complementary Therapies for Vaginitis

An alternative approach to treating VVC is the use of *Lactobacillus* preparations. The rationale for use of these preparations is to reestablish normal vaginal flora and inhibit overgrowth of *Candida* organisms. Data on the effectiveness of this approach are limited; one study that treated five women with positive vaginal cultures for *C. albicans* found 4 of the 5 women had negative cultures after administration of *Lactobacillus* GG suppositories for 7 days.[25] However, another study examining the usefulness of *Lactobacillus* and other probiotic bacteria administered orally, vaginally, and by both routes found that none of the regimens protected against the development of postantibiotic VVC.[33] However, eating yogurt with live cultures (8 ounces daily) may be of some benefit in preventing recurrent VVC.[25] (For more information on probiotics, see Chapter 24.)

Home remedies such as vaginal douches of yogurt or vinegar have also been used to treat this condition but are generally not effective. However, use of a sodium bicarbonate sitz bath may provide prompt relief of vulvar irritation associated with a candidal vaginal infection before antifungal agents can provide benefit[21,34]:

- Add 1 teaspoon sodium bicarbonate to 1 pint of water.
- Add 2 to 4 tablespoons of the solution to 2 inches of bath water.
- Sit in the sitz bath or bathtub for 15 minutes as needed for symptom control.

Some women may prefer herbal products to manage VVC. An herbal product used for the treatment of VVC is tea tree oil (vaginal preparations).[35,36] Tea tree oil has antibacterial and antifungal properties, and *Lactobacillus* organisms are more resistant to tea tree oil than are organisms associated with BV. A 200 mg vaginal suppository containing tea tree oil is also available commercially. It is used nightly for 6 nights. The possibility of allergic dermatitis exists. (For an in-depth discussion on tea tree oil, see Chapter 54.)

Gentian violet (a dye available in community pharmacies) is an old treatment for VVC, which is generally used today as therapy for resistant candidal infections. It is available on the nonprescription market and can be used as topical therapy; a tampon can be soaked in the dye and inserted into the vagina. The tampon is left in the vagina for several hours or overnight. Often a single application is adequate, but tampons saturated with gentian violet can be used once or twice a day for up to 5 consecutive days. The major disadvantage of using gentian violet is that it can stain fabrics and skin.[20]

Another option for the treatment of VVC is boric acid. The regimen is boric acid 600 mg in a size 0 gelatin capsule inserted vaginally once or twice daily for 14 days. Boric acid 5% in lanolin can be applied topically for vulvar irritation.[2,3,37] Boric acid therapy is particularly useful for non–*C. albicans* infections, which are more likely to be resistant to the azole antifungals. High short–term cure rates have been reported (85%–95%) when boric acid is used following treatment failure with another antifungal.[37,38] For resistant cases, the therapy is used twice weekly for longer durations. Boric acid can be toxic and teratogenic; human fatalities have been reported from oral ingestion.[37] Boric acid capsules may be compounded in community pharmacies, and counseling should be provided to explain

TABLE 8-4 Selected Products for Vaginal Itching and Irritation	
Primary Ingredients	**Trade Names**
Benzocaine Products[a]	
Benzocaine 6%; benzethonium chloride 0.1%	Lanacane Crème
Benzocaine 5%; resorcinol 2%	Vagi-Gard Advanced Sensitive Cream
	Vagisil Anti-itch Original Formula
Benzocaine 20%; resorcinol 3%	Vagisil Maximum Strength
	Vagi-Gard Maximum Strength Cream
Benzocaine 5%; benzalkonium chloride 0.13%	Vagi-Gard Cream
Hydrocortisone Products[b]	
Hydrocortisone 0.5%	Cortef Feminine Itch Cream
	Massengill Medicated Towelette
Hydrocortisone 1%	Gyne-cort Female Cream
Povidone/Iodine Products	
Povidone/iodine 10%	Betadine Medicated Suppository[c]
Povidone/iodine 0.3% (in disposable bottles)	Betadine Premixed Medicated Disposable Douche
	Massengill Medicated Disposable Douche
	Summer's Eve Special Care Medicated Douche
Homeopathic Products	
Pulsatilla (28X); Candida albicans (28X)	Yeast-Gard Suppository[d]
Candida parapsilosis (28X)	
Pulsatilla (28X)	Yeast-X Suppository[e]
Other Products	
Cornstarch; aloe; mineral oil	Summer's Eve Feminine Powder[f]
	Vagisil Feminine Powder[f]
Tripelennamine	Vaginex[g]

[a] Apply benzocaine products externally.
[b] Apply hydrocortisone products externally; avoid prolonged use; may use concomitantly with antifungal products.
[c] Use 1 povidone/iodine suppository nightly for 7 days.
[d] Use 1 Yeast-Gard suppository daily for 7 days.
[e] Use 1 Yeast-X suppository daily as needed.
[f] Apply feminine powders externally to absorb moisture.
[g] Apply Vaginex externally 3 or 4 times/day.

that the capsule should not be ingested and that pregnant women should not use boric acid.

Assessment of Vulvovaginal Candidiasis: A Case-Based Approach

Many episodes of VVC are uncomplicated and can be effectively treated by topical antifungal agents.[3,21] In particular, women who experience episodes that are sporadic and uncomplicated (i.e., healthy women who are not immunocompromised and have no predisposing drug therapy) and women who predictably experience VVC following a course of antibiotic therapy are the best candidates for self-treatment.[21,23]

Determining the appropriateness of self-care and ascertaining the likelihood of the presence of a candidal infection are important initial steps in advising a patient about the management of vaginal symptoms with nonprescription therapy.

Practitioners can advise patients when it is appropriate to self-treat for vaginal symptoms consistent with VVC, and when medical evaluation, including pelvic examination and laboratory examination of vaginal secretions, is indicated. Self-treatment is most appropriate when the woman meets the following four criteria:

1. Vaginal symptoms are infrequent (i.e., no more than three vaginal infections per year and no vaginal infection within the past 2 months).
2. At least one previous episode of VVC was medically diagnosed.
3. Current symptoms are mild to moderate, and consistent with the characteristic signs and symptoms of VVC—in particular, a nonmalodorous discharge.
4. If measured, vaginal pH should be 4.5 or lower.

Case 8-1 is an example of assessment of a patient with VVC.

Relevant Evaluation Criteria	Scenario/Model Outcome
Information Gathering	
1. Gather essential information about the patient's symptoms, including:	
a. description of symptom(s) (i.e., nature, onset, duration, severity, associated symptoms)	Patient is experiencing vulvar redness and itching with a noticeable white, thick discharge.
b. description of any factors that seem to precipitate, exacerbate, and/or relieve the patient's symptom(s)	Patient experienced an onset of symptoms after waking up this morning.
c. description of the patient's efforts to relieve the symptoms	She washed the perineal area, which relieved the itching for a short time.
2. Gather essential patient history information:	
a. patient's identity	Jillian Augusta, administrative assistant
b. age, sex, height, and weight	23-year-old female, 5 ft 5 in, 129 lb
c. concurrent medical conditions, prescription and nonprescription medications, and dietary supplements	Yasmin 1 daily, multivitamin 1 daily, calcium (600 mg) twice daily, ibuprofen 2 tablets (200 mg) every 4–6 hours as needed
d. allergies/other adverse reactions to medications	NKDA
e. other (describe) _____	The patient has been diagnosed with VVC infections twice before (per her medical history). Her last vaginal infection was 2 years ago. Her current symptoms are similar to her previous VVC infections.
Assessment and Triage	
3. Differentiate patient's signs/symptoms and correctly identify the patient's primary problem(s) (see Table 8-1).	She has vulvar redness, itching, and a white, thick discharge without malodor, which are consistent with a vaginal candidal infection.
4. Identify exclusions for self-treatment (see Figure 8-1).	None
5. Formulate a comprehensive list of therapeutic alternatives for the primary problem to determine if triage to a medical practitioner is required and share this information with the patient.	Options include: (1) Refer patient for medical evaluation. (2) Recommend self-treatment with a nonprescription vaginal antifungal product. (3) Suggest that patient consider the use of an OTC vaginal preparation for relief of her itching and irritation until she can see her PCP. (4) Take no action.
Plan	
6. Select an optimal therapeutic alternative to address the patient's problem, taking into account patient preferences.	The patient has classic symptoms associated with VVC. She has had two previous VVC infections. She has no chronic medical problems. She is also a good candidate for self-treatment, because she is in a monogamous relationship and not at risk for STIs. (See Figure 8-1.)
7. Describe the recommended therapeutic approach to the patient.	You have several choices of nonprescription vaginal antifungal products. Because you have vulvar itching, a cream preparation or a combination pack will probably provide the best relief of your symptoms. See the box Patient Education for Vulvovaginal Candidiasis, or VVC, for instructions on proper use.
8. Explain to the patient the rationale for selecting the recommended therapeutic approach from the considered therapeutic alternatives.	This treatment is appropriate because you have the characteristic symptoms of VVC, your symptoms are mild to moderate, you have no contraindications to self-treatment, and you have infrequent vaginal infections. See your PCP if your symptoms do not improve within 3 days or are not gone within a week, if the vaginal discharge changes (particularly if it becomes malodorous), or if symptoms return within the next 2 months.

C A S E   8 - 1 *(continued)*

Relevant Evaluation Criteria	Scenario/Model Outcome
Patient Education	
9. When recommending self-care with non-prescription medications and/or nondrug therapy, convey accurate information to the patient:	
a. appropriate dose and frequency of administration	Miconazole cream: Insert vaginally once daily for 3 days; apply externally to the vulva as needed for itching.
b. maximum number of days the therapy should be employed	3 days
c. product administration procedures	See Table 8-3.
d. expected time to onset of relief	Relief should occur in 24–48 hours; often some relief occurs within hours of the first application.
e. degree of relief that can be reasonably expected	All symptoms should be resolved within a week after beginning treatment.
f. most common side effects	Vulvovaginal burning and itching
g. side effects that warrant medical intervention should they occur	Significant stinging, burning, or itching that persists beyond the first 48 hours of treatment
h. patient options in the event that condition worsens or persists	See your PCP if symptoms do not improve in 3 days or worsen.
i. product storage requirements	Product should be stored in a cool area; storage in the bathroom or bedside is appropriate for ease of use.
j. specific nondrug measures	None
10. Solicit follow-up questions from patient.	(1) Are any of the nonprescription vaginal antifungal products better than any others? Are some regimens more effective than others?
	(2) Is yogurt consumption helpful in reducing VVC infections?
11. Answer patient's questions.	(1) No. All of the products and regimens are equally effective.
	(2) Daily intake of yogurt can be beneficial. It may have a prophylactic benefit against VVC infections.

Key: NKDA, no known drug allergy; OTC, over-the-counter; PCP, primary care provider; STI, sexually transmitted infection; VVC, vulvovaginal candidiasis.

Patient Counseling for Vulvovaginal Candidiasis

Providers counseling patients who are considering self-treatment with vaginal antifungals should emphasize the importance of (1) limiting self-treatment to appropriate circumstances (e.g., presence of mild-to-moderate classic symptoms, infrequent vaginal symptoms, and predictable antibiotic–associated VVC) and (2) seeking medical evaluation if symptoms persist beyond a week after treatment, if symptoms recur within 2 months, or if vaginal symptoms occur more than three times in a 12-month interval. For patients concurrently taking warfarin, the risk–benefit of temporarily reducing the dose of warfarin needs to be carefully considered; patients should be referred to the practitioner who monitors their warfarin therapy.

Patients should be informed that a short course of a nonprescription vaginal antifungal product will kill the "yeast" organisms that caused the infection. Label instructions should also be reviewed with the patient, stressing that the antifungal is to be used only once a day for the length of time specified on the label. The provider should advise the patient that symptomatic relief will likely begin within a day or so but that it may take a week for complete resolution of symptoms. The patient should also be advised of signs and symptoms that indicate medical attention is needed. The box Patient Education for Vulvovaginal Candidiasis lists specific information to provide patients.

Evaluation of Patient Outcomes for Vulvovaginal Candidiasis

Symptoms of VVC should improve within 2 to 3 days of initiation of therapy and resolve within 1 week. The length of treatment (particularly for 1- to 3-day treatments) does not directly correspond to the time of resolution of symptoms.

The practitioner should advise the patient to call to discuss treatment effectiveness (continued or altered symptoms) and the importance of adherence to the course of treatment. Persistent symptoms or new-onset symptoms that are incompatible with

PATIENT EDUCATION FOR
Vulvovaginal Candidiasis

The goals of self-treatment are to (1) cure the vaginal fungal infection and (2) reestablish normal vaginal flora. Carefully following the product instructions and the self-care measures listed here will help ensure optimal therapeutic outcomes.

Nondrug Measures

- If significant irritation of the vulva is present, use a sodium bicarbonate sitz bath to provide relief and give the antifungal medication time to become effective.
- If you have recurrent infections, try eating yogurt (1 cup per day of live culture yogurt), and decreasing sugar and refined carbohydrates in your diet.

Nonprescription Medications

- Insert the antifungal product into the vagina once a day, preferably at bedtime to minimize leakage from the vagina. Use a sanitary pad or panty liner to avoid staining of underwear.
- See Table 8-3 for instructions on administering vaginal antifungals. You should have significant relief of symptoms within 24–48 hours. Some relief is often apparent within hours after the first dose. However, the length of treatment (particularly for 1- to 3-day treatments) does not directly correspond to the time of resolution of symptoms.
- Continue the therapy for the recommended length of time, even if your symptoms are gone. Stopping treatment early is one of the most common reasons for recurrence of vaginal symptoms and, possibly, occurrence of difficult-to-treat organisms.
- Note that vaginal antifungals can be used during a menstrual period. If desired, wait and treat the infection after menses ends. Do not, however, interrupt a course of therapy because your period begins.
- Do not use tampons or douche while using a vaginal antifungal product and for 3 days after use.

- Although side effects are uncommon, the first dose of the antifungal may cause some vaginal burning and irritation, and a few women (about 1 in 10) experience a headache.
- Refrain from sexual intercourse during treatment with the vaginal antifungal. Vaginal lubricants and vaginal spermicides should not be used at the same time as the vaginal antifungal. Vaginal antifungals can damage latex condoms and diaphragms, and may result in unreliable contraceptive effects. Do not use these contraceptives during therapy or for 3 days after therapy, because the antifungal medication remains in the vagina for several days.

Consult Physician First

- Do not use vaginal antifungals if
  —You are less than 12 years old.
  —You are pregnant.
  —You have diabetes mellitus, are HIV-positive or have AIDS, or have impaired immune function, including use of medications that may impair function of the immune system.
- If you are breast-feeding, consult a primary care provider before using a vaginal antifungal.

 Seek medical attention if symptoms do not improve within 3 days, or if symptoms persist beyond 7 days.

 Seek medical attention if vaginal symptoms worsen or change, especially if the vaginal secretions begin to smell bad, become frothy, or discolored; or other symptoms (e.g., abdominal tenderness) occur. These events may indicate that the *Candida* (yeast) organisms are resistant to the nonprescription therapy or that another type of vaginal infection is present.

VVC are reasons for advising the patient to see her primary care provider.

ATROPHIC VAGINITIS

Atrophic vaginitis is inflammation of the vagina related to atrophy of the vaginal mucosa secondary to decreased estrogen levels.

An estimated 10% to 40% of postmenopausal women have symptomatic atrophic vaginitis, but only 20% to 25% of symptomatic women seek treatment.[39] Dyspareunia, a symptom sometimes related to inadequate vaginal lubrication or atrophic vaginitis, is common. In one primary care study, 46% of sexually active women of all ages reported dyspareunia; this value compares with other studies that reported a prevalence of 17% to 34% (a result of varying definitions of dyspareunia).[40]

Pathophysiology of Atrophic Vaginitis

During menopause, the postpartum period, and breast-feeding, the vaginal epithelium becomes thin, and vaginal lubrication declines secondary to a decrease in estrogen levels. Women may experience atrophic vaginitis and associated dyspareunia during these intervals.[20,39] The most common cause of dyspareunia is a lack of adequate vaginal lubrication. Atrophic vaginitis may also occur among women with a decrease in ovarian estrogen production (e.g., radiation therapy or chemotherapy), or in women who are taking antiestrogenic medications such as clomiphene, medroxyprogesterone, tamoxifen, raloxifene, danazol, leuprolide, and nafarelin.[20,39] Rarely, a low-estrogen oral contraceptive may cause atrophic vaginitis secondary to a nonphysiologic/undesirable estrogen–progestin balance.[8]

Clinical Presentation of Atrophic Vaginitis

Generally, a long-term decrease in estrogen levels is required for atrophic vaginitis to occur. An early symptom of atrophic vaginitis is a decrease in vaginal lubrication;[39] other symptoms include vaginal irritation, dryness, burning, itching, leukorrhea, and dyspareunia. A thin, watery (occasionally bloody), or yellow malodorous vaginal discharge or "spotting" may also be present.[3,7,39] Sexual activity may result in vaginal bleeding or spotting. Any postmenopausal vaginal bleeding needs to be evaluated, because it is presumed to be endometrial cancer until proven otherwise. Dyspareunia may result in emotional distress.

Treatment of Atrophic Vaginitis

Self-treatment of atrophic vaginitis is limited to alleviating the primary symptom, vaginal dryness, with lubricant products. Preventing vaginal dryness requires prescription estrogen therapy, a measure often recommended for women at menopause. Women who are breast-feeding or have recently given birth often have temporary declines in estrogen levels. Vaginal lubricants may be needed only until estrogen levels return to normal.

Treatment Goals

The goals of therapy are to (1) reduce or eliminate the symptoms of vaginal dryness, burning, and itching, and (2) eliminate dyspareunia, if vaginal dryness causes discomfort during or interferes with sexual intercourse.

General Treatment Approach

Vaginal dryness can often be treated with nonprescription topical lubricants such as those listed in Table 8-5. One study found that about half of women with vaginal dryness tried "something," including substances such as butter, baby oil, and petroleum jelly (Vaseline), before seeking medical attention.[41,42] Among women with dyspareunia in one primary care study,[40] 10% had tried a nonprescription analgesic and 62% had done nothing; there was little use of personal lubricant products.

TABLE 8-5 Selected Vaginal Lubricants

Primary Ingredients	Trade Name
Glycerin; propylene glycol	Astroglide; K-Y Personal Lubricant Liquid; Surgel; Vagisil Intimate Moisturizer Lotion[a]
Hydroxypropyl methylcellulose	H-R Lubricating Jelly
Glycerin; hydroxyethyl-cellulose	K-Y Jelly
Vitamin E; propylene glycol gel	K-Y Silk-E Vaginal Moisturizer
Propylene glycol; glycerin; acacia honey type O	K-Y Warming Liquid Personal Lubricant
Glycerin; mineral oil	Replens Gel

[a] Fragrance-free formulation.

Many women are likely to be inadequately treating dyspareunia, given the apparent lack of knowledge about personal lubricant products.[40] Sexual arousal and intercourse can improve atrophic vaginitis, and women who are sexually active have fewer symptoms of atrophic vaginitis.[39]

Self-treatment is appropriate when the symptoms are mild to moderate and confined to the vaginal area, and no bleeding is present. Self-treatment is most appropriate for women who have previously been able to maintain adequate vaginal lubrication. Severe vaginal dryness, dyspareunia, or bleeding warrants medical evaluation (Figure 8-2). In addition, products that may aggravate vaginal symptoms (e.g., irritants and allergens such as powders, perfumes, spermicides, and panty liners) should be avoided.[39]

Figure 8-2 outlines the treatment of vaginal dryness associated with atrophic vaginitis.

Pharmacologic Therapy

Vaginal Lubricants

A number of water-soluble products for vaginal lubrication (e.g., Astroglide, K-Y Jelly, and Replens) are available on the nonprescription market. Personal lubricant products act to temporarily moisten vaginal tissues. These products provide short-term improvement in atrophic vaginal symptoms, such as relief from burning and itching. Personal lubricants can also provide adequate vaginal lubrication to facilitate sexual intercourse.

Vaseline should not be used because it is difficult to remove from the vagina. If the patient is using a latex condom or diaphragm, only water-soluble lubricants should be used because other products (e.g., Vaseline) may damage the latex and impair the efficacy of these contraceptive methods. Water-soluble lubricant gels can be applied both externally and internally. Initially, the patient should be instructed to use a liberal quantity of lubricant (up to 2 teaspoons), and then to tailor the quantity and frequency of use to her specific needs. Most lubricant products provide an improvement in symptoms for less than 24 hours.[39] If the patient is treating dyspareunia, the lubricant should be applied to both the vaginal opening and the penis. If the use of nonprescription lubricants does not produce adequate benefit or is esthetically unappealing to the patient, she should be referred for medical evaluation.

Assessment of Atrophic Vaginitis: A Case-Based Approach

When discussing symptoms of vaginal dryness, patient assessment should include obtaining a description of symptoms (including the association with sexual intercourse) and their severity, as well as information about whether the woman has recently given birth, is lactating, or is perimenopausal or postmenopausal. The practitioner should question patients about the use of any vaginal or feminine hygiene products, because such products may cause or worsen vaginal irritation and dyspareunia.

Case 8-2 gives an example of assessment of patients with atrophic vaginitis.

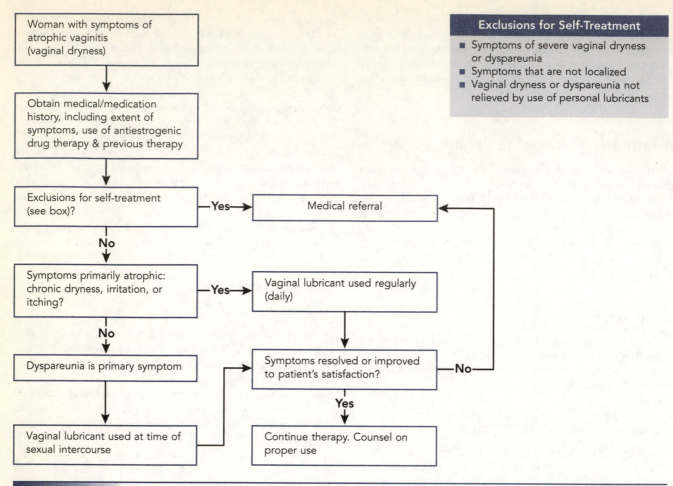

FIGURE 8-2 Self-care of atrophic vaginitis.

CASE 8-2

Relevant Evaluation Criteria	Scenario/Model Outcome
Information Gathering	
1. Gather essential information about the patient's symptoms, including:	
a. description of symptom(s) (i.e., nature, onset, duration, severity, associated symptoms)	Patient is experiencing significant vaginal irritation, dryness, and dyspareunia.
b. description of any factors that seem to precipitate, exacerbate, and/or relieve the patient's symptom(s)	She is postmenopausal; she was taking oral estrogen but stopped because of concern about possible side effects.
c. description of the patient's efforts to relieve the symptoms	Previous use of oral estrogen
2. Gather essential patient history information:	
a. patient's identity	Vicky Mosley, insurance agent
b. age, sex, height, and weight	65-year-old female, 5 ft 5 in, 149 lb
c. concurrent medical conditions, prescription and nonprescription medications, and dietary supplements	Hypertension: hydrochlorothiazide 50 mg daily; hypercholesterolemia: Lipitor 20 mg daily; arthritis: glucosamine and chondroitin 250 mg/200 mg (3 tablets) twice daily
d. allergies/other adverse reactions to medications	NKDA
e. other (describe) _____	Discontinuation of Premarin 0.625 mg about 6 months ago

CASE 8-2 (continued)

Relevant Evaluation Criteria	Scenario/Model Outcome
Assessment and Triage	
3. Differentiate patient's signs/symptoms and correctly identify the patient's primary problem(s).	The patient is postmenopausal. She has vaginal irritation and dryness with no symptoms indicative of other vaginal infections. She had these symptoms previously; they were treated with oral estrogen, which she recently discontinued. These symptoms and her history are consistent with atrophic vaginitis.
4. Identify exclusions for self-treatment (see Figure 8-2).	None
5. Formulate a comprehensive list of therapeutic alternatives for the primary problem to determine if triage to a medical practitioner is required and share this information with the patient.	Options include: (1) Recommend self-treatment with a vaginal lubricant. (2) Refer patient to her PCP for possible vaginal estrogen therapy. (3) Suggest that patient consider use of a vaginal lubricant for symptom improvement until she can see her PCP. (4) Take no action.
Plan	
6. Select an optimal therapeutic alternative to address the patient's problem, taking into account patient preferences.	Because the patient has decided not to use oral estrogens, she should try a vaginal lubricant product. A lubricant product may provide adequate relief for generalized vaginal dryness. If it does not provide adequate relief, then she will have to discuss prescription (vaginal) estrogen with her PCP.
7. Describe the recommended therapeutic approach to the patient.	See the box Patient Education for Atrophic Vaginitis.
8. Explain to the patient the rationale for selecting the recommended therapeutic approach from the considered therapeutic alternatives.	A vaginal lubricant may relieve your symptoms. If it does not, you will likely have to consider use of a topical (vaginal) estrogen product (e.g., a vaginal ring). These vaginal estrogen products have limited systemic estrogenic effects.
Patient Education	
9. When recommending self-care with nonprescription medications and/or nondrug therapy, convey accurate information to the patient:	
a. appropriate dose and frequency of administration	See the box Patient Education for Atrophic Vaginitis.
b. maximum number of days the therapy should be employed	No limitations on length or dosing (quantity used) of lubricant therapy
c. product administration procedures	See the box Patient Education for Atrophic Vaginitis.
d. expected time to onset of relief	For generalized vaginal dryness, some relief should be apparent initially, but optimal effect will likely be noted only after the product has been used regularly for several weeks.
e. degree of relief that can be reasonably expected	Vaginal lubricants may decrease symptoms. However, these products are often unable to provide adequate relief of generalized vaginal dryness.
f. most common side effects	Leakage of product from vagina
g. side effects that warrant medical intervention should they occur	None
h. patient options in the event that condition worsens or persists	Referral for medical evaluation
i. product storage requirements	Product should be stored in a cool dry place.
j. specific nondrug measures	None
10. Solicit follow-up questions from patient.	How often can I apply the lubricant? If this doesn't work for me, will I have to take oral estrogen?
11. Answer patient's questions.	Vaginal lubricants can be applied as often as required in the quantity needed to keep you comfortable. Oral estrogen therapy is usually not necessary for the treatment of atrophic vaginitis; vaginal estrogen products (creams or tablets) are options. Vaginal products are often effective when used only intermittently (e.g., twice a week).

Key: NKDA, no known drug allergy; PCP, primary care provider.

Patient Counseling for Atrophic Vaginitis

The practitioner should stress the short-term nature of atrophic vaginitis to women who are breast-feeding or who recently gave birth. Women who are perimenopausal or postmenopausal should know that long-term treatment with vaginal lubricants may be necessary. In either case, the practitioner should explain the proper use of the lubricants for treatment of vaginal dryness or dyspareunia. The box Patient Education for Atrophic Vaginitis lists specific information to provide to patients.

Evaluation of Patient Outcomes for Atrophic Vaginitis

Symptoms of atrophic vaginitis should improve within a week. The practitioner should advise the patient to call to discuss treatment effectiveness if she has any questions or concerns, and to call after 1 week of treatment to report progress in resolution of the symptoms. Symptoms that persist or the presence of bleeding requires medical evaluation.

VAGINAL DOUCHING

Prevalence of Douching

The 1995 National Survey of Family Growth reported that 27% of U.S. women douche on a regular basis. Douching rates were influenced by race, geographic region, socioeconomic status, and education. Race and education are important predictors of douching practices: Among black women, 70% of those who had not completed high school douched compared with 40% of those with a college degree, whereas among white women, 53% of those who had not completed high school douched compared with only 9% of women with a college degree.[43] Geographic region was another strong predictor of douching. A telephone survey of southern U.S. women 18 to 88 years of age found that almost 80% had douched at some point during their lives, and 60% had begun the practice before or at age 20.[44] Most women

who report douching state that they began the practice as adolescents. A recent study of 250 black adolescents found that the mean age at which douching was initiated was 16 years.[45] Similar to the data for older women, adolescents residing in the South are more likely to douche. A study of Texas adolescents (mean age 18 years) found that 70% had douched and 51% douched at least once a week.[44]

The most frequently stated reason for douching is to achieve good vaginal hygiene. Because vaginal douches mechanically irrigate the vagina, clearing away mucus and other accumulated debris, they may be used as cosmetic cleansing agents. Among the women in a focus group study,[43] most considered it part of normal feminine hygiene, and most reported douching after menstruation and sexual intercourse. These women also stated that douching was done to ensure vaginal cleanliness and eliminate odors. Another reported reason for douching is to enhance the sexual experience. Over half of adolescents in one survey had heard that douching could dry and tighten the vagina for sexual purposes.[46]

Potential Adverse Effects of Douching

Studies have not shown douching to be either safe or desirable. Conversely, although many studies have found an association between douching and adverse health outcomes, it is unclear if this is a causal relationship.[47] Frequent douching has been associated with an increased risk for PID, reduced fertility, ectopic pregnancy, vaginal infections (e.g., bacterial vaginosis), sexually transmitted infections, low birth weight, and cervical cancer.[43,45] Less frequent douching (less than once a week) was not associated with an increased risk of BV in a recent study.[48] Additional possible problems include irritation or sensitization from douche ingredients and disruption of normal vaginal flora and pH. Local irritation, sensitization, and contact dermatitis are also possible with many antimicrobial agents found in douches.

The effect of douches on vaginal flora varies depending on the douche ingredients and douching frequency. The most commonly used douche is a commercially prepared water/vinegar solution.[44,48] Studies have found that water/vinegar douches had little to no effect on lactobacilli, but inhibited some vaginal pathogens, whereas douches containing antiseptics inhibited all

---

PATIENT EDUCATION FOR
Atrophic Vaginitis

The objective of self-treatment with vaginal lubricants is to relieve vaginal dryness or pain during sexual intercourse related to atrophic vaginitis. Carefully following product instructions and the self-care measures listed here will help ensure optimal therapeutic outcomes.

- Apply the vaginal lubricant as frequently as needed for relief of atrophic symptoms (vaginal dryness, irritation, burning, or itching) or inadequate vaginal lubrication.
- Begin treatment of atrophic symptoms with a liberal quantity of lubricant (2 teaspoons); tailor subsequent doses to the quantity and frequency of use needed to provide relief.
- If using lubricants at the time of sexual intercourse, apply the lubricant to the vagina, particularly at the vaginal opening, and to the penis.

- Some leakage of product will occur. If desired, use a sanitary napkin or panty liner to avoid staining of underwear.
- Relief of symptoms may be apparent within hours after the first dose. Regular application of a lubricant can reverse atrophic symptoms to some extent.

 If no improvement is noticeable within a week, or if symptoms worsen or there is any vaginal bleeding, see a primary care provider.

vaginal flora.[48,49] Povidone/iodine (e.g., Betadine) has a greater potential than acetic acid douches to reduce total bacteria but may allow pathogenic species to proliferate, increasing the risk for vaginal infection.[50] Although few allergic reactions have been reported with intravaginal povidone/iodine, it may be systemically absorbed and should not be used by individuals allergic to iodine-containing products. Absorption poses a particular hazard to pregnant women; repeated vaginal applications may result in iodine-induced goiter and hypothyroidism in the fetus. Table 8-4 lists examples of douche products that contain povidone/iodine. Numerous nonmedicated douches are also available.

Proper Use of Douche Equipment

Two types of syringes are available for douching purposes: douche bags and bulb douche syringes. The douche bag (fountain syringe or folding feminine syringe) holds 1 to 2 quarts of fluid, and comes with tubing and a shutoff valve. Two types of tips are supplied: one for enema use (the shorter rectal nozzle) and one for douching. The two tips are not interchangeable; vaginal infections may occur if a single tip is used for both douching and enemas.

Bulb douche syringes are available as both disposable and nondisposable products. The nondisposable units hold 8 to 16 ounces of fluid, whereas the disposable units contain 3 to 9 ounces. The flow rate is regulated by the amount of hand pressure exerted when the bulb is squeezed. Gentle pressure is recommended, because excess pressure may force fluid through the cervix, causing uterine inflammation. Instructions for the proper use of these devices are found in Table 8-6.

Patient Counseling for Douching

Practitioners should discuss a woman's reasons for douching. Women should be informed that douching is not necessary for cleansing of the vagina and that douching has potential adverse consequences. Douching for routine hygienic purposes should be discouraged, and douching is contraindicated during pregnancy. Douching should be delayed at least 6 to 8 hours after sexual intercourse if a vaginal spermicide was used as a contraceptive agent.

An alternative cleansing method for vaginal and perineal areas should be suggested, such as gently washing the vagina and the vulvar, perineal, and anal regions with the fingers using lukewarm water and mild soap. If a woman is douching to prevent or treat symptoms of a vaginal infection (e.g., an abnormal vaginal discharge), she should be counseled about more effective therapy or referred for medical evaluation, as appropriate.

Patients for whom douches have been prescribed or those who insist on douching for other reasons should be instructed on how to use these products safely, appropriately, and effectively. The box Patient Education for Douching lists specific information to provide these patients.

TABLE 8-6 Administration Guidelines for Douches

Bulb Douche Syringe Method
- Choose a douching position that is comfortable for you. Two positions are recommended: (1) sitting on the toilet or (2) standing in the shower. Whichever position you choose, remember that douching is easier when you are relaxed.
- Gently insert the nozzle about 3 inches into your vagina. Avoid closing the lips of the vagina.
- Squeeze bottle gently, letting the solution cleanse the vagina and then flow freely from the body.
- After douching, throw away bottle and nozzle, if disposable.

Douche Bag Method
- Fill the douche bag with the prescribed solution or with a warm water and vinegar solution.
- Lie back in the tub with knees bent. Place the douche bag about 1 foot above the height of your hips. Do not place or hang the bag any higher, because such height will cause the pressure of fluid entering the vagina to be too high.
- Insert the nozzle several inches into the vagina. Aim the nozzle up and back toward the small of the back. While holding the labia closed around the nozzle, release the clamp slowly to allow fluid to enter the vagina. Rotate the tip and allow fluid to enter the vagina until the vagina feels full. Stop the flow of fluid; then hold the fluid in the vagina for about 30–60 seconds. Release and allow the fluid to flow out; repeat until the douche bag is empty.
- Wash the nozzle with mild soap and water.

PATIENT EDUCATION FOR Douching

Improper methods of douching or too frequent douching can cause vaginal irritation. Douching can also increase the risk for pelvic inflammatory disease, ectopic pregnancy, and sterility. Strictly following the product instructions and the self-care measures listed here will help avoid these problems.

- Keep all douche equipment clean.
- Use lukewarm water to dilute products.
- Follow the appropriate instructions in Table 8-6 for the method of douching being used.
- Never instill a douche with forceful pressure.
- Do not use these products for birth control.
- Do not douche until at least 8 hours after intercourse during which a diaphragm, cervical cap, or contraceptive jelly, cream, or foam was used.

- Do not douche for at least 3 days after the last dose of vaginal antifungal medication.
- Do not douche for 48 hours before any gynecologic examination.
- Do not douche during pregnancy unless under the advice and supervision of a primary care provider.
- Use douches only as directed for routine cleansing.
- Do not douche more often than twice a week, except on the advice of a primary care provider.
- If vaginal dryness or irritation occurs, discontinue use of the douche.

Key Points for Vaginal and Vulvovaginal Disorders

➤ Vaginal symptoms are often nonspecific, and it may be difficult to distinguish the three common vaginal infections. The symptom most likely to differentiate a candidal infection from BV and trichomoniasis is the absence of an offensive odor to the vaginal secretions. Measurement of vaginal pH (pH > 4.5 indicates a noncandidal infection) may also help to distinguish *Candida* and reduce inappropriate use of nonprescription antifungals.

➤ Vaginal candidal infections are typically caused by *C. albicans,* but recently non–*C. albicans* infections have increased. These species of *Candida* may be more resistant to azole antifungals.

➤ Self-treatment for a vaginal candidal infection is most appropriate when the woman's symptoms are mild to moderate, there are no predisposing illnesses or medications, and symptoms are not recurrent. Recurrent infections are defined as four or more infections within a 12-month period and symptoms occurring within 2 months of previous vaginal symptoms.

➤ All of the azole antifungals are equally effective. Selection of length of regimen or time of day of administration can be determined by patient preference. For patients concurrently taking warfarin, the risk–benefit of temporarily reducing the dose of warfarin needs to be carefully considered; patients should be referred to the practitioner monitoring their warfarin therapy.

➤ Patients should be informed that symptoms typically improve shortly after application of the vaginal antifungals; symptoms should improve within 2 to 3 days after initiation of therapy and be resolved within a week. The length of the treatment regimen does not directly correspond to resolution of symptoms.

➤ Use of a sodium bicarbonate sitz bath can provide relief of itching and irritation prior to onset of benefit from the antifungal.

➤ Eating yogurt with live cultures (8 ounces daily) may be of some benefit to patients in preventing recurrent VVC infections.

➤ Atrophic vaginitis, inflammation of the vagina secondary to decreased estrogen levels, can occur after menopause, postpartum, during breast-feeding, or as a result of antiestrogenic medications. Vaginal dryness and dyspareunia can be relieved by use of topical personal lubricant products. If symptoms do not improve within a week, medical evaluation is needed.

➤ Atrophic vaginitis may cause vaginal bleeding; however, any postmenopausal bleeding needs to be evaluated to rule out endometrial cancer.

➤ Douching is not necessary for vaginal cleansing, and adverse consequences of douching can occur. Douching is contraindicated during pregnancy and should be postponed until at least 8 hours after sexual intercourse if a vaginal spermicide was used for contraception.

REFERENCES

1. Reed B. Vaginitis In: Sloane PD SL, Ebell MH, et al., eds. *Essentials of Family Medicine.* Philadelphia: Lippincott Williams & Wilkins; 2002.
2. Haefner H. Current evaluation and management of vulvovaginitis. *Clin Obstet Gynecol.* 1999;42:184–95.
3. Mashburn J. Etiology, diagnosis and management of vaginitis. *J Midwifery Women's Health.* 2006;51:423–30.
4. Cullins VA, Dominguez L, Guberski T, et al. Treating vaginitis. *Nurse Pract.* 1999;24:46–58.
5. Benjamin F. Anatomy, physiology, growth, and development. In: Seltzer VL Pearse WH, eds. *Women's Primary Health Care.* New York: McGraw-Hill, Inc; 1995.
6. Cleveland A. Vaginitis: finding the cause prevents treatment failure. *Cleve Clin J Med.* 2000;67:634–46.
7. Quan M. Vaginitis: meeting the clinical challenge. *Clin Cornerstone.* 2000; 3:36–47.
8. Ledger W, Monif G. A growing concern: inability to diagnose vulvovaginal infections correctly. *Obstet Gynecol.* 2004;103:782–4.
9. Anderson MR, Klink K, Cohrssen A, et al. Evaluation of vaginal complaints. *JAMA.* 2004;291:1368–79.
10. Soper D. Trichomoniasis: under control or undercontrolled? *Am J Obstet Gynecol.* 2004;190:281–90.
11. Holzman C, Leventhal JM, Qui H, et al. Factors linked to bacterial vaginosis in nonpregnant women. *Am J Pub Health.* 2001;91:1661–70.
12. Foxman B, Barlow R, D'Arcy H, et al. Candida vaginitis: self-reported incidence and associated costs. *Sex Transm Dis.* 2000;27:230–5.
13. Sobel JD, Chaim W, Nagappan V, et al. Treatment of vaginitis caused by Candida glabrata: use of topical boric acid and flucytosine. *Am J Obstet Gynecol.* 2003;189:1297–300.
14. Ferris DG, Dekle C, Litaker MS. Women's use of over-the-counter antifungal medications for gynecologic symptoms. *J Fam Pract.* 1996;42:595–600.
15. Moraes PSA, Taketomi EA. Allergic vulvovaginitis. *Ann Allergy Asthma Immunol.* 2000;85:253–67.
16. Coco A, Vandenbosche M. Infectious vaginitis: an accurate diagnosis is essential and attainable. *Postgrad Med.* 2000;107:63–74.
17. Roy S, Caillouette JC, Faden, JS, et al. Improving use of antifungal medications: the role of an over-the-counter vaginal pH self-test device. *Infect Dis Obstet Gynecol.* 2003;11:209–16.
18. Owen MK, Clenney TL. Management of vaginitis. *Am Fam Physician.* 2004;70:2125–32, 2139–40.
19. Klebanoff M, Schwebke J, Zhang J, et al. Vulvovaginal symptoms in women with bacterial vaginosis. *Obstet Gynecol.* 2004;104:267–72.
20. Suess JA, Holzman C. Vulvar and vaginal disease. In: Smith MA, Shimp LA, eds. *20 Common Problems in Women's Health Care.* New York: McGraw-Hill, Inc; 2000.
21. Sobel JD, Faro S, Force RW, et al. VVC: epidemiologic, diagnostic, and therapeutic considerations. *Am J Obstet Gynecol.* 1998;178:203–11.
22. Castelo-Branco C, Cancelo MJ, Villero J, et al. Management of postmenopausal vaginal atrophy and atrophic vaginitis. *Maturitas Eur Menopause J.* 2005;52S:S46–S52.
23. Sobel J. Candida vulvovaginitis. *Semin Dermatol.* 1996;15:17–28.
24. American College of Obstetricians and Gynecology. Vaginitis. ACOG Technical Bulletin Number 226. *Int J Gynaecol Obstet.* 1996;54: 293–302.
25. Falagas ME, Betsi GI, Athanasiou S. Probiotics for prevention of recurrent vulvovaginal candidiasis: a review. *J Antimicrob Chemother.* 2006;58: 266–72.
26. Singh SI. Treatment of vulvovaginal candidiasis. *CPJ.* 2003;136(9):26–30.
27. Elmer GW, Surawicz CM, McFarland LV. Biotherapeutic agents: a neglected modality for the treatment and prevention of selected intestinal and vaginal infections. *JAMA.* 1996;275:870–6.
28. Upmalis DH, Cone FL, Lamia CA, et al. Single-dose miconazole nitrate vaginal ovule in the treatment of vulvovaginal candidiasis: two single-blind, controlled studies versus miconazole nitrate 100 mg cream for 7 days. *J Womens Health Gend Based Med.* 2000;9:421–9.
29. Brown D, Henzl MR, Kaufman RH; Gynazole Study Group. Butoconazole nitrate 2% for vulvovaginal candidiasis: new, single-dosed vaginal cream formulation vs. seven-day treatment with miconazole nitrate. *J Reprod Med.* 1999;44:933–8.
30. Barnhart K. Safety and efficacy of bedtime versus daytime administration of the miconazole nitrate 1200 mg vaginal ovule insert to treat vulvovaginal candidiasis. *Curr Med Res Opin.* 2005;21:127–34.
31. Kohlberger P, Bancher-Todesca D. Bacterial colonization in suspected sexually abused children. *J Pediatr Adolesc Gynecol.* 2007;20:289–92.

32. American College of Obstetricians and Gynecology. Vaginitis. ACOG Practice Bulletin. *Obstetr Gynecol.* 2006;107:1195–206.

33. Pirotta M, Gunn J, Chondros P, et al. Effect of lactobacillus in preventing post-antibiotic vulvovaginal candidiasis: a randomized controlled trial. *BMJ.* 2004;329:548–51.

34. Korenek P, Britt R, Hawkins C. Differentiation of the vaginosis-bacterial vaginosis, lactobacillosis, and cytolytic vaginosis. *Internet J Adv Nurs Pract.* 2003;6(1).

35. Van Kessel K, Assefi N, Marrazzo J, et al. Common complementary and alternative therapies for yeast vaginitis and bacterial vaginosis: a systematic review. *Obstet Gynecol Survey.* 2003;58:351–8.

36. Reid G, Bocking A. The potential for probiotics to prevent bacterial vaginosis and preterm labor. *Am J Obstet Gynecol.* 2003;189:1202–8.

37. Allen-Davis JT, Beck A, Parker R, et al. Assessment of vulvovaginal complaints: accuracy of telephone triage and in-office diagnosis. *Obstet Gynecol.* 2002;99:18–22.

39. Ferris DG, Nyirjesy P, Sobel JD, et al. Over-the-counter antifungal drug misuse associated with patient-diagnosed vulvovaginal candidiasis. *Obstet Gynecol.* 2002;99:419–25.

39. Bachmann GA, Nevadunsky N. Diagnosis and treatment of atrophic vaginitis. *Am Fam Physician.* 2000;61:3090–6.

40. Jamieson DJ, Steege JF. The prevalence of dysmenorrhea, dyspareunia, pelvic pain, and irritable bowel syndrome in primary care practices. *Obstet Gynecol.* 1996;87:55–8.

41. Sarazin SK, Seymour SF. Causes and treatment options for women with dyspareunia. *Nurse Pract.* 1991;16:30–41.

42. MacNeil C. Dyspareunia. *Obstet Gynecol Clin North Am.* 2006;33:565–77, viii.

43. Lichtenstein B, Nansel TR. Women's douching practices and related attitudes: findings from four focus groups. *Womens Health.* 2000;31:117–31.

44. Oh MK, Merchant JS, Brown P. Douching behavior in high-risk adolescents: what do they use, when and why do they douche? *J Pediatr Adolesc Gynecol.* 2002;15:83–8.

45. Schwebke JR, Desmond RA, Oh MK. Predictors of bacterial vaginosis in adolescent women who douche. *Sex Transm Dis.* 2004;31:433–6.

46. Simpson T, Merchant J, Grimley Dm, et al. Vaginal douching among adolescents and young women: more challenges than progress. *J Pediatr Adolesc Gynecol.* 2004;17:249–55.

47. Martino JL, Vermund SH. Vaginal douching: evidence for risks or benefits to women's health. *Epidemiol Rev.* 2002;24:109–24.

48. Zhang J, Hatch M, Zhang D, et al. Frequency of douching and risk of bacterial vaginosis in African American women. *Obstet Gynecol.* 2004;104:756–60.

49. Pagvlova SI, Tao L. In vitro inhibition of commercial douche products against vaginal microflora. *Infect Dis Obstet Gynecol.* 2000;8:99–104.

50. Onderdonk AB, Delaney ML, Hinkson PL, et al. Quantitative and qualitative effects of douche preparations on vaginal microflora. *Obstet Gynecol.* 1992;80:333–8.

Disorders Related to Menstruation

Leslie A. Shimp

The menstrual cycle is a regular physiologic event for women beginning during adolescence and usually continuing through late middle age. Women are able to self-treat for two common menstrual disorders: primary dysmenorrhea and premenstrual syndrome. Many women use nonprescription products and seek advice from health care professionals on how best to manage symptoms of these disorders, including abdominal pain and cramping, irritability, and fluid retention. An understanding of the menstrual cycle will help both patients and health care professionals make informed and appropriate decisions about self-care. Health care professionals should also be familiar with common menstrual symptoms and disorders, as well as with the risks associated with some menstrual products (e.g., toxic shock syndrome [TSS]).

Menstruation results from the monthly cycling of female reproductive hormones. A single menstrual cycle is the time between the onset of one menstrual flow (menstruation or menses) and the beginning of the next.

The average age at which menarche (the initial menstrual cycle) occurs in U.S. women is 12 years; however, normal menarche may occur as early as age 10 or as late as age 16.[1] The onset of menstruation is influenced by a number of factors such as race, genetics, nutritional status, and body mass.

The menstrual cycle, on average, lasts 28 days; however, only 15% of women have a 28-day cycle.[2] Menstrual cycle length varies between 21 and 40 days.[2] Menses lasts, on average, 4 days (plus or minus 2 days).[3] Most of the blood loss occurs during days 1 and 2. The major components of menstrual fluid are endometrial cellular debris and blood. Average whole blood loss per cycle is 30 to 80 mL.[2] A loss of more than 80 mL per cycle or bleeding lasting longer than 7 days is considered abnormal and is associated with anemia.[2]

Two principal reproductive events, each hormonally controlled, occur during each menstrual cycle. The first event is the maturation and release of an ovum (egg) from the ovaries; the second is the preparation of the endometrial lining of the uterus for the implantation of a fertilized ovum. The events of the menstrual cycle (Figure 9-1) can be described in phases that reflect changes in either the ovary (follicular/ovulatory and luteal phases) or the uterine endometrium (menstrual/proliferative and secretory phases).[3] The follicular/ovulatory phase correlates with the menstrual/proliferative phase, and the luteal phase correlates with the secretory phase.

The menstrual cycle results from the hormonal activity of the hypothalamus, pituitary gland, and ovaries (hypothalamic-pituitary-ovarian axis). The hypothalamus plays the key role in regulating the menstrual cycle by producing gonadotropin-releasing hormone (GnRH). Low levels of both estradiol and progesterone, present at the end of the previous menstrual cycle, stimulate the hypothalamus to release GnRH, which stimulates pituitary gonadotroph cells to synthesize and secrete luteinizing hormone (LH) and follicle-stimulating hormone (FSH).

The first day of the menstrual flow is called day 1 of the cycle. Day 1 is the beginning of the follicular phase in the ovary and of the menstrual/proliferative phase in the uterus. The follicular phase can range in length from several days to several weeks but lasts an average of 14 days. During the follicular phase, FSH stimulates the maturation of a group of ovarian follicles. These maturing follicles secrete the estrogen estradiol, which promotes the growth of the uterine endometrium.

By about cycle day 8, a single ovarian follicle becomes dominant. The usual development of a single dominant follicle results in the ovulation of only one egg. The ovulatory phase of the cycle is approximately 3 days in length. During this phase, the LH surge (a 48-hour period when the pituitary secretes high levels of LH) occurs. The LH surge catalyzes the final steps in the maturation of the ovum, as well as stimulates production of prostaglandins and proteolytic enzymes necessary for ovulation (release of a mature ovum). Estradiol levels also decrease during the LH surge, sometimes with midcycle endometrial bleeding. Ovulation typically occurs 12 hours after the LH surge.[4] Ovulation releases 5 to 10 mL of follicular fluid, which contains the oocyte mass and prostaglandins; this event may cause abdominal pain (mittelschmerz) for some women. In adolescents, the LH surge does not occur until 2 to 5 years after menarche; as a result, 50% to 80% of cycles are anovulatory (i.e., no ovulation occurs) and irregular during the first 2 years after menarche.[4]

The luteal phase is the time between ovulation and the beginning of menstrual blood flow. After the follicle ruptures, it is referred to as the corpus luteum. The luteal phase length is more constant, about 14 days (plus or minus 2 days), and is consistent with the functional period (about 10–12 days) of the corpus luteum.[3] The corpus luteum secretes progesterone, estradiol, and androgens. The increased levels of estrogen and progesterone alter the uterine endometrial lining; glands mature, proliferate, and become secretory (secretory phase) as the uterus prepares for the implantation of a fertilized egg. Progesterone and estrogen levels reach their peaks in the middle of the luteal phase, whereas levels of LH and FSH decline in response to the increased hormone levels. If pregnancy occurs, human chorionic

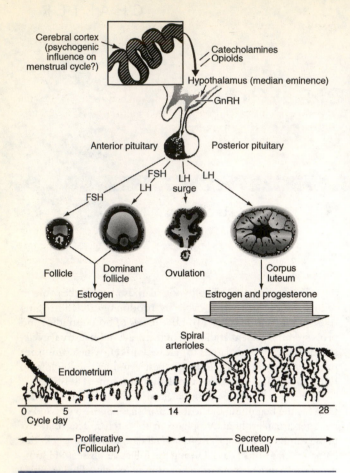

FIGURE 9-1 Hormonal and anatomic relationships during menstrual cycle. There is also feedback from ovarian hormones estradiol and progesterone to the pituitary and the hypothalamus. (Reprinted with permission from Mattox JH. Normal and abnormal uterine bleeding. In: Mattox JH, ed. *Core Textbook of Obstetrics and Gynecology.* St Louis: Mosby-Yearbook; 1998:397.)

gonadotropin released by the developing embryo supports the function of the corpus luteum until the placenta develops enough to begin secreting estrogen and progesterone. If pregnancy does not occur, the corpus luteum ceases to function. Estrogen and progesterone levels then decline, causing the endometrial lining of the uterus to become edematous and necrotic. The decrease in progesterone also allows prostaglandin synthesis. Following prostaglandin-initiated vasoconstriction and uterine contractions, sloughing of the outer two endometrial layers occurs. The decline in estrogen and progesterone results in an increase in GnRH and in the renewed production of LH and FSH, which begins a new menstrual cycle.[3]

DYSMENORRHEA

Dysmenorrhea (difficult or painful menstruation) is one of the most common gynecologic problems in the United States. Dysmenorrhea is divided into primary and secondary disorders by etiology. Primary dysmenorrhea is idiopathic and associated with cramp-like abdominal pain at the time of menstruation in the absence of pelvic disease. Secondary dysmenorrhea is usually associated with pelvic pathology. The prevalence of dysmenorrhea is highest in adolescence with up to 90% of young women being affected.[5] Primary dysmenorrhea usually develops within 6 to 12 months of menarche, generally affecting women during their teens and early 20s. Primary dysmenorrhea occurs only during ovulatory cycles; therefore, its prevalence increases between early and older adolescence as the regularity of ovulation increases.[6,7] Its prevalence decreases after the age of 25 years.

Approximately 15% of young women report that the pain associated with dysmenorrhea is severe.[6,7] Dysmenorrhea has been described as the single greatest cause of school absenteeism and lost working hours among adolescent girls and young women. Two large studies of adolescents found that 10% to 15% of girls reported missing school because of dysmenorrhea,[8] whereas a study of about 700 Hispanic girls found that 38% had missed school days because of dysmenorrhea.[9] Those reporting moderate or severe pain were two or four times as likely to miss school as those with mild pain. A study of freshman college women found that 25% of this group reported missing school, and 42% reported that at some time they had missed an activity because of dysmenorrhea.[8] In addition to school absence, girls with dysmenorrhea reported that it limited classroom concentration (59%), sports participation (51%), and going out with friends (46%).[9] Similarly, an estimated 600 million work hours are lost annually because of dysmenorrhea.[7]

The decrease in prevalence and severity in women in their late 20s and older may be partially explained by oral contraceptive use and pregnancy. Oral contraceptive use is more common after adolescence and is known to be an effective therapy for dysmenorrhea. The amount of endometrium is greatly reduced, by as much as two-thirds, in women using combined oral contraceptives, which results in a much lower prostaglandin production. During the last trimester of pregnancy, uterine adrenergic nerves virtually disappear and only a portion regenerate after childbirth.[7] This is believed to explain the disappearance of dysmenorrhea following childbirth for many women.

Factors that can increase risk for or severity of dysmenorrhea include tobacco smoking, obesity, low fish consumption, alcohol consumption, and stress, anxiety, and depression.[4]

Pathophysiology of Primary Dysmenorrhea

The cause of primary dysmenorrhea is not fully understood, but it is known that prostaglandins and, possibly, leukotrienes are involved.[7,8] After ovulation, fatty acids accumulate in cell membranes. Because the U.S. diet is high in intake of omega-6 fatty acids, there is a predominance of omega-6 fatty acids such as arachidonic acid, a precursor to both prostaglandins (notably $PGF_{2\alpha}$) and leukotrienes.[4] At the end of the luteal phase of the menstrual cycle, progesterone levels decrease, and prostaglandins and leukotrienes are released. Prostaglandin levels are two to four times greater in women with dysmenorrhea than in women without dysmenorrhea and are highest during the first 2 days of menses, when dysmenorrhea commonly occurs.[4,8] Leukotrienes, inflammatory mediators known to cause vasoconstriction and uterine contractions, have also been found to be elevated in women with dysmenorrhea. It has been suggested that leukotrienes may contribute significantly to dysmenorrhea in women who do not respond to therapy with prostaglandin inhibitors (i.e., nonsteroidal anti-inflammatory drugs [NSAIDs]).[7] Similarly, vasopressin (a substance that can produce dysrhythmic uterine contractions) may play a role in the etiology of primary dysmenorrhea; circulating levels of vasopressin are fourfold higher in women with dysmenorrhea than in asymptomatic women.[7]

Prostaglandins stimulate uterine contractions. Normal contractions and vasoconstriction help expel menstrual fluids and control bleeding as the endometrium sloughs.[6] However, the increased levels of prostaglandins, leukotrienes, and vasopressin present with dysmenorrhea can lead to strong uterine contractions and significant vasoconstriction, resulting in uterine ischemia and pain. In women without dysmenorrhea, uterine contractions are rhythmic and contraction pressure reaches 120 mm Hg. In women with dysmenorrhea, contractions occur more often and pressures can reach 180 mm Hg.[10] Both intrauterine pressure and the frequency of uterine contractions contribute to ischemia and tissue hypoxia and, thus, to pain.

Clinical Presentation of Primary Dysmenorrhea

Primary dysmenorrhea pain is cyclic pain directly related to the onset of menstruation. It is typically experienced as a continuous dull aching pain with spasmodic cramping in the lower midabdominal or suprapubic region, which may radiate to the lower back and upper thighs. Uterine contractions can force prostaglandins into the systemic circulation, causing additional symptoms such as nausea, vomiting, fatigue, dizziness, irritability, diarrhea, and headache. The onset of pain is several hours prior to or coincident with the onset of menses and usually lasts less than 48 hours, but pain may persist up to 72 hours.[7] For this reason, women with regular periods may wish to prophylax against dysmenorrhea before the onset of menses. Primary dysmenorrhea usually initially occurs within the first 6 to 12 months after menarche, when ovulatory cycles begin; dysmenorrhea occurs only during cycles in which ovulation occurs.[5,7] This clinical presentation can be adequate for the diagnosis of primary dysmenorrhea, if the pain is mild to moderate and the patient responds to NSAID therapy.

Secondary dysmenorrhea is suggested if dysmenorrhea initially begins years after menarche (at age 25 years or older); if pelvic pain occurs at times other than during menses and is not related to the first day of menses; or if the patient experiences irregular menstrual cycles, or has menorrhagia (excessively prolonged or profuse menses), or a history of pelvic inflammatory disease (PID), dyspareunia, or infertility.[5,7] Causes of secondary dysmenorrhea include endometriosis, PID, ovarian cysts, uterine tumors, uterine fibroids, cervical os stenosis, inflammatory bowel disease, and congenital abnormalities.[7,11] Secondary dysmenorrhea may also be caused by the presence of an intrauterine contraceptive (IUC).

Treatment of Primary Dysmenorrhea

Many women believe they are able to self-treat dysmenorrhea with nonprescription products. In one study,[12] 66% of women with dysmenorrhea did not see a clinician despite having moderate-to-severe symptoms, and 92% were satisfied with self-treatment. In contrast, only 14% of adolescents sought medical care for dysmenorrhea. Many are undertreated (use of low or mistimed doses) or use less-effective medications, thus increasing the likelihood of school absence and other activity limitations.[13]

Treatment Goals

The goals of treating primary dysmenorrhea are to (1) provide relief or a significant improvement in symptoms and (2) minimize the disruption of usual activities.

General Treatment Approach

An important initial step in managing dysmenorrhea is distinguishing between primary and secondary disease. Self-care is appropriate for an otherwise healthy young woman who has a history consistent with primary dysmenorrhea and is not sexually active, or a woman who has been diagnosed with primary dysmenorrhea.[4,5,6] Adolescents with pelvic pain who are sexually active (at risk for PID) and women with characteristics indicating secondary dysmenorrhea should be referred for medical evaluation. Table 9-1 compares primary and secondary dysmenorrhea. Essentially all patients with primary dysmenorrhea can obtain adequate relief of symptoms with nondrug interventions, or nonprescription or prescription drug therapy. Approximately 80% to 90% of women with primary dysmenorrhea can be successfully treated with NSAIDs, oral contraceptives, or both. Other treatment options include nonpharmacologic measures, such as use of topical heat, dietary supplementation with omega-3 fatty acids from fish or fish oil, and discontinuation of tobacco smoking. These measures often serve as adjuncts to drug therapy, although topical heat may be adequate as sole therapy for some women.

Figure 9-2 presents an algorithm for managing primary dysmenorrhea.

The patient with more severe dysmenorrhea, a change in the pattern or intensity of pain, intolerance to NSAIDs, or dysmenorrhea that does not respond to nonprescription therapy should be referred to her primary care provider. (Figure 9-2 lists exclusions for self-care.)

Nonpharmacologic Therapy

Many women use nonpharmacologic measures to help manage dysmenorrhea and menstrual discomfort. A study of adolescents found common nondrug measures were sleep (84% of respondents), hot baths or a heating pad (75% and 50%, respectively), and exercise (30%).[13] The use of heat is a commonly recommended nondrug therapy. An abdominal heat patch (i.e., ThermaCare) has been developed and tested for the treatment of dysmenorrhea.[14] The heat patch was significantly better (14% greater pain relief) than placebo and acetaminophen in relieving pain and cramping. The analgesic effect of the heat patch had a faster onset than drug therapy, and it added to the relief provided by ibuprofen. Evidence regarding the benefit of exercise is conflicting. Participation in regular exercise may lessen the symptoms of primary dysmenorrhea for some women.[5] Nondrug therapy may be especially useful for the estimated 15% of women who cannot tolerate or do not respond to nonprescription medications.

Lifestyle alterations may alleviate symptoms to varying degrees. Smoking and exposure to secondhand smoke have been associated with more severe dysmenorrhea.[5] The severity reportedly increases with the number of cigarettes smoked per day. The basis for this effect is unknown, but it has been hypothesized that nicotine-induced vasoconstriction is involved. Increased consumption of fish rich in omega-3 fatty acids (e.g., tuna, salmon,

TABLE 9-1 Differentiation of Primary and Secondary Dysmenorrhea

	Primary Dysmenorrhea	Secondary Dysmenorrhea
Age at onset of dysmenorrhea symptoms	Typically 6–12 months after menarche—age 12–13 years for most girls	Mid to late 20s or older; usually 30s and 40s for women with secondary dysmenorrhea
Menses	More likely to be regular with normal blood loss	More likely to be irregular; menorrhagia more common
Pattern and duration of dysmenorrhea pain	Onset just prior to or coincident with onset of menses; pain with each or most menses, lasting only 2–3 days	Pattern and duration vary with cause; change in pain pattern or intensity also may indicate secondary disease
Pain at other times of menstrual cycle	No	Yes, may occur before, during, or after menses
Response to NSAIDs and/or oral contraceptives	Yes	No
Other symptoms	Nausea, vomiting, fatigue, dizziness, irritability, diarrhea, and headache may occur at same time as dysmenorrhea pain	Vary according to cause of the secondary dysmenorrhea; may include dyspareunia, pelvic tenderness

Key: NSAID, nonsteroidal anti-inflammatory drug.
Source: References 5, 6, and 11.

sardines, herring, mackerel, trout) or use of fish oil may reduce symptoms.[4]

Pharmacologic Therapy

The three nonprescription analgesic medications most commonly used by women to treat dysmenorrhea are acetaminophen, aspirin, and ibuprofen. A study of adolescents found that 91% used nonprescription medications to manage dysmenorrhea compared with only 21% who used prescription analgesics.[13] Ibuprofen was the most commonly used agent, but the doses used were typically less than the recommended dose for dysmenorrhea.

Unfortunately, many women and adolescents with dysmenorrhea remain untreated or are inadequately treated. They continue to experience the pain and limitations on activity this condition imposes. The following sections outline the uses and properties of aspirin, acetaminophen, and the nonsalicylate NSAIDs as agents in the treatment of dysmenorrhea; Table 9-2 lists their dosages for dysmenorrhea. Chapter 5 provides further discussion of the adverse effects, contraindications, and drug interactions of these agents, as well as a table describing all nonprescription internal analgesic products.

Aspirin

Aspirin may be adequate for treating mild symptoms of dysmenorrhea. However, in low doses, aspirin has only a limited effect on prostaglandin synthesis and is, therefore, only moderately effective in treating women with more than minimal symptoms of dysmenorrhea.[11] Aspirin may increase menstrual flow. In addition, adolescent girls should not use aspirin because of the association with Reye's syndrome in this age group.

Acetaminophen

Similar to aspirin, acetaminophen may be adequate for treating only mild symptoms of dysmenorrhea. Acetaminophen is a weak inhibitor of prostaglandin synthesis; the reduction of PGF2a levels is much greater with nonsalicylate NSAIDs than with acetaminophen.[15] Acetaminophen may be useful in managing dysmenorrhea in doses of 1000 mg four times daily, but lower doses are less apt to be effective. Even in doses of 4 grams daily, acetaminophen is less effective than ibuprofen.[15]

Nonsalicylate NSAIDs

Nonsalicylate NSAIDs are the principal nonprescription agents for treating primary dysmenorrhea. Two nonsalicylate NSAIDs are available as nonprescription products: ibuprofen 200 mg and naproxen sodium 220 mg. In clinical trials, these NSAIDs were found to be effective in 66% to 90% of patients. However, clinical trial doses and currently recommended prescription doses for the treatment of dysmenorrhea are often higher than the labeled nonprescription doses. Therefore, prescription therapy may be required if the maximum nonprescription dose does not provide adequate symptom relief.

Therapy with nonsalicylate NSAIDs should begin at the onset of menses or pain; if inadequate pain relief occurs, treatment beginning 1 to 2 days before expected menses may improve symptomatic relief.[2] If the possibility of pregnancy exists, then therapy should be initiated only after menses begins. Patients should be instructed that the NSAID is used as much to prevent cramps as to relieve pain. Optimal pain relief is achieved when these agents are taken on a scheduled rather than an as-needed basis. Therefore, ibuprofen should be taken every 4 to 6 hours and naproxen sodium every 8 to 12 hours for the first 48 to 72 hours of menstrual flow, because that time frame correlates with maximum prostaglandin release (Table 9-2). The therapeutic effect of these drugs is usually apparent within 30 to 60 minutes, and benefit will be optimal with continued regular dosing.

A patient with dysmenorrhea may respond better to one nonsalicylate NSAID than to another. If an adequate dose (or the maximum nonprescription dose) of one agent does not

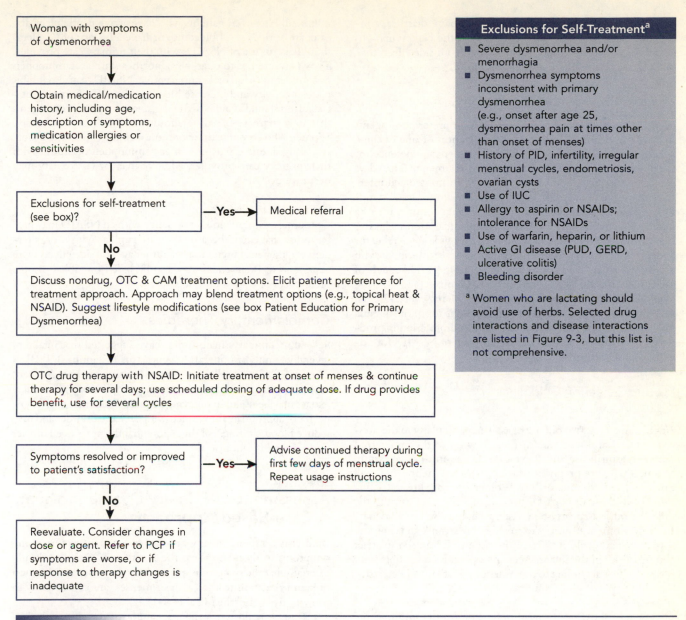

Exclusions for Self-Treatment[a]

- Severe dysmenorrhea and/or menorrhagia
- Dysmenorrhea symptoms inconsistent with primary dysmenorrhea (e.g., onset after age 25, dysmenorrhea pain at times other than onset of menses)
- History of PID, infertility, irregular menstrual cycles, endometriosis, ovarian cysts
- Use of IUC
- Allergy to aspirin or NSAIDs; intolerance for NSAIDs
- Use of warfarin, heparin, or lithium
- Active GI disease (PUD, GERD, ulcerative colitis)
- Bleeding disorder

[a] Women who are lactating should avoid use of herbs. Selected drug interactions and disease interactions are listed in Figure 9-3, but this list is not comprehensive.

FIGURE 9-2 Self-care of primary dysmenorrhea. Key: CAM, complementary and alternative medicine; GERD, gastro-esophageal reflux disease; GI, gastrointestinal; IUC, intrauterine contraceptive; NSAID, nonsteroidal anti-inflammatory drug; OTC, over-the-counter; PID, pelvic inflammatory disease; PCP, primary care provider; PUD, peptic ulcer disease.

TABLE 9-2 Treatment of Dysmenorrhea with Nonprescription Medications

Agent	Recommended Nonprescription Dosage (Maximum Daily Dosage)
Acetaminophen	650–1000 mg every 4–6 hours (4000 mg)
Aspirin	650–1000 mg every 4–6 hours (4000 mg)
Ibuprofen	200–400 mg every 4–6 hours[a] (1200 mg)
Naproxen sodium	220–440 mg initially; then 220 mg every 8–12 hours (660 mg)

[a] If 200 mg every 4–6 hours is ineffective, the recommended dosage for dysmenorrhea of 400 mg every 6 hours should be taken.

provide adequate benefit, then switching to another agent is recommended. The analgesic effect for most of these NSAIDs plateaus, so further dose increases may increase the risk of adverse drug effects rather than provide more benefit. Therapy with nonsalicylate NSAIDs should be undertaken for three to six menstrual cycles, with changes made in the agent, dosage, or both before judging the effectiveness of these agents for a particular patient. If nonprescription NSAID therapy does not provide an adequate therapeutic effect, prescription NSAIDs; prescription doses of the nonprescription NSAIDs; or use of a combined oral contraceptive, medroxyprogesterone acetate (Depo-Provera), or the levonorgestrel IUC (Mirena) may provide relief from dysmenorrhea.

Side effects from a few days of intermittent use are limited and usually include gastrointestinal (GI) symptoms (e.g., upset stomach, vomiting, heartburn, abdominal pain, diarrhea, constipation, and anorexia) and side effects of the central nervous system (e.g., headache and dizziness). Some GI side effects may be decreased by taking the drugs with food.

Pharmacotherapeutic Comparison

Nonsalicylate NSAIDs are the preferred nonprescription agents for treating primary dysmenorrhea. Selection of one of these agents should be based on cost and the patient's preference for the number of doses and tablets to take. A regimen of 2 to 3 days is usually adequate, and adverse effects with limited and intermittent use are uncommon and are typically limited to GI symptoms. Women at risk of GI ulceration should consider use of a gastroprotective agent or another therapeutic option such as an oral contraceptive. Acetaminophen may provide some relief for patients who are hypersensitive or intolerant to aspirin, or who are intolerant to the GI and platelet-inhibition side effects of aspirin and the nonsalicylate NSAIDs. Choline (435–870 mg every 4 hours) or sodium salicylate (325–650 mg every 4 hours) may also be an option in patients hypersensitive to aspirin, because no cross-sensitivity has been seen. These nonprescription products are, however, less effective than aspirin or NSAIDs for primary dysmenorrhea.

Product Selection Guidelines

SPECIAL POPULATIONS

Adolescents should avoid use of aspirin, particularly in the presence of a viral illness and/or fever, owing to the association between aspirin use and Reye's syndrome in this age group. Women who are pregnant or those who are menopausal will not experience dysmenorrhea. Women who are breast-feeding should avoid use of NSAIDs because of a potential harm to the infant's cardiovascular system. Aspirin should also be avoided by lactating women. Aspirin is excreted in breast milk and exposure through breast milk may result in rashes, bleeding, or platelet abnormalities in the infant. Acetaminophen is compatible with breast-feeding according to the American Academy of Pediatrics.

PATIENT FACTORS

Given that NSAIDs are used only short-term and intermittently, the risk for GI toxicity (irritation, bleeding, or ulceration) is limited. However, patients who have active peptic ulcer disease, are at risk for GI bleeding, or have a history of GI ulcers should discuss use of NSAIDs with their primary care provider. They may attempt to treat dysmenorrhea with acetaminophen or consider use of an oral contraceptive. NSAIDs can also inhibit platelet activity and increase bleeding time. Women on anticoagulants should avoid NSAID use, and women on other agents that may increase bleeding should use NSAIDs cautiously. Women who consume three or more alcohol-containing beverages daily should discuss use of acetaminophen or aspirin with their primary care provider; additive liver or GI toxicity may occur, respectively.

PATIENT PREFERENCES

Consumers with previous experience with an NSAID may prefer to use that agent, because they are familiar with it or, alternatively, they may prefer to try another agent if side effects were experienced. Preferences may also be based on tablet/capsule preferences or cost of products.

Complementary Therapies

Several preliminary small studies have suggested that intake of several vitamins or minerals (magnesium,[16] vitamins B_1,[17] B_{12},[18] vitamin E,[19,20] or zinc[21]) may decrease dysmenorrhea. A recent report also suggested that sweet fennel (*Foeniculum vulgare dulce*) extract may be useful in relieving primary dysmenorrhea.[22] Fennel is not appropriate for women with a seizure disorder and may reduce blood clotting. All these potential therapies need further study and verification.

Assessment of Primary Dysmenorrhea: A Case-Based Approach

Before recommending any product to a patient experiencing symptoms of dysmenorrhea, the health care provider should ascertain that the symptoms, particularly the onset and duration of pain in relation to the onset of menses, are consistent with primary dysmenorrhea (Table 9-1).

Case 9-1 illustrates the assessment of patients with dysmenorrhea.

CASE 9-1

Relevant Evaluation Criteria	Scenario/Model Outcome
Information Gathering	
1. Gather essential information about the patient's symptoms, including:	
a. description of symptom(s) (i.e., nature, onset, duration, severity, associated symptoms)	Patient is experiencing painful menstrual cramps. She began menses about 4 years ago and has had cramping before, but now it occurs almost every month. She has also started to have backaches and headaches. These symptoms begin as soon as her menses begins and last for about 2 days. If the cramps are really bad, she may stay home from school or skip soccer practice.
b. description of any factors which seem to precipitate, exacerbate, and/or relieve the patient's symptom(s)	Patient tries to sleep when the symptoms are worst. A hot bath or use of a heating patch helps.

Relevant Evaluation Criteria	Scenario/Model Outcome
c. description of the patient's efforts to relieve the symptoms	She uses a heat patch if she stays home. She also takes either acetaminophen 325 mg or ibuprofen 200 mg (2 tablets 2–3 times a day).
2. Gather essential patient history information:	
a. patient's identity	Erin McTavish
b. age, sex, height, and weight	17-year-old female, 5 ft 7 in, 120 lb
c. concurrent medical conditions, prescription and nonprescription medications, and dietary supplements	No major or chronic illnesses; multivitamin 1 daily, acetaminophen 325 mg or ibuprofen 200 mg as needed for headaches
d. allergies/other adverse reactions to medications	NKDA

Assessment and Triage

3. Differentiate patient's signs/symptoms and correctly identify the patient's primary problem(s) (see Table 9-1).	Ms. McTavish has symptoms and a history consistent with primary dysmenorrhea.
4. Identify exclusions for self-treatment (see Figure 9-2).	None; she is not sexually active.
5. Formulate a comprehensive list of therapeutic alternatives for the primary problem to determine if triage to a medical practitioner is required and share this information with the patient	Options include: (1) Refer her for medical evaluation. (2) Recommend self-treatment with a nonprescription NSAID. (3) Take no action.

Plan

6. Select an optimal therapeutic alternative to address the patient's problem, taking into account patient preferences.	Ms. McTavish has symptoms and a pattern of symptoms indicating primary dysmenorrhea. She has no chronic medical problems and has used NSAIDs previously with some relief. She is a good candidate for self-treatment (see Figure 9-2).
7. Describe the recommended therapeutic approach to the patient.	You have two choices of nonprescription NSAID products. Because you have used ibuprofen previously with some pain relief, I suggest you try using this agent every 6 hours at the recommended dose, starting when your menses begins and continuing for the first 2 days of your menses. You may also continue use of hot baths and heat patches. See the box Patient Education for Primary Dysmenorrhea for instructions on proper use.
8. Explain to the patient the rationale for selecting the recommended therapeutic approach from the considered therapeutic alternatives.	Your symptoms are typical of primary dysmenorrhea, and there are no reasons why you should not use self-treatment. NSAIDs are the drugs of choice for the treatment of primary dysmenorrhea, because they are usually very effective and well tolerated. Heat and acetaminophen can be helpful, but NSAIDs are more effective for most women.

Patient Education

9. When recommending self-care with nonprescription medications and/or nondrug therapy, convey accurate information to the patient:	
a. appropriate dose and frequency of administration, maximum number of days the therapy should be employed	Ibuprofen 200 mg: Take 2 tablets at the onset of menses and every 6 hours for the first 2 days of menses.
b. expected time to onset of relief	Relief should begin within 30–60 minutes. The best approach to preventing cramps is to take ibuprofen every 6 hours on a regular schedule.
c. degree of relief that can be reasonably expected	Symptoms should be improved or alleviated by treatment.
d. most common side effects	Nausea or heartburn-like pain is possible; take with food.
e. side effects which warrant medical intervention should they occur	Significant nausea or heartburn that persists beyond the first 48 hours of treatment

C A S E   9 - 1   (continued)

Relevant Evaluation Criteria	Scenario/Model Outcome
f. patient options in the event that condition worsens or persists	If ibuprofen therapy is unsuccessful, naproxen sodium may be tried. If you use nonprescription NSAIDs for several menstrual cycles and your symptoms do not improve to where they are tolerable and do not disrupt your activities, you should see your primary care provider.
g. product storage requirements	Product should be stored in a cool area.
h. specific nondrug measures	Heat (hot baths, heating patch) can be used.
10. Solicit patient's follow-up questions.	(1) Why are my menstrual cramps worse now? (2) Why do I have to take the ibuprofen every 6 hours?
11. Answer patient's questions.	(1) As women mature, the body ovulates every month rather than just some months. Dysmenorrhea occurs only if ovulation has occurred. (2) Taking the medication regularly provides better pain relief and can prevent cramping, which is the cause of the pain.

Key: NKDA, no known drug allergies; NSAID, nonsteroidal anti-inflammatory drug.

Patient Counseling for Primary Dysmenorrhea

Adolescents and young women who experience primary dysmenorrhea symptoms should be educated about this condition so they (1) realize primary dysmenorrhea is normal, (2) recognize typical symptoms and symptoms that are inconsistent with primary dysmenorrhea and when to seek medical evaluation, (3) understand that NSAIDs are preferred therapy because of their proven greater efficacy, and (4) know how to use these agents for greatest benefit. Patients should also be advised that nonprescription nonsalicylate NSAIDs can be appropriate for initial therapy, but not all women will respond to these agents. If response to the first agent is not adequate, the other nonsalicylate NSAIDs, as well as nondrug interventions, can be tried. The health care provider should explain the proper use of these agents and their potential adverse effects. The box Patient Education for Primary Dysmenorrhea lists specific information to provide patients.

PATIENT EDUCATION FOR **Primary Dysmenorrhea**

The objective of self-treatment is to relieve or significantly improve symptoms of dysmenorrhea so as to limit discomfort and disruption of usual activities. For most patients, carefully following product instructions and the self-care measures listed here will help ensure optimal therapeutic outcomes.

Nondrug Measures

- If effective, apply topical heat to the abdomen, lower back, or other painful area.
- Stop smoking cigarettes.
- Consider eating more types of fish that are high in omega-3 fatty acids or taking a fish oil supplement.
- Participate in regular exercise if it lessens the symptoms.

Nonprescription Medications

- Nonprescription nonsalicylate NSAID medications (ibuprofen and naproxen sodium) are the best type of nonprescription medication to treat primary dysmenorrhea. These medications stop or prevent the strong contractions (cramping) of the uterus.
- Start taking the medication when the menstrual period begins or when menstrual pain or other symptoms begin. Then take the medication at regular intervals following the product instructions, rather than just when the symptoms are present. See Table 9-2 for recommended dosages of nonprescription nonsalicylate NSAIDs.

- Take a nonsalicylate NSAID with food to limit the most common side effects: upset stomach and heartburn.
- Do not take nonsalicylate NSAIDs if you are allergic to aspirin or any nonsalicylate NSAID, or if you have peptic ulcer disease, gastroesophageal reflux disease, colitis, or any bleeding disorder.
- If you have hypertension, asthma, or congestive heart failure, watch for early symptoms that the nonsalicylate NSAID is causing fluid retention.
- Do not take a nonsalicylate NSAID if you are also taking anticoagulants or lithium.

 If abdominal pain occurs at times other than just before or during the first few days of a menstrual period, seek medical attention.

 Seek medical attention if the pain intensity increases or if new symptoms occur.

Evaluation of Patient Outcomes for Primary Dysmenorrhea

Patient monitoring is accomplished by having the patient report whether the symptoms are resolved. Symptoms should improve within an hour or so of taking an NSAID. The optimal effect of drug therapy may not be seen, however, until the woman has used the medication on a scheduled basis. The woman should be encouraged to contact her health care provider to report on treatment effectiveness (i.e., continued or altered symptoms). The patient with persistent symptoms should be advised to try another nonprescription nonsalicylate NSAID, to add adjunct therapy, or to see a primary care provider for evaluation.

PREMENSTRUAL SYNDROME

Premenstrual syndrome (PMS) is defined as a cyclic disorder composed of a combination of physical and emotional (mood) symptoms that occur during the luteal phase of the menstrual cycle, improve significantly or disappear within the first several days of menstrual flow, and are absent during the first week following menses. The diagnosis of PMS can be made on the basis of physical or mood symptoms that occur cyclically. Premenstrual dysphoric disorder (PMDD) is a severe form of PMS; the diagnosis of this condition requires that a specific constellation of symptoms occurs on a cyclic basis, and that symptoms are severe enough to cause functional impairment (interfere with social and/or occupational functioning).[23]

Almost all women experience some physical or mood changes before the onset of menses that are[24] normal signs of ovulatory cycles; these symptoms are referred to medically as "molimina."[25] Symptoms vary among women but are typically constant for an individual woman. They may include physical symptoms, food cravings, and emotional lability or lowered mood. In addition, some women report positive changes, such as increased energy, creativity, work productivity, and sexual desire.[23,24]

The majority of women with premenstrual symptoms experience only mild, primarily physical symptoms that do not interfere with their lives. An estimated 40% of women with premenstrual symptoms describe them as bothersome, 10% to 15% report their symptoms as severe, and 3% to 5% report symptoms that cause significant impairment in daily life that interferes with relationships, lifestyle, or work.[24] The number and severity of symptoms and the extent to which they interfere with functioning distinguish typical premenstrual symptoms, PMS, and PMDD[24,26,27] (Table 9-3).

PMS can occur any time after menarche; symptoms usually originate when women are in their early 20s, but typically women wait to seek care until they are over age 30.[24,26,28] PMS symptoms occur only during ovulatory cycles. Symptoms disappear during events that interrupt ovulation, such as pregnancy and breast-feeding, and PMS symptoms disappear at menopause. However, use of hormone therapy postmenopausally may result in recurrence of PMS symptoms.[29]

Among women, Caucasians and African Americans have a similar symptom experience. Asian women report a lower severity of PMS symptoms, whereas Hispanic women report more severe PMS symptoms.[30] Factors that predict severe PMS or PMDD are a past history of depression, working outside the home, less education, and use of tobacco.[31] Current smokers are four times more likely to have a diagnosis of PMDD than nonsmokers.[31] Similarly, symptoms may also be more severe for current smokers.[30] This finding parallels the correlation between tobacco smoking and depression.[31]

Women with PMDD tend to be high utilizers of health care; use of both mental health practitioners and primary care providers is greater in women with PMDD than in the general population. Women with PMDD also have a significant rate of suicide attempts (15% report at least one attempt).[32]

TABLE 9-3 Differentiation of PMS and PMDD from Other Conditions with Luteal Phase Symptoms

Typical premenstrual symptoms (molimina)	Mild physical (breast tenderness, bloating, lower backache, food cravings) or mood (emotional lability, lowered mood, increased energy or creativity) changes before the onset of menses that do not interfere with normal life functions
Premenstrual syndrome	At least one mood (e.g., depression, irritability, anger, anxiety) or physical (e.g., breast tenderness, abdominal bloating) symptom during the 5 days prior to menses. Symptoms are virtually absent during cycle days 5–10. The symptom or symptoms have a negative effect on social functioning or lifestyle, but the severity is mild to moderate.
Premenstrual dysphoric disorder	Five or more symptoms (mood or physical) are present the last week of the luteal phase of the menstrual cycle, with at least one symptom being significant depression, anxiety, affective lability, or anger. The intensity of the symptoms interferes with work, school, social activities, and social relationships. Symptoms should be absent the week after menses and must not be an exacerbation of the symptoms of another disorder such as depression, panic disorder, or personality disorder.
Premenstrual exacerbation	A worsening of the symptoms of other, typically psychiatric disorders such as depression and anxiety or panic disorders. Conditions such as endometriosis, hypothyroidism, attention deficit disorder, diabetes mellitus, migraine headaches, and perimenopause can also worsen premenstrually. However, symptoms do not occur only during the luteal phase of the menstrual cycle; there is no symptom-free interval.

Source: References 24, 26, and 27.

Pathophysiology of PMS

The etiology of PMS is unknown. The current consensus is that normal ovarian function (and the consequent fluctuation of estrogen and progesterone levels) is the cyclic trigger for PMS/PMDD symptoms. There is no known hormonal imbalance in women with PMS. It appears that some women are biologically vulnerable or predisposed to experience PMS because of a neurotransmitter sensitivity to physiologic changes in hormone levels.[28] Women with PMS/PMDD may be predisposed to mood and anxiety symptoms caused by a difference in the sensitivity of the serotonin system. The neurotransmitter serotonin is affected by estrogen and progesterone levels, and is involved in the pathogenesis of premenstrual irritability and dysphoria. Other neurotransmitters and systems that may be of potential importance are gamma-aminobutyric acid (GABA), opiates (endorphins) and the beta-adrenergic receptors.[28] Thys-Jacobs[33] suggests that a difference in the cyclicity of calcium and of substances influencing calcium levels in the body (i.e., vitamin D or parathyroid hormone) may explain why some women experience PMS symptoms. PMS symptoms are quite similar to symptoms of hypocalcemia. There is evidence of a genetic predisposition, and sociocultural factors may also influence PMS symptoms.[23] A recent study of twins found evidence for a genetic predisposition, but environmental influences (external stressors) correlated more strongly with symptoms.[34]

PMS does not appear to be simply a variant of depression: It is cyclic; it does not spontaneously remit; symptoms are not relieved by all types of antidepressants; and its primary symptoms are irritability and anxiety, not depression.[35] Early studies found an association between PMDD and mood disorders such as major depression; in one study, 58% of women with PMDD had a history of depression.[31] However, this association has been disputed except for evidence of an increased likelihood of postpartum depression among women with PMDD.[35]

Exogenous hormones may influence premenstrual symptoms. Women taking either oral contraceptives or postmenopausal hormone replacement therapy may experience adverse effects similar to PMS symptoms as a result of altered hormone levels.[23,29] Conversely, oral contraceptive use may also protect against emotional symptoms. PMS scores for women using oral contraceptives were lower than those for nonusers.[30,34]

Fluctuations in ovarian hormones (estrogen and progesterone) give rise to biochemical changes in neurotransmitters. Serotonin levels are decreased in women with PMS.[29] A decrease in serotonin levels is associated with irritability, dysphoria, and food cravings; these symptoms are also associated with PMS/PMDD.

Central nervous system metabolism of steroids may also be different in women with PMS/PMDD. Levels of allopregnanolone, a progesterone metabolite that interacts with the GABA system, have been found to be lower during the luteal phase in women with PMS than in women without these symptoms.[23] A decrease in allopregnanolone could increase anxiety. Also, selective serotonin reuptake inhibitors (SSRIs), which are known to relieve PMS/PMDD, have been found to affect the synthesis of allopregnanolone. Therefore, for symptoms severe enough to warrant prescription drug therapy, treatment is based on medications that affect the levels of serotonin or suppress ovulation and interrupt hormonal cycling.

Clinical Presentation of PMS

None of the symptoms of PMS or PMDD is unique to these conditions; however, the occurrence of specific symptoms and their fluctuation with the phases of the menstrual cycle are diagnostic. Premenstrual symptoms typically begin or intensify about a week prior to the onset of menses, peak the day before or on the first day of menses, and resolve within several days after the beginning of menses.[24] A woman with PMS or PMDD should experience essentially a symptom-free interval during days 4 to 12 of her menstrual cycle. Symptoms may also be experienced for 1 day at the time of ovulation.[25,26] Symptoms of PMS/PMDD appear to be worse early in reproductive life and tend to improve toward menopause, when ovulation may be intermittent and hormonal fluctuations perhaps lessen.[30]

Common symptoms of PMS are listed in Table 9-4. In a recent study, the two most common premenstrual symptoms were bloating/weight gain and breast swelling/tenderness. Aside from these physical symptoms, affective symptoms (e.g., fatigue, anxiety, and irritability) were more common than other physical symptoms.[34] For an individual woman, symptoms remain consistent across cycles.[25,26] Among women experiencing at least one PMS symptom frequently over the past 12 months, 55% reported that the symptom was present in almost all cycles.[32] The majority of women rate their symptoms as mild or moderate and do not feel the symptoms interfere in their life or are limiting. Mood symptoms tend to cause more impairment than physical symptoms.[26]

Symptoms of PMDD are similar to those of PMS; however, compared with women who have PMS, women with PMDD experience more of the symptoms, more severe symptoms, and symptoms that impair personal relationships and the ability to function well at work to a greater extent. Among women with PMDD, the most common symptoms are affective: depressed mood/hopelessness/self-depreciation (90.5%), affective lability (89.7%), irritability/anger (81.5%), fatigability (78.6%), physical complaints (78.1%), anxiety/tension (67%), and decreased

---

TABLE 9-4 Occurrence Rate of Common PMS Symptoms

Most Common Negative Symptoms

Fatigue, lack of energy
Irritability
Labile mood with alternating sadness and anger
Depression
Anxiety, feeling stressed
Crying spells, oversensitivity
Difficulty concentrating
Abdominal bloating, edema of extremities
Breast tenderness
Appetite changes and food cravings
Headache
Gastrointestinal upset

Most Common Positive Symptoms

Increased energy, more efficient at work
Increased libido, more affectionate
Increased sense of control, more self-assured

Source: Adapted from reference 23.

interest (63.3%).[32] Other symptoms of PMDD include difficulty concentrating, lethargy, hypersomnia or insomnia, and physical symptoms (e.g., breast tenderness and bloating). The severity of symptoms results in an average of 2.6 days of impairment or disability per month.[32] A daily rating of symptoms for several cycles establishes a diagnosis of PMDD, and these types of symptoms should have occurred during most menstrual cycles over the past year. PMDD symptoms during the late luteal phase (last 7 days of the cycle) should be at least 30% worse than those experienced during the mid-follicular phase (days 3–9 of the menstrual cycle).

It is important to distinguish PMS/PMDD from typical premenstrual symptoms (molimina) and also from premenstrual exacerbations (PMEs) of other disorders, particularly mood disorders. A number of medical conditions can be aggravated during the premenstrual phase, including major depression, panic attacks, migraine headaches, asthma, and seizure disorders.[35] In addition, mood disorders not occurring solely during the luteal phase must be distinguished from cyclic mood symptoms (Table 9-3).

Lack of a symptom-free interval suggests that the patient has a psychiatric disorder (e.g., anxiety or panic disorder) or another health condition (e.g., perimenopause) rather than PMS.

Treatment of PMS

PMS is a multisymptom disorder, involving behavioral and physical symptoms. A single therapeutic agent is unlikely to address all symptoms; thus, agents should be selected to address the patient's most bothersome symptoms. A symptom log/calendar is a very useful tool to document the most bothersome symptom(s) and the cyclic nature of this disorder. This information will also be useful in evaluating the efficacy of treatment. Patients with severe symptoms are less likely to have symptoms alleviated solely by use of nonprescription therapies. In addition, PMS symptoms are chronic and in most cases will continue until menopause. Therefore, the cost of therapy, the fact that a woman may become pregnant, and the likelihood of adverse effects from therapy are important considerations in selecting therapy.[24,25]

Treatment Goals

Two outcomes are desirable for women with PMS or PMDD: (1) to understand PMS and (2) to improve or resolve symptoms to reduce the impact on activities and interpersonal relationships. Typically, therapy is considered effective if symptoms are reduced by 50% or more.

General Treatment Approach

The initial treatment of PMS symptoms is generally conservative, consisting of education and nondrug measures such as dietary modifications, physical exercise, and stress management. Women with symptoms of PMS should be educated about the syndrome and encouraged to identify techniques for coping with PMS symptoms and stress. Many women are engaged in multiple social roles, which can increase stress. Knowledge of this disorder can allow a woman to exert some control over her symptoms by anticipating and planning. For example, she might schedule more challenging tasks during the first half of the cycle, thus limiting the influence of this condition on her social and occupational functioning.

For symptoms unresponsive to nondrug therapy, several nonprescription or complementary agents that are relatively nontoxic might be suggested. These agents include calcium, magnesium, vitamin E, pyridoxine, and chasteberry (*Vitex agnus*).

Prescription drug therapy should be considered if the treatments outlined in Figure 9-3 fail or the patient suffers from severe PMS or PMDD. Prescription therapy includes psychotropic medications (e.g., alprazolam and SSRIs) and menstrual cycle modifiers (e.g., oral contraceptives, danazol, and GnRH agonists).

Nonpharmacologic Therapy

Several nonpharmacologic therapies may provide some amelioration of PMS symptoms. These include aerobic exercise, dietary modifications, and cognitive-behavioral therapy.[27] Women who exercise may have fewer and less severe PMS symptoms compared with nonexercisers.[27,36] Although the benefit of nutritional therapy for PMS is largely unproven, many clinicians recommend a balanced diet combined with avoiding salty foods and simple sugars (which may cause fluid retention) as well as caffeine and alcohol (which can increase irritability). Consumption of caffeine-containing beverages has been associated with increased PMS symptoms.[36] Cravings for foods high in carbohydrates, which contain the serotonin precursor tryptophan, are common in women with PMS. A study of a carbohydrate-rich beverage, which increased tryptophan levels, demonstrated an improvement in mood scores (depression, tension, anger, and confusion) for women with PMDD.[37] Consuming foods that are rich in complex carbohydrates (e.g., whole-grain foods) during the premenstrual interval may reduce symptoms. A strict low-fat diet may decrease breast pain.[35]

Stress is reported to increase PMS symptoms. Cognitive-behavioral therapy, which emphasizes relaxation techniques and coping skills, can help reduce PMS symptoms. These approaches may be helpful used singly or as adjuncts to other therapies.

Pharmacologic Therapy

Surveys of women have found that 20% to 50% use some nonprescription medication for premenstrual symptoms, primarily analgesics and vitamins.[38] One study[39] of more than 1000 women ages 21 to 64 years found that 42% of those who had PMS-type symptoms (feeling more emotional, bloating, food cravings, and pain) took medication for their symptoms; 80% were taking a nonprescription product. Among women taking a nonprescription product, the medications most commonly cited were Midol (24% of women), acetaminophen (19%), ibuprofen (16%), and Pamprin (14%). Other nonprescription therapies that may be effective are vitamins, minerals, and NSAIDs.

Pyridoxine

Vitamin B_6 has been suggested as a therapy for PMS. Many trials have found this agent to be ineffective. However, a meta-analysis found that B_6 was more effective than placebo in relieving overall PMS symptoms (mastalgia, irritability, fatigue, bloating, and tension) and depression associated with PMS,[40] although no dose-response correlation was shown. It is recommended that the dose of pyridoxine be limited to 100 mg daily because of the potential for neuropathy. Risk of neuropathy is usually associated with high doses (2–6 g daily) but can occur with daily doses greater than 200 mg, although with lower doses the neuropathy

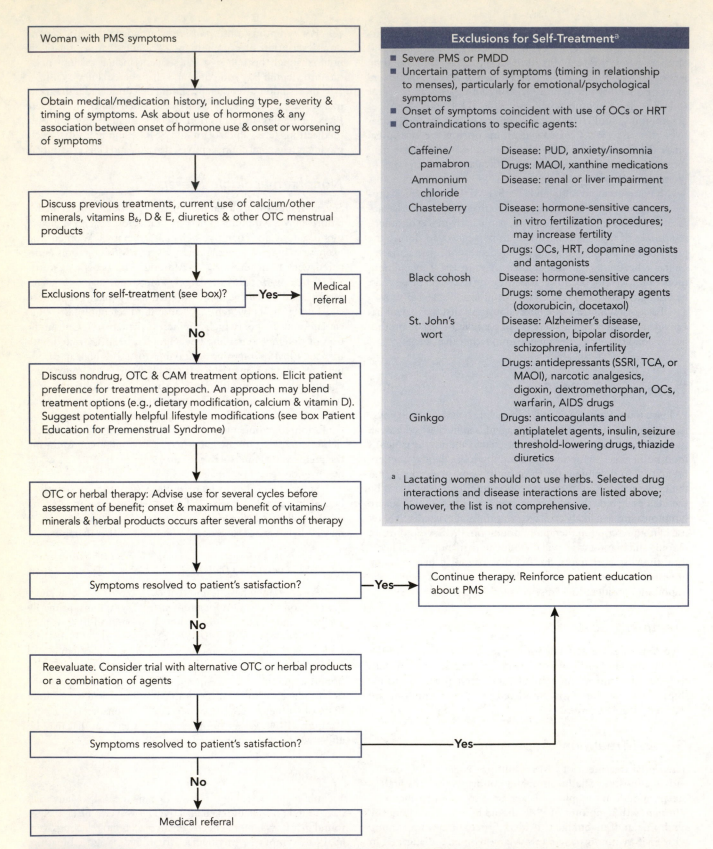

Woman with PMS symptoms

Obtain medical/medication history, including type, severity & timing of symptoms. Ask about use of hormones & any association between onset of hormone use & onset or worsening of symptoms

Discuss previous treatments, current use of calcium/other minerals, vitamins B₆, D & E, diuretics & other OTC menstrual products

Exclusions for self-treatment (see box)? —Yes→ Medical referral

No

Discuss nondrug, OTC & CAM treatment options. Elicit patient preference for treatment approach. An approach may blend treatment options (e.g., dietary modification, calcium & vitamin D). Suggest potentially helpful lifestyle modifications (see box Patient Education for Premenstrual Syndrome)

OTC or herbal therapy: Advise use for several cycles before assessment of benefit; onset & maximum benefit of vitamins/minerals & herbal products occurs after several months of therapy

Symptoms resolved to patient's satisfaction? —Yes→ Continue therapy. Reinforce patient education about PMS

No

Reevaluate. Consider trial with alternative OTC or herbal products or a combination of agents

Symptoms resolved to patient's satisfaction? —Yes→ (Continue therapy)

No

Medical referral

Exclusions for Self-Treatment[a]

- Severe PMS or PMDD
- Uncertain pattern of symptoms (timing in relationship to menses), particularly for emotional/psychological symptoms
- Onset of symptoms coincident with use of OCs or HRT
- Contraindications to specific agents:

Caffeine/ pamabron	Disease: PUD, anxiety/insomnia
	Drugs: MAOI, xanthine medications
Ammonium chloride	Disease: renal or liver impairment
Chasteberry	Disease: hormone-sensitive cancers, in vitro fertilization procedures; may increase fertility
	Drugs: OCs, HRT, dopamine agonists and antagonists
Black cohosh	Disease: hormone-sensitive cancers
	Drugs: some chemotherapy agents (doxorubicin, docetaxol)
St. John's wort	Disease: Alzheimer's disease, depression, bipolar disorder, schizophrenia, infertility
	Drugs: antidepressants (SSRI, TCA, or MAOI), narcotic analgesics, digoxin, dextromethorphan, OCs, warfarin, AIDS drugs
Ginkgo	Drugs: anticoagulants and antiplatelet agents, insulin, seizure threshold-lowering drugs, thiazide diuretics

[a] Lactating women should not use herbs. Selected drug interactions and disease interactions are listed above; however, the list is not comprehensive.

FIGURE 9-3 Self-care of premenstrual syndrome. Key: AIDS, acquired immunodeficiency syndrome; CAM, complementary and alternative medicine; HRT, hormone replacement therapy; MAOI, monoamine oxidase inhibitor; OC, oral contraceptive; OTC, over-the-counter; PMDD, premenstrual dysphoric disorder; PMS, premenstrual syndrome; PUD, peptic ulcer disease; SSRI, selective serotonin reuptake inhibitor; TCA, tricyclic antidepressant.

is usually reversible.[40] Symptoms of this toxicity include paresthesia (a sensation of pricking, tingling, or creeping on the skin), bone pain, muscle weakness, and hyperesthesia (stinging, burning, or itching sensations).

Vitamin E

Vitamin E (400 IU daily) is sometimes recommended for the symptom of breast tenderness. However, data on its effectiveness are unconvincing.

Calcium and Vitamin D

Three randomized trials have evaluated the effect of calcium supplementation on PMS symptoms. A well-designed trial studied the effect of calcium (600 mg twice daily) in 466 women with moderate-to-severe PMS.[41] Symptoms were significantly reduced by the second month of therapy; by the third month, calcium had reduced overall symptoms by 48%. Emotional (e.g., mood swings, depression, and anger), behavioral (e.g., food cravings), and physical symptoms (e.g., fluid retention, breast tenderness, backaches, and abdominal cramping) were all reduced. More than 50% of the women taking calcium had a greater than 50% improvement in symptoms; 29% had a greater than 75% improvement in symptoms. Few women experienced adverse effects from calcium, five withdrew from the study because of nausea, and one woman in each group (calcium and placebo) developed kidney stones. The dose of calcium used in the trial is consistent with the recommended daily calcium intake for women of reproductive age. Similarly, a study[42] of women with PMS taking 1000 mg of calcium daily found that 73% reported fewer symptoms (negative affect or fluid retention) while taking calcium. A third study[43] comparing two doses of dietary calcium (587 or 1336 mg) found that women experienced less severe mood symptoms and fluid retention on the higher calcium diet. Recently, it was reported that high dietary intake of both calcium (1200 mg/day) and vitamin D (400 IU) may prevent the development of PMS symptoms.[44] Importantly, all health care providers should be reinforcing adequate calcium and vitamin D intake in women to help prevent osteoporosis and some cancers.[45]

Magnesium

One small trial has shown that magnesium (360 mg daily administered during the luteal phase) can relieve affective symptoms of PMS.[46] It has been hypothesized that magnesium deficiency may lead to PMS-type symptoms (e.g., irritability), and low magnesium levels in red blood cells have been found in women with PMS.[46] The dose of magnesium used in the trial was similar to the recommended dietary allowance of magnesium for women (280–300 mg). About one-half of women regularly consume less than that amount and obtaining adequate magnesium from food may be difficult. Side effects from magnesium are uncommon; diarrhea is the most common side effect.

Nonsteroidal Anti-Inflammatory Drugs

Prostaglandin inhibitors (e.g., NSAIDs) have also been studied for treating PMS. NSAIDs have been shown to reduce some of the physical symptoms (e.g., headache, fatigue, and other pain) and mood symptoms associated with PMS when taken for 1 week prior to and during the first several days of menses. It has been suggested that the benefit from these agents may be a result of the coexistence of dysmenorrhea and PMS.

Diuretics

One of the most common premenstrual complaints is the subjective sensation of fluid accumulation, particularly abdominal bloating. However, the majority of women do not experience any true water or sodium retention and do not experience weight gain.[47] Two factors may explain the sense of abdominal bloating. First, a distinction must be made between fluid redistribution and fluid retention (detected by weight gain). The bloating and swelling observed with PMS are primarily caused by a fluid shift; therefore, diuretics—indicated for relieving fluid retention—are unlikely to be helpful for most PMS patients. Second, abdominal distension may occur secondary to relaxation of the gut muscle caused by progesterone.[47] For women who have true water retention and resultant weight gain, a diuretic may be useful.

The Food and Drug Administration (FDA) has approved three diuretics as useful for relieving water retention, weight gain, bloating, swelling, and feeling of fullness, while being safe for nonprescription use. These diuretics are ammonium chloride, caffeine, and pamabrom. Pamabrom is the diuretic most commonly contained in commercially available menstrual products (Table 9-5).

Ammonium chloride is an acid-forming salt with a short duration of effect; it is taken in oral doses of up to 3 g/day (divided into three doses) for no more than 6 consecutive days. Larger doses of ammonium chloride (412 g/day) can produce significant adverse effects of the GI and central nervous systems. Ammonium chloride is contraindicated in patients with renal or liver impairment, because metabolic acidosis may result.

Caffeine, a xanthine, promotes diuresis by inhibiting the renal tubular reabsorption of sodium and water. It is safe and

---

TABLE 9-5 Selected Menstrual Products

Trade Name	Diuretic	Other Ingredients
AquaBan Diuretic Maximum Strength Tablets	Pamabrom 50 mg	
Diurex PMS Pre-menstrual Relief, Midol PMS Multisymptom Formula; Pamprin Multisymptom, Premsyn PMS	Pamabrom 25 mg	Acetaminophen 500 mg; pyrilamine maleate 15 mg
Midol Maximum Strength Multisymptom Menstrual Formula	Caffeine 60 mg	Acetaminophen 500 mg; pyrilamine maleate 15 mg

effective as a diuretic in dosages of 100 to 200 mg every 3 to 4 hours. Patients may develop tolerance to the diuretic effect. Caffeine may also cause anxiety, restlessness, or insomnia or worsen PMS by causing irritability. Additive side effects (nervousness, irritability, or tachycardia) might occur if other caffeine-containing beverages (especially "energy drinks"), foods, or medications are consumed concurrently. Caffeine may also cause GI irritation, so patients with a history of peptic ulcer disease should avoid it. Patients taking monoamine oxidase inhibitors or xanthine medications (e.g., theophylline) should avoid diuretics that contain caffeine.

Pamabrom, a derivative of theophylline, is contained in combination products (along with analgesics and antihistamines) marketed for the treatment of PMS. It is taken in doses of up to 200 mg/day (50 mg four times daily).

Combination Products

Multi-ingredient nonprescription products are marketed for women with PMS-type symptoms. Two of the most commonly used products are Midol and Pamprin (acetaminophen, pamabrom, and pyrilamine; Table 9-5). Pain is a relatively uncommon feature of PMS, and no evidence exists that the sedative effect of an antihistamine (e.g., pyrilamine) will provide benefit to women experiencing the emotional symptoms of PMS. Therefore, these types of nonprescription products should not be recommended. More appropriate therapeutic recommendations are use of more definitive agents, such as those previously discussed, and referral for prescription drug therapy.

Pharmacotherapeutic Comparison

Calcium, because it has overall health benefits and is generally well tolerated, can be suggested for the initial treatment of PMS symptoms. If this agent provides inadequate relief, another agent or a combination of two or more agents may be tried. Women who experience bloating with documented weight gain might try pamabrom, caffeine, or ginkgo. Caffeine and pamabrom may not be an appropriate choice for a woman who experiences irritability as a PMS symptom. Both xanthines (caffeine and pamabrom) are contraindicated in patients who have a history of peptic ulcer disease or are taking monoamine oxidase inhibitors or other xanthine medications (e.g., theophylline). NSAIDs should be reserved for women who experience both PMS and dysmenorrhea or headache symptoms. Use of combination products containing antihistamines should be discouraged; drowsiness may impair job performance, schoolwork, and driving.

Product Selection Guidelines

SPECIAL POPULATIONS

PMS does not occur during pregnancy or after menopause. Adolescents and adult women can be treated similarly, and they should initially attempt management of symptoms with lifestyle changes and use of low-risk therapies such as calcium supplementation. Adolescents should avoid combination products containing aspirin (see Dysmenorrhea, Product Selection Guidelines). Women who are breast-feeding should avoid all herbal products, because there is limited information about their safety for the infant. Vitamins and minerals in the doses used for PMS are generally compatible with breast-feeding; magnesium use may cause diarrhea in infant. Diuretic products should be avoided during breast-feeding; caffeine is excreted in breast milk.

PATIENT FACTORS

Patients using medications that increase stomach pH (e.g., proton pump inhibitors and H_2-blockers) should use calcium citrate rather than calcium carbonate products, because the carbonate products are not soluble in low-stomach-acid conditions.

PATIENT PREFERENCES

Patient preferences (i.e., herbal or nondrug approach) about the approach to PMS treatment can be accommodated. Women preferring to use herbal products should discuss their use with a health care provider to be sure no drug–drug or drug–disease contraindications exist.

Complementary Therapies

Trials have been conducted on several alternative therapies. Herbs studied for the treatment of PMS include evening primrose oil, St. John's wort (*Hypericum perforatum*), chaste tree or chasteberry (*Vitex agnus-castus*), black cohosh (*Cimicifuga racemosa*), and ginkgo (*Ginkgo biloba*) (Table 9-6).[48]

Vitex (chasteberry) has been used traditionally for managing menstrual cycle symptoms. Two trials using a standardized fruit extract ZE 440 of *Vitex* found a significant reduction in the symptoms of mood, irritability/anger, pain/headache, breast tenderness, and fluid retention.[49,50] Symptoms were progressively reduced over several cycles, some benefit persisted for a few months after discontinuation, and therapy was well tolerated with few side effects. Another uncontrolled trial of the *Vitex* preparation Femicur in 1634 patients found much or very much reduced symptoms for 80% of women; only 6% reported no improvement.[51] In a trial in women diagnosed with PMDD, *Vitex* was compared with fluoxetine, an SSRI antidepressant known to be effective for the treatment of severe PMS and PMDD. A similar percentage of patients improved on both agents. *Vitex* was shown to decrease the following symptoms by more than 50%— irritability, breast tenderness, swelling, food cravings, and cramps. In contrast, fluoxetine improved more mood symptoms; those with a 50% reduction included depression, irritability, insomnia, nervous tension, feeling out of control, breast tenderness, and aches. *Vitex* was well tolerated; nausea and headache were the most common side effects of therapy. *Vitex* may offer more benefit for patients with less severe symptoms—mild-to-moderate PMS.[52] This herb may have estrogenic or progestogenic activity; use should be avoided by women who may be pregnant or who are not using reliable contraception.

A placebo-controlled randomized trial of ginkgo (165 women) found it improved all PMS-related symptoms. Benefit was greatest for breast pain and fluid retention symptoms.[36,48] Ginkgo may increase the risk of bleeding. (See Chapter 54 for more detailed information on ginkgo.)

Assessment of PMS: A Case-Based Approach

The health care provider should obtain a complete description of the patient's symptoms and their timing to determine whether the patient has PMS/PMDD or another disorder with PMS-type symptoms. The severity of PMS symptoms is another factor in self-treatment. As with any disorder, the health care provider should explore the use of medications that might be causing the symptoms or that might potentially interact with nonprescription agents used to treat PMS. Previous treatments of the symptoms should also be explored.

Case 9-2 illustrates the assessment of a patient with PMS.

TABLE 9-6 Complementary Therapies for the Treatment of PMS

Agent	Effectiveness	Comments
Vitamin B$_6$	Likely effective	Limit dose to 100 mg to avoid neuropathy; insufficient evidence on effectiveness from high-quality studies; not first-line therapy
Vitamin E	Possibly effective for mastalgia	Minimal evidence of benefit; nontoxic in usual dose (400 IU/day)
Calcium (elemental)	Effective	Good evidence on effectiveness from large randomized trials; improvement in both mood and physical symptoms; onset of benefit across several cycles; usual dose 1200–1500 mg/day
Magnesium (elemental)	Likely effective	Limited data on effectiveness but biological rationale exists; usual dose 200–400 mg day
Manganese	Insufficient evidence	One small trial (10 women); used along with calcium
Potassium	Insufficient evidence	Uncontrolled case reports; dose: 600 mg of potassium gluconate
Evening primrose oil[a]	Not effective	Controlled trials did not show a benefit; use unwarranted
St. John's wort[a]	Possibly effective	Only one small study to date using 300 mg (0.3% standardized hypericin) daily; showed improvement in mood scores; herb may be beneficial because MOA is similar to SSRI antidepressants
Vitex (chasteberry)[a]	Likely effective	Several trials (some using 20–40 mg Ze440 extract) have shown that herb reduces PMS symptoms, onset of benefit occurs over several cycles, and is well tolerated; GI symptoms and headache are possible side effects; dosing depends on product
Black cohosh[a]	Possibly effective	Often beneficial for menopausal symptoms; may relieve PMS symptoms because of similarity of symptoms; dosing depends on product; Remifemin, enzymatic therapy, and phytopharmica products are standardized to 1 mg triterpene per 20 mg tablet; 40–80 mg twice daily used in many studies
Ginkgo[a]	Likely effective	Ginkgo shown in randomized trial to improve PMS symptoms, particularly breast tenderness and fluid retention; ginkgo's antiplatelet effects may increase risk for bleeding; interacts with a number of drugs including anticoagulants, antiplatelet agents, anticonvulsants, fluoxetine, omeprazole, trazodone, buspirone, and St. John's wort; usual dose is 80 mg twice daily beginning cycle day 16 until day 5 of the next cycle

Key: GI, gastrointestinal; MOA, mechanism of action; PMS, premenstrual syndrome; SSRI, selective serotonin reuptake inhibitor.

[a] See Chapter 54 for more information.

CASE 9-2

Relevant Evaluation Criteria	Scenario/Model Outcome
Information Gathering	
1. Gather essential information about the patient's symptoms, including:	
a. description of symptom(s) (i.e., nature, onset, duration, severity, associated symptoms)	The patient cries easily and becomes irritable the week before her menses begins. But she also feels more energetic and can accomplish home or work projects. She also notices abdominal bloating that week.
b. description of any factors that seem to precipitate, exacerbate, and/or relieve the patient's symptom(s)	If she feels stressed—deadlines at work or an argument with her husband—then the irritability and/or sadness is worse. Getting to her yoga class helps lessen the irritability.
c. description of the patient's efforts to relieve the symptoms	Gets adequate sleep; goes to yoga class. For the bloating, she tries to cut back on salty foods.

Relevant Evaluation Criteria	Scenario/Model Outcome
2. Gather essential patient history information:	
a. patient's identity	Peggy Yee
b. age, sex, height, and weight	30-year-old female; 5 ft 1 in, 100 lb
c. dietary habits	She easts lots of tofu, vegetables, and noodles, and drinks green tea; her favorite snack food is nuts.
d. concurrent medical conditions, prescription and nonprescription medications, and dietary supplements	Healthy, no major or chronic illnesses; lactose intolerance; occasional headaches and muscle aches after gardening; no regular medicine use
e. allergies/other adverse reactions to medications	NKDA

Assessment and Triage

3. Differentiate patient's signs/symptoms and correctly identify the patient's primary problem(s).	Symptoms are consistent with PMS (see Tables 9-3 and 9-4).
4. Identify exclusions for self-treatment (see Figure 9-3).	None
5. Formulate a comprehensive list of therapeutic alternatives for the primary problem to determine if triage to a medical practitioner is required and share this information with the patient.	Options include: (1) Refer Ms. Yee for medical evaluation. (2) Recommend self-treatment with a nonprescription product, vitamin and/or mineral, or an herb. (3) Take no action.

Plan

6. Select an optimal therapeutic alternative to address the patient's problem, taking into account patient preferences.	Symptoms are consistent with PMS and are bothersome but not severe. Nonprescription options are safe and often effective. Self-treatment if reasonable; there are no contraindications to self-care. Ms. Yee has expressed an interest in a "natural approach." (See Figure 9-3.)
7. Describe the recommended therapeutic approach to the patient.	Learn about PMS, or premenstrual syndrome. Begin lifestyle changes, and use of calcium and vitamin D. (See the box Patient Education for Premenstrual Syndrome.)
8. Explain to the patient the rationale for selecting the recommended therapeutic approach from the considered therapeutic alternatives.	Adequate intake of calcium and vitamin D can relieve PMS symptoms and also prevent osteoporosis and some cancers. Intermittent use of ginkgo might be tried for relief of abdominal bloating (see Table 9-6) if calcium does not adequately manage this symptom; caffeine and pamabrom should be avoided because you experience irritability.

Patient Education

9. When recommending self-care with nonprescription medications and/or nondrug therapy, convey accurate information to the patient:	
a. appropriate dose and frequency of administration	See the box Patient Education for Premenstrual Syndrome.
b. maximum number of days the therapy should be employed	Calcium and vitamin D: Take every day. Ginkgo: Begin use on day 16 of the month and continue use until day 5 of menses.
c. expected time to onset of relief	An optimal benefit will occur only after about 3 months of use.
d. degree of relief that can be reasonably expected	Symptoms are often reduced by about 50%.
e. most common side effects	Calcium and vitamin D typically cause no side effects, but nausea and constipation are possible adverse effects of calcium.
f. patient options in the event that condition worsens or persists	Other nonprescription and herbal products might be tried (see Table 9-6).
g. specific nondrug measures	See the box Patient Education for Premenstrual Syndrome.
10. Solicit patient's follow-up question.	How long does it take for calcium and vitamin D to work?
11. Answer patient's question.	Calcium and vitamin D will reduce symptoms after 2–3 months of use.

Key: NKDA, no known drug allergies; PMS, premenstrual syndrome.

PATIENT EDUCATION FOR
Premenstrual Syndrome

The objective of self-treatment is to achieve relief from or significant improvement in symptoms to limit discomfort, distress, and the disruption of personal relationships or usual activities. For most patients, carefully following product instructions and the self-care measures listed here will help ensure optimal therapeutic outcomes.

Nondrug Measures

- Try to avoid stress, develop effective coping mechanisms for managing stress, and learn relaxation techniques.
- If possible, participate in regular aerobic exercise.
- During the 7–14 days before your menstrual period, reduce or eliminate intake of salt, caffeine, chocolate, and alcoholic beverages. Eating foods rich in carbohydrates and low in protein during the premenstrual interval may also reduce symptoms.

Nonprescription Medications

- Nonprescription medications and lifestyle modifications may not improve symptoms for all women, and it may take several months to determine whether these therapies are working.
- Therapy with one nonprescription medication may improve only some of the symptoms; several medications may be needed for optimal symptom control. However, it is best to add one agent at a time so that it is possible to determine which agent causes benefit or side effects.

- Follow the guidelines here for the agents that best control your symptoms:
  - Take 1200 mg of elemental calcium daily in divided doses. Take no more than 500 mg at one time. Calcium may cause stomach upset (if this occurs, take with food) or constipation.
  - Take at least 400 IU of vitamin D daily.
  - Take 360 mg of elemental magnesium daily during the premenstrual interval only. Magnesium may cause diarrhea.
  - Take 400 IU of vitamin E daily.
  - Take up to 100 mg of pyridoxine (vitamin B_6) daily. Do not exceed this daily dosage, or neurologic symptoms caused by vitamin B_6 toxicity may occur.

 If you are taking vitamin B_6 and develop neurologic symptoms, such as a sensation of pricking, tingling, or creeping on the skin; bone pain; muscle weakness; or stinging, burning, or itching sensations, stop taking the vitamin and seek medical attention.

 If the symptoms do not improve or if they worsen, a medical evaluation is suggested.

Patient Counseling for PMS

Educating women with PMS about the timing of symptoms (symptom log/calendar) and what might control them may increase compliance with recommended therapies. Health care providers should be prepared to discuss treatment of behavioral as well as physical symptoms of mild-to-moderate PMS. If the patient wants to use nonprescription medications or vitamins, the proper use and potential adverse effects of these agents should be explained. The patient should also be advised that treatment measures must be implemented during every menstrual cycle, because it may take several cycles for symptomatic relief to occur. The box Patient Education for Premenstrual Syndrome lists specific information to provide patients.

Evaluation of Patient Outcomes for PMS

Patient monitoring is accomplished by having the patient (or household members or coworkers, with the patient's permission) report whether the symptoms are resolved. It may take several menstrual cycles to ascertain if lifestyle changes or nonprescription therapies are reducing the symptoms of PMS. Comparing the occurrence of symptoms (as recorded on the log/calendar) for pre- and post-vitamin or medication use can help determine the usefulness of a therapy. The woman should be encouraged to contact her health care provider to discuss treatment effectiveness (continued or altered symptoms) and to clarify information or answer any questions. Reasons for advising the patient to see a primary care provider are either persistent symptoms, or symptoms that the patient reports as disruptive to personal relationships, or that affect the patient's ability to engage in usual activities or function productively at work.

TOXIC SHOCK SYNDROME

Toxic shock syndrome was a term originally coined in 1978 to describe a severe multisystem illness characterized by high fever, profound hypotension, severe diarrhea, mental confusion, renal failure, erythroderma, and skin desquamation. In 1980, these symptoms were recognized as affecting a relatively large number of young, previously healthy, menstruating women, and the term *toxic shock syndrome* was applied to their illness. TSS is commonly divided into menstrual and nonmenstrual cases.

Menstrual TSS has been found to affect primarily young women between 15 and 19 years of age; about 40% of cases of menstrual TSS still occur in women 13 to 19 years of age.[53] Menstrual TSS is associated with menstruation and tampon use (98% of cases), and is strongly linked to the use of high-absorbency tampons.[53]

During the TSS epidemic of 1979 to 1980, menstrual TSS accounted for 91% of TSS cases. More recently (1987–1996), menstrual TSS accounted for only 59% of all TSS cases.[53,54] Incidence rates have declined to two to four cases per 100,000 women ages 15 to 44 years old.[53,54] The decrease in cases of menstrual TSS has been attributed to several factors: removal of superabsorbent tampons from the market, a change in the composition of tampons, an increased awareness of the recommendations on the frequency of tampon changing and the need to alternate tampon and pad use, and FDA-required standardized labeling of tampons.[53]

Risk factors for menstrual TSS have been identified. The strongest predictor of risk is the use of tampons. Since the early 1980s, when the association between tampon usage and TSS was first noted, the absorbency and composition of tampons have changed dramatically. Certain compositions were associated with a higher risk, and tampons with cross-linked carboxymethylcellulose and polyester foam were removed from the market. In addition, FDA changed the requirement for labeling of tampons so that terms used to indicate the absorbency of tampons have a uniform meaning and indicate a specific range of fluid absorbed per tampon. Nonetheless, women who currently use tampons still have a 33-fold greater risk for TSS than nonusers. The greatest risk is associated with the use of higher absorbency tampons; for every 1 gram increase in absorbency, the risk for TSS increases 34% to 37%. Continuous use of tampons for at least 1 day of menses has also been shown to correlate with an increased risk for menstrual TSS. Besides tampons, TSS has been associated with the use of barrier contraceptives, including diaphragms, cervical caps, and cervical sponges, and with IUCs.[55]

Pathophysiology of Menstrual TSS

TSS is caused by the toxin-producing strains of *Staphylococcus aureus* or *Streptococcus pyogenes*. TSS is an inflammatory immune response to the enterotoxins produced by these bacteria. *S. aureus* is the cause of almost all cases of menstrual TSS.[55] Toxin-producing strains of *S. aureus* produce the superantigen toxin TSST-1. Most adults have a protective level of antibodies against the TSST-1 toxin. Younger people who lack this antibody protection and who become infected with a toxin-producing strain of *S. aureus* may develop TSS.[55]

TSS develops in three phases: proliferation of toxin-producing bacteria, production of toxin, and engagement of the immune system. Menstrual blood can serve as a medium for bacterial growth, and the retention of blood in the vagina by the tampon can increase bacterial proliferation. Also, some tampons contain fibers that inhibit lactobacilli, thereby diminishing their ability to limit the proliferation of *S. aureus*. Four conditions promote toxin production: (1) elevated protein levels, (2) neutral pH, (3) elevated carbon dioxide levels, and (4) elevated oxygen levels.[53] During menses, menstrual blood provides an increase in protein and also increases vaginal pH to 7, or neutral pH. Tampon use may create the environment for TSS by introducing oxygen into the vagina.[53] It takes hours for the vagina to return to its anaerobic state with elevated carbon dioxide levels after the introduction of a tampon. In addition, tampons, IUCs, and contraceptive sponges have been shown to create microtrauma, which may increase exposure of the toxins to the circulation and immune system. Exposure of immune cells to TSST-1 initiates the inflammatory cascade involving interleukin-1 and tumor necrosis factor. This inflammatory response results in the signs and symptoms of TSS.[55]

Clinical Presentation of Menstrual TSS

By definition, menstrual TSS occurs within 2 days of the onset of menses, during menses, or within 2 days after menses.[54] Prodromal symptoms (malaise, myalgias, and chills) occur for 2 to 3 days prior to TSS.[55] GI symptoms (vomiting, diarrhea, and abdominal pain) typically occur early in the illness and affect almost all patients. After that period of time, TSS characteristically evolves quite rapidly. Full-blown TSS includes high fever, myalgias, vomiting and diarrhea, erythroderma, decreased urine output, severe hypotension, and shock. Neurologic manifestations (headache, confusion, agitation, lethargy, and seizures) also occur in almost all cases. Acute renal failure, cardiac involvement, and adult respiratory distress syndrome are also common.

Dermatologic manifestations are characteristic of TSS; both early rash and subsequent skin desquamation are required for a definite diagnosis (Table 9-7). The early rash is often described as a sunburn-like, diffuse, macular erythroderma that is not pruritic. About 5 to 12 days after the onset of TSS, desquamation of the skin on the patient's face, trunk, and extremities, including the soles of the feet and the palms of the hands, occurs.

Prevention of Menstrual TSS

Women can reduce the risk of menstrual TSS to nearly zero by using sanitary pads instead of tampons during their menstrual cycle. Women who use tampons can reduce the risk by following the guidelines in the box Patient Education for Toxic Shock Syndrome.

Women who have had TSS are at risk for recurrence; TSS recurs in about 28% to 64% of women with menstrual TSS.[55] Recurrence rates are lower for women who are treated with antibiotics during TSS. Prevention of TSS for these patients includes avoiding tampons, IUCs, diaphragms, and contraceptive sponges.

TABLE 9-7 CDC Clinical Case Definition of TSS

- Fever: oral temperature ≥ 102°F (38.9°C)
- Rash: diffuse macular erythroderma
- Desquamation: 1–2 weeks after onset of illness, particularly on palms and soles
- Hypotension: systolic blood pressure ≤ 90 mm Hg, ≥ 15 mm Hg orthostatic drop in diastolic blood pressure, orthostatic syncope or dizziness
- Involvement of three or more of the following organ systems:
  — Gastrointestinal: vomiting or diarrhea at onset of illness
  — Muscular: severe myalgia or twice-normal creatine phosphokinase
  — Mucous membranes: vaginal, oropharyngeal, or conjunctival hyperemia
  — Renal: twice-normal blood urea nitrogen or creatinine; pyuria (≥5 white blood cells in a high-power field)
  — Hepatic: twice-normal bilirubin or transaminases
  — Hematologic: platelets <1,000,000/mm³
- Central nervous system: disorientation or alterations in consciousness without focal neurologic signs when fever and hypotension are absent
- Negative results on the following tests, if obtained:
  — Blood, throat, or cerebrospinal fluid cultures (blood culture may be positive for *S. aureus*)
  — Serologic tests for Rocky Mountain spotted fever, leptospirosis, or measles

Key: CDC, Centers for Disease Control and Prevention.

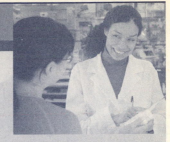

PATIENT EDUCATION FOR
Toxic Shock Syndrome

The objective of self-treatment is to reduce the risk of developing toxic shock syndrome (TSS) associated with the use of tampons or contraceptive devices. For most patients, carefully following product instructions and the self-care measures listed here will help ensure optimal therapeutic outcomes.

- To reduce the risk of toxic shock syndrome to almost zero, use sanitary pads instead of tampons during your period.
- To lower the risk while using tampons, use the lowest-absorbency tampons compatible with your needs. Also, alternate the use of menstrual pads with the use of tampons (e.g., use pads at night).
- Change tampons four to six times a day and at least every 6 hours; overnight use should be no longer than 8 hours.
- Wash your hands with soap before inserting anything into the vagina (e.g., tampon, diaphragm, contraceptive sponge, or vaginal medication). The bacteria causing TSS is usually found on the skin.

- Do not leave a contraceptive sponge, diaphragm, or cervical cap in place in the vagina longer than recommended; do not use any of them during menstruation.
- Do not use tampons, contraceptive sponges, or a cervical cap during the first 12 weeks after childbirth. It may also be best to avoid using a diaphragm.
- Read the insert on TSS enclosed in the tampon package, and familiarize yourself with the early symptoms of this disorder. If you develop symptoms of TSS (a high fever, muscle aches, a sunburn-like rash appearing after a day or two, weakness, fatigue, nausea, vomiting, and diarrhea), remove the tampon or contraceptive device immediately and seek emergency medical treatment. If left untreated, TSS can cause shock and even death.

Assessment of Menstrual TSS: A Case-Based Approach

Obtaining prompt medical attention is a very important aspect of care for patients with symptoms consistent with TSS. A health care provider can be alert to symptoms of TSS when patients seek nonprescription therapy for a severe "flu" (e.g., fever, vomiting, diarrhea, and dizziness) or an unusual skin rash that occurs in conjunction with the previously described symptoms. If TSS is suspected, the patient should be advised to seek medical care immediately and avoid use of NSAIDs for fever and myalgias, because these agents may increase the progression of TSS by increasing the production of tumor necrosis factor.

Patient Counseling for Menstrual TSS

Tampons are used by most (81%) women of all ages during the reproductive years.[56] Health care providers should counsel patients about the prevention of TSS as outlined in the box Patient Education for Toxic Shock Syndrome. In particular, the importance of washing the hands (organisms causing TSS are found on the skin) before inserting a tampon should be emphasized; only about half of women report doing so.[56] Similarly, about 18% to 36% of women report that they do not always change a tampon at least every 6 hours. The health care provider should emphasize, however, that the risk for this condition is quite small. If a patient presents with early symptoms of TSS, she should be advised to remove the tampon or any barrier contraceptive device and to seek emergency medical treatment.

KEY POINTS FOR DISORDERS RELATED TO MENSTRUATION

➤ Self-care is appropriate for an otherwise healthy young woman whose history is consistent with primary dysmenorrhea and who is not sexually active, or for a woman diagnosed with

primary dysmenorrhea. Adolescents with pelvic pain who are sexually active (at risk for PID) and women with characteristics indicating secondary dysmenorrhea should be referred for medical evaluation.

➤ NSAIDs are the drugs of choice for the management of primary dysmenorrhea. These medications should be taken at the onset, or just prior to menses, and be used in scheduled doses for several days for optimum reduction in pain and cramping.

➤ The use of local topical heat can also provide relief from dysmenorrhea. Its analgesic effect had a faster onset than drug therapy, and it can add to the relief provided by an NSAID. Nondrug therapy may be especially useful for women who cannot tolerate or who do not respond to nonprescription NSAIDs.

➤ It is important to distinguish PMS/PMDD from typical premenstrual symptoms and also from premenstrual exacerbations (PMEs) of other disorders, particularly mood disorders.

➤ PMS/PMDD symptoms typically begin or intensify about a week prior to the onset of menses, peak the day before or on the first day of menses, and resolve within several days after the beginning of menses. A woman with PMS or PMDD experiences a symptom-free interval during days 4 to 12 of her menstrual cycle.

➤ PMS symptoms are chronic and, in most cases, will continue until menopause. Therefore, the cost of therapy, the fact that a woman may become pregnant, and the likelihood of adverse effects from therapy are important considerations in selecting therapy.

➤ Several nonprescription or complementary agents (calcium, vitamin D, magnesium, vitamin E, pyridoxine, and chasteberry [*Vitex agnus*]) might be suggested to reduce the symptoms of PMS. PMDD symptoms warrant prescription drug therapy.

➤ TSS has been linked to tampon use. To lower the risk for TSS while using tampons, women should use the lowest-absorbency tampons compatible with their needs and alternate the use of sanitary pads with the use of tampons (e.g., at night).

REFERENCES

1. Yussman SM, Klein JD. Adolescent health care. In: Leppert PC, Peipert JF, eds. *Primary Care for Women*. 2nd ed. Philadelphia: Lippincott Williams & Wilkins; 2004.

2. Griswold D. Menstruation and related problems and concerns. In: Youngkin EQ, Davis MS, eds. *Women's Health: A Primary Care Clinical Guide*. 3rd ed. Upper Saddle River, NJ: Prentice Hall; 2004.

3. Letterie GS. Disorders of menstruation: from amenorrhea to menorrhagia. In: Lemcke DP, Pattison J, Marshall LA, et al., eds. *Current Care of Women Diagnosis and Treatment*. New York: Lange Medical Books McGraw-Hill, Inc; 2004.

4. Harel A. Dysmenorrhea in adolescents and young adults: etiology and management. *J Pediatr Adolesc Gynecol*. 2006;19:363–71.

5. Durain D. Primary dysmenorrhea: assessment and management update. *J Midwifery Women's Health*. 2004;49:520–8.

6. Slap GB. Menstrual disorders in adolescents. *Best Pract Res Clin Obstet Gynaecol*. 2003;17:75–92.

7. Howard FM. Dysmenorrhea. In: Leppert PC, Peipert JF, eds. *Primary Care for Women*. 2nd ed. Philadelphia: Lippincott Williams & Wilkins; 2004.

8. Davis AR, Westhoff CL. Primary dysmenorrhea in adolescent girls and treatment with oral contraceptives. *J Pediatr Gynecol*. 2001;14:3–8.

9. Banikarim C, Chacko MR, Kelder SH. Prevalence and impact of dysmenorrhea on Hispanic female adolescents. *Arch Pediatr Adolesc Med*. 2000;154:1226–9.

10. Daywood MY. Primary dysmenorrhea advances in pathogenesis and management. *Obstet Gynecol*. 2006;108:428–41.

11. Mazza D. *Women's Health in General Practice*. Edinburgh: Butterworth Heinemann; 2004.

12. Hewison A, van den Akker OB. Dysmenorrhea, menstrual attitude, and GP consultation. *Br J Nurs*. 1996;5:480–4.

13. O'Connell K, Davis AR, Westhoff C. Self-treatment patterns among adolescent girls with Dysmenorrhea. *J Pediatr Adolesc Gynecol*. 2006;19:285–9.

14. Akin M, Price W, Rodriguez G Jr, et al. Continuous, low-level, topical heat wrap therapy as compared to acetaminophen for primary dysmenorrhea. *J Reprod Med*. 2004;49:739–45.

15. Dawood MY, Khan-Dawood FS. Clinical efficacy and differential inhibition of menstrual fluid prostaglandin F 2a in a randomized, double-blind, crossover treatment with placebo, acetaminophen, and ibuprofen in primary dysmenorrhea. *Am J Obstet Gynecol*. 2007;196:35e1–e5.

16. Benassi L, Barletta FP, Baroncini L, et al. Effectiveness of magnesium pindolate in the prophylactic treatment of primary dysmenorrhea. *Clin Exp Obstet Gynecol*. 1992;19:176–9.

17. Wilson ML, Murphy PA. Herbal and dietary therapies for primary and secondary dysmenorrhea. *Nurs Times*. 2001;97(36):44.

18. Deutch B, Jorgensen EB, Hansen JC. Menstrual discomfort in Danish women reduced by dietary supplements of omega-3 PUFA and B-12 (fish oil or seal oil capsules). *Nutr Res*. 2000;20:621–31.

19. Ziaei S, Faghihzadeh F, Sohrabvand M, et al. A randomized placebo-controlled trial to determine the effect of vitamin E in treatment of primary dysmenorrhea. *Br J Obstet Gynaecol*. 2001;108:1181–3.

20. Ziaei S, Zakeri M, Kazemnejad A. A randomized controlled trial of vitamin E in the treatment of primary dysmenorrhea. *BJOG*. 2005;112:466–9.

21. Eby GA. Zinc treatment prevents dysmenorrhea. *Med Hypotheses*. 2007; 69:297–301.

22. Jahromi BN, Tartifizadeh A, Khabnadideh S. Comparison of fennel and mefenamic acid for the treatment of primary dysmenorrhea. *Int J Gynaecol Obstet*. 2003;80:153–7.

23. Campagne DM, Campagne G. The premenstrual syndrome revisited. *Eur J Obstet Gynecol Reprod Biol*. 2007;130:4–17.

24. Johnson SR. Premenstrual syndrome, premenstrual dysphoric disorder, and beyond: a clinical primer for practitioners. *Obstet Gynecol*. 2004;104845–59.

25. Ryden JR. Premenstrual syndrome. In: Ryden JR, Blumenthal PD, eds. *Practical Gynecology: A Guide for the Primary Care Physician*. Philadelphia: American College of Physicians; 2002.

26. Dell DL. Premenstrual syndrome, premenstrual dysphoric disorder, and premenstrual exacerbation of another disorder. *Clin Obstet Gynecol*. 2004; 47:568–75.

27. Dickerson LM, Mazyck PJ, Hunter MH. Premenstrual syndrome. *Am Fam Physician*. 2003;67:1743–52.

28. Grady-Weliky TA, Lewis V. Premenstrual syndrome. In: Leppert PC, Peipert JF, eds. *Primary Care for Women*. 2nd ed. Philadelphia: Lippincott Williams & Wilkins; 2004.

29. Indusekhar R, Usman SB, O'Brien S. Psychological aspects of premenstrual syndrome. *Best Pract Res Clin Obstetr Gynaecol*. 2007;21:207–20.

30. Sternfeld B, Swindle R, Chawla A, et al. Severity of premenstrual symptoms in a health maintenance organization population. *Obstet Gynecol*. 2002;99:1014–24.

31. Cohen LS, Soares CN, Otto MW, et al. Prevalence and predictors of premenstrual dysphoric disorder (PMDD) in older premenopausal women: the Harvard study of moods and cycles. *J Affect Disord*. 2002; 70:125–32.

32. Wittchen HU, Becker E, Lieb R, Krause P. Prevalence, incidence and stability of premenstrual dysphoric disorder in the community. *Psychol Med*. 2002;32:119–32.

33. Thys-Jacobs S. Micronutrients and the premenstrual syndrome: the case for calcium. *J Am Coll Nutr*. 2000;19:220–7.

34. Treloar SA, Heath AC, Martin NG. Genetic and environmental influences in premenstrual symptoms in an Australian twin sample. *Psychol Med*. 2002;32:25–38.

35. Ulman KH, Carlson KJ. Premenstrual syndrome. In: Carlson KJ, Eisenstat SA, eds. *Primary Care of Women*. 2nd ed. St Louis: Mosby; 2002.

36. Dog TL. Integrative treatments for premenstrual syndrome. *Altern Ther Health Med*. 2001;7:32–9.

37. Sayegh R, Wurtman J, Spiers P, et al. The effect of a carbohydrate-rich beverage on mood, appetite, and cognitive function in women with premenstrual syndrome. *Obstet Gynecol*. 1995;86:520–8.

38. Steiner M, Pearlstein T. Premenstrual dysphoria and the serotonin system: pathophysiology and treatment. *J Clin Psychiatry*. 2000;61(suppl 12):17–21.

39. Singh B, Berman BM, Simpson RL, et al. Incidence of premenstrual syndrome and remedy usage: a national probability sample study. *Altern Ther Health Med*. 1998;4:75–9.

40. Wyatt KM, Dimmock PW, Jones PW, et al. Efficacy of vitamin B_6 in the treatment of premenstrual syndrome: systematic review. *BMJ*. 1999;318: 1375–81.

41. Thys-Jacobs S, Starkey P, Bernstein D, et al. Calcium carbonate and the premenstrual syndrome: effect on premenstrual and menstrual symptoms. *Am J Obstet Gynecol*. 1998;179:444–52.

42. Thys-Jacobs S, Ceccarelli S, Bierman A, et al. Calcium supplementation in premenstrual syndrome. *J Gen Intern Med*. 1989; 4:183–9.

43. Penland JG, Johnson PE. Dietary calcium and manganese effects on menstrual cycle symptoms. *Am J Obstet Gynecol*. 1993;168:1417–23.

44. Bertone-Johnson ER, Hankinson SE, Bendich A, et al. Calcium and vitamin D intake and risk of incident premenstrual syndrome. *Arch Intern Med*. 2005;165:1246–52.

45. Holick MF, Chen TC. Vitamin D deficiency: a worldwide problem with health consequences. *Am J Clin Nutr*. 2008; 87(suppl):1080S–6S.

46. Facchinetti F, Borella P, Sances G, et al. Oral magnesium successfully relieves premenstrual mood changes. *Obstet Gynecol*. 1991;78:177–81.

47. O'Brien PMS, Ismail KMK, Dimmock P. Premenstrual syndrome. In: Shaw RW, Soutter WP, Stanton SL, eds. *Gynecology*. 3rd ed. Edinburgh: Churchill Livingstone; 2003.

48. Girman A, Lee R, Kligler B. An integrative medicine approach to premenstrual syndrome. *Am J Obstet Gynecol*. 2003;188:S56–S65.

49. Schellenberg R. Treatment for the premenstrual syndrome with agnus castus fruit extract: prospective, randomized, placebo-controlled study. *BMJ*. 2001;322:134–7.

50. Berger D, Schaffner W, Schrader E, et al. Efficacy of *Vitex agnus* L. extract Ze 440 in patients with premenstrual syndrome (PMS). *Arch Gynecol Obstet*. 2000;264:150–3.

51. Loch EG, Selle H, Boblitz N. Treatment of premenstrual syndrome with a phytopharmaceutical formulation containing Vitex agnus castus. *J Women's Health Gend Based Med*. 2000;9:315–20.

52. Atmaca M, Kumru S, Tezcan E. Fluoxetine versus Vitex agnus castus extract in the treatment of premenstrual dysphoric disorder. *Hum Psychopharmacol Clin Exp*. 2003;18:191–5.

53. McCormick JK, Yarwood JM, Schlievert PM. Toxic shock syndrome and bacterial superantigens: an update. *Annu Rev Microbiol*. 2001;55:77–104.

54. Schlievert PM, Tripp TJ, Perterson ML. Reemergence of staphylococcal toxic shock syndrome in Minneapolis-St. Paul, Minnesota, during the 2000–2003 surveillance period. *J Clin Microbiol*. 2004;42:2875–6.

55. Reiss MA. Toxic shock syndrome. *Prim Care Update Obstet Gynecol*. 2000;7:85–90.

56. Czerwinski BS. Variation in feminine hygiene practices as a function of age. *J Obstet Gynecol Neonatal Nurs*. 2000;29:625–33.

Prevention of Pregnancy and Sexually Transmitted Infections

Louise Parent-Stevens and Jennifer L. Hardman

Unprotected sexual activity can result in unintended pregnancy and sexually transmitted infections (STIs), either of which can exact a high physical, psychological, and financial toll on those affected. This chapter discusses how nonprescription contraceptive products or methods, when properly used, can reduce the risks of these adverse outcomes.

According to the 2002 National Survey of Family Growth (NSFG), approximately 90% of sexually active 15- to 44-year-old U.S. women at risk for unintended pregnancy use some form of birth control (Table 10-1).[1,2] Some women use more than one method simultaneously. Approximately half of women using condoms do so in conjunction with another method such as hormonal or chemical agents.[1]

Approximately 50% of pregnancies in the United States are unintended.[3] A survey of women with unintended pregnancies found that more than half had used a method of contraception during the month in which they conceived; however, fewer than 20% of these women reported using it correctly and consistently.[4]

In the United States alone, an estimated 15 million persons are infected annually with one or more STIs, and 65 million persons are living with STIs.[5,6] The economic, social, and personal costs of STIs are staggering. The direct and indirect costs associated with STIs, excluding human immunodeficiency virus (HIV) and acquired immunodeficiency syndrome (AIDS), are estimated to exceed $10 billion yearly.[5]

Of particular concern is the high risk of pregnancy and STIs in the adolescent population. The NSFG found that about one-half of high-school students had experienced sexual intercourse.[7] Although the teenage pregnancy rate in the United States decreased by approximately 25% between 1995 and 2001, it remains the highest among developed countries.[8] Among sexually active female teenagers, about one-fifth engage in unprotected intercourse or use contraceptives only sporadically.[1] The reasons for low levels of contraceptive use in this population include lack of knowledge and planning, denial, and infrequent or unpredictable intercourse. Of teenage pregnancies, 78% are unintended.[3] Repeat pregnancies are common and are often associated with inadequate contraceptive use after the first pregnancy.[9] Adolescents are particularly vulnerable to STIs, with one in four teenage girls infected with one or more STIs.[10] Reasons include having multiple sexual partners, unprotected intercourse, an inherent biological susceptibility to infection, and barriers to health care utilization.[11]

Perimenopausal women are at risk of unintended pregnancies. The NSFG found that, among women ages 40 years or older, 38% of pregnancies were unplanned.[3] Postmenopausal women and older men in sexual relationships that are not mutually monogamous are also at increased risk of STIs.[12]

In the United States and worldwide, reliance on nonprescription methods of contraception for pregnancy and STI prevention is widespread. These readily accessible and relatively inexpensive products are very important for those who are unwilling or unable to access family-planning services or use prescription contraceptives. Even if a prescription product is chosen as the primary contraceptive method, low-cost and low-risk nonprescription methods may be appropriate at different times during a person's sexually active life.

Pathophysiology of Pregnancy and Sexually Transmitted Infections

Pregnancy can result only when a viable egg is available for fertilization by a sperm. (See Chapter 9 for a discussion of the reproductive process.) It is estimated that conception can occur during a 6-day window that begins 5 days before ovulation through the day of ovulation. The estimated risk of pregnancy from an unprotected coital act during this 6-day period in the middle of the menstrual cycle ranges from 5% to 45%, with peak risk occurring with intercourse the day before ovulation.[13] Pregnancy can occur even with the use of contraceptive products if the product is used incorrectly or it fails (e.g., condom breakage).

STIs are acquired through contact with infected genital tissues, mucous membranes, and/or body fluids. Table 10-2 summarizes the major infections. Whereas STIs affect both genders, women are more likely to develop reproductive consequences including pelvic inflammatory disease, chronic pelvic pain, ectopic pregnancy, malignancies, and infertility. Intrauterine and perinatal morbidity and mortality also increase as a consequence of STIs during pregnancy.[6] Gender-biased complications may result from difficulties in diagnosis, lack of patient recognition of symptoms, and high probability of asymptomatic infection.[6] Women are also more likely than men to acquire an STI after a single unprotected coital act: Approximately 50% of women will become infected with gonorrhea after a single exposure with an infected man, whereas only 25% of men contract gonorrhea from a single exposure with an infected woman.[6]

TABLE 10-1 Failure and Use Rates of Various Contraceptive Methods

Method	Accidental Pregnancy in the First Year of Use (%)		% of Women Using Method[c]
	Typical Use[a]	Perfect Use[b]	
No method	85		10.2
Withdrawal	27	4	3.4
Fertility Awareness Methods			12.4
Calendar method	25	9	
Cervical mucus method	25	3	
Symptothermal method	25	2	
Basal body temperature method	25	1	
Lactational amenorrhea method (first 6 months postpartum)	2	0.5	
Standard days method	12	5	
TwoDay method	13.7	3.5	
Spermicides (foam, gel, vaginal suppositories, vaginal film)	29	18	<0.8
Contraceptive sponge	32 (parous women) 16 (nulliparous women)	20 (parous women) 9 (nulliparous women)	<0.8
Male condom (without spermicide)	15	2	15.3
Female condom (without spermicide)	21	5	<0.8
Prescription methods	0.05–8	≤0.6	33.6
Sterilization (male/female)	≤0.5	≤0.5	35.2

[a] Among typical couples who initiate use of a method (not necessarily for the first time), the percentage who experience an accidental pregnancy during the first year if they do not stop use for any other reason.

[b] Among typical couples who initiate use of a method (not necessarily for the first time) and who use it consistently and correctly, the percentage who experience an accidental pregnancy during the first year if they do not stop use for any other reason.

[c] Percentage of sexually active 15- to 44-year-old women who are not pregnant, postpartum, or attempting to become pregnant. If a woman is using more than one method, only the most effective method is listed.

Source: References 1 and 2.

TABLE 10-2 Sexually Transmitted Infections

Disease [Scientific Name] (Type)	Incubation Period	Symptoms	Diagnosis/ Treatment	Complications	Congenital Transmission/ Neonatal Complications
Non-Curable but Vaccine-Preventable STIs					
Genital warts [Human papillomavirus[a]] (DNA virus)	2–4 months (average)	Asx infections common; warts on external genitalia, rectum, anus, perineum, mouth, larynx, vagina, urethra, cervix	Colposcopy; serology; molecular-based assays/cytoablation (chemical or physical); antivirals; antimetabolites; immunomodulators	Cervical dysplasia/ neoplasia	Yes
Hepatitis B [Hepatitis B virus] (virus)	6 weeks– 6 months	Acute, self-limited, mild	Serology/antivirals	Cirrhosis, hepatocellular cancer	Yes
Curable STIs					
Genital chlamydia [*Chlamydia trachomatis*] (bacterium)		M: range from asx to urethritis, proctitis, urogenital discharge, itching, dysuria F: range from asx to vaginal discharge, postcoital bleeding, cervicitis	NAAT/antibiotics	PID, ectopic pregnancy, infertility	Yes/ophthalmia neonatorum, pneumonia

TABLE 10-2 Sexually Transmitted Infections *(continued)*

Disease [Scientific Name] (Type)	Incubation Period	Symptoms	Diagnosis/ Treatment	Complications	Congenital Transmission/ Neonatal Complications
Gonorrhea [*Neisseria gonorrhea*] (bacterium)	Up to 10 days	Urethritis, cervicitis, proctitis, pharyngitis M: mucopurulent urethral discharge F: often asx	Gram stain; EIA; culture; NAAT/ antibiotics	Septic arthritis, perihepatitis, endocarditis, meningitis, PID, infertility, ectopic pregnancy	Yes/sepsis, meningitis, arthritis, ocular infections
Nongonococcal urethritis (males) [Various, including *Chlamydia trachomatis*, *Ureaplasma urealyticum*, *Mycoplasma* sp.] (bacteria)	1–2 weeks	M: nonspecific urethritis, discharge, dysuria, pruritus	NAAT; culture/ antibiotics	Epididymitis, proctitis, proctocolitis, Reiter syndrome	—
Syphilis [*Treponema pallidum*] (spirochete)	3 weeks	Primary syphilis: chancre	Darkfield microscopy; direct fluorescent antibody exam of tissue; serology; EIA; PCR assay; treponomal/ non-treponomal tests/antibiotics	Secondary syphilis: rash, lymphedema, hepatosplenomegaly, alopecia Tertiary syphilis: syphilitic tumors of vasculature, CNS, skin and skeleton	Yes/stillbirth, preterm labor, intrauterine growth restriction, hepatosplenomegaly, failure to thrive, progression to neurosyphilis as adult
Trichomoniasis [*Trichomonas vaginalis*] (flagellated anaerobic protozoan)		M: commonly asx F: ~50% asx, malodorous, frothy green vaginal discharge, itching, dyspareunia, postcoital bleeding	Microscopic exam of vaginal fluids/ antibiotics	Pregnancy: preterm labor, low birth weight, premature rupture of membranes	No

Non-Curable STIs

Disease [Scientific Name] (Type)	Incubation Period	Symptoms	Diagnosis/ Treatment	Complications	Congenital Transmission/ Neonatal Complications
AIDS [HIV] (virus)	Up to 10 years	After initial flu-like illness, asx until OIs occur	Serologic antibody testing/antivirals; prophylaxis for OIs	OIs, malignancies, death	Yes, also transmitted via breast milk
Genital herpes [HPV] (virus)[a]	6 days (average)	Vesicular/ulcerative lesions on mucous membranes	Culture; serology; PCR assay/ antivirals	Disseminated infection, pneumonitis, hepatitis, meningitis/encephalitis	Yes
Hepatitis C [Hepatitis C virus] (virus)[b]	8–9 weeks	Asx or mild clinical illness	Serology/antivirals	Cirrhosis, hepatocellular cancer	Yes

Key: asx, asymptomatic; F, female; EIA, enzyme immunoassay; HIV, human immunodeficiency virus; HPV, human papillomavirus; HSV, herpes simplex virus; M, male; NAAT, nucleic acid amplification test; OI, opportunistic infection; PCR, polymerase chain reaction; PID, pelvic inflammatory disease.

[a] Self-clearance of HPV virus may occur.

[b] Compared with transmission through blood exposure, sexual transmission of hepatitis C is inefficient but may still occur.

Prevention of Pregnancy and Sexually Transmitted Infections

The goal of contraceptive use is to prevent unintended pregnancy and STIs with a minimum of adverse effects. No method of birth control is perfect. Contraceptive choices may change during a person's sexually active life. Major points to consider in selecting a contraceptive method are safety (including potential adverse effects on future fertility and on the fetus, if unintended conception occurs), effectiveness, accessibility, and acceptability to each sexual partner.

The effectiveness of a contraceptive method in preventing pregnancy is reported in two ways: the accidental pregnancy rate in the first year of *perfect* use (method-related failure rate), and the rate in the first year of *typical* use (use-related failure rate; Table 10-1). The pregnancy rate with perfect use is very difficult to measure and indicates the method's theoretical effectiveness. It assumes accurate and consistent use of the method every time intercourse occurs. The more realistic rate of typical use includes pregnancies that may have occurred because of inconsistent or incorrect use of the method. Reported use-related failure rates vary, depending on the population studied. Effectiveness increases the longer a particular method is used. Decreased coital frequency and declining fertility in older users may contribute to increased effectiveness rates in this population.[2]

The best way for an individual to avoid contracting an STI is either to abstain from risky sexual activity or to be involved in a long-term mutually monogamous sexual relationship with an uninfected partner.[11] In the absence of these options, preventive strategies in conjunction with use of selected contraceptives may provide the best method for reducing risk of infection (Table 10-3, Table 10-4, and Figure 10-1).

TABLE 10-3 Prevention Strategies for STIs

- Abstain from sexual activity.
- Avoid intercourse with a known infected partner.
- Avoid intercourse with an individual having multiple sex partners.
- Use a new condom with each episode of anal, oral, or vaginal intercourse.
- Seek a mutually monogamous relationship with an uninfected partner.
- Discuss partner's past sexual experiences.
- Examine partner for genital lesions.
- Practice genital self-examination.
- Avoid sexual activity involving direct contact with blood, semen, or other body fluids.
- Avoid sharing sexual devices that come in contact with semen or other body fluids.
- Choose safe and effective methods (e.g., mechanical barriers) to reduce the risk of STIs (consider adding more effective methods of pregnancy prevention when necessary).
- Avoid sexual activity if signs/symptoms of an STI are present.
- Consider vaccination if at high risk for a vaccine-preventable STI (e.g., HBV and HPV).

Key: HBV, hepatitis B virus; HPV, human papillomavirus; STI, sexually transmitted infection.

Source: References 6 and 11.

TABLE 10-4 Contraceptive Methods and STI Risk

Method	Effect on STI Risk
Latex male condoms	Protective[a]
Polyurethane male condoms	Probably protective[a]
Natural membrane condoms	Protective against bacterial STI, not protective against viral STI[a]
Female condoms	Protective[a]
Spermicides	Possibly increased risk
Diaphragms (with spermicide)	Possibly protective against cervical infection/dysplasia/cancer[a]
Contraceptive sponge	Possibly protective against bacterial STI, not protective against viral STI[a]
Intrauterine devices	Not protective: risk of PID during first month following insertion
Hormonal methods	Not protective: increase in cervical *Chlamydia*
Fertility awareness-based methods	Not protective

Key: PID, pelvic inflammatory disease; STI, sexually transmitted infection.

[a] Improper or inconsistent use will significantly decrease the protection these contraceptive products provide against transmission of STIs.

Selection of a Contraceptive Method

Acceptability of any given contraceptive method is vital for correct and consistent use of the method. Factors that affect acceptability include the user's religious beliefs and future reproductive plans, effectiveness, the partner's supportiveness, complexity of the method, degree of interruption of spontaneity, "messiness," and cost. To help patients make informed decisions, practitioners should be aware of the safety, effectiveness, accessibility, and relative cost of different contraceptive methods. The algorithm in Figure 10-1 can assist the practitioner in making appropriate contraceptive recommendations.

Nonprescription Contraceptive Products

MALE CONDOMS

Condoms—also known as rubbers, sheaths, prophylactics, safes, skins, or pros—are the most important barrier contraceptive device in an era of STIs, second only to abstinence in their effect on disease prevention. Condoms are available in latex, polyurethane, and lamb cecum (natural membrane or skin; Table 10-5).

Latex condoms come in various sizes, colors, styles, shapes, and thicknesses (ranging from 0.03 mm to approximately 0.11 mm). Other features include reservoir tips, ribs, studs, and lubrication. Spermicide-treated condoms are also available, but the amount of spermicide they contain is much less than that of a vaginal spermicide.[14] Latex condoms range in price from $0.25 to $1.50 each.

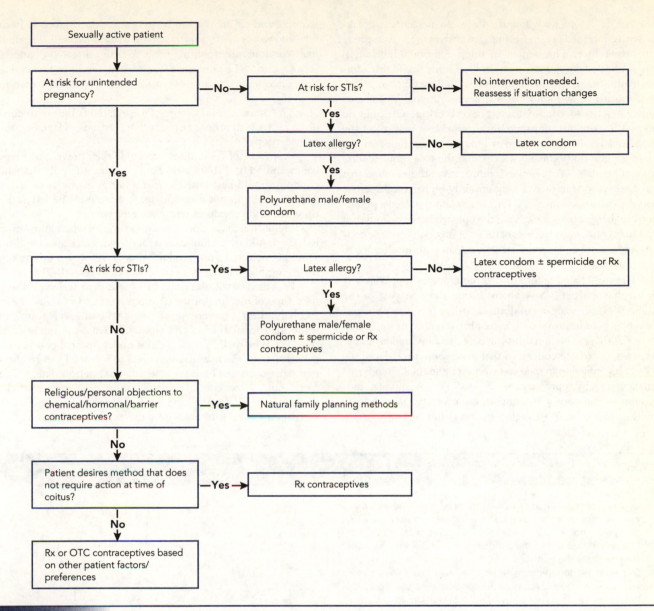

FIGURE 10-1   Prevention of unintended pregnancy and sexually transmitted infections. Key: OTC, over-the-counter; Rx, prescription; STI, sexually transmitted infection.

Polyurethane condoms conduct heat well, come prelubricated, and are not subject to degradation by oil-based products.[15] However, they are less stretchy and, at $1.50 to $2.00 each, are more expensive than latex condoms.

Condoms made from lamb cecum are labeled only for pregnancy prevention, because the presence of pores in the membrane may allow passage of viral organisms, including HIV and hepatitis B virus.[16] These condoms conduct heat well and are very strong. With a price of about $3.00 each, they are also more expensive than latex condoms.

The Food and Drug Administration (FDA) is responsible for monitoring condom quality, and uses a water-leak test and an air-burst test as the standards for latex condoms. The failure rate per batch cannot exceed 0.25%.[17] There is currently no standard test for polyurethane condoms.

The true incidence of condom breakage is unknown, and breakage rates from studies vary widely, ranging from 0.4% to 2.3%.[17] In some studies, a limited group of study patients reported multiple incidences of breakage, indicating that breakage may be related as much to the individual user as it is to manufacturing defects. Behaviors that have been associated with an increased risk of condom breakage are (1) incorrect placement of the condom; (2) use of an oil-based lubricant with latex condoms; (3) reuse of condoms; (4) increased duration, intensity, or frequency of coitus; and (5) prior history of condom

TABLE 10-5 Selected Male Condoms	
Polyurethane condoms	Durex Avanti, Trojan Supra
Natural membrane condoms	Trojan Naturalamb
Latex condoms	Beyond Seven, Crown, Durex, 4Play, Inspiral, Kimono, LifeStyles, Trojan

breakage.[16,18,19] One study found a decreased incidence of breakage with continued use, indicating that correct use may improve with experience. The benefit of using additional lubrication with lubricated condoms is unclear. One study found that additional lubricant use increased the risk of condom slippage. However, another study found that use of an additional water-based lubricant was associated with decreased breakage rates, but no increase in condom slippage rates. Factors that may affect the impact of additional lubrication include the type of lubricant, the site of application (vaginal or rectal), and the type of intercourse (vaginal or anal).[19] A review of comparative studies found that polyurethane condoms had a significantly higher breakage rate than the latex condom.[15,20,21] One study also reported a significantly higher pregnancy rate with the polyurethane condom than with latex condoms.[22] Because of these reports, polyurethane condom use should be reserved for individuals with intolerance to latex condoms.

The use-related failure rate for condoms is approximately 15 pregnancies per 100 women during the first year of use (Table 10-1). Efficacy of condoms regarding pregnancy prevention appears to improve with increasing duration of use.

In 2001, the National Institutes of Health Condom Effectiveness Conference concluded that male condoms reduced the risk of HIV infection in men and women by about 85% and gonorrhea in men by approximately 25% to 75%.[17] Additional studies support that consistent condom use protects against human papillomavirus, bacterial vaginosis, and gonorrhea infection in women, and chlamydia and herpes simplex infections in both men and women.[23–26] Studies suggest that nonoxynol-9–coated male condoms are no more effective than untreated condoms at preventing STIs, and use of the treated condoms as such has been discouraged because of possible increased risk of irritation and infection.[27]

The most common cause of use-related failure with condoms, as with all other contraceptive methods, is lack of consistent, proper use.

Proper use of condoms is essential to their preventing pregnancy and STIs (Table 10-6). Patients using the polyurethane condom should be advised that it is not as elastic as the latex condom and will not fit as snugly. A space must be left at the tip when using condoms without a reservoir.

Prelubricated condoms are a good choice when lubrication is desired. Additional lubrication for use with any latex condom should be selected from products that do not harm or weaken the strength and integrity of the condom (Table 10-7).

Packaged condoms should be kept in their sealed packages until time of use, and protected from light and excessive heat. Excessive heat or overexposure to ozone at levels found in some metropolitan areas will rapidly decrease the integrity of the latex. The shelf life of condoms under optimal conditions, as packaged by the manufacturers, is 3 to 5 years. FDA requires that latex condoms be labeled with an expiration date.[17] The user should always check for discoloration, brittleness, or stickiness, and should discard condoms displaying any of these characteristics, even if they are within the expiration date.

TABLE 10-6 Usage Guidelines for Male Condoms

- Use only condoms that are fresh (not previously opened), that are within their expiration date, and that have been stored in a dry, cool place (not a wallet or car glove compartment).
- Do not attempt to test the condom for leaks before using; this step weakens the condom.
- Be aware that long fingernails or jewelry may easily tear condoms.
- As shown in drawing A, unroll the condom onto the erect penis before the penis comes into any contact with the vagina. If you start to put the condom on backward, discard that condom and use a fresh one. (*Note:* Preejaculate secretions may contain sperm.)
- If you are not using a reservoir-tipped condom, leave one-half inch of space between the end of the condom and the tip of the penis by pinching the top of the condom as you unroll it (drawing B). This method leaves space for the ejaculate (drawing C) and decreases the risk of breakage.
- If your partner has vaginal dryness, use additional lubrication, if desired. This step will help decrease the risk of tears and breakage. Use only water-based lubricants; oil-based lubricants weaken latex condoms and increase the chance of breakage. Spermicidal agents may be used as lubricants with condoms (Table 10-9) and may also increase the effectiveness of the condom.
- After ejaculation, withdraw the penis immediately. To prevent the condom from slipping off, hold on to the rim of the condom as you withdraw.
- Check the condom for tears and then discard.
- If a tear or break occurs, immediately insert spermicidal foam or jelly containing a high concentration of spermicide into the vagina. Do not use suppositories or a vaginal film in these cases, because the delay time for dissolution may decrease the product's efficacy. Do not douche because this may force sperm that are present into the cervical canal.

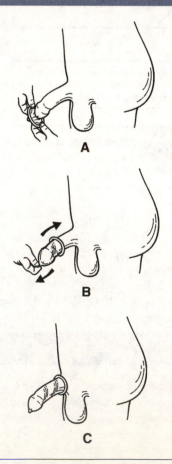

TABLE 10-7 Selected Lubricants/Products That Are Safe or Unsafe to Use with Latex Condoms

Safe	Unsafe
Contraceptive foams/gels	Topical oils (e.g., baby oil, mineral oil, massage oil)
Personal lubricants such as KY Jelly	Edible oils/fats (e.g., olive, peanut, corn, canola, safflower, butter, margarine)
Egg white	
Glycerin (USP)	Hemorrhoidal ointments
Replens Inserts	Petroleum jelly (e.g., Vaseline)
Saliva	Vaginal creams (e.g., Monistat, Estrace, Vagisil, Premarin)
Water	

The most frequent complaint about condoms is decreased sensitivity of the glans penis, resulting in decreased sexual pleasure for the male. Contact dermatitis caused by latex allergy can occur in the male or female partner, and may be characterized by immediate localized itching and swelling (urticarial reaction) or by a delayed eczematous reaction. In patients with severe sensitivity, the reaction may include systemic symptoms. The spermicide in spermicide-treated condoms may enhance latex allergy or cause sensitivity reactions itself.[28]

Product Selection Guidelines For most people, condoms are an effective, acceptable, inexpensive, safe, and nontoxic method of birth control. Given the wide variety of condoms available, patients should be encouraged to try a different style or brand if they are dissatisfied with the condom used previously. Before recommending a latex condom, health care providers should assess for latex allergy. The sensitizers in latex condoms are usually antioxidants or accelerators used in processing the rubber. Because different manufacturers use different processes, changing brands may alleviate the problem of allergic contact dermatitis. Some patients may be sensitized to components of the lubricant or spermicide. Changing brands or using a condom without spermicide may resolve the problem.[16] If switching brands does not eliminate the irritation, the patient may use polyurethane condoms. Natural skin condoms may also be used if the patient recognizes their limitations in preventing STIs.

The use of very thin condoms, ridged condoms, polyurethane condoms, or natural membrane condoms—in a monogamous relationship with an HIV-negative individual—may alleviate complaints of decreased sensitivity.

FEMALE CONDOMS

The F.C. Female Condom is made of polyurethane rather than latex. It is prelubricated, comes with additional lubricant, and resists degradation by oil-based lubricants. The female condom consists of an outer ring, a sheath or pouch that fits over the vaginal mucosa, and an inner ring that secures the sheath by fitting like a diaphragm over the cervix. The female condom is designed for one-time use only and, at a cost of $3 to $3.50 each, is significantly more expensive than the latex male condom. Although one study has shown that the female condom retains its integrity after multiple cycles of disinfection and washing,[29] reuse of female condoms is not recommended.

The breakage rate of the female condom has been shown to be lower than that of latex male condoms, but slippage rates may be higher, especially with initial uses.[18] The 6-month pregnancy failure rate among all users of the female condom is 12.4%, similar to that for users of diaphragms and cervical caps. Among perfect users, however, 6-month pregnancy failure rates of 0.8 to 2.5% have been documented. The extrapolated annual pregnancy failure rate for the female condom is 21% for all users and 5% for perfect users (Table 10-1).[3,30]

The female condom has been shown to be an effective barrier to sexually transmitted bacteria and viruses, and it appears to be similar in efficacy to latex male condoms in decreasing the risk of STIs.[29]

Table 10-8 provides step-by-step instructions for proper use of the female condom. A high proportion of women report difficulty inserting the female condom during initial use; this problem resolves with practice and continued use.[29] The condom may be inserted up to 8 hours before intercourse, but it is effective immediately on insertion.

Fresh condoms can be stored at room temperature in their unopened package. Before inserting the female condom, the woman should ensure that the product is within its expiration date.

The most common complaints about the female condom are vaginal irritation and increased noise ("squeaking"). Additional lubrication may resolve these problems. Some women may complain of decreased sensation or discomfort caused by the outer ring during intercourse.

Product Selection Guidelines The female condom provides a method for women to protect themselves against pregnancy. It is thinner than many latex condoms and has a lower breakage rate than the male condom.[18] Compared with vaginal spermicides, the female condom can be inserted much earlier before intercourse and is less messy to use. However, some women find the female condom cumbersome and unattractive.

VAGINAL SPERMICIDES

Vaginal spermicides use surface-active agents to immobilize (kill) sperm. For gels and foams, the spermicide vehicle also acts as a physical barrier against sperm. The effective spermicides include nonoxynol-9, octoxynol-9, and menfegol. In the United States, all currently available products contain nonoxynol-9 (Table 10-9). The cost of vaginal spermicides ranges from $1.00 to $3.00 per dose.

Vaginal spermicide products differ in application method, and onset and duration of action (Table 10-10).

Vaginal gels (jellies) provide additional lubrication and are safe to use with latex condoms. For convenience, applicators may be prefilled before use. Prefilled unit-dose applicators are also available for some products. Some vaginal gels are labeled for use only in conjunction with a diaphragm or cervical cap. When selecting an agent to use without a diaphragm or cervical cap, the person should choose a product with a higher concentration of spermicide, rather than one with a lower concentration designed for use with barrier methods. Products with a higher concentration of spermicide may be used alone or with a diaphragm or cervical cap.

Vaginal foams distribute more evenly and adhere better to the cervical area and vaginal walls, but provide less lubrication than jellies. A new canister should always be available as it is difficult to know when the canister is nearly empty.

Vaginal suppositories are solid or semisolid dosage forms that are activated by moisture in the vaginal tract. Incomplete dissolution of the suppository may result in an unpleasant,

TABLE 10-8 Usage Guidelines for Female Condoms

- Remove the condom from the package. One end of the condom is closed to form a pouch, as shown in drawing A.
- Gently rub the sides together to evenly distribute the lubricant. If needed, add additional lubrication at this point.
- Add a drop of lubricant on the outside of the pouch to improve the ease of insertion. Oil- or water-based lubricants can be used with this condom.
- To place the pouch properly, grasp the inner ring between the thumb and middle finger of one hand. Place the index finger on the sheath between the other two fingers. (See drawing B.)
- Be careful that sharp fingernails or jewelry do not tear the condom.
- Squeeze the inner ring. Then insert the condom into the vagina as far as possible. (See drawing C.)
- Be sure that the inner ring is placed beyond the pubic (pelvic) bone, that the pouch is not twisted, and that the outer ring is outside the vagina, as shown in drawing D.
- During intercourse, make sure that the penis enters the vagina inside the pouch and that the outer ring remains outside the vagina.
- If desired, add more lubricant during intercourse, without removing the condom.
- Remove the pouch before standing by twisting the outer ring and pulling gently. (See drawing E.)
- Discard the used condom in a trash can, not a toilet.
- Insert a new condom for each act of intercourse.
- Do not use a male condom with the female condom. The increased friction could cause displacement of the female condom.[30]

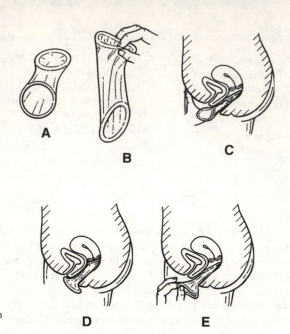

gritty sensation. Although vaginal suppositories do not require refrigeration, in warmer climates, it may be desirable to prevent softening.

Vaginal contraceptive film contains nonoxynol-9, 28% in paper-thin, 2-inch-square sheets. The film is activated by vaginal secretions. One film is used for each act of intercourse. The practice of inserting the film by placing it over the penis should be avoided, because this method does not ensure proper placement and does not allow adequate time for dissolution. In one comparison of spermicide dosage formulations, the film was rated the most difficult to use but the least messy.[31] A similarly designed vaginal cleansing film does not contain spermicide and should not be used for contraception. Patients should be advised to verify that they are using the correct vaginal film product if they desire contraception.

Spermicides used alone have a relatively high typical usage failure rate among first-year users (Table 10-1). A comparative trial of five vaginal spermicidal dosage forms found a similar pregnancy rate between two gels, a suppository, and film, each containing 100 to 150 mg nonoxynol-9 per dose. However, a gel containing 52.5 mg nonoxynol-9 per dose was significantly less effective at preventing pregnancy than the higher-dose formulations.[32] (The 52.5 mg product is not currently available in the United States.)

Efficacy improves greatly if spermicides are used in conjunction with barrier methods such as diaphragms, cervical caps, or condoms.

Although nonoxynol-9 can inactivate many sexually transmitted pathogens in vitro, clinical studies do not support a protective effect of vaginal spermicides against STI transmission, including gonorrhea, chlamydia, and HIV.[33,34] Higher rates of genital lesions, especially in frequent users, has been reported, raising concerns about an increased risk of STI transmission.[35] Diaphragms with spermicide offer no protection against HIV infection, but they may guard against cervical gonorrhea and chlamydia.[11,30] In 2007, FDA ruled that vaginal spermicide products must carry a label stating that the product does not protect against AIDS and other STIs.[36] On the basis of current knowledge, if a risk of STIs exists, use of spermicides alone should not be recommended.

Table 10-10 provides guidelines for the proper administration of vaginal spermicides. Regardless of the dosage formulation used, women should delay douching for at least 6 hours after intercourse when using a vaginal spermicide.

TABLE 10-9 Selected Vaginal Spermicides Containing Nonoxynol-9

Spermicidal foams	Delfen Foam 12.5%, 85 mg
	VCF Vaginal Contraceptive Foam 12.5%, 85 mg
Spermicidal gels/jellies	Encare Contraceptive Gel 4%, 100 mg
	Ortho Options Gynol II Vaginal Contraceptive Jelly[a] 2%, 100 mg
	Ortho Options Gynol II Extra Strength Vaginal Contraceptive Jelly 3%, 150 mg
Spermicidal suppositories	Encare Vaginal Contraceptive Inserts 100 mg
Spermicidal film	Ortho Options Vaginal Contraceptive Film 100 mg
	VCF Vaginal Contraceptive Film 28%, 72 mg

[a] Product formulated for use with a diaphragm or cervical cap; it should not be used alone.

TABLE 10-10 Administration Guidelines for Vaginal Spermicides

Dosage Form	Application Method	Onset/Duration of Action	Application Time before Intercourse	Reapplication Requirements
Vaginal gel alone	Insert full dose near cervix.	Immediate/1 hour	Up to 30–60 minutes	Reapply for each coital act.
Vaginal gel used with diaphragm/cervical cap	Fill barrier device one-third full with gel and place it near cervix. Leave barrier in place for at least 6 hours after intercourse.	Immediate/diaphragm: 6 hours; cervical cap: 48 hours	Up to 1 hour	Diaphragm: for each coital act that occurs within 6 hours of initial insertion of device, reapply spermicide without removing device; for coitus after 6 hours of initial insertion, remove and wash device, fill with new spermicide, and reinsert device. Cervical cap: remove and wash device; then reapply spermicide for each coital act that occurs 48 hours after initial insertion of device.
Vaginal foam	Insert full dose near cervix.	Immediate/1 hour	Up to 1 hour	Reapply for each coital act.
Vaginal suppository	Insert suppository near cervix.	10–15 minutes/1 hour	10–15 minutes	Reapply for each coital act.
Vaginal contraceptive film	Drape film over fingertip; place film near cervix.	15 minutes/1–3 hours (brand-dependent)	15 minutes	Reapply for each coital act.

Although allergic reactions are rare, either partner may experience such reactions to spermicides. Couples having oral–genital sex may find the taste of some products unpleasant. Frequent use or use of high-concentration products may irritate or damage vaginal and cervical epithelium,[35] which may be associated with an increased risk for STIs. Despite concerns about a possible association between spermicide use and birth defects or miscarriage should an unintended pregnancy occur, currently available data do not support an increased risk of birth defects attributable to spermicides.[37]

Product Selection Guidelines   The relatively low effectiveness of spermicides when used alone is their major disadvantage. However, studies suggest that simultaneous use of condoms and spermicides have efficacy rates similar to those of oral contraceptives and intrauterine contraceptives (IUCs).[2] Their availability and ease of use make spermicides a good choice for women who need a backup method. Spermicides are not recommended for women with anatomic abnormalities that would preclude proper placement of the spermicide near the cervical opening. Product selection can be based on patient preference and specific product characteristics.

CONTRACEPTIVE SPONGE

The contraceptive sponge is a small, circular, disposable sponge made of polyurethane permeated with spermicide (Table 10-11). The sponge is believed to act as a contraceptive by (1) serving as a mechanical barrier, (2) providing a spermicide, and (3) absorbing semen. The contraceptive sponge ranges in price from $3 to $7 per sponge.

In two large trials, the failure rate for the contraceptive sponge ranged from 17.4 to 24.5 pregnancies per 100 women in the first year of use.[38] Women who had given birth previously (parous women) had a significantly higher pregnancy rate while using the sponge, compared with women who had never given birth (nulliparous women); this finding may be related to poor fit in women who have delivered vaginally. If the sponge becomes dislodged during intercourse, its efficacy may be decreased.

Use of a contraceptive sponge has been associated with a decreased risk of cervical infections with chlamydia and gonorrhea. However, protection against HIV infection has not been shown with use of the contraceptive sponge, and one study found an increased risk of HIV infection in women with frequent sponge use, possibly because of an increased incidence of vaginal ulceration from the spermicide.[39]

A woman must be able to locate her cervix and must be comfortable in doing so to correctly place the sponge. Table 10-11 provides instructions for properly using these products. The sponges have slits or a loop attached to the convex side to facilitate removal. Some women have difficulty removing the sponge, and it has been known to fragment on removal. The sponge should be stored in its unopened package in a cool place and used before its expiration date.

Vaginal dryness is reported among sponge users. Although the incidence is rare, the contraceptive sponge has been associated with an increased risk of toxic shock syndrome (TSS).[30] Women should take special care to wash their hands before inserting the sponge, should not use the sponge during menstruation or for 6 weeks postpartum, and should not exceed the maximum recommended retention time. Women should also be advised to make sure the entire sponge is removed, because fragments left in the vagina may serve as a focus for infection.

Product Selection Guidelines   The contraceptive sponge is convenient, safe, and portable. Contraindications for use include spermicide sensitivity, anatomic abnormalities of the vagina, and a history of TSS. At this time, it may be prudent not to routinely

		TABLE 10-11 Contraceptive Sponges		
Product	**Spermicide**	**Instructions for Use**	**Onset/Duration**	**Removal**
Today	Nonoxynol-9, 100 mg	Moisten with tap water, insert convex side against cervix; can be inserted up to 24 hours before intercourse.	Immediate onset/ 24 hours	Leave in for >6 hours after intercourse, no longer than 30 hours total; polyester loop to facilitate removal.
Protectaid[a]	F-5 gel[b] (nonoxynol-9, 6.25 mg; benzalkonium chloride 6.25 mg; sodium cholate 25 mg)	Does not need to be moistened before insertion; can be inserted up to 6 hours before intercourse.	15 minutes/12 hours	Leave in for >6 hours after intercourse; has finger slots to facilitate removal.
Pharmatex	Benzalkonium chloride 60 mg[a]	Does not need to be moistened before insertion; can be inserted up to 22 hours before intercourse.	Immediate onset/ 24 hours	Leave in for >2 hours after intercourse, no longer than 24 hours total.

[a] Available through the Internet from sources outside the United States.

[b] Spermicide not approved by Food and Drug Administration.

recommend the contraceptive sponge to parous women because of possible problems with adequate cervical coverage.

Fertility Awareness Methods

Contraceptive methods that do not use a chemical or barrier to prevent conception include the basal body temperature (BBT) method, cervical mucus method, lactational amenorrhea method, and withdrawal. Many couples select these methods because they pose no health risks to the couple (or to the fetus should pregnancy occur). Others use these methods for financial or religious reasons. Most natural contraceptive methods cost little to no money, so they can be significantly less expensive than prescription methods. In some cases, natural contraceptive methods are used because of a lack of access to or knowledge of other methods of contraception. A disadvantage of fertility awareness methods (FAM) is a lack of STI protection. Most of these methods require periods of abstinence or the use of another method of contraception (such as condoms) during fertile days.

FAM involves use of various techniques to determine a woman's period of fertility. The information provided by these techniques helps identify the fertile phase of the menstrual cycle. A couple can choose to abstain from sexual intercourse during that period to avoid pregnancy.

CALENDAR METHOD

The calendar method uses a woman's monthly menstrual cycle length to calculate the fertile period. The viabilities of ova (1 day) and sperm (up to 7 days) are factored into this method.[13,40] Because a woman's menstrual cycles may vary, menstrual cycle lengths should be recorded for 6 to 12 cycles to predict the likely range of fertile days. The first fertile day in a woman's menstrual cycle is calculated by subtracting 18 from the number of days in her shortest cycle. The last fertile day is calculated by subtracting 11 from the number of days in her longest cycle.

BASAL BODY TEMPERATURE METHOD

The BBT method is most effective at calculating the end of the fertile phase and therefore should be used only with another fertility awareness method (see Symptothermal Method below). In the BBT method, the woman measures and charts her body temperature every morning.[40] She takes her temperature, preferably with a digital thermometer calibrated in increments of 0.1°F (0.05°C), to detect small changes in body temperature. She must obtain her temperature before getting out of bed and at the same time every day. Daily temperatures should be recorded on a chart (Figure 10-2).

In some but not all women, onset of ovulation may be detected by a drop in BBT 12 to 24 hours before ovulation. At the time of ovulation, BBT rises by at least 0.4°F (0.2°C) above the lowest point (the nadir).[40] This sharp rise, called the thermal shift, is caused by high progesterone levels. The safe (infertile) period begins once there have been 3 consecutive days of rising temperature and lasts until the end of menses.

For patients with difficulty interpreting shifts in their BBT, a computerized monitor (e.g., Bioself SymptoTherm and OvuTherm) registers and stores the BBTs (see Chapter 51).[13] The monitors use the collected data to predict periods of infertility and fertility. However, these products are only as good as the information they record. A woman must still take her temperature at the same time every morning before any physical activity. Anything that affects her BBT will interfere with the computer's ability to generate an accurate indicator of her fertility levels.

Some women do not have a definite or significant temperature dip or rise with ovulation. Stress, inadequate sleep, travel, fever, or lactation may affect BBT.[40] Also, temperature changes are difficult to interpret just before and during menopause. For women who work rotating shifts, it may be difficult to maintain an accurate record of BBT.[40] At such times, it is best for couples to use an alternative method of contraception.

CERVICAL MUCUS METHOD

The cervical mucus method uses the rather consistent changes in cervical mucus that take place during a normal menstrual

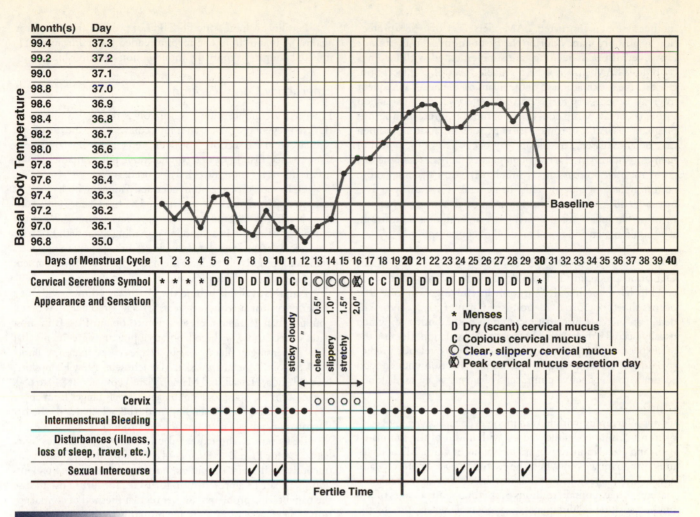

FIGURE 10-2 Symptothermal variations during a model menstrual cycle. (Reprinted with permission from Jennings VH, Arevalo M, Kowal D. Fertility awareness-based methods. In: Hatcher RA, Trussell J, Stewart F, et al., eds. *Contraceptive Technology*. 18th rev ed. New York: Ardent Media; 2004:327.)

cycle.[40] Every day, the woman observes the cervical mucus; she charts its character and quantity (Figure 10-2). After menstruation, most women notice a sensation of vaginal dryness on some days. About 5 to 6 days before ovulation, estrogen levels rise, causing the cervical mucus to increase in quantity and elasticity and to become clear, resembling raw egg white. The peak symptom, the last day of the clear, stretchy, estrogenic mucus, has been shown to occur within a day of ovulation for most women. With the postovulatory rise in progesterone, the mucus becomes thick and sticky or is absent. The woman is considered fertile from the first day after menstruation on which mucus is detected until 4 days after appearance of the peak symptom.[40] This interval is when intercourse should be avoided. Most women can learn this method after three cycles. With experience, a woman learns to differentiate other vaginal secretions, such as seminal fluid or an infectious discharge, from normal mucus, enabling her to seek early treatment for an infection. Women should be informed that vaginal foams, gels, creams, and douches will interfere with cervical mucus.

Another method of monitoring cervical secretions is called the TwoDay method.[41,42] On a day a woman is considering intercourse, she should think about whether she noticed any secretions that day or the day before. If she did not, she is probably not fertile. If she did notice secretions on either day, then she is likely to be fertile. The TwoDay method is a simple method that does not require keeping records or logs. Unfortunately, the exact effectiveness of this method is unknown and it should be used with caution.

SYMPTOTHERMAL METHOD

The symptothermal method combines methods of fertility awareness to determine the fertile period. Usually BBT charting is combined with notations of changes in cervical mucus (Figure 10-2).[13,40] This method may also combine changes in libido or cervical texture, for example.[40]

STANDARD DAYS METHOD

The standard days method is recommended for only women with cycles between 26 and 32 days in length. Counting the first day of menstruation as day 1, a woman should avoid intercourse on days 8 to 19 of her menstrual cycle or use another method of contraception such as condoms during this time.[40]

LACTATIONAL AMENORRHEA METHOD

In many developing countries, the lactational amenorrhea method (LAM; i.e., breast-feeding) is used as a contraceptive method for spacing the birth of children. When an infant receives at least 90% of his nutrition from breast-feeding and the mother has not menstruated, LAM offers more than 98% protection against pregnancy during the first 6 months postpartum.[43] However, if breast-feedings are supplemented with feedings by bottle, LAM may not be a reliable form of contraception. Because the suckling action of the infant on the breast at frequent intervals is necessary for LAM to be effective, milk extraction through a breast pump does not offer the same protection against pregnancy.[44] Although menstrual periods in lactating women may be anovulatory, ovulation may occur before the return of menses. With LAM, the risk of pregnancy increases after the initial 6 months postpartum as supplementation becomes more commonplace in older infants. In general, if a sexually active, breast-feeding woman is having menstrual periods, is supplementing her infant's diet, or is more than 6 months postpartum, she should use an additional method of contraception.[43,44]

HOME TESTS FOR OVULATION PREDICTION

Ovulation prediction tests are designed to aid couples in conceiving by detecting the surge in luteinizing hormone that occurs shortly before ovulation (see Chapter 51).[40] These kits detect an increase in urinary excretion of the hormone, which usually occurs 8 to 40 hours before actual ovulation. Because the life expectancy of sperm is up to 7 days, these ovulation predictors do not give warning of impending ovulation with enough accuracy to be effective contraceptive agents when used alone.

WITHDRAWAL

Coitus interruptus (withdrawal) involves coital activity until ejaculation is imminent, followed by withdrawal of the stimulated penis and ejaculation away from the vagina or vulva. Method failures (pregnancy even when the method is used correctly and consistently) occur in part because involuntary preejaculation secretions may contain millions of sperm. Disadvantages of this method include requirement of considerable self-control by the man and the potential for diminished pleasure for the couple because of interrupted lovemaking.

DOUCHING

Vaginal douches should never be considered a method of contraception. Under favorable conditions in the female reproductive tract, active sperm have been found in the cervical crypts and oviducts within minutes after ejaculation. Postcoital douching has no effect in removing sperm from the upper reproductive tract and could, in fact, force or propel sperm higher up in the tract.

EFFECTIVENESS OF FERTILITY AWARENESS METHODS

Overall, the pregnancy rate for typical use of FAM is approximately 25% (Table 10-1).[2] The risk of pregnancy is far higher with any of these methods alone compared with condoms, hormonal methods, or the nonhormonal intrauterine device. Consequently, family planners do not recommend using a single method alone; instead they suggest using a combination of methods. Methods that specifically identify preovulatory and postovulatory changes, such as the symptothermal method, have much better outcomes. Table 10-1 shows that combinations of these methods have good predicted effectiveness; with perfect use, the annual failure rate is 2%.

For a woman who is breast-feeding an infant almost exclusively, studies have reported pregnancy rates of 0.5% to 2% for the 6-month period after delivery. However, once supplemental feedings begin, the efficacy rate falls significantly.[44] Efficacy rates on using home ovulation prediction tests are not available. For couples who rely on withdrawal, accidental pregnancy rates range from 4 to 27 pregnancies per 100 couples in the first year of use.[2]

Fertility awareness methods do not provide any protection against STIs and should be recommended solely for non–STI-infected couples in mutually monogamous relationships.

Emergency Contraception

Emergency contraception (EC) involves the use of pills or an IUC to prevent pregnancy after intercourse. Only the use of pills is discussed in this section. The dedicated emergency contraceptive product, Plan B, or oral contraceptive pills containing levonorgestrel or D,L-norgestrel may be used.

ECPs should be recommended for patients who had recent unprotected intercourse or experienced method failure (e.g., condom breakage).[43,45] Some patients may be seeking ECPs in the case of sexual assault. In addition to providing them with ECPs for immediate use, pharmacy staff should refer the patient to providers who can appropriately evaluate them for STIs as well as document the incident for possible inclusion in legal proceedings.

Plan B is available behind the pharmacy counter without a prescription for anyone 18 years of age or older.[43] Women younger than 18 need a prescription to obtain Plan B in most states except those with collaborative practice agreements that allow dispensing in pharmacies to all ages (Washington, California, Vermont, Montana, Alaska, Massachusetts, New Hampshire, New Mexico, Hawaii, and Maine). Plan B costs about $40 to $50. The cost for EC using oral contraceptive pills ranges from about $25 to more than $50, depending on the pill selected and whether the patient receives a brand or generic product.

ECPs reduce the expected number of pregnancies by at least 89% for Plan B users and 74% for combination oral contraceptive pill users. Providers should consider giving patients younger than 18 a prescription for ECPs for future use in case the patient has a problem with her regular method of contraception. The efficacy of ECPs is due primarily to the suppression of ovulation.[46] Other possible mechanisms of action include interference with transport of sperm or egg, including thickening of cervical mucus.

Progestin-only EC (Plan B) is usually given as a single dose of two tablets.[43,45] The package labeling for Plan B instructs patients to take one pill every 12 hours for two doses. Both methods of administration have equal effectiveness; the first method is preferred because of simplicity.[47] Emergency contraception using combined oral contraceptive pills is given in two doses. For optimal efficacy, the first dose should be given as soon as possible after unprotected intercourse, and the second dose 12 hours later. Although the initial recommendations were to give the first dose of ECPs (progestin-only and oral contraceptive pills) within 72 hours of unprotected intercourse, several studies have shown that ECPs are still effective if given within 5 days.[47,48] Therefore, women presenting within 120 hours of unprotected sex should be offered ECPs. Patients presenting between 5 to 7 days after unprotected intercourse should be referred to a physician for possible IUC insertion. Table 10-12 lists the available products used for emergency contraception.

The most common adverse effects reported are nausea and vomiting.[43,45] Nausea occurs in about 50% of women using combination EC and 25% of women using progestin-only EC. Vomiting occurs in about 20% and 5% of combination and progestin-only EC users, respectively. An antiemetic is usually not necessary for progestin-only EC but may be recommended 30 to 60 minutes before each dose when using combination oral contraceptive pills. Headaches, breast tenderness, and dizziness have also been reported. Progestin-only EC has been found to

TABLE 10-12 Oral Contraceptive Pills That May Be Used for Emergency Contraception		
Trade Name	**No. of Pills** *per Dose*	**Color of Pills to Take**
Alesse, Lessina, Levlite	5	Pink
Aviane	5	Orange
Cryselle, Levora, Lo-Ovral, Low-Ogestrel, Quasense	4	White
Enpresse	4	Orange
Jolessa, Portia, Seasonale, Trivora	4	Pink
Levlen, Nordette	4	Light orange
Lutera	5	White
Lybrel	6	Yellow
Ogestrel, Ovral	2	White
Seasonique	4	Light blue-green
Tri-Levlen, Triphasil	4	Yellow

TABLE 10-13 Counseling Points for Emergency Contraception
■ Identify patient who has had recent unprotected sex or is at risk for unprotected sex and does not want to get pregnant.
■ Explain how to take emergency contraception: Both doses of Plan B may be given at the same time or as two doses. It is best if emergency contraception is taken as soon as possible after unprotected intercourse; however, the method is effective when taken up to 120 hours after unprotected intercourse.
■ Recommend an antiemetic for women using combination oral contraceptive pills.
■ Emphasize that emergency contraception is not to be used as a regular contraceptive method.
■ Recommend that a sexually active woman begin using regular contraception after taking ECPs. Barrier methods should be used with each subsequent act of intercourse. Hormonal methods may be started with next menses or may be started the day after taking ECPs, including 7 days of a back-up method.
■ Explain that ECPs do not protect against STIs.
■ Explain that emergency contraception is not 100% effective. Recommend using a pregnancy test if menses is more than 21 days late.
■ Provide written instructions.

Key: ECP, emergency contraceptive pill; STI, sexually transmitted infection.

Source: References 37 and 41.

be more effective and better tolerated than combination pills. Table 10–13 provides patient counseling information on ECPs.

Complementary Therapies

At this time, there is insufficient evidence to recommend any complementary therapies for the prevention of pregnancy and STIs.

Assessment of the Prevention of Pregnancy and Sexually Transmitted Infections: A Case-Based Approach

Before advising a patient on contraception and STI prevention, the practitioner must identify first the patient's level of knowl-edge about these issues. Before they can select a product or method that is appropriate, patients must understand their risk for pregnancy and STIs. Patients who prefer FAM methods must understand the reproductive cycle before they can use these methods effectively. Patients who prefer nonprescription contraceptive products must know how to use them properly and be prepared to use them with every act of intercourse. The practitioner should identify the patient's preferences for prod-ucts or methods on the basis of the timing of use or on religious or cultural practices.

Case 10–1 illustrates the assessment of a patient who is seeking advice on contraception, whereas Case 10–2 deals with the use of emergency contraceptives.

C A S E   1 0 - 1

Relevant Evaluation Criteria	Scenario/Model Outcome
Information Gathering	
1. Gather essential information about the patient's symptoms, including:	
a. description of symptom(s) (i.e., nature, onset, duration, severity, associated symptoms)	Patient has been having recurrent vaginal itching after sexual intercourse. There is no vaginal discharge, and she does not have any lesions or blisters when the itch-ing occurs. The symptoms occur only after intercourse.
b. description of any factors that seem to precipitate, exacerbate, and/or relieve the patient's symptom(s)	Patient uses latex condoms with spermicide for prevention of pregnancy and STIs. Symptoms resolve in 2–3 days with or without intervention.

Relevant Evaluation Criteria	Scenario/Model Outcome
c. description of the patient's efforts to relieve the symptoms	She tried a different brand of condoms but experienced a similar reaction. She also used an OTC antifungal product for yeast vaginitis, but it did not clear her symptoms more rapidly than no intervention.
2. Gather essential patient history information:	
a. patient's identity	Jo Harding
b. patient's age, sex, height, and weight	31-year-old female, 5 ft 5 in, 160 lb
c. concurrent medical conditions, prescription and nonprescription medications, and dietary supplements	None; pregnancy test done yesterday is negative.
d. allergies	NKA
e. history of STIs	History of chlamydia and trichomonas last year with previous partner
	Current partner with history of genital herpes

Assessment and Triage

3. Differentiate the patient's signs/symptoms and correctly identify the patient's primary problem(s).	Risk for undesired pregnancy and STI
	Possible latex or spermicide allergy
4. Identify exclusions for self-treatment.	None, but patient should be referred to her PCP if she develops symptoms consistent with an STI, such as vaginal discharge or blisters.
5. Formulate a comprehensive list of therapeutic alternatives for the primary problem to determine if triage to a medical practitioner is required, and share this information with the patient.	Options include: (1) Recommend use of a spermicide-free latex condom, latex-free male or female condom. (2) Recommend use of spermicide alone (with or without barrier method). (3) Recommend use of FAM. (4) Refer patient to PCP for a prescription method of contraception. (5) Take no action.

Plan

6. Select an optimal therapeutic alternative to address the patient's problem, taking into account patient preferences.	Polyurethane female condom because patient prefers female-controlled method
7. Describe the recommended therapeutic approach to the patient.	Use polyurethane female condom with each act of sexual intercourse.
8. Explain to the patient the rationale for selecting the recommended therapeutic approach from the considered therapeutic alternatives.	Your symptoms may be due to spermicide or latex allergy. Because you have not obtained relief by trying a different brand of latex condoms, use of nonlatex (polyurethane) condoms (either male or female) should eliminate the adverse reaction while still providing comparable prevention of pregnancy and sexually transmitted infections. Natural membrane condoms should not be used, because they are not as effective as other condoms in preventing sexually transmitted infections.

Patient Education

9. When recommending self-care with nonprescription medications and/or nondrug therapy, convey accurate information to the patient:	
a. appropriate dose and frequency of administration	Use fresh condom with each act of sexual intercourse.
b. product administration procedures	See Table 10-8.
c. expected time to onset of relief	Female condoms are effective immediately once correctly inserted, and they can be inserted up to 8 hours prior to intercourse.
d. degree of relief that can be reasonably expected	See Table 10-1.

Relevant Evaluation Criteria	Scenario/Model Outcome
e. most common side effects	Vaginal irritation, increased noise (squeaking)
f. patient options in the event that condition worsens or persists	Consult your primary care provider.
g. product storage guidelines	See Table 10-8.
10. Solicit follow-up questions from patient.	May I use lubricants or vaginal spermicides with the female condom?
11. Answer patient's questions.	Yes. The female condom comes with its own lubricant, but additional lubrication can also be used. Polyurethane condoms are not affected by oil-based lubricants. Use of a vaginal spermicide may enhance the contraceptive effectiveness of condoms, but discontinue spermicide use if itching recurs.

Key: FAM, fertility awareness methods; NKA, no known allergies; OTC, over-the-counter; PCP, primary care provider; STI, sexually transmitted infection.

Relevant Evaluation Criteria	Scenario/Model Outcome
Information Gathering	
1. Gather essential information about the patient's symptoms, including:	
a. description of symptom(s) (i.e., nature, onset, duration, severity, associated symptoms)	Patient recently missed 5 doses of her oral contraceptive pills. Yesterday she had intercourse with her boyfriend and did not use a backup method of contraception. She is worried about becoming pregnant.
2. Gather essential patient history information:	
a. patient's identity	Lydia James
b. patient's age, sex, height, and weight	24-year-old female, 5 ft 4 in, 125 lb
c. patient's occupation	Graduate student
d. concurrent medical conditions, prescription and nonprescription medications, and dietary supplements	Ortho-Cyclen 1 tablet daily (last dose 5 days ago), multivitamin 1 tablet daily
e. allergies	NKA
f. history of other adverse reactions to medications	None
Assessment and Triage	
3. Differentiate the patient's signs/symptoms and correctly identify the patient's primary problem(s).	Elevated risk of pregnancy due to missed doses of oral contraceptive pill
4. Identify exclusions for self-treatment.	Patient would be unable to purchase emergency contraception without a prescription if she were younger than 18 years. Patient has no exclusions for self-treatment.
5. Formulate a comprehensive list of therapeutic alternatives for the primary problem to determine if triage to a medical practitioner is required, and share this information with the patient.	Options include: (1) Recommend purchasing emergency contraception at her local pharmacy. (2) Recommend obtaining a prescription for an oral contraceptive pill that can be used as emergency contraception (see Table 10-12). (3) Recommend she see her provider for evaluation and possible insertion of a copper intrauterine contraceptive. (4) Take no action.

CASE 10-2 *(continued)*

Relevant Evaluation Criteria	Scenario/Model Outcome
Plan	
6. Select an optimal therapeutic alternative to address the patient's problem, taking into account patient preferences.	The patient prefers to purchase emergency contraception at her local pharmacy.
7. Describe the recommended therapeutic approach to the patient.	You should take Plan B, 2 tablets by mouth at one time within 120 hours of unprotected intercourse. You may also prefer to follow the directions on Plan B's packaging and take 1 tablet as soon as possible and a second tablet 12 hours later. Both regimens offer similar efficacy and have similar side effect profiles.
8. Explain to the patient the rationale for selecting the recommended therapeutic approach from the considered therapeutic alternatives.	Because you are 24 years of age, you do not need to see your provider to obtain a prescription for emergency contraception.
Patient Education	
9. When recommending self-care with non-prescription medications and/or nondrug therapy, convey accurate information to the patient.	See Table 10-13.
10. Solicit follow-up questions from patient.	(1) How effective is Plan B? (2) May I start taking birth control pills after I use Plan B?
11. Answer patient's questions.	See Table 10-13.

Key: NKA, no known allergies.

Patient Counseling for Prevention of Pregnancy and Sexually Transmitted Infections

As the most accessible health care provider, pharmacists are in a distinctive position to impact the incidence and consequences of unintended pregnancy and STIs in their communities. The pharmacist should seek opportunities to discuss specific diseases or prevention strategies with individuals who may be at high risk for unintended pregnancy and STIs.

Practitioners should thoroughly familiarize themselves with the proper use of currently available nonprescription contraceptive products and provide opportunities for consultation with patients by removing barriers that may prevent dialogue. In pharmacies, contraceptive products and information as well as STI–related consumer information should be available in an area where the patient can browse and the pharmacist can easily interact with the patient, such as next to or directly in front of the prescription counter.

In addition to the educational role, the practitioner may be able to assist an individual in gaining access to other needed medical and social supportive services. In cases of suspected domestic violence or sexual abuse, pharmacists should act on their role as mandatory reporters. A private area for education and counseling is important if adequate discussion is to take place.

Special efforts should be made to offer contraceptive information and services to adolescents. Clinicians who are uncomfortable discussing reproductive health in a nonjudgmental manner with young people should refer adolescents to a clinic that specializes in services to young people, if one is available. Adolescents need clear, accurate information on all aspects of reproductive health. The practitioner should keep in mind that misconceptions about STI and pregnancy risk and proper contraceptive use are common, especially among adolescents; therefore, adequate education is very important. Particularly useful nonprescription methods for the sometimes impulsive adolescent might include condoms and contraceptive foam in prefilled applicators.

FAM may be best recommended for a couple in a stable relationship. FAM, especially the BBT and cervical mucus methods, require extensive training and support from health care professionals who have experience and training with these methods. The provider should be supportive and available to answer questions regarding such techniques. Besides stocking spermicidal products, BBT thermometers, and monitoring charts, the pharmacist may serve as a referral center for patients who want to use these methods of family planning. A pharmacist with the proper training might consider counseling patients on FAM as a unique practice possibility.

Evaluation of Patient Outcomes for Prevention of Pregnancy and Sexually Transmitted Infections

Many sexually active patients are at risk for unintended pregnancy or STIs. Efficacy rates of contraceptives vary, but the most important factor affecting their ability to prevent pregnancy and STIs is correct and consistent use with each sexual encounter. Although any of the methods can be used for pregnancy prevention, the latex male condom and the female condom are the preferred methods for prevention of STIs. Individuals who experience an adverse reaction after use of a nonprescription contraceptive should switch to an alternative brand or agent. If the symptoms do not resolve or recur with the use of other agents, the patient should seek medical attention. A sexually active woman who misses a menstrual period should be encouraged to perform a home pregnancy test or seek medical attention. Symptoms of an STI in a sexually active individual require medical referral (Table 10-2).

Key Points for Prevention of Pregnancy and Sexually Transmitted Infections

➤ No method of contraception is completely effective at preventing unintended pregnancy and STIs.

➤ Selection of a contraceptive product or method must be based on patient risk for undesired outcomes (pregnancy and STI) and efficacy, safety, and patient acceptability.

➤ Efficacy of nonprescription contraceptives is significantly increased by correct and consistent use of the product/ method with each sexual encounter (Tables 10-6, 10-8, 10-10, and 10-11).

➤ Latex male condoms and female condoms are the preferred contraceptive products for patients at risk for STIs. The polyurethane condom may be used in persons with latex hypersensitivity.

➤ Currently available spermicides decrease risk of unintended pregnancy but may increase risk of STIs.

➤ Vaginal spermicides are available in a variety of dosage forms to improve patient acceptability.

➤ Fertility awareness methods are an inexpensive, modestly effective method of contraception that can be used by non–STI-infected couples in a mutually monogamous relationship.

➤ Emergency contraception is an effective method of postcoital contraception that can decrease risk of unintended pregnancy, but it does not decrease risk of STIs.

REFERENCES

1. Mosher WD, Martinez GM, Chandra A, et al. Use of contraception and use of family planning services in the United States: 1982–2002. *Advance Data*. 2004;350:1–36.

2. Trussell J. The essentials of contraception: efficacy, safety, and personal considerations. In: Hatcher RA, Trussell J, Stewart F, et al., eds. *Contraceptive Technology*. 18th rev ed. New York: Ardent Media; 2004:221–52.

3. Finer LB, Henshaw SK. Disparities in rates of unintended pregnancy in the United States, 1994 and 2001. *Perspect Sex Reprod Health*. 2006;38:90–6.

4. Jones RK, Darroch JE, Henshaw SK. Contraceptive use among U.S. women having abortions in 2000–2001. *Perspect Sex Reprod Health*. 2002;34:294–303.

5. Cason C, Orrock N, Schmitt K, et al. The impact of laws on HIV and STD prevention. *J Law Med Ethics*. 2002;30(3 suppl):139–45.

6. Cates W. Reproductive tract infections. In: Hatcher RA, Trussell J, Stewart F, et al., eds. *Contraceptive Technology*. 18th ed. New York: Ardent Media; 2004:191–220.

7. Biddlecom AE. Trends in sexual behaviours and infections among young people in the United States. *Sex Transm Infect*. 2004; 80(suppl):ii74–9.

8. Miller FC. Impact of adolescent pregnancy as we approach the new millennium. *J Pediatr Adolesc Gynecol*. 2000;13:5–8.

9. Paukku M, Quan J, Barney P, et al. Adolescent's contraceptive use and pregnancy history: is there a pattern? *Obstet Gynecol*. 2003;101:534–8.

10. Centers for Disease Control and Prevention. Nationally Representative CDC Study Finds 1 in 4 Teenage Girls Has a Sexually Transmitted Disease. Available at: http://www.cdc.gov/stdconference/2008/media/release-11march2008.htm. Last accessed September 9, 2008.

11. Centers for Disease Control and Prevention. Sexually transmitted diseases treatment guidelines 2006. *MMWR Morb Mortal Wkly Rep*. 2006; 51(RR-11):1–94.

12. Sherman AC, Harvey SM, Noell J. 'Are they still having sex?' STIs and unintended pregnancy among mid-life women. *J Women Aging*. 2005; 17(3):41.

13. Sanford JB, White GL Jr, Hatasaka H. Timing intercourse to achieve pregnancy: current evidence. *Obstet Gynecol*. 2002;100:1333–41.

14. Condoms: Extra protection. *Consumer Rep*. 2005;70:34–5.

15. Nonlatex vs latex condoms: an update. *Contracept Rep*. 2003;14:10–3.

16. Warner DL, Hatcher RA, Steiner MJ. Male condoms. In: Hatcher RA, Trussell J, Stewart F, et al., eds. *Contraceptive Technology*. 18th rev ed. New York: Ardent Media; 2004:331–53.

17. Workshop Summary: Scientific Evidence on Condom Effectiveness for Sexually Transmitted Disease (STD) Prevention. July 20, 2001. Washington, DC: National Institute of Allergy and Infectious Diseases, National Institutes of Health, Department of Health and Human Services. Available at: http://www.premaritalsex.info/docs/condomreport.pdf. Last accessed October 19, 2008.

18. Valappil T, Kelaghan J, Macaluso M, et al. Female condom and male condom failure among women at high risk of sexually transmitted diseases. *Sex Transm Dis*. 2005;32:35–43.

19. Golombok S, Harding R, Sheldon J. An evaluation of a thicker versus a standard condom with gay men. *AIDS*. 2001;15:245–50.

20. Potter WD, de Villemeur M. Clinical breakage, slippage and acceptability of a new commercial polyurethane condom: a randomized, controlled study. *Contraception*. 2003;68:39–45.

21. Gallo MF, Grimes DA, Lopez LM, et al. Non-latex versus latex condoms for contraceptive (review). *Cochrane Database Syst Rev*. 2006;1: CD003550.

22. Steiner MJ, Dominik R, Rountree W, et al. Contraceptive effectiveness of a polyurethane condom and a latex condom. *Obstet Gynecol*. 2003; 101:539–47.

23. Winer RL, Hughes JP, Feng Q, et al. Condom use and the risk of genital human papillomavirus infection in young women. *N Engl J Med*. 2006;354:2645–54.

24. Warner L, Stone KM, Macaluso M, et al. Condom use and risk of gonorrhea and chlamydia: a systematic review of design and measurement factors assessed in epidemiologic studies. *Sex Transm Dis*. 2006; 33:36–51.

25. Wald A, Langenberg AGM, Krantz E, et al. The relationship between condom use and herpes simplex virus acquisition. *Ann Inter Med*. 2005; 143:707–13.

26. Hutchinson KB, Kip KE, Ness RB. Condom use and its association with bacterial vaginosis and bacterial vaginosis–associated vaginal microflora. *Epidemiology* 2007;18:702–8.

27. Farley T. WHO/CONRAD technical consultation on nonoxynol-9, World Health Organization, Geneva, 9–10 October 2001: summary report. *Reprod Health Matter*. 2002;10:175–81.

28. Liccardi G, Senna G, Rotiroti G, et al. Intimate behavior and allergy: a narrative review. *Ann Allergy Asthma Immunol*. 2007;99:394–400.

29. Hoffman S, Mantell J, Exner T, et al. The future of the female condom. *Perspect Sex Reprod Health*. 2004;3:120–6.

30. Cates W Jr, Stewart F. Vaginal barriers: the female condom, diaphragm, contraceptive sponge, cervical cap, Lea's shield and femcap. In: Hatcher, RA, Trussell J, Stewart F, et al., eds. *Contraceptive Technology*. 18th rev ed. New York: Ardent Media; 2004: 365–89.

31. Raymond EG, Chen PL, Condon P, et al. Acceptability of five nonoxynol-9 spermicides. *Contraception*. 2005;71:438–42.

32. Raymond E, Chen PL, Luoto J. Contraceptive effectiveness and safety of five nonoxynol-9 spermicides: a randomized trial. *Obstet Gynecol*. 2004; 103:430–9.

33. Roddy RE, Zekeng L, Ryan KA, et al. Effect of nonoxynol-9 gel on urogenital gonorrhea and chlamydial infection. *JAMA*. 2002; 287:1117–22.

34. Wilkinson D, Tholandi M, Ramjee G, et al. Nonoxynol-9 spermicide for the prevention of vaginally acquired HIV and other sexually transmitted infections: systematic review and meta-analysis of randomized controlled trials including more than 5000 women. *Lancet*. 2002;2:613–7.

35. Wilkinson D, Ramjee G, Tholandi M, et al. Nonoxynol-9 for preventing vaginal acquisition of sexually transmitted infections by women from men. *Cochrane Database Syst Rev*. 2002;4:CD003939.

36. Over-the-counter vaginal contraceptive and spermicide drug products containing nonoxynol-9, required labeling. Final rule. *Fed Regist*. 2007; 72:71769–85.

37. Briggs G, Freeman RK, Yaffe SJ. *Drugs in Pregnancy and Lactation*. 6th ed. Philadelphia: Lippincott Williams & Wilkins; 2002:1010–3.

38. Kuyoh MA, Toroitich-Ruto C, Grimes DA, et al. Sponge versus diaphragm for contraception: a Cochrane review. *Contraception*. 2003;67:15–8.

39. Kreiss J, Ngugi E, Holmes K, et al. Efficacy of nonoxynol-p contraceptive sponge use in the prevention of heterosexual acquisition of HIV in Nairobi prostitutes. *JAMA*. 1992;268:477–82.

40. Jennings VH, Arevalo M, Kowal D. Fertility awareness-based methods. In: Hatcher RA, Trussell J, Stewart F, et al., eds. *Contraceptive Technology*. 18th rev ed. New York: Ardent Media; 2004:317–29.

41. Jennings V, Sinai I. Further analysis of the theoretical effectiveness of the TwoDay method of family planning. *Contraception*. 2001;64:149–53.

42. Arévalo M, Jennings V, Nikula M, et al. Efficacy of the new TwoDay Method of family planning. *Fertil Steril*. 2004;82:885–92.

43. Zieman M, Hatcher RA, et al. *A Pocket Guide to Managing Contraception*. Tiger, Ga: Bridging the Gap Foundation; 2007.

44. Kennedy KI, Trussell J. Postpartum contraception and lactation. In: Hatcher RA, Trussell J, Stewart F, et al., eds. *Contraceptive Technology*. 18th rev ed. New York: Ardent Media; 2004:575–600.

45. Stewart F, Trussell J, Van Look PFA. Emergency contraception. In: Hatcher RA, Trussell J, Stewart F, et al., eds. *Contraceptive Technology*. 18th rev ed. New York: Ardent Media; 2004:279–303.

46. Croxatto HB, Brache V, Pavez M, et al. Pituitary-ovarian function following the standard levonorgestrel emergency contraceptive dose or a single 0.75-mg dose given on the days preceding ovulation. *Contraception*. 2004;70:442–50.

47. Ellertson C, Webb A, Blanchard K, et al. Modifying the Yuzpe regimen of emergency contraception: a multicenter, randomized controlled trial. *Obstet Gynecol*. 2003;101:1160–7.

48. Rodrigues I, Grou F, Joly J. Effectiveness of emergency contraceptive pills between 72 and 120 hours after unprotected sexual intercourse. *Am J Obstet Gynecol*. 2001;184:531–7.

Respiratory Disorders

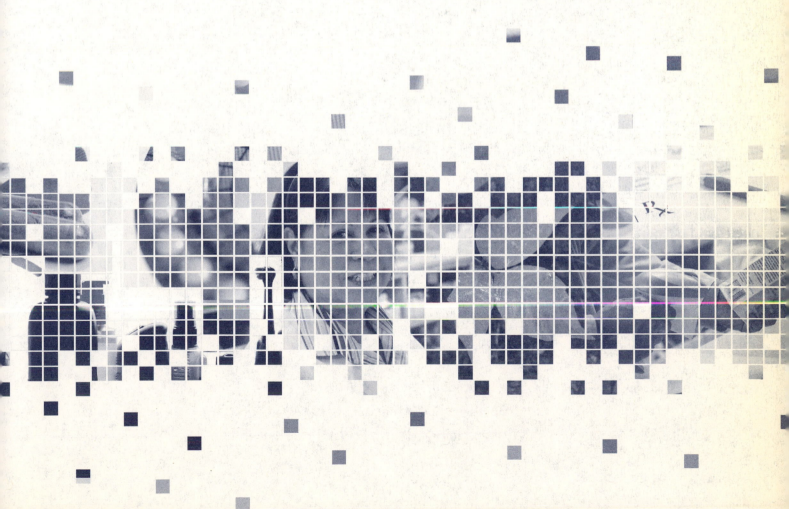

Disorders Related to Colds and Allergy

Kelly L. Scolaro

Colds and allergic rhinitis are two of the most common conditions for which patients access the health care system. This chapter reviews the role of the plethora of nonprescription products that patients may use to self-treat symptoms associated with these two disorders.

COLDS

A cold, also known as the common cold, is a viral infection of the upper respiratory tract. According to some estimates, 1 billion cases of colds occur annually in the United States, making this illness one of the top five diagnosed in the United States.[1] Children usually have 6 to 10 colds per year but may have as many as 12 colds annually, especially if they attend day care.[1] Adults younger than 60 years typically have 2 to 4 colds per year, whereas adults older than 60 have 1 cold per year.[1] Women, especially ages 20 to 30 years, tend to have more colds than men do, possibly because of more frequent contact with preschool or school-age children.[1] Colds may occur at any time, but in the United States cold season is from late August through early April.[1]

Colds are the leading cause of work and school absenteeism. Colds are usually self-limiting; however, because symptoms are bothersome, patients frequently self-medicate and spend approximately $2.6 billion annually on nonprescription cold products.[2]

Pathophysiology of Colds

Colds are limited to the upper respiratory tract and primarily affect the following respiratory structures: pharynx, nasopharynx, nose, cavernous sinusoids, and paranasal sinuses. Usually the respiratory tract's intricate host defense system (Table 11-1) protects the body from infections and foreign particles. The respiratory tract, especially the nose, is well perfused and innervated. The nose contains sensory, cholinergic, and sympathetic nerves. When stimulated by an infectious (i.e., a cold) or allergic process (i.e., allergic rhinitis), these nerves play a role in the resultant symptoms and are also targets for some nonprescription therapies. Sensory fibers respond to mechanical and thermal stimuli, and to mediators such as histamine and bradykinin. Cholinergic stimulation dilates whereas sympathetic stimulation constricts arterial blood flow. Sympathetic nerves also innervate veins and venules. Cholinergic and sympathetic nerves innervate glands as well as

the arteries that supply the glands. The cavernous sinusoids contain erectile tissue that engorges when the sympathetic tone is reduced or when the cholinergic system is stimulated. The sensory, cholinergic, and sympathetic nerves also respond to a variety of neuropeptide neurotransmitters.

More than 200 viruses cause colds. The majority of colds in children and adults are caused by rhinoviruses.[1] Other pathogens shown to cause colds include coronaviruses, influenza viruses, parainfluenza viruses, adenoviruses, echoviruses, respiratory syncytial virus, and coxsackieviruses. Viral and bacterial coinfection (usually with group A beta-hemolytic streptococci) occurs but is rare. Rhinoviruses bind to intercellular adhesion molecule-1 receptors on respiratory epithelial cells in the nose and nasopharynx. Once inside the epithelial cells, the virus replicates and infection spreads to other cells.[3] Peak viral concentrations occur 2 to 4 days after initial infection, and viruses are present in the nasopharynx for 16 to 18 days. Infected cells release chemokine "distress signals" and cytokines activate inflammatory mediators and neurogenic reflexes. The activation processes result in recruitment of additional inflammatory mediators; vasodilatation; transudation of plasma; glandular secretion; and stimulation of pain nerve fibers, and sneeze and cough reflexes. Inflammatory mediators and parasympathetic nervous system reflex mechanisms cause hypersecretion of watery nasal fluid. Viral infection ends once enough neutralizing antibody (secretory immunoglobulin A [IgA] or serum IgG) leaks into the mucosa to end viral replication.

The most efficient mode of transmission is self-inoculation of the nasal mucosa or conjunctiva following contact with viral-laden secretions on animate (hands) or inanimate (doorknobs and telephones) objects. Aerosol transmission is also important. Smoking, allergic disorders affecting the nose or pharynx, increased population density, a sedentary lifestyle, less diverse social networks, and chronic (e.g., ≥1 month) psychological stress increase susceptibility to colds.[4] Contrary to common belief, cold environments, sudden chilling, exposure to central heating, walking outside barefoot, teething, or enlarged tonsils or adenoids do not increase susceptibility to viral upper respiratory infections.[5,6]

Clinical Presentation of Colds

A predictable sequence of symptoms appears 1 to 3 days after infection.[7] Sore throat is the first symptom to appear, followed by nasal symptoms, which dominate by day 2 or 3. Cough, although

TABLE 11-1 Respiratory Defense System

Structure	Location	Function
Vibrissae (coarse hairs)	Nose	Removes large particles from inspired air
Mucus layer	Outer layer of respiratory mucosa	Thick, sticky layer traps foreign and infectious particles
Ciliated epithelial cells	Inner layer of respiratory mucosa	Sweeps outer layer of mucus/trapped particles to larynx where the mucus is swallowed
Mucus-secreting glands	Respiratory mucosa	Secretes enzymes, immunoglobulins, and immunomodulatory factors to manage infectious particles; produces mucus for outer layer

an infrequent symptom (<20%), appears by day 4 or 5. Physical assessment of a patient with a cold may yield the following findings: slightly red pharynx with evidence of postnasal drainage, nasal obstruction, and mildly to moderately tender sinuses on palpation. During the first 2 days of a cold, patients may report clear, thin and/or watery nasal secretions. As the infection progresses, the secretions become thicker, and the color may change to yellow or green. When the cold begins to resolve, the secretions again become clear, thin, and/or watery. Patients may have low-grade fever, but colds are rarely associated with a fever above 100°F (37.8°C). Rhinovirus cold symptoms persist for about 7 to 14 days.[7] Signs and symptoms of a cold may be confused with influenza and other respiratory illness (Table 11-2). However, a new test approved by the Food and Drug Administration (FDA), xTAG Respiratory Viral Panel by Luminex Molecular Diagnostics, rapidly identifies 12 respiratory viruses, including rhinovirus, and may help clinicians better differentiate between illnesses.[8]

Most people do not have complications from colds. However, complications of colds may be severe and, rarely, life threatening. Complications include sinusitis, middle ear infections, bronchitis, bacterial pneumonia, and exacerbations of asthma or chronic obstructive pulmonary disease.

Treatment of Colds

Treatment Goals

Because there is no known cure for colds, the goal of therapy is to prevent transmission of cold viruses and reduce bothersome symptoms.

General Treatment Approach

Studies show proper hand hygiene reduces the transmission of cold viruses, and the Centers for Disease Control and Prevention (CDC) encourages frequent hand cleansing with soap or soap substitutes (e.g., hand sanitizers) to help prevent colds.[1] Hand sanitizers have gained popularity owing to their convenience and quick action. However, not all hand sanitizers are effective at eradicating rhinoviruses from hands. Products containing the following ingredients have been proven effective: ethyl alcohol (62%–95% concentration); benzalkonium chloride; salicylic acid; pyroglutamic acid; and triclosan.[9] Studies conducted in the 1980s found that use of antiviral disinfectants such as Lysol (kills >99% of rhinoviruses after 1 minute) and antiviral tissues such as Kleenex Anti-Viral (10% fewer respiratory infections than in

TABLE 11-2 Differentiation of Colds and Other Respiratory Disorders

Illness	Signs and Symptoms
Allergic rhinitis	Watery eyes; itchy nose, eyes, or throat; repetitive sneezing; nasal congestion; watery rhinorrhea; red, irritated eyes with conjunctival injection
Asthma	Cough, dyspnea, wheezing
Bacterial throat infection	Sore throat (moderate-to-severe pain), fever, exudate, tender anterior cervical adenopathy
Colds	Sore throat (mild-to-moderate pain), nasal congestion, rhinorrhea, sneezing common; low-grade fever, chills, headache, malaise, myalgia, and cough possible
Croup	Fever, rhinitis, and pharyngitis initially, progressing to cough (may be "barking" cough), stridor, and dyspnea
Influenza	Myalgia, arthralgia, fever ≥100°F–102°F (37.8°C–38.9°C), sore throat, nonproductive cough, moderate-to-severe fatigue
Otitis media	Ear popping, ear fullness, otalgia, otorrhea, hearing loss, dizziness
Pneumonia or bronchitis	Chest tightness, wheezing, dyspnea, productive cough, changes in sputum color, persistent fever
Sinusitis	Tenderness over the sinuses, facial pain aggravated by Valsalva's maneuver or postural changes, fever >101.5°F (38.6°C), tooth pain, halitosis, upper respiratory tract symptoms for >7 days with poor response to decongestants
West Nile virus infection	Fever, headache, fatigue, rash, swollen lymph glands, and eye pain initially, possibly progressing to GI distress, CNS changes, seizures, or paralysis
Whooping cough	Initial catarrhal phase (rhinorrhea, mild cough, sneezing) of 1–2 weeks, followed by 1–6 weeks of paroxysmal coughing

Key: CNS, central nervous system; GI, gastrointestinal.

placebo group) may also help prevent colds.[10] Antibiotics, often prescribed for patients with colds, are ineffective against viral infections. The mainstay of treatment is nonpharmacologic therapy. If a patient desires to self-treat, symptom-specific therapy with single-entity products over combination products is recommended (Figure 11-1), given that symptoms appear, peak, and resolve at different times.[11] Patient education regarding the administration of intranasal (Table 11-3) and ocular (see Chapter 28) drugs is important. Not all patients should self-treat colds (see the exclusions for self-treatment listed in Figure 11-1).

Nonpharmacologic Therapy

Nondrug therapy includes maintenance of fluid intake, adequate rest, a nutritious diet as tolerated, and increased humidification with steamy showers, humidifiers, or vaporizers. Humidifiers use fans or ultrasonic technology to produce a cool mist, whereas vaporizers superheat water to produce steam. Saline nasal sprays or drops soothe irritated mucosal membranes and loosen encrusted mucus; saline gargles may ease sore throats. Simple, inexpensive foods such as tea with lemon and honey, chicken soup, and hot broths are soothing and increase fluid intake. Limited evidence suggests that chicken soup could have anti–inflammatory activity.[12] Milk products should not be withheld, because there is no evidence that milk increases cough or congestion. Medical devices, such as Vicks Breathe Right nasal strips, are marketed for temporary relief from nasal congestion and stuffiness resulting from colds and allergies. These devices lift the nares open, enlarging the anterior nasal passages. A variety of aromatic products, (Sudacare Shower Soothers Vaporizing Shower Tablets, Triaminic Flowing Vapors fan, Theraflu Vapor Patch, and Vicks VapoRub) claim to ease nasal congestion by producing soothing odors. Children should be supervised closely when using these products; aromatic oils, such as camphor and eucalyptus, are toxic if ingested. Menthol, in large quantities, can also be toxic if absorbed or ingested.

Nondrug therapy for infants includes upright positioning to enhance nasal drainage, maintaining an adequate fluid intake, increasing the humidity of inspired air, and irrigating the nose with saline drops. Also, because children typically cannot blow their own noses until about 4 years of age, carefully clearing the nasal passageways with a bulb syringe may be necessary if accumulation of mucus interferes with sleeping or eating. To use the syringe, the caregiver should squeeze the large end of the bulb, continue to squeeze the bulb while gently inserting the tip into the infant's nose, and then slowly release the squeezing pressure to draw out the fluid. After the pressure is completely released, the syringe is removed from the infant's nose and the fluid expelled from the syringe.

Pharmacologic Therapy

Decongestants

Decongestants specifically treat sinus and nasal congestion. Decongestants are adrenergic agonists (sympathomimetics). Stimulation of alpha-adrenergic receptors constricts blood vessels, thereby decreasing sinusoid vessel engorgement and mucosal edema. There are three types of decongestants. Direct-acting decongestants (phenylephrine, oxymetazoline, and tetrahydrozoline) bind directly to adrenergic receptors. Indirect-acting decongestants (ephedrine) displace norepinephrine from storage vesicles in prejunctional nerve terminals. Indirect-acting sympathomimetics have the slowest onset and longest duration of action; however, tachyphylaxis develops as stored neurotransmitter is depleted. Mixed decongestants (pseudoephedrine) have both direct and indirect activity.

The systemic nonprescription decongestants include pseudoephedrine and phenylephrine. The ophthalmic nonprescription decongestants include naphazoline, oxymetazoline, phenylephrine, and tetrahydrozoline (see Chapter 28). The intranasal nonprescription decongestants include the short-acting decongestants ephedrine, epinephrine, levmetamfetamine (L-desoxyephedrine), naphazoline, phenylephrine, propylhexedrine, and tetrahydrozoline; the intermediate-acting decongestant xylometazoline; and the long-acting decongestant oxymetazoline.

Systemic decongestants are rapidly metabolized by monoamine oxidase (MAO) and catechol-O-methyltransferase in the gastrointestinal (GI) mucosa, liver, and other tissues. Pseudoephedrine is well absorbed after oral administration; phenylephrine has a low oral bioavailability (approximately 38%). Both pseudoephedrine and phenylephrine have large volumes of distribution (2.6–5 L/kg) and short half-lives (pseudoephedrine, 6 hours; phenylephrine, 2.5 hours); peak concentrations for both drugs occur at 0.5 to 2 hours following oral administration.

Decongestants are indicated for temporary relief of nasal and eustachian tube congestion, and cough associated with postnasal drip. Nonprescription decongestants are not approved by FDA to self-treat nasal congestion associated with sinusitis.

FDA-approved dosages for decongestants are listed in Tables 11-4[13–16] and 11-5.[13] Nonprescription decongestants are marketed in a variety of dosage formulations, and many combination products are available (Table 11-6).

Adhering to FDA-approved doses of decongestant products is very important, given that acute overdose, especially in children, can be life threatening. Systemic decongestant overdoses cause excessive central nervous system (CNS) stimulation, paradoxical CNS depression, cardiovascular collapse, shock, and coma. Treatment is supportive.

Adverse effects associated with decongestants include cardiovascular stimulation (elevated blood pressure, tachycardia, palpitation, or arrhythmias) and CNS stimulation (restlessness, insomnia, anxiety, tremors, fear, or hallucinations). Children and older adults are more likely to experience adverse effects than other age groups. These adverse effects are more common with systemic decongestants, because topical decongestants are minimally absorbed. Adverse effects specifically related to topical decongestants include propellant- or vehicle-associated side effects (burning, stinging, sneezing, or local dryness) and trauma from the tip of the administration device. Rhinitis medicamentosa (RM; i.e., rebound congestion) has been associated with topical decongestants. The exact cause is unknown but short-acting products, preservative agents (e.g., benzalkonium chloride), and long duration of therapy have been suspected to contribute to the problem.[17] Currently, 3 to 5 days are the accepted duration of therapy to avoid RM. However, controversy exists and some studies showed that durations of 10 days to 8 weeks appear to be safe and do not cause RM.[17] Further investigation is needed to determine the optimal duration of treatment. Treatment of RM consists of slowly withdrawing the topical decongestant (one nostril at a time); replacing the decongestant with topical normal saline, which soothes the irritated nasal mucosa; and, if needed, using topical corticosteroids and systemic decongestants. The mucous membrane returns to normal within 1 to 2 weeks. A nonprescription kit, RhinoStat, has been advertised to assist clinicians and patients with colds with management of RM. The product creates a patient-specific mixture of the patient's topical decongestant product and a diluent; however, the kit is not FDA-approved.

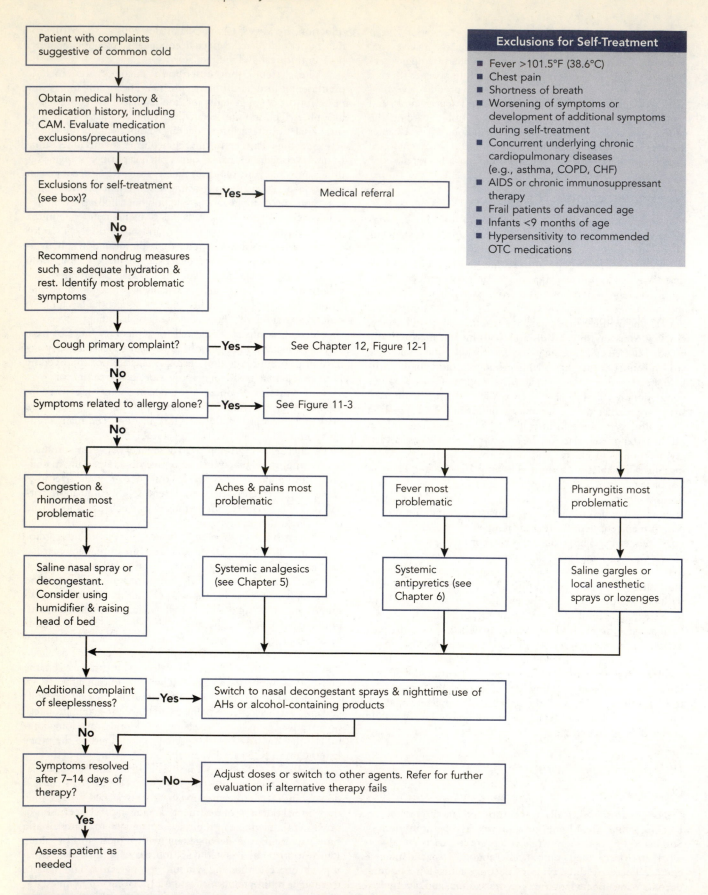

FIGURE 11-1 Self-care of the common cold. Key: AH, antihistamine; AIDS, acquired immunodeficiency syndrome; CAM, complementary and alternative medicine; CHF, congestive heart failure; COPD, chronic obstructive pulmonary disorder. (*Source:* Adapted from reference 11.)

TABLE 11-3 Administration Guidelines for Nasal Dosage Formulations

Nasal Sprays

- Gently insert the bottle tip into one nostril, as shown in drawing A.
- Keep head upright. Sniff deeply while squeezing the bottle. Repeat with other nostril.

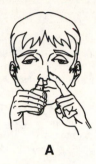

A

Pump Nasal Sprays

- Prime the pump before using it the first time. Hold the bottle with the nozzle placed between the first two fingers and the thumb placed on the bottom of the bottle.
- Tilt the head forward.
- Gently insert the nozzle tip into one nostril (see drawing B). Sniff deeply while depressing the pump once.
- Repeat with other nostril.

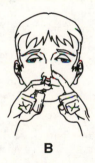

B

Nasal Inhalers

- Warm the inhaler in hand just before use.
- Gently insert the inhaler tip into one nostril, as shown in drawing C. Sniff deeply while inhaling.
- Wipe the inhaler after each use. Discard after 2–3 months even if the inhaler still smells medicinal.

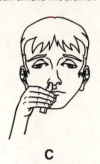

C

Nasal Drops

- Squeeze the bulb to withdraw medication from the bottle.
- Lie on bed with head tilted back and over the side of the bed, as shown in drawing D.
- Place the recommended number of drops into one nostril. Gently tilt head from side to side.
- Repeat with other nostril. Lie on bed for a couple of minutes after placing drops in the nose.
- Do not rinse the dropper.

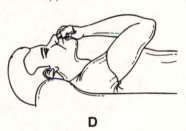

D

Note: Do not share the drug with anyone. Discard solutions if discolored or if contamination is suspected. Remove caps before use and replace tightly after each use. Do not use expired products. Clear nasal passages before administering the dose. Gently depress the other side of the nose with finger to close off the nostril not receiving the medication. Aim tip of products away from nasal septum to avoid accidental damage to the septum. Wait a few minutes after using the drug before blowing the nose.

TABLE 11-4 Dosage Guidelines for Nonprescription Systemic Nasal Decongestants

Drug	Dosage (Maximum Daily Dosage)		
	Adults/Children ≥12 Years	**Children 6 to <12 Years**	**Children 2 to <6 Years[a]**
Phenylephrine HCl	10 mg every 4 hours (60 mg)	5 mg every 4 hours (30 mg)	2.5 mg every 4 hours (15 mg)
Phenylephrine bitartrate[b]	15.6 mg every 4 hours (62.4 mg)	7.8 mg every 4 hours (31.2 mg)	Not recommended for children <6 years except under advice of PCP
Pseudoephedrine	60 mg every 4–6 hours (240 mg)	30 mg every 4–6 hours (120 mg)	15 mg every 4–6 hours (60 mg)

[a] The Consumer Health Care Products Association announced in October 2008 that manufacturers were voluntarily updating cough and cold product labels to state "do not use" in children under 4 years of age.[14] FDA announced that it would not object to the more restrictive labeling.[15] These actions have not changed the official monograph for cold, cough, allergy, bronchodilator, and antiasthmatic drug products.[16]

[b] Effervescent tablet formulation approved in 2005.

Source: Reference 13.

TABLE 11-5 Dosage Guidelines for Nonprescription Topical Nasal Decongestants

Drug	Concentration (%)	Adults/Children ≥12 Years	Children 6 to <12 Years	Children 2 to <6 Years[a]
Sprays/Drops				
Ephedrine	0.5	2–3 drops/sprays not more often than every 4 hours	1–2 drops/sprays not more often than every 4 hours	Not recommended for children <6 years except under advice of PCP
Naphazoline	0.05	1–2 drops/sprays not more often than every 6 hours	Not recommended for children <12 years except under advice of PCP	Not recommended for children <6 years except under advice of PCP
	0.025	—	1–2 drops/sprays not more often than every 6 hours	Not recommended for children <6 years except under advice of PCP
Oxymetazoline	0.05	2–3 drops/sprays not more often than every 10–12 hours (max: 2 doses/24 hours)	2–3 drops/sprays not more often than every 10–12 hours (max: 2 doses/24 hours)	Not recommended for children <6 years except under advice of PCP
	0.025	—	—	2–3 drops/sprays not more often than every 10–12 hours (max: 2 doses/24 hours)
Phenylephrine	1.0	2–3 drops/sprays not more often than every 4 hours	Not recommended for children <12 years except under advice of PCP	Not recommended for children <6 years except under advice of PCP
	0.5	2–3 drops/sprays not more often than every 4 hours	Not recommended for children <12 years except under advice of PCP	Not recommended for children <6 years except under advice of PCP
	0.25	2–3 drops/sprays not more often than every 4 hours	2–3 drops/sprays not more often than every 4 hours	Not recommended for children <6 years except under advice of PCP
	0.125	—	—	2–3 drops not more often than every 4 hours
Xylometazoline	0.1	2–3 drops/sprays not more often than every 8–10 hours	Not recommended for children <12 years except under advice of PCP	Not recommended for children <6 years except under advice of PCP
	0.05	—	2–3 drops/sprays not more often than every 8–10 hours	2–3 drops/sprays not more often than every 8–10 hours

Key: max, maximum; N/A, not applicable; PCP, primary care provider.

[a] No recommended dosages exist for children younger than 2 years, except under the advice and supervision of a PCP.

Source: Reference 13.

Decongestants interact with numerous drugs, as summarized in Table 11-7. Decongestants are contraindicated in patients receiving concomitant MAO inhibitors (MAOIs).

Decongestants may exacerbate diseases sensitive to adrenergic stimulation, such as hypertension, hyperthyroidism, diabetes mellitus, coronary heart disease, ischemic heart disease, elevated intraocular pressure, and prostatic hypertrophy. Patients with hypertension should use decongestants only with medical advice. No clear evidence exists that any one agent is safer in patients with hypertension. Products specifically marketed for patients with hypertension (e.g., Coricidin HBP) do not contain decongestants. These products usually contain a combination of ingredients that may or may not be appropriate, depending on the patients' symptoms.

Clinicians should be aware of patients wishing to purchase large quantities of pseudoephedrine that may be used illegally to produce methamphetamine. In 2005, passage of the Combat Methamphetamine Epidemic Act changed the classification of pseudoephedrine and ephedrine to "scheduled listed chemical products."[18] This change in classification allowed limits to be placed on sales of these products. All pseudoephedrine products must be kept in secure areas of the store (e.g., behind a pharmacy counter or in a locked cabinet), and quantities are now limited to 3.6 grams per day and 9 grams per month per patient.[18] The following information from each sale must be entered into a logbook (written or electronic): product name, quantity sold, patient's name and address, and time and date of sale.[18] Patients must show valid identification to purchase pseudoephedrine and then sign the logbook. Some states and corporations have enacted stricter guidelines regarding sales of pseudoephedrine. The Consumer Healthcare Products Association and the National Association of Chain Drug Stores created Meth Watch (www.methwatch.com/index.aspx) to provide assistance to clinicians.

Antihistamines

Recent reviews have shown that monotherapy with nonprescription antihistamines is not effective in reducing rhinorrhea

TABLE 11-6 Selected Products for Nasal Decongestion	
Trade Name	**Primary Ingredients**
Topical Decongestants	
Afrin Original Nasal Spray	Oxymetazoline HCl 0.05%
Mucinex Nasal Spray	Oxymetazoline HCl 0.05%
Vicks Early Defense Nasal Gel	Oxymetazoline HCl 0.05%
4-Way Fast Acting	Phenylephrine HCl 1%
Vicks Sinex Nasal Spray	Phenylephrine HCl 0.5%
Neo-Synephrine	Phenylephrine HCl 0.25%
Little Noses Decongestant Nose Drops	Phenylephrine HCl 0.125%
Otrivin Nasal Spray (Canada)	Xylometazoline 0.1%
Nasal Decongestant Inhalers	
Benzedrex Inhaler	Propylhexedrine 250 mg
Vicks Vapor Inhaler	Levmetamfetamine (l-desoxyephedrine) 50 mg
Systemic Decongestants	
Sudafed PE	Phenylephrine HCl 10 mg
Triaminic Thin Strips Cold with Stuffy Nose	Phenylephrine HCl 2.5 mg
Sudafed 24 Hour Long Acting	Pseudoephedrine HCl 240 mg
Sudafed 12-Hour	Pseudoephedrine HCl 120 mg
Sudafed Non-Drowsy Maximum Strength	Pseudoephedrine HCl 30 mg
Combination Products	
Alka-Seltzer Plus Cold and Sinus	Phenylephrine HCl 5 mg; acetaminophen 250 mg
Robitussin Head and Chest Congestion PE	Phenylephrine HCl 5 mg/5 mL; guaifenesin 100 mg/5 mL
Vicks Dayquil Liquicaps	Phenylephrine HCl 5 mg; acetaminophen 325 mg; dextromethorphan hydrobromide 10 mg
Triaminic Chest & Nasal Congestion Liquid	Phenylephrine HCl 2.5 mg/5 mL; guaifenesin 50 mg/5 mL
Aleve-D Sinus & Cold	Pseudoephedrine HCl 120 mg; naproxen sodium 220 mg
Sudafed Sinus & Cold	Pseudoephedrine HCl 30 mg; acetaminophen 325 mg
Other Products	
Ocean Premium Saline Nasal Spray	Sodium chloride 0.65%

and sneezing due to colds.[19] However, a combination of first-generation (sedating) antihistamines and decongestants showed some benefit in adults, but the significance of the data is questionable.[19] Apart from questions of efficacy, an important issue is whether potential benefits of sedating antihistamines outweigh known risks associated with these drugs. (See the discussion of antihistamines in the Allergic Rhinitis section of this chapter.)

Local Anesthetics

A variety of products containing local anesthetics (e.g., benzocaine or dyclonine hydrochloride) are available for the tempo-rary relief of sore throats (Table 11-8). Local anesthetic products may be used every 2 to 4 hours. Some products contain local antiseptics (cetylpyridinium chloride or hexylresorcinol) and/or menthol or camphor. Local antiseptics are not effective for viral infections. The clinical efficacy of menthol or camphor is not well documented. Clinicians should counsel patients with a history of allergic reactions to anesthetics to avoid products with benzocaine.

Systemic Analgesics

Systemic analgesics (e.g., aspirin, acetaminophen, ibuprofen, or naproxen) are effective for aches or fever sometimes associated with colds. Concerns that use of aspirin and acetaminophen may increase viral shedding and prolong illness have not been proven.[20] Aspirin–containing products should not be used in children with viral illnesses because of the risk of Reye's syndrome (see Chapters 5 and 6).

Antitussives and Protussives (Expectorants)

When present, cough associated with colds is usually nonproductive. The use of antitussives (codeine or dextromethorphan) have questionable efficacy in colds and are not recommended.[21] Guaifenesin, an expectorant, has not been proven effective in natural colds.[22] (See Chapter 12 for a complete discussion of these products.)

Combination Products

Decongestants and antihistamines are marketed in many combinations, including decongestant/antihistamine combinations and various combinations with analgesics, expectorants, and antitussives. Products are also marketed for daytime or night-time use. Products for nighttime use usually contain a sedating antihistamine, whereas daytime products do not. Combination products are convenient, but the convenience must be weighed against the risks of taking unnecessary drugs.

Pharmacotherapeutic Comparison

As stated earlier, evidence does not support the use of antihistamines, antitussives, and expectorants for treatment of symptoms related to colds. Local anesthetics and systemic analgesics have good evidence for treatment of pain due to sore throat or fever related to colds.

Topical decongestants are convenient dosage forms and are effective in relieving nasal congestion; however, their use is limited to 3 to 5 days owing to concerns about RM. When comparing the topical decongestants, the major differences are duration of action, dosage formulation (e.g., mist vs. spray), moisture content, and preservative content. Although many manufacturers have reformulated products with phenylephrine as a response to the pseudoephedrine regulations, controversy exists with regard to comparison of the efficacy and safety of the systemic decongestants. The efficacy of oral dosage forms of phenylephrine is questionable, whereas strong evidence supports the efficacy of oral dosage forms of pseudoephedrine.[23,24] Questions about the current approved dose of phenylephrine have also been raised, and a citizen's petition was filed with FDA in 2007 to change the recommended adult dose from 10 mg every 4 hours to 25 mg every 4 hours.[24,25] Clear evidence that oral phenylephrine is safer than pseudoephedrine has yet to be presented.[24,25]

TABLE 11-7 Decongestant and Antihistamine Drug Interactions

Drug	Effect
Decongestants	
MAOIs (phenelzine, tranylcypromine, isocarboxazid, furazolidone, procarbazine)	Increased blood pressure
Methyldopa	Increased blood pressure
TCAs (amitriptyline, nortriptyline, imipramine)	Increased blood pressure (direct-acting decongestant) Decreased decongestant activity (indirect-acting decongestants)
Antacids/alkalinizers (potassium acetate, sodium acetate, sodium bicarbonate, sodium citrate, sodium lactate, potassium citrate, citric acid)	Decreased elimination (pseudoephedrine)
Antihistamines	
CNS depressants (alcohol, sedatives)	Increased sedation (sedating antihistamines)
MAOIs (phenelzine, tranylcypromine, isocarboxazid, furazolidone, procarbazine)	Prolonged and intensified anticholinergic and CNS depressive effects (sedating antihistamine) Decreased blood pressure (dexchlorpheniramine)
Phenytoin	Decreased phenytoin elimination (chlorpheniramine)
Ketoconazole, erythromycin, cimetidine	Increased loratadine plasma concentration
Theophylline (doses >400 mg)	Increased cetirizine plasma concentration

Key: CNS, central nervous system; MAOI, monoamine oxidase inhibitor; TCA, tricyclic antidepressant.

Product Selection Guidelines

SPECIAL POPULATIONS

Drug use during pregnancy and lactation is a balance between risk and benefit. Because most colds are self-limiting, with bothersome rather than life-threatening symptoms, many clinicians recommend nondrug therapy. When drugs are considered, those with a long record of safety in animals and humans are preferred. To minimize possible adverse effects on the fetus or newborn, pregnant or nursing mothers should be advised to avoid products labeled as "extra strength," "maximum strength," or "long-acting," as well as combination products. Most of the active ingredients in FDA-approved cold medications are Pregnancy Category B or C. There is no clear association between birth defects and the use of systemic or intranasal decongestants during pregnancy.[26] However, systemic decongestants theoretically decrease fetal blood flow and should be avoided. Pseudoephedrine has also been linked to abdominal wall defects (gastroschisis) in newborns.[26] Oxymetazoline is poorly absorbed following intranasal administration and is the preferred topical decongestant during pregnancy. The American Academy of Pediatrics has found pseudoephedrine to be compatible with breast-feeding and to be the preferred decongestant.[27] Intranasal phenylephrine usually is safe in nursing mothers. Nasal preparations containing xylometazoline and naphazoline should be avoided in lactating mothers.[27] Because decongestants may decrease milk production, mothers should monitor their milk production and drink extra fluids as needed. Analgesics do not increase the risk for birth defects when taken in the first trimester, but analgesics with prostaglandin–inhibiting properties (aspirin and nonsalicylate nonsteroidal anti-inflammatory drugs [NSAIDs]) are associated with an increased risk for intracranial hemorrhage and premature closure of the patent ductus arteriosus and should be avoided during the third trimester. Aspirin should be avoided during lactation. Acetaminophen is safe for use during pregnancy and lactation. Dextromethorphan, guaifenesin, benzocaine, dyclonine, camphor, and menthol have low risks for birth defects and have been found to be compatible with breast-feeding.[27]

Using nonprescription cold products in children is controversial owing to the lack of clinical evidence of safety and efficacy in this age group. In January 2008, FDA issued a public advisory stating that nonprescription cold medications should not be given to children younger than 2 years because of the lack of efficacy and high risk for adverse events and death.[28] Manufacturers vol-

TABLE 11-8 Selected Products for Sore Throat

Trade Name	Primary Ingredients
Lozenges	
Cepacol Sore Throat Sugar Free + Coating	Benzocaine 15 mg; pectin 5 mg
Chloraseptic Sore Throat	Benzocaine 6 mg; menthol 10 mg
Halls Fruit Breezers	Pectin 7 mg
Sucrets Maximum Strength	Dyclonine HCl 3 mg
Throat Sprays	
Cepacol Dual Relief Spray	Benzocaine 5%; glycerin 33%
Chloraseptic Sore Throat	Phenol 1.4%
Oral Disintegrating Strips	
Chloraseptic Sore Throat Relief Strips	Benzocaine 3 mg; menthol 3 mg
Orajel Kids Sore Throat Relief Strips	Menthol 2 mg; pectin 30 mg

untarily recalled nonprescription products targeted at this age group. In October 2008, manufacturers decided to voluntarily update product labeling to include the following statement: "Do not use in children under four years of age."[14] Antihistamine-containing products were also relabeled with a warning against use for sedation purposes.[14] These changes were not mandated by FDA, so a mandatory recall of products with the old labeling was not issued.[15] Therefore, clinicians should be aware that pharmacy shelves may contain pediatric products that have the same strength and dosage form but bear different labeling for minimum age of use. FDA continues to monitor and review the use of nonprescription cold medications in children between the ages of 2 and 11 years.[15] Clinicians should emphasize nonprescription measures in children and, if pharmacotherapy is deemed necessary, parents should follow dosing instructions carefully and avoid combination products to avoid overdosage.

PATIENT FACTORS

As discussed earlier, it may be difficult to differentiate cold symptoms from some chronic disorders (Table 11-2). If a chronic condition is suspected or if duration of symptoms is longer than 7 to 14 days, patients should not self-treat. Patients with chronic conditions exacerbated by, or those overly sensitive to, adrenergic stimulation should avoid decongestants. Clinicians should educate patients who participate in organized sports that oral decongestants are considered "doping" products and should be used with caution.

PATIENT PREFERENCES

Oral disintegrating strips, soft chews, and nasal drug delivery forms may be preferred for patients who have difficulty swallowing or when access to water is not convenient. However, nasal delivery forms may be difficult to use in patients with severe arthritis or coordination problems.

For patients who prefer a nasal delivery form, each form has distinct advantages and disadvantages. Nasal sprays are simple to use, cover a large surface area, are relatively inexpensive, and have a fast onset of action. The disadvantages include imprecise dosage, a tendency for the tip to become clogged with repeated use, and a high risk of contamination from aspiration of nasal mucus into the bottle. Metered pump sprays deliver a more precise dose. Nasal drops are preferred for small children but are awkward to use, cover a limited surface area, and pass easily into the larynx. There is also a high risk of contamination because of the tendency to touch the dropper to the nose during administration. Nasal inhalers are small and unobtrusive, but they require an unobstructed airway and sufficient airflow to distribute the drug to the nasal mucosa. Nasal inhalers lose efficacy after 2 to 3 months even when tightly capped because of dissipation of the active ingredient. Nasal polyps, enlarged turbinates, and abnormalities such as septal deviation may reduce the efficacy of topical dosage forms.

Complementary and Alternative Therapies

Numerous complementary therapies are marketed for the treatment of colds (Table 11-9; see also Chapter 54).[29–31] Some of the most popular therapies are echinacea, high–dose vitamin C, and zinc lozenges. In addition to the more traditional complementary therapies for colds, new products that claim to help strengthen the immune system are gaining popularity.

Conflicting evidence exists regarding the ability of echinacea to significantly decrease the incidence, severity, or duration of colds (see Chapter 54).

TABLE 11-9 Complementary Therapies for Colds and Allergies

Agent	Risks	Effectiveness
Botanical Natural Products (Scientific Name)		
Butterbur (*Petasites hybridus*)	Drowsiness, GI disturbances, long-term use may cause hepatotoxicity and renal toxicity due to PAs	Some evidence of anti-inflammatory/antihistaminic effects in allergic rhinitis; safety not established with use >2 weeks
Echinacea (*Echinacea angustifolia, Echinacea pallida, Echinacea purpurea*)	Hepatotoxicity; metabolic disturbances; immuno-suppression (with prolonged use); aggravation of autoimmune disorders (e.g., multiple sclerosis, rheumatoid arthritis, lupus)	Controversial evidence of immunostimulant effects in prevention or treatment of colds and influenza
English Ivy (*Hedera helix*)	Nausea/vomiting, uterine contractions, skin irritation	Some evidence for use in treating coughs associated with colds
Ephedra [ma huang] (*Ephedra sinica*)	Tachycardia, hypertension, heart attack, stroke, seizure	Effective decongestant
Goldenseal (*Hydrastis canadensis*)	Potentially toxic, especially in patients with gluocose-6-dehydrogenase deficiency	Some evidence of anti-inflammatory effects of active ingredient berberine for treatment of pulmonary inflammation
Indian echinacea [active ingredient in Kan Jang] (*Andrographis paniculata*)	Gall bladder contraction; aggravation of auto-immune disorders (e.g., multiple sclerosis, rheumatoid arthritis, lupus)	Some evidence for treating and preventing colds
North American ginseng [active ingredient in Cold FX] (*Panax quinquefolium*)	Insomnia, restlessness, hot flashes	Some evidence for preventing and reducing severity/duration of colds

Key: GI, gastrointestinal; PA, pyrrolizidine alkaloid.

High local concentrations of zinc ions purportedly block the adhesion of human rhinovirus to the nasal epithelium and are also thought to inhibit viral replication by disrupting viral capsid formation. However, in vitro studies have shown only a modest antiviral effect. Formulations include tablets, capsules, chewing gums, lozenges, and various nasal gels, sprays, and swabs. The effectiveness of zinc has been highly debated. Clinical trials that concluded zinc decreased severity and/or duration of symptoms in adults used a rigorous administration schedule that started within 24 to 48 hours of symptom onset (i.e., one lozenge every 2 hours or one spray in each nostril every 4 hours for the duration of the cold).[29] GI side effects (e.g., nausea, upset stomach, and bitter taste) are common with the lozenges. Adverse effects related to intranasal zinc include headache, nasal tenderness, dry mouth, nasal stinging or burning, and anosmia (loss of smell).[32]

A recent meta-analysis of 14 trials concluded that zinc lozenges were not effective in reducing cold symptoms or duration of the cold.[33] The analysis also concluded that intranasal zinc had questionable efficacy and called for further studies.[33]

The efficacy and safety of high-dose (e.g., ≥2 g/day) vitamin C (ascorbic acid) supplementation for prophylaxis and treatment of colds has been debated for more than 60 years. A recent analysis of 30 trials showed that, although high-dose vitamin C does not appear to prevent colds in the general population, it did reduce the duration by 8% in adults and 13.6% in children.[34] In contrast, high-dose vitamin C prophylaxis was effective in preventing colds in a subgroup of patients subjected to severe physical stress (e.g., marathon runners).[34] Using vitamin C as treatment after the onset of a cold was not effective at reducing severity or duration of symptoms.[34] The clinical significance and risk–benefit ratio of these results are debatable. Doses of 4 g/day or greater are associated with diarrhea and other GI symptoms and, therefore, should not be recommended.

Several new products that claim to strengthen the immune system are available. Larch arabinogalactan, traditionally used as a food additive, is now marketed as Natrol My Defense Immune Support. This product is thought to have probiotic properties and to increase the activity of natural killer cells. Airborne effer-

vescent tablets are a combination of 17 active ingredients including high doses of vitamins A and C; herbs (echinacea, ginger, and Chinese vitex); and amino acids (glutamine and lysine). The marketing for Airborne is unique. Patients are urged to take the product before entering crowded environments such as airplanes, offices, and classrooms. Despite the popularity of these new products, their safety and efficacy have not been proven.

Assessment of Colds: A Case-Based Approach

After asking questions about the patient's symptoms, medical history, medication use (current and past), efficacy of past self-treatment of colds, the practitioner should conduct a brief physical assessment (Table 11-10). If the assessment and patient's answers do not reveal exclusions for self-treatment, the practitioner should recommend medications that target the patient's most troublesome symptoms.

Case 11-1 is an example of assessment of patients with a cold.

TABLE 11-10 Physical Assessment of Patient Presenting with Cold Symptoms

1. Observe patient (look and listen for signs of chronic conditions, such as red, watery eyes; wheezing; productive cough; barrel chest; poorly perfused areas; enlarged lymph nodes; rash).

If equipment and privacy allow, conduct the following:

2. Obtain vitals (temperature, respiratory rate, pulse, and blood pressure).
3. Palpate sinuses and neck, and observe any pain/tenderness.
4. Visually examine throat for redness or exudates. If bacterial pharyngitis suspected, run rapid strep test.
5. Auscultate chest to detect wheezing, crackles, and rapid or irregular heartbeat.

CASE 11-1

Relevant Evaluation Criteria	Scenario/Model Outcome
Information Gathering	
1. Gather essential information about the patient's symptoms, including:	
a. description of symptom(s) (i.e., nature, onset, duration, severity, associated symptoms)	Patient complains of severe congestion and rhinorrhea for 3 days. He also has a headache and is tired.
b. description of any factors that seem to precipitate, exacerbate, and/or relieve the patient's symptom(s)	Symptoms appeared 3 days ago after a trip to Chicago. Congestion and headache are worse in the morning. No symptom relief has been noted.
c. description of the patient's efforts to relieve the symptoms	Patient has tried hot showers, warm compresses, and acetaminophen 500 mg this morning for the headache.
2. Gather essential patient history information:	
a. patient's identity	John Roberts
b. patient's age, sex, height, and weight	41-year-old male, 5 ft 8 in, 225 lb

CASE 1 1 - 1 *(continued)*

Relevant Evaluation Criteria	Scenario/Model Outcome
c. patient's occupation	Business executive
d. patient's dietary habits	He eats healthy, low-carbohydrate, low-fat diet when home but eats fast food when traveling.
e. patient's sleep habits	Erratic due to frequent travel
f. concurrent medical conditions, prescription and nonprescription medications, and dietary supplements	Lisinopril 40 mg 1 tablet every day, metformin 1000 mg twice a day, Centrum multivitamin once a day, echinacea 1 tablet twice a day
g. allergies	NKA
h. history of other adverse reactions to medications	None
i. other (describe) _____	Patient's temperature at the pharmacy is 100°F (37.8°C), and blood pressure is 125/80 mm Hg. His fasting blood glucose was 117 mg/dL at home.

Assessment and Triage

3. Differentiate the patient's signs/symptoms and correctly identify the patient's primary problem(s) (see Table 11-2).	The recent onset and short duration of the patient's congestion and lack of high fever are indicative of a cold.
4. Identify exclusions for self-treatment (see Figure 11-1).	None
5. Formulate a comprehensive list of therapeutic alternatives for the primary problem to determine if triage to a medical practitioner is required, and share this information with the patient.	Options include: (1) Recommend separate OTC products for each symptom: nasal saline or decongestant (topical or systemic) for congestion; analgesic for headache; antihistamine for rhinorrhea, or because the patient has multiple symptoms, a combination product may be appropriate. (2) Recommend that John see his PCP for further evaluation and treatment. (3) Recommend self-care until John can consult his PCP. (4) Take no action.

Plan

6. Select an optimal therapeutic alternative to address the patient's problem, taking into account patient preferences.	Self-care with a nonprescription product for congestion and headache is appropriate. Diabetes is not an exclusion for self-treatment, but the patient should check his blood glucose more frequently and see his PCP if his blood glucose becomes uncontrolled. John prefers nasal sprays.
7. Describe the recommended therapeutic approach to the patient.	For your congestion, use a topical decongestant such as oxymetazoline HCl 0.05%. Your headache is most likely related to the congestion and will resolve when the congestion does. If needed, continue to use acetaminophen 500 mg, 1–2 tablets every 4–6 hours for headache and fever. Do not take more than 8 tablets per day.
8. Explain to the patient the rationale for selecting the recommended therapeutic approach from the considered therapeutic alternatives.	Because you have diabetes, topical decongestants have less systemic absorption and, therefore, will not raise your blood pressure or blood glucose as much.

Patient Education

9. When recommending self-care with non-prescription medications and/or nondrug therapy, convey accurate information to the patient:	
a. appropriate dose and frequency of administration	Use 2–3 sprays of oxymetazoline in each nostril every 10–12 hours.
b. maximum number of days the therapy should be employed	Do not use the nasal spray longer than 5 days.
c. product administration procedures	See Table 11-3.
d. expected time to onset of relief	Nasal congestion should significantly diminish in 10 minutes, and relief should last 10–12 hours after each administration.

CASE 11-1 *(continued)*

Relevant Evaluation Criteria	Scenario/Model Outcome
e. degree of relief that can be reasonably expected	Nasal congestion will be temporarily relieved but may persist for 7–14 days.
f. most common side effects	Nasal stinging or burning, sneezing, dryness
g. side effects that warrant medical intervention should they occur	Rebound congestion if oxymetazoline is used longer than 5 days; increased heart rate, blood pressure, or blood glucose
h. patient options in the event that condition worsens or persists	Your primary care provider should be consulted if congestion, headache, or fever worsens with treatment or lasts longer than 7–14 days.
i. product storage requirements	Store at room temperature with the cap tightly closed.
j. specific nondrug measures	Dress normally, maintain clear fluids and healthy diet, and rest as much as possible. Wash your hands frequently, and clean surfaces with antiviral products, such as Lysol, to prevent spreading your cold to others.
10. Solicit follow-up questions from patient.	Should I increase the dose of my echinacea supplement while I am sick?
11. Answer patient's questions.	No. Increasing the dose of echinacea will not help you get well and will increase your risk of suffering unwanted adverse effects.

Key: NKA, no known allergies; OTC, over-the-counter; PCP, primary care provider.

Patient Counseling for Colds

Nondrug measures may be effective in relieving the discomfort of cold symptoms. The practitioner should explain the appropriate nondrug measures for the patient's particular symptoms. For patients who prefer to self-medicate, the purpose of each medication should be described, and the patient should be counseled to use only medications that target their specific symptoms. Patients need an explanation of possible side effects, drug interactions, and precautions or warnings. Finally, the practitioner should explain the signs and symptoms that indicate the disorder is worsening and that medical care should be sought. (See the box Patient Education for Colds.)

PATIENT EDUCATION FOR Colds

The objectives of self-treatment are to (1) reduce symptoms, (2) improve functioning and the sense of well-being, and (3) prevent the spread of the disease. For most patients, carefully following product instructions and the self-care measures listed here will help ensure optimal therapeutic outcomes.

Nondrug Measures

- To prevent spreading a cold to others, follow these steps:
  — Frequently wash your hands with soap for at least 15 seconds.
  — Use facial tissues to cover your mouth and nose when coughing or sneezing, and then promptly throw the tissues away.
  — Use antiviral products, such as Lysol to clean surfaces (e.g., door knobs or telephones) that you may have touched.
- The following measures may provide relief or speed up recovery from a cold:
  — Getting adequate rest may help you recover more quickly.
  — Drinking more fluids and using a humidifier or vaporizer may loosen mucus and promote sinus drainage.
  — Sucking on hard candy, gargling with salt water (1 teaspoon of salt per 8 ounces of warm water), or drinking fruit juices or hot tea with lemon may soothe a sore throat.

Nonprescription Medications

- Ask a clinician to help you select medications that target the most bothersome symptoms.

Sore Throat and Cough

- Sore throat may be treated with anesthetic products and/or systemic pain relievers:
  — Allow lozenges, troches, and orally disintegrating strips to dissolve slowly in the mouth; do not chew or bite these products.
  — Benzocaine and dyclonine may numb the mouth and tongue. If these effects occur, do not eat or drink until they go away.
- Cough related to a runny nose (postnasal drip) may be treated with a sedating antihistamine and decongestant combination.

Rhinorrhea (Runny Nose) and Sneezing

- See the box Patient Education for Allergic Rhinitis for treatment of rhinorrhea (runny nose) and sneezing.

Nasal Congestion

- Nasal congestion may be treated with topical or systemic decongestants, which constrict blood vessels in the nose to reduce congestion.
  — Systemic decongestants include pseudoephedrine and phenylephrine. Dosages are listed in Table 11-4.
  — Topical decongestants include ephedrine, naphazoline, oxymetazoline, phenylephrine, and xylometazoline. Dosages are listed in Table 11-5.

- Decongestants have the following side effects:
  - The most common side effects caused by systemic decongestants are cardiovascular stimulation (i.e., elevated blood pressure, rapid heart rate, palpitations, arrhythmias) and central nervous system stimulation (i.e., restlessness, insomnia, anxiety, tremors, fear, hallucinations).
  - Topical decongestants may cause any of the side effects listed for systemic decongestants; however, less of the topical medication gets into the body, so side effects are less common.
  - Topical decongestants may irritate the nose, or the bottle tip can injure the nose if used forcefully.
  - Topical decongestants may cause rebound congestion if used longer than 3–5 days.
- Note the following precautions for use of decongestants in persons with other medical conditions:
  - Persons with high blood pressure should use decongestants only with medical advice.
  - Persons with thyroid disorders, heart disease, glaucoma, or an enlarged prostate may experience worsening symptoms of their underlying disease if they take decongestants.
  - Persons with diabetes may need to adjust their dose of insulin if they take decongestants.
  - Blood glucose concentrations need to be monitored closely.
- Note the following drug interactions for decongestants:
  - Persons taking MAOIs (e.g., tranylcypromine or phenelzine), the antibacterial furazolidone, and the anticancer drug procarbazine, should not take decongestants.

- Persons taking rauwolfia alkaloids, methyldopa, and tricyclic antidepressants should use decongestants with caution. These medications interact with decongestants to increase blood pressure, sometimes to the point of causing strokes. Tricyclic antidepressants may increase or decrease blood pressure, depending on the specific decongestant.
- Large amounts of some antacids or medicines that increase pH decrease the elimination of pseudoephedrine.

⚠ Seek medical attention for the following situations:
  - Sore throat persists more than several days, is severe, or is associated with persistent fever, headache, or nausea or vomiting.
  - Cough does not improve within 7–14 days.
  - Symptoms worsen while nonprescription medications are being taken.
  - Signs and symptoms of bacterial infections develop (e.g., thick nasal or respiratory secretions that are not clear; temperature higher than 101.5°F [38.6°C]; shortness of breath; chest congestion; wheezing, rash, or significant ear pain).
  - Store all medications according to the manufacturer's recommendations. Do not use expired medications.

Evaluation of Patient Outcomes for Colds

Given that most colds are self-limiting, symptoms will usually resolve on their own in 7 to 14 days. For the majority of patients, targeted nonprescription therapy will relieve their cold symptoms. Patients should be monitored for worsening symptoms and progression of complications by measuring their temperature, assessing nasal secretions, assessing respirations for wheezing or shortness of breath, identifying productive cough, and asking about facial or neck pain. If complications are suspected, medical referral is necessary. Referral to a primary care provider (PCP) is also required for patients who meet the exclusions for self-treatment in Figure 11-1 or the warnings listed in the box Patient Education for Colds. Follow-up usually is not necessary for patients with uncomplicated colds, but a clinician may deem telephone follow-up in 7 to 14 days to be appropriate.

ALLERGIC RHINITIS

Allergic rhinitis, a systemic disease with prominent nasal symptoms, is a worldwide problem that affects adults and children. An estimated 20% of adults and 40% of children in the United States have this disease, and the number of newly diagnosed cases in the country has been steadily increasing over the past 3 decades.[35] Approximately 9% of adults and 10% of children in the United States were newly diagnosed with allergic rhinitis in 2005–2006.[36] Annual direct costs (e.g., medications and office visits)

and indirect costs (e.g., lost school and work days) are estimated to be $2 to $5 billion.[37] Impaired quality of life creates additional significant, but yet to be quantified, intangible costs. An estimated $1 billion is spent annually on nonprescription allergy/sinus medications in the U.S.[2]

Symptoms of allergic rhinitis generally begin after the second year of life, and the disease is prevalent in children and adults ages 18 to 64 years.[38] After age 65, the number of cases decreases. The prevalence of allergic rhinitis is higher in the southern United States.[38]

Pathophysiology of Allergic Rhinitis

Allergic rhinitis affects the upper respiratory system. (The section Colds provides a detailed discussion of the respiratory anatomy and physiology.) Risk factors for developing allergic rhinitis include family history of atopy (allergic disorders) in one or both parents, elevated serum IgE greater than 100 IU/mL before age 6, higher socioeconomic class, and positive reaction to allergy skin tests.[39] Allergic rhinitis is triggered by indoor and outdoor environmental allergens. Common outdoor aeroallergens (airborne environmental allergens) include pollen and mold spores. Other non-airborne pollens have also been implicated. Pollutants (e.g., ozone and diesel exhaust particles) are considered environmental triggers and are becoming more of a concern in highly populated areas. Common indoor aeroallergens include house dust mites, cockroaches, mold spores, cigarette smoke, and pet dander. Occupational aeroallergens include the following: wool dust; latex; resins; biologic enzymes; organic dusts (e.g., flour); and various chemicals (e.g., isocyanate and glutaraldehyde).

The pathogenesis of allergic rhinitis is complex, involving numerous cells and mediators, and consists of four phases.[40] First is the sensitization phase, which occurs on initial allergen exposure. The allergen stimulates beta-lymphocyte–mediated IgE production. Second is the early phase, occurring within minutes of subsequent allergen exposure. The early phase consists of rapid release of preformed mast cell mediators (e.g., histamine and proteases), as well as the production of additional mediators (e.g., prostaglandins, kinins, leukotrienes, neuropeptides). Figure 11-2 shows mediator-specific symptoms. The third phase is cellular recruitment. Circulating leukocytes, especially eosinophils, are attracted to the nasal mucosa and release more inflammatory mediators. Fourth is the late phase, which begins 2 to 4 hours after allergen exposure; symptoms include mucus hypersecretion secondary to submucosal gland hypertrophy and congestion. Continued persistent inflammation "primes" the tissue, resulting in a lower threshold for allergic- and nonallergic-mediated (e.g., cold air and strong odors) triggers.

Clinical Presentation of Allergic Rhinitis

Allergic rhinitis has been classified as seasonal allergic rhinitis ("hay fever") and perennial allergic rhinitis. New classifications, intermittent allergic rhinitis (IAR) and persistent allergic rhinitis (PER), were proposed in the late 1990s and are now the more accepted terminology.[39] Classification depends on the timing and duration of symptoms. Symptoms can be further classified as mild or moderate-to-severe (Table 11-11).[39] Symptoms of allergic rhinitis and common physical findings in these patients are summarized in Table 11-12[39,41] and can be used to differentiate allergic from nonallergic rhinitis. Table 11-13 lists causes of nonallergic rhinitis.[39] Systemic symptoms include fatigue, irritability, malaise, and cognitive impairment.

Acute complications of allergic rhinitis include sinusitis and otitis media with effusion. Chronic complications include nasal polyps, sleep apnea, and hyposmia (diminished sense of smell).[39,42] Allergic rhinitis and asthma share a common pathology, and allergic rhinitis has been implicated in the development of asthma and exacerbations of preexisting asthma in children and adults. Depression, anxiety, delayed speech development, and facial or dental abnormalities also have been linked to allergic rhinitis.[39,42]

Treatment of Allergic Rhinitis
Treatment Goals

Allergic rhinitis cannot be cured. The goals of therapy are to reduce symptoms and improve the patient's functional status and sense of well-being. Treatment is individualized to provide optimal symptomatic relief and control of symptoms.

General Treatment Approach

Allergic rhinitis is treated in three steps: allergen avoidance, pharmacotherapy, and immunotherapy.[39,40] Clinicians should maximize each step before going on to the next intervention. Patient education is an important part of all three steps, especially regarding the administration of nonprescription medications (see Table 11-3 for intranasal preparations and Chapter 28 for ocular drugs). The algorithm in Figure 11-3 outlines the self-treatment of IAR and PER and lists exclusions for self-treatment.[39] Because allergen avoidance is usually not sufficient to provide complete relief of allergic rhinitis, targeted therapy with single-entity drugs usually is initiated. Nonprescription therapy with antihistamines or decongestants usually will treat most symptoms. Drugs with different mechanisms of action or delivery systems may be added if

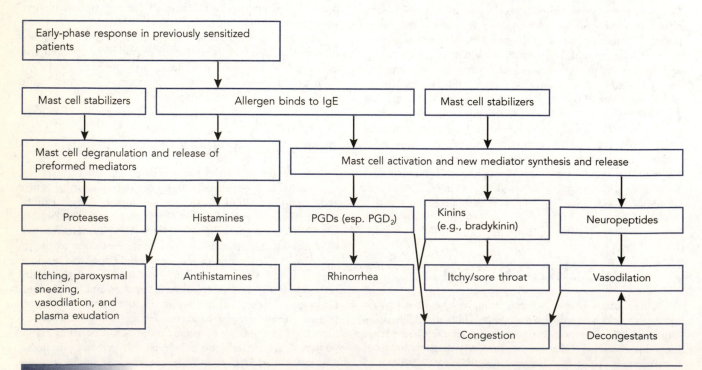

FIGURE 11-2 Mediator-specific symptoms and targeted drug therapy. Key: Ig, immunoglobulin; PGD, prostaglandin. (*Source:* Reference 40.)

TABLE 11-11 Classification of Allergic Rhinitis	
Duration	**Severity**
Intermittent	**Mild**
Symptoms occur ≤4 days per week OR ≤4 weeks	Symptoms do not impair sleep or daily activities[a]; no troublesome symptoms
	Moderate-to-Severe
	One or more of the following occurs: impairment of sleep; impairment of daily activities[a]; troublesome symptoms
Persistent	**Mild**
Symptoms occur >4 days per week AND >4 weeks	Symptoms do not impair sleep or daily activities[a]; no troublesome symptoms
	Moderate-to-Severe
	One or more of the following occurs: impairment of sleep; impairment of daily activities[a]; troublesome symptoms

[a] Daily activities include work, school, sports, and leisure.
Source: Reference 39.

the single-drug therapy does not provide adequate relief, or if the symptoms are already moderately severe, particularly intense, or long lasting.

Nonpharmacologic Therapy

Allergen avoidance is the primary nonpharmacologic measure for allergic rhinitis. Avoidance strategies depend on the specific allergen. House-dust mites (*Dermatophagoides* spp.), found in all but the driest regions of the United States, thrive in warm, humid household environments. The main allergen is a fecal glycoprotein, but other mite proteins and proteases are also allergenic. Avoidance strategies, targeted at reducing the mite population, include lowering the household humidity to less than 40%, application of acaricides, and reduction of mite-harboring dust by removing carpets, upholstered furniture, stuffed animals, and bookshelves from the patient's bedroom and other areas of the house if possible. Mite populations in bedding are reduced by encasing the mattress, box springs, and pillows with mite-impermeable materials. Bedding that cannot be encased should be washed at least weekly in hot (130°F [54.4°C]) water. Bedding that cannot be encased or laundered should be discarded.

Outdoor mold spores are prevalent in late summer and fall, especially on calm, clear, dry days. *Alternaria* and *Cladosporium* are common outdoor mold allergens; *Penicillium* and *Aspergillus* are

TABLE 11-12 Differentiation of Allergic Rhinitis from Nonallergic Rhinitis		
Symptoms/Findings	**Allergic Rhinitis**	**Nonallergic Rhinitis**[a]
Symptom presentation	Bilateral symptoms; worse upon awakening, improves during the day, then may worsen at night	Unilateral symptoms common but can be bilateral; constant day and night
Sneezing	Frequent, paroxysmal	Little or none
Rhinorrhea	Anterior, watery	Posterior, watery or thick and/or mucopurulent (associated with an infection)
Pruritus (itching) of eyes, nose, and/or palate	Frequent	Not present
Nasal obstruction	Variable	Usually present and often severe
Conjunctivitis (red, irritated eyes with prominent conjunctival blood vessels)	Frequent	Not present
Pain	Not present	Variable
Anosmia	Rare	Frequent
Epistaxis	Rare	Recurrent
Facial features	"Allergic shiners" (periorbital darkening secondary to venous congestion) "Dennie's lines" (wrinkles beneath the lower eyelids) "Allergic crease" (horizontal crease just about bulbar portion of the nose secondary to the "allergic salute") "Allergic salute" (patient will rub the tip of the nose upward with the palm of the hand) "Allergic gape" (open-mouth breathing secondary to nasal obstruction) Nonexudative cobblestone appearance of posterior oropharynx	Nasal polyps Nasal septal deviation Enlarged tonsils and/or adenoids

[a] Depending on the cause of the nonallergic rhinitis, not all symptoms may be exhibited.
Source: References 39 and 41.

TABLE 11-13 Causes of Nonallergic Rhinitis

Hormonal
Pregnancy, puberty, thyroid disorders

Structural
Septal deviation, adenoid hypertrophy

Drug-Induced
Cocaine, beta blockers, ACEIs, chlorpromazine, clonidine, reserpine, hydralazine, oral contraceptives, aspirin or other NSAIDs, or overuse of topical decongestants

Systemic Inflammatory
Vasomotor, eosinophilic nonallergic rhinitis (NARES)

Lesions
Nasal polyps, neoplasms

Traumatic
Recent facial or head trauma

Key: ACEI, angiotensin-converting enzyme inhibitor; NSAID, nonsteroidal anti-inflammatory drug.
Source: Reference 39.

common indoor molds. Avoiding activities that disturb decaying plant material (e.g., raking leaves) lessens exposure to outdoor mold. Indoor mold exposure is minimized by lowering household humidity, removing houseplants, venting food preparation areas and bathrooms, repairing damp basements or crawl spaces, and frequently applying fungicide to obviously moldy areas.

Cat-derived allergens (Fel d1; proteins secreted through sebaceous glands in the skin) are small and light, and stay airborne for several hours. Cat allergens can be found in the house months after the cat is removed. Although unproven, weekly cat baths may reduce the allergen load.

Cockroaches are major urban allergens. To eliminate cockroaches, patients should be encouraged to keep areas clean, keep food stored tightly sealed, and treat infested areas with baits or pesticides. Infestations in multiple-family dwellings are difficult to eliminate.

Pollutants (e.g., ozone and diesel fumes) are an additional concern in urban environments. Pollutants such as diesel exhaust particles are especially irritating to the respiratory tract and have been shown to increase the severity of allergic rhinitis.[41] Patients whose allergies are triggered by air pollutants should be aware of the air quality index (AQI; a measure of five major air pollutants per 24 hours) and plan outdoor activities when the AQI is low.

Trees pollinate in March and April, grasses in May and June, and ragweed from mid-August to the first fall frost. Pollen counts (the number of pollen grains per cubic meter per 24 hours) help patients plan outdoor activities. Most patients are symptomatic when pollen counts are very high, and only very sensitive patients have symptoms when pollen counts are low. Pollen counts are highest early in the morning and in the evening, and lowest after rainstorms clear the air. Avoiding outdoor activities when pollen counts are high and closing house and car windows reduce pollen exposure.

Ventilation systems with high-efficiency particulate air (HEPA) filters remove pollen, mold spores, and cat allergens from household air but not fecal particles from house-dust mites, which settle to the floor too quickly to be filtered. HEPA filtration systems are expensive and not effective for all patients. Patients should be encouraged to rent a HEPA filtration device before investing in freestanding or permanently installed systems. HEPA filters are also found in some vacuum cleaners. Weekly vacuuming of carpets, drapes, and upholstery with a HEPA filter-equipped vacuum cleaner may help reduce household allergens, including dust mites.[43]

Nasal wetting agents (e.g., saline, propylene, and polyethylene glycol sprays or gels) or nasal irrigation with warm saline (isotonic or hypertonic) delivered via a syringe or neti pot may relieve nasal mucosal irritation and dryness, thus decreasing nasal stuffiness, rhinorrhea, and sneezing. This process also aids in the removal of dried, encrusted, or thick mucus from the nose. No significant side effects have been noted with nasal wetting agents. Mild stinging or burning has been noted with saline irrigation.

Pharmacologic Therapy

Pharmacotherapy is symptom-specific and depends on the severity of the illness. There is no single ideal medication, and combination drug regimens are commonly used. Nonprescription options include ocular and oral antihistamines, topical and oral decongestants, and mast cell stabilizers. Antihistamines and mast cell stabilizers should be used regularly rather than episodically. Patients should start taking antihistamines and/or mast cell stabilizers at least 1 week before symptoms typically appear or as soon as possible before known allergen exposures. Length of therapy with antihistamines and mast cell stabilizers should be individualized according to duration and severity of symptoms, pattern of allergen exposure (episodic or continuous), and geographical location.

Antihistamines

Antihistamines are one of the top choices for treating allergic rhinitis. The use of antihistamines in the United States has increased 35% since 1995.[44] These drugs are classified as sedating (first-generation, nonselective) or nonsedating (second-generation, peripherally selective). The role of sedating antihistamines in treating allergic rhinitis is controversial. Sedating antihistamines are effective, readily available without a prescription, and relatively inexpensive. However, these antihistamines expose patients to risks of sedation, impaired performance, and anticholinergic effects, and should be used with caution.

Antihistamines compete with histamine at central and peripheral histamine$_1$-receptor sites, preventing the histamine–receptor interaction and subsequent mediator release. In addition, second-generation antihistamines inhibit the release of mast cell mediators and may decrease cellular recruitment.

Differences among antihistamines relate to the rapidity and degree to which they penetrate the blood–brain barrier as well as to their receptor specificity. Sedating antihistamines are highly lipophilic molecules that readily cross the blood–brain barrier. Nonsedating antihistamines, large protein-bound lipophobic molecules with charged side chains, do not readily cross the blood-brain barrier. Both types of antihistamines are highly selective for histamine$_1$ receptors but have little effect on histamine$_2$ or histamine$_3$ receptors. The sedating antihistamines activate 5-hydroxytryptamine (serotonin) and alpha–adrenergic receptors, and block cholinergic receptors.

Each antihistamine chemical class (Table 11-14) differs slightly in terms of its activity and side effect profile.[45,46]

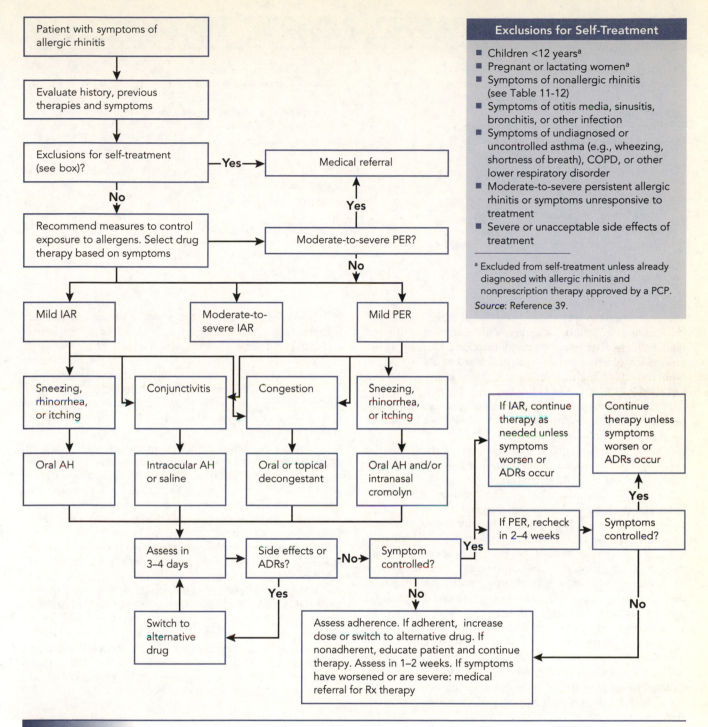

FIGURE 11-3 Self-care of allergic rhinitis. Key: ADR, adverse drug reaction; AH, antihistamine; IAR, intermittent allergic rhinitis; PER, persistent allergic rhinitis; Rx, prescription.

Most sedating antihistamines are well absorbed after oral administration with time to peak plasma concentrations in the 1.5- to 3-hour range. Protein binding is in the range of 78% to 99%, and sedating antihistamines undergo significant first-pass metabolism through the cytochrome P450 system. Half-lives range from approximately 9 hours for diphenhydramine to 28 hours for chlorpheniramine.

Loratadine is rapidly absorbed after oral administration and hepatically metabolized to descarboethoxyloratadine, an active metabolite. Time to peak concentrations for loratadine and descarboethoxyloratadine are 1.3 and 2.5 hours, respectively. The half-lives of loratadine and descarboethoxyloratadine are 8.4 and 28 hours, respectively. Loratadine and its metabolites are eliminated renally and in the feces.

Cetirizine is rapidly absorbed after oral administration and reaches peak concentration in 1 to 2 hours with a half-life of 8.3 hours. Cetirizine is highly protein bound (93%), hepatically metabolized, and primarily eliminated in the urine.

TABLE 11-14 Antihistamine Classes

Alkylamines
  Brompheniramine, chlorpheniramine, dexbrompheniramine,
  dexchlorpheniramine, triprolidine, pheniramine
	Most potent antihistamines, sedating, higher risk of paradoxical CNS
	stimulation compared with other classes

Ethanolamines Clemastine, diphenhydramine, doxylamine	Strong anticholinergic effects, highly sedating, large doses cause seizures and arrhythmias
Ethylenediamines Pyrilamine, tripelennamine, thonzylamine	Weak CNS effects, increased GI effects
Phenothiazines Promethazine	Blocks alpha-adrenergic receptors, more likely to cause hypotension, strong anticholinergic effects, highly sedating
Piperidines Fexofenadine, loratadine, phenindamine	Nonsedating
Piperazines Cetirizine, chlorcyclizine, levocetirizine, meclizine	Minimally to moderately sedating

Source: References 45 and 46.

Antihistamines are indicated for relief of symptoms of allergic rhinitis (e.g., itching, sneezing, and rhinorrhea) and other types of immediate hypersensitivity reactions. FDA-approved dosages for systemic antihistamines are listed in Table 11-15.[13] Nonprescription antihistamines are marketed as immediate- and sustained-release tablets and capsules, chewable tablets, oral disintegrating tablets and strips, solutions, and syrups. Alcohol-, sucrose-, and dye-free formulations are available. (See Chapter 28 for ocular antihistamines.)

Sedating antihistamine overdoses are characterized by excessive histamine$_1$-receptor and cholinergic-receptor blockade, and by alpha-adrenergic and serotonergic activity.[45] Overdoses also cause excessive blockade of fast sodium channels and potassium channels, leading to cardiac symptoms.[45] CNS symptoms (toxic psychosis, hallucinations, agitation, lethargy, tremor, insomnia, or tonic-clonic seizures) predominate, with children being more sensitive to the CNS excitatory effects and adults more likely to experience CNS depression.[45] Peripheral symptoms include tachycardia, hyperpyrexia, mydriasis, vasodilation, decreased exocrine secretion, urinary retention, decreased GI motility, dystonic reactions, rhabdomyolysis, and cardiac tachyarrhythmias and conduction abnormalities, including torsades de pointes (a dysrhythmia). Overdoses of nonsedating antihistamines are characterized by headache, somnolence, and tachycardia. Extrapyramidal signs have been reported in children. Treatment is supportive for antihistamine overdoses.

The side effect profile of systemic antihistamines varies widely and depends on the receptor activity, chemical structure, and lipophilicity of the drug. The primary side effects are CNS effects (depression and stimulation) and anticholinergic effects. These side effects are common with first-generation antihistamines but are rarely seen with second-generation agents. CNS depressive effects include sedation and impaired performance (impaired driving performance, poor work performance, incoordination, reduced motor skills, and impaired information processing).[46] CNS stimulatory effects include anxiety, hallucinations, appetite stimulation, muscle dyskinesias, and activation of epileptogenic foci. High doses of first-generation antihistamines cause nervousness, tremor, insomnia, agitation, and irritability. Side effects associated with cholinergic blockage include dryness of the eyes and mucous membranes (mouth, nose, vagina); blurred vision; urinary hesitancy and retention; constipation; and tachycardia.

Side effects reported with ocular antihistamines include burning, stinging, itching, foreign body sensation, dry eye, hyperemia, and lid edema. Patients with a history of narrow-angle glaucoma may need to contact their eye care provider before choosing to self-treat with ocular antihistamines.

Antihistamines interact with numerous drugs (Table 11-7). All antihistamines decrease or prevent immediate dermal reactivity and should be discontinued at least 4 days before scheduled allergy skin testing.

The sedating antihistamines are contraindicated in newborns or premature infants, lactating women, and patients with narrow-angle glaucoma. Additional contraindications include acute asthma exacerbation, stenosing peptic ulcer, symptomatic prostatic hypertrophy, bladder neck and pyloroduodenal obstruction, and concomitant use of MAOIs. Formulations of 12- and 24-hour sustained-release loratadine/pseudoephedrine combination products are contraindicated in patients with esophageal narrowing, abnormal esophageal peristalsis, or a history of difficulty swallowing tablets.

Patients with lower respiratory tract diseases (e.g., emphysema and chronic bronchitis) should use sedating antihistamines with caution. Patients requiring mental alertness should not use sedating antihistamines and should use cetirizine with caution. Patients may be impaired even if they do not feel drowsy or if they have taken the dose the evening before. The sedating antihistamines are photosensitizing drugs. Patients should be advised to use sunscreens and wear protective clothing.

Combination Products

Antihistamines are marketed in combination with decongestants and analgesics. These combinations are also available in sustained-release formulations, allowing for convenient dosage regimens. However, these combination products should be used with caution because of the increased risk of side effects, especially insomnia, which compounds daytime fatigue already associated with this disease.

Decongestants

Congestion is a common allergic rhinitis symptom controllable with systemic decongestants or short-term (≤5 days) topical nasal decongestants. (See discussion of decongestants in the section Colds.)

TABLE 11-15   Dosage Guidelines for Systemic Nonprescription Antihistamines

Drug	Dosage (Maximum Daily Dosage)		
	Adults/Children ≥12 Years	**Children 6–<12 Years**	**Children 2–<6 Years**[a]
Brompheniramine maleate	4 mg every 4–6 hours (24 mg)	2 mg every 4–6 hours (12 mg)	
Cetirizine HCl[b]	10 mg every 24 hours	5–10 mg every 24 hours (10 mg)	2.5–5 mg every 24 hours (5 mg)
Chlorcyclizine HCl	25 mg every 6–8 hours (75 mg)	Not recommended for children <12 years except under advice of PCP	
Chlorpheniramine maleate	4 mg every 4–6 hours (24 mg)	2 mg every 4–6 hours (12 mg)	
Clemastine fumarate	1.34 mg every 12 hours (2.68 mg)	Not recommended for children <12 years except under advice of PCP	
Dexbrompheniramine maleate	2 mg every 4–6 hours (12 mg)	1 mg every 4–6 hours (6 mg)	
Dexchlorpheniramine maleate	2 mg every 4–6 hours (12 mg)	1 mg every 4–6 hours (6 mg)	
Diphenhydramine citrate	38–76 mg every 4–6 hours (456 mg)	19–38 mg every 4–6 hours (228 mg)	
Diphenhydramine HCl	25–50 mg every 4–6 hours (300 mg)	12.5–25 mg every 4–6 hours (150 mg)	
Doxylamine succinate	7.5–12.5 mg every 4–6 hours (75 mg)	3.75–6.25 mg every 4–6 hours (37.5 mg)	
Loratadine	10 mg every 24 hours	10 mg every 24 hours	5 mg every 24 hours
Phenindamine tartrate	25 mg every 4–6 hours (150 mg)	12.5 mg every 4–6 hours (75 mg)	
Pheniramine	12.5–25 mg every 4–6 hours (150 mg)	6.25–12.5 mg every 4–6 hours (75 mg)	
Pyrilamine maleate	25–50 mg every 6–8 hours (200 mg)	12.5–25 mg every 6–8 hours (100 mg)	
Thonzylamine HCl	50–100 mg every 4–6 hours (600 mg)	25–50 mg every 4–6 hours (300 mg)	
Triprolidine HCl	2.5 mg every 4–6 hours (10 mg)	1.25 mg every 4–6 hours (5 mg)	

Key: PCP, primary care provider.

[a] With the exception of cetirizine and loratadine, these products are not recommended for children younger than 6 years, except with the advice and supervision of a PCP.

[b] For adults older than 65 years, 10 mg cetirizine is not recommended, except with the advice and supervision of a PCP.

Source: Reference 13.

Cromolyn Sodium

Intranasal cromolyn is an anti-inflammatory drug indicated for preventing and treating the symptoms of allergic rhinitis. Cromolyn stabilizes mast cells, thereby preventing mediator release; the exact mechanism of action is not known. Cromolyn protects mast cells from immune-mediated (i.e., antigen–antibody) and nonimmune-mediated (e.g., cold air, hyperventilation, and exercise) triggers. Less than 7% of an intranasal cromolyn dose is absorbed systemically, and what little is absorbed has no systemic activity. The absorbed drug is rapidly excreted unchanged in the urine and bile, with a half-life of 1 to 2 hours. Swallowed cromolyn is excreted unchanged in the feces.

Cromolyn is approved for patients older than 5 years; the recommended dosage is one spray in each nostril three to six times daily at regular intervals.[13] Treatment is more effective if started before symptoms begin. It may take 3 to 7 days for initial treatment efficacy to become apparent and 2 to 4 weeks of continued therapy before achieving maximal therapeutic benefit. Sneezing is the most common side effect reported for intranasal cromolyn. Other adverse effects include nasal stinging and burning. No drug interactions have been reported with intranasal cromolyn.

Pharmacotherapeutic Comparison

Sedating antihistamines are effective, and some evidence does suggest that this group of drugs may be more effective than nonsedating antihistamines in treating symptoms of allergic rhinitis.[47] However, this evidence is based on trials using the maximum daily dose of diphenhydramine.[47] Sedating antihistamines have a quick onset of action but also have shorter duration of action and require multiple daily doses. The risks of cognition impairment and sedation have been well established with this class of drugs.[48] The World Health Organization and numerous clinicians now recommend nonsedating antihistamines as first-line therapy on the basis of their efficacy and safety profile, quick onset of action, and long duration, which allows once–daily dosing.[39]

Comparisons of cetirizine and loratadine have shown cetirizine to be a more potent antihistamine.[49] However, unlike loratadine, cetirizine causes sedation (in approximately 10% of patients).

Product Selection Guidelines

SPECIAL POPULATIONS

Because pregnancy is a common cause of nonallergic rhinitis, pregnant women should be referred for differential diagnosis. If allergic rhinitis is confirmed and nonprescription therapy is approved by a PCP, several treatment choices are available.[26,50] Intranasal cromolyn (Pregnancy Category B) has a wide margin of safety and is considered a first-line option.[26] Pregnancy Category B nonprescription antihistamines include cetirizine, chlorpheniramine, clemastine, diphenhydramine, and loratadine. Chlorpheniramine is the first–generation antihistamine of choice in pregnancy because of its long history of safety.[26] If chlorpheniramine is not tolerated, loratadine and cetirizine are preferred alternatives.[26,50] Although immunotherapy should not be initiated during pregnancy, maintenance therapy may be continued.[26,51]

Lactating women diagnosed with allergic rhinitis and approved for self-treatment by a PCP have fewer options. Because of its limited systemic absorption, intranasal cromolyn is a good choice, and there are no reports of adverse effects on nursing infants.[27] Antihistamines are contraindicated during lactation because of their ability to pass into breast milk. There have been reports of drowsiness and irritability in infants after mothers took clemastine.[27] Short-acting chlorpheniramine or loratadine seems to be the best option if an oral antihistamine is needed, but they should be used with caution and under the supervision of a PCP. If an oral antihistamine is used during lactation, the mother should avoid long-acting and high-dose antihistamines, and take the dose at bedtime after the last feeding of the day.[27]

Because of concerns of undiagnosed asthma, children younger than 12 years should be referred to a PCP for a differential diagnosis.[39] If nonprescription therapy is approved by a PCP, several treatment choices are available for children.[52] Loratadine is the initial nonprescription drug of choice followed by cetirizine. Sedating antihistamines should be avoided in children because of paradoxical excitation. Intranasal mast cell stabilizers are safe for children older than 5 years but may be difficult for children to self-administer. Immunotherapy may be used in children older than 5 years.

Patients of advanced age may experience paradoxical excitation with sedating antihistamines and are more likely than younger adults to have CNS depressive side effects, including confusion as well as hypotension. These side effects contribute to a higher risk of falling in the elderly. Loratadine and intranasal cromolyn are drugs of choice in the older population.

Dosages of loratadine and cetirizine should be adjusted in patients with renal or hepatic impairment.

PATIENT FACTORS AND PREFERENCES

The duration of treatment and the presence of concomitant symptoms will determine which product is selected (Table 11–16). Product selection may also be based on side effect profiles and cost. For example, all first-generation antihistamines are sedating but the degree of sedation depends on chemical class (Table 11–14). Loratadine and cetirizine are more expensive, but their lack of sedation and impairment may justify the additional cost. Some patients report that antihistamines are less effective after prolonged use. This decline is most likely not true tolerance but

rather stems from several factors, including patient nonadherence, an increase in antigen exposure, worsening of disease, the limited effectiveness of antihistamines in severe disease, or the development of similar symptoms from unrelated diseases. Although antihistamines induce their own metabolism, tolerance has not been clinically demonstrated.[46] Chemical class differences make it reasonable to suggest switching to a different

TABLE 11-16 Selected Products for Allergic Rhinitis

Trade Name	Primary Ingredients
Systemic First-Generation Antihistamine Products	
Chlor-Trimeton Allergy (4, 8, or 12 Hour) Tablets	Chlorpheniramine 4 mg, 8 mg, or 12 mg
Tavist Allergy Tablets	Clemastine fumarate 1.34 mg
Benadryl Allergy Tablets	Diphenhydramine HCl 25 mg
TheraFlu Thin Strips Multisymptom	Diphenhydramine HCl 25 mg
Children's Benadryl Allergy Relief Syrup	Diphenhydramine HCl 12.5 mg/5 mL
Triaminic Thin Strips Cough & Runny Nose	Diphenhydramine 12.5 mg
Systemic Second-Generation Antihistamine Products	
Zyrtec tablets	Cetirizine 10 mg
Children's Zyrtec Syrup	Cetirizine 5 mg/5 mL
Claritin Non-Drowsy Tablets	Loratadine 10 mg
Alavert Orally Disintegrating Tablets[a]	Loratadine 10 mg
Children's Dimetapp ND Tablets[a]	Loratadine 10 mg
Combination Systemic Products	
Dimetapp Cold and Allergy Elixir	Brompheniramine 1 mg/5 mL; phenylephrine 2.5 mg/5 mL
Zyrtec D tablets	Cetirizine 5 mg; pseudoephedrine 120 mg
Actifed Cold and Allergy Tablets	Chlorpheniramine 4 mg; phenylephrine 10 mg
Advil Allergy Sinus Caplets	Chlorpheniramine 2 mg; pseudoephedrine HCl 30 mg; ibuprofen 200 mg
Drixoral Cold and Allergy Tablets	Dexbrompheniramine 6 mg; pseudoephedrine 120 mg
Tylenol Severe Allergy Tablets	Diphenhydramine HCl 12.5 mg; acetaminophen 500 mg
Claritin-D 24 Hour Tablets Tablets	Loratadine 10 mg; pseudoephedrine sulfate 240 mg
Nasal Products	
Ayr Saline Nasal Gel	Sodium chloride; aloe; propylene glycol; glycerin
NasalCrom Spray	Cromolyn sodium 5.2 mg/spray
Ocean Spray	Sodium chloride 0.65%

[a] Contains phenylalanine; use with caution in phenylketonurics.

class of antihistamine if the patient has a less than optimal response to one class of antihistamine.

Immunotherapy

Immunotherapy, a series of subcutaneous injections with patient-specific allergens, is indicated for refractory allergic rhinitis in patients with moderate-to-severe symptoms. The exact mechanism of action is not known, but many theories have been proposed, including reduced elevations in IgE, decreased circulating eosinophils, and reduced mast cells.[40,51] Immunotherapy is the only therapy shown to modify the immune system and therefore the disease process; it is most effective for pollen-related allergens. Under clinician supervision, injections are initially given weekly, with concentrations of the allergen increased gradually. The maintenance dose is generally reached within 4 to 8 months. Maintenance injections are repeated every 3 to 4 weeks for 3 to 5 years. Relative contraindications to immunotherapy include autoimmune disease, unstable coronary artery disease, unstable asthma, and concurrent therapy with beta-adrenergic–blocking drugs.[51] Clinicians should have resuscitative equipment available in case of anaphylactic reaction.

Complementary Therapies

Ephedra (ma huang) and feverfew are commonly suggested herbal remedies for allergic rhinitis. Ephedra-containing products are banned by FDA owing to their serious adverse effects. Parthenolide, feverfew's biologically active component, may have anti-inflammatory properties, but its safety and efficacy in allergic rhinitis are unproven. (For further discussion of these types of products, see Chapter 54.) Homeopathic practitioners stress avoidance techniques but limit symptomatic treatment. Some homeopathic products actually contain known allergens (e.g., bioAllers Animal Hair and Dander Allergy Relief Liquid contains cat, cattle, dog, horse, and sheep wool extracts); these products claim to induce long-term resistance by repeated exposure to controlled amounts of allergen. These products should be used with extreme caution. Symptom-specific homeopathic remedies include sabadilla for nasal and ocular symptoms (red watery eyes) and wyethia for itching. The effectiveness and value of homeopathic products are highly questionable.

Assessment of Allergic Rhinitis: A Case-Based Approach

Asking the patient for a detailed description of the symptoms, and obtaining the patient's medical and medication use (previous and current) history are essential to determining whether the patient has allergic rhinitis or rhinitis related to other causes and is eligible for self-care (Tables 11-12 and 11-13).

The medical history may uncover other respiratory illnesses that complicate treatment of allergic rhinitis. The patient's current medication use will also alert the practitioner to possible interactions with nonprescription allergy medications. The practitioner should also ask whether nonprescription products used to treat intermittent or persistent rhinitis were effective and without adverse effects.

Case 11-2 presents an example of the assessment of a patient with allergic rhinitis.

C A S E   1 1 - 2

Relevant Evaluation Criteria	Scenario/Model Outcome
Information Gathering	
1. Gather essential information about the patient's symptoms, including:	
a. description of symptom(s) (i.e., nature, onset, duration, severity, associated symptoms)	Patient's mother says that patient has been complaining of a runny nose, mild congestion, headache, and itchy eyes for 1 week.
b. description of any factors that seem to precipitate, exacerbate, and/or relieve the patient's symptom(s)	Symptoms appeared about the same time the family moved into a new home.
c. description of the patient's efforts to relieve the symptoms	Patient's parents have not tried anything.
2. Gather essential patient history information:	
a. patient's identity	Christy Bates
b. patient's age, sex, height, and weight	4-year-old female, 3 ft 5 in, 40 lb
c. patient's occupation	N/A
d. patient's dietary habits	Normal healthy diet with occasional junk food
e. patient's sleep habits	Patient sleeps 5–6 hours at night; takes 1-hour nap during the day. Sleep is disturbed by symptoms.
f. concurrent medical conditions, prescription and nonprescription medications, and dietary supplements	Flintstone's vitamins 1 tablet every morning

C A S E 1 1 - 2 *(continued)*

Relevant Evaluation Criteria	Scenario/Model Outcome
g. allergies	NKA
h. history of other adverse reactions to medications	None
i. other (describe) _____	Patient has mild wheezing when breathing.

Assessment and Triage

3. Differentiate the patient's signs/symptoms and correctly identify the patient's primary problem(s) (see Tables 11-2 and 11-12).	Allergic rhinitis symptoms (runny nose, mild congestion, itchy eyes) seem to be associated with the move to a new location. Headache may be due to congestion. Wheezing may indicate new onset of asthma.
4. Identify exclusions for self-treatment (see Figure 11-3).	Patient is younger than 12 years and has symptoms of undiagnosed asthma (wheezing).
5. Formulate a comprehensive list of therapeutic alternatives for the primary problem to determine if triage to a medical practitioner is required, and share this information with the parent.	Options include: (1) Recommend a separate OTC product for each symptom: nonsedating or sedating antihistamine for runny nose and itchy eyes; topical or systemic decongestant for congestion; analgesic for headache. (2) Refer Christy to PCP for evaluation and treatment. (3) Recommend self-care until Christy's parents can consult PCP. (4) Take no action.

Plan

6. Select an optimal therapeutic alternative to address the patient's problem, taking into account patient preferences.	Refer Christy to PCP for differential diagnosis.
7. Describe the recommended therapeutic approach to the parent.	N/A
8. Explain to the patient the rationale for selecting the recommended therapeutic approach from the considered therapeutic alternatives.	Christy needs to see her PCP, because she has symptoms of asthma and is not eligible for self-care.

Patient Education

9. When recommending self-care with non-prescription medications and/or nondrug therapy, convey accurate information to the parent.	Criterion does not apply in this case.
10. Solicit follow-up questions from parent.	Is there anything we can do to help prevent these symptoms?
11. Answer parent's questions.	Yes. Inspect the house for indoor allergens (mold and cockroaches) and take steps to remove them if needed. Find out if the previous owners had pets, because pet dander may be present in the home even after the pet is removed.
	Wash Christy's bed linens in hot water every week. Encase her pillows and mattress in mite-impermeable materials. Change air filters, dust, and vacuum frequently. Consider removing carpets, upholstered furniture, books, and stuffed toys from Christy's bedroom.

Key: NKA, no known allergies; OTC, over-the-counter; PCP, primary care provider.

Patient Counseling for Allergic Rhinitis

The practitioner should stress that the best method of treating allergic rhinitis is to avoid allergens. Many patients, however, have no control over their work environment or are unable to implement all the preventive measures at home. These patients usually rely on allergy medications for symptom control. The patient should be advised about proper use of the recommended medications and about the possible adverse effects, drug–drug and drug–disease interactions, and other precautions and warnings. Patients should also know the signs and symptoms that indicate the disorder has progressed to the point where medical care is needed. The box Patient Education for Allergic Rhinitis lists specific information to provide patients.

PATIENT EDUCATION FOR
Allergic Rhinitis

The primary objective of self-treatment is to prevent or reduce symptoms, which in turn will improve functioning and sense of well-being. For some patients, prescription therapy such as short-course oral corticosteroids may help control symptoms while other therapy is initiated or when symptoms are especially severe. For most patients, carefully following instructions for nonprescription allergy medications and the self-care measures listed here will help ensure optimal therapeutic outcomes.

Nondrug Measures

- Avoidance of allergens is important regardless of whether allergy medications are being taken.
- For symptoms that develop mainly when outdoors:
  — Frequently check local pollen counts and air quality index.
  — Keep house and car windows shut on days with high levels of pollen (spring/summer), mold (late summer/fall), or pollution.
- Try not to do yard work or engage in outdoor sports.
- For symptoms that occur mainly when indoors:
  — Try to remove the symptom trigger(s) (e.g., cats, dust mites, tobacco smoke, molds) from the house.
  — Lower the humidity in the home to reduce molds. Use lower settings on humidifiers, repair damp basements and crawl spaces, vent kitchens and bathrooms, and remove house plants.
  — Wash bedding in hot water (130°F [54.4°C]) every week, and encase mattresses and pillows in dust mite–resistant coverings.

Nonprescription Medications

- Ask a clinician for help in selecting an allergy medication that treats the most bothersome symptoms. If needed, additional medications can be added for other symptoms:
  — Antihistamines are effective for itching, sneezing, and rhinorrhea but have little effect on nasal congestion.
  — Decongestants are effective for nasal congestion but have little effect on other symptoms.
  — Combination therapy with an antihistamine and a decongestant is common.
  — Intranasal and ocular preparations are available to reduce nasal and eye symptoms, respectively.
- Allergy medications are more effective if they are used regularly rather than episodically:
  — If you have intermittent allergies, start allergy medications as soon as possible, before exposure to allergen.
  — If you have persistent allergies, take allergy medications on a regular basis.

Nasal Congestion

- See the box Patient Education for Colds for information about relieving nasal congestion.

Rhinorrhea (Runny Nose) and Sneezing

- Many factors cause a runny nose. Nonprescription antihistamines or prescription medications only partially treat this symptom. Because some nonprescription antihistamines may make you very drowsy, the potential benefits of the medication must be weighed against the potential risks.
- Sneezing may be reduced with nonprescription antihistamines. Sneezing is a common and sometimes bothersome symptom. The potential benefits of using these medications must be weighed against the potential risks.

- Antihistamines are the preferred initial treatment for runny nose and sneezing in persons who are eligible for self-care (see exclusions in Figure 11-3).
- There are two types of antihistamines, sedating and nonsedating. Cetirizine and loratadine are nonsedating antihistamines and usually do not cause significant drowsiness.
- Nasal saline solutions may relieve nasal irritation and dryness, and aid in the removal of dried, encrusted, or thick mucus from the nose.
- Intranasal cromolyn is the preferred initial drug of choice during pregnancy and lactation. This medication is not absorbed into the body.
- Follow the dosing and administration directions carefully. See Table 11-3.
- The most common side effects of nasal preparations include nasal stinging and burning.
- Note the following side effects for antihistamines:
  — The sedating antihistamines cause drowsiness and impair mental alertness. Mental alertness is impaired even if you do not feel drowsy or if you took the dose the prior evening. While taking these medications, do not drive a vehicle, operate machinery, or engage in other activities that require alertness.
  — Sedating antihistamines may cause sensitivity to sunlight. Use sunscreens and wear protective clothing when outdoors.
  — Use of sedating antihistamines may cause dryness in your mouth, nose, and other areas of your body.
  — Children and persons of advanced age may experience unexpected excitement with sedating antihistamines.
  — Persons of advanced age may need lower doses of antihistamines, because they are more sensitive to the effects these medications have on the brain and heart.
- Do not use antihistamines:
  — If you are allergic to antihistamines or similar medications.
  — If you are breast-feeding.
- Do not give antihistamines to newborns or premature infants unless directed to do so by a primary care provider.
- Note the following precautions for use of nonprescription antihistamines:
  — Persons with glaucoma, stenosing peptic ulcer, symptomatic enlarged prostate, bladder-neck obstruction, or stomach-intestinal blockage should not use sedating (first-generation) antihistamines.
  — Persons with lower respiratory tract disease (e.g., emphysema, chronic bronchitis) should use sedating antihistamines with caution.
  — Persons with esophageal narrowing, abnormal esophageal peristalsis, or problems swallowing tablets should not take the 12- or 24-hour sustained-release dosage forms of loratadine combined with pseudoephedrine. There have been reports of esophageal obstruction and perforation with these sustained-release dosage forms.
- Sedating antihistamines interact with the following drugs:
  — Alcohol, sedatives, and other CNS depressants may cause additive depressive effects when taken with sedating antihistamines.

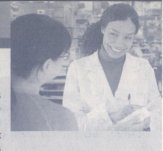

PATIENT EDUCATION FOR
Allergic Rhinitis *(continued)*

— Monoamine oxidase inhibitors such as tranylcypromine and phenelzine, the antibacterial furazolidone, and the anti-cancer drug procarbazine prolong and intensify some of the side effects of the sedating antihistamines.

— Decreased blood pressure may occur when MAOIs are taken with dexchlorpheniramine.

— Chlorpheniramine may increase the side effects of phenytoin.

■ Sedating antihistamines interact with the following drugs:

— Loratadine interacts with the following drugs: ketoconazole, erythromycin, and cimetidine.

— Cetirizine interacts with high doses of theophylline.

■ Store all medications according to the manufacturer's instructions.

 Seek medical attention in the following situations:

— Your allergy symptoms worsen while you are taking nonprescription medications or do not improve after 2–4 weeks of treatment.

— You develop signs or symptoms of secondary bacterial infections (i.e., thick nasal or respiratory secretions that are not clear, temperature higher than 101.5°F [88.6°C], shortness of breath, chest congestion, wheezing, significant ear pain, rash).

Evaluation of Patient Outcomes for Allergic Rhinitis

Many patients achieve symptomatic relief with initial nonprescription drug therapy in 3 to 4 days, but complete relief of symptoms may take 2 to 4 weeks. After this time frame, the clinician should follow up with a telephone call or a scheduled appointment to determine whether symptom control has been achieved or the patient is encountering any side effects or problems. Patients who respond poorly to treatment should be assessed to determine whether they are complying with allergen avoidance strategies and medication regimens. Options for patients who do not achieve relief include increasing current medications to maximally effective dosages or changing to a different medication or dosage formulation. Patients who do not respond to nonprescription therapy should be referred back to their PCP for prescription medications such as inhaled or systemic corticosteroids, leukotriene inhibitors, anticholinergics, or immunotherapy. Patients should also be reassessed, and the diagnosis of allergic rhinitis may need to be reconsidered. Patients who develop any of the warning signs or symptoms listed in the box Patient Education for Allergic Rhinitis should be referred to a PCP.

Key Points for Disorders Related to Colds and Allergic Rhinitis

➤ Colds are self-limiting, viral infections characterized by initial sore throat followed by nasal symptoms and nonproductive cough.

➤ Medical referral is appropriate for patients with suspected colds who are immunocompromised, have underlying cardiopulmonary diseases, or have alarm symptoms (high fever, chest pain, shortness of breath, or wheezing).

➤ Treatment for colds is symptomatic and targeted at the most bothersome symptoms.

➤ Decongestants are the most common nonprescription treatment for congestion related to colds and allergic rhinitis, but they should be used cautiously in patients with hypertension, diabetes, and other chronic diseases.

➤ Medical referral is appropriate for patients with symptoms suggestive of nonallergic rhinitis, otitis media, sinusitis, or lower respiratory tract problems such as pneumonia, asthma, or bronchitis, and those who fail to respond to nonprescription medications.

➤ Therapy for allergic rhinitis is sequential and consists of allergen avoidance, pharmacotherapy, and allergen immunotherapy.

➤ No single medication is ideal for treating allergic rhinitis, but initial therapy should target the most dominant symptom.

➤ In treating allergic rhinitis, multiple drug formulations may be added or used initially if the patient presents with moderately severe, particularly intense, or long-lasting symptoms, or if the patient is at risk for exacerbation of an underlying disease.

REFERENCES

1. National Institutes of Health, National Institute of Allergy and Infectious Diseases. Common Cold. December 2007. Available at: http://www3.niaid.nih.gov/topics/commoncold. Last accessed October 24, 2008.

2. Kline & Company. 2006 Fact Sheet. Nonprescription Drugs USA 2006. Little Falls, NJ: Kline & Company; June 2006.

3. Gwaltney JM. Clinical significance and pathogenesis of viral respiratory infections. *Am J Med*. 2002;112:13S–8S.

4. Cohen S, Doyle WJ, Turner R, et al. Sociability and susceptibility to the common cold. *Psychol Sci*. 2003;14:389–95.

5. Eccles R. Acute cooling of the body surface and the common cold. *Rhinology*. 2002;40:109–14.

6. Lee GM, Friedman JF, Ross-Degnan D, et al. Misconceptions about colds and predictors of health service utilization. *Pediatrics*. 2003;111:231–6.

7. Anzueto A, Niederman MS. Diagnosis and treatment of rhinovirus respiratory infections. *Chest*. 2003;123:1664–72.

8. Mahony J, Chong S, Merante F, et al. Development of a respiratory virus panel test for detection of twenty human respiratory viruses by use of multiplex PCR and a fluid microbead-based assay. *J Clin Microbiol*. 2007; 45:2965–70.

9. Salcido AL. Newer Insights into the Prevention of the Common Cold. *US Pharm*. 2007 November. Available at: http://www.uspharmacist.com/index.asp?page=ce/105608/default.htm#tbl1. Last accessed October 24, 2008.

10. Can antiviral tissues prevent the spread of colds? *Consum Rep*. 2004;69:56.

11. Self-care of the common cold. In: Albrant DH, ed. *The American Pharmaceutical Association's Drug Treatment Protocols*. Washington, DC: American Pharmaceutical Association; 2001:403–15.

12. Rennard BO, Ertl RF, Gossman GL, et al. Chicken soup inhibits neutrophil chemotaxis *in vitro*. *Chest*. 2000;118:1150–7.

13. Cold, cough, allergy, bronchodilator, and antiasthmatic drug products for over-the counter human use [serial online]. *CFR*. Revised April 1, 2007; Title 21, Vol 5, Pt 341. Available at: http://www.fda.gov. Last accessed October 24, 2008.

14. Statement from CHPA on the Voluntary Label Updates to Oral OTC Children's Cough and Cold Medicines. Available at: http://www.chpa-info.org. Last accessed October 24, 2008.

15. FDA Statement Following CHPA's Announcement on Nonprescription Over-the-Counter Cough and Cold Medicines in Children [news release]. Available at: http://www.fda.gov/bbs/topics/NEW/2008/NEW01899.html. Last accessed October 24, 2008.

16. Cold, cough, allergy, bronchodilator, and antiasthmatic drug products for over-the-counter human use. *CFR*. 2006; Title 21, Vol. 5, Pt 342. Available at: http://www.fda.gov. Last accessed October 24, 2008.

17. Ramey JT, Bailen E, Lockey RF. Rhinitis medicamentosa. *J Investig Allergol Clin Immunol*. 2006;16:148–55.

18. United States 109th Congress. Combat Methamphetamine Epidemic Act. Title VII of Public Law 109-177. USA Patriot Improvement Reauthorization Act 2005. March 9, 2006.

19. Sutter AI, Lemiengre M, Campbell H, et al. Antihistamines for the common cold. *Cochrane Database Syst Rev*. 2003;3:CD001267.

20. Eccles R. Efficacy and safety of over-the-counter analgesics in the treatment of common cold and flu. *J Clin Pharm Ther*. 2006;31:309–19.

21. Irwin RS, Baumann MH, Bolser DC, et al. Diagnosis and management of cough. ACCP evidence-based clinical practice guidelines. *Chest*. 2006; 129:1S–292S.

22. Bosler DC. Cough suppressant and pharmacologic protussive therapy: ACCP evidence-based clinical practice guidelines. *Chest*. 2006;129: 238S–49S.

23. Eccles R. Substitution of phenylephrine for pseudoephedrine as a nasal decongestant. An illogical way to control methamphetamine abuse. *Br J Clin Pharmacol*. 2007;63:10–4.

24. Hatton RC, Winterstein AG, McKelvey RP, et al. Efficacy and safety of oral phenylephrine: systematic review and meta-analysis. *Ann Pharmacother*. 2007;41:381–90.

25. Guthrie EW. The decongestant shuffle. *Pharm Today OTC Supplement*. April 2007;13(4 suppl 1):12–3.

26. Gilbert C, Mazzotta P, Loebstein R, et al. Fetal safety of drugs used in the treatment of allergic rhinitis. *Drug Saf*. 2005;28:707–19.

27. Nice FJ, Snyder JL, Kotansky BC. Breastfeeding and over-the-counter medications. *J Hum Lact*. 2000;16:319–31.

28. US Food and Drug Administration, Center for Drug Evaluation and Research. FDA Recommends that Over-the-Counter (OTC) Cough and Cold Products not be used for Infants and Children under 2 Years of Age. Rockville, Md: Center for Drug Evaluation and Research; January 17, 2008.

29. Roxas M, Jurenka J. Colds and influenza a review of diagnosis and conventional, botanical and nutritional considerations. *Alt Med Rev*. 2007; 12:25–48.

30. National Center for Complementary and Alternative Medicine. Herbs at a Glance. Available at http://nccam.nih.gov/health/herbsataglance.htm. Last accessed October 24, 2008.

31. Guo R, Pittler MH, Ernst E. Herbal medicines for the treatment of allergic rhinitis: a systematic review. *Ann Allergy Asthma Immunol*. 2007; 99:483–95.

32. Alexander TH, Davidson TM. Intranasal zinc and anosmia: the zinc-induced anosmia syndrome. *Laryngoscope*. 2006;116:217–20.

33. Caruso TJ, Prober CG, Gwaltney JM. Treatment of naturally acquired common colds with zinc: a structured review. *CID*. 2007;45:569–74.

34. Douglas RM, Hemila H, Chalker E, et al. Vitamin C for preventing and treating the common cold. *Cochrane Database Syst Rev*. 2007;3: CD000980.

35. Fineman SM. The burden of allergic rhinitis; beyond dollars and cents. *Ann Allergy Asthma Immunol*. 2002;88:S2–S7.

36. *Fastats—Allegies and Hay Fever*. Hyattsville, Md: National Center for Health Statistics; December 2007.

37. Reed SD, Lee TA, McCrory DC. The economic burden of allergic rhinitis: a critical evaluation of the literature. *Pharmacoeconomics*. 2004;22:345–61.

38. Pleis JR, Lethbridge-Çejku M. Summary health statistics for U.S. adults: National health interview survey, 2005. National Center for Health Statistics. *Vital Health Stat*. 2006;10(232):5, 19–20.

39. Bousquet J, Khaltev N, Cruz AA, et al. Allergic rhinitis and its impact on asthma (ARIA) 2008. *Allergy*. 2008;63(suppl 86):8–160.

40. Quraishi SA, Davies MJ, Craig TJ. Inflammatory responses in allergic rhinitis: traditional approaches and novel treatment strategies. *JAOA*. 2004;104:S7–S15.

41. Marshall GD. Internal and external environmental influences in allergic diseases. *JAOA*. 2004;104:S1–S6.

42. Skoner DP. Complications of allergic rhinitis. *J Allergy Clin Immunol*. 2000;105:S605–9.

43. National Institutes of Allergy and Infectious Disease. Airborne allergens: something in the air. Bethesda, Md: US Department of Health and Human Services, National Institutes of Allergy and Infectious Disease (NIAID); April 2003. NIH Publication No. 03-7045.

44. Cherry DK, Woodwell DA, Rechtsteiner EA. National Ambulatory Medical Care Survey: 2005 Summary. Hyattsville, Md: National Center for Health Statistics; 2007. Advance Data from Vital and Health Statistics, No. 387.

45. McCann DJ, Roth B. Toxicity, antihistamine. E-medicine. June 21, 2007. Available at: http://www.emedicine.com/EMERG/topic38.htm. Last accessed October 24, 2008.

46. Simons FER. Advances in H_1 antihistamines. *N Engl J Med*. 2004; 351:2203–17.

47. Raphael GD, Angello JT, Wu MM, et al. Efficacy of diphenhydramine vs desloratadine and placebo in patients with moderate-to-severe seasonal allergic rhinitis. *Ann Allergy Asthma Immunol*. 2006;96:606–14.

48. Kay GG. The effects of antihistamines on cognition and performance. *J Allergy Clin Immunol*. 2000;105:S622–7.

49. Curran MP, Scott LJ, Perry CM. Cetirizine a review of its use in allergic disorders. *Drugs*. 2004;64:523–61.

50. The American College of Obstetricians and Gynecologists (ACOG), The American College of Allergy, Asthma and Immunology (ACAAI). The use of newer asthma and allergy medications during pregnancy. *Ann Allergy Asthma Immunol*. 2000;84:475–80.

51. Huggins JL, Looney RJ. Allergen immunotherapy. *Am Fam Physician*. 2004;70:689–96.

52. Fireman P. Therapeutic approaches to allergic rhinitis: treating the child. *J Allergy Clin Immunol*. 2000;105:S616–21.

Cough

Karen J. Tietze

Cough is an important defensive respiratory reflex with potentially significant adverse physical and psychological consequences, as well as economic impact. Cough is the most common symptom for which patients seek medical care.[1] Approximately one in five ambulatory care visits to physician offices, hospital outpatient departments, and emergency departments is for disease associated with cough (acute upper respiratory tract infections, allergic rhinitis, chronic rhinitis, asthma, or chronic bronchitis).[2] Because many patients self-treat cough, the true incidence of cough is likely much higher. It has been estimated that Americans spend several billion dollars annually on nonprescription cough and cold medications.[3] The six cough products listed in the top 100 nonprescription medications by sales in 2006 accounted for more than $370 million in sales.[4]

Pathophysiology of Cough

Cough is elicited by stimulation of sensory receptors located throughout the larynx and the proximal portion of the tracheobronchial tree.[5] Cough is primarily vagally mediated.[6] Reflex cough (involuntary cough) is controlled by the "cough control center" in the medulla oblongata of the brainstem, whereas voluntary cough is controlled by the cerebral cortex.[7] Receptors in the larynx and proximal large airways are more sensitive to mechanical stimulation, whereas laryngeal receptors are more sensitive to chemical stimulation.[8] Efferents to expiratory respiratory muscles are carried by the vagus, phrenicus, laryngeal, and spinal motor nerves. The cough threshold may be influenced by the number of afferent nerves activated and the intensity of activation.[9] Viruses appear to increase cough receptor sensitivity.[10]

Cough consists of three phases: inspiratory, compressive, and expulsive.[11] A cough starts with a deep inspiration followed by closure of the glottis and forceful contraction of the chest wall, abdominal wall, and diaphragmatic muscles against the closed glottis; pressure in the thoracic cavity may reach 300 mm Hg with expiratory air velocities up to 500 mph. Mucus, cellular debris, and foreign material are propelled out of the respiratory system when the glottis opens. Cough typically occurs in epochs ("coughing fits").

Cough, classified as acute (i.e., duration of less than 3 weeks), subacute (i.e., duration of 3–8 weeks), or chronic (i.e., duration of longer than 8 weeks), is a symptom of diverse infectious and noninfectious disorders (Table 12-1).[3] Acute cough is most commonly caused by viral upper respiratory tract infection (URTI; e.g., the common cold). Subacute cough is commonly caused by infection, bacterial sinusitis, and asthma. The most common causes of chronic cough in adult nonsmokers are upper airway cough syndrome (UACS; previously known as postnasal drip syndrome), asthma, and gastroesophageal reflux disease (GERD). In children, cough may be a symptom of viral or bacterial respiratory infection, heart disease, foreign body aspiration, aspiration caused by poor coordination of sucking and swallowing, or esophageal motility disorders. Angiotensin-converting enzyme inhibitors cause dry cough in 20% or more of treated patients.[12] Systemic and ophthalmic beta-adrenergic blockers may cause cough in patients with obstructive airway diseases (e.g., asthma or chronic obstructive pulmonary disease [COPD]).

Clinical Presentation of Cough

Coughs are described as productive or nonproductive. A productive cough (e.g., a wet or "chesty" cough) expels secretions from the lower respiratory tract that, if retained, could impair ventilation and the lungs' ability to resist infection. Productive coughs may be effective (secretions easily expelled) or ineffective (secretions present but difficult to expel). Although the appearance of the secretions is not always a reliable diagnostic indicator, the secretions may be clear (e.g., bronchitis); purulent (e.g., bacterial infection); discolored (e.g., yellow with inflammatory disorders); or malodorous (e.g., anaerobic bacterial infection). A nonproductive cough (e.g., a dry or "hacking" cough) serves no useful physiologic purpose. Nonproductive coughs are associated with viral respiratory tract infections, atypical bacterial infections, GERD, cardiac disease, and some medications.

Complications secondary to high intrathoracic pressures and expiratory velocities occur regardless of the cause or type of cough. Common complications include exhaustion, insomnia, musculoskeletal pain, hoarseness, excessive perspiration, and urinary incontinence. Less common complications include cardiac dysrhythmias, syncope, stroke, and rib fractures. Cough may cause prolonged absence from work or school, withdrawal from social activities, and fear that the cough is a symptom of a serious illness such as cancer or tuberculosis.

TABLE 12-1   Etiology of Cough

Classification	Etiology
Acute	Viral URTI, pneumonia, acute left ventricular failure, asthma, foreign body aspiration
Subacute	Postinfectious cough, bacterial sinusitis, asthma
Chronic	UACS, asthma, GERD, COPD (chronic bronchitis), ACEIs, bronchogenic carcinoma, carcinomatosis, sarcoidosis, left ventricular failure, aspiration secondary to pharyngeal dysfunction

Key: ACEI, angiotensin-converting enzyme inhibitor; COPD, chronic obstructive pulmonary disease; GERD, gastroesophageal reflux disease; UACS, upper airway cough syndrome; URTI, upper respiratory tract infection.
Source: Reference 3.

Treatment of Cough

Treatment Goals

The primary goal of self-treatment of cough is to reduce the number and severity of cough episodes. The second goal is to prevent complications. Cough treatment is symptomatic; the underlying disorder must be treated to stop the cause of the cough (e.g., antibiotics for bacterial pneumonia, acid-suppressive therapy and lifestyle modifications for GERD, and decongestants for UACS).

General Treatment Approach

Selection of a medication for self-care of cough depends on the nature and etiology of the cough.[13] Figure 12-1 lists exclusions for self-care. Antitussives (cough suppressants) control or eliminate cough and are the drugs of choice for nonproductive coughs. Protussives (expectorants) change the consistency of mucus and increase the volume of expectorated sputum. Protussives are the drugs of choice for coughs that expel thick, tenacious secretions from the lungs with difficulty. Antitussives should not be taken by patients with productive coughs unless absolutely necessary (e.g., exhaustion from lack of sleep). Suppression of productive coughs may lead to retention of lower respiratory tract secretions and potentially adverse consequences (e.g., airway obstruction or secondary bacterial lower respiratory tract infection).

Cough medications are marketed in a variety of dosage forms (syrups, liquids, tablets, capsules, lozenges, oral disintegrating strips, oral granules, oral sprays, topical ointments and creams, and vaporizer solutions). In general, the newer convenience-oriented dosage forms (oral disintegrating strips, oral sprays, extended-release tablets, and granules) cost more per dose than older dosage forms. Products containing various combinations of antitussives, protussives, analgesics, decongestants, and

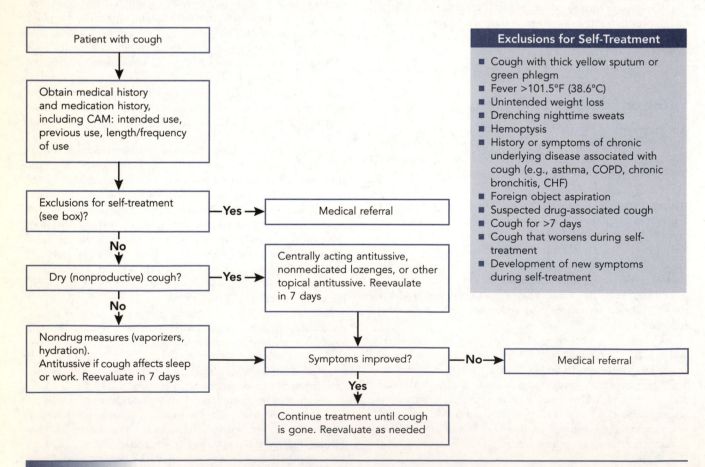

FIGURE 12-1   Self-care of cough. Key: CAM, complementary and alternative medicine; CHF, congestive heart failure; COPD, chronic obstructive pulmonary disease. (Adapted from reference 13.)

antihistamines are available. Although convenient, cost per dose of combination products may be higher than that of single-entity products. In addition, products containing both an antitussive and a protussive are irrational and should be avoided.

Nonpharmacologic Therapy

Nonpharmacologic therapy includes nonmedicated lozenges, humidification, and hydration. Hard candies and other non-medicated lozenges reduce throat irritation and may decrease coughing. Humidifiers (ultrasonic, impeller, and evaporative) increase the amount of moisture in inspired air, which may soothe irritated airways. However, high humidity may increase the amount of mold and dust mites in the house, thus worsening allergies. Humidifiers and vaporizers also disperse minerals and microorganisms into the air. Vaporizers are humidifiers with a medication well or cup for volatile inhalants that combine with the mist to produce a medicated vapor. Cool-mist humidifiers and vaporizers are preferable to warm-mist humidifiers and vaporizers, because fewer bacteria grow at the cooler temperatures and there is less risk of scalding if they are tipped over. Humidifiers and vaporizers must be cleaned daily and disinfected weekly. Babies and young children to about 2 years of age cannot blow their noses; a rubber bulb nasal syringe may be used to clear the nasal passages and reduce cough if postnasal drip causes cough.

Less viscous and thus easier-to-expel secretions are formed when a person is well hydrated. Most people need approximately eight 8-ounce glasses of water daily. However, water cannot be incorporated into previously formed mucus, and there are theoretical risks of over hydration during respiratory infections. Excessive fluid intake may cause fluid overload and hyponatremia in patients with lower respiratory tract infections; it is not known whether these effects occur with URTIs.[14] Cautious hydration is recommended for patients with lower respiratory tract infections, heart failure, renal failure, or other conditions potentially exacerbated by over hydration.

Pharmacologic Therapy

Table 12-2 lists examples of products that contain oral antitussives, expectorants, and topical antitussives.

Systemic Antitussives

Nonprescription systemic antitussives approved by the Food and Drug Administration (FDA) include codeine, dextromethorphan, and diphenhydramine.[15]

CODEINE

Codeine is the gold standard antitussive. At antitussive dosages, codeine is a Schedule C-V narcotic available without a prescription in 30 states (9 of the 30 states limit sales to products sold by a pharmacist in a pharmacy).[16] Codeine-containing Schedule C-V products must contain one or more noncodeine active ingredients and no more than 200 mg of codeine per 100 milliliters. Hydrocodone and hydromorphone have similar efficacy, but they are associated with a greater risk of dependency and are available only by prescription. Abuse of the combination of codeine and promethazine hydrochloride, known by the street names of "lean" and "purple stuff," has been popularized by the hip-hop culture.[17]

Codeine acts centrally on the medulla to increase the cough threshold. Codeine is methylmorphine; morphine may be the active antitussive. Codeine is well absorbed orally with a 15- to 30-minute onset of action and a 4- to 6-hour duration of effect. The elimination half-life is 2.5 to 3 hours. Ten percent of a codeine dose is demethylated in the liver to form morphine. Approximately 3% to 16% of codeine is eliminated unchanged in the urine.

Codeine is indicated for the suppression of nonproductive cough caused by chemical or mechanical respiratory tract irritation. Although widely available, codeine's efficacy and safety as an antitussive drug in children have not been established.[18] Table 12-3 lists FDA-approved codeine dosages and updated labeling information.[15,19-21] Pediatric dosage guidelines are extrapolated from the adult literature.[18] Reduced doses are appropriate for patients of advanced age and the debilitated. Codeine is available as oral solutions and syrups in combination with other active ingredients, including guaifenesin, antihistamines, and decongestants. Alcohol-, dye-, and sucrose-free formulations are available. The lethal dose of codeine in adults is 0.5 to 1 gram, with death from marked respiratory depression and cardiopulmonary collapse.

Usual antitussive codeine dosages have low toxicity and little risk of addiction. The most common side effects associated with antitussive codeine dosages are nausea, vomiting, sedation, dizziness, and constipation. Concomitant use of codeine and central nervous system (CNS) depressants (e.g., barbiturates, sedatives, or alcohol) causes additive CNS depression. Codeine is contraindicated in patients with known codeine hypersensitivity and during labor when a premature birth is anticipated. Patients with impaired respiratory reserve (e.g., asthma or COPD) or preexisting respiratory depression, addicts, and those who take other respiratory depressants or sedatives, including alcohol, should use codeine with caution.

TABLE 12-2 Selected Products for Cough

Primary Ingredients	Trade Name
Single-Ingredient Products	
Dextromethorphan	Delsym, Triaminic Long Acting Cough, Vicks Formula 44
Guaifenesin	Humibid Maximum Strength, Mucinex, Robitussin
Menthol	Robitussin Cough Drops, Vicks Cough Drops
Combination Products	
Dextromethorphan and guaifenesin	Cheracol D, Mucinex DM, Robitussin Cough DM
Codeine and guaifenesin	Cheracol, Cheratussin AC, Guaituss AC
Camphor and menthol	Mentholatum Ointment

TABLE 12–3 Dosage Guidelines for Nonprescription Oral Antitussives and Expectorants

Drug	Dosage (Maximum Daily Dosage)		
	Adults/Children ≥12 Years	**Children 6 to <12 Years**	**Children 2 to <6 Years**[a]
Codeine[b–d]	10–20 mg every 4–6 hours (120 mg)	5–10 mg every 4–6 hours (60 mg)	1 mg/kg/day in 4 equal divided dosages or by average body weight
Dextromethorphan hydrobromide[b]	10–20 mg every 4 hours or 30 mg every 6–8 hours (120 mg)	5–10 mg every 4 hours or 15 mg every 6–8 hours (60 mg)	2.5–5 mg every 4 hours or 7.5 mg every 6–8 hours (30 mg)
Diphenhydramine citrate[b,c]	38 mg every 4 hours (228 mg)	19 mg every 4 hours (114 mg)	9.5 mg every 4 hours (57 mg)
Diphenhydramine HCl[b,c]	25 mg every 4 hours (150 mg)	12.5 mg every 4 hours (75 mg)	6.25 mg every 4 hours (37.5 mg)
Guaifenesin[b]	200–400 mg every 4 hours (2.4 g)	100–200 mg every 4 hours (1.2 g)	50–100 mg every 4 hours (600 mg)

[a] The Consumer Health Care Products Association announced in October 2008 that manufacturers were voluntarily updating cough and cold product labels to state "do not use" in children under 4 years of age.[19] FDA announced that it would not object to the more restrictive labeling.[20] These actions have not changed the official monograph for cold, cough, allergy, bronchodilator, and antiasthmatic drug products.[21]

[b] Not recommended for use in children younger than 2 years.

[c] FDA recommends that the labels on nonprescription products not provide dosage information for children younger than 6 years.

[d] Codeine may be dosed by average body weight: 2 years of age (average body weight of 12 kg) = 3 mg every 4–6 hours (maximum in 24 hours: 12 mg); 3 years of age (average body weight of 14 kg) = 3.5 mg every 4–6 hours (maximum in 24 hours: 14 mg); 4 years of age (average body weight of 16 kg) = 4 mg every 4–6 hours (maximum in 24 hours: 16 mg); 5 years of age (average body weight of 18 kg) = 4.5 mg every 4–6 hours (maximum in 24 hours: 18 mg). A dispensing device such as a dropper calibrated for age or weight should be dispensed along with the product when it is intended for use in children 2 to younger than 6 years, to prevent possible overdose from improperly measured dose.

Source: Reference 15.

DEXTROMETHORPHAN

Considered approximately equipotent with codeine, dextromethorphan is a nonopioid with no analgesic, sedative, respiratory depressant, or addictive properties at usual antitussive doses. Dextromethorphan is the methylated dextrorotatory analogue of levorphanol, a codeine analogue. Dextromethorphan acts centrally in the medulla to increase the cough threshold. It is well absorbed orally with a 15- to 30-minute onset of action and a 3- to 6-hour duration of effect. Dextromethorphan exhibits polymorphic metabolism, with a usual elim-ination half-life of 1.2 to 2.2 hours. However, the half-life may be as long as 45 hours in people with a poor metabolism phenotype.

Dextromethorphan is indicated for the suppression of nonproductive cough caused by chemical or mechanical respiratory tract irritation. As with codeine, the efficacy and safety of dextromethorphan as an antitussive drug in children have not been established.[18] Table 12-3 lists FDA-approved dextromethorphan dosages.[15] This agent is marketed in the form of syrups, liquids, extended-release oral suspensions, liquid-filled gelcaps, oral disintegrating strips, oral sprays, and lozenges. Alcohol-, sucrose-, and dye-free formulations are available. Dextromethorphan overdoses cause confusion, excitation, nervousness, irritability, restlessness, drowsiness, and severe nausea and vomiting; respiratory depression may occur with very high doses.

Dextromethorphan has a wide margin of safety. Side effects with usual doses are uncommon but may include drowsiness, nausea or vomiting, stomach discomfort, or constipation. Dextromethorphan is abused for its phencyclidine-like euphoric effect[22]; abuse may be associated with psychosis and mania.

Additive CNS depression occurs with alcohol, antihistamines, and psychotropic medications. Dextromethorphan blocks serotonin reuptake; the combination of monoamine oxidase inhibitors (MAOIs) and dextromethorphan may cause serotonergic syndrome (e.g., increased blood pressure, hyperpyrexia, arrhythmias, and myoclonus). Patients who have known hypersensitivity to dextromethorphan or who have a prior history of dextromethorphan dependence should not take it. If the patient takes MAOIs, dextromethorphan should not be administered for at least 14 days after the MAOIs are halted.

DIPHENHYDRAMINE

Diphenhydramine is a nonselective (first-generation) antihistamine with significant sedating and anticholinergic properties. Although diphenhydramine is an FDA-approved antitussive, it is not a first-line antitussive. Diphenhydramine acts centrally in the medulla to increase the cough threshold. The antitussive effect is most likely related to anticholinergic activity and not competitive histamine antagonism; second-generation antihistamines (e.g., loratadine and fexofenadine) lack antitussive activity.[23] Diphenhydramine is well absorbed following oral administration, with a bioavailability of 40% to 70% and an onset of action of about 15 minutes. The volume of distribution is 3.3 to 4.5 L/kg. Diphenhydramine is hepatically metabolized to n–dealkylated and acidic metabolites with a clearance of 0.4 to 0.7 L/kg per hour. Less than 4% is excreted unchanged in the urine.

Diphenhydramine is indicated for the suppression of nonproductive cough caused by chemical or mechanical respiratory tract irritation. Table 12-3 lists FDA-approved diphenhydramine dosages.[15] Diphenhydramine's antitussive dose is lower than its antihistaminic dose. Antitussive diphenhydramine formulations include syrups, liquids, and oral disintegrating strips. Alcohol-, sucrose-, and dye-free formulations are available. Symptoms of diphenhydramine overdose include mild-to-severe CNS depression (e.g., mental confusion, sedation, or respiratory depression), hypotension, and CNS stimulation (e.g., hallucinations or convulsions).

Side effects of diphenhydramine include drowsiness, disturbed coordination, respiratory depression, blurred vision, urinary retention, dry mouth, and dry respiratory secretions. Uncommon side effects reported with diphenhydramine include acute dystonic reactions such as oculogyric crisis (rotation of the eyeballs), torticollis (contraction of neck muscles), and catatonia-like states, as well as allergic and photoallergic reactions. Diphenhydramine may cause excitability, especially in children. Diphenhydramine potentiates the depressant effects of narcotics, nonnarcotic analgesics, benzodiazepines, tranquilizers, and alcohol on the CNS, and intensifies the anticholinergic effect of MAOIs and other anticholinergics. Diphenhydramine is contraindicated in patients with known hypersensitivity to diphenhydramine or structurally similar antihistamines. Diphenhydramine should be used with caution in patients with diseases potentially exacerbated by drugs with anticholinergic activity, including narrow-angle glaucoma, stenosing peptic ulcer, pyloroduodenal obstruction, symptomatic prostatic hypertrophy, bladder-neck obstruction, asthma and other lower respiratory disease, elevated intraocular pressure, hyperthyroidism, cardiovascular disease, or hypertension. Because of the increased risk of toxicity, diphenhydramine-containing antitussives should not be used with any other diphenhydramine-containing product, including external products.

Protussives (Expectorants)

Guaifenesin (glyceryl guaiacolate), the only FDA-approved expectorant, is indicated for the symptomatic relief of acute, ineffective productive coughs.[15] Guaifenesin is not indicated for chronic cough associated with chronic lower respiratory tract diseases such as asthma, chronic obstructive lung disease, emphysema, or smoker's cough. Guaifenesin should not be used to treat effectively productive coughs. Guaifenesin loosens and thins lower respiratory tract secretions, making minimally productive coughs more productive. However, few data support its efficacy, especially at nonprescription dosages.[24] The pharmacokinetics of guaifenesin are not well described.

Table 12-3 lists FDA-approved dosages of guaifenesin.[15] Guaifenesin is marketed as oral liquids, syrups, and immediate-release and extended-release tablets. Alcohol-, sucrose-, and dye-free formulations are also available. Most reports of guaifenesin overdosages involve combinations of drugs and therefore are difficult to assess. However, signs and symptoms of overdosages appear to be extensions of the adverse effects.

Guaifenesin is generally well tolerated, but its side effects may include nausea, vomiting, dizziness, headache, rash, diarrhea, drowsiness, and stomach pain. Guaifenesin may have a mild uricosuric effect and large dosages may cause urolithiasis. There are no reported drug interactions with guaifenesin. Guaifenesin is contraindicated in patients with a known hypersensitivity to guaifenesin.

Topical Antitussives

Camphor and menthol are the only two FDA-approved topical antitussives.[15] Other volatile oils (e.g., eucalyptus), common in many cough and cold preparations, impart a strong medicinal odor to products, but they are not FDA-approved antitussives. Although the mechanism of action is not well described, inhaled camphor and menthol vapors stimulate sensory nerve endings within the nose and mucosa, creating a local anesthetic sensation and a sense of improved airflow. However, there is little objective evidence of clinical efficacy. Topical antitussive ointments and creams contain camphor (4.7%–5.3%) or menthol (2.6%–2.8%). Steam inhalants contain 6.2% camphor or 3.2% menthol. Lozenges each contain 5 to 10 mg of menthol. Many lozenges contain one or more of the volatile oils. Table 12-4 provides administration guidelines for these agents.

Camphor- and menthol-containing products may splatter and cause serious burns if used near an open flame or placed in hot water or in a microwave oven. Ointments, creams, and solutions containing camphor or menthol are toxic if ingested. Toxicities include burning sensations in the mouth, nausea and vomiting, epigastric distress, restlessness, excitation, delirium, seizures, and death. Ingestion of as little as 4 teaspoons of products containing 5% camphor may be lethal for children.[25]

Product Selection Guidelines

EFFICACY

Although antitussives and expectorants have been marketed for decades, efficacy has been difficult to prove and may depend on

TABLE 12-4	Administration Guidelines for Nonprescription Topical Antitussives (Adults and Children ≥2 Years[a])
Formulation	**Administration**
Ointments and creams	Rub on the throat and chest as a thick layer; application may be repeated up to 3 times daily or as directed by primary care provider; loosen clothing around throat and chest so vapors reach the nose and mouth; cover with a warm, dry cloth (optional). Do not use in the nostrils, under the nose, by the mouth, on damaged skin, or with tight bandages.
Lozenges	Allow lozenge to dissolve slowly in mouth; repeat hourly or as needed or directed by a primary care provider.
Inhalation	For products to be added directly to cold water for use in a steam vaporizer: Add measured solution to cold water, place the mixture in the vaporizer, breathe in the medicated vapors up to 3 times daily. For products to be placed in medication chamber of hot steam vaporizer: Place water in vaporizer; place solution in medication chamber; breathe in the medicated vapors up to 3 times daily.

[a] For children ages ≤ 2 years, consult a primary care provider.
Source: Reference 15.

the etiology of the cough. Effective in models of experimentally induced cough and in chronic cough, neither codeine nor dextromethorphan has been shown to be effective for acute coughs associated with viral URTI in either adults or children.[26–28] Coughs associated with URTIs involves the voluntary and brainstem reflex pathway,[29] which may partially explain the ineffectiveness of brainstem-active antitussives as well as the large placebo response (up to 85%).[30,31] Factors such as taste, smell, color, viscosity, sugar content, and personal expectation may contribute to the placebo response. Efficacy will remain unproven until data are available from well-designed trials of subjects with natural disease who are assessed with standardized objective outcome parameters.

The American College of Chest Physicians published updated evidence-based diagnosis and management of cough guidelines in 2006[32]; similar international guidelines are available.[33] The guidelines state that central cough suppressants are ineffective in cough associated with the common cold and recommend a combination of first-generation antihistamine plus decongestant to treat the virus-induced postnasal drip that is most likely the cause of the cough.[34] Given that viral infection increases upper airway afferent nerve sensitivity, the guidelines suggest that the anti-inflammatory naproxen may reduce viral-associated cough.[34] Although the etiology of cough associated with chronic UACS is unclear, the guidelines recommend empiric treatment with a first-generation antihistamine/decongestant combination.[35] The guidelines recommend codeine or dextromethorphan for the short-term symptomatic relief of cough associated with acute and chronic bronchitis, and postinfectious (subacute) cough. The guidelines do not recommend guaifenesin for any indication.

SPECIAL POPULATIONS

In response to a March 2007 citizen's petition from 16 pediatric specialists, FDA is investigating the efficacy and safety of nonprescription cough and cold medicine in children under 6 years of age.[36] In January 2008, FDA issued a public health advisory recommending that nonprescription cough and cold medicines ". . . not be used to treat infants and children under 2 years of age because several serious and potentially life-threatening side effects can occur."[37] In response to this action, many products intended for infants, babies, and young children were voluntarily withdrawn from the market. In October 2008, the Consumer Healthcare Products Association announced that manufacturers were voluntarily updating cough and cold product labels to state "do not use" in children under 4 years of age.[19] FDA announced that it would not object to the more restrictive labeling.[20] The Agency will continue to assess the safety and efficacy of nonprescription cough and cold medications in children.

Codeine is a Pregnancy Category C drug and should be used during pregnancy only if the potential benefits outweigh the risks. Nonteratogenic concerns include the risk of neonatal respiratory depression if codeine is taken close to the time of delivery and neonatal withdrawal if codeine is used regularly during the pregnancy. Although codeine is excreted in breast milk, the American Academy of Pediatrics lists codeine as a maternal medication usually compatible with breast-feeding.[38] Because the elderly may be more susceptible to the sedating effects of codeine, the dose should be started at the lower end of the dosage range and titrated as tolerated with careful monitoring.

Although listed as a Pregnancy Category C drug, dextromethorphan is viewed by some clinicians as probably safe for use during pregnancy.[39,40] It is not known whether dextromethorphan is excreted in breast milk. The American Academy of Pediatrics' current drugs and breast-feeding policy statement makes no recommendation regarding dextromethorphan and breast-feeding.[38] Because the elderly may be more susceptible to the sedating effects of dextromethorphan, the dose should be started at the lower end of the dosage range and titrated as tolerated with careful monitoring.

Diphenhydramine is a Pregnancy Category B drug. It is excreted in breast milk and may cause unusual excitation and irritability in the infant; it may also decrease the flow of milk. Persons of advanced age are more likely to experience dizziness, excessive sedation, syncope, confusion, and hypotension with diphenhydramine compared with the general population. Children and persons of advanced age may experience paradoxical excitation, restlessness, and irritability with diphenhydramine. Dosing for the latter group should be started at the lower end of the dosage range and titrated as tolerated with careful monitoring.

PATIENT FACTORS

Cough is a symptom of many acute and chronic diseases; self-treatment may delay effective treatment of the underlying disease. Patients with known, or signs and symptoms of, chronic diseases associated with cough (Table 12-5) should not attempt to self-treat cough, even cough caused by an acute viral URTI, because the acute infection may exacerbate the underlying disease. Patients with smoker's cough should be counseled regarding smoking cessation options (see Chapter 50). Patients with identified exclusions for self-care (Figure 12-1) should be referred for further evaluation.

Codeine or dextromethorphan are the drugs of choice for nonproductive coughs. Neither dextromethorphan nor diphenhydramine should be taken by patients on MAOIs. Diphenhydramine is highly sedating and should be avoided by

---

TABLE 12-5 Signs and Symptoms of Diseases Associated with Cough

Disease	Signs and Symptoms
Asthma	Wheezing or chest tightness; coughing predominantly at night; cough in response to specific irritants such as dust, smoke, or pollen
CHF	Fatigue, dependent edema, breathlessness
COPD	Productive cough most days of the month at least 3 months of the year for at least 2 consecutive years
GERD	Heartburn, worsening of symptoms when supine, improvement with acid-lowering drugs
Lower respiratory tract infection	Oral temperature > 101.5°F (38.6°C); thick, purulent, discolored phlegm; drenching night sweats
UACS	Mucus drainage from nose, frequent throat clearing
Viral URTI	Sneezing, sore throat, rhinorrhea, low-grade temperature

Key: CHF, congestive heart failure; COPD, chronic obstructive pulmonary disease; GERD, gastroesophageal reflux disease; UACS, upper airway cough syndrome; URTI, upper respiratory tract infection.

patients at risk from the anticholinergic properties of the drug. First-generation antihistamines and decongestants should be used only if the potential benefit outweighs the risk (see Chapter 11).

Complementary Therapies

Hundreds of herbal and other complementary therapies are marketed for cough. However, evidence does not support the use of complementary therapies for treating cough, and some products have potential safety issues. Honey is a common home remedy but should not be given to children under 1 year of age owing to the risk of botulism.[41]

Assessment of Cough: A Case-Based Approach

Before recommending any treatment, the practitioner needs to know how long the patient has been coughing, whether the cough is productive, and whether it is associated with a chronic illness (Table 12-5). It is also important to obtain a list of all the patient's current medications to identify possible drug–drug or drug–disease interactions. In addition, the practitioner should find out how the patient has treated the current cough as well as previous coughs, and whether these treatments were satisfactory or effective.

Case 12-1 provides an example of the assessment of a patient with cough.

CASE 12-1

Relevant Evaluation Criteria	Scenario/Model Outcome
Information Gathering	
1. Gather essential information about the patient's symptoms, including:	
a. description of symptom(s) (i.e., nature, onset, duration, severity, associated symptoms)	Patient has had a cold for several days. The rhinorrhea is resolving, but the cough persists, waking the patient, her siblings, and parents at night. The cough is dry and hacking. The patient had a fever the first couple days of the cold but has not had a fever since then.
b. description of any factors that seem to precipitate, exacerbate, and/or relieve the patient's symptom(s)	The cough is worse when she is put down for naps and at bedtime. She does not cough as much when she is sitting in her car seat/carrier.
c. description of the patient's efforts to relieve the symptoms	Samantha's mom says that she looked for Infant Triaminic Thin Strips but could not find them in the pharmacy or grocery store.
2. Gather essential patient history information:	
a. patient's identity	Samantha Miller
b. patient's age, sex, height, and weight	1-year-old female, 29 inches, 21 lb
c. patient's occupation	N/A
d. patient's dietary habits	Regular table foods supplemented with breast milk
e. patient's sleep habits	Beginning to sleep through the night
f. concurrent medical conditions, prescription and nonprescription medications, and dietary supplements	None
g. allergies	NKDA
h. history of other adverse reactions to medications	None
i. other (describe)	N/A
Assessment and Triage	
3. Differentiate the patient's signs/symptoms and correctly identify the patient's primary problem(s).	The cough appears to be due to a viral URTI.
4. Identify exclusions for self-treatment (see Figure 12-1).	None
5. Formulate a comprehensive list of therapeutic alternatives for the primary problem to determine if triage to a medical practitioner is required, and share this information with the caregiver.	Options include: (1) Refer Samantha to her pediatrician. (2) Recommend nondrug therapy. (3) Take no action.

CASE 12-1   (continued)

Relevant Evaluation Criteria	Scenario/Model Outcome
Plan	
6. Select an optimal therapeutic alternative to address the patient's problem, taking into account patient preferences.	Samantha's mom prefers to try your nondrug therapy recommendations before calling the pediatrician.
7. Describe the recommended therapeutic approach to the caregiver	Use a nasal bulb syringe to clear the nasal passages and reduce the post-nasal drip that is the most likely cause of Samantha's cough. Place Samantha in her car seat/carrier, and let her sleep in an upright position to reduce the postnasal drip.
8. Explain to the caregiver the rationale for selecting the recommended therapeutic approach from the considered therapeutic alternatives.	Cough and cold medications are no longer recommended for infants and children under 2 years of age. Manufacturers voluntarily stopped marketing these products in response to FDA concerns about the lack of information about the safety and dosing of these produces in this age group.
Patient Education	
9. When recommending self-care with nonprescription medications and/or nondrug therapy, convey accurate information to the caregiver:	
a. appropriate dose and frequency of administration	N/A
b. maximum number of days the therapy should be employed	N/A
c. product administration procedures	N/A
d. expected time to onset of relief	N/A
e. degree of relief that can be reasonably expected	N/A
f. most common side effects	N/A
g. side effects that warrant medical intervention should they occur	N/A
h. patient options in the event that condition worsens or persists	A pediatrician should be consulted if the cough worsens or does not improve in a few days.
i. product storage requirements	N/A
j. specific nondrug measures	See step 8.
10. Solicit follow-up questions from caregiver.	Samantha's mom asks if it is safe to give cough medicine to her other children (ages 4 and 7 years).
11. Answer caregiver's questions.	Some questions have been raised about the safety and dosing of cough medications in children under 6 years of age, but the FDA advisory applies to only children under 2 years of age. Follow the labeled dosage guidelines or consult your pediatrician if you have questions

Key: FDA, Food and Drug Administration; N/A, not applicable; URTI, upper respiratory tract infection.

Patient Counseling for Cough

The practitioner should explain the appropriate drug and nondrug measures for treating the patient's type of cough. After recommending a product, the dosage guidelines, drug administration techniques (for topical drugs), and possible side effects, drug–drug interactions, and precautions or warnings should be fully explained. The practitioner should ensure that the patient understands when self-care of cough should be discontinued and medical care sought. For patients with underlying medical disorders, the practitioner should explain which nonprescription medications are contraindicated and what symptoms indicate the need to seek medical care. The box Patient Education for Cough lists specific information for patients.

PATIENT EDUCATION FOR
Cough

The goal of self-treatment is to reduce the number and severity of cough episodes and prevent complications. For most patients, carefully following product instructions and the self-care measures listed here will help ensure optimal therapeutic outcomes.

Nondrug Measures

- Stay well hydrated. Most adults need about eight 8-ounce glasses of water per day.
- Reduce throat irritation by slowly dissolving nonmedicated lozenges and candies in mouth.
- Humidifiers and vaporizers increase the moisture in the air and may soothe irritated airways.
- Treat the underlying cause of cough (e.g., nasal congestion).

Nonprescription Medications

- Cough is a symptom of an underlying disorder. Contact your primary care provider if you have any of the exclusions for self-care listed in Figure 12-1.
- Slowly dissolve medicated lozenges in your mouth; do not chew.
- Swallow tablets and capsules whole; do not crush or chew.
- Slowly dissolve oral disintegrating strips on your tongue; do not chew.
- Hold the oral spray bottle close to your mouth. Depress the sprayer fully and swallow the medication. Do not inhale the mist.
- Follow the recommended dosing guidelines for each medication.
- Store all these medications according to the manufacturer's recommendations. Do not use any expired drug.

Cough Suppressants (Antitussives)

- Cough suppressants control or eliminate cough and are the drugs of choice for nonproductive coughs.
- Oral nonprescription cough suppressants include codeine (available without a prescription in some states), dextromethorphan, and diphenhydramine.
- Topical nonprescription antitussives include camphor and menthol.
- Do not heat, microwave, or add topical antitussives to hot water. Do not use topical antitussives near an open flame. Topical antitussive ointments, creams, and liquids are toxic if ingested.
- The most common side effects of codeine include nausea, vomiting, sedation, dizziness, and constipation.
- Dextromethorphan's side effects are uncommon but may include drowsiness, nausea, vomiting, stomach discomfort, and constipation.

- The most common diphenhydramine side effects include drowsiness, disturbed coordination, decreased respiration, blurred vision, difficult urination, and dry mouth.
- Codeine, dextromethorphan, and diphenhydramine interact with all drugs that cause drowsiness (e.g., narcotics, sedatives, some antihistamines, and alcohol).
- Dextromethorphan also interacts with monoamine oxidase inhibitors (e.g., phenelzine, tranylcypromine, and isocarboxazid). Do not take dextromethorphan within 14 days of taking one of these medications.
- Diphenhydramine also interacts with drugs that have anticholinergic activity, such as monoamine oxidase inhibitors.
- Patients with impaired respiratory reserve (e.g., asthma or chronic obstructive pulmonary disease) should use codeine and diphenhydramine with caution.
- Patients with narrow-angle glaucoma, stenosing peptic ulcer, pyloroduodenal obstruction, symptomatic prostatic hypertrophy, bladder-neck obstruction, elevated intraocular pressure, hyperthyroidism, heart disease, or hypertension should use diphenhydramine with caution.
- Talk with your doctor before using any medication while pregnant.
- Codeine and diphenhydramine are excreted in breast milk and may cause side effects in the child.
- Older adults and children may have paradoxical excitation, restlessness, and irritability with diphenhydramine. Older adults are more likely than the general population to have side effects from diphenhydramine.

Expectorants (Protussives)

- Guaifenesin is the only available nonprescription protussive.
- Guaifenesin is generally well tolerated, but side effects may include nausea, vomiting, dizziness, headache, rash, diarrhea, drowsiness, and stomach pain.
- There are no reported drug interactions with guaifenesin.
- Guaifenesin is contraindicated in patients with a known hypersensitivity to the medication.
- Guaifenesin is not indicated for chronic cough associated with chronic lower respiratory tract diseases such as asthma, chronic obstructive lung disease, emphysema, or smoker's cough.

Evaluation of Patient Outcomes for Cough

For most patients, 7 days of nonprescription drug therapy should relieve cough. If the cough persists but has improved at follow-up, the patient should continue the therapy until the cough is resolved. If the cough has worsened or the patient has developed other exclusions for self-treatment (Figure 12-1), the patient should be referred for further medical evaluation.

Key Points for Cough

- ➤ Cough is an important respiratory defensive reflex.
- ➤ Antitussives (cough suppressants) are the drugs of choice for nonproductive coughs.
- ➤ Protussives (expectorants) are the drugs of choice for coughs that expel thick, tenacious secretions from the lungs with difficulty.
- ➤ Refer patients who have a cough with thick yellow or green sputum, fever greater than 101.5°F, unintended weight loss, drenching night sweats, hemoptysis, underlying chronic disease associated with cough, foreign object aspiration, suspected drug-associated cough, cough lasting more than 7 days, or cough that worsens or is associated with new symptoms during self-treatment to their primary care provider.
- ➤ Neither codeine nor dextromethorphan has been shown to be effective for acute coughs associated with viral URTI in either adults or children.
- ➤ In response to a 2007 FDA public health advisory, many manufacturers voluntarily withdrew cough and cold prod-

ucts intended for infants and young children from the market. In 2008, manufacturers voluntarily updated labels for the remaining cough and cold products to state "do not use" in children under 4 years of age.

➤ Combination products are convenient but generally more expensive per dose and increase the risk of undesirable side effects.

➤ Convenience dosage forms (e.g., oral disintegrating strips) are generally more expensive per dose than standard dosage forms.

➤ Refer patients with cough and a history of or symptoms of chronic underlying disease associated with cough (e.g., asthma, COPD, chronic bronchitis, or heart failure) to their primary care provider.

REFERENCES

1. Cherry DK, Woodwell DA, Rechsteiner EA. *National Ambulatory Medical Care Survey: 2005 Summary*. Hyattsville, Md: National Center for Health Statistics; 2007. Advance Data from Vital and Health Statistics, No. 387. Available at: http://www.cdc.gov/nchs/data/ad/ad387.pdf. Last accessed August 3, 2008.

2. Burt CW, Schappert SM. Ambulatory care visits to physician offices, hospital outpatient departments, and emergency departments: United States, 1999–2000. National Center for Health Statistics. *Vital Health Stat*. 2004; 13(157):30.

3. Irwin RS. Introduction to the diagnosis and management of cough. *Chest*. 2006;129:25S–7S.

4. Top 200 OTC/HBC brands in 2006. *Drug Top*. May 2007;51:42–3.

5. Widdicombe J, Eccles, R, Fontana G. Supramedullary influences on cough. *Respir Physiol Neurobiol*. 2006;152:320–8.

6. Canning BJ. Anatomy and neurophysiology of the cough reflex. *Chest*. 2006;129:33S–47S.

7. Mazzone SB. Sensory regulation of the cough reflex. *Pulm Pharmacol Ther*. 2004;17:361–8.

8. Chang AB. The physiology of cough. *Paediatric Respir Rev*. 2006;7:2–8.

9. Canning BJ. Encoding of the cough reflex. *Pulm Pharmacol Ther*. 2007; 20:396–401.

10. Jacoby DB. Pathophysiology of airway viral infections. *Pulm Pharmacol Ther*. 2004;17:333–6.

11. Fontana GA, Widdicombe J. What is cough and what should be measured? *Pulm Pharmacol Ther*. 2007;20:307–12.

12. Dykewicz MS. Cough and angioedema from angiotensin-converting enzyme inhibitors: new insights into mechanisms and management. *Curr Opin Allergy Clin Immunol*. 2004;4:267–70.

13. Self-care of coughing. In: Albrant DH, ed. *The American Pharmaceutical Association Drug Treatment Protocols*. Washington, DC: American Pharmaceutical Association; 2001:417–22.

14. Guppy MPB, Mickan SM, Del Mar CB. "Drink plenty of fluids": a systematic review of evidence for this recommendation in acute respiratory infections. *BMJ*. 2004;328:499–500.

15. Food and Drug Administration. Cold, cough, allergy, bronchodilataor, and antiasthmatic drug products for over-the-counter human use. *CFR*. 2006; Title 21, Vol 5, Pt 341. Available at: http://www.gpoaccess.gov/CFR/INDEX.HTML. Last accessed August 23, 2008.

16. 2007 Survey of Pharmacy Law. Mount Prospect, Ill: National Association of Boards of Pharmacy, 2007:65–7.

17. Peters RJ, Kelder SH, Markham CM, et al. Beliefs and social norms about codeine and promethazine hydrochloride cough syrup (CPHCS) onset and perceived addiction among urban Houstonian adolescents: an addiction trend in the city of lean. *J Drug Educ*. 2003;33:415–25.

18. American Academy of Pediatrics. Committee on Drugs. Use of codeine- and dextromethorphan-containing cough remedies in children. *Pediatrics*. 1997;99:918–20.

19. Statement from CHPA on the Voluntary Label Updates to Oral OTC Children's Cough and Cold Medicines. Available at: http://www.chpa-info.org. Last accessed October 24, 2008.

20. FDA Statement Following CHPA's Announcement on Nonprescription Over-the-Counter Cough and Cold Medicines in Children [news release]. Available at: http://www.fda.gov/bbs/topics/NEW/2008/NEW01899.html. Last accessed October 24, 2008.

21. Cold, cough, allergy, bronchodilator, and antiasthmatic drug products for over-the-counter human use. *CFR*. 2006; Title 21, Vol. 5, Pt 342. Available at: http://www.fda.gov. Last accessed October 24, 2008.

22. Banerji S, Anderson IB. Abuse of Coricidin HBP cough and cold tablets: episodes recorded by a poison center. *Am J Health-Syst Pharm*. 2001;58:1811–4.

23. Dicpinigaitis PV, Gayle YE. Effect of the second-generation antihistamine, fexofenadine, on cough reflex sensitivity and pulmonary function. *Br J Clin Pharmacol*. 2003;56:501–4.

24. Over-the-counter (OTC) cough remedies. *Med Lett Drug Ther*. 2001; 43:23–5.

25. American Academy of Pediatrics. Committee on Drugs. Camphor revisited: focus on toxicity. *Pediatrics*. 1994;94:127–8.

26. Schroeder K, Fahey T. Systematic review of randomized controlled trials of over-the-counter cough medicines for acute cough in adults. *BMJ*. 2002;324:329–34.

27. Schroeder K, Fahey T. Should we advise parents to administer over-the-counter cough medicines for acute cough? Systematic review of randomized controlled trials. *Arch Dis Child*. 2002;86:170–5.

28. Schroeder K, Fahey T. Over-the-counter medications for acute cough in children and adults in ambulatory settings. *Cochrane Database Syst Rev*. 2004;4:CD001831.

29. Lee PCL, Jawad MSN, Eccles R. Antitussive efficacy of dextromethorphan in cough associated with acute upper respiratory tract infection. *J Pharmacol Ther*. 2000;52:1137–42.

30. Eccles R. The powerful placebo in cough studies? *Pulm Pharmacol Ther*. 2002;15:303–8.

31. Eccles R. Mechanisms of the placebo effect of sweet cough syrups. *Respir Physiol Neurobiol*. 2006;152:340–8.

32. Irwin RS, Baumann MH, Boulet L-P, et al. Diagnosis and management of cough. Executive summary. *Chest*. 2006;129:1S–23S.

33. Morice AH, McGarvey L, Pavord I. Recommendations for the management of cough in adults. *Thorax*. 2006;61(suppl 1):i1–i24.

34. Pratter MR. Cough and the common cold. *Chest*. 2006;129:72S–4S.

35. Pratter MR. Chronic upper airway cough syndrome secondary to rhinosinus diseases (previously referred to as postnasal drip syndrome). *Chest*. 2006;129:63S–71S.

36. Traynor K. FDA investigating nonprescription cough and cold products. *Am J Health-Syst Pharm*. 2007;64:802–3.

37. Public Health Advisory. Nonprescription Cough and Cold Medicine Use in Children. January 17, 2008. Available at: http://www.fda.gov/cder/drug/advisory/cough_cold_2008.htm. Last accessed August 23, 2008.

38. American Academy of Pediatrics. Committee on Drugs. The transfer of drugs and other chemicals into human milk. *Pediatrics*. 2001;108:776–89.

39. Koren G, Pastuszak A, Ito S. Drugs in pregnancy. *N Engl J Med*. 1998; 338:1128–37.

40. Einarson A, Lyszkiewicz D, Koren G. The safety of dextromethorphan in pregnancy. *Chest*. 2001;119:466–9.

41. Paul IM, Beiler J, McMonagle A, et al. Effect of honey, dextromethorphan, and no treatment on nocturnal cough and sleep quality for coughing children and their parents. *Arch Pediatr Adolesc Med*. 2007;161:1140–6.

Asthma

Suzanne G. Bollmeier and Theresa R. Prosser

Asthma is the fourth most common chronic health condition in the United States.[1] In 2004, there were 13.6 million asthma visits to private physician offices and hospital outpatient departments compared with just 5.9 million visits in 1980.[2] Asthma is one of the 10 most common diagnoses seen in emergency departments and is responsible for 500,000 hospitalizations per year.[1] In 2004, 1.8 million emergency department visits were related to asthma symptoms.[3] The death rate from asthma in the United States for children ages 5 to 14 years increased from 1.5 to 3.7 deaths per million children during the periods of 1979–1980 and 1993–1995, respectively.[1] Currently, the death rate overall is 1.4 deaths per 100,000 adults.[2]

Ideally, most treatment for asthma should be in the ambulatory setting and should focus on preventing symptoms, rather than treating asthma exacerbations. Patients with asthma need to know how to take their medications, monitor for worsening symptoms, manage environmental triggers, and recognize when to seek medical care. Fortunately, asthma is usually responsive to comprehensive treatment. Adequately treated patients with asthma can have a normal life span and quality of life. Developing an optimal, comprehensive, and individualized asthma care plan, however, requires a partnership between individuals with asthma and their health care providers. Therefore, self-*care* is a critical part of management. However, isolated self-*treatment* of asthma-like symptoms is potentially dangerous. Other serious conditions, such as heart failure, can cause similar symptoms. In addition, mild asthma symptoms may escalate into serious exacerbations, if inadequately treated.

An estimated 22.2 million people in the United States have asthma.[2] The number of people with asthma doubled between 1979–1980 and 1993–1994. The asthma rate is increasing more rapidly in children than in adults.[1] Asthma affects more than 6 million children in the United States.[4] A family history of asthma increases the risk of developing asthma, but those with atopy have an even greater risk.[4] Being exposed to irritants such as tobacco smoke and allergens early in life has also been shown to increase the incidence of asthma.[4]

Asthma more negatively affects some subsets of the population.[1] Children younger than 5 years of age and women are more likely to be hospitalized for asthma. Nonwhite people are twice as likely to be hospitalized for or die from asthma despite similar asthma rates.[2] Poverty also appears to be a factor in increasing disability and death rates, possibly because of inadequate access to health care, a greater exposure to environmental allergens and pollutants, and inadequate financial and other resources.[1]

The major role of the lungs is the exchange of oxygen and carbon dioxide between inspired air and the blood. The trachea divides into bronchi for each lung. Progressive branching of the bronchi forms increasingly smaller bronchioles, terminal bronchioles, and finally the acinus, where gas exchange takes place. Stimulation of beta$_2$-receptors in bronchial smooth muscle results in bronchodilation, whereas stimulation of cholinergic, and alpha-adrenergic receptors causes bronchoconstriction. Release of substance P and vasoactive intestinal peptide, (neuromediators from the noncholinergic, nonadrenergic nervous system) can also decrease airway diameter. Goblet cells, intermixed throughout the pulmonary tree, are stimulated by the vagal nerve to increase mucus production. Small hairs lining the airways called cilia move the mucus toward the pharynx, thus keeping dust, bacteria, and other foreign matter out of the lower lungs.

The airflow and the relative diameter of the larger airways can be assessed by the forced expiratory volume at 1 second (FEV_1) and the peak expiratory flow (PEF). FEV_1 measures the amount of air expired in the first second as the subject forcefully exhales from a maximum inspiration. The PEF is the maximum flow at the outset of forced expiration. PEF meters are relatively inexpensive and portable, which makes PEF monitoring suitable for home assessment of asthma. Home monitoring of PEF is recommended for patients who have moderate-to-severe persistent asthma, a history of a severe exacerbation, an unexplained response to environmental or occupational exposures, and for those who may not correctly perceive airflow obstruction and worsening symptoms.[4]

Predicted values for PEF and FEV_1 are determined in part by the individual's age, gender, and height. A value greater than 80% of the predicted value is considered within normal limits. However, there is significant individual variation based on body type and ethnic background. Therefore, "personal best" PEF is recommended for use in asthma self-care plans.[4] The personal best PEF is the highest PEF achieved by the patient over a 2-week period of monitoring when the patient is well. To determine the PEF, patients check their PEF twice daily, once in the morning and again in the late afternoon or early evening hours, 15–20 minutes after using the quick-relief inhaler.[4] For routine home PEF monitoring, patients check their PEF daily in the morning when they first wake up and before taking their asthma medication.

Pathophysiology of Asthma

The exact etiology of asthma is unknown.[5] A positive family history of asthma or concurrent atopy increases the risk of developing asthma. Atopy, a predisposition to produce abnormally high amounts of immunoglobulin E (IgE) after exposure to environmental allergens, may play a role in 50% of those with asthma. Smoking by the mother during pregnancy or exposure to secondhand smoke after birth increases the risk of asthma. It is unclear whether smoking is a direct cause of asthma, but exposure to smoke can precipitate asthma symptoms, increases the rate of decline in lung function, and can decrease the response to asthma therapy. A higher body mass index and obesity also may increase the risk of developing asthma. Severe viral respiratory infections in the first 3 years of life and especially infections with respiratory syncytial viruses may increase the risk of developing asthma and atopy.

Once asthma develops, various stimuli (often called "triggers"; Table 13-1) can precipitate asthma symptoms. Not all patients with asthma have the same triggers and the response of an individual to a particular trigger can change over time.

Although bronchoconstriction may be responsible for some acute asthma symptoms, inflammation is largely responsible for severe and persistent asthma symptoms.[6] Once exposed to a trigger, an immediate or early asthmatic response occurs within minutes. The mechanism includes degranulation of mast cells to release histamine and leukotrienes, which cause bronchoconstriction. In atopic individuals, IgE binding to the mast cells may cause the initial mediator release. As the airways narrow, the peak expiratory flow decreases. If clinically significant bronchoconstriction occurs, symptoms such as wheezing, chest tightness, cough, and shortness of breath occur. Symptoms either resolve spontaneously with clearance of the mediators or in response to bronchodilator treatment.

Mast cells also release chemotactic factors that recruit other inflammatory cells (e.g., eosinophils, neutrophils, and macrophages) to the lungs. Several hours later these cells release their own mediators, which contribute to microvascular leakage, airway edema, and an increase in mucus. This process results in progressive airway obstruction and symptoms.

Bronchial hyperresponsiveness (BHR), an exaggerated airway bronchoconstriction and inflammation in response to triggers, may develop with repeated trigger exposure. BHR is expressed clinically as either frequent-to-continuous symptoms over a period of weeks (persistent asthma) or as a significant worsening of asthma symptoms over several days (asthma exacerbations).

Allergic rhinitis, gastroesophageal reflux disease (GERD), and tobacco smoking all can cause airway hyperreactivity and therefore worsen asthma symptoms.

Because allergic rhinitis is an IgE-mediated atopic disease, it is frequently found in conjunction with asthma (see Chapter 11). Triggers for patients' allergy symptoms are often the same as those for their asthma symptoms. Improvement of allergy symptoms may also improve upper airway hyperreactivity and asthma symptoms. Labels on first-generation antihistamines (e.g., diphenhydramine) caution people with asthma against using these agents, because of concern that the anticholinergic properties may thicken mucus and decrease mucociliary clearance. These effects are generally minor and are outweighed by the benefits when treating allergic rhinitis in asthma patients. Newer antihistamines (e.g., loratadine) do not have anticholinergic properties and do not carry this labeling precaution.

Upper airway hyperreactivity, the risk of asthma-related hospitalization, and the need for oral corticosteroid therapy are increased in people with asthma and concurrent GERD. Approximately 77% of patients with asthma report heartburn, a potential trigger of asthma.[7] Proton pump inhibitor therapy may improve symptoms and pulmonary function in 30% to 50% of patients with GERD and asthma.[8] Antacids and histamine$_2$-receptor–blocking agents may also slowly improve asthma symptoms (see Chapter 14).

Patients with asthma and their family members should be urged not to smoke because tobacco smoke may trigger an asthma exacerbation. Mothers who smoke during pregnancy increase their children's risk of acquiring asthma.[9] Children exposed to tobacco smoke are more likely to develop asthma and have poorer asthma control. Practitioners should educate all patients who use tobacco products about options for cessation (see Chapter 50). All commercially available forms of nicotine replacement therapy may be effective as part of a comprehensive tobacco cessation plan. However, the prescription nicotine nasal spray and inhaler are not recommended for people with asthma, because nicotine could irritate the airways and trigger an exacerbation.

Certain medications can also worsen asthma. Specifically, patients with asthma should be cautious about the use of nonprescription nonsteroidal anti-inflammatory drugs (NSAIDs) used to treat fever and/or pain and inflammation because of an increased risk of aspirin sensitivity (see Chapters 5 and 6). Symptoms of aspirin sensitivity can be severe and life-threatening, and may include itchy or watery eyes, itchy rashes, rashes around

---

TABLE 13-1 Examples of Asthma Triggers

Environmental	Drugs or Chemicals	Conditions or Events
Cold air	Beta-adrenergic blockers	Gastroesophageal reflux
House dust mites	Aspirin	Allergic rhinitis
Cockroaches	Nonsteroidal anti-inflammatory agents	Panic attacks
Animals (e.g., cats, dogs, rodents)	Food or drug preservatives (e.g., metabisulfite)	Menstruation, pregnancy
Indoor irritants (e.g., wood burning stoves)	Seafood, shellfish	Viral respiratory infections
Outdoor air pollution (e.g., vehicle emissions, sulfur dioxide, ozone, nitrogen oxides)	Occupational exposure to dust, chemicals, irritants	Emotional stress, excitement
Indoor or outdoor molds and fungi	Household cleaning agents	Exercise
Tobacco smoke	Perfumes	
Pollen (e.g., grass, weeds, trees)		

the mouth, nasal congestion, hives, worsening asthma, cough or wheezing, and anaphylaxis.[10] There is a significant potential for cross-sensitivity to other NSAIDs such as ibuprofen and naproxen. If a person has aspirin sensitivity, they can usually tolerate acetaminophen. Patients sensitive to aspirin should be cautioned to check the labels of headache and pain relief medications before use to see if they contain NSAIDs. Aspirin-sensitive patients should also be cautioned to avoid other agents that contain salicylates such as oil of wintergreen.

Although some asthma patients insist that certain foods make them wheeze or experience shortness of breath, confirmed asthmatic reactions to food are uncommon.[11] Questionnaires may help identify these triggers (Table 13-6). Eggs and milk are commonly implicated, but other food allergies include wheat, soy, peanuts, fish, and shellfish. Some patients report an allergy to food additives such as tartrazine (FD&C Yellow No. 5), a yellow food colorant, or sulfite, an antioxidant used to preserve food. Soy lecithin, an additive, may worsen asthma in patients allergic to legumes. Those allergic to latex may have cross-reactions with fruits such as avocados, kiwis, and pineapples. Even when the trigger is known, it can be challenging to prospectively identify and avoid foods containing these compounds.

Chronic inflammation can cause permanent airway remodeling. This process involves scar tissue deposition, increased bronchial smooth muscle mass, and increased mucus gland mass.[6] A fixed airway obstruction develops, and symptoms become less responsive to treatment with either anti-inflammatory or bronchodilatory medications.[4,5]

The current understanding of asthma pathophysiology has affected the approach to acute and chronic asthma treatment. Asthma exacerbations can be prevented by avoiding repeated trigger exposure or by pretreating with medications prior to exposure to a known trigger. Inhaled corticosteroids are used daily in persistent asthma to prevent chronic inflammation. Severe symptoms, a longer duration of symptoms, and a partial or poor response of symptoms to bronchodilators imply that inflammation is likely present and that anti-inflammatory medications are needed. Only bronchodilator medications are available without a prescription. Therefore, an individual with asthma needs to recognize when significant airway inflammation is present and to seek appropriate medical care.

Clinical Presentation of Asthma

Key features of asthma are recurrent bouts of wheezing, shortness of breath, chest tightness, and cough, especially at night and in the early morning hours. Asthma symptoms vary in duration, severity, and frequency (Table 13-2). The severity of asthma

TABLE 13-2 Classifying Asthma Severity and Stepwise Approach for Managing Asthma in Youths ≥12 Years of Age and Adults

Classification	Components	Lung Function	Preferred Therapy
Severe persistent	Symptoms: throughout the day Nighttime awakenings: often 7 times a week Short-acting beta-agonist use: several times per day Interference with normal activity: extremely limited	FEV_1 less than <60% predicted FEV_1/FVC reduced by >5%	Medium dose inhaled corticosteroid AND long-acting beta-agonist Short-acting bronchodilator: inhaled $beta_2$-agonists as needed for symptoms
Moderate persistent	Symptoms: daily Nighttime awakenings: >1 time a week but not nightly Short-acting beta-agonists use: daily Interference with normal activity: some limitation	FEV_1 >60% but <80% predicted FEV_1/FVC reduced 5%	Low dose inhaled corticosteroids AND long-acting beta-agonist OR medium dose inhaled corticosteroid Short-acting bronchodilator: inhaled $beta_2$-agonists as needed for symptoms
Mild persistent	Symptoms: >2 days a week but not daily Nighttime awakenings: 3–4 times a month Short-acting beta-agonists use: >2 days a week but not daily, and not more than 1 time on any day Interference with normal activity: minor limitation	FEV_1 >80% predicted FEV_1/FVC normal	Low dose inhaled corticosteroid Short-acting bronchodilator: inhaled $beta_2$-agonists as needed for symptoms
Intermittent	Symptoms: ≤2 days a week Nighttime awakenings: ≤2 times a month. Short-acting beta-agonists use: ≤2 days a week Interference with normal activity: none	Normal FEV_1 between exacerbations FEV_1 >80% predicted FEV_1/FVC normal	No daily controller medication needed Short-acting bronchodilator: inhaled $beta_2$-agonists as needed for symptoms

Key: FEV_1, forced expiratory volume at 1 second; FVC, forced vital capacity.
Source: Reference 4.

exacerbations is assessed on the basis of the severity of the symptoms (Table 13-3). Patients with asthma need to monitor for worsening control and identify the onset of acute asthma exacerbations. A drop in PEF can be the first sign of an impending exacerbation and may precede the onset of significant symptoms. A drop in PEF of 20% warrants a change in drug therapy. Patients who have moderate-to-severe persistent asthma or a history of a severe exacerbation should have an asthma self-care plan (Figure 13-1), which provides guidance for symptom treatment and when to seek immediate medical attention. Early treatment with systemic anti-inflammatory agents may decrease the need for emergency department visits and hospitalizations for asthma.

Other conditions may present with asthma-like symptoms (Table 13-4). In assessing someone who presents with shortness of breath, it is important to inquire about a prior diagnosis of asthma, tobacco use, and onset and duration of symptoms. It is also important to inquire about other associated signs (e.g., edema) or symptoms (e.g., feverishness). If the individual does not have a prior diagnosis of asthma or if the symptoms are different or more severe than usual, a medical referral is necessary for further evaluation (Table 13-5).

Symptoms usually respond to medications; however, severe asthma exacerbations may require emergent care and systemic corticosteroids. Even patients with mild asthma can develop life-threatening exacerbations. Risk factors for death from asthma include[4]:

- A history of severe asthma exacerbations.
- Previous intubation or admission to an intensive care unit for asthma.

- Two or more hospitalizations, or three or more emergency department visits for asthma within the past year.
- A hospitalization or emergency department visit within the past month.
- Use of more than two canisters per month of inhaled short-acting beta$_2$-agonist.
- A recent or current withdrawal from systemic corticosteroids.
- Low socioeconomic status.
- Urban residence.
- Illicit drug use.

Treatment of Asthma
Treatment Goals

Most patients realize that severe symptoms requiring the need for urgent medical care represents uncontrolled asthma. However, optimal therapy implies that *all* goals are met. The goals include achieving and maintaining control of symptoms, having normal activity levels, infrequently using an inhaled short-acting beta-agonist (less than twice per week), maintaining pulmonary function as close to normal as possible, preventing recurrent exacerbations and the need for urgent care visits, providing optimal pharmacologic therapy with minimal or no adverse effects, and meeting the patient's and their family's expectations of asthma care.[4] Even relatively mild-to-moderate symptoms of asthma can significantly impair the quality of life. Because most symptoms are readily responsive to medications, it is important for the patient to understand that frequent symptoms (even mild ones) can

TABLE 13-3 Classification Scheme for Asthma Exacerbations and Warning Symptoms in Adults

	Mild	Moderate	Severe	Respiratory Arrest Imminent
Symptoms				
Breathlessness	Occurs while walking Can lie down	Occurs while at rest Prefers sitting	Occurs while at rest Sits upright	
Talks in . . .	Sentences	Phrases	Words	
Alertness	May be agitated	Usually agitated	Usually agitated	Drowsy or confused
Signs				
Respiratory rate	Increased	Increased	Often >30/min	
Use of accessory muscles: suprasternal retractions	Usually not	Commonly	Usually	Paradoxical thoracoabdominal movement
Wheeze	Moderate, often only end expiratory	Loud, throughout exhalation	Usually loud, throughout inhalation and exhalation	Absence of wheeze
Pulse/minute	<100	100–120	>120	Bradycardia
Functional Assessment				
PEF	≥70%	Approx. 40%–69%, or response lasts <2 hours	<40%	<25% *Note:* PEF assessment may not be needed in very severe attacks.

Key: PEF, peak expiratory flow.
Source: Reference 4.

ASTHMA ACTION PLAN

St. Louis Regional *Asthma Consortium*

Sponsored by the American Lung Association of Eastern Missouri

Name: _____

Provider: _____

Date: _____

Phone for doctor or clinic: _____

After office hours call: _____

GREEN ZONE

- Breathing is good
- No cough or wheeze
- Can work and play

YOU'RE OK! TAKE ALL OF THESE MEDICATIONS EVERY DAY!

Medicine	How much to take	When to take it
_____	_____	_____
_____	_____	_____
_____	_____	_____
_____	_____	_____

20 minutes before physical activity, use this medicine: _____

YELLOW ZONE

- You are feeling sick or it's harder to breathe

CAUTION! TAKE 2 PUFFS (OR 1 NEBULIZER TREATMENT) OF YOUR QUICK RELIEVER MEDICINE NOW: _____
YOU MAY REPEAT THIS EVERY 20 MINUTES FOR 2 MORE TIMES.
IF YOU ARE NO BETTER CALL YOUR DOCTOR
IMMEDIATELY AT _____ !

Cough	Wheeze	Tight chest	Wake up at night

Medicine	How much to take	When to take it
_____	_____	_____
_____	_____	_____

RED ZONE

- Medicine is not helping
- Breathing is hard and fast
- Nose opens wide
- Can't walk or talk well
- Ribs show

DANGER!
TAKE 4 MORE PUFFS (OR 1 NEBULIZER TREATMENT)
OF YOUR QUICK RELIEVER MEDICINE NOW.
CALL 9-1-1 OR GO DIRECTLY TO THE NEAREST HOSPITAL!

Medicine	How much to take	When to take it
_____	_____	_____
_____	_____	_____
_____	_____	_____

FIGURE 13-1 Sample asthma self-care plan. (Reprinted with the permission of the St. Louis Regional Asthma Consortium.)

TABLE 13-4 Comparison of Selected Conditions That May Present with Respiratory Symptoms

	Asthma	Chronic Obstructive Pulmonary Disease	Respiratory Infection	Heart Failure
Signs	Decreased PEF Increased heart rate Increased respiratory rate	Progressive decline in PEF and FEV_1 Polycythemia Signs of right heart failure Pulmonary hypertension Decreased oxygen saturation Pursed lip breathing Increased heart rate Increased respiratory rate	Increased heart rate Increased respiratory rate Fever Increased white blood cell count	Ejection fraction <40% Lower extremity edema, S_3 heart sound Positive hepatojugular reflex Jugular venous distension
Symptoms	Wheezing Cough Chest tightness	Progressive dyspnea on exertion Productive cough Wheezing	Productive cough Nasal congestion Rhinorrhea	Dyspnea on exertion Orthopnea
Onset	Often occurs in childhood, but can develop in adults	Usually the forth or fifth decade of life Progressive; symptoms develop over years	Any age Symptoms acute, sudden	Older adults
Etiology	Often atopy	Most commonly tobacco smoking	Viruses Bacteria	Hypertension Coronary artery disease
Exacerbating factors	Trigger exposure	Continued smoking		Heavy salt intake, Myocardial infarction Nonadherence with medications

Key: FEV_1, forced expiratory volume at 1 second; PEF, peak expiratory flow.

TABLE 13-5 Comparison of Indications for Self-Treatment with Nonprescription Medications versus Medical Care for Asthma

Self-treatment *may* be appropriate when:	Referral for medical care *should* be made when:
■ A prior diagnosis of intermittent asthma has been made by a health care provider AND ■ The individual knows the warning symptoms indicating the need for urgent medical care AND ■ The individual does not have any other serious concurrent diseases that might impair oxygenation or breathing (e.g., chronic obstructive pulmonary disease, coronary artery disease) AND ■ The individual is age 5 years or older and not pregnant AND ■ The current asthma symptoms are consistent with previous symptoms AND ■ The current symptoms are mild, intermittent (less than twice weekly), and of short duration (e.g., <24 hours) OR ■ The nonprescription medications are for short-term (<24 hours) treatment of mild symptoms until the individual can be seen by a health care provider	■ The individual does not have a previous diagnosis of asthma OR ■ The individual has a concurrent condition with symptoms (e.g., cough, wheeze, or shortness of breath) that may be similar to asthma (e.g., heart failure, chronic obstructive pulmonary disease, vocal cord dysfunction) OR ■ The individual has a history of asthma episodes severe enough to require systemic corticosteroids or urgent medical care OR ■ The individual is taking (or nonadherent to) other prescription long-term controller medications for asthma OR ■ The individual does not have an asthma care provider or has not seen their asthma care provider in the last year OR ■ The individual is pregnant or a child younger than 5 years OR ■ The individual perceives that the prescription medications are not effective OR ■ The symptoms are of moderate severity (e.g., affect activities or sleep) or are more frequent than twice weekly OR ■ The symptoms have lasted more than 24 hours OR ■ The symptoms do not respond to nonprescription asthma medications within 24 hours OR ■ The symptoms differ in quality or severity from that in previous episodes OR ■ There are also signs or symptoms of a respiratory or sinus infection (e.g., fever, purulent nasal discharge)

and should be prevented. Patients with asthma also need to be confident that they can successfully prevent escalation of symptoms into significant asthma exacerbations.

General Treatment Approach

Asthma medications are categorized into two groups. Quick-relief medications are used as needed to treat symptoms. This group includes short-acting beta-agonists (e.g., albuterol), a short-acting anticholinergic (ipratropium), and systemic corticosteroids (e.g., prednisone) to treat inflammation in moderate-to-severe asthma exacerbations. Long-term control medications are used daily to prevent symptoms. This group includes inhaled corticosteroids (e.g., fluticasone), leukotriene modifiers (e.g., montelukast), mast cell stabilizers (e.g., cromolyn), and long-acting bronchodilators (e.g., salmeterol). Either inhaled beta-agonists or mast cell stabilizers can be used prior to exposure to known triggers (e.g., exercise and cigarette smoke) to prevent symptoms. All patients with asthma should have a short-acting beta-agonist available for as-needed treatment of acute symptoms. Patients with persistent asthma, regardless of severity, should preferably be treated with an inhaled corticosteroid (Table 13-2).

Inhaled medications have fewer adverse reactions compared with systemic medications. However, the effectiveness of inhaled medications is severely limited when poor device technique decreases drug delivery to the lungs. Interested readers are referred to the guidelines from the Global Initiative for Asthma[5] and the National Asthma Education Prevention Program[4] for a detailed discussion of the therapeutic options and rationale for the treatment of asthma in adults and children.

A comprehensive, individualized *asthma self-care plan* includes when to utilize long-term control medications and quick-relief medications, how to use asthma devices to optimally deliver medications, how to avoid and minimize affects of asthma triggers, how to prevent the escalation of asthma symptoms into exacerbations, and how to recognize warning signs that require emergent medical treatment. Specific recommendations are provided for when to use quick-relief medications (e.g., prior to exposure to known triggers) and how much to use (e.g., 2 puffs every 2 hours). Figure 13-1 is an example of a symptom-based asthma self-care plan. Some self-care plans include recommendations based on the patient's personal best PEF.

Nonpharmacologic Therapy

Because exposure to triggers can lead to worsening asthma symptoms and because each patient's asthma triggers are different, a comprehensive, individualized trigger management plan should be developed. A screening tool can be utilized to help identify asthma triggers (Table 13-6). Once triggers are identified, suggestions are incorporated into the self-care plan to minimize exposure to triggers at home, work, or school (see Chapter 11).

Nonprescription Pharmacologic Therapy

Few nonprescription medications are available to treat asthma (Table 13-7).[12–15] Nonprescription medications are generally indicated for only mild infrequent symptoms. Patients who have more frequent or serious symptoms should be referred for a prescription long-term controller. Figure 13-2 lists additional

---

TABLE 13-6 Example of a Trigger Screen Tool[a]

Thinking about how you have felt in the past month, please answer the following questions. . . .

Do you ever have problems with wheezing or catching your breath when exposed to cold air?

Do you wheeze when dusting, vacuuming, or using cleaning solvents in the home?

Do you wheeze, cough, or sneeze, or become short of breath when around household pets such as cats or dogs?

Do you have problems breathing when exposed to high levels of stress or excitement?

Have you ever noticed wheezing or worsening shortness of breath before or during your menstrual period?

Have you ever had a reaction such as shortness of breath, swollen throat, lips, or tongue after you took medications such as aspirin or ibuprofen?

Do you have breathing problems after eating shellfish, peanuts, or any other foods?

Do you have breathing problems when exposed to latex (e.g., rubber gloves or balloons)?

Does it take you a long time to get over a viral cold?

Do you have chronic heartburn?

Do you have problems breathing at work, yet are fine during holidays or weekends spent at home?

Does anyone else at work appear to have similar symptoms?

Do you typically have a runny nose and watery eyes, and experience repetitive sneezing during outdoor activities?
Are these symptoms worse during:
    Early spring?
    Late spring?
    Late summer to fall?
    Summer and fall?

Do you experience shortness of breath during or after exercise?

If you answered yes to any of the above questions, please show this questionnaire to your health care provider.

---

[a] See Chapter 11 for more information on allergies and triggers.

TABLE 13-7 Medications Included in Nonprescription Products for the Treatment of Asthma

Drug	Mechanism	Dosage and Administration				Safety Considerations
Epinephrine (e.g., Primatene Mist Inhaler)	Bronchodilator	Adults and children older than 4 years: 1 puff at onset of symptoms. If symptoms are not relieved in 1 minute, repeat 1 puff. Do not use again for 3 hours.				Seek medical assistance if symptoms are not relieved or worsen in 20 minutes. Adverse drug reactions include increased heart rate, arrhythmias, and nervousness. Do not use with concomitant MAOI therapy. Contraindications include pregnancy, cardiac arrhythmias, coronary insufficiency, poorly controlled hypertension, and seizures, hypokalemia, angina, hyperglycemia, and uncontrolled hyperthyroidism.
Racepinephrine (e.g., microNefrin)	Bronchodilator	Adults and children 4 years and older (microNefrin) 2.25% racepinephrine HCl (1.125% epinephrine base): Pour 0.5 mL (10 drops) racepinephrine into nebulizer reservoir; add 3 mL diluent; administer for 15 minutes every 3–4 hours.				Relative contraindications include pregnancy, hyperthyroidism, hypertension, heart disease, use of other medications (prescription, nonprescription, or herbal therapy). Do not use this product if it is brown in color or cloudy.
Ephedrine/ guaifenesin combination products	Bronchodilator + expectorant	Bronkaid Dual Action Formula	Ephedrine 25 mg	Guaifenesin 400 mg	1 tablet every 4 hours as needed; do not exceed 6 tablets per day	Ephedrine side effects include palpitations, tachycardia, arrhythmias, seizures, hypokalemia, angina, hyperglycemia, hypotension, and hypertension. Guaifenesin: Case reports have linked nephrolithiasis to guaifenesin alone and in combination with ephedrine.
		Primatene Tablets	Ephedrine 12.5 mg	Guaifenesin 200 mg	2 tablets every 4 hours as needed; do not exceed 12 tablets per day	
		Mini Two Way Action Tablets	Ephedrine 12.5 mg	Guaifenesin 200 mg	1–2 tablets every 4 hours as needed; do not exceed 12 tablets per day	
		Dynafed Asthma Relief Tablets	Ephedrine 25 mg	Guaifenesin 200 mg	1/2 to 1 tablet every 4 hours as needed; do not exceed 6 tablets per day	
		Mini Two Way Action Tablets	Ephedrine 25 mg	Guaifenesin 200 mg	1/2 to 1 tablet every 4 hours as needed; do not exceed 6 tablets per day	

Key: MAOI, monoamine oxidase inhibitor.
Source: References 12–15.

exclusions for self-care. All patients with asthma should be followed closely by a primary care practitioner.

Bronchodilators

Two nonselective beta-agonists, epinephrine and ephedrine, are available without a prescription (Table 13-7). Because nonselective beta-agonists also act on alpha-receptors, they can constrict blood vessels and increase blood pressure, thus having the potential to cause arrhythmias, nervousness, and palpitations. Generally, nonprescription beta-agonists have a shorter duration of action requiring more frequent administration, and they have a greater potential for side effects compared with similar prescription medications.

The Food and Drug Administration (FDA) has ruled that the sale of chlorofluorocarbon (CFC)-containing nonprescription

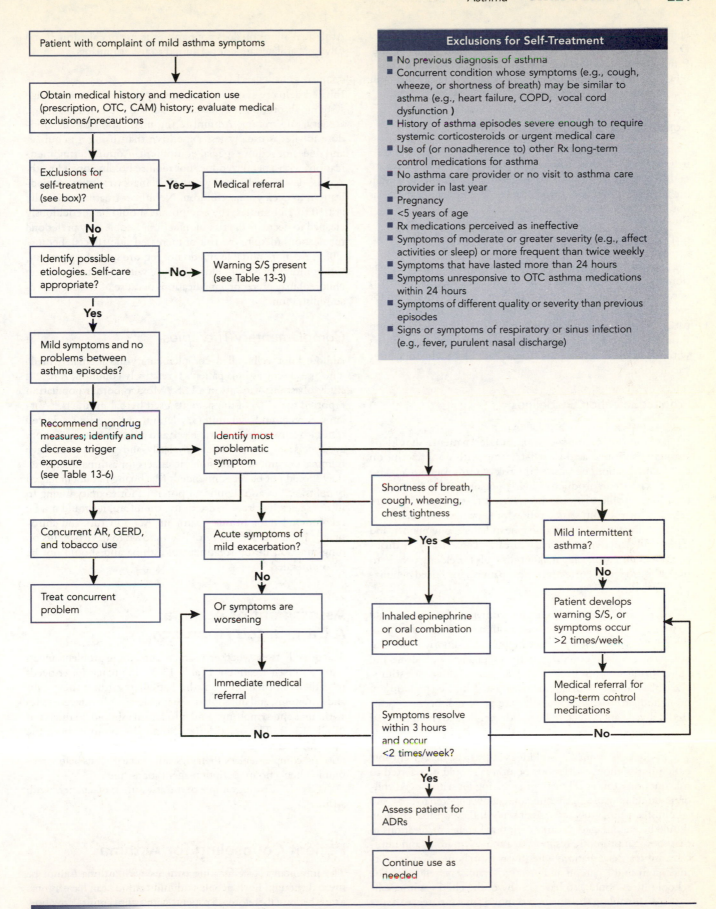

Patient with complaint of mild asthma symptoms

Obtain medical history and medication use (prescription, OTC, CAM) history; evaluate medical exclusions/precautions

Exclusions for self-treatment (see box)? —**Yes**→ Medical referral

No

Identify possible etiologies. Self-care appropriate? —**No**→ Warning S/S present (see Table 13-3)

Yes

Mild symptoms and no problems between asthma episodes?

Recommend nondrug measures; identify and decrease trigger exposure (see Table 13-6)

Identify most problematic symptom

Concurrent AR, GERD, and tobacco use

Treat concurrent problem

Acute symptoms of mild exacerbation?

Shortness of breath, cough, wheezing, chest tightness

Mild intermittent asthma?

Yes

No

Or symptoms are worsening

Inhaled epinephrine or oral combination product

Patient develops warning S/S, or symptoms occur >2 times/week

Immediate medical referral

Medical referral for long-term control medications

Symptoms resolve within 3 hours and occur <2 times/week? —**No**— ... —**No**—

Yes

Assess patient for ADRs

Continue use as needed

Exclusions for Self-Treatment

- No previous diagnosis of asthma
- Concurrent condition whose symptoms (e.g., cough, wheeze, or shortness of breath) may be similar to asthma (e.g., heart failure, COPD, vocal cord dysfunction)
- History of asthma episodes severe enough to require systemic corticosteroids or urgent medical care
- Use of (or nonadherence to) other Rx long-term control medications for asthma
- No asthma care provider or no visit to asthma care provider in last year
- Pregnancy
- <5 years of age
- Rx medications perceived as ineffective
- Symptoms of moderate or greater severity (e.g., affect activities or sleep) or more frequent than twice weekly
- Symptoms that have lasted more than 24 hours
- Symptoms unresponsive to OTC asthma medications within 24 hours
- Symptoms of different quality or severity than previous episodes
- Signs or symptoms of respiratory or sinus infection (e.g., fever, purulent nasal discharge)

FIGURE 13-2 Self-care of asthma. Key: ADR, adverse drug reaction; AR, allergic rhinitis; CAM, complementary and alternative medicine; COPD, chronic obstructive pulmonary disease; GERD, gastroesophageal reflux disease; OTC, over-the-counter; Rx, prescription; S/S, signs and symptoms.

epinephrine metered-dose inhalers shall be phased out by December 31, 2010. The manufacturer of inhaled epinephrine, Primatene Mist, will comply with the final FDA ruling, but a CFC-free product may become available before the phaseout is complete.[16]

Combination Bronchodilator Products

Compared with inhaled medications, nonprescription oral products (Table 13-7) have a greater potential for side effects because of their systemic absorption. An expectorant, guaifenesin, is often included in combination products, but its efficacy in asthma has not been shown (see Chapter 12).

Influenza Vaccine

All patients with asthma should receive an influenza vaccination yearly.[4] An intranasal form of influenza vaccine (FluMist) is available. This prescription-only live vaccine is indicated for patients ages 2 to 49 years. FluMist is not recommended for patients with a history of asthma or reactive airways disease and should not be administered to children younger than 5 years with recurrent wheezing because of the risk of wheezing after vaccination.[17]

Product Selection Guidelines

SPECIAL POPULATION CONSIDERATIONS

Persons of Advanced Age Older patients should be strongly cautioned against self-treating with nonprescription asthma medications because of the risk of cardiovascular adverse effects with these products. Elderly persons with a new-onset breathing problem should be referred to their primary care provider to rule out other causes of shortness of breath that mimic asthma, such as congestive heart failure, pneumonia, and chronic obstructive pulmonary disease (Table 13-4). Arthritis and impaired vision may make it difficult for elderly people to use asthma devices correctly. These patients may need nebulizers to deliver medications.

Pregnant Patients Pregnant women with asthma should be urged not to use nonprescription asthma medications without the knowledge of their health care provider. Poorly controlled asthma can worsen outcomes of the pregnancy. Ephedrine and epinephrine are both Pregnancy Category C drugs that stimulate alpha- and beta-adrenergic receptors.[18] Inhaled prescription bronchodilators (e.g., albuterol)[19] are preferred, because localized delivery and selective beta$_2$-adrenergic activity limit fetal drug exposure.

Pediatric Patients Children with wheezing or a chronic cough but without a diagnosis of asthma should be referred to rule out other causes.[20] Practitioners caring for school-aged children should know local laws that may allow children to carry and administer asthma medications at school. Responsible children should be encouraged to carry their quick-relief medications so that they can promptly respond to asthma symptoms and minimize asthma exacerbations when away from home. Written permission from the parents and practitioner may be required. The school nurse should also have a copy of the child's asthma self-care plan, enabling the nurse to respond appropriately to acute asthma exacerbations that develop at school. Student athletes should check with school administrators before self-administering nonprescription asthma medications. The National Collegiate

Athletic Association does not permit the use of ephedrine[21] and Olympic athletes are not permitted to use stimulants.

PATIENT PREFERENCES

Inhaled delivery systems are generally preferred to minimize systemic absorption and side effects such as increased heart rate, anxiety, and tremor. Administering medication by metered-dose inhaler is usually less expensive than using a nebulizer and does not require special equipment. Administering medications with a nebulizer does not require holding one's breath, and the device can be used with a facial mask to administer medications to even young children. Nebulizer treatments usually last 10 to 15 minutes; the equipment should be meticulously cleaned to decrease the risk of infection. People may prefer oral medications (despite the risk of increased side effects), because tablets are more portable and do not require special equipment. Other individuals (e.g., elderly, those with arthritis, or young children) may prefer oral medications because of relative ease of administration.

Complementary Therapies

Although not well studied, complementary and alternative medicine use among asthma patients is relatively common. A recent study of asthma patients in a U.S./Mexico border population reported that 42% of the patients used herbal products.[22] Vitamin A, vitamin E, vitamin C, selenium, magnesium, selected omega-3 fatty acids, as well as black and oregano teas, cinnamon, eucalyptus and peppermint oil, royal jelly, and cayenne chiles have minimal documented physiologic effects for asthma; therefore, they should not be recommended. Ma-huang has documented benefits[23,24] but also significant potential for toxicity owing to its nonselective adrenergic activity; therefore, it should not be recommended for asthma treatment. Acupuncture and chiropractic manipulation have not been shown to have benefits on lung function in the treatment of asthma and should not be recommended.[25]

Assessment of Asthma: A Case-Based Approach

To correctly assess whether a patient's breathing problems meets criteria for self-treatment (Table 13-5), the practitioner needs to gather information from the patient regarding their signs and symptoms, and duration of the problem. Other disease states with signs and symptoms similar to asthma should be ruled out (Table 13-4). The practitioner should also inquire about the patient's current use of prescription and nonprescription medications, complementary therapies, and dietary habits before recommending a nonprescription agent for asthma.

Case 13-1 is an example of the assessment of a patient with asthma.

Patient Counseling for Asthma

The importance of educating patients with asthma cannot be stressed enough. Even people with mild asthma can have asthma exacerbations; therefore, all patients with asthma must know how to self-monitor and recognize asthma symptoms, and what action to take if they have symptoms that do not respond to quick-relief medications.[26] Practitioners should assess each patient's readiness

CASE 13-1

Relevant Evaluation Criteria	Scenario/Model Outcome

Information Gathering

1. Gather essential information about the patient's symptoms including:

  a. description of symptom(s) (i.e., nature, onset, duration, severity, associated symptoms)

  Patient describes trouble sleeping due to wheezing, which is worse at night in the hotel room. Patient is in town for a 3-day business meeting and was unable to get a no-smoking room.

  b. description of any factors that seem to precipitate, exacerbate, and/or relieve the patient's symptom(s)

  Patient's symptoms are rare when at home but usually respond to 2 puffs of his prescribed quick-relief medication. He did not bother to bring it with him, because he has not used it in about a year. His asthma has not caused him to miss any work in the past 2 years. He states that secondhand smoke is a known trigger.

  c. description of the patient's efforts to relieve the symptoms

  He rested and drank water, and requested clean sheets from housekeeping last night. Hotel sprayed deodorizer on carpet and drapes per his request.

2. Gather essential patient history information:

  a. patient's identity

  Jay Booker

  b. patient's age, sex, height, and weight

  39-year-old male, 6 ft 0 in, 195 lb

  c. patient's occupation

  Accountant for large law firm. Patient's place of employment is a smoke-free building.

  d. patient's dietary habits

  Eats in the firm's cafeteria for lunch, has cereal for breakfast, and wife cooks dinner nightly.

  e. patient's sleep habits

  Sleeps 8 hours a night. He reports feeling rested and denies daytime drowsiness when at home. Last night in the hotel, however, he had problems sleeping because of his cough and is tired today.

  f. concurrent medical conditions, prescription and nonprescription medications, and dietary supplements

  Past medical history includes allergic rhinitis and eczema.

  Fluticasone (Flonase) prescription nasal spray, nonprescription loratadine (Claritin) 10 mg every day as needed, One-A-Day Men's Multivitamin

  Herbal products or alternative therapies: none

  g. allergies

  Sulfa: hives and shortness of breath

  h. history of other adverse reactions to medications

  N/A

  i. other (describe) ____

  He does not have runny nose or congestion if he takes his Flonase and Claritin.

  Tobacco use: none

  Street drug use: none

  Caffeine use: one cup of coffee a day

Assessment and Triage

3. Differentiate the patient's signs/symptoms and correctly identify the patient's primary problem(s) (see Table 13-4).

  Intermittent asthma

  Triggers: secondhand smoke

4. Identify exclusions for self-treatment (see Table 13-5 and Figure 13-2).

  None

5. Formulate a comprehensive list of therapeutic alternatives for the primary problem to determine if triage to a medical practitioner is required, and share this information with the patient.

  Options include:

  (1) Recommend nonprescription Primatene Mist Inhaler before bedtime.
  (2) Recommend nonprescription Primatene Mist Inhaler as needed for signs and symptoms of wheezing and chest tightness.
  (3) Recommend oral nonprescription combination product as needed for wheezing and chest tightness.
  (4) Recommend a medical referral for follow-up or adequate diagnosis.
  (5) Recommend a medical referral for refill of his prescription quick-relief medication as an alternative to Primatene Mist Inhaler.
  (6) Recommend a medical referral for a long-term controller prescription agent to use prior to trigger exposure (e.g., cromolyn).
  (7) Recommend a medical referral for a prescription long-term controller medication (e.g., inhaled corticosteroid).
  (8) Recommend urgent care visit.
  (9) Take no action.

CASE 13-1 *(continued)*

Relevant Evaluation Criteria	Scenario/Model Outcome
Plan	
6. Select an optimal therapeutic alternative to address the patient's problem, taking into account patient preferences.	The patient cannot see a health care practitioner at this time because of the time of day and his location. His symptoms likely do not require an urgent care visit. His primary doctor is more than 500 miles away in his hometown, and he does not have the office phone number. Given that it is evening and Jay's hometown pharmacy is closed (and is not a national chain), a refill on his albuterol inhaler is impossible.
	Jay would prefer a nonprescription alternative. Primatene Mist inhaler can prevent symptoms if taken before exposure to smoke, and can treat his symptoms of wheezing and chest tightness should they occur after he has been in the hotel room for an extended period of time.
7. Describe the recommended therapeutic approach to the patient.	OTC Primatene Mist Inhaler: 1–2 puffs 15 minutes before exposure to hotel room AND
	1–2 puffs as needed for chest tightness and wheezing
	May repeat 1 time. Do not use again for 3 hours.
8. Explain to the patient the rationale for selecting the recommended therapeutic approach from the considered therapeutic alternatives.	Seeking emergent care may not be necessary if Jay's mild symptoms can be controlled with this therapy. However, he should be encouraged to discuss his symptoms at his next health care practitioner visit.
	It usually takes less medication to prevent symptoms than to treat symptoms once they occur. It is better to use the inhaled, rather than oral, route of medication, because the chance of side effects is reduced.
Patient Education	
9. When recommending self-care with non-prescription medications and/or nondrug therapy, convey accurate information to the patient:	
a. appropriate dose and frequency of administration	See step 7.
b. maximum number of days the therapy should be employed	Jay can use this medication long term if he does not need more than 2 doses per week. If symptoms increase in frequency, he should see his health care provider. Jay will most likely be using this therapy for the short term, because he is returning home tomorrow.
c. product administration procedures	See Figure 13-3.
d. expected time to onset of relief	Inhaler should adequately prevent symptoms for up to 1–2 hours (if taken before exposure to secondhand smoke) and should provide relief within 3–5 minutes if symptoms occur.
e. degree of relief that can be reasonably expected	Adequate prevention and relief from acute symptoms of wheezing and chest tightness are expected.
f. most common side effects	Increased heart rate, tremor, nervousness, insomnia
g. side effects that warrant medical intervention should they occur	Palpitations, irregular heart beat
h. patient options in the event that condition worsens or persists	Seek medical help if you experience an increase in frequency or severity of symptoms, or if symptoms no longer respond to therapy.
i. product storage requirements	Store at room temperature (68°F–77°F). Do not store near open flame or heat above 120°F.
j. specific nondrug measures	Avoid tobacco smoke as much as possible.
10. Solicit follow-up questions from patient.	Should I continue to take my Claritin tablet and Flonase nasal spray while using this inhaler?
11. Answer patient's questions.	Yes. The Claritin may actually help prevent symptoms of wheezing and chest tightness, because allergy symptoms may worsen asthma symptoms in some people. The Flonase should also be used and will not interfere with the Primatene Mist Inhaler.

Key: N/A, not available; OTC, over-the-counter.

Closed Mouth Technique

- Step 1
  — Remove dust cap from inhaler.
  — Attach inhaler to spacer/holding chamber if you have one.
  — Shake the inhaler well, as shown in drawing A.

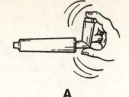

A

- Step 2
  — Blow out all the air in your lungs. (See drawing B.)

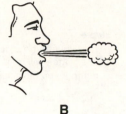

B

- Step 3
  — Seal lips tightly around the mouthpiece.
  — Press down on the inhaler to release medicine as you breathe in slowly until your lungs are full. (See drawing C.)
  — If using a spacer/holding chamber press down on the inhaler and then wait 5 seconds before breathing in. (See drawing C.)

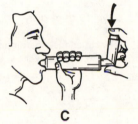

C

- Step 4
  — Hold your breath for 10 seconds to allow medicine to reach deeply into your lungs. (See drawing D.)

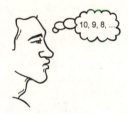 10, 9, 8, ...

D

- Step 5
  — Blow out the air in your lungs. (See drawing E.)

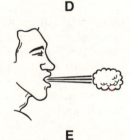

E

Open Mouth Technique

- Step 1
  — Take off the cap.
  — Shake the inhaler.
  — See drawing F.

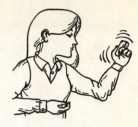

F

- Step 2
  —Stand up and tilt head back a little.
  — See drawing G.

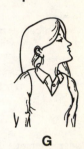

G

- Step 3
  — Place your hand between your mouth and the inhaler. This will help measure how far away the inhaler should be from your mouth. (See drawing H.)

- Step 4
  —Take a cleansing breath, in and out.

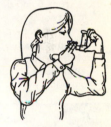

H

- Step 5
  — Open your mouth wide.
  — Start to breathe in slowly.
  — Push down on the medicine and continue to breathe in. (See drawing I.)

- Step 6
  — Hold your breath.
  — Count to 10 and then breathe out.

- Step 7
  — If asthma care plan instructs you to use 2 puffs, wait 15–30 seconds and repeat steps 1–6.

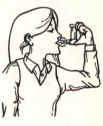

I

FIGURE 13-3 Guidelines for using a metered-dose inhaler.

---

to learn about asthma, identify individualized goals for each patient, and identify and correct any misconceptions about asthma or medications. Any individual concerns or fears about asthma or asthma medications should be elicited and addressed.

Peak Flow Meters

Peak flow meters are hand-held devices, available by prescription. PEF measures the amount of airway obstruction (Figure 13-4); a decrease in the PEF can precede symptoms of a significant asthma exacerbation. Some people with moderate-to-severe persistent asthma may monitor PEF daily as part of their asthma self-

care plan. The green, yellow, and red zone method discussed in the next section is often used. The green zone is a PEF reading of at least 80% of predicted or personal best, the yellow zone is 50% to 79%, and the red zone is less than 50%. Readings are recorded in a diary that is brought to each primary care visit.

Asthma Self-Care Plans

Asthma self-care plans are written instructions detailing how to manage both chronic and acute symptoms (Figure 13-1). Written self-care plans are recommended for all patients with moderate-to-severe persistent asthma and those with a history

- **Step 1**
  — Get your peak flow meter, a pencil, and your asthma care plan ready.
- **Step 2**
  — Some peak flow meters have a mouthpiece.
  — Put the mouthpiece on the meter, as shown in drawing A.

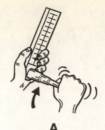

A

- **Step 3**
  — Move the indicator to the bottom of the numbered scale to set the meter to zero, as shown in drawing B.

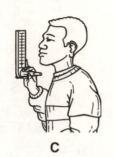

B

- **Step 4**
  — Stand up.
  — Keep the meter upright so the numbers run up and down.
  — Do not cover the hole in the back of the meter or the numbers in the front with your fingers. (See finger positions in drawing C.)
  — Take a deep breath, filling your lungs completely.

C

- **Step 5**
  — Place the mouthpiece in your mouth and close your lips tightly around it, as shown in drawing D.
  — Do not put your tongue inside the hole or your teeth on the mouthpiece.
  — Blow out as hard and as fast as you can in a single blow.

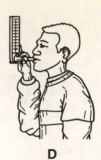

D

- **Step 6**
  — Find your number on the scale.
  — The button will go up and stay at the number you blew. (See drawing E.)
- **Step 7**
  — Repeat steps 1–6 two more times.
  — Record the best of the three blows in your asthma diary.
  — Check your asthma care plan for further instructions regarding the number you blew (the red, yellow, and green zones).

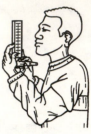

E

FIGURE 13-4 Guidelines for using peak expiratory flow meters.

of severe exacerbations. Self-care plans are developed with a health care practitioner, and encourage communication and partnership between individuals and their providers. The self-care plan should be concise, easily understandable, and empower the patient to take charge of their asthma.

Self-care plans allow patients to make decisions regarding when to seek medical care. Typically, self-care plans are divided into several sections based on the PEF zones. Green zone plans focus on what to do when the patient feels well and has normal lung function. Green zone directions encourage adherence with long-term controller medications. Yellow zone directions provide guidance when PEF readings fall or symptoms begin or persist. The red zone section details management of an episode that is severe or does not improve with initial treatment. Even patients with intermittent asthma can still experience significant asthma exacerbations, so they should learn how to recognize and manage severe symptoms.[27] Copies of self-care plans should be given to school nurses, teachers, and day care providers to ensure prompt treatment of asthma episodes that occur when children are away from the home.

Nonadherence to Prescription Asthma Medications

Nonadherence to long-term control medications is a significant problem. Adherence ranges from 34% to 68% depending on the medication.[26] Inhalers are the mainstay of therapy, but these items tend to be bulky to carry to school or work. The most effective controller medications are the inhaled corticosteroids, which possess anti-inflammatory properties. Because it may take several days to weeks to see the full anti-inflammatory effects and symptom improvement, patients often perceive that long-term control medications are ineffective.[28] Confusion among the lay public about the potential toxicity of anabolic steroids misused by athletes versus corticosteroids used for asthma, as well as concerns about the long-term effects of medications can discourage adherence. Compliance can usually be increased if the person (1) accepts the diagnosis of asthma, (2) believes that asthma may be dangerous or is a problem, (3) believes that he or she is at risk, (4) believes that the treatment is safe, (5) feels in control, and (6) feels that there is good communication with their health care provider.[5] Therefore, education regarding asthma and asthma medications can improve adherence with medications and self-care plans.

The box Patient Education for Asthma provides specific information to provide patients.

Evaluation of Patient Outcomes for Asthma

Acute asthma symptoms should respond to inhaled bronchodilators quickly (within 1 hour). Medical attention should be sought if symptoms worsen or keep returning for longer than 24 to 48 hours, or if PEF readings remain in the yellow zone for 2 or more days. If any symptoms of severe asthma exacerbations or imminent respiratory arrest develop, then immediate medical attention should be sought (Table 13-3).

Patients with persistent asthma should be scheduled for follow-up appointments at least every 6 months with their health care practitioner to assess the adequacy of their self-care plan and assess achievement of their goals (Table 13-8). Patients with asthma-like symptoms who are not candidates for self-care should be referred to their health care practitioners (Table 13-5).

The objectives of self-treatment are to (1) identify candidates for self-care (Table 13-5), (2) prevent acute asthma exacerbations with quick-relief medications, and (3) have tools available to manage acute exacerbations (Figure 13-1).

Asthma is an inflammatory disorder characterized by periods of stable lung function coupled with acute exacerbations. Symptoms of an acute exacerbation include wheezing, chest tightness, shortness of breath, and cough.

Nondrug Measures

- Identify and control environmental triggers (Table 13-6).
- Stop smoking cigarettes.
- Control concomitant disease states (e.g., GERD, allergic rhinitis, and tobacco use).

Nonprescription Medications

- See Table 13-7 for examples of available medications.
- Two types of nonprescription asthma medications are available: inhaled and oral.
  - Inhaled medications contain epinephrine or racepinephrine.
  - Possible adverse drug effects of inhaled medications include nervousness and rapid heart beat.
  - Oral medications include ephedrine and guaifenesin.
  - Possible adverse drug effects of oral medications include nervousness, tremor, sleeplessness, nausea, and loss of appetite.
- Precautions and contraindications for inhaled and oral asthma medications include:
  - Do not use unless a diagnosis of asthma has been made.
  - Do not take with monoamine oxidase inhibitors (MAOIs).

  - Do not use if you have heart disease, high blood pressure, thyroid disease, diabetes, or difficulty with urination due to enlargement of the prostate gland unless the use is directed by a health care professional.
  - Do not use if you have been hospitalized for asthma or if you are taking a prescription medication for asthma.
- Monitoring parameters include relief of symptoms and occurrence of adverse effects:
  - If acute symptoms do not improve or become worse within 20 minutes of use of nonprescription bronchodilator medications, seek immediate medical attention.
  - Monitor continuously for adverse effects such as palpitations, angina, anxiety, nervousness, tremor, agitation, dizziness, insomnia, and restlessness. Discontinue use and notify provider if experiencing unwanted adverse effects.
- See Figure 13-1 for safe administration of medication.
- See Table 13-7 for recommended daily dose.
- Warning signs and symptoms include drowsiness, confusion, absence of wheeze, and slow heart beat.
- Store epinephrine inhalers at room temperature (68°F–77°F). Do not store near open flame or heat above 120°F.
- Store combination oral products in a cool, dry place. Do not take products after expiration date on packaging.

 Seek a medical referral if symptoms occur or nonprescription bronchodilator is used more than twice a week.

Key Points for Asthma

➤ Candidates for self-care of asthma are few. Medical referral is appropriate for those with concurrent diseases but no prior diagnosis of asthma, or those with persistent asthma (Table 13-5).

➤ Nonprescription medications should be used for mild infrequent symptoms or exacerbations lasting less than 2 days.

➤ All patients with asthma need to know warning symptoms of severe asthma exacerbations to recognize when to seek urgent care.

➤ Education regarding asthma, medications, and self-monitoring is a crucial part of asthma self-care.

➤ Self-care plans should be developed in a partnership with health care practitioners. All patients with moderate-to-severe persistent asthma should have a written self-care plan.

TABLE 13-8 Asthma Therapeutic Goals and Monitoring Parameters

Therapeutic Goal	Monitoring Parameter
Control of symptoms	Symptoms 1–2 times per week; symptoms resolve within several minutes after bronchodilator
Normal pulmonary function	>80% of personal best PEF *consistently* every day
Normal activity levels	Few missed school/workdays, able to do desired activities (play, activities of daily living, etc.)
Prevention of recurrent episodes of asthma (minimize the need for urgent care visits)	No hospitalizations or emergency department visits, regular follow-ups for asthma
Prevention of adverse effects	No increased heart rate, insomnia, palpitations, nervousness, anxiety
Meeting expectations of asthma care	Achievement of patient's goals (e.g., able to do desired activities): participates in care, is comfortable asking questions, is confident in dealing with symptoms and triggers

Key: PEF, peak expiratory flow.

➤ Environmental and trigger control can help reduce symptoms of asthma.

➤ Concomitant conditions (e.g., GERD, allergic rhinitis, and tobacco use) can worsen asthma symptoms and should be treated individually.

REFERENCES

1. US Department of Health and Human Services, Office of Minority Health. Respiratory diseases. In: *Healthy People 2010*. Rockville, Md: US Department of Health and Human Services; 2000. Available at: http://www.healthypeople.gov. Last accessed August 29, 2008.

2. Centers for Disease Control and Prevention. National surveillance for asthma—United States, 1980–2004. *MMWR Surveill Summ*. 2007; 56(SS-08):1–14, 18–51. Available at: http://www.cdc.gov. Last accessed September 3, 2008.

3. Akinbami L. Asthma Prevalence, Health Care Use and Mortality: United States, 2003–05. National Center for Health Statistics. Available at: http://www.cdc.gov. Last accessed August 29, 2008.

4. National Heart, Lung, and Blood Institute, National Asthma Education and Prevention Program. *Expert Panel Report 3. Guidelines for the Diagnosis and Management of Asthma. Full Report 2007*. Bethesda, Md: US Department of Health and Human Services; August 28, 2007. Available at: http://www.nhlbi.nih.gov/guidelines/asthma/asthgdln.pdf. Last accessed August 29, 2008.

5. *Global Strategy for Asthma Management and Prevention, 2007*. Global Initiative for Asthma (GINA). Available at: http://www.ginasthma.org. Last accessed August 29, 2008.

6. Bousquet J, Jeffery PK, Busse WW, et al. Asthma. From bronchoconstriction to airways inflammation and remodeling. *Am J Respir Crit Care Med*. 2000;161:1721–45.

7. Harding SM. Gastroesophageal reflux: a potential asthma trigger. *Immunol All Clin North Am*. 2005:25:131–48.

8. Kiljander T. The role of proton pump inhibitors in the management of gastroesophageal reflux disease-related asthma and chronic cough. *Am J Med*. 2003;115(3A):65S–71S.

9. Gilliland FD, Islam T, Berhane K, et al. Regular smoking and asthma incidence in adolescents. *Am J Respir Crit Care Med*. 2006;174:1094–100.

10. Parmet S. Asprin sensitivity. *JAMA*. 2004;292:3098.

11. James JM. Respiratory manifestations of food allergy. *Pediatrics*. 2003; 111:1625–30.

12. Drug Enforcement Administration. Retail sales of scheduled listed chemical products; self-certification of regulated sellers of scheduled listed chemical products. Interim final rule with request for comment. *Fed Regist*. 2006;71:56008–27.

13. Upper respiratory combinations. In: Novak KK, Corrigan CA, Scott JA, et al., eds. *Drug Facts and Comparisons 2008*. St Louis, Mo: Wolters Kluwer Health; 2008:1022–3.

14. Expectorants. In: Novak KK, Corrigan CA, Scott JA, et al., eds. *Drug Facts and Comparisons 2008*. St Louis, Mo: Wolters Kluwer Health; 2008:1066–7.

15. Drugs@FDA. FDA Approved Drug Products. Available at: http://www.accessdata.fda.gov. Last accessed August 29, 2008.

16. Food and Drug Administration. FDA Proposing Phase Out of CFCs in Metered-Dose Inhalers for Epinephrine. Available at: http://www.fda.gov/bbs/topics/NEWS/2007/NEW01706.html. Last accessed September 3, 2008.

17. Agents for Active Immunization In: Novak KK, Corrigan CA, Scott JA, et al., eds. *Drug Facts and Comparisons 2008*. St Louis, Mo: Wolters Kluwer Health; 2008:1238.

18. Briggs GG, Freeman RK, Yaffe SJ. Epinephrine and ephedrine. In: Sydor AM, ed. *Drugs in Pregnancy and Lactation*. 7th ed. Philadelphia: Lippincott Williams & Wilkins; 2005:568–70.

19. American College of Gynecology. ACOG practice bulletin no. 90: Asthma in pregnancy. *Obstet Gynecol*. 2008;111(2 pt 1):457–64.

20. Gibson PG, Simpson JL, Chalmers AN, et al. Airway eosinophilia is associated with wheeze but is uncommon in children with persistent cough and frequent chest colds. *Am J Respir Crit Care Med*. 2001;164:977–81.

21. National Collegiate Athletic Association. NCAA Banned-Drug Classes 2008–09. Available at: http://www.ncaa.org. Last accessed August 29, 2008.

22. Rivera JO, Hughes HW, Stuart AG. Herbals and asthma: usage patterns among a border population. *Ann Pharm*. 2004;38:220–5.

23. Graham M, Blaiss, M. Complementary/alternative medicine in the treatment of asthma. *Ann All Asthma Immun*. 2000;85:438–49.

24. Theoharides T, Bielory L. Mast cells and mast cell mediators as targets of dietary supplements. *Ann All Asthma Immun*. 2004;93:S24–S34.

25. Markham, AW, Wilkinson JM. Complementary and alternative medicines (CAM) in the management of asthma: an examination of the evidence. *J Asthma*. 2004;41:131–9.

26. Jones C, Santanello JC, Boccuzzi SJ, et al. Adherence to prescribed treatment for asthma: evidence from pharmacy benefits data. *J Asthma*. 2003;40: 93–101.

27. Naureckas E, Solway J. Mild asthma. *New Engl J Med*. 2001;345:1257–62.

28. Farber HJ, Capra AM, Finkelstein JA, et al. Misunderstanding of asthma controller medications: association with non-adherence. *J Asthma*. 2003; 40:17–25.

Gastrointestinal Disorders

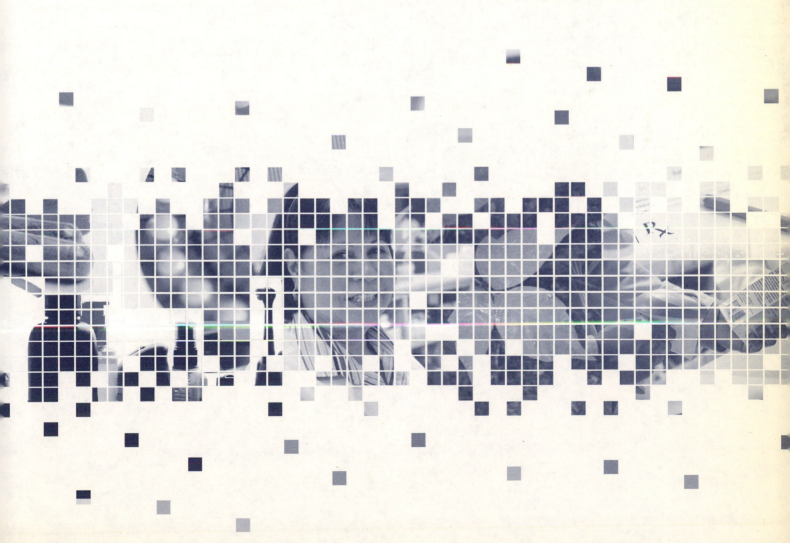

Heartburn and Dyspepsia

Ann Zweber and Rosemary R. Berardi

Heartburn and dyspepsia are common symptoms that originate in the upper gastrointestinal (GI) tract. These symptoms are frequently treated with nonprescription medications. Heartburn (pyrosis) is a burning sensation that usually arises from the substernal area (lower chest) and moves up toward the neck or throat.[1] Postprandial heartburn usually occurs within 2 hours after eating or when bending over or lying down. Nocturnal heartburn occurs during sleep and often awakens the individual. Most patients experience "simple" heartburn, which is typically mild, infrequent, episodic, and often associated with diet or lifestyle.[1] Others have frequent heartburn (defined as heartburn that occurs 2 or more days a week). Heartburn that is frequent and persistent (3 or more months) is the most common typical symptom of gastroesophageal reflux disease (GERD). Patients with this chronic disease present with symptoms, esophageal damage, or both, which result from the abnormal reflux of gastric contents into the esophagus.[2] About 20% to 30% of patients with GERD are diagnosed with endoscopic erosive esophagitis, whereas 60% to 70% suffer from heartburn, even when esophageal injury is not present at endoscopy (nonerosive gastroesophageal reflux disease; NERD).[3] Although it is not life-threatening, patients with frequent heartburn limit their food choices and often suffer from disruptions in sleep and work.[4,5] In 2000, the treatment of GERD ranked the highest in total direct and indirect costs (9.8 billion) among 17 selected GI diseases, with drug costs responsible for 63% of the direct costs.[6]

Dyspepsia (bad digestion) is a consistent or recurrent discomfort located primarily in the upper abdomen (epigastrium).[7] The discomfort is a subjective feeling that does not reach the level of pain and is usually characterized by bloating, belching, postprandial fullness, nausea, and early satiety. The discomfort, however, is not necessarily restricted to meal-related symptoms. Patients with GERD, peptic ulcer disease (PUD), gastritis, delayed gastric emptying (e.g., gastroparesis), and irritable bowel syndrome (IBS) may complain of dyspeptic symptoms.[7] Although the symptoms of IBS technically differ from those of dyspepsia, there is considerable overlap in the patient's clinical description of these symptoms.

The Rome II consensus definition and regulatory agencies in the United States have adopted definitions of dyspepsia for research purposes that exclude heartburn, whereas other definitions consider heartburn an accompanying symptom of dyspepsia.[8] Dyspepsia may be associated with an underlying cause such as PUD and GERD or may not have any known cause.[7,9] Dyspepsia may be described as uninvestigated (no endoscopy has been performed) or investigated (endoscopy has been performed). Nonulcer dyspepsia is a diagnosis made at endoscopy, which indicates that "ulcerlike" dyspeptic symptoms are not related to a peptic ulcer. About 18 million adults in the United States take nonprescription medications for "indigestion."[2] The most widely used nonprescription medications include antacids, histamine$_2$–receptor antagonists (H$_2$RAs), and proton pump inhibitors (PPIs).

In clinical practice, it is not always possible to predict the cause of heartburn or dyspepsia on the basis of symptom assessment alone, because individuals may not describe adequately what they actually feel. In addition, there is considerable overlap of symptoms. Heartburn and dyspepsia may also occur in association with other acid-related disorders, such as GERD and PUD, and may overlap with symptoms related to IBS. However, empirical treatment with nonprescription medications is appropriate and reasonable for most patients who have symptoms suggestive of heartburn and/or dyspepsia. Thus, assessment of the patient is most important in determining if the condition is self-treatable or if the individual should be referred for further evaluation. Medical referral is indicated if the patient is unresponsive to nonprescription medications, symptoms are severe, alarm symptoms are present, or symptoms suggest complicated disease.

This chapter focuses on the self-treatment and prevention of heartburn and dyspepsia. Emphasis is placed on distinguishing individuals who are appropriate candidates for self-treatment from those who require further medical evaluation. Specific recommendations for self-treatment, including dietary and lifestyle modifications and nonprescription medications, are provided.

The overall prevalence of heartburn in the United States is approximately 45% (about 110 million people), with an equal distribution between men and women of all age groups.[1] Among individuals who experience heartburn, 45% report heartburn 2 or more days a week, whereas 7% to 10% report heartburn daily.[10] Sixty-five percent of adults who experience heartburn at least once a week indicate that they have both daytime and nighttime heartburn.[4] Most women who are pregnant experience heartburn during the course of their pregnancy.[1]

Approximately 25% of adults in the United States report having dyspeptic symptoms, with equal prevalence between men and women.[7] A peptic ulcer is found in about 5% to 15% of patients with dyspepsia in North America, whereas esophagitis is identified in an additional 5% to 15% of cases at endoscopy.[7] Gastric and esophageal cancer are less common causes but may also be associated with dyspeptic symptoms. Less than 50% of patients in the United States seek medical care for their dyspeptic symtoms.[7]

Pathophysiology of Heartburn and Dyspepsia

The lower esophageal sphincter (LES) permits the passage of food into the stomach and serves as the primary antireflux barrier by preventing backflow of stomach contents upward into the esophagus (Figure 14-1). Although the LES is contracted at rest, healthy individuals experience relaxations of the LES throughout the day, often in association with swallowing.[1] When reflux occurs, the refluxate is cleared from the esophagus through peristaltic contractions brought on by swallowing, through neutralization of the refluxate by bicarbonate in the swallowed saliva and, when in the upright position, through gravity. Esophageal mucosal resistance minimizes epithelial damage from noxious stomach contents. Thus, transient episodes of gastroesophageal reflux in healthy persons usually go unnoticed and do not damage the esophagus.

The stomach contains parietal cells that secrete hydrochloric acid and intrinsic factor (necessary for vitamin B_{12} absorption), G cells that secrete gastrin, mucus-secreting cells, and chief cells that secrete pepsinogen.[11,12] The parietal cells have receptors for histamine, acetylcholine, and gastrin, all of which stimulate hydrochloric acid secretion. When these substances come into contact with their receptors on the parietal cell, intracellular calcium and cyclic adenosine monophosphate (cAMP) concentrations increase.[11] The increased levels of calcium and cAMP activate the proton pump, adenosine triphosphatase ($H^+/K^+/ATPase$), located in the membranes of the parietal cell. When stimulated, the proton pump secretes hydrogen ions into the stomach lumen in exchange for potassium. Thus, the proton pump is the final common path-

way for gastric acid secretion. The gastric mucosa withstands the acidic environment of the stomach through a combination of defense and repair mechanisms that are collectively called the gastric mucosal barrier.[11]

Risk factors that contribute to heartburn include diet, lifestyle, medications, and certain diseases (Table 14-1).[1,13–15] However, evidence to support each of the proposed risk factors is limited.[14] Foods and beverages including coffee, tea, chocolate, and citrus; the regular use of aspirin and nonsteroidal anti-inflammatory drugs (NSAIDs); life stress; and tobacco smoking are widely recognized as precipitators of individual heartburn episodes.[15] Heartburn may also occur during certain types of exercise (e.g., weight lifting, cycling, or sit-ups). Obesity and pregnancy contribute to reflux by a direct physical effect (e.g., disrupting the intra-abdominal pressure). Genetic factors may predispose to neurologic dysfunction of the LES.[15] Diseases such as gastroparesis and scleroderma increase intra-abdominal pressure and lower LES pressure, respectively.

NSAIDs, including aspirin and cyclooxygenase-2 inhibitors, are very important causes of drug-induced dyspepsia.[7] Bisphosphonates, potassium or iron supplements, digoxin, theophylline, and certain antibiotics (e.g., erythromycin, ampicillin) are often

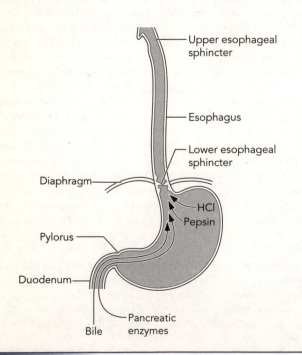

FIGURE 14-1 Esophageal defense mechanisms and offensive factors associated with heartburn.

Upper esophageal sphincter

Esophagus

Lower esophageal sphincter

Diaphragm

HCl
Pepsin

Pylorus

Duodenum

Bile

Pancreatic enzymes

TABLE 14-1 Risk Factors That May Contribute to Heartburn

Dietary	Medications
Fatty foods	Bisphosphonates
Spicy foods	Aspirin/NSAIDs
Chocolate	Iron
Salt and salt substitutes	Potassium
Garlic or onions	Quinidine
Mint (e.g., spearmint, peppermint)	Tetracycline
	Zidovudine
Alcohol (ethanol)	Anticholinergic agents
Caffeinated beverages	Alpha-adrenergic antagonists
Carbonated beverages	Barbiturates
Citrus fruit or juices	$Beta_2$-adrenergic agonists
Tomatoes/tomato juice	Calcium channel blockers
	Benzodiazepines
Lifestyle	Dopamine
Exercise	Estrogen
Smoking (tobacco)	Narcotic analgesics
Obesity	Nitrates
Stress	Progesterone
Supine body position	Prostaglandins
Tight-fitting clothing	Theophylline
	TCAs
Diseases	Chemotherapy
Motility disorders (e.g., gastroparesis)	
Scleroderma	**Other**
PUD	Genetics
Zollinger-Ellison syndrome	Pregnancy

Key: NSAID, nonsteroidal anti-inflammatory drug; PUD, peptic ulcer disease; TCA, tricyclic antidepressant.
Source: References 1 and 13–15.

associated with dyspeptic symptoms. Alcohol ingestion, tobacco, caffeine, and stress may contribute to dyspepsia.

Heartburn arises from the sensory nerve endings in the esophageal epithelium and is most likely stimulated by spicy foods or by the reflux of acidic gastric contents into the esophagus.[1] The noxious quality of the refluxate (acid, pepsin) is central to the development of symptoms, esophageal damage, and complications (Figure 14-1). Individuals with an incompetent pylorus may reflux duodenal contents (bile, pancreatic enzymes) into the stomach, which increases the noxious quality of the gastric refluxate. Most patients with heartburn do not secrete excessive amounts of gastric acid. Esophageal tissue damage is caused primarily by gastric acid, pepsin, and bile salts. The esophageal epithelium is not as tolerant as that of the stomach to repetitive exposure of gastric acid. What usually distinguishes individuals with heartburn from those with normal physiologic reflux is the increased frequency and duration of reflux episodes, which may result in esophageal tissue damage that ranges from inflammation (esophagitis) to erosions and ulcers. However, there is no direct correlation between heartburn severity and underlying esophageal injury. The refluxed acidic contents also may damage the oropharynx, larynx, and respiratory system.

Many patients with heartburn have transient LES relaxations.[1] In these patients, the higher pressure in the stomach creates enough force to overcome the decreased LES pressure, allowing reflux of gastric contents into the lower esophagus (Figure 14-1). Hiatal hernia (a weakening in the diaphragmatic muscles resulting in the protrusion of the upper portion of the stomach into the thoracic cavity) may also contribute to heartburn by disrupting the gastroesophageal junction and lowering the LES pressure.[1] Delayed gastric emptying increases the volume of the noxious refluxate and increases intra-abdominal pressure. A sudden increase in intra-abdominal pressure (e.g., straining, coughing, or bending over) may also be associated with reflux. Impaired esophageal acid–clearing mechanisms (peristalsis, saliva, gravity) prolong the duration of contact between the refluxate and the esophageal epithelium and are less operative during sleep or when the patient is lying down. Age-related decreases in saliva production, esophageal motility (resulting in decreased acid clearance), and a reduction in esophageal sensitivity to refluxed gastric acid contributes to increased severity of esophageal mucosal injury.[16] However older patients tend to present with less severe typical symptoms (e.g., heartburn) than younger individuals.[16] Although this issue is controversial, *Helicobacter pylori* infection does not appear to play a pathogenic role but potentially may be protective.[1,17]

The pathophysiology of dyspepsia remains unclear. Acute, infrequent dyspepsia is often associated with food, alcohol, smoking, or stress. Chronic dyspeptic symptoms may be associated with PUD, GERD, gastric cancer, *H. pylori,* GI dysmotility (e.g., delayed gastric emptying), or may lack any identifiable cause (endoscopy-negative, functional, idiopathic dyspepsia). It is possible that the esophagus, stomach, duodenum, and other regions of the GI tract are hypersensitive and may be associated with IBS.[7] Some suggest that psychological disturbances are an important contributing factor.

Clinical Presentation of Heartburn and Dyspepsia

Heartburn may occur alone or be associated with acid-related disorders such as dyspepsia, GERD, and PUD (Table 14-2). Heartburn is highly specific for GERD and may suggest esophageal complications.[1] However, the frequency and severity of heartburn are not predictive of esophageal injury, because many patients with frequent and severe heartburn may not have esophageal damage (e.g., NERD). Upper endoscopy is the standard for determining the type and extent of esophageal mucosal damage. Patients with esophageal injury may have varying grades of severity as well as strictures (a narrowing of the esophageal lumen).[1] Symptomatic GERD is the strongest risk factor for the development of esophageal adenocarcinoma.[18] Barrett's esophagus, a precancerous condition, develops in the lower esophagus and is related to long-standing (greater than 5 years) moderate-to-severe erosive/ulcerative esophagitis.[1,19] This condition is more prevalent in men and increases with age. Barrett's esophagus is associated with an increased risk of esophageal adenocarcinoma with an annual incidence of less than 1%.[1,18,19]

Alarm symptoms can result from complications associated with GERD (Table 14-2). Dysphagia (difficulty in swallowing) occurs initially with the ingestion of solid foods such as toast or crackers and may be related to severe erosive esophagitis, esophageal stricture, or cancer.[1] Odynophagia (painful swallowing) is less common but may also result from severe ulcerative esophagitis or esophageal cancer. However, the presence of odynophagia should raise questions about other causes of esophagitis including pill-induced (e.g., tetracycline, potassium chloride, quinine, vitamin C, aspirin, NSAIDs, or bisphosphonates) and infections (e.g., herpes or fungal candidiasis).[1] Upper GI bleeding (e.g., hematemesis, melena, occult bleeding, or anemia) may also result from esophageal complications.

Abnormal gastric reflux of stomach contents may also cause atypical (extra-esophageal) manifestations of GERD (Table 14-2).[20] The atypical symptoms may or may not be accompanied by heartburn, making recognition of GERD difficult. GERD-related chest pain is usually substernal, but it may mimic ischemic cardiac pain, radiating to the back, neck, jaw, or arms. It often worsens after meals and during periods of emotional stress, and may awaken the patient from sleep. Severe, crushing chest pain—especially if accompanied by nausea, vomiting, sweating, and shortness of breath—suggests ischemic pain and possibly myocardial infarction, and should be considered a medical emergency. However, the "typical" crushing chest pain usually associated with a myocardial infarction is more common in men than in women. Because women with ischemic cardiac pain may present differently than men, and because it is not possible clinically to differentiate cardiac pain from noncardiac pain, patients with these complaints should be referred to the emergency department. Other atypical symptoms result from the aspiration of refluxate into the upper airways and lungs.

Treatment of Heartburn and Dyspepsia
Treatment Goals

The goals of self-treatment of heartburn are to render the patient symptom-free, prevent meal- or exercise-related symptoms, improve quality of life, and prevent complications by using the most cost-effective therapy. The primary goal of self-treatment of dyspepsia is aimed at relieving abdominal discomfort.

General Treatment Approach

The approach to self-treatment of heartburn and dyspepsia requires an initial assessment to determine whether the patient

TABLE 14-2 Differentiation of Simple Heartburn from Other Acid-Related Disorders

	Simple Heartburn	**GERD**	**Dyspepsia**	**PUD**
Etiology	See Table 14-1	See Table 14-1	Food, alcohol caffeine, stress, and medications contribute to dyspepsia. Chronic dyspepsia is associated with PUD, GERD, and gastric cancer or may lack an identifiable cause (functional dyspepsia).	Gastric or duodenal ulcer is caused most commonly by *H. pylori* infection and/or NSAIDs.
Typical symptoms	Burning sensation behind the breastbone that may move upward toward the neck or throat	Heartburn, acid regurgitation (acid taste in the mouth), hypersalivation	Primary: epigastric discomfort Other: belching or burping, bloating, nausea, early satiety; may be accompanied by heartburn and acid regurgitation.	Gnawing or burning epigastric pain, occurring during day and frequently at night; may be accompanied by heartburn and dyspepsia.
Complications		Erosive esophagitis, strictures, bleeding, Barrett's esophagus, esophageal cancer		Perforation, obstruction, penetration, or bleeding may occur.
Alarm symptoms		Dysphagia; odynophagia; chest pain; upper GI bleeding; unexplained weight loss; continuous nausea, vomiting, and diarrhea		Upper GI bleeding; unexplained weight loss; continuous nausea, vomiting, and diarrhea may occur.
Atypical symptoms		Asthma, chronic laryngitis, hoarseness, cough, globus sensation (sensation of a lump in the throat), noncardiac chest pain, dental erosions, sleep apnea		

Key: GERD, gastroesophageal reflux disease; GI, gastrointestinal; NSAID, nonsteroidal anti-inflammatory drug; PUD, peptic ulcer disease.

is a candidate for self-treatment (Figure 14-2). Individuals with exclusions for self-treatment should be referred for further medical evaluation. If the individual is a candidate for self-treatment, nondrug measures should be recommended and continued throughout treatment (see the box Patient Education for Heartburn and Dyspepsia). If appropriate, a recommendation should also be made for a nonprescription medication. Antacids and nonprescription H$_2$RAs should be recommended for individuals with mild, infrequent heartburn and dyspepsia. Antacids are advantageous because they provide rapid relief of symptoms (Table 14-3). The use of antacids, however, is limited by their short duration when taken on an empty stomach. The duration of relief may be prolonged for several hours by taking the antacid after a meal. When used in recommended dosages, the antacids are interchangeable despite differences in antacid salts and potency. Products that contain antacids plus alginic acid are also effective in relieving heartburn and may be superior to antacids alone.[2] Antacid/alginic acid products are usually more expensive than

antacids and therefore are considered second-line agents for treating mild, occasional heartburn.

A nonprescription H$_2$RA is preferred to an antacid when individuals with mild-to-moderate, episodic heartburn require more prolonged relief of symptoms. Although H$_2$RAs do not relieve heartburn or dyspepsia as rapidly as an antacid (Table 14-3), onset of action may not be important to some individuals.[2] The H$_2$RAs may also be used to prevent heartburn and acid indigestion when given 30 minutes to 1 hour prior to a heavy or spicy meal and exercise. When rapid relief and longer duration are desirable, taking an antacid initially followed by an H$_2$RA or taking a combination antacid/H$_2$RA product (Table 14-3) may be recommended. Nonprescription H$_2$RA products containing the lower doses (e.g., famotidine 10 mg twice daily) should be recommended for patients with mild, infrequent heartburn, whereas higher nonprescription dosages (e.g., famotidine 20 mg twice daily) should be reserved for moderate symptoms. When used in recommended and comparative dosages, the H$_2$RAs are

Exclusions for Self-Treatment

- Frequent heartburn for more than 3 months
- Heartburn while taking recommended dosages of nonprescription H_2RA or PPI
- Heartburn that continues after 2 weeks of treatment with a nonprescription H_2RA or PPI
- Heartburn and dyspepsia that occur when taking a prescription H_2RA or PPI
- Severe heartburn and dyspepsia
- Nocturnal heartburn
- Difficulty or pain on swallowing solid foods

- Vomiting up blood or black material or black tarry stools
- Chronic hoarseness, wheezing, coughing, or choking
- Unexplained weight loss
- Continuous nausea, vomiting, or diarrhea
- Chest pain accompanied by sweating, pain radiating to shoulder, arm, neck, or jaw, and shortness of breath
- Pregnancy
- Nursing mothers
- Children younger than 12 years (for antacids, H_2RAs) or younger than 18 years (for omeprazole)

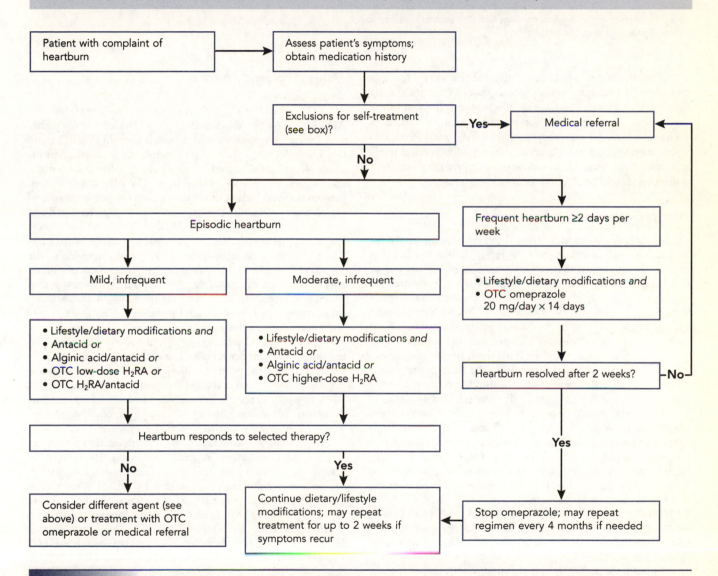

FIGURE 14-2 Self-care of heartburn. Key: H_2RA, histamine$_2$-receptor antagonist; OTC, over-the-counter; PPI, proton pump inhibitor.

interchangeable despite minor differences in potency, onset, and duration of action. Patients should not exceed 14 days of self-treatment with an H_2RA without consulting their primary care provider.

Nonprescription PPIs are the drugs of choice for treatment of individuals with frequent heartburn occurring 2 or more days a week and for those who do not respond to nonprescription H_2RAs. The onset of symptomatic relief follow-ing an oral dose of omeprazole is slower than that of an H_2RA (Table 14-3), and complete relief of symptoms may take several days after initiating treatment. However, compared with the nonprescription H_2RAs, the PPIs provide superior symptomatic relief and a prolonged duration of action. Patients should not take a nonprescription PPI for more than 14 days and should not re-treat more often than every 4 months unless under medical supervision.

TABLE 14-3 Effectiveness of Nonprescription Medications in Relieving Heartburn

Medication	Onset of Relief	Duration of Relief	Symptomatic Relief
Antacids	<5 minutes	20–30 minutes[a]	Excellent
H₂RAs	30–45 minutes	4–10 hours	Excellent
H₂RA + antacid	<5 minutes	8–10 hours	Excellent
PPIs	2–3 hours	12–24 hours	Superior

Key: H₂RA, histamine₂-receptor antagonist; PPI, proton pump inhibitor.
[a] Food prolongs duration of relief.

The selection of a nonprescription medication for the self-treatment of heartburn and dyspepsia should be based on the frequency, duration, and severity of symptoms; the cost of the medication; potential drug–drug interactions; and the patient's preference. Antacids, nonprescription H₂RAs, and PPIs should not be used beyond 2 weeks unless the individual is under medical supervision. Individuals with severe, recurrent, or persistent symptoms should be referred for medical evaluation.

Nonpharmacologic Therapy

Dietary and lifestyle modifications should be recommended for all patients with heartburn and dyspepsia despite the fact that evidence supporting their effectiveness is either lacking or equivocal.[2,14,15,21,22] These measures may benefit many individuals, but such changes alone are unlikely to completely relieve symptoms in the majority of patients.[2,14,22] Nonpharmacologic approaches to reducing the frequency and severity of heartburn include actions to increase the LES pressure, decrease the intragastric pressure, and assist in the movement of gastric contents. A complete and accurate history will assist in identifying contributing factors. Recommendations should be tailored to the individual on the basis of specific dietary and lifestyle patterns.

Individuals should be asked to keep a diary to track dietary, lifestyle, and medication "triggers" (Table 14-1). Weight loss should be encouraged, although there is some controversy as to whether this will significantly decrease symptoms.[15,21] For nocturnal symptoms, relief may be attained from elevating the head of the bed by placing 6-inch blocks underneath the legs of the head of the bed, or placing a foam wedge (e.g., GERD pillow) beneath the patient's upper torso and head.[14,21,23] Use of traditional pillows may worsen symptoms, because it causes the individual to bend at the waist, which contributes to an increase in intragastric pressure.

Individuals should be educated about factors that contribute to heartburn and how to manage them (see the box Patient Education for Heartburn and Dyspepsia). Most importantly, heartburn sufferers should be counseled to eat smaller meals, to reduce intake of dietary fat, and to refrain from eating at least 3 hours before going to bed or lying down. Prescription and nonprescription medications should be evaluated for potential effects on heartburn and dyspepsia. When possible, individuals should be advised to switch to less troublesome nonprescription medications or consult their prescriber about prescription drugs that may be exacerbating their symptoms. Use of tobacco products should be discouraged. If alcohol or caffeine consumption is a contributing factor, individuals should be advised to limit or discontinue use.

Pharmacologic Therapy

Antacids

Antacids relieve heartburn and dyspepsia by neutralizing gastric acid. Nonprescription antacid products contain at least one of the following salts: magnesium (hydroxide, carbonate, trisilicate); aluminum (hydroxide, phosphate); calcium carbonate; and sodium bicarbonate (Table 14-4). Over the last few years, many pharmaceutical manufacturers have reformulated antacid products that had long-standing trade names (e.g., Mylanta) and introduced new products (e.g., Mylanta Supreme) and dosage forms (e.g., Mylanta Ultimate Strength Chewables) with similar trade names. Many of these modifications have led to the addition of calcium to the formulation or replacement of another antacid salt with calcium (e.g., Maalox Total Stomach Relief Maximum Strength). Most antacids are relatively inexpensive, making them desirable products for the temporary relief of mild and infrequent heartburn and dyspepsia.

Antacids act as buffering agents in the lower esophagus, gastric lumen, and duodenal bulb. The cations react with chloride, whereas the anionic portion of the molecule reacts with hydrogen ions to form water and other compounds. As a result, a small, but noticeable, increase in intragastric pH occurs.[24] Increasing the intragastric pH above 5 blocks the conversion of pepsin to pepsinogen.[24] Antacids may also increase LES pressure.[1]

Sodium bicarbonate rapidly reacts with gastric acid to form sodium chloride, carbon dioxide, and water. Its duration of action is shortened by its quick elimination from the stomach.[24] Of the magnesium salts, magnesium hydroxide is used most often. Magnesium hydroxide rapidly reacts with gastric acid to form magnesium chloride and water. Its duration of action is shorter than that of calcium carbonate and aluminum hydroxide. Calcium carbonate is a potent antacid that dissolves slowly in gastric acid to form calcium chloride, carbon dioxide, and water. Its onset of action is slower, but its duration of effect is longer than that of magnesium hydroxide or sodium bicarbonate. Aluminum hydroxide reacts with hydrochloric acid to form aluminum chloride and water. This agent has a slower onset but a longer duration than those of magnesium hydroxide.

Because they are already dissolved or suspended, liquid antacids usually have a faster onset than tablets and provide a maximal surface area for action. Of the tablet dosage forms, the quick-dissolve antacid tablets may provide the most rapid relief of symptoms. The duration of action for all antacids is transient, lasting only as long as the antacid remains in the stomach. The presence of food affects the duration of action of antacids. When administered within 1 hour after a meal, antacids may remain in the stomach for up to 3 hours.[24]

TABLE 14-4 Selected Antacid and Bismuth Products and Dosage Regimens

Trade Name	Primary Ingredients	Adult Dosage (Maximum Daily Dosage)
Alka-Mints Chewable Antacid	Calcium carbonate 850 mg	Chew 1 or 2 tablets every 2 hours as needed (8 tablets)
Alka-Seltzer Heartburn Relief	Sodium bicarbonate 1940 mg; citric acid 1000 mg	Dissolve 2 tablets in 4 oz of water every 4 hours as needed (8 tablets)
Alka-Seltzer Original	Sodium bicarbonate 1916 mg; citric acid 1000 mg; aspirin 325 mg	Dissolve 2 tablets in 4 oz of water every 4 hours as needed (8 tablets)
AlternaGEL Liquid	Each 5 mL contains aluminum hydroxide 600 mg	1–2 tsp between meals and at bedtime (18 tsp)
Gaviscon Extra Strength Liquid	Each 5 mL contains[a] aluminum hydroxide 254 mg; magnesium carbonate 237 mg	2–4 tsp 4 times a day, after meals and at bedtime (16 tsp)
Gelusil Tablets	Aluminum hydroxide 200 mg; magnesium hydroxide 200 mg; simethicone 25 mg	Chew 2 to 4 tablets; repeat hourly if symptoms return (12 tablets)
Maalox Liquid Regular Strength Antacid/Anti-Gas	Each 5 mL contains aluminum hydroxide 200 mg; magnesium hydroxide 200 mg; simethicone 20 mg	2–4 tsp 4 times a day (16 tsp)
Maalox Quick Dissolve Regular Strength Chewable Antacid Tablets	Calcium carbonate 600 mg	Chew 2–3 tablets as symptoms occur (12 tablets)
Mylanta Ultimate Strength Chewables	Calcium carbonate 700 mg; magnesium hydroxide 300 mg	Chew 2–4 tablets between meals and at bedtime as needed (10 tablets)
Mylanta Maximum Strength Liquid	Each 5 mL contains aluminum hydroxide 400 mg; magnesium hydroxide 400 mg; simethicone 40 mg	2–4 tsp between meals and at bedtime (12 tsp)
Mylanta Supreme Liquid	Each 5 mL contains calcium carbonate 400 mg; magnesium hydroxide 135 mg	2–4 tsp between meals and at bedtime (18 tsp)
Pepto-Bismol Maximum Strength Liquid	Each 15 mL contains bismuth subsalicylate 525 mg	2 tbsp every 1 hour as required (4 doses or 8 tbsp)
Pepto-Bismol Original Liquid	Each 15 mL contains bismuth subsalicylate 262 mg	2 tbsp every 1/2–1 hour as required (8 doses or 16 tbsp)
Phillips Milk of Magnesia Original	Each 5 mL contains magnesium hydroxide 400 mg	1–3 tsp every 4 hours (4 times/day or 12 tbsp)
Rolaids Original Antacid Tablets	Calcium carbonate 550 mg; magnesium hydroxide 110 mg	Chew 2–4 tablets hourly as needed (12 tablets)
Tums E-X 750 Tablets	Calcium carbonate 750 mg	Chew 2–4 tablets as needed for symptoms (10 tablets)
Tums Regular Strength Tablets	Calcium carbonate 500 mg	Chew 2–4 tablets as needed for symptoms (15 tablets)

[a] Sodium alginate (alginic acid) is listed as an inactive ingredient.

Differences in antacids are determined primarily by the cation, specific salt, and potency. Antacid potency is based on the number of milliequivalents of acid neutralizing capacity (ANC), which is defined as the amount of acid buffered per dose over a specified period of time. Factors that contribute to ANC include product formulation, ingredients, and concentration.[24] As a result, ANC is product-specific, which means equal volumes of liquid antacids or the same number of tablets is not necessarily equal in potency.

Most antacids are minimally absorbed into the systemic circulation. About 90% of calcium is converted to insoluble calcium salts; the remaining 10% is absorbed systemically.[24] Approximately 15% to 30% of magnesium and 17% to 30% of aluminum may be absorbed and then excreted renally; therefore, accumulation may occur in patients with renal insufficiency.[24] In contrast, sodium bicarbonate is readily absorbed and eliminated.

Antacids are indicated for the treatment of mild, infrequent heartburn, sour stomach, and acid indigestion. Combination products containing aspirin or acetaminophen are indicated for overindulgence in food and drink, and hangover. Individuals with mild dyspepsia may experience some relief with antacids, but no studies demonstrate their effectiveness.[9,24]

Antacids are administered orally. The effective dose of an antacid varies depending on product ingredients, milliequivalents of ANC, formulation, and the frequency and severity of symptoms. Individuals should be instructed to take product-specific recommended dosages at the onset of symptoms. Dosing may be repeated in 1 to 2 hours, if needed, but should not exceed the maximum daily dosage for a particular product (Table 14-4). Individuals should be reevaluated if antacids are used more than twice a week or regularly for over 2 weeks. Frequent antacid users may need to be switched to a longer-acting product such as an H_2RA, an H_2RA plus an antacid, or a PPI.

Antacids are usually well tolerated. Side effects are generally associated with the cation. The most common side effect associated with magnesium-containing antacids is dose-related diarrhea. Diarrhea may be reduced by combining magnesium-containing antacids with aluminum hydroxide. However, when higher dosages are used, the predominating effect is diarrhea. Magnesium excretion is impaired in patients with renal disease and may result in systemic accumulation of magnesium. Magnesium-containing antacids should not be used in patients with a creatinine clearance of less than 30 mL/minute.[24]

Aluminum-containing antacids are associated with dose-related constipation. Aluminum hydroxide binds dietary phosphate in the GI tract, increasing phosphate excretion in the feces. Frequent and prolonged use of aluminum hydroxide may lead to hypophosphatemia.[24] Chronic use of aluminum-containing antacids in renal failure may lead to aluminum toxicity and should be avoided.

Calcium carbonate may cause belching and flatulence as a result of carbon dioxide production. Patients may complain of constipation when taking calcium antacids, but there is little evidence to support this side effect.[23] Calcium stimulates gastric acid secretion and is hypothesized to cause acid rebound when calcium-containing antacids are used to treat acid-related disorders. The clinical importance of this finding, however, remains uncertain.[1,25] If renal elimination is impaired, hypercalcemia may occur and accumulation of calcium may result in the formation of renal calculi. Because many antacids have been reformulated to contain calcium, the risk of hypercalcemia exists when high and frequent dosages of calcium-containing antacids are taken with other calcium supplements or foods such as milk or orange juice with added calcium. Up to 2500 mg/day of elemental calcium can be ingested safely in individuals with normal renal function.[26] (See Chapter 23 for discussion of calcium supplementation.)

Sodium bicarbonate frequently causes belching and flatulence resulting from the production of carbon dioxide.[24] The high sodium content (274 mg sodium/gram sodium bicarbonate) may cause fluid overload in patients with congestive heart failure, renal failure, cirrhosis, pregnancy, and in those on sodium-restricted diets. In individuals with normal renal function, additional bicarbonate is excreted, whereas in patients with impaired renal function, retained bicarbonate may cause systemic alkalosis. A high intake of calcium along with an alkalinizing agent (such as sodium bicarbonate or calcium carbonate) may produce a condition referred to as milk-alkali syndrome. Signs and symptoms include hypercalcemia, alkalosis, irritability, headache, nausea, vomiting, weakness, and malaise.[24,25] Individuals who take calcium supplements should avoid using sodium bicarbonate as an antacid.

All antacids may potentially increase or decrease the absorption of other oral medications when given concomitantly, by adsorbing or chelating the other drug or increasing intragastric pH.[24,27] Medications such as tetracyclines, azithromycin, and fluoroquinolones bind to divalent and trivalent cations, potentially decreasing antibiotic absorption. The absorption of medications such as itraconazole, ketoconazole, and iron, which depend on a low intragastric pH for disintegration, dissolution, or ionization, may also be decreased. Specific antacids, such as aluminum

hydroxide, may decrease the absorption of isoniazid. The absorption of enteric-coated products may be increased with concurrent administration of antacids. The intraluminal interactions of antacids with other oral medications can usually be avoided when potentially interacting drugs are separated by at least 2 hours. Antacid-induced alkalization of the urine may increase urinary excretion of salicylates and decrease blood concentrations.[27] In contrast, an increase in urine pH may decrease urinary excretion and increase blood concentrations of amphetamines and quinidine.[24]

Alginic acid reacts with sodium bicarbonate in saliva to form a viscous layer of sodium alginate that floats on the surface of gastric contents, theoretically forming a protective barrier against esophageal irritation.[1] Alginic acid by itself does not neutralize acid. Because there is insufficient evidence supporting its efficacy as a single agent, the Food and Drug Administration (FDA) has not granted alginic acid category I status. However, alginic acid may be found as an inactive ingredient in several antacid products (Table 14-4). Combination products of alginic acid and an antacid may be superior to an antacid alone.[2] Several antacid products contain simethicone to decrease discomfort related to intestinal gas. (See Chapter 15 for a more detailed description of simethicone.)

Histamine₂-Receptor Antagonists

Cimetidine, ranitidine, famotidine, and nizatidine are available for nonprescription use (Table 14-5) in one-half of the prescription dose and in the higher prescription dose. These H_2RAs are considered interchangeable, despite differences in onset and duration of symptomatic relief, side effects, and the potential for drug–drug interactions. The H_2RAs decrease fasting and food-stimulated gastric acid secretion and gastric volume by inhibiting histamine on the histamine₂ receptor of the parietal cell. Therefore, the H_2RAs are effective in relieving fasting and nocturnal symptoms.[1] Their bioavailability is not affected by food but may be reduced modestly by antacids. Onset of symptomatic relief is not as rapid as with antacids, but the duration of effect is longer (Table 14-3).[1,28] Cimetidine is the shortest-acting (4–8 hours), whereas ranitidine, famotidine, and nizatidine have a somewhat longer duration. Tolerance to the gastric antisecretory effect may develop when H_2RAs are taken daily (versus as needed) and may be responsible for diminished efficacy.[29] Therefore, it is preferable to take an H_2RA on an as-needed basis rather than continuously every day. All four H_2RAs are eliminated by a combination of renal and hepatic metabolism, with renal elimination being the most important. Consideration should be given to reducing the daily H_2RA dose in patients with renal failure and patients of advanced age.[12,30]

Nonprescription H_2RAs are indicated for the treatment of mild-to-moderate, infrequent, episodic heartburn and for the prevention of heartburn associated with acid indigestion and sour stomach. H_2RAs are more effective than placebo for relief of mild-to-moderate heartburn[2,4] and provide moderate improvement in patients with mild dyspeptic symptoms.[9,31] The combined antacid (magnesium hydroxide and calcium carbonate) and H_2RA (famotidine) product is indicated for individuals with postprandial heartburn who have not premedicated with an H_2RA. H_2RAs may be used at the onset of symptoms or 30 minutes to 1 hour prior to an event (meal or exercise) in which heartburn is anticipated. Self-treatment dosing should be limited to no more than two times a day. If the H_2RA is used for more than 2 weeks, a medical referral is recommended. The combined

TABLE 14-5 Selected Nonprescription H$_2$RA and PPI Products and Dosage Regimens

Trade Name	Primary Ingredients	Adult Dosage (Maximum Daily Dosage)
Tagamet HB	Cimetidine 200 mg	1 tablet with a glass of water (2 tablets)
Axid AR	Nizatidine 75 mg	1 tablet with a glass of water (2 tablets)
Pepcid AC	Famotidine 10 mg	1 tablet with a glass of water (2 tablets)
Pepcid AC Maximum Strength	Famotidine 20 mg	1 tablet with a glass of water (2 tablets)
Zantac 75	Ranitidine 75 mg	1 tablet with a glass of water (2 tablets)
Zantac 150	Ranitidine 150 mg	1 tablet with a glass of water (2 tablets)
Pepcid Complete	Famotidine 10 mg; calcium carbonate 800 mg; magnesium hydroxide 165 mg	Chew and swallow 1 tablet (2 tablets)
Prilosec OTC	Omeprazole magnesium 20.6 mg	1 tablet with a glass of water 30 minutes before morning meal; take daily for 14 days (1 tablet)
Various pharmacy brands	Omeprazole 20 mg	1 tablet with a glass of water 30 minutes before morning meal; take daily for 14 days (1 tablet)

antacid and H$_2$RA product provides immediate relief and a longer duration of effect.

H$_2$RAs are well tolerated and have a low incidence of side effects. The most common side effects reported with all four H$_2$RAs include headache, diarrhea, constipation, dizziness, and drowsiness.[11,12] Thrombocytopenia is less common and may occur with all four H$_2$RAs, but it is reversible upon discontinuation of the drug. Cimetidine is associated with a weak anti-androgenic effect that, when taken in high dosages, may result in decreased libido, impotence, or gynecomastia in men.[12]

Cimetidine binds to hepatic cytochrome P450 (3A4, 2D6, 1A2, and 2C9), inhibiting the metabolism of numerous drugs including phenytoin, warfarin, theophylline, tricyclic antidepressants, and amiodarone.[27,32] Ranitidine binds to the cytochrome P450 system to a lesser extent, so interactions are uncommon at nonprescription doses. Famotidine and nizatidine do not interact with the cytochrome P450 system. Medications such as ketoconazole, itraconazole, indinavir and atazanavir, and iron salts are dependent on an acidic environment for absorption.[11,27,33] When administered with an acid-reducing product, their absorption may be reduced. Cimetidine may inhibit the renal tubular secretion of drugs such as procainamide.

Proton Pump Inhibitors

PPIs are potent antisecretory drugs that relieve heartburn and dyspepsia by decreasing gastric acid secretion. Omeprazole magnesium 20.6 mg (Prilosec OTC) was the first PPI to become available for nonprescription use in the United States. It is converted in the body to omeprazole 20 mg. Nonprescription omeprazole 20 mg is also available as specific pharmacy-branded nonprescription products. Other PPIs are currently under consideration for a prescription-to-nonprescription switch and may soon be available. The PPIs inhibit hydrogen potassium ATPase (the proton pump), irreversibly blocking the final step in gastric acid secretion; therefore, they have a more potent and prolonged antisecretory effect than that of the H$_2$RAs (Table 14-3).[34,35] The relative bioavailability of the prescription dosage form (enteric-coated granules contained in a capsule) increases from 35% to 65% with continued daily dosing. Nonprescription omeprazole is formulated as a tablet containing multiple enteric-coated pellets and has a similar oral bioavailabilty.[36] Omeprazole is almost completely absorbed after oral administration, regardless of the presence of food. The tablet should not be chewed or crushed, because the effectiveness of the drug may be decreased.

Onset of symptomatic relief following an oral dose occurs in 2 to 3 hours, but complete relief may take 1 to 4 days.[34,35] A recent study indicates that on day 1, the percentage of time the intragastric pH was greater than 4 with Prilosec OTC taken once daily was higher than with Pepcid AC taken twice a day and was comparable to famotidine 20 mg twice daily.[37] In addition, the intragastric pH with Prilosec OTC was consistently higher than that of both famotidine regimens on subsequent treatment days.

Nonprescription PPIs are indicated for the treatment of frequent heartburn in patients who have symptoms 2 or more days a week. It is not intended for immediate relief of dyspepsia, or occasional or acute episodes of heartburn. Because PPIs inhibit only those proton pumps that are actively secreting acid, they are most effective when taken 30 minutes before a meal.[38]

Nonprescription PPIs should be taken every morning for 14 days. Treatment of heartburn may be repeated after 4 months if symptoms recur.[36] If heartburn continues while taking a nonprescription PPI, persists for more than 2 weeks, or recurs within 4 months, further medical evaluation is recommended.

The most common short-term side effects of PPIs are similar to those reported for the H$_2$RAs (i.e., diarrhea, constipation, and headache).[34] Recent retrospective case-controlled studies of large databases have shown an association between PPIs and community-acquired pneumonia,[39] *Clostridium difficile* infection,[40-43] and an increased risk for hip fractures in individuals older than 50 years.[44] Possible increased risk of pneumonia may result from a decrease in the antibacterial action of gastric juice, which when aspirated may lead to an overgrowth of pathogens. Risk factors include asthma, chronic obstructive pulmonary disease, young or old age (e.g., children and elderly), and immunocompromised state. Although an increased risk of bacterial gastroenteritis and *C. difficile* infection has been reported, another population-based study showed no association between PPI use and hospitalizations for *C. difficile* infection.[45] Although these associations are of interest, there is insufficient evidence to confirm that they resulted from a cause and effect. The clinical importance of these findings for ambulatory patients taking recommended dosages of nonprescription PPIs short-term is questionable.

The safety of nonprescription antisecretory medications, when used appropriately, is well established. Self-treatment with PPIs and H$_2$RAs should be limited to short-term use at nonprescription doses. Patients developing symptoms of gastroenteritis or moderate-to-severe diarrhea should be referred for medical attention. Long-term use and high doses of acid-suppressing medications should take place only under medical supervision.

Omeprazole may interact with other medications that depend on the hepatic CYP2C19 for metabolism.[34,35] Although clinically important drug interactions are minimal given the widespread use of omeprazole, patients taking medications such as diazepam, phenytoin, and warfarin should be warned about the potential for a drug interaction.[36] Similar to antacids and H$_2$RAs, PPIs increase intragastric pH and may decrease the absorption of pH-dependent drugs (see previous discussion of drug–drug interactions for antacids and H$_2$RAs). PPIs may increase the bioavailability of digoxin, but the clinical importance of this effect is unknown.

Bismuth Subsalicylate

Bismuth subsalicylate (BSS) is indicated for heartburn, upset stomach, indigestion, nausea, and diarrhea. FDA has tentatively determined that BSS is safe and effective for the relief of upset stomach associated with belching and gas associated with overindulgence in food and drink.[46] It is uncertain how BSS relieves heartburn, but for upset stomach, it is believed to act by a topical effect on the stomach mucosa. When used to treat acid-related symptoms, the adult dose of BSS is 262 to 525 mg every one-half to 1 hour as needed (Table 14-4). Recently, numerous nonprescription products have been reformulated to contain BSS. In the past, common trade-name products, such as Maalox, contained only antacids. Today, product line extensions, such as Maalox Total Stomach Relief, contain BSS and no antacid (Table 14-4). Therefore, health care providers and patients are often confused and may not know what they are recommending or purchasing, respectively. Individuals taking these products need to know that bismuth salts may cause the stool and tongue to turn black. Dark-colored stools may be interpreted as an upper GI bleed, prompting needless medical procedures. (For a complete discussion of BSS, see Chapter 17.)

Product Selection Guidelines

SPECIAL POPULATIONS

Careful consideration should be given to the elderly before recommending self-treatment for new onset of heartburn or dyspepsia. Older patients are more likely to take medications that can contribute to heartburn and dyspepsia. In addition, they are at higher risk for developing complications and may have a more severe underlying disorder.[1,16] If self-treatment is appropriate, an assessment should be made to determine if the individual has renal impairment and to identify potentially interacting medications. Patients with decreased renal function should be cautioned about using aluminum- and magnesium-containing antacids. The daily H$_2$RA dose should also be reduced, especially in those taking the higher nonprescription dosages. Omepra-

zole may be used in patients with renal impairment. Sodium bicarbonate should be avoided in patients taking cardiovascular medications.

Antacid selection for eligible patients should be based, in part, on potential side effects. For example, if a patient has a tendency toward constipation, a less constipating antacid, such as magnesium hydroxide, may be more appropriate, whereas constipating antacids, such as aluminum hydroxide, should be avoided.

Children under 12 years of age with heartburn or dyspepsia should be referred to their primary care provider for further evaluation.[47] Nonprescription antacids such as calcium carbonate and magnesium hydroxide are labeled for children 12 years and older. If antacids are recommended, an assessment of the child's average daily intake of calcium may help guide the recommendation. The recommended daily intake of calcium for children 9 to 18 years old is 1300 mg.[26] Nonprescription H$_2$RAs are labeled for patients 12 years and older, and nonprescription omeprazole is indicated for patients 18 years and older.

Infrequent and mild heartburn in pregnant women should be treated initially with dietary and lifestyle modifications.[23] Calcium- and magnesium-containing antacids are Pregnancy Category B agents; they may be used safely if the recommended daily dosages are not exceeded.[24] Special attention should be given to the recommended intake of calcium during pregnancy (1000–1300 mg/day).[26] If a woman is meeting the recommendations, the addition of a calcium-containing antacid may cause her to exceed the upper limit of 2500 mg of calcium per day. Pregnant women with frequent and moderate-to-severe heartburn should be referred for medical evaluation. Although cimetidine, famotidine, ranitidine, and nizatidine are listed as Pregnancy Category B and have been used during pregnancy, women should seek medical advice prior to self-treating with an H$_2$RA. Omeprazole is a Pregnancy Category C drug and should not be used by pregnant women without medical supervision.

Magnesium hydroxide and aluminum hydroxide are not secreted into breast milk in substantial amounts.[48] Therefore, these antacids may be safely recommended for self-treatment of heartburn in nursing mothers. The American Academy of Pediatrics considers cimetidine to be compatible with breast-feeding.[49] However, ranitidine and famotidine are less concentrated in the breast milk and may be preferable. There is insufficient information regarding the use of omeprazole in women who are breast-feeding, so it cannot be recommended for nursing mothers at this time.[48]

PATIENT PREFERENCES

Antacids and antisecretory drugs are available in a wide range of prices, flavors, and dosage forms. Once the most appropriate nonprescription medication is determined, the individual should be involved in selecting a product that is affordable, palatable, and practical to administer. Other nonactive ingredients such as dyes, sodium, and sugar should be considered for individuals with allergies, sensitivities, or dietary restrictions.

Complementary and Alternative Therapies

There is no evidence that botanical natural products increase intragastric pH and relieve heartburn. A few studies have shown an improvement in dyspeptic symptoms with a combination of herbs. Limited studies of products containing various combinations of iberis, peppermint, chamomile, bitter candy tuft, matricaria flower, caraway, licorice root, and lemon balm demonstrated some relief of dyspeptic symptoms.[50–52,53] Products identical to those studied, however, are not widely available. A combination of peppermint oil and caraway oil was shown to be effective for dyspepsia.[54] (See Chapter 54 for a more thorough discussion of ginger, peppermint oil, and chamomile.)

Assessment of Heartburn and Dyspepsia: A Case-Based Approach

Cases 14-1 and 14-2 illustrate the assessment of patients with heartburn and dyspepsia.

Patient Counseling for Heartburn and Dyspepsia

Many cases of uncomplicated heartburn and dyspepsia are self-treatable. For optimal outcomes, individuals need to understand how to treat symptoms appropriately and when to seek additional care. This information is provided in the box Patient Education for Heartburn and Dyspepsia.

Evaluation of Patient Outcomes for Heartburn and Dyspepsia

Individuals taking antacids or an H_2RA for infrequent heartburn and dyspepsia should obtain symptomatic relief within 30 minutes to 1 hour. Patients taking omeprazole may require up to 4 days for complete relief of symptoms, but most individuals are asymptomatic within 1 or 2 days. Self-treating individuals should be encouraged to contact their health care provider to report on the effectiveness of therapy and problems, such as side effects, that may arise during treatment. In some cases, the clinician may provide a follow-up phone call to assess therapeutic outcomes. Patients should be asked to describe the change in frequency and severity of symptoms since they initiated therapy. They should be questioned regarding side effects and any new symptoms that may have developed. If an inadequate response is noted, the individual should be reevaluated to determine if a different product is suitable or if medical referral is necessary. Side effects may be managed by adjusting dosage or switching to another product. Development of atypical or alarm symptoms (Table 14-2) should be referred to a primary care provider.

CASE 14-1

Relevant Evaluation Criteria	Scenario/Model Outcome
Information Gathering	
1. Gather essential information about the patient's symptoms, including:	
a. description of symptom(s) (i.e., nature, onset, duration, severity, associated symptoms)	Patient complains of recurring substernal burning sensation after eating heavy meals. It occurs once a week. The discomfort is rated a 4 on a scale of 1–10. It is associated with a feeling of fullness and occasional acid regurgitation. Symptoms typically last 2–4 hours after eating.
b. description of any factors that seem to precipitate, exacerbate, and/or relieve the patient's symptom(s)	Symptoms occur after eating at restaurants or at potluck events at work.
c. description of the patient's efforts to relieve the symptoms	Patient has tried drinking chamomile tea to help relieve the symptoms but has not noticed an improvement.
2. Gather essential patient history information:	
a. patient's identity	Jane Young
b. patient's age, sex, height, and weight	36-year-old female, 5 ft 5 in, 165 lb
c. patient's occupation	Office manager
d. patient's dietary habits	Normal balanced diet; drinks 4–5 cups of coffee each day; drinks 3–4 alcoholic drinks when she goes out for dinner
e. patient's sleep habits	6–8 hours uninterrupted sleep each night
f. concurrent medical conditions, prescription and nonprescription medications, and dietary supplements	Ethinyl estradiol/norgestimate contraceptive, venlafaxine 75 mg for depression, multivitamin every day, calcium citrate 630 mg with vitamin D 400 IU twice daily
g. allergies	NKA
h. history of other adverse reactions to medications	None

CASE 14-1 *(continued)*

Relevant Evaluation Criteria	Scenario/Model Outcome
Assessment and Triage	
3. Differentiate the patient's signs/symptoms and correctly identify the patient's primary problem(s) (see Table 14-2).	Infrequent postprandial substernal burning is consistent with uncomplicated heartburn.
4. Identify exclusions for self-treatment (see Figure 14-2).	None
5. Formulate a comprehensive list of therapeutic alternatives for the primary problem to determine if triage to a medical practitioner is required, and share this information with the patient.	Options include: (1) Refer Jane to her primary care provider. (2) Recommend lifestyle modifications. (3) Recommend an OTC antacid or acid-suppressing product. (4) Take no action.
Plan	
6. Select an optimal therapeutic alternative to address the patient's problem, taking into account patient preferences.	An OTC acid-suppressing product should be effective. Patient will consider lifestyle modifications.
7. Describe the recommended therapeutic approach to the patient.	Take famotidine 20 mg 30–60 minutes prior to a type of meal that precipitates symptoms (restaurant or potluck). See directions in Table 14-5.
8. Explain to the patient the rationale for selecting the recommended therapeutic approach from the considered therapeutic alternatives.	Seeking a PCP may not be necessary if symptoms remain mild and infrequent. An antacid will not provide long-lasting relief, and symptoms are not frequent enough to meet the criteria for a PPI at this time. Follow the administration guidelines in Table 14-5.
Patient Education	
9. When recommending self-care with nonprescription medications and/or nondrug therapy, convey accurate information to the patient:	
a. Appropriate dose and frequency of administration	See Table 14-5.
b. Maximum number of days the therapy should be employed	See the box Patient Education for Heartburn and Dyspepsia.
c. Product administration procedures	See Table 14-5.
d. Expected time to onset of relief	See Table 14-3.
e. Degree of relief that can be reasonably expected	Complete prevention of symptoms if taken before meals; relief if taken at onset of symptoms
f. Most common side effects	Side effects are uncommon. Some patients report headache, diarrhea, or constipation.
g. Side effects that warrant medical intervention should they occur	None
h. Patient options in the event that condition worsens or persists	A PCP should be consulted if symptoms occur despite appropriate use of an H_2RA, or if alarm symptoms occur. See Table 14-2.
i. Product storage requirements	See the box Patient Education for Heartburn and Dyspepsia.
j. Specific nondrug measures	Eat smaller meals. Reduce caffeine and alcohol consumption. See the box Patient Education for Heartburn and Dyspepsia for other measures.
10. Solicit follow-up questions from patient.	Can I take an antacid for immediate relief of symptoms?
11. Answer patient's questions.	Yes, taking a product that contains magnesium hydroxide after symptoms occur will provide faster relief. Avoid calcium-containing products, because you currently take calcium supplements.

Key: NKA, no known allergies; OTC, over-the-counter; PCP, primary care provider.

CASE 14-2

Relevant Evaluation Criteria	Scenario/Model Outcome
Information Gathering	
1. Gather essential information about the patient's symptoms, including:	
a. description of symptom(s) (i.e., nature, onset, duration, severity, associated symptoms)	Patient suffers from recurrent upper abdominal discomfort. Pain is described as a gnawing or burning sensation, fluctuating throughout the day. Pain rating varies from 2–6 on a scale of 10. Symptoms started 2 months ago; they affect his appetite, resulting in a 10-lb weight loss.
b. description of any factors that seem to precipitate, exacerbate, and/or relieve the patient's symptom(s)	Symptoms seem to be relieved temporarily with food.
c. description of the patient's efforts to relieve the symptoms	Patient has tried eating smaller meals, and has tried herbal teas and ranitidine 150 mg as needed. Improvement was not noticeable.
2. Gather essential patient history information:	
a. patient's identity	Yen Xu Wang
b. patient's age, sex, height, and weight	64-year-old male, 5 ft 8 in, 185 lb
c. patient's occupation	Grocery clerk
d. patient's dietary habits	Traditional Chinese food
e. patient's sleep habits	Averages 4 hours per night
f. concurrent medical conditions, prescription and nonprescription medications, and dietary supplements	Indomethacin 75 mg as needed and allopurinol 300 mg every day for gout, atenolol 50 mg every day, HCTZ 25 mg every day, verapamil ER 120 mg every day for hypertension, ginseng supplements every day
g. allergies	Codeine
h. history of other adverse reactions to medications	None
Assessment and Triage	
3. Differentiate the patient's signs/symptoms and correctly identify the patient's primary problem(s) (see Table 14-2).	Late onset, ongoing and frequent GI symptoms, loss of appetite, and unintended weight loss may be an indication of PUD or another more serious condition, rather than a self-treatable condition. Alarm symptoms indicate medical referral. Calcium channel blocker may provoke GERD symptoms. See Table 14-2.
4. Identify exclusions for self-treatment (see Figure 14-2 and Table 14-2).	Alarm symptoms
5. Formulate a comprehensive list of therapeutic alternatives for the primary problem to determine if triage to a medical practitioner is required, and share this information with the patient.	Options include: (1) Refer Yen to a PCP for a differential diagnosis. (2) Recommend an OTC product with lifestyle modifications. (3) Take no action.
Plan	
6. Select an optimal therapeutic alternative to address the patient's problem, taking into account patient preferences.	Refer the patient to a PCP for a differential diagnosis.
7. Describe the recommended therapeutic approach to the patient.	N/A
8. Explain to the patient the rationale for selecting the recommended therapeutic approach from the considered therapeutic alternatives.	You need to see a PCP because symptoms indicate a more serious medical condition that needs evaluation. Treatment with an antisecretory medication has failed. OTC therapy may not be effective or appropriate.
Patient Education	
9. When recommending self-care with non-prescription medications and/or nondrug therapy, convey accurate information to the patient.	Criterion does not apply in this case.

Relevant Evaluation Criteria	Scenario/Model Outcome
10. Solicit follow-up questions from patient.	Is there an herbal medication that would relieve the symptoms?
11. Answer patient's questions.	There is insufficient evidence for effective herbal treatments for this condition. Your current symptoms indicate a need for prompt medical attention.

Key: N/A, not applicable; NKA, no known allergies; OTC, over-the-counter; PCP, primary care provider.

PATIENT EDUCATION FOR
Heartburn and Dyspepsia

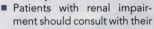

Heartburn and dyspepsia (indigestion) are often self-treatable conditions. Heartburn is characterized by a burning sensation in the chest, usually occurring after meals. Dyspepsia is characterized by discomfort in the upper abdomen. The objectives of self-treatment are to (1) provide complete relief of symptoms, (2) reduce frequency of intermittent episodes, (3) manage factors that contribute to the development of symptoms, (4) prevent and manage side effects of selected treatment, and (5) improve quality of life.

Nondrug Measures

- Avoid food, beverages, and activities associated with an increased frequency and severity of symptoms.
- If possible, avoid the use of medications that may aggravate heartburn or dyspeptic symptoms.
- Avoid eating large meals.
- Stop or reduce smoking.
- Lose weight if overweight and not pregnant.
- Wear loose-fitting clothing.
- If nocturnal symptoms are present:
  — Avoid lying down within 3 hours of a meal.
  — Elevate the head of the bed using 6-inch blocks, or use a foam pillow wedge.

Nonprescription Medications

- Store all medications at 68°F to 77°F (20°C–25°C), and protect them from heat, humidity, and moisture. Discard after expiration date.

Antacids

- Antacids (sodium bicarbonate, calcium carbonate, magnesium hydroxide, and aluminum hydroxide) are available alone and in combination with each other and other ingredients.
- Antacids work by neutralizing acid in the stomach.
- Antacids may be used for relief of mild, infrequent heartburn or dyspepsia (indigestion).
- Antacids are usually taken at the onset of symptoms. Relief of symptoms begins within 5 minutes.
- Because antacids come in a variety of strengths and concentrations, it is essential to consult the label of an individual product for correct dosing quantities and frequencies. Generally antacids should not be used more than four times a day, or regularly for more than 2 weeks.
- If symptoms are not relieved with recommended dosages, consult a health care provider.
- Diarrhea may occur with magnesium- or magnesium/aluminum–containing antacids; constipation may occur with aluminum- or

calcium-containing antacids. Consult with a heath care provider if these effects are severe or do not resolve in a few days.

- Patients with renal impairment should consult with their primary care provider prior to self-treatment with antacids.
- Patients taking tetracyclines, fluoroquinolones, azithromycin, digoxin, ketoconazole, itraconazole, and iron supplements should not take antacids within 2 hours of taking any of these medications.

Histamine$_2$-Receptor Antagonists

- H$_2$RAs (cimetidine, famotidine, nizatidine, and ranitidine) may be used to prevent heartburn and indigestion associated with meals.
- H$_2$RAs are usually taken at the onset of symptoms or 1 hour before symptoms are expected. Relief of symptoms can be expected to begin within 30–45 minutes. A combination product that contains both an antacid and an H$_2$RA provides more rapid relief of symptoms.
- H$_2$RAs generally relieve symptoms for 4–10 hours. H$_2$RAs can be taken when needed up to twice daily for 2 weeks
- H$_2$RAs work by decreasing acid production in the stomach.
- H$_2$RAs should be used for relief of mild-to-moderate, infrequent, and episodic heartburn and indigestion when a longer effect is needed; use lower dosages for mild infrequent heartburn and higher dosages for moderate infrequent symptoms.
- If symptoms are not relieved with recommended doses or persist after 2 weeks of treatment, consult a primary care provider.
- Side effects are uncommon. Consult a primary care provider if side effects are severe or do not resolve within a few days.
- Cimetidine may interact with certain prescription medications. Consult your primary care provider if you are taking a blood thinner such as warfarin, an antifungal such as ketoconazole, antidepressants, anticonvulsants, theophylline, or amiodarone.

Proton Pump Inhibitors

- Proton pump inhibitors (omeprazole) work by decreasing acid production in the stomach.
- Omeprazole is indicated for mild-to-moderate frequent heartburn that occurs 2 or more days a week. It is not intended for the relief of mild, occasional heartburn.
- Omeprazole should be taken with a glass of water every morning 30 minutes before breakfast for 14 days. Make sure that you take the full 14-day course of treatment.

PATIENT EDUCATION FOR
Heartburn and Dyspepsia (continued)

- Do not take more than 1 tablet a day.
- Complete resolution of symptoms should be noted within 4 days of initiating treatment.
- If symptoms persist, are not adequately relieved after 2 weeks of treatment, or recur before 4 months has elapsed since treatment, consult your primary care provider.
- Do not crush or chew tablet, or crush tablet in food or beverage; this may decrease omeprazole's effectiveness.
- Side effects are uncommon. Consult with a health care provider if side effects are severe or do not resolve with a few days.
- Ask a health care provider if you are also taking blood thinners such as warfarin, antifungals such as ketoconazole, or anti-anxiety medications such as diazepam or digoxin.

 Consult your primary care provider if you experience:
— Heartburn or dyspepsia for more than 3 months
— Heartburn or dyspepsia while taking recommended dosages of nonprescription medications
— Heartburn or dyspepsia after 2 weeks of continuous treatment with a nonprescription medication
— Heartburn that awakens you during the night
— Difficulty or pain on swallowing foods
— Light-headedness, sweating, dizziness accompanied by vomiting blood or black material or black tarry bowel movements
— Chest pain or shoulder, arm, neck pain, with shortness of breath
— Chronic hoarseness, cough, choking, or wheezing
— Unexplained weight loss
— Continuous nausea, vomiting, or diarrhea
— Severe stomach pain

Key Points for Heartburn and Dyspepsia

➤ Limit the self-treatment of heartburn and dyspepsia to mild or moderate symptoms including postprandial burning in the upper abdomen or centralized abdominal discomfort.
➤ Refer patients with atypical or alarm symptoms (Table 14-2) for further evaluation.
➤ Refer children younger than 12 years with heartburn or dyspepsia to their primary care provider.
➤ Counsel patients with heartburn on nondrug measures such as dietary and lifestyle modifications (see the box Patient Education for Heartburn and Dyspepsia).
➤ Advise self-treating individuals of the advantages and disadvantages of various antacids and acid-reducing products so they can select a product that is best suited for them.
➤ Antacids provide temporary relief for mild and infrequent heartburn and dyspepsia. Dosages are product-specific because of variability in antacid ingredients and concentrations.
➤ H_2RAs are indicated for mild, infrequent heartburn or dyspepsia. They may be taken at the onset of symptoms or 1 hour prior to an event (meal or exercise) that causes symptoms.
➤ Combining an antacid with an H_2RA provides immediate relief of heartburn and a longer duration of action.
➤ The nonprescription PPI omeprazole is indicated for the treatment of frequent heartburn (heartburn that occurs 2 or more days a week) and is not intended for immediate relief of infrequent symptoms.
➤ Advise individuals with self-treatable symptoms that if symptoms worsen or do not improve after 14 days of effective self-treatment, they should contact their primary care provider.

REFERENCES

1. Richter JE. Gastroesophageal reflux disease. In: Yamada T, Alpers DH, Kaplowitz N, et al., eds. *Textbook of Gastroenterology*. 4th ed. Philadelphia: Lippincott Williams & Williams; 2003:1196–224.
2. DeVault KR, Castell DO. Updated guidelines for the diagnosis and treatment of gastroesophageal reflux disease. *Am J Gastroenterol*. 2005;100:190–200.
3. Fass R, Shapiro M, Dekel R, et al. Systematic review; proton-pump inhibitor failure in gastro-oesophageal reflux disease—where next? *Aliment Pharmacol Ther*. 2005;22:79–94.
4. Peterson WL, Berardi RR, El-Serag H, et al. American Gastroenterological Association Consensus Development Panel. In: *Improving the Management of GERD: Evidence-based Therapeutic Strategies*. Bethesda, Md: AGA Press; 2002:1–21.
5. Rivicki DA., Wood M, Maton PN, et al. The impact of gastroesophageal reflux disease on health-related quality of life. *Am J Med*. 1998;104:252–8.
6. Sandler RS, Everhart JE, Donowitz M, et al. The burden of selected digestive diseases in the United States. *Gastroenterology*. 2002;122:1500–11.
7. Talley NJ, Vakil NB, Moayyedi P. American Gastroenterologic Association technical review on the evaluation of dyspepsia. *Gastroenterology*. 2005;129:1756–80.
8. Vakil N. Dyspepsia and GERD: breaking the rules. *Am J Gastroenterol*. 2005;100:1489–90.
9. Erstad BL. Dyspepsia: initial evaluation and treatment. *J Am Pharm Assoc*. 2002;42:460–8.
10. Procter & Gamble. Data on file. Cincinnati, Ohio; 2002.
11. Del Valle J, Chey WD, Scheiman JM. Acid-peptic disorders. In: Yamada T, Alpers DH, Kaplowitz N, et al., eds. *Textbook of Gastroenterology*. 4th ed. Philadelphia: Lippincott Williams & Williams; 2003:1321–76.
12. Berardi RR, Welage LS. Peptic ulcer disease. In: DiPiro JT, Talbert RL, Yee GC, et al., eds. *Pharmacotherapy: A Pathophysiologic Approach*. 7th ed. McGraw-Hill, Inc; 2008.
13. Oliveria SA, Christos PJ, Talley NJ, et al. Heartburn risk factors, knowledge, and prevention strategies: a population-based survey of individuals with heartburn. *Arch Intern Med*. 1999;159:1592–8.
14. Kaltenbach T, Crockett S, Gerson LB. Are lifestyle measures effective in patients with gastroesophageal reflux disease? Arch Intern Med. 2006; 166:965–71.
15. Nandurkar S, Locke III GR, Fett S, et al. Relationship between body mass index, diet, exercise and gastro-oesophgeal reflux symptoms in a community. *Aliment Pharmacol Ther*. 2004;20:497–505.
16. Pilotto A, Franceschi M, Leandro G, et al. Clinical features of reflux esophagitis in older people: a study of 840 consecutive patients. *J Am Geriatr Soc*. 2006;54:1537–42.
17. McColl KEL. Review article: Helicobacter pylori and gastro-oesophageal reflux disease—the European perspective. *Aliment Pharmacol Ther*. 2004; 20(suppl 8):36–9.
18. Lagergren J, Bergstrom R, Lindgren A, et al. Symptomatic gastroesophageal reflux as a risk factor for esophageal adenocarcinoma. *N Engl J Med*. 1999;11:825–31.
19. Spechler SJ. Barrett's esophagus. *N Engl J Med*. 2002;346:836–42.

20. Richter JE. Review article: extraeosophageal manifestations of gastro-oesophageal reflux disease. *Aliment Pharmacol Ther* 2005;22(suppl 1):70.

21. Howden CW, Chey WD. Gastroesophageal reflux disease. *J Fam Pract.* 2003;52:240–7.

22. Moayyedi P, Talley NJ. Gastro-oesophageal disease. *Lancet.* 2006;367:2086–100.

23. Richter JE. Review article: the management of heartburn in pregnancy. *Aliment Pharmacol Ther.* 2005;22:749–57.

24. Maton PN, Burton ME. Antacids revisited: a review of their clinical pharmacology and recommended therapeutic use. *Drugs.* 1999;57:855–70.

25. Hade JE, Spiro HM. Calcium and acid rebound: a reappraisal. *J Clin Gastroenterol.* 1992;15:37–44.

26. National Institute of Health, Office of Dietary Supplements. Dietary Supplement Fact Sheet: Calcium. Available at: http://dietary-supplements.info.nih.gov/factsheets/calcium.asp. Last accessed August 5, 2008.

27. Welage LS, Berardi RR. Drug interactions with antiulcer agents: considerations in the treatment of acid-peptic disease. *J Pharm Pract.* 1994;7:177–95.

28. Marsh TD. Nonprescription H2-receptor antagonists. *J Am Pharm Assoc.* 1997;37:552–6.

29. Furuta K, Adachi K, Komazawa Y, et al. Tolerance to H2-receptor antagonist correlates well with the decline in efficacy against gastroesophageal reflux in patients with gastroesophageal reflux disease. *J Gastroenterol Hepatol* 2006;21:1581–5.

30. Rodgers PT, Brengel GR. Famotidine-associated mental status changes. *Pharmacotherapy.* 1998;18:404–7.

31. Bytzer P. H2 receptor antagonists and prokinetics in dyspepsia: a critical review. *Gut.* 2002;50(suppl IV):iv58–62.

32. Michalets EL. Update: clinically significant cytochrome P-450 drug interactions. *Pharmacotherapy.* 1998;18:84–112.

33. Fulco PP, Vora UB, Bearman GM. Acid suppressive therapy and the effects on protease inhibitors. *Ann Pharmacother* 2006;40:1974–83

34. Berardi RR. Proton pump inhibitors: an effective, safe approach to GERD management. *Postgrad Med Spec Rep.* 2001;25–35.

35. Welage LS, Berardi RR. Evaluation of omeprazole, lansoprazole, pantoprazole, and rabeprazole in the treatment of acid-related diseases. *J Am Pharm Assoc.* 2000;40:52–62.

36. Prilosec OTC [package insert]. Cincinnati, Ohio: Proctor & Gamble; September 2003.

37. Miner PP, Graves MR, Grender JM, et al. Comparison of gastric acid pH with omeprazole magnesium 20.6 mg (Prilosec OTC) qd, famotidine 10 mg bid (Pepcid AC) and famotidine 20 mg bid over 14-days of treatment [abstract]. *Am J Gastroenterol.* 2004;99(suppl):S8.

38. Hatlebakk JG, Katz PO, Camacho-Lobato L, et al. Proton pump inhibitors: better acid suppression when taken before a meal than without a meal. *Aliment Pharmacol Ther.* 2000;14:1267–72.

39. Laheij RJF, Sturkenboom MCJM, Hassing R, et al. Risk of community acquired pneumonia and use of gastric acid suppressive drugs. *JAMA.* 2004;292:1955–60.

40. Garcia Rodriguez LA, Ruigomez A, Panes J. Use of acid suppressing drugs and the risk of bacterial gastroenteritis. *Clin Gastroenterol Hepatol.* 2007;5:1418–23

41. Canani RB, Cirillo P, Roggero P, et al. Therapy with gastric acidity inhibitors increases the risk of acute gastroenteritis and community-acquired pneumonia in children. *Pediatrics.* 2006;117:e81720

42. Dial S, Delaney C, Schneider V, et al. Proton pump inhibitor use and the risk of community-acquired *Clostridium difficile*-associated disease defined by prescription for oral vancomycin therapy. *CMAJ* 2006;175:745–8

43. Dial S, Delaney JA, Barkun AN, et al. Use of gastric-acid suppressive agents and the risk of community-acquired *Clostridium difficile*-associated disease. *JAMA* 2005;294:2989–95

44. Yang YX, Lewis JD, Epstein S, et al. Long-term proton pump inhibitor therapy and risk of hip fracture. *JAMA* 2006;296:2947–53

45. Lowe DO, Mamdani MM, Kopp A, et al. Proton pump inhibitors and hospitalization for Clostridium difficile-associated disease: a population based study. *Clin Infect Dis* 2006;43:1272–6

46. US Food and Drug Administration. Orally administered drug products for relief of symptoms associated with overindulgence in food and drink for over-the-counter human use; proposed amendment of the tentative final monograph. *Fed Regist.* 2005;70:741–2.

47. Gremse DA. Gastroesophageal reflux disease in children: an overview of pathophysiology, diagnosis, and treatment. *J Ped Gastroenterol Nutr.* 2002;35:S297–9.

48. Briggs GG, Freeman RK, Yaffe SJ. *Drugs in Pregnancy and Lactation.* 6th ed. Baltimore: Williams & Wilkins; 2002.

49. American Academy of Pediatrics, Committee on Drugs. The transfer of drugs and other chemicals into human milk. *Pediatrics.* 2001;108:776–89.

50. Thompson CJ, Ernst E. Systematic review: herbal medicinal products for non-ulcer dyspepsia. *Aliment Pharmacol Ther.* 2002;16:1689–99.

51. Madisch A, Holtmann G, Mayr G, et al. Treatment of functional dyspepsia with a herbal preparation. A double-blind, randomized, placebo-controlled, multicenter trial. *Digestion.* 2004;69:45–52.

52. Melzer J, Rosch J, Reichling R, et al. Meta-analysis: phytotherapy of functional dyspepsia with the herbal drug preparation STW 5 (Iberogast). *Aliment Pharmacol Ther.* 2004;20:1279–87.

53. Koretz RL, Rotblatt M. Complementary and alternative medicine in gastroenterology: the good, the bad, and the ugly. *Clin Gastroenterol Hepatol.* 2004;2:957–67.

54. May B, Kohler S, Schneider B. Efficacy and tolerability of a fixed combination of peppermint oil and caraway oil in patients suffering from functional dyspepsia. *Aliment Pharmacol Ther.* 2000;14:1671–7.

Intestinal Gas

Patrick D. Meek

Intestinal gas symptoms and conditions that predispose patients to intestinal gas are common, and may cause considerable discomfort and lifestyle impairment. The most frequent symptoms are eructation (belching of swallowed air), bloating (excessive gas particularly after eating), and flatulence (excessive passage of air from the stomach or intestines). Patients may also complain of recurrent "gas pains" or abdominal distention. Differentiation of healthy individuals with temporary symptoms from those with a chronic gastrointestinal (GI) condition such as irritable bowel syndrome (IBS), lactose intolerance, or celiac disease is important in recommending appropriate nonprescription treatment.

The primary categories of nonprescription pharmacologic therapies for intestinal gas symptoms are antiflatulent medications (simethicone and activated charcoal), digestive enzymes (lactase replacement and alpha–galactosidase products), and probiotic products (*Bifidobacterium, Lactobacillus, Saccharomyces,* and *Streptococcus* species). Sales of antiflatulent and probiotic products account for a significant portion of the nonprescription drug and dietary supplement markets. In 2007, a leading antiflatulent/antacid combination product ranked among the top 200 nonprescription medications, with annual sales of $50 million, a 10% increase over 2006 sales figures.[1] Several probiotic products have recently entered the market as dietary supplements for patients with digestive problems and have garnered blockbuster sales. In 2007, annual sales of some probiotic products grew by nearly 50% and exceeded $100 million.[2]

A significant portion of the population of the United States is affected by conditions that may cause intestinal gas symptoms, such as lactose malabsorption (29% of the population), IBS (10%–15%), and other less common medical conditions, such as celiac disease (0.4%).[3-6] The prevalence of bloating and other intestinal gas symptoms in patients with one of these conditions may be as high as 80% to 90%.[4,7] In the general population, abdominal distention and bloating are reported by approximately 10% and 20% of individuals in the United States, respectively.[8] An earlier survey of the U.S. population conducted in 1997 evaluated the prevalence and impact of abdominal pain, bloating, and other digestive complaints from any cause: Approximately 40% of survey respondents reported having one or more digestive symptoms in the past month, 20% reported abdominal pain or discomfort, and 15% reported bloating or distention.[9] More than half of symptomatic respondents rated symptoms as moderate to severe in nature, and most indicated that symptoms resulted in some limitation in their ability to conduct usual activities, with 10% reporting that their activities were reduced by half or more.

Pathophysiology of Intestinal Gas

The pathophysiology of intestinal gas symptoms is poorly understood; however, minor disruptions of normal physiologic processes of the GI tract appear to play a role. Each time food, liquid, and saliva are swallowed, a small amount of air from the atmosphere passes into the stomach. In the stomach, the swallowed food is mixed with gastric acid, pepsin, and other substances; churned into small fragments; and then emptied into the small intestine, where most of the absorption of vitamins, minerals, and digestion products (e.g., food-derived monosaccharides such as glucose) occurs.[10] The rate at which the stomach empties varies but generally takes about 1 to 2 hours. Smooth muscle contractions in the small intestine move the liquid food fragments and air downstream toward the large intestine, where the indigestible liquid waste is mixed with the bacterial flora of the colon. In the colon, most of the remaining liquid is absorbed from the mixture of liquid waste, bacteria, and intestinal gas as it is transported toward the rectum and temporarily stored as stool prior to a bowel movement. During a bowel movement, stool is eliminated and intestinal gas is expelled from the rectum as flatus.

Gas is produced and removed by various mechanical and biochemical processes during the transport, digestion, and elimination of food, nutrients, and waste from the GI tract (Figure 15-1). At any given time, approximately 200 mL of gas resides in the GI tract of most individuals and is excreted at a rate ranging from 500 to 1500 mL/day. The primary gases present in the intestine are nitrogen (N_2), hydrogen (H_2), methane (CH_4), carbon dioxide (CO_2), and oxygen (O_2), accounting for more than 99% of gas passed through the rectum (Figure 15-1).[11] None of these principal gases causes odor. The remaining 1% of colonic gas consists of volatile gases, such as hydrogen sulfide (H_2S) and other sulfur-based gases (e.g., methanethiol and dimethyl sulfide), which are produced by bacteria in the colon. These trace gases have an unpleasant smell and are noticeable in quantities as low as a few parts per million.

The source and composition of intestinal gas vary throughout the GI tract. Gas in the upper GI tract arises from the swallowing of atmospheric air, which consists primarily of N_2 (78% by volume) and O_2 (20.8% by volume). Most swallowed air in the stomach is subsequently eliminated through belching. In the first portion of the small intestine, CO_2 is produced when bicarbonate is secreted to neutralize gastric acid, and from metabolism of dietary substrates (such as fat and protein).[11] Most of the CO_2 that is formed in the upper GI tract beyond the stomach

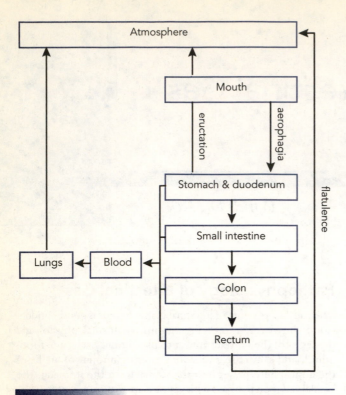

FIGURE 15-1   Pathways of intestinal gas elimination.

diffuses rapidly from the small intestine into the blood and does not contribute significantly to the volume of gas passed through the rectum.

Compared with the gas composition of the upper GI tract, the colon and rectum contain less O_2, more CH_4, a similar amount of N_2, and variable amounts of H_2 and CO_2. N_2 from atmospheric air remains in the intestinal lumen, whereas most of the O_2 diffuses into the bloodstream. Significant volumes of H_2, CH_4, and other trace gases result from the fermentation or bacterial metabolism of ingested materials by bacteria that reside naturally in the distal small bowel and colon (Figure 15-1). The site of gas formation is closely related to the location of intestinal bacteria. The intestinal content of bacteria is typically very low in the initial portions of the small bowel, and the duodenum, jejunum, and proximal ileum are often sterile. In the distal small bowel and colon, the intestinal bacterial content increases from $1 \times 10^{5-8}$ in the last portion of the small intestine (terminal ileum) to $1 \times 10^{10-12}$ in the first portion of the large intestine (cecum). Virtually all H_2 production in the GI tract results from the fermentation of dietary carbohydrates (simple sugars, polysaccharides, and starches) that escape digestion earlier in the GI tract and enter the colon; dietary modification may lessen the amount of H_2 produced.[12,13] Similarly, levels of CO_2 in flatus are believed to be produced almost entirely by bacterial fermentation of indigestible carbohydrates in the colon. Because both result from the process of bacterial fermentation, the concentrations of H_2 and CO_2 are closely related. Although the volume of flatus due to CO_2 formed in the upper GI tract is insignificant, CO_2 formed in the lower GI tract accounts for close to 60% of the volume of flatus.

As with H_2, CH_4 is also formed almost exclusively in the colon by bacterial metabolism. In the case of CH_4, anaerobic organisms (methanogens) use H_2 and CO_2 to form CH_4 (and water) in the colon through a process called methanogenesis. The rate of CH_4 production is only minimally influenced by food

ingestion; however, some people consistently excrete large quantities of CH_4, whereas others excrete little or none.[14]

Diet, underlying medical conditions, alterations in intestinal flora, and drugs may precipitate or aggravate symptoms attributed to intestinal gas.[15] Recent studies have revealed new theories of the pathophysiology of intestinal gas symptoms.[14,16–19] Although the exact mechanisms are not fully known, the origin of gas retention and symptoms appears to be affected by alterations in visceral perception and intestinal transit that vary at different physiologic locations along the GI tract.[17] In patients with IBS, these alterations may be under ridden in part by an overgrowth of bacteria in the small bowel.[7]

Certain foods can increase intestinal gas production and lead to bothersome symptoms (Tables 15-1[20,21] and 15-2[22]). Dietary sugars (e.g., lactose in dairy products and prepared foods; fructose in fruits, vegetables, candies, and soft drinks; sucrose from "table sugar"; and glucose from the breakdown of starches) may be incompletely absorbed in the healthy human small intestine.[23] These sugars are the principal substrates for H_2 production in the colon. Similarly, foods rich in complex carbohydrates (e.g., whole wheat, oats, potatoes, and corn); indigestible oligosaccharides (e.g., raffinose, stachyose, and verbascose); or fatty foods are also malabsorbed. These substances remain in the intestinal lumen, are passed into the colon, and provide substrate for bacterial

---

TABLE 15-1   Gas-Producing Foods

Foods that produce a normal amount of gas:
- Meats: lean cuts of meat and poultry, fish
- Vegetables: asparagus, avocado, lettuce, okra, olives, peas, tomato, zucchini
- Fruit: cantaloupe (and other melons), grapes, berries
- Carbohydrates: rice, chips, popcorn, graham crackers
- All nuts, eggs, gelatin, fruit juice

Foods that cause moderate amounts of excessive gas:
- Root vegetables: potatoes, rutabaga, turnips
- Other vegetables: broccoli, cauliflower, cucumbers, eggplant, peppers, radishes
- Citrus fruits, apples
- Carbohydrates: pastries, non-wheat breads (e.g., breads made from non-wheat flours, such as rice or potato flour)

Foods that cause major amounts of excessive gas:
- Vegetables: onions, celery, carrots, brussel sprouts, cabbage, kohlrabi, sauerkraut
- Legumes: most beans, especially dried beans and peas, baked beans, soy beans, lima beans
- Fruit: raisins, bananas, apricots, prunes
- Carbohydrates: all foods that contain wheat and wheat products, including cereals, breads, bagels, and pretzels
- Liquids: carbonated beverages, beer, red wine
- Dairy products: milk, ice cream, cheese in people who have trouble digesting lactose (check food labels of processed foods for added lactose or milk-derived ingredients)
- Fatty foods: pan fried or deep fried foods, fatty meats; rich cream sauces and gravies (although fatty foods are not carbohydrates, these foods can also contribute to intestinal gas)
- Foods with high sugar content (e.g., soft drinks)
- Products containing sorbitol and mannitol (e.g., sugar-free candies, sugar-free brownie and cake mixes, diet foods, and chewing gum)

Source: References 21 and 22.

TABLE 15-2 Oligosaccharide-Containing Foods That Alpha-Galactosidase Might Affect

Vegetables

Beets
Broccoli
Brussel sprouts
Cabbage
Carrots
Cauliflower
Corn
Cucumbers
Leeks
Lettuce
Onions
Parsley
Peppers, sweet

Legumes

Black-eyed peas
Bog beans
Broad beans
Chickpeas
Field beans
Lentils
Lima beans
Mung beans
Peanuts
Peas
Pinto beans
Red kidney beans
Soybeans

Grains, Cereals, Seeds, and Nuts

Bagels
Barley
Breakfast cereals
Granola
Oat bran
Oat flour
Pistachios
Rice bran
Rye
Sesame flour
Sorghum, grain
Sunflower flour
Wheat bran
Whole-grain breads
Whole-grain flour

Other Foods

Baked beans
Bean salads
Chili
Lentil soup
Pasta
Peanut butter
Soy milk
Split-pea soup
Stir-fried vegetables
Stuffed cabbage
Tofu

Source: Reference 23.

fermentation and colonic production of H_2 and CO_2.[14] Fermentation in the colon is the primary source of intestinal gas. The quantity of gas produced by fermentation of these substances in the colon is influenced by the quantity of foods ingested.

Diets high in dietary fiber may also lead to bloating and flatulence. Terminology, recommended intake, and potential benefits associated with fiber are discussed in Chapter 24. Fiber is a valuable component of a balanced diet and may be beneficial in the treatment of constipation (see Chapter 16). A systematic review of fiber use in patients with IBS-related constipation noted an overall favorable effect of fiber on constipation and global symptoms; however, bloating and abdominal pain were not improved.[24] Although wheat bran and psyllium were among the fibers showing favorable results in this systematic review, the coarseness of such insoluble fiber is a potential drawback and may trigger painful attacks in some patients with bloating caused by IBS. Soluble fiber absorbs water and stabilizes intestinal contractions; however, results of soluble fiber supplementation on IBS symptoms are conflicting.[24–26] Some studies and systematic reviews have failed to show a benefit of soluble fiber supplementation in improving bloating, abdominal discomfort, and global symptoms in patients with IBS, whereas others have shown favorable results for constipation and global symptoms without improving bloating.[24–26] A soluble semisynthetic fiber supplement such as calcium polycarbophil may be preferred to natural fibers such as psyllium for patients who experience gas-related symptoms (bloating and flatulence) from other fiber forms. However, in patients with IBS, slow intestinal transit, and diverticulosis,

fiber may increase intestinal gas symptoms.[26,27] Slowly increasing the intake of fiber or using a variety of fiber-containing foods may help reduce symptoms in these groups of patients.

The odor attributed to flatulence may be worsened by the ingestion of sulfate-containing foods such as cruciferous vegetables (e.g., broccoli and cabbage), breads and beers containing sulfate additives, and proteins with a high sulfur-containing amino acid (e.g., methionine and cysteine) content. Sulfur-based gases (e.g., H_2S, methanethiol, and dimethyl sulfide) are produced through the action of sulfate-reducing bacteria on sulfate.[16] Rating foods by their potential to cause intestinal gas symptoms is difficult, but clinical experience suggests that certain foods are generally more problematic than others (Table 15-1).

Intestinal gas symptoms may also be related to the amount of air that enters the GI tract upon swallowing. Smoking, chewing gum, sucking on hard candies, drinking carbonated beverages, wearing poor-fitting dentures, and hyperventilating or being overly anxious may cause individuals to swallow larger amounts of air.[14,28,29] Poor eating habits such as gulping food or beverages too rapidly may also cause larger amounts of air to enter the stomach.

A number of medical conditions cause or predispose patients to the formation of intestinal gas. Some conditions, such as carbohydrate malabsorption, lead to an increased amount of gas produced from bacterial fermentation in the colon. The most common cause of carbohydrate malabsorption is lactase deficiency. Lactase is the enzyme that normally breaks down lactose in the intestinal lumen so that it can be absorbed. Approximately 50 million people in the United States are lactose maldigesters. The condition is more common in black (90%) and Asian populations (75%) than in eastern Europeans (6%). In patients with lactase deficiency, the lactase enzyme is not available in sufficient quantities to break down lactose in dairy products before it reaches the colon.

In the colon, the malabsorbed lactose remains in the intestinal lumen where it is available to colonic bacteria for fermentation to H_2 and other substances. Individuals with lactase deficiency experience GI symptoms such as gas pains, bloating, nausea, and diarrhea upon exposure to dairy and other products with milk or milk-derived carbohydrate (e.g., caramel).[30] Milk-derived protein (e.g., whey powder, caseinate, and other lactoproteins) does not cause lactose-associated GI symptoms unless the product is contaminated with milk-derived carbohydrate (i.e., lactose). Bacterial fermentation in the small intestine resulting from bacterial overgrowth may also lead to excessive amounts of intestinal gas. Effects of probiotics on bloating symptoms associated with small-bowel bacterial overgrowth and lactose intolerance are uncertain (see Chapter 24). Some suggest probiotics improve bloating associated with lactose intolerance by producing lactic acid, which in turn improves lactose digestion.[30]

Other conditions such as IBS may predispose patients to intestinal gas symptoms.[15] Gas pains and bloating are very common in patients with IBS and may be caused by a number of interrelated factors, including heightened sensation of the GI tract to intestinal stretch (or visceral hypersensitivity), altered intestinal motility, activated intestinal immunity, altered brain–gut interaction, and autonomic dysfunction.[7,31,32] Small-bowel bacterial overgrowth has recently been proposed as a unifying theory linking each of these factors, and has stimulated exciting research that aims to further define the relationship between intestinal bacterial overgrowth and the onset of symptoms of IBS. As this research evolves, the role of therapies that affect the bacterial flora of the intestinal tract, such as probiotics, will become more clearly defined. Probiotics, such as lactobaccilli and bifidobacteria, are part of the normal "healthy" flora of the intestinal tract; they are thought to maintain intestinal health through a variety of mechanisms: by shifting the intestinal bacterial content in favor of nonpathologic organisms; by producing beneficial substances, such as short-chain fatty acids; and by acting primarily as carbohydrate-fermenting bacteria, thereby producing a favorable effect on intestinal gas production (see Chapter 24). Substances such as oligofructose (a "prebiotic") are used as nutrients by the normal intestinal bacterial flora and by probiotic organisms; however, the normal flora produces greater amounts of CO_2 and H_2, which may result in increased symptoms of intestinal gas.[33,34]

Intestinal gas symptoms may also result from other less common medical conditions, such as celiac disease or diabetic gastroparesis. Patients with celiac disease have intolerance to gluten (a protein contained in wheat, rye, barley, and oats) and must follow a gluten-free diet. Intestinal gas symptoms may result from the inflammatory response that occurs in the GI tract after exposure to gluten. The most common sources of gluten are baked goods that contain the causative grains, wheat and oat cereals, noodles, and pastas; however, many other food products, especially any processed foods with thickeners, and some medications contain gluten. Successful adherence to a diet free of gluten requires rigorous label reading and close scrutiny of the gluten content of foods and nonprescription medications. There are a number of valuable resources for individuals seeking information about celiac disease.[35-44] In addition, referral to a registered dietitian may be beneficial because *all* gluten must be removed from the diet to avoid symptoms.

A variety of drugs may cause intestinal gas symptoms. These drugs can be broadly categorized by the mechanisms that cause symptoms: drugs that affect the intestinal flora (lactulose and antibiotics); drugs that affect the metabolism of glucose and other dietary substances (alpha-glucosidase inhibitors including acarbose and miglitol); and the GI lipase inhibitor orlistat. Drugs that affect GI motility (narcotics, anticholinergics, and calcium channel blockers); drugs that are high in fiber (psyllium) or nonabsorbable polymers (cholestyramine); and drugs that contain or release gas (effervescent solutions such as Alka-Seltzer) may also cause intestinal gas symptoms.

Clinical Presentation of Intestinal Gas

Patients with symptoms of intestinal gas complain most commonly of excessive belching, abdominal discomfort or cramping, bloating, and flatulence. Gas pains and belching appear to be more common complaints than flatulence. Other less common symptoms associated with "gaseousness" include nausea; audible bowel sounds, called borborygmi; and dyspepsia or indigestion. Some patients may experience multiple symptoms concurrently.

Everyone experiences belching, especially after eating. Belching is the easiest way for air to leave the stomach after it is swallowed. Some people have excessive belching, which may be annoying and embarrassing because of its frequency and/or unexpected occurrence. The more frequently a person swallows, the greater is the potential for air to enter the stomach. Drinking carbonated beverages or eating food too quickly is an easy way to inadvertently increase the amount of air that is swallowed, which may then cause excessive belching.

Gas pains are often described as a generalized, crampy discomfort associated with gaseousness; passing gas or having a bowel movement may relieve gas pains. In some patients, symptoms may be brought on by stress or anxiety. In others, the size of a meal may be associated with the onset and severity of gas pains, with larger meals causing more bothersome symptoms. Patients who complain of recurrent gas pains (occurring at least 3 days per month in the last 3 months) that are associated with either diarrhea or constipation may have IBS. Because gas pains can mimic other conditions, such as gallbladder, diabetic gastroparesis, or heart disease, a primary care provider should be consulted prior to initiating self-management.

Bloating may be characterized by patients as a sensation of tension in the abdominal area after eating or as a subjective sensation that the abdomen is larger than normal. Patients with bloating may observe that clothes fit more tightly or are difficult to fit into comfortably. The ingestion of certain foods (Tables 15-1 and 15-2), especially high-fiber diets and eating too rapidly or too much may contribute to bloating. The onset of bloating may be associated with periods of stress and anxiety. In women, bloating is one of the most frequent menstrual symptoms and may be related to hormonal effects during the menstrual cycle.[45] Similar to chronic gas pains, chronic bloating accompanied by a change in bowel function is suggestive of IBS. Patients with diabetes who complain that symptoms of bloating are accompanied by a sensation of early satiety or fullness after the ingestion of a small amount of food may be experiencing diabetic gastroparesis and should be referred to a primary care provider.

Most patients who complain of flatulence are referring to the passage of intestinal gas through the rectum. Passing gas is normal and occurs either consciously or unconsciously between 20 and 40 times a day, even while sleeping. Sometimes patients complain that flatulence occurs more frequently than expected, or occurs unexpectedly or uncontrollably. Certain foods (Tables 15-1 and 15-2), especially those that contain fiber, fructose, lactose, or oligosaccharides, are more likely to cause gas and therefore can contribute to flatulence. Sorbitol or mannitol from commonly used sweeteners in low-calorie foods and liquid medications can also contribute to flatulence.

Intestinal gas symptoms are rarely a serious problem and can occasionally be treated with medications. However, intestinal gas complaints may be symptoms of an underlying chronic condition such as inflammatory bowel disease, celiac disease, bacterial overgrowth, or IBS. In rare cases, gas complaints may be a sign of a more serious problem such as peptic ulcer disease, intestinal obstruction, or neoplastic disease. To avoid an unnecessary delay in the initiation of therapy, patients should be referred to a primary care provider for medical evaluation if any of the criteria for exclusion for self-management are met (Figure 15-2). Patients with lactose intolerance are at risk for the development of low bone density and osteoporosis because of reduced dietary intake; they should be counseled to supplement their diets to achieve the recommended daily intake of 1000 to 1200 mg of elemental calcium per day.

Treatment of Intestinal Gas

Most patients will be able to control the symptoms by understanding how they occur, by following steps to reduce predisposing factors, and by making informed decisions regarding the use of nonprescription medications. Symptoms that are related to eating habits or diet often will subside quickly once the source of the problem is identified and the necessary changes are made. Self-treatment of intestinal gas symptoms (Figure 15-2) should begin

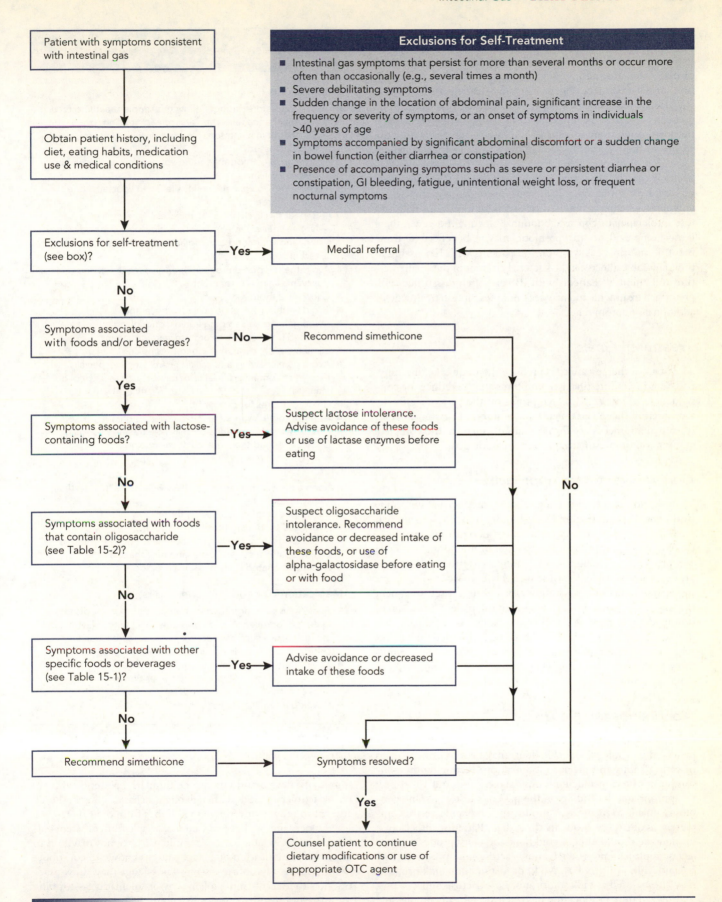

FIGURE 15-2 Self-care of intestinal gas symptoms. Key: GI, gastrointestinal; OTC, over-the-counter.

with an assessment of the patient's history of symptoms, diet, eating habits, medication use, and relevant medical conditions. Patients who associate symptoms with foods containing lactose or oligosaccharide and who do not meet the criteria for exclusion for self-treatment (Figure 15-2) may use digestive enzymes (i.e., lactase replacement or alpha–galactosidase products). Antiflatulents such as activated charcoal and simethicone may also be used, although there is contradictory evidence supporting the ability of these agents to reduce the amount of intestinal gas formation. Probiotics (see Chapter 24) maintain gastrointestinal health by protecting against pathologic GI flora,[46] and they may be useful for some individuals with intestinal gas. There is no consensus whether probiotics are beneficial in patients with lactose intolerance or chronic abdominal bloating; however, there is increasing evidence that probiotics may be beneficial for treatment of intestinal gas symptoms in patients with IBS owing to their favorable affects on the bacterial content of the small intestine and colon.[7,47] Patients with IBS are often dissatisfied with prescribed treatments and may seek nonprescription treatment for additional symptom relief.

Treatment Goals

The goals of therapy are to (1) reduce the frequency, intensity, and duration of intestinal gas symptoms and (2) reduce the consequences of intestinal gas symptoms on the patient's lifestyle. Considering that a certain amount of intestinal gas production is normal and necessary for normal GI function, the complete elimination of intestinal gas is not a realistic goal.

General Treatment Approach

Identification of the underlying cause of intestinal gas will guide treatment decisions (Figure 15-2). Inquiry into the patient's diet, including a review of eating habits and rate of food ingestion, can often lead to appropriate suggestions in attempting to reduce the problem. Although several nonprescription antiflatulent products are available, their use is largely empiric, and evidence supporting their benefit is limited. Exclusions for self-treatment (Figure 15-2) should be reviewed with the patient prior to recommending therapy. Referral of the patient to a primary care provider for further evaluation should be considered for patients with exclusions for self-treatment, and for patients whose symptoms persist after initiating simple treatment options, such as dietary modification, and nonprescription medications.

Nonpharmacologic Therapy

General information for controlling intestinal gas symptoms is provided in Table 15-3.[48,49] Patients may benefit from changes in eating habits and dietary modification. Reducing the consumption of gas-producing foods (Tables 15-1 and 15-2) may be appropriate, depending on the patient's history. Some people are unable to tolerate gas-producing foods and need to completely avoid these foods in their diet. Patients with lactose intolerance should either avoid milk and dairy products or use lactase replacement products. Low-lactose milk products (e.g., Lactaid Milk or Dairy Ease Milk) or fortified soy milk products may also be used as milk substitutes. Low-lactose milk is a prehydrolyzed milk product in which lactose is already predigested and contains the same nutrients as regular milk, but the product is not entirely lactose-free. Fortified soy products are palatable lactose-free milk alternatives, which are low in fat and a good

| TABLE 15-3 Useful Information to Decrease Symptoms of Intestinal Gas |

Eating Habits

- Relax a bit before eating. Follow this simple breathing technique to enhance relaxation and release tension:
  - Sit straight in a comfortable position with your arms and legs uncrossed.
  - Breathe in comfortably, using your abdomen. Pause briefly before exhaling.
  - Each time you exhale, count silently to yourself, "one . . . two . . . three . . . four."
  - Repeat this cycle for 5–10 minutes.
  - Notice your breathing gradually slowing, your body relaxing, and your mind calming as you practice this breathing technique.
- Avoid the temptation to rush through a meal. Eat and drink slowly in a calm environment.
- Chew food thoroughly.
- Avoid washing solids down with a beverage.
- Avoid gulping and sipping liquids, or drinking out of small-mouthed bottles, straws, or from water fountains.
- Eliminate pipe, cigar, and cigarette smoking.
- Avoid gum chewing and sucking hard candy, especially those that contain artificial sweeteners, such as sorbitol or mannitol.
- Check dentures for proper fit.
- Attempt to be aware of and avoid deep sighing.
- Do not attempt to induce belching or strain to pass gas.
- Do not overload the stomach at any one meal.

Diet

- Keep a dietary diary for a few days while tracking intestinal gas symptoms.
- Avoid foods that cause gas symptoms.
- Avoid gas-producing foods (Table 15-1).
- Avoid foods with air whipped into them, such as whipped cream, soufflés, sponge cake, and milk shakes.
- Avoid carbonated beverages, such as sodas and beer.

Medication Use and Lifestyle Habits

- Avoid long-term or frequent intermittent use of medications intended for relief of cold symptoms (e.g., anticholinergic antihistamines such as brompheniramine, carbinoximine, chlorpheniramine, clemestine, diphenhydramine).
- Avoid tight-fitting garments, girdles, and belts.
- Do not lie down or sit in a slumped position immediately after eating.
- Develop a regular routine of exercise and rest.

Source: References 48 and 49.

source of calcium and vitamin D. Similarly, patients who are unable to tolerate foods with high oligosaccharide content should attempt to reduce or remove these foods from their diet.

Understanding the food values of people from different cultures, ethnicities, and socioeconomic backgrounds may lead to improved identification of dietary patterns known to contribute to intestinal gas symptoms.[50] This knowledge may allow practitioners to identify and explain why problematic gas-forming foods are not healthy options in a culturally sensitive manner. Addressing dietary issues with family members may be a better approach for developing healthy eating habits over time, especially for children experiencing intestinal gas symptoms.

Pharmacologic Therapy

Simethicone and activated charcoal may relieve symptoms after intestinal gas has formed. Alpha-galactosidase and lactase enzymes are taken with foods to prevent gas from forming. Lactase replacement products may be beneficial for the treatment of intestinal gas and diarrhea associated with lactose intolerance, and they are also used as digestive aids, allowing individuals with lactose intolerance to incorporate dairy foods into their diet without producing intolerable symptoms. Most lactose maldigesters can tolerate up to 1 cup of milk, so these products should be used when more than that amount is ingested in one sitting. Osmotic laxatives may be used for patients with abdominal cramps, bloating, and gas associated with constipation (see Chapter 16).

Simethicone

Simethicone, a mixture of inert silicon polymers, is used as a defoaming agent to relieve gas. Simethicone acts in the stomach and intestine to reduce the surface tension of gas bubbles embedded in mucus in the GI tract. As surface tension changes, the gas bubbles are broken or coalesced and then eliminated more easily by belching or passing gas through the rectum.[51]

FDA considers simethicone safe and effective as an antiflatulent agent. In patients with acute, nonspecific diarrhea, the combination of simethicone with loperamide produced quicker relief from gas-related discomfort than either agent alone.[52] However, the ability of simethicone to reduce intestinal gas symptoms for all patients with symptoms is questionable.[53] The use of simethicone may be encouraged on a trial basis because some patients report benefit from it. The usual adult and pediatric dosages for simethicone are provided in Table 15-4.

Many antacid products contain a combination of simethicone and antacids; therefore, patients should follow the label instructions for dosages of these products. However, use of both agents is often unnecessary, and the efficacy of such combination products has not been well studied. Furthermore, single-ingredient antiflatulent products (Table 15-5) usually contain a higher concentration of simethicone than that of the combination products.

Because simethicone is not absorbed from the GI tract, it has no known systemic side effects and its safety has been well documented. Simethicone is contraindicated in patients with a known hypersensitivity to simethicone products or suspected intestinal perforation and obstruction.

Many antacid products contain a combination of simethicone and antacids; patients should follow the label instructions for dosages. However, use of both agents is often unnecessary, and the efficacy of such combination products is unknown. Combination products containing simethicone and activated charcoal are also available; these products aim to provide relief from intestinal gas symptoms by combining the gas-reducing activity of each of the individual components.

Activated Charcoal

Activated charcoal is also promoted for relief of intestinal gas; however, it is neither approved nor shown to be effective for this indication.[54] The usual adult dosages for this agent are provided in Table 15-4. The proposed antiflatulent properties of activated charcoal are related to the adsorbent effects of the substance and its potential to facilitate the elimination of intestinal gas from the GI tract. Activated charcoal has been purported to be beneficial for the elimination of malodorous, sulfur-based gases.[55] This substance also has poor palatability. External devices containing activated charcoal are also available to reduce the odor of flatus in patients with ostomies (see Chapter 22).

Table 15-5 lists examples of commercially available products, including products containing activated charcoal and simethicone.

TABLE 15-4 Dosage Guideline for Intestinal Gas Products

Agent	Adults	Dosage (Maximum Daily Dose) Children >12 Years	Children 2 to ≤12 Years	Children <2 Years
Simethicone	125–250 mg four times daily (500 mg)	40–125 mg four times daily (500 mg)	40 mg four times daily (240 mg)	20 mg four times daily (240 mg)
Activated charcoal	520 mg (2 capsules) orally after meals as needed, may repeat hourly (4.16 g)	Specific guidelines not available		
Alpha-galactosidase	150 units per serving of food (450 units)	Not recommended		
Lactase enzyme	3000–9000 units at first bite of food or drink containing lactose (18,000 units)	Specific guidelines not available (18,000 units)		
Bifidobacterium infantis 35624	1 capsule (1×10^9 bacteria) per day (manufacturer's recommended dose)	Specific guidelines not available		
Lactobacillus acidophilus *Bifidobacterium* *Lactobacillus paracasei* *Streptococcus thermophilus*	1 capsule (consisting of an aggregate of 16×10^9 bacteria) per day (manufacturer's recommended dose)	Specific guidelines not available		

TABLE 15-5 Selected Antiflatulent Products

Trade Name	Primary Ingredients
Single-Entity Simethicone Products	
Gas-X Extra Strength Chewable Tablets	Simethicone 125 mg
Gas-X Regular Strength Chewable Tablets	Simethicone 80 mg
Gas-X Thin Strips	Simethicone 62.5 mg per (edible film) strip
Mylicon Infant's Drops	Simethicone 40 mg/0.6 mL
Activated Charcoal Products	
Activated Charcoal Tablets	Activated charcoal 250 mg
CharcoCaps Capsules	Activated charcoal 260 mg
Combination Charcoal Product	
Charcoal Plus	Activated charcoal 250 mg
	Simethicone 80 mg
Alpha-Galactosidase Replacement Products	
Beano Drops	Alpha-galactosidase 150 units (5 drops)
Beano Tablets	Alpha-galactosidase 150 units (1 tablet)
Gaz Away Caplets	Alpha-galactosidase 150 units (1 caplet)
Lactase Replacement Products	
Dairy Ease Tablets	Lactase 3000 units
Lactaid Original Strength Caplets	Lactase 3000 units
Lactase Fast Act Chewable Tablets	Lactase enzyme 9000 units
Lactase Fast Act Tablets	Lactase enzyme 9000 units
Lactrase Capsules	Lactase enzyme 250 mg = 3750 lactase enzyme units
Probiotic Products	
Activia Probiotic Yogurt	*Lactobacillus bulgaricus*
	Streptococcus thermophilus
	Bifidobacterium animalis DN173010
	(1×10^8 live bacteria per gram[a])
Align Capsules	*Bifidobacterium infantis* 35624, 4 mg = 1×10^9 live bacteria
DanActive Probiotic Dairy Drink	*Lactobacillus bulgaricus*
	Streptococcus thermophilus
	Lactobacillus casei DN-114 001
Danimals Yogurt Smoothie Drinks	*Lactobacillus bulgaricus*
	Streptococcus thermophilus
	Lactobacillusrhamnosus GG
	(1×10^8 live bacteria per gram[a])
FloraQ	*Lactobacillus acidophilus*
	Bifidobacterium
	Lactobacillus paracasei
	Streptococcus thermophilus
	(230 mg = an aggregate of a minimum of 8×10^9 freeze-dried bacteria)
Florastor	*Saccharomyces boulardi* freeze-dried capsules
	250 mg

[a] Meets National Yogurt Association criteria for live and active culture yogurt.

Alpha-Galactosidase

Another FDA–approved product for use as an antiflatulent is the enzyme alpha–galactosidase. This enzyme, which is derived from the *Aspergillus niger* mold and classified as a food, hydrolyzes oligosaccharides into their component parts before they can be metabolized by colonic bacteria. The usual adult and pediatric dosages for alpha-galactosidase are provided in Table 15-4.[51]

Because high-fiber foods contain large amounts of oligosaccharides, alpha-galactosidase is recommended as a prophylactic treatment of intestinal gas symptoms produced by high-fiber diets or foods that contain oligosaccharides (Table 15-2). Two controlled trials of alpha–galactosidase demonstrated that the agent significantly reduced symptoms of intestinal gas in healthy individuals fed oligosaccharide-containing foods.[22,56]

The safety of alpha-galactosidase remains to be determined. Although this enzyme has been used in food processing for years and is regarded as safe by FDA, the amount contained in available products is probably much greater than that in processed foods. One patient developed an intestinal perforation after taking Beano for several weeks, but a causal relationship was not established and there have been no similar reports. Because the enzyme produces galactose, this product should not be used by patients with galactosemia (an inherited metabolic disorder in which galactose accumulates in the blood owing to deficiency of an enzyme that catalyzes galactose's conversion to glucose). Similarly, diabetic patients should be cautioned about the use of the enzyme, which may produce 2 to 6 grams of carbohydrates per 100 grams of food. Allergic reactions are also possible in patients allergic to molds.

Lactase Replacement Products

Lactase replacement products are used in patients with lactose intolerance (see Chapter 17). Lactase enzymes break down lactose, a disaccharide, into the monosaccharides glucose and galactose, which are absorbed. Lactase replacement products should be used in patients with lactose intolerance to aid in the digestion of dairy products. There are no adverse effects listed for lactase replacement products. The usual adult dose for lactase enzymes is provided in Table 15-4.

Product Selection Guidelines

SPECIAL POPULATIONS

Several pediatric formulations of simethicone are indicated for the relief of intestinal gas. These products, which contain simethicone 40 mg per 0.6 mL suspension, are often promoted and used to relieve gas associated with colic. Because many infants suffer from infantile colic, simethicone is sometimes recommended. However, simethicone was not found to be superior to placebo for intestinal gas and/or infantile colic in a recent study.[57] Although its efficacy is questionable, simethicone is not absorbed from the GI tract and is considered safe for use in infants and children.[26] There are no reports linking simethicone to congenital defects.[26] Simethicone is a Pregnancy Category C drug and is considered to be safe for use by nursing mothers. For alpha-galactosidase products, safety and efficacy have not been evaluated in infants and children. Therefore, this product should not be used in pediatric patients until data are available to support such use. Manufacturers recommend that pregnant or nursing patients first consult with a primary care provider before using alpha-galactosidase. No special population considerations are listed for lactase replacement products. Patients should consult a primary care provider if symptoms continue after using a product or if symptoms are unusual and seem unrelated to eating dairy products.

PATIENT FACTORS

Alpha-galactosidase and lactase replacement products are used to prevent the onset of symptoms in patients unable to tolerate problematic foods. Patients with symptoms of gas who need immediate relief or patients who cannot associate their symptoms with certain foods should receive simethicone. Activated charcoal may be an alternative to simethicone for patients with gas symptoms and may be beneficial for patients who also experience malodorous gas production. If used on a regular basis, alpha-galactosidase is more cost-effective than simethicone. Because alpha-galactosidase produces carbohydrates, patients with galactosemia or diabetes mellitus should avoid this product and use simethicone instead. Lactase replacement products should be considered for patients with lactose intolerance when ingesting dairy products.

PATIENT PREFERENCES

Most products for intestinal gas are available in a variety of strengths and dosage forms. A liquid formulation of simethicone is available for infants. Simethicone is also available as chewable tablets or an edible filmstrip. Liquid dosage forms and alternative solid dosage forms are generally more expensive than standard solid oral dosage forms, such as tablets and capsules, but may be more palatable. Activated charcoal is available in two solid oral dosage forms (tablets or capsules), as well as a combination product with simethicone. Alpha-galactosidase is available as tablets, caplets, and liquid drops. Patients may either take the tablet or caplets orally, or use the liquid drops with problematic foods. There is no difference in onset of symptomatic relief between the tablets and liquid drops, so the choice between dosage forms is left entirely to personal preference and convenience. Both forms of alpha-galactosidase are equally potent and need to be administered at the same time that the problematic food is ingested. Similarly, a variety of products is available for patients with lactose intolerance. Lactase replacement products can be either added to milk or dairy products to reduce the amount of lactose in the product, or ingested along with dairy products in an effort to reduce the amount of lactose in the food. Alternatively, patients may elect to use one of the available milk alternatives, such as low-lactose milk or a fortified soy milk product. Because both alternatives would be effective in supplementing dietary calcium and vitamin D, and in reducing lactose exposure, patients may use a combination of the available alternatives in an effort to prevent symptoms while maintaining a healthy diet.

Probiotic Therapies

A variety of probiotic dietary supplements (see Chapter 24) is widely used for GI complaints including intestinal gas and bloating.[58] The most common formulations for intestinal gas (Table 15-5) are capsules with one bacterium (e.g., *Bifidobacterium infantis*) or multiple bacteria (e.g., *Lactobacillus acidophilus* and *Lactobacillus paracasei*, *Bifidobacterium*, and *Streptococcus thermophilus*). Functional food products with active cultures of probiotic species (e.g., *Bifidobacterium animalis* DN173010, also known as *Bifidus regularis*) are also available. *Lactobacillus* and *Bifidobacterium* species are found in many fermented foods, are normal colonizers of the intestinal tract, and when consumed as food or a dietary supplement, are considered to have low-level infection risk.[59] Serious complications of probiotic therapies have been noted in patients with severe pancreatitis.[60] In patients with IBS and those with lactose intolerance, there is increasing, but limited, evidence that specific probiotics provide temporary relief from GI symptoms.[61-65] Further clinical research is needed to define the optimal dose and duration of probiotics before these agents can be recommended for routine use as self-management of these conditions. Probiotic bacteria leave the intestine soon after therapy is discontinued. When using probiotic therapy, daily administration is required to maintain bacterial populations in the intestinal flora. An adequate trial of 14 days is generally recommended for patients interested in using probiotic therapy. If no benefit is obtained within this time frame, further use should be discontinued. Concurrent administration of probiotics with antibiotics will inactivate the probiotic bacteria, removing any possible benefit.

Complementary Therapies

Natural products commonly used for intestinal gas are known as carminatives.[66] Examples include fennel, Japanese mint, peppermint, and spearmint. These agents are widely used for the treatment of intestinal gas despite insufficient evidence.[26,67] Carminatives may reduce the tone of the lower esophageal sphincter and are among the foods that should be minimized

TABLE 15-6 Differentiation of Intestinal Gas Discomfort and Irritable Bowel Syndrome

Criterion	Intestinal Gas Discomfort	Irritable Bowel Syndrome (IBS)
Location	Generalized discomfort in the upper, mid, or lower abdomen.	Generalized discomfort, bloating, and or pain in the area of the abdomen or colon.
Signs	Eructation (upper abdomen): belching of air. Bloating (mid abdomen): the perception of accumulated intestinal gas. Flatulence (lower abdomen, colon): excessive air or other gas in the stomach and intestines.	There may be no physical signs of disease in IBS. Symptoms are relieved with defecation or associated with a change in frequency or consistency of stools.
Symptoms	May present as minimal physical discomfort but significant, negative psychosocial effects.	Symptoms of IBS vary widely from one person to another. Patients with IBS typically have abdominal pain that is relieved after a bowel movement, and is accompanied by either diarrhea or constipation usually lasting at least 3 months.
Onset	May occur at any age.	Begins in early adulthood; rarely occurs after the age of 60.
Etiology	Symptoms commonly believed to be caused by an excessive amount of gas in the stomach (eructation) and intestines (bloating, flatulence). Other causes: lactase deficiency, overgrowth of intestinal bacteria, and excessive air swallowing (aerophagia).	The cause of IBS is still unknown. Altered gastrointestinal motility, heightened visceral perception, and overgrowth of intestinal bacteria appear to contribute to the condition.
Exacerbating factors	Diet, underlying medical conditions, and certain drugs (e.g., lactulose, antibiotics, alphaglucosidase inhibitors, orlistat, narcotics, anticholinergics, calcium channel blockers, psyllium or cholestyramine, and effervescent solutions).	Stress, overeating, problem foods (alcohol, chocolate, caffeinated beverages, dairy products, and sugar-free products that contain sorbitol or mannitol). Foods high in fats also may aggravate symptoms.
Modifying factors	Minimization of exacerbating factors.	Minimization of exacerbating factors; physician evaluation and treatment.

or avoided by patients with gastroesophageal reflux disease (see Chapter 14)[68,69]; however, the effect of carminatives on lower esophageal sphincter tone in healthy individuals with intestinal gas symptoms may be less problematic.[70] Fennel can cause photodermatitis, is contraindicated during pregnancy, and enters breast milk in lactating women. If fennel is used, patients should be advised to avoid excessive sunlight, and avoid use during pregnancy and lactation. In addition, coadministration of fennel with ciprofloxacin may lead to reduced ciprofloxacin levels through a chelation mechanism, so doses should be spaced appropriately in patients using both agents.[71]

Assessment of Intestinal Gas: A Case-Based Approach

When a patient complains of intestinal gas, it is important to try to discern the causes, duration, and frequency of the symptoms (Table 15-6). Items noted that produce relief may provide clues as to the cause. A thorough review of dietary habits, medical problems, and use of prescription and nonprescription medications may provide other clues.

Cases 15-1 and 15-2 are examples of the assessment of patients with intestinal gas.

CASE 15-1

Relevant Evaluation Criteria	Scenario/Model Outcome
Information Gathering	
1. Gather essential information about the patient's symptoms, including:	
a. description of symptom(s) (i.e., nature, onset, duration, severity, associated symptoms)	Patient has been experiencing mild diffuse abdominal bloating and occasional flatulence over the past month, especially after a meal. Her bowel function is normal, which she describes as being somewhat infrequent (usually 3 stools per week), but she does not feel constipated. She states that her stools are well formed and easily passed.

C A S E   1 5 - 1 (continued)

Relevant Evaluation Criteria	Scenario/Model Outcome
b. description of any factors that seem to precipitate, exacerbate, and/or relieve the patient's symptom(s)	When symptoms started, it was the beginning of the summer, and she recalls one episode quite vividly. The incident occurred during a summer picnic after eating her second serving of fruit salad (prepared with grapes, orange slices, and water-melon). She felt quite self-conscious and embarrassed when her belly became visibly distended, and she experienced uncomfortable flatulence.
	She denies having any dietary intolerances that she knows of, and she tries to eat a high-fiber, low-fat diet with sufficient dairy to maintain adequate dietary calcium intake.
	Onset of symptoms also seemed to coincide with the initiation of a new medication for her overactive bladder.
c. description of the patient's efforts to relieve the symptoms	She has used a probiotic supplement in the past with no relief of her symptoms.
2. Gather essential patient history information:	
a. patient's identity	Mrs. Laura Forrist
b. patient's age, sex, height, and weight	73-year-old female, 4 ft 11 in, 138 lb
c. patient's occupation	Retired human resource manager
d. patient's dietary habits	Healthy diet with up to three servings of dairy each day. Her daily fiber intake consists of a dish of bran cereal in the morning, and multiple servings of fruits and vegetables throughout the day.
	Mrs. Forrist tries to exercise routinely (walks daily, swims at local community pool at least once a week).
e. patient's sleep habits	She gets a restful 6–8 hours of sleep each night, and awakens by 6 am each morning to her alarm clock to start the day.
f. concurrent medical conditions, prescription and nonprescription medications, and dietary supplements	Fexofenadine 180 mg 1 tablet by mouth in the morning for allergic rhinitis; daily multiple vitamin 1 tablet daily (with no iron); solifenacin 10 mg 1 tablet by mouth in the morning for overactive bladder symptoms
g. allergies	NKA
h. history of other adverse reactions to medications	None
i. other (describe) _____	N/A

Assessment and Triage

3. Differentiate the patient's signs/symptoms and correctly identify the patient's primary problem(s) (see Table 15-6).	Intestinal gas symptoms are most likely related to a recent increase in dietary intake of high-fiber foods that are also high in simple sugars (i.e., fruits and vegetables). Her symptoms are not associated with lactose or gluten intolerance. Symptoms appear to be mild and predictable in nature, occurring after eating fruits and vegetables. No alarm symptoms are noted.
	Although her stools are well formed and easily passed, and she is not constipated, her new medication for overactive bladder may be contributing to her symptoms by decreasing GI motility.
4. Identify exclusions for self-treatment (see Figure 15-2).	None
5. Formulate a comprehensive list of therapeutic alternatives for the primary problem to determine if triage to a medical practitioner is required, and share this information with the patient.	Options include: (1) Recommend reducing the intake of fruits and vegetables, and substituting other fiber-containing foods (such as breads, whole-wheat foods) in an effort to reduce symptoms while maintaining adequate fiber intake from a variety of foods (see Chapter 24). (2) If constipation becomes a problem, maintain adequate fluid intake, exercise, and increase dietary fiber (see Chapter 16). If faster relief is desired, discuss the use of a stool softener or laxative with the PCP. (3) Suggest that Mrs. Forrist talk with her PCP to discuss possible side effects of solifenacin and possible alternatives for the treatment of her overactive bladder symptoms. (4) Recommend self-care with an OTC antiflatulent until she can consult with her PCP. (5) Take no action.

Relevant Evaluation Criteria	Scenario/Model Outcome
Plan	
6. Select an optimal therapeutic alternative to address the patient's problem, taking into account patient preferences.	Reduce the number of servings of fruits and vegetables, and add additional servings of other fiber-containing foods (i.e., breads, brown rice) to achieve an adequate intake of dietary fiber, as well as relief of intestinal gas symptoms.
	OTC treatment with simethicone (125 mg) is appropriate.
7. Describe the recommended therapeutic approach to the patient.	Chew 1 tablet as needed.
8. Explain to the patient the rationale for selecting the recommended therapeutic approach from the considered therapeutic alternatives.	Decreasing dietary fruits and vegetables may relieve symptoms by reducing intake of simple sugars that may be poorly absorbed. Intestinal gas is produced when these sugars are metabolized by intestinal bacteria in the colon.
	Use of simethicone as needed until symptoms resolve may offer additional relief.
Patient Education	
9. When recommending self-care with non-prescription medications and/or nondrug therapy, convey accurate information to the patient:	
a. appropriate dose and frequency of administration	Chew 1 or 2 tablets after meals and at bedtime.
b. maximum number of days the therapy should be employed	Use only if symptoms are present. If symptoms persist longer than 3 days or no relief is gained, discontinue the medication and contact your PCP.
c. product administration procedures	Tablets should be chewed and then swallowed.
d. expected time to onset of relief	Within hours of first dose
e. degree of relief that can be reasonably expected	The medication may provide minor relief of symptoms.
f. most common side effects	None. Simethicone is generally well tolerated.
g. side effects that warrant medical intervention should they occur	None. Simethicone is contraindicated in patients with a known hypersensitivity to simethicone products or suspected intestinal perforation and obstruction.
h. patient options in the event that condition worsens or persists	Contact your primary care provider if the condition does not improve after modifying your diet by reducing the number of servings of fruits or vegetables and by substituting other high-fiber foods.
	If constipation becomes a problem, maintain adequate fluid intake, exercise, and increase dietary fiber (see Chapter 16).
	If faster relief is desired, discuss the use of a stool softener, or bulk-forming laxative with the PCP.
i. product storage requirements	Store at room temperature. Protect from moisture.
j. specific nondrug measures	Maintain a well-rounded diet. Avoid other foods that may cause intestinal gas symptoms (see Tables 15-1 and 15-2). Practice eating behaviors that may decrease intestinal gas symptoms (see Table 15-3).
10. Solicit follow-up questions from patient.	May I double the dose of simethicone to get relief more quickly?
11. Answer patient's questions.	Yes. Up to 2 tablets can be used at one time. No more than 6 tablets should be used in a 24-hour period.

Key: N/A: not applicable; NKA, no known allergies; OTC, over-the-counter; PCP, primary care provider.

CASE 15-2

Relevant Evaluation Criteria	Scenario/Model Outcome
Information Gathering	
1. Gather essential information about the patient's symptoms, including:	
a. description of symptom(s) (i.e., nature, onset, duration, severity, associated symptoms)	Patient has a 12-month history of multiple abdominal complaints, including diarrhea, bloating, and a 42-pound weight loss. He has not noticed blood in his stool; however, he complains of signs and symptoms consistent with anemia (lightheadedness, palpitation, general malaise).
b. description of any factors that seem to precipitate, exacerbate, and/or relieve the patient's symptom(s)	Patient's symptoms are closely related to his diet. He attempts to exclude all dairy products owing to the onset of severe symptoms. Other foods, including pastas and breads, also cause similar symptoms.
c. description of the patient's efforts to relieve the symptoms	He has tried several nonprescription products for his symptoms on different occasions without success, including simethicone 125 mg 4 times a day for 1 week; alpha-galactosidase 150-unit tablets, 3 with each meal for 3 days; and lactase enzymes as chewable tablets, 9000 units at first bite of dairy-containing foods for 14 days. The only activity that seems to provide relief is a reduction in his overall dietary intake and avoidance of problematic foods.
2. Gather essential patient history information:	
a. patient's identity	John McNutt
b. patient's age, sex, height, and weight	46-year-old male, 5 ft 11 in, 130 lb
c. patient's occupation	Law enforcement
d. patient's dietary habits	Avoids all dairy products and any foods containing wheat/oat cereals, noodles, and pastas. His diet primarily includes meats including chicken and beef, fruits, vegetables, and legumes, such as baked beans, soybeans, and lima beans.
e. patient's sleep habits	Averages 8 hours per night
f. concurrent medical conditions, prescription and nonprescription medications, and dietary supplements	Triamterene/hydrochlorothiazide 37.5 mg/25 mg 1 capsule daily for hypertension; Motrin 400 mg 1 tablet every 6 hours as needed for arthritis pain; daily multiple vitamin 1 tablet daily
g. allergies	NKA
h. history of other adverse reactions to medications	None
i. other (describe) _____	
Assessment and Triage	
3. Differentiate the patient's signs/symptoms and correctly identify the patient's primary problem(s) (see Table 15-3).	Abdominal symptoms are consistent with multiple food intolerances. Patient's complaints suggest that significant lactose intolerance and gluten sensitivity (celiac disease) may be present.
4. Identify exclusions for self-treatment (see Figure 15-2).	Significant, unintentional weight loss; anemia symptoms; and onset after the age of 40
5. Formulate a comprehensive list of therapeutic alternatives for the primary problem to determine if triage to a medical practitioner is required, and share this information with the patient.	Options include: (1) Refer Mr. McNutt to a PCP or gastroenterologist for a differential diagnosis. (2) Recommend an OTC antiflatulent product with continued dietary modifications. (3) Take no action.
Plan	
6. Select an optimal therapeutic alternative to address the patient's problem, taking into account patient preferences.	Refer the patient to a PCP or gastroenterologist for a differential diagnosis. The available OTC medications are unlikely to relieve Mr. McNutt's symptoms. Medical evaluation for underlying GI disorders and subsequent treatment is warranted.
7. Describe the recommended therapeutic approach to the patient.	You should consult your primary care provider or a gastroenterologist, as scheduled. Until then, you should continue selecting foods that you can tolerate and reducing foods that may cause gas symptoms (see Tables 15-1 and 15-2).
8. Explain to the patient the rationale for selecting the recommended therapeutic approach from the considered therapeutic alternatives.	See a primary care provider or gastroenterologist as necessary because OTC products may not be appropriate. Your symptoms may be related to an underlying GI condition and are unlikely to be relieved by OTC remedies. Further evaluation and prescription therapy may provide beneficial relief of symptoms.

CASE 15-2 *(continued)*

Relevant Evaluation Criteria	Scenario/Model Outcome
Patient Education	
9. When recommending self-care with non-prescription medications and/or nondrug therapy, convey accurate information to the patient.	Criterion does not apply in this case.
10. Solicit follow-up questions from patient.	Is there an OTC medication that might work?
11. Answer patient's questions.	No OTC medications are approved and/or appropriate to recommend without a definite diagnosis from a PCP or gastroenterologist. If left untreated, gastrointestinal conditions that affect your diet and nutrition may cause persistent symptoms and significant complications.

Key: N/A, not applicable; NKA, no known allergies; OTC, over-the-counter; PCP, primary care provider.

Patient Counseling for Intestinal Gas

Patient counseling is important to ensure the appropriate selection and use of nonprescription medications for intestinal gas. Patients should be encouraged to keep a diary of foods in an effort to identify problematic foods. Avoidance of foods or other substances that cause intestinal gas is the best advice to give patients suffering from this disorder. This advice is often difficult to follow, causing patients to resort to pharmacologic agents. The practitioner should explain the proper use of these medications and should warn the patient of possible adverse effects. (See the box Patient Education for Intestinal Gas.)

Evaluation of Patient Outcomes for Intestinal Gas

The practitioner should ask the patient to return or call after 1 week of self-treatment with either dietary measures or with nonprescription antiflatulents or digestive enzymes. If symp-

---

PATIENT EDUCATION FOR
Intestinal Gas

The objectives of self-treatment are to (1) reduce the symptoms of intestinal gas and (2) reduce the chance of its recurrence. For most patients, carefully following product instructions and the self-care measures listed below will help ensure optimal therapeutic outcomes.

Nondrug Measures
- If possible, avoid foods known to cause intestinal gas.
- Avoid activities known to introduce gas into the digestive system, such as drinking carbonated beverages.

Nonprescription Medications
- Lactase replacement products and alpha-galactosidase should be taken with foods to prevent intestinal gas from forming.
- Simethicone is used to treat intestinal gas after it has occurred.

Alpha-Galactosidase
- Do not cook with this product. Add to food after it has cooled, because food temperatures higher than 130°F may inactivate the enzyme.
- If using drops, add drops to the first bite of the problem foods.
- If using tablets, swallow, chew, or crumble tablets with the first bite of problem foods.

- An average meal may contain three servings of a problem food. If needed, use more tablets for larger meals, up to the maximum recommended dose.

Lactase Replacement Products
- Take at first bite of dairy or lactose-containing food.
- Dosing of the medication may vary according to the amount of lactase in the product and the level of lactose intolerance.
- Do not take more than the recommended maximum daily dose.
- Low-lactose milk, or fortified soy milk products may also be used to supplement dietary intake of calcium.
- Calcium and vitamin D supplements may also be used to obtain the recommended daily allowance for your specific age and sex.

Simethicone
- For infants, to ease administration, mix the suspension with 1 ounce of cool water, infant formula, or other liquid.
- Discontinue simethicone if adequate relief is not obtained within 24 hours.
- Seek medical attention if symptoms do not improve or worsen.

toms persist or have worsened, the patient should seek medical attention. Patients who achieve symptomatic relief should be advised to continue the self-care measures as needed.

Key Points for Intestinal Gas Complaints

➤ Limit the self-treatment of intestinal gas symptoms to minor symptoms and to cases in which exclusions for self-treatment (Figure 15-2) do not exist.

➤ Counsel patients on dietary measures that may reduce the amount of intestinal gas. Certain foods (Tables 15-1 and 15-2) are more likely to cause gas and contribute to symptoms.

➤ Patients who associate symptoms with foods containing lactose or oligosaccharide and who do not meet criteria for exclusion for self-treatment may use digestive enzymes (lactase replacement or alpha-galactosidase products).

➤ Probiotics may be helpful for patients with lactose intolerance who experience bloating, or for patients with bloating associated with irritable bowel syndrome.

➤ Antiflatulents such as activated charcoal and simethicone may also be used, although there is contradictory evidence supporting the ability of these agents to reduce the amount of intestinal gas formation.

➤ Referral of the patient to a primary care provider for further evaluation should be considered for patients with exclusions for self-treatment, and for patients whose symptoms persist after initiating simple treatment options, such as dietary modification and nonprescription medications.

REFERENCES

1. Top 200 OTC/HBC Brands in 2007. Available at: http://drugtopics. modernmedicine.com. Last accessed September 17, 2008.
2. Brendan Borrell. A boom in edible bacteria; Probiotic products claim to improve digestion with microorganisms. And sales are up—way up. *Los Angeles Times.* May 12, 2008;sect F:1.
3. Jackson KA, Savaiano DA. Lactose maldigestion, calcium intake and osteoporosis in African-, Asian-, and Hispanic-Americans. *J Am Coll Nutr.* 2001;20(2 suppl):198S–207S.
4. Hungin AP, Chang L, Locke GR, et al. Irritable bowel syndrome in the United States: prevalence, symptom patterns and impact. *Aliment Pharmacol Ther.* 2005;21:1365–75.
5. Sandler RS, Everhart JE, Donowitz M, et al. The burden of selected digestive diseases in the United States. *Gastroenterology.* 2002;122:1500–11.
6. Nelsen DA Jr. Gluten-sensitive enteropathy (celiac disease): more common than you think. *Am Fam Physician.* 2002;66:2259–66.
7. Lin HC. Small intestinal bacterial overgrowth: a framework for understanding irritable bowel syndrome. *JAMA.* 2004;292:852–8.
8. Jiang X, Locke GR 3rd, Choung RS, et al. Prevalence and risk factors for abdominal bloating and visible distention: a population-based study. *Gut.* 2008;57:756–63.
9. Sandler RS, Stewart WF, Liberman JN, et al. Abdominal pain, bloating, and diarrhea in the United States: prevalence and impact. *Dig Dis Sci.* 2000;45:1166–71.
10. Johnson LR. *Gastrointestinal Physiology: Regulation.* 7th ed. Philadelphia: Mosby; 2007:107–26.
11. Sleisenger MH, Feldman M, Friedman LS, et al. *Sleisenger & Fordtran's Gastrointestinal and Liver Disease: Pathophysiology, Diagnosis, Management.* 8th ed. Philadelphia: Saunders; 2006.
12. Shepherd SJ, Gibson PR. Fructose malabsorption and symptoms of irritable bowel syndrome: guidelines for effective dietary management. *J Am Diet Assoc.* 2006;106:1631–9.
13. Barrett JS, Gibson PR. Clinical ramifications of malabsorption of fructose and other short-chain carbohydrates. *Pract Gastroenterol.* 2007:51–65.
14. Suarez F. Intestinal gas. *Clin Perspect Gastroenterol.* 2000 July/August:209–18.
15. Houghton LA, Whorwell PJ. Towards a better understanding of abdominal bloating and distension in functional gastrointestinal disorders. *Neurogastroenterol Motil.* 2005;17:500–11.
16. Azpiroz F. Intestinal gas dynamics: mechanisms and clinical relevance. *Gut.* 2005;54:893–5.
17. Salvioli B, Serra J, Azpiroz F, et al. Origin of gas retention and symptoms in patients with bloating. *Gastroenterology.* 2005;128:574–9.
18. Harder H, Serra J, Azpiroz F, et al. Intestinal gas distribution determines abdominal symptoms. *Gut.* 2003;52:1708–13.
19. Serra J, Azpiroz F, Malagelada JR. Mechanisms of intestinal gas retention in humans: impaired propulsion versus obstructed evacuation. *Am J Physiol Gastrointest Liver Physiol.* 2001;281:138–43.
20. Foods and flatus. January 2002. University of Michigan Health System. Available at: http://www.med.umich.edu/1libr/aha/aha_gas_sha.htm. Last accessed September 17, 2008.
21. Di Stefano M, Miceli E, Gotti S, et al. The effect of oral alpha-galactosidase on intestinal gas production and gas-related symptoms. *Dig Dis Sci.* 2007; 52:78–83.
22. Gassy Food List. Research Triangle Park, NC: GlaxoSmithKline; 2003. Available at: http://www.beanogas.com/BeanoFoods.aspx. Last accessed September 17, 2008.
23. Choi YK, Johlin FC, Jr., Summers RW, Jackson M, Rao SS. Fructose intolerance: an under-recognized problem. *Am J Gastroenterol.* 2003;98: 1348–53.
24. Bijkerk CJ, Muris JWM, Knottnerus JA, et al. Systematic review: the role of different types of fibre in the treatment of irritable bowel syndrome. *Aliment Pharmacol Ther.* 2004;19:245–51.
25. Toskes PP, Connery KL, Ritchey TW. Calcium polycarbophil compared with placebo in irritable bowel syndrome. *Aliment Pharmacol Ther.* 1993; 7:87–92.
26. Brandt LJ, Bjorkman D, Fennerty MB, et al. Systematic review on the management of irritable bowel syndrome in North America. *Am J Gastroenterol.* 2002;97(11 suppl):S7–S26.
27. Korzenik JR. Case closed? Diverticulitis: epidemiology and fiber. *J Clin Gastroenterol.* 2006;40(suppl 3):S112–6.
28. Azpiroz F, Malagelada JR. The pathogenesis of bloating and visible distension in irritable bowel syndrome. *Gastroenterol Clin North Am.* 2005;34: 257–69.
29. Dua K, Bardan E, Ren J, et al. Effect of chronic and acute cigarette smoking on the pharyngo-upper oesophageal sphincter contractile reflex and reflexive pharyngeal swallow. *Gut.* 1998;43:537–41.
30. Lomer MC, Parkes GC, Sanderson JD. Review article: lactose intolerance in clinical practice—myths and realities. *Aliment Pharmacol Ther.* 2008;27:93–103.
31. Zar S, Benson MJ, Kumar D. Review article: bloating in functional bowel disorders. *Aliment Pharmacol Ther.* 2002;16:1867–76.
32. Chang L, Lee OY, Naliboff B, et al. Sensation of bloating and visible abdominal distension in patients with irritable bowel syndrome. *Am J Gastroenterol.* 2001;96:3341–7.
33. Macfarlane S, Macfarlane GT, Cummings JH. Review article: prebiotics in the gastrointestinal tract. *Aliment Pharmacol Ther.* 2006;24:701–14.
34. Cummings JH, Macfarlane GT. Gastrointestinal effects of prebiotics. *Br J Nutr.* 2002;87(suppl 2):S145–51.
35. Green PHR, Jones R. *Celiac Disease: A Hidden Epidemic.* 1st ed. New York: Collins; 2006.
36. Gluten Free Drugs. Available at: http://www.glutenfreedrugs.com. Last accessed September 17, 2008.
37. Gluten Intolerance Group of North America. Available at: http://www. gluten.net. Last accessed September 17, 2008.
38. Celiac Sprue Association (CSA/USA). Available at: http://www.csaceliacs. org. Last accessed September 17, 2008.
39. Celiac Disease Foundation (CDF). Available at: http://www.celiac.org. Last accessed September 17, 2008.
40. American Celiac Society. Available at: http://www.americanceliac society.org. Last accessed September 17, 2008.
41. The University of Chicago Celiac Disease Program. University of Chicago Children's Hospital. Available at: http://www.uchospitals.edu/specialties/ celiac. Last accessed September 17, 2008.

42. Beth Israel Deaconess Medical Center-Boston Celiac Center. Available at: http://www.bidmc.harvard.edu. Last accessed September 17, 2008.

43. Hill ID, Dirks MH, Liptak GS, et al. Guideline for the diagnosis and treatment of celiac disease in children: recommendations of the North American Society for Pediatric Gastroenterology, Hepatology and Nutrition. *J Pediatr Gastroenterol Nutr.* 2005;40:1–19.

44. England CY, Nicholls AM. Advice available on the Internet for people with celiac disease: an evaluation of the quality of websites. *J Hum Nutr Diet.* 2004;17:547–59.

45. Huerta-Franco MR, Malacara JM. Association of physical and emotional symptoms with the menstrual cycle and life-style. *J Reprod Med.* 1993;38:448–54.

46. Guarner F, Malagelada JR. Gut flora in health and disease. *Lancet.* 2003;36:512–9.

47. Di Stefano M, Miceli E, Armellini E, et al. Probiotics and functional abdominal bloating. *J Clin Gastroenterol.* 2004;38(6 suppl):S102–3.

48. American College of Gastroenterology. Common Gastrointestinal Problems: Intestinal Gas Problems. August 2001. Available at: http://www.acg.gi.org/patients/cgp/cgpvol3.asp#gas. Last accessed September 17, 2008.

49. Mayer EA. The Neurobiology of Stress and Emotions. Available at: http://www.iffgd.org/store/viewproduct/106. Last accessed September 17, 2008.

50. Nitzke S, Freeland-Graves J. Position of the American Dietetic Association: total diet approach to communicating food and nutrition information. *J Am Diet Assoc.* 2007;107:1224–32.

51. McEvoy GK. *American Hospital Formulary Service, AHFS Drug Information.* Bethesda, Md: American Society of Health-System Pharmacists; 2004.

52. Hanauer SB, DuPont HL, Cooper KM, et al. Randomized, double-blind, placebo-controlled clinical trial of loperamide plus simethicone versus loperamide alone and simethicone alone in the treatment of acute diarrhea with gas-related abdominal discomfort. *Curr Med Res Opin.* 2007;23:1033–43.

53. Friis H, Bode S, Rumessen JJ, et al. Effect of simethicone on lactulose-induced H2 production and gastrointestinal symptoms. *Digestion.* 1991;49:227–30.

54. Suarez FL, Furne J, Springfield J, et al. Failure of activated charcoal to reduce the release of gases produced by the colonic flora. *Am J Gastroenterol.* 1999;94:208–12.

55. Quigley EM. Aerophagia and intestinal Gas. *Curr Treat Options Gastroenterol.* 2002;5:259–65.

56. Ganiats TG, Norcross WA, Halverson AL, et al. Does Beano prevent gas? A double-blind crossover study of oral alpha-galactosidase to treat dietary oligosaccharide intolerance. *J Fam Pract.* 1994;39:441–5.

57. Metcalf TJ, Irons TG, Sher LD, et al. Simethicone in the treatment of infant colic: a randomized, placebo-controlled, multicenter trial. *Pediatrics.* 1994;94:29–34.

58. Barbara G, Stanghellini V, Cremon C, et al. Probiotics and irritable bowel syndrome: rationale and clinical evidence for their use. *J Clin Gastroenterol.* 2008;42(suppl 3 pt 2):S214–7.

59. Borriello SP, Hammes WP, Holzapfel W, et al. Safety of probiotics that contain lactobacilli or bifidobacteria. *Clin Infect Dis.* 2003;36:775–80.

60. Besselink MG, van Santvoort HC, Buskens E, et al. Probiotic prophylaxis in predicted severe acute pancreatitis: a randomised, double-blind, placebo-controlled trial. *Lancet.* 2008;371:651–9.

61. Guyonnet D, Chassany O, Ducrotte P, et al. Effect of a fermented milk containing Bifidobacterium animalis DN-173 010 on the health-related quality of life and symptoms in irritable bowel syndrome in adults in primary care: a multicentre, randomized, double-blind, controlled trial. *Aliment Pharmacol Ther.* 2007;26:475–86.

62. Nobaek S, Johansson ML, Molin G, et al. Alteration of intestinal microflora is associated with reduction in abdominal bloating and pain in patients with irritable bowel syndrome. *Am J Gastroenterol.* 2000;95:1231–8.

63. O'Mahony L, McCarthy J, Kelly P, et al. Lactobacillus and bifidobacterium in irritable bowel syndrome: symptom responses and relationship to cytokine profiles. *Gastroenterology.* 2005;128:541–51.

64. Whorwell PJ, Altringer L, Morel J, et al. Efficacy of an encapsulated probiotic Bifidobacterium infantis 35624 in women with irritable bowel syndrome. *Am J Gastroenterol.* 2006;101:1581–90.

65. Kajander K, Hatakka K, Poussa T, et al. A probiotic mixture alleviates symptoms in irritable bowel syndrome patients: a controlled 6-month intervention. *Aliment Pharmacol Ther.* 2005;22:387–94.

66. Jellin JM. *Natural Medicines Comprehensive Database.* 9th ed. Stockton, Calif: Therapeutic Research Faculty; 2006.

67. Zhu M, Wong PY, Li RC. Effect of oral administration of fennel (Foeniculum vulgare) on ciprofloxacin absorption and disposition in the rat. *J Pharm Pharmacol.* 1999;51:1391–6.

68. Castell DO, Brunton SA, Earnest DL, et al. GERD: management algorithms for the primary care physician and the specialist. *Pract Gastroenterol.* 1998;4:18–46.

69. Creamer B. Oesophageal reflux and the action of carminatives. *Lancet.* 1955;268:590–2.

70. Bulat R, Fachnie E, Chauhan U, et al. Lack of effect of spearmint on lower oesophageal sphincter function and acid reflux in healthy volunteers. *Aliment Pharmacol Ther.* 1999;13:805–12.

71. Brinker FJ. *Herb Contraindications & Drug Interactions: With Extensive Appendices Addressing Specific Conditions, Herb Effects, Critical Medications, and Nutritional Supplements.* 3rd ed. Sandy, Ore: Eclectic Medical Publications; 2001.

Constipation

Clarence E. Curry, Jr., and Demetris M. Butler

Constipation is a common gastrointestinal (GI) complaint. However, the complaint is viewed differently by health care providers and patients. Medical practitioners generally describe constipation as a decrease in the frequency of fecal elimination characterized by the difficult passage of hard, dry stools.[1] It usually results from the abnormally slow movement of feces through the colon, resulting in their accumulation in the descending colon. Patients may describe constipation as (1) straining to have a stool; (2) the passage of hard, dry stool; (3) the passage of small stools; (4) feelings of incomplete bowel evacuation; or (5) bloating or decreased stool frequency.

Although constipation is a common reason for visiting a primary care provider, it also is a common reason for undertaking self-care. A laxative is often the treatment of choice for constipation. Laxative sales in the United States exceed $750 million and are projected to top $850 million by 2010.[2] Despite numerous recognized indications for when to use laxatives, many patients use them inappropriately to alleviate what they incorrectly consider to be constipation.

Constipation is a heterogeneous disorder that occurs throughout the age continuum in both men and women. It is reported more often in women than in men.[3] The prevalence in the general population ranges from 2% to 28% and is higher in older adults (>65 years), possibly affecting over half of elderly residents in nursing homes.[4-7] Constipation is also a frequent complaint during pregnancy and after childbirth.

All of the structures shown in Figure 16-1 contribute to the process of digestion. For example, the pharynx and esophagus serve as entryway to the system, the stomach serves as a storage depot and an initiator of the digestive process, and the liver provides bile for fat emulsification, whereas nearly all absorption of solids (>94%) occurs in the small intestine. The colon allows for the orderly elimination of nonabsorbed food products from the body, along with desquamated cells from the gut lumen and detoxified and metabolic end products. The colon functions to conserve fluid and electrolytes, so the quantity eliminated represents about 10% of what enters it in a 24-hour period. The colon also has the capacity (as does the kidney) to absorb certain electrolytes because of differences in osmotic pressure.

Tonic contractions of the stomach churn and knead food, and large peristaltic waves start at the fundus and move food toward the duodenum. Autonomic reflexes and hormones influence the time it takes the stomach contents to empty into the duodenum.

The mixture and passage of the contents of the small and large intestines are the result of four muscular movements: pendular, segmental, peristaltic, and vermiform (worm-like). Pendular movements result from contractions of the longitudinal muscles of the intestine, which pass up and down small segments of the gut at the rate of about 10 contractions per minute. Pendular movements mix rather than propel the contents. Segmental movements resulting from contractions of the circular muscles occur at about the same rate as pendular movements. Their primary function is also mixing. Pendular and segmental movements are caused by the intrinsic contractility of smooth muscle and occur in the absence of innervation of intestinal tissue.

Peristaltic movements propel intestinal contents by circular contractions that form behind a point of stimulation and pass along the GI tract toward the rectum. The contraction rate ranges from 2 to 20 cm per second. These contractions require an intact myenteric (Auerbach's) nerve plexus. Peristaltic waves move the intestinal contents through the small intestine in about 3.5 hours. Vermiform movements occur mainly in the large intestine. In the cecum and ascending colon, the contents retain a fluid consistency. Peristaltic and antiperistaltic waves occur frequently, but activity is very irregular in the transverse, descending, and sigmoid segments of the colon, where—through further water absorption—the contents become semisolid.

Three or four times a day, a strong peristaltic wave (mass movement) propels the contents about one-third (38 cm) the length of the colon. When initiated by a meal, the mass movement is referred to as the gastrocolic reflex. This normal reflex seems to be associated with the entrance of food into the stomach and the subsequent distention of the stomach; the reflex is very strong in infants. The sigmoid colon serves as a storage place for fecal matter until defecation occurs.

The act of defecation involves the rectal passage of accumulated fecal material. This material is propelled from the sigmoid colon into the rectum by a mass peristaltic movement. This movement results in a desire to defecate as somatic impulses are sent to the defecation center in the sacral spinal cord. The defecation center then sends impulses to the internal anal sphincter, causing it to relax and intra-abdominal pressure to increase as the muscles of the abdominal wall tighten; a Valsalva maneuver forces the stool down. Voluntary relaxation of the external anal sphincter occurs, followed by elevation of the pelvic diaphragm, which lifts the anal sphincter over the fecal mass, allowing the mass to be expelled. Defecation, a spinal reflex, is either voluntarily inhibited by keeping the external sphincter contracted or

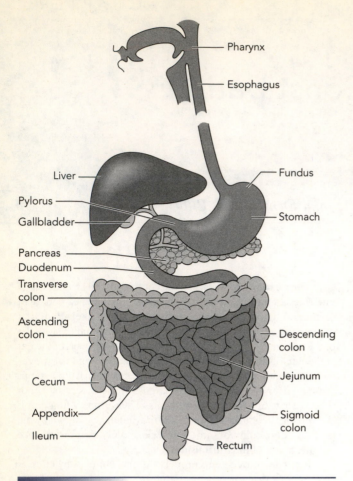

Pharynx

Esophagus

Liver

Fundus

Pylorus

Gallbladder

Stomach

Pancreas

Duodenum

Transverse colon

Ascending colon

Descending colon

Cecum

Jejunum

Appendix

Sigmoid colon

Ileum

Rectum

FIGURE 16-1 Anatomy of the digestive system.

facilitated by relaxing the sphincter and contracting the abdominal muscles. Children usually defecate after meals; in adults, however, habits and cultural factors may determine the "proper" time for defecation.

Pathophysiology of Constipation

Causes of constipation are numerous and include various medical conditions and medications; psychological and physiologic conditions (e.g., menopause or dehydration); and lifestyle characteristics. Some population groups are more susceptible to developing constipation as a result of one or more of the defined causes. Two distinct disorders of colorectal motility are characterized by constipation: slow-transit constipation (slower than normal movement of fecal contents) and pelvic floor dysfunction (storage of fecal contents for prolonged time in the rectum).[5]

Constipation of recent onset suggests a possible disease-related or drug-induced cause (Table 16-1).[5-7] If a disease is the underlying cause, referral for proper diagnosis and medical treatment will be necessary.

Painful lesions of the anal canal such as ulcers, fissures, and thrombosed hemorrhoidal veins can lead to constipation if patients suppress defecation to avoid pain. Pain from various causes, including gallbladder disease, appendicitis, and regional ileitis, may inhibit GI reflexes, leading to functional and acute symptomatology.

Drugs with constipating side effects may counteract the therapeutic effects of laxatives or may require use of a laxative (Table 16-2).[7-9]

A clinical condition known as the narcotic bowel syndrome is characterized by chronic abdominal pain, nausea and vomiting, abdominal distention, and constipation. Such a condition might occur in a cancer patient or in other patients who require chronic administration of large doses of narcotics.

Constipation can also be related to psychologic conditions. Depression, eating disorders such as anorexia nervosa, and conscious efforts to withhold stool are frequently responsible.

A diet that is low in calories, carbohydrates (e.g., Atkins diet), or fiber may lead to diet-related constipation. Dietary fiber dissolves or swells in the intestinal fluid, which increases the bulk of fecal mass and, in turn, aids in stimulating peristalsis and eliminating stools. Increasing dietary fiber and reducing consumption of soft foods and foods that harden stools (e.g., processed cheese) help relieve constipation in many individuals. Some fiber-based foods (e.g., certain breakfast cereals) could actually contribute to constipation because of the processed sugar they contain.

Inadequate intake of fluids may also contribute to the development of constipation in some persons. Intestinal fluids are essential for eliminating stools and must be replenished from dietary sources. Gravity and good abdominal muscle tone also aid in proper bowel function. Exercise increases muscle tone and promotes bowel motility. Immobility and sedentary lifestyles can contribute to the development of constipation as well.

Avoiding the urge to empty the bowel can eventually lead to constipation. When this stimulus is ignored or suppressed, rectal muscles can lose tonicity and become less effective in eliminating stool. Nerve pathways may degenerate and stop sending the signal to defecate. Bowel retraining will be necessary for most patients to establish a pattern of regular bowel movements.

Clinical Presentation

If frequency of bowel movements decreases or difficult passage of hard stools occurs, other symptoms of varying degrees of severity may develop, including anorexia, dull headache, lassitude, low back pain, abdominal discomfort, and abdominal distention

The frequency of bowel movements in humans is quite variable but generally ranges from three times a day to three times a week.[10] Persons in the latter category can be symptom-free and do not have any specific abnormality related to their individual pattern of defecation. Therefore, constipation cannot be defined solely in terms of the number of bowel movements in any given period. Regularity is what is "regular" or typical for the individual who experiences none of the classic symptoms of constipation.

In some instances, self-care is inappropriate and medical referral is necessary, including all situations typified by so-called red flag or alarm symptoms: (1) sudden changes in stool, (2) recent weight loss, (3) presence of abdominal pain, (4) blood in the stool, (5) fever, (6) anorexia, (7) nausea and vomiting. Other factors suggesting more than simple constipation include the possibility of fecal impaction or obstruction, ineffectiveness of self-medication with nonprescription laxatives, and presence of a disorder known to be accompanied by constipation.

Constipation can occur in infants who have one to two daily bowel movements and often is unrecognized. Infants whose frequency of bowel movements is less than average in the first

TABLE 16-1	Selected Conditions Associated with Constipation

Metabolic Disorders

Amyloidosis
Diabetic ketoacidosis
Diabetic neuropathy
Hypokalemia
Hypomagnesemia
Porphyria
Uremia

Endocrine Disorders

Hypercalcemia
  Pseudohypoparathyroidism
  Hyperparathyroidism
  Milk alkali syndrome
  Carcinomatosis
Hypothyroidism
Panhypopituitarism
Pheochromocytoma

Neurologic Disorders

Aganglionosis (Hirschsprung's disease)
Autonomic neuropathy (paraneoplastic, pseudo-obstruction)
Cauda equina tumor
Cerebrovascular accidents
Chagas' disease
Dementia
Ganglioneuromatosis
Multiple sclerosis

Parkinson's disease
Shy-Drager syndrome
Tumors

Disorders of the Large Intestine, Rectum, and Anus

Anal fissure
Chronic amebiasis
Colonic inertia
Corrosive enemas
Diverticulitis
Hernias
Internal rectal prolapse
Irritable bowel syndrome
Ischemic colitis
Mucosal prolapse
Pelvic floor dysfunction and lesions
Rectocele
Stenotic obstruction
Strictures
Surgical stricture (end-to-end anastomosis)
Tumors
Ulcerative proctitis

Muscular Disorders

Dermatomyositis
Myotonic dystrophy
Segmental dilatation of the colon
Systemic sclerosis

Source: References 5–7.

TABLE 16-2	Selected Drugs That May Induce Constipation

Analgesics (including nonsteroidal anti-inflammatory drugs)
Antacids (e.g., calcium and aluminum compounds, bismuth)
Anticholinergics (e.g., benztropine)
Anticonvulsants (e.g., carbamazepine)
Antidepressants (specifically, tricyclics such as amitriptyline)
Antihistamines (e.g., diphenhydramine)
Antimotility (e.g., diphenoxylate, loperamide)
Barium sulfate
Benzodiazepines (especially alprazolam and estazolam)
Calcium channel blockers (e.g., verapamil)
Calcium supplements
Diuretics (e.g., thiazides)
Hematinics (especially iron)
Hyperlipidemia agents (e.g., cholestyramine, pravastatin, simvastatin)
Hypotensives (e.g., angiotensin-converting enzyme inhibitors, beta-blockers)
Memantine
Monoamine oxidase inhibitors (e.g., phenelzine)
Opiates (e.g., morphine, codeine)
Parasympatholytics (e.g., atropine)
Parkinsonism agents (e.g., bromocriptine)
Psychotherapeutic drugs (e.g., phenothiazines, butyrophenones)
Polystyrene sodium sulfonate
Sucralfate
Vinca alkaloids (e.g., vincristine)

Source: References 7–9.

weeks of life may be prone to developing chronic constipation in later years.[11]

Patients of advanced age often strain to pass hard stools, which may predispose them to complications, including cardiovascular problems and hemorrhoids. Because defecation has been found to alter hemodynamics, straining to defecate may result in blood pressure surges or cardiac rhythm disturbances. Occasionally, straining may lead to rectal prolapse.

Treatment of Constipation

The patient should attempt nondrug measures initially to relieve constipation and help prevent recurrences. Constipation associated with an underlying medical condition or use of medications should be referred to a primary care provider to evaluate the need for further medical treatment or to adjust therapy of constipating medications.

At a minimum, successful therapy for constipation should return the patient to the preconstipation frequency, consistency, and quantity of stool. Pharmacotherapy should restore usual function using the lowest effective dosage without producing adverse effects.

Treatment Goals

The primary goals of treatment are to (1) relieve constipation and reestablish normal bowel function, (2) establish dietary and exercise habits that aid in preventing recurrences, (3) promote the safe and effective use of laxative products, and (4) avoid the overuse of laxative products.

General Treatment Approach

In general, constipation should be initially managed by adjusting the diet to include foods high in fiber and increasing fluid intake, accompanied by some form of exercise. Pharmacologic intervention can be used in conjunction with lifestyle modifications if more immediate relief is desired. Laxatives should be selected according to the age and health status of the patient, as well as the mechanism of action of the individual product. The Food and Drug Administration (FDA) has long mandated labeling of laxatives to stress only short-term (i.e., less than 1 week) use

without medical referral. This use is thought to be sufficient for most cases of occasional simple or acute constipation. When constipation continues over several weeks to months, it can be referred to as chronic. Chronic constipation, as described in the Rome criteria, may require more sustained and aggressive therapy directed by a medical practitioner.[12,13] The Rome criteria are a set of guidelines developed primarily to aid researchers in classifying chronic constipation. They are used to some extent by clinicians in routine practice. Most patients who develop constipation will self-medicate and consult a health care provider only after a nonprescription preparation or dietary manipulation has failed. Treatment success is enhanced when likely causes of constipation have been identified and therapeutic modalities are tailored to the individual. The treatment algorithm in Figure 16-2 provides

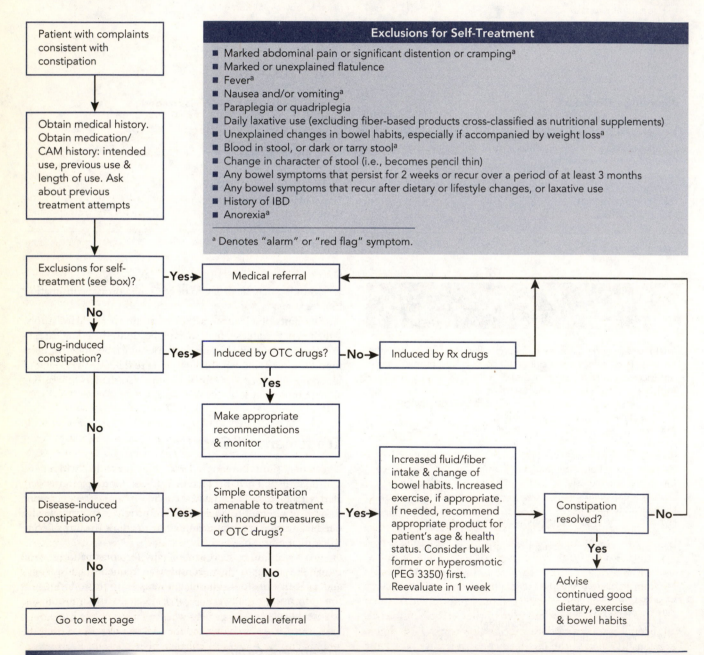

Exclusions for Self-Treatment

- Marked abdominal pain or significant distention or cramping[a]
- Marked or unexplained flatulence
- Fever[a]
- Nausea and/or vomiting[a]
- Paraplegia or quadriplegia
- Daily laxative use (excluding fiber-based products cross-classified as nutritional supplements)
- Unexplained changes in bowel habits, especially if accompanied by weight loss[a]
- Blood in stool, or dark or tarry stool[a]
- Change in character of stool (i.e., becomes pencil thin)
- Any bowel symptoms that persist for 2 weeks or recur over a period of at least 3 months
- Any bowel symptoms that recur after dietary or lifestyle changes, or laxative use
- History of IBD
- Anorexia[a]

[a] Denotes "alarm" or "red flag" symptom.

FIGURE 16-2 Self-care of constipation. Key: CAM, complementary and alternative medicine; IBD, inflammatory bowel disease; OTC, over-the-counter; PCP, primary care provider; PEG, polyethylene glycol; Rx, prescription. *(continued on next page)*

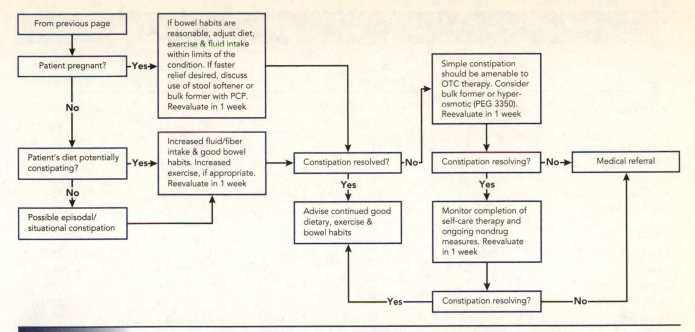

FIGURE 16-2 *(Continued)* Self-care of constipation. Key: CAM, complementary and alternative medicine; IBD, inflammatory bowel disease; OTC, over-the-counter; PCP, primary care provider; PEG, polyethylene glycol; Rx, prescription.

a systematic approach to the self-care of constipation[14] and lists exclusions for self-treatment.

Nonpharmacologic Therapy

Constipation that does not have an organic etiology (i.e., metabolic or disease-related) can often be alleviated with lifestyle modifications such as increased fiber in the diet, adequate fluid intake, and exercise. Patients should adhere to a balanced diet that incorporates recommendations from the U.S. Department of Agriculture's Food Guide Pyramid (see Chapter 23) including daily servings of grains, cereals, fruit, and vegetables to prevent constipation.[15] The American Dietetic Association recommends an adult daily dietary fiber intake of 20 to 35 grams, not to exceed 50 grams.[16] Adequate intake for fiber as published by the Institute of Medicine is discussed in Chapter 24, along with actual fiber intake documented in several large surveys. In addition, Chapter 24 provides information on terms used to describe fiber, types and sources of fiber, potential fiber benefits besides laxation effects, and recommended methods of increasing fiber intake.

It is commonly believed that increasing dietary fiber enhances regularity; fiber improves bowel function by adding bulk and softening the stool. Both insoluble fiber (e.g., whole-grain breads and soy polysaccharide) and soluble fiber (e.g., oat bran, barley, peas, carrots, citrus fruits, and apples) are believed to be instrumental in this regard (Table 16-3).[16,17] However, some people may not be able to consume sufficient amounts of fiber because of GI intolerance. The clinician should inform patients that increasing dietary fiber may lead to erratic bowel habits, flatulence, and abdominal discomfort during the first few weeks. Fiber should be gradually added to the diet to increase tolerance. For some patients it may take several weeks before tolerance develops, so beneficial effects may not be immediately achieved. Remedies containing natural fiber such as whole grains, or oat or wheat bran may help relieve symptoms; however, some patients find

them unpalatable. Excessive fiber should be avoided in patients with hypocalcemia or low serum iron, because the phytates found in some foods associated with high-fiber content (e.g., bran) may inhibit absorption of minerals and aggravate these conditions. Patients with slow-transit constipation or functional outlet obstruction may respond poorly to fiber supplementation.[18] An increase in dietary fiber and use of fiber supplements should be avoided in patients with fecal impaction to avoid worsening the condition. A sugar-free bulk-forming fiber supplement containing psyllium may help minimize constipation associated with low-carbohydrate diets (e.g., Atkins), but adequate fluid intake to avoid the development of paradoxical constipation is also required.[19] Although increasing dietary fiber is generally recommended, its overall effectiveness remains controversial; therefore, its use is not a panacea for all cases of constipation.[6]

In conjunction with fiber, an increase in the intake of fluids, especially water, helps alleviate constipation in most patients. Physiologically, water also helps to prevent constipation.[20] Recommendations for daily fluid consumption vary widely, from 1 to 4 liters. In general, 2 liters of fluid per day is recommended. This approach may be limited in patients who are fluid-restricted or who have renal insufficiency. Fluid requirements increase for pregnant and lactating females; an additional 300 mL and 750 to 1000 mL of fluid, respectively, should be added to daily requirements. Most investigators generally believe the additional fluid expands and softens the fiber, although water-insoluble fiber is said to be primarily responsible for producing a laxative effect.[16]

Concentrated fiber sources, referred to as functional fibers, are available for use by patients who find it difficult to get enough fiber from their usual diet and for addition to foods during the manufacturing process to enhance fiber content. Examples of mostly soluble functional fibers include various gums (guar, locust bean, and karaya), pectin, and psyllium (ispaghula seed husk); insoluble functional fibers include primarily calcium polycarbophil, methylcellulose, powdered cellulose, and soy

TABLE 16-3 Dietary Fiber[a]

Food	Fiber (g/100 g)	Calories (per 100 g)	Serving Size	Fiber (g/serving)	Calories (per serving)
Breakfast Cereals					
All-Bran	29.9	249	1/3 cup (1 oz)	8.5	71
Cheerios	3.8	391	1 1/4 cups (1 oz)	1.1	111
Cornflakes	1.1	389	1 1/3 cups (1 oz)	0.3	110
Grape-Nuts	4.8	357	1/4 cup (1 oz)	1.4	101
Rice Krispies	0.2	395	1 cup (1 oz)	0.1	112
Shredded Wheat	9.3	359	2/3 cup (1 oz)	2.6	102
Fruits					
Apple (with skin)	2.5	59	1 med	3.5	81
Banana	2.1	92	1 med	2.4	105
Orange	2.0	47	1	2.6	62
Peach (with skin)	2.1	43	1	1.9	37
Pineapple	1.4	49	1/2 cup	1.1	39
Prunes	11.9	239	3	3.0	60
Strawberries	2.0	30	1 cup	3.0	45
Juices					
Apple	0.3	47	1/2 cup (4 oz)	0.4	56
Grape	0.5	51	1/2 cup (4 oz)	0.6	64
Orange	0.4	45	1/2 cup (4 oz)	0.5	56
Vegetables, Cooked					
Asparagus, cut	1.5	20	1/2 cup	1.0	15
Beans, string, green	2.6	25	1/2 cup	1.6	16
Kale, leaves	2.6	34	1/2 cup	1.4	22
Sweet potatoes	2.4	141	1/2 med	1.7	80
Vegetables, Raw					
Onions, sliced	1.3	23	1/2 cup	0.8	33
Tomato	1.5	22	1 med	1.5	20
Legumes					
Baked beans, tomato sauce	7.3	121	1/2 cup	8.8	155
Dried peas, cooked	4.7	115	1/2 cup	4.7	115
Lentils, cooked	3.7	97	1/2 cup	3.7	97
Breads and Flours					
Bran muffins	6.3	263	1 muffin	2.5	104
Pita bread (5 inch)	0.9	273	1 piece	0.4	123
White bread	1.6	279	1 slice	0.4	78
Pasta and Rice, Cooked					
Macaroni	0.8	111	1 cup	1.0	144
Rice, brown	1.2	119	1/2 cup	1.0	97
Spaghetti (regular)	0.8	111	1 cup	1.1	155

[a] The values are literature-derived averages. Also, cereals vary greatly in their fiber content, so consumers should read labels to determine fiber content per serving.

Source: References 16 and 17.

polysaccharide. Inulin and fructooligosaccharides are other functional fibers with interesting characteristics. They function as prebiotics, promoting growth of beneficial bifidobacteria in the digestive system. Inulin is found in supplements such as FiberChoice and Fibersure; natural sources, including bananas, onions, garlic, artichokes, and asparagus, contain low concentrations. Wheat dextrin is another natural soluble fiber. It is now the active ingredient in Benefiber products; however, Benefiber Plus Calcium Chewables still contains soluble fiber from partially hydrolyzed guar gum. (See Chapter 24 and www.nationalfibercouncil.org for more information on fiber.)

As with adults, increasing both fluids and the bulk content of a child's diet may improve bowel habits and decrease frequency of constipation. Simply increasing the amount of fluid or sucrose in infant formulas may be corrective during the first few months of life (see Chapter 26). Once solid foods are introduced, adding or increasing the amount of high-fiber cereals, vegetables, and fruits to the diet may relieve symptoms of constipation. For children older than 2 years, the recommended dietary fiber intake should equal or exceed their age plus 5 g/day.[16] Unbuttered popcorn is a good bulk-containing snack for children older than 4 years. Water should be incorporated into the diets of children older than 7 months. Although milk is the primary fluid consumed by most young children, milk intake should not be considered a substitute for water. In addition to dietary changes, some children may need to establish regular bowel habits including promptly responding to the urge to toilet as well as toileting in an unhurried manner.[21]

Because constipation often afflicts those with sedentary lifestyles, the importance of exercise to the body cannot be discounted. Although any concentrated regular exercise is good, aerobic exercise is best. Regular walking, running, or swimming, among other forms of exercise, may help alleviate constipation.

Finally, for people who achieve a beneficial effect from one of these measures, promptly heeding the urge to pass the stool is paramount, or the beneficial effect will be lost. Allowing sufficient time for toileting, particularly after a meal when the gastrocolic reflexes are greatest, helps to promote defecation consistent with the body's normal physiologic response. Toileting 30 to 40 minutes after the morning meal has been suggested as the best time to attempt to have a bowel movement.[20] For patients who are confined to bed, defecation can be facilitated by having the patient lie on the left side to facilitate movement of feces.[20] The use of a bedpan should be avoided, because the urge to defecate may be reduced or inhibited.[20] When nondrug measures prove ineffective, a laxative may be indicated.

Pharmacologic Therapy

The ideal laxative would (1) be nonirritating and nontoxic, (2) act on only the descending and sigmoid colon, and (3) produce a normally formed stool within a few hours, after which its action would cease and normal bowel activity would resume. Because no currently available laxative precisely meets these criteria, proper selection of a laxative depends on the etiology of the constipation.

Agents used to treat constipation have been classified according to their chemical structure and site, intensity, or mechanism of action. The most meaningful classification is by mechanism of action, including bulk-forming, emollient, lubricant, saline, hyperosmotic, and stimulant agents (Table 16-4). None of these laxative agents should be taken for more than 1 week without consulting a primary care provider.

Bulk-Forming Agents

Most bulk-forming laxatives are derived from natural sources such as agar, plantago (psyllium) seed, kelp (alginates), and plant gums (e.g., tragacanth, chondrus, karaya [*Sterculia*]). Guar gum is a natural product found in the bean cluster plant (*Cyamopsis tetragonolobus*); it is most useful today as partially hydrolyzed guar gum. The synthetic cellulose derivatives—methylcellulose and carboxymethyl cellulose sodium—are also used, with methylcellulose products being more prominent. Another agent is calcium polycarbophil, the calcium salt of a synthetic polyacrylic resin. These synthetic colloidal materials have a high degree of uniformity and can be readily compressed into tablets. They are also less troublesome in that they tend to cause less intestinal gas than natural fiber produces.[4]

Bulk-forming products are the recommended choice for the treatment of most instances of constipation, because they most closely approximate the physiologic mechanism in promoting evacuation. These agents dissolve or swell in the intestinal fluid, forming emollient gels that facilitate passage of the intestinal contents and stimulate peristalsis. Calcium polycarbophil has a marked capacity for binding water and is a quite useful agent of this class. Another bulk-forming agent, malt soup extract, is obtained from barley and contains maltose protein, potassium, and amylolytic enzymes. An interesting aspect of this agent is that it reduces fecal pH, which may contribute to its laxative activity.

These hydrophilic colloidal bulk-forming agents are not absorbed systemically and do not seem to interfere with the absorption of nutrients. The usual onset of action is from 12 to 24 hours but may be delayed as long as 72 hours.

Bulk-forming agents are indicated as short-term therapy to relieve constipation, and they may be indicated for (1) patients on low-fiber (also referred to as low-residue) diets that cannot be corrected; (2) postpartum women; (3) older adult patients; and (4) patients with colostomies, irritable bowel syndrome, or diverticular disease. They are also indicated prophylactically in patients who should refrain from straining during a bowel movement.

Dosages vary according to the type of product. Table 16-4 lists dosing information for the various agents. Exceeding the recommended doses for a bulk-forming agent could lead to increased flatulence and obstruction if appropriate fluid intake is not maintained.

Common adverse effects include abdominal cramping and flatulence. Esophageal obstruction has occurred in older adults, in patients who have difficulty swallowing, and in patients with strictures of the esophagus after they ingested a bulk laxative that had been chewed or taken in dry form. Symptoms of esophageal obstruction include chest pain, vomiting, excessive salivation, and an inhibited swallowing reflex that may precipitate choking. Because of its concern for continued reports of esophageal obstruction, FDA has established that nonprescription, granular-type laxatives containing psyllium, psyllium hydrophilic mucilloid, psyllium seed, blond psyllium seed, psyllium seed husks, plantago ovata husks, and plantago seed are not generally recognized as safe and effective and are therefore misbranded. This final order does not apply to psyllium-containing laxative products in other dosage forms, including powders, tablets, or wafers.[22] Practitioners should advise patients to use extra care to observe administration guidelines regarding fluid use with such products. There have also been reports of acute bronchospasm associated with inhalation of dry hydrophilic mucilloid, as well as hypersensitivity reactions characterized by anaphylaxis.[23]

TABLE 16-4 Classification and Properties of Laxatives

| Agent | Dosage Form^a | Daily Dosage Range | | Site of Action | Approximate Onset of Action | Systemic Absorption |
		Adults	Children			
Bulk-Forming						
Methylcellulose	Solid	4–6 g	1–1.5 g (>6 years)	Small and large intestines	12–72 hours	No
Malt soup extract	Solid, liquid, powder	12–64 g	6–32 mL (1 month to 2 years)	Small and large intestines	12–72 hours	—
Partially hydrolyzed guar gum	Powder	1–6 g	None identified	Small and large intestines	12–72 hours	No
Polycarbophil	Solid	1–6 g	0.5–1.0 g (<2 years) 1–1.5 g (2–≤6 years) 1.5–3.0 g (6–12 years)	Small and large intestines	12–72 hours	No
Plantago seeds (psyllium)	Solid	2.5–30 g	1.25–15 g (>6 years)	Small and large intestines	12–72 hours	No
Emollient						
Docusate calcium	Solid	50–360 mg	20–50 mg (<2 years) 50–150 mg (≥2 years)	Small and large intestines	24–72 hours	Yes
Docusate sodium	Solid	50–360 mg	20–50 mg (<2 years) 50–150 mg (≥2 years)	Small and large intestines	24–72 hours	Yes
	Liquid	50–500 mg	10–40 mg (<3 years) 20–60 mg (3–<6 years) 40–150 mg (6–12 years)	Small and large intestines	—	—
Lubricant						
Mineral oil	Liquid	14–45 mL	10–15 mL (>6 years)	Colon	6–8 hours	Yes, a minimal amount
Saline						
Magnesium citrate	Liquid	150–300 mL	2–4 mL/kg given once or in divided doses (<6 years) 100–150 mL (6–12 years)	Small and large intestines	0.5–3 hours	Yes
Magnesium hydroxide	Liquid	30–60 mL	0.5 mL/kg per dose (<2 years) 5–15 mL (2–<6 years) 15–30 mL (6–12 years)	Small and large intestines	0.5–3 hours	Yes
	Liquid (concentrate)	15–30 mL	2.5–7.5 mL (2–<6 years) 7.5–15 mL (6–12 years)	Small and large intestines	0.5–3 hours	Yes
	Solid	6–8 tablets	1–2 tablets (2–<6 years) 3–4 tablets (6–11 years) 6–8 tablets (>12 years)	Small and large intestines	0.5–3 hours	Yes
Magnesium sulfate	Solid	10–30 g	2.5–5.0 g (2–<6 years) 5.0–10.0 g (≥6 years)	Small and large intestines	0.5–3 hours	Yes
Dibasic sodium phosphate	Solid	1.9–3.8 g	1/4 adult dose (5–<10 years) 1/2 adult dose (10 years)	Small and large intestines	0.5–3 hours	Yes
	Solution (rectal)	6.84–7.56 g once daily	1/2 adult dose (2–11 years)	Colon	2–15 minutes	Yes
Monobasic sodium phosphate	Solid	8.3–16.6 g	1/4 adult dose (5–<10 years) 1/2 adult dose (10 years)	Small and large intestines	0.5–3 hours	Yes
	Solution (rectal)	18.24–20.16 g once daily	1/2 adult dose (2–11 years)	Colon	2–15 minutes	Yes
Sodium biphosphate	Solid	9.6–19.2 g	1/2 adult dose (5–<10 years) 1/2 adult dose (10 years)	Small and large intestines	0.5–3 hours	Yes

TABLE 16-4 Classification and Properties of Laxatives *(continued)*

Agent	Dosage Form[a]	Daily Dosage Range		Site of Action	Approximate Onset of Action	Systemic Absorption
		Adults	**Children**			
Hyperosmotic						
Glycerin	Solid (rectal)	3 g	1–1.5 g (<6 years)	Colon	0.25–1 hour	—
	Liquid (rectal)	5–15 mL	2–5 mL (<6 years)	—	—	—
Polyethylene glycol 3350	Powder	17 g in 8 oz of water once daily		Colon	24–72 hours	Yes, a minimal amount
Stimulants (Anthraquinones)						
Senna	Solid	187–374 mg standardized senna concentrate 8.6–17.2 mg sennosides	187 mg standardized senna concentrate (BW >27 kg)	Colon	6–10 hours	Yes
	Granules	326 mg (1 tsp) standardized senna concentrate	163 mg (1/2 tsp) standardized senna concentrate (BW >27 kg)	Colon	6–10 hours	Yes
	Syrup	436–654 mg standardized senna extract	218–436 mg standardized senna extract (5–15 years) 109–218 mg standardized senna extract (1–5 years) 54.5–109 mg standardized senna extract (1 month to 1 year)	Colon	6–10 hours	Yes
	Solid (rectal)	652 mg standardized senna concentrate 30 mg sennosides	326 mg standardized senna concentrate (BW >27 kg)			
Stimulants (Diphenylmethane)						
Bisacodyl	Solid	10–30 mg	5–10 mg (>6–11 years) 10 mg (>11 years)	Colon	6–10 hours	Yes
Miscellaneous						
Castor oil	Liquid	15–60 mL	1–5 mL (2 years) 5–15 mL (2–11 years)	Small intestine	2–6 hours	Yes

Key: BW, body weight.

[a] All doses are oral unless indicated otherwise.

Note: Em dash (—) indicates information could not be identified.

Calcium polycarbophil may decrease the absorption of oral tetracylines because of the possible formation of nonabsorbable calcium complexes. In general, concurrent use of bulk-forming agents with other medications may reduce the desired effect of the co-administered medications because of physical binding or other mechanisms, which hinder absorption. Caution should be exercised by advising patients not to take a bulking agent within 1 to 2 hours of taking other medications.

Because of the danger of fecal impaction or intestinal obstruction, individuals with intestinal ulcerations, stenosis, or disabling adhesions should not take bulk-forming products. Diarrhea, abdominal discomfort, flatulence, and excessive loss of fluid can also occur. However, when taken properly, these agents have few systemic side effects because they are not absorbed.

Bulk-forming products may be inappropriate for patients who must severely restrict their fluid intake, such as those with significant renal dysfunction or heart failure. Patients who have demonstrated a previous hypersensitivity or who may be susceptible to an allergic reaction should exercise caution when considering a bulk-forming laxative, especially psyllium. Psyllium has a history of triggering hypersensitivity reactions.[18]

Bulk-forming agents should not be recommended for children younger than 6 years of age. Failure to consume sufficient fluid (at least 8 ounces) with a bulk laxative decreases drug efficacy and may result in intestinal or esophageal obstruction. Intestinal obstruction is a particular risk for patients suffering from opiate-induced constipation who have inadequate fluid intake.

The maximum calcium content of calcium polycarbophil is approximately 150 mg (7.6 mEq) per tablet. Susceptible patients (patients who are elderly, or have a malignancy, renal disease, or AIDS) who ingest the recommended therapeutic doses of calcium polycarbophil may have increased risk of hypercalcemia.

The dextrose content of some of the commercial products should be evaluated before use by diabetic patients and other patients on carbohydrate-restricted diets. Furthermore, sugar-free, bulk-forming agents that contain aspartame should be avoided by patients suffering from phenylketonuria.

Emollient Agents

Emollients commonly used include docusate sodium and docusate calcium. Emollients are anionic surfactants. When administered orally, they increase the wetting efficiency of intestinal fluid and facilitate a mixture of aqueous and fatty substances to soften the fecal mass. These agents are commonly known as "stool softeners."

Docusate has an onset of action after oral administration of between 24 and 72 hours. In the typical patient, effectiveness is achieved within 48 hours, but some patients may require as long as 3 to 5 days. These agents are not believed to be appreciably absorbed from the GI tract. In addition, docusate does not retard absorption of nutrients from the intestinal tract.

Orally administered emollients are most useful to prevent constipation. They can be used to treat occasional constipation but are of little or no value in treating long-standing constipation. Emollients soften stool and prevent painful defecation when the patient has undergone or is about to undergo surgery for hemorrhoids or other anorectal disorders, or when it is desirable for the patient to avoid straining at the stool (e.g., after abdominal surgery, immediately postpartum, or in patients with severe hypertension or cardiovascular disease). The patient should increase fluid intake to facilitate softening the stool. Because of the stool-softening effect of docusate, it is frequently used along with a stimulant (senna or bisacodyl) as a long-term treatment for opiate-induced constipation. Stool softeners are also useful agents in colostomy patients requiring a laxative product (see Chapter 22).

Table 16-4 lists dosing information for emollient agents. Children younger than 6 years old should not use emollients except as prescribed by a primary care provider. Doses above those recommended by the manufacturer may result in weakness, sweating, muscle cramps, and an irregular heartbeat in some patients.

Docusate can potentially cause diarrhea and mild abdominal cramping. Emollients facilitate the absorption of other poorly absorbed substances such as mineral oil and may increase the toxicity of these substances.[12] Docusate and its congeners are claimed to be nonabsorbable, relatively nontoxic (when administered alone), and pharmacologically inert. Caution should be exercised, however, because the detergent (surfactant) properties of docusate are believed to facilitate transport of other substances (e.g., increased absorption of mineral oil) across cell membranes.

No additional drug–drug interactions of clinical importance are noted.

Emollient use should be avoided if nausea and vomiting, symptoms of appendicitis (e.g., abdominal pain, nausea, and vomiting), or undetermined abdominal pain exist.

Lubricant Agent

Mineral oil (liquid petrolatum) is the only nonprescription lubricant. Heavy mineral oil is used enterally, whereas light mineral oil is used to prepare topical products.

Mineral oil and certain digestible plant oils such as olive oil soften fecal contents by coating them, thereby preventing colonic absorption of fecal water. Emulsified products increase palatability. Emulsions also penetrate and soften fecal matter more effectively than nonemulsified preparations.

The onset of action of mineral oil is about 6 to 8 hours after oral administration and 5 to 15 minutes after rectal administration. Nonemulsified mineral oil is minimally absorbed after oral or rectal doses.

Mineral oil is widely available and is often chosen by some older patients to self-treat constipation. Mineral oil has been used in cases requiring the maintenance of a soft stool to avoid straining (e.g., when there has been hernia, aneurysm, hypertension, myocardial infarction, or cerebrovascular accident, or after a hemorrhoidectomy or abdominal surgery). However, an emollient such as docusate is a better choice. Generally, mineral oil can be used for an occasional bout of constipation; however, because other safer agents are available, its use in self-care is strongly discouraged.

Table 16-4 lists dosing information for mineral oil. This product should never be taken by children younger than 6 years. Mineral oil use increases the possibility of loss of fat-soluble nutrients from the GI tract and enhances the likelihood of product aspiration and anal leakage.

Lipid pneumonia may result from the oral ingestion and subsequent aspiration of mineral oil, especially when the patient reclines. The pharynx may become coated with the oil, and droplets may reach the trachea and the posterior part of the lower lobes of the lungs. Because aspiration into the lungs is possible, mineral oil should not be administered at bedtime or to patients who are very young, of advanced age, or debilitated. When a patient takes large doses of mineral oil, the oil may leak through the anal sphincter and produce anal pruritus (pruritus ani), cryptitis, or other perianal conditions. The patient can avoid this leakage by reducing or dividing the dose, or by using a stable emulsion of mineral oil.

Mineral oil should never be used by a patient who is bedridden and if any of the following are present: appendicitis or its symptoms, undiagnosed rectal bleeding, or dysphagia.

The adverse effects and toxicity of mineral oil are associated with its repeated and prolonged use. The oil droplets may reach the mesenteric lymph nodes and may also be present in the intestinal mucosa, liver, and spleen, where they elicit a typical foreign-body reaction.

Mineral oil may impair the absorption of vitamins A, D, E, and K. Patients should not take mineral oil with meals because of potential delayed gastric emptying. In addition, it should not be given to pregnant women, because it can decrease the availability of vitamin K to the fetus. Patients taking oral anticoagulants should use mineral oil with caution; the potentially decreased absorption of vitamin K may increase the blood-thinning property of the anticoagulant. As indicated, mineral oil may reduce the absorption of oral anticoagulants, oral contraceptives, and digitalis glycosides. Because surfactants may increase absorption of other nonabsorbable drugs such as mineral oil, concomitant use with emollients (e.g. docusate) should be avoided.

Saline Laxative Agents

Saline laxative agents include magnesium citrate, magnesium hydroxide, magnesium sulfate, dibasic sodium phosphate, monobasic sodium phosphate, and sodium biphosphate

The active constituents of saline laxatives are relatively nonabsorbable cations and anions such as magnesium and sulfate ions. Sulfate salts are considered to be the most potent of this category of laxatives. The wall of the small intestine, which acts as a semipermeable membrane to the magnesium, sulfate, tartrate, phosphate, and citrate ions, retains the highly osmotic ions in the intestine. The presence of these ions draws water into the intestine, increasing intraluminal pressure. This increased pressure exerts a mechanical stimulus that increases intestinal motility.

Mechanisms independent of the osmotic effect may be partially responsible for the laxative properties of these salts. Saline laxatives produce a complex series of reactions, both secretory and motor, on the GI tract. For example, the action of magnesium sulfate on the GI tract is similar to that of cholecystokinin/pancreozymin and may be due to the release of this hormone when the laxative is administered. This release favors accumulation of fluid and electrolytes within the intestinal lumen.

Saline laxatives have an onset of action of 30 minutes to 3 hours for oral doses and 2 to 5 minutes for rectal doses. Up to 20% of an orally administered dose may be absorbed.

Saline laxatives are primarily indicated for use when acute evacuation of the bowel is required, as when preparing for endoscopic examination or eliminating drugs in suspected poisonings. When used for constipation, they should be used for no more than 1 week before seeing a primary care provider. These agents have no place in the long-term management of constipation. In some cases of food or drug poisoning, saline laxatives are used in purging doses. Rectal phosphate products are used to prepare the bowel for a barium enema and eliminate fecal impaction.

Table 16-4 lists dosing information for saline laxative agents. Rectal agents should not be used in children younger than 2 years. Oral products should not be used in children younger than 5 years. Any of the magnesium-containing products may lead to hypermagnesemia in both adults and children. Hypotension, muscle weakness, and electrocardiographic changes may indicate a toxic effect of magnesium. In addition, excessive levels of serum magnesium exert a depressant effect on the central nervous system and neuromuscular activity.

As much as 20% of the administered magnesium ion may be absorbed from magnesium salts. With normal renal function, elimination is largely unaffected. However, in marked renal impairment, or in newborns or older adults, toxicity may result. Other adverse effects include abdominal cramping, excessive diuresis, nausea, vomiting, and dehydration. Phosphate laxatives may lead to hyperphosphatemia when dosed excessively. Careful monitoring is required in renal impairment.

Saline laxatives can interact with oral anticoagulants, digitalis glycosides, and some phenothiazines (especially chlorpromazine). Magnesium-containing laxatives may interfere with the absorption of oral tetracycline products. If used concurrently with a magnesium salt, sodium polystyrene sulfonate may bind with magnesium and lead to systemic alkalosis.

Saline laxatives are contraindicated in patients with ileostomy or colostomy, dehydration syndromes, renal function impairment, or congestive heart failure.

Phosphate salts are available in oral and rectal dosage forms. The typical oral dose contains 96.5 mEq of sodium and should be administered with caution to patients on sodium-restricted diets. When phosphate salts are given as an enema, up to 10% or more of the sodium content may be absorbed. FDA has issued a final rule that amends the regulations regarding sodium labeling for nonprescription products. This rule applies to products for oral ingestion and mandates that they must include the sodium content and a general warning that persons who are on a sodium-restricted diet should not take the product except under medical supervision. Sodium phosphate and sodium bisphosphate products, among others, fall within the rule. This action was taken to protect patients who may be at risk for electrolyte imbalance while using such products.[24] Cathartics containing sodium may be toxic to individuals with edema, congestive heart disease, or renal failure; phosphates will accumulate with impaired renal function and should be avoided in these patients. Because dehydration may occur with the repeated use of hypertonic solutions of saline cathartics, patients who cannot tolerate fluid loss should not use phosphate salts. In patients who are not fluid-restricted, oral phosphate salts should be followed by at least one full glass of water to prevent dehydration.

At press time, FDA had ordered that a boxed warning be added to prescription-only oral sodium phosphate products. Acute kidney injury has been reported in some patients who received these products for bowel cleansing. FDA is also requiring that manufacturers develop and implement a risk evaluation and mitigation program. Further, FDA recommends that nonprescription versions of these products not be used for bowel cleansing (www.fda.gov/cder/drug/infopage/OSP_solution/default.htm). In response, Fleet products are being voluntarily removed from the market.

Hyperosmotic Agents

Glycerin was the only nonprescription hyperosmotic agent available until the approval of polyethylene glycol 3350 (PEG 3350) on October 6, 2006. PEG 3350 is available for oral use without electrolytes. Other commonly used agents in this class are prescription-only products and include lactulose, sorbitol, and PEG solutions with electrolytes (e.g., Colyte and Golytely).

Glycerin's cathartic capability is caused by combining an osmotic effect with the local irritant effect of sodium stearate. The combination acts by drawing water into the rectum to stimulate a bowel movement.

Glycerin is poorly absorbed after rectal administration. Use of glycerin suppositories in infants and adults usually produces a bowel movement within 30 minutes. Glycerin has been available for many years in suppository form to be used for lower bowel evacuation.

Table 16-4 lists dosing information for glycerin. The rectal dose of glycerin considered safe and effective for adults and children older than 6 years is 3 grams. Use of liquid glycerin as an enema is not recommended in adults and older children; this use may cause considerable rectal irritation. For infants and children younger than 6 years, the dose is 1 to 1.5 grams as a suppository. Overdosage with glycerin might cause additional rectal irritation that would not be expected to lead to serious sequelae.

Adverse reactions and side effects from glycerin suppositories are minimal. Some rectal irritation may occur. The irritation can be attributed to the sodium stearate component.

Interactions between glycerin and other drugs are not clinically important. Use of glycerin may be inappropriate in patients with a previous condition involving rectal irritation. Chronic use or overuse may lead to reduced serum potassium concentrations.

PEG solutions consist of very large poorly absorbable ethylene glycol molecules that cause an osmotic effect, resulting in distension and catharsis. Following oral administration, the PEG 3350 dose remains almost entirely within the GI tract and is not subject to degradation by intestinal enzymes or bacterial metabolism. The very small amount that is systemically absorbed (0.2%) is rapidly excreted in the urine.

PEG 3350 is useful in the treatment of occasional constipation. It is usually taken as 17 grams (about 1 heaping tablespoon) of powder per day in 4 to 8 ounces of water. One to 3 days (24–72 hours) may be required to produce a bowel movement. PEG 3350 is more costly than glycerin. The cost of a 4.1 ounce bottle of MiraLAX is about $8 per bottle in a typical pharmacy. It contains approximately seven doses, so the cost per ounce is about $1.00. The cost of a 17.9 oz bottle is around $22, lowering the per-dose cost to about $0.75. Patients with occasional constipation may find these products acceptable. Those with more chronic constipation problems may find them expensive.

PEG 3350 is safe for short-term therapy of constipation. Bloating, abdominal discomfort, cramping, and flatulence may occur. Higher doses (e.g., 34 g/day) might lead to diarrhea and excessive stool frequency. Patients who have renal disease should be cautioned to consult with their primary care provider before using PEG 3350. It has no documented drug–drug interactions.

Stimulant Agents

Stimulants are believed to increase the propulsive peristaltic activity of the intestine by local irritation of the mucosa or by a more selective action on the intramural nerve plexus of intestinal smooth muscle, thereby increasing motility. It has been suggested that these laxative agents stimulate secretion of water and electrolytes in either the small or large intestine or both, depending on the specific laxative.[7] Intensity of action is proportional to dosage, but individual effective doses vary.

Stimulants are classified according to their chemical structure and pharmacologic activity. The two classifications of stimulant laxatives are anthraquinone and diphenylmethane. Anthraquinones are aromatic organic compounds derived from anthracene and sometimes are known as anthracene cathartics. Diphenylmethanes are organic compounds from which a number of widely used products have been derived.

The cathartic activity of anthraquinones is limited primarily to the colon. Anthraquinones usually produce their action 6 to 12 hours after administration but may require up to 24 hours. The properties of each anthraquinone laxative varies somewhat, depending on the anthraquinone content and the speed with which the active principles are liberated. The anthraquinones are hydrolyzed by colonic bacteria into active compounds and are minimally absorbed. The precise mechanism by which anthraquinones increase peristalsis is unknown.

Anthraquinones include aloe, cascara sagrada, casanthranol, senna (including the sennosides, which are hydroanthracene glycosides derived from senna leaves), aloin, danthron, rhubarb, and frangula. The drugs of choice in this group are senna compounds. Not long ago, FDA reclassified several stimulants used as

nonprescription laxatives as "misbranded," including the long-time favorites cascara, casanthranol, and aloe.[25] Manufacturers were invited to submit data that supported the effectiveness of these agents, but they declined. All products containing these ingredients have since been reformulated. The banned substances have largely been replaced by ingredients such as sennosides, standardized senna, or senna. Patients should be informed that products containing the banned substances have not been proven to be unsafe, so the risk associated with taking products that may have already been purchased is minimal. Although rhubarb and aloin were not affected by the FDA ruling, practitioners should not recommend these very irritating substances.

Senna's active constituents include sennosides A and B. Sennosides are metabolized to an active byproduct called rhein. Senna and the sennosides appear to inhibit water and electrolyte absorption from the large intestine, resulting in increased intestinal volume and pressure that stimulates colonic motility.

The most commonly used diphenylmethane laxatives have been bisacodyl and phenolphthalein. However, after a review of reports of the development of carcinogenic tumors and genetic damage in rats, FDA determined that phenolphthalein posed a risk and subsequently placed it on the list of misbranded substances.[26] Phenolphthalein-containing products are no longer available in the United States.

Bisacodyl acts in the colon on contact with the mucosal nerve plexus. Stimulation is segmented and axonal, producing contractions of the entire colon. Bisacodyl's action is independent of intestinal tone, and the drug is minimally absorbed systemically (approximately 5%).[27]

The activity of diphenylmethanes is limited to the colon, and a cathartic effect is usually produced within 6 to 10 hours after administration. Bisacodyl is minimally absorbed whether given by oral or rectal administration. Action on the small intestine is negligible. A soft, formed stool is usually produced 6 to 10 hours after oral administration and 15 to 60 minutes after rectal administration.

Stimulants such as bisacodyl are used before radiologic or endoscopic examination of the GI tract and GI surgery, when thorough evacuation of the bowel is crucial. Both bisacodyl and senna are finding wide use as treatment for chronic constipation induced by opiates.[28] Bisacodyl may be administered orally or rectally and may be used in combination with or instead of an enema or suppository for emptying the colon and rectum before proctologic or colonic examination or GI surgery. Because of its thoroughness in evacuating the bowel, bisacodyl is effective in patients with colostomies, and it may reduce or eliminate the need for irrigations.

Traditionally, castor oil has been classified as a third category of stimulant but is viewed by some as an anionic surfactant.[27] Castor oil's laxative action is produced by ricinoleic acid, which is produced when castor oil is hydrolyzed in the small intestine by pancreatic lipase. Its exact mechanism of action is unknown.

Castor oil has an oral onset of action of about 2 to 6 hours. It is metabolized to ricinoleic acid, which is absorbed to a small extent. Metabolism of castor oil, a glyceride, is probably similar to that of other fatty acids. Because the main site of action is the small intestine, prolonged use of castor oil may result in excessive loss of fluid, electrolytes, and nutrients. This agent is most effective when administered on an empty stomach. Because a laxative effect occurs quickly, castor oil should not be given at bedtime.

In general, stimulants may be used in patients with simple constipation, but the bulk-forming agents or the hyperosmotic PEG 3350 should be tried first. The dose should be within the recommended dosage range listed in Table 16-4. However, listed doses and dosage ranges are only guides when determining the optimal individual dose. Overdoses of stimulants, especially anthraquinones, may lead to sudden vomiting, nausea, diarrhea, or severe abdominal cramping, requiring prompt medical attention.

Major hazards of stimulant laxative use are severe cramping, electrolyte and fluid deficiencies, enteric loss of protein, malabsorption resulting from excessive hypermotility and catharsis, and hypokalemia. All stimulants may produce cramping, colic, increased mucus secretion and, in some people, excessive evacuation of fluid. Stimulants can be effective but should be recommended cautiously. Because the intensity of their activity is proportional to the dose used, a large enough dose of any stimulant laxative can produce unwanted and sometimes dangerous adverse effects. Nevertheless, these laxatives are frequently used by those who self-medicate for constipation. Because of their perceived effectiveness, stimulant laxatives may be subject to overuse (i.e., that is, indiscriminate or excessive routine use beyond accepted limits). Such use was once thought to contribute to "cathartic colon," described as a poorly functioning colon (see the box A Word about Laxative Abuse). However, data seem unconvincing regarding the ability of stimulants to induce this alleged disorder.[4]

The prolonged use of anthraquinones can result in a harmless, reversible melanotic pigmentation of the colonic mucosa (melanosis coli), which is usually found on sigmoidoscopy, colonoscopy, or rectal biopsy.

Senna may color urine pink to red, red to violet, or red to brown, affecting the accurate interpretation of the phenolsulfonphthalein test. Chrysophanic acid, a component of rhubarb and senna that is excreted in urine, colors acidic urine yellowish brown and colors alkaline urine reddish violet.

Adverse effects of diphenylmethanes, which come with chronic, regular use (abuse), include metabolic acidosis or alkalosis, hypocalcemia, tetany, loss of enteric protein, and malabsorption. The suppository form may produce a burning sensation in the rectum. No systemic or adverse effects on the liver, kidney, or hematopoietic system have been observed after administration.

The administration of bisacodyl tablets within 1 hour of antacids, cimetidine, famotidine, ranitidine, or milk results in

---

A WORD ABOUT   Laxative Abuse

Routine, chronic use of most laxative preparations is considered laxative abuse, or at least laxative overuse, and should be avoided if at all possible. Some believe that the risk of abuse has been overemphasized. Although the laxative abuser may commonly be thought of as an older adult, this is not an accurate view. Some adolescents, college students, and young adults (especially women) may misuse laxatives for weight control.[29,30] Such abuse is often part of a pattern of "purging behavior," which may also include self-induced vomiting. These individuals may suffer from bulimia nervosa or anorexia nervosa.[31]

Excessive use of laxatives can cause diarrhea and vomiting, leading to fluid and electrolyte losses, especially hypokalemia, which may result in a general loss of tone of smooth and striated muscle. Clinical features of laxative abuse may include (1) factitious diarrhea (a severe chronic watery diarrhea, frequently occurring at night and accompanied by abdominal pain, weight loss, nausea, and vomiting)[32]; (2) electrolyte imbalance (e.g., hypokalemia, hypocalcemia, and hypermagnesemia); (3) osteomalacia; (4) protein-losing enteropathy (intestinal disease); (5) steatorrhea; and (6) liver disease.

The association of cathartic colon with laxative abuse is now largely dismissed owing to lack of evidence.[33] Although past literature offered a few case reports, the recent literature offers no support; some suggest that recent case reports are lacking, because currently used products are less capable of producing cathartic colon than were older, out-of-favor products.[7]

Laxative abuse can usually be classified as either habitual or surreptitious. The habitual abuser often believes that a daily bowel movement is a necessity and uses a laxative to accomplish this end. These patients may freely admit to this practice, because they believe regular laxative use to be entirely correct and natural. Conversely, surreptitious abuse is similar to other illnesses. Surreptitious abusers tend to manifest various psychiatric disturbances. Confronting this type of abuser does not usually help resolve the problem, and psychiatric intervention should be encouraged. Practitioners should be alert to the possibility of laxative abuse when making a patient assessment. The diagnosis of laxative abuse may include a stool osmolarity test to detect salines and a colonoscopy to detect melanosis coli. Urine samples may be analyzed for the presence of the most commonly used laxatives.

Once the abuse has been adequately substantiated, it may be possible to (1) wean the patient off the laxative before permanent bowel damage occurs and (2) regularize the patient's bowel habits with a high-fiber diet supplemented by bulk-forming laxatives as needed. After an abuser is withdrawn from one or more laxatives, several months may be required to retrain the bowel to work in regular, unaided function. Affected patients should be educated about laxative abuse. The information provided should describe types of laxatives and their harmful effects. Patients should be advised that constipation, weight gain, bloating, or abdominal distention may occur after laxative abuse ceases. These patients should be encouraged to exercise, increase dietary fiber, and maintain adequate fluid intake. The practitioner should also encourage them to discuss their attitudes about laxative abuse and be prepared to answer any questions that arise in such discussions.

rapid erosion of the enteric coating, which may lead to gastric or duodenal irritation. Enteric-coated bisacodyl tablets prevent irritation of the gastric mucosa and, therefore, should not be broken, crushed, chewed, or administered with agents that increase gastric pH such as antacids, histamine$_2$-receptor antagonists, or proton pump inhibitors.

Stimulants should not be used for patients with undiagnosed rectal bleeding, signs of intestinal obstruction, or presence of appendicitis. Pregnant women should use stimulants under the direction of a medical practitioner, especially during the third trimester.

Practitioners should exercise caution when recommending magnesium-containing products to patients with renal failure because of the risk of hypermagnesemia. A practitioner should be similarly cautious when recommending sodium-containing products to patients with cardiovascular disease because of the potential for sodium overload. As a rule, laxative products whose maximum daily dose contains more than sodium 345 mg (15 mEq), potassium 975 mg (25 mEq), magnesium 600 mg (50 mEq), or calcium 1800 mg (90 mEq) should not be used in kidney or liver disease, heart failure, hypertension, or other conditions requiring sodium, potassium, magnesium, or calcium restriction.

Combination Products

Many combination laxative products are available (Table 16-5). Companies attempt to take advantage of multiple mechanisms of action and other factors to create a product that better meets the criteria for an ideal laxative. For example, several combination products contain a stimulant and a second entity. Emollients do not stimulate bowel movements when used alone, but they do support this purpose when combined with stimulant laxatives. A popular combination is docusate sodium with senna, which takes advantage of both a cathartic action and a stool-softening effect.

In many cases of fecal impaction, a solution of docusate is often added to the enema fluid. Some products incorporate senna with psyllium. The desired effect is for the senna to act quickly and the bulk-forming agent to aid in producing easier stools beyond the initial movement. Other available combination oral products include various agents such as psyllium, bisacodyl, or docusate as the principal ingredient and glycerin as an adjunctive agent. It is unlikely that the contributing effect of glycerin is significant to the overall laxative action of the product. The amount of oral glycerin necessary to produce laxation would lead to appreciable glycerin absorption from the small intestine.

Because a common ingredient in most combination products is a stimulant, it is important to remember that combining laxative entities has the potential for greater adverse impact if administration and dosing guidelines are not closely followed. If a stimulant and a stool softener are combined, the potential for adversity depends largely on the stimulant. However, if a stimulant and a saline are combined, the potential for adverse effects is enhanced, because both agents have significant effects on the intestine.

Bowel evacuant kits are designed for use to prepare the bowel for endoscopic examination or surgery (Table 16-5). The kit usually contains separate dosages of the specific laxatives rather than a single dosage form containing all the ingredients. Although a patient may experience adverse effects from the use of preparation kits, they are intended for single use before a procedure, unlike the usual treatment for constipation.

Pharmacotherapeutic Comparison

Head-to-head comparison studies of solely nonprescription laxatives are largely unavailable. Much of what is practiced has been learned through observation after laxative use. If used properly, a bulk-forming product should soften the stool by its normal action. Because both a traditional stool softener and a bulk-forming agent take about the same length of time to work, a bulk-forming agent may be the correct choice for some patients who require stool softening.

Very few new-entity laxative products have been introduced into the nonprescription marketplace in recent years. Most principal ingredients were brought into being before the current era of rigorous comparative studies. Although stimulants and saline-type laxatives have been used widely for self-care, it is important to recommend a product with the lowest likelihood of untoward effects.

Product Selection Guidelines

When considering the use of any laxative to treat constipation, the clinician should remember that normal defecation empties only the rectum and the descending and sigmoid branches of the colon. The preparation chosen should duplicate the normal physiologic process as nearly as possible. Most stimulant products have the potential to promote catharsis, that is, a complete emptying of the entire colon. However, the laxative user who is unaware of this effect may take another laxative dose on the first or second post-laxative day, thereby maintaining a completely empty colon. Therefore, when it is necessary to use a laxative to treat constipation, the recommended initial choice is most often a bulk-forming product.

Acute constipation is the primary indication for self-treatment with a nonprescription laxative. In most cases, laxative selection for simple constipation should begin with a bulk-forming agent unless it is contraindicated or the need exists for a more rapid effect. Should it prove ineffective, the hyperosmotic PEG 3350 should be considered. If PEG 3350 is unable to produce a satisfactory response, a stimulant (e.g., a senna product or bisacodyl) should be considered. In each case, the lowest effective dose should be used and the dose reduced once symptoms improve.

Nonprescription laxative products are also prescribed or indicated for patients preparing for diagnostic GI procedures and radiography. A primary care diagnostician should supervise the use of laxatives (1) during treatment for perianal disease (preoperatively or postoperatively); (2) with conditions in which straining is undesirable (e.g., postoperative or post–myocardial infarction); or (3) for chronic constipation. Although bulk-forming and emollient laxatives may be suitable for such problems, therapy in these situations is highly individualized.

SPECIAL POPULATIONS

Children A number of factors can alter a child's bowel habits, including unavailable toilet facilities; emotional distress; febrile illness; chronic medical conditions (e.g., cystic fibrosis and hypothyroidism); family conflict; dietary changes (e.g., switching from human to cow's milk); or a change in daily routine or environment.[21] Some children are poor or picky eaters, which may contribute to the development of constipation due to inadequate bulk and fluids in the diet. Constipation associated with an organic or pathologic etiology is uncommon in children.[34] Bowel movement patterns vary widely in children; therefore,

TABLE 16-5 Selected Laxative Products

Trade Name	Primary Ingredients
Bulk-Forming Laxatives	
Citrucel Powder	Methylcellulose 2 g/tsp
Citrucel Sugar Free Powder	Methylcellulose 2 g/tsp
FiberCon Tablets	Calcium polycarbophil 625 mg
Maltsupex Liquid	Barley malt extract 750 mg/tsp
Metamucil Fiber Wafer	Psyllium hydrophilic mucilloid 3.4 g/2 wafers
Metamucil Smooth Texture, Sugar Free Orange Flavor Powder/Individual Packets	Psyllium hydrophilic mucilloid 3.4 g/tsp
Emollient Laxatives	
Colace Liquid	Docusate sodium 20 mg/5 mL
Correctol Stool Softener Softgels	Docusate sodium 100 mg
Lubricant Laxatives	
Fleet Mineral Oil Enema	Mineral oil 100%
Kondremul Emulsion	Mineral oil 55%
Saline Laxatives	
Citroma Solution	Magnesium citrate 1.745 g/oz
Fleet Ready-to-Use Enema	Monobasic sodium phosphate 19 g/133 mL; dibasic sodium phosphate 7 g/133 mL
Fleet Ready-to-Use Enema for Children	Monobasic sodium phosphate 9.5 g/59 mL; dibasic sodium phosphate 3.5 g/59 mL
Phillips' Milk of Magnesia Suspension	Magnesium hydroxide 400 mg/5 mL
Hyperosmotic Laxatives	
Fleet Babylax Liquid	Glycerin 2.3 g
Fleet Glycerin Suppository (Adult/Child Size)	Glycerin 5.6 g
MiraLAX	Polyethylene glycol 3350 17g
Stimulant Laxatives	
Dulcolax Tablets	Bisacodyl 5 mg
Ex-Lax Regular Strength Chocolate Tablets	Sennosides 15 mg
Purge Liquid	Castor oil 95%
Senokot Tablets	Standardized senna concentrate 8.6 mg sennosides
X-Prep Liquid	Senna concentrate 3.7 g/75 mL standardized extract of senna fruit
Combination Laxatives	
Perdiem Granules	Senna (cassia pod concentrate) 0.74 g/tsp; psyllium 3.25 g/tsp
Senokot-S Tablets	Senna concentrate 8.6 mg sennosides; docusate sodium 50 mg
Bowel Evacuant Kits	
Evac-Q-Kwik System Liquid/Suppository/Tablets	Tablets: bisacodyl 15 mg/3 tablets Suppository: bisacodyl 10 mg Liquid: magnesium citrate 25 mEq/30 mL

constipation can be a complex problem that is often difficult to detect and manage. Children typically describe constipation as a difficulty in passing stools. Straining to pass large or hard stools can be painful. The child may then avoid or withhold bowel movements, resulting in worsening symptoms and fear of toileting. Normal frequency of bowel movements varies with the age of a child, making it difficult to recognize abnormal bowel habits. Because stooling becomes less frequent with increasing age, what may be a normal stooling pattern may be misdiagnosed as constipation. Parents seek advice for children of all ages when stooling patterns differ from what the parent perceives to be normal. Laxatives are often administered to children in an attempt to facilitate the passage of stools and to reestablish a normal stooling pattern. As a result, indiscriminate use of laxatives may result if the child has a stooling pattern that is changing or when other constipating factors are present. Children should be encouraged to establish a regular pattern of bowel movements and to avoid withholding of stools when the urge to have a bowel movement occurs. The clinician should do a thorough assessment of possible causes for constipation, and always consider a child's age and any previous laxative use when recommending laxative products. The route of administration and the taste of oral products may be especially significant in children. Laxative use can be avoided in older children by encouraging them to adhere to suggested dietary guidelines to improve stool regularity.

If medications are indicated in children younger than 5 years, glycerin suppositories may initiate the defecation reflex with onset usually within 15 to 60 minutes. Barley malt extract (malt soup extract) is relatively safe for infants younger than 2 months. Breast-fed infants may receive 6 to 10 mL in 2 to 4 ounces of water or fruit juice twice daily. Bottle-fed infants may receive 7.5 to 32 mL in a day's total formula, or 5 to 10 mL every second feeding. Mineral oil is not recommended because of the risk of aspiration. Stimulant laxatives and phosphate enemas should be avoided.[35]

In children who have fecal impaction, disimpaction can usually be achieved by the use of oral medications, enemas, or a combination of both.[36] For infants younger than 1 year, glycerin suppositories or an enema can be used.[11] However, some experts suggest avoiding enemas in infants younger than 1 year; if an enema is necessary, it should be done under the direction of a primary care provider.[35] For children 1 year and older, bisacodyl, magnesium citrate, PEG electrolyte solutions (e.g., Colyte and Golytely) or PEG solutions without electrolytes (MiraLAX in an initial dose of 1–1.5 g/kg/day for 3 days) are oral medications that may be useful for fecal impaction.[21,35] Enemas containing phosphate soda or saline can also achieve disimpaction, although the oral route is less invasive.[21] Parents should be cautioned that enemas act fast but can be traumatic for children. Saline agents can lead to salt and water retention. Use in children younger than 2 years may lead to electrolyte abnormalities, such as hypocalcemia, tetany, hypernatremia, dehydration, and hyperphosphatemia. Electrolyte levels in these patients require careful monitoring.

When fecal impaction is not present, treatment of constipation in infants should consist of glycerin suppositories or oral juices containing light or dark corn syrup (1–3 mL/kg/day divided into two feedings per day). In children older than 1 year, milk of magnesia or PEG 3350 without electrolytes can be given according to age-appropriate dosage recommendations.[11] In general, stimulants should be avoided, as should excessive use of enemas.

Patients of Advanced Age   Constipation is more common in adults as they advance in age. Older adults (e.g., >65 years old) frequently describe constipation as straining to move bowels and report fewer stools per week. The aging process is associated with physiologic changes that prolong the transit time through the colon, which decreases the perception of the urge to defecate. Constipation in older adults can be precipitated or aggravated by conditions such as neuromuscular disorders, confusion, dementia, and depression.[4–6] In addition, the older population tends to have multiple medical conditions and take multiple medications that may contribute to the development of constipation. Constipating medications commonly used by older adults include narcotic analgesics; sedatives; hypnotics; antidepressants; anticholinergics; some antacids and vitamins that contain calcium, aluminum, or iron; and calcium channel blockers.[7,8] Laxative use increases with age.[7] Abuse of stimulant laxatives, in an attempt to regulate bowel activity, was thought to lead paradoxically to worsening symptoms of constipation. However, lack of evidence supporting this view suggests otherwise.[33]

Lifestyle factors that can contribute to or worsen constipation in older adults include failure to establish a schedule for bowel movements; emotional stress; inadequate chewing of foods, which is often a result of poor dentition; a diet that is insufficient in calories and fiber; inadequate fluid intake; and limited exercise. Elderly patients who are sedentary or confined to the bed have an increased risk for developing constipation, because walking has a positive impact on gut peristalsis.

If any of these factors exist, the health care provider should consider lifestyle modifications or an adjustment to current drug therapy before recommending a laxative.

Dietary considerations are especially important in the evaluation of constipation in the elderly. Maintaining a balanced diet with adequate fiber and fluids is important but often difficult to sustain for many older adults. Daily consumption of foods high in fiber or fiber supplements along with six to eight 8-ounce glasses of noncaffeinated, nonalcoholic liquids is recommended. Constipation is often an indication of dehydration in the elderly; therefore, fluid status should be monitored closely.[20]

Chronic laxative use is common among the older population. The aging process can cause the colon to lack normal tone, resulting in an overreliance on oral laxatives or rectal enemas to produce defecation. However, because of the physiologic effects of chronic laxative use on the intestine, laxative dependency is often difficult to manage. Some researchers have found an increased risk for colorectal cancer among laxative abusers.[20] Laxative preparations can also increase the rate at which other drugs pass through the GI tract by increasing GI motility, which then decreases absorption and the effectiveness of concurrently administered medications.

Older patients are particularly sensitive to shifts in fluid and electrolytes. Use of any laxative that alters the fluid and electrolyte balance, particularly saline-type laxatives, may be inappropriate in certain patients of advanced age. These laxatives can place older patients, particularly those who are on diuretics or have decreased fluid intake, at risk for adverse effects.

An acute episode of constipation may be treated with plain water or saline enemas. Although not available over the counter, soapsuds enemas and enemas using detergents should be avoided; they can be irritating and can cause serious complications.[8,37] Sodium phosphate and biphosphate enemas are effective but can result in hyperphosphatemia in patients with renal disease.

Bulk-forming agents are generally preferred for older patients who are able to tolerate adequate fluid intake. The onset of effect is usually 12 to 72 hours. Sugar-free products are recommended for patients with diabetes. Adequate fluid intake is necessary with bulk-forming agents to avoid worsening constipation. Glycerin suppositories and the oral administration of lactulose or sorbitol (prescription-only products) are safe and have been used successfully in patients of advanced age. Although considerably more costly than sorbitol, lactulose may be of particular benefit to those who are bedridden, and it is preferred in patients with hepatic encephalopathy. Mineral oil should be avoided in older adults because of the risk of developing lipid pneumonia, particularly in patients who are bedridden. For patients with cardiac and renal disease, PEG–electrolyte solutions, which are poorly absorbed, have been safely used for acute management of constipation.

Some health care providers may recommend chronic stimulant laxatives in certain situations, but these products should not be generally recommended for all older patients. The recommendation to use laxatives in this population should be patient-specific. Older individuals can have complicating pathology, multiple medical complaints, and are vulnerable to the effects of medications. A complete and thorough history should aid in selecting the most appropriate product.

Pregnancy   Constipation is common during pregnancy and after childbirth or surgery. It is estimated that one in every three pregnant women experiences constipation during the first and third trimesters.[38] The increasing size of the uterus compresses the colon, affecting the emptying of fecal material. In addition, reduced intestinal muscle tone, which can contribute to a decrease in peristalsis, is likely the primary reason.[39] Other contributing factors in pregnancy include the use of prenatal vitamin and mineral supplements that contain iron and calcium, a decease in dietary fiber and fluid, and a reduction in physical activity.[38] Constipation in pregnancy can lead to backaches, hemorrhoids, and fecal impaction.

The main goal of treatment of constipation in pregnancy is to achieve soft stools without the use of laxatives. Dietary measures that include natural remedies such as prunes or prune juice should be attempted as an initial measure in most patients. However, laxatives may be necessary postpartum in some women to reestablish normal bowel function that was lost because of perineal pain. Other indications for laxative use may include ileus secondary to colonic dilatation in a decompressed abdomen, laxness of the anal sphincter and abdominal musculature, low fluid intake, hemorrhoids, and administration of enemas during labor. Consultation with a woman's health care provider is recommended prior to laxative use in more severe cases and when the safety of certain laxative products is questionable.

Because of the potential for adverse effects of several products, such as (1) decreased vitamin absorption caused by mineral oil, (2) premature labor brought on by the irritant effects of castor oil, or (3) possible dangerous electrolyte imbalances with osmotic agents, pregnant women should be very selective in choosing a laxative. Bulk-forming laxatives are the common first-line choice in pregnancy because of their safety and effectiveness.[7] These products require liberal amounts of fluid intake. Usual recommendations are at least 1500 mL/day. If bulk-forming laxatives are ineffective or intolerable, an emollient, senna, or bisacodyl may relieve symptoms. Senna and bisacodyl have also been used safely during breast-feeding.[40] Senna and bisacodyl have not been shown to be present in significant concentrations in breast milk, or no data are available to suggest that infants may experience any potential toxicity. If these products are used, the infant should be carefully observed for diarrhea. Saline cathartics should be avoided during pregnancy and lactation, because appreciable GI absorption can occur in the mother. Toxicity occurring from excessive use of a saline cathartic such as magnesium sulfate could be significant, resulting in diarrhea, drowsiness, respiratory difficulty, and hypotonia. These products may promote sodium retention and edema. Pregnant patients who are suspected of using these products should be monitored for increases in serum sodium and weight gain.

PATIENT FACTORS

Laxative products are available in a wide array of dosage forms, most of them for oral use. This variety probably yields the most benefits for pediatric and geriatric patients. Many of the dosage forms enhance patient acceptability and perhaps make laxative use more pleasant. However, laxatives available as chewing gum, wafers, effervescent granules, and chocolate tablets may not be thought of as drug products; therefore, they are more likely to be misused and abused. Enemas and suppositories are popular nonoral dosage forms used for laxative administration.

Routine use of laxative enemas includes preparing patients for surgery, child delivery, and GI radiologic or endoscopic examinations, as well as for treating certain cases of constipation. The enema fluid determines the mechanism by which evacuation is produced. Tap water and normal saline create bulk through an osmotic volume effect; vegetable oils lubricate, soften, and facilitate the passage of hardened fecal matter; and the irritant action of soapsuds produces defecation. However, prolonged rectal irritation may occur after soap enemas and may result in proctitis or colitis.[4,8] Therefore, soap enemas are not recommended.

The popular sodium phosphate/sodium biphosphate enemas (e.g., Fleet) fall into the category of saline laxatives. These agents are more efficient and effective than tap water, soapsuds, or saline enemas. Because they can alter fluid and electrolyte balance significantly with prolonged use, chronic use of these products is not warranted for controlling constipation.

A properly administered enema cleans only the distal colon, most nearly approximating a normal bowel movement. Proper administration requires that the diagnosis, the enema fluid, and the technique of administration be correct. Improperly administered, an enema can produce fluid and electrolyte imbalances. Enema fluids have caused mucosal changes or spasm of the intestinal wall. Water intoxication has resulted from the use of tap water or soapsuds enemas in the presence of megacolon. A misdirected or inadequately lubricated nozzle may cause abrasion of the anal canal and rectal wall or may cause colonic perforation.

Patients should be advised to follow all directions carefully when using these products (Table 16-6). The patient should lie or be placed either on the left side with knees bent or in the knee-to-chest position. If the patient is in a sitting position, use of an enema clears only the rectum of fecal material. The solution should be allowed to flow into the rectum slowly; if the patient is uncomfortable, the flow is probably too fast. One pint (500 mL) or less of properly introduced fluid usually produces adequate evacuation if it is retained until definite lower abdominal cramping is felt. As long as 1 hour may be needed for the entire procedure.

Bisacodyl-containing suppositories are promoted as replacements for enemas when the distal colon requires cleaning. Suppositories that contain bisacodyl are used for postoperative, antepartum, and postpartum care, and are adequate in preparing for proctosigmoidoscopy. Although bisacodyl suppositories are

TABLE 16-6 Administration of Rectal Suppositories or Enemas

Enemas

1. If someone else is administering the enema, lie on your left side with knees bent or in the knee-to-chest position (see drawings A and B). Position A is preferred for children older than 2 years. If self-administering the enema, lie on your back with your knees bent and buttocks raised (see drawing C). A pillow may be placed under the buttocks.
2. If using a concentrated enema solution, dilute solution according to the product instructions. Prepare 1 pint (500 mL) for adults and 1/2 pint (250 mL) for children.
3. Lubricate the enema tip with petroleum jelly or other nonmedicated ointment/cream. Apply the lubricant to the anal area as well.
4. Gently insert the enema tip 2 (recommended depth for children) to 3 inches into the rectum.
5. Allow the solution to flow into the rectum slowly. If you experience discomfort, the flow is probably too fast.
6. Retain the enema solution until definite lower abdominal cramping is felt. The parent/caregiver may have to gently hold a child's buttocks closed to prevent the solution from being expelled too soon.

Suppositories

1. Gently squeeze the suppository to determine if it is firm enough to insert. Chill a soft suppository by placing it in the refrigerator for a few minutes or by running it under cool running water.
2. Remove the suppository from its wrapping.
3. Dip the suppository for a few seconds in lukewarm water to soften the exterior.
4. Lie on your left side with knees bent or in the knee-to-chest position (see drawings A and B). Position A is best for self-administration of a suppository. Small children can be held in a crawling position.
5. Relax the buttock just before inserting the suppository to ease insertion. Gently insert the tapered end of the suppository high into the rectum. If the suppository slips out, it was not inserted past the anal sphincter (the muscle that keeps the rectum closed).
6. Continue to lie down for a few minutes, and hold the buttocks together to allow the suppository to dissolve in the rectum. The parent/caregiver may have to gently hold a child's buttocks closed.
7. Remember that the medication is most effective when the bowel is empty. Try to avoid a bowel movement after insertion of the suppository for up to 1 hour so that the intended action can occur.

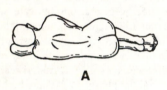 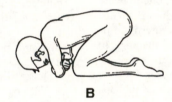 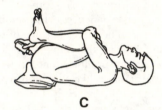

A   **B**   **C**

prescribed and are used more often than other suppositories, some clinicians still prefer enemas as agents for cleaning the lower bowel. Glycerin suppositories are useful in initiating the defecation reflex in children and in promoting rectal emptying in adults (Table 16-6).

PATIENT PREFERENCES

Liquid formulations of emollients may be made more palatable if mixed with juices or milk. The most commonly used products that contain castor oil are the more palatable emulsions. When plain castor oil is used, it may be administered with fruit juice or a carbonated beverage to mask its unpleasant taste. Chilling the oral form of a sodium phosphate–type product or taking it with ice seems to make it more palatable. Palatability may also be improved by drinking the product with a citrus fruit juice or with a citrus–flavored carbonated beverage.

Alternative and Complementary Therapies

Patients frequently treat constipation with a botanical product (Table 16-7).[41-43] Common dietary supplements include buckthorn, flaxseed, plantago, and senna. Although many of the commercially available stimulant and bulk-forming laxatives are derived from plants, some consumers prefer to use a "more natural" version of these products. In recent years, FDA has banned the use of aloe and cascara in nonprescription stimulant laxatives. Both agents are classified as generally unsafe and not effective. However, they are commonly found in many herbal teas, extracts, and pills. Individuals should either limit or avoid use of these products. They should also be cautioned against the use of botanical laxatives during pregnancy or breast-feeding, and in children.

Consumers are increasingly selecting dietary supplements that contain probiotics to promote regularity of the digestive tract. Fermented dairy products containing *Bifidobacterium animalis* DN-173 010 (in Activa yogurt) can usually be found in the refrigerated dairy section of the supermarket. Other products containing *Bifidobacterium infantis* 35624 (contained in Aligh) are available as oral capsules. These probiotics interact with the bacteria in the digestive tract and are marketed to improve the transit of food through the system and regulate digestion. Users should be cautioned that increased bloating and gas are common with consumption of these products. Probiotics, in general, are regarded as well tolerated and safe; however, the beneficial effects in preventing or relieving constipation have not been substantiated.[43]

Assessment of Constipation: A Case-Based Approach

The practitioner should obtain as much lifestyle and medical information as possible before making any recommendations for preventing or treating constipation. Appropriate information allows the practitioner to make rational recommendations based on knowledge of the patient, the problem, and the product,

TABLE 16-7 Selected Botanical Natural Products That May Act as Laxatives or Cathartics

Product (Scientific Name)	Risks	Effectiveness in Constipation
Buckthorn (*Rhamnus catharticus*)	Significant adverse effects with chronic use or abuse, including abdominal pain, anxiety, decreased respirations, trembling, vomiting, and excessive diarrhea Contraindicated in children younger than 12 years, or during pregnancy or lactation	Harsh cathartic laxative that stimulates contraction of large intestine; contains anthraquinones, which are known to produce laxative effects; effectiveness appears to be dose-related.
Flaxseed (*Linum usitatissimum*)	Generally regarded as safe when taken orally Use with caution in patients with history of bleeding, and diabetes Significant drug interactions with warfarin, antiplatelets, lithium, antihypertensives, antidiabetic agents	Bulk-forming laxative that may have beneficial effects for chronic symptoms of constipation; adequate fluid must be consumed to avoid paradoxical constipation or intestinal blockage.
Rhubarb (*Rheum palmatum*)	Prolonged use not recommended Use during pregnancy not recommended Should be used only on the advice of PCP because of potential toxicity	Strong stimulant laxative properties; effectiveness appears to be dose-related but is not sufficiently proven.
Senna leaves (*Cassia* sp.)	Safe for short-term use; laxative dependence possible with prolonged use Medical supervision recommended in children, or during pregnancy or lactation	Stimulant laxative for constipation and as an adjunct to evacuation for diagnostic tests of the GI tract; short-term oral use is generally recognized as effective.

Key: GI, gastrointestinal; PCP, primary care provider.

as well as on the practitioner's own judgment and experience. Evaluation of all drug use is critical in selecting appropriate laxatives. A patient who presents with constipation should initially be evaluated for any signs of significant GI problems that may warrant medical evaluation, such as severe abdominal pain, nausea and vomiting, or rectal bleeding. The practitioner must recognize the situations in which laxative use is inappropriate. For example, laxatives are not recommended to treat constipation associated with intestinal pathology or secondary to laxative abuse unless bowel retraining has been successful. Laxatives also are not a cure for functional constipation and, therefore, are of only secondary importance in treating this condition. Attention should be directed first to questions relating to diet, fluid intake, physical activity, and any underlying pathology that may be producing constipation as a symptom.

Patients should then be questioned regarding the characteristics of bowel movements including the caliber, color, and texture of stools as well as the frequency of elimination. Additional assessment should include questions about use of medications, both prescription and nonprescription, as well as previous laxative use. Adequate patient assessment is essential to effective management of constipation. For older patients without a history of constipation, a thorough investigation should be conducted to determine whether acute cases of constipation have resulted from new or old diseases or from the use of medications. When information is insufficient to assess the cause of the symptoms or any doubt exists regarding the patient's disease status, medical referral is appropriate.

Cases 16-1 and 16-2 are examples of the assessment of patients presenting with constipation.

CASE 16-1

Relevant Evaluation Criteria	Scenario/Model Outcome
Information Gathering	
1. Gather essential information about the patient's symptoms, including:	
a. description of symptom(s) (i.e., nature, onset, duration, severity, associated symptoms)	Patient indicates a decrease in frequency of bowel movements over the last several months since she began trying to lose weight. She admits to straining to pass hard stools.
b. description of any factors that seem to precipitate, exacerbate, and/or relieve the patient's symptom(s)	Patient recalls having problems with constipation in the past during class examinations. Her symptoms typically resolve after several weeks but usually require several doses of stool softeners and occasionally a laxative.

CASE 16-1 *(continued)*

Relevant Evaluation Criteria	Scenario/Model Outcome
c. description of the patient's efforts to relieve the symptoms	Patient has increased her water intake, because she began dieting, but she has not seen a notable difference in frequency or hardness of stools. She has also tried stool softeners in an attempt to alleviate straining but without success. Within the last couple of days, she admits to taking Milk of Magnesia and an enema.
2. Gather essential patient history information:	
a. patient's identity	Jasmine
b. patient's age, sex, height, and weight	28-year-old female, 5 ft 8 in, 180 lb
c. patient's occupation	Engineering student
d. patient's dietary habits	Usual diet contains fast foods and red meat. She has been on a low-carbohydrate diet for the last month.
e. patient's sleep habits	Sleeps 5–6 hours nightly
f. concurrent medical conditions, prescription and nonprescription medications, and dietary supplements	Oscal 1200 mg by mouth daily; Centrum with iron 1 tablet by mouth daily since start of diet
g. allergies	NKA
h. history of other adverse reactions to medications	None
i. other (describe) _____	Recent travel to China for spring break

Assessment and Triage

3. Differentiate the patient's signs/symptoms and correctly identify the patient's primary problem(s).	Constipation during periods of dieting and stress is common. Although the patient's constipation may be associated with her dietary changes, it could also be related to her use of an iron-containing multivitamin and calcium supplements, or perhaps it is related to her recent travel.
4. Identify exclusions for self-treatment (see Figure 16-2)	None
5. Formulate a comprehensive list of therapeutic alternatives for the primary problem to determine if triage to a medical practitioner is required, and share this information with the patient.	Options include: (1) Recommend a balanced diet with adequate fiber, fruits, and vegetables. (2) Recommend at least 2 liters of fluid daily during dieting and on a routine basis. (3) Recommend incorporating a regular exercise routine, along with increased hours of sleep to decrease the effect of stress. (4) Recommend adding a fiber supplement given the constipating effects of calcium and iron. (5) Refer patient to a PCP if lifestyle changes do not alleviate symptoms. (6) Take no action.

Plan

6. Select an optimal therapeutic alternative to address the patient's problem, taking into account patient preferences.	Jasmine has had recurrent problems with constipation during periods of stress. The introduction of a low-calorie, high-protein diet coupled with her decrease in fluid intake may be contributing to her acute constipation. She has been taking calcium and iron supplements while dieting to support her nutrition. Because both calcium and iron have constipating side effects, these supplements may be contributing to her symptoms. Jasmine has experienced short periods of constipation in the past during class examinations, which may be brought on by an increase in stress during these periods. Her problem is likely exacerbated by the fact that she has been traveling for 2 weeks and has had long periods of immobility due to her long flights to and from China. Because she has been unsuccessful at self-management and is committed to her diet program and school, a referral is appropriate.

CASE 16-1 *(continued)*

Relevant Evaluation Criteria	Scenario/Model Outcome
7. Describe the recommended therapeutic approach to the patient.	You should modify your diet to include more fiber, fruits, and vegetables. A fiber supplement should also be added, along with an increase in fluid intake. A regular exercise routine is recommended. Because your constipation is a recurrent problem, you should consider a bulk-forming laxative if dietary changes and exercise do not improve your symptoms. If such measures do not successfully relieve your constipation or if the frequency of symptoms increases, you should obtain an appointment with your PCP, that is, primary care provider, to discuss preventive measures and treatment options for recurrences.
8. Explain to the patient the rationale for selecting the recommended therapeutic approach from the considered therapeutic alternatives.	The recommended dietary adjustments should continue to support your weight loss and provide the needed nutrients. Regular exercise should improve your metabolism and digestive activity. Short-term use of a mild laxative is generally safe and effective, and may give you more immediate relief of symptoms. Readjusting after recent travel and examinations should also promote regularity. A visit to your PCP for further assessment can rule out a possible organic cause.

Patient Education

9. When recommending self-care with nonprescription medications and/or nondrug therapy, convey accurate information to the patient:	Bulk-forming laxatives are recommended for short-term treatment, but they can also be used prophylactically. Avoid their use if you have a history of any gastrointestinal obstruction, or if fluid intake is inadequate.
a. appropriate dose and frequency of administration	Daily administration of laxative during each recurrence, if necessary
b. maximum number of days the therapy should be employed	Dietary modifications and daily intake of at least 2 liters of fluids should continue indefinitely. Use the laxative for no more than 7 days.
c. product administration procedures	Powder mixed with fruit juice or soda, or wafers chewed followed by liberal fluid intake
d. expected time to onset of relief	12–72 hours
e. degree of relief that can be reasonably expected	Easier passage of stools and more frequent bowel movements
f. most common side effects	An increase in gas when fiber is introduced in the diet and more frequent urination as water intake increases; worsening constipation, if fiber is increased without adequate fluid intake; abdominal bloating and gas with bulk-forming laxative
g. side effects that warrant medical intervention should they occur	Allergic reaction, vomiting, choking or difficulty with swallowing
h. patient options in the event that condition worsens or persists	Contact your PCP.
i. product storage requirements	N/A
j. specific nondrug measures	Consider implementing stress-relieving measures during class examinations.
10. Solicit follow-up questions from patient.	When should I resume dietary supplements?
11. Answer patient's questions.	Consult your PCP who will evaluate your need for supplements.

Key: N/A, not applicable; NKA, no known allergies; PCP, primary care provider.

Relevant Evaluation Criteria	Scenario/Model Outcome

Information Gathering

1. Gather essential information about the patient's symptoms, including:

   a. description of symptom(s) (i.e., nature, onset, duration, severity, associated symptoms)

   Patient says that his bowel movements have gone from 1–2 times daily to once every 2–3 days over the past 10–12 weeks. His stool is described as "normal looking" but harder to pass.

   b. description of any factors that seem to precipitate, exacerbate, and/or relieve the patient's symptom(s)

   Patient notes that he never had problems during the 18 years that he walked his postal route. Coincidental to his developing lower back pain, he took an administrative position 6 months ago as a promotion. His symptoms have also included periods of lassitude and have been rather consistent in recent weeks.

   c. description of the patient's efforts to relieve the symptoms

   His wife got him to increase his dietary fiber, and he takes a fiber supplement when he remembers. He admits that he does not drink as much water as he used to when he worked outside.

2. Gather essential patient history information:

   a. patient's identity

   Edgar

   b. patient's age, sex, height, and weight

   40-year-old male, 5 ft 11 in, 199 lb

   c. patient's occupation

   Postal office supervisor

   d. patient's dietary habits

   Usual diet consists of some vegetables, occasional fruit, whole-grain breads, meat and fish, fruit juices, sodas, and candy.

   e. patient's sleep habits

   Sleeps 7 hours nightly

   f. concurrent medical conditions, prescription and nonprescription medications, and dietary supplements

   Hypertension, lower back pain; Ziac 5 mg 1 tablet daily, Tylenol with codeine #3 1 to 2 tablets as needed, Metamucil 2 capsules daily with water

   g. allergies

   Peanuts

   h. history of other adverse reactions to medications

   None

   i. other (describe) _____

   N/A

Assessment and Triage

3. Differentiate the patient's signs/symptoms and correctly identify the patient's primary problem(s).

   The patient has changed jobs during the past 6 months. The former job was outside and required a lot of physical activity, mainly through walking. Contrast the former job to the current one in which he probably spends a great deal of time indoors and at a desk using a computer. In addition, the patient admits to ingesting more dietary fiber and sometimes taking Metamucil capsules. He further indicates that his water intake has decreased because he changed jobs and he no longer walks a lot.

4. Identify exclusions for self-treatment (see Figure 16-2).

   None

5. Formulate a comprehensive list of therapeutic alternatives for the primary problem to determine if triage to a medical practitioner is required, and share this information with the patient.

   Options include:

   (1) Recommend the patient incorporate a regular exercise regimen into his lifestyle.
   (2) Recommend that he consume 48–64 ounces of fluid daily.
   (3) Recommend a short-term course of docusate.
   (4) Assess his use of Tylenol with codeine and Ziac.
   (5) Refer patient to a PCP if lifestyle changes do not alleviate symptoms.
   (6) Take no action.

Plan

6. Select an optimal therapeutic alternative to address the patient's problem, taking into account patient preferences.

   Edgar did not experience problems prior to beginning the new administrative position; he had worked in a physically active position for the previous 18 years. He has taken some measures to address the change in frequency of his bowel movements, but he has not been successful in restoring his former function. A short course (1 week) of docusate should be recommended. In addition, adequate hydration is very important for his continued intake of dietary and supplemental fiber, and to counteract mild fluid loss that he may be experiencing from Ziac.

C A S E   1 6 - 2 (continued)

Relevant Evaluation Criteria	Scenario/Model Outcome
7. Describe the recommended therapeutic approach to the patient.	A short course (1 week) of docusate should soften your stools and make their passage more comfortable. At the same time, you must adjust your fluid intake to ensure that your hydration is adequate to help the fiber facilitate more normal frequency of bowel movements and to assist the docusate in softening your stools. Finally, you must leave your office on a regular basis to engage in some form of physical exercise.
8. Explain to the patient the rationale for selecting the recommended therapeutic approach from the considered therapeutic alternatives.	Lifestyle changes seem to be largely responsible for the change in your bowel movements. When coupled with increased fiber intake without adequate fluid intake, constipation might be made worse rather than better. Although the pain medication can also lead to constipation, the usage pattern and the description of the condition do not suggest that the medication is to blame. Ziac contains a small dose of a diuretic or "water pill." It does cause the body to lose fluid and may play a role in your constipation, along with the fiber and reduced fluid intake.

Patient Education

9. When recommending self-care with nonprescription medications and/or nondrug therapy, convey accurate information to the patient:	
a. appropriate dose and frequency of administration	Docusate 100 mg
b. maximum number of days the therapy should be employed	Daily for no more than 7 days
c. product administration procedures	By mouth
d. expected time to onset of relief	24–72 hours
e. degree of relief that can be reasonably expected	Within 3 days, a more comfortable stool should be achieved. In 1–2 weeks, dietary and exercise modifications should yield the desired effect, and frequency of bowel movements should be improved.
f. most common side effects	Docusate may cause mild abdominal cramping. An increase in gas can be expected when fiber is introduced in the diet. More frequent urination results as fluid intake increases. Expect worsening or no change in constipation if fiber is increased without adequate fluid intake.
g. side effects that warrant medical intervention should they occur	Weakness or irregular heartbeats
h. patient options in the event that condition worsens or persists	PCP should be contacted.
i. product storage requirements	Store docusate at room temperature.
j. specific nondrug measures	Follow the directions carefully when adding fiber supplements. Fluid intake cannot be neglected if bowel frequency is to be maintained. Institute an exercise program and be consistent.
10. Solicit follow-up questions from patient.	What is it about my pain medicine that could make constipation worse?
11. Answer patient's questions.	Your pain medication contains two ingredients. Codeine is one of the ingredients. It is a member of a family of medications that include morphine; all members of the family have a tendency to cause constipation.

Patient Counseling for Constipation

Because laxative products are both widely used and abused, clinicians can provide a valuable service by educating patients about the appropriate use of laxatives. Proper education about laxative products and wise advice on product selection and use are particularly crucial for children and older patients. Before recommending a laxative product, the clinician should first discuss the nondrug measures for treating constipation. Pregnant women and children, especially, should be counseled on proper diet, adequate fluid intake, and reasonable exercise. Individuals may not understand the importance of these factors in the development of constipation and how simple lifestyle changes can restore relatively normal bowel function without laxative use. If a laxative is needed, the health care provider should explain why a particular type of laxative is appropriate for the present situation, how to use the laxative, when to expect to see results, what adverse effects could occur, and what precautions to take. The box Patient Education for Constipation lists specific information to provide patients.

PATIENT EDUCATION FOR
Constipation

The objectives of self-treatment are to relieve constipation and restore "normal" bowel functioning by implementing (1) dietary and lifestyle measures and/or (2) the safe use of laxative products. For most patients, carefully following the product instructions and the self-care measures listed here will help ensure optimal therapeutic outcomes.

Nondrug Measures

- Use nonpharmacological methods such as a high-fiber diet (goal is 25–35 grams per day), adequate fluid intake, and exercise to foster regular bowel movements.
- Increase dietary fiber by eating foods containing wheat grains, oats, fruits, and vegetables.
- Avoid constipating foods such as processed cheeses and concentrated sweets.
- Drink plenty of fluids (six to eight 8-ounce glasses a day) to aid in stool softening and to facilitate fecal evacuation.
- Develop and maintain a routine exercise program. Walking can be beneficial if your cardiovascular system is healthy and if you have no other apparent health risks.
- Establish a regular pattern for bathroom visits. Do not delay responding to the urge to defecate; allow adequate time for elimination in a relaxed, unhurried atmosphere.
- Maintain general emotional well-being and avoid stressful situations.

Nonprescription Medications

- Do not routinely take laxatives if your bowel habits are interrupted for a day or two, or to routinely "clean your system."
- Do not give laxatives to children younger than 6 years unless the use is recommended by a primary care provider.
- If you have kidney or liver disease, heart failure, hypertension, or other conditions requiring sodium, potassium, magnesium, or calcium restriction, do not use laxative products whose maximum daily dose contains more than 345 mg (15 mEq) of sodium, 975 mg (25 mEq) of potassium, 600 mg (50 mEq) of magnesium, or 1800 mg (90 mEq) of calcium.
- Consult your primary care provider before using laxatives if you currently have or have a history of any of the following conditions: colectomy, ileostomy, diabetes, heart disease, kidney disease, or swallowing difficulties.
- Consult a primary care provider or pharmacist before using a laxative product if you are taking anticoagulants (blood thinners), digoxin (a heart medicine), sodium polystyrene sulfonate (a treatment for high potassium levels), or tetracycline antibiotics.
- Avoid taking laxatives within 2 hours of taking other medications.
- Take most laxatives at bedtime, especially if more than 6–8 hours are required to produce results.
- Discard any medications that are outdated, that appear to have been tampered with, or that have an unusual appearance.

Bulk-Forming Laxatives

- Unless a rapid effect, such as cleaning out the bowel for a diagnostic procedure or X-ray, is needed, take a bulk-forming laxative. Be sure to drink at least 8 ounces of fluid with each dose to prevent intestinal obstruction.
- Use bulk-forming agents with caution if you have diabetes or are on a carbohydrate-restricted diet. These agents have a high caloric content per dose and contain sugar.
- Do not give sugar-free bulk-forming products to patients with phenylketonuria. Such products may contain aspartame, which contributes excessive levels of phenylalanine, an amino acid these patients cannot metabolize.

Lubricant Laxatives

- Do not give mineral oil to children younger than 6 years of age, pregnant patients, older patients, or patients taking anticoagulants.
- Do not take mineral oil with emollient laxatives.
- To avoid delaying the absorption of foods, nutrients, and vitamins, do not take mineral oil within 2 hours of eating.

Saline Laxatives

- Take saline laxatives on an empty stomach; the presence of food will delay action.
- Do not take saline laxatives every day.
- Do not give these laxatives orally to children younger than 6 years of age or rectally to infants younger than 2 years of age.

Hyperosmotic Laxatives

- Do not take the medication in larger than recommended amounts.
- When using PEG 3350 (MiraLAX), use the provided cap to measure the prescribed dose. Mix the powder with a full glass (8 ounces or 240 milliliters) of liquid such as water, juice, soda, coffee, or tea.
- Use of glycerin may be inappropriate in patients with a previous condition that caused rectal irritation.

Stimulant Laxatives

- Do not use castor oil to treat constipation except under the advice of a primary care provider.

 Do not take laxatives if you have any symptoms of appendicitis (i.e., abdominal pain, nausea, vomiting), rectal bleeding, painful anal or rectal conditions, bloating, or cramping. See a primary care provider immediately.

 If symptoms of constipation are unrelieved by nondrug measures or by 1 week of any laxative treatment, see a primary care provider. Chronic constipation may be a symptom of an underlying medical condition.

Note: For an additional resource, access the *OTC Advisor: Self-Care for Gastrointestinal Disorders, Module 4* at www.pharmacist.com/otcadvisor.

Evaluation of Patient Outcomes for Constipation

Constipation often presents with a great degree of variability among individuals. Although a decrease in frequency of bowel movements is typically associated with constipation, difficulty in passing stools and a decrease in the amount passed are also common complaints. The type, severity, and chronicity of symptoms are important determinants in selecting the most appropriate treatment modality. Once therapy has been selected, effectiveness is determined by how rapidly constipation is relieved and to what degree normal bowel habits have been restored. For acute constipation, dietary changes and exercise or the use of bulk-forming laxatives may take several days to weeks to provide relief. Stimulant laxatives usually provide results within 24 hours; osmotic laxatives provide more immediate relief, usually within 15 minutes to 3 hours for oral preparations. Laxative enemas, often used when fecal impaction accompanies constipation, can produce evacuation within minutes. If initial treatment of constipation is ineffective, therapy should be repeated according to product-specific directions.

If an adequate response is not achieved after a short period of laxative use, usually within 1 week, chronic constipation should be considered. Follow-up should be attempted to assess whether the patient should receive further evaluation by a primary care provider.

Self-medication with laxatives can be safe and effective if used as directed and not used excessively. Close monitoring of the frequency and duration of laxative use can be beneficial in determining whether normal bowel habits are actually re-established between bouts of constipation or if a more severe condition exists. If a laxative must be continued for an extended period such as in chronic constipation, bulk-forming agents are preferred. However, the need for frequent laxative use should be discussed with a primary care provider, because frequent use may be a sign of (1) a more severe form of constipation, (2) a side effect of a medication, or (3) an underlying medical problem. Overuse or extended use of some laxatives can alter the normal physiologic functioning of the gut and, in some persons, may lead to a dependence on laxatives for bowel function. Adhering to a diet high in fiber and drinking plenty of fluids can aid in preventing constipation and should be continued even during periods when bowel habits are normal.

Key Points for Constipation

➤ Constipation is a decrease in frequency of fecal elimination characterized by the difficult passage of hard, dry stool.

➤ Successful treatment of constipation depends on careful identification of the cause.

➤ In determining whether self-treatment or medical referral is appropriate, the clinician also needs to know the case history and current symptoms as well as the patient's reason for desiring to purchase a laxative.

➤ If the case history discloses a sudden change in bowel habits that has persisted for 2 weeks, the patient should be immediately referred to a primary care provider.

➤ For most cases of simple constipation, a balanced diet, exercise, and adequate fluid intake should be helpful.

➤ In addition, patients should always be encouraged to establish a regular pattern for bathroom visits and never delay responding to the urge to defecate.

➤ Special circumstances and patient characteristics (i.e., pregnancy or age) should be considered when assessing the need for self-medication.

➤ Therapy with any laxative product should be limited, in most cases, to short-term use.

➤ Laxative treatment for constipation should not be recommended if the patient exhibits "red flag" or "alarm" symptoms (sudden changes in stool, recent weight loss, presence of abdominal pain, blood in the stool, fever, anorexia, and nausea and vomiting), painful anal or rectal conditions, bloating, or cramping.

➤ Patients should be advised to avoid taking laxatives within 2 hours of other medications to reduce the potential for drug interactions.

➤ The cost of laxative products is variable; however, concomitant use of nonpharmacologic measures may lead to lower expenditures on laxative products for the patient with simple constipation.

REFERENCES

1. Lembo A, Camilleri M. Chronic constipation. *N Engl J Med*. 2003; 349:1360–8.
2. Levy S. Drug outlets remain leader in laxative sales. *Drug Topics*. 2002;146:8.
3. Talley NJ. Definitions, epidemiology, and impact of chronic constipation. *Rev Gastroenterol Disord*. 2004;4(suppl 2):S3–S10.
4. Bossard W, Dreher R, Schnegg JF, et al. The treatment of chronic constipation in elderly people: an update. *Drugs Aging*. 2004;21:911–30.
5. Locke GR III, Pemberton JH, Phillips SF. AGA medical position statement: guideline on constipation. *Gastroenterology*. 2000;119:1761–6.
6. DeLillo AR, Rose S. Functional bowel disorders in the geriatric patient: constipation, fecal impaction and fecal incontinence. *Am J Gastroenterol*. 2000;95:901–5.
7. Patel SM, Lembo AJ. Constipation. In: Feldman M, Friedman LS, Brandt LJ, et al., eds. *Sleisenger & Fordtran's Gastrointestinal and Liver Disease: Pathophysiology, Diagnosis, Management*. 8th ed. Philadelphia: Elsevier Science; 2006:221–47.
8. Spruill WJ, Wade WE. Diarrhea, constipation, and irritable bowel syndrome. In: DiPiro JT, Talbert RL, Yee GC, et al., eds. *Pharmacotherapy: A Pathophysiologic Approach*. 7th ed. New York: McGraw-Hill, Inc; 2008: 617–32.
9. Wald A. Chronic constipation: advances in management. *Neurogastroenterol Motil*. 2007;19:4–10.
10. Locke GR III, Pemberton JH, Phillips SF. AGA technical review on constipation. *Gastroenterology*. 2000;119:1766–78.
11. Felt B, Brown P, Coran A, et al. Functional Constipation and Soiling in Children. University of Michigan Health System Guidelines for Clinical Care; 2003. Available at http://cme.med.umich.edu/pdf/guideline/peds03.pdf. Last accessed October 14, 2008.
12. Berardi RR. Clinical update on the treatment of constipation in adults. *Pharm Times*. 2004;70:99–108.
13. Johanson JF. Review of the treatment options for chronic constipation. *MedGenMed*. 2007;9(2):25.
14. Self-care for constipation. In: Albrant DH, ed. *The American Pharmaceutical Association Drug Treatment Protocols*. Washington, DC: American Pharmaceutical Association; 1999.
15. US Department of Agriculture. *U.S. Nutrition and Your Health: Dietary Guidelines for Americans*. 5th ed. Washington, DC: US Government Printing Office; 2000. Home and Garden Bulletin no. 232.
16. Marlett JA, McBurney MI, Slavin JL. Position of the American Dietetic Association: health implications of dietary fiber. *J Am Diet Assoc*. 2002; 102:993–1000.
17. USDA Agricultural Research Service. Nutritive Value of Food. Washington, DC: US Government Printing Office. 2002;72:20–95. Home and Garden Bulletin. Publication No. 001-000-04703-5.
18. Schiller LR. Review article: the therapy of constipation. *Aliment Pharmacol Ther*. 2001;15:749–61.

19. Bouchez C. The Down Low on Low-Carb Diets. Available at http://www.medicinenet.com/script/main/art.asp?articlekey=50291. Last accessed October 14, 2008.

20. Folden SL, Backer JH, Maynard F et. al., *Practice Guidelines for the Management of Constipation in Adults*. Glenview, Ill: Rehabilitation Nursing Foundation; 2002.

21. Baker SS, Liptak GS, Colletti RB, et al. Constipation in infants and children: evaluation and treatment. *J Pediatr Gastroenterol Nutr.* 2000;30:109.

22. Laxative drug products for over-the-counter human use; psyllium ingredients in granular dosage forms. *Fed Regist.* 2007;72:14669–74.

23. Khalili B, Bardana EJ, Yunginger JW. Psyllium-associated anaphylaxis and death: a case report review of the literature. *Ann Allergy Asthma Immunol.* 2003;91:579–84.

24. Drug labeling; sodium labeling for over-the-counter drugs; technical amendment; termination of delay of effective date; compliance dates. *Fed Regist.* 2004;69:13717–25.

25. Status of certain additional over-the-counter drug category II and III active ingredients. *Fed Regist.* 2002;67:31125–7.

26. Laxative drug products for over-the-counter human use. *Fed Regist.* 1999;64:4535–40.

27. Wald A. Is chronic use of stimulant laxatives harmful to the colon? *J Clin Gastroenterol.* 2003;36:386–9.

28. Herndon CM, Jackson KC, Hallin PA. Management of opioid-induced gastrointestinal effects in patients receiving palliative care. *Pharmacotherapy.* 2002;22:240–50.

29. Kovacs D. The associations between laxative abuse and other symptoms among adults with anorexia nervosa. *Int J Eat Disord.* 2004; 36:224–8.

30. Becker AE, Look A. Eating disorders. In: Feldman M, Friedman LS, Brandt LJ, et al., eds. *Sleisenger & Fordtran's Gastrointestinal and Liver Disease: Pathophysiology, Diagnosis, Management.* 8th ed. Philadelphia: Elsevier Science; 2006:383–403

31. Favaro A, Santonastaso P. Self-injurious behavior in anorexia nervosa. *J Nerv Ment Dis.* 2000;188:537–42.

32. Semrad CE, Powell DW. Approach to the patient with diarrhea and malabsorption. In: Goldman L, Ausiello D, eds. *Goldman: Cecil Medicine.* 23rd ed. Philadelphia: WB Saunders; 2007:1019–41.

33. Muller-Lissner SA, Kamm MA, Scarpignato C, et al. Myths and misconceptions about chronic constipation. *Am J Gastroenterol.* 2005;100: 232–42.

34. National Digestive Diseases Information Clearinghouse. Constipation. June 2003. NIH Publication No. 07–2754. Available at: http://digestive.niddk.nih.gov/ddiseases/pubs/constipation/index.htm. Last accessed October 14, 2008.

35. Clinical practice guideline: evaluation and treatment of constipation in infants and children: recommendations of the North American Society of Pediatric Gastroenterology, Hepatology and Nutrition, *J Ped Gastroenterol Nutr.* 2006;43:e1–e13.

36. Biggs WS, Dery WH. Evaluation and treatment of constipation in infants and children, *Am Fam Physician.* 2006;73:469–77, 479–80, 481–2.

37. Wald A. Constipation. *Med Clin North Am.* 2000;84:1231–46.

38. Bonapace ES Jr, Fisher RS. Constipation and diarrhea in pregnancy. *Gastroenterol Clin North Am.* 1998;27:197–211.

39. Reinus JF, Riely CA. Gastrointestinal and hepatic disorders in the pregnant patient. In: Feldman M, Friedman LS, Brandt LJ, et al., eds. *Sleisenger & Fordtran's Gastrointestinal and Liver Disease: Pathophysiology, Diagnosis, Management.* 8th ed. Philadelphia: Elsevier Science; 2006:795–807.

40. Briggs GG, Freeman RK, Yaffe SJ. *Drugs in Pregnancy and Lactation: A Reference Guide to Fetal and Neonatal Risk.* 8th ed. Baltimore: Lippincott Williams & Wilkins; 2008.

41. National Center for Complementary and Alternative Medicine (NCCAM). Health Information. Available at: http://nccam.nih.gov/health. Last accessed October 14, 2008.

42. National Institutes of Health, Office of Dietary Supplements. International Bibliographic Information on Dietary Supplements. Available at: http://dietary-supplements.info.nih.gov/Health_Information/IBIDS.aspx. Last accessed October 14, 2008.

43. Jonkers D, Stockbrugger R. Review article: probiotics in gastrointestinal and liver diseases. *Aliment Pharmacol Ther.* 2007;26(suppl 2):133–48.

Diarrhea

Paul C. Walker

Diarrhea is a symptom characterized by an abnormal increase in stool frequency, liquidity, or weight. Although the normal frequency of bowel movements varies with each individual, more than three bowel movements per day are considered abnormal. The mean daily fecal weight loss is 100 to 150 grams; an increase in stool weight above 200 grams is generally interpreted as diarrhea.

Diarrhea may be acute, persistent, or chronic in nature. Acute diarrhea, defined as an episode of less than 14 days duration, can generally be managed with fluid and electrolyte replacement, dietary interventions, and nonprescription drug treatment. Persistent diarrhea is diarrhea of 14 days to 4 weeks duration. Chronic diarrhea, by definition, lasts more than 4 weeks. Chronic and persistent diarrheal illnesses are often secondary to other chronic medical conditions or treatments and need medical care; therefore, these illnesses are outside the scope of this book.

Diarrhea is a common cause of morbidity. Between 200 million and 211 million episodes of diarrheal illness (diarrhea that lasts more than 1 day or impairs normal activities) occur in the United States annually.[1] Estimates of the overall prevalence of acute gastroenteritis range from 5% to 11% of the general population, which results in an incidence rate ranging from 0.6 to 1.4 episodes per person per year.[1,2] The prevalence of diarrheal disease is highest in children younger than 5 years and lowest in adults; prevalence rates are estimated to be 8% to 10% for young children and 2% to 3% for persons of advanced age.[1,2] Most patients experience illness without seeking medical attention; however, approximately 936,726 cases per year result in hospitalization. Each year, acute gastroenteritis and its complications account for approximately 8200 deaths in the United States.[3]

Pathophysiology of Diarrhea

The specific causes of acute diarrhea differ between developing and developed countries. In the United States, viral and foodborne diarrheal illnesses are common; however, in the majority of cases, the causes cannot be determined. In developing countries, poor sanitation and poor hygiene lead to infectious diarrhea caused by parasites, bacteria, and viruses. Bacterial causes are as common as viral infections in these countries. Table 17-1 highlights some of the common viral, bacterial, and protozoal diarrheas and their treatment.[4–6]

Epidemiologic factors that increase the risk for particular infectious diarrheal diseases or their spread include attendance or employment at day care centers, occupation as a food handler or caregiver, congregate living conditions (e.g., nursing homes, prisons, and multifamily dwellings), consumption of unsafe foods (e.g., raw meat, eggs, and shellfish), and presence of medical conditions, such as acquired immunodeficiency syndrome (AIDS), that predispose to infectious diarrhea.[7]

Acute diarrhea may also be caused by poisoning, medications, intolerance of certain foods, or various non–gastrointestinal (GI) acute or chronic illnesses.

Viral Gastroenteritis

Noroviruses are the most common viral pathogens, accounting for approximately 70% to 75% of viral gastroenteritis. The symptoms and clinical course are described in Table 17-1. The virus is usually transmitted by contaminated water or food. Community-wide outbreaks may result when municipal water supplies become contaminated. Recent outbreaks of norovirus gastroenteritis on cruise ships have received attention, although 60% to 80% of all outbreaks occur on land.[8] Contaminated food is the most frequently identified vehicle of infection in this setting.[8] Person-to-person transmission may also be important, and it has been suggested that infected cruise ship crew members may serve as reservoirs of infection for passengers.[8]

Rotaviruses account for about 12% of all acute gastroenteritis and up to 50% of infantile gastroenteritis. The incidence of rotavirus infection is highest among children between 3 to 24 months of age. The peak infectious period is during the winter months (November to February). Spread is by the fecal–oral route. Clinical features are presented in Table 17-1. Treatment is usually restricted to fluid and electrolyte therapy. Severe dehydration and electrolyte disturbances, however, can occur and may result in death. In 2006, a live, oral vaccine to prevent rotavirus gastroenteritis was licensed by the Food and Drug Administration (FDA) for routine use in healthy infants. In clinical trials, this vaccine prevented 74% of all rotavirus gastroenteritis cases and 98% of the severe cases, and reduced the need for hospitalization attributable to rotavirus gastroenteritis by 96%.[9]

Other, less frequent viral causes of gastroenteritis include adenoviruses, astroviruses, and hepatitis A virus.

Bacterial Gastroenteritis

Bacterial pathogens cause approximately 5 million episodes of acute gastroenteritis in the United States each year. Pathogens

TABLE 17-1 Common Infectious Diarrheas and Their Treatment

Type	Epidemiologic/ Etiologic Factors	Symptoms	Treatment	Usual Prognosis
Viral				
Rotaviruses	Infects infants; oral–fecal spread	Onset of 24–48 hours; vomiting, fever, nausea, acute watery diarrhea	Vigorous fluid and electrolyte replacement; no antibiotics	Self-limiting; usually lasts 5–8 days
Norovirus	Infects all ages; frequently spread person to person by the fecal–oral route; causes "24-hour stomach flu"	Onset of 24–48 hours; sudden-onset vomiting, nausea, headache, myalgia, fever, watery diarrhea	Fluid and electrolytes; no antibiotics	Self-limiting; usually lasts 12–60 hours
Bacterial				
Campylobacter jejuni	Ingestion of contaminated food or water; oral–fecal spread; immunocompromised host	Onset of 24–72 hours; nausea, vomiting, headache, malaise, fever, watery diarrhea	Fluid and electrolytes; in severe or persistent diarrhea, antibiotics may be required[a]	Self-limiting, usually <7 days
Salmonella	Ingestion of improperly cooked or refrigerated poultry and dairy products; immunocompromised host	Onset of 12–24 hours; diarrhea, fever, and chills	Fluid and electrolytes for mild cases; antibiotics reserved for complicated cases[b]	Self-limiting
Shigella	Ingestion of contaminated vegetables or water; frequently spread person to person; immunocompromised host	Onset of 24–48 hours; nausea, vomiting, diarrhea	Fluid and electrolytes; antibiotics	Self-limiting
Escherichia coli Enterotoxigenic *E. coli*, Enteroaggregative *E. coli*	Ingestion of contaminated food or water; recent travel outside the United States or to a U.S. border area	Onset of 8–72 hours; watery diarrhea, fever, abdominal cramps, bloating, malaise, occasional vomiting	Fluid and electrolytes; antibiotics[c]	Self-limiting, usually within 3–5 days
Shigatoxin-producing *E. coli* (STEC)	Ingestion of contaminated food or water, direct person-to-person spread	Onset of 8–72 hours; watery, often bloody, diarrhea, abdominal cramps, hemolytic uremic syndrome	Fluid and electrolytes	Self-limiting, usually within 5–10 days
Clostridium difficile	Antibiotic-associated diarrhea leading to pseudomembranous colitis	Onset during or up to several weeks after antibiotic therapy; watery or mucoid diarrhea, high fever, cramping	Fluid and electrolytes; discontinuation of offending agent; antibiotics (metronidazole, vancomycin)	Self-limiting
Clostridium perfringens	Ingestion of contaminated food, especially meat and poultry	Onset of 8–14 hours; watery diarrhea without vomiting, cramping, midepigastric pain	Fluid and electrolytes; no antibiotics	Self-limiting, usually resolves within 24 hours
Staphylococcus aureus	Ingestion of improperly cooked or stored food	Onset of 1–6 hours; nausea, vomiting, watery diarrhea	Fluid and electrolytes; no antibiotics	Self-limiting
Yersinia enterocolitica	Ingestion of contaminated food	Onset within 16–48 hours; fever, abdominal pain, diarrhea, vomiting	Fluid and electrolytes; antibiotics may be needed in severe cases	Self-limiting, although diarrhea may persist for up to 3 weeks

TABLE 17-1 Common Infectious Diarrheas and Their Treatment (*continued*)

Type	Epidemiologic/ Etiologic Factors	Symptoms	Treatment	Usual Prognosis
Vibrio cholera	Ingestion of contaminated food, including undercooked or raw seafood; recent travel outside the United States	Onset within 24–48 hours; painless, watery, often voluminous, diarrhea, vomiting	Fluid and electrolytes; antibiotics needed in moderate-to-severe cases	Self-limiting, although *V. cholera* may cause severe, fatal illness
Bacillus cereus	Ingestion of contaminated food	Onset within 10–12 hours; abdominal pain, watery diarrhea, tenesmus, nausea, vomiting	Fluid and electrolytes; no antibiotics	Self-limiting
Protozoal				
Giardia lamblia	Ingestion of water contaminated with human or animal feces; frequently spread person to person; immunocompromised host	Onset of 1–3 weeks; acute or chronic watery diarrhea, nausea, vomiting, anorexia, flatulence, abdominal bloating, epigastric pain	Fluids and electrolytes; antimicrobial therapy[d]	Good, if treated
Cryptosporidium sp.	Frequently spread person to person; travel outside the United States; AIDS, immunocompromised host	Onset of 2–14 days; acute or chronic watery diarrhea, abdominal pain, flatulence, malaise	Fluid and electrolytes; antimicrobial therapy[e]	Self-limiting, lasting up to 3 weeks, except in patients with AIDS or other immunosuppressive diseases
Entamoeba histolytica	Travel outside the United States; fecal-soiled food or water, immunocompromised host	Chronic watery diarrhea, abdominal pain, cramps	Fluid and electrolytes; antibiotics[f]	Good, except for immunocompromised host
Isospora belli	Ingestion of contaminated food or water; immunocompromised host	Onset of approximately 1 week; profuse watery diarrhea, malaise, anorexia, weight loss, abdominal cramps	Fluid and electrolytes; antibiotics	Self-limited, remitting in 2–3 weeks

Key: AIDS, acquired immunodeficiency syndrome.

[a] Empirical therapy with prescription antibiotics (azithromycin, erythromycin) should be considered for patients with febrile diarrheal illness, especially if moderate-to-severe invasive disease is suspected, and for patients in whom supportive therapy fails to manage symptoms. Ciprofloxacin has been recommended, but it is no longer considered a first-line agent, because many *Campylobacter* strains are resistant to fluoroquinolones.

[b] Antibiotics are not indicated routinely for *Salmonella* gastroenteritis; antibiotic therapy is used in young infants and children who fail to respond to supportive treatment, who do not spontaneously remit, or who are at increased risk of disseminated disease. Antibiotic therapy is also indicated for suspected bacteremia in patients at high risk for this complication. These include patients who appear to be toxic with high fever (>102.2°F [39°C]); infants (<3 months); older adult patients (>65 years); patients with cancer, immunodeficiency (e.g., AIDS), or hemoglobinopathy (e.g., sickle cell disease); patients receiving corticosteroids or on hemodialysis; and patients with vascular grafts or prosthetic joints. Duration of antimicrobial therapy is usually 7–10 days.

[c] Antibiotic treatment with fluoroquinolones, azithromycin, or rifaximin (prescription antibiotics) is given for travelers' diarrhea caused by *E. coli*. Trimethoprim/sulfamethoxazole is no longer an optimal choice because of increasing worldwide resistance. Antibiotic treatment is not recommended for gastroenteritis caused by *E. coli* 0157:H7, because the treatment is likely to enhance toxin release and may increase risk for hemolytic uremic syndrome.

[d] Self-treatment of giardiasis is not appropriate; metronidazole, nitazoxanide, tinidazole, quinacrine, furazolidone, and paromomycin are effective prescription alternatives for treating giardiasis.[4,6]

[e] Self-treatment of cryptosporidiosis is not appropriate. Symptomatic relief of cryptosporidiosis may be achieved in AIDS patients by adding paromomycin and azithromycin (both prescription antimicrobial agents) to the patient's antiretroviral therapy.[4]

[f] Self-treatment of amebiasis is not appropriate; prescription therapy with metronidazole followed by either paromomycin or iodoquinol is the preferred treatment.[4]

Source: Adapted from references 4–6.

most commonly responsible for these cases, in order of decreasing incidence, are *Campylobacter* sp., *Salmonella* sp., *Shigella* sp., *Escherichia coli* (including O157:H7, non–O157:H7 Shigatoxin-producing *E. coli* [STEC], enterotoxigenic *E. coli,* and other diarrheagenic strains), *Staphylococcus* sp., *Clostridium* sp., *Yersinia enterocolitica,* and *Bacillus cereus. Aeromonas* sp. are being increasingly recognized as enteropathogens, particularly in food-borne disease; *Bacteroides fragilis, Klebsiella oxytoca,* and *Laribacter honkongensis* are newly identified causes of acute diarrhea.[7,10] *Campylobacter* is identified as the etiologic agent two to seven times more frequently than *Salmonella, Shigella,* or *E. coli.*[11]

Bacteria cause diarrhea through elaboration of an enterotoxin (e.g., toxigenic *E. coli* and *Staphylococcus aureus*) or by directly invading the mucosal epithelial cells (e.g., *Shigella, Salmonella, Yersinia, Campylobacter jejuni,* and invasive *E. coli*). Patients with diarrhea caused by toxin-producing agents have a watery diarrhea, which primarily involves the small intestine. If the large intestine is the site of attack, invasive organisms produce a dysentery-like (bloody diarrhea) syndrome characterized by fever, abdominal cramps, tenesmus (straining), and the frequent passage of small-volume stools that may contain blood and mucus. Clinical features of common bacterial diarrheas are presented in Table 17-1.

Food-borne transmission of pathogens accounts for 36% of acute gastroenteritis episodes in the United States; of these infections, 30% are due to bacteria, 67% to viruses, and 3% to protozoa. Recent surveillance statistics on the incidence of food-borne illnesses in the United States document that *Salmonella* and *Campylobacter,* which caused 14.81 and 12.71 cases of illness per 100,000 population in 2006, respectively, are the most frequently diagnosed bacterial pathogens, followed by *Shigella* (6.09 cases per 100,000 population), Shigatoxin-producing *E. coli* O157:H7 (1.31 cases per 100,000 population), *Yersinia* (0.35 cases per 100,000 population), *Vibrio* (0.34 cases per 100,000 population), and *Listeria* (0.31 cases per 100,000 population).[12]

Outbreaks of food-borne bacterial infection have been traced to poor sanitary conditions in meat-processing plants and various retail outlets (e.g., grocery stores and restaurants). Outbreaks of infection have also been associated with specific foods, such as milk (*Campylobacter*), raw eggs (*Salmonella*), chicken (*Campylobacter, Salmonella*), melons (*Listeria*), hummus (*Listeria*), and raspberries (*Cyclospora*). Therefore, an attentive and thorough history regarding food intake before the onset of diarrhea is essential in identifying a probable cause. For example, toxin-producing *S. aureus* grows rapidly in food (especially salads, custard, sausage, ham, dairy products, and poultry). Upon ingestion, the enterotoxin provokes nausea and vomiting with diarrhea within 6 hours. In contrast, the incubation period for *Salmonella,* which is harbored on raw foods and particularly on eggs, is 12 to 24 hours. These microbes invade the mucosal layer of the GI tract and disrupt the normal absorptive–secretory mechanisms. Fever, malaise, muscle aches, and profound epigastric or periumbilical discomfort with severe anorexia suggest an infectious, inflammatory disease of the large intestine. Abdominal pain, vomiting, and diarrhea suggest viral gastroenteritis, and symptoms usually persist for 2 to 3 days before gradually subsiding.

A major public health issue is contamination of food, especially undercooked hamburger and unpasteurized apple cider, with *E. coli* O157:H7 and other STECs. Recently, outbreaks of STEC O157 have been caused by consumption of contaminated spinach, lettuce, and raw milk.[12,13] The toxins produced by these organisms cause an acute bloody diarrhea, but they may also be associated with serious, potentially fatal systemic complications, such as hemolytic uremic syndrome or thrombotic thrombocytopenic purpura.

Other causes of food-borne gastroenteritis include *Listeria monocytogenes, Cyclospora cayetanensis,* and viruses. Noroviruses and rotavirus have also been implicated in food-borne disease.

Travelers' diarrhea is a secretory diarrhea acquired, for the most part, through ingestion of contaminated food or water. This acute diarrhea is usually caused by bacterial enteropathogens. It affects millions of tourists visiting foreign countries or U.S. border areas with poor sanitation. Although *Salmonella, Shigella, Campylobacter, Entamoeba histolytica, Giardia,* and rotavirus have all been implicated in the disease, *E. coli* is the most common infecting organism in travelers' diarrhea. Two strains, enterotoxigenic *E. coli* (ETEC) and enteroaggregative *E. coli* (EAEC), are responsible for most cases. ETEC is found in up to 40% of travelers with diarrhea in various areas around the world; EAEC is almost as common, causing approximately 25% of cases.[12] The causative organisms are found most often on foods such as fruits, vegetables, raw meat, seafood, and even hot sauces; less commonly, pathogens are found in the local water, including ice cubes. After ingestion, ETEC produces two plasmid-mediated enterotoxins that cause symptoms; one of these enterotoxins is structurally, functionally, and immunologically closely related to cholera toxin. The pathogenic mechanisms underlying diarrhea caused by EAEC are not well understood; these organisms may produce disease through elaboration of an enterotoxin, a cytotoxin, or some other means.[14] The diarrheal disorder caused by these organisms is characterized in Table 17-1. Patients may experience between three and eight (or more) watery stools per day, with symptoms usually subsiding over 3 to 5 days.

Bacterial pathogens not only cause acute illness, they can also cause functional bowel disorders, including postinfectious irritable bowel syndrome (IBS), for 6 months or longer after a bout of acute gastroenteritis. In 10% to 30% of patients, bowel dysfunction persisted 6 months after infectious diarrhea caused by *Campylobacter, Shigella, Salmonella,* and diarrheagenic *E. coli* (ETEC and EAEC).[15,16] IBS is diagnosed in 4% to 10% of patients 1 to 2 years after an episode of acute bacterial gastroenteritis.[16]

Protozoal Diarrhea

Diarrhea may also be caused by protozoa, including *Giardia lamblia, E. histolytica, Isospora belli,* and *Cryptosporidium* sp. (Table 17-1). No nonprescription therapies are available to manage diarrhea caused by these pathogens and self-management is inappropriate.

Food-Induced Diarrhea

Food intolerance can provoke diarrhea and may result from a food allergy or ingestion of foods that are excessively fatty or spicy, or contain a high amount of roughage or many seeds. Carbohydrates in the diet commonly include the disaccharides lactose and sucrose, which are normally hydrolyzed to monosaccharides by the enzyme lactase. When these disaccharides are not hydrolyzed, they pool in the lumen of the intestine, where they not only ferment but also produce an osmotic imbalance and pH change. The resulting hyperosmolarity draws fluid into the intestinal lumen, causing diarrhea. Lactase enzymatic activity may be reduced in intestinal disorders such as infectious diarrhea and GI allergy. Acute viral diarrhea may cause temporary milk intolerance in patients of all ages. Lactase deficiency resulting from viral gastroenteritis is short-lived and is particularly problematic during the first few days of the disease. Infants born with lactase deficiency and adults who develop lactase deficiency are intolerant of cow's milk and milk-based products. Lactase enzyme products are effective treatments for some patients (see Treatment of Diarrhea).

Clinical Presentation of Diarrhea

The most common signs and symptoms of acute infectious diarrheal illnesses are shown in Table 17-1. Variability in the causes of diarrhea makes identification of the pathophysiologic mechanisms difficult. The etiology, and subsequently the pathophysiology, can be determined by a thorough medical history in most cases. However, a complete medical assessment, including clinical laboratory evaluation, may be required to identify the cause in a subset of patients with severe or persistent diarrhea.

Diarrhea can be classified as osmotic, secretory, inflammatory, or motor, depending on the underlying pathophysiologic mechanisms that disrupt normal intestinal function. The common mechanisms of acute diarrhea are osmotic and secretory, whereas motor and exudative mechanisms commonly underlie chronic diarrheal illnesses. Table 17-2 correlates the clinical groups and mechanism with their most common causes.

Bacterial and viral enterotoxins play a role in the pathophysiology of secretory diarrheas. Enterotoxins elaborated by *E. coli* and *Vibrio cholera* evoke the release of endogenous secretagogues that mediate secretory reflexes, including serotonin, substance P, and vasoactive intestinal peptide. Some enterotoxins, such as cholera toxin, can directly stimulate GI secretomotor neurons to increase intestinal secretion. *C. difficile* enterotoxin A also injures enterocytes to evoke a necroinflammatory response that causes a secretory diarrhea. Rotaviruses produce an enterotoxin that causes a calcium-mediated secretory diarrhea. In addition, inflammatory mediators (e.g., interleukins 1 and 6, prostaglandins, substance P, tissue necrosis factor-alpha, and platelet-activating factor) evoked by enteric infection stimulate a characteristic GI motility pattern that leads to the urgent defecation associated with diarrhea. This altered motility also causes abdominal cramps.

Stool characteristics give valuable information about the diarrhea's pathophysiology. For example, undigested food particles in the stool suggest disease of the small intestine. Black, tarry stools may indicate upper GI bleeding, and red stools suggest possible lower bowel or hemorrhoidal bleeding or simply recent ingestion of red food (e.g., beets) or drug products (e.g., rifampin). Diarrhea originating from the small intestine is characterized by a marked outpouring of fluid high in potassium and bicarbonate. Passage of many small-volume stools suggests diarrhea with a colonic disorder. Yellowish stools may suggest the presence of bilirubin and a potentially serious pathology of the liver. A whitish tint to the stool suggests a fat malabsorption disease. Patients who have stool containing blood or mucus need medical evaluation.

Fluid and electrolyte imbalance is the major complication of diarrheal illness. Therefore, assessment of the patient's risk for dehydration and the degree of dehydration present is key in determining the appropriateness of self-care and the need for medical referral. The specific signs and symptoms of dehydration are associated with the severity of the diarrhea, as well as the etiology and degree of fluid and electrolyte losses (Table 17-3).[17]

Healthy patients with uncomplicated acute diarrhea usually improve clinically within 24 to 48 hours. If the condition remains the same or worsens after 48 hours of onset, medical referral is necessary to prevent complications. Certain medical conditions can increase the risk for dehydration. Referral for medical care should be considered for patients with diabetes mellitus, severe cardiovascular or renal diseases, or multiple unstable chronic medical conditions. Specifically, medical evaluation is indicated for[18,19]:

- Severe vomiting or dehydration.
- Passage of multiple small-volume stools containing blood and mucus.
- Fever of 38.5°C (101.3°F) or higher.

TABLE 17-2 Clinical Classification of Diarrhea

Type	Mechanism	Common Causes
Osmotic	Unabsorbed solutes in intestines increase luminal osmotic load, retarding fluid absorption. Decreased fluid absorption of even a few hundred milliliters may cause diarrhea. Decreased absorption of solutes and fluid can be secondary to brush border damage caused by lactase deficiency or bacterial/viral infection. Viral-induced damage to epithelial cells accelerates migration of immature crypt cells to the tip of the villus; altered epithelial turnover also decreases absorption.	Noroviruses, rotaviruses, *E. coli*, *C. jejuni*, lactase deficiency, magnesium antacid excess
Secretory	Stimulation of crypt cells produces net flow of electrolytes (most notably chloride) and fluids into intestinal lumen. Tumors can secrete GI hormones and peptides that act as secretagogues.	*C. jejuni*, *C. difficile*, *E. coli*, *Salmonella*, *Shigella*, *Vibrio*, rotaviruses, *G. lamblia*, *Cryptosporidium* sp. *Isospora*, ileal resection, thyroid cancer
Inflammatory	Impaired fluid absorption and leaking of mucus, blood, and pus into lumen caused by inflammation of intestinal mucosa (e.g., IBD) or bacterial infection (i.e., dysentery).	*C. jejuni*, *E. coli*, *Salmonella*, *Shigella*, *Yersinia*, *E. histolytica*, ulcerative colitis, Crohn's disease
Motor	Abnormally rapid intestinal transit time reduces contact time between luminal contents and absorptive areas of intestinal wall.	IBS, diabetic neuropathy

Key: GI, gastrointestinal; IBD, inflammatory bowel disease; IBS, irritable bowel syndrome.

TABLE 17-3 Assessment of Dehydration and Severity of Acute Diarrhea

	Self-Treatable		Not Self-Treatable
	Minimal or No Dehydration	**Mild-to-Moderate Dehydration/Diarrhea**	**Severe Dehydration/Diarrhea**
Degree of dehydration (loss of body weight)	<3%	3%–9%	>9%
Signs of dehydration[a]			
Mental status	Good, alert	Normal, fatigued or restless, irritable	Apathetic, lethargic, unconscious
Thirst	Drinks normally, might refuse liquids	Thirsty, eager to drink	Drinks poorly, unable to drink
Heart rate	Normal	Normal to increased	Tachycardia, bradycardia in most severe cases
Quality of pulses	Normal	Normal to decreased	Weak, thready, impalpable
Breathing	Normal	Normal, fast	Deep
Eyes	Normal	Slightly sunken[b]	Deeply sunken[b]
Tears	Present	Decreased[b]	Absent
Mouth and tongue	Moist	Dry	Parched
Skin fold	Instant recoil	Recoil in <2 seconds	Recoil in >2 seconds
Capillary refill	Normal	Prolonged	Prolonged, minimal
Extremities	Warm	Cool	Cold, mottled, cyanotic
Urine output	Normal to decreased	Decreased[b]	Minimal[b]
Number of unformed stools/day	<3	≤5	6–9
Other signs/symptoms	Afebrile, normal blood pressure, no orthostatic changes in blood pressure/pulse	May be afebrile or may develop fever >102.2°F (39°C); normal blood pressure; mild orthostatic blood pressure/pulse changes with or without mild orthostatic-related symptoms may be present; sunken fontanelle[c]	Fever >102.2°F (39°C), low blood pressure, dizziness, severe abdominal pain

[a] If signs of dehydration are absent, rehydration therapy is not required. Maintenance therapy and replacement of stool losses should be undertaken.

[b] Signs and symptoms experienced especially by young children.

[c] Signs and symptoms of concern for young infants.

Source: Adapted from reference 17.

- Passage of six or more unformed stools in 24 hours or illness lasting 48 hours or longer.
- Diarrhea accompanied by severe abdominal pain in a patient older than 50 years.

Patients with severe abdominal pain, particularly those older than 50 years, may have a complicating illness such as ischemic bowel disease. Immunocompromised patients, such as those receiving cancer treatment, organ transplant recipients, and patients with AIDS, also need medical evaluation, because their diarrhea will often be complicated and difficult to manage. Self-care medication may also be inappropriate for diarrhea during pregnancy, and pregnant women should consult with a primary care provider before self-treating.

Children younger than 5 years and adults older than 65 years are at greater risk for complications than other age groups. In developed countries, most children experience complete recovery, although some die of complications. In the United States, approximately 300 to 450 children die annually from acute gastroenteritis; most of these deaths occur in infants.[3,17] Children 2 years of age or younger are likely to suffer complications that require hospitalization. In newborns, water may comprise up to 75% of total body weight; severe diarrhea may cause water loss equal to 10% or more of body weight. After 8 to 10 bowel movements within a 24-hour period, a 2-month-old infant could lose enough fluid to cause circulatory collapse and renal failure. Moderate-to-severe diarrhea in infants requires evaluation by a primary care provider.

In recent years, deaths from viral and bacterial GI infection have increased most sharply among people 65 years of age and older whose diarrhea is likely to be more severe than in other adults; older adults currently experience the highest rate of death from enteric infections.[3]

Treatment of Diarrhea

Treatment Goals

The goals of self-treatment are to (1) prevent or correct fluid and electrolyte loss and acid–base disturbance, (2) relieve symptoms, (3) identify and treat the cause, and (4) prevent acute morbidity and mortality.

General Treatment Approach

Infectious diarrhea is often self-limiting. Symptomatic relief and correction of fluid and electrolyte loss are generally adequate for mild-to-moderate, uncomplicated diarrhea. Initial self-management for adults and children should focus on fluid and electrolyte replacement by administering commercially available oral solutions (e.g., Pedialyte) in adequate doses (Table 17-4). Simultaneous implementation of oral rehydration and specific dietary measures is appropriate for treating mild-to-moderate diarrheal illness. Symptomatic relief can also be achieved by using nonprescription antidiarrheal drugs, such as loperamide, in carefully selected patients. Normal function of the alimentary tract is often restored in 24 to 72 hours without additional treatment. Exclusions for self-treatment are listed in Figure 17-1. Severe diarrhea constitutes a medical emergency, especially in young children, and requires immediate referral for medical evaluation and treatment. Initial management with intravenous (IV) fluid therapy is necessary until perfusion and mental status improve.

Nonpharmacologic Therapy

Fluid and Electrolyte Management

Correction of fluid loss and electrolyte imbalances is important, and can be accomplished by oral or IV therapy. Rehydration using oral rehydration solution (ORS) is the preferred treatment for mild-to-moderate diarrhea. This approach is as effective as IV therapy in managing fluid and electrolytes in children with mild-to-moderate dehydration secondary to diarrhea.[20] Because the GI glucose–sodium cotransport mechanism is not adversely affected by most diarrheal diseases, ORSs containing low concentrations of glucose or dextrose (2%–2.5%) can be useful in managing fluid and electrolyte balance. The sugar molecules provide very little caloric support, but they facilitate intestinal sodium and water absorption. Maximal sodium absorption occurs at a molar glucose-to-sodium ratio close to 1. In mild-to-moderate diarrhea, practitioners can safely recommend an ORS.

According to the patient's fluid and electrolyte status, oral treatment may be carried out in two phases: rehydration therapy and maintenance therapy. Rehydration over 3 to 4 hours quickly replaces water and electrolyte deficits to restore normal body composition. In the maintenance phase, electrolyte solutions are given to maintain normal body composition, and adequate dietary intake is reestablished. Figures 17-1 and 17-2 outline rehydration and maintenance therapies, including fluid and electrolyte recommendations, for children and adults. Although ORSs generally are recommended for use in adults with diarrhea, there is scant evidence to support this recommendation. ORSs may not provide any real benefit to otherwise healthy adults with mild diarrhea who can maintain an adequate fluid intake during the episode of diarrhea; for these patients, fluid and electrolyte status can be maintained by increasing intake of fluids, such as clear juices, soups, or sports drinks.[18] Rehydration using an ORS has no effect on the duration of diarrhea.

A variety of ORSs are available (Table 17-4). Most products are premixed solutions; a few are available as dry powders of glucose and electrolytes that require addition of water. The premixed products are preferred for use in children because they are safe and convenient; improper mixing of dry powders by caregivers has led to patient fluid and electrolyte complications and injury. The World Health Organization (WHO) and United Nations Children's Fund (UNICEF) recommend use of an ORS containing 75 mEq/L of sodium.[21] This ORS significantly reduces the need for unscheduled IV therapy, stool output, and the incidence of vomiting in children with noncholera diarrhea; this formulation is also as effective as the previous formulation in children with cholera.[21,22] This ORS is also effective in adults with cholera, although transient, asymptomatic hyponatremia may develop. Rehydration solutions available in the United States contain 75 to 90 mEq/L of sodium; maintenance ORSs contain 40 to 60 mEq/L of sodium.

ORSs have been improved with the development of cereal-based products that use complex carbohydrates (e.g., rice syrup solids) instead of glucose. Complex carbohydrates are

TABLE 17-4 Selected Oral Rehydration Products

Trade Name	Osmolarity	Calories	Carbohydrate	Electrolytes
WHO–ORS	245 mOsm/L	46 cal/L	Glucose 13.5 g/L	Sodium 75 mEq/L; chloride 65 mEq/L; citrate 30 mEq/L; potassium 20 mEq/L
CeraLyte 50 Powder Packets	<200 mOsm/L	160 cal/L	Rice starch polymers 40 g/L; sucrose 10 g/L	Sodium 50 mEq/L; chloride 40 mEq/L; citrate 30 mEq/L; potassium 20 mEq/L
CeraLyte 70 Powder Packets	<230 mOsm/L	160 cal/L	Rice starch polymers 40 g/L	Sodium 70 mEq/L; chloride 60 mEq/L; citrate 30 mEq/L; potassium 20 mEq/L
CeraLyte 90 Powder Packets	260 mOsm/L	160 cal/L	Rice starch polymers 40 g/L	Sodium 90 mEq/L; chloride 80 mEq/L; citrate 30 mEq/L; potassium 20 mEq/L
Enfalyte Solution	167 mOsm/L	126 cal/L	Rice syrup solids 30 g/L	Sodium 50 mEq/L; chloride 45 mEq/L; citrate 34 mEq/L; potassium 25 mEq/L
Pedialyte	249 mOsm/L	100 cal/L	Dextrose 20 g/L; fructose 5 g/L	Sodium 45 mEq/L; chloride 35 mEq/L; citrate 30 mEq/L; potassium 20 mEq/L
Pedialyte Freezer Pops[a]		6.25 cal/L	Dextrose 25 g/L	Sodium 45 mEq/L; chloride 35 mEq/L; citrate 30 mEq/L; potassium 20 mEq/L
Rehydralyte Solution	304 mOsm/L	100 cal/L	Dextrose 25 g/L	Sodium 75 mEq/L; chloride 65 mEq/L; citrate 30 mEq/L; potassium 20 mEq/L

Key: WHO, World Health Organization; ORS, oral rehydration solution.

[a] Product to be used with appropriate maintenance ORS.

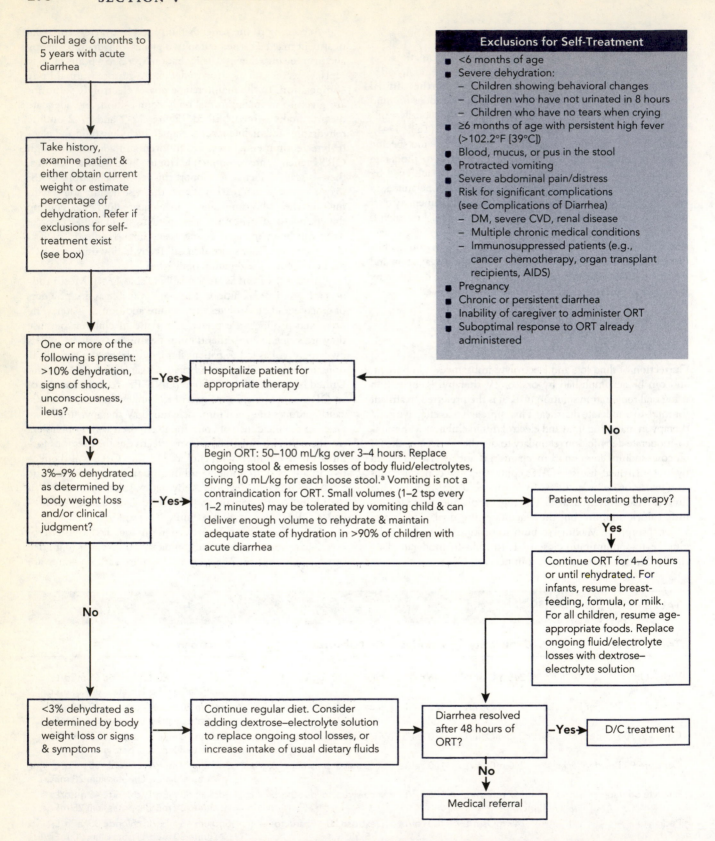

Child age 6 months to 5 years with acute diarrhea

Take history, examine patient & either obtain current weight or estimate percentage of dehydration. Refer if exclusions for self-treatment exist (see box)

Exclusions for Self-Treatment
- <6 months of age
- Severe dehydration:
  - Children showing behavioral changes
  - Children who have not urinated in 8 hours
  - Children who have no tears when crying
- ≥6 months of age with persistent high fever (>102.2°F [39°C])
- Blood, mucus, or pus in the stool
- Protracted vomiting
- Severe abdominal pain/distress
- Risk for significant complications (see Complications of Diarrhea)
  - DM, severe CVD, renal disease
  - Multiple chronic medical conditions
  - Immunosuppressed patients (e.g., cancer chemotherapy, organ transplant recipients, AIDS)
- Pregnancy
- Chronic or persistent diarrhea
- Inability of caregiver to administer ORT
- Suboptimal response to ORT already administered

One or more of the following is present: >10% dehydration, signs of shock, unconsciousness, ileus? —Yes→ Hospitalize patient for appropriate therapy

No

3%–9% dehydrated as determined by body weight loss and/or clinical judgment? —Yes→ Begin ORT: 50–100 mL/kg over 3–4 hours. Replace ongoing stool & emesis losses of body fluid/electrolytes, giving 10 mL/kg for each loose stool.[a] Vomiting is not a contraindication for ORT. Small volumes (1–2 tsp every 1–2 minutes) may be tolerated by vomiting child & can deliver enough volume to rehydrate & maintain adequate state of hydration in >90% of children with acute diarrhea

Patient tolerating therapy? →No→ (to Hospitalize)

Yes

Continue ORT for 4–6 hours or until rehydrated. For infants, resume breast-feeding, formula, or milk. For all children, resume age-appropriate foods. Replace ongoing fluid/electrolyte losses with dextrose–electrolyte solution

No

<3% dehydrated as determined by body weight loss or signs & symptoms → Continue regular diet. Consider adding dextrose–electrolyte solution to replace ongoing stool losses, or increase intake of usual dietary fluids → Diarrhea resolved after 48 hours of ORT? —Yes→ D/C treatment

No

Medical referral

[a] Alternatively: <10 kg BW, give 60–120 mL ORS for each diarrheal stool or vomiting episode; ≥10 kg BW, give 120–240 mL ORS.

FIGURE 17-1 Self-care of acute diarrhea in children 6 months to 5 years. Key: AIDS, acquired immunodeficiency syndrome; BW, body weight; CVD, cardiovascular disease; D/C, discontinue; DM, diabetes mellitus; ORT, oral rehydration therapy.

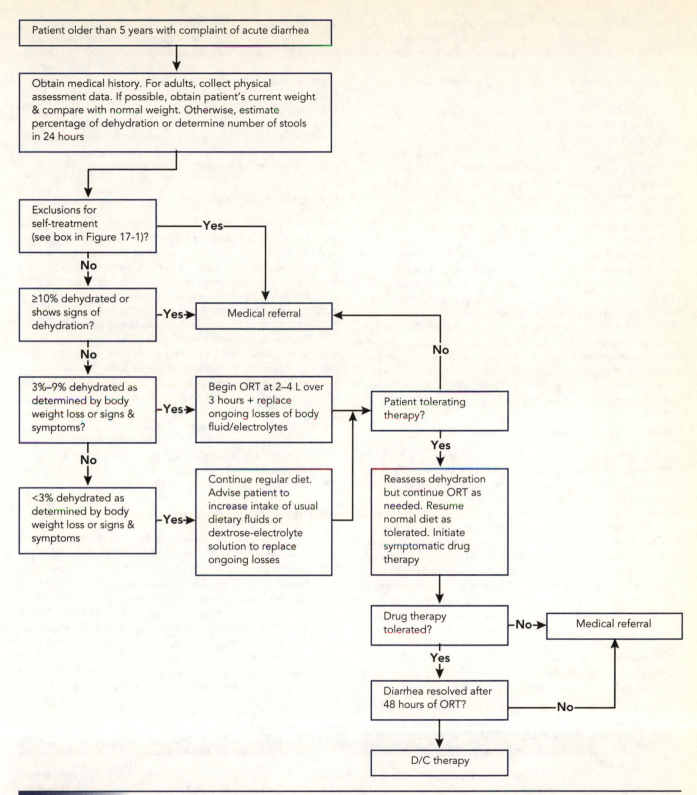

FIGURE 17-2 Self-care of acute diarrhea in children older than 5 years, adolescents, and adults. Key: D/C, discontinue; ORT, oral rehydration therapy.

converted into glucose at the intestinal brush border and provide more cotransport molecules while reducing the osmotic load of the ORS. Cereal-based ORS therapy potentially reduces stool volume by 20% to 30% in children with cholera, but this therapy may not significantly alter stool volume in children with noncholera acute diarrhea.[23]

All available premixed solutions are equally safe and effective; there is no evidence that one product is clinically superior to another in effecting rehydration.

A variety of common household oral solutions have also been used for oral rehydration and maintenance (Table 17-5). Although these solutions may be sufficient to manage mild, self-limiting diarrhea in some patients, they should be avoided if dehydration or moderate-to-severe diarrhea is present. Unlike commercial ORSs, these remedies are not formulated on the basis of the physiology of acute diarrhea. The inappropriately high carbohydrate content and osmolality of these solutions can worsen diarrhea, and their low sodium content can contribute to the development of hyponatremia. Sports drinks may be used in older children (older than 5 years) and adults if additional sources of sodium, such as crackers or pretzels, are used concomitantly. Colas, ginger ale, apple juice, sports drinks, and similar products are not recommended for infants and young children (6 months to 5 years of age) with diarrhea. Tea, another popular household remedy, is also inappropriate for children because of its low sodium content. Chicken broth is not recommended because of its inappropriately high sodium content.

Dietary Management

The traditional dietary approach to acute diarrhea has been the withdrawal of feedings and initiation of clear liquids, with a slow reintroduction of feedings over several days. However, oral intake does not worsen the diarrhea, clinically significant nutrient malabsorption is uncommon in acute diarrhea, and bowel rest is generally not necessary.[17] On the contrary, during acute diarrhea, patients are able to absorb 80% to 95% of dietary carbohydrates, 70% of fat, and 75% of the nitrogen from protein. Early refeeding, in combination with maintenance oral rehydration, improves outcomes of acute diarrhea in children by reducing duration of the diarrhea, reducing stool output, and improving weight gain.

It is inappropriate to withhold food for longer than 24 hours.[17] A normal, age-appropriate diet should be reintroduced once the patient has been rehydrated, which should take no longer than 3 to 4 hours to accomplish. Most infants and children with acute diarrhea can tolerate full-strength breast milk and cow milk. The familiar BRAT diet (bananas, rice, apple-

sauce, and toast) is not recommended; it provides insufficient calories, protein, and fat, especially in situations of strict or prolonged use.[17] Patients (or their parents) should be advised to avoid fatty foods, foods rich in simple sugars that can cause osmotic diarrhea, and spicy foods that may cause GI upset. Caffeine-containing beverages should also be avoided, given that caffeine can increase cyclic adenosine monophosphate levels, which promote fluid secretion and may worsen diarrhea. There is no evidence that fasting or dietary modification influences outcomes of acute diarrhea in adults; however, similar guidelines can be applied if a normal diet is not tolerated.[18]

Preventive Measures

Infectious diarrhea, especially acute viral gastroenteritis, often occurs in congregate living conditions such as day care centers and nursing homes through person-to-person transmission. Isolating the individual with diarrhea, washing hands, and using sterile techniques are basic preventive measures that reduce the risk among such populations and their caregivers. Strict food handling, sanitation, and other hygienic practices help control transmission of bacteria and other infectious agents.

Short-term bismuth subsalicylate (BSS) prophylaxis is frequently recommended to provide protection against travelers' diarrhea; however, FDA has deemed available data insufficient to support prophylactic use of BSS.[4,24] Antibiotics with reliable activity against enteropathogens in the region of travel provide effective prophylaxis. However, prophylactic antimicrobial agents are not currently recommended for most travelers.[25,26] Prophylactic antibiotics may be considered for short-term travelers who are high-risk hosts (e.g., immunosuppressed patients) or for those critical trips during which even a short bout of diarrhea could impact the purpose of the trip.[25]

Pharmacologic Therapy

Although most acute nonspecific diarrhea in the United States is self-limiting, nonprescription antidiarrheal products may provide relief and will usually do no harm when used according to label instructions. Table 17-6 lists dosage and administration guidelines for these agents. Scientific evidence that pharmacologic agents, with the exception of loperamide and BSS, reduce stool frequency or duration of disease in adults is lacking. Likewise, antidiarrheal drugs have not been shown to significantly improve clinical outcomes of acute nonspecific diarrhea in infants and children. Importantly, a change in stool consistency toward more formed stools does not necessarily indicate that antidiarrheal

TABLE 17-5 Comparison of Electrolyte and Dextrose Concentrations of Household Fluids

Clear Liquids	Sodium (mEq/L)	Potassium (mEq/L)	Bicarbonate (mEq/L)	Dextrose (g/L)	Osmolarity (mOsm/L)
Cola	2	0.1	13	50–150 dextrose and fructose	550
Ginger ale	3	1	4	50–150 dextrose and fructose	540
Apple juice	3	20	0	10–150 dextrose and fructose	700
Chicken broth	250	5	0	0	450
Tea	0	0	0	0	5
Gatorade	20	3	3	45 dextrose and other sugars	330
Seven Up	7.5	0.2	0	80 dextrose and fructose	564

TABLE 17-6   Recommended Dosages of Antidiarrheal Agents for Acute Diarrhea

Medication	Dosage Forms	Adult Dosages (Maximum Daily Dosage)	Pediatric Dosages	Duration of Use
Loperamide	Caplets (2 mg), liquid (1 mg/7.5 mL)	4 mg initially, then 2 mg after each loose stool (not to exceed 8 mg/day)[a]	Consult product instructions; not recommended for children < 6 years except under medical supervision	48 hours
Bismuth subsalicylate	Tablets (262 mg), caplets (262 mg), liquids (262 mg/ 15 mL, 525 mg/ 15 mL)	525 mg every 30–60 minutes up to 4200 mg/day; (8 doses/day)	Not recommended for children < 12 years except under medical supervision	48 hours
Digestive enzymes (lactase)	Chewable tablets, caplets, liquids	5–15 drops placed in or taken with dairy product; 1–3 tablets or 1–2 capsules with first bite of dairy product	Same as adult dosage	Taken with each consumption of dairy product

[a] For self-care, maximum dose is 8 mg/day. If patient is under medical supervision, up to 16 mg/day may be administered by prescription.

therapy has successfully treated the underlying problem. Formed stools can have high water content, and substantial water losses may continue despite the change in consistency. Moreover, reliance on drugs shifts the focus away from management of fluids and electrolytes and dietary measures, increasing the risk for potentially dangerous side effects, such as toxic megacolon, without offering additional benefits. Because intestinal viruses are the leading cause of self-limiting acute gastroenteritis, antibiotics are not routinely recommended.

Loperamide

Loperamide is a popular, effective, and safe nonprescription antidiarrheal agent. It is a synthetic opioid agonist that produces antidiarrheal effects by stimulating micro-opioid receptors located on the intestinal circular muscles. This action slows intestinal motility, allowing absorption of electrolytes and water through the intestine. Stimulation of GI micro-opioid receptors also decreases GI secretion, which may contribute to the drug's antidiarrheal effects. Loperamide is approximately 50-fold more potent than morphine and two to three times more potent than diphenoxylate in its effects on GI motility. However, loperamide penetrates the central nervous system (CNS) poorly and therefore has a lower risk for CNS side effects. Other pharmacologic mechanisms for loperamide's antidiarrheal effects may include disruption of cholinergic and noncholinergic mechanisms involved in the regulation of peristalsis, inhibition of calmodulin function, and inhibition of voltage-dependent calcium channels. The effects on calmodulin and calcium channels may contribute to loperamide's antisecretory effects.

Loperamide is used to provide symptomatic relief for acute, nonspecific diarrhea. Its therapeutic effects include reduction of daily fecal volume, increased viscosity, bulk volume, and reduced fluid and electrolyte loss. It may be used when the patient is afebrile or has a low-grade fever and does not have bloody stools. Current product information provides directions for use in children as young as 2 years. However, its use in children younger than 6 years is not recommended, because it produces only modest, clinically insignificant effects on stool volume and duration of illness, with an unacceptably high risk

of side effects (including life-threatening side effects such as ileus and toxic megacolon).[17]

Loperamide is also indicated as an antidiarrheal agent in travelers' diarrhea (in combination with antibiotics), for chronic diarrhea associated with IBS and inflammatory bowel disease, and for reduction of the volume of discharge from high-output ileostomies. Off-label uses of loperamide include control of chronic diarrhea secondary to diabetic neuropathy and other conditions, as well as control of toddler diarrhea (defined as diarrhea of at least 1 month duration in an otherwise healthy, active, well-nourished child, and in whom stool examination has revealed no bacterial, viral, or protozoal pathogens). All of these uses require medical supervision.[27]

At usual doses (Table 17-6), loperamide has few side effects other than occasional dizziness and constipation. Other infrequently occurring adverse effects include abdominal pain, abdominal distention, nausea, vomiting, dry mouth, fatigue, and hypersensitivity reactions. Loperamide is generally not recommended for use in patients with invasive (enteroinvasive *E. coli, Salmonella, Shigella,* or *C. jejuni*) bacterial diarrhea or antibiotic-associated diarrhea (*C. difficile*), because it may (rarely) worsen diarrhea or cause toxic megacolon or paralytic ileus. However, there is no evidence that these complications occur in actual practice when loperamide is used with appropriate antimicrobial therapy. Patients with symptoms suggestive of infection with invasive organisms or antibiotic-associated diarrhea (i.e., fecal leukocytes, high fever, or blood or mucus in the stool) require evaluation by a primary care provider for proper management. If abdominal distention, constipation, or ileus occurs, loperamide should be discontinued. No significant drug–drug interactions are reported for loperamide.

Bismuth Subsalicylate

BSS is effective in the treatment of acute diarrhea, including travelers' diarrhea, significantly reducing the number of diarrheal stools.[24,28]

BSS reacts with hydrochloric acid in the stomach to form bismuth oxychloride and salicylic acid. Bismuth oxychloride is insoluble and poorly absorbed from the GI tract; less than 1%

of the administered dose is absorbed systemically. The salicylate is readily and efficiently absorbed. Both moieties are pharmacologically active; each produces effects that reduce frequency of unformed stools, increase stool consistency, relieve abdominal cramping, and decrease nausea and vomiting in children and adults. In travelers' diarrhea, the bismuth moiety exerts direct antimicrobial effects against ETEC and EAEC, *C. jejuni,* and other diarrheal pathogens, whereas the salicylate moiety exerts antisecretory effects that reduce fluid and electrolyte losses in acute diarrhea. The antisecretory effects may be mediated by several mechanisms, including inhibition of prostaglandin synthesis, inhibition of intestinal secretion through stimulation of sodium and chloride reabsorption, or disruption of calcium-mediated processes that regulate intestinal ion transport. BSS also directly binds to enterotoxins produced by *E. coli* and other diarrheal pathogens; however, the clinical significance of this effect in the treatment of diarrhea is not clear.

BSS is FDA-approved for management of acute diarrhea, including travelers' diarrhea, in adults and children 12 years of age or older.[24,28] Although previously labeled for children as young as 3 years, the product is not recommended for use in young children and no longer carries labeling for children younger than 12 years. BSS is also indicated for indigestion and as an adjuvant to antibiotics for treating *H. pylori*–associated peptic ulcer disease (see Chapter 14).

Table 17-6 provides dosing information for BSS.

BSS dosage forms contain various amounts of salicylate. Methyl salicylate (oil of wintergreen) is used as a flavoring agent in the suspension dosage form and the original tablet formulation. The original suspension and cherry-flavored suspension dosage forms (262 mg/15 mL) contain 130 mg of salicylate, whereas the original tablets (262 mg) contain 102 mg of salicylate. The caplets (262 mg) and cherry-flavored tablets (262 mg) contain 99 mg of salicylate. If a patient is taking aspirin or other salicylate-containing drugs, toxic levels of salicylate may be reached even if the patient follows dosing directions on the label for each drug.

Mild tinnitus is a dose-related side effect that may be associated with moderate-to-severe salicylate toxicity. If tinnitus occurs, the product should be discontinued and the patient referred for medical evaluation. Salicylates may cause adverse effects that are independent of the dose. Children and adolescents who have or are recovering from chicken pox or influenza are at risk of Reye's syndrome, a rare but serious illness associated with salicylates. These patients should not use BSS. In susceptible patients, salicylate-induced gout attacks have occurred. Patients who are sensitive to aspirin (resulting in asthmatic bronchospasm) should not use BSS.

Overdosage of bismuth products can cause neurotoxicity. Blood concentrations of bismuth greater than 50 mg/L have been associated with encephalopathy characterized by slow onset of tremors, postural instability, ataxia, myoclonus, and poor concentration. Confusion, memory impairment, seizures, visual and auditory hallucinations, psychosis, delirium, and depression may also develop. Most patients gradually recover after discontinuation of the bismuth preparation; however, some develop a permanent tremor and the encephalopathy has resulted in fatality. AIDS patients with acute diarrhea may be at particular risk for bismuth encephalopathy, perhaps resulting from altered GI absorption.

Harmless black staining of stool may occur, which should not be confused with melena; in addition, harmless darkening of the tongue may also occur. These frequent effects occur in more than 10% of patients treated with BSS. Bismuth salts react with hydrogen sulfide produced by bacteria in the mouth and colon. The resulting compound, bismuth sulfide, imparts the black discoloration. It is easily removed from the surface of the tongue by brushing the tongue with a soft-bristled brush; it may also be treated by discontinuing the bismuth product.

BSS is contraindicated for nursing or pregnant women and should therefore not be used without medical advice. It also should not be used in patients with AIDS because of the risk for neurotoxicity. Bismuth is radiopaque and may interfere with radiographic intestinal studies.

BSS may interact adversely with a number of other drugs, particularly those that potentially interact with aspirin. The salicylate moiety can increase the risk of toxicity with warfarin, valproic acid, and methotrexate by significantly decreasing plasma protein binding of these drugs in vivo. Salicylate can also increase the plasma concentration of methotrexate by decreasing its renal clearance. The uricosuric effects of probenecid may be inhibited by salicylate; the exact mechanism underlying this interaction is not known. The bismuth moiety is a trivalent cation and may decrease absorption of other medications, such as tetracycline and quinolone antibiotics, by forming complexes with them in the GI tract. When ciprofloxacin is used to treat travelers' diarrhea, the patient should be instructed to discontinue BSS. Solid dosage forms of BSS contain calcium carbonate, which may enhance the cation complex interaction.

Adsorbents

GI adsorbents (attapulgite, kaolin, and pectin) are no longer used to treat diarrhea. Evidence supporting the safety and effectiveness of attapulgite and pectin is lacking; products containing these adsorbents have either been reformulated or withdrawn from the market. Sufficient data support the effectiveness of kaolin in improving stool consistency within 24 to 48 hours, although it does not reduce the number of stools passed. Kaolin has been deemed to be a safe and effective antidiarrheal agent by the FDA, but no single-ingredient kaolin products are currently available in the United States.[24]

Digestive Enzymes

For patients with lactase deficiency who are intolerant of milk products, lactase enzyme preparations (Table 17-7) may be taken with milk or other dairy products to prevent osmotic diarrhea.

TABLE 17-7 Selected Lactase Enzyme Products

Trade Name	Primary Ingredient
Lactaid Caplets	Lactase enzyme 3000 FCC units[a]/caplet
Lactaid Fast Act Caplets	Lactase enzyme 9000 FCC units[a]/caplet
Lactrase Capsules	Lactase enzyme 250 mg/capsule

[a] FCC units are standardized units established by The Food Chemicals Codex (FCC), a compendium of internationally recognized standards for purity and identity of food ingredients published by the United States Pharmacopeia.

Product Selection Guidelines

Table 17-6 provides a quick reference for recommended dosages and durations of therapy for selected antidiarrheal agents. Tables 17-7 and 17-8 list dosage forms and primary ingredients of selected trade-name products.

SPECIAL POPULATIONS

For young children (5 years or younger), self-treatment is limited to treating dehydration with ORSs; antidiarrheal medications are not recommended. If ORSs are ineffective, a primary care provider must be consulted.

Elderly patients (65 years or older) should be strongly cautioned against self-treatment with antidiarrheal medications. Diarrhea in these patients is more likely to be severe, possibly fatal; therefore, these patients should be referred for medical evaluation.

Use of nonprescription antidiarrheals may be inappropriate during pregnancy; therefore, pregnant women should consult with a primary care provider before self-treating. Loperamide is a Pregnancy Category B drug. Although BSS does not have an FDA Pregnancy Category rating, BSS-containing products should be used sparingly or not at all during pregnancy because of concerns that the salicylate component may inhibit platelet function and, in the third trimester, cause premature closure of the fetal ductus arteriosus.[27,29]

PATIENT FACTORS AND PREFERENCES

Selection of antidiarrheal products for older children and adults should be based on factors such as the etiology of the diarrhea, if known, prominent symptoms, potential interactions with prescribed medications, and the applicable contraindications. For example, BSS is suggested to be the preferred agent when vomiting is the important clinical symptom of acute gastroenteritis.[19] Furthermore, BSS should not be used to treat diarrhea in an immunocompromised patients (e.g., AIDS and transplant recipients), because they are at increased risk for bismuth encephalopathy.

A patient's preference for a particular dosage form or a product that requires fewer doses is another selection criterion.

Complementary and Alternative Therapies

Probiotics, including several *Lactobacillus* species, *Bifidobacteria lactis,* and *Saccharomyces boulardii,* are commonly used to manage or prevent acute, uncomplicated diarrhea. (See Chapter 24 for discussion of probiotics.) As normal inhabitants of the human GI tract, these lactic acid–producing bacteria help maintain normal GI flora and reduce colonization by pathogenic bacteria. The exact mechanisms underlying the effects of these bacteria are not clear; *Lactobacillus* is suggested to enhance immune responses, produce antimicrobial substances, and compete with bacteria for intestinal mucosal binding sites.[30]

Evidence demonstrates that probiotic therapy, especially with *Lactobacillus rhamnosus* GG (but also *Lactobacillus casei, Lactobacillus acidophilus,* and *Lactobacillus reuteri*), prevents or shortens the course of mild viral diarrhea in infants and young children.[31-33] *L. rhamnosus* GG therapy can shorten duration of acute infectious diarrhea in children by an average of 0.7 days and reduce diarrhea frequency on day 2 of treatment by an average of 1.6 stools.[34] Therapy with *L. rhamnosus* GG, *L. acidophilus,* and *S. boulardii* may also offer clinical benefit in antibiotic-associated diarrhea; a recent meta-analysis reported odds ratios favoring active treatment with these live organisms over placebo in preventing this condition.[33] Probiotics appear to be safe; major side effects, such as *Lactobacillus* sepsis, have been reported only rarely.[34] The role of probiotics in bacterial gastroenteritis and moderate-to-severe diarrhea is not supported conclusively by available evidence. The Food and Agriculture Organization of the United Nations and WHO have recognized the benefits of probiotics in the prevention and treatment of acute diarrhea.[35] However, probiotics are not recognized as medications by FDA; their classification as dietary supplements or components of functional foods limits the health claims that can be made. Therefore, probiotics cannot be recommended to treat or prevent acute, uncomplicated diarrhea, but they can be recommended for maintenance of GI tract function.

TABLE 17-8 Selected Antidiarrheal Products

Loperamide Products

Imodium A-D Caplets	Loperamide HCl 2 mg
Imodium EZ Chews (Tablets)	Loperamide HCl 2 mg
Imodium Advanced Caplets	Loperamide HCl 2 mg; simethicone 125 mg
Imodium Advanced Chewable	Loperamide HCl 2 mg; simethicone 125 mg
Tablets	Loperamide HCl 1 mg/7.5 mL
Imodium A-D Liquid	

Bismuth Subsalicylate Products

Kaopectate Regular Flavor Liquid	Bismuth subsalicylate 262 mg/15 mL
Kaopectate Extra Strength Peppermint Flavor Liquid	Bismuth subsalicylate 525 mg/15 mL
Kaopectate Peppermint Flavor Liquid	Bismuth subsalicylate 62 mg/15 mL
Kaopectate Cherry Flavor Liquid	Bismuth subsalicylate 262 mg/15 mL
Kaopectate Antidiarrheal Caplets	Bismuth subsalicylate 262 mg
Pepto-Bismol Caplets	Bismuth subsalicylate 262 mg
Pepto-Bismol Chewable Tablets	Bismuth subsalicylate 262 mg
Pepto-Bismol Cherry Chewable Tablets	Bismuth subsalicylate 262 mg
Pepto-Bismol Original Liquid	Bismuth subsalicylate 262 mg/15 mL
Pepto-Bismol Cherry Liquid	Bismuth subsalicylate 262 mg/15 mL
Pepto-Bismol Maximum Strength Liquid	Bismuth subsalicylate 525 mg/15 mL

Note: Pepto-Bismol adult formulations contain BSS, but the product for children contains calcium carbonate as the active ingredient.

Several large studies performed in developing countries have shown that daily zinc supplementation in young children with acute diarrhea reduces total stool output, frequency of watery stools, and duration and severity of diarrhea.[36–38] These children who are at risk for diarrheal disease are zinc–deficient because of poor nutrition; in addition, diarrhea increases intestinal losses of zinc considerably, further compromising zinc status, even in those with normal plasma zinc concentrations. Zinc deficiency is associated with impaired cellular and humoral immunity, as well as adverse GI effects such as impaired water and electrolyte absorption, increased secretion in response to bacterial endotoxin, and decreased brush border enzymes (see Chapter 23). WHO/UNICEF recommend that children with acute diarrhea also receive zinc (10 mg of elemental zinc/day for infants younger than 6 months; 20 mg of elemental zinc/day for older infants and children) for 10 to 14 days.[21] The role of zinc supplementation in young children with diarrhea in developed countries is not yet defined.

There is no evidence to substantiate the safety and effectiveness of herbal and homeopathic therapies in the treatment of acute diarrheal diseases; their use cannot be recommended.

Assessment of Diarrhea: A Case-Based Approach

To evaluate a patient with diarrhea, the practitioner differentiates symptoms and makes clinical judgments. This triage function is based on the patient's responses to questions designed to help determine the cause of the specific signs and symptoms, their characteristics, and their severity (Tables 17-1 and 17-3). The practitioner should therefore ask the patient about vomiting, high and/or prolonged fever, and other symptoms to determine the patient's susceptibility to complications. Persistent diarrhea, chronic diarrhea, or presence of high fever (greater than 102.2°F [39°C]), protracted vomiting, abdominal pain in patients older than 50 years, or blood or mucus in the stool precludes self-treatment and requires immediate medical referral. If none of these significant findings is present, the degree of dehydration is the next important assessment (Table 17-3); the practitioner should ask about the nature and amount of fluid intake. Severity of dehydration can be accurately assessed by evaluating changes in body weight. For example, in children, mild dehydration is associated with a 3% to 5% loss of body weight, whereas severe dehydration is associated with a loss of more than 9%. However, the patient (or the parent) seldom knows the exact premorbid weight for comparison, and distinguishing between mild and moderate dehydration may be difficult.

The initial assessment of a pediatric patient should also seek to determine plausible causes of the symptoms. The common symptoms of acute gastroenteritis (e.g., vomiting, loose stools, and fever) are nonspecific findings associated with many other childhood diseases (e.g., acute otitis media, bacterial sepsis, meningitis, pneumonia, and urinary tract infections). This information is key to recommending a proper course of action, which may include self-treatment or referral to a primary care provider. A complete medication history must be assessed before a product is selected.

Physical assessment of a patient with complaints of diarrhea can provide information useful in assessing severity of the diarrhea (Table 17-3). Checking skin turgor and moistness of oral mucous membranes will help determine the degree of dehydration. Vital signs (e.g., pulse, temperature, respiration, and blood pressure) are important indicators of illness severity and should be routinely measured. Symptoms of moderate-to-severe dehydration may include postural (orthostatic) hypotension, defined as a drop in the systolic and/or diastolic pressure of greater than 15 to 20 mm Hg on moving from a supine to an upright position. Normally, the diastolic pressure remains the same or increases slightly, and the systolic pressure drops slightly on rising. If the blood pressure drops, the pulse should be checked simultaneously; the pulse rate should increase as blood pressure drops. Failure of the pulse to rise suggests the problem is neurogenic (e.g., diabetic patients with peripheral neuropathy) or the patient is taking a beta-blocker. The presence of orthostatic hypotension suggests that the patient has lost 1 liter or more of vascular volume, and referral for medical care is necessary.

Cases 17-1 and 17-2 provide examples of assessment of patients with diarrhea.

CASE 17-1

Relevant Evaluation Criteria	Scenario/Model Outcome
Information Gathering	
1. Gather essential information about the patient's symptoms, including:	
a. description of symptom(s) (i.e., nature, onset, duration, severity, associated symptoms)	Mother reports that patient experienced the sudden onset of watery diarrhea, vomiting, low-grade fever (38.3°C or 101.1°F), and general muscle aches 24 hours earlier. The patient has had 2 episodes of emesis and 3 loose stools in the last 12 hours. Mother says that the patient was healthy prior to the onset of this illness. She reports that the patient's mouth is dry and he had been complaining of thirst. There is no blood or mucus in the stool. Breathing is normal and there is no complaint of dizziness.
b. description of any factors that seem to precipitate, exacerbate, and/or relieve the patient's symptom(s)	The patient's father had a bout of acute diarrhea that lasted approximately 48 hours and resolved 2 days ago without medical treatment.

CASE 17-1 (continued)

Relevant Evaluation Criteria	Scenario/Model Outcome
c. description of the patient's efforts to relieve the symptoms	No efforts have been made to relieve the symptoms.
2. Gather essential patient history information:	
a. patient's identity	Peter Mathews
b. patient's age, sex, height, and weight	5-year-old male, 3 ft 5 in, 45 lb
c. patient's occupation	N/A
d. patient's dietary habits	Patient eats a normal, healthy diet. Since the onset of the illness, the patient has not had much appetite and has eaten very little. He has been able to eat some soup and crackers and, at the mother's request, he has taken some water and apple juice.
e. patient's sleep habits	Usually sleeps 9 hours per night. Since onset of illness, he has been sleeping more.
f. concurrent medical conditions, prescription and nonprescription medications, and dietary supplements	None
g. allergies	None
h. history of other adverse reactions to medications	None
i. other (describe) _____	N/A

Assessment and Triage

3. Differentiate the patient's signs/symptoms and correctly identify the patient's primary problem(s) (see Tables 17-1 and 17-3).	Peter appears to have acute gastroenteritis, most likely of viral etiology, with mild-to-moderate dehydration.
4. Identify exclusions for self-treatment (see Figure 17-1).	There are no exclusions for self-treatment.
5. Formulate a comprehensive list of therapeutic alternatives for the primary problem to determine if triage to a medical practitioner is required, and share this information with the parent.	Options include: (1) Recommend continuation of a normal diet with an increased intake of usual dietary fluids. (2) Recommend self-care with an appropriate OTC product (e.g., loperamide) and nondrug therapies (ORSs). (3) Recommend self-care until a PCP can be consulted. (4) Refer Peter for medical evaluation and treatment. (5) Take no action.

Plan

6. Select an optimal therapeutic alternative to address the patient's problem, taking into account patient preferences.	Because dehydration is mild to moderate, it is appropriate to recommend self-care with an ORS. Pharmacologic intervention with OTC antidiarrheal products is not appropriate for young children (≤5 years of age) with acute diarrheal illness and should not be recommended.
7. Describe the recommended therapeutic approach to the parent.	See Figure 17-1 and the box Patient Education for Diarrhea. To make up his fluid deficit, Peter should drink at least 50 mL/kg of ORS over 3–4 hours. At his current weight, that amounts to approximately 1100 mL of ORS (about 4.5 cups). After each loose stool or episode of vomiting, he should be given 10 mL/kg (approximately 6–7 ounces).
8. Explain to the parent the rationale for selecting the recommended therapeutic approach from the considered therapeutic alternatives.	The recommended plan is appropriate for Peter because (1) acute gastroenteritis is usually self-limiting, (2) mild-to-moderate dehydration can be appropriately managed with ORSs, and (3) Peter has no risk factors for significant complications. If the condition does not resolve in 48–72 hours or it worsens, you should take Peter to his PCP for evaluation.

CASE 17-1 *(continued)*

Relevant Evaluation Criteria	Scenario/Model Outcome
Patient Education	
9. When recommending self-care with non-prescription medications and/or nondrug therapy, convey accurate information to the parent:	ORS may be used as a maintenance fluid and to replace ongoing fluid losses resulting from acute gastroenteritis.
a. appropriate dose and frequency of administration	See the box Patient Education for Diarrhea.
b. maximum number of days the therapy should be employed	ORS may be used as a supplement to a normal diet and as maintenance fluids until the illness resolves.
c. product administration procedures	See Figure 17-1 and the box Patient Education for Diarrhea. Vomiting is not a contraindication to ORS use. If Peter continues to vomit, ORS can be administered in 5 mL portions every 1–2 minutes.
d. expected time to onset of relief	N/A
e. degree of relief that can be reasonably expected	N/A
f. most common side effects	N/A
g. side effects that warrant medical intervention should they occur	N/A
h. patient options in the event that condition worsens or persists	If the diarrhea does not resolve in 48–72 hours, high fever develops, or blood or mucus appears in the stool, seek medical attention.
i. product storage requirements	N/A
j. specific nondrug measures	Maintain a normal diet. Do not use the BRAT diet (bananas, rice, apple juice, toast); its nutrient content is inadequate.
10. Solicit follow-up questions from parent.	May I give Peter something like Imodium or Pepto-Bismol to stop the diarrhea and vomiting?
	What should I give him for his fever?
11. Answer parent's questions.	The vomiting and diarrhea should resolve on their own. Although both are uncomfortable for Peter, OTC antiemetics or antidiarrheal products such as these should not be used to treat these symptoms in young children. Antidiarrheal products do not have any proven benefit in children and actually increase the likelihood of serious side effects and complications.
	Acetaminophen or ibuprofen would be appropriate for his fever, if it needs to be reduced.

Key: N/A, not applicable; ORS, oral rehydration solution; OTC, over-the-counter; PCP, primary care provider.

CASE 17-2

Relevant Evaluation Criteria	Scenario/Model Outcome
Information Gathering	
1. Gather essential information about the patient's symptoms, including:	
a. description of symptom(s) (i.e., nature, onset, duration, severity, associated symptoms)	Patient complains of sudden onset of watery diarrhea, nausea, vomiting, and abdominal cramps that began approximately 48 hours earlier. Patient reports having 5 unformed stools in the last 24 hours with several episodes of emesis since the onset of the illness. She has a low-grade fever (37.8°C or 100.2°F). She also complains of thirst, slight dizziness when she stands up quickly, and increased frequency of urination.

Relevant Evaluation Criteria	Scenario/Model Outcome
b. description of any factors that seem to precipitate, exacerbate, and/or relieve the patient's symptom(s)	Patient returned 3 days ago from a 2-week business trip to Costa Rica.
c. description of the patient's efforts to relieve the symptoms	Patient reports taking 5 or 6 doses of loperamide (Imodium A-D, 2 mg/dose) over the last 48 hours without relief. She has been drinking Gatorade as desired since the onset of symptoms but has had difficulty keeping it down.
2. Gather essential patient history information:	
a. patient's identity	Joan Tenney
b. patient's age, sex, height, and weight	46-year-old female, 5 ft 3 in, 186 lb (current weight), 195 lb (before onset of symptoms)
c. patient's occupation	Industrial engineer
d. patient's dietary habits	Patient is on a diabetic diet.
e. patient's sleep habits	Sleeps well, averaging 7 hours a night
f. concurrent medical conditions, prescription and nonprescription medications, and dietary supplements	Type 2 diabetes mellitus, hypertension
	Metformin 1000 mg daily; lisinopril 10 mg daily; hydrochlorothiazide 12.5 mg daily; pravastatin 40 mg daily; aspirin 81 mg daily
	You ask if she monitors her blood glucose concentrations at home and learn that her blood glucose has been elevated (between 200–230 mg/dL) at least since the onset of GI symptoms.
	You measure her blood pressure; it is 125/80 mm Hg.
g. allergies	NKA
h. history of other adverse reactions to medications	None
i. other (describe) _____	N/A

Assessment and Triage

3. Differentiate the patient's signs/symptoms and correctly identify the patient's primary problem(s) (see Tables 17-1 and 17-3).	Her history of recent travel to Central America suggests she likely has travelers' diarrhea caused by bacterial enteropathogens, which typically occurs during travel. Onset of symptoms may occur after return if contracted on the last day of travel to high-risk areas. Travelers' diarrhea usually occurs during the trip with its peak onset during the first 7–10 days of the trip. On the basis of her symptoms (approximately 5% weight loss, orthostatic hypotension, increased thirst), she is moderately dehydrated.
4. Identify exclusions for self-treatment (see Figure 17-1).	Uncontrolled type 2 diabetes mellitus with urinary frequency increases her risk for dehydration and potential complications. The lack of response to self-treatment with loperamide, as evidenced by ongoing diarrhea for ≥48 hours (although therapy may not have been maximized) is also an indication for medical referral.
5. Formulate a comprehensive list of therapeutic alternatives for the primary problem to determine if triage to a medical practitioner is required, and share this information with the patient.	Options include: (1) Recommend continuation of her regular diabetic diet with an increased intake of usual dietary fluids. (2) Recommend self-care with an appropriate OTC product, such as BSS, and nondrug therapies, such as an ORS. (3) Recommend self-care with OTC products, such as BSS, and nondrug therapies, such as an ORS, until a PCP can be consulted. (4) Refer Ms. Tenney for medical evaluation and treatment. (5) Take no action.

Plan

6. Select an optimal therapeutic alternative to address the patient's problem, taking into account patient preferences.	Refer Ms. Tenney to a PCP, urgent care center, or emergency department for evaluation and treatment.
7. Describe the recommended therapeutic approach to the patient.	You need to seek urgent medical care from your primary care provider, urgent care center, or emergency department right away.

CASE 17-2 (continued)

Relevant Evaluation Criteria	Scenario/Model Outcome
8. Explain to the patient the rationale for selecting the recommended therapeutic approach from the considered therapeutic alternatives.	Your symptoms suggest that you are dehydrated from the diarrhea, and your risk for complications from the diarrhea may be increased because your diabetes is out of control. Furthermore, prescription antibiotics may be needed to treat your gastrointestinal infection.
Patient Education	
9. When recommending self-care with non-prescription medications and/or nondrug therapy, convey accurate information to the patient.	Criterion does not apply in this case.
10. Solicit follow-up questions from patient.	Patient has no further questions.
11. Answer patient's questions.	N/A

Key: BSS, bismuth subsalicylate; GI, gastrointestinal; N/A, not applicable; NKA, no known allergies; ORS, oral rehydration solution; OTC, over-the-counter; PCP, primary care provider.

Patient Counseling for Diarrhea

Patients with diarrhea may focus on the need for a nonprescription medication to stop the frequent bowel movements. The practitioner should remind them that most episodes of acute diarrhea stop after 48 hours, and that preventing dehydration is the most important component of treating the problem. Counseling on the two-step treatment of dehydration and the need for dietary management should follow. For infants and children, educating parents and caregivers on the appropriate use of an ORS (including appropriate volumes to administer, rates of administration, and use in vomiting) and of dietary management is very important in preventive care. For patient safety reasons, premixed solutions are preferred. Importantly, if dry powder ORS is selected, the practitioner should give parents (or caregivers) explicit directions for mixing and verify that they

understand the directions. For families with infants, the Centers for Disease Control and Prevention recommends a home supply of ORS, because early administration of an ORS at home is vital if hospitalization is to be avoided. If travelers are using ORS dry powder in developing countries, potable water should be used to reconstitute the powder.

If a nonspecific antidiarrheal is recommended, the practitioner should review label instructions with the patient. The practitioner should stress an appropriate dosage on the basis of the patient's age and weight, the maximum number of doses per 24 hours, and the auxiliary administration instructions. The practitioner should also explain potential drug interactions, side effects, contraindications, and the maximum duration of treatment before seeking medical help. The box Patient Education for Diarrhea contains specific information to provide patients.

PATIENT EDUCATION FOR
Diarrhea

The primary objective of self-treatment is to prevent excessive fluid and electrolyte losses. For most patients, carefully following product instructions and the self-care measures listed here will help ensure optimal outcomes.

Nondrug Measures

Infants and Children 6 Months to 5 Years

- For mild-to-moderate diarrhea, indicated by three to five unformed bowel movements per day, give the child or infant an oral rehydration solution (ORS) at a volume of 50–100 mL/kg of body weight over 2–4 hours to replace the fluid deficit. Give additional ORS to replace ongoing losses. Continue to give the solution for the next 4 to 6 hours or until the child is rehydrated.
- If the child is vomiting, give 1 teaspoon of ORS every few minutes.

- If the child is not dehydrated, give 10 mL/kg or one-half to 1 cup of the ORS for each bowel movement, or 2 mL/kg for each episode of vomiting. As an alternative, to replace ongoing fluid losses, children weighing less than 10 kg should be given 60–120 mL of ORS for each episode of vomiting or diarrheal stool, and children weighing more than 10 kg should be given 120–240 mL for each episode of vomiting or diarrheal stool.
- After the child is rehydrated, reintroduce food appropriate for the child's age, while also administering an ORS as maintenance therapy.

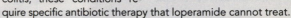

- If breast-feeding an infant with diarrhea, continue the breast-feeding. If the infant is bottle-fed, consult your doctor or pediatrician about substituting a milk-based formula with a lactose-free formula.
- Give children complex carbohydrate–rich foods, yogurt, lean meats, fruits, and vegetables. Do not give them fatty foods or sugary foods. Sugary foods can cause osmotic diarrhea.
- Do not withhold food for more than 24 hours.

Adults and Children Older Than 5 Years
- For mild-to-moderate dehydration, indicated by a 3%–9% drop in body weight or three to five unformed stools per day, drink 2–4 liters of an ORS over 4 hours.
- If not dehydrated, drink one-half to 1 cup of ORS or fluids after each unformed bowel movement.
- If you have no medical conditions, you may consume sport drinks, diluted juices, salty crackers, soups, and broths until the diarrhea stops.
- Do not withhold food for more than 24 hours.

Nonprescription Medications
- See Table 17-6 for dosages of loperamide and bismuth subsalicylate.

Loperamide
- Note that loperamide can cause dizziness and constipation.
- Do not take this agent if you are taking sedatives, antianxiety drugs, or other antidepressants.
- Do not give this agent to children 2 years of age or younger. Loperamide is not recommended for children younger than 6 years, except under the supervision of a primary care provider.
- If loperamide is not effective in treating your diarrhea (if no clinical improvement is observed in 48 hours), check with your

primary care provider or pharmacist about using a different nonprescription medication. You may have a bacterial diarrhea or pseudomembranous colitis; these conditions require specific antibiotic therapy that loperamide cannot treat.

Bismuth Subsalicylate
- Note that bismuth subsalicylate can cause a dark discoloration of the tongue and stool.
- Do not take this agent if you are taking tetracyclines, quinolones, or medicines for gout (uricosurics).
- Do not give this agent to children younger than 12 years.
- Do not give this agent to children or teenagers who have or are recovering from influenza or chicken pox. Reye's syndrome, a rare but serious condition, could occur.
- Do not give this agent to patients with AIDS.
- Do not take this agent if you are sensitive to aspirin, have a history of gastrointestinal bleeding, or have a history of problems with blood coagulation.

 If the diarrhea has not resolved after 72 hours of initial treatment, see your primary care provider.

 Monitor for excessive number of bowel movements, signs of dehydration, high fever, or blood in the stool. If any of these complications are present, discontinue bismuth subsalicylate and consult your primary care provider.

Evaluation of Patient Outcomes for Diarrhea

Many patients have mild-to-moderate diarrhea that is generally self-limiting within 48 hours. Mild-to-moderate diarrhea is managed with oral rehydration therapy, symptomatic drug therapy, and dietary measures. The patient should be monitored for dehydration by measuring body weight, vital signs, and mental alertness. With effective symptomatic relief, the patient can expect reduced frequency and normal consistency of stools, as well as relief of generalized symptoms such as lethargy and abdominal pain. As the diarrheal episode clears, the appetite will return to normal and the diet can be advanced to a regular diet.

Medical referral is necessary if any of the following signs and symptoms occur before or during treatment: high fever, worsening illness, bloody or mucoid stools, diarrhea continuing beyond 48 hours, or signs of worsening dehydration (e.g., low blood pressure, rapid pulse, or mental confusion). Also, medical referral is advised for infants, young children, frail patients of advanced age, and patients with chronic illness at risk from secondary complications (e.g., diabetes mellitus).

Key Points for Diarrhea

➤ Limit the self-treatment of diarrhea to patients with acute diarrhea who have minimal, mild, or moderate dehydration. Patients who appear volume-depleted, weak, dizzy,

or hypotensive should be referred for evaluation, as should all patients with severely acute, uncontrolled, or chronic complaints involving the GI tract.
➤ Oral rehydration solutions are the mainstay of therapy and should be used to rehydrate patients with minimal, mild, or moderate dehydration.
➤ Rehydration should be performed rapidly (i.e., within 3–4 hours; Figures 17-1 and 17-2).
➤ Additional ORS should be given to maintain hydration and replace ongoing fluid losses through diarrheal stools and/or vomiting (Figures 17-1 and 17-2).
➤ Instruct patients or their caregivers how to prepare and administer an ORS.
➤ Older children and adults may use sports drinks instead of an ORS, if additional sources of sodium (e.g., crackers and pretzels) are used concomitantly.
➤ An age-appropriate, unrestricted diet should be initiated as soon as the patient is rehydrated. Food should be withheld for no more than 24 hours.
➤ Loperamide and BSS may be used to help control acute diarrhea in carefully selected patients.
➤ Antibiotic therapy is generally not indicated for patients with acute diarrhea unless it is travelers' diarrhea.

REFERENCES
1. Herikstad H, Yang S, Van Gilder TJ, et al. A population-based estimate of the burden of diarrhoeal illness in the United States: FoodNet, 1996–7. *Epidemiol Infect.* 2002;129:9–17.

2. Jones TF, McMillian MB, Scallan E, et al. A population-based estimate of the substantial burden of diarrhoeal disease in the United States; Food-Net, 1996–2003. *Epidemiol Infect.* 2007;135:293–301.

3. Peterson CA, Calderon RL. Trends in enteric disease as a cause of death in the United States, 1989–1996. *Am J Epidemiol.* 2003;157:58–65.

4. Gilbert DN, Moellering RC, Eliopoulos GM, et al. *The Sanford Guide to Antimicrobial Therapy.* 37th ed. Hyde Park, Vt: Antimicrobial Therapy; 2007:15–17, 122.

5. American Academy of Pediatrics. *AAP 2006 Red Book Online: Report of the Committee on Infectious Diseases.* Available at: http://aapredbook.aappublications.org. Last accessed October 17, 2008.

6. Huang DB, White AC. An updated review on Cryptosporidium and Giardia. *Gastroenterol Clin N Am.* 2006;35:291–314.

7. Guerrant RL, Van Gilder T, Steiner TS, et al. Practice guidelines for the management of infectious diarrhea. *Clin Infect Dis.* 2001;32:331–50.

8. Centers for Disease Control and Prevention. Outbreaks of gastroenteritis associated with noroviruses on cruise ships–United States, 2002. *MMWR Morb Mortal Wkly Rep.* 2002;51:1112–5.

9. Centers for Disease Control and Prevention. Prevention of Rotavirus Gastroenteritis Among Infants and Children. *MMWR Morb Mortal Wkly Rep.* 2006;55:1–13

10. Marcos LA, DuPont HL. Advances in defining etiology and new therapeutic approaches in acute diarrhea. *J Infect.* 2007;55:385–93.

11. Allos BM. Campylobacter jejuni infections: update on emerging issues and trends. *Clin Infect Dis.* 2001;32:1201–6.

12. Centers for Disease Control and Prevention. Preliminary FoodNet data on the incidence of infection with pathogens transmitted commonly through food—10 States, 2006. *MMWR Morb Mortal Wkly Rep.* 2007;56:336–9.

13. Centers for Disease Control and Prevention. Escherichia coli O157:H7 infection associated with drinking raw milk—Washington and Oregon, November 2005. *MMWR Morb Mortal Wkly Rep.* 2007;56:165–7.

14. Adachi JA, Zhi-Dong J, Mathewson JJ, et al. Enteroaggregative Escherichia coli as a major etiologic agent in traveler's diarrhea in 3 regions of the world. *Clin Infect Dis.* 2001;32:1706–9.

15. Connor BA. Sequelae of traveler's diarrhea: focus on postinfectious irritable bowel syndrome. *Clin Infect Dis.* 2005;41(suppl 8);s577–86.

16. Wang LH, Fang XC, Pan GZ. Bacillary dysentery as a causative factor of irritable bowel syndrome and its pathogenesis. *Gut.* 2004;53:1096–101.

17. King CK, Glass R, Bresee JS, et al. Managing acute gastroenteritis among children: oral rehydration, maintenance, and nutritional therapy. *MMWR Morb Mortal Wkly Rep.* 2003;52:1–16.

18. Wingate D, Phillips SF, Lewis SJ, et al. Guidelines for adults on self-medication for the treatment of acute diarrhea. *Aliment Pharmacol Ther.* 2001;15:773–82.

19. DuPont HL. Guidelines on acute infectious diarrhea in adults. The Practice Parameters Committee of the American College of Gastroenterology. *Am J Gastroenterol.* 1997;92:1962–75.

20. Hartling L, Bellemare S, Wiebe N, et al. Oral versus intravenous rehydration for treating dehydration due to gastroenteritis in children. *Cochrane Database Syst Rev.* 2006;3:CD004390.

21. World Health Organization, United Nations Children's Fund. WHO/UNICEF Joint Statement: Clinical Management of Acute Diarrhoea. Available at: http://www.unicef.org/publications/files/ENAcute_Diarrhoea_reprint.pdf. Last accessed October 17, 2008.

22. Hahn S, Kim Y, Garner P. Reduced osmolarity oral rehydration solution for treating dehydration due to diarrheoa in children: systematic review. *BMJ.* 2001;323:81–5.

23. World Health Organization, United Nations Children's Fund. Expert Consultation on Oral Rehydration Salts (ORS) Formulation. WHO/FCH/CAH/01.22. 2001. Available at: http://rehydrate.org/ors/expert-consultation.html. Last accessed October 17, 2008.

24. Antidiarrheal drug products for over-the-counter human use: final monograph. *Fed Regist.* 2003;68:18869–82.

25. Centers for Disease Control. Traveler's Diarrhea. Available at: http://wwwn.cdc.gov/travel/yellowBookCh4-Diarrhea.aspx. Last accessed October 17, 2008.

26. Hill DR, Ericsson CD, Pearson RD, et al. The practice of travel medicine: guidelines by the Infectious Diseases Society of America. *Clin Infect Dis.* 2006;43:1499–539.

27. Micromedex® Healthcare Series, version 5.1. Greenwood Village, Col: Thomson Micromedex. Available at: http://www.thomsonhc.com. Last accessed October 17, 2008.

28. Antidiarrheal drug products for over-the-counter human use; amendment of final monograph. *Fed Regist.* 2004;69:26301–2.

29. Conover E. Over-the-counter products: nonprescription medications, nutraceuticals, and herbal agents. *Clin Obstet Gynecol.* 2002;45:89–98.

30. Isolauri E, Sutas Y, Kankaanpaa P, et al. Probiotics: effects on immunity. *Am J Clin Nutr.* 2001;73(suppl):444S-50S.

31. Guandalini S, Pensabene L, Zikri MA, et al. *Lactobacillus* GG administered in oral rehydration solution to children with acute diarrhea: a multicenter European trial. *J Pediatr Gastroenterol Nutr.* 2000;30:54–60.

32. Van Neil CW, Feudtner C, Garrison MM, et al. Lactobacillus therapy for acute infectious diarrhea in children: a meta analysis. *Pediatrics.* 2002;109:678–84.

33. D'Souza AL, Rajkumar C, Cooke J, et al. Probiotics in prevention of antibiotic associated diarrhea: meta-analysis. *BMJ.* 2002;324:1361–6.

34. Land MH, Rouster-Stevens K, Woods, CR, et al. Lactobacillus sepsis associated with probiotic therapy. *Pediatrics.* 2005;115:178–81.

35. Food and Agriculture Organization of the United Nations, World Health Organization. Health and Nutritional Properties of Probiotics in Food Including Milk with Live Lactic Acid Bacteria. Food and Agriculture Organization of the United Nations and the World Health Organization Expert Consultation Report. Available at: http://www.who.int/foodsafety/publications/fs_management/probiotics/en/index.html. Last accessed October 17, 2008.

36. Bahl R, Bhandari N, Saksena M, et al. Efficacy of zinc-fortified oral rehydration solution in 6- to 35-month-old children with acute diarrhea. *J Pediatr.* 2002;141:677–82.

37. Bhandari N, Bahl R, Taneja S, et al. Substantial reduction in severe diarrheal morbidity by daily zinc supplementation in young north Indian children. *Pediatrics.* 2002;109:e86.

38. Lukacik M, Thomas RL, Aranda JV. A meta-analysis of the effects of oral zinc in the treatment of acute and persistent diarrhea. *Pediatrics.* 2008;121:326–36.

Anorectal Disorders

Juliana Chan and Rosemary R. Berardi

Anorectal disorders involve the perianal area, anal canal, and lower rectum. Many signs and symptoms associated with hemorrhoids may be related to nonhemorrhoidal anorectal disorders.[1] Hemorrhoids, also known as piles, can often be self-treated, whereas other anorectal disorders may require immediate medical attention. A number of nonprescription products are available for the symptomatic treatment of anorectal disorders. It is estimated that pharmacists recommend a hemorrhoidal preparation at least once every 30 days.[2] Total dollar sales for nonprescription hemorrhoidal remedies reached $83 million in 2001, up 18% from the previous year.[3,4]

More than 10 million people in the United States complain of hemorrhoid symptoms, a prevalence of about 5%.[2] However, the true prevalence of hemorrhoids is unknown as fewer than one-third seek medical attention.[2] Hemorrhoids are more common in men than in women and increase with advancing age, peaking between the ages of 45 and 74 years.[2] In the United States, whites self-report symptoms 1.6 times more often than blacks.[2] Although epidemiologic data are lacking, the incidence is higher among pregnant than nonpregnant women of similar childbearing age, particularly in the postpartum period.[5,6]

Pathophysiology of Anorectal Area

Anorectal disorders occur in the perianal area (portion of the skin immediately surrounding the anus), anal canal, and lower portion of the rectum (Figure 18-1). Sensory nerve endings make this area very sensitive to pain. Perianal tissue differs from exposed skin tissue in that it is normally moister. The anal canal (about 4 cm long) connects the end of the gastrointestinal (GI) tract (rectum) with the outside of the body.[7] Two different types of epithelium line the anal canal and are defined by the dentate line (also known as the pectinate line). The dentate line divides squamous epithelium from columnar epithelium, thus delineating where sensory pain fibers are located in the anal canal. Anorectal disorders occurring below the dentate line may be associated with pain, whereas disorders above the line rarely cause any discomfort. The epithelium above the dentate line forms longitudinal folds known as the columns of Morgagni. In between and next to these columns are small pockets or crypts. The pockets may be obstructed by foreign material, possibly causing infections (i.e., abscesses or fistulas). The lower two-thirds of the canal is covered by modified anal skin, which is structurally similar to skin covering other parts of the body.

The external anal sphincter is a voluntary muscle located at the bottom of the anal canal that remains closed under normal conditions to prevent involuntary passage of feces. The internal sphincter is an involuntary muscle innervated by the autonomic nervous system. When the sphincters are relaxed, defecation occurs. In healthy individuals, skin covering the anal canal serves as a barrier against absorption of substances into the body. Therefore, topical agents applied to the area may manifest primarily local effects. If the protective barrier breaks, then the absorptive character of the anal skin may be altered, diminishing the skin's protective capabilities and permitting systemic absorption of medications applied to the area.

The rectum, which lies above the anal canal, is about 12 cm long and is the terminal portion of the large intestine. The highly vascular rectal mucosa is lined with a semipermeable membrane to protect the body from invasion by fecal bacteria. Although the rectum contains pressure receptors, it does not have sensory pain receptors. Three hemorrhoidal arteries and their accompanying veins are the most prominent parts of the vasculature in this area. The arteries and veins lying above the dentate line are referred to as internal and those below as external. Because of the path followed by blood returning to the heart through the hemorrhoidal veins, rectally administered medications may be absorbed and enter the systemic circulation without passing through the liver.[7]

Hemorrhoids are abnormally large, bulging, symptomatic conglomerates of hemorrhoidal vessels, supporting tissues, and overlying mucous membranes or skin in the anorectal region. Many factors have been implicated in the etiology of hemorrhoids, including erect posture, pregnancy, prolonged standing or sitting, lack of dietary fiber, constipation, diarrhea, and heavy lifting with straining. Symptomatic hemorrhoids develop in susceptible individuals. Although data are conflicting, heredity may play a role. Socioeconomics, cultural factors (e.g., diet, number of meals a day, and lifestyle), and geographic location may be related to hemorrhoid formation.[2,8] Although insufficient evidence supports a relationship between dietary fiber intake and development of hemorrhoids, increasing dietary fiber may reduce pain and bleeding associated with defecation with hemorrhoids.[9] Bowel habits, such as straining at defecation or prolonged sitting on the toilet, may increase pressure within the hemorrhoidal vessels.[7] Alternatively, constipation may follow the onset of hemorrhoidal symptoms and improve with prolapse (protrusion into the anal canal).[10,11] Hormonal changes and the

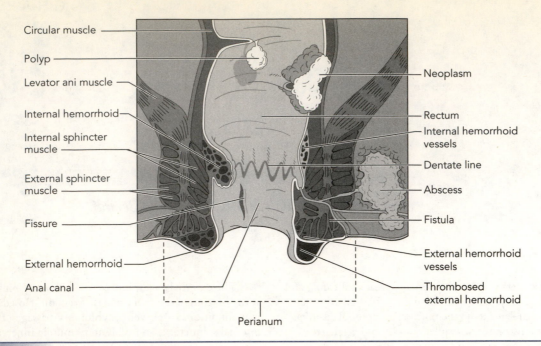

Circular muscle
Polyp
Levator ani muscle
Internal hemorrhoid
Internal sphincter muscle
External sphincter muscle
Fissure
External hemorrhoid
Anal canal

Neoplasm
Rectum
Internal hemorrhoid vessels
Dentate line
Abscess
Fistula
External hemorrhoid vessels
Thrombosed external hemorrhoid

Perianum

FIGURE 18-1 Disorders of the anorectal canal.

gravid uterus may increase pressure in the hemorrhoidal veins, leading to hemorrhoid formation during pregnancy.[5,7]

The most widely accepted pathophysiologic theory for the development of hemorrhoids is that vascular cushions are part of the normal anatomy and are located circumferentially around the anal canal above the dentate line. The cushions present at birth in three discrete masses and, by partially occluding the anus, contribute to continence. The cushions contain blood vessels, smooth muscle, and supportive connective tissue projecting into the lumen, causing a downward pressure during defecation. Younger individuals have muscle fibers anchoring the cushions and supporting the venous sinusoidal vessels.

Hemorrhoids develop with increasing age, when muscle fibers become weakened. Vascular cushions slide, become congested, bleed, and eventually protrude.[7] Downward pressure during defecation and a high resting anal pressure are common in the development of hemorrhoids.[7] These may originate either from the superior hemorrhoidal vein, producing internal hemorrhoids, or from the inferior hemorrhoidal vein, forming external hemorrhoids (Figure 18-1).[12] Internal hemorrhoids occur above the dentate line and are covered with columnar epithelium and lack sensory fibers.[12]

Internal hemorrhoids are graded by severity of prolapse into the anal canal using a degree system: First-degree hemorrhoids are enlarged but do not prolapse into the anal canal, second-degree protrude into the anal canal and return spontaneously on defecation, third-degree protrude into the anal canal on defecation but can be returned manually, and fourth-degree are permanently prolapsed and cannot be reintroduced into the anus.[12] External hemorrhoids develop below the dentate line and are covered with squamous epithelium. These are frequently visible as bluish lumps at the external or distal boundary of the anal canal (known as the anal verge). The blue color may be caused by thrombosed blood vessels, causing symptoms ranging from minimal discomfort to severe pain.[10,12]

Nonhemorrhoidal Anorectal Disorders

Potentially serious nonhemorrhoidal anorectal disorders, including abscesses, fistulas, fissures, neoplasms, polyps, pruritus ani, and inflammatory bowel disease (IBD), may present with hemorrhoid-like symptoms and should not be self-treated (Table 18-1).[1,12–18] Patients should be referred for medical evaluation if any of the conditions are suspected.

Clinical Presentation of Anorectal Disorders

The Food and Drug Administration (FDA) Advisory Panel identified specific signs and symptoms associated with hemorrhoidal complaints.[1] These common signs and symptoms of minor anorectal disorders include itching, discomfort, irritation, burning, inflammation, and swelling. In contrast, pain, bleeding, seepage, change in bowel patterns, prolapse, and thrombosis may indicate a more serious condition requiring medical referral (Table 18-2).[1,12,18]

Treatment of Anorectal Disorders
Treatment Goals

The goals of treatment for patients with anorectal itching, irritation, burning, inflammation, discomfort, and swelling are to (1) alleviate and maintain remission of anorectal symptoms and (2) prevent complications that lead to adverse consequences.

General Treatment Approach

Figure 18-2 presents an algorithm for treating minor anorectal signs and symptoms, and lists exclusions for self-treatment. If the

TABLE 18-1 Nonhemorrhoidal Anorectal Disorders

Disorder	Definition/Etiology	Common Signs and Symptoms	Comments
Anal abscess	Obstruction of anal glands, resulting in painful swelling in perianal or anal canal; usually leads to bacterial infection	Fever, local swelling, redness, tenderness, and a continuously painful bulge in the rectal or gluteal regions	Usually identified on history and physical examination; possible life-threatening sepsis if not identified and treated promptly
Anal fistula (or groove)	Unhealed or incomplete drainage of anorectal abscess located between internal and external opening of fistula tract, and manifested as hollow fibrous area lined with granulation tissue	Chronic, persistent drainage; pain; possible bleeding on defecation	Surgical repair required
Anal fissure	Slit-like ulcer in the anal canal resulting from a traumatic tear during passage of a large, hard stool (primary); may also occur secondary to underlying diseases such as IBD (especially Crohn's disease) or a neoplasm	Pain (usually out of proportion to the clinical finding) during and after defecation, lasting several minutes to hours; blood may be seen on the toilet tissue.	Primary anal fissures are usually found in young and middle-aged individuals and occur equally in women and men
Anal neoplasms	Comprises a variety of histologic types classified as epidermoid carcinomas	Bleeding, changes in bowel habits, constipation, diarrhea, anal discharge, an internal or external mass, pain, pruritus, rash; asymptomatic in 25% of patients	Relatively uncommon, accounting for 1%–2% of all GI malignancies; most are curable, but poor prognosis with anorectal melanomas (approx. 20% 5-year survival rate)
Polyps	Pedunculated growth (attached to its base by a small stalk) that arises from GI mucosa and extends into lumen of body cavity; usually found in colon but may also be present in anal canal	Bleeding	May be benign or malignant
Pruritus ani	An annoying itching sensation that may be idiopathic or associated with a primary underlying condition (e.g., anorectal or dermatologic disorder); other causes: diet (e.g., caffeinated or dairy products), lifestyle preferences (e.g., dyed, scented toilet paper, soaps, tight clothing), or medications (e.g., mineral oil, antibiotics)	Persistent itching in perianal region; more bothersome at bedtime or when patient not preoccupied	Affects men more often than women

Key: GI, gastrointestinal; IBD, inflammatory bowel disease.
Source: References 1 and 12–18.

complaint is self-treatable, the clinician may recommend non-pharmacologic measures and a nonprescription preparation to treat specific symptoms. The patient should be advised to maintain a well-balanced diet (preferably high in fiber and bulk) and good perianal hygiene, as well as to avoid prolonged sitting on the toilet. Table 18-3 outlines guidelines for applying anorectal products.[1,19]

Nonpharmacologic Therapy

Nondrug measures for treating anorectal disorders include dietary measures, improvement of hygiene practices, and possibly surgical and nonsurgical methods. In addition, patients diagnosed with or suspected of having hemorrhoids should be advised to avoid lifting heavy objects; discontinue foods that irritate or aggravate symptoms (e.g., caffeinated beverages); and increase dietary fiber. Nonsteroidal anti-inflammatory drugs or aspirin should be avoided; they may promote bleeding.

Dietary fiber softens stool and may prevent further irritation or formation of small symptomatic hemorrhoids. Adding 25 to 30 grams of fiber to a low-fiber diet may permit the passage of softer stools, thus reducing or preventing irritation and straining at defecation.[7,9] Fiber should be introduced slowly and accompanied by increasing fluid intake. If the amount of dietary fiber intake cannot be increased, fiber supplements such as psyllium or methylcellulose may be added to the treatment regimen (see Chapter 16).

TABLE 18-2 Signs and Symptoms of Anorectal Disorders

Sign/Symptom	Definition/Etiology
Usually Self-Treatable	
Itching (pruritus)	Mild stimulation of sensory nerve fibers; associated with many anorectal disorders, including hemorrhoids (typically with a mucoid discharge from prolapsing internal hemorrhoids).
	Common causes include poor hygiene (incomplete wiping/cleaning after defecation); diarrhea; parasitic or fungal infections; allergies (sensitivity to fabrics, soaps, laundry detergents, dyes, perfumes in toilet tissue); anorectal lesions; moisture in anal area.
	May be secondary to swelling, diet (caffeinated beverages, chocolate, citrus fruits), and use of oral broad-spectrum antibiotics.
	Rare cause: psychogenic origins.
Discomfort	May result from burning, itching, pain, irritation, inflammation, and swelling.
Irritation	Uncomfortable feeling associated with stimulation of sensory nerve fibers.
Burning	Greater degree of irritation of sensory nerve fibers than seen in anal itching; often associated with hemorrhoids; sensation of warmth or intense heat may be constant or occur only at defecation.
Inflammation	Tissue reaction characterized by heat, redness or discoloration, pain, and swelling; often associated with trauma, allergy, or infection.
Swelling	Temporary enlargement of cells and/or tissue resulting from excess fluid; may be accompanied by pain, burning, and itching.
Requires Medical Referral	
Pain	Intense stimulation of sensory nerve fibers caused by inflammation or irritation. Internal hemorrhoids usually painless; external hemorrhoids often cause mild pain; acute, severe perianal pain may be from thrombosed external hemorrhoid; pain from anal fissure during bowel movement often described as "being cut with sharp glass."
	Abscess, fistula, or anorectal neoplasm may also cause pain.
Bleeding	Hemorrhoids most common cause (from straining or passage of hard stool, or ulceration of perianal skin overlying thrombosed external hemorrhoid) of minor anorectal disorders.
	Often appears as bright red spots or streaks on toilet tissue, or bright red blood around stool or in toilet.
	Black or tarry stools (melena) may indicate a possible upper GI bleed (e.g., PUD, erosive esophagitis, or gastric varices).
	Large amounts of red blood (hematochezia) in toilet bowl may be indicative of lower GI bleeding (anorectal fissure, IBD, polyps, malignant disease of the colon or rectum).
	Possible indications of large-volume blood loss include shortness of breath, dizziness, fatigue, or light-headedness, especially on standing (orthostatic hypotension).
Seepage	Involuntary passage of fecal material or mucus caused by an anal sphincter not closed completely; may include discharge of pus or feces from a fistula connecting the rectum to the anal canal.
Change in bowel pattern	Unexplained change in bowel frequency or in stool form; may signal serious underlying GI disorder (e.g., IBD), colorectal cancer.
Prolapse (protrusion)	Protrusion of hemorrhoidal or rectal tissue of variable size into anal canal; usually appears after defecation, prolonged standing, unusual physical exertion, or swelling of hemorrhoidal tissue with loss of muscular support; painless except when accompanied by thrombosis, infection, or ulceration.
Thrombosis	Strangulation of protruded (external) hemorrhoid by anal sphincter possibly leading to thrombosis; associated pain is most acute during first 48–72 hours, but usually resolves after 7–10 days.
	Minimal pain with thrombosed internal hemorrhoids; likely to be unaware of condition unless sudden change in bowel habits occurs.
	If a thrombosed hemorrhoid persists, ulcers or gangrene may develop on the hemorrhoid's surface causing bleeding, especially during defecation.

Key: GI, gastrointestinal; IBD, inflammatory bowel disease; PUD, peptic ulcer disease.
Source: References 1, 12, and 18.

Proper bowel habits should be encouraged. The patient should avoid sitting on the toilet for longer than 10 minutes to reduce straining and decrease pressures on the hemorrhoidal vessels. Avoiding urges to defecate may lead to constipation and the formation of hemorrhoids.[7] Good anal hygiene may relieve symptoms and prevent the recurrence of perianal itching. The patient should clean the anal area regularly and after each bowel movement by using mild, unscented soap and water, or commercially available hygienic and lubricated wipes or pads. Avoiding excessive scrubbing of the anorectal area minimizes aggravation to the sensitive region.[1] Sitz baths promote good anal hygiene and often relieve hemorrhoidal symptoms, especially after bowel movements. When possible, the individual should sit in warm water (110°F to 115°F [43.3°C–46.1°C]) two to three times a day for about 15 minutes. Plastic sitz tubs fitting over the toilet rim are convenient, easily cleaned, and available at pharmacies and medical supply vendors.

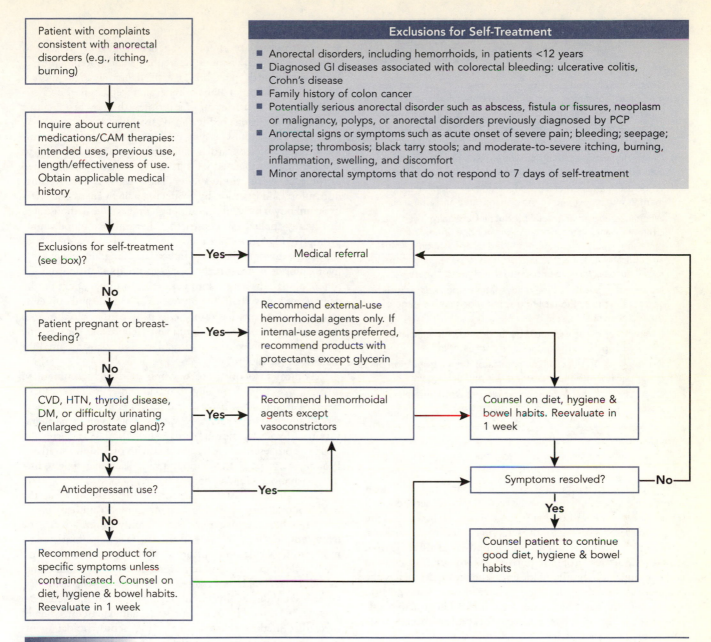

FIGURE 18-2 Self-care of hemorrhoids. Key: CAM, complementary and alternative medicine; CVD, cardiovascular disease; DM, diabetes mellitus; GI, gastrointestinal; HTN, hypertension; PCP, primary care provider.

Large and prolapsed hemorrhoids are often treated with surgery. A surgical procedure that involves excising one or more of the three hemorrhoidal masses is called a hemorrhoidectomy. Nonsurgical procedures for treating internal hemorrhoids include injection of sclerosing agents, rubber band ligation, dilation of the anal canal and lower rectum, cryosurgery, electrocoagulation, infrared photocoagulation, and local anal hypothermia.[7,20,21]

Pharmacologic Therapy

Pharmacologic agents used to relieve anorectal symptoms include local anesthetics, vasoconstrictors, protectants, astringents, keratolytics, analgesics/anesthetics/antipruritics, and corticosteroids. However, only certain astringents, protec-

tants, and vasoconstrictors may be used for internal hemorrhoidal symptoms. The remaining agents are for external use only. None of these agents are approved by FDA for the relief of anorectal pain, bleeding, seepage, prolapse, or thrombosis. Table 18-4 provides FDA–approved dosages for anorectal drug products.[19,22,23]

Local Anesthetics

Local or topical anesthetics temporarily relieve itching, irritation, burning, discomfort, and pain by reversibly blocking transmission of nerve impulses. Although there is minimal absorption with intact skin, the effects are more pronounced in areas with abraded skin. Local anesthetics should be used with caution; they may mask the pain of more severe anorectal disorders. Use of

TABLE 18-3 Guidelines for Applying or Inserting Anorectal Products

- Cleanse the affected area after bowel movement with mild, non-medicated, unscented soap and warm water; rinse thoroughly.
- Clean the anorectal area prior to applying products containing aluminum hydroxide gel or kaolin. Be sure to remove any previously used petrolatum-containing or greasy ointment.
- Gently dry area by patting or blotting with unscented and uncolored toilet tissue or a soft cloth prior to product application.
- When using an anorectal product externally, apply the ointment as a thin covering to the perianal area and anal canal.
- When inserting an anorectal product intrarectally, insert the ointment using an intrarectal applicator or a finger. Intrarectal applicators are preferred to digital application, because an applicator enables the drug product to be applied to the rectal mucosa (which cannot be reached with a finger).
- Intrarectal applicators should have lateral openings, as well as a hole in the tip, to facilitate application and coverage of the rectal mucosa.
- Intrarectal applicators should be lubricated before insertion by spreading ointment around the applicator tip.
- Do not use a product with an applicator if the introduction of the applicator into the rectum causes additional pain.
- Do not exceed the recommended daily dosage unless increase is directed by primary care provider.

Source: References 1 and 19.

these products should be limited to the perianal region or areas below the dentate line, because the rectum is not innervated with sensory nerve fibers.[1] Local anesthetics listed in Table 18-4 are approved for external use for the temporary relief of external anal symptoms.[1,19,22] These agents are composed of three distinct structure moieties: aromatic portion, intermediate chain, and amine group.[24] Categories of local anesthetics are defined by the nature of the chemical linkage between the aromatic portion and the intermediate chain, ester, or amide.[25] The structural differences give rise to different allergenicity and absence of cross-reactivity among agents.[26,27]

Contact dermatitis may be more common with benzocaine than with other topical anesthetics because of its chemical structure.[28] Patients who had an adverse reaction to benzocaine should use a different local anesthetic with a different chemical structure (e.g., pramoxine).[28] Preparations containing local anesthetics must carry a warning stating that allergic reactions may occur in some individuals.[1,19] Local anesthetics may produce local allergic reactions (e.g., burning and itching), which are indistinguishable from the anorectal symptoms being treated.

Local anesthetics should not be used internally, because pain receptors are not present in the rectal mucosa and because the agents may be rapidly absorbed through the rectal mucosa, potentially causing toxic systemic effects. Systemic reactions including cardiovascular and central nervous system effects may occur because of the abundant vasculature in the anal area. Accidental ingestion of dibucaine-containing anorectal products has been reported in children, resulting in lethargy, seizures, and cardiorespiratory arrest.[1] All anorectal products that contain local anesthetics (regardless of type) should be kept out of the reach of children.[29]

Vasoconstrictors

Vasoconstrictors are chemical agents structurally related to endogenous catecholamines: epinephrine and norepinephrine. When ephedrine or epinephrine is applied topically to the anorectal area, stimulation of alpha-adrenergic receptors in the vascular beds causes constriction of arterioles, thereby producing a modest and transient reduction of swelling. If absorbed systemically, beta-agonist activity may increase cardiac contractility, heart rate (tachycardia), and bronchodilation, leading to adverse effects associated with its anorectal use. When applied to the anal region, these agents (Table 18-4) relieve itching, discomfort, and irritation by producing a slight anesthetic effect by an unknown mechanism. Although studies have demonstrated that locally applied vasoconstrictors alter mucosal blood supply promptly, FDA does not recognize or approve of the use of such agents to control minor anorectal bleeding.[1] Phenylephrine hydrochloride is structurally related to norepinephrine and is a potent alpha-adrenergic stimulant with minimal effect on the central nervous system. In contrast to ephedrine and epinephrine, phenylephrine has minor effects on cardiac rhythm and, therefore, does not cause significant tachycardia.[1] Ephedrine sulfate and phenylephrine hydrochloride may also be used for internal hemorrhoids.[19,22]

Topical vasoconstrictors, when used in recommended dosages, may be systemically absorbed and cause nervousness, tremor, sleeplessness, nausea, and loss of appetite.[1] However, serious adverse effects such as elevation of blood pressure, aggravation of hyperthyroidism, cardiac arrhythmias, and irregular heart rate are less likely to occur than with oral administration.[1] Prolonged use may lead to rebound vasodilatation, anxiety, and, rarely, paranoia. Contact dermatitis may occur.

Rectally administered vasoconstrictors may attenuate the effects of oral antihypertensive agents and may increase blood pressure when administered concomitantly. Alternatively, the hypertensive effects of vasoconstrictors may be potentiated by monoamine oxidase inhibitors and tricyclic antidepressants. Concomitant use may lead to serious and even lethal outcomes including cerebral hemorrhage or stroke.[1,19] Patients with diabetes, thyroid disease, hypertension, angina pectoris, or enlarged prostate, and those taking antidepressants, antihypertensive agents, or cardiac medications should not use hemorrhoidal agents with vasoconstrictors without first consulting their primary care provider.[1,19]

Protectants

Protectants prevent irritation of the anorectal area and water loss from the stratum corneum by forming a physical barrier on the skin. These agents act as a protective coat over the affected areas and soften the dry anal area by decreasing water loss. Perianal irritation by fecal matter may be reduced by applying protectants to minimize discomfort in the affected anal area.[19] The protectant drug class includes absorbents, adsorbents, demulcents, and emollients. These agents listed in Table 18-4 are approved for the temporary relief of discomfort, itching, irritation, and burning associated with external and internal hemorrhoids, with the exception of glycerin, which is for external use only.[22] Products containing kaolin or aluminum hydroxide gel are indicated for the temporary relief of anorectal itching.

Systemic absorption of protectants is minimal; therefore, adverse reactions to these agents as a class are uncommon.

TABLE 18-4 Dosage Guidelines for Anorectal Products		
Ingredient	**Concentration per Dosage Unit (%)**	**Frequency of Use (Maximum Daily Dosage)**
Local Anesthetics		
Benzocaine	5–20	Up to 6 times/day (2.4 g)
Benzyl alcohol	1–4	Up to 6 times/day (480 mg)
Dibucaine, dibucaine hydrochloride	0.25–1	Up to 3–4 times/day (80 mg)
Dyclonine hydrochloride	0.5–1	Up to 6 times/day (100 mg)
Lidocaine	2–5	Up to 6 times/day (500 mg)
Pramoxine hydrochloride[a]	1	Up to 5 times/day (100 mg)
Tetracaine, tetracaine hydrochloride	0.5–1	Up to 6 times/day (100 mg)
Vasoconstrictors		
Ephedrine sulfate	0.1–1.25	Up to 4 times/day (100 mg)
Epinephrine hydrochloride/epinephrine	0.005–0.01	Up to 4 times/day (800 mg)
Phenylephrine hydrochloride	0.25	Up to 4 times/day (2 mg)
Protectants		
Aluminum hydroxide gel, cocoa butter, glycerin, hard fat, kaolin, lanolin, mineral oil, white petrolatum, petrolatum, shark liver oil, zinc oxide, topical starch, calamine, cod liver oil	See footnote b.	Petrolatum/white petrolatum: as often as needed; other protectants: up to 6 times/day or after each bowel movement
Astringents		
Calamine[c]	5–25	Up to 6 times/day or after each bowel movement
Zinc oxide	5–25	Up to 6 times/day or after each bowel movement
Witch hazel	10–50	Up to 6 times/day or after each bowel movement
Keratolytics		
Alcloxa	0.2–2	Up to 6 times/day
Resorcinol	1–3	Up to 6 times/day
Analgesics/anesthetics/antipruritics		
Menthol	0.1–1	Up to 6 times/day
Juniper tar	1–5	Up to 6 times/day
Camphor	0.1–3	Up to 6 times/day
Corticosteroids		
Hydrocortisone	0.25–1	Up to 3–4 times/day

[a] External dosage forms may include aerosol foams, ointments, creams, and jellies (water-miscible base).

[b] If a single protectant ingredient is used, it must comprise at least 50% of the product. Aluminum hydroxide gel and kaolin may not be combined with other protectants when the combined percentage by weight of all protectants in the combination is at least 50% of the final product. Aqueous solutions of glycerin cannot contain less than 20% or more than 45% glycerin (weight-to-weight).[1,19]

[c] Concentration of calamine is not to exceed 25% by weight/dosage unit (based on zinc oxide content of calamine).

Source: References 1 and 19.

Lanolin is a natural product obtained from the fleece of sheep. Wool alcohols are the principle components of lanolin in which allergens are found and are considered to be the main sensitizers. Chemically modified lanolin is available and may be less sensitizing.

Preparations containing aluminum hydroxide gel and kaolin are required to contain a warning that states petrolatum or greasy ointments should be removed before these agents are applied, because greasy substances interfere with the ability of aluminum hydroxide gel and kaolin to adhere properly to the skin.[19]

Astringents

Astringents applied to the anorectal area promote coagulation of skin cells, thereby protecting the underlying tissue while decreasing cell volume. In addition to coagulating the surface proteins, astringents form a thin layer protecting the underlying tissue from further irritation. Astringents cause contracting, wrinkling, and blanching of the affected area and decrease secretions, making the region drier.[19] Astringents listed in Table 18–4 are approved for the temporary relief of itching, irritation, and burning symptoms associated with anorectal disorders.[19] Witch hazel (hamamelis water, the original name prior to January 1, 1995) is indicated for external use, whereas calamine and zinc oxide may be used for both external and internal anorectal disorders.[19]

Adverse effects associated with the topical use of calamine, zinc oxide, and witch hazel are uncommon. Witch hazel may cause a slight stinging sensation when applied because of the alcohol used to prepare the compound. Contact dermatitis may occur with witch hazel owing to the small amount of volatile oil.[1] If calamine or zinc oxide is used for prolonged periods of time, especially for internal anorectal disorders, systemic zinc toxicity (nausea, vomiting, lethargy, and/or severe pain) may develop.

Keratolytics

Keratolytics cause desquamation and debridement, or sloughing, of epidermal surface cells. By fostering cell turnover and loosening surface cells, keratolytics may help expose underlying tissue, allowing local application of other medications. Keratolytics used externally in low concentrations are somewhat useful in reducing itching and discomfort, yet the exact mechanism of action is unknown. Because mucous membranes do not contain a keratin layer, intrarectal use of keratolytics is not justified and may be harmful.[19] Keratolytics approved for the temporary relief of external anorectal discomfort and itching in the perianal area are listed in Table 18-4.[19]

With repeated dosing, the absorption of resorcinol has led to methemoglobinemia, exfoliative dermatitis, and death in infants, and myxedema in adults.[1] Other adverse effects range from ringing in the ears, increased pulse rate, sweating, and shortness of breath to methemoglobinemia, circulatory collapse, unconsciousness, and convulsions. Preparations containing resorcinol must list the following warnings: (1) "Certain persons can develop allergic reactions to ingredients in this product. If the symptoms being treated do not subside or if redness, irritation, swelling, pain or other symptoms develop or increase, discontinue use and consult a doctor." (2) "Do not use on open wounds near the anus" to minimize absorption through abraded mucosal lining and decrease potential for systemic toxicity.[19] Although keratolytics are available in selected anorectal preparations, their use must be weighed against their potentially serious adverse effects.

Analgesics/Anesthetics/Antipruritics

Formerly classified as "counterirritants," menthol, juniper tar, and camphor are safe and effective when used externally in the perianal area. Such agents relieve pain, itching, burning, or discomfort by producing a local sensation that distracts from these complaints. Local sensations include cool, warm, or tingling relief. The agents should not be used internally, because the rectum has no identifiable nerve fibers. The products listed in Table 18-4 are approved for the temporary relief of itching, discomfort, pain, and burning associated with perianal disorders when applied to the involved area.[1,19,22] Menthol-containing products must bear the following warning: "Certain persons can develop allergic reactions to ingredients in this product. If the symptoms being treated do not subside or if redness, irritation, swelling, pain, or other symptoms develop or increase, discontinue use and consult a doctor."[19] In addition, extensive application of menthol to the trunk of the body has caused laryngospasm, dyspnea, and cyanosis; it is important to use these preparations sparingly.[1]

Corticosteroids

Topical hydrocortisone acts as a vasoconstrictor and antipruritic. This agent has the potential to reduce itching and pain by producing lysosomal membrane stabilization and antimitotic activity. Its onset of action may require up to 12 hours, but its effect has a longer duration than most other agents (e.g., local anesthetics). Hydrocortisone is the only corticosteroid approved for nonprescription use in anorectal preparations. The maximum permitted concentration is 1%. Hydrocortisone is indicated for the temporary relief of minor external anal itching caused by minor irritation or rash. Hydrocortisone may mask the symptoms of bacterial and fungal infections.

Combination Products

Federal regulations state that a nonprescription product may combine two or more safe and effective active ingredients, and generally be recognized as safe and effective when (1) each active ingredient contributes to the claimed effect; (2) the combination of active ingredients does not decrease the safety or effectiveness of any individual active ingredient; and (3) the combination, when listing adequate directions for use and warning against unsafe use, provides rational, concurrent therapy for a significant proportion of the target population.[23] FDA restrictions on the number and type of agents that may be combined in nonprescription anorectal preparations can be found elsewhere.[19]

Combination products are reasonable given that some self-treatable anorectal disorders may have concurrent symptoms. However, there is no evidence that an anorectal preparation with a combination of active ingredients is more effective than a preparation with a therapeutic amount of a single ingredient. Theoretically, restricting the number of ingredients in the anorectal preparation should decrease the risk of interactions and adverse drug reactions, and lessen the likelihood of altering the product's effectiveness.

Product Selection Guidelines

Table 18-5 contains examples of products that the clinician can recommend.

Knowledge of a patient's medical history, medication profile, and relevant socioeconomic factors is necessary to determine how an individual may respond to self-treatment. The clinician should decide on a suitable anorectal product, while taking into account the following patient history: (1) the type, location, and severity of the anorectal disorder; (2) diseases or significant past medical history; (3) medications or allergies; (4) ability to apply or insert the medication (physical, mental, and emotional limitations); and (5) any other factors, such as diet, daily activities, or cost of the product, that may affect treatment.

SPECIAL POPULATIONS

Pregnant and breast-feeding women should use products recommended for external use except for the recommended protectants, which may be used internally. Children younger than 12 years of age with hemorrhoids or any other anorectal disorder should be referred to a primary care provider.[1,19]

PATIENT FACTORS

FDA does not require comparison trials between combination and individual products, so therapeutic differences are unknown. However, combination products containing

TABLE 18-5 Selected Products for Hemorrhoids

Trade Name	Primary Ingredients
Local Anesthetics	
Americaine Ointment	Benzocaine 20%
Fleet Pain-Relief Pads	Pramoxine HCl 1%; glycerin 12%
Nupercainal Ointment	Dibucaine 1%; lanolin; white petrolatum; light mineral oil
Tronolane Cream	Pramoxine HCl 1%; zinc oxide 5%; glycerin
TUCKS Hemorrhoidal Ointment	Pramoxine HCl 1%; zinc oxide 12.5%; mineral oil 46.6%; cocoa butter; kaolin
Vasoconstrictors	
Hemorid Crème	Phenylephrine HCl 0.25%; pramoxine HCl 1%; white petrolatum 30%; mineral oil 20%
Hemorid Ointment	Phenylephrine HCl 0.25%; pramoxine HCl 1%; white petrolatum 82.15%; light mineral oil 12.5%
Preparation H Cooling Gel	Witch hazel 50%; phenylephrine HCl 0.25%
Preparation H Suppositories	Phenylephrine HCl 0.25%; cocoa butter 85.5%; shark liver oil 3%; starch
Skin Protectants	
Balneol Lotion	Mineral oil; lanolin oil
Preparation H Ointment	Mineral oil 14%; petrolatum 71.9%; phenylephrine HCl 0.25%; shark liver oil 3%; glycerin; lanolin
TUCKS Topical Starch Hemorrhoidal Suppositories	Topical starch 51%
Hydrocortisone Products	
Preparation H Anti-Itch Cream with Hydrocortisone 1%	Hydrocortisone 1%; glycerin; lanolin; methylparaben; petrolatum
TUCKS Hydrocortisone Anti-Itch Ointment	Hydrocortisone acetate 1.12% (equivalent to hydrocortisone 1%); mineral oil; white petrolatum
Miscellaneous Combination Products	
Preparation H Cream with Maximum Strength Pain Relief	Glycerin USP 14.4%; phenylephrine HCL 0.25%; pramoxine HCL 1%; white petrolatum 15%; mineral oil
TUCKS Medicated Pads	Witch hazel 50%; glycerin
TUCKS Take Alongs Medicated Towelettes	Witch hazel 50%; glycerin

approved ingredients in appropriate dosages are most likely therapeutically similar to individual drug products when used to treat indicated anorectal symptoms. Any perceived differences by patients are most likely related to personal preference for a specific product or dosage form. Using more than one product or products containing multiple ingredients is reasonable, because patients may have multiple different symptoms that may not be treated by one product alone.

Medications used to treat anorectal disorders are available in many dosage forms including ointments, creams, suppositories, and gels. Applicators, intrarectal applicators, or the patient's fingers are used to facilitate applying and instilling the preparations. Creams, ointments, gels, pastes, liquids, and foams are used externally. Although considerable pharmaceutical differences exist among ointments, creams, pastes, and gels, therapeutic differences do not appear to be clinically different. This discussion uses the term *ointment* to refer to all semisolid preparations designed for intrarectal or external use in the anorectal area. The primary function of an ointment is to provide a vehicle for the safe and efficient delivery of the active ingredients, yet some ointments also possess inherent protectant and emollient properties.

Suppositories provide a lubricating effect, which eases straining at defecation, thereby alleviating hemorrhoidal symptoms. However, suppositories should not be recommended as an initial dosage form, because they may leave the affected anal region and ascend into the rectum and lower colon when the patient is in a prone (lying with the face downward) position. If the patient remains prone after inserting a suppository or an ointment, the active ingredients may not distribute evenly over the anal mucosa. Also, suppositories are relatively slow acting given that they must dissolve to release the active ingredients (see Chapter 16).

Foam products should theoretically provide more rapid release of active ingredients than ointments. However, foam dosage forms are more expensive than ointments and do not offer any important advantage. In addition, foams may not remain in the affected area, and differences in the size of the foam bubbles may result in different concentrations of the active ingredient.

Complementary Therapies

Dietary supplements used to treat hemorrhoids have been poorly researched, although several have evidence of efficacy to support their use.[30,31] The combination of diosmin and hesperidin, a micronized purified flavonoid fraction, has been used to stop acute hemorrhoidal bleeding and decrease the intensity of hemorrhoidal symptoms.[32] The mechanism of action is still in question, but in animal models it is thought to inhibit prostaglandin and thromboxane mediators, thus decreasing the inflammatory processes. The combination appears safe when both are taken orally for less than 6 months, with the most common adverse effects being abdominal pain, diarrhea, and gastritis.[32] Purified diosmin without hesperidin administered orally or topically has also been shown to be effective in reducing pain, bleeding, and swelling associated with hemorrhoids.[31] Butcher's broom combined with other dietary supplements such as flavonoids has been found effective for the treatment of hemorrhoids.[30] Horse chestnut seed extract (HCSE) has been used to treat hemorrhoids effectively and is considered relatively safe when processed properly; the most common side effects include itching, nausea, and vomiting.[33] However, improperly prepared HCSE preparations may be poisonous and may lead to death. (See Chapter 54 for further discussion of HCSE.)

Assessment of Anorectal Disorders: A Case-Based Approach

The clinician should obtain a thorough description of the patient's signs and symptoms to accurately assess whether the anorectal disorder is self-treatable. If the condition is self-treatable, targeted questions should be asked about the presence of specific diseases (e.g., hypertension, diabetes mellitus, and benign prostatic hyperplasia), prescription and non-prescription medications, complementary and alternative medicines, as well as diet and lifestyle, before recommending self-treatment.

Cases 18-1 and 18-2 illustrate assessment of patients with anorectal disorders.

CASE 18-1

Relevant Evaluation Criteria	Scenario/Model Outcome
Information Gathering	
1. Gather essential information about the patient's symptoms, including:	
a. description of symptom(s) (i.e., nature, onset, duration, severity, associated symptoms)	Patient complains of itching and discomfort in the anal area that has lasted 3 days. The itching occurs mostly after having a bowel movement and diminishes throughout the day. She reports blood is present on the stool with each bowel movement.
b. description of any factors that seem to precipitate, exacerbate, and/or relieve the patient's symptom(s)	Discomfort and bleeding are associated with each bowel movement.
c. description of the patient's efforts to relieve the symptoms	Taking a shower after each bowel movement for the past 3 days somewhat helps relieve the itching. Scratching the anal area also helps the discomfort.
2. Gather essential patient history information:	
a. patient's identity	Jackie Smither
b. patient's age, sex, height, and weight	36-year-old female, 5 ft 6 in, 134 lb
c. patient's occupation	Stay-at-home mom who gave birth 7 days ago. (She gave birth to a 6.8-lb, 15.1-inch baby girl via vaginal delivery with no complications.)
d. patient's dietary habits	Normal diet includes fruits, vegetables and meats. (She is not breastfeeding her daughter.)
e. patient's sleep habits	Lack of sleep because she has to be awake frequently to tend to the newborn; sleeps about 5 hours each night, interrupted
f. concurrent medical conditions, prescription and nonprescription medications, and dietary supplements	Prenatal vitamin; Colace (She stopped taking it after giving birth 7 days ago.)
g. allergies	NKDA
h. history of other adverse reactions to medications	None
i. other (describe) family history _____	Mom died of colon cancer at the age of 49.
Assessment and Triage	
3. Differentiate the patient's signs/symptoms and correctly identify the patient's primary problem(s) (see Tables 18-1 and 18-2).	Jackie complains of itching, discomfort, and bleeding with each bowel movement for the past 3 days. She recently gave birth to a baby and stopped taking her stool softener, yet she continues the prenatal vitamin. Her stools may be harder now, causing the passage of hard stools, bleeding, and essentially the formation of hemorrhoids.
4. Identify exclusions for self-treatment (see Figure 18-2).	Blood on the stool

CASE 18-1 (continued)

Relevant Evaluation Criteria	Scenario/Model Outcome
5. Formulate a comprehensive list of therapeutic alternatives for the primary problem to determine if triage to a medical practitioner is required, and share this information with the patient.	Options include: (1) Recommend self-care with an appropriate nonprescription anorectal product and advise on nondrug measures. (2) Recommend self-care with an appropriate anorectal product and advise on nondrug measures until Jackie contacts her PCP. (3) Refer Jackie to her PCP for medical evaluation. (4) Take no action.

Plan

6. Select an optimal therapeutic alternative to address the patient's problem, taking into account patient preferences.	See Table 18-5 and Figure 18-2. Jackie should be referred for medical evaluation to rule out bleeding from a source other than a hemorrhoid, considering that she has a family history of colon cancer. An appropriate anorectal product from Table 18-5 should be recommended to relieve the symptoms until she can be seen by her PCP.
7. Describe the recommended therapeutic approach to the patient.	You should contact your PCP as soon as possible so that he or she is aware of the bleeding. In the meantime, you can take some steps to relieve your itching and discomfort. Apply an anorectal ointment listed in Table 18-5 as described in Tables 18-3 and 18-4. Continuing your prenatal vitamin and stopping the stool softener for the past week may be contributing to your hard stools. Consider increasing fiber intake and drinking plenty of water, or resume the stool softener. See Chapter 16.
8. Explain to the patient the rationale for selecting the recommended therapeutic approach from the considered therapeutic alternatives.	Although your symptoms, including blood in the stools, may be related to hemorrhoids, it is important for you to contact your PCP for further evaluation, because other conditions may also cause similar symptoms and rectal bleeding.

Patient Education

9. When recommending self-care with nonprescription medications and/or nondrug therapy, convey accurate information to the patient:	
a. appropriate dose and frequency of administration	See Table 18-4.
b. maximum number of days the therapy should be employed	Contact your PCP as soon as possible even if your symptoms resolve with treatment. Be sure to let your PCP know what self-care measures you have taken, and ask whether you should continue with your self-treatment program if your symptoms do not resolve after 7 days.
c. product administration procedures	See Table 18-3.
d. expected time to onset of relief	Itching, irritation, and discomfort may be relieved within a few days of applying the topical agent as directed. Straining may be relieved with adequate fluids and a healthy diet, or with a stool softener or fiber supplement. Although bleeding may stop with treatment, still contact the PCP.
e. degree of relief that can be reasonably expected	Complete relief of itching, discomfort, and bleeding is possible.
f. most common side effects	Most products applied to the anal area are usually well tolerated.
g. side effects that warrant medical intervention should they occur	If you develop an allergic reaction (e.g., redness, swelling, increased irritation, or pain) to the ointment, discontinue use and contact your PCP as soon as possible.
h. patient options in the event that condition worsens or persists	If your symptoms worsen, contact your PCP as soon as possible.
i. product storage requirements	Store medication out of the reach of children and at a controlled room temperature.
j. specific nondrug measures	Practice good anal hygiene, take sitz baths, and consider modifying your diet to increase fluids and fiber to soften stools and decrease straining. See Chapter 16.
10. Solicit follow-up questions from patient.	Do I need surgery?
11. Answer patient's questions.	Probably not. The hemorrhoidal symptoms should resolve with good anal hygiene and proper diet.

Key: PCP, primary care provider.

Relevant Evaluation Criteria	Scenario/Model Outcome
Information Gathering	
1. Gather essential information about the patient's symptoms, including:	
a. description of symptom(s) (i.e., nature, onset, duration, severity, associated symptoms)	Patient complains of mild discomfort and itching in the anal area over the past few weeks after having a bowel movement. Symptoms remained the same over this period of time and have not worsened. The stool firmness has not changed and no blood is present in the toilet or on the toilet paper.
b. description of any factors that seem to precipitate, exacerbate, and/or relieve the patient's symptom(s)	Symptoms are worse when he sits for prolonged periods of time. Exercising prior to bedtime makes the anal discomfort less irritating. There is no change in soaps or detergents.
c. description of the patent's efforts to relieve the symptoms	None
2. Gather essential patient history information:	
a. patient's identity	Mark Blaine
b. patient's age, sex, height and weight	51-year-old white male, 5 ft 10 in, 211 lb
c. patient's occupation	Software programmer
d. patient's dietary habits	Moderate-carbohydrate, moderate-protein, low-fat, low-cholesterol diet
e. patient's sleep habits	Averages 10 hours per night
f. concurrent medical conditions, prescription and nonprescription medications, and dietary supplements	Gemfibrozil 600 mg twice daily for hypertriglyceridemia for 10 years, OTC omeprazole as needed for acid reflux
g. allergies	NKA
h. history of other adverse reactions to medications	None
i. other (describe) _____	None
Assessment and Triage	
3. Differentiate patient's signs/symptoms and correctly identify the patient's primary problem(s) (see Tables 18-1 and 18-2).	Mark complains of mild discomfort and itching in the anal area that has occurred over the past few weeks, mostly after having a bowel movement. Symptoms remained the same over this period of time and have not worsened. Patient denies any changes in stool hardness, or noticing any blood in the toilet or on the toilet paper. These symptoms are most likely associated with hemorrhoids.
4. Identify exclusions for self-treatment (see Figure 18-2).	Mark does not appear to have any exclusions for self-care. No constipation or rectal bleeding was noted.
5. Formulate a comprehensive list of therapeutic alternatives for the primary problem to determine if triage to a medical practitioner is required and share this information with the patient.	Options include: (1) Recommend self-care with an appropriate nonprescription anorectal product and advise on nondrug measures. (2) Recommend self-care with an appropriate anorectal product and advise on nondrug measures until he contacts his PCP. (3) Refer to his PCP for medical evaluation of his symptoms. (4) Take no action.
Plan	
6. Select an optimal therapeutic alternative to address the patient's problem, taking into account patient preferences.	The optimal anorectal product should relieve the patient's discomfort and anal itching. Figure 18-2 lists appropriate therapeutic options. Table 18-5 lists specific products. Mark states that he prefers an ointment-containing hydrocortisone.
7. Describe the recommended therapeutic approach to the patient.	Apply the hydrocortisone 1% ointment to the external anal area up to 3 to 4 times a day, preferably after a bowel movement and at bedtime as described in Table 18-3.
8. Explain to the patient the rationale for selecting the recommended therapeutic approach from the considered therapeutic alternatives.	You do not need to see your PCP at this time, because your symptoms are relatively mild and may be related to hemorrhoids, which are usually treated with nonprescription products. Hydrocortisone 1% ointment, when applied to the anal area, should provide temporary relief of the itching, burning, and discomfort that you describe.

CASE 18-2 *(continued)*

Relevant Evaluation Criteria	Scenario/Model Outcome

Patient Education

9. When recommending self-care with nonprescription medications and/or nondrug therapy, convey accurate information to the patient:

   a. appropriate dose and frequency of administration — See Table 18-4.

   b. maximum number of days the therapy should be employed — 7 days

   c. product administration procedures — See Table 18-3.

   d. expected time to onset of relief — Symptom relief should be evident within a few days of applying the ointment as directed.

   e. degree of relief that can be reasonably expected — Complete relief of your itching, burning, and discomfort is possible.

   f. most common side effects — Hydrocortisone ointment, when applied to the anal area, is usually well tolerated.

   g. side effects that warrant medical intervention should they occur — Hydrocortisone ointment may mask the symptoms of an infection. If this occurs, you may notice worsening or recurrence of your symptoms when you discontinue this medication.

   h. patient options in the event that condition worsens or persists — Contact your PCP if your symptoms worsen or persist beyond 7 days of self-treatment. See the box Patient Education for Hemorrhoids.

   i. product storage requirements — Store medication out of the reach of children and at a controlled room temperature.

   j. specific nondrug measures — See the box Patient Education for Hemorrhoids.

10. Solicit follow-up questions from patient. — Will the hydrocortisone cause me to have diabetes?

11. Answer patient's questions — No. The hydrocortisone is administered topically; therefore, the amount of hydrocortisone absorbed should be minimal. Also, the treatment duration is for a very short time; therefore, it should not cause diabetes.

Key: OTC, over-the-counter; PCP, primary care provider.

Patient Counseling for Anorectal Disorders

The clinician should explain the most appropriate drug and nondrug measures for treating patient-specific anorectal signs and symptoms. Patient counseling should include information on dosage and frequency of administration, administration technique, possible adverse effects, precautions or warnings, and product storage. In addition, clinicians should be sure the patient understands when self-care of anorectal disorders should be discontinued and when to consult the primary care provider. The box Patient Education for Anorectal Disorders lists specific information to provide patients.

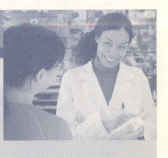

PATIENT EDUCATION FOR
Anorectal Disorders

The objectives of self-treatment are to relieve specific signs and symptoms and prevent complications leading to serious problems. For most patients, carefully following product instructions and self-care measures listed here will help ensure relief of symptoms.

Nondrug Measures

- Maintain hydration and a healthy diet. If experiencing hard stools, straining, or constipation, increase amount of fiber and fluids in the diet to reduce or prevent straining during bowel movements (see Chapter 16).

- If possible, avoid medications that cause constipation (see Chapter 16).
- Clean anorectal area after each bowel movement with a moistened, unscented, white toilet tissue or a wipe.
- A sitz bath or a soak in the bathtub two to three times a day may help mild anal itching, burning, irritation, and discomfort.

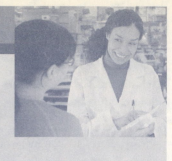

PATIENT EDUCATION FOR
Anorectal Disorders (continued)

Nonprescription Medications

- Anorectal products contain local anesthetics, vasoconstrictors, protectants, astringents, keratolytics, and/or analgesics/anesthetics/antipruritics. Select products containing only ingredients needed to relieve specific symptoms.
- See Table 18-3 for guidelines for applying anorectal products.
- See Table 18-4 for recommended dosages.
- Use only selected vasoconstrictors (ephedrine and phenylephrine), protectants (not glycerin), and astringents (calamine and zinc oxide) inside the rectum.
- Use only products approved for external use if patient is pregnant. If internal use is required, protectants with the exception of glycerin, may be used.
- If patient has a history of cardiovascular disease, diabetes, hyperthyroidism, hypertension, or difficulty urinating due to prostate problems, avoid topical products containing vasoconstrictors.
- If patients are taking medications to treat hypertension or depression, then avoid the use of any anorectal product containing vasoconstrictors without first consulting your primary care provider.
- Anorectal products containing ephedrine sulfate or phenylephrine may cause nervousness, tremor, sleeplessness, nausea, and loss of appetite.
- Appropriate use of anorectal products should reduce or relieve symptoms within a few days of self-treatment.

- Patient preferences should be considered, especially when specific products may be used to treat the same symptoms, when there is a choice between an ointment and a suppository, and when generic products are available.

 Stop using the anorectal product and contact a primary care provider as soon as possible if insertion of a product into the rectum causes pain.

 Contact a primary care provider if symptoms worsen, new symptoms such as bleeding develop, or symptoms do not improve after 7 days of self-treatment.

 Certain people may develop allergic or hypersensitivity reactions to products containing recommended concentrations of approved ingredients. Discontinue product and contact a primary care provider as soon as side effects develop, such as a rash or increased itching, redness, burning, or swelling in the anorectal area.

Evaluation of Patient Outcomes for Anorectal Disorders

Self-treatment of anorectal disorders should be limited to minor symptoms. If serious or severe symptoms are present or become progressively worse, then the patient should be advised to contact his or her primary care provider. In addition, if alarm signs or symptoms are present, including blood in the stool and severe anal pain, or if symptoms persist beyond 7 days of self-treatment, the patient should be counseled to seek immediate medical attention.[19] If symptoms resolve, the patient should be encouraged to maintain a well-balanced diet, good personal hygiene, and good bowel habits.

Key Points for Anorectal Disorders

➤ Limit self-treatment of anorectal disorders to minor symptoms such as burning, itching, discomfort, swelling, and irritation.

➤ Refer patients with anorectal seepage, bleeding, thrombosis, severe pain, or a change in bowel patterns.

➤ Advise patients with self-treatable symptoms that, if symptoms worsen or do not improve after 7 days, they should contact their primary care provider.

➤ Use only products for external use (except for protectants) in pregnant and breast-feeding women.

➤ Refer children younger than 12 years with anorectal disorders to their primary care provider.

➤ Advise patients to select an anorectal product containing the fewest number of ingredients necessary to treat specific symptoms to minimize undesirable effects.

➤ Instruct patients on how to use or apply specific anorectal products (Table 18–3).

➤ Counsel patients with hemorrhoids on nondrug measures such as dietary measures and perianal hygiene (see the box Patient Education for Anorectal Disorders).

➤ Do not use anorectal products containing vasoconstrictors in patients with conditions such as diabetes, hypertension, and cardiac disease because of the possibility of systemic adverse effects.

➤ Advise patients of the advantages and disadvantages of various anorectal dosage forms so they can select a product that is best suited for them

REFERENCES

1. US Food and Drug Administration. Anorectal drug products for over-the-counter human use: establishment of a monograph. *Fed Regist.* 1980; 45:35576–7.
2. Johanson JF. Hemorrhoids. In: Everhart JE, ed. *Digestive Diseases in the United States: Epidemiology and Impact.* US Department of Health and Human Services, Public Health Service, National Institutes of Health, National Institutes of Diabetes, Digestive and Kidney Diseases. Washington, DC: US Government Printing Office; 1994:271–98. NIH Publication No. 94-1447.
3. Fleming H. OTCs pharmacists recommend most. *Drug Top.* 2000;14:24.
4. Levy S. Hemorrhoidal remedies category up across all outlets. *Drug Top.* August 6, 2001. Available at: http://www.drugtopics.com/drugtopics/article/articleDetail.jsp?id=118857. Last accessed August 24, 2008.
5. Madoff RD, Fleshman JW, Clinical Practice Committee, American Gastroenterological Association. American Gastroenterological Association technical review on the diagnosis and treatment of hemorrhoids. *Gastroenterology.* 2004;126:1463–73.
6. Abrameowitz L, Sobhani I, Benifla JL, et al. Anal fissure and thrombosed external hemorrhoids before and after delivery. *Dis Colon Rectum.* 2002; 45:650–5.

7. Hull T. Examination and diseases of the anorectum. In: Feldman M, Friedman LS, Sleisenger MH, eds. *Sleisenger & Fordtran's Gastrointestinal and Liver Disease: Pathophysiology/Diagnosis/Management.* 7th ed. Philadelphia: WB Saunders; 2002:2277–93.

8. Ahmed SK, Thomson HJ. The effect of breakfast on minor anal complaints: a matched case-control study. *J R Coll Surg Edinb.* 1997;42:331–3.

9. Johanson JF. Nonsurgical treatment of hemorrhoids. *J Gastrointest Surg.* 2002;6:290–4.

10. Delco F, Sonnenberg A. Associations between hemorrhoids and other diagnoses. *Dis Colon Rectum.* 1998;41:1534–41.

11. Barnett JL. Anorectal diseases. In: Yamada T, Alpers DH, Powell DW, et al., eds. *Textbook of Gastroenterology.* 4th ed. Philadelphia: JB Lippincott; 2003:1990–2012.

12. Lunniss PJ, Mann CV. Classification of internal haemorrhoids: a discussion paper. *Colorectal Dis.* 2004;6:226–32.

13. Pfenninger JL, Zainea GG. Common anorectal conditions: part II, lesions. *Am Fam Physician.* 2001;64:77–88.

14. Hyman N. Anorectal abscess and fistula. *Prim Care.* 1999; 26:69–80.

15. Madoff RD, Fleshman JW. AGA technical review on the diagnosis and care of patients with anal fissure. *Gastroenterology.* 2003;124:235–45.

16. Moore HG, Guillem JG. Anal neoplasms. *Surg Clin North Am.* 2002; 82:1233–51.

17. Vincent C. Anorectal pain and irritation—anal fissure, levator syndrome, proctalgia fugax, and pruritus ani. *Prim Care.* 1999;26:53–68.

18. Pfenninger JL, Zainea GG. Common anorectal conditions: part I, symptoms and complaints. *Am Fam Physician.* 2001;63:2391–8.

19. US Food and Drug Administration. Anorectal drug products for over-the-counter human use. *Fed Regist.* 2002;5:265–70.

20. Hussain JN. Hemorrhoids. *Prim Care.* 1999;26:35–51.

21. El Ashaal Y, Chandran V, Prem V, et al. Short note: local anal hypothermia with a frozen finger: a treatment for acute painful prolapsed piles. *Br J Surg.* 1998;85:520–1.

22. US Food and Drug Administration. Anorectal drug products for over-the-counter human use: tentative final monograph. *Fed Regist.* 1988;53: 30756–8.

23. US Food and Drug Administration. Anorectal drug products for over-the-counter human use. *CFR.* 2004; Title 21, Vol 5, Pt 346. Available at: http://www.fda.gov/search/databases.html. Last accessed August 24, 2008.

24. Skidmore RA, Patterson JD, Tomsick RS. Local anesthetic. *Dermatol Surg.* 1996;22:511–22.

25. Eggleston ST, Lush LW. Understanding allergic reactions to local anesthetics. *Ann Pharmacother.* 1996;30:851–7.

26. Sanchez-Perez J, Cordoba S, Cortizas CF, et al. Allergic contact balanitis due to tetracaine (amethocaine) hydrochloride. *Contact Dermat.* 1998; 39:268.

27. Young Lee AI. Allergic contact dermatitis from dibucaine in proctosedyl ointment without cross-sensitivity. *Contact Dermatitis.* 1998;39:261.

28. Lodi A, Ambonati M, Coassini A, et al. Contact allergy to 'caines' by anti-hemorrhoidal ointments. *Contact Dermat.* 1999;41:221–2.

29. US Food and Drug Administration. Requirements for child-resistant packaging; requirements for products containing lidocaine or dibucaine. *Fed Regist.* 1995; 60:17992–8005.

30. Abascal K, Yarnell E. Botanical treatments for hemorrhoids. *Altern Complement Ther.* 2005;11:285–9.

31. Misra MC, Imlitemus. Drug treatment of haemorrhoids. *Drugs.* 2005; 65:1481–91.

32. Misra MC, Parshad R. Randomized clinical trial of micronized flavonoids in the early control of bleeding from acute internal haemorrhoids. *Br J Surg.* 2000;87:868–72.

33. National Center for Complementary and Alternative Medicine Herbs at a Glance: Horse Chestnut. Update June 2008. Available at: http://nccam.nih.gov/health/horsechestnut. Last accessed August 15, 2008.

Pinworm Infection

Jeffery A. Goad and Joycelyn Mallari

Parasitic helminth (worms) infections cause significant morbidity and mortality worldwide. This chapter will focus on the detection and management of pinworm (*Enterobius vermicularis*) infection, because it is the most common worm infestation in the United States and is the only helminthic infection for which a nonprescription medication has been approved for treatment. Although pinworms are a nuisance, the infection presents little risk to the infected individual or the public. Rarely, infestations involving the genitourinary tract may occur. Table 19-1 is a summary of the sources of infection, common signs and symptoms, and treatment options for pinworms.[1–3]

Enterobiasis is also known as oxyuriasis or "pinworm," "seatworm," and "threadworm" infection. In the United States, pinworm infection is the most common of all worm infections, occurring in an estimated 42 million people, with the greatest infection rate in children ages 5 to 14 years.[4] Humans are the only hosts of *E. vermicularis*. Unlike most other worm infections, pinworms do not live in the soil or water and are not transmitted through animal feces. However, animal fur of household dogs and cats may be carriers of infective eggs.[5] Enterobiasis is associated with all socioeconomic levels and, in contrast to other helminthic infections, does not affect any particular race or culture. *E. vermicularis* is more often spread among individuals in institutionalized groups, child care facilities, hospitals, and family members.[4,5]

Pathophysiology of Pinworm Infection

The most common pinworm transmission route is through ingestion of infective eggs by direct anus-to-mouth transfer by fingers or fomites. Reinfection may occur readily, because eggs often are found under fingernails of infected children who have scratched the anal area. Finger sucking may be considered a source of infection, particularly in children with recurring symptoms.[5] Nail biting and nose picking, however, have not been associated with the initial infection but can certainly contribute to reinfection.[1] Embryonated eggs also can be transferred from the perianal region to clothes, bedding, or bathroom fixtures and dust. The eggs can remain viable for 20 days, especially under humid conditions, and can spread within a microcommunity, such as a household or school.[6]

The adult pinworm is small, white, and thread-like with a pin-shaped pointed tail (from which the name is derived; see Color Plates, photograph 1A).[4,6] Adult male and female worms inhabit the first portion, or ileocecum, of the large intestine and seldom cause damage to the intestinal wall. The mature female, approximately 8 to 13 mm in length, usually stores approximately 11,000 eggs in her body (see Color Plates, photograph 1B). After migrating down the colon and out the anus, she deposits her sticky eggs in the perianal region and dies shortly afterward. Males are smaller (2.5 mm), live only approximately 2 weeks, and do not migrate.[5,7] If eggs are not washed off, they hatch within a few hours, and larvae may return to the large intestine through the anus (retroinfection) or, rarely, in female patients, may mistakenly crawl into the urogenital tract where they may cause pelvic inflammatory disease or urinary tract infections.[8] Up to 36% of young girls with a urinary tract infection may be infected with pinworms, and the pinworm infection is harder to treat owing to the low absorption of the antiparasitic agents.[6] Within 2 to 6 weeks of egg ingestion, larvae are released and mature into gravid females, thus continuing the cycle indefinitely unless appropriate behavioral and pharmacotherapeutic interventions are instituted.

Clinical Presentation of Pinworm Infection

Patients with minor pinworm infections are often asymptomatic. The most frequent symptom is usually an irritating perianal or perineal itch that typically occurs at night when the female deposits eggs. Major infections may produce symptoms ranging from abdominal pain, insomnia, and restlessness, to anorexia, diarrhea, and intractable localized itching.[1,5,6] Less common clinical features may include vaginitis, pelvic inflammatory disease, urethritis, dysuria, urinary tract infection, and hives.[1,6] Patients with these symptoms should be referred to a primary care provider for further evaluation. Depending upon the age of the patient, the pharmacist should rule out other common pediatric conditions, such as diaper dermatitis and constipation, before recommending treatment or referral.

In addition to physical signs and symptoms, psychological trauma (i.e., pinworm neurosis) to patients and parents can also occur when worms are found near a child's anus. Patients and parents need to be assured that pinworms are common and curable, and that no social stigma is attached to their occurrence.

Scratching to relieve itching from pinworm infection may lead to secondary bacterial infection of the perianal and perineal

TABLE 19-1	Pinworm Infection and Treatment			
Common Name (Scientific Name)	**Source of Infection**	**Clinical Features**	**Treatment**	**Comments**
Pinworm (*Enterobius vermicularis*)	Autoinoculation with eggs by anus-to-mouth transfer; retroinfection: larvae return to rectum; transmission: egg-contaminated fomites and aerosolized eggs	Minor infections asymptomatic; most frequent symptoms: irritating itch in perianal and perineal regions, usually at night; children: nervousness, inability to concentrate, lack of appetite	Drugs of choice: Rx: mebendazole (Vermox); adult/pediatric (>2 years) dose: 100 mg once; repeat in 2 weeks if symptoms do not resolve OTC: pyrantel (Pin-X, Reese's Pinworm); adult/pediatric dose: 11 mg/kg once (max: 1 g); repeat in 2 weeks if symptoms do not resolve Rx alternatives: albendazole (Albenza); adult/pediatric dose: 400 mg once; repeat in 2 weeks if symptoms do not resolve	Mebendazole is available as chewable tablets. Pyrantel is OTC, and available as oral suspension, liquid, chewable tablets, caplets. High rate of reinfection often necessitates re-treatment.

Source: References 1–3.

regions. Helminthic infections in the genital tract may lead to endometritis, salpingitis, tubo-ovarian abscess, pelvic inflammatory disease, vulvovaginitis, and possibly infertility.[6,8] Pinworms may also migrate into the peritoneal cavity and form granulomas. Rarely, they may cause appendicitis in children.[9]

Treatment of Pinworm Infection

Treatment Goals

The goal of self-treatment is to eradicate pinworms from the patient and the household, thereby preventing reinfection.

General Treatment Approach

The management of pinworm infection includes drug treatment with pyrantel for the patient and for every household member, as well as prevention of reinfection. Strict hygiene (e.g., washing linens and disinfecting toilet seats) is an integral part of the treatment. Figure 19-1 outlines self-care of this infection and lists exclusions for self-treatment. Although pyrantel is not indicated for self-treatment of hookworm, it can treat both parasites if necessary (Table 19-1).

Nonpharmacologic Therapy

Once pinworm infection is suspected, the patient or caregiver should follow the nondrug measures in Table 19-2 to minimize family and household infections and reinfections. Children can usually return to school after the first dose of an appropriate anthelminthic agent, and after their fingernails are cut and cleaned. Practitioners are in an ideal position to inform patients of behaviors that may increase their risk of helminthic infections.

Pharmacologic Therapy

At one time, gentian violet was the only nonprescription medication available to treat pinworm infections. The Food and Drug Administration (FDA) has since declared gentian violet a nonmonograph ingredient, and it can no longer be marketed as an anthelminthic. Pyrantel is the only nonprescription medication approved for pinworm infection.

Pyrantel

Pyrantel was first used in veterinary practice as a broad-spectrum drug for pinworms, roundworms, and hookworms. Although a contemporary formal evaluation of efficacy has not been published, pyrantel is considered to be 90% to 100% effective with a relative lack of toxicity.[2,10] It has become an important drug for treating certain helminthic infections in humans (Table 19-1).

Although this product is readily available in a nonprescription form, helminthic infections other than those caused by pinworms should be diagnosed and treated by a primary care provider.

Pyrantel is a depolarizing neuromuscular agent that paralyzes adult worms, causing them to loosen their hold on the intestinal wall and subsequently be passed out in the stool before they can lay eggs. It is poorly absorbed and 50% of the drug is excreted unchanged in the feces. It is effective in treating pinworm infections without a primary care provider visit, but treatment of other

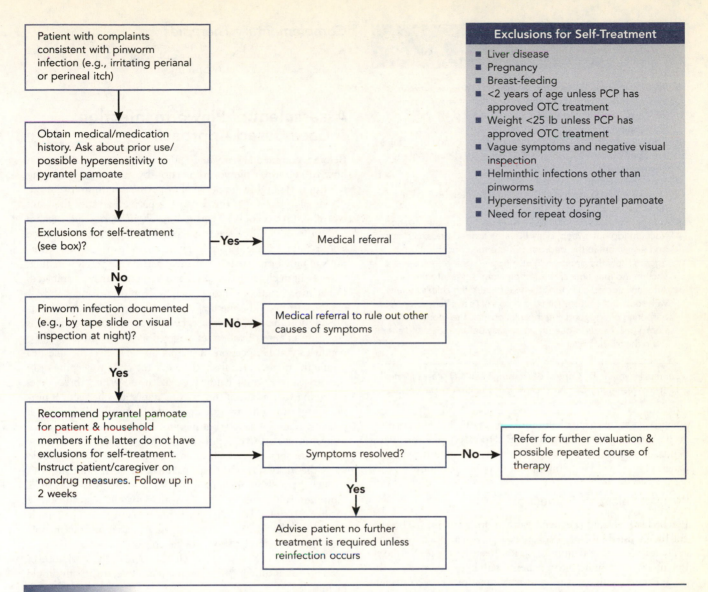

FIGURE 19-1 Self-care of pinworm infection. Key: OTC, over-the-counter; PCP, primary care provider.

roundworm infections such as hookworm requires a medical referral (Table 19-1).

A single oral dose of pyrantel (liquid, caplet, or chewable tablet) is based on the body weight (11 mg/kg) of adults and children. The maximum single dose is 1 gram. The recommended dosage is the same for children younger than 2 years or weighing less than 25 pounds; however, they should not be treated without first consulting a primary care provider. The product includes a schedule of recommended dosages based on body weight, which should not be exceeded. The dose should be repeated in 2 weeks if symptoms do not resolve because reinfection is common; however, the repeat dose should be administered only under the guidance of a primary care provider. Reinfection may be due to the drug's lack of effect on eggs and larvae, and to the eggs being viable up to 20 days. Pyrantel may be taken at any time of the day with or without food. A special diet, fasting, or purging before or after administration is not necessary. The liquid formulation, containing 50 mg/mL, should be shaken well before the dose is measured.

Side effects are usually mild, infrequent, and transient. The most common adverse effects involve the gastrointestinal (GI) tract and include nausea, vomiting, tenesmus, anorexia, diarrhea, and abdominal cramps.[10] However, a patient who experiences severe or persistent abdominal symptoms or other side effects after taking the first or second dose of this medication should be referred to a primary care provider for further evaluation. Less commonly, headache, dizziness, drowsiness, insomnia, rash, fever, and weakness may occur. In very rare circumstances, transient increases in aspartate aminotransferase, ototoxicity, optic neuritis, and hallucinations with confusion and paresthesia have been reported.[2]

Other medications are available by prescription to treat pinworms. Mebendazole (Vermox) is considered by experts[3,11] to be the drug of choice to treat pinworm infection, but there is little recent evidence to suggest that its efficacy differs from that of nonprescription pyrantel, and obtaining the medication requires a primary care provider visit. Alternative prescription agents include albendazole (Albenza) and thiabendazole (Mintezol). Albendazole

TABLE 19-2 Nondrug and Preventive Measures for Treating Pinworm Infection

- Wash bed linens, bedclothes, towels, and underwear of the infected individual and the entire family in hot water (131°F [55°C]) daily during treatment period. Do not shake these items; shaking can spread eggs into the air.
- Eggs are destroyed by sunlight, so ensure blinds or curtains are open in the affected room to enhance cleaning of the environment.
- Have the infected individual take daily morning showers to remove eggs deposited in the perianal region during the night (avoid tub baths).
- Use disinfectants on toilet seats daily during treatment period.
- Vacuum (do not sweep) daily the area around beds, curtains, and elsewhere in the bedroom where the concentration of eggs is likely the greatest. Wet-mopping before or instead of vacuuming may limit spread of pinworm eggs into the air.
- After an infected child uses the toilet, scrub the child's fingers with soap and a brush. Trim the child's nails regularly to prevent harboring of eggs and autoinoculation (hand-to-mouth reinfection). Wash hands frequently, especially before meals and after using the toilet.

Source: Heymann D. *Control of Communicable Diseases Manual.* 18th ed. Washington DC: American Public Health Association; 2004.

is approved to treat other helminthic infections, but FDA considers it an investigational drug when used to treat pinworms. Thiabendazole is not a first-line agent but may be considered when patients are infected with multiple susceptible helminths.

Product Selection Guidelines

Pyrantel is a safe and effective treatment for pinworms. The several brands listed in Table 19-3 are comparatively priced and generally less expensive than prescription treatment (e.g., Vermox). Pyrantel is contraindicated in patients with hypersensitivity to the drug. Patients with preexisting liver dysfunction or severe malnutrition should not self-medicate without first consulting a primary care provider. Pyrantel is a Pregnancy Category C drug and has not been studied in pregnant women; therefore, it should be used during pregnancy only when the benefits clearly outweigh the risks and only under the direction of a primary care provider.[12] Pyrantel should also not be used in patients younger than 2 years or those weighing less than 25 pounds, unless they are under the direction of a primary care provider.

TABLE 19-3 Selected Nonprescription Anthelminthic Products

Trade Name	Primary Ingredient
Pin-X Liquid/Chewable Tablet	Pyrantel 50 mg/mL (base) and 250 mg/tablet (base)
Pyrantel Suspension	Pyrantel 50 mg/mL (base)
Reese's Pinworm Caplet	Pyrantel 180 mg (equals 62.5 mg pyrantel base)
Reese's Pinworm Liquid	Pyrantel 144 mg/mL (equals 50 mg/mL base)

Complementary Therapies

Evidence does not support the use of complementary therapies for the eradication of pinworm infections

Assessment of Pinworm Infection: A Case-Based Approach

Before recommending treatment, the practitioner should explain how to confirm a pinworm infection by any of the following methods: (1) nighttime perianal or perineal itching in a child, (2) visual inspection of the perianal or perineal area for the adult worm, or (3) a cellophane tape test. Adult pinworms and eggs are seldom found in the feces; therefore, looking for worms in the stool is not a reliable way to diagnose enterobiasis.[7] When symptoms of pinworms, such as nocturnal perianal or perineal itching, are present in children, nonprescription therapy may be initiated. Other more vague symptoms such as sleep disturbances and GI complaints should be medically evaluated before initiating nonprescription therapy. However, because asymptomatic disease is common in enterobiasis, visual inspection may be necessary. To conduct a visual inspection, the parent should inspect the anal area during the night with a flashlight while the child is sleeping or in the very early morning before the child arises. White, thread-like, wriggling worms about the size of a staple may be seen. If pinworms are present, treatment should be initiated. Finally, if pinworms are suspected, but symptoms are vague and/or visual inspection is negative, a primary care provider may instruct the patient to obtain a cellophane tape sample. The parent should apply the sticky side of the tape to the perianal area (usually with a tongue depressor) and affix it sticky side down on a glass slide. Commercially available kits use a sticky paddle instead of tape to affix to a slide (see Color Plates, photograph 1C). The sample should then be taken to a primary care provider for microscopic examination. Samples should be taken over 3 consecutive days upon the child's awakening, which may increase the likelihood of detection to around 90%.[1] If this test is positive, treatment should be initiated.

Cases 19-1 and 19-2 illustrate the assessment of patients with pinworm infections.

Patient Counseling for Pinworm Infection

After making the decision to treat a pinworm infection, the practitioner should review the package insert material for pyrantel with the patient/caregiver. This material explains the pinworm life cycle, symptoms of pinworm infection, and methods of transmitting the infection. The practitioner should calculate the doses for the patient and all family members, being sure to emphasize the need to treat the whole family. The patient/caregiver should be advised to implement strict hygienic measures to prevent reinfection or transmission of the infection to other family members (Table 19-2). The practitioner should explain that the side effects of pyrantel are usually mild and infrequent, but if more severe effects occur, medical referral may be necessary. The most common adverse effects involve the GI tract and include nausea, vomiting, tenesmus, anorexia, diarrhea, and abdominal cramps. Patients who experience severe or persistent abdominal cramps, nausea, vomiting, anorexia, diarrhea, headache, drowsiness, or dizziness after taking this medication

Relevant Evaluation Criteria	Scenario/Model Outcome
Information Gathering	
1. Gather essential information about the patient's symptoms, including:	
a. description of symptom(s) (i.e., nature, onset, duration, severity, associated symptoms)	A father presents to the pharmacy requesting assistance in selecting an OTC product to treat himself and his son. The father reports his daughter had intense perianal itching over the last few days, particularly at night, and was diagnosed with pinworms. The daughter was given a prescription medication, and the father was told by the physician to purchase medications to also treat his son and himself. The son also reports perianal itching that is most intense at night, but his symptoms are not as intense as those of the daughter. The father has no current symptoms.
b. description of any factors that seem to precipitate, exacerbate, and/or relieve the patient's symptom(s)	No precipitating factors
c. description of the patient's efforts to relieve the symptoms	The son tried diphenhydramine topical cream for itching with no relief
2. Gather essential patient history information:	
a. patient's identity	Son: Don Young; father: Michael Young
b. patient's age, sex, height, and weight	Son: 5-year-old male, 42 inches, 43 lb
	Father: 38-year-old male, 69 inches, 178 lb
c. patient's occupation	The father is a self-employed gardener and the family has no health insurance.
d. patient's dietary habits	Normal diet for father and son; son frequently eats using his hands.
e. patient's sleep habits	Son: frequent awakenings at night due to perianal itching
	Father: normal sleep habits
f. concurrent medical conditions, prescription and nonprescription medications, and dietary supplements	Son: none
	Father: none
g. allergies	NKA for father or son
h. history of other adverse reactions to medications	None for father or son
Assessment and Triage	
3. Differentiate the patient's signs/symptoms and correctly identify the patient's primary problem(s).	Mild-to-moderate perianal itching, which interferes with normal sleep habits for the son.
4. Identify exclusions for self-treatment (see Figure 19-1).	Consider patients to be excluded for self-treatment if they (1) are allergic to the OTC product, (2) are younger than 2 years (unless treatment approved by PCP), (3) weigh less than 25 lb (unless treatment approved by PCP), or (4) have liver disease.
	The patients do not have exclusions for self-treatment.
5. Formulate a comprehensive list of therapeutic alternatives for the primary problem to determine if triage to a medical practitioner is required, and share this information with the patient.	Options include:
	(1) Recommend an appropriate OTC product such as pyrantel at appropriate doses for the father and son, along with nondrug therapies.
	(2) Recommend that father and son see a health care provider for a prescription medication.
	(3) Counsel on only environmental control measures.
	(4) Take no action.
Plan	
6. Select an optimal therapeutic alternative to address the patient's problem, taking into account patient preferences.	OTC treatment with pyrantel is appropriate for the son and father. The child prefers a liquid to a tablet; therefore, pyrantel is a good choice.

C A S E   1 9 - 1   *(continued)*

Relevant Evaluation Criteria	Scenario/Model Outcome
7. Describe the recommended therapeutic approach to the patient.	Mebendazole and pyrantel are both effective in the treatment of pinworms. However, pyrantel is available without a prescription and mebendazole requires a prescription. Because one of the family members was recently diagnosed with *E. vermicularis* and the physician instructed that other family members be treated, pyrantel is a reasonable option.
8. Explain to the patient the rationale for selecting the recommended therapeutic approach from the considered therapeutic alternatives.	Pinworms are not life threatening and may resolve on their own. However, if untreated, patients may reinfect themselves or other family members and may experience some complications; therefore treatment is recommended. Pyrantel is a reasonable option because it is available without a prescription, so the other family members do not need to visit a primary care provider, which may increase the cost of treatment and delay its initiation. It is also available as an oral suspension, which offers flexible dosing based on weight for multiple family members; other formulations such as tablets and caplets are available for patient preference.

Patient Education

9. When recommending self-care with non-prescription medications and/or nondrug therapy, convey accurate information to the patient:	
a. appropriate dose and frequency of administration	The son weighs 19.5 kg (43 lb); the dose of pyrantel is 11 mg/kg, so he should receive 214.5 mg. The oral suspension and Pin-X liquid are available in 50 mg/mL (base); therefore, he should receive 4.3 mL (or 5 mL as rounded up for measurement convenience). He could also take 5 mL of Reese's Pinworm liquid. If desired, he could also take the chewable tablets, which come as a 250 mg/tablet. Therefore, the son could take 1 chewable tablet.
	The father is 80.9 kg and should receive 889.9 mg of pyrantel, which would be approximately 3.5 chewable tablets.
b. maximum number of days the therapy should be employed	A single dose is required. If symptoms persist after 2 weeks, a repeat dose may be necessary and a health care provider contacted.
c. product administration procedures	Shake the oral suspension well before administering. Measure the dose using an oral medication dosing syringe or spoon for accuracy. Verify that other family members who need to be treated do not meet criteria for exclusion for self-treatment prior to administering medication. Doses will need to be calculated for the other family members.
d. expected time to onset of relief	It may take several days for relief of symptoms; the repeat dose should not be administered until 2 weeks have elapsed.
e. degree of relief that can be reasonably expected	Perianal itching should decrease after several days with complete pinworm eradication after at least 2 weeks.
f. most common side effects	The side effects are usually mild and may consist of nausea, vomiting, loss of appetite, diarrhea, or abdominal cramps.
g. side effects that warrant medical intervention should they occur	Severe or persistent abdominal symptoms
h. patient options in the event that condition worsens or persists	The patients should contact their health care provider if their conditions worsen or any severe side effects occur after taking the medication. Reinforce with the parents that pinworms are very common and rarely cause serious problems, but the condition will continue and potentially spread to others if not treated.
i. product storage requirements	Store at room temperature away from direct light with container sealed tightly.
j. specific nondrug measures	See Table 19-2.
10. Solicit follow-up questions from patient.	(1) Should my daughter who had the initial pinworm diagnosis receive an additional dose of a nonprescription antihelminthic medication along with the prescribed drug?
	(2) May my son also receive the same medication prescribed for my daughter?

CASE 19-1 (continued)

Relevant Evaluation Criteria	Scenario/Model Outcome
11. Answer patient's questions.	(1) The daughter with the initial infection should receive only one medication for treatment. Because both medications are equally effective in treating pinworms, either the prescription medication or nonprescription pyrantel may be used according to patient preferences such as costs.
	(2) If the prescription medication is desired for the son, he would also need to be evaluated by his primary care provider first.

Key: NKA, no known allergies; OTC, over-the-counter; PCP, primary care provider.

CASE 19-2

Relevant Evaluation Criteria	Scenario/Model Outcome
Information Gathering	
1. Gather essential information about the patient's symptoms, including:	
a. description of symptom(s) (i.e., nature, onset, duration, severity, associated symptoms)	A woman presents to the pharmacy requesting help in choosing a product to help with her itching. She states the itching, which began approximately 4 days ago, is mostly in her perineal and vaginal area. She also has some mild stomach pain, nausea, and dysuria.
b. description of any factors that seem to precipitate, exacerbate, and/or relieve the patient's symptom(s)	No precipitating factors
c. description of the patient's efforts to relieve the symptoms	She has not yet tried any OTC medications.
2. Gather essential patient history information:	
a. patient's identity	Rachel Smith
b. patient's age, sex, height, and weight	21 year-old female, 5 ft 3 in, 138 lb
c. patient's occupation	College student who lives in the dorms; works as a waitress
d. patient's dietary habits	Normal diet
e. patient's sleep habits	Frequent awakenings at night due to perineal itching
f. concurrent medical conditions, prescription and nonprescription medications, and dietary supplements	No concurrent medical conditions; current medications include daily birth control pills.
g. allergies	NKA
h. history of other adverse reactions to medications	None
Assessment and Triage	
3. Differentiate the patient's signs/symptoms and correctly identify the patient's primary problem(s).	Patient's symptoms, such as perianal itching at night, are consistent with pinworms, but vaginal itching, dysuria, and nausea are unusual symptoms and should be medically evaluated.
4. Identify exclusions for self-treatment (see Figure 19-1).	Consider the patient to be excluded from self-treatment if she (1) is allergic to the OTC product, (2) is less than 2 years of age (unless treatment approved by PCP), (3) weighs less than 25 lb (unless treatment approved by PCP), (4) has liver disease, (5) is pregnant, (6) is breast-feeding, or (7) has vague symptoms and negative visual inspection.

Relevant Evaluation Criteria	Scenario/Model Outcome
5. Formulate a comprehensive list of therapeutic alternatives for the primary problem to determine if triage to a medical practitioner is required, and share this information with the patient.	Options include: (1) Recommend an appropriate OTC product at appropriate doses for the patient, along with nondrug therapies. (2) Refer the patient to a health care provider for further evaluation, diagnosis, and recommended treatment. (3) Counsel on only environmental control measures. (4) Take no action.
Plan	
6. Select an optimal therapeutic alternative to address the patient's problem, taking into account patient preferences.	Medical evaluation by a health care provider is warranted for the perineal and vaginal symptoms and subsequent treatment.
7. Describe the recommended therapeutic approach to the patient.	You should see your primary care provider for further evaluation of your symptoms, appropriate diagnosis, and recommended treatment.
8. Explain to the patient the rationale for selecting the recommended therapeutic approach from the considered therapeutic alternatives.	Because you have no documented pinworm infection, either by visual inspection or by tape slide, and have vague symptoms, self-treatment is not appropriate. Your symptoms may be consistent with pinworm infection, but other possibilities need to be ruled out.
Patient Education	
9. When recommending self-care with nonprescription medications and/or nondrug therapy, convey accurate information to the patient.	Self-treatment is not appropriate, but you should institute environmental control measures and seek medical care. See Table 19-2.
10. Solicit follow-up questions from patient.	(1) What are some of the complications associated with pinworms? (2) How are pinworms normally treated?
11. Answer patient's questions.	(1) If untreated, pinworms may possibly lead to secondary bacterial infections in the perianal and perineal regions. Pinworms can also lead to pelvic inflammatory disease, endometritis, and possibly infertility. In addition, other possible symptoms associated with pinworm infection include insomnia, restlessness, and anorexia. (2) Patients may be treated with a single dose of various nonprescription (pyrantel) or prescription medications (mebendazole, albendazole). Along with medications, patients must also follow specific nondrug measures to prevent reinfection.

Key: NKA, no known allergies; OTC, over-the-counter; PCP, primary care provider.

should be referred for medical evaluation. Practitioners should also explain that the symptoms of pinworm infection (e.g., nocturnal perianal itching) should improve within 2 weeks with treatment. However, if symptoms persist or worsen to include systemic complaints (e.g., abdominal discomfort, insomnia, and nervousness), medical referral may be necessary.

Evaluation of Patient Outcomes for Pinworm Infection

The patient/caregiver should be instructed to contact a primary care provider, if anal itching persists beyond 2 weeks or recurs, or if new symptoms develop. A second dose of pyrantel should be given 2 weeks after the first dose. If hygienic measures are not being followed, the practitioner should again stress their importance for preventing reinfection.

Key Points for Pinworm Infection

➤ The practitioner should be familiar with common helminthic infections, their symptoms, and their treatment.
➤ Although pyrantel is used in treating other helminthic infections, only pinworm infection should be evaluated for self-treatment with a nonprescription drug.
➤ A medical referral may be necessary when helminths other than pinworms are suspected.

PATIENT EDUCATION FOR
Pinworm Infection

The objectives of self-treatment are to (1) eradicate pinworms in the infected patient, (2) prevent reinfection, and (3) prevent transmission of the infection to others. For most patients, carefully following product instructions and the self-care measures listed here will help ensure optimal therapeutic outcomes.

Nondrug Measures

- See Table 19-2 for nondrug/preventive measures.

Nonprescription Medications

- Read package insert for pyrantel information carefully; this information will help prevent reinfection or transmission of the infection.
- Consult a primary care provider before giving the medication to a person with liver disease, or for a child who is younger than 2 years and/or weighs less than 25 pounds, or to a woman who is pregnant or breast-feeding.
- Treat all household members to ensure elimination of the infection. Medical referral may be necessary if household members meet criteria for exclusion for self-treatment.

- Take only one dose as shown on the dosing schedule included with this product. For adults and children older than 2 years, dosing is the same: 11 mg/kg, taken orally. The maximum dose is 1 gram.
- Shake the liquid formulation well and use a measuring spoon to ensure an accurate dose.
- If desired, pyrantel may be taken with food, milk, or fruit juices on an empty stomach any time during the day. The liquid formulation may be mixed with milk or fruit juice.
- Note that fasting, laxatives, special diets, or purging is not necessary to aid treatment.
- If abdominal cramps, nausea, vomiting, anorexia, rash, diarrhea, headache, drowsiness, or dizziness occurs and persists after taking the medication, medical referral may be necessary.
- If symptoms of the pinworm infection persist beyond 2 weeks, medical referral may be necessary

---

➤ Pinworms are common in the United States and rarely cause significant morbidity.

➤ Practitioners can aid patients and caregivers in the self-diagnosis, counseling, and self-treatment with nonprescription anthelminthic medication.

REFERENCES

1. Kucik CJ, Martin GL, Sortor BV. Common intestinal parasites. *Am Fam Physician.* 2004;69:1161–8.
2. American Society of Health-System Pharmacists. *AHFS Drug Handbook. STAT!Ref Online Electronic Medical Library.* Bethesda, Md: Lippincott Williams & Wilkins; 2008.
3. Drugs for parasitic infections [serial online]. *Med Lett Drugs Ther.* 2007; 5(suppl):e1–e15.
4. Cappello M, Hotez P: Intestinal nematodes. In: Long S, ed. *Principles and Practice of Pediatric Infectious Diseases,* 2nd ed. New York: Churchill Livingstone; 2003.
5. St Georgiev V. Chemotherapy of enterobiasis (oxyuriasis). *Expert Opin Pharmacother.* 2001;2:267–75.
6. Burkhart CN, Burkhart CG. Assessment of frequency, transmission, and genitourinary complications of enterobiasis (pinworms). Int J Dermatol. 2005;44:837–40.
7. Liu LX. Enterobiasis. In: Guerrant RL, Walker DH, Weller PF, eds. *Tropical Infectious Diseases: Principles, Pathogens & Practice.* Philadelphia: Churchill Livingstone; 1999:949–53.
8. Tandan T, Pollard AJ, Money DM, et al. Pelvic inflammatory disease associated with Enterobius vermicularis. *Arch Dis Child.* 2002;86:439–40.
9. Arca MJ, Gates RL, Groner JI, et al. Clinical manifestations of appendiceal pinworms in children: an institutional experience and a review of the literature. *Pediatr Surg Int.* 2004;20:372–5.
10. Bagheri H, Simiand E, Montastruc J-L, et al. Adverse drug reactions to anthelmintics. *Ann Pharmacother.* 2004;38:383–8.
11. Jacobson CC, Abel EA. Parasitic infestations. *J Am Acad Dermatol.* 2007; 6:1026–43.
12. Briggs G, Freeman R, Sumner J. *Drugs in Pregnancy and Lactation.* 7th ed. Philadelphia: Lippincott Williams & Wilkins; 2005.

Nausea and Vomiting

Laura Shane-McWhorter and Lynda Oderda

Nausea and vomiting (N/V) may occur in a variety of benign circumstances, but these symptoms are also associated with several important medical disorders. Nonprescription antiemetics are used to prevent or control the symptoms of N/V that are primarily caused by motion sickness, pregnancy, and mild infectious diseases. Some nonprescription antiemetics are promoted for the relief of vague symptoms such as "upset stomach," indigestion, and distention associated with overeating. Although accurate statistics are lacking, it is estimated that billions of dollars are spent on nonprescription products to treat N/V. (Information on the 200 top-selling nonprescription products in 2007 is available at drugtopics.modernmedicine.com/drugtopics/data/articlestandard//drugtopics/082008/492702/article.pdf.)

N/V occurs in adults and children and in a variety of circumstances. Accurate statistics on the epidemiology of N/V are not available, because these symptoms occur in many conditions, and many individuals do not report these disturbances to a health care provider. Three common conditions that involve N/V are motion sickness, N/V of pregnancy (NVP), and viral gastroenteritis.

The severity of N/V related to motion sickness is difficult to quantify because of interindividual variability and susceptibility to this malady. Motion sickness rarely occurs in children under 2 years of age or those over 50.[1] Compared with men, women are more susceptible to motion sickness.[1]

NVP may occur in 80% of women and usually subsides by the 16th week of pregnancy.[2] It may persist throughout the pregnancy in 15% of women.[2] Half of all women have both nausea and vomiting, one-fourth have nausea only, and it is rare for only vomiting to occur.[3,4] A very severe form of pregnancy-related vomiting, hyperemesis gravidarum, occurs in less than 1% of women and may require rehydration and hospitalization.[2]

Another cause of N/V is viral gastroenteritis.[5] Acute transient attacks of vomiting in conjunction with diarrhea are frequently observed during these episodes. This acute infectious disease may affect any age group and is usually self-limiting, but pediatric patients may experience serious consequences.[5] Two common pathogens are rotavirus and norovirus.[5] According to the Centers for Disease Control and Prevention (CDC), it is difficult to quantify the epidemiology of gastroenteritis because of inaccurate reporting, especially underreporting of mild cases. In the United States, approximately 3.5 million cases of rotavirus-induced gastroenteritis occur each year; N/V and diarrhea are prominent symptoms.[5] Norovirus may cause up to 70% of gastroenteritis cases.[5] In children, acute gastroenteritis associated with diarrhea accounts for more than 1.5 million outpatient visits, 200,000 hospitalizations, and an estimated 300 deaths per year.[6] The CDC reports that in children, rotavirus infections result in approximately 400,000 physician visits, up to 272,000 emergency room visits, and 55,000 to 70,000 annual hospitalizations, with total costs approximating $1 billion.[7] A rotavirus vaccine is also available as part of the childhood immunization schedule.[7]

Pathophysiology of Nausea and Vomiting

The pathophysiology of N/V involves both the brain and gastrointestinal tract (GI). Four different areas—the chemoreceptor trigger zone (CTZ), vestibular apparatus, cerebral cortex, and visceral GI tract afferent nerves—provide input to an area composed of a complex system of neurons in the medulla oblongata in the brain stem, known as the vomiting center (VC).[1,8,9]

The CTZ is located in the area postrema at the floor of the fourth ventricle. Neurons in the CTZ may be stimulated by many emetogenic toxins. Because the CTZ is outside the blood–brain barrier, it responds to stimuli from either the blood or the cerebral spinal fluid.[1] The vestibular apparatus is located in the bony labyrinth of the temporal lobe. It detects motion and body position, including changes in equilibrium. Direct input to the VC is through cholinergic pathways. The cortex and limbic system provide direct input to the VC through different neuroreceptors. Sensory input, including sight, smell, different toxins, or memory may elicit a strong sensation of nausea.[1,8,9] Finally, vagal nerve pathways from the GI tract also provide input to the VC. Gut distention and decreased GI emptying may stimulate mechanoreceptors and may be responsible for eliciting nausea and emesis.[1,9]

The VC receives different stimuli from these areas and sends impulses to the salivation center, vasomotor center, respiratory center, cranial nerves, and then to the pharynx and GI tract, after which nausea and/or vomiting may occur.[1,8,9]

N/V may be caused by many stimuli: travel (i.e., motion sickness), pregnancy, drug therapy, stress, viral gastroenteritis, overeating, food poisoning, bulimia, abdominal distention, certain diseases, and other factors. Most occurrences of N/V are self-limiting and require minimal therapy. Table 20-1 lists several causes of N/V; however, many of these are not self-limiting and require extensive medical evaluation and treatment.[7–12]

TABLE 20-1 Primary Causes of Nausea and Vomiting

Visceral Afferent Stimulation	CNS Disorders
Mechanical Obstruction	**Vestibular Disorders**
Gastric outlet obstruction (i.e., PUD, gastric carcinoma, pancreatic disease); small intestinal obstruction	Labyrinthitis; Ménière's syndrome; motion sickness
Motility Disorders	**Increased Intracranial Pressure**
Gastroparesis (i.e., DM, drug-induced, postviral); chronic intestinal pseudo-obstruction; IBS; anorexia nervosa; idiopathic gastric stasis	CNS tumor; subdural or subarachnoid hemorrhage; pseudotumor cerebri
Peritoneal Irritation	**Infections**
Appendicitis; bacterial peritonitis	Meningitis; encephalitis
Infections	**Psychogenic**
Viral gastroenteritis (i.e., norovirus, rotavirus); food poisoning (i.e., toxins from *Bacillus cereus*, *Staphylococcus aureus*, *Clostridium perfringens*); hepatitis A or B; acute systemic infections	Anticipatory vomiting; bulimia; psychiatric disorders
	Other CNS Disorders
	Migraine headache
Topical Gastrointestinal Irritants	**Irritation of CTZ**
Alcohol; NSAIDs; antibiotics	*Initiated/Withdrawn Drugs*
	Cytotoxic chemotherapy; opiates; theophylline or digoxin toxicity; antibiotics; radiation therapy; drug withdrawal (i.e., opiates, BDZs)
Other	*Systemic Conditions*
Cardiac disease (i.e., MI, HF); urologic disease (i.e., stones, pyelonephritis); overeating	DM (i.e., DKA); renal disease (i.e., uremia); adrenocortical crisis (i.e., Addison's disease); pregnancy

Key: BDZ, benzodiazepines; CNS, central nervous system; CTZ, chemotrigger receptor zone; DKA, diabetic ketoacidosis; DM, diabetes mellitus; HF, heart failure; IBS, irritable bowel syndrome; MI, myocardial infarction; NSAIDs, nonsteroidal anti-inflammatory drugs; PUD, peptic ulcer disease.
Source: References 7-12.

Emesis is thought to be a complicated defense response secondary to a variety of different mechanisms. Certain processes may evoke this response and may include toxic substances, psychogenic causes, cancer chemotherapy or radiation, myocardial infarction, motion sickness, pregnancy, or infections.[1,8,9] The abdominal and diaphragmatic musculature may contract or relax, and the associated coordinating circuitry involves other areas such as the laryngeal or pharyngeal muscles. The epiglottis closes (to prevent aspiration), the soft palate is elevated, a retrograde contraction occurs while the gastric fundus relaxes, and the stomach contents move into the esophagus and are expelled as vomiting begins.[9]

Major neurotransmitters and receptors involved in vomiting include serotonin (5-HT$_3$), dopamine (D$_2$), histamine type 1 (H$_1$), muscarinic (M$_1$), benzodiazepine, opioid, and neurokinin (NK$_1$) receptors.[8,9,11] In cancer chemotherapy, serotonin 5-HT$_3$ receptors are implicated in emesis,[10] whereas the cyclic vomiting syndrome may be affected by substance P and its receptor, neurokinin-1 (NK$_1$).[8,9]

N/V of motion sickness is produced by overstimulation of the labyrinth (inner ear) apparatus.[1] The three semicircular canals in the labyrinth on each side of the head are responsible for maintaining equilibrium. Postural adjustments are made when the brain receives nerve impulses initiated by the movement of fluid in the canals. When the head is rotated on two axes simultaneously, unusual motion patterns may produce motion sickness. Inaccurate interpretation of visual stimuli while standing or sitting motionless may also produce motion sickness. For instance, a person may experience motion sickness when watching a film taken from a roller coaster or watching an airplane performing aerobatics, or when extending the head upward while standing on a rotating platform.[1] Individuals differ in their response to motion sickness stimuli, such as flying and boating, but no one is immune. Regardless of the type of stimulus-producing event, motion sickness is easier to prevent than to treat.

Clinical Presentation of Nausea and Vomiting

N/V consists of three different processes: (1) nausea (characterized by a person's subjective feeling of a need to vomit); (2) retching (involuntary rhythmic diaphragmatic and abdominal contractions); and (3) vomiting (rapid, forceful expulsion of the GI tract contents).[8,11] Although most cases of N/V are self-limiting, a patient may show evidence of dehydration or esophageal tears, manifested by blood in the vomitus, in which case the patient needs medical referral.

Possible acute complications of vomiting include dehydration, aspiration, malnutrition, electrolyte and/or acid–base abnormalities, diaphragmatic herniation, as well as Mallory-Weiss syndrome, which causes esophageal tears, typically at the gastroesophageal junction, and thus blood may appear in the vomitus.[13] Dehydration and electrolyte imbalances are the major concerns associated with vomiting. Signs and symptoms of dehydration include dry mouth, decreased skin turgor, excessive thirst, little or no urination, dizziness, lightheadedness, fainting, and reduced blood pressure.[13] These symptoms warrant further evaluation by a PCP.

In infants and small children, recurrent or protracted N/V (with accompanying diarrhea) may lead to marked dehydration and electrolyte imbalance that should not be ignored. Parents should be educated to recognize signs and symptoms of dehydration such as dry mucous membranes, decreased skin turgor, irritability, altered mental status, and weight loss (Table 20-2).[6,14,15] Weight loss as an objective measure of dehydration should be emphasized, and an accurate infant weight scale is an essential tool to measure weight. The child should be referred for further evaluation in the following situations[6,14,15]:

- Dehydration is present.
- Child is younger than 3 months and has a fever greater than 100.4°F (38°C).
- Child is 3- to 36-months-old and has a fever greater than 102.2°F (39°C).
- Child is younger than 6 months or weighs less than 8 kg.[6]
- Exclusions for self-treatment apply to N/V (Figure 20-2).

TABLE 20-2 Signs and Symptoms of Dehydration in Children

- Dry mouth and tongue
- Sunken and/or dry eyes
- Sunken fontanelle
- Decreased urine output (dry diapers for several hours)
- Dark urine
- Fast heartbeat
- Thirst (drinks extremely eagerly)
- Absence of tears when crying
- Decreased skin turgor
  —Increased axillary skinfolds
  —"Doughy" skin (may indicate hypernatremia)
  —When "pinched," skin returns to normal very slowly (prolonged skin tenting)
- Unusual listlessness, sleepiness, decreased alertness, or tiredness
  —Body is "floppy"
  —Lightheadedness when sitting or standing up (in older children)
  —Difficulty in waking up the child (may indicate severe dehydration)
- Weight loss
  —Noticeable decrease in abdominal ("tummy") size
  —Clothes or diaper fit loosely
  —<3% body weight loss indicating minimal or no dehydration
  —3%–9% body weight loss indicating mild-to-moderate dehydration
  —>9% body weight loss indicating severe dehydration

Source: References 6, 14, and 15.

Treatment of Nausea and Vomiting

Treatment Goals

Treatment of N/V should focus on identifying and correcting the underlying cause. However, most acute vomiting cases are mild and self-limiting, resolve spontaneously, and require only symptomatic treatment. Acute severe vomiting necessitates further evaluation and may require hospitalization. Decisions should be made to determine whether a patient is a candidate for self-treatment. Figures 20-1 and 20-2 list exclusions for self-care for adults[12,13,16,17] and children, respectively.[6,14,15]

General Treatment Approach

Treatment of N/V may involve both nonpharmacologic and pharmacologic treatments. The population affected and the causes and severity of N/V determine whether pharmacologic or nonpharmacologic therapy should be used. Symptomatic relief may not be possible until the underlying cause has been identified and corrected. The algorithms in Figures 20-1 and 20-2 outline the self-care of N/V in adults and children, respectively.

Nausea and Vomiting in Adults

In adults, N/V may be associated with a variety of diseases, certain medications, or conditions including gastroenteritis, food poisoning, or overeating. Females of childbearing age may experience NVP and self-treatment should be approached cautiously. Another condition warranting caution is self-treatment of N/V in women who are breast-feeding.

Nausea and Vomiting in Children

Children warrant special consideration. In newborns, serious abnormalities may cause vomiting. These include GI tract obstruction, neurologic disorders, and neuromuscular control disorders. Vomiting may rapidly lead to acid–base disturbances and dehydration. Infants and young children may become dehydrated very quickly and, if not appropriately managed, dehydration may lead to death. Thus, referral for medical evaluation is always recommended.

Simple regurgitation or spitting up is common in infants and does not require medical attention. Esophageal sphincter blockage (pyloric stenosis) occurs when an infant forcefully vomits large amounts of fluid; this condition requires medical referral.

Although N/V may occur secondary to head trauma, toxic ingestion, or central nervous system infection, the most common cause is acute viral gastroenteritis. Treatment is primarily directed at preventing and correcting dehydration and electrolyte disturbances. Fluid loss should generally be replaced within 24 hours. An oral rehydration solution (ORS) may be used to treat even minimal or mild-to-moderate cases. Antiemetic use in children may be controversial, and some clinicians question the value of using antiemetics to treat acute, self-limiting disorders.[15,18] Recently the Food and Drug Administration (FDA) has cautioned that, because of severe adverse effects, certain ingredients found in cough and cold products, including antihistamines (also used as antiemetics), should not be used in children younger than 2 years. Therefore, FDA is examining information to determine safety of these products in children up to 11 years of age.[18]

Exclusions for Self-Treatment

- Urine ketones and/or high BG with signs of dehydration in patients with DM (may indicate DKA or HHS)
- Suspected food poisoning that is severe and/or does not clear up after 12 hours
- Severe abdominal pain in the middle or right lower quadrant (may indicate appendicitis or bowel obstruction)
- N/V with fever and/or diarrhea (may indicate infectious disease)
- Severe right upper quadrant pain, especially after eating fatty foods (may indicate cholecystitis or pancreatitis)
- Blood in the vomitus (may indicate ulcers, esophageal tears, or severe nosebleed)
- Yellow skin or eye discoloration and dark urine (may indicate hepatitis)
- Stiff neck with or without headache and sensitivity to brightness of normal light (may indicate meningitis)

- Head injury with N/V, blurry vision, or numbness and tingling
- Persons with glaucoma, BPH, chronic bronchitis, emphysema, or asthma (may react adversely to OTC antiemetics)
- Pregnancy (moderate-to-severe symptoms) or breast-feeding
- N/V caused by cancer chemotherapy; radiation therapy; serious metabolic disorders; CNS, GI, or endocrine disorders
- Drug-induced N/V: adverse effects of drugs used therapeutically (e.g., opioids, NSAIDs, antibiotics, estrogens); toxic doses of drugs used therapeutically (e.g., digoxin, theophylline, lithium); ethanol
- Psychogenic-induced N/V: bulimia, anorexia
- Chronic disease-induced N/V: gastroparesis with DM; DKA or HHS with DM; GERD

Source: References 11–13, 16, and 17.

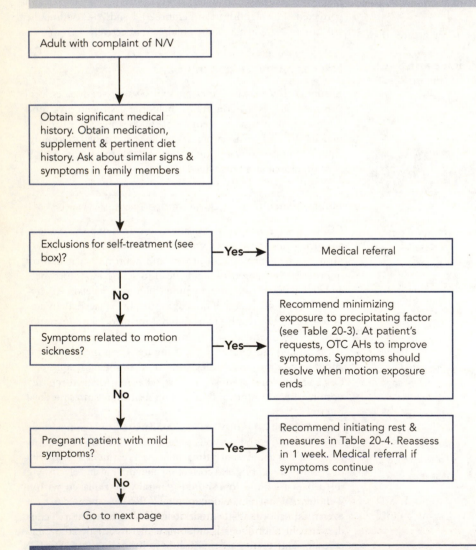

FIGURE 20-1 Self-care of N/V in adults. Key: AH, antihistamine; BG, blood glucose; BPH, benign prostatic hyperplasia; CNS, central nervous system; DKA, diabetic ketoacidosis; DM, diabetes mellitus; GERD, gastroesophageal reflux disease; GI, gastrointestinal; HHS, hyperosmolar hyperglycemic syndrome; H$_2$RA, histamine$_2$-receptor antagonist; NSAID, nonsteroidal anti-inflammatory drug; OTC; over-the-counter; PCP, primary care provider. *(continued on next page)*

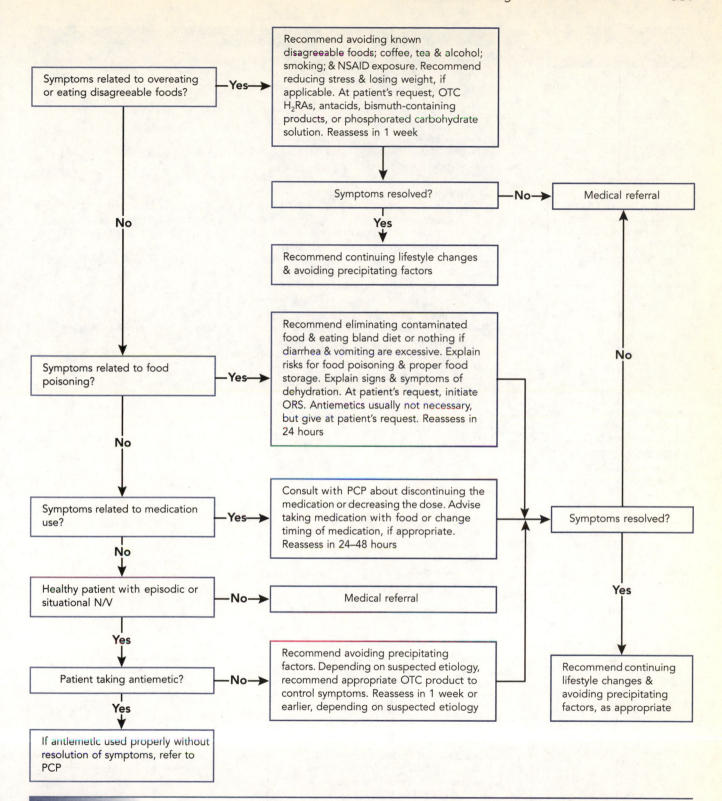

FIGURE 20-1 *(Continued)* Self-care of N/V in adults. Key: AH, antihistamine; BG, blood glucose; BPH, benign prostatic hyper-plasia; CNS, central nervous system; DKA, diabetic ketoacidosis; DM, diabetes melli-tus; GERD, gastroesophageal reflux disease; GI, gastrointestinal; HHS, hyperosmolar hyperglycemic syndrome; H₂RA, histamine₂-receptor antagonist; NSAID, nonsteroidal anti-inflammatory drug; OTC; over-the-counter; PCP, primary care provider.

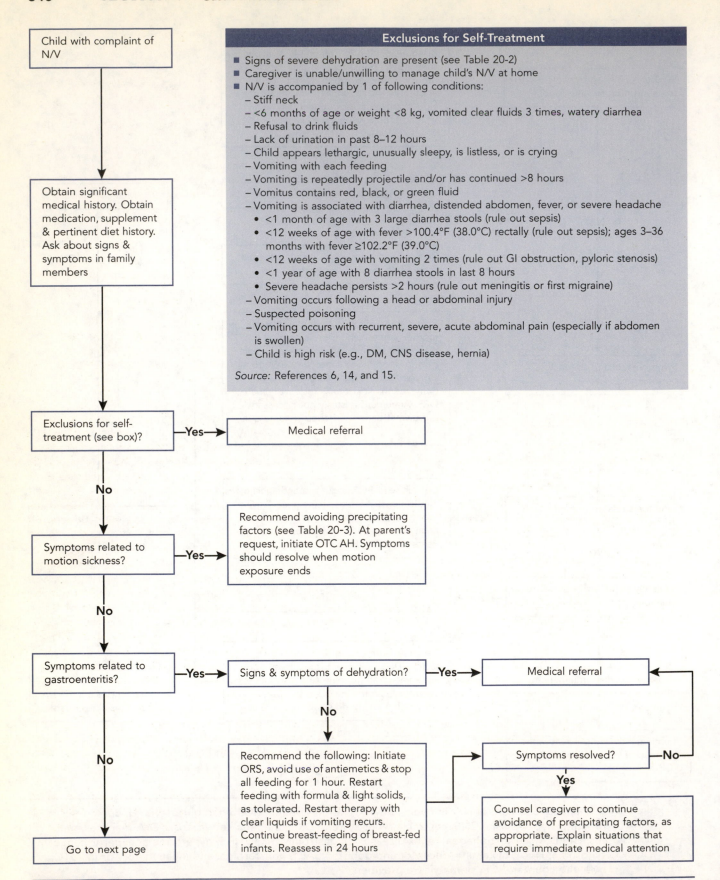

FIGURE 20-2 Self-care of N/V in children. Key: AH, antihistamine; CNS, central nervous system; DM, diabetes mellitus; GI, gastrointestinal; ORS, oral rehydration solution; OTC, over-the-counter. *(continued on next page)*

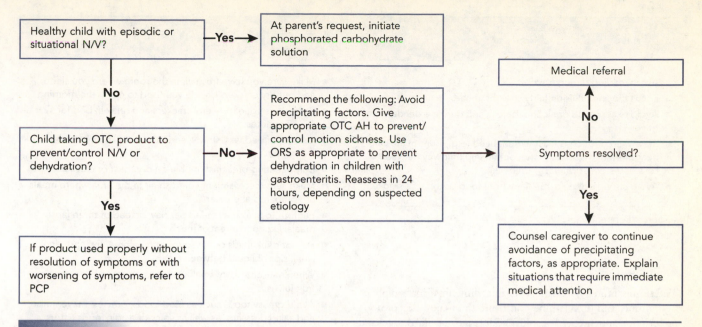

FIGURE 20-2 *(Continued)* Self-care of N/V in children. Key: AH, antihistamine; CNS, central nervous system; DM, diabetes mellitus; GI, gastrointestinal; ORS, oral rehydration solution; OTC, over-the-counter.

Nonpharmacologic Therapy

Nonpharmacologic treatments may be used to treat a variety of different causes of N/V. Acupressure wristbands are used to treat the symptoms of NVP, motion sickness, and overeating.[19–21] Acupressure therapy to treat N/V is based on the ancient Eastern theory that the body is activated by the vital force Chi. Chi energy travels along meridians known as "acu" points. For centuries, the Chinese have used stimulation of the Neiguan–or pericardium 6 (P6)–point, located bilaterally on the inner forearm three finger widths up from the first wrist crease, to relieve N/V symptoms. Acupressure wristbands are indicated to prevent motion sickness, NVP, and N/V associated with chemotherapy and anesthesia.[19–21] Acupressure wristbands offer an alternative to medications and may be considered by patients who want to avoid the adverse effects of pharmacologic agents. According to one manufacturer, children as young as 2 years of age have used these wristbands safely (www.sea-band.com/faqs.htm#q10).

Another device that stimulates the P6 point is a battery-powered acustimulation band. This device is approved by FDA for nonprescription use in treating N/V related to motion sickness, as well as mild-to-moderate (but not severe) NVP.[20] The device is also available by prescription to treat N/V related to chemotherapy and as an adjunct to antiemetics in reducing post-operative nausea. Mechanism of action is believed to be stimulation of the P6 acupuncture point by means of electricity.[20] Individuals may choose from five power settings. The prescription product has a higher power output than the device available for nonprescription use. The only reported adverse effect has been a mild, transient rash at the application site after use of the band. In addition, the wristband contains latex, which may cause allergic reactions in some individuals. It is important for clinicians to advise patients that the device must be worn on the wrist to prevent interference with pacemakers. The manufacturer states that product use in children is not contraindicated.

A meta-analysis that evaluated P6 acustimulation points determined that acupressure is effective in reducing postoperative vomiting in children and is as effective as medications.[19] A Cochrane systematic review has determined that, for nausea, P6 stimulation is superior to antiemetic medications and, for vomiting, the two modalities are equivalent.[21] For pregnancy the meta-analysis indicated that results are mixed; some trials show benefit but others do not.[21]

Motion sickness occurs when there is a neural mismatch between visual and vestibular stimuli. Acupressure and acustimulation bands may have some advantages over nonprescription emetics, because they are not sedating and they may be used before the onset of anticipated motion sickness or when symptoms first occur. In contrast, nonprescription antiemetics such as dimenhydrinate must be taken at least 30 to 60 minutes before beginning the activity that causes motion sickness. These antiemetics also cause drowsiness, which may not be acceptable to some travelers. Acupressure and acustimulation devices may be used concomitantly with antiemetics. The original acupressure band was worn on both wrists, but new products are available that may be worn on only one wrist. The acustimulation device is also worn on only one wrist. Cost may be a factor in selection of the products; the acustimulation device costs approximately eight times more than an acupressure band.

To minimize motion sickness in a young child, parents may seat the child in a safe position that allows vision out of the car windows. Other nonpharmacologic measures are included in Table 20-3.[1]

Because teratogenicity is a major consideration, many physicians are reluctant to prescribe any medication for a pregnant woman. A number of nonpharmacologic approaches may be recommended, although they are not evidence-based (Table 20-4).[22–24]

Pharmacologic Therapy

Selection of a nonprescription medication is determined by the potential cause of N/V. Myriad causes account for the numerous medications used to treat these symptoms.

TABLE 20-3 Nonpharmacologic Measures to Decrease Motion Sickness

- Avoid reading during travel.
- Focus the line of vision fairly straight ahead.
- Avoid excess food or alcohol before and during extended travel.
- Stay where motion is least experienced (e.g., front of the car, near the wings of an airplane, or midship [midway between bow and stern], preferably on deck).
- Avoid strong odors, particularly from food or tobacco smoke.

Source: Reference 1.

Antihistamines

The antihistamines meclizine, cyclizine, dimenhydrinate, diphenhydramine, and doxylamine constitute the major class of nonprescription antiemetics.[25] Table 20-5 lists age-specific dosages and maximum daily limits for these FDA-approved antiemetics.[25,26] Although used for N/V, doxylamine is not approved for antiemetic use.

Histamine levels increase in the hypothalamus, pons, and medulla oblongata in response to certain motions commonly associated with N/V. Neural centers for salivation, vomiting, and other symptoms associated with motion sickness contain histaminic neurons. Antihistamines that cross the blood–brain barrier depress labyrinth excitability and may prevent, as well as control, motion sickness to varying degrees.[25,27]

Nonprescription antihistamines are classified as safe and effective for prevention and treatment of nausea, vomiting, or dizziness associated with motion sickness. However, there are age-specific limits.[26] Antihistamines are not recommended in children younger than 2 years. Meclizine should not be used in children younger than 12 years, and cyclizine should not be given to children younger than 6 years. Although FDA has approved dosages of diphenhydramine and dimenhydrinate for children ages 2 to 6 years, pharmacists should be extremely cautious in recommending these products for young children.

TABLE 20-4 Nonpharmacologic Measures to Prevent NVP

- Make sure you have fresh air in the room where you sleep, and put dry crackers beside your bed to eat in the morning.
- Before arising, eat several crackers and relax in bed for 10–15 minutes.
- Get out of bed very slowly, and do not make any sudden movements.
- Before eating breakfast, nibble on dry toast or crackers.
- Make sure there is plenty of fresh air in the area where meals are prepared and eaten.
- Eat four to five small meals per day instead of three large meals. Do not overeat at meals.
- Do not drink fluids or eat soups at mealtime. Instead, drink small sips of liquid between meals.
- When nauseated, try small sips of carbonated beverages or fruit juices.
- Avoid greasy foods such as fried foods, gravies, mayonnaise, and salad dressing, as well as spicy or acidic foods (citrus fruits and beverages, tomatoes).
- If necessary, eat food that is chilled rather than warm or hot (cold foods tend to be less nauseating).

Source: References 22–24.

Because it is easier to prevent than treat motion sickness-related N/V, antihistamines are taken before boarding the vehicle that elicits motion sickness. These agents should be taken at least 30 to 60 minutes before departure to allow ample time for onset of effect; their use should be continued during travel.

Drowsiness is the most common side effect and may occur even with therapeutic doses. Patients should be cautioned not to combine antihistamines with alcohol-containing products, drive a vehicle, operate hazardous machinery, or engage in tasks requiring a high degree of physical dexterity or mental alertness. One study reported that 50 mg of diphenhydramine caused greater impairment than alcohol intoxication.[28] Anticholinergic adverse effects may occur, including blurred vision, dry mouth,

TABLE 20-5 Dosage Guidelines for Antiemetic Antihistamines[a]

Agent	Dosage (Maximum Daily Dosage)		
	Adults and Children ≥12 Years	**Children 6 to <12 Years**	**Children 2 to <6 Years**
Cyclizine	50 mg 30 minutes before travel, then 50 mg every 4–6 hours (200 mg)	25 mg every 6–8 hours (75 mg)	Not recommended
Dimenhydrinate	50–100 mg every 4–6 hours (400 mg)	25–50 mg every 6–8 hours (150 mg)	12.5–25 mg every 6–8 hours (75 mg)
Diphenhydramine	25–50 mg every 4 hours (300 mg)	12.5–25 mg every 4 hours (150 mg)	6.25 mg every 4 hours (37.5 mg)
Meclizine	25–50 mg 1 hour before travel (50 mg)	Not recommended	Not recommended

[a] Take antihistamines at least 30 to 60 minutes before travel; then take continuously for the duration of travel.

Source: References 25 and 26.

urinary retention, and constipation. Paradoxical stimulatory reactions such as insomnia, nervousness, and irritability may also occur. In acute overdose, doxylamine and diphenhydramine have been reported to produce rhabdomyolysis.[29,30] The 2006 National Poison Data System reported 66,448 cases of overdoses secondary to antihistamines.[31] These cases included 31,816 secondary to diphenhydramine, with the remainder attributable to other antihistamines. Serious toxicities have included cardiac arrhythmias and seizures; the most common autopsy finding was pulmonary congestion.[32] Psychiatric reactions have also been reported, including hallucinations and psychosis. Persons of advanced age may be particularly vulnerable to side effects of antihistamines.[33] Lactating women should not use antihistamines, because these agents may be excreted in the milk and potentially cause adverse effects in the nursing infant.[34]

When combined with other CNS depressants (e.g., alcohol, tranquilizers, hypnotics, and sedatives), antihistamines may result in additive sedation. A small study[35] conducted in vitro and in vivo in 16 subjects found that diphenhydramine interfered with the biotransformation of metoprolol by inhibiting the polymorphic P450 enzyme CYP2D6. Metoprolol clearance was decreased twofold in 10 of 16 subjects. The effects of metoprolol on decreasing heart rate and systolic blood pressure were also more pronounced. A similar study[36] in 15 subjects found that diphenhydramine increased venlafaxine plasma concentration more than twofold. Diphenhydramine use warrants caution, particularly if a person is taking medications metabolized by CYP2D6 isoenzymes (e.g., opiates, certain psychiatric medications, beta-blockers, and certain antiarrhythmics). Additive sedation or anticholinergic effects may occur when antihistamines are combined with tricyclic antidepressants.[25]

Specific warnings require that persons be advised not to use the antihistamine, except under medical supervision, if they have respiratory conditions (chronic bronchitis or emphysema), glaucoma, or difficulty with urination attributable to prostate gland enlargement. These agents should be used with caution in children or elderly patients because of the increased possibility of side effects.[26,33]

FDA issued a final rule, effective December 8, 2003, amending labeling for oral nonprescription antiemetics, antihistamines, antitussives, and nighttime sleep-aid drug products that contain diphenhydramine citrate or hydrochloride.[37] The label reads, "Do not use with any other product containing diphenhydramine, even one used on skin." Cases of toxic psychosis reported in children prompted this ruling.

A final precaution is that practitioners should be aware that nonprescription antihistamines such as cyclizine, diphenhydramine, or dimenhydrinate may be used and/or abused for psychiatric effects.[38,39]

Overall, nonprescription antihistamines are generally effective and safe to treat N/V. Results from comparisons many years ago indicate that equal doses of dimenhydrinate may be more effective than meclizine in the treatment of N/V of motion sickness.[40]

Pharmacologic Agents Used to Treat Nausea Associated with Food or Beverages

Nausea and/or vomiting may be associated with excessive or disagreeable food or beverage intake. The exact prevalence of gastric upset associated with overindulgence is unknown, but symptoms may include heartburn, indigestion, and upset stomach. Antacids, histamine₂-receptor antagonists, bismuth subsalicylate, and phosphorated carbohydrate solution have been used to relieve the symptoms associated with dietary overindulgence.

ANTACIDS

Antacids contain various combinations of ingredients, including magnesium hydroxide, aluminum hydroxide, calcium carbonate, and magnesium carbonate. Antacids neutralize gastric acidity, increasing the pH of the stomach and duodenum.[25] These agents are indicated for complaints of infrequent heartburn, dyspepsia, acid indigestion, and the symptomatic relief of upset stomach associated with gastric acidity.[25] The patient should take 15 mL of most antacids 30 minutes after meals and at bedtime. However, the efficacy of antacids for N/V associated with overeating has been marginal.[41] (See Chapter 14 for further discussion of antacids.)

HISTAMINE₂-RECEPTOR ANTAGONISTS

Histamine₂-receptor antagonists include cimetidine, ranitidine, famotidine, and nizatidine. These agents decrease acid secretion by competing with histamine for binding at H₂-receptor sites on parietal cells.[25] FDA has approved nonprescription use of these agents for infrequent heartburn and indigestion. However, the efficacy of histamine₂-receptor antagonists for N/V associated with overeating remains uncertain. (See Chapter 14 for further discussion of histamine₂-receptor antagonists.)

PROTON PUMP INHIBITORS

Proton pump inhibitors (PPI) such as omeprazole decrease gastric acid by shutting down the acid (or proton) pumps in the stomach.[25] These agents are not intended to provide immediate heartburn relief or protection before eating a spicy meal. Data are insufficient to support the use of PPIs for treating N/V associated with overeating. (See Chapter 14 for further discussion of PPIs.)

BISMUTH PRODUCTS

Bismuth subsalicylate (Pepto-Bismol) has been used to treat various GI complaints, including nausea associated with indigestion, heartburn, and fullness (gas) caused by overindulgence in food and drink.[25] It has also been used to treat diarrhea. Pepto-Bismol for adults contains bismuth subsalicylate, but Children's Pepto has been reformulated to contain calcium carbonate (www.childrenspepto.com). Salicylate-containing products should never be used in children with fever of unknown origin. (See Chapters 14 and 17 for further discussion of bismuth products.)

PHOSPHORATED CARBOHYDRATE SOLUTION

Phosphorated carbohydrate solution is a mixture of levulose (fructose), dextrose (glucose), and phosphoric acid[25] (Table 20-6). Phosphoric acid is added to adjust the pH of the commercial product to between 1.5 and 1.6. Hyperosmolar solutions with phosphoric acid are believed to relieve N/V by a direct local action on the GI tract wall that may decrease smooth muscle contraction and delay gastric emptying time. This product is believed to have a dose-related effect.[25] Phosphorated carbohydrate solution is indicated for nausea associated with upset stomach caused by intestinal or stomach influenza, and by food or drink indiscretions. This product has also been used in attempts to alleviate NVP and for motion sickness.[25]

The usual adult dosage of phosphorated carbohydrate solution is 15 to 30 mL (1–2 tablespoons) at 15-minute intervals until vomiting ceases.[25] Patients should be told not to take this

TABLE 20-6 Selected Antiemetic Products	
Trade Name	**Primary Ingredients/Features**
Bonine Chewable Tablets	Meclizine HCl 25 mg
Bonine Chewable Anti-Emetic Travel Tablets for Kids	Cyclizine HCl 25 mg
Dramamine Orange Chewable Tablets	Dimenhydrinate 50 mg
Dramamine Less Drowsy Formula Tablets	Meclizine HCl 25 mg
Marezine for Motion Sickness	Cyclizine HCl 50 mg
Emetrol Cherry Flavor Liquid	Phosphoric acid 21.5 g/5 mL; dextrose 1.87 g/5 mL; fructose 1.87 g/5 mL
Children's Pepto Chewable Tablets	Calcium carbonate 400 mg
Bio Band	Acupressure band worn on one hand
ReliefBand NST (Nerve Stimulation Technology)	Acustimulation band worn on one hand
Sea-Band	Acupressure band worn on both hands

Source: Reference 25.

agent for more than 1 hour and not to exceed five doses. The solution should not be diluted, and the patient should not consume other liquids for 15 minutes after taking a dose. If symptoms do not cease after five doses, the patient should be referred for medical evaluation.[25] For NVP the dose is 15 to 30 mL on arising and repeated every 3 hours or if nausea threatens.[25] Because of the product's high fructose and glucose content, phosphorated carbohydrate solution should not be used by individuals with hereditary fructose intolerance or diabetes.[25]

Probiotics

These products may improve microflora balance in the GI tract and may help to prevent or treat diarrhea. The role or exact strain(s) and doses of various probiotics for the treatment or prevention of N/V have not been determined. However, there is evidence that some products may help diarrhea secondary to rotavirus, infection, or antibiotic use.[42] (See Chapters 17 and 24 for further discussion of probiotics.)

Product Selection Guidelines

When considering use of certain products, several factors should be considered, including whether the patient is a woman who is pregnant or lactating, whether the patient is a child or of advanced age, and whether the patient has any limitations such as hepatic or renal impairment. These factors may affect dosing. Furthermore, the product should also be compatible with the patient's lifestyle, sensitivity to certain product ingredients such as dyes or fructose, and preference for frequency of dosing (Table 20-5). Hence, product selection guidelines should be compatible with special populations and patient factors, and should consider patient preferences, such as whether the product is chewable or contains alcohol (Table 20-6).

PREGNANCY

Nonpharmacologic modalities for NVP include diet and environmental changes, acupressure, and acustimulation. Pharmacologic treatment includes antihistamines, pyridoxine, combinations of antihistamines and pyridoxine, phosphorated carbohydrate solutions, and ginger (see the Complementary Therapies section). A number of evidence-based guidelines make recommendations for the treatment of NVP.[2,43,44] These guidelines state that taking a multivitamin at conception may help decrease the severity

of NVP.[43] Hence, the clinician may wish to suggest this in preconception counseling.

Antihistamines None of these agents has an FDA-approved indication for managing NVP, although all antihistamines appear to have a low risk of teratogenicity. Meclizine, cyclizine, dimenhydrinate, and diphenhydramine are classified as Pregnancy Category B.[25] However, use should be reserved for pregnant women with severe N/V unresponsive to nonpharmacologic measures.[2,43,44] Pregnant women should always consult their medical provider before taking any medication.

Pyridoxine Pyridoxine (vitamin B_6) is a water-soluble B complex essential vitamin. Uncontrolled studies in the 1940s suggested that pyridoxine might be effective in treating NVP. In 1979 the American Medical Association Council on Drugs found no conclusive evidence that pyridoxine was effective for treating NVP. According to a Cochrane review, one controlled study of 25 mg of pyridoxine given orally every 8 hours produced significant improvement in women who complained of severe NVP.[4] Another study showed that 30 mg/day relieved nausea but not vomiting.[4] The specific mechanism of action of pyridoxine is unknown. Evidence-based guidelines from the American College of Obstetrics and Gynecologists (ACOG) suggest starting NVP treatment with pyridoxine 10 to 25 mg three or four times a day.[43] The Cochrane review indicates that pyridoxine is the product least likely to result in adverse reactions.[4] Side effects are rare but may include peripheral sensory neuropathic disturbances at high doses, although such disturbances have been reported with daily doses as low as 50 mg.[25] Extremely high doses (200–600 mg/day) have inhibited prolactin secretion.[25] Pyridoxine is Pregnancy Category A.[34]

Doxylamine and Pyridoxine Doxylamine 10 mg was originally in the combination prescription product Bendectin, which also contained pyridoxine 10 mg (see previous section Pyridoxine). Although FDA had approved this product for treating NVP, the manufacturer withdrew Bendectin from the market in 1983 because of the high cost of litigation regarding teratogenicity. Analysis of data describing Bendectin use in large numbers of women indicates no evidence of teratogenicity.[45,46] However, the ingredients–doxylamine and pyridoxine–remain available as nonprescription products, and physicians continue to recommend these agents, in combination, for NVP when nonpharmacologic measures do not work. Pyridoxine and doxylamine are both classified as Pregnancy Category A.[34] The ACOG guidelines have suggested doxylamine 12.5 mg three or four times a day as second-line treatment for NVP.[43] In Canada, a sustained-release combination of 10 mg pyridoxine and 10 mg doxylamine is available under the trade name Diclectin.[2,44] Canadian guidelines suggest taking up to four tablets a day of this product (one in the morning, one in the afternoon, and two at bedtime) to treat NVP.[2,44] Updated Canadian guidelines confirm safety and efficacy of the combination of doxylamine and pyridoxine.[2]

Other Products   Other agents that have been used in pregnancy include antacids, phosphorated carbohydrate solution, and ginger. Acupressure and acustimulation bands have also been used successfully,[19–21] although results have been mixed.[3,4] Use of these devices should be considered for only cases of mild-to-moderate NVP. Histamine$_2$-receptor antagonists should not be used during pregnancy without consulting a medical provider. Bismuth subsalicylate (BSS) is contraindicated during pregnancy. Probiotics may be considered for diarrhea that may accompany NVP.[47]

LACTATING WOMEN

Most antiemetic products may be used except for antihistamines, because they may adversely affect the nursing infant. BSS is also contraindicated in breast-feeding. No studies evaluating ginger in lactating women are available.

CHILDREN

Agents used to treat N/V in children include antihistamines, phosphorated carbohydrate solution, and oral rehydration solutions. Antacids and histamine$_2$-receptor antagonists should be used only when recommended by medical providers. BSS is not recommended for use in children because of the possibility of Reye's syndrome.[26]

Antihistamines have been used to treat N/V associated with motion sickness and other causes in children. However, it is important for clinicians to counsel parents that these products may cause paradoxical stimulation and agitation.[26] Certain age limitations apply to antihistamines for cough and cold products (Table 20-5; see also Chapter 11); the same cautions should apply when considering an agent to treat N/V in children.

For phosphorated carbohydrate solution, children 12 years and older may use the same dose as adults (Table 20-6). In children 2 to 12 years, the dose is 5 to 10 mL (1–2 teaspoons) every 15 minutes. Parents should be told not to give the product for more than 1 hour and not to exceed five doses. As in adults, the solution should not be diluted, and other liquids should not be consumed for 15 minutes after taking a dose. Infants may also receive this product for regurgitation.[25] The dose is 5 to 10 mL (1–2 teaspoons) administered 10 to 15 minutes before each feeding or, for refractory cases, 10 to 15 mL (2–3 teaspoons) administered 30 minutes before feeding.[25,26]

Pediatric gastroenteritis is an important disorder that warrants close monitoring. In 1996, the American Academy of Pediatrics published practice parameters on acute gastroenteritis in children, but the academy has recently endorsed and accepted guidelines from the CDC on managing gastroenteritis.[6] The CDC treatment is supportive care while continuing diet and fluids. ORSs, which contain electrolyte mixtures, are the primary treatment for minimal or mild-to-moderate dehydration. CDC guidelines recommend that parents have ORS on hand in the home in case a child experiences diarrhea secondary to gastroenteritis.[6] Available products include Enfalyte, LiquiLytes, Pedialyte, and Rehydralyte. (See Chapter 17 for further discussion of ORSs.)

Use of sports drinks, gelatin water, fruit juices, and carbonated beverages is discouraged, because they are hyperosmolar and may worsen diarrhea; they are also deficient in electrolytes such as sodium, potassium, and chloride, which produce a rapid and significant therapeutic response to severe dehydration and electrolyte depletion.[6] Furthermore, use of homemade sugar-water or salt-water solutions should be discouraged, because they may lack certain electrolytes, such as bicarbonate and potassium.[15]

Administration of an ORS is based on severity of dehydration, as measured by weight loss.[6] The child is considered to have minimal or no dehydration if body weight loss is less than 3%. In this case, if the child weighs less than 10 kg, the parent should administer 60 to 120 mL ORS for each diarrheal stool or vomiting episode and 120 to 240 mL ORS if weight is over 10 kg.[6] For mild-to-moderate dehydration (3%–9% body weight loss), 50 to 100 mL/kg ORS over 2 to 4 hours is administered.[6] Limited fluid volumes starting with 5 mL aliquots should be given every 1 to 2 minutes, increasing the amount gradually as tolerated. Severe dehydration (>9% body weight loss) is a medical emergency and requires intravenous fluid replacement (see Chapter 17).[6] For all levels of dehydration, maintenance calories should be administered through breast-feeding or by providing the amount of formula that is usually consumed; there is no need for special or diluted formula.[6] Certain situations are best handled on an in-patient basis, such as the caregiver being unable to provide adequate care at home, substantial difficulty with ORS administration or ORS refusal, intractable vomiting, or inadequate intake or failure of ORS treatment. In cases of severe dehydration, the child should be admitted for in-patient care.[6]

ORS and other products (Table 20-6) are sometimes flavored to improve palatability in consideration of childrens' preferences.

PATIENTS OF ADVANCED AGE

Antiemetic use warrants caution in patients of advanced age, because they are at increased risk of adverse effects such as drowsiness, falls secondary to orthostasis, or anticholinergic effects such as constipation, urinary retention, or dry eyes that may occur with antihistamine use. These patients may also experience confusion or cognitive dysfunction when taking antihistamines.[33]

Many older patients take multiple medications, which increases the possibility of drug interactions with certain products such as antacids, certain histamine$_2$-receptor antagonists (cimetidine), PPIs, and BSS. For use of these agents, medical referral is always suggested.

Phosphorated carbohydrate solution may be used safely if the patient does not have diabetes or hereditary fructose intolerance. Acupressure bands may be safely used, although acustimulation devices should not be used if the patient has a pacemaker.

SUMMARY OF PRODUCT SELECTION GUIDELINES

Nonprescription antihistamines and phosphorated carbohydrate solutions are suitable to prevent or control self-limiting N/V, such as that associated with motion sickness or overindulgence in food and drink. Patients with hereditary fructose intolerance, however, should not take phosphorated carbohydrate solutions. Young children, persons of advanced age, and lactating women should avoid antihistamines.

Antacids, histamine$_2$-receptor antagonists, and BSS are appropriate for treating nausea related to overeating or consumption of disagreeable foods. Patients taking medications that may interact with salicylates should not take BSS. Children and teenagers recovering from chickenpox or viral influenza also should not take this agent, nor should pregnant or lactating women. Chapter 14 discusses possible drug interactions with antacids and histamine$_2$-receptor antagonists. Persons of advanced age and pregnant or lactating women may take either drug class.

Vomiting related to food poisoning or other self-limiting causes should be treated with ORSs to prevent dehydration and electrolyte disturbances. Inability to eat or drink because of nausea may cause dehydration, which also may be treated with ORSs. All age groups, including pregnant or lactating women, may safely use ORSs. Probiotics are also safe to use for diarrhea secondary to N/V in all age groups. Table 20-6 lists a variety of antiemetic products.

Complementary Therapies

Popular products for N/V include ginger, chamomile, and peppermint, but other products include lemon balm and artichoke. Table 20-7 lists selected complementary therapies for N/V. (See Chapter 54 for additional information about these products.)

Ginger (*Zingiber officinale*) is a botanical product that has been used to relieve nausea associated with motion sickness, pregnancy, and surgery. Ginger is used in different forms and contains gingerols and shogaols, which may work at the level of the digestive tract to inhibit N/V.[48] Unlike antihistamines, ginger does not produce CNS depression.

Two other herbal products commonly used for GI disorders are chamomile and peppermint. In GI disorders, chamomile (*Matricaria recutita*) is thought to have antispasmodic and mild sedative activities; it has GRAS (Generally Recognized as Safe by FDA) status in the United States.[48] Peppermint oil (*Mentha piperita*) is thought to have antispasmodic effects from direct action on digestive tract smooth muscle. It has GRAS status and is unsafe only when used in high doses or in very young children, because bronchospasm and respiratory arrest may occur.[48] Other products used to treat N/V are listed in Table 20-7.

Assessment of Nausea and Vomiting: A Case-Based Approach

Vomiting is a symptom produced not only by benign processes but also by serious illnesses. Vomiting may cause various complications. Physical assessment of the patient may help to determine whether some of the complications of N/V listed under Clinical Presentation of Nausea and Vomiting have occurred. Physical assessment should include the patient's general appearance, mental status, volume status, and the presence of any abdominal pain. Evaluation of vital signs such as blood pressure, heart rate, temperature, and weight (to determine whether recent weight loss has occurred) is also pertinent. Evaluation of concurrent signs and symptoms is useful in determining the potential cause of vomiting. Preexisting disease is an important factor to rule out. Detailed information about the patient's medical history related to the GI tract is especially helpful in determining potential causes.

A major concern with vomiting is the loss of fluids and the inability to eat or drink. This situation may result in dehydration and electrolyte disturbances. Self-care is inappropriate for patients with dehydration, severe anorexia, weight loss, or poor nutritional status. Medical evaluation for dehydration should be provided when severe vomiting or diarrhea persists for more than several hours in children or 48 hours in adults.[12-14,16,17]

Practitioners should be aware that some patients might use nonprescription antiemetics to self-treat the early stages of a serious illness. Therefore, to avoid potential additive toxicity, they should ask patients what they have already used to treat the symptoms. Many patients choose to self-medicate N/V with various nonprescription products to avoid a medical office visit. However, the practitioner should be cautious about recommending self-medication for these symptoms and ask appropriate questions to determine whether medical referral is indicated.

Cases 20-1 and 20-2 give examples of the assessment of patients with vomiting.

TABLE 20-7 Selected Complementary Therapies for Nausea and Vomiting

Botanical Agent (Scientific Name)	Risks	Uses/Properties
Artichoke (*Cynara scolymus*)	Possible allergic reactions and cross-reactions with members of Asteraceae family (chrysanthemums, arnica, pyrethrum)	Used for dyspeptic problems and nausea
Chamomile (*Matricaria recutita*)	Allergic reactions with members of Asteraceae family; coumarin content may interact with antiplatelet agents; additive sedation with CNS depressants	Has spasmolytic properties; used for gastric complaints and sedation
Ginger (*Zingiber officinale*)	Heartburn, worsening colic in persons with gallstones, possible bleeding reactions	Efficacy for N/V, NVP, and motion sickness shown in several trials
Lemon balm (*Melissa officinalis*)	Hypersensitivity reactions	Has spasmolytic and carminative effects for digestive disorders; used for different gastric complaints including vomiting
Peppermint (*Mentha piperita*)	Bronchial spasms in high doses; may worsen heartburn	Has spasmolytic properties; used for dyspepsia

Key: N/V, nausea and vomiting; NVP, nausea and vomiting of pregnancy.
Source: Reference 48.

CASE 20-1

Relevant Evaluation Criteria	Scenario/Model Outcome
Information Gathering	
1. Gather essential information about the patient's symptoms, including:	
a. description of symptom(s) (i.e., nature, onset, duration, severity, associated symptoms)	Patient has had frequent episodes of nausea and occasional vomiting; the episodes last a few hours during the main part of the day. She has maintained her appetite.
b. description of any factors that seem to precipitate, exacerbate, and/or relieve the patient's symptom(s)	Symptoms seem to worsen when the patient is preparing breakfast for her husband and 3-year-old child. She usually cooks bacon and eggs, but recently the smell of cooking bacon has nauseated her. She has tried to cut back to cooking bacon only a few times a week.
c. description of the patient's efforts to relieve the symptoms	The patient eats some dry toast and takes a few sips of ginger ale or water. She does not like the idea of taking "drugs" for her malady.
2. Gather essential patient history information:	
a. patient's identity	Amy Benson
b. patient's age, sex, height, and weight	28-year-old female, 5 ft 5 in, 135 lb
c. patient's occupation	Loan officer
d. patient's dietary habits	Balanced diet with plenty of fruits and vegetables; occasional alcohol (1–2 glasses of wine per month)
e. patient's sleep habits	Averages 7–8 hours per night
f. concurrent medical conditions, prescription and nonprescription medications, and dietary supplements	Patient found out that she is 7 weeks pregnant, is taking a prenatal vitamin, and denies use of dietary supplements.
g. allergies	Rash when given sulfa-containing medications
h. history of other adverse reactions to medications	Stomach upset with ibuprofen
i. other _____	N/A
Assessment and Triage	
3. Differentiate the patient's signs/symptoms and correctly identify the patient's primary problem(s).	Nausea lasting a few hours during the main part of the day; occasional vomiting. She does not like the smell of certain foods; NVP is likely.
4. Identify exclusions for self-treatment (see Figure 20-1).	None
5. Formulate a comprehensive list of therapeutic alternatives for the primary problem to determine if triage to a medical practitioner is required, and share this information with the patient.	Options include: (1) Recommend self-care with: —Nondrug strategies (dietary and environmental changes; see Table 20-4). —Acupressure or acustimulation bands. —OTC pyridoxine. —OTC doxylamine. —OTC phosphorated carbohydrate solution. —Ginger. (2) Recommend lifestyle modifications until medical provider may be consulted. (3) Make a medical referral. (4) Take no action.
Plan	
6. Select an optimal therapeutic alternative to address the patient's problem, taking into account patient preferences.	Because AB does not appear dehydrated and can drink small amounts of ginger ale and water, and she can tolerate dry toast, you encourage her to continue to take sips of liquids and eat toast. She does not have signs/symptoms of dehydration such as fast heartbeat, decreased skin turgor, noticeable weight loss, or clothes that fit loosely. A therapeutic alternative is the use of acupressure bands, because the patient has stated that she would prefer not to use "drugs" if possible. If symptoms persist, then she can try doxylamine 12.5 mg 3–4 times a day and vitamin B_6 10 mg 3–4 times a day. Other nonpharmacologic suggestions in Table 20-4 should be followed. If symptoms persist, she should consult her medical provider.

C A S E 2 0 - 1 (continued)

Relevant Evaluation Criteria	Scenario/Model Outcome
7. Describe the recommended therapeutic approach to the patient.	You probably have NVP. The acupressure bands may work but if they do not, then a combination of an antihistamine such as doxylamine and vitamin B_6 may help. These products should be taken 3–4 times a day. You may also benefit from other nonpharmacologic techniques (see Table 20-4) such as continuing the dry toast or eating bland foods and crackers in the morning before arising, sleeping in a well-ventilated room, and avoiding strong odors. If you do not feel better, you may want to contact your medical provider.
8. Explain to the patient the rationale for selecting the recommended therapeutic approach from the considered therapeutic alternatives.	Published information regarding acupressure bands has shown that they may help with NVP. However, the evidence-based guidelines of the American College of Obstetricians and Gynecologists and the Canadian Family Physician state that doxylamine and vitamin B_6, up to 4 tablets daily, may help your symptoms. Because you are able to drink fluids and are not dehydrated, seeking medical care may not be necessary at this time. However, if nausea and/or vomiting worsens, medical attention is necessary for further evaluation.

Patient Education

9. When recommending self-care with non-prescription medications and/or nondrug therapy, convey accurate information to the patient:	
a. appropriate dose and frequency of administration	Wear the acupressure bands continually.
b. maximum number of days the therapy should be employed	No limitations
c. product administration procedures	Wear the band on each wrist, 3 finger widths up from the first wrist crease.
d. expected time to onset of relief	Variable
e. degree of relief that can be reasonably expected	Variable
f. most common side effects	None expected
g. side effects that warrant medical intervention should they occur	None expected
h. patient options in the event that condition worsens or persists	Add vitamin B_6 10 mg combined with 12.5 mg of doxylamine (one-half of a 25 mg tablet). Take these with a small glass of water 3–4 times a day. Doxylamine is available in the United States as an OTC sleep aid (Unisom Sleeptabs 25 mg). There are no limits on the number of days these medications can be taken. Expected time to onset of relief and degree of relief are variable.
	Vitamin B_6 likely will not cause any side effects. Drowsiness is the most common side effect of doxylamine; therefore, it is important not to drive or operate machinery while taking doxylamine. Other possible side effects include dry mouth, dry eyes, nasal congestion, urinary retention, and constipation. Medical attention is necessary if the N/V does not improve or if side effects from the OTC product occur.
i. product storage requirements	Store at 59°F–86°F (15°C–30°C).
j. specific nondrug measures	See Table 20-4 for dietary and other measures.
10. Solicit follow-up questions from patient.	Will any of these products hurt my baby? What other products could I use instead?
11. Answer patient's questions.	These products have been used by many other pregnant women and have not caused harm to the mother or baby. They are considered Pregnancy Category A, which is the safest class. You should talk to your medical provider about these products and obtain information from the resources listed on this handout (see Table 20-8). Another product used for NVP is an acustimulation device, worn as a wristwatch on a single wrist, but this product is expensive. Other products include ginger or phosphorated carbohydrate solution. If these products do not work, then medical attention is necessary to consider a prescription product for the NVP.

Key: N/A, not applicable; NKA, no known allergies; NVP, nausea and vomiting of pregnancy; OTC, over-the-counter.

CASE 20-2

Relevant Evaluation Criteria	Scenario/Model Outcome

Information Gathering

1. Gather essential information about the patient's symptoms, including:

   a. description of symptom(s) (i.e., nature, onset, duration, severity, associated symptoms)

   Patient has had six episodes of nausea, vomiting, and diarrhea in the past 10 hours. The patient seems somnolent and quiet except for violent episodes of emesis or diarrhea.

   b. description of any factors that seem to precipitate, exacerbate, and/or relieve the patient's symptom(s)

   Symptoms worsen when the patient's mother attempts to provide small sips of Gatorade.

   c. description of the patient's efforts to relieve the symptoms

   Patient's mother tried to get the child to eat a few bites of soda crackers or sips of fluid.

2. Gather essential patient history information:

   a. patient's identity

   Megan Moore

   b. patient's age, sex, height, and weight

   18-month-old female, 25 inches, 23 lb (26 lb on previous day)

   c. patient's occupation

   N/A

   d. patient's dietary habits

   Normal healthy diet, consisting of cereals, mashed vegetables, pasta, rice, chicken, yogurt, milk, and juice

   e. patient's sleep habits

   Up at 7:00 am; in bed at 7:30 pm; naps for 2 hours from 1 to 3 pm

   f. concurrent medical conditions, prescription and nonprescription medications, and dietary supplements

   Children's multivitamin

   g. allergies

   NKA

   h. history of other adverse reactions to medications

   None

   i. other _____

   N/A

Assessment and Triage

3. Differentiate the patient's signs/symptoms and correctly identify the patient's primary problem(s).

   Patient has had several episodes of nausea, vomiting, and diarrhea. The patient appears drowsy, unusually lethargic, and her body appears floppy. The child appears dizzy when she stands up and her abdomen seems somewhat flat. She has had a dry diaper for several hours. Although the child appears to cry, few tears are noted.

   Patient appears dehydrated and may have viral gastroenteritis.

4. Identify exclusions for self-treatment (see Figure 20-2).

   Based on signs/symptoms, patient appears dehydrated.

5. Formulate a comprehensive list of therapeutic alternatives for the primary problem to determine if triage to a medical practitioner is required, and share this information with the caregiver.

   Options include:

   (1) Recommend that patient's mother administer:
   —OTC oral rehydration solution.
   —OTC phosphorated carbohydrate solution.
   —An acupressure band.
   (2) Recommend patient's mother administer self-care modalities until a medical practitioner can be consulted.
   (3) Refer patient for further medical evaluation.
   (4) Take no action.

Plan

6. Select an optimal therapeutic alternative to address the patient's problem, taking into account patient preferences.

   Megan is unable to drink small amounts of fluid or eat small bites of crackers. She also has signs/symptoms of dehydration (appears drowsy and lethargic; has a floppy body, dizziness, flat abdomen; has lost 3 pounds since the previous day; has a dry diaper and sheds few tears). Based on the signs/symptoms, the patient's mother should immediately take the child for medical evaluation and attempt to administer small sips of ORS on the way to the emergency room.

CASE 20-2 (continued)

Relevant Evaluation Criteria	Scenario/Model Outcome
7. Describe the recommended therapeutic approach to the caregiver.	Your child needs to be seen by a medical provider because she appears dehydrated. Please have someone drive you and your child to the emergency room at the hospital. On the way, administer 1 teaspoonful of ORS every 1 to 2 minutes.
8. Explain to the caregiver the rationale for selecting the recommended therapeutic approach from the considered therapeutic alternatives.	Your child's symptoms (floppy body, flat abdomen, weight loss, dry diaper, few tears) indicate that she is dehydrated. Because she has been unable to drink sufficient fluids or eat anything to counter the dehydration, she needs medical attention.
Patient Education	
9. When recommending self-care with nonprescription medications and/or nondrug therapy, convey accurate information to the caregiver.	Criterion does not apply in this case.
10. Solicit follow-up questions from caregiver.	Is there an OTC medication that might work so that I don't have to take her to the emergency room?
11. Answer caregiver's questions.	No. Your child is dehydrated; she needs urgent medical care so that she can feel better and get well.

Key: N/A, not applicable; NKA, no known allergies; ORS, oral rehydration solution; OTC, over-the-counter.

Patient Counseling for Nausea and Vomiting

The practitioner should stress that treatment of N/V must focus on identifying and, if possible, correcting the underlying cause. Patients prone to overeating, eating disorders, or motion sickness should try to avoid behaviors or situations that cause N/V. The patient should be advised that acute vomiting requires only symptomatic treatment, because it is usually self-limiting and will resolve spontaneously. If the cause of the symptoms is known and self-treatment is appropriate, the practitioner should explain the proper use of the recommended product. Patient education should include information about possible adverse effects, as well as signs and symptoms that indicate medical attention is warranted.

Telling patients about information resources for N/V may help provide reassurance (Table 20-8). The box Patient Education for Nausea and Vomiting lists specific information to provide patients.

TABLE 20-8 Information Resources on Nausea and Vomiting

- Information from the American Academy of Family Physicians on nausea and vomiting is available at www.familydoctor.org/online/famdocen/home/tools/symptom/529.html.
- The National Organization of Teratology Information Services refers patients to a teratology information service in their area. Toll-free phone: 1-866-626-6847; Web site: www.otispregnancy.org.
- A help line for patients with NVP is available at 1-800-436-8477.
- Information on NVP is available at www.motherisk.org.
- The American Academy of Family Physicians (AAFP) provides tips about "morning sickness" at its Web site (www.familydoctor.org).
- Information on "morning sickness" is available at www.my.webmd.com (click on Pregnancy health center and search on "morning sickness").
- Evidence-based guidelines for NVP are available in the ACOG (American College of Obstetrics and Gynecology)

Practice Bulletin: nausea and vomiting of pregnancy. *Obstet Gynecol.* 2004;103:803–14.
- Canadian updated evidence-based guidelines for NVP are available in Einarson A, Maltepe, C, Boskovic R, Koren G. Treatment of nausea and vomiting in pregnancy—an updated algorithm. *Can Fam Physician.* 2007;53:2109–11.
- Information on telephone triage for specific referral recommendations is available in Schmitt BD. *Pediatric Telephone Protocols: Office Version.* 10th ed. Elk Grove Park, Ill: American Academy of Pediatrics; 2004.
- The CDC provides information on acute gastroenteritis in children in King CB, Glass R, Bresee JS, Duggan C. Managing acute gastroenteritis among children: oral rehydration, maintenance, and nutritional therapy from the Centers for Disease Control and Prevention. *MMWR Recomm Rep.* 2003;52 (RR-16):1–16. Available at: www.cdc.gov/mmwr/PDF/RR/RR5216.pdf.

Key: NVP, nausea and vomiting of pregnancy.

The objectives of self-treatment are to (1) prevent or control symptoms of occasional mild, self-limiting nausea and vomiting, (2) improve the symptoms and the patient's overall sense of well-being, and (3) avoid unnecessary emergency health care visits. For most patients, carefully following product instructions and the self-care measures listed here will help ensure optimal therapeutic outcomes.

Nondrug Measures

- To prevent NVP, eat small, frequent meals that are low in fat content. Sleep in a room with fresh air. Also, try eating crackers before getting up in the morning. Try lying down to relieve the symptoms once they occur. (See Tables 20-4 and 20-8.)
- To prevent motion sickness in young children, place them in a car seat that allows them to look out the windows (see Table 20-3). Try acupressure wristbands to prevent motion sickness in adults or older children.
- To prevent nausea associated with overeating, avoid foods or beverages known to cause nausea; consume foods and beverages in moderation.

Nonprescription Medications

Antacids, Histamine₂-Receptor Antagonists, and Bismuth Subsalicylate

- Take antacids, histamine₂-receptor antagonists (e.g., ranitidine, famotidine, cimetidine, or nizatidine), or bismuth subsalicylate (Pepto-Bismol) for nausea caused by overeating. Follow product instructions for dosages. (See Chapters 14 and 17 for additional information on these medications.)

Phosphorated Carbohydrate Solution

- Take phosphorated carbohydrate solutions for nausea and vomiting associated with upset stomach caused by viral gastroenteritis, food indiscretions, and emotional upset. (See Table 20-6 for selected brand-name products.)
- Give 1–2 tablespoonfuls (15–30 mL) of the solution to adults at 15-minute intervals until vomiting stops. For children ages 2–12 years old, give 1–2 teaspoonfuls (5–10 mL). Do not give more than five doses in 1 hour.

- Do not dilute the solution, and do not allow the patient to consume other liquids for 15 minutes after taking a dose.
- Patients with hereditary fructose intolerance should not take this product.
- Patients with diabetes should consult their medical provider before taking this product.
- Seek medical attention if vomiting does not stop after five doses of a phosphorated carbohydrate solution.

Antihistamines

- Take antihistamines for self-treatment of nausea and vomiting caused by motion sickness.
- To prevent motion sickness, take antihistamines at least 30–60 minutes before departure. Continue taking the medication during travel. Follow the dosage guidelines in Table 20-5.
- While using antihistamines, avoid driving or operating hazardous machinery or engaging in tasks that require a high degree of mental alertness. Drowsiness is the most common adverse effect of these medications.
- Patients with asthma, narrow-angle glaucoma, obstructive disease of the GI or genitourinary tract, or benign prostatic hypertrophy should consult a medical provider before using antihistamines.
- Caution patients that antihistamines may increase the sedative effects of alcohol, tranquilizers, hypnotics, and sedatives. Antihistamines may produce excitability in children or mental confusion in persons of advanced age.
- Do not take oral diphenhydramine products if topical or external diphenhydramine preparations are being used.

Oral Rehydration Solutions

- If needed, take an oral rehydration solution to prevent dehydration secondary to vomiting and diarrhea.

 Seek medical attention if there are signs and symptoms of serious dehydration associated with nausea and vomiting.

Evaluation of Patient Outcomes for Nausea and Vomiting

There are many causes of N/V including overeating, motion sickness, an acute illness, or pregnancy. In most cases this condition is self-limiting. Depending on the cause, various treatments or medications are used to treat N/V. After a clinician has provided information or suggestions for treatment of N/V, a follow-up assessment of the patient should occur within 24 hours of the initial encounter. This contact allows the clinician to determine whether symptoms have improved, changed, or worsened. This evaluation may best be accomplished by a follow-up phone call and then a scheduled appointment if desired by the patient. The follow-up should include an assessment of whether the N/V has diminished or abated, whether there are any residual related symptoms such as signs or symptoms of dehydration, whether vital signs such as racing heart or delayed capillary refill have returned to normal, and whether the patient is febrile. If the patient had prolonged N/V (longer than 24–48 hours) or a

change in or worsening of symptoms that required immediate referral to a medical provider, it is important for the clinician to follow up with the patient by telephone to determine whether the patient sought medical help and what type of treatment was administered. It is also important for the clinician to assess whether he or she needs to provide any further counseling or answer further patient questions. The clinician should also use this opportunity to provide reassurance and support.

Key Points for Nausea and Vomiting

- ➤ N/V are symptoms of an underlying disorder; therefore, treatment should focus on identifying and correcting the underlying cause.
- ➤ Nonprescription antiemetic medications are suitable for preventing and controlling the symptoms of occasional self-limiting N/V.
- ➤ Overeating, food poisoning, and motion sickness may cause self-limiting cases of these symptoms.

➤ Overeating may be treated with antacids, nonprescription histamine$_2$-blockers, or phosphorated carbohydrate solution.

➤ Antihistamines are agents of choice to treat N/V of motion sickness.

➤ Agents that may be used safely to treat N/V in all persons 2 years of age and older, as well as NVP, include acupressure/acustimulation devices and phosphorated carbohydrate solution.

➤ Uncomplicated NVP may be treated with pyridoxine, doxylamine, phosphorated carbohydrate solution, or acupressure/acustimulation devices.

➤ Loss of fluids and the inability to eat or drink because of N/V may result in dehydration and electrolyte disturbances. This primary complication of N/V should be treated with ORSs.

➤ Diarrhea secondary to N/V may be treated with probiotics at all ages.

➤ A patient who presents with complicated issues relating to N/V may not be a candidate for self-treatment but instead should be referred.

REFERENCES

1. Amdipharm. Nausea and vomiting. Available at: http://www.nauseaandvomiting.co.uk. Last accessed August 8, 2008.

2. Einarson A, Maltepe C, Boskovic R, Koren G. Treatment of nausea and vomiting in pregnancy—an updated algorithm. *Can Fam Physician*. 2007;53:2109–11.

3. Badell ML, Ramin SM, Smith JA. Treatment options for nausea and vomiting during pregnancy. *Pharmacotherapy*. 2006;26:1273–87.

4. Jewell MD, Young G. Interventions for nausea and vomiting in early pregnancy. *Cochrane Database System Rev* 2003;4:CD000145.

5. Dishkin AA. Gastroenteritis. Available at: http://www.emedicine.com/emerg/TOPIC213.HTM. Last accessed August 8, 2008

6. King CB, Glass R, Bresee JS, et al. Managing acute gastroenteritis among children: oral rehydration, maintenance, and nutritional therapy from the Centers for Disease Control and Prevention. *MMWR Recomm Rep*. 2003;52(RR-16):1–16. Available at: http://www.cdc.gov/mmwr/PDF/RR/RR5216.pdf. Last accessed August 8, 2008.

7. Parashar UD, Alexander JP, Glass RI. Advisory Committee on Immunization Practices (ACIP), Centers for Disease Control and Prevention (CDC): prevention of rotavirus gastroenteritis among infants and children. Recommendations of the Advisory Committee on Immunization Practices (ACIP). *MMWR Recomm Rep*. 2006;55(RR-12):1–13.

8. Wilhelm SM, Dehoorne-Smith ML, Kale-Pradhan PB. Prevention of postoperative nausea and vomiting. *Ann Pharmacother*. 2007;41:68–78.

9. Hornby PJ. Central neurocircuitry associated with emesis. *Am J Med*. 2001;111(8A):106S–12S.

10. Quigley EM, Hasler WL, Parkman HP. AGA technical review on nausea and vomiting. *Gastroenterology*. 2001;120:263–86.

11. DiPiro CV, Taylor AT. Nausea and vomiting. In: Dipiro JT, Talbert RL, Yee GC, et al., eds. *Pharmacotherapy: A Pathophysiologic Approach*. 6th ed. New York. McGraw-Hill, Inc; 2005:665–76.

12. Arnold MS, Trence DL. Hyperglycemia. In: Mensing C, ed. *The Art and Science of Diabetes Self-Management Education—A Desk Reference for Healthcare Professionals*. Chicago: American Association of Diabetes Educators, 2006:163–85.

13. Kuver R, Sheffield JV, McDonald GB. Nausea and vomiting in adolescents and adults. Available at: http://www.uwgi.org/guidelines/ch_01/ch01txt.htm. Last accessed August 8, 2008.

14. Schmitt BD. *Pediatric Telephone Protocols: Office Version*. 10th ed. Elk Grove Park, Ill: American Academy of Pediatrics; 2004.

15. Armon K, Stephenson T, MacFaul R, et al. An evidence and consensus based guideline for acute diarrhoea management. *Arch Dis Child*. 2001;85:132–42.

16. Thielman NM, Guerrant RL. Acute infectious diarrhea. *N Engl J Med*. 2004;350:38–47.

17. Helton T, Rolston DD. What adults with acute diarrhea should be evaluated? What is the best diagnostic approach? *Cleve Clin J Med*. 2004;71:778–9, 783–5.

18. US Food and Drug Administration, Center for Drug Evaluation and Research. Public Health Advisory: Nonprescription Cough and Cold Medicine Use in Children. Available at: http://www.fda.gov/cder/drug/advisory/cough_cold_2008.htm. Last accessed August 8, 2008.

19. Dune LS, Shiao SY. Meta-analysis of acustimulation effects on postoperative nausea and vomiting in children. *Explore* (NY). 2006;2:314–20.

20. Rosen T, de Veciana M, Miller HS, et al. A randomized controlled trial of nerve stimulation for relief of nausea and vomiting in pregnancy. *Obstet Gynecol*. 2003;102:129–35.

21. Ezzo J, Streitberger K, Schneider A. Cochrane systematic reviews examine P6 acupuncture-point stimulation for nausea and vomiting. *J Altern Complement Med*. 2006;12:489–95.

22. Quinlan JD, Hill DA. Nausea and vomiting of pregnancy. *Am Fam Physician*. 2003;68:121–8.

23. Kaiser LL, Allen L. Position of the American Dietetic Association: nutrition and lifestyle for a healthy pregnancy outcome. *J Am Diet Assoc*. 2002;102:1479–90.

24. American Academy of Family Physicians. Morning sickness. Available at: http://familydoctor.org/online/famdocen/home/women/pregnancy/basics/154.html. Last accessed August 8, 2008.

25. Wickersham RM, Novak KK, eds. *Drug Facts and Comparisons*. St. Louis, Mo: Wolters Kluwer Health, Inc; 2007.

26. Taketomo CK, Hodding JH, Krause DM, eds. *Pediatric Dosage Handbook*. 14th ed. Hudson, Ohio: Lexi-Comp, Inc; 2007.

27. Pasricha PJ. Treatment of disorders of bowel motility and water flux; antiemetics; agents used in biliary and pancreatic disease. In: Brunton LL, Lazo JS, Parker KL, eds. *The Pharmacological Basis of Therapeutics*. 11th ed. New York: McGraw-Hill, Inc; 2005:983–1008.

28. Weiler JM, Bloomfield JR, Woodworth GG, et al. Effects of fexofenadine, diphenhydramine, and alcohol on driving performance: a randomized, placebo-controlled trial in the Iowa driving simulator. *Ann Intern Med*. 2000;132:354–63.

29. Khosla U, Ruel KS, Hunt DB. Antihistamine-induced rhabdomyolysis. *South Med J* 2003;10:1023–6.

30. Jo Y-I, Song J-O, Park J-H, et al. Risk factors for rhabdomyolysis following doxylamine overdose. *Hum Exp Toxicol* 2007;26:617–21.

31. Bronstein AC, Spyker A, Cantilena LR, et al. 2006 annual report of the American Association of Poison Control Centers' National Poison Data System (NPDS). *Clin Toxicol*. 2007;45:815–917.

32. Nine JS, Rund CR: Fatality from diphenhydramine monointoxication—a case report and review of the infant, pediatric, and adult literature. *Am J Forensic Med Pathol*. 2006;27:36–41.

33. Fick DM, Cooper JW, Wade WE, et al. Updating the Beers criteria for potentially inappropriate medication use in older adults. *Arch Intern Med*. 2003;163:2716–24.

34. Briggs GG, Freeman RK, Yaffe SJ, eds. *Drugs in Pregnancy and Lactation*. 7th ed. Philadelphia: Lippincott William & Wilkins; 2005.

35. Hamelin BA, Bouayad A, Methot J, et al. Significant interaction between the nonprescription antihistamine diphenhydramine and the CYP2D6 substrate metoprolol in healthy men with high or low CYP2D6 activity. *Clin Pharmacol Ther*. 2000;67:466–77.

36. Lessard E, Yessine MA, Hamelin BA, et al. Diphenhydramine alters the disposition of venlafaxine through inhibition of CYP2D6 activity in humans. *J Clin Psychopharmacol*. 2001;21:175–84.

37. Food and Drug Administration, Department of Health and Human Services. Labeling of diphenhydramine-containing drug products for over-the-counter human use: final rule. *Fed Regist* physician. 2002;67:72555–9.

38. Barsoum A, Kolivakis TT, Margolese HC, et al. Diphenhydramine (Unisom), a central anticholinergic and antihistaminic: abuse with massive ingestion in a patient with schizophrenia. *Can J Psychiatry*. 2000;45:846–7.

39. Halpert AG, Olmstead MC, Beninger RJ. Mechanisms and abuse liability of the antihistamine dimenhydrinate. *Neurosci Biobehav Rev*. 2002;26:61–7.

40. Zajonc TP, Roland PS: Vertigo and motion sickness. Part II: pharmacologic treatment. *ENT*. 2006;85:25–35.

41. Dickerson LM, King DE. Evaluation and management of nonulcer dyspepsia. *Am Fam Physician*. 2004;70:107–14.

42. Ouwehand A, Vesterlund S: Health aspects of probiotics. *Idrugs*. 2003; 6:573–80.

43. ACOG (American College of Obstetrics and Gynecology) Practice Bulletin: nausea and vomiting of pregnancy. *Obstet Gynecol*. 2004;103:803–14.

44. Levichek Z, Atanackovic G, Oepkes D, et al. Nausea and vomiting of pregnancy. Evidence-based treatment algorithm. *Can Fam Physician*. 2002; 48:267–8, 277.

45. Brent R. Bendectin and birth defects: hopefully, the final chapter. *Birth Defects Res Part A Clin Mol Teratol* 2003;67:79–87.

46. Kutcher JS, Engle A, Firth J, et al. Bendectin and birth defects II: ecological analyses. *Birth Defects Res A Clin Mol Teratol* 2003;67:88–97.

47. Reid G, Kirjaivanen P: Taking probiotics during pregnancy. Available at: http://www.motherisk.org. Last accessed August 8, 2008.

48. Fetrow CW, Avila JR (Eds.). *Professional's Handbook of Complementary and Alternative Medicines*. 3rd ed. Springhouse, Pa: Lippincott Williams & Wilkins; 2004.

Poisoning

Wendy Klein-Schwartz and Barbara Insley Crouch

Poisoning is a common and potentially life-threatening injury. Although unintentional poisoning is responsible for most toxic exposures in young children, poisonings in other age groups may be unintentional or intentional, that is, caused by suicide attempts, substance abuse, or drug misuse. The majority of poisonings are a result of ingestion of a substance, but poisonings may also occur after a toxin is inhaled or comes in contact with the skin and eyes. Bites and envenomations are other potential sources of toxin exposures. First aid for poisonings focuses on minimizing the extent of the exposure. For inhalation exposure, the person is removed to fresh air, and, for topical exposures, the skin or eye is irrigated to remove the toxic substance. Gastrointestinal (GI) decontamination reduces absorption of ingested toxins, thereby minimizing toxicity. Ipecac syrup, a nonprescription emetic, has been used to induce vomiting for some poisonings managed at home, but this agent is rarely recommended. Alternatively, activated charcoal may be used to adsorb substances in the GI tract, although it is not universally accepted as a self-treatment. A poison control center should be contacted for assessment and treatment of poisonings, as well as for educational materials on poison prevention. Figure 21-1 shows the nationwide poison control center number and logo.

Unintentional poisonings are one of the leading causes of injury-related hospitalizations in preschool children, even though fatalities among preschoolers have declined significantly since the early 1970s. According to a recent analysis of the National Electronic Injury Surveillance System—All Injury Program (NEISS-AIP), an estimated 50,000 children younger than 5 years are evaluated in emergency departments annually for unintentional medication-related exposures.[1] Hospitalization or specialized medical care was required in nearly 10% of cases. The most common categories of medications were acetaminophen, antidepressants and mood stabilizers, cough and cold medications, nonsteroidal anti-inflammatory medications, and other central nervous system medications.

The National Center for Health Statistics mortality data for 2004 reports 31 deaths caused by unintentional poisoning in children younger than 5 years.[2] Only 29 of the 1229 fatalities reported by poison control centers in 2006 involved children younger than 6 years.[3] Medications and illicit drugs (excluding ethanol) were the primary substances responsible for 1000 (81.4%) of the 1229 fatalities, and they were involved in 27 additional deaths in which a nonpharmaceutical substance was the primary agent. In 2006, 61 poison control centers serving the United States and territories reported 2,403,539 cases to the National Poison Data System (formerly the Toxic Exposure Surveillance System) of the American Association of Poison Control Centers.[3]

The majority of poison exposures (50.9%) occur in children younger than 6 years, of which 89% involve children 3 years of age and younger.[3] Nonprescription and prescription medications are frequently responsible for potentially toxic exposures reported to poison control centers. Nonprescription products, such as analgesics and cough and cold preparations, are among the most common substances ingested by young children. The large number of nonprescription medications involved in pediatric exposures reflects the common use and availability of these products in the home. Other substances include cleaning substances, cosmetics and personal care products, plants, pesticides, food products/poisoning, alcohols, hydrocarbons (e.g., gasoline), and chemicals.

Child-resistant closures help prevent unintentional poisonings. These closures have been responsible for a decline in mortality related to childhood poisoning with regulated substances such as aspirin, prescription drugs, and some household chemicals. A 34% reduction in the aspirin-related mortality rate in children younger than 5 years is associated with the use of child-resistant closures.[4] Similarly, the decline in iron poisonings from 2370 cases in 1996 to 790 cases in 1999, as reported to the National Electronic Injury Surveillance System, has been attributed to unit-dose packaging requirements for products containing 30 mg or more of elemental iron; the Food and Drug Administration (FDA) enacted these requirements, which were in effect from 1997 to 2003.[5] The impact of the reversal of this FDA decision on childhood iron poisonings has not been evaluated.

Nearly 73% of poison exposures reported to poison control centers are managed onsite, usually in a residence. Only 11.5% of children younger than 6 years are managed in a health care facility, and major effects or fatal outcomes occur in less than 1%.[3] However, unintentional childhood poisonings remain a common cause of injury-related morbidity, requiring significant expenditures of health care dollars for inpatient and outpatient care. Pediatric admissions to urban hospitals related to poisoning accounted for almost $1 million in hospital charges in 1995.[6] Alternatively, unnecessary economic costs are incurred when an emergency department is used as the initial means of intervention for unintentional pediatric ingestions, rather than a poison control center.[7] In a survey conducted by one regional poison control center that served 60% of the counties in one state, the staff estimated that their center prevented more than

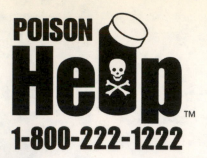

$3.6 million in unnecessary emergency department visits, including more than $1 million to the state medical assistance program.[8] A benefit–cost analysis for poisonings in the United States found that poison control centers reduce medical spending by $355 million (1992 dollars) and cost $65 million (1992 dollars) for their operation.[9] A significant portion of the cost savings results from home observation and decontamination, as well as the reduction of unnecessary emergency medical transport and treatment costs.

Clinical Presentation of Poisoning

Poisons can affect every organ system. Signs and symptoms of poisoning can range in severity from mild to life threatening. For some drugs, toxicity after overdose is similar to the drug's adverse effect profile with therapeutic use. For example, ibuprofen overdose is characterized primarily by nausea, vomiting, and abdominal pain. Patients with diphenhydramine overdose may exhibit sedation or stimulation (agitation, hallucinations), tachycardia, hypertension, dry mouth, and dilated pupils from its anticholinergic properties. Overdoses of other drugs, such as aspirin, result in multiorgan system effects including GI, central nervous system, metabolic, cardiovascular, pulmonary, and hematologic toxicity. A lack of symptoms immediately after a poison exposure does not preclude toxicity. Patients may be asymptomatic initially, but they can develop severe toxicity hours later after ingestion of some sustained-released or enteric-coated products or products that delay gastric emptying and/or slow GI motility (e.g., diphenoxylate/atropine). For other drugs, such as levothyroxine and sulfasalazine and some chemicals (e.g., methanol and acetonitrile), clinical effects are delayed while the substance is being metabolized to active or toxic metabolites. The time course of acetaminophen overdose is related to formation and covalent binding of a toxic metabolite to hepatic cells. As a result, a relatively mild initial clinical course characterized by nausea, vomiting, anorexia, and malaise can be followed by severe hepatic and renal toxicity 3 to 5 days later. Some poisons may produce no symptoms or they may be delayed. Any symptoms may require attention, because they may due to causes other than poisoning. Regardless of the cause of symptoms, if they are serious enough, they warrant medical attention.

Treatment of Poisoning

Most unintentional poison exposures in small children result in minimal, if any, effects and require no treatment other than observation. Although self-treatment may be appropriate, practitioners, caregivers, and patients are encouraged to seek counsel from the nearest poison control center before attempting any treatment.

Treatment Goals

The primary goal of home or prehospital therapy is to prevent absorption of toxins or stem the progression of toxicity, thus minimizing morbidity and mortality.

General Treatment Approach

The first step in assessing a potential poison exposure is to determine whether the patient has symptoms and whether the exposure puts the patient at risk of toxicity. Many exposures are, in fact, nontoxic or minimally toxic, because either the substance has a very low inherent toxicity or the amount consumed is too low to cause toxicity. A decision regarding the option for self-treatment depends on the nature of the poison exposure, toxicity of the agent, and general health status of the patient. Self-treatment should be considered only if the ingestion is unintentional and the potential for toxicity is assessed as minor. Any exposure to a toxin that can potentially result in moderate-to-severe toxicity, as well as all intentional exposures, should be referred immediately to a hospital. If the patient exhibits potentially life-threatening clinical effects (e.g., coma, convulsions, or syncope), transportation to an emergency department should be arranged immediately through the emergency 911 system. Additional exclusions for self-treatment can be found in Figure 21-2. Hospital care includes observing the patient, supporting vital functions (airway, breathing, and circulation), preventing absorption, enhancing elimination, and using antidotes.

The majority of individuals who do not require immediate hospital referral are managed with onsite observation only and no specific treatment.[3] In some instances, the approach is to attenuate the exposure by irrigating or preventing further absorption. The nonprescription drugs ipecac syrup and activated charcoal may prevent or reduce the absorption of some ingested substances. However, their routine use is not recommended without consultation with a poison control center. In the past, nonprescription cathartics have been recommended to decrease absorption of substances by facilitating their elimination through the GI tract. However, cathartics by themselves are not beneficial in the treatment of a poisoned patient. Figure 21-2 outlines self-care of exposure to poisons.

Nonpharmacologic Therapy

Inhalation exposures are managed by removing the patient from the toxic fumes to fresh air. Irrigation may be beneficial to decrease the contact time of a chemical with the skin or mucosal surface. Skin surfaces should be washed with soap and water (usually twice) to decrease the contact time of a chemical exposure. Irrigation of the eye with water should be initiated immediately after an ocular exposure to a chemical or drug not intended for ocular use (e.g., inadvertent ocular administration of an otic preparation). If an irritating chemical has been swallowed, the administration of a small amount of fluids may decrease the con-

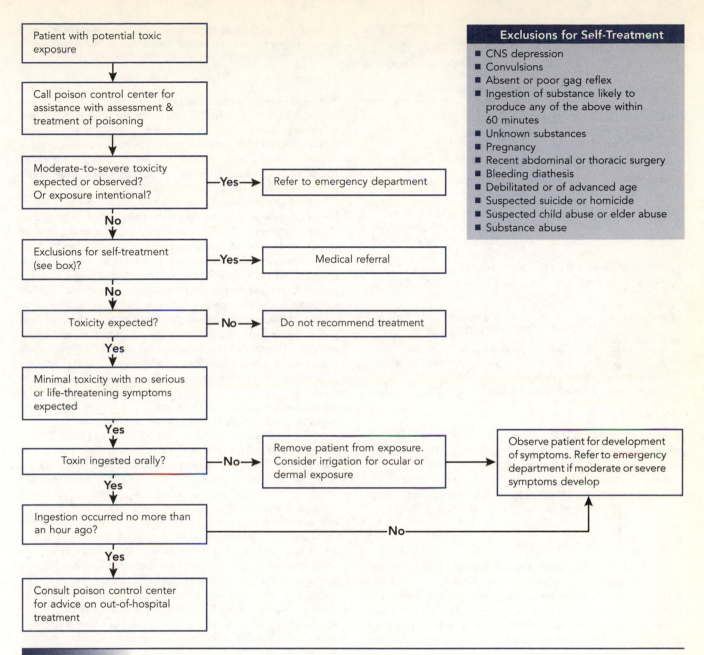

FIGURE 21-2 Self-care for poisoning. Key: CNS, central nervous system.

tact time of the chemical with the mucosal surface. Neutralization after a chemical contacts skin or eyes, or for ingested substances is not recommended. The administration of a large amount of fluids should be discouraged, because the fluids are likely to result in spontaneous vomiting. The administration of oral fluids after an ingestion of a drug is not recommended, because the fluids theoretically may facilitate dissolution of a solid dosage form, thereby enhancing its absorption. The only exception would be administering fluids after ingestions of drugs that are known to have a high risk of esophageal impaction, such as bisphosphonates. Manually stimulating the gag reflex at the back of the throat with either a blunt object or a finger may induce vomiting, but this practice is not recommended and can lead to soft palate injury.

Gastric lavage, a procedure in which fluids are instilled into a tube placed into the stomach through the mouth or nose and then removed by suction or aspiration, is not an option for self-treatment. Improvement of patient outcome from use of this procedure has not been definitively demonstrated and lavage is not without risks. Use of activated charcoal as the primary method of GI decontamination in health care facilities has further limited the role of lavage in the management of poisoning.

Pharmacologic Therapy

Ipecac syrup, an emetic, and activated charcoal, an adsorbent, are the only approved self-treatments for ingested poisons. Table 21-1 lists selected trade-name products. Despite the availability of these agents for the self-treatment of poisoning, they are used to only a limited extent. In 2006, ipecac syrup was used in less than 0.1% of cases reported to poison control centers, and activated charcoal was used in just under 4.5% of cases.[3]

TABLE 21-1	Selected Nonprescription Agents for Treatment of Poisoning[a]

Trade Name	Primary Ingredients
Emetics	
Ipecac syrup[b]	Emetine; cephaeline
Activated Charcoal Products	
Actidose-Aqua	Activated charcoal 25 g/120 mL or 50 g/240 mL
Liqui Char	Activated charcoal 12.5 g/60 mL, 15 g/75 mL, 25 g/120 mL, 30 g/120 mL, or 50 g/240 mL
Activated Charcoal Cathartic Products	
Actidose with Sorbitol	Activated charcoal 25 g/120 mL, or 50 g/240 mL; sorbitol
CharcoAid	Activated charcoal 15 g/120 mL or 30g/150 mL; sorbitol

[a] Ipecac is rarely recommended; activated charcoal is not universally accepted as a self-treatment (see text).

[b] Labeling states a dose for only children ages 1 year and older.

Controversy surrounds the use of either treatment in the outpatient setting, because there is no evidence that either therapy improves the medical outcome. In addition, there are concerns that the therapy may be used when treatment is contraindicated or is not necessary; therefore, the risk outweighs the benefit. Activated charcoal may also be poorly tolerated.

Emetic Treatment with Ipecac Syrup

Ipecac syrup is FDA-approved as an emetic for use in some poisonings. Serious toxicity after acute administration of ipecac syrup is rare; however, there is no evidence that ipecac improves outcome. Persistent vomiting, lethargy, and diarrhea are adverse consequences of ipecac use. Ipecac syrup is no longer routinely recommended. It should not be administered without consultation with a poison control center.

In November 2003, the American Academy of Pediatrics (AAP) Committee on Injury, Violence and Poison Prevention removed ipecac syrup from its anticipatory guidance during prenatal and well-child visits; the committee also recommended that ipecac no longer be used routinely.[10] The primary reason for the change was the lack of documented benefit with several potential risks. The risks include the unpleasant experience of vomiting, the possibility of persistent vomiting and other adverse effects, and the potential for misuse. Chronic ipecac poisoning has been reported in patients who suffer from bulimia and from intentional administration of ipecac to small children, also referred to as Münchausen syndrome by proxy.[11] In addition to chronic vomiting and diarrhea, chronic exposure to ipecac syrup is associated with muscle weakness, cardiomyopathies, and electrolyte imbalances. In 2003, an FDA panel recommended that ipecac syrup be removed from the market. At this time, FDA has not made a decision and ipecac syrup remains available for purchase. Pharmacists should question any person who frequently purchases ipecac syrup to ascertain whether chronic misuse is occurring. Key contraindications to ipecac syrup include ingestions of substances likely to produce CNS depression or seizures, as well as ingestions of corrosive substances or hydrocarbons.

Treatment with Activated Charcoal

Activated charcoal is a tasteless, gritty, fine, black insoluble powder made from the pyrolysis of various organic materials.[12] Wood or other carbon-containing compounds are "activated" by an oxidizing gas at high temperatures to produce a product with a very large surface area, resulting in a highly effective adsorbent for many drugs and chemicals. The surface area usually ranges from 950 to 2000 m^2/g.[12]

Activated charcoal has been shown to adsorb a large number of commonly ingested drugs and many other toxic agents. These substances are bound in the internal surface of the pores of the charcoal molecule, thereby preventing their absorption. Activated charcoal is incapable of being digested, so is not absorbed from the GI tract. As the ratio of activated charcoal to toxin increases, the proportion of bound toxin increases.[12] Highly ionized substances, such as potassium and lithium, are poorly adsorbed by activated charcoal. Activated charcoal does not bind well to alcohols or glycols (e.g., ethanol, methanol, and ethylene glycol), hydrocarbons, mineral acids and alkali, heavy metals (e.g., iron, lead, and arsenic), or cyanide (Table 21-2). The presence of food in the GI tract may reduce the efficacy of activated charcoal.

Activated charcoal is FDA-approved for use as an emergency antidote in the treatment of an ingested poison.

The usual dose of activated charcoal is 1 g/kg (Table 21-3).[12] Activated charcoal is available premixed with water, sorbitol (for catharsis), or water and carboxymethylcellulose (Table 21-1). Activated charcoal slurries are prone to settling, so these products should be vigorously shaken before administration. Activated charcoal is also available as a powder for reconstitution into an oral suspension just before use; this product should be stirred thoroughly or vigorously shaken after water is added. Flavoring agents have been used to try to increase the palatability of activated charcoal but these agents are generally avoided, because they may reduce the adsorptive capacity of charcoal. Activated charcoal is most effective if given within 1 hour after ingestion. Repeat doses of activated charcoal (given in a health care facility setting only) may enhance the elimination of some drugs (e.g., phenobarbital and theophylline) after they are absorbed into the systemic circulation.

Activated charcoal combined with sorbitol is also available to improve palatability and act as a cathartic. The cathartic is intended to speed the transit of the activated charcoal complex through the GI tract and prevent constipation; however, the need for cathartics has been questioned.[13] Sorbitol-containing activated charcoal products are not recommended in children younger than 1 year or when multiple doses of activated charcoal are administered; in these situations, the risk of fluid and electrolyte disturbances and hypotension is higher. Most activated charcoal products marketed specifically for home use do not contain sorbitol. Activated charcoal capsules marketed as a dietary supplement for gastrointestinal complaints or other ailments should not be used for management of poisonings, because the surface area of charcoal in these products is too small to effectively adsorb toxins.

Activated charcoal is used primarily for patients managed in a health care facility. Although this agent is available as a nonprescription drug, it is not available in most homes. A study evaluating the administration of activated charcoal in the home to manage potentially toxic ingestions in children reported that

TABLE 21-2 Contraindications to GI Decontamination with Activated Charcoal as Self-Treatment

Category	Inclusion Criteria	Recommendation
Patient condition	Coma, convulsions, syncope, airway or breathing problems, blood pressure or pulse irregularities, hallucinations, and severe agitation	Refer to hospital for evaluation.
Ingestion of low-viscosity hydrocarbons and terpenes	Gasoline; kerosene; mineral seal oil (furniture polish); naphtha (lighter fluid); pine oil (cleaners); turpentine (paint removers); mineral oil	Contact poison control center.
Ingestion of caustic substances	Methacrylic acid (artificial nail primers); sodium silicate and carbonate (automatic dishwashing detergents); sulfuric acid (automotive battery, drain cleaners, toilet bowl cleaners); sodium hydroxide (Clinitest tablets, drain cleaners, oven cleaners, hair relaxers); hypochlorites (bleach, pool chlorine); thioglycolates (hair relaxers); hydrofluoric acid (rust removers); hydrochloric acid (toilet bowl cleaner)	Contact poison control center.
Ingestion of substances not adsorbed by charcoal	Ethanol (alcoholic beverages, colognes, mouthwashes, aftershaves); isopropyl alcohol (rubbing alcohol); methanol (windshield washer fluid); ethylene glycol (antifreeze); ionized substances (potassium); metals (iron, lithium, lead, arsenic); cyanide (potassium cyanide, acetonitrile artificial nail remover, laetrile)	Contact poison control center.

Key: GI, gastrointestinal.

90% of parents did not have activated charcoal in their home, requiring them to obtain it from their local pharmacy for the poisoning incident.[14] Following a professional education program targeted at pharmacists, pediatricians, and family practice physicians in one state, a telephone survey found that 72% of 203 randomly selected pharmacies had activated charcoal on their shelves.[15] Practitioners should consult their poison control center to determine whether to promote routine availability of activated charcoal in the home.

The most common adverse effects of activated charcoal are vomiting and black stools. Vomiting occurs in 12% to 20% of patients receiving activated charcoal.[12,16,17] One-fifth of children younger than 18 years who were given activated charcoal for poisoning vomited a median time of 10 minutes after initiation of charcoal administration.[17] Previous vomiting was a significant risk factor for vomiting after activated charcoal administration. More serious complications, such as pulmonary aspiration and GI obstruction, are associated more often with administration of multiple doses of activated charcoal. In 878 patients who received two or more doses of activated charcoal, clinically significant complications were infrequent and included five pulmonary aspirations, eight electrolyte abnormalities, and one

TABLE 21-3 Activated Charcoal Dosing Information

Age	Dose
0–12 months[a]	10–25 g
10–12 years	25–50 g
>12 years	25–100 g

[a] Used primarily in a health care setting in this age group.

Source: Reference 12.

corneal abrasion.[18] Sorbitol-containing activated charcoal products increase the risk of vomiting, diarrhea, abdominal cramps, and electrolyte abnormalities. Hypernatremic dehydration has been reported with multiple-dose sorbitol-containing activated charcoal regimens.[16]

Activated charcoal is contraindicated in patients in whom the GI tract is not anatomically (e.g., following caustic injury) or functionally (e.g., ileus) intact. Activated charcoal is also contraindicated in patients at high risk for aspiration without airway protection (Table 21-2). Activated charcoal should not be administered after ingestion of substances that it does not adsorb, unless the presence of other ingestants that are adsorbed by charcoal is suspected.

PHARMACOTHERAPEUTIC CONSIDERATIONS FOR ACTIVATED CHARCOAL

Studies have demonstrated that the effectiveness of GI decontamination decreases significantly with increasing time interval since ingestion. For most overdoses, GI decontamination with activated charcoal should be performed early, usually within an hour of the ingestion.

There is no convincing evidence that activated charcoal improves patient outcomes, and its utility in adults with intentional overdoses has been questioned.[19] Some toxicologists question whether the risk–benefit ratio supports the administration of activated charcoal in the patient with mild-to-moderate poisoning.[20,21] A position statement by the American Academy of Clinical Toxicology and the European Association of Poison Control Centers and Clinical Toxicologists concluded that activated charcoal may be considered for a potentially toxic amount of a poison ingested up to 1 hour before treatment. There are insufficient data to support or exclude use of charcoal when poison ingestion occurred more than 1 hour previously.[12] The majority of studies upon which the position statement was based were conducted in a controlled research or hospital environment. An American Academy of Pediatrics position statement against the use of ipecac in the home did not endorse the use of activated charcoal in lieu of ipecac because of lack of data that demonstrate improved outcome with charcoal.[10]

Poison control centers vary by region in recommending home use of activated charcoal. Home administration of activated charcoal is usually intended for patient management outside a health care facility, but sometimes the agent is given to provide early prehospital GI decontamination in patients who subsequently are transported to an emergency department. Data on prehospital administration provide insight into the potential difficulty in administering activated charcoal in the home. A study of prehospital emergency medical technicians or paramedics reported that charcoal was not given to 15.4% of patients in whom administration was attempted; in 71% of these cases the reason was patient refusal.[22] A pediatric emergency department found that 32% of young children offered oral-activated charcoal refused the treatment or were intolerant.[23]

Consideration of home use of activated charcoal requires addressing the following questions: What are the benefits? Will children take it at home? Does home administration shorten the interval between the overdose and charcoal administration? Is it safe to give at home?[24] Eldridge et al.[24] cited two studies (21 children total) that questioned whether activated charcoal can be successfully administered at home after finding that most children did not drink a full dose administered by parents. Three other studies (217 children total) reported that a full dose was administered in 64% of children and a partial dose was ingested in 16% of 157 children.[24] In a study evaluating home management of poisoning with activated charcoal in 115 children (median age, 2 years; range, 1–14 years), parents reported administering a mean of 12.1 grams of activated charcoal.[14] Although all parents successfully administered charcoal, 25.9% reported some difficulty, which is a commonly reported complaint. Problems with these studies include reliance on parental reports and lack of validation of the accuracy of the amount of charcoal administered.

Home administration shortens time to charcoal administration. Lamminpaa et al.[25] found that the average time to administration of activated charcoal was 24.5 minutes when charcoal was available in the home compared with 41.6 minutes when charcoal was not in the home. Spiller and Rodgers[14] found that home use significantly reduced time to charcoal administration compared with its administration in the emergency department (average of 38 versus 73 minutes, respectively).

To date, experience with home administration of activated charcoal has shown that it is relatively safe. Gastrointestinal effects have been reported, with the main adverse effect being vomiting.[25] There is concern that if home use of activated charcoal becomes more prevalent and parents administer charcoal when it is contraindicated (e.g., altered mental status with compromised airway, or hydrocarbon ingestion), serious adverse effects such as aspiration may increase.[24] Consultation with a poison center is recommended before a practitioner recommends use of activated charcoal.

Assessment of Poisoning: A Case-Based Approach

Assessment of airway, breathing, circulation, and mental status are the primary concerns in a poisoned patient:

- Determine whether the airway is open.
- Determine whether the patient is breathing.

- Determine cardiovascular status by assessing blood pressure and pulse.
- Determine whether the patient's mental status is altered. Specifically, determine whether the patient is experiencing:
  — Coma or stupor.
  — Convulsions.
  — Agitation, disorientation, or hallucinations.

After obtaining the history regarding the exposure and performing an initial assessment of the patient's condition, it must be decided whether to refer the patient directly to an emergency treatment facility, manage him or her at home, or not provide any specific treatment. Involving the poison control center in this triage and treatment decision is important, because poison control centers have considerable experience managing poisoned patients and specialized resources that are not usually available to practitioners. The nationwide toll-free poison control center number, 1-800-222-1222, connects callers to the center in their geographic area (Figure 21-1).

Obtaining a reliable history, identifying the drug or toxin, and accurately assessing the patient's condition are critical steps in determining appropriate treatment for a poisoned patient. Self-treatment at home is primarily intended for unintentional poison exposures in children younger than 6 years in whom no or, at most, minimal toxicity is expected. In addition, unintentional inhalation or skin or eye exposures in any age group, with possible minimal toxicity, can often be self-treated.

If an individual inquires about purchasing ipecac syrup or activated charcoal, the pharmacist must determine whether these drugs are being purchased for an acute situation, in which case the poison control center should be contacted to assess the appropriateness of self-treatment. The poison control center will need information about the patient (age, weight, past medical history, and whether the patient is currently experiencing clinical effects), the toxin (name of the toxin, dose, route of exposure, and time since exposure), and what treatment, if any, has already been administered.

Cases 21-1 and 21-2 provide examples of assessment of patients who have been poisoned.

Patient Counseling for Poisoning

After removal from toxic fumes, patients should be counseled about when to seek medical attention (e.g., difficulty breathing, worsening or persistent symptoms). In the home or other non-industry setting, fumes are often soluble, irritant gases (e.g., chlorine), so clinical effects are evident immediately and usually resolve soon after exposure stops. Patients also should be counseled about ventilating the room to facilitate dispersion of the vapor. If the exposure resulted from mixing products such as bleach and ammonia, the patient should be warned not to mix household products in the future. If carbon monoxide is suspected, the patient should be instructed to have the source turned off or removed (e.g., malfunctioning furnace, stove, or vehicle). The poison control center should be contacted to assess severity and expected duration of clinical effects in symptomatic patients and the possibility of delayed onset in asymptomatic patients.

Patients with eye exposures should be counseled on how to irrigate the eye at home under the faucet. Contacts should be removed before irrigation. Instructions should include running the water at a comfortable temperature (room temperature) and

CASE 21-1

Relevant Evaluation Criteria	Scenario/Model Outcome

Information Gathering

1. Gather essential information about the patient's symptoms, including:

   a. description of symptom(s) (i.e., nature, onset, duration, severity, associated symptoms)

   To rid her dorm room of insects, the patient used an aerosol house and garden bug killer that contained a hydrocarbon and pyrethrin. She used the entire can and got the product on her hands. Shortly after using the product, she began to feel dizzy. She called the pharmacy for advice. She complained of headache, scratchy throat, and mild cough. Her hands felt irritated and were slightly erythematous.

   b. description of any factors that seem to precipitate, exacerbate, and/or relieve the patient's symptom(s)

   N/A

   c. description of the patient's efforts to relieve the symptoms

   She opened windows to air out the room.

2. Gather essential patient history information:

   a. patient's identity — Allison Summerson

   b. patient's age, sex, height, and weight — 20-year-old female, 5 ft 4 in, 125 lb

   c. patient's occupation — College student

   d. patient's dietary habits — N/A

   e. patient's sleep habits — N/A

   f. concurrent medical conditions, prescription and nonprescription medications, and dietary supplements — Healthy; multiple vitamins with iron daily; no other medications

   g. allergies — No history of asthma, reactive airway disease, or ragweed sensitivity

   h. history of other adverse reactions to medications — None

   i. other (describe) _____ — N/A

Assessment and Triage

3. Differentiate the patient's signs/symptoms and correctly identify the patient's primary problem(s).

   Allison did not read the directions for use on the product and is experiencing toxicity as a result of inhalation and dermal exposure to the insecticide, as well as the hydrocarbon solvent.

4. Identify exclusions for self-treatment (see Figure 21-2).

   None

5. Formulate a comprehensive list of therapeutic alternatives for the primary problem to determine if triage to a medical practitioner is required, and share this information with the patient.

   Options include:
   (1) Opening windows provides sufficient ventilation. Recommend washing skin with water.
   (2) Recommend that Allison leave the room so that she is no longer exposed to the fumes and that she wash her hands twice with soap and water; contact the poison center for consultation regarding whether referral for additional irrigation and respiratory support is needed.
   (3) Refer Allison to the emergency department for pulmonary and skin evaluation, skin irrigation, and therapy with oxygen and inhaled beta-adrenergic agonists.
   (4) Take no action.

Plan

6. Select an optimal therapeutic alternative to address the patient's problem, taking into account patient preferences.

   Advise patient to leave the room, wash her hands twice with soap and water, and then reassess her symptoms. She should contact the poison control center for advice after irrigating her skin.

7. Describe the recommended therapeutic approach to the patient.

   Removing yourself from the room will eliminate your exposure to the fumes and allow you to breath fresh air. Washing with soap and water will remove both the hydrocarbon and the insecticide from your skin. These measures should shorten the duration of exposure and limit local injury caused by both the hydrocarbon and the pyrethrin.

CASE 21-1 (continued)

Relevant Evaluation Criteria	Scenario/Model Outcome
8. Explain to the patient the rationale for selecting the recommended therapeutic approach from the considered therapeutic alternatives.	Seeking medical attention immediately is not necessary. You should first terminate the exposure to the insecticide by getting fresh air and thoroughly washing your skin with soap and water. The soap will break down the hydrocarbon and improve its removal from the skin. Washing the skin with only water is inadequate, because the hydrocarbon solvent is lipophilic and does not mix well with water. After removing yourself to fresh air and irrigating your skin, the poison control center may recommend referral to a PCP (primary care provider) or emergency department if symptoms persist or worsen.

Patient Education

9. When recommending self-care with non-prescription medications and/or nondrug therapy, convey accurate information to the patient:	
a. appropriate dose and frequency of administration	Wash skin twice with soap and water.
b. maximum number of days the therapy should be employed	N/A
c. product administration procedures	N/A
d. expected time to onset of relief	Clinical effects should resolve within 15–30 minutes after removal to fresh air and skin irrigation. If not, medical referral may be appropriate, and the poison center can help facilitate the referral.
e. degree of relief that can be reasonably expected	Complete relief is possible. Skin may continue to be slightly irritated and/or red.
f. most common side effects	N/A
g. side effects that warrant medical intervention should they occur	N/A
h. patient options in the event that condition worsens or persists	A PCP should be consulted or you may be referred to the emergency department by the poison control center if clinical effects do not resolve within a relatively short period of time (see 9d).
i. product storage requirements	N/A
j. specific nondrug measures	Fresh air; irrigation with soap and water
10. Solicit follow-up questions from patient.	(1) May I use a moisturizing lotion on my skin if it is still red or dry after the irrigation? (2) May I use a throat lozenge for the scratchy throat?
11. Answer patient's questions.	(1) Yes. A moisturizing lotion may help the irritation caused by the defatting effects of the hydrocarbon. (2) Sucking on a throat lozenge or hard candy can provide symptomatic relief of the scratchy throat.

Key: N/A, not applicable; PCP, primary care provider.

CASE 21-2

Relevant Evaluation Criteria	Scenario/Model Outcome
Information Gathering	
1. Gather essential information about the patient's symptoms, including:	
a. description of symptom(s) (i.e., nature, onset, duration, severity, associated symptoms).	A grandmother asks the pharmacist about treatment options for her 2-year-old granddaughter who was found with a pill minder that contains alprazolam 1 mg tablets. No more than 3 tablets are missing. The exposure happened 30 minutes ago. The child is sleepy but it is her normal nap time.

Relevant Evaluation Criteria	Scenario/Model Outcome
b. description of any factors that seem to precipitate, exacerbate, and/or relieve the patient's symptom(s).	N/A
c. description of the patient's efforts to relieve the symptoms	N/A
2. Gather essential patient history information:	
a. patient's identity	Sarah Jones
b. patient's age, sex, height, and weight	2-year-old female, 34 inches tall, 20 lb
c. patient's occupation	N/A
d. patient's dietary habits	Last meal was 1 hour before the exposure
e. patient's sleep habits	N/A
f. Concurrent medical conditions, prescription and nonprescription medications, and dietary supplements	Healthy; takes no medications
g. Allergies	NKA
h. History of other adverse reactions to medications	None
i. other (describe) _____	

Assessment and Triage

3. Differentiate the patient's signs/symptoms and correctly identify the patient's primary problem(s).	Sarah is sleepy but can be aroused. It is her normal nap time, so she is normally sleepy at this time.
4. Identify exclusions for self-treatment (see Figure 21-2).	CNS depression is an exclusion for self-treatment. Child is drowsy.
5. Formulate a comprehensive list of therapeutic alternatives for the primary problem to determine if triage to a medical practitioner is required, and share this information with the caregiver.	Options include: (1) The pharmacist should contact the poison control center for recommendations to determine whether to refer Sarah to an emergency department for GI decontamination and evaluation. (2) Have grandmother administer an OTC treatment to decrease absorption at home. (3) Take no action.

Plan

6. Select an optimal therapeutic alternative to address the patient's problem, taking into account patient preferences.	The poison control center should be contacted immediately. The poison center will determine whether it is safe to manage the child at home.
7. Describe the recommended therapeutic approach to the caregiver.	No treatment should be provided at home because the child is already drowsy. The poison control center recommends that Sarah be treated in the hospital.
8. Explain to the caregiver the rationale for selecting the recommended therapeutic approach from the considered therapeutic alternatives.	Sarah has ingested up to 3 alprazolam tablets and is drowsy. It is not known whether she is drowsy because it is her nap time or because she absorbed some of the alprazolam. It is not safe to give an OTC treatment in this case.

Patient Education

9. When recommending self-care with nonprescription medications and/or nondrug therapy, convey accurate information to the caregiver.	Criterion does not apply in this case.
10. Solicit follow-up questions from caregiver.	How should I transport Sarah to the hospital, which is 30 minutes away? No transportation is available.
11. Answer caregiver's questions.	Contact 911 for transport to the hospital.

Key: CNS, central nervous system; GI, gastrointestinal; N/A, not applicable; NKA, no known allergies; OTC, over-the-counter.

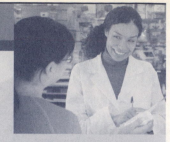

The objectives of self-treatment are to (1) minimize exposure by removing the patient to fresh air, irrigating the skin or eyes, or preventing absorption of potentially toxic agents in the GI tract; and (2) treat patients with minimally toxic ingestions at home under the supervision of a poison control center. For most patients, carefully following the self-care measures listed here will help ensure optimal therapeutic outcomes.

Treatment

- For eye exposures, immediately irrigate with water for 10–15 minutes.
- For skin exposures, immediately wash with soap and water.
- For inhalation exposures, immediately remove the patient to fresh air.
- Contact the poison control center to obtain a consultation, or refer the patient to the poison control center (see Figure 21-1

for toll-free number) for advice on the appropriateness of self-treatment of the toxic exposure, including ingested toxins.

 Refer the patient to a health care facility through 911 if the patient:
- —Is lethargic or comatose or is having convulsions or hallucinations.
- —Has decreased respirations or is having difficulty breathing.
- —Has abnormal blood pressure or pulse.
- —Has taken medications that may produce a rapid decline in consciousness or convulsions.

---

at a low pressure. Irrigating the eyes in the shower or using a clean cup to pour water into the eyes may be an easier alternative in children. Placing a damp washcloth on the eye or irrigating with small volume nonprescription eyewashes is ineffective. Finally, eye drops, including topical vasoconstrictors, should not be used after irrigation. Patients with skin exposures should be counseled to remove clothing, if necessary, and wash affected areas thoroughly (Case 21-1). For eye and skin exposures, counseling should stress the importance of immediate irrigation or washing.

If the poison control center in a region is recommending activated charcoal for home use, pharmacies in that area should stock the appropriate product, and practitioners should educate parents that activated charcoal should never be used without first consulting a poison control center staff member or a primary care provider. Patients who purchase activated charcoal for immediate use following the recommendation of a poison control center should be counseled to ensure appropriate drug use. The practitioner should also explain potential adverse effects, as well as signs and symptoms that indicate medical attention should be sought.

Patients who are taking multiple prescriptions and using a regular pill minder should be advised to purchase a locking pill minder if they are around young children. When loading the device, there should be paper or cardboard underneath to catch stray pills that may fall on the floor. Pharmacists can also prevent therapeutic 10-fold error types of poisonings by always dispensing 1 mL oral syringes for prescription medications that are dosed in infants at less than 1 mL, such as metoclopramide. The box Patient Education for Poisoning lists specific information to provide parents, caregivers, or patients.

Counseling should include providing the nationwide toll-free number for the poison control center (Figure 21-1) and promoting poison prevention practices, including purchase of nonprescription drugs and household products with child-resistant packaging. If parents or caregivers choose to purchase a product without a child-resistant closure, the practitioner should advise them to place the container in a locked cabinet or store the container out of sight and out of reach of young children to avoid an unintentional poisoning.

Evaluation of Patient Outcomes for Poisoning

Patients who have inhaled potentially toxic fumes, or spilled or splashed a substance on their skin or in their eye should be reassessed for symptoms after removal to fresh air or irrigation. If clinical effects are minimal and resolve within a relatively short period of time (e.g., under 30 minutes), the patient may be observed at home. If symptoms persist or worsen, the patient should be referred to a health care provider or the emergency department, depending on the severity of symptoms and immediacy of need for medical evaluation. The poison control center can facilitate referral to the appropriate health care facility and provide treatment recommendations to the health care provider.

Patients who receive activated charcoal should be contacted at least once to determine whether any symptoms related to the exposure develop. The time of the call depends on the substance ingested, how rapidly it is absorbed, and when symptoms would be anticipated. If clinical effects develop and are minor, the patient may be observed at home. If more significant effects develop, the patient should be referred to an emergency department for treatment. If the poison control center recommended self-treatment with activated charcoal, the center staff should remain involved in subsequent decisions regarding the appropriateness of continued home treatment of these patients.

Key Points for Poisoning

➤ Poison exposures are a common pediatric injury.
➤ Minimizing the duration or limiting the extent of the exposure is the rationale for most self-treatment practices.
➤ There are no data demonstrating that self-treatment for poisoning with activated charcoal improves patient outcomes.
➤ Self-treatment should be considered for only unintentional poison exposures that are likely to cause no or minimal toxicity (i.e., no serious or life-threatening symptoms; Figure 21-2).

➤ Practitioners should consult with the poison control center for input regarding patient assessment and decisions regarding the appropriateness of self-treatment.

➤ All patients who exhibit potentially life-threatening clinical effects (e.g., convulsions or coma) should be referred to an emergency department through the emergency 911 system.

➤ Because poison control centers vary by region regarding when to recommend self-treatment and what options are available for self-treatment, health care practitioners should contact their poison control center to discuss regional preferences for self-treatment, as well as to obtain patient education materials.

REFERENCES

1. Burt A, Annest JL, Budnitz DS. Nonfatal, unintentional medication exposures among young children—United States, 2001–2003. *MMWR Morb Mortal Wkly Rep.* 2006;55:1–5.

2. Minino AM, Heron MP, Murphy SL, et al. Deaths: final data for 2004. National Center for Health Statistics. *Natl Vital Stat Rep.* 2007;55(19):1–120.

3. Bronstein AC, Spyker DA, Cantilena LR, et al. 2006 annual report of the American Association of Poison Control Centers' National Poison Data System. *Clin Toxicol.* 2007;45:815–917.

4. Rodgers GB. The effectiveness of child-resistant packaging for aspirin. *Arch Pediatr Adolesc Med.* 2002;156:929–33.

5. Morris CC. Recent trends in pediatric iron poisonings. *South Med J.* 2000;93:1229.

6. Woolf A, Wieler J, Greenes D. Costs of poison-related hospitalizations at an urban teaching hospital for children. *Arch Pediatr Adolesc Med.* 1997;151:719–23.

7. Stremski ES. Accidental pediatric ingestion, hospital charges and failure to utilize a poison control center. *West J Med.* 1999;98:29–33.

8. Darwin J, Seger D. Reaffirmed cost-effectiveness of poison centers [letter]. *Ann Emerg Med.* 2003;41:159–60.

9. Miller T, Lestina DC. Costs of poisoning in the United States and savings from poison control centers: a benefit–cost analysis. *Ann Emerg Med.* 1997;29:239–45.

10. American Academy of Pediatrics Committee on Injury, Violence, and Poison Prevention. Poison treatment in the home. *Pediatrics.* 2003;112:1182–5.

11. Schneider DJ, Perez A, Knilans TE, et al. Clinical and pathologic aspects of cardiomyopathy from ipecac administration in Munchausen's syndrome by proxy. *Pediatrics.* 1996;97:902–6.

12. Chyka PA, Seger D, Krenzelok EP, Vale JA; American Academy of Clinical Toxicology; European Association of Poisons Centers and Clinical Toxicologists. Position paper: single-dose activated charcoal. *Clin Toxicol* (Phila). 2005;43:61–87.

13. American Academy of Clinical Toxicology, European Association of Poison Control Centers and Clinical Toxicologists. Position statement: cathartics. *J Toxicol Clin Toxicol.* 1997;35:743–52.

14. Spiller HA, Rodgers GC. Evaluation of administration of activated charcoal in the home. *Pediatrics.* 2001;108:E100.

15. Spiller HA, Revolinski DH, Rodgers GC. Evaluation of professional education program to have activated charcoal available in local pharmacies [abstract]. *J Toxicol Clin Toxicol.* 1997;35:485.

16. McFarland AK, Chyka PA. Selection of activated charcoal products for the treatment of poisonings. *Ann Pharmacother.* 1993;27:358–61.

17. Osterhoudt KC, Durbin D, Alpern ER, et al. Risk factors for emesis after therapeutic use of activated charcoal in acutely poisoned children. *Pediatrics.* 2004;113:806–10.

18. Dorrington CL, Johnson DW, Brant R, et al. The frequency of complications associated with the use of multiple-dose activated charcoal. *Ann Emerg Med.* 2003;41:370–7.

19. Merigian KS, Blaho KE. Single-dose oral activated charcoal in the treatment of the self-poisoned patient: a prospective, randomized, controlled trial. *Am J Ther.* 2002;9:301–8.

20. Seger D. Single-dose activated charcoal-backup and reassess. *J Toxicol Clin Toxicol.* 2004;42:101–10.

21. Bond GR. Activated charcoal in the home: helpful and important or simply a distraction? *Pediatrics.* 2002;109:145–6.

22. Alaspaa AO, Kuisma MJ, Hoppu K, et al. Out-of-hospital administration of activated charcoal by emergency medical services. *Ann Emerg Med.* 2005;45:207–12.

23. Osterhoudt KC, Alpern ER, Durbin D, et al. Activated charcoal administration in a pediatric emergency department. *Pediatr Emerg Care.* 2004;20:493–8.

24. Eldridge DL, Van Eyk J, Kornegay C. Pediatric toxicology. *Emerg Med Clin N Am.* 2007;15:283–308.

25. Lamminpaa A, Vilska J, Hoppu K. Medical charcoal for a child's poisoning at home: availability and success of administration in Finland. *Hum Exp Toxicol.* 1993;12(1):29–32.

Ostomy Care and Supplies

Joan Lerner Selekof and Sharon Wilson

An ostomy is an opening or outlet through the abdominal wall created surgically for the purpose of eliminating waste. It is usually made by bringing a portion of the bladder, colon, small intestine, or ureters through the abdominal wall. The opening of the ostomy is called the *stoma* (from the Latin word for mouth).

The creation of an ostomy may be a dramatic life-changing event. Therefore, it is important for clinicians to provide reassurance, support, and education for the patient and family. An understanding of improvements in surgical procedures, ostomy supplies, and outcomes can allay much of a patient's fear and anxiety. The goal in ostomy care is to enable the individual to resume his or her lifestyle—to be a person, not a patient. A person with an ostomy carefully notes the reactions of health care professionals to the disorder; any negative response may reinforce the patient's negative feelings about the ostomy.

An estimated 750,000 Americans are currently living with an ostomy, and 75,000 new surgeries are performed annually.[1] Ostomy surgery is performed in individuals of all ages and for many reasons, both acquired and congenital.

Indications for Ostomies

Ostomies may be permanent or temporary, and they are performed in individuals ranging from neonates to persons of advanced age. Reasons for performing ostomies include congenital anomalies (e.g., imperforate anus, Hirschsprung's disease), inflammatory bowel disease, familial polyposis, cancer, radiation damage, pressure ulcers, trauma, and any other reason to divert the urinary or fecal stream.[2,3] The type of ostomy depends on the condition being treated.

The two most common disorders leading to ileostomy surgery are (1) ulcerative colitis, which affects the large intestine and rectum, and (2) Crohn's disease, which may involve any part of the gastrointestinal (GI) tract. Other conditions that may require an ileostomy include traumatic injury, cancer, familial polyposis, and necrotizing enterocolitis.

The most common reasons for colostomy surgery are (1) cancer of the colon or rectum, (2) diverticulitis, and (3) trauma. Other indications include obstruction of the colon or rectum, genetic malformation, radiation colitis, and loss of anal muscular control. In some cases, a temporary colostomy may be performed to protect areas of the colon that have been surgically repaired. Healing of a diseased or damaged bowel may take several weeks, months, or years, but eventually the colon and

rectum are reconnected and bowel continuity is restored. Figure 22-1 shows the location of various types of colostomies.

Urinary diversions are created to correct bladder loss or dysfunction, which can be caused by cancer, neurogenic bladder, genetic malformation, or interstitial cystitis.

Types of Ostomies

The three basic types of ostomies are (1) ileostomy, (2) colostomy (the most common type), and (3) urinary diversion (see Color Plates, photographs 2A-I). Each type of ostomy has several variations, depending on the location of the stoma, reason for surgical procedure, or whether the procedure renders a patient continent.

Ileostomy

An ileostomy is surgically created by bringing a portion of the ileum through the abdominal wall (see Color Plates, photograph 2A.) Initially, the discharge is liquid, but as the ileum adapts, it assumes some of the absorptive functions of the colon and the discharge may become semisoft. The discharge is continuous and contains intestinal enzymes that may irritate the peristomal skin.

Several types of continent ileostomies exist (see Color Plates, photograph 2B). An internal pouch is created from the ileum, and an intussusception (a slipping of a length of intestine into an adjacent portion) of the bowel is used to create a "nipple" that renders the patient continent for stool and flatus. The pouch is periodically emptied by inserting a catheter through the nipple into the pouch. At first, the pouch holds about 75 mL, but it stretches with use so that, at 6 months postoperatively, it may hold 600 to 800 mL and can be drained three to five times daily. Patients do not need to wear an external pouching system, but they often wear a gauze pad or stoma cap.

The restorative proctocolectomy (S pouch or J pouch) ileoanal reservoir spares the rectum of patients with ulcerative colitis or familial polyposis. Diseased mucosa is stripped from the rectum, and an internal pouch is created from the ileum. The distal end is pulled through the rectum and attached. The sphincter is preserved and ostomy pouching systems are unnecessary. However, a patient undergoing this procedure may have a temporary (about 3 months) stoma to protect the healing pouch. Patients will have more frequent bowel movements and may experience perianal skin irritation.

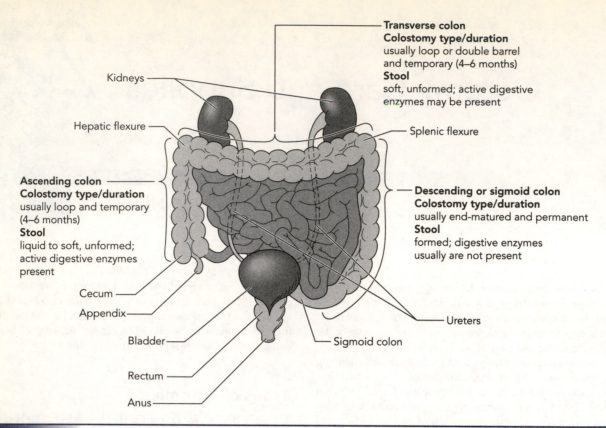

Transverse colon
Colostomy type/duration
usually loop or double barrel
and temporary (4–6 months)
Stool
soft, unformed; active digestive
enzymes may be present

Kidneys

Hepatic flexure

Splenic flexure

Ascending colon
Colostomy type/duration
usually loop and temporary
(4–6 months)
Stool
liquid to soft, unformed;
active digestive enzymes
present

Descending or sigmoid colon
Colostomy type/duration
usually end-matured and permanent
Stool
formed; digestive enzymes
usually are not present

Cecum

Appendix

Ureters

Bladder

Sigmoid colon

Rectum

Anus

FIGURE 22-1 Anatomic drawing of the lower digestive and urinary tracts depicting the location and permanence of colostomies. (Adapted with permission from *Am J Nurs.* 1977;77:443.)

Colostomy

A colostomy is created by bringing a portion of the large bowel (colon) through the abdominal wall. The discharge may be semisoft, paste-like, or formed, depending on the portion of bowel used (Figure 22-1).

Ascending colostomies are uncommon. The ascending colon is retained, but the rest of the large bowel is removed or bypassed (see Color Plates, photograph 2C). The stoma is usually on the right side of the abdomen. The discharge is semisoft and a pouch must be worn at all times.

The transverse colon is the site of most temporary colostomies (Figure 22-1). A loop of the transverse colon is lifted through the abdominal incision, and a rod or bridge (which is removed within 1-2 weeks) is placed under the loop to give it support while it heals. The discharge is usually semiliquid or very soft.

Loop colostomies have one large opening but two tracts (see Color Plates, photograph 2D). The proximal tract discharges fecal material, and the distal tract secretes small amounts of mucus. An appliance must be worn at all times. A patient with a loop colostomy may also pass a minimal amount of stool or mucus through the rectum. This is a normal occurrence.

For a *double-barrel transverse colostomy,* the bowel is completely divided by bringing both the proximal end and the distal end through the abdominal wall, and then suturing it to the skin (see Color Plates, photograph 2E). The distal stoma may also be called the mucous fistula.

Descending and sigmoid colostomies are fairly common; generally the stoma is on the left side of the abdomen (see Color Plates, photograph 2F). The fecal discharge has a paste-like consistency

and at times may consist of formed stool. This type of colostomy may be regulated by irrigation; therefore, a pouching system may not be needed. However, many patients prefer a pouch to irrigation; not everyone with a descending or sigmoid colostomy is a good candidate for irrigation or prefers irrigation. Factors to consider in making the decision to irrigate include the presence or absence of stomal complications, as well as the patient's normal stooling pattern, psychomotor ability, and willingness to commit the time required to be successful.

Urinary Diversions

Urinary diversion surgery diverts the urine through an opening in the abdominal wall. Urinary stomas should function immediately after surgery.

The *ileal conduit* is the most common type of urinary diversion (see Color Plates, photograph 2G). After the bladder is removed, ileal and colon conduits are created by implanting the ureters into an isolated loop of bowel; one end of the bowel loop is sutured and the distal end is brought to the surface of the abdomen. The stoma looks similar to the stoma in an ileostomy or colostomy. A pouching system must be worn continuously. Mucous shreds will be present in the urine if the bowel is used to create the diversion (see Color Plates, photograph 2H). Because the ileum is used to create an ileal conduit, some people incorrectly refer to the ileal conduit as an ileostomy. Clarification of the type of effluent (stool or urine) will help in selecting the correct type of pouch.

In an *ureterostomy,* one or both ureters are detached from the bladder and brought to the outside of the abdominal wall, where a stoma is created. This procedure is used less frequently, because the ureters tend to narrow unless they have been dilated permanently by previous disease (see Color Plates, photograph 2I).

A *cystostomy* is performed when blockage or narrowing of the urethra occurs. Urine is diverted from the bladder to the abdominal wall. A pouch must be worn continuously. An infant may use diapers instead of a pouch.

The *continent urinary diversion* is available for selected patients but it requires certain criteria. An Indiana pouch is a type of continent urostomy in which a pouch is created from part of the cecum, and a portion of the ileum is then brought through the abdominal wall. The ureters are attached to the cecum pouch. The remaining ileum is reattached to the colon for normal digestive flow. The ileocecal valve is left intact and becomes part of the continence mechanism. The pouch is emptied by inserting a catheter into the stoma to drain the urine. Patients are usually placed on a strict schedule and will eventually catheterize the stoma often enough to avoid leakage. The new pouch may hold up to 600 mL of urine. An external pouching system is not necessary. Most patients wear a gauze pad or stoma cap. The orthotopic neobladder procedure includes connecting the newly created bladder to the urethra, which allows the patient to void through the urethra. The neobladder is an internal urinary reservoir (pouch) usually constructed of a detubularized segment of the ileum to which the ureters and urethra are sewn.

Complications of Ostomies

Patients with ostomies may experience both psychological and physical complications. The clinician should be prepared to address these complications or to refer patients to their primary care provider or a wound ostomy continence nurse (WOC Nurse). WOC Nurses are often based in hospitals or home health care agencies. The United Ostomy Associations of America is an organization that provides peer support for patients. To alleviate any anxiety, patients should receive a thorough explanation before surgery that describes what procedure will be performed, what to expect during the postsurgical recovery period, and what pouching and supplies the patient will use. The clinician can use the following information on potential complications to assist patients seeking advice after their surgery.

Psychological Complications

Some patients anticipating ostomy surgery fear that they will not be able to continue their former job, participate in sports, perform sexually, or have children. These patients need reassurance that an ostomy will not impair their ability to carry out such activities. Contacting the local United Ostomy Associations of America is of utmost importance in assisting with the rehabilitation of these patients; both clinicians and patients may contact this organization. Patients may also want to find a local WOC Nurse. Patient education and counseling on ostomy care provides information and support before and after ostomy surgery. Literature is available from the major ostomy product manufactures.

Physiologic Complications

The major physiologic consequence of a GI ostomy is fluid and electrolyte imbalance, which is most problematic in patients with a liquid or semisoft stoma discharge, such as ileostomies or ascending and transverse colostomies. Patients with these types of ostomies must maintain adequate fluid intake to compensate for loss of the absorptive function of the colon and loss of ileocecal valve function. Patients with ileostomies lose about 500 to 1000 mL of fluid daily through the stoma, compared with a loss of 100 to 200 mL daily by individuals with a normally functioning colon.[3] During illnesses, patients with ileostomies, especially infants, are particularly vulnerable to fluid and electrolyte imbalance caused by vomiting and diarrhea. They should be counseled regarding common signs and symptoms of imbalance (Table 22-1).[3–5]

Because the GI tract is the site of nutrient absorption, some patients with ostomies may experience deficiencies. For example, iron and vitamins D_2 and D_3 are absorbed in the small intestine; riboflavin is absorbed in the upper GI tract; vitamin B_{12} is absorbed in the terminal ileum; phytonadione is absorbed in the proximal small intestine; menadione is absorbed in the distal small intestine; and calcium, pyridoxine, pantothenic acid, biotin, choline, inositol, carnitine, vitamins C and E, and thiamin are absorbed in various sites within the intestinal tract (specific sites not identified). Vitamin A deficiency may be seen in individuals with disease of the terminal ileum (e.g., Crohn's disease). Hypophosphatemia and hypomagnesemia are present in individuals with calcium deficiency caused by malabsorption. In addition, copper deficiency, which interferes with the absorption of iron, has been reported in individuals who have undergone intestinal bypass surgery. Folic acid absorption requires interaction with enzymes present in the upper part of the jejunum; therefore, most absorption of folic acid takes place in the proximal part of the small intestine.[6–9] The effect of ostomy surgery on absorption of vitamins and minerals has not been well studied; patients with ileostomies or colostomies should be monitored for signs and symptoms of deficiencies.

TABLE 22-1 Signs and Symptoms of Fluid and Electrolyte Imbalance	
Adults	**Infants**
Increased thirst	Depressed fontanel
Dry mouth and mucous membranes	Lethargy
Orthostatic hypotension	Sunken eyes
Decreased urine volume	Weak cry
Increased urine concentration (dark in color)	Decreased frequency of wet diaper
Sunken eyes	Increased urine concentration (dark in color)
Extreme weakness	
Flaccid muscles	
Diminished reflexes	
Muscle cramps (abdominal and leg)	
Lethargy	
Tingling or cramping in feet and hands	
Confusion	
Nausea and vomiting	
Shortness of breath	

Source: References 3–5.

Patients with urostomy, ileostomy, or ascending colostomy must include an adequate amount of fluid in their diets to prevent the precipitation of crystals or kidney stones in the urine. They also may have an increased incidence of gallbladder stone formation. Patients with urostomies should adjust their diet to produce acidic urine, thereby reducing the risk of infection and crystal formation around the stoma. These patients are at risk of urine reflux onto the stoma, which increases the risk of infection and skin breakdown. Some evidence suggests that cranberries in the form of juice or tablets may assist in maintaining a healthy urinary tract. However, more data are needed to provide evidence of cranberry's role in urinary health.[10–13]

Systemic Complications

Constipation is caused by the regular use of constipating analgesics or other medications, or by a patient's eating habits. Patients should be encouraged to avoid the foods listed in Table 22-2 that can thicken the stool.[3,5,11,12] Constipation may be a problem in patients with descending and sigmoid colostomies. Treatment depends on the cause and may include dietary changes or medication adjustment.

Certain foods can cause diarrhea in ostomy patients (Table 22-2).[3,5,11,12] Gut pathology (ulcerative colitis, Crohn's disease, and *Clostridium difficile* colitis) or obstruction caused by a food bolus can also cause diarrhea. Medications, influenza, and food poisoning are other potential causes. Diarrhea is a special problem in patients with ileostomies and ascending colostomies, causing impaired fluid and electrolyte reabsorption. Patients with chronically loose stools may want to use an absorptive agent (Ileosorb and Par-Sorb) designed for use in the pouch. Absorptive agents do not correct the problem; they assist in coping with the problem. Increased fiber (e.g., Metamucil and Citrucel) may be used to help correct the diarrhea. Antidiarrheals may be ordered to decrease output. Also, an unexpected high output or decreased output or no output in a patient with an ileostomy may represent a partial small-bowel obstruction. In this case, the patient needs to seek emergency medical attention.

Intestinal gas may be related to food. Eliminating foods that cause gas from the diet may solve the problem (Table 22-2).

Odor is not normal except when the pouching system is changed or emptied. Otherwise, odor may be an indication of poor hygiene or leakage, failure to properly connect the pouch to the skin barrier, or use of a pouch with small holes that allow gas to escape. The clinician should review proper care and connection of the pouching system with patients who are concerned about odor. Oral deodorants are also available that will act in the digestive system to eliminate odors from digested foods (see the section Deodorizers).

Local Complications

The normal stoma is shiny, moist, and either pink or red. The stoma does not contain nerve fibers, so it does not transmit pain or other sensations. In an adult, the stoma size is approximately one-eighth to 3 inches, depending on the portion of the bowel or urinary tract used. The stoma gradually shrinks after surgery and reaches its permanent size within 6 weeks.

Skin irritation around the stoma can result from output from an ostomy, either stool or urine. Ostomy pouching systems and accessories can also irritate skin because of materials used in their composition or poor fit. The peristomal skin may look weepy or erythematous and have papules and macules. The patient may use a skin barrier powder, ostomy cream, or barrier to protect the skin, although a properly fitting pouching system should be the first priority.

Denuded peristomal skin is caused by erosion of the epidermis by digestive enzymes. The eroded or denuded epidermis may bleed, and is painful when touched and when the pouch is applied. Denuded peristomal skin occurs when an improper pouch is worn, when the pouch opening is too big or too small, or when the pouch has leaked and not been promptly replaced. These problems can allow the output to come in contact with the skin. The output produced by patients with ileostomies is particularly irritating. The patient should be referred to a WOC Nurse or primary care provider for treatment. Once the etiology of the denuded skin is determined, a skin barrier powder may be applied to the peristomal skin before the pouch is applied. The pouch should be changed more often to reduce the risk of further irritation. Treatment should be continued until the skin is clear.

TABLE 22-2 Effects of Food on Stoma Output

Foods That Thicken Stool

Applesauce; bananas; bread; buttermilk; cheese; marshmallows; milk, boiled; pasta; peanut butter, creamy; potatoes; pretzels; rice; tapioca; toast; yogurt

Foods That Loosen Stool

Beer and other alcoholic beverages; chocolate; dried or string beans; fried foods; greasy foods; highly spiced foods; leafy green vegetables (lettuce, broccoli, spinach); prune or grape juice; raw fruits (except bananas); raw vegetables

Foods That Cause Stool Odor

Asparagus; beans; cabbage-family vegetables (onions, cabbage, brussels sprouts, broccoli, cauliflower); cheese; eggs; fish; garlic; some spices; turnips

Foods That Cause Urine Odor

Asparagus; seafood; some spices

Foods That Combat Urine Odor

Buttermilk; cranberry juice; yogurt

Foods That Cause Gas

Beans (dried, string, or baked); beer; cabbage-family vegetables (onions, cabbage, brussels sprouts, broccoli, cauliflower); carbonated beverages; corn; cucumbers; dairy products; mushrooms; peas; radishes; spinach

Foods That Color Stool

Beets; berries; chocolate; fats; fish; meat (large amounts of red meat); milk; red gelatin; vegetables

Source: References 3, 5, 11, and 12.

Contact dermatitis is characterized by burning, stinging, itching, and red or denuded skin. This complication usually results from an allergic reaction to the pouching system or an accessory. A patch test will identify the allergen in patients who have a history of allergy, reaction to adhesive tape, eczema, or psoriasis, as well as in those who have very fair skin. Patients exhibiting sensitivity may need to change products. A fabric pouch cover may be helpful if the allergy is to the pouch itself. Special precautions are necessary in patients with a latex allergy. On request, a manufacturer will provide written information regarding the natural latex rubber content of its products and packaging (check the manufacturer's Web site). In some cases, the latex source is a dry, natural latex rubber, which is used to seal blister packs that contain nonlatex products.

Alkaline dermatitis (encrustation) may occur in patients with urinary diversions because of the alkaline nature of the output. The skin around the stoma may feel gritty, like sandpaper. Alkaline dermatitis, which renders the stoma extremely friable, is a common cause of blood in the pouch. A cloth soaked with a solution of one-third white vinegar to two-thirds water should be applied to the involved area for 5 to 10 minutes at least once weekly before the pouching system is put on. Patients who use a two-piece system can apply the solution as often as three to four times daily. The vinegar may cause the stoma to blanch, but blanching is not indicative of damage.

Treatment for alkaline dermatitis is acidification of the urine. Patients should avoid alkaline ash foods, such as citrus fruits and juices; paradoxically these foods are acidic when consumed but are excreted in alkaline form. Increasing fluid intake to between 2 and 3 quarts daily may reduce alkalinity. Use of a urinary appliance with an antireflux feature is recommended, because this feature prevents urine from contacting the skin when the patient is lying down.

Hyperplasia (an overgrowth of skin) occurs when the pouch opening is too large. There is no pain in the early stages, but later the affected skin cells multiply and cause agonizing pain. The condition resembles a mucosal polyp and may also be called *hyperkeratosis* or *pseudoverrucous lesion.* Treatment entails ensuring that the pouch has the correct size opening and that the seal is secure. The seal is achieved with paste, paste strips, or a moldable seal or skin barrier ring that will mold into the irregular surfaces. Other management approaches include cauterization using silver nitrate sticks and/or surgical removal.

Mechanical injury is caused by a poorly fitting appliance, a skin barrier, a stoma that is difficult to access, or tight-fitting clothing. A poorly fitting pouching system can be corrected by measuring the stoma before each purchase of supplies, selecting a skin barrier of the proper size, and adjusting the size of the skin barrier opening, if necessary. The opening should be one sixteenth to one-eighth inch larger than the stoma. Patients experiencing mechanical injury should be encouraged to contact a WOC Nurse.

Skin stripping refers to inadvertent sloughing or removal of the top layer of skin around the stoma. The skin around the stoma may be irritated from use of a strong adhesive or removal of the skin barrier in a rough manner. The skin barrier should be removed by pushing the skin away from the barrier, not by pulling the barrier away from the skin. Adhesive removers are useful in preventing skin damage if the stoma is new or the peristomal skin is fragile. After use of adhesive removers, the peristomal skin must be cleaned to remove all adhesive remover residue, because blistering, irritation, or ineffective adhesion of a new pouching system may occur.

Stenosis of the stoma results from the formation of scar tissue. Excessive scar tissue is usually caused by improper surgical construction, postoperative ischemia, active disease, or alkaline stomatitis or dermatitis. Although dilation of the stoma is often advocated to prevent or palliate this problem, the only cure is revision of the stoma.

Excessive sweating under the pouch can decrease wearing time and cause monilial infection. A skin sealant or cement plus a belt may be necessary to hold the pouching system in place. Purchasing or making a cover or bib to keep the pouch material from touching the skin can alleviate discomfort from perspiration underneath the collection pouch.

Folliculitis, an inflammation of the hair follicles, is characterized by redness at the base of the hair follicles around the stoma. Aggressive removal of any adhesive around the stoma can remove hairs, resulting in irritation and infection. Using an electric razor to shave the areas on which adhesive will be applied may help prevent folliculitis. Because folliculitis is related to an overgrowth of staphylococci on the skin, the use of an antibacterial wash should be considered; in some advanced cases, use of an oral antibiotic may be considered.

Infections are not more frequent in patients with ostomies, with the possible exceptions of patients with Crohn's disease, diabetes, or ruptured diverticulitis, or those undergoing radiation or chemotherapy. In some cases, however, infections under the pouching system can be problematic. Candidal infection may be a problem in patients who wear a pouch continuously. A dark, warm, moist environment promotes the growth of *Candida* species. The primary symptoms are itching and rash. If the infection is allowed to continue unchecked, the skin will become denuded, the pouching system will not stick, and additional skin irritation will result from the output.

If the skin is indurated, swollen, and red, it may need incision and draining. Culture and susceptibility testing should be performed, and an appropriate antibiotic should be prescribed for topical use, systemic use, or both. Patients should be encouraged to contact a WOC Nurse for assistance. Minor candidal infections may be treated with nystatin powder or miconazole 2% powder. Excessive powder should be brushed off before the pouch is applied. Antifungal preparations are generally used every other day for 1 week after the skin has become clear. In treatment of candidal infections, it is important to ascertain whether the patient is taking antibiotics. Any antibiotic, but especially a broad-spectrum agent, changes the flora of the skin, and the entrenched *Candida* can become difficult to eradicate. Therefore, it is often helpful to continue using nystatin powder or 2% miconazole powder for 1 month after all signs of candidal infection are gone in ostomy patients being treated with antibiotics.[16,17]

A *peristomal hernia* is a protrusion of the colon or ileum through a defect in the fascia in the area around the stoma. It usually occurs if the abdominal wall is weak or the stoma was placed lateral to the rectus muscle. The patient may complain of a bulge when standing or sitting. Modification of the pouching system or technique, clothing, or diet may help alleviate a peristomal hernia. An ostomy support belt/binder may be used to provide comfort and possibly prevent further herniation. The patient should be referred to the WOC Nurse for a plan of care. Surgery may be required if the patient has increased pain at the site or increased herniation, or develops signs of stoma obstruction.

A *fistula* is formation of an opening between two internal organs or from inside the body to the skin. Enterocutaneous fistulas can occur in patients with or without an ostomy. This complication is most often a manifestation of inflammatory bowel disease. Other causes include cancer, abscess formation, foreign body retention, radiation, tuberculosis, and trauma. If a fistula has excessive drainage, an ostomy pouching system may be applied to contain the drainage and prevent the skin from becoming denuded.

Prolapse is a telescoping of the bowel through the stoma. This problem results when the opening in the abdominal wall is too large. Women with ileostomies may experience prolapse of the ileostomy during pregnancy. Other causes include inadequate fixation of the bowel to the abdominal wall; poorly developed fascial support; or increased abdominal pressure associated with tumors, coughing, or crying (the latter being of special concern in infants). The danger of prolapse is the resulting decrease in blood supply to the bowel outside the abdominal cavity.

A prolapse may be reduced by having the patient lie on his or her back and apply continuous pressure on the most distal part of the stoma. Once the prolapse is reduced, a rigid pouching system should be avoided because of the risk of strangulation. The patient should apply a flexible pouch with resized opening, while lying on his or her back. A support belt may also be used. Surgical correction may be required if the stoma becomes purple, ecchymotic, or continues to prolapse.

Retraction, a recession of the stoma to a subnormal length at or below skin level, is caused by several factors. Active Crohn's disease and weight gain may lead to this damage of the skin surface. If it is not severe, a convex pouching system and use of an elastic belt may be adequate. In other cases, treatment may require surgical correction.

Organic impotence results from a radical resection of the rectum or bladder caused by disruption of nerves and vascular supply. Male patients who are impotent should be referred to a urologist for evaluation and treatment.

Management of Ostomies

Management Goals

The ideal ostomy pouching system should be leak-proof, odor-proof, comfortable, easily manipulated, inconspicuous, safe, and as inexpensive as possible. The patient has lost a normal body function. The pouching system assists the patient in managing that loss and becomes almost a part of the body. It is common for patients and their families to find discussing ostomy needs difficult or embarrassing, especially during the first several weeks or months after surgery.

The ostomy industry is highly specialized and rapidly changing in an effort to improve designs, resulting in a wide range of choices. Pouch selection is extremely personal and is based on the patient's specific needs, abilities, and cost.

General Management Approach

Adult and adolescent patients must be taught self-care skills to manage the ostomy, including (1) sizing the stoma, (2) cutting a pouch or skin barrier to fit the stoma, (3) cleaning the skin, (4) applying paste or powder if necessary, (5) applying the pouch, (6) removing the pouch, and (7) emptying the pouch. Patients must be prepared for effluent from the stoma at any time during the pouch-changing procedure.

One- and two-piece pouching systems are available for the younger child. The Hollister, Convatec, and Coloplast companies have excellent teaching booklets for children. The Hollister Company will also provide ostomy dolls for children with ostomies. Table 22-3 lists contact information for these companies.

Patients are most likely to achieve optimal outcomes if a pouching system is properly fitted (Figure 22-2), and the stoma is cared for appropriately. The clinician should always be aware of the sensitive nature of the topic and ensure that privacy is respected during all discussions. Failure to provide a comfortable environment in which to discuss problems, concerns, and alternatives may cause patients to avoid such discussions and result in less than optimal outcomes. Follow-up assessment and care may be through a telephone or scheduled appointment, or during the patient's routine visits to purchase supplies or medications.

Frequent changes in the pouching system and accessories should signal a potential problem, as should the use of multiple products intended for the same purpose. In many cases, patients may be referred to a primary care provider or WOC Nurse for follow-up of problems identified by the clinician. Complications such as impotence, peristomal hernia, and stenosis, prolapse, retraction, or excoriation of the stoma require medical referral. In some cases, however, self-care is appropriate, particularly by experienced ostomy patients.

The presence of an ostomy and its location should always be noted on the patient's profile to minimize medication-related risks. It is helpful to maintain a record of current and past ostomy products that the patient has used and any problems that the patient has experienced. This information can be useful in making future recommendations.

Types of Ostomy Pouches

The surgical technique used to create the stoma influences the pouching system required, the complexity of the pouching procedure, and the risks of stomal and peristomal complications (e.g., necrosis, stenosis, or hernia). In the past, most ostomy pouches were reusable. The advantages of reusable pouching systems were their durability, availability in numerous configurations, and relatively low cost. Their disadvantages were that they required cleaning before each use, and they were heavy, tended to retain odor, and often required a separate skin barrier.

Ostomy patients are now fitted with odor-proof, lightweight, disposable pouching systems. Most pouches incorporate a solid skin barrier in each flange or one-piece pouch, which eliminates the need for a separate skin barrier. Disposable equipment is available in one- and two-piece systems (Figure 22-3). The one-piece system, in which the skin barrier and the pouch are available in one piece, is easy to apply, especially for patients with impaired manual dexterity. The two-piece system, in which the skin barrier is separate from the pouch, allows patients to access the flange easily and change the pouch, if desired, without having to remove the flange from the skin. It is easy to apply and is generally more pliable and adaptable to different abdominal contours.

Although pouches are available for infants, some ostomies are managed with a diaper instead. If a diaper is used, care must be taken to avoid skin irritation from a caustic effluent. Barriers and creams are required for neonates and infants who are only diapered. The decision to diaper or pouch is based on the

TABLE 22-3   Sources of Ostomy Support and Information

Organization/Manufacturer	Telephone Number	Web Site[a]
American Cancer Society	800-ACS-2345	www.cancer.org
ConvaTec	800-422-8811	www.convatec.com
Crohn's and Colitis Foundation of America, Inc.	800-343-3637	www.ccfa.org
Cymed Ostomy Company	800-582-0707	www.cymed-ostomy.com
Dansac (Incutech, Inc., is the importer)	800-699-4232	www.incutech.com www.dansac.dk
Hollister, Inc.	800-323-4060	www.hollister.com
Hy-Tape Corporation	800-248-0101	www.hytape.com
International Ostomy Association		www.ostomyinternational.org
Kem-Osto EZ-Vent		www.kemOnline.com
Marlen Manufacturing		www.marlenmfg.com
Nu-Hope Laboratories, Inc.	800-899-5017	www.nu-hope.com
Options Ostomy Support Barrier, Inc.	800-736-6555	www.options-ostomy.com
The Parthenon Company, Inc.	800-453-8898	www.parthenoninc.com
Torbot Group, Inc.	800-545-4254	www.torbot.com
United Ostomy Associations of America, Inc. ■ Pull-Thru Network ■ Parents of Ostomy Children ■ Continent Diversion Network ■ Young Adult Network ■ Gay and Lesbian Ostomates Youth Rally	800-826-0826	www.uoaa.org
United Ostomy Association of Canada, Inc.	416-595-5452 888-969-9698 (Canadian residents only)	www3.ns.sympatico.ca/canada.ostomy
Wound Ostomy and Continence Nurses Society (WOCN)	888-224-WOCN	www.wocn.org

[a] Some Web sites may copyright their information. People who access a site should read and follow the instructions in the copyright statement, if one is given.

location of the stoma, type and amount of effluent, and the child's activity. Once a child is crawling or exploring, it is difficult to keep stool contained in a diaper.

Both one- and two-piece pouch systems are available in drainable, high-output, closed-end, and urostomy styles. Drainable styles are used when bowel regulation cannot be established; they allow for easy and frequent emptying. Closed-end systems are used by patients who have regulated colostomies, have one or two formed bowel movements within 24 hours, or routinely irrigate the ostomy to remove output. The goal is to avoid output between irrigations; however, this outcome may not occur immediately, and it can also be impacted by the patient's diet, activity, and illness. Urostomy systems allow a constant output of urine and easy emptying throughout the day through a narrow valve opening.

Fitting and Application

Reusable and disposable pouches are available in transparent and opaque styles and various sizes. The pouch opening may be cut to fit or presized. If it is cut to fit, the stoma pattern is traced onto the skin barrier of the pouch and then cut out before the barrier is applied. Skin barriers on one- and two-piece pouching systems are available in cut-to-fit or presized openings. Other options in skin barriers include a flat or convex skin barrier. When convex barriers are indicated, they are available with oval or moldable openings that fit flush to the skin.

Measuring the stoma to determine the proper fit of a pouch is an important part of ostomy care. The diameter of the round stoma is measured at the base, where the mucosa meets the skin; this area is considered the widest measurement. Oval stomas should be measured at both their widest and narrowest diameters. A stoma may swell if the pouch fits too tightly or slips, or if the patient falls or experiences a hard blow to the stoma. It is important to reassess the size for proper fitting.

Other considerations in fitting the pouch include body contour, stoma location, skin creases and scars, and type of ostomy. The lack of uniformity in types of ostomies and ostomy equipment makes it difficult to give standard instructions for application. Also, the stoma and the contour of the area surrounding it change over time, necessitating continuous adjustments to pouches and accessories. In general, when a rigid barrier is used, the opening should provide a clearance of one-sixteenth to one-eighth inch around the stoma. Less clearance (0–1 mm) is required with a flexible barrier. A WOC Nurse is an excellent source of assistance in custom fitting these pouching systems.

Wearing Time

The pouch should be emptied when it is one-third to one-half full to prevent leakage. With a two-piece system, the closed-end pouch is simply removed from the flange and thrown away. Patients who want to save on pouch costs may use the two-piece drainable system and alternate the use of two pouches. The

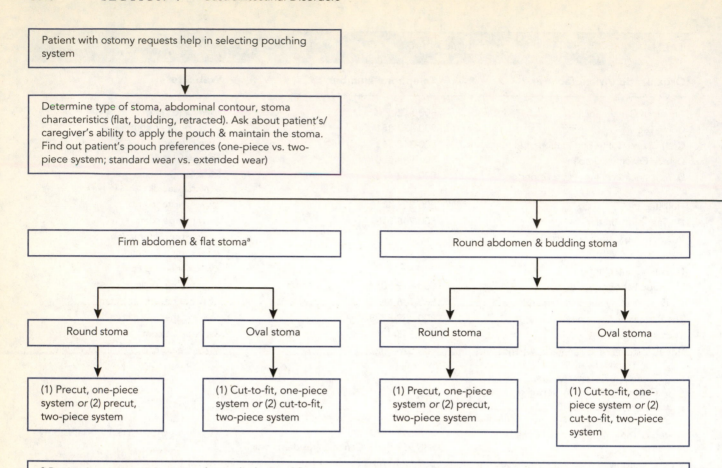

FIGURE 22-2 Selection of ostomy pouching system. Key: WOC, wound ostomy and continence. *(continued on next page)*

full pouch is removed, replaced by a second pouch, emptied, washed, and then reused when the second pouch is changed. One-piece, closed-end systems are removed and disposed of once or twice daily; those that can be drained can be left in place as long as they are comfortable and there is no leakage. The flange and skin barrier may be left in place for 3 to 7 days, depending on the condition of the skin and skin barrier. The skin barrier is constructed from a material called a hydrocolloid. The hydrocolloid softens in the presence of moisture. As the hydrocolloid softens, less adhesive is present to secure the seal. Therefore a person with a high liquid output or very moist skin (i.e., sweat) may find that the skin barrier must be changed in 3 to 4 days. A person with solid to semisolid stool may be able to wear the skin barrier for longer than 4 days. Although activities such as swimming or playing tennis may decrease the wear time of the pouch, this decreased time should not discourage participation in physical activities. New pouch adhesives can effectively keep the system in place during such activities. Because water will not enter the stoma, it is not necessary to cover it while swimming, bathing, or showering. However, the pouching system can be secured with waterproof tape (e.g., Hy-Tape and Pink Tape) by taping around the edges of the wafer/flange to prevent leakage of output from the stoma.

Product Selection Guidelines

The selection of products must be tailored to the patient's activity level and, if present, specific disabilities. Some systems require manipulation that a patient with arthritis may not be able to perform. Special products are also available to assist patients who have poor vision. In general, patients with visual or physical impairments will do best with one-piece systems, because they are precut and require minimal manipulation. Waterproof materials or a stoma cover should be included. Selection of these and other options depends on how the stoma functions. Table 22-3 lists examples of ostomy manufacturers. The Web sites

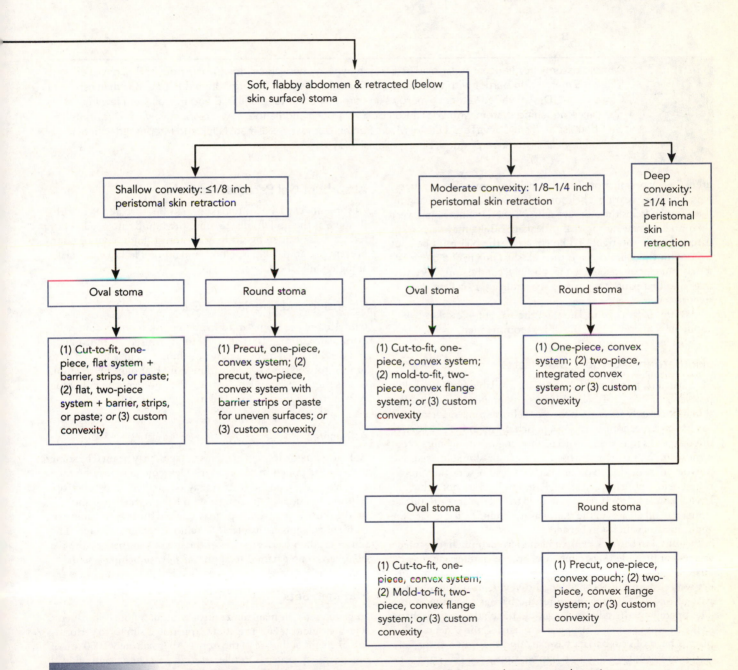

FIGURE 22-2 *(Continued)* Selection of ostomy pouching system. Key: WOC, wound ostomy and continence.

list all available products and product information. No particular device will prevent patients who are confused (e.g., with Alzheimer's disease) from reaching and dislodging the pouching system. It may be helpful to dress such patients in garments that make it difficult for the patient to reach the pouch. With infants, dressing them in one-piece clothing will help prevent them from exploring and pulling off their pouches.

Ostomy Accessories

Belts

Special elastic belts that attach to various pouching systems provide additional support. However, not all ostomy patients need to wear belts. Indications for their use are a deeply convex faceplate, poor wearing time, high activity level (especially in chil-

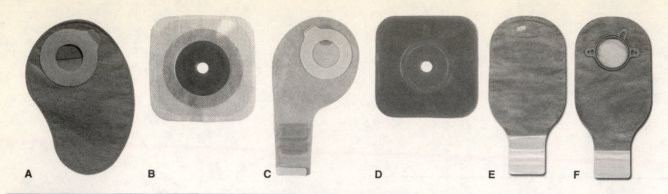

Sample ostomy appliances: **A,** ConvaTec Esteem Synergy two-piece closed-end pouch; **B,** ConvaTec Esteem Synergy skin barrier with tape collar; **C,** ConvaTec Esteem Synergy drainable pouch with Invisi-Close outlet; **D,** ConvaTec Esteem Synergy skin barrier without tape collar; **E** and **F,** Hollister New Image two-piece pouching system with Lock'n Roll closure: pouch and flange views, respectively. (A-D reprinted with permission from ConvaTec, a Bristol Myers Squibb Company, Skillman, NJ; E and F reprinted with permission from Hollister Incorporated, Libertyville, Illinois.)

dren), heavy perspiration, and personal preference. Some patients may find that wearing a belt for just a few hours after changing their pouch helps the adhesive adhere, thereby increasing wear time and decreasing the risk of leakage. Belts may cause skin ulcers if worn too tight. To be effective, the belt must be kept even with the belt hooks. If the belt slips up around the waist, it may cause poor adherence and, possibly, cut the stoma. Women may find that pantyhose or a panty girdle are excellent alternatives to a belt.

Many belts contain latex, so the patient should be asked about latex allergy before a belt is recommended.

Skin Barriers, Powders, and Pastes

Skin barriers, powders, and pastes are available for special skin problems (Table 22-4). Skin barriers are intended to protect the skin immediately adjacent to the stoma from stoma discharge and to serve as a means of attaching a pouching system. They correct imperfections in the skin surface, allowing the pouching system to fit securely. Powders are used on weeping skin, but excessive powder must be dusted off or sealed with a no-sting skin preparation before pouch application. Pastes (which are not a glue but have a paste-like consistency) are used to seal the area around the stoma and fill creases in the skin. Pastes produce a flat surface for application of other skin barriers.

Solid skin barriers are preattached to the pouch (one-piece system) or provided separately (two-piece system) and may be custom-cut (sizable) or precut (presized). Some manufacturers will custom cut the barriers; however, in most cases, the patient or WOC Nurse modifies the barrier to fit the stoma. The opening in the skin barrier should match the size and shape of the patient's stoma. To apply a skin barrier, the patient should place a bead of skin barrier paste around the stoma or directly to the inside edge of the skin barrier, apply the skin barrier to wrinkle-free skin, and then press the skin barrier around the stoma to improve adherence. Newer moldable seals are now available from major manufacturers.

Solid skin barriers may melt if exposed to high temperatures. Therefore, during the summer and especially when traveling, the solid skin barrier should be put in an insulated box (ice is not required) to minimize the risk of melting. Pouches should not be left in the car during the day, unless the car is completely shaded and the outside temperature is not extremely high.

Absorbent Gel Packets and Flakes

Absorbent gel packets and flakes (e.g., Ileosorb and Par-Sorb) dissolve as the pouch fills, turning the liquid into a gel. They reduce noise caused by sloshing of stomal fluids, control odor, prevent peristomal skin irritation, and prevent leakage, especially at night while the patient sleeps.

Cleansing and Special Skin Care Products

Cleansing of the stoma and surrounding skin is best done with plain water. If soap is used, it should be rinsed off thoroughly and the skin dried before a new pouching system is applied. Use of moisturizers and products containing lanolin, petrolatum, or oils should be avoided, because they prevent the pouching system from adhering to the skin.

Adhesives

Adhesives, in the form of cements or tapes, may be used by some to keep the pouch in place. Hypoallergenic tape may be used to support the pouch. A strip may be applied across the top, bottom, and sides of the flange, with half on the flange and half on the skin. Waterproof tape may be used during swimming or bathing. Solvents are available to remove adhesive residue. The skin must then be cleansed after the use of solvents or adhesive removers in preparation to apply the new pouching system.

Irrigating Sets

Irrigating sets can maintain control without a pouch in patients who are candidates for irrigation. Irrigation is similar to performing an enema at the site of the stoma. Approximately 1000 mL of lukewarm tap water is instilled through a cone into the bowel through the stoma. The bowel then expands, causing peristalsis and elimination of waste through the stoma. A good candidate for irrigation is an adult patient who has a colostomy distal to the splenic flexure and does not have a history of irritable bowel syndrome, is not undergoing chemotherapy, and does not have a disability. For the process to be safe and effective, the patient should use a colostomy irrigation set, rather than a standard enema set.

Frequency of irrigation depends somewhat on a patient's normal bowel habits. It is recommended to irrigate at the same

TABLE 22-4 Selected Ostomy Skin Barriers, Adhesives, Adhesive Removers, Belts, Powders, Cleaners, and Air Vent System

HollisterAdapt Lubricating Deodorant	Available in 8 oz bottle or 8 mL packs
Coloplast Strip Paste	Moldable strips to fill in uneven surfaces
ConvaTec Allkare Protective BarrierWipes	Thin film protects against skin stripping; excellent barrier for adhesives, tapes, and self-adhesive dressings
ConvaTec AllKare Adhesive Remover Wipes	Helps prevent skin damage by easing removal of all adhesives; has oily residue; skin should be washed after use
ConvaTec Eakin Cohesive Seals	Moldable, double-sided adhesive seals designed to help prevent skin damage; absorbs moisture and forms a gel to further protect skin; adheres to moist, sore skin; suitable for all types of ostomies (especially hard to fit stomas); can be used with pastes and all skin barriers and pouching systems
ConvaTec Stomahesive Paste	Pectin product; helps prevent leakage and skin irritation by filling in uneven surfaces; new easy-to-squeeze tube
ConvaTec Stomahesive Powder	Pectin base; light dusting applied to excoriated skin to promote healing
Hollister Adapt Barrier Rings, Strips, Paste	Custom (molded, bent, shaped, and stacked) convex barrier rings; barrier strips can mold and stack; paste in easy-to-squeeze tube
Hollister Medical Adhesive	Improves adhesive contact between skin and barrier
Hollister M9 Cleaner/Decrystallizer	Cleans urinary drainage systems; pH balanced and nonacidic
Hollister M9 Odor Eliminator	Available in spray or drops, scented or unscented
Hollister Adapt Powder	Light dusting applied to excoriated skin to promote healing
Hollister Universal Remover Wipes	Removes adhesives and barriers; available as spray and wipes
KEM Air VENT System (OSTO-EZ-VENT)	Quickly and easily releases gas buildup in ostomy pouches
Nu-Hope Barrier Rings and Strips	Karaya/pectin; moldable rings and strips
Nu-Hope Cement	Natural rubber; hexane; excellent adherence for difficult pouching
Nu-Hope Support Belt	Standard 2 3/8 inch opening; 3–9 inch widths; customized belts available; provides excellent support to prevent parastomal herniation; prolapse overbelt and custom openings available
Torbot Skin Cement	4 oz can; natural rubber; hexane; excellent adherence for difficult pouching
Smith & Nephew Adhesive Remover	Helps prevent skin damage by easing removal of all adhesives
3M No Sting Wipes	Does not contain alcohol; thin film protects against skin stripping; excellent barrier for adhesives, tapes, and self-adhesive dressings

time every day and eventually regulate to every other day. It takes approximately 6 weeks to become regulated. After achieving control, the patient may wear a security pouch or a piece of gauze, a stoma cover, or a cap over the stoma. Irrigation is not necessary for health; it is merely one method of colostomy management. Patients should use this procedure only if instructed to do so by a WOC Nurse or primary care provider.

Deodorizers

Deodorizers are available as liquids or tablets; however, regular emptying/changing of the pouch is all that is needed to prevent odor. However, liquid concentrates are available as companion products to most ostomy pouches; they can be placed directly into the pouch to neutralize odor. DevKo external tablets may also be placed into the pouch to decrease odor. Derifil internal deodorant tablets (active ingredient is 100 mg chlorophyllin copper complex sodium) may also be used.

In addition to local methods of odor control, many pouches have charcoal filters built into the pouch devices, which fit directly on the pouch to control gas and odor (Osto–EZ-vent).

Changes in Diet

Diet does not generally play an important role in ostomy management. Most patients can eat their usual diet, including all the food they ate before surgery, if they chew their food well. However, it is wise to remain on a diet low in fiber for the first 6 weeks after surgery to allow the intestine to heal and swelling to resolve. The usual diet can be resumed after that time.

The effects of various foods on ostomy output are summarized in Table 22-2. Patients with a urostomy may want to avoid foods that cause odor. Patients with colostomies, especially those who irrigate, should avoid foods that cause loose stools. (This problem varies among individuals.) If they have no control over gas passage, patients with a fecal ostomy may prefer to reduce their intake of gas-forming foods. Products such as alpha-D-galactosidase may be used to control gas (see Chapter 15). Patients with ileostomies are more prone to intestinal obstruction from high-fiber foods eaten in large quantities or eaten exclusive of other foods (Table 22-5). Chewing high-fiber foods well and eating them in small amounts and with other types of food will help prevent food blockage. The patient should be instructed how to manage food blockage, if it occurs. Table 22-6 lists signs and symptoms of blockage; Table 22-7 describes its management.[3]

Precautions for Medication Use

Because part of or the entire colon has been removed and intestinal transit time may be altered, the patient may experience adverse effects from taking prescription or nonprescription medications, or the medications may be ineffective. Table 22-8 lists a broad selection of medications and their potential to cause

TABLE 22-5 High-Fiber Foods[a]

Apple skins	Hot dogs
Apricots	Mushrooms
Asparagus	Nuts
Beans and lentils	Oranges and orange rinds
Bologna	Pineapples
Bran	Popcorn
Celery	Potato peels
Chinese vegetables	Raisins
Coconut	Raw vegetables
Corn	Sausage
Dried figs	Seeds
Grapefruits	Shrimp
Grapes	Tomatoes

[a] To be consumed cautiously by persons with ileostomies.
Source: References 3–5.

adverse effects, which vary with different dosage forms.[16–30] Ostomy patients should be instructed to check the pouch for undissolved tablets or tablet fragments whenever they take solid oral medications. Coated or sustained-release preparations may pass through the intestinal tract without being absorbed; therefore, patients may receive a subtherapeutic dose. Liquid preparations or preparations that are crushed or chewed before swallowing are preferred. Some medications are contained on a wax matrix (e.g., Slow K). The active medication is leached out as the tablet moves through the GI tract. Although inactive fragments normally pass through the intestines, the medication is fully absorbed.

Patients must be careful when taking antibiotics, diuretics, and laxatives. Antibiotics may alter the normal flora of the intestinal tract, causing diarrhea or fungal infection of the skin surrounding the stoma. Antidiarrheal and antimotility drugs may reduce ileal output. Sulfa drugs should be used with caution, given that crystallization in the kidney may occur more often in patients who have difficulty with fluid balance. To minimize this problem, patients should increase fluid intake and not acidify the urine. Because fluid and electrolyte balance is more difficult to maintain in patients who have had an ileostomy, diuretics should be given with care.

TABLE 22-6 Signs and Symptoms of Intestinal Obstruction

Partial Obstruction	Complete Obstruction
Cramping abdominal pain	Absence of output (urine and fecal)
Watery output with foul odor	Severe cramping pain
Abdominal distention (possible)	Abdominal distention
Stomal swelling (possible)	Stomal swelling
Nausea and vomiting (possible)	Nausea and vomiting
	Decreased pulse rate
	Fever (possible)

Source: References 3 and 4.

TABLE 22-7 Conservative Management of Food Blockage

1. Sit in warm tub bath to relax abdominal muscles.
2. Massage the peristomal area while in the knee-to-chest position to attempt dislodgement of fibrous mass.
3. If stoma is swollen, remove pouch and replace with a pouch that has a larger stoma opening.
4. If able to tolerate fluids (i.e., not vomiting) and passing stool, increase intake of fluid and electrolytes, but avoid solid foods. Drink one glass of liquid each time pouch is emptied. Juices such as grape juice exert a mild cathartic effect.
5. If vomiting, not passing stool, or both, do not take liquids or solid food orally.
6. Notify a primary care provider or WOC Nurse if any of the following develops:
   —Stool output stops (complete blockage).
   —Conservative measures (listed above) fail to resolve symptoms.
   —Signs of partial obstruction persist (Table 22-6).
   —Inability to tolerate fluids or replace fluids and electrolytes develops.
   —Signs and symptoms of fluid and electrolyte imbalance (Table 22-1) develop.

Source: Reference 3.

Patients with colostomies may use laxatives, but only under close supervision. Because of the risk of electrolyte imbalance and dehydration, ileostomy patients should never use laxatives unless they are ordered by their primary care provider. If the patient is constipated, the clinician may recommend a stool softener. Prokinetic agents (e.g., metoclopramide and erythromycin) and certain antacids should be taken with caution. Products that contain calcium may cause calcium stones in patients with a urostomy, products containing magnesium may cause diarrhea in patients with an ileostomy, and aluminum products may cause constipation in patients with a colostomy. Patients with ostomies should not use herbal supplements except under supervision of their doctor. Herbal supplements can also interact with medications, and cause adverse reactions and toxicities. In addition, herbal products are not regulated by the Food and Drug Administration, because they are considered dietary supplements.

To alleviate anxiety, the clinician should counsel the patient about medications that may discolor the feces. Some of these medications and the discoloration they cause are listed in Table 22-9.[31–36]

Assessment of Patients with Ostomies: A Case-Based Approach

In most cases, ostomy surgery necessitates the use of a pouching system designed to collect the waste material normally eliminated through the bowel or bladder. Because each ostomy patient is different, one patient may benefit from a particular type of pouch, accessory, or procedure, whereas another may develop problems with the same products. Moreover, pouch needs may change over time. A pouching system, accessory, or procedure that previously produced ideal outcomes may no longer be appropriate because of changes in body contour caused by aging, pregnancy,

TABLE 22-8 Potential Effects of Selected Prescription Drugs in Patients with Ostomies

Class	Type of Ostomy	Potential Effects
Histamine$_1$-receptor antagonists	Ileostomy, colostomy, urostomy	No reported problems with cetirizine, loratadine, and fexofenadine
Anti-inflammatories	Ileostomy	NSAIDs associated with GI irritation and bleeding: use with caution if history of GI ulceration or bleeding exists (COX-2 inhibitors may have lower risk profile); no reported problems with Celecoxib
Opiates	Colostomy	Tramadol's opiate agonist activity can cause constipation, similar to opiates such as oxycodone; liquids, immediate-release products, or patches preferred to avoid erratic absorption associated with ER products
Selective serotonin reuptake inhibitors	Ileostomy	No reported problems with sertraline, citalopram, or fluoxetine; hyponatremia and diarrhea reported with paroxetine, requiring close monitoring of fluid and electrolyte status
Antipsychotics	Colostomy, ileal conduit	Constipation reported with olanzapine, caused primarily by drug's anticholinergic effect; constipation possible with all anticholinergic drugs; reported delayed lithium toxicity requires close monitoring of serum levels in patients with ileal conduits
Antidiabetic	Ileostomy	Possible dose-related GI effects related to variable absorption of metformin, a weak base primarily absorbed in the small intestine; no reported problems with other antidiabetic agents
Anticonvulsants	Ileostomy	Erratic absorption reported with enteric-coated and sustained-release products; use of liquids or immediate-release products generally recommended
Antilipidemics	Ileostomy, colostomy, urostomy	No reported problems with use of HMG-CoA reductase inhibitors
Cardiac/antihypertensive drugs	Ileostomy	Fluid and electrolyte abnormalities common; careful monitoring recommended during use of ACE inhibitors; hyperkalemia may be a particular problem
GI medications	Ileostomy, colostomy	Diarrhea associated with all PPIs, requiring careful monitoring of fluid and electrolyte status; no reported problems with H$_2$RAs
Antimicrobial agents	Ileostomy, urostomy, colostomy	Altered normal bowel flora and diarrhea related to broad-spectrum antibiotics can be a significant problem for patients with ileostomies; high doses of ciprofloxacin associated with alkaline urine (if used, urinary acidification to avoid bacterial overgrowth in urostomy patients requires close monitoring)
Other drugs	End jejunostomy, ileostomy	Some reports of drug failure associated with malabsorption of warfarin in patients with short-bowel syndrome Length of functionally intact proximal small bowel important in cyclosporine dosing (if liquid formulation or IV is required, more frequent monitoring is recommended) Variable volume of distribution and increased clearance of gentamicin reported in patients with ileostomies, possibly requiring more frequent monitoring Highly variable bioavailability of digoxin (depends on length of remaining bowel) requires monitoring for drug failure

Key: ACE inhibitors, angiotensin-converting enzyme inhibitors; COX-2, cyclooxygenase-2; ER, extended-release; GI, gastrointestinal; HMG-CoA, hydroxymethyl glutaryl coenzyme A; H$_2$RAs, histamine$_2$-receptor antagonists; NSAID, nonsteroidal anti-inflammatory drug; PPI, proton pump inhibitor.
Source: References 16–30.

weight change, or concurrent medical conditions. As the obesity epidemic continues, so do the challenges in caring for that ostomy population.

Patients who have an ostomy are often apprehensive about how the surgery will proceed, how to manage the ostomy, and how they will be perceived by others. A patient's self-esteem may also be affected. Therefore, a special effort should be made to ensure the patient's privacy and to gain the patient's confidence during the assessment encounter.

Cases 22–1 and 22–2 illustrate assessment of patients with ostomies.

Patient Counseling for Ostomy Care

The pharmaceutical care needs of a patient with an ostomy include procurement and distribution of ostomy supplies and selection of appropriate products. Monitoring a patient's manage-

TABLE 22-9 Selected Drugs That Discolor Feces and Urine

Drugs That Discolor Feces

Black		**Blue**	**Orange-Red**	**White or Speckled**
Acetazolamide	Hydralazine	Manganese dioxide	Phenazopyridine	Aluminum hydroxide
Aluminum hydroxide	Iodide-containing drugs	Chloramphenicol	Rifampin	Barium
Aminophylline	Iron	Methylene blue	Rifapentine	Oral antibiotics
Amphetamine	Levodopa			
Amphotericin B[a]	Melphalan	**Gray**	**Orange-Brown**	**Yellow or Yellow-Green**
Anticoagulants[a]	Methotrexate	Colchicine	Rifabutin	Senna
Aspirin[a]	Nitrates			
Barium	Nonsteroidal	**Green**	**Pink-Red**	
Bismuth	anti-inflammatory drugs[a]	Indomethacin	Anticoagulants[a]	
Chloramphenicol	Phenylephrine	Iron	Aspirin	
Chlorpropamide	Potassium salts[a]	Medroxyprogesterone	Barium	
Cholestyramine	Procarbazine		Cefdinir[b]	
Corticosteroids	Sulfonamides	**Green-Gray**	Nonsteroidal	
Cyclophosphamide	Tetracycline	Oral antibiotics	anti-inflammatory drugs[a]	
Cytarabine	Thallium		Tetracycline syrup	
Ethacrynic acid	Theophylline		Clofazimine	
Fluorouracil	Thiotepa[a]			

Drugs That Discolor Urine

Black	**Dark**	**Pink-Red**	**Red-Brown**	**Yellow-Brown**
Ferrous salts	Aminosalicylic acid	Phenothiazines	Aloe	Cascara
Phenacetin	Metronidazole	Phenytoin	Levodopa	Nitrofurantoin
	Phenacetin		Phenytoin	Primaquine
Blue or Green		**Purplish Red**	Quinine	Senna
Amitriptyline	**Orange**	Chlorzoxazone	Warfarin	Sulfonamides
Cimetidine (injection)	Chlorzoxazone			
Flutamide	Warfarin	**Red**	**Violet**	**Yellow-Orange**
Indomethacin		Carbidopa/levodopa	Senna	Vitamin A
Methocarbamol	**Orange-Red**	Daunorubicin		
Methylene blue	Phenazopyridine	Dimethylsulfoxide	**Yellow**	**Yellow-Pink**
Mitoxantrone	Rifampin	Doxorubicin	Aloe	Cascara
Promethazine (injection)		Idarubicin	Riboflavin	
Propofol (injection)			Sulfasalazine	
Triamterene			Vitamin B_{12}	

[a] Discoloration may be caused by bleeding.

[b] Discoloration caused by nonabsorbable complex between cefdinir or metabolites and iron in the GI tract.

Source: References 31–36.

ment of the ostomy and counseling on special needs (e.g., skin care, diet, fluid intake, and drug therapy) are other important components of pharmaceutical care for these patients.

When counseling an ostomy patient, the clinician should provide services in a sensitive and caring manner. An ostomy patient's self-esteem is often damaged; therefore, when assisting a patient with ostomy needs, the clinician must take special care to avoid verbal or facial expressions that might convey negative feelings regarding the procedure. Peer support can be especially helpful to such patients. The clinician should consider providing patients with a list of local and national ostomy associations, as well as a list of product manufacturers who can supply information about product use (Table 22-3). Patients who want to contact a WOC Nurse in their area should be

advised to check the Web site at www.wocn.org. The following self-help books should also be recommended to patients with ostomies:

- Barrie B. *Second Act*. New York: Scribner; 1997.
- Benirschke R. *Alive & Kicking*. San Diego: Rolf Benirschke Enterprises; 1999.
- Benirschke R. *Great Comebacks*. San Diego: Rolf Benirschke Enterprises; 2002.
- Elsagher B. *I'd like to Buy A Bowel Please! Ostomy A to Z.* Andover, Minn: Expert Publishing; 2006.
- Elsagher B. *If The Battle Is Over Why am I Still In Uniform? Humor as a Survival Tactic to Combat Cancer.* Andover, Minn: Expert Publishing; 2005.

CASE 22-1

Relevant Evaluation Criteria	Scenario/Model Outcome
Information Gathering	
1. Gather essential information about the patient's symptoms, including:	
a. description of symptom(s) (i.e., nature, onset, duration, severity, associated symptoms)	The patient's symptoms began during the summer, when he was perspiring a lot.
b. description of any factors that seem to precipitate, exacerbate, and/or relieve the patient's symptom(s)	The patient applied pectin-based powder before appliance changes, but his symptoms have not resolved.
c. description of the patient's efforts to relieve the symptoms	He has experienced itching and rash underneath his urostomy for the past week, and now the skin is becoming denuded. His pouch has started to leak more often. He usually wears his pouching system for 1 week but can keep it on for only 24 hours.
2. Gather essential patient history information:	
a. patient's identity	Kevin Sabato
b. patient's age, sex, height, and weight	60-year-old male, 5 ft 10 in, 220 lb
c. patient's occupation	Computer analyst
d. patient's dietary habits	Diabetic diet
e. patient's sleep habits	N/A
f. concurrent medical conditions, prescription and nonprescription medications, and dietary supplements	Glucophage 500 mg twice daily, Flovent 220 mg 2 puffs twice daily, albuterol 2 puffs every 6 hours as needed; underwent ileal loop for bladder cancer 2 years earlier
g. allergies	Aspirin
h. history of other adverse reactions to medications	None
i. other (describe) _____	N/A
Assessment and Triage	
3. Differentiate the patient's signs/symptoms and correctly identify the patient's primary problem(s).	Since the summer, Kevin has developed a rash and itching. The rash appears to be caused by *Candida*, which thrives in dark, damp areas (caused by Kevin's leaking pouching system, perspiration, and denuded skin). Kevin's diabetes is another related factor.
4. Identify exclusions for self-treatment.	None
5. Formulate a comprehensive list of therapeutic alternatives for the primary problem to determine if triage to a medical practitioner is required, and share this information with the patient.	Options include: (1) Refer Kevin to a WOC Nurse. (2) Recommend application of miconazole 2% powder to affected area with each pouch change. (3) Have Kevin see his clinician for a prescription for nystatin powder to apply to the affected area with each pouch change if 2% miconazole is not effective. (4) Take no action.
Plan	
6. Select an optimal therapeutic alternative to address the patient's problem, taking into account patient preferences.	OTC treatment with a powder containing 2% miconazole is appropriate for Kevin. He should also change his pouching system more frequently.
7. Describe the recommended therapeutic approach to the patient.	You can use an OTC powder to get rid of the rash and itching. You should change your pouching system more often and apply the powder at each change to prevent these symptoms from occurring again.
8. Explain to the patient the rationale for selecting the recommended therapeutic approach from the considered therapeutic alternatives.	Seeing a WOC Nurse (wound ostomy and continence nurse), or your primary care provider will not be necessary, because rash and itching are quite common in this situation. A referral is necessary only if the symptoms do not resolve.

CASE 22-1 *(continued)*

Relevant Evaluation Criteria	Scenario/Model Outcome
Patient Education	
9. When recommending self-care with non-prescription medications and/or nondrug therapy, convey accurate information to the patient.	Wash peristomal skin per your usual routine. Apply 2% miconazole powder sparingly, and massage it into the peristomal skin. Dust off excess powder. A sealant (3M No Sting, etc.) may be applied to enhance the pouch seal. Apply the pouch. Use the miconazole powder with each pouch change until 1 week after the rash has resolved. You should change the appliance every other day until the rash clears; then you can return to once-a-week appliance changes. If rash and itching continue, consult a WOC Nurse or your primary care provider.
10. Solicit follow-up questions from patient.	How long should I continue using the 2% miconazole or the Nystatin powder?
11. Answer patient's questions.	Use for 1 week after rash has resolved. You may use it as needed if the rash develops again.

Key: N/A, not applicable; OTC, over-the-counter; WOC, wound ostomy continence.

CASE 22-2

Relevant Evaluation Criteria	Scenario/Model Outcome
Information Gathering	
1. Gather essential information about the patient's symptoms, including:	
a. description of symptom(s) (i.e., nature, onset, duration, severity, associated symptoms)	Patient has developed leakage from her ileostomy pouching system in the past few weeks. She also noticed redness and denuded skin around her ileostomy. Pain at the site is also frustrating the patient.
b. description of any factors that seem to precipitate, exacerbate, and/or relieve the patient's symptom(s)	Since her surgery 6 months ago, the patient has gained 30 pounds. She usually changes her pouch every 4 days, but now she has to change it every 2 days and continues to have leakage and redness.
c. description of the patient's efforts to relieve the symptoms	Patient applied skin barrier powder and skin sealant to protect skin, but she continues to have skin irritation and leakage.
2. Gather essential patient history information:	
a. patient's identity	Sharon Lipinski
b. patient's age, sex, height, and weight	22-year-old female, 5 ft 4 in, 160 lb
c. patient's occupation	Sales consultant
d. patient's dietary habits	High-fiber diet with junk food
e. patient's sleep habits	N/A
f. concurrent medical conditions, prescription and nonprescription medications, and dietary supplements	Nasonex 2 sprays once daily or 1 spray in each nostril once daily; Imodium A-D 2 mg taken after each unformed stool, not to exceed 16 mg/day

Sharon developed ulcerative colitis 5 years earlier. After a major bleeding episode and failure of medical management, she underwent total colectomy and ileostomy. |
g. allergies	Latex
h. history of other adverse reactions to medications	None
i. other (describe) _____	Patient has been nervous about her job and has been constantly eating, which has increased her weight.

Relevant Evaluation Criteria	Scenario/Model Outcome

Assessment and Triage

3. Differentiate the patient's signs/symptoms and correctly identify the patient's primary problem(s).

Leakage, burning sensation, and denuded skin around her ileostomy are caused by abdominal creases from increased weight.

4. Identify exclusions for self-treatment.

None

5. Formulate a comprehensive list of therapeutic alternatives for the primary problem to determine if triage to a medical practitioner is required, and share this information with the patient.

Options include:
(1) Refer Sharon to a WOC Nurse for further assessment and treatment.
(2) Recommend use of a skin barrier powder to improve peristomal skin, followed by application of a skin sealant.
(3) Recommend use of pouch convexity and belt for support.
(4) Take no action.

Plan

6. Select an optimal therapeutic alternative to address the patient's problem, taking into account patient preferences.

Assessment of the stoma and skin indicates that a convex pouch with a belt for support is needed. Upon further discussion, Sharon says she prefers a one-piece convex pouch with belt versus a two-piece pouch.

7. Describe the recommended therapeutic approach to the patient.

Because your stoma has retracted to skin level, you will need a convex pouch with a belt for support. Treat skin around the stoma with a skin barrier powder, such as Stomahesive powder, and a skin sealant, such as 3M No Sting, before applying the pouch. Change the pouching system twice a week until the peristomal skin is free of burning and is no longer denuded; then resume pouch changes every 4 days.

Losing some weight will also decrease the retraction of the stoma.

8. Explain to the patient the rationale for selecting the recommended therapeutic approach from the considered therapeutic alternatives.

Pouch leakage, denuded skin, and pain will decrease with proper follow-up with your WOC Nurse (wound ostomy and continence nurse) to modify the pouching technique.

Refer to the local chapter of the United Ostomy Associations of America for peer support to improve your self-esteem and body image (see Table 22-3).

Patient Education

9. When recommending self-care with non-prescription medications and/or nondrug therapy, convey accurate information to the patient:

a. appropriate dose and frequency of administration

See Figure 22-2 for proper assessment of convexity, and Figure 22-3 and Table 22-4 for proper pouching and skin accessories.

b. maximum number of days the therapy should be employed

Change pouch twice a week.

c. product administration procedures

Wash peristomal skin as usual. Apply thin layer of powder. Massage powder into skin well and dust off excess powder. Apply skin sealant before the pouch application.

d. expected time to onset of relief

With proper convexity and powder application, leakage and excoriation should decrease within 24 hours. You will notice a decrease in the burning sensation.

e. degree of relief that can be reasonably expected

Deceased intensity of symptoms within 24–48 hours

f. most common side effects

Allergic reaction to the powder or pouch adhesive

g. side effects that warrant medical intervention should they occur

Burning, stinging, local irritation

h. patient options in the event that condition worsens or persists

Consult a WOC Nurse or your primary care provider if leakage or burning continues after 1 week of treatment.

i. product storage requirements

Store away from heat.

j. specific nondrug measures

Change pouch every 2 days until peristomal skin is clear.

10. Solicit follow-up questions from patient.

What happens if I can't lose weight, develop more creases, and my stoma retracts more?

11. Answer patient's questions.

Consult a WOC Nurse; you may need another type of pouching system.

Obesity is now epidemic; consult a nutritionist for a proper diet program.

Key: N/A, not available; WOC, wound ostomy and continence.

PATIENT EDUCATION FOR
Ostomy Care

The objectives of self-care of ostomies are to (1) understand how the stoma functions and how to manage it; (2) understand the proper use of the pouching system and accessories, and avoid complications that result from improper use; and (3) reduce the risk of other types of complications. For most patients, carefully following the product instructions and the self-care measures listed here will help to ensure optimal therapeutic outcomes.

Pouching System Selection and Use

- Use only the type of pouching system recommended for your type of ostomy.
- If your system no longer fits well, consult your WOC Nurse or clinician before changing to a different type of pouching system.
- Do not consider skin irritation to be inevitable; identify the cause and treat it as soon as it occurs.
- If possible, identify the cause for leakage around the pouching system and correct the problem immediately. Consult your WOC Nurse or primary care provider if you cannot determine the cause.
- Establish a routine for ostomy care. Keep the routine simple; use as few accessories as possible.

Effects of Medication Use

- Sustained- or extended-release medicines may undergo erratic absorption, which makes their effect unpredictable. These medications should be used with caution. Coated medications, as well as sustained- or extended-release medications should not be crushed or chewed.
- Use caution when taking antibiotics and diuretics. Antibiotics can cause diarrhea or fungal infections of the skin around the stoma. Diuretics can cause dehydration or electrolyte imbalance in individuals with ileostomies.
- Use caution when taking laxatives, antidiarrheals, or other medications that alter gastrointestinal motility. Laxatives can

increase fecal output in individuals with ileostomies, whereas antidiarrheals decrease the fecal output.
- Know which medications will discolor the urine or feces (Table 22-9).

Complications

- To prevent urine crystals from forming around a urostomy and causing skin irritation, apply a cloth soaked with a vinegar solution (one-third white vinegar to two-thirds water) for 5–10 minutes to the stoma at least once weekly before putting on the pouching system. If you use a two-piece system, apply the solution as often as three to four times daily. The vinegar may cause the stoma to turn white, but this effect does not indicate the stoma is being harmed.
- Consult your clinician about using nonprescription medications to treat diarrhea or constipation. Return for reevaluation of the problem after 1 week of treatment.

⚠ See your WOC Nurse if you experience any of the following complications:
  —Depression and anxiety
  —Sexual dysfunction
  —Abdominal pain
  —Narrowing of the stoma
  —A bulge near the stoma
  —An extension of the bowel through the stoma
  —Recession of the stoma to a subnormal length
  —Bleeding from or around the stoma
  —Pain when touching the skin around the stoma or when applying the appliance
  —Overgrowth of the skin around the stoma

- Kupfer B, Foley-Bolch K, Kasouf MF, et al. *Yes We Can.* Worchester, Mass: Chandler House Press; 2000.
- Ruggieri P. *Colon & Rectal Cancer. A Patient's Guide For Treatment.* Omaha, Neb: Addicus Books; 2001.

The patient should be encouraged to express problems and concerns so the clinician can better assess the patient's ability to achieve self-treatment objectives. Moreover, the clinician must maintain an awareness of the patient's special needs when managing conditions unrelated to the ostomy. The box Patient Education for Ostomy Care lists specific information to provide a patient with an ostomy.

Key Points for Ostomy Care

➤ Patients with ostomies may experience both psychological and physical complications after ostomy surgery. It is the obligation of the clinician to address these issues and refer patients to their primary care provider, WOC Nurse, and/or United Ostomy Associations of America.

➤ The objectives of self-care of an ostomy are to understand how the stoma functions and how to manage it, to understand proper use of the pouching system and accessories, to

avoid complications that result from improper use, and to reduce the risks of other complications.

➤ Patients should be advised about the effects of food on stomal output and the need to monitor for signs and symptoms of dehydration.

➤ The selection of appropriate pouching depends on the patient's body contour, manual dexterity, and type of ostomy.

➤ The ideal ostomy pouching system should be leak-proof, odor-proof, comfortable, and easy to use. The clinician as well as the WOC Nurse can assist the patient in achieving these outcomes.

➤ Patients should be counseled on the effects of medications:
  —Use of liquid, crushed, or chewed medications is preferable.
  —Coated or sustained-release medications should be used with caution, because most should not be crushed or chewed.
  —Caution is warranted with use of antibiotics and diuretics. Antibiotics can cause diarrhea or fungal infections of the skin around the stoma. Diuretics can cause dehydration or electrolyte imbalance in patients with ileostomies.
  —Use caution when taking laxatives, antidiarrheals, or other medications that alter GI motility. Laxatives can

increase fecal output in patients with ileostomies, whereas antidiarrheals decrease the fecal output.

REFERENCES

1. United Ostomy Association Fact Sheet. Available at: http://www.uoaa.org/ostomy_info/faq.shtml. Last accessed September 18, 2008.

2. Wise B, McKenna, Gavin G, et al. *APSNA Nursing Care of the General Pediatric Surgical Patient*. Gaithersburg, Md: Aspen Publishers; 2000.

3. Colwell JC, Goldberg MT, Carmel JE. *Fecal & Urinary Diversions Management Principles*. St Louis: Mosby; 2004:224.

4. Colwell JC, Goldberg MT, Carmel JE. *Fecal & Urinary Diversions Management Principles*. St Louis: Mosby; 2004.

5. Krenta KS. *Living with Confidence after Ileostomy Surgery*. Princeton, NJ: ConvaTec, a Bristol Myers Squibb Co; 2003.

6. Hillman RS. Hematopoietic agents: growth factors, minerals, and vitamins. In: Hardman JG, Limbird LE, eds. *Goodman and Gilman's The Pharmacological Basis of Therapeutics*. 10th ed. New York: McGraw-Hill, Inc; 2001:1487–517.

7. Marcus R. Agents affecting calcification and bone turnover: calcium, phosphate, parathyroid hormone, vitamin D, calcitonin, and other compounds. In: Hardman JG, Limbird LE, eds. *Goodman and Gilman's The Pharmacological Basis of Therapeutics*. 10th ed. New York: McGraw-Hill, Inc; 2001:1715–43.

8. Marcus R, Coulston AM. Water-soluble vitamins: the vitamin B complex and ascorbic acid. In: Hardman JG, Limbird LE, eds. *Goodman and Gilman's The Pharmacological Basis of Therapeutics*. 10th ed. New York: McGraw-Hill, Inc; 2001:1753–71.

9. Marcus R, Coulston AM. Fat-soluble vitamins: vitamins A, K, and E. In: Hardman JG, Limbird LE, eds. *Goodman and Gilman's The Pharmacological Basis of Therapeutics*. 10th ed. New York: McGraw-Hill, Inc; 2001:1773–91.

10. Gray M. Are cranberry juice or cranberry products effective in the prevention or management of urinary tract infection? *J WOCN*. 2002;29:122–6.

11. Raz R, Chazan B, Dan M. Cranberry juice and urinary tract infection. *CID*. 2004;38:1413–9.

12. Jepson RG, Mihaljevicl, Craig J. Cranberries for treating urinary tract infections. *Cochrane Database Syst Rev*. 2002;2:CD001322.

13. Jepson RG, Mihaljevicl, Craig J. Cranberries for preventing urinary tract infections. *Cochrane Database Syst Rev*. 2004;2:CD001321.pub3.

14. Hollister, Inc. *Patient Education Series: What's right for me?* Libertyville, Ill: Hollister, Inc; 2003.

15. Krenta KS. *Living with Confidence after Urostomy Surgery*. Princeton, NJ: ConvaTec, a Bristol-Myers Squibb Co; 2003.

16. Aly R, Forney R, Bayes C. Treatment for common superficial fungal infections. *Dermatol Nurs*. 2001;13:91–9.

17. Erwin-Toth P. Caring for a stoma. *Nursing 2001*. 2001;31(5):36–40.

18. Colwell JC, Goldberg MT, Carmel JE. *Fecal & Urinary Diversions Management Principles*. St Louis: Mosby; 2004:345–8.

19. *AHFS Drug Information*. Bethesda, Md: American Society of Health-System Pharmacists; 2003.

20. Colwell JC, Goldberg MT, Carmel JE. *Fecal & Urinary Diversions Management Principles*. St Louis: Mosby; 2004:345–8.

21. Severijnen R, Bayat N, Bakker H, et al. Enteral drug absorption in patients with short small bowel—a review. *Clin Pharmacokinet*. 2004;43:951–62.

22. Tewari A, Ward RG, Sells RA, et al. Reduced bioavailability of cyclosporine A capsules in a renal transplant patient with partial gastrectomy and ileal resection. *Ann Clin Biochem*. 1993;30:587–9.

23. Gaskin TL, Duffull SB. Enhanced gentamicin clearance associated with ileostomy fluid loss. *Aust N Z J Med*. 1997;27:196–7.

24. Ritchie HA, Duggull SB. Another case of high gentamicin clearance and volume of distribution in a patient with high output ileostomy. *Aust N Z J Med*. 1998;28:212–3.

25. Al-Habet S, Kinsella HC, Rogers HJ, et al. Malabsorption of prednisolone from enteric-coated tablets after ileostomy. *BMJ*. 1980;281:843–4.

26. Owens JP, Mirtallo JM, Murphy CC. Oral anticoagulation in patients with short-bowel syndrome. *DICP*. 1990;24:585–9.

27. Lutomski DM, LaFrance RJ, Bower RH, et al. Warfarin absorption after massivesmall bowel resection. *Am J Gastroenterol*. 1985; 80:99–102.

28. Chen JP. Ileostomy and ramipril-induced acute renal failure and shock. *Heart Lung*. 2007 July/August:298–99.

29. Brophy DF, Ford SL, Crouch MA. Warfarin resistance in a patient with short bowel syndrome. *Pharmacotherapy*. 1998;18:1375–6.

30. Roberts R, Sketris IS, Abraham I, et al. Cyclosporine absorption in two patients with short-bowel syndrome. *DICP*. 1988;22:570–2.

31. Knoben JE, Anderson PO. *Handbook of Clinical Drug Data*. 7th ed. Hamilton, Ill: Drug Intelligence Publications; 1998.

32. Allen J, Burson SC. Drug discoloration of the urine. Document 150907. *Pharm Lett*. September 1999.

33. *Physicians' Desk Reference Electronic Library*. Montvale, NJ: Medical Economics; 2003.

34. Fecal discoloration induced by drugs, chemicals, and disease states. In: Gelman CR, Rumack BH, Hutchison TA, eds. *DRUGDEX System*. Englewood, NJ: Micromedex; 2003.

35. Alhasso A, Bryden AA, Neilson D. Lithium toxicity after urinary diversion with ileal conduit. *BMJ*. 2000;320:1037.

36. Urinary discoloration—drug and disease induced. In: *DRUGDEX System*. Englewood, NJ: Micromedex; 2003.

Nutrition and Nutritional Supplementation

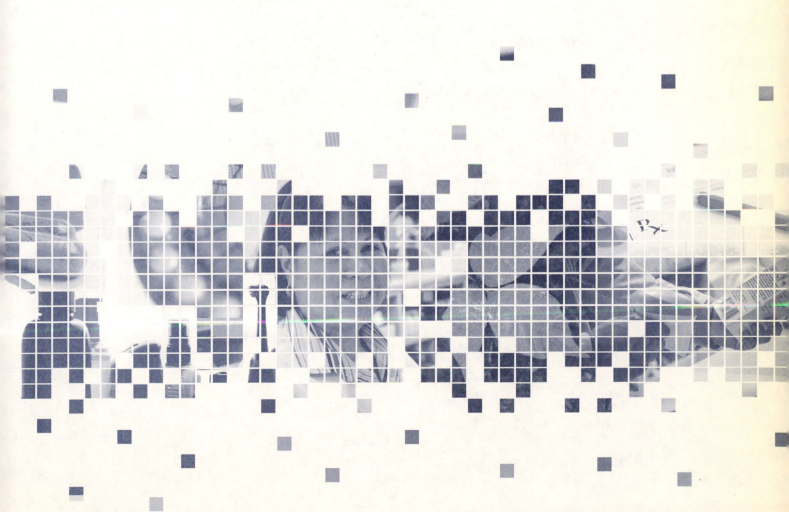

CHAPTER

23

Essential and Conditionally Essential Nutrients

Yvonne Huckleberry and Carol J. Rollins

Approximately 40% to 50% of Americans consume a vitamin, dietary, or mineral supplement daily, accounting for estimated annual sales in excess of $14 billion.[1] Nutrition experts agree that foods are the preferred source of vitamins and minerals, and that most individuals can easily meet their requirements by eating a balanced diet. There is less agreement, however, about the extent to which the U.S. population consumes a balanced diet. Many believe that most Americans receive adequate levels of vitamins and minerals from their diet; the lack of deficiency symptoms in this country supports this position. However, there is growing concern that subclinical deficiencies may be contributing to chronic diseases such as arteriosclerosis, osteoporosis, and cancer.[2] This finding suggests primary attention should be directed toward improving the selection of nutrient-dense foods. Despite such attention, some individuals are unlikely to consume adequate amounts of vitamins and minerals; therefore, a multivitamin supplement may be appropriate.

The issue of who will benefit from or be harmed by oral supplements is complex. For example, one study evaluated the role of dietary supplements in improving the overall nutrient intake of adults.[3] These authors found that regular use of dietary supplements helps patients meet dietary requirements. However, many supplement users exceeded the tolerable upper intake levels (ULs) of some nutrients, thereby increasing the risk of adverse effects.

Consumers are eager to be proactive with self-treatment for prevention and treatment of different ailments. Product marketing and natural product enthusiasts encourage them to do so with promotions for supplementation of various nutrients in doses well above those recommended as safe. However, often little data are available to support safety and efficacy of such claims. Even benefits speculated as potentially beneficial by the medical community have often been disproven once evaluated by randomized trials. For example, the United States Preventive Services Task Force (USPSTF) evaluated randomized trials of vitamin supplementation with beta-carotene, vitamins A, C, and E, folic acid, or antioxidants in the prevention of cancer or cardiovascular disease.[4] Evidence was conflicting and insufficient to support regular supplementation for this purpose. Furthermore, the USPSTF found potential harm associated with beta-carotene supplementation in certain populations and recommends avoiding its use.

One of the greatest dangers of food fads, multiple supplements, and large doses of single vitamins is that they are sometimes used in place of sound medical care. The lure of superior health or freedom from disease may attract desperate or uninformed patients who have cancer, heart disease, arthritis, or other serious illnesses. This may place them at greater risk by causing a delay in seeking and receiving appropriate medical attention.

Epidemiology/Etiology of Nutritional Deficiencies

Although overt nutrient deficiency is rare in the United States, the prevalence of subclinical deficiencies is unknown. Specific patient populations may be at higher risk of deficient nutrient intakes because of the following pathophysiologic, physiologic, behavioral, or economic situations:

- *Inadequate dietary intake:* patients who are alcoholics, impoverished, or on severe calorie-restricted or fad diets, or those who have eating disorders
- *Increased metabolic requirements:* pregnant and breast-feeding women, infants, children undergoing periods of accelerated growth, postsurgical patients, and patients with cancer, severe injury, infection, or trauma
- *Poor absorption:* patients of advanced age or those with conditions such as prolonged diarrhea, severe gastrointestinal (GI) disorders or malignancy, surgical removal of a section of the GI tract (including gastric bypass for weight reduction), celiac disease, obstructive jaundice, or cystic fibrosis
- *Iatrogenic situations:* patients taking prolonged broad-spectrum antibiotics, those with drug–nutrient interactions, or those who are receiving parenteral nutrition

Although several factors increase the risk of malnutrition in patients of advanced age (Table 23-1), vitamin and mineral deficiency among noninstitutionalized older patients is uncommon. This finding has been attributed to an increasing number of healthy, active individuals older than 65 years, better nutrition, and an increase in self-treatment with vitamin and mineral supplements.[5] Although clinical deficiency is rare, dietary intakes for some older patients may still be below optimum levels. Because foods contain numerous other compounds that are important for health maintenance and disease prevention, health care professionals play an important role in educating these patients on nutrient-dense food choices before vitamin and/or mineral supplementation is recommended.

TABLE 23-1 Factors Contributing to Nutritional Deficiency in Patients of Advanced Age

- Mastication or swallowing difficulty, or xerostomia
- Loss of taste, smell, or sight perception
- Constipation or diarrhea
- Decreased absorption of some nutrients such as lactose
- Gastric hypochlorhydria, atrophic gastritis, or use of medications that raise gastric pH
- Inability to buy or prepare meals because of tremor, fatigue, or arthritic pain
- Anorexia caused by reduced physical activity, social isolation, pain, or depression
- Dementia
- Lack of knowledge about balanced nutrition
- Poverty
- Substance abuse
- Inadequate exposure to sunlight
- Medications affecting judgment, coordination, memory, appetite, nutrient absorption, or GI tract function

Source: Reference 5.

Pathophysiology of Nutritional Deficiencies

A comprehensive discussion of the pathophysiology of vitamin and mineral deficiencies is outside the scope of this chapter. The reader is referred to standard medical and nutrition textbooks for such information.

Clinical Presentation of Nutritional Deficiencies

A vitamin deficiency may evolve in several stages (Table 23-2).[6] Signs and symptoms of vitamin and mineral deficiencies are discussed in the individual micronutrient sections.

Poor nutrition increases the risks of chronic disease, infection, and complications from surgery and chemotherapy. In addition, wound-healing time and mortality may be increased. For the pediatric population, growth, development, and learning may be compromised as well. Balanced nutrition with adequate protein, calories, vitamins, and minerals is essential for health through all stages of the life cycle.

Nutrient Supplementation

Nutritional supplements should be used as adjuncts to a balanced diet and not as substitutes for nutritious food. Nutritional

TABLE 23-2 Stages in Evolution of Vitamin Deficiency

1. Inadequate nutrient delivery, synthesis, or absorption
2. Depletion of nutrient stores
3. Biochemical changes
4. Physical manifestations of deficiency
5. Morbidity and mortality

Source: Reference 6.

supplements are often self-prescribed. Although nutritional supplements can be obtained without a prescription, they are complex agents with specific indications. Medical assessment should precede their use, especially if intakes exceed the dietary reference intakes (DRIs) for vitamins and/or minerals. Furthermore, the patient should be reminded that vitamins and minerals are often better absorbed from food sources than supplements. The practitioner may refer patients to a registered dietitian for personalized counseling on diet modification as well as nutritional supplementation.

Intent of Use

Nutritional supplement use is intended to prevent nutritional deficiencies, replenish compromised stores, or maintain the present nutritional status. Nonprescription nutritional supplements are not intended for the self-treatment of vitamin deficiencies.

General Approach to Use

If a patient's diet is not providing the required levels of micronutrients, supplementation with vitamins and minerals is appropriate, as long as the patient has no underlying pathology and is not taking megadoses of micronutrients. A once-daily multivitamin providing no more than 100% of the DRIs should suffice in most cases. Patients should be reminded that there is no established benefit for healthy individuals to supplement nutrients in doses above the DRI.[7]

Practitioners should counsel patients regarding the potential disparity of product contents versus the label. Several studies have reported significant discrepancies when supplements were analyzed for the labeled dietary ingredient.[8] This potential for labeling inaccuracy exists, because dietary supplements are not assessed for compliance by any government agency. Unlike prescription drugs, dietary supplements do not need proof of safety, efficacy, or production under good manufacturing practices at this time. However, the U.S. Pharmacopeia (USP) provides a Dietary Supplement Verification Program that allows product labeling with the USP mark if the tested product meets specific requirements. These requirements include verification of product ingredients and amounts, effective disintegration and dissolution for absorption, absence of harmful contaminants, and safe, sanitary, well-controlled manufacturing.[9] Practitioners should advise patients to look for this USP mark on vitamin and mineral supplement labels.

Some patients need supplemental macronutrients (e.g., fat, protein, and carbohydrate), because they are unable to consume all the nutrients they need. Liquid nutritional supplements (e.g., Ensure and Boost) are discussed in Chapter 24.

Nonpharmacologic Therapy

The best method to avoid nutritional deficiencies is to eat a balanced diet that includes foods from sources high in several essential nutrients each day. To guide consumers in selection of a balanced diet while allowing for individual preferences, the U.S. Department of Health and Human Services recently released Dietary Guidelines for Americans 2005.[10] In these guidelines, consumers are advised to regularly choose a variety of nutrient-dense foods, as exemplified in the Food Guide Pyramid (Figure 23-1). Each food group in the pyramid represents a significant source of one or more essential and conditionally essential nutrients. For example, the milk group is a major source of calcium, whereas the

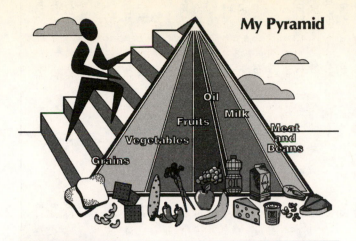

FIGURE 23-1 The Food Guide Pyramid. (Image from Mini-Poster Download at mypyramid.gov.)

fruits and vegetables groups are sources of fiber and the primary sources of antioxidant vitamins. By selecting a variety of foods within the various groups and eating the appropriate number of servings from each food group daily, consumers can "balance" their diet relative to essential and conditionally essential nutrients. In terms of portion size, approximately one-half cup of fruit, vegetable, rice, pasta, or cereal; 3 ounces of meat, fish, or poultry; or 1 cup of milk typically counts as one serving. Avoidance of "hidden" servings (e.g., the fat and bread servings in addition to the poultry serving of a batter-coated fried chicken breast) is a key to calorie control (see Chapter 27). Several alternative food pyramids and various other plans, such as food selection by color, are reported in the popular press, but few of these plans have been adequately evaluated for the balance of nutrients they provide. Thus, the Food Guide Pyramid remains the most appropriate tool for assessing the need for nutrient supplementation, and practitioners should inquire about the patient's intake from these food groups.[7]

Pharmacologic Therapy

Although there are situations in which high doses of specific vitamins and minerals are reported to be of therapeutic benefit, the claims of megavitamin enthusiasts have not been objectively confirmed. Those vitamins and minerals that have therapeutic value in the treatment of medical conditions (e.g., niacin therapy for hyperlipidemia) are actually being used as drugs rather than supplements for disease prevention or health maintenance. Deficiency states should be treated under medical supervision. Furthermore, prolonged ingestion of vitamin and mineral supplements has not been tested for safety. Some vitamins, such as A, D, niacin, and pyridoxine, and minerals, such as iron and fluoride, are known to be toxic in high doses. Therefore, patients should be cautioned against initiating high-dose self-medication with vitamins and minerals. Practitioners should discourage chronic, high-dose ingestion of any nutrient without proper medical supervision.

Vitamins

Vitamins are nutrients that cannot be synthesized in the body in sufficient quantities and must be obtained through the diet. Vita-

mins can be conditionally essential, meaning that under most circumstances endogenous production may be adequate, but there are conditions in which dietary intake is essential to meet requirements. Vitamins are used as both dietary supplements and therapeutic agents to treat deficiencies or other pathologic conditions.

DRIs have replaced the traditional recommended dietary allowances (RDAs) as reference values of daily nutrient intake that are recommended by the Food and Nutrition Board of the Institute of Medicine, National Academy of Science[11,12] (Tables 23-3 and 23-4). The DRIs include four reference categories: estimated average requirements (EARs), RDAs, adequate intakes (AIs), and ULs. EARs are values obtained after a careful review of the literature on specific nutrients. The EARs provide nutrient intake values that are estimated to meet the requirements of half of the healthy individuals in a specific gender and age group. An RDA value is set at 2 standard deviations above the EAR as an estimate of daily nutrient intake sufficient to meet requirements of nearly all individuals of a specified age group and gender. AIs are used as recommended intakes for nutrients when adequate scientific data are lacking and an EAR cannot be established with confidence. Finally, the ULs are the highest dose of nutrient intake that may be consumed daily without risk of adverse effects in the general population. ULs are also based on current literature, but they are not available for all nutrients (Table 23-5).[11–15] DRIs should be used as guidelines for nutritional assessment. The application of DRIs to individuals may require adjustment according to strenuous physical activity or the presence of disease.

The Food and Drug Administration (FDA) has published a less comprehensive set of values to be used for food and dietary supplement labeling.[16] Nutrients are listed as a percentage of daily value (%DV). These values are based on the recommended intakes for a 2000-calorie diet for adults older than 18 years. The vitamin or mineral supplement label includes a box with the heading Supplement Facts. In addition to information on serving size and servings per container, the label lists all required nutrients that are present in the dietary supplement in significant amounts and the %DV, if a reference has been established. It also lists all other dietary ingredients that are present in the product, including botanicals and amino acids, for which no %DV has been established. The %DV is based on DRI values for adults and for children ages 4 years and older, unless the product is designed for children younger than 4 years, for pregnant women, or for lactating women.

Frequently, "natural" vitamin products are supplemented with synthetic vitamins. For example, because the amount of vitamin C that can be acquired from rose hips (the fleshy fruit of a rose) is relatively small, synthetic vitamin C is added to prevent too large a tablet size. However, this addition may not be noted on the label, and the price of the partially natural product is often considerably higher than that for the completely synthetic, but equally effective, product. Patients should be informed that the body cannot distinguish between a vitamin molecule derived from a synthetic source and one derived from a natural source, and that most synthetic vitamins are equal to the more expensive "natural" vitamins. One exception may be vitamin E, in which the natural RRR-alpha-tocopherol form of the vitamin appears to have improved biologic activity compared with synthetic forms of the vitamin.[17]

TABLE 23-3 Recommended Intakes for Individuals: Vitamins Food and Nutrition Board, Institute of Medicine, National Academies

Life Stage Group	Vitamin A (mcg/day)[a]	Vitamin C (mg/day)	Vitamin D (mcg/day)[b,c]	Vitamin E (mg/day)[d]	Vitamin K (mcg/day)	Thiamin (mg/day)	Riboflavin (mg/day)	Niacin (mg/day)[e]	Vitamin B6 (mg/day)	Folate (mcg/day)[f]	Vitamin B12 (mcg/day)	Pantothenic Acid (mg/day)	Biotin (mcg/day)	Choline[g] (mg/day)
Infants														
0–6 months	400*	40*	5*	4*	2.0*	0.2*	0.3*	2*	0.1*	65*	0.4*	1.7*	5*	125*
7–12 months	500*	50*	5*	5*	2.5*	0.3*	0.4*	4*	0.3*	80*	0.5*	1.8*	6*	150*
Children														
1–3 years	300	15	5*	6	30*	0.5	0.5	6	0.5	150	0.9	2*	8*	200*
4–8 years	400	25	5*	7	55*	0.6	0.6	8	0.6	200	1.2	3*	12*	250*
Males														
9–13 years	600	45	5*	11	60*	0.9	0.9	12	1.0	300	1.8	4*	20*	375*
14–18 years	900	75	5*	15	75*	1.2	1.3	16	1.3	400	2.4	5*	25*	550*
19–30 years	900	90	5*	15	120*	1.2	1.3	16	1.3	400	2.4	5*	30*	550*
31–50 years	900	90	5*	15	120*	1.2	1.3	16	1.3	400	2.4	5*	30*	550*
51–70 years	900	90	10*	15	120*	1.2	1.3	16	1.7	400	2.4[h]	5*	30*	550*
>70 years	900	90	15*	15	120*	1.2	1.3	16	1.7	400	2.4[h]	5*	30*	550*
Females														
9–13 years	600	45	5*	11	60*	0.9	0.9	12	1.0	300	1.8	4*	20*	375*
14–18 years	700	65	5*	15	75*	1.0	1.0	14	1.2	400[i]	2.4	5*	25*	400*
19–30 years	700	75	5*	15	90*	1.1	1.1	14	1.3	400[i]	2.4	5*	30*	425*
31–50 years	700	75	5*	15	90*	1.1	1.1	14	1.3	400[i]	2.4	5*	30*	425*
51–70 years	700	75	10*	15	90*	1.1	1.1	14	1.5	400	2.4[h]	5*	30*	425*
>70 years	700	75	15*	15	90*	1.1	1.1	14	1.5	400	2.4[h]	5*	30*	425*
Pregnancy														
≤18 years	750	80	5*	15	75*	1.4	1.4	18	1.9	600[j]	2.6	6*	30*	450*
19–30 years	770	85	5*	15	90*	1.4	1.4	18	1.9	600[j]	2.6	6*	30*	450*
31–50 years	770	85	5*	15	90*	1.4	1.4	18	1.9	600[j]	2.6	6*	30*	450*
Lactation														
≤18 years	1200	115	5*	19	75*	1.4	1.6	17	2.0	500	2.8	7*	35*	550*
19–30 years	1300	120	5*	19	90*	1.4	1.6	17	2.0	500	2.8	7*	35*	550*
31–50 years	1300	120	5*	19	90*	1.4	1.6	17	2.0	500	2.8	7*	35*	550*

Note: This table (taken from the DRI reports; see www.nap.edu) presents recommended dietary allowances (RDAs) in **bold type** and adequate intakes (AIs) in regular type followed by a *single asterisk* (*). RDAs and AIs may both be used as goals for individual intake. RDAs are set to meet the needs of almost all (97%–98%) individuals in a group. For healthy breast-fed infants, AI is the mean intake. AI for other life stage and gender groups is believed to cover needs of all individuals in the group, but lack of data or uncertainty in the data prevents being able to specify with confidence the percentage of individuals covered by this intake.

a As retinol activity equivalents (RAEs). 1 RAE = retinol 1 mcg, beta-carotene 12 mcg, alpha-carotene 24 mcg, or beta-cryptoxanthin 24 mcg. To calculate RAEs from REs of provitamin A carotenoids in foods, divide REs by 2. For preformed vitamin A in foods or supplements and for provitamin A carotenoids in supplements, 1 RE = 1 RAE.

b As cholecalciferol. Cholecalciferol 1 mcg = vitamin D 40 IU.

c In the absence of adequate exposure to sunlight.

d As alpha-tocopherol. Alpha-tocopherol includes *RRR*-alpha-tocopherol, the only form of alpha-tocopherol that occurs naturally in foods, and the 2*R*-stereoisomeric forms of alpha-tocopherol (*RRR*-, *RSR*-, *RRS*-, and *RSS*-alpha-tocopherol) that occur in fortified foods and supplements. It does not include the 2*S*-stereoisomeric forms of alpha-tocopherol (*SRR*-, *SSR*-, *SRS*-, and *SSS*-alpha-tocopherol), also found in fortified foods and supplements.

e As niacin equivalents (NE). Niacin 1 mg = tryptophan 60 mg; 0–6 months = preformed niacin (not NE).

f As dietary folate equivalents (DFE). 1 DFE = food folate 1 mcg = folic acid 0.6 mcg from fortified food or as a supplement consumed with food = supplement 0.5 mcg taken on an empty stomach.

g Although AIs have been set for choline, there are few data to assess whether a dietary supply of choline is needed at all stages of the life cycle; the choline requirement may be met by endogenous synthesis at some of these stages.

h Because 10%–30% of people of advanced age may malabsorb food-bound B$_{12}$, it is advisable for those older than 50 years to meet their RDA mainly by consuming foods fortified with B$_{12}$ or a supplement containing B$_{12}$.

i In view of evidence linking folate intake with neural tube defects in the fetus, it is recommended that all women capable of becoming pregnant consume folate 400 mcg from supplements or fortified foods, in addition to intake of food folate from a varied diet.

j It is assumed that women will continue consuming folic acid 400 mcg from supplements or fortified food until their pregnancy is confirmed and they enter prenatal care, which ordinarily occurs after the end of the periconceptional period, the critical time for formation of the neural tube.

Source: Reprinted with permission from references 11–14. Copyright 2001 by the National Academy of Sciences.

TABLE 23-4 Recommended Intakes for Individuals: Elements Food and Nutrition Board, Institute of Medicine, National Academies

Life Stage Group	Calcium (mg/day)	Chromium (mcg/day)	Copper (mcg/day)	Fluoride (mg/day)	Iodine (mcg/day)	Iron (mg/day)	Magnesium (mg/day)	Manganese (mg/day)	Molybdenum (mcg/day)	Phosphorus (mg/day)	Selenium (mcg/day)	Zinc (mg/day)
Infants												
0–6 months	210*	0.2*	200*	0.01*	110*	0.27*	30*	0.003*	2*	100*	15*	2*
7–12 months	270*	5.5*	220*	0.5	130*	11	75*	0.6*	3*	275*	20*	3
Children												
1–3 years	500*	11*	340	0.7*	90	7	80	1.2*	17	460	20	3
4–8 years	800*	15*	440	1*	90	10	130	1.5*	22	500	30	5
Males												
9–13 years	1300*	25*	700	2*	120	8	240	1.9*	34	1250	40	8
14–18 years	1300*	35*	890	3*	150	11	410	2.2*	43	1250	55	11
19–30 years	1000*	35*	900	4*	150	8	400	2.3*	45	700	55	11
31–50 years	1000*	35*	900	4*	150	8	420	2.3*	45	700	55	11
51–70 years	1200*	30*	900	4*	150	8	420	2.3*	45	700	55	11
>70 years	1200*	30*	900	4*	150	8	420	2.3*	45	700	55	11
Females												
9–13 years	1300*	21*	700	2*	120	8	240	1.6*	34	1250	40	8
14–18 years	1300*	24*	890	3*	150	15	360	1.6*	43	1250	55	9
19–30 years	1000*	25*	900	3*	150	18	310	1.8*	45	700	55	8
31–50 years	1000*	25*	900	3*	150	18	320	1.8*	45	700	55	8
51–70 years	1200*	20*	900	3*	150	8	320	1.8*	45	700	55	8
>70 years	1200*	20*	900	3*	150	8	320	1.8*	45	700	55	8
Pregnancy												
≤18 years	1300*	29*	1000	3*	220	27	400	2.0*	50	1250	60	13
19–30 years	1000*	30*	1000	3*	220	27	350	2.0*	50	700	60	11
31–50 years	1000*	30*	1000	3*	220	27	360	2.0*	50	700	60	11
Lactation												
≤18 years	1300*	44	1300	3*	290	10	360	2.6*	50	1250	70	14
19–30 years	1000*	45*	1300	3*	290	9	310	2.6*	50	700	70	12
31–50 years	1000*	45*	1300	3*	290	9	320	2.6*	50	700	70	12

Note: This table presents recommended dietary allowances (RDAs) in **bold type** and adequate intakes (AIs) in regular type followed by a *single* asterisk (*). RDAs and AIs may both be used as goals for individual intake. RDAs are set to meet the needs of almost all (97%–98%) individuals in a group. For healthy breast-fed infants, AI is the mean intake. AI for other life stage and gender groups is believed to cover needs of all individuals in the group, but lack of data or uncertainty in the data prevents ability to specify with confidence the percentage of individuals covered by this intake.

Source: Reprinted with permission from references 11–14. Copyright 2001 by the National Academy of Sciences.

TABLE 23-5	Adult Tolerable Upper Intake Levels of Selected Micronutrients

Nutrient	Tolerable UL (mg/day)
Vitamin A	3
Vitamin D	0.05
Vitamin E	1000
Vitamin C	2000
Folate	1
Niacin	35
Vitamin B$_6$	100
Choline	3500
Calcium	2500
Iron	45
Magnesium	350
Phosphorus	4000
Copper	10
Fluoride	10
Iodine	1.1
Manganese	11
Molybdenum	2
Selenium	0.4
Zinc	40

Source: References 11–14.

Vitamins are grouped into two broad classifications: fat soluble and water soluble. Vitamins A, D, E, and K are fat-soluble vitamins. They are soluble in lipids, and are usually absorbed into the lymphatic system of the small intestine and subsequently pass into the general circulation. Their absorption is facilitated by bile. These vitamins are stored in body tissues, so ingestion of excessive quantities may be toxic. Deficiencies occur when fat intake is limited or fat absorption is compromised. Examples of disease states that may cause malabsorption of fat-soluble vitamins include celiac disease, cystic fibrosis, obstructive jaundice, cirrhosis of the liver, and short-bowel syndrome. These deficiencies may also be precipitated by drugs that affect lipid absorption, such as cholestyramine (which binds bile acids, thereby hindering lipid emulsification), orlistat (which inhibits gastric and pancreatic lipases in the intestinal lumen), and mineral oil (which is an unabsorbed oil that increases the fecal loss of fat-soluble vitamins). Consumption of snack foods that contain olestra, a fat substitute that is neither digested nor absorbed, has been associated with a decreased absorption of fat-soluble vitamins. However, this effect may be offset by the supplementation of fat-soluble vitamins in olestra-containing foods. A daily multivitamin supplement is recommended by the manufacturer for those taking orlistat. Use of Orlistat for weight loss is discussed in Chapter 27.

Vitamin C and the B-complex vitamins (riboflavin, thiamin, B$_6$, B$_{12}$, niacin, pantothenic acid, biotin, and folic acid) are water-soluble vitamins. These vitamins are generally not stored in the body, and excessive quantities tend to be excreted in the urine. Therefore, daily intake of these vitamins is desirable for optimal health.

As nutritional supplements, vitamins are usually dosed at 50% to 150% of the DRI values. Practitioners should advise caution with high-dose supplements that provide greater than 200% of the DRI. As therapeutic agents, vitamins should be recommended for only specific evidence-based medical indications.

VITAMIN A

The designation *vitamin A* refers to a large group of compounds that includes the retinoids (e.g., retinol) and the carotenoids (e.g., alpha-carotene and beta-carotene). Biochemical changes occur in some of these compounds during absorption in the intestine to form active vitamin A. Other compounds, such as the carotenoids lutein and lycopene, are not converted to the active vitamin but have other health-promoting properties. These compounds can be found in dark green vegetables and red, orange, or deep yellow vegetables and fruits.

In healthy adults, more than 90% of the body's supply of vitamin A is stored in the liver. Because of this generous reserve, there is minimal risk of deficiency with short-term periods of inadequate intake or fat malabsorption. Infants and young children, however, are more susceptible to vitamin A deficiency, because they have not established the necessary reserves.

Function Vitamin A is essential for normal growth and reproduction, normal skeletal and tooth development, and proper functioning of most organs of the body, notably the specialized functions involving the conjunctiva, retina, and cornea of the eye. It is thus indicated in preventing and treating symptoms of vitamin A deficiency, such as xerophthalmia (dry eye) and nyctalopia (night blindness). Synthesis of the glycoproteins necessary to maintain normal epithelial cell mucous secretions also requires vitamin A. This barrier is vital to the body's defense against bacterial infections in the upper respiratory system.

Dietary Sources See Table 23-6.[18]

Deficiency Vitamin A deficiency is rare in well-nourished populations. However, approximately 500,000 children worldwide develop blindness each year because of vitamin A deficiency.[19] Conditions such as cancer, tuberculosis, pneumonia, chronic nephritis, urinary tract infections, and prostate disease, as well as therapy with corticosteroids, may cause excessive excretion of vitamin A. Fat malabsorption may impair vitamin A absorption. Neomycin, cholestyramine, or orlistat may cause significant malabsorption of vitamin A and other fat-soluble vitamins, and may precipitate deficiencies with long-term use. In the United States, vitamin A deficiency occurs more often from diseases of fat malabsorption than from malnutrition.

One of the earliest symptoms of vitamin A deficiency is night blindness.[18,19] Other characteristic clinical findings include follicular hyperkeratosis, loss of appetite, impaired taste and smell, and impaired equilibrium. Some of these findings may be masked by concurrent deficiencies of other nutrients. Notable, however, is the drying and hyperkeratinization of the skin, because disruption of vitamin A–dependent epithelial integrity predisposes patients to infections.

Dose/DRI Vitamin A is FDA-approved for use in the treatment and prevention of vitamin A deficiency.[20] To avoid toxicity, the patient's dietary intake of vitamin A should be estimated when determining a dose for supplementation.

The DRI values for vitamin A are measured in micrograms of retinol activity equivalents (RAEs). The Food and Nutrition

TABLE 23-6 Food Sources Rich in Selected Nutrients

Vitamin	Food Sources
Vitamin A	Liver, milk fat, egg yolk, yellow and dark green leafy vegetables, apricots, cantaloupe, peaches
Vitamin D	Vitamin D–supplemented milk, egg yolk, liver, salmon, tuna, sardines, milk fat
Vitamin E	Wheat germ, vegetable oils, margarine, green leafy vegetables, milk fat, egg yolks, nuts
Vitamin K	Liver, vegetable oil, spinach, kale, cabbage, cauliflower
Vitamin C	Green and red peppers, broccoli, spinach, tomatoes, potatoes, strawberries, citrus fruit, kiwi
Vitamin B_{12}	Liver, meat, poultry, oysters, clams, dairy products
Folate	Liver, lean beef, wheat, whole-grain cereals, eggs, fish, dry beans, lentils, green leafy vegetables
Niacin	Lean meats, fish, liver, poultry, many grains, eggs, peanuts, milk, legumes
Pantothenic acid	Eggs, kidney, liver, salmon, yeast, some present in all foods
Vitamin B_6	Meats, cereals, lentils, legumes, nuts, egg yolk, milk
Riboflavin	Meats, poultry, fish, dairy products, green leafy vegetables, enriched cereals and breads, eggs
Thiamin	Legumes, whole-grain and enriched cereals and breads, wheat germ, pork, beef
Biotin	Liver, egg yolk, mushrooms, peanuts, milk, most vegetables, bananas, yeast
l-Carnitine	Dairy products, meat
Choline	Egg yolks, cereal, fish, meats
Calcium	Dairy products, sardines, clams, oysters, turnip greens, mustard greens
Iron	Liver, meat, egg yolk, legumes, whole or enriched grains, dark green vegetables, shrimp
Magnesium	Whole-grain cereals, tofu, nuts, legumes, green vegetables
Phosphorus	Milk, meat, poultry, fish, seeds, nuts, egg yolk
Chromium	Liver, fish, clams, meats, whole-grain cereals, milk, corn oil
Cobalt	Organ meats, oysters, clams, poultry, milk, cream, cheese
Copper	Liver, shellfish, whole grains, cherries, legumes, poultry, oysters, chocolate
Manganese	Vegetables, fruits, nuts, legumes, whole-grain cereals
Molybdenum	Legumes, cereals, dark green leafy vegetables, organ meats, milk
Selenium	Meat, grains, onions, milk
Silicon	Cereal products, root vegetables
Vanadium	Shellfish, mushrooms, parsley, dill seed, black pepper
Zinc	Oysters, shellfish, liver, beef, lamb, pork, legumes, milk, wheat bran

Source: Reference 18.

Board recommended RAEs as a way to determine the amount of absorption of the carotenoids, as well as their degree of conversion to vitamin A in the body. RAEs replace the former designation of retinol equivalents (REs) used to calculate total vitamin A values from various dietary sources. These RAEs are listed in Table 23-7.

The DRI values for vitamin A are listed in Table 23-3. A UL of 3 mg has been established for vitamin A, on the basis of risks of physical birth defects in the young and liver abnormalities in adults that are associated with vitamin A toxicity.[14] Recent evidence suggests that vitamin A intake below the established UL may be associated with an increased risk of bone fractures.[21]

Clearly, if the practitioner determines that a vitamin A supplement is appropriate, the recommendation should be a nonprescription multivitamin that contains no more than the DRI value of vitamin A. Preferably, a significant percentage of total vitamin A content should be contributed by beta-carotene, because beta-carotene intake is not associated with the risk of fractures or vitamin A toxicity. The improved safety profile of beta-carotene may be related to limitations in absorption and conversion to retinol.[21] However, the increased cancer risk associated with beta-carotene supplementation in those who smoke should be kept in mind (see subsequent text). High-dose vitamin A or beta-carotene therapy should never be undertaken without close medical supervision.

Safety Considerations Because vitamin A is stored in the body, high doses of it can lead to a toxic syndrome known as hypervitaminosis A. The incidence of hypervitaminosis A is increasing because of publicity regarding the potential ther-

TABLE 23-7 Retinol Activity Equivalents

1 retinol activity equivalent	= 1 retinol equivalent
	= 1 mcg retinol
	= 12 mcg beta-carotene
	= 24 mcg alpha-carotene
	= 24 mcg beta-cryptoxanthin
	= 3.33 IU vitamin A activity from retinol
	= 10 IU vitamin A activity from beta-carotene

apeutic benefits of vitamin A in cancer, skin disorders, and wound healing. A single megadose of retinol (25,000 IU/kg; 7507 RAE/kg) may precipitate acute toxicity 4 to 8 hours after ingestion. Chronic daily ingestion of 4000 IU/kg (approximately 1200 RAE/kg) has resulted in toxicity in adults.[20] Headache is a predominant symptom, but it may be accompanied by diplopia (double vision), nausea, vomiting, vertigo, fatigue, or drowsiness. Treatment consists of discontinuing vitamin A supplementation and the prognosis is good. Although beta-carotene toxicity is not likely, eating large amounts of carrots daily may result in carotenemia, which can produce a yellow skin hue. Pregnant women or women of childbearing age should avoid vitamin A doses above the DRI because of the teratogenic risk. For this reason, women of childbearing age should carefully evaluate the total vitamin A content of all dietary supplements and fortified foods consumed regularly. These patients should be reminded not to take other dietary supplements when a prescription prenatal vitamin is dispensed.

The potential role of Vitamin A as a cancer-preventing antioxidant prompted large randomized, controlled trials evaluating supplementation for patients at risk of lung cancer. In the Alpha-Tocopherol, Beta Carotene Cancer Prevention Study (ATBC), more than 29,000 male smokers were randomized to receive 50 mg alpha-tocopherol, 20 mg beta-carotene, both supplements, or placebo. Findings after 5 to 8 years of study suggested no benefit to supplementation.[22] Furthermore, there appeared to be greater risk of lung cancer in those who received beta-carotene supplementation.

Similar results were shown in a subsequent study, the Beta-Carotene and Retinol Efficacy Trial (CARET).[23] This study included more than 18,000 participants randomized to receive either 30 mg beta-carotene and 25,000 IU of retinyl palmitate or placebo. Enrollees were either smokers or previously smokers, or those exposed to asbestos. After an average of 4 years of participant enrollment, the CARET trial was prematurely terminated because of the association of higher rates of lung cancer, cardiovascular disease, and death in those receiving supplementation. Furthermore, these effects were observed for years after the exposure to supplementation, although the increased risks of disease were not statistically significant. Such trials confirm that vitamin supplementation cannot provide the same health benefits as that of a diet rich in fruits and vegetables.

Potential drug–nutrient interactions are listed in Table 23-8.

VITAMIN D (CALCIFEROL)

A number of chemicals are associated with vitamin D activity. Cholecalciferol (vitamin D$_3$) is the naturally occurring form of vitamin D. It is synthesized in the skin from endogenous or dietary cholesterol on exposure to ultraviolet radiation (sunlight). Ergocalciferol (vitamin D$_2$), which differs structurally only slightly from cholecalciferol, is used as a food additive. Activation of vitamin D requires both the liver and the kidney. One metabolite, 25-hydroxycholecalciferol, is formed by the liver and then hydroxylated by the kidney to its active form, 1,25-dihydroxycholecalciferol. Therefore, both renal and hepatic dysfunction may result in clinical manifestations of vitamin D deficiency. In patients with renal failure, impaired vitamin D hydroxylation may cause hypocalcemia that persists despite massive doses of vitamin D. Administration of 1,25-dihydroxycholecalciferol (available as calcitriol) to these patients has been successful. Similarly, supplementation can be used to prevent or treat vitamin D deficiency in patients with hepatic failure.

Function Vitamin D, which has properties of both a hormone and a vitamin, is necessary for the proper formation of bone and for mineral homeostasis. It is closely involved with parathyroid hormone, phosphate, and calcitonin in the homeostasis of serum calcium. Adequate vitamin D intake reportedly reduces the risk of osteoporosis, heart disease, and some cancers.[24–26] In fact, recent studies have suggested that doses above the current DRI, up to 1000 to 2000 IU daily, may have greater benefits in reducing falls, reducing risk of breast and colon cancer, and preventing fractures.[27,28] However, there are no recommendations from the Institute of Medicine to adjust the UL or DRI levels at this time.

Dietary Sources Milk and milk products are the major sources of preformed vitamin D in the United States, given that milk is routinely supplemented with 100 IU (30 RAE) of vitamin D per cup. Other sources of vitamin D are listed in Table 23-6.

Deficiency Vitamin D deficiency may result from inadequate intake, GI disease (hepatobiliary disease, malabsorption, or chronic pancreatitis), chronic renal failure, inadequate sunlight exposure, hereditary disorders of vitamin D metabolism, or long-term phenytoin therapy. The aging skin of older patients may not synthesize vitamin D as efficiently, and the converting process in the liver and kidney may also be compromised. These altered physiologic actions, in addition to reduced sun exposure, and absorption and dietary intake of vitamin D, leave this age group at higher risk of vitamin D deficiency.

The signs and symptoms of vitamin D deficiency are reflected as calcium abnormalities, specifically those involved with bone formation. The classic deficiency state is rickets, but osteoporosis with increased risk of fractures can also occur. Vitamin D increases calcium and phosphate absorption from the small intestine, mobilizes calcium from bone, permits normal bone mineralization, improves renal reabsorption of calcium, and maintains serum calcium and phosphorus levels. As serum calcium decreases, compensatory mechanisms attempt to increase calcium levels. Parathyroid hormone secretion increases, possibly leading to secondary hyperparathyroidism. If physiologic mechanisms fail to make the appropriate adjustments in levels of calcium and phosphorus, demineralization of bone will ensue to maintain essential plasma calcium levels. During growth, demineralization leads to a failure of bone matrix mineralization. The epiphyseal plate may widen because of the weight load on softened bone structures during growth. As a result, rickets is manifested by soft bones and deformed joints. In adults, such demineralization may lead to severe osteomalacia.

The incidence of rickets in the United States is low, but the increasing popularity of vegetarian diets has led to rickets in some children who abstain from milk and infants breast-fed by mothers who do not drink milk, who fail to take prenatal vitamins, who have inadequate exposure to sunlight, or who otherwise receive inadequate intake of vitamin D.[29] Vitamin D deficiency has also been associated with muscle weakness, an increased risk of falls, and an increased risk of certain types of cancer such as colon, prostate, and breast.[27]

Dose/DRI Most people obtain the AI for vitamin D from dietary sources and exposure to sunlight (Table 23-3). People regularly exposed to sunlight will generally have no dietary requirement for vitamin D. However, a substantial part of the U.S. population is exposed to very little sunlight, especially during the winter.

TABLE 23-8 Micronutrient–Drug and Micronutrient–Micronutrient Interactions

Micronutrient	Drug/Micronutrient	Effect	Precautionary Measures
Vitamins			
Vitamins A, E (large doses)	Warfarin	Increased anticoagulation through vitamin K antagonism	Take only recommended U.S. DRIs.
Vitamins A, E, D, K, C	Cholestyramine, colestipol, or mineral oil (unabsorbed)	Decreased vitamin absorption	Avoid prolonged use of cholestyramine, colestipol, or mineral oil.
Vitamin D	Phenytoin, carbamazepine, barbiturates	Increased metabolism of vitamin D	Ensure adequate dietary intake of vitamin D.
	Corticosteroids	May impair metabolism of vitamin D	Ensure adequate dietary intake of vitamin D.
Vitamin K	Broad-spectrum antibiotics (long-term therapy)	Vitamin K deficiency induced by decreased gut flora	Ensure adequate dietary intake of vitamin K.
Vitamin K	Warfarin	Decreased anticoagulation	Keep daily intake of vitamin K consistent.
Vitamin K	Vitamin E (large doses)	Antagonizes function of vitamin K	Avoid chronic supplementation with high-dose vitamin E.
	Vitamin A (large doses)	May interfere with vitamin K absorption	Avoid chronic supplementation of high-dose vitamin A.
Vitamin B_{12}	Metformin, colchicine, anticonvulsants, ascorbic acid supplements, antiulcer agents, and antibiotics	Potential decreased absorption of cyanocobalamin	Clinical significance is unknown.
Folic acid	Phenytoin and possibly other related anticonvulsants (chronic use)	Possible inhibition of folic acid absorption, leading to megaloblastic anemia	Monitor for megaloblastic anemia. Consult with neurologist regarding supplementation, if possible.
		Subsequent increased folic acid supplementation may decrease serum phenytoin levels and complicate seizure control	
	Trimethoprim	Weak folic acid antagonism; decreased activity/effectiveness	Monitor for megaloblastic anemia.
		Rare occurrence of megaloblastic anemia in patients with low folic acid level at onset of trimethoprim therapy	
	Pyrimethamine (large doses)	Possible megaloblastic anemia	Monitor for megaloblastic anemia.
	Methotrexate	Folic acid antagonism; decreased activity/effectiveness	Monitor use of folic acid in patients on maintenance regimens for psoriasis or rheumatoid arthritis.
	Sulfasalazine	Decreased folic acid absorption when these agents are administered together	Separate dosing of these agents.
Niacin	Oral hypoglycemics	Decreased hypoglycemic effects	Monitor blood glucose with regular finger sticks.
	Sulfinpyrazone and probenecid	Possible inhibited uricosuric effects	
Vitamin B_6	Isoniazid	Pyridoxine antagonism, manifested as perioral numbness resulting from peripheral neuropathy	Routinely take 50 mg/day of pyridoxine hydrochloride with isoniazid, or 10 mg of pyridoxine for each 100 mg of isoniazid.
	Phenobarbital and phenytoin	Decreased serum drug levels	Consider monitoring levels in patients taking high-dose pyridoxine.
	Levodopa	Levodopa antagonism Decreased effectiveness	Avoid supplemental pyridoxine or, if possible, substitute levodopa carbidopa for levodopa.

| TABLE 23-8 Micronutrient–Drug and Micronutrient–Micronutrient Interactions *(continued)* |

Micronutrient	Drug/Micronutrient	Effect	Precautionary Measures
Minerals			
Calcium	Iron, zinc, magnesium	Inhibited nutrient absorption caused by high calcium intake	Separate dosing by at least 2 hours.
	Corticosteroids	Inhibited calcium absorption from gut; increased bone fractures and osteoporosis	Consider calcium supplementation.
	Aluminum-containing antacids, phosphates, cholestyramine	Decreased calcium absorption	Separate dosing by at least 2 hours.
	H_2-blockers, proton pump inhibitors	Decreased absorption of calcium carbonate, which requires an acidic environment	Consider calcium citrate supplementation.
	Levothyroxine	Reduced drug absorption	Separate dosing by 4 hours.
	Tetracyclines, fluoroquinolones	Decreased antibiotic absorption	Separate dosing by 2 hours before or 6 hours after the antibiotic.
	Phenytoin, carbamazepine, phenobarbital	Decreased calcium absorption by increasing metabolism of vitamin D	Consider calcium and vitamin D supplementation.
Magnesium	Tetracyclines, fluoroquinolones	Decreased antibiotic absorption	Separate dosing by 2 hours before or 6 hours after the antibiotic.
Phosphorus	Sucralfate or antacids containing magnesium, calcium, or aluminum	Decreased absorption of phosphorus	Ensure adequate intake of dietary phosphorus.
Iron	Antacids	Decreased iron solubility and absorption	Separate dosing by at least 2 hours.
	Tetracyclines, fluoroquinolones	Decreased antibiotic and iron absorption	If concurrent administration is medically necessary, take tetracycline or fluoroquinolone 2 hours before or 6 hours after taking iron.
	Levothyroxine	Decreased drug absorption	Separate dosing by 4 hours.
Trace Elements			
Copper	Zinc, high-dose vitamin C	Copper antagonism	Micronutrients may compete for absorption and utilization.
Fluoride	Magnesium, aluminum, calcium	Decreased effect and absorption of fluoride	Separate supplementation by at least 2 hours.
Iodine (potassium iodide)	Lithium salts	Possible additive hypothyroid effects	Monitor thyroid function tests.
Zinc	Copper	Possible decreased copper levels	High-dose, prolonged zinc supplementation may require copper supplementation.
	Tetracyclines, fluoroquinolones	Possible decreased antibiotic absorption	Separate dosing by 2 hours before or 6 hours after the antibiotic.

Key: DRI, dietary reference intake.

Vitamin D is FDA–approved for treating hypocalcemia associated with hypoparathyroidism and secondary hyperparathyroidism in patients with chronic renal failure.[20]

If the practitioner determines that vitamin D supplementation is appropriate on the basis of poor dietary intake or inadequate exposure to sunlight, a multivitamin supplement containing cholecalciferol 5 to 15 mcg (200–600 IU) should be recommended. Some evidence suggests that daily intakes of up to 1000 IU of vitamin D may have health benefits. At this time, however, the Food and Nutrition Board has not made recommendations to increase requirements for the general population. The UL for vitamin D is 50 mcg (2000 IU) daily.

Safety Considerations   Taking more than the UL of vitamin D daily may lead to adverse effects, including anorexia, hypercalcemia, soft-tissue calcification, kidney stones, and renal failure.[11] Patients receiving treatment for rickets should be closely monitored for these adverse effects.

Potential drug interactions with vitamin D are listed in Table 23-8.

VITAMIN E (TOCOPHEROL)

The term *vitamin E* refers to the tocopherols and the tocotrienols, which are naturally occurring compounds in plants.

Function Vitamin E functions primarily as an antioxidant, protecting cellular membranes from oxidative damage or destruction. This process may be aided by selenium and vitamin C. Vitamin E may also have a role in heme biosynthesis, steroid metabolism, and collagen formation.

Vitamin E supplements have been used for treatment of claudication, atherosclerosis, diabetes, cancer, Parkinson's disease, and Alzheimer's disease with inconclusive results. Moderate consumption of dietary sources of vitamin E may reduce the risk of diseases such as Parkinson's disease and diabetes.[30]

Dietary Sources See Table 23-6.

Deficiency Vitamin E deficiency is extremely rare but may occur in two groups: premature, very-low-birth-weight infants, and patients who do not absorb fat normally. For example, neurologic abnormalities responsive to supplemental vitamin E have been reported in some patients with biliary disease and cystic fibrosis. Vitamin E deficiency has also been associated with symptoms of peripheral neuropathy, intermittent claudication, muscle weakness, and hemolytic anemia.

Dose/DRI The recommended dietary allowance for vitamin E is reported as milligrams of alpha-tocopherol. However, most food and nutrient supplement labels list vitamin E content in IU. In converting recommendations from one to the other, it is important to note that one milligram of alpha-tocopherol vitamin E is equivalent to 1.49 IU.

The average diet contains approximately 3 to 15 mg of vitamin E daily; therefore, large doses (i.e., in excess of the DRI) are not necessary unless the patient is experiencing fat malabsorption. The FDA-approved use of vitamin E is for prevention and treatment of hemolytic anemia associated with deficiency.[20]

Vitamin E requirements may vary in proportion to the amount of polyunsaturated fatty acids in the diet. The polyunsaturated fatty acid content of the U.S. diet has increased, and the plant oils responsible for the increase are rich in tocopherol. The lack of evidence of deficiency at the present intake supports the current adult DRI of 15 mg/day. The UL for vitamin E is 1000 mg daily.

Safety Considerations Vitamin E is relatively nontoxic. Most adults tolerate 100 to 800 mg daily without adverse effects. However concerns have been raised over long-term, high-dose supplementation. A meta-analysis of trials with doses greater than 400 IU daily suggested an increase in all-cause mortality compared with controls, although the increase was not statistically significant.[31] A recent prospective cohort study of more than 77,000 men and women evaluated the impact of an average of 10-year supplementation with multivitamins, vitamin C, vitamin E, or folate on the incidence of lung cancer.[32] Only vitamin E showed an influence on lung cancer risk, with a small increase in those taking supplementation.

Vitamin E has been reported to enhance warfarin anticoagulation, possibly by inducing vitamin K deficiency.[20] This and other potential drug–nutrient interactions are listed in Table 23-8.

VITAMIN K

Phytonadione (vitamin K$_1$) is present in many vegetables. Menaquinone (vitamin K$_2$) is a product of bacterial metabolism; colonic bacteria may be able to synthesize about 2 mcg/kg of body weight per day of the vitamin. Menadione (vitamin K$_3$) is a synthetic compound that is two to three times as potent as the natural vitamin K.

Function Vitamin K has important roles in normal physiology. First, it promotes the synthesis of clotting factors II, VII, IX, and X in the liver. Second, it activates these factors, along with the anticoagulation proteins C and S. The clotting factors remain inactive in the liver in the presence of warfarin or in the absence of vitamin K. When vitamin K is administered, normal activity of the clotting factors resumes. Third, vitamin K is key in the activation of osteocalcin, which appears to play a role in bone mineralization and the prevention of osteoporosis.[33]

Dietary Sources See Table 23-6.

Deficiency The mean dietary intake of vitamin K is approximately 90 mcg daily.[34] Moreover, microbiologic flora of the normal gut synthesize enough menaquinone to supply a significant part of the body's requirement for vitamin K. Therefore, there is a low incidence of deficiency among healthy, well-nourished individuals. Interference with bile production or secretion may contribute to a vitamin K deficiency, because the absorption of vitamin K requires bile in the small intestine. Malabsorption syndromes and bowel resections may decrease vitamin K absorption. Liver disease may also cause symptoms of vitamin K deficiency if hepatic production of the prothrombin-clotting factor is decreased. Other potential causes of deficiency include intestinal disease or resection and chronic, broad-spectrum antibiotic therapy. A deficiency may be evidenced by unusual bleeding and demonstrated by a prolonged prothrombin time (PT). There is also some evidence that lower dietary intakes of vitamin K may be associated with higher risk of osteoporotic fractures as opposed to those taking higher amounts. However, well-designed trials are needed to confirm this association.[35]

Dose/DRI The 2001 DRI values for vitamin K are listed in Table 23-3. Vitamin K$_1$ (phytonadione) is FDA-approved for use in neonates at birth (one dose of 1 mg) to prevent hemorrhaging. This dose is necessary because placental transport of vitamin K is low and the neonate has yet to acquire the intestinal microflora that produce the vitamin. Other approved uses include the prevention and treatment of hypoprothrombinemia caused by drug-induced deficiency and the treatment of hemorrhage.[20] A UL for vitamin K has not been established.

Safety Considerations Even in large amounts over an extended period, vitamin K does not produce toxic manifestations. Consistent dietary intake of vitamin K (70–140 mcg daily) does not usually interfere with warfarin anticoagulant activity. However, sudden changes in the dietary intake of vitamin K can significantly alter the patient's PT and international normalized ratio. Other potential drug interactions with this vitamin are listed in Table 23-8.

VITAMIN C (ASCORBIC ACID)

Vitamin C is the most easily destroyed of all the vitamins given its sensitivity to heat, oxygen, and alkaline environments. Although a relatively simple compound, it is a powerful reducing agent that serves to protect the capillary basement membrane.

Function Vitamin C is necessary for the biosynthesis of hydroxyproline, a precursor of collagen, osteoid, and dentin. It also assists in the absorption of nonheme iron from food by reducing the ferric iron in the stomach. However, use of vitamin C supplementation with iron is generally not necessary for patients taking adequate iron supplementation.

Large doses of vitamin C (500–1000 mg daily) have been promoted to prevent and treat the common cold. However, such claims are largely unsupported by well-designed controlled clinical studies.[13,19] Consumption of five servings or more of fruits and vegetables daily (≥200 mg vitamin C) has been associated with a lower incidence of cancer, heart disease, stroke, and certain eye diseases.[36] However, there is currently inadequate data to support vitamin C supplementation above the DRI for the prevention or treatment of these chronic conditions.[37]

Dietary Sources   Vitamin C has been called the "fresh-food" vitamin, and most of the daily intake is derived from vegetables and fruit sources (Table 23-6).

Deficiency   Characteristics of vitamin C deficiency include fatigue, capillary hemorrhages and petechiae, swollen hemorrhagic gums, and bone changes. A deficiency may also impair wound healing. A profound dietary deficiency can eventually lead to scurvy, producing widespread capillary hemorrhaging and a weakening of collagenous structures.

Scurvy is rare in the United States. It develops with only chronically inadequate consumption of vitamin C. Infants who are fed artificial formulas without vitamin supplements may develop symptoms of scurvy. In adults, however, scurvy occurs after only 3 to 5 months on a diet free of vitamin C.

Dose/DRI   Practitioners are rarely confronted with overt symptoms of vitamin C deficiency. Only 10 mg/day of vitamin C prevents scurvy; a normal diet containing fresh fruits and vegetables contains many times this amount. The DRI values for vitamin C are listed in Table 23-3. Supplementation of 100 to 125 mg daily is recommended for smokers, on the basis of higher daily ascorbic acid losses observed in these individuals.[13,37] The UL for vitamin C is 2 g/day.

Most adult multivitamin supplements contain 60 to 100 mg of vitamin C, an appropriate level to consume if supplements are required. A dose greater than 400 mg/day is rarely indicated, because the body will excrete most of a dose above this level.[38] In patients with a severe vitamin C deficiency, as evidenced by clinical signs of scurvy, 100 to 300 mg of vitamin C daily for at least 2 weeks is recommended to replenish body stores.[20] Infants who do not have vitamin C supplements in their formula should receive 40 to 50 mg/day; those who are breast-fed by well-nourished mothers will receive a sufficient amount. If a supplement is warranted, the practitioner may recommend a multivitamin product containing 60 to 200 mg of vitamin C to be taken once a day. Vitamin C is FDA-approved for use in the prevention and treatment of scurvy and to acidify the urine.[20]

Safety Considerations   The practitioner is urged to weigh the relative risks and benefits of ascorbic acid therapy. Short-term use to promote healing in potentially deficient patients may warrant a trial of ascorbic acid with medical supervision. Megadoses, however, may cause nausea, stomach cramps, diarrhea, and nephrolithiasis. Ascorbic acid toxicity can also lead to hemolysis in patients deficient in glucose 6-phosphate dehydrogenase. Rebound scurvy has occurred on sudden withdrawal of ascorbic acid in infants whose mothers took megadoses of vitamin C during pregnancy. Patients with diabetes mellitus, recurrent renal calculi, or renal dysfunction should avoid prolonged use of high-dose vitamin C supplementation.

Vitamin C therapy causes acidification of the urine, resulting in enhanced reabsorption of acidic drugs from the renal tubules and higher, more prolonged blood levels of these agents. Conversely, basic drugs such as tricyclic antidepressants and amphetamines may be excreted more rapidly from acidified urine, and their effect may be reduced by ascorbic acid therapy. Because the ascorbic acid–induced decrease in urine pH has been shown to be small, the clinical significance of the effects of ascorbic acid on the reabsorption and elimination of acidic and basic drugs is controversial. Nevertheless, patients who are on medications eliminated by renal excretion should be monitored if megadose ascorbic acid therapy is initiated.

VITAMIN B$_{12}$ (CYANOCOBALAMIN)

Cyanocobalamin contains a single atom of cobalt and is the most complex vitamin molecule. The term *vitamin B$_{12}$* refers to all cobalamins that have vitamin activity in humans. Cyanocobalamin, the common pharmaceutical form of the vitamin, is also the most stable of the cobalamins.

Function   Vitamin B$_{12}$ is active in all cells, especially those in the bone marrow, the central nervous system (CNS), and the GI tract. It is also involved in fat, protein, and carbohydrate metabolism. A cobalamin coenzyme functions in the synthesis of DNA, and in the synthesis and transfer of single-carbon units (e.g., the methyl group in the synthesis of methionine and choline). Vitamin B$_{12}$ participates in methylation reactions and cell division, usually in concert with folic acid. It is necessary for the metabolism of folates; therefore, a folate deficiency may be observed as a feature of vitamin B$_{12}$ deficiency. Vitamin B$_{12}$ is also necessary for the metabolism of lipids and formation of myelin.

Vitamin B$_{12}$ has been studied in relation to elevated levels of homocysteine, an amino acid that requires vitamins B$_{12}$, B$_6$, and folate as cofactors for metabolism. Hyperhomocysteinemia has been identified as an independent risk factor for Alzheimer's disease (promoted by cerebrovascular disease) as well as cardiovascular disease.[38] Although vitamin B$_{12}$ supplementation has not shown a significant effect on homocysteine levels in healthy volunteers, it may be effective in some patients with low vitamin B$_{12}$ levels.[39] However, it remains unclear whether reducing homocysteine levels will result in a lower risk of these chronic diseases.

Dietary Sources   Vitamin B$_{12}$ is found almost exclusively in animal protein (Table 23-6).

Deficiency   In healthy individuals who have not restricted their diets, cyanocobalamin deficiency is rare. Vitamin B$_{12}$ deficiency may be caused by poor absorption or utilization, or by an increased requirement or excretion of this vitamin. Because the body conserves vitamin B$_{12}$, approximately 3 years is required for the deficiency to develop. In patients with malabsorption (e.g., those with ileal diseases, intestinal resection, or gastrectomy), the reabsorption phase of the enterohepatic cycle is affected, and the deficiency may occur much earlier. Patients with atrophic gastritis, a condition that occurs in 10% to 30% of those 50 years or older, are at increased risk of pernicious anemia caused by inadequate production of intrinsic factor, which is essential for vitamin B$_{12}$ absorption. A more common cause of B$_{12}$ deficiency in older adults is the inability to absorb food-bound B$_{12}$. In addition, reduced intestinal motility, achlorhydria, and gastric acid–lowering agents contribute to bacterial overgrowth in the small intestine, and these microorganisms utilize available vitamin B$_{12}$.[40] For these reasons, vitamin B$_{12}$ supplementation is recommended from either fortified foods or a dietary supplement for this age group.[7,12]

Vegetarians who do not consume any animal products, including infants breast-fed by vegetarian mothers, are also at risk for developing a vitamin B_{12} deficiency. Vitamin B_{12} supplementation should be encouraged for these patients.

The symptoms of a vitamin B_{12} deficiency mimic those of a folate deficiency and are manifested in organ systems with rapidly duplicating cells. Therefore, one effect of such a deficiency on the hematopoietic system is macrocytic anemia. The GI tract is also affected, with glossitis and epithelial changes occurring along the entire digestive tract. Some people lack the glycoprotein (intrinsic factor) necessary for absorbing vitamin B_{12}, resulting in pernicious anemia. Because vitamin B_{12} is necessary for the maintenance of myelin, deficiency states produce many neurologic symptoms: paresthesia, peripheral neuropathy, unsteadiness, poor muscular coordination, mental confusion, agitation, hallucinations, and overt psychosis.

The practitioner should caution patients that an accurate diagnosis of the causes of a suspected anemia is essential in selecting effective treatment. For example, anemia resulting from a folic acid deficiency should be treated with folic acid, pernicious anemia should be treated with vitamin B_{12}, and iron-deficiency anemia should be treated with iron. Practitioners should avoid use of a "shotgun" antianemia preparation that contains multiple hematinic factors.

Dose/DRI   The DRI values for vitamin B_{12} are listed in Table 23-3. Oral forms can be used if the deficiency is caused by inadequate intake; intramuscular or deep subcutaneous administration is often necessary for deficiencies caused by malabsorption. Vitamin B_{12} is FDA-approved for use in the treatment of pernicious anemia and vitamin B_{12} deficiency. Other approved uses include supplementation during periods of increased requirements such as pregnancy, thyrotoxicosis, hemorrhage, malignancy, liver disease, or kidney disease.[20] A UL has not been established for cyanocobalamin.

Hydroxocobalamin is a longer-acting form equal in hematopoietic effect to cyanocobalamin. Because it is more extensively bound to proteins at the site of injection and in plasma, renal excretion is slower, and the vitamin remains in the body for a longer period.

Safety Considerations   Excessive doses have not resulted in toxicity, nor has any benefit been reported from nondeficient patients taking large quantities of the vitamin. Certain drugs may impair absorption of vitamin B_{12} (Table 23-8). In fact, vitamin B_{12} deficiency has been reported after 3 months of metformin therapy.[40]

FOLIC ACID (PTEROYLGLUTAMIC ACID, FOLATE)

Function   Folates are reduced in vivo to the bioactive form, tetrahydrofolic acid, and are involved in the biosynthesis of purines and pyrimidines. Folic acid is further biotransformed in the body, and is involved in DNA synthesis and red blood cell maturation. The function of folic acid is closely related to that of vitamin B_{12}. A folic acid deficiency can occur as a consequence of vitamin B_{12} deficiency. Low plasma levels of folate, vitamin B_6, and vitamin B_{12} have been linked with elevated levels of homocysteine, which may increase the risk of coronary artery disease and Alzheimer's disease.[38] Folate supplementation in particular has been shown to reduce homocysteine levels.[19,39] More studies evaluating the relationship between homocysteine levels and vascular disease are currently underway.

Dietary Sources   Folates are present in nearly all natural foods. Primary food sources are listed in Table 23-6. Folates are heat labile, so the folic acid content of food depends on how the food is processed. Canning, long exposure to heat, and extensive refining may destroy 50% to 100% of naturally occurring folic acid in a given food. Many commercially prepared carbohydrate foods (e.g., breads and pasta) are now fortified with folic acid.

Deficiency   The requirements for folic acid are related to metabolic rate and cell turnover, and increased amounts of folic acid are needed during pregnancy, lactation, and infancy. Infection, hemolytic anemias, and blood loss (in which red blood cell production must be increased to replenish blood supply), and hypermetabolic states such as hyperthyroidism also increase folic acid requirements. Because folic acid deficiency has been associated with an increased risk of neural tube defects in newborns, supplementation for all women anticipating a pregnancy is recommended.

Causes of folic acid deficiency include alcoholism, malabsorption, food faddism, and liver disease. Iatrogenic causes are associated with the administration of various therapeutic agents such as dihydrofolate reductase inhibitors (e.g., methotrexate or trimethoprim), anticonvulsants, and sulfasalazine.[20]

A deficiency of folic acid results in impaired cell division and protein synthesis. Symptoms of folic acid deficiency are similar to those of vitamin B_{12} deficiency, including sore mouth, diarrhea, and CNS symptoms such as irritability and forgetfulness. The most common laboratory-identified feature of folic acid deficiency is megaloblastic anemia, an anemia characterized by large erythroblasts circulating in the blood.

Because vitamin B_{12} is essential for the metabolism of folates, a megaloblastic anemia responsive to folic acid administration is a feature of pernicious anemia. Folic acid given without vitamin B_{12} to patients with pernicious anemia will correct the anemia but will have no effect on the more insidious damage to the CNS, characterized by lack of coordination, impaired sense of position, and various behavioral disturbances. Because of the potential for folic acid to mask the signs—but not the progression—of pernicious anemia (which is caused by a vitamin B_{12} deficiency), patients should receive an appropriate medical evaluation for the cause of anemia rather than an empiric vitamin supplement.

Dose/DRI   The DRI values for folic acid are listed in Table 23-3. Folate is FDA-approved for use in the treatment of megaloblastic anemias caused by folate deficiency that is associated with tropical and nontropical sprue, nutritional anemias, pregnancy, infancy, or lactation. Folate is also approved for prophylactic use against neural tube defects of the newborn.[20]

The absorption of folate from food is significantly lower than that of synthetic folic acid.[7,15] Recommendations for women of childbearing age are synthetic folic acid 400 mcg daily from fortified foods and/or dietary supplementation in addition to the folate obtained from food.[15]

The supplemental dose of folic acid for correction of a deficiency is usually 1 mg/day, particularly if the deficiency occurs with conditions that may increase the folate requirement or suppress red blood cell formation (e.g., pregnancy, hypermetabolic states, alcoholism, or hemolytic anemia). Doses larger than the UL of 1 mg/day are not necessary except in some life-threatening hematologic diseases. Maintenance therapy for deficiencies may be stopped after 1 to 4 months if the diet contains at least one fresh fruit or vegetable daily. For chronic malabsorption diseases, folic acid treatment may be lifelong and parenteral doses may be required.

Safety Considerations   Folic acid toxicity is virtually non-existent because of its water solubility and rapid excretion. Doses up to 15 mg have been given daily without toxic effect. Several drugs taken chronically may increase the need for folic acid (Table 23-8).

NIACIN (NICOTINIC ACID)

The physiologically active form of niacin is niacinamide. Niacin and niacinamide are constituents of the coenzymes nicotinamide adenine dinucleotide and nicotinamide adenine dinucleotide phosphate.

Function   The niacin coenzymes are electron transfer agents; that is, they accept or donate hydrogen in the aerobic respiration of all body cells. Niacin is unusual as a vitamin in that humans can synthesize it from dietary tryptophan, with about 60 mg of tryptophan being equivalent to 1 mg of niacin. Most individuals receive about 50% of their niacin requirement from tryptophan-containing proteins and the rest as preformed niacin or niacinamide. In therapeutic doses, niacin will lower triglycerides and low-density lipoprotein cholesterol by mechanisms unrelated to its function as an essential micronutrient.

Dietary Sources   See Table 23-6.

Deficiency   The classic and only described niacin deficiency state is pellagra. Pellagra is rare, occurring most often in alcoholics, poorly nourished persons of advanced age, and individuals on bizarre diets that restrict sources of niacin. It may occur in areas where much corn is eaten, because niacin in corn may be bound to undigestible constituents, making it unavailable. Other causes of pellagra include isoniazid therapy and decreased tryptophan conversion, as in Hartnup disease and carcinoid tumors.

Clinical findings of niacin deficiency include the "three D's" of *d*ermatitis, *d*iarrhea, and *d*ementia, often accompanied by neuropathy, glossitis, stomatitis, and proctitis. Patients manifest a characteristic rash. The skin over the face and on pressure points may become thickened or hyperpigmented, or it may appear burned. Secondary infections may occur in such lesions. The entire GI tract is generally affected, with angular fissures around the mouth and atrophy of the epithelium. Inflammation of the small intestine may be associated with episodes of occult bleeding and/or diarrhea.

Dose/DRI   The DRI values for niacin are listed in Table 23-3. The recommended UL for this vitamin is 35 mg/day.[12]

Niacin requirements are increased when the patient has an acute illness; when the patient is convalescing after a severe injury, infection, or burn; when the patient has substantially increased caloric expenditure or dietary caloric intake; or when the patient has a low tryptophan intake (e.g., a low-protein diet or a high intake of corn as a staple in the diet). The FDA-approved use of niacin, but not niacinamide, is for adjunctive treatment of hyperlipidemia and hypercholesterolemia. Both niacin and niacinamide are approved for the prevention and treatment of pellagra.[20]

Treatment of pellagra involves the ingestion of niacinamide or niacin 150 to 500 mg daily in divided doses. Niacin has been used in daily dosages of 1 to 2 grams three times per day, up to 8 g/day, to treat hypercholesterolemia and hyperlipidemias. Niacin treatment increases beneficial high-density lipoprotein cholesterol and decreases levels of potentially harmful triglycerides, total cholesterol, and low-density lipoprotein cholesterol. Niacin treatment of hyperlipidemias requires close medical supervision for evidence of effectiveness and manifestations of drug-induced toxicity.

Safety Considerations   Niacin toxicity can involve GI symptoms (e.g., nausea, vomiting, and diarrhea), hepatotoxicity, skin lesions, tachycardia, and hypertension. Patients should be forewarned that therapeutic doses of niacin may cause flushing and a sensation of warmth, especially around the face, neck, and ears. This reaction, which many people experience especially on initiation of therapy, may be diminished if they take aspirin 325 mg or ibuprofen 200 mg 30 minutes before the niacin dose, provided there are no contraindications. Alternatively, the extended-release formulation may cause less flushing but potentially a greater risk of gastric and hepatic side effects. Itching or tingling and headache may also occur with niacin supplementation. These effects will usually subside or decrease in intensity within 2 weeks of continued therapy. If niacin causes GI upset, it should be taken with meals. Niacinamide does not produce the discomforting side effects associated with therapeutic doses of niacin; however, it does not have a beneficial lowering effect on plasma lipids.

Potential drug–nutrient interactions with niacin are listed in Table 23-8.

Because of the adverse effects on the GI tract, high doses of niacin are contraindicated in patients with gastritis or peptic ulcer disease. Niacin can provoke the release of histamine, so its use in patients with asthma should be undertaken carefully. Niacin may also impair liver function, disturb glucose tolerance, and cause hyperuricemia. Patients prescribed therapeutic doses of this nutrient must be monitored regularly for potential adverse effects.

PANTOTHENIC ACID

Pantothenic acid is a water-soluble vitamin of the B-complex family.

Function   Pantothenic acid is a precursor of coenzyme A (CoA), a product that is active in many biologic reactions and plays a primary role in cholesterol, steroid, and fatty acid synthesis. Pantothenic acid is important for acetylation reactions and the formation of citric acid for the Krebs cycle, and it is crucial in the intraneuronal synthesis of acetylcholine. It is also important in gluconeogenesis; in the synthesis and degradation of fatty acids; in the synthesis of sterols, steroid hormones, and porphyrins; and in the release of energy from carbohydrates.

Dietary Sources   Pantothenic acid is widely distributed in foods (Table 23-6).

Deficiency   Because pantothenic acid is contained in many foods, deficiency states are rare and hard to detect. In malabsorption syndromes, it is difficult to separate pantothenic acid deficiency symptoms from those of other deficiencies. Symptoms of pantothenic acid deficiency include somnolence, fatigue, cardiovascular instability, abdominal pain, and paresthesia of hands and/or feet followed by hyperreflexia and muscular weakness in the legs. Administration of pharmacologic doses of pantothenic acid reverses these symptoms and has even been used to eliminate burning feet syndrome.

Dose/DRI   AI values for this vitamin are listed in Table 23-3. There is no established UL for pantothenic acid.

Safety Considerations   Pantothenic acid is generally considered nontoxic, even in large doses. Doses as high as 10 grams of calcium pantothenate daily have been given to young men for 6 weeks with no toxic symptoms. However, ingestion of more than 20 grams has been reported to result in diarrhea and water retention.

Significant drug–nutrient interactions with pantothenic acid have not been reported.

VITAMIN B$_6$ (PYRIDOXINE)

This water-soluble vitamin exists in three forms: pyridoxine (vitamin B$_6$), pyridoxal, and pyridoxamine. Although all three forms are equally effective in nutrition, pyridoxine hydrochloride is the form most often used in vitamin formulations.

Function Vitamin B$_6$ serves as a cofactor for more than 60 enzymes, including decarboxylases, synthetases, transaminases, and hydroxylases. It is important in heme production and in the metabolism of homocysteine. As previously stated, hyperhomocysteinemia is a potential risk factor for coronary artery and cerebrovascular disease, and it has been shown to respond particularly to folic acid supplementation but also to vitamin B$_6$. Whether the impact of these nutrients on homocysteine levels results in improved outcomes has yet to be determined.[38] Vitamin B$_6$ has also been suggested as a potential treatment of carpal tunnel syndrome, premenstrual syndrome (PMS), depression, and migraine. Unfortunately, no clinical research evidence supports use of vitamin B$_6$ for these ailments.[41]

Dietary Sources See Table 23-6 for food sources; cooking destroys some vitamin B$_6$.

Deficiency Causes of vitamin B$_6$ deficiency include alcoholism, severe diarrheal syndromes, food faddism, malabsorption syndromes, drugs (isoniazid and penicillamine,), and genetic diseases (cystathioninuria and xanthinuric aciduria).

The symptoms of severe vitamin B$_6$ deficiency in infants include irritability and convulsive disorders. Treatment with vitamin B$_6$ hydrochloride (2 mg/day for infants) generally normalizes the electroencephalogram and resolves clinical symptoms. Symptoms in adults whose diets are deficient in vitamin B$_6$ or who have been given a vitamin B$_6$ antagonist are difficult to distinguish from symptoms of niacin and riboflavin deficiencies. These symptoms include pellagra-like dermatitis; oral lesions; peripheral neuropathy; scaliness around the nose, mouth, and eyes; and dulling of mentation. Serious deficiency symptoms include convulsions, peripheral neuritis, and sideroblastic anemia.

Dose/DRI DRI values for vitamin B$_6$ are listed in Table 23-3. The FDA-approved use of this vitamin is for treatment of vitamin B$_6$ deficiency, including drug-induced deficiency as seen with isoniazid.[20] Daily doses up to 250 mg of vitamin B$_6$ have been used in the treatment of hyperhomocysteinemia.[39] However, the UL for this vitamin is 100 mg/day for adults and patients of advanced age.[15]

Treatment of sideroblastic anemia requires 50 to 200 mg/day of pyridoxine hydrochloride to aid production of hemoglobin and erythrocytes. At least five vitamin B$_6$–dependent inborn errors of metabolism have been shown to respond to large doses of vitamin B$_6$.

Safety Considerations Vitamin B$_6$ may be toxic in high doses. A severe sensory neuropathy, similar to that observed with the deficiency state, has been reported when gram quantities were taken to relieve symptoms of PMS. Similar symptoms have been reported in women taking doses as small as 50 mg/day for PMS. Recovery occurred on withdrawal of vitamin B$_6$ but it was slow.

High daily doses of vitamin B$_6$ (200–600 mg) inhibit prolactin. Prenatal vitamins, which contain 1 to 10 mg per dosage unit, do not appear to have a significant antiprolactin effect.

Potential drug–nutrient interactions are listed in Table 23-8.

RIBOFLAVIN (VITAMIN B$_2$)

Riboflavin is a water-soluble vitamin essential for cellular growth and maintenance of vision, mucous membranes, skin, nails, and hair.

Function Riboflavin is a constituent of two coenzymes: flavin adenine dinucleotide and flavin mononucleotide. It is involved in numerous oxidation and reduction reactions, including the cytochrome P-450 reductase enzyme system involved in drug metabolism.

Dietary Sources See Table 23-6.

Deficiency Riboflavin deficiency, although rare, may be caused by inadequate intake, alcoholism, or malabsorption syndromes. Deficiency of this vitamin may occur in association with other vitamin B-complex deficiency states (e.g., pellagra) or during pregnancy. Early signs of riboflavin deficiency may involve ocular symptoms as the eyes become light sensitive and easily fatigued. The patient may develop blurred vision; itching, watering, sore eyes; and corneal vascularization, which causes a bloodshot appearance of the eye. Clinical findings of more advanced deficiency include stomatitis, seborrheic dermatitis, and magenta tongue.

Dose/DRI The DRI values for riboflavin are listed in Table 23-3. The need for riboflavin appears to increase during periods of increased cell growth, such as during pregnancy and wound healing. Absorption is enhanced when taken with food. Alternatively, riboflavin may be injected intramuscularly or given intravenously as a component of an injectable multivitamin. The FDA-approved use of riboflavin is in the prevention of riboflavin deficiency and the treatment of ariboflavinosis.[27] No UL has been determined for this vitamin.

High-dose riboflavin (400 mg daily) may be effective in the prevention of migraine. One randomized controlled trial in 55 adult patients showed significantly reduced incidence and duration of migraine attacks compared with placebo after 3 months of prophylactic therapy.[42] Another small study suggested this same high-dose riboflavin therapy was equal to beta-blockers in reducing the frequency of migraines.[43] Further study on riboflavin therapy for migraine prevention is warranted.

Safety Considerations The use of riboflavin may cause a yellow-orange fluorescence or discoloration of the urine. Patients who report this effect should be reassured that this color is normal. There is no known toxicity level, and no significant drug interactions have been reported for riboflavin.

THIAMIN (VITAMIN B$_1$)

Thiamin is a water-soluble, B-complex vitamin available in oral tablet and injectable dosage forms.

Function Thiamin's active form, thiamin pyrophosphate (formerly known as cocarboxylase), plays a vital role in the oxidative decarboxylation of pyruvic acid; in the formation of acetyl CoA, which enters the Krebs cycle; and in other important biochemical conversion cycles. Thiamin is necessary for myocardial function, nerve cell function, and carbohydrate metabolism. The amount of thiamin required increases with increased carbohydrate consumption.

Dietary Sources   Dietary sources highest in thiamin are listed in Table 23-6. The thiamin content of food can be destroyed by heat, oxidation, and an alkaline environment but is stable through frozen storage.

Deficiency   The primary causes of thiamin deficiency are generally inadequate diet, alcoholism, malabsorption syndromes, prolonged diarrhea, increased requirements (pregnancy), or food faddism.

Thiamin deficiency in the United States is found primarily in alcoholics. Not only is their diet often nutritionally deficient, but alcohol ingestion also impairs thiamin absorption and transport across the intestine, and increases the rate of destruction of thiamin diphosphate. Thiamin deficiency, also known as beriberi, may present with neuromuscular symptoms such as peripheral neuritis, weakness, and Wernicke's encephalopathy. Cardiac dysfunction may also be observed, possibly accompanied by edema, tachycardia on minimal exertion, enlarged heart, and electrocardiographic abnormalities. Because of these risks, a vitamin supplement containing thiamin should be prescribed for the alcoholic patient.

Dose/DRI   The DRI values for thiamin are listed in Table 23-3. To treat the symptoms of heart failure caused by a thiamin deficiency, the patient should take thiamin 5 to 10 mg three times daily. At this dosage, the failure is rapidly corrected, but the neurologic signs correct much more slowly. The FDA-approved use of thiamin is for the treatment of thiamin deficiency.[20]

Safety Considerations   The kidney easily clears excessive thiamin intake, and oral doses of 500 mg have been found to be nontoxic.

Diuretics have been shown to increase the urinary excretion of thiamin. Therefore, patients on chronic diuretic therapy, such as those with congestive heart failure or hypertension, may be at risk of subclinical thiamin deficiency and its associated cardiovascular complications. Although the effect of thiamin supplementation in this patient population has yet to be evaluated, recommending supplementation with 100% of the DRI for this vitamin would be reasonable.[44]

BIOTIN (VITAMIN H)

Biotin is included in several multivitamin preparations.

Function   Biotin, a member of the B-complex group of vitamins, is required for various metabolic functions, including carbohydrate, fat, and amino acid metabolism. Several biotin-dependent enzymes are now known to exist.

Dietary Sources   Food sources of biotin are listed in Table 23-6. In addition to food sources, colonic flora probably synthesize a considerable amount of biotin, which is then absorbed from the large intestine into the bloodstream.

Deficiency   Deficiency states of biotin are rare but appear to result in symptoms of nausea, vomiting, lassitude, muscle pain, anorexia, anemia, and depression. Dermatitis, a grayish color of the skin, and glossitis may be among the physical findings; hypercholesterolemia and cardiac abnormalities may also occur.

Biotin deficiency in humans can be caused by ingesting a large number of raw egg whites. Raw egg white contains avidin, a protein that binds biotin, thereby preventing its absorption. Individuals undergoing a rapid weight-loss program with intense caloric restriction or those with chronic malabsorption may not be obtaining adequate biotin and should receive supplementation.

Dose/DRI   See Table 23-3.

Safety Considerations   Adverse effects have not been reported with biotin therapy.

Vitamin-Like Compounds and Pseudovitamins

Vitamin-like compounds, or pseudovitamins, are substances that have a chemical structure very similar to that of vitamins but lack the usual physiologic or biochemical actions. That is, they are not essential for specific body functions of growth, maintenance, and reproduction.

CHOLINE

Choline is contained in most living cells and in foods. It is usually present in the form of phosphatidylcholine, commonly known as lecithin, and in several other phospholipids found in cell membranes. Intestinal mucosal cells and pancreatic secretions contain enzymes capable of splitting phospholipids to release choline. Choline is also found in sphingomyelin and is highly concentrated in nervous tissue.

Function   Choline, a precursor in the biosynthesis of acetylcholine, is an important donor of methyl groups used in the biochemical formation of other substances in vivo. It can be biosynthesized in humans. Furthermore, choline and inositol are considered to be lipotropic agents (i.e., agents involved in the mobilization of lipids). They have been used to treat fatty liver and abnormal fat metabolism, but their efficacy has not been established.

Dietary Sources   Although choline is found in food sources, it is also synthesized in the body. Therefore, it is doubtful that choline is a vitamin. Choline is obtained from the diet as either choline or lecithin. Food sources are listed in Table 23-6.

Deficiency   A deficiency state has not been identified in humans, possibly because choline is readily available in the diet and synthesized in the body.

Dose/DRI   See Table 23-3 for DRI values. An average diet furnishes 400 to 900 mg of choline daily. The recommended UL for choline is 3.5 g/day.[12,15]

Safety Considerations   The administration of large doses of lecithin has been associated with sweating, GI distress, vomiting, and diarrhea. No drug interactions have been reported.

Minerals

Minerals constitute about 4% of body weight. These micronutrients are present in the body in a diverse array of organic compounds (e.g., phosphoproteins, phospholipids, hemoglobin, and thyroxine). They function as constituents of many enzymes, hormones, vitamins, and inorganic compounds (e.g., sodium chloride, potassium chloride, calcium, and phosphorus), which are present as free ions. Different body tissues contain various quantities of different minerals. For example, bone has a high content of calcium, phosphorus, and magnesium; soft tissue has a high quantity of potassium. Minerals are involved in regulating cell membrane permeability, osmotic pressure, and acid–base and water balance. In addition, certain ions act as the mediators of action potential conduction and neurotransmitter action.

A well-balanced diet is required to maintain proper mineral balance. Optimal mineral intake values for humans are still imprecise; only AIs are available for trace element minerals such as chromium, fluoride, and manganese. Similarly, the possible adverse effects of long-term ingestion of high-dose mineral supplements are often unknown, and high doses of one mineral can decrease the bioavailability of other minerals and vitamins.

CALCIUM

The most abundant cation in the body is calcium (about 1200 grams). Approximately 99% of calcium is present in the skeleton, and the remaining 1% is present in the extracellular fluid, intracellular structures, and cell membranes. Calcium is a major component of bones and teeth. The calcium content in bone is continuously undergoing a process of resorption and formation. In people of advanced age, the resorption process predominates over formation, and a decrease in calcium absorption efficiency results in a gradual loss of bone density that leads to osteoporosis. This effect can be minimized by encouraging optimal calcium intake throughout the life cycle as well as regular participation in weight-bearing exercise.

Function Calcium is important for several reasons. It activates a number of enzymes and is required for acetylcholine synthesis. Calcium increases cell membrane permeability, aids in vitamin B_{12} absorption, regulates muscle contraction and relaxation, and catalyzes several steps in the activation of plasma-clotting factors. Calcium is also necessary for the functional integrity of many cells, especially those of the neuromuscular and cardiovascular system.

The small intestine controls calcium absorption. Patients ingesting relatively low amounts of calcium absorb proportionately more calcium than those with adequate intake, and patients taking large amounts of calcium excrete more as fecal calcium.

Dietary Sources Dietary sources of calcium are listed in Table 23-6. Teenagers experiencing rapid growth and bone maturation need to consume adequate calcium through dairy products, especially milk, or through a nutritional supplement. Most adults can easily meet calcium AI levels by incorporating dairy products into their diets daily. Nonfat milk contains about 300 mg of calcium per 8 ounces. As an alternative, calcium supplements are usually well tolerated in daily doses of less than 2 grams. Table 23-9 lists selected trade-name calcium supplements.

Practitioners should evaluate the dietary intake of calcium, including calcium-fortified foods, before recommending daily calcium supplementation. Calcium fortification is found in numerous nontraditional sources such as juices, breads, and breakfast bars. Dietary factors that increase calcium absorption from supplements or foods include avoiding intake with bran, whole-grain cereals, or high-oxalate foods (e.g., cocoa, soybeans, or spinach) and obtaining adequate vitamin D.

Deficiency Decreased calcium levels may have profound and diverse consequences, including convulsions, tetany, behavioral and personality disorders, mental and growth retardation, and bone deformities (the most common being rickets in children and osteomalacia in adults). Changes that occur in osteomalacia include softening of bones, rheumatic-type pain in the bones of the legs and lower back, general weakness with difficulty walking, and spontaneous fractures. Common causes of hypocalcemia and

TABLE 23-9 Selected Calcium Supplements	
Trade Name	**Primary Ingredients**
Caltrate 600 + D High Potency Tablets	Elemental calcium 600 mg (as carbonate); vitamin D 200 IU
Citracal + D Caplets	Elemental calcium 315 mg (as citrate); vitamin D 200 IU
Os-Cal 500 + D Tablets	Elemental calcium 500 mg (as carbonate); vitamin D 125 IU
Tums 500 Chewable Tablets	Elemental calcium 200 mg (as carbonate)
Viactiv Calcium Soft Chews	Elemental calcium 500 mg (as carbonate); vitamin D 100 IU; vitamin K 40 mcg

associated skeletal disorders are as follows: malabsorption syndromes; hypoparathyroidism; vitamin D deficiency; renal failure with impaired activation of vitamin D; long-term anticonvulsant therapy (with increased breakdown of vitamin D); and decreased dietary intake of calcium, particularly during periods of growth, pregnancy, and lactation and among people of advanced age.

Dose/DRI The AIs for calcium are listed in Table 23-4. Oral calcium supplements are FDA-approved for use in the treatment and prevention of calcium deficiency, which may result in rickets, osteomalacia, or osteoporosis. Other FDA-approved uses include treatment of acid indigestion and hyperphosphatemia associated with end-stage renal disease.[20] The recommended UL for calcium is 2.5 g/day for all individuals older than 1 year.[20]

Calcium supplementation may be effective in the prevention of PMS. One randomized, controlled multicenter trial showed that supplementation of elemental calcium 1200 mg daily for three menstrual cycles resulted in a significant reduction in PMS symptoms.[45] The American College of Obstetrics and Gynecology recommends regular calcium supplementation for women with PMS.

Numerous studies have evaluated the relationship between calcium intake and the risk of colon cancer; however, the results of these studies have been inconsistent. Further research to better define this relationship is currently underway.

Calcium intake has also been suggested to influence risk of prostate cancer. Previous observational studies have showed conflicting results, with some suggesting higher calcium intakes may increase prostate cancer risks, and others showing no influence or an opposite effect. However, a recent prospective trial suggests an increased risk for advanced and fatal prostate cancer with calcium intakes greater than 1500 mg daily from either supplements or dietary sources.[46] It would seem reasonable to recommend calcium intakes closer to the DRI for those at risk of prostate cancer until further evidence clarifies this association.

Practitioners should counsel patients regarding potential constipation associated with calcium supplementation, and the importance of adequate hydration, dietary fiber, and physical activity. In addition, calcium absorption is improved by dividing the dose into 500 mg or less to be taken two to three times daily with meals.

Recommendations for calcium intake are based on elemental calcium, not the calcium salt. Because labels can be misleading, practitioners should be familiar with the many salt forms and the different percentages of calcium in each, including carbonate (40%), citrate (21%), lactate (18%), gluconate (9%), and phosphate salts (23%–39%).[47] Calcium carbonate and calcium phosphate salts are insoluble and should be taken with meals to enhance absorption, which is optimal in a low pH. Patients requiring supplementation who have achlorhydria or who are on histamine₂ antagonists or proton pump inhibitors may need to take a soluble salt (e.g., calcium citrate, calcium lactate, or calcium gluconate). In conjunction with adequate calcium and vitamin D, weight-bearing exercise is essential in maintaining bone mass.

Safety Considerations   Calcium in doses greater than 2 g/day can be harmful. Large amounts taken as dietary supplements or antacids can lead to high levels of calcium in the urine and to renal stones; the latter development may result in renal damage. Hypercalcemia—with associated anorexia, nausea, vomiting, constipation, and polyuria—is also possible, particularly in patients taking high-dose vitamin D preparations. Hypercalcemia can also result in an increased deposition of calcium in soft tissue.

Calcium supplementation and calcium-fortified foods may alter the absorption of several drugs. Examples of drug–nutrient interactions with calcium are listed in Table 23-8.

IRON

Iron is widely available in the U.S. diet. Iron absorption from the intestinal tract is controlled by the body's need for iron, the intestinal lumen conditions, the food source of iron, and the food components of the meal, such as the vitamin C content.

Function   Iron plays an important role in oxygen and electron transport. In the body, it is either functional or stored. Functional iron is found in hemoglobin, myoglobin, heme-containing enzymes, and transferrin, which is the transport form of iron. Stored iron is primarily found in the hemoglobin of red blood cells, which contain 60% to 70% of total body iron. The rest is stored primarily in the form of ferritin and hemosiderin in the intestinal mucosa, liver, spleen, and bone marrow.

Dietary Sources   Dietary iron is available in two forms. Heme iron is found in meats and is reasonably well absorbed. Nonheme iron, such as that found in enriched grains and dark green vegetables, constitutes most of the dietary iron but is poorly absorbed. Therefore, the published values of iron content in foods are misleading, because the amount absorbed depends on the nature of the iron. Although there are specific ways to calculate the iron absorption from a given meal, the available iron content of foods is often estimated by assuming that about 10% of the total iron (heme plus nonheme) is absorbed if no iron deficiency exists. In the iron-deficient state, iron absorption improves, so as much as 20% may be absorbed and used from an average diet. However, this estimate would not be valid in the absence of heme iron.

Ingested nonheme iron, which is mostly in the form of ferric hydroxide, is solubilized in gastric juice to ferric chloride, then reduced to the ferrous form and chelated to substances such as ascorbic acid, sugars, and amino acids. Chelates have a low molecular weight and can be solubilized and absorbed before they reach the alkaline medium of the distal small intestine, where precipitation may occur. In intestinal mucosal cells, iron is stored in a protein-bound form known as ferritin. As needed, it is released into the plasma, where it is oxidized to the ferric state and bound to a beta-globulin to form transferrin. When

released at the spleen, liver, bone marrow, intestinal mucosa, and other iron storage sites, the iron is combined with apoferritin to form ferritin or hemosiderin. Iron is used in all cells of the body; however, most of it is incorporated into the hemoglobin of red blood cells. The major source of iron loss is through blood loss (e.g., hemorrhagic loss and menstruation). Iron is also lost from the body by the sloughing of skin cells and GI mucosal cells, and by excretion of urine, sweat, and feces.

Deficiency   Early symptoms of iron deficiency are vague. Pallor and easy fatigability cannot in themselves be easily related to iron deficiency. Other signs and symptoms of iron-deficiency anemia include split or "spoon-shaped" nails, sore tongue, angular stomatitis, and dyspnea on exertion. Coldness and numbness of the extremities may be reported. Hypochromic microcytosis, as evidenced by a decreased mean corpuscular volume and low hemoglobin concentrations (decreased mean corpuscular hemoglobin concentration), characterizes iron deficiency.

Iron-deficiency anemia is a widespread clinical problem and the most common form of anemia in the United States. Although it causes few deaths, it does contribute to the poor health and suboptimal performance of many people. Iron deficiency results from inadequate diet, malabsorption, pregnancy and lactation, or blood loss. Treatment with epoetin alfa combined with inadequate iron supplementation can also cause iron deficiency. Because normal iron losses through the urine, feces, and skin are minimal, and because the majority of total body iron is efficiently stored and conserved (recycled), iron deficiency caused by poor diet or malabsorption develops very slowly over the course of several months.

Despite fortification of flour and educational efforts regarding proper nutrition, iron deficiency remains a problem, especially during the following four life periods:

- *During childhood (under 2 years of age):* Children obtain low iron content from cow's milk.
- *During adolescence:* In addition to blood loss during menses, young women experience rapid growth, which entails an expanding red cell mass and the need for iron in myoglobin.
- *During and after pregnancy:* Women face the expanding blood volume of pregnancy, the demands of the fetus and placenta, and the blood loss of childbirth.
- *During later years:* Persons of advanced age often consume inadequate dietary iron, demonstrate compromised absorption caused by achlorhydria, and experience an increased incidence of GI tract blood loss resulting from malignancy, gastric ulceration, or use of nonsteroidal anti-inflammatory drugs. However, the prevalence of elevated iron stores may be significantly greater than iron deficiency in this age group.[19] It has been suggested that high iron stores may contribute to chronic diseases such as cancer and heart disease, although research to date has been inconclusive. In the absence of a confirmed diagnosis of iron-deficiency anemia, routine supplementation for this age group is not recommended.

Supplemental iron may be warranted for women with heavy and/or prolonged menstrual blood loss or patients who frequently donate blood. In addition, iron may be indicated during recovery from disease- and injury-associated blood loss. Examples include peptic ulcer disease, esophageal varices, cancer, and traumatic injury such as motor vehicle accidents.

Chronic use of drugs such as salicylates, nonsteroidal anti-inflammatory drugs, corticosteroids, or anticoagulants may cause drug-induced blood loss. This effect may be the result of direct irritation of the gastric mucosa or the increased bleeding tendency these medications cause. Iron supplementation should be used cautiously, if at all, with patients at high risk of GI bleeding.

Medications such as aspirin or ibuprofen may not be included on a medication record. Therefore, the practitioner should routinely question the patient regarding the use of nonprescription drugs and ascertain whether the patient's problem is chronic, whether self-treatment has been tried, and whether medical evaluation for anemia or conditions that could contribute to anemia has been sought or received. Anemia in patients who are not pregnant, lactating, or menstruating, or who are not on a meat-restricted diet may be a symptom of a more serious medical disorder. Such patients require further evaluation to determine the cause of anemia and should not simply be treated empirically. Patients who report bleeding should be immediately referred to a primary care provider. Abnormal blood loss may be indicated by (1) hematemesis or "coffee-ground" vomitus; (2) bright red blood in the stool or black, tarry stools; (3) large clots or an abnormally heavy flow during the menstrual period; or (4) cloudy or pink-red urine (if the use of drugs that may cause urine discoloration has been ruled out).

Blood loss, particularly through the stool, is not always obvious. Even when abnormal blood loss occurs, the patient may not notice or report it. Periodic testing using home occult blood test kits may be considered for certain high-risk patients.

Dose/DRI   The DRI values for iron are listed in Table 23-4. Because of the GI side effects associated with oral iron supplementation, the UL for elemental iron has been set at 45 mg/day.[14] Oral iron supplements are FDA-approved for the prevention and treatment of iron-deficiency anemia.[20]

In a ferrous sulfate 325 mg tablet, 20% (about 60 mg) is elemental iron. In patients with iron deficiency, 20% of the elemental iron (12 mg) may be absorbed. Because iron 36 to 48 mg daily is enough to support maximum incorporation into red blood cells and replace iron stores, the usual therapeutic dose of two to four tablets daily for 3 months is probably reasonable in treating a deficiency. If the patient has an inadequate response or if symptoms worsen during this time, the patient should consult a primary care provider. In cases of severe or chronic iron deficiency, when serious medical conditions have been ruled out, continuous maintenance doses of three to four tablets daily for approximately 3 to 6 months should normalize hemoglobin and replace iron stores, in the absence of ongoing bleeding.

If iron supplementation is appropriate, the practitioner will need to evaluate which iron product is best. The choice should be based on how well the iron preparation is absorbed and tolerated, on the amount of elemental iron per dose, and on its price. Because ferrous salts are more efficiently absorbed than ferric salts, an iron product of the ferrous group is usually appropriate. Ferrous sulfate is the standard against which other iron salts are compared. Table 23-10 lists selected trade-name iron products.

Ferrous salts may be given in combination with ascorbic acid to improve iron absorption. The practitioner can encourage the consumption of fruit or juice high in ascorbic acid or a vitamin C supplement to be taken with the iron, if necessary. Combination products with iron and ascorbic acid are also available, but these products can be expensive. Chemicals that may decrease iron absorption include phosphates in eggs and milk, phytates in cereals, carbonates, oxalates, and tannins.

Iron is available in numerous salt forms and as immediate- and controlled-release products. The enteric-coated and delayed-release products are generally more expensive but may cause fewer

TABLE 23-10 Selected Iron Supplements

Trade Name	Primary Ingredients
Femiron Daily Iron Supplement Tablets	Elemental iron 20 mg (as fumarate)
Feosol Tablets	Elemental iron 65 mg (as sulfate)
Fer-In-Sol Drops	Elemental iron 15 mg/0.6 mL (as sulfate)
Fer-In-Sol Syrup	Elemental iron 18 mg/5 mL (as sulfate)
Fergon Tablets	Elemental iron 27 mg (as gluconate)
Slow Fe Tablets	Elemental iron 50 mg (as sulfate)

symptoms of gastric irritation. However, because progressively less iron is absorbed as it is passed from the duodenum (the site of maximum absorption) to the ileum of the small intestine, overall iron absorption is decreased by delaying the time of release.

Safety Considerations   All iron products tend to irritate the GI mucosa and may produce nausea, abdominal pain, and diarrhea. These adverse effects may be minimized by reducing the dose or by giving iron with meals; however, food may decrease the amount of iron absorbed by as much as 50%. Practitioners may want to recommend that iron be initiated on an empty stomach, and instruct the patient to change this routine and take the iron with food if GI side effects occur.

A frequent side effect of iron therapy is constipation. This adverse effect has prompted the formulation of iron products that also contain a stool softener (e.g., docusate). During iron therapy, stools commonly have a black, tarry appearance because of the presence of unabsorbed iron in the feces. Unfortunately, this symptom may also indicate GI blood loss and a serious medical problem. Medical evaluation is indicated if an underlying GI condition is suspected or if there is a history of GI disease. If the stool does not darken somewhat during iron therapy, however, the iron product may not have disintegrated properly or released the iron.

Iron must be dispensed and stored in a child-resistant container. Accidental poisoning with iron occurs most often in children, who are attracted to the sugar-coated, colored tablets. It can also occur from an overdose of chewable multivitamins containing iron. Such poisoning is considered a medical emergency. As few as 15 tablets of ferrous sulfate 325 mg have been lethal to children; however, recovery has followed the ingestion of as many as 70 such tablets. The clinical outcome depends on the speed and adequacy of treatment.

Symptoms of acute iron poisoning include abdominal pain, vomiting, diarrhea, electrolyte imbalances, and shock. In later stages, cardiovascular collapse may occur, especially if the cause has not been properly recognized and treated as a medical emergency. Treatment of iron toxicity may begin immediately at home after consultation with a poison control center or local emergency room.

Iron is chelated, or its solubility is altered, by many substances. Examples of drug interactions with iron are listed in Table 23-8.

MAGNESIUM

Magnesium, which is essential for all living cells, is the second most plentiful cation of the intracellular fluids and the fourth most abundant cation in the body. About 2000 mEq of magnesium are present in an average 70 kg adult, with about 50% of this amount in the bone, about 45% as an intracellular cation, and about 1% to 5% in the extracellular fluid.

Function   Magnesium is required for normal bone structure formation and the proper function of more than 300 enzymes, including those involved with ATP (adenosine triphosphatase)–dependent phosphorylation, protein synthesis, and carbohydrate metabolism. Extracellular magnesium is critical to both the maintenance of nerve and muscle electrical potentials and the transmission of impulses across neuromuscular junctions.

Magnesium tends to mimic calcium in its effects on the CNS and skeletal muscle. Magnesium deficiency blunts the normal response of the parathyroid glands to hypocalcemia. Therefore, tetany, caused by a lack of calcium, cannot be corrected with calcium unless the hypomagnesemia is also corrected. Similarly, magnesium deficiency impairs the renal conservation of potassium, and hypokalemia cannot be corrected in the presence of magnesium deficiency.

Dietary Sources   Individuals consuming fresh foods regularly should not develop magnesium deficiency, given that all unprocessed foods contain magnesium, albeit in widely varying amounts. Food sources highest in magnesium are listed in Table 23-6. Processing, which leads to removal of the germ and outer layers of cereal grains, results in a loss of more than 80% of the magnesium available.

Deficiency   Deficiency states are usually caused by malabsorption syndromes, general malnutrition, alcoholism, and iatrogenic causes. In addition, hypomagnesemia may result from prolonged total parenteral nutrition therapy with magnesium-free formulations, hemodialysis, diabetes mellitus, pancreatitis, diuretic-induced electrolyte imbalance, and primary aldosteronism, a condition characterized by loss of body potassium, muscular weakness, and elevated blood pressure.

Symptoms of magnesium deficiency may include neuromuscular irritability, increased CNS stimulation, delirium, and convulsions.

Dose/DRI   The DRI values for magnesium are listed in Table 23-4. Oral magnesium supplements are FDA-approved for use in treatment and prevention of hypomagnesemia.[20] The recommended UL for this nutrient is 350 mg/day.[11,15]

Controversial uses of magnesium supplements include prophylaxis of PMS, migraine, and atherosclerosis, as well as the treatment of asthma and hypertension.[49] Magnesium deficiency may potentially contribute to these ailments, but there are insufficient data to support oral magnesium supplementation for therapeutic use in a generally well-nourished population.

Safety Considerations   No evidence is available to suggest that oral intake of magnesium is harmful to individuals with normal renal function, although diarrhea may occur with large doses. Hypermagnesemia can occur with overzealous use of magnesium sulfate (Epsom salts) or magnesium hydroxide (milk of magnesia) as a laxative, or even with use of magnesium-containing antacids in patients with severe renal failure. Hypermagnesemia may cause diminished deep tendon reflexes and varying degrees of muscle weakness, lethargy, and sedation. These effects may progress to stupor and coma, especially at high serum concentrations. Cardiovascular symptoms may include hypotension and dysrhythmia.

Potential drug–nutrient interactions are listed in Table 23-8.

PHOSPHORUS

Phosphorus is present throughout the body, but approximately 85% of the body's store is located in bone.

Function   Phosphorus is essential for many metabolic processes. As calcium phosphate, it serves as an integral structural component of the bone matrix and as a functional component of phospholipids, carbohydrates, nucleoproteins, and high-energy nucleotides. Plasma phosphate levels are under tight biologic control, involving parathyroid hormone, calcitonin, and vitamin D. DNA and RNA structures contain sugar-phosphate linkages. Cell membranes contain phospholipids, which regulate the transport of solutes into and out of the cell. Many metabolic processes depend on phosphorylation. The adenosine diphosphate (ADP)–ATP system, which provides a mechanism for storage and release of energy for use in all of the body's metabolic processes, involves phosphorus compounds. An important buffer system of the body consists of inorganic phosphates.

There is a reciprocal relationship between calcium and phosphorus. Both minerals are regulated partially by parathyroid hormone. Secretion of parathyroid hormone stimulates an increase in serum calcium levels through increased bone resorption, gut absorption, and reabsorption in renal tubules. Parathyroid hormone also causes a decrease in the reabsorption of phosphate by the kidney. Therefore, when serum calcium is high, serum phosphate is generally low, and vice versa.

Dietary Sources   Phosphorus is present in nearly all foods, especially protein-rich foods and cereal grains (Table 23-6).

Deficiency   Because nearly all foods contain phosphorus, deficiency states do not usually occur unless induced. For example, patients receiving aluminum hydroxide as an antacid for prolonged periods may exhibit weakness, anorexia, malaise, pain, and bone loss. The aluminum hydroxide binds phosphorus, making it unavailable for GI absorption through formation of insoluble and poorly absorbed complexes.

Dose/DRI   The DRI values for phosphorus are listed in Table 23-4. The FDA-approved use for phosphorus is to alleviate the deficiency state. In addition, phosphates have been used to decrease serum calcium levels in hypercalcemia. The recommended UL for phosphorus is 4 g/day.[11,15]

Safety Considerations   GI side effects such as diarrhea and stomach pain have been reported with oral supplementation of phosphate salts. Potential drug–nutrient interactions with phosphorus are listed in Table 23-8.

Trace Elements

Trace elements, which are present in minute quantities in plant and animal tissue, are considered essential for numerous physiologic processes. Zinc and manganese are trace elements. "Ultratrace" minerals have been defined as those elements with an estimated dietary requirement of less than 1 mg/day. The essential ultratrace minerals include arsenic, boron, cobalt, copper, chromium, iodine, molybdenum, nickel, selenium, and silicon. Lithium and vanadium are considered probably essential minerals, but further study is required. Bromine, cadmium, fluorine, lead, and tin are not considered essential.

CHROMIUM

About 5 mg of chromium is present in the normal adult, and levels decline with age.

Function   Chromium is a component of glucose tolerance factor. This dietary organic chromium complex potentiates the activity of insulin.

Chromium combines with picolinic acid (a metabolite of tryptophan) to form chromium picolinate (a form of chromium with enhanced bioavailability). Chromium picolinate, in doses of 200 mcg/day, has been promoted for the general population as an aid in controlling diabetes, lowering cholesterol, producing weight loss, and increasing muscle mass. However, reliable data are insufficient to support any therapeutic value of chromium supplementation in the absence of a diagnosed deficiency.

Dietary Sources   See Table 23-6.

Deficiency   Deficiency of trivalent chromium (the chemical form present in diets) is manifested by glucose intolerance, elevated circulating insulin, glycosuria, fasting hyperglycemia, elevated serum cholesterol and triglycerides, neuropathy, and encephalopathy.

Dose/DRI   Chromium intake in the United States is low (about 50 mcg/day) compared with that of other countries. The estimated DRI values for chromium are listed in Table 23-4. Oral administration of trivalent chromium has a relatively high margin of safety, and there is no UL for chromium.[14]

Safety Considerations   Oral chromium has not been reported to be toxic. However, the hexavalent forms of chromium can be toxic and carcinogenic. These forms, which are encountered through industrial exposure, may enter the body through inhalation or cutaneous absorption.

Drug interactions have not been reported for chromium.

COBALT

Cobalt is an essential component of vitamin B_{12}, but ingested cyanocobalamin is metabolized in vivo to form the B_{12} coenzymes.

Function   Cobalt's nutritional functions are the same as those for cyanocobalamin (see Cyanocobalamin [Vitamin B_{12}]).

Dietary Sources   Cobalt is an integral part of vitamin B_{12} and, therefore, the normal dietary sources of cobalt are the same as for vitamin B_{12} (Table 23-6).

Deficiency   No deficiency state for cobalt is reported to exist in humans.

Dose/DRI   No DRI values exist for cobalt.

Safety Considerations   Large doses of cobalt may result in goiter, congestive heart failure, and myxedema. Cardiomyopathy has also been described. Cyanosis and coma may result from accidental ingestion by children. There are no known drug–nutrient interactions with cobalt.

COPPER

Copper ions exist in two states: the cuprous and the cupric (a potent oxidizing agent). Copper is similar to zinc in the complexes it forms with a number of the same chelating agents. Copper is found in virtually all tissues of the body, but concentrations are highest in the liver, brain, heart, and kidney.

Function   Copper is essential for the proper structure and function of the CNS, and it plays a major role in iron metab-olism. Ceruloplasmin, one of the copper metalloenzymes, is especially important in converting absorbed ferrous iron to transported ferric iron. Other copper-containing enzymes are cytochrome oxidase, dopamine beta-hydroxylase, and super-oxide dismutase.

Dietary Sources   See Table 23-6.

Deficiency   Copper deficiency is uncommon in humans, even though many individuals may consume less than the recommended intake. Contemporary diets provide about 1.2 mg/day for men and 0.9 mg/day for women; these amounts approximate the suggested AI for this nutrient. Deficiencies have been observed in premature infants; in severely malnourished infants fed milk-based, low-copper diets; and in patients receiving parenteral nutrition with inadequate copper.

One of the prominent features of copper deficiency is impaired iron absorption, which results in hypochromic anemia. In copper-deficient animals, bone cortices are fragile and thin, resulting from the failure of collagen cross-linking. Spontaneous rupture of major vessels may also be observed in deficiency states.

Dose/DRI   The DRI values for copper are listed in Table 23-4. For protection against possible hepatoxicity, the recommended UL for this nutrient is 10 mg/day.[14]

Safety Considerations   Copper sulfate doses in excess of 250 mg produce vomiting. However, copper salts should not be used for this purpose.

Wilson's disease is an inborn error of metabolism that causes failure to eliminate copper. These individuals must avoid any copper supplementation. Wilson's disease results in CNS, kidney, and liver damage. Acute symptoms of copper toxicity include nausea, vomiting, diarrhea, hemolysis, convulsions, and GI bleeding. Symptoms respond to treatment with penicillamine.

Supplementation should be avoided in patients with severe hepatic dysfunction or cholestasis caused by compromised biliary clearance of copper.

Potential drug–nutrient interactions are listed in Table 23-8.

FLUORIDE

Available therapeutic forms of fluoride include sodium fluoride, acidulated phosphate fluoride, and stannous fluoride. Sodium fluoride contains about 45% fluoride ion, whereas stannous fluoride contains about 24% fluoride ion.

Function   Fluoride occurs normally in bones and tooth enamel as a calcium salt. Intake of small amounts has been shown to markedly reduce tooth decay, presumably by making the enamel more resistant to the erosive action of acids produced by bacteria in the oral cavity.

Dietary Sources   Fluoride is present in soil and water, but the content varies widely from region to region. Most municipal water supplies are fluoridated to 1 ppm of fluoride, a level that has been shown to be safe and to reduce caries in children by about 50%. Estimates of fluoride intake from food, beverages, and water vary greatly, depending on the presence of fluoridated drinking water.

Deficiency   Fluoride deficiency states in humans, other than potential dental decay, have not been described.

Dose/DRI   The DRI values for fluoride are listed in Table 23-4. The recommended UL for this trace element is 10 mg/day for adults.[11,15]

Fluoride is FDA-approved for use in the prevention of dental caries.[20] Fluoride is a normal constituent of the diet, given that it occurs in soils, water supplies, plants, and animals. All sources of fluoride should be evaluated before supplementation is recommended for children whose home water supply is low in fluoride. Children may obtain fluoride from other water sources (e.g., day care or school) or from other beverages such as soft drinks, juices, and bottled water that may contain varying amounts of fluoride.[50]

Sodium fluoride is available by prescription as oral tablets and solutions, topical solutions, and gels, as well as in combination products. Nonprescription topical rinses containing fluoride 0.01% to 0.02%, such as sodium fluoride, and gels containing 0.4% stannous fluoride (e.g., Gel-Kam) are brushed onto the teeth to reduce sensitivity and prevent dental cavities.

Safety Considerations   Excessive fluoride can be toxic. Acute toxicity should not result from the low levels present in drinking water but may result from the administration of excessive doses of fluoride supplements. Because acute toxicity affects the GI system and the CNS, it can be life threatening. Symptoms include salivation, GI distress, muscle weakness, tremors, and (rarely) seizures. Because of the calcium-binding effect of fluoride, symptoms of calcium deficiency, including tetany, may be seen. Eventually, respiratory and cardiac failure may occur. The dose that causes acute toxicity in adults is approximately 5 grams. Death has occurred after ingestion of 2 grams in adults, but much larger overdoses have been treated successfully. In children, 0.5 gram of sodium fluoride may be fatal. Treatment includes precipitation of the fluoride by using gastric lavage with calcium hydroxide 0.15% solution, intravenous dextrose and saline for hydration, and treatment with calcium to prevent tetany.

Chronic fluoride toxicity is manifested as changes in the structure of bones and teeth. Tooth enamel, if still under development, acquires a mottled appearance consisting of white, patchy plaques occurring with pitting brown stains. Prolonged ingestion of water that contains more than 2 ppm of fluoride has resulted in a significant incidence of mottling. Extremely large doses (e.g., 20–80 mg/day) have resulted in chalky, brittle bones that tend to fracture easily, a condition known as crippling skeletal fluorosis.

Potential drug–nutrient interactions are listed in Table 23-8.

IODINE

The thyroid gland contains about one-third of the iodine in the body, stored in the form of a complex glycoprotein, thyroglobulin. The only known function of thyroglobulin is to provide thyroxine and triiodothyronine, which are hormones that regulate the metabolic rate of cells and, therefore, influence physical and mental growth, nervous and muscle tissue function, circulatory activity, and use of nutrients.

Function   Iodine is an essential micronutrient required to synthesize thyroxine and triiodothyronine. High concentrations of iodine inhibit the release of these hormones. In the absence of iodine, thyroid hypertrophy occurs, resulting in goiter. The iodine content of produce reflects that of the soil in which it is grown. The consumption of foods from diverse locations and the addition of iodide to table salt have essentially eliminated goiter as a health problem in the United States.

Dietary Sources   The primary dietary source of iodine is iodized salt, which contains 1 part of sodium or potassium iodide per 10,000 parts (0.01%) of salt. A dose of about 95 mcg of iodine can be obtained from about one-fourth teaspoon of salt (1.25 grams). In the United States, most of the table salt sold is iodized; however, salt used in food processing and for institutional use is not. Additional dietary sources of iodine include saltwater fish and shellfish.

Deficiency   A moderate deficiency of iodine can result in goiter; severe deficiency results in hypothyroidism.

Dose/DRI   Because of the fortification of salt, the iodine content of typical diets in the United States is still well above the DRI values for adults (Table 23-4). Iodine supplements are unwarranted for most individuals. Potassium iodide is available as a tablet, syrup, and solution, and is included in various combination products.

Safety Considerations   Some individuals are allergic to iodide or organic preparations containing iodine and may develop a rash. Symptoms of chronic iodism (iodide intoxication) may include an unpleasant taste and burning in the mouth or throat, along with soreness of the teeth or gums. Increased salivation, sneezing, irritation of the eyes, and swelling of the eyelids commonly occur. In addition, prolonged use of iodine supplementation can result in hypothyroidism.[19] A UL of iodine 1.1 mg/day has been recommended.[14]

Potential drug–nutrient interactions are listed in Table 23-8.

MANGANESE

The body concentrates its stores of manganese in the liver, pancreas, kidney, muscle, and bone.

Function   Manganese is required for the utilization of glucose; the synthesis of mucopolysaccharides of cartilage; the biosynthesis of steroids, cholesterol, and fatty acids; and the biologic activity of pyruvate carboxylase.

Dietary Sources   Manganese is widely available in foods; primary dietary sources are listed in Table 23-6.

Deficiency   Manganese deficiency is extremely rare, and the only theorized method of manganese deficiency is insufficient dietary intake.

Dose/DRI   Even though manganese is poorly absorbed after oral administration (3%), sufficient quantities are present in the average diet to maintain appropriate levels. A dose or dietary intake of 2 to 5 mg/day is considered safe and adequate. The estimated AIs for manganese are listed in Table 23-4. The recommended UL of 11 mg/day is based on data that showed no adverse effects with long-term consumption at this level.[14]

Safety Considerations   Toxicity is rare for orally administered manganese. Toxicity has been observed, however, from inhalation of dust and industrial fumes containing manganese. Because of the reduced biliary clearance of manganese in patients with severe liver dysfunction or cholestasis, supplementation should be avoided under these conditions.

Significant drug interactions with manganese have not been reported.

MOLYBDENUM

Molybdenum is an ultratrace mineral that has only rarely been associated with deficiency. Practitioners monitoring patients on long-term parenteral nutrition must be aware of the potential for deficiency in this population.

Function   Molybdenum readily changes its oxidation state and acts as an electron transfer agent in oxidation–reduction reactions. It may also function as an enzyme cofactor, and is involved in the metabolism of sulfur and purines.

Dietary Sources   The molybdenum content of food varies, depending on the growth environment. Dietary sources of molybdenum are listed in Table 23-6.

Deficiency   Molybdenum is a cofactor for several flavoprotein enzymes and is found in xanthine oxidase. Because xanthine oxidase is involved in the oxidation of xanthine to uric acid, high molybdenum intake has been associated with goutlike symptoms. Parenteral nutrition without molybdenum has resulted in an acquired molybdenum deficiency, which has been treated with ammonium molybdate. Symptoms of molybdenum deficiency may include tachycardia, tachypnea, headache, lethargy, and disorientation. Congenital deficiency of specific molybdenum cofactors results in severe neurologic dysfunction and mental retardation.

Dose/DRI/Safety Considerations   The human molybdenum requirement is low and is easily furnished by the average diet (Table 23-4). Supplements are rarely warranted.

On the basis of animal studies showing impaired reproduction and growth with prolonged intake of excessive molybdenum, a UL of 2 mg/day is recommended.[14]

No significant drug interactions have been reported with molybdenum.

SELENIUM

Selenium is present in all tissues and is generally incorporated into organic compounds involving amino acids such as methionine or cysteine. Selenium compounds are about 80% absorbed. The highest concentrations are in the kidneys and liver; the lowest are in the lungs and brain. The kidney is the primary route of excretion, although losses can also occur through the GI tract.

Function   Selenium is an antioxidant that serves as part of glutathione peroxidase. This enzyme protects cells from the peroxidase-induced oxidative damage that occurs with cellular metabolism.

The antioxidant properties of selenium have prompted evaluation for its use in cancer prevention. For example, a recent randomized, controlled trial evaluated the effect of 200 mcg selenium daily on the risk of various types of cancer. Selenium was found to significantly reduce the incidence of prostate cancer but not of lung or colorectal cancer.[51] Additional trials evaluating the role of selenium in cancer risk reduction are warranted.

Dietary Sources   See Table 23-6. The selenium content of foods depends on the soils in which the plants are grown.

Deficiency   Selenium is an essential trace element in humans, but deficiencies are not common in the general population. Selenium deficiency has been reported in patients with alcoholic cirrhosis, probably because of an insufficient diet or the altered metabolism of selenium. It has been reported rarely in patients on long-term parenteral nutrition. Limited evidence in humans suggests that deficiency results in cardiomyopathy, musculoskeletal pain, bleaching of the hair and skin, and abnormal nail beds. Epidemiologic studies suggest that cancer and heart disease may be common in areas of low selenium availability. Keshan disease, a cardiomyopathy that occurs almost exclusively in children, has been shown to respond to selenium.

Dose/DRI   The DRI values for selenium are listed in Table 23-4. The UL for this mineral is 400 μg/day.[13]

Safety Considerations   Toxic effects of selenium may include loss of hair and nails, skin lesions, muscular weakness, fatigue, and CNS abnormalities. No significant drug interactions with selenium have been reported.

ZINC

Zinc is an integral part of at least 70 metalloenzymes, including carbonic anhydrase, lactic dehydrogenase, alkaline phosphatase, carboxypeptidase, aminopeptidase, and alcohol dehydrogenase.

Function   Zinc is a cofactor in the synthesis of DNA and RNA. It is involved in the mobilization of vitamin A from the liver, and in the enhancement of follicle-stimulating hormone and luteinizing hormone. Zinc is essential for normal cellular immune functions, as well as for spermatogenesis and normal testicular function. It is also important in the stabilization of membrane structure.

The divalent ion is most commonly found and used in the body. Zinc has a relatively rapid turnover rate. The balance between zinc absorption from the small intestine and excretion through the feces is efficiently regulated by the body. Vegetarians may require higher amounts of zinc, because diets high in fiber and phytates hinder zinc absorption.[14]

Dietary Sources   Most dietary zinc (about 70%) is derived from animal products (Table 23-6).

Deficiency   Although zinc deficiencies are not widespread in the United States, marginally low zinc values have been associated with growth retardation in children, slow wound healing in adults, and birth defects. Additional symptoms include immunologic abnormalities, impaired taste and smell, delayed sexual maturation, hypogonadism, hypospermia, and dermatitis.

Malabsorption syndromes, infection, major surgery, alcoholism, pregnancy, lactation, and high-fiber diets rich in phytate predispose an individual to a suboptimal zinc status. Zinc depletion is relatively rare but may be seen in patients on long-term parenteral nutrition and in patients with GI tract abnormalities, such as fistulas and prolonged, severe diarrhea.

Zinc deficiencies adversely affect DNA, RNA, carbohydrate, and protein metabolism. Iron supplements decrease zinc absorption just as zinc supplements decrease iron absorption, probably resulting from competition for the same transport system. If these minerals are taken with a meal, the adverse interaction is less pronounced. In patients with impaired wound healing, zinc supplementation may be marginally beneficial.

Dose/DRI   The DRI values for zinc are listed in Table 23-4. Typical Western diets supply 10 to 15 mg of zinc per day.

Because only 10% to 40% of zinc is absorbed from the GI tract, ingestion of zinc sulfate 220 mg (50 mg of elemental zinc) will supply 5 to 20 mg of zinc. Treatment of suspected deficiencies usually involves short-term administration of elemental zinc 150 mg in three divided doses daily. Patients with large GI losses through fistulas, ostomies, or stool require larger supplemental doses of zinc. At doses above 40 mg elemental zinc per day, copper deficiency may be induced. On the basis of this interaction, the UL for elemental zinc is 40 mg daily if therapy with zinc is going to be long term.[14] Absorption of zinc supplements may be reduced if taken with foods high in calcium or phosphorus.[27]

Zinc has been evaluated in numerous studies as a potential treatment for the common cold. However, zinc formulations and doses have varied, and trial results have been conflicting. A meta-analysis on the use of zinc lozenges concluded that insufficient evidence exists for routine use of these products in the treatment of the cold.[52]

Safety Considerations   Because ingestion of zinc sulfate 2 grams or more has resulted in GI irritation and vomiting, zinc should be taken with food. Zinc is also toxic; however, the emetic effect that occurs after consumption of large amounts may minimize problems with accidental overdose. Reported signs of zinc toxicity in humans include vomiting, dehydration, muscle incoordination, dizziness, and abdominal pain.

Potential drug–nutrient interactions are listed in Table 23-8.

Assessment of Nutritional Adequacy: A Case-Based Approach

Assessing a patient's nutritional status is difficult in the ambulatory environment. Clinical impressions are often erroneous, given that the stages between well-nourished and poorly nourished states are not readily evident. There are guidelines, however, that may help provide a more objective assessment of a patient's nutritional sta-

tus. Practitioners should exercise good observational skills, know which questions yield helpful information, and know which population groups tend to be poorly nourished. By asking key questions, the practitioner may detect cultural, physical, environmental, and social conditions that suggest inadequate vitamin intake. The more specific the information obtained from the patient is, the more helpful the practitioner can be in determining the need for nutritional supplementation. Questions about food generally not included in the diet and about previous treatment of similar symptoms may also be important.

Although most nutritional assessment measures are beyond the scope of routine pharmacy practice, the pharmacist can observe the physical status of the patient. For example, a patient's fingernails may indicate malnutrition if they are not lustrous and are dark at the upper ends. The texture, amount, and appearance of hair may indicate the patient's nutritional status. The eyes, particularly the conjunctiva, may indicate vitamin A and iron deficiencies. The mouth may show stomatitis, glossitis, or hypertrophic or pale gums. Poor dentition may limit the foods that a patient is able to eat, thereby compromising intake from certain food groups such as protein. Visible goiter, poor skin color and texture, obesity or thinness relative to bone structure, and the presence of edema may also indicate malnutrition. The pharmacist should be able to recognize overt but nonspecific symptoms of vitamin and mineral deficiencies for which prompt referral to a primary care provider may be crucial.

Checking a patient's medication history is important because of the number of potential drug–micronutrient interactions (Table 23-8). It is also the practitioner's responsibility to refer patients with a suspected serious illness to a primary care provider. Just as nutritional deficiencies may lead to disease, disease may lead to nutritional deficiencies. Patients may present with one or more deficiencies, which may be very difficult to identify. Rarely in the United States do practitioners encounter patients with severe deficiencies resulting in diseases such as scurvy, pellagra, or kwashiorkor. However, milder forms of malnutrition may be seen.

Cases 23-1 and 23-2 are examples of the assessment of patients with nutritional inadequacy.

CASE 23-1

Relevant Evaluation Criteria	Scenario/Model Outcome
Information Gathering	
1. Gather essential information about the patient's symptoms, including:	
a. description of symptom(s) (i.e., nature, onset, duration, severity, associated symptoms)	Patient inquires about information found on the Internet recommending supplementation with various vitamins to prevent cancer and aging. He states he currently takes Centrum Silver plus extra vitamin C to prevent colds and gingko biloba for his memory.
b. description of any factors that seem to precipitate, exacerbate, and/or relieve the patient's symptom(s)	N/A
c. description of the patient's efforts to relieve the symptoms	N/A

Relevant Evaluation Criteria	Scenario/Model Outcome
2. Gather essential patient history information:	
a. patient's identity	Bruce Trappers
b. patient's age, sex, height, and weight	79-year-old male, 6 ft 1 in, 190 lb
c. patient's occupation	Retired professor of agriculture
d. patient's dietary habits	Eats only two meals daily to help maintain weight: typically cereal and fruit or 3–4 eggs, starch, and fruit for breakfast; balanced meals for dinner with salad, protein, starch, vegetable, and a glass of wine
e. patient's sleep habits	N/A
f. concurrent medical conditions, prescription and nonprescription medications, and dietary supplements	Patient has a history of hyperlipidemia with family history of myocardial infarction in his brother. Every morning he takes 325 mg aspirin, atorvastatin 10 mg, 2 omega-3 fish oil capsules, 1 Centrum Silver multivitamin, 500 mg vitamin C, and 120 mg of gingko biloba.
g. allergies	Sulfa
h. history of other adverse reactions to medications	N/A

Assessment and Triage

3. Differentiate the patient's signs/symptoms and correctly identify the patient's primary problem(s).	Taking multiple supplements can increase the risk of exceeding the UL for various nutrients. There is no evidence to suggest that this practice is beneficial, and evidence is mounting that supplementation of certain nutrients can potentially be harmful.
4. Identify exclusions for self-treatment.	None
5. Formulate a comprehensive list of therapeutic alternatives for the primary problem to determine if triage to a medical practitioner is required, and share this information with the patient.	Options include: (1) Assess the client's perceived need for the nutrient supplements. (2) Evaluate dietary intake from food groups, encouraging at least 5 servings of produce daily, 3 servings of low-fat dairy products, 2 servings of protein, and 6 servings of whole-grain food sources daily. (3) Discuss which nutrients may need supplementation, on the basis of the patient's patterns of dietary intake. Evaluate Centrum Silver for adequacy, while avoiding intakes above the UL. (4) Discuss the lack of data and potential harm associated with megadoses of vitamin. (5) Take no action.

Plan

6. Select an optimal therapeutic alternative to address the patient's problem, taking into account patient preferences.	Encourage a well-balanced diet, emphasizing that studies repeatedly demonstrate that good nutrition is associated with multiple health benefits, including a lower risk of some cancers and other age-related diseases. Evaluate the Centrum Silver multivitamin with the client, comparing the level of supplementation of each nutrient compared with the DRI. Point out that the product contains gingko biloba and vitamin C; therefore, additional supplementation of these substances is not necessary.
7. Describe the recommended therapeutic approach to the patient.	See step 6.
8. Explain to the patient the rationale for selecting the recommended therapeutic approach from the considered therapeutic alternatives.	See step 6.

Patient Education

9. When recommending self-care with nonprescription medications and/or nondrug therapy, convey accurate information to the patient:	
a. appropriate dose and frequency of administration	Consider one USP-approved multivitamin daily that contains no more than 100% of DRI for nutrients.

Relevant Evaluation Criteria	Scenario/Model Outcome
b. maximum number of days the therapy should be employed	N/A
c. product administration procedures	You may take your multivitamin with your current medications in the morning. However, check with your pharmacist on coadministration of any newly prescribed medications.
10. Solicit follow-up questions from patient.	What about antioxidant vitamins?
11. Answer patient's questions.	Data from well-designed trials do not support antioxidant supplementation for the prevention or treatment of cancer. In fact, some trials have suggested potential harm is associated with supplementation of vitamins A, E, and C, selenium, and other nutrients in relation to cancer risk. Therefore, dosing of these nutrients above the DRI cannot be recommended at this time.

Key: DRI, dietary reference intake; N/A, not applicable; UL, upper intake level; USP, United States Pharmacopeia.

Relevant Evaluation Criteria	Scenario/Model Outcome
Information Gathering	
1. Gather essential information about the patient's symptoms, including:	
a. description of symptom(s) (i.e., nature, onset, duration, severity, associated symptoms)	Patient does not have any complaints. However, on inquiry of supplementation taken at home, patient says she regularly takes a multivitamin with extra nutrients to reduce stress, an antioxidant supplement plus beta-carotene once daily for vision, and calcium tablets twice daily for osteoporosis prevention.
b. description of any factors that seem to precipitate, exacerbate, and/or relieve the patient's symptom(s)	N/A
c. description of the patient's efforts to relieve the symptoms	N/A
2. Gather essential patient history information:	
a. patient's identity	Katherine Forest
b. patient's age, sex, height, and weight	37-year-old female, 5 ft 8 in, 130 lb
c. patient's occupation	Postal worker and mother of 4 children
d. patient's dietary habits	Cereal or toast and fruit for breakfast; soup or frozen meal for lunch; dinner varies between fast-food meals and easy-to-prepare meals at home.
e. patient's sleep habits	N/A
f. concurrent medical conditions, prescription and nonprescription medications, and dietary supplements	Ibuprofen 400 mg twice daily, levothyroxine 88 mcg daily
g. allergies	No known allergies
h. history of other adverse reactions to medications	Family history of glaucoma and osteoporosis
Assessment and Triage	
3. Differentiate the patient's signs/symptoms and correctly identify the patient's primary problem(s).	Taking multiple supplements can increase the risk of exceeding the UL for various nutrients. No evidence exists that this practice is beneficial, and concern exists that long-term supplementation of certain nutrients in doses exceeding the UL may potentially have negative effects.

Relevant Evaluation Criteria	Scenario/Model Outcome
4. Identify exclusions for self-treatment.	None
5. Formulate a comprehensive list of therapeutic alternatives for the primary problem to determine if triage to a medical practitioner is required, and share this information with the patient.	Options include: (1) Focus on only potential drug–nutrient interactions. (2) Discuss the role of balanced nutrition as the ideal route of taking vitamins and minerals. Identify nutritional needs unique to this geriatric client and where supplementation may be recommended. (3) Take no action.

Plan

6. Select an optimal therapeutic alternative to address the patient's problem, taking into account patient preferences.	Assess the client's perceived need for the nutrient supplements. Evaluate dietary intake from food groups, encouraging at least 5 servings of produce daily, 3 servings of low-fat dairy products, 2 servings of protein, and 6 servings of whole grain food sources daily. Discuss the vitamin and mineral content of the various supplements and the total intake in comparison with the DRIs. Conversion of units of measure for vitamin A may be necessary to assess total intake. For example, if the multivitamin provides 3500 IU of vitamin A and the antioxidant supplement plus beta-carotene provides 25,000 IU of beta-carotene, the patient's intake of vitamin A is likely excessive. The DRI for this client is 700 mcg as RAE (2330 IU) with a UL of 3 mg (9990 IU) daily. To convert the client's supplemented intake to micrograms of RAE per day, you note that 1 mcg as RAE = 10 IU vitamin A activity as beta-carotene = 3.33 IU vitamin A activity as retinol. This calculates to 3551 mcg as RAE daily in supplements alone. Suggest limiting vitamin supplementation to a USP-approved multivitamin with no more than 100% of DRI for vitamins and minerals.
7. Describe the recommended therapeutic approach to the patient.	Unless specifically recommended by your primary care provider or ophthalmologist, reconsider taking the supplement for vision if you are taking a USP-approved multivitamin with minerals. Take the multivitamin and the calcium supplement at different times. Separate both of these supplements from the levothyroxine (see Table 23-9).
8. Explain to the patient the rationale for selecting the recommended therapeutic approach from the considered therapeutic alternatives.	Your current supplemental intake for vitamin A well exceeds the DRI. Instead of taking multiple supplements, optimize your nutrient intake by eating whole grains, fruits, and vegetables. In addition to fiber and many commonly recognized vitamins and minerals, fruits and vegetables provide lutein, a carotenoid associated with reduced risk of age-related macular degeneration when consumed regularly. Also choose low-fat dairy products and protein sources daily. Complementing a balanced diet with a daily multivitamin with minerals is reasonable to ensure adequate nutrient intake when the regular intake of healthy meals becomes difficult. If vitamin D intake is not sufficient between dietary sources and the multivitamin, a calcium product with vitamin D may be recommended.

Patient Education

9. When recommending self-care with nonprescription medications and/or nondrug therapy, convey accurate information to the patient.	Criterion does not apply in this case.

Key: DRI, dietary reference intake; N/A, not applicable; RAE, retinol activity equivalent; UL, upper intake level; USP, United States Pharmacopeia.

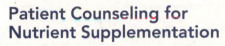

PATIENT EDUCATION FOR
Nutritional Deficiencies

The objective of self-treatment is to prevent nutritional deficiencies or maintain present nutritional status. For most patients, carefully following product instructions and the self-care measures listed here will help ensure optimal therapeutic outcomes.

Vitamins, Minerals, and Trace Elements

- To ensure proper nutrition, eat a varied diet as recommended in the Food Guide Pyramid (see Figure 23-1). Vitamin supplements are not a substitute for a well-balanced diet.
- Read labels on all vitamin and mineral preparations carefully before taking them. Note the quantity of vitamins and minerals required to meet the DRI, or dietary reference intake, values.
- Do not take doses of vitamins and minerals higher than the recommended DRIs. High doses of vitamins or minerals may be dangerous and should not be taken indiscriminately.
- Take vitamins and mineral supplements with meals if you experience gastrointestinal symptoms.
- Women of childbearing age should take 400 mcg supplemental folic acid in addition to a well-balanced diet. This has been shown to reduce the risk of neural tube defects in the fetus.

- Be aware that iron supplements or vitamins with iron may turn the stool black. This occurrence is not a cause for alarm, unless it is associated with other symptoms involving the digestive system.
- As with any medicine, store vitamin and combination vitamin/mineral supplements out of the reach of children, especially if the product contains iron. Teach children that vitamins are drugs and potential poisons, and that vitamins cannot be taken indiscriminately.
- Be aware that therapeutic use of niacin-containing products may cause a flushing, itching, or tingling sensation, which should decrease in intensity with continued therapy. Taking an aspirin or nonsteroidal anti-inflammatory agent 30–60 minutes before taking niacin may help decrease these effects.
- Do not self-medicate if you suspect a vitamin deficiency; consult a health care practitioner instead.

Patient Counseling for Nutrient Supplementation

The public is often exposed to exaggerated and fraudulent claims concerning vitamin products. The practitioner can help expose such claims by keeping up with medical and pharmaceutical literature, and by not supporting or appearing to support the claims until they are substantiated by reliable clinical studies. Patients inquiring about such claims should be educated about the increased potential risk of the nontraditional use of vitamins. They should be told, for example, about adverse drug reactions that might occur with such products when used in alternative doses or in combination with prescription and nonprescription drug products. This advice, however, becomes difficult to give when patients purchase nutritional supplements from health food stores or from online and mail-order vendors.

Patients purchasing a nonprescription liquid dietary supplement should be instructed on its proper use and storage, including dilution and preparation techniques. In addition, the practitioner should offer to discuss with the patient possible adverse effects such as diarrhea.

The box Patient Education for Nutritional Deficiencies lists specific information to provide patients. The practitioner could also refer the consumer to Web sites and printed literature with evidence-based recommendations for vitamin and mineral supplementation, such as those listed in the reference section of this chapter.

Evaluation of Patient Outcomes for Nutritional Adequacy

Nutritional therapy should involve a diet based on the Food Guide Pyramid and possibly the use of nutritional supplements. The practitioner should advise patients to return after 30 days

of implementing nutritional therapy, or sooner if the symptoms worsen. Patients whose symptoms have worsened should be referred to a primary care provider. Patients whose symptoms have improved while taking nutritional supplements should be encouraged to eat a healthful diet and not to rely on supplements as the primary source for vitamins and minerals.

Key Points for Nutritional Adequacy

➤ The benefits of a varied, balanced diet in terms of health maintenance and disease prevention have been demonstrated repeatedly. However, the same benefits have not been observed when suboptimal dietary intake is augmented with vitamin and mineral supplementation.

➤ Practitioners can assess the variety of food choices by comparing the patient's typical food pattern to that recommended in the Food Guide Pyramid. The practitioner may refer patients to a registered dietitian for personalized and/or more complete counseling on diet modification as well as nutritional supplementation.

➤ Overt vitamin or mineral deficiencies are rare in this country; however, subclinical deficiencies may be contributing to chronic disease.

➤ Vitamin and/or mineral supplementation may be appropriate on the basis of the practitioner's assessment of the patient's dietary intake, metabolic requirements, absorptive capability, and potential drug–micronutrient interactions.

REFERENCES

1. US Department of Health and Human Services, National Institutes of Health. Biologically Based Practices: An Overview. March 2007. Available at: http://nccam.nih.gov/ health/backgrounds/D237.pdf. Last accessed July 2, 2008.
2. Fairfield KM, Fletcher RH. Vitamins for chronic disease prevention in adults: scientific review. *JAMA*. 2002;287:3116–26.

3. Troppmann L, Gray-Donald K, Johns T. Supplement use: is there any nutritional benefit? *J Am Diet Assoc.* 2002;102:818–25.

4. US Preventive Services Task Force. *Routine Vitamin Supplementation to Prevent Cancer and Cardiovascular Disease: Recommendations and Rationale.* Rockville, Md: Agency for Healthcare Research and Quality; June 2003. Available at: http://www.ahrq.gov/clinic/3rduspstf/vitamins/vitaminsrr.htm. Last accessed August 16, 2008.

5. Zawada, ET. Malnutrition in the elderly: is it simply a matter of not eating enough? *Postgrad Med.* 1996;100:207–8, 211–4, 220–2.

6. Fuhrman, MP. Identifying your patient's risk for a vitamin deficiency. *Nutr Clin Pract.* 2001;16:S8–S11.

7. American Dietetic Association. Position of the American Dietetic Association: food fortification and dietary supplements. *J Am Diet Assoc.* 2001; 101:115–25.

8. Cooperman T, Obermeyer W. Do all supplements contain what their labels say they contain? *US Pharm.* October 2002;68, 71–2, 74.

9. US Pharmacopeia Dietary Supplement Verification Program. Available at: http://www.usp.org. Last accessed June 21, 2008.

10. *Dietary Guidelines for Americans 2005.* Washington, DC: US Department of Health and Human Services, US Department of Agriculture; January 12, 2005. HHS Publication HHS-ODPHP-2005-01-DGA-A.

11. Food and Nutrition Board, Institute of Medicine. *Dietary Reference Intakes for Calcium, Phosphorus, Magnesium, Vitamin D, and Fluoride.* Washington, DC: National Academy Press; 1997.

12. Food and Nutrition Board, Institute of Medicine. *Dietary Reference Intakes for Thiamin, Riboflavin, Niacin, Vitamin B6, Folate, Vitamin B12, Pantothenic Acid, Biotin, and Choline.* Washington, DC: National Academy Press; 2000.

13. Food and Nutrition Board, Institute of Medicine. *Dietary Reference Intakes for Vitamin C, Vitamin E, Selenium, and Carotenoids.* Washington, DC: National Academy Press; 2000.

14. Food and Nutrition, Board Institute of Medicine. *Dietary Reference Intakes for Vitamin A, Vitamin K, Arsenic, Boron, Chromium, Copper, Iodine, Iron, Manganese, Molybdenum, Nickel, Silicon, Vanadium, and Zinc.* Washington, DC: National Academy Press; 2002.

15. Yates AA, Schlicker SA, Suitor CW. Dietary reference intakes: the new basis for recommendations for calcium and related nutrients, B vitamins, and choline. *J Am Diet Assoc.* 1998;98:699–708.

16. Hathcock J. Dietary supplements: how they are used and regulated. *J Nutr.* 2001;131:1114S-7S.

17. Stone WL, LeClair I, Ponder T, et al. Infants discriminate between natural and synthetic vitamin E. *Am J Clin Nutr.* 2003; 77:899–906.

18. Combs GF. Vitamins. In: Mahan LK, Escott-Stump S, eds. *Krause's Food, Nutrition, and Diet Therapy.* 10th ed. Philadelphia: WB Saunders; 2000:168–9.

19. Balint JP. Physical findings in nutritional deficiencies. *Ped Clin North Am.* 1998;45:245–60.

20. Lacy CF, Armstrong LL, Goldman MP, et al. *Drug Information Handbook.* 15th ed. Hudson, Ohio: Lexi-Comp; 2007.

21. Feskanich D, Singh V, Willett W, et al. Vitamin A intake and hip fractures among postmenopausal women. *JAMA.* 2002;287:47–54.

22. The Alpha-Tocopherol, Beta Carotene Cancer Prevention Study Group. The effect of vitamin E and beta carotene on the incidence of lung cancer and other cancers in male smokers. *N Engl J Med.* 1994;330:1029–35.

23. Goodman GE, Thornquist MD, Balmes J, et al. The Beta-Carotene and Retinol Efficacy Trial: incidence of lung cancer and cardiovascular disease mortality during 6-year follow-up after stopping beta-carotene and retinol supplements. *J Natl Cancer Inst.* 2004;96:1743–50.

24. Papadimitropoulos E, Wells G, Shea B, et al. VIII: meta-analysis of the efficacy of vitamin D treatment in preventing osteoporosis in postmenopausal women. *Endocr Rev.* 2002;23:560–9.

25. Osborne JE, Hutchinson PE. Vitamin D and systemic cancer: is this relevant to malignant melanoma? *Br J Dermatol.* 2002;147: 197–213.

26. Zittermann A, Schleithoff SS, Tenderich G, et al. Low vitamin D status: a contributing factor in the pathogenesis of congestive heart failure? *J Am Coll Cardiol.* 2003;41:105–12.

27. Holick MF. Vitamin D deficiency. *N Engl J Med.* 2007;357:266–81.

28. Garland CF. The role of vitamin D in cancer prevention. *Am J Pub Health.* 2006; 96:9–18.

29. Hartman JJ. Vitamin D deficiency rickets in children: prevalence and need for community education. *Orthoped Nurs.* 2000;19:63–7.

30. Zhang SM Hernan MA, Chen H, et al. Intakes of vitamins E and C, carotenoids, vitamin supplements, and PD risk. *Neurology.* 2002;59:1161–9.

31. Miller ER, Pastor-Barriuso R, Dalal D, et al. Meta-analysis: high-dosage vitamin E supplementation may increase all-cause mortality. *Ann Intern Med.* 2005;142:37–46.

32. Slatore CG, Littman AJ, Au DH, et al. Long-term use of supplemental multivitamins, vitamin C, vitamin E, and folate does not reduce the risk of lung cancer. *Am J Respir Crit Care Med.* 2008; 177:524–30.

33. Pearson DA. Bone health and osteoporosis: the role of vitamin K and potential antagonism by anticoagulants. *Nutr Clin Pract.* 2007;22:517–44.

34. Bialostosky K, Wright JD, Kennedy-Stephenson J, et al. Dietary intake of macronutrients, micronutrients and other dietary constituents: United States 1988–94. National Center for Health Statistics. *Vital Health Stat.* 2002;11(245). Available at: http://www.cdc.gov/nchs/data/series/sr_11/sr11_245.pdf.

35. Feskanich D, Weber P, Willett WC, et al. Vitamin K intake and hip fractures in women: a prospective study. *Am J Clin Nutr.* 1999;69:74–9.

36. Jacob RA, Sotoudeh G. Vitamin C function and status in chronic disease. *Nutr Clin Care.* 2002;5:47–9.

37. Levine M, Wang Y, Padayatty SJ, et al. A new recommended dietary allowance of vitamin C for healthy young women. *Proc Natl Acad Sci U S A.* 2001;98:9842–6.

38. LeBoeuf R. Homocysteine and Alzheimer's disease. *J Am Diet Assoc.* 2003;103:304–7.

39. Desouza C, Keebler M, McNamara, et al. Drugs affecting homocysteine metabolism: impact on cardiovascular risk. *Drugs.* 2002;62:605–16.

40. Dharmarajan TS, Adiga GU, Norkus EP. Vitamin B_{12} deficiency: recognizing subtle symptoms in older adults. *Geriatrics.* 2003;58:30–38.

41. Bender DA. Non-nutritional uses of vitamin B6. *Br J Nutr.* 1999;81:7–20.

42. Schoenen J, Jacquy J, Lenaerts M. Effectiveness of high-dose riboflavin in migraine prophylaxis: a randomized controlled trial. *Neurology.* 1998;50:466–70.

43. Sandor PS, Afra J, Ambrosini A, et al. Prophylactic treatment of migraine with beta-blockers and riboflavin: differential effects on the intensity dependence of auditory evoked cortical potentials. *Headache.* 2000;40:30–5.

44. Suter PM, Vetter W. Diuretics and vitamin B_1: are diuretics a risk factor for thiamin malnutrition? *Nutr Rev.* 2001;58:319–23.

45. Thys-Jacobs S, Starkey P, Bernstein D, et al. Calcium carbonate and the premenstrual syndrome: effects on premenstrual and menstrual symptoms. Premenstrual Syndrome Study Group. *Am J Obstet Gynecol.* 1998; 179:444–52.

46. Giovannucci E, Lui Y, Stampfer MJ. A prospective study of calcium intake and incidence of fatal prostate cancer. *Cancer Epidemiol Biomarkers Prev.* 2006;15:203–10.

47. Straub DA. Calcium supplementation in clinical practice: A review of forms, doses, and indications. *Nutr Clin Prac.* 2007;22:286–96.

48. Fleming DJ, Jacques PF, Tucker KL, et al. Iron status of the free-living, elderly Framingham Heart Study cohort: an iron-replete population with a high prevalence of elevated iron stores. *Am J Clin Nutr.* 2001; 73:638–46.

49. Saris NL, Mervaala E, Karppanen H, et al. Magnesium: an update on physiological, clinical and analytical aspects. *Clin Chem Acta.* 2000;294:1–26.

50. Levy SM. An update on fluorides and fluorosis. *J Can Dent Assoc.* 2003;69:286–91.

51. Duffield-Lillico AJ, Reid ME, Turnbull BW, et al. Baseline characteristics and the effect of selenium supplementation on cancer incidence in a randomized clinical trial: a summary report of the Nutritional Prevention of Cancer Trial. *Cancer Epidemiol Biomarkers Prev.* 2003;11:630–9.

52. Jackson JL, Lesho E, Peterson C. Zinc and the common cold: a meta-analysis revisited. *J Nutr.* 2000;130:1512S-5S.

Functional and Meal Replacement Foods

Carol J. Rollins

Foods serve many purposes in our lives. Foremost is their role in survival, providing us with the sustenance needed to maintain metabolism and be physically active. Scientific research suggests foods may also impact health and wellness, and consumers believe so. Among 1000 consumers in a 2007 survey, 77% believed foods and beverages provide benefits for maintaining overall health and wellness; other benefits consumers believed in were improving heart health (80%) and reducing the risk of developing specific diseases (65%).[1] An earlier Web-based survey of 1012 consumers found that 88% believed certain foods may reduce the risk of disease or other health issues.[2] More than 80% of Americans consume, or are interested in consuming, foods for added health benefits, and consumption appears to be fairly evenly distributed across all age groups.[1,3] More consumers are citing healthfulness as a factor in food purchases, although taste and price are still the most important factors, and convenience is cited nearly as frequently as healthfulness.[1] Lack of time to plan and prepare meals leads health-conscious consumers to seek convenient methods to optimize nutrition for wellness and health promotion, including fast yet healthy alternatives to traditional "sit-down" meals. In addition, more individuals with conditions or impairments that affect their ability to obtain adequate nutrients through a regular diet are living independently and may seek convenient methods to supplement or replace conventional meals. Although dietitians are the recognized food and nutrition experts, it is important for all health care practitioners to be aware of the role that foods may play in an overall plan to improve or maintain health, especially foods that may have benefits beyond those of their basic nutrients or that may help patients reach nutrient goals when healthy meals are not readily available or cannot be ingested. (See Chapter 23 for a discussion of basic nutrition.) This chapter provides an introduction to foods that are used for their potential health benefits (functional foods), as well as foods that are intended to replace regular meals (meal replacement foods).

DRUGS, DIETARY SUPPLEMENTS, AND FOODS

The Food and Drug Administration (FDA) is charged with regulation of drugs, dietary supplements, and foods. (See Chapter 4 for a discussion of regulatory issues.) Foods are defined as articles used for food or drink or components of any such article, or substances providing taste, aroma, or nutritive value.[4,5] Specific FDA regulations pertain to food safety and labeling. FDA requires all regulated foods to provide assurance in advance (premarket) that ingredients are safe and claims are substantiated, truthful, and not misleading. Particular forms or uses of foods, such as infant formulas (see Chapter 26) and medical foods, are required to meet additional criteria to ensure the safety of somewhat vulnerable groups.

FUNCTIONAL FOODS

Functional foods may blur the distinction between drugs, dietary supplements, and foods, as defined by FDA. The term *functional food* is not sanctioned officially by FDA, and there is no legal definition to determine if a foodstuff is a functional food.[4–7] This lack of validation makes it difficult to determine which foods should be included in the sales figures and market estimates for functional foods. Nonetheless, sales of functional foods in the United States were reported as nearly $25 billion in 2006, and sale are estimated to reach nearly $39 billion by 2011, indicating strong consumer support for the development of such products.[8] In fact, in slightly more than a year after introduction to the U.S. market, sales of one probiotic yogurt were estimated as more than $100 million in grocery stores alone.[3] Functional foods are clearly entering the food supply at an ever-increasing rate and are therefore becoming a significant contributing factor in our diets. Health care practitioners should be familiar with functional foods to fully evaluate their patient's diet.

"Health benefits beyond those of basic nutrition" is a broad definition of functional foods, encompassing unmodified whole foods (fruits, vegetables, and whole-grain products) and "designer" foods such as purple carrots.[4,6,7] A somewhat narrower definition, which restricts the definition to unmodified foods with naturally occurring bioactive components, is used by the International Life Sciences Institute.[6,7] Examples include tomatoes for their lycopene content and soybeans, which provide isoflavones. The Institute of Medicine (IOM) Food and Nutrition Board, restricts the definition of functional food to those in which the concentration of one or more ingredients has been altered to enhance the food's contribution to a healthful diet.[6,7] This definition includes foods enriched or fortified with nutrients, phytochemicals, or botanical products, including foods such as orange juice with added calcium. Elements isolated from non-traditional food sources and added to traditional foods, such as stanol esters added to margarine-type spreads, also fit this definition of functional foods.

Categories of Foods Classified as Functional Foods

Functional foods typically fit into one of five categories on the basis of statutory definitions and regulatory guidelines for label claims on foods:

1. Foods associated with health claims recognized by FDA
2. Foods that carry structure or function claims
3. Foods for special dietary use
4. Medical foods
5. Certain conventional foods

Practitioners should have a basic understanding of these categories, because the need for medical supervision varies between categories. All labeling claims require prior approval by FDA; however, the required level of supporting science varies depending on the category under which the functional food is marketed (i.e., greater supporting science is required for medical foods than for structure and function claims).

Foods with Health Claims

Health claims characterize the relationship between a substance (food, food component, dietary ingredient, or dietary supplement) and a disease or health-related condition.[4–7,9] (See Chapters 53 and 54 for discussion of dietary supplements.) Only claims about disease risk reduction are allowed; no claim about "diagnosis, cure, mitigation, or treatment of disease" can be made. Three types of health claims can be made for conventional foods: authorized, authoritative, and qualified. Each type of claim is associated with specific levels of supportive data and specified labeling criteria. *Authorized* health claims require publication of an FDA regulation after an extensive review of the scientific literature, along with significant scientific agreement that the food/nutrient and disease relationship is well established. Of the health claims allowed for foods, authorized claims undergo the most thorough FDA review. The exact wording of the claim statement is not specified, although the statement appearing on the food label must meet specific criteria.

Statements for authorized health claims cannot quantify the degree of risk reduction, and the terms *may* or *might* must be used to qualify the relationship between a food or dietary component and disease. The label must state that the disease or health-related condition depends on many factors, implying that diet is not the only consideration in disease management. It also must indicate that the benefit related to a disease or health-related condition is a part of a total dietary pattern; thus, the need for an overall healthy diet is enforced. No health claims are permitted for foods containing more than 13 grams of fat, 4 grams of saturated fat, 60 mg of cholesterol, or 480 mg of sodium per reference amount customarily consumed (RACC).[9] Up to double the amount of these components associated with negative health risks are allowed for main dishes and meal products. The RACC is typically one serving as defined on the product label. Health claims cannot be indicated for children under 2 years of age. Table 24-1 lists authorized health claims, requirements

for foods listing these health claims, and sample statements that might be used on a food label.[4–7,9] Table 24-2 shows amounts of soy in various foods, although not all of the foods listed meet all qualifications for a health claim related to soy protein and risk of coronary heart disease (CHD).[10]

Certain health claims for foods, food components, or dietary ingredients (but not dietary supplements) can be made through notification to FDA by the manufacturer after a statement is received from an authoritative scientific body of the U.S. government that has responsibility to protect public health or conduct research related to human nutrition (an *authoritative* claim).[4,6,9] The National Institutes of Health, the Centers for Disease Control and Prevention, and the National Academy of Sciences are sources for authoritative claims. Significant scientific evidence supports such health claims, although FDA itself does not complete an extensive review of the data. Specific wording is required on the claims statement. The four authoritative health claims currently recognized by FDA and required label statements are listed in Table 24-1.[4–6,9]

The third type of health claim is a *qualified* claim. Qualified health claims are appropriate for use when evidence of health benefits for a food, food component, or dietary supplement is still emerging; scientific research supporting the claim tends to be limited or preliminary; and the "significant scientific agreement" level of evidence required for authorized and authoritative health claims cannot be met. Qualified claims are currently allowed for several foods in association with heart disease and cancer, as shown in Table 24-3. FDA-issued health claims for such products require specific wording that includes "qualifying" terms to indicate evidence for the claim is limited.[4–7,9,11] Labeling guidance issued by FDA for qualified health claims intermixes information regarding labeling of dietary supplements and conventional foods.[11] The reader is referred to Chapter 53 for further discussion of qualified health claims and labeling.

Structure and function claims are commonly associated with dietary supplements but can also appear on food labels. These claims indicate the effect of consuming the product on a body structure or function, such as building strong bones or supporting the immune system (versus referencing disease risk). They differ from health claims in that FDA validation or authorization is not required before use, although prior notification of FDA regarding the structure-function claim is required. These claims cannot make reference regarding reduced risk of disease.[4–7,9] Foods that carry a structure or function claim are considered functional foods; they are not dietary supplements when they are represented as a conventional food. For instance, margarine-type spreads with added stanol esters are a food, with the stanol ester considered a food additive. Of interest, dietary supplements in food form (drinks and bars) that are labeled and marketed as dietary supplements are regulated as dietary supplements (see Chapter 53). Distinguishing functional foods from dietary supplements can therefore be confusing.

Foods for Special Dietary Use

Foods for special dietary use, as defined by FDA, include foods used to supply *particular dietary needs,* or to supplement or fortify the usual diet and are marketed as such; they do not meet general dietary needs (see Chapter 23).[4,5,9] Particular dietary needs may exist because of physical, physiologic, pathologic, or other conditions, such as disease, convalescence, pregnancy, lactation, underweight, overweight, infancy, or need for sodium restriction. Foods intended for use as the only nutrient source in the

TABLE 24-1 Authorized and Authoritative Health Claims

Health Claim	Requirements for Foods	Sample Claim Statement Containing Required Components	Selected Foods Meeting Claim Requirements
Authorized Health Claims			
Calcium—osteoporosis	High in calcium Bioavailable Phosphorus content no more than calcium content	Regular exercise and healthy diet with enough calcium helps teens, and white and Asian women maintain good bone health, and may reduce their high risk of osteoporosis later in life.	Milk Orange juice with added calcium
Sodium—hypertension	Low sodium content	Diets low in sodium may reduce the risk of high blood pressure, a disease associated with many factors.	Fruits and vegetables, canned or frozen with no added salt, fresh
Dietary fat—cancer	Low fat "Extra lean" fish and game meat	Development of cancer depends on many factors. A diet low in total fat may reduce the risk of some cancers.	Fruits and vegetables, fresh, frozen, or canned Most cereals Nonfat and low-fat milk and dairy products
Dietary saturated fat and cholesterol—risk of coronary heart disease	Low saturated fat Low cholesterol Low fat "Extra lean" fish and game meat	Although many factors affect heart disease, diets low in saturated fat and cholesterol may reduce the risk of this disease.	Fruits and vegetables, fresh, frozen, or canned Most cereals Nonfat and low-fat milk and dairy products
Fiber-containing grain products, fruits, and vegetables—cancer	Grain product, fruit, or vegetable containing dietary fiber Low fat Good source of fiber without fortification	Low-fat diets rich in fiber-containing grain products, fruits, and vegetables may reduce the risk of some types of cancer, a disease associated with many factors.	Fruits and vegetables, fresh, frozen, or canned Whole-grain breads, cereals, and pasta Brown rice
Fruits, vegetables, and grain products that contain fiber, particularly soluble fiber—risk of coronary heart disease	Fruit, vegetable, or grain product containing fiber Low saturated fat Low cholesterol Low fat Minimum of 0.6 g soluble fiber per RA without fortification	Diets low in saturated fat and cholesterol and rich in fruits, vegetables, and grain products that contain some types of dietary fiber, particularly soluble fiber, may reduce the risk of heart disease, a disease associated with many factors.	Fruits and vegetables, fresh, frozen, or canned Whole-grain breads, cereals, and pasta Brown rice
Fruits and vegetables—cancer	Fruit or vegetable Low fat Good source of vitamin A or C, or dietary fiber without fortification	Low-fat diets rich in fruits and vegetables (foods that are low in fat and may contain dietary fiber, vitamin A, or vitamin C) may reduce the risk of some types of cancer, a disease associated with many factors. [X food is high in vitamin A, vitamin C, and/or is a good source of fiber.]	Broccoli Berries Green beans Carrots Cantaloupe Citrus fruit Most dark green leafy vegetables
Folate—neural tube defects	Contains at least 40 mcg folate per serving Good source without fortification Contains not more than the RDI for vitamin A as retinol, or preformed vitamin A or D	Healthful diets with adequate folate may reduce a woman's risk of having a child with a brain or spinal cord defect.	Most dark green leafy vegetables (see Chapter 23)
Dietary noncarcinogenic carbohydrate sweeteners—dental caries	Sugar-free Eligible substances listed in 21 *CFR* 101.80; examples include xylitol, sorbitol, mannitol, erythritol, D-tagatose, and sucralose Does not lower plaque pH below 5.7 when fermentable carbohydrate is present	Frequent between-meal consumption of foods high in sugars and starches promotes tooth decay. The sugar alcohols in [name of food] do not promote tooth decay. Short claim for small packages: Does not promote tooth decay	Many "dietetic" sugar-free products marketed for people with diabetes Many low-calorie products marketed for weight loss

(continued)

TABLE 24-1 Authorized and Authoritative Health Claims *(continued)*

Health Claim	Requirements for Foods	Sample Claim Statement Containing Required Components	Selected Foods Meeting Claim Requirements
Soluble fiber from certain foods—risk of coronary heart disease	Low saturated fat Low cholesterol Low fat Includes one or more: (1) an eligible source of whole oat or barley with ≥0.75 g soluble fiber per RACC (2) Oatrim containing ≥0.75 g beta-glucan per RACC (3) psyllium husk containing ≥1.7 g soluble fiber per RACC	Soluble fiber from foods such as [name of soluble fiber source (optional—name of food product)], as part of a diet low in saturated fat and cholesterol, may reduce the risk of heart disease. A serving of [name of food product] supplies [X] grams of the [necessary daily dietary intake for the benefit] soluble fiber from [name of soluble fiber source] necessary per day to have his effect.	Rolled oats Oatmeal Whole oats cold cereals Barley Cereals with added psyllium
Soy protein—risk of coronary heart disease	Contains ≥6.25 g soy protein per RACC Low saturated fat Low cholesterol Low fat, unless fat is from whole soybeans	Example 1: 25 g of soy protein a day, as part of a diet low in saturated fat and cholesterol, may reduce the risk of heart disease. A serving of [name of food] supplies [X] grams of soy protein. Example 2: Diets low in saturated fat and cholesterol that include 25 g of soy protein a day may reduce the risk of heart disease. One serving of [name of food] provides [X] grams of soy protein.	See Table 24-2 for soy protein content of some foods
Plant sterol/stanol esters—risk of coronary heart disease	Spreads and salad dressings must contain ≥0.65 g plant sterol esters per RACC Spreads, salad dressings, and snack bars must contain ≥1.7 g plant stanol esters per RACC Low saturated fat Low cholesterol	Example 1: Foods containing at least 0.65 g per serving of vegetable oil sterol esters, eaten twice a day with meals for a total intake of at least 1.3 g, as part of a diet low in saturated fat and cholesterol, may reduce the risk of heart disease. A serving of [name of food] supplies [X] grams of vegetable oil sterol esters. Example 2: Diets low in saturated fat and cholesterol that include two servings of foods that provide a daily total of at least 3.4 g of plant stanol esters in two meals may reduce the risk of heart disease. A serving of [name of food] supplies [X] grams of plant stanol esters.	Margarine spreads with added sterol/stanol esters Orange juice with added sterol/stanol esters

Authoritative Health Claims[a]

Health Claim	Requirements for Foods	Sample Claim Statement Containing Required Components	Selected Foods Meeting Claim Requirements
Whole-grain foods—risk of heart disease and certain cancers	Must contain 51% or more whole-grain ingredients by weight per RACC Low fat Must meet specified dietary fiber content: 3 g/RACC of 55 g; 2.8 g/RACC of 50 g; 2.5 g/RACC of 45 g; 1.7 g/RACC of 35 g	Diets rich in whole-grain foods and other plant foods and low in total fat, saturated fat, and cholesterol may reduce the risk of heart disease and some types of cancer.	Low-fat whole-grain breads and cereals Whole-grain cereals and pasta Brown rice
Potassium—risk of high blood pressure and stroke	Good source of potassium Low sodium Low total fat Low saturated fat Low cholesterol	Diets containing foods that are a good source of potassium and that are low in sodium may reduce the risk of high blood pressure and stroke.	Many fruits and vegetables (see Chapter 23)

TABLE 24-1 Authorized and Authoritative Health Claims *(continued)*

Health Claim	Requirements for Foods	Sample Claim Statement Containing Required Components	Selected Foods Meeting Claim Requirements
Fluoridated water—reduced risk of dental caries	Total fluoride >0.6–1 mg/L Bottled water must meet standards of identity and quality Excludes bottled water for infants	Drinking fluoridated water may reduce the risk of dental caries or tooth decay.	Bottled water containing fluoride
Saturated fat, cholesterol, and trans fat—reduced risk of heart disease	Low saturated fat Low cholesterol Quantity of trans fat on label and < 0.5 g trans fat per RACC Total fat < 6.5 g	Diets low in saturated fat and cholesterol, and as low as possible in trans fat, may reduce the risk of heart disease.	Fruits and vegetables, fresh, frozen, or canned Most cereals Nonfat and low-fat milk and dairy products

Key: RACC, reference amount customarily consumed (usually one serving as listed on label); RDI, recommended dietary intake.

[a] Wording in sample claim statement is required by FDA.

Source: References 4–7 and 9.

diet and those intended to supplement the diet by increasing total dietary intake of a specific ingredient (vitamin, mineral, or other nutrient) are also considered to meet a particular dietary need. These foods are subject to general labeling requirements for foods, and medical supervision of their use is not required. By some definitions, foods for special dietary use are considered functional foods; however, this approach to marketing functional foods is much less broadly seen in the food supply than is structure-function labeling.

Medical Foods

Medical foods are defined in the Orphan Drug Acts Amendments of 1988 and must meet specific criteria before use and distribution. These foods are to be recommended or prescribed by a physician and used under continued medical supervision; however, they are not "prescription-only" products in the same manner as prescription drugs, because they can be sold without a physician's order. Medical foods do not occur naturally; rather, they are specially formulated and processed to meet *distinctive nutritional requirements* of the disease or condition for which they are intended.[4,5] The distinctive requirements for a select medicinal component in the food (or the food product as a whole) must be established by prior medical evaluation on the basis of recognized scientific principles. An example is food products developed with low phenylalanine content for patients with phenylketonuria. Enteral nutrition products are classified as medical foods; however, many products are marketed directly to the

TABLE 24-2 Soy Protein Content of Selected Foods

Food	Amount	Soy Protein (g)	Comments/Uses
Soy burger	1 patty	11–16	
Soybeans, green, cooked/boiled	1/2 cup	13	
Soybeans, sprouted	1 cup	8	
Soy milk, plain or vanilla	8 oz	8	Lactose-free; milk substitute; chocolate or other flavors sometimes available
Soy nuts	1/4 cup	15	Used alone or combined in snack mix
Protein powder, soy	1 tbsp	3.4	Added to other foods to increase protein content
Protein bar, soy	1 bar	10–14	Snack or meal replacement
Tempeh	4 oz (1/2 cup)	16	Used as a meat substitute
Tofu, soft	4 oz (1/2 cup)	16	Blends to cream cheese consistency; used in dips or as cream cheese
Tofu, firm	4 oz (1/2 cup)	13 20	Takes on flavor of what it is cooked with; works well in stir fry and soups

Source: Reference 10.

TABLE 24-3 Qualified Health Claims for Conventional Foods

Food/Nutrient	Disease/Condition	Level of Evidence	Comments
Claims Related to Cardiovascular Disease			
Omega-3 fatty acids: EPA and DHA	CHD	Supportive but not conclusive research	Total fat, saturated fat, cholesterol, and sodium maximum limits apply
Walnuts	Heart disease	Supportive but not conclusive research	1.5 oz of whole or chopped walnuts per day
Nuts	Heart disease	Supportive but not conclusive research	Limited to almonds, hazelnuts, peanuts, pecans, some pine nuts, pistachio nuts, walnuts; 1.5 oz per day
Monounsaturated fat from olive oil	CHD	Limited and not conclusive evidence	Suggested intake of about 2 tbsp (23 g) daily; replaces a similar amount of saturated fat and does not increase the total number of calories
Unsaturated fatty acids from canola oil	CHD	Limited and not conclusive evidence	Suggested intake of about 1.5 tbsp (19 g) daily; replaces a similar amount of saturated fat and does not increase the total number of calories
Corn oil	Heart disease	Very limited and preliminary	Suggested intake of about 1 tbsp (16 g) daily; replaces a similar amount of saturated fat and does not increase the total number of calories
Claims Related to Cancer Risk			
Green tea	Cancer	Highly unlikely to reduce risk	Breast cancer and prostate cancer studies evaluated
Tomatoes, tomato sauce	Prostate, ovarian, gastric, and pancreatic cancers	Unlikely, uncertain, or little scientific evidence	Few studies; major study limitations and conflicting results

Key: CHD, coronary heart disease; DHA, docosahexaenoic acid; EPA, eicosapentaenoic acid.
Source: References 4–7, 9, and 11.

consumer as regular foods, often as meal replacement products, and are readily available without medical supervision. Practitioners should be able to distinguish between medical foods that require physician supervision and those that can be safely used as "nutritional self-care" by the public; for that reason, medical foods are discussed with meal replacement foods in this chapter.

Conventional Foods

Conventional foods that do not fit into any of the preceding four categories can also be classified as functional foods. These foods typically are associated with health benefits in epidemiologic studies, and specific compounds within the foods may have been identified as the functional component. The strength of published research and scientific agreement, however, may not be adequate to support even a qualified health claim at this time. In general, the strength of evidence supporting a functional role for these foods is weak to moderate, and clinical trials tend to be lacking.[6,7] Table 24-4 provides examples of conventional foods and the components likely responsible for their role as functional foods.[6,7,12–17] Some of these foods, such as fruits, vegetables, and whole-grain foods, do have an FDA-recognized health claim, but the claim does not specify a functional component.

Fiber, Prebiotics, and Probiotics

Fiber, prebiotics, and probiotics are components of functional foods that have generated considerable interest in both medical and popular literature during the past decade because of their potential influence on health, particularly gastrointestinal (GI) tract health. In some cases, beneficial effects may extend beyond the GI tract, including improved glucose control, lower serum cholesterol, and reduced inflammation. However, epidemiologic studies generally rely on people recalling their food intake—a challenge that sometimes obscures true associations between selected food components and disease risk. Clinical studies commonly isolate the food component, administering it as a dietary supplement rather than a functional food, and for many studies only a small number of subjects are enrolled. Because isolated components may not have the same effect as a whole food, this approach may produce conflicting results between clinical studies and epidemiologic research.

Fiber

Fiber consists of fruit, vegetable, grain, nut, and legume components that humans cannot digest. Plant cell walls, nonstarch polysaccharides from sources other than plant cell walls (seaweed, microorganisms, or seed husks [psyllium]), resistant starches, and

TABLE 24-4   Examples of Conventional Foods Classified as Functional Foods

Food	Functional Component	Potential Health Benefit	Comments
Apples	Flavonols, phenols, proanthocyanidins, soluble fiber (pectin)	Decreased risk of certain types of cancer; improved glucose and cholesterol concentrations; may contribute to maintenance of heart health	Recommend one a day but amount for health benefit not defined
Banana, ripe	Prebiotics, FOS	Decreased hypertension and hyper-cholesterolemia	Weak evidence for 3–10 g/day
Berries	Anthocyanidins	Antioxidant functions; may contribute to healthy immune system	Recommend ½–1 cup/day but amount for health benefit not defined
Cherries	Anthocyanidins	Antioxidant functions; may contribute to healthy immune system; anti-inflammatory effect	Recommend ½–1 cup/day but amount for health benefit not defined
Cinnamon	Proanthocyanidins	May contribute to maintenance of urinary tract and heart health	Weak evidence; amount for health benefit not well researched
Citrus fruits	Ascorbic acid, zeaxanthin, limonene	Decreased risk of age-related macular degeneration; decreased cancer risk	Weak-to-moderate evidence for decreased macular degeneration with 6 mg/day as lutein; rodent studies with limonene and cancer
Cocoa, chocolate	Flavonols	Antioxidant functions, decreased risk of coronary heart disease	Dark chocolate appears to be best
Corn	Lutein, zeaxanthin, free stanols/sterols	Decreased risk of age-related macular degeneration; may decrease risk of CHD	Weak-to-moderate evidence for 6 mg/day as lutein; health claim for stanol/sterol esters added to foods
Cranberry juice	Proanthocyanidins	Decreased UTI from decreased adherence of bacteria to cell walls; may also prevent adhesion of plaque-forming bacteria in the mouth	Moderate evidence for 300 mL/day to decrease UTI (58% reduction in bacteriuria in 150 elderly women in the first randomized controlled trial [1994])
Cruciferous vegetables: broccoli, brussels sprouts, cauliflower, cabbage	Glucosinolates, indoles, isothiocyanates (sulphoraphane); organosulfur compounds, thiols	Decreased risk of certain types of cancer	Weak-to-moderate evidence for greater than ½ cup/day
Dairy products, including some cheese	Conjugated linoleic acid	Decreased risk of breast cancer; possible role in improved body composition	Weak evidence for breast cancer link; animal studies suggest role in decreased body fat; necessary amount not determined for health effects
Dairy products, fermented (acidophilus milk, buttermilk, kefir, yogurt)	Probiotic organisms (lactobacilli, bifidobacteria)	Maintenance of GI tract health; decreased colon cancer risk; decreased cholesterol	See discussion of probiotics in this chapter
Eggs (yolk)	Lutein, zeaxanthin	Decreased risk of age-related macular degeneration	Weak-to-moderate evidence for 6 mg/day as lutein
Eggs, enriched with DHA	DHA	Decreased risk of CHD, increased HDL cholesterol	Chickens are fed fish oils or algae as a source of DHA
Fatty fish (wild salmon, herring)	Omega-3 fatty acids	Decreased triglycerides and risk of heart disease, including fatal and nonfatal MI	Recommend 2 meals/week with fatty fish; supportive but not conclusive evidence per qualified health claim

(continued)

TABLE 24-4 Examples of Conventional Foods Classified as Functional Foods *(continued)*

Food	Functional Component	Potential Health Benefit	Comments
Flax	Phytoestrogens (lignans); alpha-linoleic acid	Decreased risk of CHD by decreasing cholesterol and platelet aggregation; weak estrogenic activity may decrease hormone-related cancers; maintenance of a healthy immune system; alpha-linoleic acid may contribute to maintenance of visual function	Weak evidence for CHD association; very weak evidence for cancer risk; amounts necessary for health benefit from flax is not defined
Garlic	Organosulfur compounds, thiols	Decreased total and LDL cholesterol; may decrease the risk of gastric cancer; promotes healthy immune function	Weak-to-moderate evidence for about one fresh clove daily for cholesterol; epidemiologic evidence for decreased cancer is equivocal; considerable variation exists in the amount of active compounds for available products
Grapes, red and black	Anthocyanidins; phenolic compounds	Antioxidant functions; decreased cardiovascular risk	Epidemiologic evidence suggesting inverse association with cardiovascular disease risk
Grape juice	Resveratrol	Decreased risk of MI caused by decreased platelet aggregation	Moderate-to-strong evidence for 8–16 oz/day
Greens: spinach, kale, collards	Lutein, zeaxanthin	Decreased risk of age-related macular degeneration	Weak-to-moderate evidence for 6 mg/day as lutein
Jerusalem artichoke	Prebiotics, FOS	Decreased hypertension; decreased hypercholesterolemia	Weak evidence for 3–10 g/day
Meat (beef, lamb, turkey) and milk	Conjugated linoleic acid	Antitumor effect proposed; possible role in improved body composition	Effect suppression of cancer cell growth in rat studies; animal studies suggest role in decreased body fat; necessary amount not determined for health effects
Onions, leeks, scallions	Organosulfur compounds, thiols	Decreased total and LDL cholesterol	Weak-to-moderate evidence
Onion powder	Prebiotics, FOS	Decreased hypertension; decreased hypercholesterolemia	Weak evidence for 3–10 g/day
Rye	Phytoestrogens (lignans)	May contribute to maintenance of heart health and healthy immune system	
Tea, black	Polyphenols; flavonoids	Decreased risk of coronary heart disease	Evidence is not conclusive
Tea, green	Catechins (epigallocatechin-3-gallate, epigallocatechin, epicatechin-3-gallate, epicatechin)	Decreased risk of certain types of cancer; improved CV health; weight control	Qualified health claim evaluation concluded it is highly unlikely that green tea (not specifically catechins) reduces risk for cancer; prevention of CV and obesity weak (intake estimates of >4 cups/day)
Tomatoes and processed tomato products	Lycopene	Antioxidant that efficiently decreased singlet oxygen in biologic systems; possible decreased risk of certain cancers (prostate) and MI	Weak evidence based on inverse associations of tissue lycopene and cancers or MI; qualified health claim evaluation concluded it is unlikely or uncertain that tomatoes/sauce (not specifically lycopene) reduce risks
Tree nuts	Monounsaturated fatty acids, vitamin E	Decreased risk of CHD	Moderate evidence for 1–2 oz/day; some nuts have qualified health claim

Key: CFU, colony-forming units; CHD, coronary heart disease; CV, cardiovascular; DHA, docosahexaenoic acid; FOS, fructooligosaccharides, GI, gastrointestinal; MI, myocardial infarction; UTI, urinary tract infection.

Adapted from references 6, 7, and 12–17.

undigestible oligosaccharides are components of dietary fiber.[18–20] Resistant starches, such as those in legumes and partially milled cereal grains and seeds, withstand the enzymatic activity in the small bowel, reaching the colon relatively intact. Physiologic definitions of dietary fiber generally include fermentation in the colon and evidence of effects on stool bulking, softening, and frequency; on cholesterol lowering; or on glucose control.[18] On the basis of chemical analysis, fibers are defined by solubility in water and buffer solutions as either soluble or insoluble. Different fiber components may have different health effects, and effects of fiber extracted from cell walls may differ from those of in situ fiber because of altered chemical and physical properties. These factors likely contribute to the conflicting results sometimes reported for studies related to health benefits of fiber.

The terms *dietary fiber* and *functional fiber* are related to dietary reference intakes (DRI; see Chapter 23) and distinguish sources of fiber.[19,20] Total fiber is the sum of dietary and functional fiber. Dietary fiber is defined as nondigestible carbohydrates and lignin that are naturally occurring (intrinsic and intact) in plants. Functional fiber is defined as isolated nondigestible carbohydrates that have beneficial physiologic effects in humans. Fiber extracted or modified from plants or animal sources, including chitin and chitosan from the shells of crustaceans, is included as functional fiber. Because of their current widespread use in both professional and nonprofessional literature, the terms *soluble fiber* and *insoluble fiber* are used here. However, gradual replacement of these terms by the specific fibers has been recommended, because viscosity and fermentability may be more important correlates with health effects.[20]

RECOMMENDED AND ACTUAL INTAKE

Adequate intakes (AIs) have been published by the IOM for total fiber as shown in Table 24-5.[21] (See Chapter 23 for general information on AI.) The AIs are based on usual caloric intake in each age group and 14 grams of dietary fiber per 1000 calories, which appears to be the amount needed to promote heart health.[19] Unfortunately, as Table 24-5 shows, actual mean and median fiber intakes of adults in the United States fall considerably below the AI, as determined from national surveys of several thousand participants. The surveys include NHANES 2003–2004[22] the Continuing Survey of Food Intakes by Individuals (CSFII),[19] and the 2000 National Health Interview Survey (NHIS).[23] Data from the third NHANES (NHANES III; 1988–1994) are included for their analysis of soluble and insoluble fiber, and to demonstrate the lack of progress toward meeting goals for fiber intake.[24] Only 38.5% of men and 16.2% of women among the NHIS participants older than 18 years met recommended intakes for fiber.[23]

TABLE 24-5 Adequate Intakes and Actual Intakes for Fiber (g/day)

	Younger Age[a]	Older Age[b]	Data Source
Men			
AI, total fiber	38	30	IOM[21]
Actual intake			
Total fiber, mean	17.5–18.3	16–16.2	NHANES 2003–2004[22]
Total fiber, median	17	16	NHANES III[24]
Soluble fiber	7.1	6.5	NHANES III[24]
Insoluble fiber	13.1	12.7	NHANES III[24]
Mean intake (50th percentile)	17.4–17.9	17.5–16.5	CSFII[19]
Median intake	18.8–20.3	17.7	NHIS[23]
Women			
AI, total fiber	25	21	IOM[21]
Actual intake			
Total fiber, mean	13.2–13.8	14–14.1	NHANES 2003–2004[23]
Total fiber, median	13	13	NHANES III[24]
Soluble fiber	4.9	5.3	NHANES III[24]
Insoluble fiber	9.4	10.3	NHANES III[24]
Mean intake (50th percentile)	12.1–13.1	13.3–13.8	CSFII[19]
Median intake	14.1–14.8	14.1	NHIS[23]
Pregnancy/Lactation			
AI	28/29	N/A	IOM[21]
Actual intake	ND	N/A	

Key: AI, adequate intake; CSFII, Continuing Survey of Food Intakes by Individuals; IOM, Institute of Medicine; N/A, not applicable; ND, no data available; NHANES, National Health and Nutrition Survey; III, third; NHIS, 2000 National Health Interview Survey.

[a] Younger age (years) = 19–50 for AI and CSFII; 18–59 for NHIS; 20–59 for NHANES 2003–2004 and III.

[b] Older age (years) = 51 and older for AI and CSFII; 60 and older for NHIS, and NHANES 2003–2004 and III.

Source: References 19 and 21–24.

The AIs do not specify amounts of fiber on the basis of solubility. Different methods can be used to determine solubility; therefore, different amounts of soluble and insoluble fiber are reported for the same foods. In addition, determination of AI relied heavily on epidemiologic data that correlate fiber intake from foods to health benefits. Foods nearly always provide a mixture of soluble and insoluble fiber along with other potentially beneficial ingredients; however, the ratios differ among foods and health effects may vary. Examples of soluble-to-insoluble fiber ratios include 15%:85% in whole-wheat flour and brown rice; 35%:65% in broccoli, spinach, and tomatoes; 50%:50% in dried fruit and oatmeal; and 60%:40% in oranges.[10]

SOLUBLE AND INSOLUBLE FIBERS

Soluble fibers typically undergo substantial degradation and fermentation in the colon; negligible degradation and fermentation occur with most insoluble fibers.[18-20] Table 24-6 outlines the components and sources typically attributed to soluble and insoluble fibers. The food sources listed are good-to-excellent sources of total dietary fiber and are listed under the heading that exemplifies their predominant health effects. Terms indicating the fiber content of foods are defined by FDA.[25] Excellent sources of fiber are classified as "high fiber," and one serving provides 5 grams or more of fiber. Foods providing 2.5 to 4.9 grams of fiber per serving are considered a "good source" of fiber.

METHODS OF INCREASING FIBER INTAKE

Table 24-7 lists ideas for increasing fiber content in the diet. Caution is advised for the use of fiber-containing products in patients with poor GI motility or underlying GI dysfunction, including narcotic-associated dysmotility. Inadequate fluid intake may also contribute to GI distress from a high-fiber diet. It is advisable to increase fiber intake gradually, because a sudden increase can cause GI distress, including bloating, gas, and occasionally diarrhea.[18,20] A reasonable approach is to add one or two servings of foods that are abundant in fiber, as listed in Table 24-6, to the diet every few days until the AI or other goal for fiber intake is reached. Reading ingredient labels is essential to ensure adequate fiber content, especially for breads and cereals in which a *whole* grain should be the first ingredient listed.

BENEFITS OF FIBER

The generally accepted benefits of fiber are laxation effects, normalization of blood lipid concentrations, and attenuation of blood glucose response.[20] These are the accepted measures of efficacy for fiber sources as required for label claims of fiber content in Canada; only evidence of safety is required in the United States but there must be appropriate evidence to support any health claim made. Other possible benefits of fiber such as cancer risk reduction and weight control have been suggested in humans; however, results are limited and conflicting.

Laxation Stool characteristics associated with laxation, or improved bowel function, include increased stool bulk, weight, and water content; decreased stool transit time and normalization of stool frequency to once daily; reduced symptoms of constipation (see Chapter 16); and an overall improvement in ease of defecation. Epidemiologic studies strongly support the positive role of fiber from whole grains, fruits, and vegetables in laxation. Most studies show strong correlations between dietary fiber intake and increased stool weight and decreased transit time. In a meta-analysis of approximately 100 studies, stool weight increased by 5.4 grams per gram of wheat bran fiber, compared with 4.9 grams per gram of fruits and vegetables, 3 grams per gram of cellulose, and only 1.3 grams per gram of pectin.[19] The first three sources of fiber are associated with improved laxation, whereas the highly fermentable and soluble fiber, pectin, is not. Caution must be used in interpreting stool weight alone, however, because an increase in bacteria within the stool could increase weight without affecting transit time. Also, stool weight is highly variable even with rigidly controlled study diets and some soluble fibers do increase stool bulk.[19,20]

The role of functional fibers in laxation is well accepted, and adequate scientific evidence exists to support FDA approval of some fibers as nonprescription bulking agents for treatment of *occasional* constipation, as discussed in Chapter 16. Studies sup-

---

TABLE 24-6 Components and Sources of Soluble and Insoluble Fiber

	Soluble Fiber	Insoluble Fiber
Food component	Pectins, gums, mucilages, algal substances, and some hemicellulose	Cellulose, lignin, and most hemicellulose
Food with ≥2.5 g of total fiber per serving[a]	Cereals: oat bran (uncooked, 2/3 cup), oatmeal (cooked, 1 cup) Fruits: apples and pears with skin on, oranges (1 medium), figs and prunes (3 small) Vegetables: broccoli, carrots, cauliflower, corn, kale and other greens, dark green or loose leaf lettuce, peas, squash, zucchini (cooked, 3/4–1 cup)	Bran and whole-grain (corn, rye, wheat) products: bran cereals (dry cereal, 1/3–1 cup), brown rice (cooked, 1 cup), whole-wheat bread (2 slices) Dried beans: lima, kidney, pinto, white (cooked, 1/4–1/2 cup) Dried peas: green, split (cooked, 1/4–1/2 cup)
Functional fiber sources	Beet fiber, FOS, guar gum (galactomannan, Benefiber), inulin, karaya gum, konjac mannan, locust bean gum, pectin, psyllium (ispaghula seed husk)	Calcium polycarbophil, methylcellulose, powdered cellulose, soy polysaccharide (also has significant soluble fiber effects)

Key: FOS, fructooligosaccharides.

[a] Serving size shown in parentheses.

TABLE 24-7 Methods for Increasing Fiber in the Diet

- Eat breads containing whole-wheat grain, whole-wheat flour, or other whole grains as the first ingredient on the label. These products should replace breads from refined flours that do not include whole grains.
- Replace part of refined-grain cereals with whole-grain cereal for persons who prefer refined cereals; or mix very high-fiber cereals into a favorite brand of cereal.
- Eat oatmeal as a hot breakfast cereal, or select a cold cereal with oats or whole grain as the primary ingredient.
- Sprinkle bran on cereal, yogurt, or other foods.
- Eat brown rice, whole-wheat pasta, and whole-grain crackers rather than white rice and products from refined grains.
- Add fruit to breakfast cereals, breads, yogurt, and salads.
- Select recipes that use whole-grain flours, and/or add rolled oats to baked goods.
- Select recipes for baked goods that include apples, applesauce, carrots, pumpkins, or other fruits or vegetables as a significant ingredient.
- Add kidney, garbanzo, navy, or other beans to salads and soups, including canned soups. Rinse and drain canned beans to reduce components prone to cause gas.
- Serve fruit and/or vegetable salads with picnic lunches instead of potato chips.
- Serve canned beans (black, kidney, white, or baked) as an alternative protein source.
- Eat fresh or dried fruit for snacks and desserts; frozen and canned fruits can also be used.
- Use a low-fat refried bean dip or humus with whole-wheat baked tortilla chips for snacks.
- Eat fruits and vegetables, including potatoes, with the skin on.
- Select snack or meal replacement bars containing at least 2.5 g fiber per serving.
- Include "finger food" vegetables (carrots, celery, cauliflower pieces, and broccoli flowerets) in lunch boxes and as snacks.
- For children, make animal or other fun shapes from vegetables pieces.
- Eat nuts and/or seeds for snacks, or add to mixed dishes, salads, breads, and cereals.

porting the efficacy of bulk-forming fibers in *chronic* constipation are less certain and tend to be of intermediate-to-low quality.

Normalization of Blood Lipid Concentrations   Data on reduced risk of CHD are sufficient for certain fibers to support an FDA-authorized health claim (Table 24-1).[4,9]

Multiple epidemiologic studies have reported a reduced risk of CHD or cardiovascular disease (CVD) with high dietary fiber intake and/or fiber-rich foods. Table 24-8 summarizes data related to risk of CHD from several large, well-designed prospective epidemiologic studies with longer-term follow-up and pooled data studies.[19,26–30] Overall, these studies indicate a strong inverse relationship between risk of CHD/CVD and intake of whole-grain cereal fiber. Fruit fiber may have a beneficial effect relative to CHD/CVD but the association is less clear. Vegetable fiber does not appear to be associated with reduced risk of CHD/CVD.

A large number of relatively small intervention studies have reported cholesterol-lowering effects with fiber intake, including trials with oats, beans, guar gum, pectin, and psyllium. A meta-analysis also supports the role of "practical" quantities (2–10 g/day) of fiber from guar gum, oat bran, pectin, or psyllium to significantly reduce both total and LDL cholesterol concentrations.[20]

The key to fiber's ability to lower cholesterol and reduce CHD risk appears to be consuming an adequate quantity of highly viscous fiber. Foods most likely to provide a positive effect include cereal grains such as oats, barley, or rye, and beans (legumes). Highly viscous functional fibers associated with lower cholesterol and/or reduced risk of CHD include guar gum, pectin, and psyllium.

Attenuation of Blood Glucose Response   Multiple, large, well-designed prospective epidemiologic and cohort studies with longer-term follow-up have reported an association between consumption of fiber and attenuation of blood glucose, improved insulin response, and/or reduced risk of diabetes, as summarized in Table 24-8.[19,26,27,31–36] The overall conclusion from these studies is that an inverse relationship exists between the risk of diabetes and intake of dietary fiber. Intake of cereal fiber appears to be most frequently related to improved glucose control and/or reduced risk of diabetes; foods most likely to provide a positive effect include cereal grains such as oats, barley, and rye. Some legumes (beans), fruits, and vegetables as well as guar gum and pectin may also have a beneficial effect on glucose control. Evidence suggests that nonviscous fibers, such as wheat bran, have little effect on glycemic control.

Weight Loss and Maintenance   Epidemiologic studies show a lower body mass in participants who eat a high-fiber diet and greater incidence of obesity in those with low intake of dietary fiber.[19] Interventional studies show mixed results with high-fiber diets and weight loss (see Chapter 27).

Colorectal Cancer   Epidemiologic evidence from the European Prospective Investigation into Cancer and Nutrition (EPIC) found an inverse relationship between fiber intake from foods and the risk of colorectal cancer among the 520,000 participants from 10 European countries.[36] However, a pooled analysis including 13 prospective cohort studies with 725,628 participants found no protective effect, whereas another large cohort study (197,623 women aged 50–71 years) found no association between total dietary fiber and colorectal cancer, although whole grain consumption was associated with a moderately reduced risk.[38,39] Despite the inconsistency in results, it is reasonable for practitioners to recommend greater fiber intake, including a variety of sources such as whole grains, fruits, and vegetables, given

TABLE 24-8 Summary of Studies Related to Fiber and Risk of CHD and Improved Glucose Control

Study	Number and Gender[a]	Age Range (years)	Follow-Up Time (years)	Results/Conclusions
Nurse's Health Study; cohort design[19,26,27]	>65,000 women	37–64	10	*CHD:* An inverse relationship between dietary fiber intake and risk of CHD evident only for dietary fiber from cereal sources, not fruits and vegetables; cereal fiber intake averaging 7.7 g/day reduced risk of CHD by 34%, compared with average intake of 2.2 g/day; RR 0.77 with higher fiber intake; 19% decrease in risk for CHD events per 10 g/day increase in dietary fiber and a 37% decrease per 5 g increase in cereal fiber. *Glucose:* RR type 2 DM 2.5 for high-GL/low-cereal-fiber diet (<2.5 g/day), compared with low-GL/high-cereal-fiber diet (>5.8 g/day); more frequent intake of dark breads, whole-grain breakfast cereals, and brown rice was associated with decreased likelihood of developing diabetes.
Health Professionals' Follow-up Study; cohort design[19,27]	>42,000 men	40–75	6–12	*CHD:* RR fatal CHD 0.45 and RR total MI 0.59 in those averaging 28.9 g dietary fiber/day, compared with those averaging 12.5 g/day; stronger association with cereal fiber than with fruits and vegetables; 19% decrease in risk of MI per 10 g/day increase in dietary fiber and a 29% decrease per 10 g/day increase in cereal fiber. *Glucose:* RR type 2 DM 2.17 for high-GL/low-cereal-fiber diet (<2.5 g/day), compared with low-GL/high-cereal-fiber diet (>5.8 g/day).
Iowa Women's Health Study; cohort design[19,27]	Nearly 36,000 women	Postmenopause	6	*CHD:* Approximately one-third decrease in risk of fatal CHD in women with ≥1 serving/day of whole grains, compared with those with little whole-grain intake; risk decreased with fiber from cereals, not fruits and vegetables; decreased likelihood of mortality from ischemic heart disease with more frequent intake of dark (whole-grain) bread and whole-grain breakfast cereals. *Glucose:* Inverse relationship of insoluble fiber intake from cereals and risk of DM; no relationship to fruit, vegetable, legume intake; RR diabetes 0.79 for median intake of 20.5 servings/week of whole-grain products, compared with median of 1 serving/week.
NHANES I epidemiologic follow-up study[29]	9776 men and women	25–74; free of CVD at baseline	19	*CHD/CVD:* Reduced risk of CHD with higher dietary fiber intake, especially soluble fiber. RR 0.88 for CHD and 0.89 for CVD events with median fiber intake of 20.7 g/day versus 5.9 g/day. RR 0.85 for CHD and 0.9 for CVD events with median soluble fiber intake of 5.9 g/day versus 0.9 g/day.

TABLE 24-8   Summary of Studies Related to Fiber and Risk of CHD and Improved Glucose Control *(continued)*

Study	Number and Gender[a]	Age Range (years)	Follow-Up Time (years)	Results/Conclusions
				Glucose: Participants with higher fiber intake reported DM more frequently, but the association was not evaluated in this study.
Cardiovascular Health Study, fiber intake analysis; cohort design[29]	3588 men and women	65 and older (average 72 at baseline), free of known CVD at baseline	8.6	*CHD/CVD:* Cereal fiber intake was inversely associated with incident CVD. Hazard ratio 0.79 (21% lower risk) in highest quintile of fiber intake versus lowest quintile. The difference was seen with about 4.6 g fiber/day (2 slices whole-grain bread). Lower risk predominantly with fiber in dark bread (whole-wheat, rye, pumpernickel). Fruit and vegetable fiber intake was not associated with incident CVD.
Alpha-tocopherol, beta-carotene cancer prevention study[19]	Nearly 22,000 men	50–69	6	*CHD:* RR CHD 0.84 for those averaging 34.5 g dietary fiber/day, compared with those averaging 16.1 g/day with fiber intake adjusted to 2000 calories; high-fiber intake: 12.9 g/1000 cal; low-fiber intake: 5.9 g/1000 cal.
Meta-analysis, diets high in soluble fibers[20]	67 controlled trials			*CHD:* Small but significant decrease in total and LDL cholesterol with intake of 2–10 g/day of viscous fibers including guar gum, oat bran, pectin, or psyllium.
Pooled data, prospective cohort studies[30]	10 studies; total of 91,058 men and 245,186 women	35–98	6–10	*CHD:* RR for all coronary events 0.86 (14% decrease) and RR 0.73 (27% decrease) for coronary death for each 10 g/day increment of total dietary fiber. For cereal fiber, RR 0.9 for all coronary events and RR 0.75 for death; fruit fiber RR 0.84 and 0.7; vegetable fiber RR 1.00 for all coronary events and death. Similar results for men and women.
Nurse's Health Studies: NHS-I and NHS-II; cohort design[31]	Total: 161,737 women; NHS-I: 73,327 NHS-II: 88,410	NHS-I: 37–64 NHS-II: 26–46	12–18	*Glucose:* For each 40 g increment in whole-grain intake, multivariate analysis indicated RR for DM of 0.54 (NHS-I) and 0.64 (NHS-II). BMI accounted for 42% and 57% of the association with RR after adjusting for BMI of 0.7 and 0.83, respectively, for NHS-I and NHS-II.
Atherosclerosis Risk in Communities (ARIC) Study[27]	12,251; white and African Americans	45–64	9	*Glucose:* Inverse relationship of cereal fiber intake and risk of DM in both African American and white subgroups, but statistically significant in only whites; no relationship to fruit and legume intake in either subgroup.
Finnish Mobile Clinic Health Examination Survey[27,30]	2286 men and 2030 women	40–69	10	*Glucose:* Inverse relationship of cereal fiber intake and risk of DM (cereal fiber predominantly from rye; little wheat).

(continued)

TABLE 24–8 Summary of Studies Related to Fiber and Risk of CHD and Improved Glucose Control *(continued)*

Study	Number and Gender[a]	Age Range (years)	Follow-Up Time (years)	Results/Conclusions
U.S. population[27]	9665	Adults	18	*Glucose:* Inverse relationship of vegetable intake with risk of DM.
Seven Countries Study[27]	338; Finnish and Dutch cohorts	Adults	20	*Glucose:* Inverse relationship of legume and vegetable intake with risk of DM.
Danish Inter99 Study[33]	5675	30–60	Baseline data	*Glucose:* Inverse relationship between dietary fiber, fruit, and vegetable intake and insulin resistance.
Insulin Resistance Atherosclerosis Study (IRAS); cohort design[34]	978	40–69, normal (67%) and impaired (33%) glucose tolerance	1-year, semi-quantitative food-frequency questionnaire	*Glucose:* High-fiber bran or granola cereals and shredded wheat showed a strong positive association with insulin sensitivity and a strong inverse relationship with fasting insulin; the associations for whole-wheat, rye, pumpernickel, and other high-fiber bread were evident, but not as strong; no associations noted for cooked oatmeal, cream of wheat, or grits.
Black Women's Health Study; cohort design[35]	59,000 black women	Adult	8	*Glucose:* Inverse relationship between cereal fiber intake and DM (IRR 0.82). GId associated with risk of DM (IRR 1.23) for the highest quartile versus lowest. Stronger associations for BMI < 25 kg/m².
Meta-analysis[36]	24 studies; average of 13–16 subjects	Adults, DM	Averaged under 45 days	*Glucose:* Significant decreases of 13%–14% in fasting, postprandial, and average daily glucose with a high-CHO/high-fiber diet, compared with a low-fiber diet; significant decrease (21%) in postprandial glucose with moderate CHO-high fiber intake; high-fiber intake: 20 g or more/1000 cal.
Pooled date from cohort studies[35]	6 studies; total of 286,125 men and women	26–75	6–18	*Glucose:* 21% decreased risk of type 2 DM with a 2-serving/day increment in whole grain (40–60 g) after adjusting for BMI and other potential confounders.

Key: BMI, body mass index; CHD, coronary heart disease; CHO, carbohydrate; CVD, cardiovascular disease; DM, diabetes mellitus; GId, glycemic index; GL, glycemic load; HDL, high-density lipoprotein; IRR, incident rate ratio; LDL, low-density lipoprotein; MI, myocardial infarction; NHANES I, first National Health and Nutrition Examination Study; RR, relative risk; VLDL, very-low-density lipoprotein.

[a] Number of participants included in the analysis is not always the entire study population; number of trials included in meta-analysis.

Source: References 19 and 26–36.

that fiber intake in most people is well below general guidelines for a healthy diet (see Chapter 23).

Diverticular Disease The Health Professionals Follow-Up Study reported a strong negative association between dietary fiber intake and the incidence of symptomatic diverticular disease.[19] The strongest inverse relationship appears to be with non-viscous dietary fiber, especially cellulose. Case–control studies also find lower dietary fiber intake among people with diverticula.[19] Recommendations for fiber intake in people with diver-

ticular disease depend on the stage of disease but typically follow general dietary recommendations for people with asymptomatic disease and no complications. Those with symptomatic disease should follow the advice of their primary care provider.

Irritable Bowel Syndrome Irritable bowel syndrome (IBS) is a chronic, relapsing GI condition associated with abdominal pain, bloating, and changes in bowel habits that manifest as intermittent constipation and/or diarrhea (see Chapters 16 and 17). Outpatient management of IBS includes increased fiber intake for patients with constipation. A systematic review including 1363 referred patients (non–primary care) noted an overall favorable effect of fiber on IBS-related constipation with relative risk (RR) of 1.56 and a 95% confidence interval (CI) of 1.21 to 2.02.[40] Wheat bran showed favorable results for constipation (RR, 1.54; 95% CI, 1.1–2.14) as did ispaghula (psyllium). Of the 17 studies in the review, 12 reported improvement in global symptoms of IBS with fiber (RR, 1.33; 95% CI, 1.19–1.5) without improvement in abdominal pain. Soluble fiber also improved global symptoms of IBS (RR, 1.55; 95% CI, 1.35–1.78) without improving abdominal pain or bloating.

Prebiotics

Some fibers act as prebiotics, and like all fibers, prebiotics enter the colon undigested. Here they serve as substrates for fermentation by bacteria, primarily bifidobacteria and lactobacilli. Fermentation products, including short-chain fatty acids (acetate, butyrate, and propionate) and lactate, produce an environment favorable to growth of these beneficial bacteria. To be considered a prebiotic, fiber must "selectively stimulate the growth and/or activity of one or a limited number of bacteria in the colon" and benefit the host.[13]

SOURCES AND INTAKE

Inulin-type fructans (ITF), including their partial hydrolysis product fructose oligosaccharides (FOS), are the most common prebiotics. They are found in low amounts in many edible plants including asparagus, bananas, chicory, Jerusalem artichoke, leek, onion, soy, and wheat.[41] The ITF are isolated from such sources and added to foods to attain concentrations that contribute to prebiotic effects. Average intake for adults in the United States is estimated at 2.6 g/day.[42]

HEALTH EFFECTS

Both ITF and FOS significantly increase bifidobacteria in humans. Doses used in studies range from 2 to 40 g/day, although 5 to 8 g/day is thought to be adequate for prebiotic effects.[42,43] The optimal dose for increasing bifidobacteria without developing GI side effects in a 7-day study involving 40 healthy subjects was 10 g/day.[41] However, others consider up to 20 g/day a reasonable amount that should not cause bloating, distention, and flatulence.[42]

Beneficial effects related to prebiotics that are supported by some human data include stool bulking and decreased constipation, better absorption of calcium and magnesium, reduced triglycerides in mildly hypercholesterolemic individuals, and stimulation of bifidobacteria growth.[42,44] Studies with prebiotics for diarrhea are conflicting and results may depend on the etiology of diarrhea.[43,44] Improved vaccine response, decreased GI infections, stimulation of intestinal hormonal peptides, improvement in IBD symptoms, and reduced tumor growth are other possible benefits of prebiotics. Some of the beneficial effects may be enhanced with synbiotics, a mixture of both prebiotics and probiotics that together improve host welfare.[13]

Probiotics

Probiotics are nonpathogenic, living microorganisms that have a beneficial effect on the host when consumed in adequate amounts.[44–48] Probiotics must withstand processing, storage, and delivery of the product, and survive gastric acidity, bile acid lysis, and pancreatic enzyme digestion. Lactic acid–producing bacteria,

especially of the genuses *Lactobacillus, Bifidobacterium,* and *Streptococcus* are most often used in foods and studies. Beyond early infancy, these microorganisms do not permanently colonize the GI tract and must be taken regularly in sufficient quantity to maintain their presence. When a sufficient number of these bacteria are present, they appear to reduce colonization by pathogenic bacteria and enhance mucosal defenses in the GI tract. Table 24-9 lists possible protective effects of probiotics and postulated mechanisms by which these effects occur.[44–46] Caution is advised in interpreting these data, because multiple species and strains of common probiotic bacteria exist and each has potentially different effects. Dosing may also influence response and variable doses are used in studies. The optimum dose for a given probiotic is not known. A minimum concentration of 10^5 colony-forming units (CFU) per gram or milliliter has been proposed for therapeutic purposes, although many factors may influence the necessary dose.[45] Studies showing efficacy typically use a minimum of 10^7 to 10^{10} CFU per dose or 10^8 to 10^{10} CFU daily.[46]

HEALTH EFFECTS

Interest in probiotics has increased dramatically in the past decade. Research covers a wide range of disease states and all ages (premature neonate to elderly). A comprehensive review is beyond the scope of this text; only a glimpse into this active area of research can be provided. Table 24-10 lists some of the uses of probiotics and associated organisms.[45–48] Results may be influenced by the dose, frequency of dose, and/or organisms comprising any individual probiotic product. Most studies have been small and have used isolated bacteria (classified as nutritional supplements) or foods with added probiotics, rather than foods that naturally contain the beneficial bacteria (functional foods).

SOURCES

Many traditional foods are fermented by bacteria and contain high concentrations of lactobacilli. Corn, cassava, millet, leafy vegetables (cabbage), and beans commonly serve as the basic food for fermentation. The vast majority of these foods are eaten primarily in developing countries and only rarely in industrialized countries. A few fermented foods are occasionally eaten in the United States, such as brined olives, Kim chi (Korean fermented cabbage), meso, sauerkraut, and tempeh; however, the major food source of probiotic bacteria is dairy foods. Many major brands of yogurt contain probiotic bacteria, although viable cultures are not required for yogurt in the United States and labels do not list the number of viable probiotic organisms. Liquid yogurt drinks (kefyr) and cultured fluid milk, such as sweet acidophilus milk and buttermilk, can contain variable amounts of viable organisms; however, most provide adequate amounts (10^8 viable organisms per gram). A few brands of cottage cheese contain active cultures, but most do not. With the interest in probiotics, new products are appearing regularly with added probiotic organisms, sometimes with little to no data on the organisms added or to support efficacy in the combinations used.

Assessment of Functional Food Use: A Case-Based Approach

Functional foods play a role in preventing disease and optimizing health. For patients with mild signs of or at risk for CHD, functional foods may be a viable option to pharmacotherapy.

TABLE 24-9 Possible Protective Effects of Probiotics

Effect of Probiotic	Possible Mechanism for the Effect
GI Barrier Function	
Induce production of protective cytokines mediating EC regeneration and inhibiting apoptosis	Action through TLRs Induction of IL-6
Redistribution and increased expression of factors involved in maintaining EC tight junctions	Altered protein kinase C signaling
Counteract effects of inflammatory cytokines associated with increased EC permeability	IL-10 upregulation (regulatory cytokine) Reduced effect of TNF-alpha and INF-gamma Stimulation of IgA secretion
Antimicrobial Activity	
Inhibit growth of potential pathogens	Decreased luminal pH Production of bactericidal proteins (bacteriocins)
Inhibit adhesion of pathogenic bacteria to EC	Increased mucin production Reduced transepithelial resistance associated with binding of some pathogens
Influence production of cryptdins by Paneth cells	Antibacterial action of cryptdins
EC Inflammatory Responses	
Alter EC cytokine production	Down-regulation of bacteria-induced protein kinase C and IL-6 Inhibition of TNF-alpha–induced IL-8 production Down-modulation of genes associated with proinflammatory signal induction
Lymphoid Cell	
Enhance antiviral activity	Inhibition of T-cell proliferation Induction of macrophages to express increased amounts of inflammatory cytokines and nitric oxide Stimulation of granulocyte colony-stimulating factor release by macrophages Increased natural killer T-cell activity
Regulatory T-Cell Induction	
Increased CD4+ (regulatory) T cells with cell-surface TGF-beta (regulatory cytokine)	Monocyte-derived dendritic cells induce IL-10 production by T cells

Key: EC, epithelial cell; IgA, immunoglobulin type A; IL, interleukin; INF, interferon; TGF, transforming growth factor; TLR, Toll-like receptor; TNF, tumor necrosis factor

Source: References 44–46.

Case 24-1 illustrates use of functional foods for a patient with a family history of CHD who wishes to reduce her risk for disease.

MEDICAL FOODS AND MEAL REPLACEMENT FOODS

Medical foods are typically semi-synthetic liquid formulas intended for oral consumption or administration through a feeding tube; these products are commonly known as enteral formulas. In addition, certain liquid diets designed for use in medically supervised very-low-calorie diets or bariatric programs (Optisource and Optifast) are classified as medical foods. Various puddings, shakes, and other solid or semisolid food forms that are specially formulated and processed to meet *distinctive* nutritional requirements of the disease or condition for which they are intended can also be classified as medical foods. Both liquid and solid medical foods replace regular meals or enhance nutrient intake to meet the distinctive nutritional requirements of patients. However, these products are also frequently used to meet general nutritional needs. Practitioners involved with self-care counseling should determine when a product is used as a medical food to meet truly *distinctive* nutritional requirements, as determined by scientific studies, and when it is used as meal replacement or enhancement to meet *general* nutritional requirements. Foods intended to meet general nutritional requirements (see Chapter 23) do not need medical oversight and can be used safely for self-care. In contrast, FDA regulations state that medical foods require

TABLE 24-10 Reported Uses of Probiotics

Condition/Disease	Probiotics Most Often Associated with Benefit[a]	Comments
Allergy		
Atopic dermatitis	*L. rhamnosus* GG, *B. lactis*	Multiple studies show decreased severity; most had <100 subjects, largest study included 230 patients.
Diarrhea		
Acute, prevention or symptomatic relief	***B. lactis* Bb12, *L. rhamnosus* GG,** *L. casei* Shirota, *L. acidophilus*, *L. reuteri*, *S. boulardii*	Studies in infants and children show decreased stool frequency, duration, incidence, and severity for watery diarrhea and viral gastroenteritis but not for invasive bacterial diarrhea; supported by meta-analysis of 34 randomized trials and many other trials.
Antibiotic-associated, prevention and treatment	***L. rhamnosus* GG,** *B. lactis*, *Strep. thermophilus* in pediatric population; *L. rhamnosus* GG, VSL#3[b] in adults	Benefit is supported by pooled data from 6 randomized, controlled trials with 766 young children and many other studies in pediatric patients. Overall, literature supports benefit in adults but not in *Clostridium difficile*–associated diarrhea.
Clostridium difficile colitis, prevention and treatment	*S. boulardii*	Mixed results for antibiotic-associated diarrhea of different etiology.
Infectious (not invasive bacterial diarrhea) and Traveler's diarrhea		Results in randomized, controlled studies are conflicting.
Lactose intolerance	Mixed cultures in fermented milk products	Microbial beta-galactosidase improves lactose hydrolysis; however, there are no studies documenting efficacy.
Radiation enteritis	*L. acidophilus* NDCO1748	Small studies provide promising results.
Rotavirus infection	***L. rhamnosus* GG,** *L. reuteri*, *L. casei* GG, *B. bifidum*, *B. lactis*	Studies in infants/children strongly support beneficial effect for prevention and treatment.
Tube feeding associated		Data from clinical trials are insufficient to recommend probiotic use.
IBD		
Crohn's disease, induce and maintain remission	*E. coli* Nissle 1917, *S. boulardii*, VSL#3	Small clinical studies, some with up to 1-year follow-up, have mixed results, but overall show promise for treatment.
Pouchitis	VSL#3	Small, randomized, double-blind, placebo-controlled study with pouchitis in remission shows benefit and was incorporated into treatment algorithm at some facilities.
Ulcerative colitis	VSL#3	No randomized, controlled trials have demonstrated benefit, but a small uncontrolled trial reported improvement in relapse.
IBS		
Motility disorders	*L. plantarum* 299v and DSM 9843 *S. boulardii* *B. infantis*	Decrease was seen in abdominal pain, bloating, flatulence, and constipation. Decrease in diarrhea, but not in other symptoms. Benefit was seen with only one dosage level of *B. infantis*; results between studies are conflicting.
Infection		
Helicobacter pylori	*L. salivarious*	Probiotic inhibits colonization.
Post-pancreatitis	*L. plantarum* 299	Decrease was seen in infected pancreatic necrosis, abscess formation, and reoperation rate.
Postsurgical	*L. plantarum* 299	Decrease was seen in bacterial infection after liver, gastric, and pancreatic resection.
Post–liver transplant	*L. plantarum* 299	Decrease was seen in cholangitis and pneumonia.
Small-bowel bacterial overgrowth	*L. acidophilus*; *L. plantarum* 299V + *L. rhamnosus* GG	Decrease was seen in inflammation in children, in toxins indicating overgrowth in very small study in hemodialysis patients, and in overgrowth in 6 short-bowel patients, but 2 prospective studies failed to find benefit.

(continued)

TABLE 24-10 Reported Uses of Probiotics *(continued)*

Condition/Disease	Probiotics Most Often Associated with Benefit[a]	Comments
Urogenital	*L. rhamnosus* GG	Prospective, double-blind study in 585 premature infants showed decreased urinary tract infection.
	L. acidophilus, other lactobacilli	Decreased vaginosis was shown in women with recurrent disease.
Intestinal Permeability		
NEC	*L. acidophilus, B. infantis, B. bifidus + B. infantis + Strep. thermophilus*	Retrospective study in >12,000 premature infants showed decreased NEC incidence and mortality; other studies (some using combinations of organisms) also showed decreased NEC.
Liver Disease		
Minimal hepatic encephalopathy	*Strep. thermophilus*, bifidobacteria, *L. acidophilus, L. plantarum, L. casei, E. faecum*, synbiotic formulation	Decrease was seen in portal pressure and bleeding risk; increase in non–urease-producing *Lactobacillus* species and decrease in potentially pathogenic organisms were seen; decreased blood ammonia and reverse encephalopathy were seen.

Key: *B., Bifidobacterium; E., Escherichia;* IBD, inflammatory bowel disease; IBS, irritable bowel syndrome; *L., Lactobacillus;* NEC, necrotizing enterocolitis; *S., Saccharomyces; Strep., Streptococcus.*
[a]Organisms with the most evidence of benefit are bolded.
[b]VSL#3 contains 4 lactobacilli strains, 3 bifidobacteria strains, and *Streptomyces thermophilus.*
Source: References 45–48.

C A S E   2 4 - 1

Relevant Evaluation Criteria	Scenario/Model Outcome
Information Gathering	
1. Gather essential information about the patient's symptoms, including:	
a. description of symptom(s) (i.e., nature, onset, duration, severity, associated symptoms)	Patient has no symptoms; older brother was recently diagnosed with coronary heart disease and her mother died from this disease. The patient wants to do what she can to avoid heart disease and is particularly interested in "functional foods" because of an article she saw in a magazine.
2. Gather essential patient history information:	
a. patient's identity	Mary Romero
b. patient's age, sex, height, and weight	33-year-old female, 5 ft 4 in, 135 lb
c. patient's occupation	Clerk at a department store
d. patient's dietary habits	Eats breakfast most mornings: usually a cup of coffee and cold cereal with reduced-fat (2%) milk
	Lunch: something from the mall's food court; often a sandwich with potato chips and soft drink
	Afternoon snack: typically a candy bar or granola bar
	Dinner: meat (beef, pork, or chicken mostly; fish every once in a while when someone has gone fishing); potatoes or pasta most nights; fresh, frozen, or canned vegetable 4–5 times per week; sweet dessert (cake, pie, baked goods) or ice cream 5–6 times a week; typically has a soft drink with dinner, occasionally an alcoholic drink
e. patient's sleep habits	Usually sleeps 7–8 hours per night

Relevant Evaluation Criteria	Scenario/Model Outcome
f. concurrent medical conditions, prescription and nonprescription medications, and dietary supplements	None; birth control pill and multivitamin
g. allergies	NKA
h. history of other adverse reactions to medications	None
i. other (describe) _____	

Assessment and Triage

3. Differentiate the patient's signs/symptoms and correctly identify the patient's primary problem(s).	Mrs. Romero has no signs/symptoms of disease but wants to follow a preventive strategy with diet.
4. Identify exclusions for self-treatment.	None
5. Formulate a comprehensive list of therapeutic alternatives for the primary problem to determine if triage to a medical practitioner is required, and share this information with the patient.	Options include: (1) Refer Mrs. Romero to her PCP for assessment of heart disease and evaluation of her risk. (2) Refer Mrs. Romero to a registered dietitian for comprehensive nutritional assessment and counseling. (3) Inform Mrs. Romero of foods that have health claims associated with reduced risk of heart disease. (4) Take no action.

Plan

6. Select an optimal therapeutic alternative to address the patient's problem, taking into account patient preferences.	Mrs. Romero may require a combination of the options. (1) Provide basic information and counseling related to functional foods with health claims associated with heart disease. Emphasize authorized and authoritative health claims (Table 24-1), because these have strong scientific evidence supporting the claim. The limited evidence for qualified claims and structure-function claims can be presented along with a discussion of where they fit, if at all, in the patient's overall plan. (2) Refer Mrs. Romero for cholesterol screening (or perform screening in the pharmacy) and assessment for heart disease. (3) Refer Mrs. Romero to a dietitian if she wants/needs more than basic counseling on nutrition or have her request a referral from her PCP (may be necessary for insurance coverage).
7. Describe the recommended therapeutic approach to the patient.	A number of foods with health claims are associated with decreased risk of heart disease. For several foods, there is significant scientific agreement regarding the potential benefits. Using these foods in place of some of your current foods may reduce your risk of heart disease. However, it would also be helpful to know what your risks are, including your cholesterol level.
8. Explain to the patient the rationale for selecting the recommended therapeutic approach from the considered therapeutic alternatives.	Given your family history, you should have your cholesterol checked periodically and be evaluated for other risk factors for heart disease. I can provide you basic information on foods that have health claims related to heart disease and may be of benefit in maintaining heart health. Dietitians are the food and nutrition experts; they can do a comprehensive assessment of your diet and provide more in-depth dietary counseling if you want that.

Relevant Evaluation Criteria	Scenario/Model Outcome

Patient Education

9. When recommending self-care with nonprescription medications and/or nondrug therapy, convey accurate information to the patient:

a. appropriate dose and frequency of administration

(1) Decreased dietary saturated fat and cholesterol: Recommend not more than 10% of calories from saturated fat and not more than 300 mg cholesterol a day, but less is better. Most people find 1% milk to be more acceptable than nonfat (skim) milk, so you might want to try it in place of 2% milk, or you could try soy milk.

(2) Fruits, vegetables, and grain products that contain fiber, particularly soluble fiber: Recommend replacement of white breads and pasta with whole grain. Total dietary fiber should be at least 25 g/day (AI for women 19–50 years of age).

(3) Soluble fiber from oat bran, rolled oats, or whole oat flour in certain foods, or barley: Incorporate these products into the diet as replacement for breads and cereals that are not whole grain.

(4) Soy protein: 25 g/day is required in conjunction with a diet low in saturated fat and cholesterol. For many people, the major dietary modifications needed to eat this much soy are very difficult to make, especially if all family members are not committed to the changes.

(5) Plant sterol and stanol esters: Total intake is at least 1.3 g/day of sterol esters or 3.4 g/day of stanol esters, as part of a diet low in saturated fat and cholesterol. You usually need to eat the products at least twice a day to get the recommended amount. Some margarines and orange juice have added plant/stanol esters.

(6) Whole-grain foods: This health claim overlaps somewhat with that for "grain products that contain fiber" (#2) but does not specify "particularly soluble fiber." Insoluble fibers are also important in health. Look for whole grain, such as whole wheat, as the first ingredient on labels.

To make these health claims, foods must generally contain a certain amount of the component. Check food labels for these claims and for ingredient amounts.

There are also health claims with less vigorous supporting data for which evidence suggests a benefit but research is not conclusive (does not prove a benefit; therefore, these claims may not be as effective or the claim might be changed if new studies are reported. Because the following foods are otherwise healthy foods when used in moderation, they can still be safely incorporated into your diet.

(1) Walnuts and several other types of nuts: 1.5 ounces a day; remember that nuts are a concentrated source of calories, so use judiciously.

(2) Omega-3 fatty acids: specifically eicosapentaenoic acid (EPA) and docosahexaenoic acid (DHA), found in salmon, lake trout, herring, and other oily fish.

(3) Monounsaturated fats from olive oil; 23 g/day (2 tablespoons) in place of a similar amount of saturated fat. A number of salad dressings and a few soft margarines now include olive oil.

(4) Canola oil, unsaturated fatty acids; 19 g/day (1.5 tablespoons) in place of a similar amount of saturated fat. Some cooking oil, a number of salad dressings, a few soft margarines, and some baked goods include canola oil.

b. maximum number of days the therapy should be employed

No limit; preferably, these foods will be incorporated as part of an ongoing healthful diet for life.

c. product administration procedures

These foods can replace other foods in your diet so that the total calories do not increase. The more "healthful" fats must replace saturated fats and not increase the total fat intake. You will need to read food labels carefully to be sure you are getting whole grains, low-saturated fats, low cholesterol, and sterol/stanol esters in the product. Also look for the amount of soy or soluble fiber.

d. expected time to onset of relief

These steps are preventive at this time; for elevated cholesterol, dietary changes typically are effective within a few weeks.

Relevant Evaluation Criteria	Scenario/Model Outcome
e. degree of relief that can be reasonably expected	Mild-to-moderate decrease in total and low-density lipoprotein cholesterol. You should be able to decrease "borderline" high cholesterol to within an acceptable range, but these foods alone would probably not be enough if you had significantly elevated cholesterol, especially considering the history of heart disease in the family.
f. most common side effects	Rapid increases in fiber content of the diet can cause gas and bloating, so it is best to gradually increase the fiber in your diet. Replace 1–2 servings of white bread and pasta with whole-grain products every few days until the refined foods are totally replaced. Also add extra fiber by gradually replacing the low-fiber cereals with a whole-grain cereal or oatmeal. Fruits and vegetables can be increased gradually as well to replace snacks and desserts. Be sure to take plenty of water when eating a high-fiber diet.
g. side effects that warrant medical intervention should they occur	Moderate-to-severe abdominal pain, nausea, vomiting; these side effects may be signs of bowel obstruction or diverticulitis.
h. patient options in the event that condition worsens or persists	Dietary changes for Mrs. Romero are preventive, unless her cholesterol is elevated at the time it is checked. Cholesterol levels should be monitored periodically; if cholesterol increases to an unacceptable level despite these dietary changes, it may be necessary for Mrs. Romero to consider drug (statin) therapy.
i. product storage requirements	See food label.
j. specific nondrug measures	N/A
10. Solicit follow-up questions from patient.	Where can I find more information on dietary changes and diet plans to prevent heart disease? May I use dietary supplements instead of changing to functional foods? Most information on the Internet is advertising for dietary supplements.
11. Answer patient's questions.	The FDA Web site (www.fda.gov) includes information on health claims and food labels that you might find helpful. You could consider making an appointment with a registered dietitian who could help develop some menus that incorporate foods you like and provide more specific plans for substituting healthier foods. Your health plan may contract with a dietitian. If not, the American Dietetic Association can provide the name(s) of private consultants and the contact information for a dietitian. The phone number for referrals is on their Web site (www.eatright.org). In general, foods are better than supplements. Many studies have shown beneficial effects from a diet containing fiber-rich foods and whole grains but not with isolated supplements. Psyllium, found in products like Metamucil, fits criteria for a health claim related to soluble fiber and risk of congestive heart disease, and could be used to increase soluble fiber. It also has the added benefit of reducing constipation, as do fibers from whole grains.

Key: AI, adequate intake; FDA, Food and Drug Administration; NKA, no known allergies; OTC, over-the-counter; PCP, primary care provider.

recommendation or prescription by a physician or authorized prescriber and ongoing medical supervision.[9] When enteral formulas are used to meet general nutritional requirements, however, third-party providers may refuse to cover the cost under insurance benefits, leaving patients with self-care responsibility.

Enteral Formula Uses

Tube Feeding

Enteral formulas are best known as complete nutritional replacements for patients requiring a feeding tube to meet their nutritional needs, such as stroke patients with severe dysphagia. Patients who cannot, should not, or will not take adequate nutrients by mouth are candidates for tube feeding. Patients requiring tube feeding should be under medical care; tube feeding is not a condition conducive to safe and effective self-care. For information related to tube feeding, the reader is referred to one of the many specialized references available, to the American Society for Parenteral and Enteral Nutrition (ASPEN; www.nutritioncare.org), the national organization that focuses on specialized nutrition support, or to the Oley foundation (www.oley.org), a consumer-oriented organization for support of individuals requiring intravenous or tube feeding.

Many enteral preparations currently are available. Most formulas provide nutritional support consistent with general dietary guidelines and are safe for use in self-care. Formulas intended for patients with impaired digestion and those designed for specific metabolic or clinical conditions require oversight by a health care provider. Common formula characteristics that are likely to result in its use as a true medical food requiring medical supervision are listed in Table 24–11, along with a few representative products.

Supplementation of Nutrition Intake

Enteral products are frequently used as an oral supplement to normal or impaired nutrient intake. Persons of advanced age are often the focus population for supplemental nutrition because of effects of chronic disease and impaired mobility on nutrient intake. Oral nutritional supplements do appear to benefit hospitalized members of this population who are undernourished at baseline; however, routine supplementation for this population at home or for those who are well nourished in any setting is not supported by available evidence.[49] Finally, enteral formulas have been increasingly marketed as "meal replacements." Marketing targets healthy individuals who perceive a meal replacement product as a healthier alternative to fast foods or skipping a meal.

Classification of Enteral Nutrition Products

Enteral products are classified as polymeric formulas, oligomeric formulas, and modular components. In addition, a growing segment of meal supplement and meal replacement products, including beverages, bars, and puddings, are designed to assist in meeting nutrient goals within an appropriate caloric intake.

Polymeric Formulas

Polymeric formulas are used most commonly. They are for individuals with normal digestive capability and contain macronutrients in the form of intact proteins, carbohydrates, and fatty acids or oils. Most individuals who require alternative nutrition support will tolerate and do well with standard polymeric formulas. The standard formulas usually (1) are 1.0 kcal/mL unless concentrated to provide less free water; (2) contain a macronutrient composition typical of the American diet (carbohydrate: 45%–70%, protein: 10%–18%, and fat: 20%–40%); and (3) are isotonic to slightly hypertonic (300–450 mOsm/kg) to reduce the risk of osmotic diarrhea; however, flavored products are often in the range of 500 to 700 mOsm/kg. These formulas are generally safe for self-care when taken orally. The formulas listed in Table 24–12 as generally safe for self-care are polymeric formulas.

Oligomeric Formulas

Oligomeric products require minimal digestion and are also known as predigested, peptide, or elemental formulas. They contain free amino acids, hydrolyzed or partially hydrolyzed protein, and less complex carbohydrates; these formulas frequently alter the fat content to improve absorption in patients with impaired absorption. They are rarely consumed orally because of very poor palatability. In general, oligomeric formulas require medical supervision.

Modular Products

Modular products supplement a single macronutrient. Examples include protein powder, medium-chain triglyceride oil, emulsified oils, and powdered, flavorless glucose polymers. These products can be incorporated into food to increase protein and calorie content. They are used to provide a more appropriate balance between macronutrient sources for an individual. For example, a protein powder may be useful in a person of advanced age who is having difficulty meeting the protein requirement with their usual oral diet.

Specialty Formulas

Specialty formulas may be either polymeric or oligomeric. They are designed to optimize the nutrient intake and improve disease management for patients with specific disease states such as renal insufficiency, diabetes mellitus, hepatic dysfunction, and carbon dioxide–retaining pulmonary dysfunction. The use of specialty formulas is controversial because data supporting improved outcomes are minimal. In general, use of specialty formulas requires medical supervision. Consultation with a registered dietitian, certified nutrition support nurse, or board-certified nutrition support pharmacist may be warranted.

Some "specialty" formulas, such as certain pulmonary and diabetic formulas, alter the ratio of fat and carbohydrate but contain no special dietary components. Although technically such products are medical foods, there would be little concern for most individuals who used them to replace a few meals per week. However, individuals must be encouraged to limit use of these products unless otherwise advised by their primary care provider or a practitioner who specializes in nutritional

TABLE 24-11 Enteral Formula Characteristics Consistent with Need for Medical Supervision

Characteristic	Examples
Protein as peptides and/or free amino acids	Peptamen, Crucial, Vivonex Plus
Alteration of the amino acid content by addition of individual amino acids, such as glutamine, arginine, or branch-chain amino acids	Impact, Hepatic Aid II
Addition of specific fatty acids to alter the inflammatory response	Oxepa
Addition of significant amounts of medium-chain triglycerides to alter absorption	Portagen
High percentage (>50%) of calories from fat	Pulmocare
Very-high-protein content (≥25% of calories as protein)	Replete
Intended for patients with organ failure	Nepro, NutriRenal, NutriHep

TABLE 24-12 Meal Replacement Products/Liquid Formulas Suitable for Self-Care

Product Name	Energy kcal/mL	Protein g/L (% kcal)	CHO g/L (% kcal)	Fat g/L (% kcal)	Fiber g/L	Comments
Routine Formula						
Boost with Benefiber	1.01	42 (17)	173 (67)	17.8 (16)	12.5 (S)	Boost Drink has similar nutrient profile without fiber.
Ensure Fiber	1.06	37 (14)	143 (64)	37 (22)	12	Fiber includes FOS; Ensure has similar nutrient profile without fiber.
Jevity 1 Cal	1.06	44 (17)	155 (54)	35 (29)	14.4	Fiber from soy; Osmolite 1 Cal has similar nutrient profile without fiber.
Routine Formula with Extra Protein						
Boost High Protein Drink	1.01	61 (24)	139 (55)	23 (21)	None	
Ensure High Protein	0.97	50 (21)	129 (55)	25 (24)	None	
Routine Concentrated (High-Calorie) Formula						
Boost Plus	1.52	59 (16)	200 (50)	58 (34)	None	
Ensure Plus	1.45	54 (15)	208 (56)	46 (29)	None	
HI-CAL	1.98	83 (17)	214 (43)	88 (40)		Use sparingly if used for self-care because of high-fat content; higher fat allows concentrated calories.
Jevity 1.5 Cal	1.5	64 (17)	216 (54)	50 (29)	22 (75% I; 25% S, FOS)	Osmolite 1.5 Cal has similar nutrient profile without fiber.
Diabetic Formula[a]						
Boost Glucose Control Drink	0.8	68 (34)	68 (33)	30 (33)	13	
Boost Diabetic	1.05	57 (22)	83 (31)	49 (42)	14 (I, S, FOS)	
Glucerna Select	1.0	50 (20)	96 (31)	54 (49)	21 (high S, FOS)	Use sparingly if used for self-care because of high-fat content; for oral use only; not intended as sole source of nutrition.
Nutren Glytrol with Prebio	1.0	45 (18)	100 (40)	48 (42)	15 (I, S)	Amylase starch (low-glycemic index); use sparingly if used for self-care because of high-fat content.
RESOURCE Diabetic TF	1.0	64 (20)	100 (36)	47 (44)	15 (I, S)	Use sparingly if used for self-care because of high-fat and high-protein content; use for tube feeding.
Pulmonary Formula[b]						
Pulmocare	1.5	63 (17)	106 (28)	93 (55)	None	Use sparingly if used for self-care because of high-fat content
Nutren Pulmonary	1.5	67 (18)	101 (27)	93 (55)	None	Use sparingly if used for self-care because of high-fat content
Other Meal Replacements and Supplements						
Resource Breeze	10.6	38 (14)	131 (86)	None		Product, a clear liquid, is not intended as sole source of nutrition.
Carnation Instant Breakfast	0.92	13 (25)	39 (13)	2.5 (4)		Put 1 packet in 1 cup skim milk; mixing with 2% or whole milk would increase calories as fat.
Glucerna Shake	0.93	42 (18)	122 (47)	36 (35)	11.7	Fiber is from FOS and soy polysaccharide; use orally, not for tube feeding; use sparingly if used for self-care because of high-fat content; product not intended as sole source of nutrition.
Myoplex Delux	340/78 g packet	53 g/ packet	28 g/ packet	4.5 g/ packet	7 g/packet	Use for meal replacement.

(continued)

TABLE 24-12 Meal Replacement Products/Liquid Formulas Suitable for Self-Care *(continued)*

Product Name	Energy kcal/mL	Protein g/L (% kcal)	CHO g/L (% kcal)	Fat g/L (% kcal)	Fiber g/L	Comments
Myoplex Lite	180/78 g packet	25 g/ packet	20 g/ packet	1.5 g/ packet	3 g/packet	Use for meal replacement.
Modular Components						
Microlipid	4.5	0	0	500 (100)		Modular component (available in 89-mL bottle) is composed of safflower oil; add to enteral formula or foods to increase calories as fat.
Moducal Powder	30/tsp	0	8/tsp (100)	0		Modular component is composed of malto-dextrin; add to enteral formula or foods to increase calories.
ProMod Powder	28	5 (71)	0.67 (10)	0.60 (19)		Listed amounts of modular component are per 6.6 g scoop; add to enteral formula or foods to increase protein.
RESOURCE Benecalorie	7	16 (9)	0	71 (91)	None	Product is a modular component; add to enteral formula or foods to increase calories.
RESOURCE Benefiber		3 per serving (100)			3 per serving	Product is soluble fiber.

Key: CHO, carbohydrate; FOS, fructose oligosaccharides; I, insoluble fiber; S, soluble fiber

[a] Data supporting improved glycemic control is lacking; therefore, the American Society of Parenteral and Enteral Nutrition (ASPEN) does not recommend the routine use of diabetic specialty formulas.[50] Fat content is higher than that recommended by general dietary guidelines and the American Diabetes Association.

[b] Data supporting excessive carbon dioxide production with appropriate caloric intake and decreased hospitalizations with use of pulmonary formulas are lacking; therefore, ASPEN does not recommend the routine use of pulmonary-specific formulas.[50] Fat content is higher than that recommended by general dietary guidelines.

Note: The most current and detailed information is available at manufacturer Web sites, including Abbott Nutrition (www.abbottnutrition.com), Novartis Nutrition (www.novartisnutrition.com), and Nestle Nutrition (www.nestle-nutrition.com).

management of their condition. They should advise their primary care provider when they use these products, because management of the underlying disease itself requires medical oversight. Table 24-12 includes examples of pulmonary and diabetic formulas.[50]

Product Use for Self-Care

All products recommended for self-care should contain basic nutrition labeling including serving size, calories, protein, fat, and other components consistent with food labeling so that nutrient intake can be determined in the same manner as with regular foods. Many formulas are available in a variety of flavors to reduce taste fatigue; slight differences in nutrient content may be noted among the flavors.

Administration and Monitoring Guidelines for Enteral Nutrition

For products taken orally, the practitioner should encourage the individual to vary the flavors to avoid taste fatigue and consume the product after an attempt to eat a well-balanced meal or a between-meal snack. Chilling may improve palatability. Once opened, the container should be kept under refrigeration to prevent bacterial growth, and all open or prepared products should be discarded after 24 hours.

When products are given as tube feeding instead of taken orally, medical supervision is recommended. Referral to a nutrition support practitioner may be appropriate. Medical referral is appropriate for individuals who develop diarrhea, nausea, or abdominal distention when taking meal replacement formulas. Formula-related diarrhea is an osmotic diarrhea that usually stops within 24 hours of discontinuing the formula; diarrhea that persists longer is unlikely to be caused by the formula per se. Lactose intolerance is seldom an issue with enteral formulas, because most formulas are lactose-free except powders prepared with milk. High-fat products can delay gastric emptying, resulting in nausea and/or bloating.

Food–Medication Interactions

Interactions between medications and enteral formulas often are complex and poorly understood. When the interaction involves a component of the formula, the interaction has the potential to occur with either oral administration or feeding tube administration. The practitioner is advised to consult specialty references for a more complete listing and explanation of such interactions. General practice for certain medications (including phenytoin, carbamazepine, and warfarin) is to hold the formula for 1 or 2 hours before and after administering the medication, especially when therapeutic levels are not achieved with typical doses. It is reasonable to suggest this same precaution to an individual who takes formula by mouth and to advise supervision of the medication response by a primary care provider. Vitamin K content of the formula should also be checked for individuals on warfarin. Although most formulas provide no more vitamin K than a typical diet, a few contain amounts that could interfere with anticoagulation. Manufacturers' Web sites, as listed at the bottom of Table 24-12, provide detailed, up-to-date information on the nutrient content of formulas.

Other Medical Foods and Meal Replacement Food

Foods designed for use in weight loss and bariatric programs require medical supervision when used as intended because of significant medical risks associated with rapid weight loss. These foods include liquid diets (Optisource High Protein Drink and Optifast 800 Ready to Drink) and various nutrition bars (Optisource Mini Nutrition Bar and Optifast Nutrition Bar). Meal replacement foods such as Slim Fast, Weight Watchers, and Jenny Craig products can help control portion size and balance nutrient intake. They can be used safely without medical supervision; however, they should be used as part of an overall weight-loss plan (see Chapter 27).

Assessment of Enteral Nutrition and Meal Replacements: A Case-Based Approach

The first step in assessing the type of meal replacement (or supplement) to recommend is to determine whether the individual has any exclusion to self-care as listed in Table 24-13. If self-care is appropriate, ascertain the reason for a meal replacement/supplement so that the most appropriate product can be selected. For instance, a person of advanced age with early satiety may benefit from a concentrated formula that provides 1.5 or 2 calories per milliliter, whereas a young person wanting a meal supplement for use with weight lifting may benefit from a higher protein formula. The selected formula should be appropriate to meet the individual's specific nutritional needs according to health status, while also avoiding excessive or contraindicated macronutrients and micronutrients.

Meal replacement products can have efficacy for the treatment of many health concerns. Traditionally, meal replacement has been considered a therapeutic intervention needed to maintain adequate nutrition in malnourished patients, to completely replace nutritional intake in patients with a physical limitation that interferes with nutritional intake such as dysphagia, or to precisely control intake of specific dietary components (calories for obesity and phenylalanine in phenylketonuria). Increasingly, nutrition products are used as lifestyle choices of self-directed therapy. This practice is particularly true of the meal replacement products used by working individuals who are too busy to prepare or eat a proper meal, or who perceive these products as healthier alternatives to fast foods. Case 24-2 illustrates assessment of a patient with dysphagia and weight loss who seeks a liquid meal replacement.

TABLE 24-13 Exclusions for Self-Care with Enteral Formulas

Condition	Example/Comment
Organ dysfunction requiring diet modification	Renal insufficiency requiring restriction of protein and electrolytes eliminated through the kidneys (potassium, phosphorus, magnesium)
Gastrointestinal dysfunction	Poor motility: Dietary modification may be required to avoid bowel obstructions; enteral formula may be appropriate under the supervision of a primary care provider or nutrition specialist, but not as self-care.
	Reduced absorption: Hydrolyzed protein, modified fats, and/or relatively simple carbohydrates may be necessary for adequate absorption; monitoring for nutrient deficiencies is required.
	Dysphagia: Referral for medical evaluation is required.
	Bariatric surgery: Medical supervision is required; recommendations of primary care provider or nutrition specialist should be followed.
Significant unintended weight loss	Refer for medical evaluation to determine the etiology.
	Life-threatening fluid and electrolyte abnormalities can occur when refeeding these individuals; medical supervision and monitoring are required.
Disease state affected by diet, such as diabetes mellitus, chronic obstructive pulmonary disease	Enteral formula may be appropriate to meet nutritional requirements; however, use should be under the supervision of a primary care provider or nutrition specialist, but not as self-care.

Relevant Evaluation Criteria	Scenario/Model Outcome
Information Gathering	
1. Gather essential information about the patient's symptoms, including:	
a. description of symptom(s) (i.e., nature, onset, duration, severity, associated symptoms)	Patient describes difficulty swallowing solid foods for several weeks and requests a "low-cost Ensure product" that she can drink. She describes solid foods as "getting stuck" in her throat.
b. description of any factors that seem to precipitate, exacerbate, and/or relieve the patient's symptom(s)	She can drink liquids, but all solid food seems to be a problem, even soft foods.
c. description of the patient's efforts to relieve the symptoms	She takes only liquids, avoids solid foods, crushes all pills and mixes them with water.
2. Gather essential patient history information:	
a. patient's identity	Abigail Quinn
b. patient's age, sex, height, and weight	74-year-old female; 5 ft 5 in; 120 lb
c. patient's occupation	Retired bookkeeper
d. patient's dietary habits	She has been taking only liquids for the past several weeks.
e. patient's sleep habits	Averages 5–6 hours per night but naps during the day
f. concurrent medical conditions, prescription and nonprescription medications, and dietary supplements	Hypertension, treated with hydrochlorothiazide/triamterene; osteoporosis, treated with calcium, vitamin D, and alendronate; multivitamin
g. allergies	NKA
h. history of other adverse reactions to medications	None
i. other (describe) _____	Weight loss over the past 2–3 months; usual weight 135 lb; history of stroke several years ago
Assessment and Triage	
3. Differentiate the patient's signs/symptoms and correctly identify the patient's primary problem(s).	Dysphagia is of unknown cause but could be related to stroke or esophageal damage related to alendronate. Weight loss of 11% over 2–3 months is significant, and may place the patient at risk of electrolyte and fluid abnormalities associated with refeeding syndrome.
4. Identify exclusions for self-treatment.	Significant weight loss
5. Formulate a comprehensive list of therapeutic alternatives for the primary problem to determine if triage to a medical practitioner is required, and share this information with the patient.	Options include: (1) Refer Mrs. Quinn to her PCP for evaluation of her dysphagia and assessment of nutritional status. (2) Recommend a liquid meal replacement product that can be used without medical supervision. (3) Take no action.
Plan	
6. Select an optimal therapeutic alternative to address the patient's problem, taking into account patient preferences.	Refer the patient to her PCP for evaluation.
7. Describe the recommended therapeutic approach to the patient.	N/A
8. Explain to the patient the rationale for selecting the recommended therapeutic approach from the considered therapeutic alternatives.	You need to see your PCP, because the swallowing problem may be related to the alendronate you take to improve your bone strength or to something more serious. Your weight loss also indicates that blood tests might be needed to monitor your electrolytes when you start taking the liquid nutrition product.

C A S E   2 4 - 2   (continued)

Relevant Evaluation Criteria	Scenario/Model Outcome
Patient Education	
9. When recommending self-care with nonprescription medications and/or nondrug therapy, convey accurate information to the patient.	Criterion does not apply in this case.
10. Solicit follow-up questions from patient.	Why is the weight loss so concerning? I thought it was good for me to weigh less.
11. Answer patient's questions.	Many people are overweight and they are encouraged to loose weight. However, your usual weight was considered a healthy weight; you had a body mass index of 22.4, which is considered normal. Any time weight loss is not planned, there are concerns about the cause. Rapid weight loss can cause changes in blood tests (your electrolytes) that could affect your heart and breathing.

Key: BMI, body mass index; N/A, not applicable; NKA, no known allergies; PCP, primary care provider.

Patient Counseling for Enteral Nutrition and Meal Replacements

Advancements in enteral products and home infusion therapy are allowing more people with serious, even terminal, illnesses to be cared for at home. Enteral products are also appropriate for ambulatory patients with metabolic or digestive diseases and for persons who want to ensure adequate nutrition for their life stage. Practitioners serve a pivotal role in helping patients to use the product best suited for their nutritional needs and to use it under medical supervision when appropriate. The patient education box lists specific information to provide patients and caregivers.

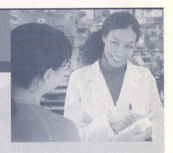

PATIENT EDUCATION FOR Enteral and Meal Replacement Products

The objective of self-treatment is to provide the appropriate amount and types of specific micronutrients and macronutrients to meet the individual's nutritional needs. For most individuals, the product instructions and self-care measures listed here will help ensure optimal therapeutic outcomes.

- Typical products provide 1 cal/mL; higher calorie products are available if you must limit your fluid intake or can drink only a small amount at a time.
- When drinking the formula, take about one-half to one can at a time. You can drink the formula at room temperature, but it may taste better if chilled or semifrozen as a slush-type drink.
- Varying the flavor of the formula may reduce taste fatigue.
- For tube feeding, the product should be used as directed by your primary care or nutrition care provider. The Oley Foundation (www.oley.org) provides consumer information on tube feeding.

- Keep opened containers refrigerated and covered to prevent bacterial growth; discard all remaining prepared products after 24 hours. Unopened product can be stored at room temperature.
- Use of meal replacement products as the sole or primary source of nutrition for more than a short time (2–3 weeks) requires medical supervision and should be discussed with your primary care provider. Periodic laboratory testing may be appropriate to detect electrolyte abnormalities in this situation.
- Monitor blood glucose levels if you have diabetes or have had high blood glucose (sugar) levels. Talk to your primary care provider if blood glucose levels are high or low.

KEY POINTS FOR FUNCTIONAL AND MEAL REPLACEMENT FOODS

➤ The definition of functional foods typically includes "health benefits beyond those of basic nutrition."

➤ Health claims are statements that describe an association between a food, food component, dietary ingredient, or dietary supplement and the risk of a disease or health–related condition.

➤ Authorized and authoritative health claims meet the significant scientific agreement level of evidence. These claims should routinely be incorporated into counseling for lifestyle changes associated with health benefits and, when appropriate, as part of an overall plan for management of diseases associated with these claims.

➤ Qualified health claims do not meet the significant scientific agreement level of evidence; claims statements must include language that indicates the "qualified" nature of the health claim.

➤ Structure and function claims lack the significant scientific agreement level of evidence and make no association between the product and risk of a disease or health-related condition; they do not require validation or authorization by FDA.

➤ Health care providers should understand the limitations of qualified health claims and structure-function claims. When counseling for lifestyle changes, the limited scientific evidence for these claims should be clearly delineated so that individuals can understand the role, or lack thereof, for these products in a healthy lifestyle.

➤ Foods for special dietary use meet *particular dietary needs* related to physical, physiologic, pathologic, or other conditions, such as disease, convalescence, pregnancy, lactation, underweight, overweight, infancy, or need for sodium restriction, or they supplement or fortify the usual diet; they are subject to general labeling requirements for foods and do not require use under medical supervision.

➤ Medical foods are specially formulated and processed to meet *distinctive nutritional requirements* (established by medical evaluation based on recognized scientific principles) of the disease or condition for which they are intended. These foods are to be recommended and used under medical supervision.

➤ Conventional foods classified as functional foods are typically associated with health benefits in epidemiologic studies; the evidence supporting a functional role for these foods is weak to moderate, with clinical trials often lacking.

➤ Epidemiologic studies strongly support the positive role of fiber from whole grains, fruits, and vegetables in laxation.

➤ Adequate intake of highly viscous fiber, including cereal grains, guar gum, pectin, and psyllium, are associated with reduced cholesterol and CHD risk.

➤ Improved glucose control and diabetes risk reduction are associated with highly viscous fiber, including cereal grains, legumes, fruits, vegetables, guar gum, and pectin.

➤ Prebiotics are fermentable fibers that selectively stimulate the growth and/or activity of one or a limited number of bacteria in the colon (bifidobacteria and lactobacilli), thereby benefiting the host.

➤ Probiotics are nonpathogenic, living microorganisms that have a beneficial effect on the host when consumed regularly in adequate amounts. They are often present in fermented products from milk (yogurt and kefir) or plants (sauerkraut and miso).

➤ Probiotics have shown beneficial effects in a number of diseases; however, the particular species and dose necessary for beneficial effects often remain controversial and may vary from condition to condition.

➤ Enteral nutrition products are classified as medical foods; however, many polymeric enteral formulas are readily available without enforcement of the provision for medical supervision and can often be used safely as a meal replacement product.

➤ Specialty enteral formulas should be used with medical supervision, not for self-treatment.

REFERENCES

1. International Food Information Council. Consumer Attitudes toward Functional Foods/Foods for Health, 2007. Available at: http://www.ific.org/research/foodandhealthsurvey.cfm. Last accessed August 10, 2008.

2. International Food Information Council. Consumer Attitudes toward Functional Foods/Foods for Health, 2005. Available at: http://www.ific.org/research/foodandhealthsurvey.cfm. Last accessed August 10, 2008.

3. Food Navigator.Com USA. Probiotics Lead Functional Category, Datamonitor. February 9, 2007. Available at: http://www.foodnavigator-usa.com/Financial-Industry/Probiotics-lead-functional-category-Datamonitor. Last accessed August 14, 2008.

4. Institute of Food Technologists. Expert Report on Functional Foods: Opportunities and Challenges, 2005. Available at: http://members.ift.org/IFT/Research/IFTExpertReports/functionalfoods_report.htm. Last accessed August 10, 2008.

5. Burdock GA, Carabin IG, Griffiths JC. The importance of GRAS to the functional food and nutraceutical industries. *Toxicology.* 2006;221:17–27.

6. Meister K. Facts About "Functional Foods." New York: American Council on Science and Health; 2002. Available at: http://www.acsh.org. Last accessed August 10, 2008.

7. Hasler CM, Bloch AS, Thomson CA, et al. Position of the American Dietetic Association: functional foods. *J Am Diet Assoc.* 2004;104:814–26.

8. Lukovitz K. Functional Food Sales Hit $25 Billion in US in 2006. Available at: http://www.mediapost.com/publications/index.cfm?fuseaction=Articles.showArticle&art_aid=55835. Last accessed August 15, 2008.

9. US Department of Health and Human Services, Food and Drug Administration, Center for Food Safety and Applied Nutrition. Guidance for Industry. A Food Labeling Guide. April 2008. Available at: http://www.cfsan.fda.gov/~dms/2lg-toc.html. Last accessed August 14, 2008.

10. Agriculture Research Service, US Department of Agriculture (USDA). Nutrient data laboratory [database online]. [Search for "standard reference."] Available at: http://www.nal.usda.gov/fnic/foodcomp/search. Last accessed August 10, 2008.

11. US Food and Drug Administration, Office of Nutritional Products, Labeling, and Dietary Supplements. Qualified Health Claims Subject to Enforcement Discretion. April 2007. Available at http://www.cfsan.fda.gov/~dms/qhc-sum.html. Last accessed August 10, 2008.

12. International Food Information Council Foundation. Functional Foods. May 2004. Available at: http://www.ific.org/nutrition/functional/index.cfm. Last accessed February 15, 2008.

13. Hasler CM. Functional foods: benefits, concerns and challenges—a position paper from the American Council on Science and Health. *J Nutr.* 2002; 132:3772–81.

14. Kiani L. Natural Miracles: What Functional Foods Can Do for You. ProQuest, October 2007. Available at: http://www.csa.com/discoveryguides/food/review2.php. Last accessed August 15, 2008.

15. Arvanitoyannis IS, Van Houwelingen-Koukalliaroglou M. Functional Foods: A Survey of Health Claims, Pros and Cons, and Current Legislation. *Crit Rev Food Sci.* 2005;45:385–404.

16. Riezzo G, Chiloiro M, Russo F. Functional foods: salient features and clinical applications. *Curr Drug Targets Immune Endocr Metabol Disord.* 2005;5:331–7.

17. International Food Information Council Foundation. Functional Food Fact Sheet: Antioxidants. March 2006. [Search for "Functional Food Fact Sheet: Antioxidants. (3/23/2006)"] Available at: http://www.ific.org/publications/factsheets/index.cfm. Last accessed August 24, 2008.

18. Bliss DZ, Jung HJG. Fiber. In: Gottschlich MM, DeLegge MH, Mattox T, et al., eds. *The A.S.P.E.N. Nutrition Support Core Curriculum: A Case-Based Approach—The Adult Patient.* Silver Spring, Md: American Society for Parenteral and Enteral Nutrition; 2007:88–103.

19. Food and Nutrition Board, Institute of Medicine, National Academy of Sciences. Dietary, functional, and total fiber. In: *Dietary Reference Intakes for Energy, Carbohydrates, Fiber, Fat, Protein and Amino Acids (Macronutrients).* Washington, DC: National Academies Press; 2002:339–421. Available at: http://books.nap.edu/catalog.php?record_id=10490#toc. Last accessed August 10, 2008.

20. Timm DA, Slavin JL. Dietary fiber and the relationship to chronic diseases. *Am J Lifestyle Med.* 2008;2:233–40.

21. Food and Nutrition Board, Institute of Medicine, National Academy of Sciences. Summary tables, dietary reference intakes. Recommended intakes for individuals, total water and macronutrients. In: *Dietary Reference Intakes for Energy, Carbohydrates, Fiber, Fat, Protein and Amino Acids.* Washington, DC: National Academies Press; 2002:1324. Available at: http://books.nap.edu/catalog.php?record_id=10490#toc. Last accessed August 15, 2008.

22. US Department of Agriculture Agricultural Research Service, 2007. Nutrient Intakes from Food: Mean Amounts Consumed per Individual, One Day, 2003–2004. Available at: http://www.ars.usda.gov/ba/bhnrc/fsrg. [Table 1 containing dietary fiber g/day. Available at: http://www.ars.usda.gov/SP2UserFiles/Place/12355000/pdf/0304/Table_1_NIF.pdf.] Last accessed February 15, 2008.

23. Thompson FE, Midthune D, Subar AF, et al. Dietary intake estimates in the National Health Interview Survey, 2000: methodology, results, and interpretation. *J Am Diet Assoc.* 2005;105:352–63.

24. Bialostosky K, Wright JD, Kennedy-Stephenson J, et al. Dietary intake of macronutrients, micronutrients and other dietary constituents: United States 1988–94. National Center for Health Statistics. *Vital Health Stat.* 2002;11(245). [Search for "Vital and Health Statistics—series 11, no. 245 (6/02)."] Available at: http://www.cdc.gov/search.do?action=search&queryText=macronutrient+intake%2C+1988–94&image.x=9&image.y=12. Last accessed August 16, 2008.

25. International Food Information Council Foundation. Food Insights. Focus on Fiber: Why Roughage Still Warrants Our Attention. July/August 2004. Available at: http://www.ific.org/foodinsight/2004/ja/fiberfi404.cfm. Last accessed August 10, 2008.

26. Lui S, Stampfer MJ, Hu FB, et al. Whole-grain consumption and risk of coronary heart disease: results from the Nurses' Health Study. *Am J Clin Nutr.* 1999;70:412–9.

27. Parillo M, Riccardi G. Diet composition and the risk of type 2 diabetes: epidemiological and clinical evidence. *Br J Nutr.* 2004;92:7–19.

28. Bazzano LA, He J, Ogden LG, et al. Dietary fiber intake and reduced risk of coronary heart disease in US men and women. The national health and nutrition examination survey I epidemiologic follow-up study. *Arch Intern Med.* 2003;163:1897–904.

29. Mozaffarian D, Kumanyika SK, Lemaitre RN, et al. Cereal, fruit, and vegetable fiber intake and the risk of cardiovascular disease in elderly individuals. *JAMA.* 2003;289:1659–666.

30. Pereira MA, O'Reilly E, Augustsson K, et al. Dietary fiber and risk of coronary heart disease. A pooled analysis of cohort studies. *Arch Int Med.* 2004;164:370–6.

31. deMunter JSL, Hu FB, Spiegelman D, et al. Whole grain, bran, and germ intake and risk of type 2 diabetes: a prospective cohort study and systematic review. *PLoS Med.* 2007;4(8):e261–75.

32. Montonen J, Kneki P, Jaarvinen R, et al. Whole-grain and fiber intake and the incidence of type 2 diabetes. *Am J Clin Nutr.* 2003;77:622–9.

33. Lau C, Faerch K, Glumer C, et al. Dietary glycemic index, glycemic load, fiber, simple sugars, and insulin resistance: the Inter99 study. *Diabetes Care.* 2005;28:1397–404.

34. Liese AD, Roach AK, Sparks KC, et al. Whole-grain intake and insulin sensitivity: the Insulin Resistance Atherosclerosis Study. *Am J Clin Nutr.* 2003;78:965–71.

35. Krishnan S, Rosenberg L, Singer M, et al. Glycemic index, glycemic load, and fiber intake and risk of type 2 diabetes in US black women. *Arch Intern Med.* 2007;167:2304–9.

36. Anderson JW, Randles KM, Kendall CWC, et al. Carbohydrate and fiber recommendations for individuals with diabetes: a quantitative assessment and meta-analysis of the evidence. *Am Coll Nutr.* 2004;23:5–17.

37. Bingham SA, Day NE, Luben R, et al. Dietary fiber in food and protection against colorectal cancer in the European Prospective Investigation into Cancer and Nutrition (EPIC): an observational study. *Lancet.* 2003;361:1496–501.

38. Park Y, Hunter DJ, Spiegelman D, et al. Dietary fiber intake and risk of colorectal cancer. A pooled analysis of prospective cohort studies. *JAMA.* 2005;294:2849–57.

39. Schatzkin A, Mouw T, Park Y, et al. Dietary fiber and whole-grain consumption in relation to colorectal cancer in the NIH-AARP diet and health study. *Am J Clin Nutr.* 2007;85:1353–60.

40. Bijkerk CJ, Muris JWM, Knottnerus JA, et al. Systematic review: the role of different types of fibre in the treatment of irritable bowel syndrome. *Aliment Pharmacol Ther.* 2004;19:245–51.

41. Kolida S, Gibson GR. Prebiotic capacity of inulin-type fructans. *J Nutr.* 2007;137:2503S–6S.

42. Roberfroid MB. Inulin-type fructans: functional food ingredients. *J Nutr.* 2007;137:2493S–502S.

43. de Vrese M, Marteau PR. Probiotics and prebiotics: effects on diarrhea. *J Nutr.* 2007;137:803S–11S.

44. Boirivant M, Strober W. The mechanisms of action of probiotics. *Curr Opin Gastroenterol.* 2007;23:679–92.

45. Lin DC. Probiotics as functional foods. *Nutr Clin Pract.* 2003;18:497–506.

46. Saavedra JM. Use of probiotics in pediatrics: rationale, mechanisms of action, and practical aspects. *Nutr Clin Pract.* 2007;22:351–65.

47. Parvez S, Malik KA, Kang A, Kim HY. Probiotics and their fermented food products are beneficial for health. *J Appl Microbiol.* 2006;100:1171–85.

48. Mataresse LE, Seidner DL, Steiger E. The role of probiotics in gastrointestinal disease. *Nutr Clin Pract.* 2003;18:507–16.

49. Milne AC, Avenell A, Potter J. Meta-analysis: protein and energy supplementation in older people. *Ann Intern Med.* 2006;14:37–48.

50. August D, Chair. ASPEN Board of Directors and the Clinical Guideline Task Force. Guidelines for the Use of Parenteral and Enteral Nutrition in Adult and Pediatric Patients. *JPEN J Parenter Enteral Nutr.* 2002;26(suppl):78SA–80SA.

Sports Nutrition and Performance-Enhancing Nutrients

Mark Newnham

Many individuals spend their leisure time pursuing a physically active hobby, such as weight lifting, yoga, or aerobics, or endurance events, such as marathon running or triathlon participation. Active individuals may spend 5 to 10 hours per week in physical activity and require a specific nutritional intake to maintain or enhance their performance. This chapter reviews macronutrient and food supplement products and their effect on these recreational activities. Food supplements and natural products have been marketed to athletes with two primary purposes: (1) as ergogenic aids that improve strength and power and (2) as endurance aids to prolong the duration of exercise by providing fuel for continued effort, and by replacing electrolytes lost from sweat to promote normal muscle contractions. Readers are referred to a joint statement of the American Dietetic Association (ADA) and the Canadian Dietetic Association for guidelines and detailed discussion of this topic.[1]

Consumers of Sports Nutrition Products

Sports nutrition products and performance-enhancing supplements have gained wide acceptance in both highly trained athletes and mildly to moderately active individuals. Electrolyte- and carbohydrate-containing sports beverages are so popular that almost all marathon and triathlon participants report experience with them. A survey of 21,225 American college students participating in sports at the division I, II, and III levels at 713 institutions was conducted in 2001.[2] This survey, conducted before the Food and Drug Administration (FDA) took action on ephedra, revealed that 3.9% of student athletes were taking ephedra, 3.3% were taking an amphetamine, and 1.5% reported using anabolic steroids. The survey also found that 57.3% of student athletes who were actively taking supplements in college started taking supplements in high school, with 5.7% reportedly starting supplements in junior high school. A similar survey was conducted among American high-school athletes.[3] This survey revealed a high rate of nutritional supplementation by the 12th grade, including 62% reporting use of a daily multivitamin, 31% reporting use of high-energy drinks, 22% reporting use of a protein powder, and 12% reporting use of creatine. There were two surprising reports from this 2005–2006 academic year survey. First, 18.6% of the female athletes reported using a "fat burner" to lose weight during their

senior year; second, 5.9% of male seniors reported using an anabolic steroid, which would be an illegal activity.

Although historical sales of these products have been driven by serious athletes who choose to exercise regularly, emerging marketing trends show that sales to nonathletes are far outweighing sales to athletes. Increasing numbers of consumers are choosing sports nutrition products as lifestyle alternatives to traditional beverages and snacks. The market has responded with advertising aimed at wellness benefits and active lifestyles. Women, children, and the Hispanic population are also sales targets.

Retail sales for sports nutrition products in 2003 are reported at more than $3 billion, with the market share driven by the sports beverage market, followed by supplements, and then energy bars and gels. The beverage market includes energy drinks, isotonic recovery drinks, and other nutrient-enhanced soft drinks, juices, and waters. The supplement market includes tablets, capsules, and powders that are based on both macronutrients and herbal supplements.

FDA, Anti-Doping Agencies, and Regulation of Performance-Enhancing Supplements

FDA does not approve dietary supplements, including those marketed for sports performance. It is important for the athlete to know that there is evidence of misbranding of nutritional supplements. Misbranding occurs when the product does not contain the ingredients listed on the label or the quantity of an ingredient differs from the quantity stated on the label. In some cases, nutritional supplements may be misbranded by contamination or adulteration with substances that are strictly prohibited by the anti-doping agencies. The anti-doping agencies state clearly that athletes are responsible for the substances that are in their systems. A positive test will result in a violation regardless of the package label. Nutritional products are tested at some independent laboratories such as ConsumerLab.com, which provides reports for a fee. Athletes can review a list of banned substances and anti-doping resources at the following Web sites: www.usantidoping.org, www.wada-ama.org, and www.consumerlab.com. Chapter 53 provides a more detailed discussion of dietary supplement regulation.

Macronutrient Aids for Athletic Performance

Clinical trials of athletic supplements use resistance training as a measure of strength, power, and muscle mass, or exercise time on a treadmill or bicycle ergometer as a measure of endurance. Largely anaerobic, resistance training is quantified either as total weight lifted over a series of exercises or the maximum weight lifted by the athlete in one repetition, referred to as 1-Repmax. Endurance training is generally quantified by the total time of exercise, also known as "time to exhaustion," or time to complete a predetermined distance. Endurance testing must be controlled for the athlete's level of aerobic versus anaerobic effort by measuring the athlete's ability to extract oxygen (O_2) from inspired air. This measure is known as the VO_2, or volume of O_2 consumed in liters per minute. Setting the VO_2 allows for a control when comparing exercise efforts between two separate athletes or even comparing one athlete's effort with a previous baseline effort. For an endurance study, the athlete might be asked to run continuously on a treadmill until exhausted while drinking a carbohydrate-containing sports drink and then return a week later to run the same trial receiving only water. The speed of the treadmill would be adjusted to the athlete's effort, as measured by oxygen extraction, to ensure that both efforts are similar. In this case, the athlete might be asked to exercise at 50% of VO_{2max}, which would represent an aerobic effort.

The lactate threshold (LT) is the exercise intensity at which lactic acid starts to accumulate in the blood stream. LT represents the point at which an athlete begins to exercise in a relative state of oxygen deprivation. The muscles' ability to produce energy in the form of adenosine triphosphate (ATP) is determined by the relative amount of oxygen available for metabolism. When oxygen is relatively deficient, the anaerobic utilization of glucose and production of ATP also leads to production of lactic acid. There is no credible evidence that any herbal supplement or ergogenic aid can improve an athlete's VO_2 or lactate threshold. The only known influence on lactate threshold is physical activity.[4-6]

Endurance athletes rely on both fat and carbohydrates for athletic performance.[4-6] At low-intensity aerobic efforts, fat metabolism will make up 70% to 80% or more of ATP production, with carbohydrate providing as little as 20% of ATP needs.[4] The human adaptation is to preserve glycogen for high-intensity efforts such as "fight or flight" reflex energy. As effort increases, the total amount of ATP contributed by fat remains relatively constant, because fatty acid metabolism is both a rate-limited and an oxygen-dependent process. Carbohydrates act as a second type of fuel for high-intensity activity.[4,5] Carbohydrate utilization is added to the baseline fat oxidation to improve total ATP production and therefore provide more energy for a more intense effort.[4-6] Training can influence this process, making athletes more efficient at fat metabolism, therefore allowing longer and/or more intense efforts before accessing vital stores of carbohydrate.[5]

The body stores carbohydrate as glycogen in the muscles and the liver. Athletes rely on muscle glycogen to provide a substrate for ATP production through the Krebs cycle.[4-6] The rate of glycogen depletion depends on the intensity and duration of exercise, and the fitness level of the athlete. In aerobic efforts, carbohydrate utilization makes up only 20% of energy needs. As intensity increases, this percentage increases to 50% for 10-km running races and 80% to 90% for sprint events (100 meters).[5]

Glycogen depletion depends on duration and rate of use. Intensity and rapid glycogen utilization can lead a football or soccer athlete to deplete muscle glycogen in as little as 30 minutes. By comparison, glycogen depletion in marathon runners is relatively slow and occurs several hours into the race, because these athletes have adapted to more efficient fatty acid metabolism. Despite the slow use of glycogen, any endurance athlete will experience muscle glycogen depletion as a sudden and dramatic decrease in performance. Marathon runners refer to muscle glycogen depletion as "hitting the wall." A similar term, "bonking," references the cognitive and mental attention deficits that the athlete can experience when hepatic glycogen depletion leads to low blood glucose levels. For most long-distance runners, this experience is relatively predictable, occurring about 2 hours, or 18 to 22 miles, into a marathon. Before sports drinks were available, marathon runners would apply the concept of carbohydrate loading in an attempt to increase muscle glycogen stores and therefore prolong their effort before hitting the wall. Carbohydrate loading involved two phases, starting 3 to 5 days prior to the event. First the athlete restricts dietary carbohydrate severely while continuing to exercise at a high-intensity, glycogen-depleting effort. The goal of this glycogen depletion is to stimulate adaptation to more efficient fat utilization and enhance natural signals for carbohydrate storage. The second phase involves oral carbohydrate loading 12 to 24 hours prior to the event to maximize glycogen stores at the start of the race.

The sports nutrition market was initially aimed at high-intensity athletes with the goal of replacing muscle glycogen, along with electrolytes and fluids, during short breaks in competition. The market then evolved toward endurance sports by replacing pre-event carbohydrate loading with provision of small amounts of carbohydrates to athletes frequently during an event, so as to preserve muscle glycogen and maintain performance. There are no reasons for these calorie-dense products to be marketed to sedentary individuals.

Carbohydrate-Based Products

Sugar content is listed separately from carbohydrates on the food label to provide the consumer with important information. Carbohydrate-based sports nutrition products should be categorized by their glycemic index. Products that contain high-glycemix-index carbohydrates, or sugars, will provide a rapid absorption and availability of carbohydrate. Sugar-containing products stimulate a larger release of insulin than that of more complex carbohydrates. This difference is important to the athlete for a number of reasons. Insulin will act to move carbohydrates into the muscle cells for energy and into the liver for conversion to glycogen. Many insulin-sensitive athletes will need to consume repeated doses of glucose at regular intervals to prevent hypoglycemia, because insulin circulates longer than available glucose, particularly in the face of rapid glucose utilization in high-intensity efforts. Insulin also creates a fat-sparing environment. Insulin inhibits lipase enzyme activity in adipose tissues, decreasing the release of free fatty acids from triglyceride molecules. The net effect is to promote energy storage and to decrease energy expenditure, a critically important effect when the athlete continues to exercise.

High-glycemic-index products are optimized for sports requiring intermediate sprint efforts such as soccer and football. As discussed above, these products will result in rapid muscle glycogen replacement in athletes that is proportionately dependent on muscle glycogen for short bursts of high-energy activities. By comparison, these products may be detrimental to endurance athletes, because the high-glycemic carbohydrate source can stimulate insulin release, which leads to a decrease in lipase activity and a decrease in serum-free fatty acid availability. The net effect is a decrease in the endurance athlete's primary fuel. In many ways, the bonk effect may actually be induced by the products that have been marketed to prevent the bonk. The sports nutrition industry has responded by providing products using complex carbohydrates with a lower glycemic index. These products should stimulate insulin release to a lesser extent and may be more appropriate for endurance athletes competing for 2 hours or longer. For these reasons, athletes should be familiar with the specific carbohydrate in their sports drinks and the relative glycemic index of that carbohydrate.

There is essentially no difference in the effectiveness of the different forms of carbohydrates (i.e., drinks, gels, and bars) other than the amount of water and electrolytes in the products and the glycemic index of the carbohydrate. One advantage of bars and gels is that they are lighter and easier to carry than an equivalent amount of calories in the form of a sports drink. The primary disadvantage is that bars and gels require a water source for proper dissolution, absorption, and gastrointestinal (GI) tolerance. Also, sports bars tend to contain other macronutrients such as fats and proteins that are often not part of a sports drink, making them more applicable to postexercise recovery than for glycogen preservation during an event.

Although the original intent of these products was to provide fuel on the go, the market has evolved to provide meal replacements for active people in a hurry, and they are frequently perceived by the public as healthier than soft drinks, candy bars, or even regular meals. It is not uncommon to see someone skip a meal and eat a prepackaged sports nutrition bar, because it is convenient and perceived as a healthful alternative. Clinicians should be aware of the caloric density and glycemic index of these sports drinks and meal replacement bars. The clinician should be prepared to read and interpret the nutrition label with patients and to calculate total calories if the package offers multiple servings. The clinician should also be aware that the consumption of high-glycemic-index carbohydrates prior to exercise may result in a decrease in fatty acid oxidation; therefore, individuals who are using exercise to lose weight or body fat percentage should be discouraged from using these products before, during, or after exercise if that activity lasts less than 2 hours.[1,4,6] Examples of these bars, gels, and drinks are presented in Table 25-1.

Triglyceride-Containing Products

Medium-chain triglycerides (MCTs) have been packaged into sports drinks and powders to provide an alternative fuel to glucose and to reduce muscle glycogen utilization.[6,7] The moderate length (8–12 carbons) of MCTs allow them to be absorbed from the GI tract directly into the bloodstream. Direct absorption allows for much more rapid utilization than occurs with long-chain triglycerides (LCTs) and accounts for the marketing claim that MCTs can spare muscle glycogen. Clinical data in athletes suggest that MCTs are absorbed and can be utilized metabolically within 30 minutes of ingestion, but no data show that these products can improve performance.[6,7] MCTs and LCTs should be avoided in exercise sports nutrition products used before and during exercise, because they tend to slow gastric emptying and may cause discomfort and bloating during intense exercise. Meals containing fat should be consumed 2 hours before exercise because of delayed gastric emptying and the risk of GI intolerance.[1]

Protein Products

Many athletes train with weights to build muscle and to develop a bigger or stronger body. These athletes see a need to consume larger quantities of protein to provide substrates for muscle development. The source of protein can vary from athlete to athlete, and includes dietary intake of meat; vegetarian sources of protein such as legumes, beans, and nuts; and prepackaged protein sources such as protein powders, amino acid supplements, and various protein-containing bars, gels, and drinks. Most adults need to consume 0.8 to 1 gram of protein per kilogram of body weight per day to maintain their muscle mass.[1,8,9] When initiating exercise, the body will require a greater proportion of protein to maintain a neutral nitrogen balance, so the ADA recommends a protein intake of 1.2 to 1.4 g/kg/day in highly active adults who participate in endurance exercise.[1] An active athlete who exercises for 5 to 10 hours per week will have an increased protein requirement, compared with the general population. ADA suggests that athlete's protein needs are increased to assist in the repair of exercise-induced muscle damage, to build and maintain increased lean body mass, and to provide an additional calorie source for energy.

Athletes who strength train have an even larger increase in lean body mass than most athletes; therefore, ADA recommends that 1.5 g/kg/day of protein may be required for those who are attempting to increase body mass. Anecdotal evidence of athletes ingesting protein in the quantities of 1.7 to 2.5 g/kg/day has been reported despite a lack of data supporting its effectiveness. A large number of protein supplement products exist in the marketplace, and they have proven quite popular with the serious body builders. Despite the large market demand, ADA indicates that simple adjustments to the athlete's diet can provide sufficient protein to meet goal dietary intake for increasing muscle mass. There is no evidence that packaged protein supplements are more effective at increasing body mass, compared with ingested whole foods with equal amounts of protein. The use of branch-chain amino acids for endurance performance is discussed later in this chapter.

Clinical Evidence of Protein Supplementation for Muscle Building

There is little clinical research on the subject of high-protein diets and muscle accumulation. Radiolabeled carbon studies could be used to quantify the amount of dietary carbon that is incorporated into muscle; however, test subjects would be required to undergo painful muscle biopsies. One small study (N = 13) used radiolabeled C^{13}-leucine to measure nitrogen balance.[10] Participants received a 13-day diet of protein, 0.86, 1.4, or 2.4 g/kg/day, prior to a nitrogen balance study and then were crossed over between groups after 14 days. The athletes achieved a zero nitrogen balance with the moderate protein intake of 1.4 g/kg/day. The high-protein diet did not affect nitrogen balance, but leucine oxidation was significantly increased, indicating that the extra protein was utilized for ATP production.

Another important consideration of high-protein diets is the lack of rapid weight gain observed in studies.[8,9] Skeletal muscle mass is approximately 70% water; therefore, incorporation of protein into muscle should also result in accumulation of water weight. Many high-protein diet studies have focused on a protein intake of 2 g/kg/day or more in an attempt to build muscle mass. If an assumption is made that all additional protein intake above the ADA-recommended 1.5 g/kg/day (i.e., 0.5 g/kg/day) is incorporated into skeletal muscle, then a 75 kg athlete should

TABLE 25-1 Sports Nutrition Products[a]

	Carbohydrate (g)	Sugars (g)	Protein (g)	Fat (g)	Sodium (mg)	Potassium (mg)	Energy (kcal)	Serving Size	Comments
Electrolyte Drinks, Capsules, and Wafers (Low-Calorie)									
Endurolytes	0	0	0	0	80	50	0	2 capsules	
Endurolytes	0	0	0	0	100	25	0	1–3 capsules	Calcium 50 mg; magnesium 25 mg
Gatorade G2	7	7	0	0	110	30	25	8 oz	Calcium 12.5 mg; magnesium 12.5 mg
Nuun Active Hydration	0	0	0	0	175	50	5	1 wafer	Calcium 12.5 mg; magnesium 25.0 mg
Powerade Option	2	2	0	0	50	35	10	8 oz	Vitamins B_6, B_{12}, C, E, niacin (B_3), and pantothenic acid (B_5)
Propel Fitness Water	3	2	0	0	35	40	10	8 oz	Vitamins B_6, B_{12}, C, E, niacin (B_3), and pantothenic acid (B_5)
Thermolyte	0	0	0	0	300	85.2	0	2 capsules	Calcium 25 mg; magnesium 12 mg
Ultima Replenisher	2	0	0	0	25	50	8	1/3 scoop	Calcium 23 mg; magnesium 8 mg; 13 vitamins and minerals
Energy Drinks (Calories and Electrolytes)									
Accelerade	21	20	5	1	190	64	140	1 scoop/ 12 oz	37 g/scoop
Cytomax	20	11	0	0	100	110	95	1 scoop/ 16 oz	25 g/scoop
E Fuel	18	6	0	0	130	50	70	1/3 pack/ 8 oz	
Gatorade	14	14	0	0	110	30	50		
Gatorade Endurance	14	14	0	0	200	90	50	8 oz	
Gu₂O	26	4	0	0	240	40	100	2 scoops/ 16 oz	Contains mal-todextrin, fructose
Recovery Drinks									
Endurox R4	53	30	14	1.5	230	140	280		Glutamine
Gatorade Shake	54	28	20	6	280	560	370	74 g/12 oz 11 oz	
GNC Distance	38	13	7	1	140	35	190		
IsoPure Endurance	60	40	20	0	210	120	320	53 g/14 oz 20 oz	
IsoPure ZeroCarb	0	0	40	0	80	45	160	20 oz	

TABLE 25-1 Sports Nutrition Products[a] (continued)

	Carbohydrate (g)	Sugars (g)	Protein (g)	Fat (g)	Sodium (mg)	Potassium (mg)	Energy (kcal)	Serving Size	Comments
MetRx Protein Shake	19	1	25	2.5	110	190	200	1 packet	
Power Dream	43	23	10	5	160	370	240	11 oz	Soy milk
Energy Gels									
Accel Gel	20	10	5	0	95	40	90	1 packet	
CarbBoom	26–27	2–4	0	0	50	50–75	110	1 packet	
Clif Shot	24–25	7–8	0	0–0.5	40	25–50	100	1 packet	
E Gel	37	7	0	0	230	85	150	1 pack	Contains maltodextrin, fructose
Gu	20–25	3–4	0	0–2	40–55	30–40	100	1 packet	
Hammer Gel	22–23	2	0	0	18–27	NA	86–93	1 packet	2 tbsp
Power Bar/ PowerGel	28	5	0	0	50	40	110	41 g	
Energy Bars									
Bakers Breakfast Cookie	52–59	19–26	6–8	4–11	180–260		270–330	1 cookie	
Balance Bar Gold	22–24	17–20	14–15	6	90–230	85–220	200	1 bar	
Cliff Bar	43–46	17–22	10–11	2.5–6	100–220	210–3270	230–250	1 bar	
Luna Bar	24–28	8–12	10	3–5	125–200	90–160	170–180	1 bar	
Power Bar Performance	45	18–20	9–10	2–3.5	90–120	105–200	230–240	1 bar	
Protein Bars									
Balance Outdoor	21	12	15	6	140	260	200	1 bar	
PowerBar Protein Plus	36	19	24	5	140	NA	110	1 bar	
Pure Fit	28	14	18	6	180	NA	240	1 bar	

Key: NA, not available.

[a] Composition per serving. Slight differences exist within products with multiple flavors or formulations. Please refer to the product nutrition label or the manufacturer's Web site for the most current information.

gain at least 3 kg of body weight over a 12-week trial. The 3-kg weight gain from protein increases to 6 kg (13 pounds) or 1 pound per week when the additional water weight is considered. Well-designed studies of high protein intake have not resulted in consistent weight gain, compared with the control groups.[1,8–10] The manufacturers of amino acid supplements claim that athletes should use specific amino acid–enriched products, because building muscle will require increased amounts of specific amino acids, the essential amino acids, or the branch–chain amino acids. No clinical research supports these marketing claims, and ADA does not make recommendations regarding supplemental amino acid intake, given that most athletes seeking to build muscle can obtain the necessary amino acids with complete proteins from their diet.

Muscle mass building is not simply a matter of increasing protein intake or adding a protein supplement to an athlete's diet. Physical activity is the most influential factor on muscle mass

development.[9,10] An athlete who desires an increase in muscle mass will need to train and provide adequate calories from non-protein calorie sources to meet maintenance energy needs as well as the increased energy requirement of exercise.

Adverse Effect of High-Protein Diets

Proteins are complex structures composed of hundreds of amino acids held together by chemical bonds. Free amino acids are separated, or in a single state, from their original protein source. There is no advantage to the consumption of whole-source complete proteins or manufactured, packaged individual amino acids, when evaluated by muscle incorporation. However, free amino acids result in a higher osmotic effect, which can cause GI distress and diarrhea. Incomplete proteins can be deficient in one or more of the essential amino acids, which may adversely affect growth and development.

Athletes seeking a high-protein diet or diet supplementation should be cautioned to closely evaluate the effects of high-protein intake on kidney function over time. Unfortunately, most of the available data are either anecdotal or limited in study duration.[11,12] The effects of high-protein diets on creatinine clearance estimates have shown no effect after 4 to 12 weeks of supplementation. However, the conclusions in these studies should be questioned. Creatinine is a breakdown product of creatine. A high-protein diet, typically high in red meat, will result in an increased dietary intake of creatine. The elevated creatine intake from the diet can result in increased creatinine in the blood and therefore affect the accuracy of the creatinine clearance measurement. This study methodology is not sufficient to prove that high-protein diets over many years are either safe or unsafe.

High protein intake may also affect hydration status or increase the risk of dehydration, because the increased protein load can lead to an increase in nitrogenous wastes that must be eliminated. The elimination of this nitrogen can cause the urine to look dark yellow to orange and alter its smell. A frequent method for predicting dehydration risk is to evaluate urine color, with pale or light yellow urine considered a good sign of adequate hydration. An athlete may mistakenly assume that dark-colored urine is related to a protein supplement or to a multivitamin product and fail to take the proper precaution to increase hydration. A second simple method to monitor for dehydration is for athletes to weigh themselves before and after exercise; any significant weight loss from a short duration of exercise is likely to be a reflection of dehydration.

Water and Electrolytes

Free Water and Dehydration

For athletes, water and electrolytes are essential to performance. A 2% decrease in total body water can affect performance, particularly in endurance events.[13] Dehydration results in increased physical strain, as measured by elevations in core body temperature, heart rate, and perceived exertion. Dehydration can also effect cognitive performance such as mental concentration and focus on skilled tasks. Dehydration does not appear to affect anaerobic performance or muscle strength. Readers are referred to the position statement of the American College of Sports Medicine for guidelines and detailed discussion of this topic.[13]

Dehydration is a multifactorial issue, specifically related to water loss and electrolyte concentrations as separate issues. Athletes will generate heat from exercise-related muscle contractions in proportion to the intensity and duration of exercise. This heat generation is transferred to the blood and then to the body core. Blood circulation through peripheral blood vessels and the skin is intended to allow radiation heat exchange with the environment. Fluid and electrolyte loss as sweat onto the skin surface facilitates evaporative cooling. Unfortunately, environmental conditions such as temperature, humidity, air motion, and layers of the athlete's clothing can influence the success of evaporative cooling. If sweat-related water and electrolyte losses are not replaced, the athlete will experience dehydration.

The significance of dehydration is dependent on the environmental conditions and exercise intensity and duration. For example, compared with a recreational runner, an elite marathon runner may demonstrate a higher sweat rate, as measured by sweat loss per hour, but both athletes will have similar total sweat losses for the event owing to the prolonged time that the recreational athlete needs to complete the event. The elite marathon runner is at an advantage because of heat acclimatization and the metabolic effects of training efficiency. By comparison, American football players may have significantly greater sweat rates than soccer players practicing in identical conditions owing to the football players' layers of clothing and equipment. The risk of dehydration in football players is further influenced by twice-daily practice sessions, where time between sessions may be inadequate for water replacement.

HEALTH CONDITIONS RELATED TO DEHYDRATION

Dehydration can affect health through water loss or water gain (overdrinking) and through the effect that this volume status has on blood sodium levels. In general, dehydration is a more common event, but overhydration and symptomatic hyponatremia can be equally life threatening. Dehydration increases the risk of heat illness such as muscle cramps, heat exhaustion, heat stroke, and exertional rhabdomyolysis.[13] Rhabdomyolysis has been reported as a result of dehydration, heat stress, and novel training. Novel training involves the introduction of new exercise patterns in athletes who have not been acclimated to the new exercise, such as military recruits at boot camp or high-school students attending preseason football camps.

PREVENTION OF DEHYDRATION

Meal consumption is the most important aspect of maintaining optimal hydration status.[13] Eating promotes fluid intake and electrolyte retention. Meals generally contain sufficient electrolytes to replace sweat losses. In general, a protracted period (8–24 hours) between workouts is usually sufficient to return to baseline water status. Athletes can also obtain a first-morning body weight to track day-to-day changes in body weight, because significant changes in body weight in less than 72 hours should approximate changes in body water and not body mass. Athletes should take an average weight measure from several daily weights when applying this method. Sports drinks can provide water and electrolytes, but when assessed 24 hours after a workout, they have not proven superior to regular diets with regard to the time to replace water or electrolyte losses.[13]

Hyponatremia Risk from Drinking Excessive Free Water

Most laboratory-based studies of dehydration have occurred on stationary treadmills in climate-controlled rooms with little to no convective airflow to help sweat evaporation.[1,13] Because of such studies, athletes have been taught that they need to drink as much water as possible to prevent dehydration. This position has been called into question following recent clinical observations of weight gain, severe hyponatremia, cerebral edema, and death from athletes who consumed free water without electrolytes during intense athletic events.[13–15] For example, increased water availability has not resulted in a decrease in athletes seeking medical care after marathon races. Clinical hyponatremia is more likely to occur in nonelite athletes, particularly women who require more than 4 hours to finish a marathon, and in long-course triathletes who require 13 to 17 hours to complete their events.[13–15] The risk of hyponatremia is increased by frequent use of nonsteroidal anti-inflammatory medications.[13] Providing pre-event athlete education and electrolyte-containing sports drinks during the event resulted in a reduction in hyponatremia cases in triathletes, but did not appear to impact the risk of hyponatremia in experienced marathon runners.[13–15]

The result of these observations is an advisory statement from the International Marathon Medical Directors Association.[15] This advisory statement suggests that heat production by an athlete is significantly affected by the effort; therefore, a 10-km race effort will generate more heat than a marathon effort (42.2 km). Because an average athlete runs slower than an elite athlete, the average athlete is at less risk of heat illness than the elite athlete and has more time to consume water at aid stations. Average athletes exercising for more than 4 hours can consume excess free water, resulting in an increased risk of hyponatremia. The recommendations suggest that athletes should choose an electrolyte replacement drink instead of free water to avoid the risk of hyponatremia when competing in events of 4 hours and longer.[15] Most importantly, dehydration during endurance events is still a significant concern; therefore, it is important for the clinician to recognize the risks associated with dehydration, including event duration, and to educate the athlete on the difference between drinking free water and water with electrolytes.

A second paradigm shift is that an athlete who collapses immediately after crossing the finish line may be suffering from postural hypotension, rather than heat-related illness or dehydration. When an athlete crosses the finish line, the sudden decrease in leg muscle contractions allows for pooling of blood in the legs and a decrease in venous return. The resulting decrease in cardiac output may leave the brain underperfused with oxygenated blood, causing the athlete to black out.[15] One of the most important recommendations of this guideline is to ensure that athletes continue walking past the finish line to prevent this reaction. Only athletes demonstrating a rectal temperature higher than 104°F (40°C) should be treated for heat illness.[15]

Carbonated, Oxygen-Enhanced, and Clustered Water

Carbonation of water is not beneficial to athletes and may be detrimental. Dissolved gases can accumulate and cause GI distress and bloating, resulting in a decrease in total fluid consumption.[15] Oxygenated water is distilled water to which pressure has been applied to increase the percentage of dissolved oxygen to a claimed rate of 30% or greater. Marketing claims have suggested that oxygenated water improves muscle endurance, benefits athletes competing in anaerobic events such as weight lifting, and assists athletes with asthma by reducing shortness of breath. Research does not substantiate these effects in humans.[16] The results are predictable given that oxygen-enhanced water, packaged in plastic bottles, may have no more dissolved oxygen than tap water, and the amount of dissolved oxygen in a 12-ounce bottle packed in glass is less than that contained in a single breath of room air.[16] Similarly, one brand of bottled water has claimed to improve hydration and physical performance in athletes by altering the structure of water to form microclusters. No published data support this claim of improved hydration and performance in humans who use microclustered water.

Electrolytes and Water without Added Carbohydrates

For events lasting longer than 4 hours, there is a clear indication for water and electrolyte replacement during the event to maintain homeostasis of electrolyte losses from sweat.[1,13] Sodium and potassium are commonly added to electrolyte replacement drinks. The absorption rate of water is improved with the addition of small amounts of electrolytes, particularly sodium, and the volume of fluid consumed improves with a small amount of added sodium.[1,13] Electrolyte replacement may be important in shorter

events (1–2 hours) that occur in hot and humid conditions, particularly for athletes who produce very high volumes of sweat and athletes who work out several times daily, such as high-school football players doing twice-daily workouts in early preseason training.[13] ADA does not recommend electrolyte replacement during an event lasting less than 1 hour, as long as the athlete consumes a salty meal or snack before or after the event.[13]

Electrolytes, Carbohydrates, and Water

The addition of carbohydrates to sports drinks is beneficial to athletes competing longer than an hour, by replacing muscle glycogen lost during periods of intense effort. ADA does not recommend sports drinks containing carbohydrates for any event lasting less than an hour, but it does support use of carbohydrate supplementation during events as a method of glycogen preservation. As exercise duration increases, muscle glycogen will be converted to carbohydrates as a source of energy. Carbohydrate supplementation during exercise provides the exercising muscle with fuel for energy while allowing the muscle to maintain its stored carbohydrate energy as glycogen. This strategy of providing fuel during exercise has been shown to prolong the time to exhaustion in football, soccer, and long-distance endurance athletes such as runners and cyclists.[1,13]

One market segment increasing in popularity includes low-calorie carbohydrate-containing sports drinks, which are formulated to provide hydration and smaller amounts of electrolytes and vitamins without the carbohydrate and caloric load of typical sports drinks. Some of these low-calorie sports drinks provide as little as 3 grams of carbohydrates per serving, or just 10 kcal, in contrast to the 14 to 26 grams of carbohydrates and 100 to 190 kcal per serving contained in most carbohydrate-containing sports drinks. Although electrolyte-containing sports drinks can be used after exercise of any duration, there is no evidence that they are superior to food sources of electrolytes that a normal postexercise meal provides. These low-calorie electrolyte waters have not been evaluated for performance benefits.

Electrolytes, Carbohydrates, Protein, and Water

The latest trend in sports nutrition products is to introduce protein, in the form of amino acids, to the existing carbohydrate- and electrolyte-containing drinks. Amino acids are added to provide an additional metabolic fuel for ATP production through the Krebs cycle. These products are marketed to long-distance endurance athletes competing at aerobic intensities for long durations, including marathon runners (2.5–5 hours), long-distance triathletes (2–17 hours), and adventure racers (12 hours to 5 days). The available data are conflicting regarding performance benefits of protein added to a carbohydrate drink during cycle ergometry, with studies showing benefit[17,18] and no improvement.[19,20] An important observation is that subjects did not receive isocaloric regimens. The added protein acts as an additional fuel, with the carbohydrate-only control groups receiving less total energy (kcal) than the carbohydrate-plus-protein groups.

Protein added to a sports beverage also has two limitations. These protein-containing drinks come in a powder and can release a significant amount of gas when mixed with water. Bubbles and foam appear on the top layer of the hydrated powder and can influence GI tolerance in athletes. This intolerance can be significant when the athlete is unfamiliar with the product; therefore, protein-containing sports drinks should be introduced as part of the training regimen so that the athlete can gain tolerance before the drinks are used to improve performance. Because hydrolysis can affect stability of some proteins once mixed with water, optimal effect may require that the athlete carry the powder unmixed and add water during the event. This practice can introduce a safety variable in triathlon events, for example, if athletes try mixing the powder while riding a bicycle. Glutamine, which has been added to sports drink powders, is an unstable compound with a half-life of 1 hour; it will rapidly break down into glutamate and ammonia. Athletes should know not to hydrate their protein-containing dry powder drinks the night before an event, as is usually done with carbohydrate-only dry powder drinks. Once mixed, all sports drinks should be consumed or stored in the refrigerator within 2 hours to prevent bacterial growth.

Postexercise Nutrition and Recovery Drinks

The goals of postexercise nutrition are to rehydrate, replace muscle glycogen, repair muscle damage, and prepare for the next activity. The addition of protein to a carbohydrate sports drink has been proposed to improve muscle glycogen restoration and has led to subsequent performance gains compared with carbohydrate-only drinks.[21] Others have found that the addition of protein to isocaloric carbohydrates has no effect on muscle glycogen levels.[22,23] This evidence needs to be critically considered because of the difficulty in providing true isocaloric comparator groups, given that the protein provides additional calories. One small study showed that low-fat milk was more effective than carbohydrate- and electrolyte-containing sports drinks for rehydration postexercise.[24] Eleven healthy, young athletes were given a sports drink that contained 6% carbohydrate or an equal volume of low-fat milk containing 2% milk-fat, 5% natural carbohydrates, and 3.6% protein. The athletes rode a cycle ergometer until they lost 1.7% of their lean body mass. They were then given 150% of the lost volume to drink over 60 minutes and asked to void. The study showed that 62% of the carbohydrate and electrolyte solution was lost as urine compared with only 31% of milk fluid lost as urine. This observation was supported by findings of lower volume urine output and greater postexercise weight gain in the milk group. Recreational athletes are likely to benefit equally by consuming an isocaloric, isonitrogenous drink or meal versus a specific "recovery" sports drink.

Specific Ergogenic Supplements

Caffeine

Several studies have suggested an ergogenic benefit from caffeine supplementation.[25] Ordinarily, this effect would result in a no-tolerance testing policy for international athletes. However, caffeine appears in nutritional products that are unrelated to exercise or performance benefit, such as soft drinks and diet aids; therefore, incidental exposure is common and complete avoidance would be problematic. The World Anti-Doping Agency does not list caffeine as a problematic substance, although it is included in the monitoring program for stimulants.

Caffeine intake at doses of 5 mg/kg (range, 3–6 mg/kg), given 1 hour before exercise testing, appears to produce improvements in time to exhaustion on a cycle ergometer.[26] Giving the caffeine dose up to 3 hours before exercise was still beneficial. It is important to compare clinical study to real-world coffee consumption. For instance, a 24-ounce cup of coffee may contain 250 mg or more of caffeine, which is 3.6 mg/kg for a 70-kg athlete. Larger doses have been tested but do not appear to be more effective. This information is confounded by the finding that caffeine intake from drinking coffee daily does not appear to enhance performance. More importantly, regular caffeine drinkers have demonstrated blunted performance improvement when compared with coffee-naive athletes.[26] Many questions remain regarding the effective use of caffeine for ergogenic benefit. Data regarding caffeine's effect on strength training are limited and inconclusive.

Creatine

Creatine is a naturally occurring substance that is found in all skeletal muscle as free creatine or high-energy phosphorylated creatine. Creatine is synthesized by the body or absorbed intact following ingestion of red meats and fish. Phosphorylated creatine (PCr) functions as an energy buffer, transferring its phosphate group to adenosine diphosphate (ADP), thereby rapidly regenerating ATP during periods of exercise. Skeletal muscle contains a limited amount of energy stored as ATP at rest. Exercise will deplete this stored ATP energy quickly, requiring the body to oxidize macronutrients through the Kreb's cycle to restore ADP to the high-energy ATP state for continuous or repeated efforts. PCr will transfer its energy to ADP in seconds, acting as a secondary fuel. However, the total amount of PCr energy in the muscle can last for only 20 to 30 seconds. Supplementation with creatine is known to increase skeletal muscle PCr concentrations and improve performance. Use among athletes has increased, with 22.2% of male athletes reporting creatine use by the 12th grade.[3]

Performance gains are limited to short bursts of anaerobic activity lasting 30 seconds or less. Supplementation with creatine can attenuate the normal decrease in force associated with repeated work applications such as lifting weights.[27] For example, a weight lifter will perform three sets of a bench press, with a goal of 10 lifts, or repetitions, per set. The lifter will take 30 seconds of rest between each set. Ordinarily, the lifter may be able to move a planned amount of weight for 10 repetitions in the first set, then for 8 repetitions in the second set, and for only 6 repetitions in the third set. The decreasing number of lifts is called attenuation and is related to decreased energy (ATP) in the muscle. Creatine can statistically and clinically improve the athletes' strength so that they can complete more repetitions in each subsequent set with 30-second rest breaks (e.g., 10, 10, and 8 repetitions rather than 10, 8, and 6) by providing ATP to the muscle.[27] Similar improvements to 1-Rep$_{max}$ have also been reported. In this application, creatine does not increase muscle mass or size but does improve ATP fuel amounts, thus making the speed of muscle recovery faster.

Creatine is also useful for athletic events that require repeated, short, explosive bursts of power such as American football, soccer, and track and field events. American football involves bursts of anaerobic activity for 10 to 20 seconds followed by 45 to 90 seconds of recovery. Creatine improves recovery such that the muscle has a larger ATP store following each recovery phase. Similarly, soccer players tend to have short anaerobic bursts followed by longer periods of aerobic recovery. Creatine has been shown to enhance performance in these applications.[27]

By comparison, there does not appear to be a benefit to creatine in sports that require more than 20 to 30 seconds of high-intensity activity. Aerobic activities as short as the 800-meter (2-minute) and 1600-meter (5-minute) run on a track have not shown performance benefits. Sustained efforts such as marathon running (180 minutes) and triathlon (60 minutes or longer) would be unlikely to benefit. When creatine supplementation is stopped, there is a rapid return to normal muscle creatine concentrations. The extra PCr energy would also wash out. There is no evidence that the benefits gained during creatine supplementation can be maintained after supplementation is stopped. Athletes will need to consume maintenance doses of creatine to maintain the increased strength.

Available data indicate that an athlete can load on creatine at 20 g/day for 5 days (or 0.3 g/kg/day) and then maintain steady-state levels of creatine by taking 5 g/day. GI tolerance has been an issue. Nausea may be related to osmotic effects or to malabsorption and may be dose-related. The daily dosage is usually divided into four doses. If nausea is reported, the dose can be reduced or taken with more water.

Adverse effects reported with creatine include GI upset, nausea, weight gain, and muscle cramping. Weight gain may be related to an osmotic gain in water mass within the muscles. Muscle cramping has also been reported, leading to concerns of increased risk of heat-related illness when using creatine. Also, similar to high-protein diets, little is known about the adverse effects of long-term creatine supplementation on renal function, although asymptomatic increases in serum creatinine have been measured. Two reports followed college football players while they took creatine supplements for as long as 3 years. Athletes were followed for reports of muscle cramping, heat illness, dehydration, muscle strains, total injury reports, and missed practices, and were compared with their teammates who were not taking creatine.[28,29] The authors concluded that there was no difference between the groups in occurrence of adverse effects.

Caffeine use with creatine should be avoided. One study, designed to determine whether caffeine would increase the benefits of creatine, found no ergogenic effect of the combination. Several caffeine-containing natural substances, such as green tea, kola nut, and guarana, should also be avoided.

The clinician can assist athletes by recommending that creatine be used only as long as necessary. For example, an athlete can consider loading creatine just prior to a specific event to maximize performance. Alternatively, an athlete may maintain creatine intake for 1 to 2 months of a sports season and then maintain a creatine-free period until the next season. The clinician should also recommend appropriate hydration during creatine exposure, because creatine is a protein that is filtered through the kidneys. If an athlete becomes significantly dehydrated, it is best to temporarily hold creatine until a proper fluid balance is established.

Ephedra and Pseudoephedrine

FDA determined in 2004 that sufficient evidence existed to determine that ephedra was unsafe for consumption, which allowed the Agency to take action and remove ephedra from the market. This action was partly a result of safety data on ephedra use published by the poison centers from Texas[30] and data supplied to FDA through MedWatch.[31] Among the reported adverse events subjectively determined to be definitely, probably, or possibly associated with ephedra use were 17 cases of hypertension, 13 cases of palpitations or tachycardia, 10 cases of stroke, and 7 cases of seizures. Ten of these events resulted in death. Many of these adverse events occurred in active, healthy young adults who were not considered at risk for heart problems, stroke, or seizure on the basis of appropriate prior health screening.

The ephedra alkaloids, which include ephedrine, pseudoephedrine, and phenylpropanolamine, are still available in many foreign markets. Pseudoephedrine is still available as a nonprescription decongestant in the United States; therefore, data are still included in this publication. Considerable controversy exists on the subject of ephedra supplementation for athletes seeking enhanced athletic performance. The authors of a recent meta-analysis screened 530 articles and reviewed 52 controlled trials of ephedra use for weight loss and athletic performance.[32] The report included eight controlled studies of ephedra, seven of which used ephedra combined with caffeine. The authors concluded that no data exist to support that ephedra alone is useful for athletic performance, and that the combination of ephedra and caffeine is unproven at this time.

There is no evidence that pseudoephedrine enhances performance when used at labeled nonprescription doses.[33] One small study of seven runners showed an average 6-second improvement in 1500-meter time following a 2.5 mg/kg dose of pseudoephedrine.[33] This dose is roughly five times the recommended nonprescription dose. Despite this evidence, pseudoephedrine is considered a sympathomimetic chemical and remains a banned substance by the anti-doping agencies. The ban has been a problem for elite athletes who are subject to random drug testing, because the product can appear in their urine for an unpredictable amount of time even when used temporarily for symptomatic improvement of nasal congestion. At this time it would be inappropriate to recommend the ephedra alkaloids for any use without direct consultation with a primary care provider.

Steroidal Precursors

The Anabolic Steroid Control Act of 2004 defined nutritional supplement steroid precursors such as dehydroepiandrosterone (DHEA) and androstenedione as precursors to testosterone. The act further defined these substances as prescription-only, controlled substances with testosterone. These nutritional supplement steroid precursors are still available in foreign markets but have been identified as misbranded ingredients of nutritional supplements sold in the United States. For these reasons, the steroidal precursors are included here.

DHEA and androstenedione have been promoted as ergogenic aids that elevate an athlete's natural testosterone levels. Well-designed studies in humans have proven that supplementation does not lead to elevations in serum testosterone levels.[34] These studies have actually demonstrated significant elevations in estradiol and estrone in men who take the supplement, because the enzyme aromatase converts these products to estrogenic hormones. Clinicians should also be aware that androstenedione supplementation has resulted in 2 mg/dL decreases in high-density lipoprotein concentrations, which may increase cardiovascular risk.[34] There is also no credibility to the claim that other herbal products can inhibit the aromatase enzyme and result in natural increased testosterone levels. Well-designed trials, using daily doses of androstenedione 300 mg and DHEA 150 mg, alone or in combination, have failed to show a performance benefit, compared with placebo in resistance-trained athletes and nonathletes beginning a training program.[34] These products should not be recommended as performance-enhancing supplements.

Stacking

It is important to point out that marketing and sales of sports nutrition products are often complicated by the combination of several agents into a single product, a process known as "stacking." A good example is the commercial product Optygen, which contains a blend of eight ingredients. In the past, androstenedione and DHEA have been combined with other compounds referred to as natural aromatization inhibitors designed to prevent the conversion of testosterone to estrone and estradiol. Stacking also results in other products being added for "general health," such as ginseng, ginkgo biloba, and vitamin C. The products frequently claim that the additives will prevent fatigue-related decreases in performance, although no data support this claim. Other products are included to reduce or prevent side effects; for example, milk thistle is included to provide detoxification properties for the liver when athletes use steroids or herbal substances intended to affect hormone levels. Stacking may also refer to the use of two separate ergogenic regimens at the same time, such as using testosterone and human growth hormone simultaneously.

Many sports nutrition products include individual vitamins, minerals, amino acids, or herbal supplements in an attempt to improve endurance and muscle strength, or reduce oxidative stress related to exercise. Products that have insufficient data for a clear positive effect on performance are reviewed in Table 25-2.[35–52]

Assessment of Performance-Enhancing Nutrients: A Case-Based Approach

Performance enhancers run the gamut from electrolyte solutions to energy bars to hormone precursor supplements. When a person needs help in selecting a product, the practitioner should find out the type of exercise or physical activity in which the person engages. The intensity and duration of the activity are also important information. The patient should also be asked if he or she has experienced any ill effects after the physical activity or after using a performance enhancer. (See Cases 25-1 and 25-2.)

Sales of sports nutrition products designed to enhance or improve performance are increasing every year. The most common self-treatments are creatine to improve muscle strength, and carbohydrate administration during exercise to preserve muscle glycogen and prolong endurance. Several herbal supplements claim to enhance performance, but evidence to support these claims is currently lacking. Although these natural herbal products are touted as safe, there is evidence that some, including androstenedione, DHEA, and conjugate linoleic acid, may have detrimental effects on long-term health by altering cardiovascular risk, high-density lipoprotein levels, and natural, sex-determined hormone levels.

TABLE 25-2 Selected Products Marketed as Ergogenic Supplements

Ingredient	Marketed Claim	Conclusion/Evidence
Antioxidants[35]	Antioxidants claim to be able to reduce oxidative stress from exercise and/or to speed recovery following exercise. Many antioxidants have been included in sports nutrition supplements, including alpha-lipoic acid, carotenoids, glutathione, n-acetylcysteine, ubiquinones (coenzyme Q10), vitamin B complex, vitamin C, and vitamin E.	Evidence does not support an effect on performance enhancement.
Arginine[36]	Arginine has been promoted to improve muscle building and cardiovascular functioning through the production of nitrous oxide, which causes cardiac vasodilatation and increased oxygen delivery to the heart. Arginine is also reported to increase muscle vascularization and volume for the "pumped" looked desired by body builders.	Evidence does not support an effect on performance enhancement.
BCAAs[37,38] (branch-chain amino acids)	BCAAs are isoleucine, leucine, and valine. Skeletal muscle cells are adapted to use BCAAs to supply energy during exercise. Supplementation may reduce fatigue and increase exercise time to exhaustion by reducing serum levels of L-tryptophan and its effect on serotonin levels in the brain.	Evidence does not consistently support an effect on performance.
Carnitine[39]	Carnitine is an essential cofactor for the transport of long-chain fatty acids into the mitochondria. Product is proposed to improve fatty acid oxidation, fat burning, and oxygen absorption, or VO_2, in athletes, and is marketed to reduce lactic acid accumulation.	Evidence does not consistently support an effect on performance.
Chromium[40]	Chromium is marketed to athletes to enhance carbohydrate utilization in the body, possibly promoting fat burning. Product is thought to improve glycemic control, endurance, and strength. It is added to protein supplements to enhance glucose utilization, allowing the protein to be metabolically spared and utilized for building muscle mass.	Evidence does not support an effect on performance enhancement.

TABLE 25-2 Selected Products Marketed as Ergogenic Supplements (continued)

Ingredient	Marketed Claim	Conclusion/Evidence
Citrulline[41]	L-Citrulline is thought to be a metabolic precursor to arginine. Although arginine supplementation is severely reduced by hepatic first-pass metabolism, citrulline is not affected by first-pass hepatic metabolism and is converted by the kidneys to arginine. Product is proposed to improve oxygen consumption and improve time to exhaustion in treadmill running.	Evidence does not support an effect on performance enhancement.
Conjugated linoleic acid[42] (CLA)	CLA is promoted as a thermogenic aid, body fat reducer, and ergogenic aid for endurance athletes that enhances fat metabolism. CLA may increase cardiac risk by lowering high-density lipoprotein and increasing lipoprotein(a) concentrations.	Evidence does not support an effect on performance enhancement.
Cordyceps sinensis[43,44]	*Cordyceps sinensis* is used in Chinese medicine to treat lung disease and fatigue. Chinese and Russian literature implies that use of the mushroom can decrease oxygen consumption, improve VO_{2max}, and improve endurance. Product is frequently combined with rhodiola. Available research published in English is limited and does not show performance benefit.	Evidence does not consistently support an effect on performance.
Eleuthero[45]	Extracts of Siberian ginseng have been reported to affect cardiorespiratory performance, fat metabolism, and improve endurance	Evidence does not support an effect on performance enhancement.
Ginseng[46]	Extracts of *Panax ginseng* have been reported to affect performance through improved lactate clearance and delay in fatigue onset.	Evidence does not support an effect on performance enhancement.
Glycerol[47]	Glycerol is reported to act as an osmotic agent to promote hyperhydration prior to exercise, therefore reducing the risk of dehydration from intensive exercise in the heat.	Evidence does not support an effect on performance enhancement.
Hydroxy-methylbutyrate[36] (HMB)	Beta-HMB is a metabolite of leucine metabolism, claimed to decrease muscle protein breakdown following a workout, and to increase muscle mass. HMB has also been proposed to improve aerobic performance.	Evidence does not support an effect on performance enhancement.
Lecithin[48]	Lecithin is a source of choline and a precursor to acetylcholine. Decreased plasma choline and acetylcholine levels have been reported in marathon runners. Supplementation of lecithin before a marathon may prevent the decline in serum acetylcholine levels, therefore affecting muscle contraction and performance.	Evidence does not support an effect on performance enhancement.
Phosphatidylserine[49]	Phosphatidylserine, a component of human cell membranes, acts as a cofactor for a variety of enzymes and neuroendocrine responses, such as the release of acetylcholine, dopamine, and norepinephrine, thus affecting muscle contractions and performance. Product may possibly act as an antioxidant.	Evidence does not consistently support an effect on performance.
Rhodiola rosea[11,50,51]	*Rhodiola rosea* is a Chinese herb used to stimulate the nervous system, improve aerobic work performance, and eliminate fatigue. *Rhodiola* is reported in Chinese and Russian literature to improve oxygenation at high altitudes and is therefore thought to be helpful for endurance athletes. Available research published in English is limited and does not show performance benefit.	Evidence does not consistently support an effect on performance.
Tyrosine[52]	Tyrosine, the amino acid precursor for dopamine, and tryptophan, the amino acid precursor for serotonin, compete for blood–brain barrier transportation. Supplementation of tyrosine is theorized to result in a lower brain serotonin-to-dopamine ratio, which would affect fatigue and performance.	Evidence does not support an effect on performance enhancement.

CASE 25-1

Relevant Evaluation Criteria	Scenario/Model Outcome
Information Gathering	
1. Gather essential information about the patient's symptoms, including:	
a. description of symptom(s) (i.e., nature, onset, duration, severity, associated symptoms)	The patient reports that he has experienced dehydration and fatigue from twice-daily, preseason football workouts. He feels a decline in leg strength when pushing a heavy sled with his legs. He is able to complete only the first 90 minutes of each 2-hour workout. Providing Gatorade and "sugar" during the workouts does not improve his performance. He also reports a weight loss of 10 pounds in the first 5 days of preseason football camp.
b. description of any factors that seem to precipitate, exacerbate, and/or relieve the patient's symptom(s)	Workouts take place in the August heat with daytime high temperatures approaching 90°F and with 75% humidity. The fatigue sets in earlier in direct sunlight but later when the sun is blocked by cloud cover. Symptoms are lessened when the afternoon practice is moved indoors to an air-conditioned gymnasium or when conducted without pads and helmets.
c. description of the patient's efforts to relieve the symptoms	The patient has consumed large quantities of carbohydrate-containing sports drink during and after practices, and at night to prevent dehydration. Volume of intake is reported at 24 ounces of Gatorade following both morning and afternoon practices (48 ounces daily).
2. Gather essential patient history information:	
a. patient's identity	Bryan Johnson
b. patient's age, sex, height, and weight	17-year-old male, 6 ft 2 in, 245 lb
c. patient's occupation	High-school student
d. patient's dietary habits	Bryan has been eating a high-calorie diet to gain weight for football season. He does not follow a specified training diet. With both parents working, Bryan is given some sort of fast food for dinner at least 3 nights a week. When meals are cooked at home, they generally meet the healthy diet consistent with the Food Guide Pyramid shown in Chapter 23.
e. patient's sleep habits	Bryan gets 8 hours or more of sleep during summer vacation.
f. concurrent medical conditions, prescription and nonprescription medications, and dietary supplements	Bryan's preseason medical examination included a nonfasting blood glucose (185 mg/dL) and a fasting blood glucose (118 mg/dL), which suggest he has glucose intolerance and is at risk for adult-onset diabetes. Bryan's blood pressure was 110/65 at the physician's office. Bryan takes no scheduled medications or supplements, although he uses ibuprofen 200 mg as needed for muscle soreness.
g. allergies	NKA
h. history of other adverse reactions to medications	None
i. other (describe) _____	Bryan comments that white lines of salt are visible on his clothing when it dries.

Assessment and Triage

3. Differentiate the patient's signs/symptoms and correctly identify the patient's primary problem(s).	Bryan is experiencing a decline in muscle endurance (over 90 minutes) associated with a loss of 4% of his body weight. Bryan is likely feeling the effects of dehydration.
4. Identify exclusions for self-treatment.	Bryan's recent diagnosis as glucose-intolerant complicates the decision to use sports drinks, because many of the drinks contain high-glycemic-index carbohydrates.
5. Formulate a comprehensive list of therapeutic alternatives for the primary problem to determine if triage to a medical practitioner is required, and share this information with the patient.	(1) Take no action. Symptoms may improve with cooler weather in September and October. (2) Recommend a daily, morning, pre-workout weighing to track daily changes in body weight as a secondary marker of hydration status. The goal is to start each day with a stable weight and hydration status. (3) Recommend increased dietary salt intake in the patient's regular meals before and after workouts, with appropriate amounts of free water to replace sweat losses, such as 3 cups of water (24 ounces) for every pound of weight loss. (4) Consider the use of a low-carbohydrate, electrolyte-containing sports drink as a replacement for the Gatorade provided by the school. (5) Take no action.

C A S E   2 5 - 1   (continued)

Relevant Evaluation Criteria	Scenario/Model Outcome
Plan	
6. Select an optimal therapeutic alternative to address the patient's problem, taking into account patient preferences.	Several sports drinks provide electrolytes without high-glycemic-index carbohydrates. Propel Fitness water and Gatorade G2 are prebottled waters. Nuun hydration wafers are convenient in that 1 tablet can be added to 8–12 ounces of water to make a carbohydrate-free electrolyte drink. Clinically, there is little to justify one product over another except for price and convenience. Pretzels are a convenient source of low-glycemic-index carbohydrate and sodium.
7. Describe the recommended therapeutic approach to the patient.	(1) Taking 1–2 days off from practice, such as a Saturday and Sunday, should help to establish euhydration and a baseline body weight.
	(2) Monitor weight daily in the morning as a secondary measure of hydration status. Weight loss of 1 kg (2.2 pounds) in a day is suggestive of water loss of 1000 mL. Attempt to start each day with a similar weight.
	(3) Monitor urine for a light yellow color. Dark yellow to brown urine is suggestive of dehydration.
	(4) Because you do not have high blood pressure, you can increase your salt intake in meals before and after workouts.
	(5) Drinking high-glycemic-index sports drinks should be avoided, because glycogen depletion is not suspected.
	(6) Use a low-carbohydrate or carbohydrate-free electrolyte water. Low-fat milk is a reasonable alternative to a sports drink once you get home.
8. Explain to the patient the rationale for selecting the recommended therapeutic approach from the considered therapeutic alternatives.	Emphasizing meal consumption and adequate salt intake within 2 hours postexercise are the most important aspects of rehydration. Sports drinks are not better than meals for salt and water replacement between workouts. Low-fat milk, which contains carbohydrates, fat, and protein, may be more effective for rehydration and equally convenient as a sports drink.
Patient Education	
9. When recommending self-care with non-prescription medications and/or nondrug therapy, convey accurate information to the patient:	
a. appropriate dose and frequency of administration	Drinking 2 cups (16 ounces) of water 15–30 minutes before exercise and 1–1.5 cups (8–12 ounces) every 15 minutes during exercise should prevent clinical dehydration during the workout. Provide sodium supplements with meals between workouts.
b. maximum number of days the therapy should be employed	The amount of salt supplementation should be reduced when cooler weather reduces the rate of sweating, and stopped altogether following football season.
c. product administration procedures	N/A
d. expected time to onset of relief	Rehydration can occur in as little as 8–12 hours with careful water and salt intake.
e. degree of relief that can be reasonably expected	With experience, you should be able to maintain your hydration status with water intake and salt supplementation from meals.
f. most common side effects	
g. side effects that warrant medical intervention should they occur	You should see your or primary care provider if you cannot return to a normal weight, or if you experience muscle cramping that is persistent despite rest and salt intake, or if you experience persistent vomiting (suggestive of heat illness). Your primary care provider can test for electrolyte deficiencies, including sodium and potassium.
h. patient options in the event that the condition worsens or persists	
i. product storage requirements	Electrolyte tablets and capsules can be stored at room temperature until mixed with water. Unopened containers of ready-to-drink products can also be stored at room temperature. Opened containers and mixed powders should be consumed within 2 hours or refrigerated immediately.
j. specific nondrug measures	N/A

Key: N/A, not applicable; NKA, no known allergies; OTC, over-the-counter; PCP, primary care provider.

Relevant Evaluation Criteria	Scenario/Model Outcome
Information Gathering	
1. Gather essential information about the patient's symptoms, including:	
a. description of symptom(s) (i.e., nature, onset, duration, severity, associated symptoms)	Patient has excellent ball-handling skills and running speed, and has been promoted to a starting midfielder on the varsity girl's soccer team. Her playing time has increased significantly this year. As a midfielder, she is called upon to use her speed to provide scoring opportunities on offense and assist the defense when needed. As a result, she is required to roam the entire field, with frequent, explosive bursts of speed. She is finding that her endurance is insufficient to play well the entire match. Late in the match, she has significantly less speed, with her power limited to 5- to 10-second bursts of speed, whereas she can sustain 20- to 25-second bursts early in the game.
b. description of any factors that seem to precipitate, exacerbate, and/or relieve the patient's symptom(s)	Symptoms appear after 45 minutes of match time. She gets significant relief from 10-minute breaks on the sideline; however, her substitute player has less experience and is less talented.
c. description of the patient's efforts to relieve the symptoms	She has used a carbohydrate sports drink during events, but she has not observed an improvement in her endurance, speed, or power. She has started an endurance training program by running a mile after each practice, and running 3 miles on weekends and days without soccer practice.
2. Gather essential patient history information:	
a. patient's identity	Christine Coffman
b. patient's age, sex, height, and weight	16-year-old female, 5 ft 1 in, 110 lb
c. patient's occupation	High-school student
d. patient's dietary habits	Normal, healthy diet with occasional junk food
e. patient's sleep habits	Stays up late during the week to finish school assignments; sleeps in on weekends
f. concurrent medical conditions, prescription and nonprescription medications, and dietary supplements	Multivitamin 1 tablet daily
g. allergies	NKA
h. history of other adverse reactions to medications	None
i. other (describe) _____	Christine is on a team with an opportunity to play for the state championship. Her team relies on her coverage of the midfield and speed to open up scoring opportunities. The team rarely scores when she is resting on the sideline. She is feeling peer pressure to compete the full match time.
Assessment and Triage	
3. Differentiate the patient's signs/symptoms and correctly identify the patient's primary problem(s).	Christine is experiencing a common effect of mixed anaerobic/aerobic exercise. She needs muscle ATP to provide energy for explosive bursts, but she also needs to have rapid recovery (conversion of ADP to ATP) to prepare for the next explosive effort. The recovery of ATP occurs through oxidative metabolism of glucose through the Kreb's cycle during her resting periods or on-field recovery jogging; however, this process is slow and she cannot perform her optimal level when recovering.
4. Identify exclusions for self-treatment.	N/A
5. Formulate a comprehensive list of therapeutic alternatives for the primary problem to determine if triage to a medical practitioner is required, and share this information with the patient.	Options include: (1) Add endurance training. Endurance training, such as running an extra mile each practice, should improve her VO_{2max}, allow her to exercise longer at a higher intensity, and stay on the field longer during the match. (2) Creatine supplementation for the duration of soccer season may improve Christine's performance by providing an additional energy store. (3) Christine should maintain adequate hydration to avoid dehydration. (4) Take no action. Christine's experience is a natural balance of athletic competition. She can improve by consistent training on the soccer field, without supplementation. She should plan rest periods off the field.

C A S E   2 5 - 2   (continued)

Relevant Evaluation Criteria	Scenario/Model Outcome
Plan	
6. Select an optimal therapeutic alternative to address the patient's problem, taking into account patient preferences.	Christine will add creatine supplementation to her regimen of soccer practice and perform additional endurance training.
7. Describe the recommended therapeutic approach to the patient.	Because the season is well under way, Christine will need to load her muscles with creatine and then provide maintenance doses until the season ends.
8. Explain to the patient the rationale for selecting the recommended therapeutic approach from the considered therapeutic alternatives.	Creatine supplementation will lead to an increase in muscle phosphocreatine (PCr). PCr can transfer its high-energy phosphate bond to ADP and restore ATP rapidly during explosive bursts of power, helping to sustain the power. Creatine acts as a secondary fuel storage area in the muscle. PCr also recovers quickly, such that the PCr is restored quickly and can repeat its transfer for energy to ADP frequently during the match.
Patient Education	
9. When recommending self-care with non-prescription medications and/or nondrug therapy, convey accurate information to the patient:	
a. appropriate dose and frequency of administration	Creatine powder can be started at 20 grams per day (0.3 g/kg/day) for 5 days as a loading dose, followed by 5 grams per day as a maintenance dose.
b. maximum number of days the therapy should be employed	Performance benefits are related to an increased supply of creatine and PCr bonds; therefore, the benefits are present only while creatine maintenance doses are provided. Creatine should be stopped after soccer season (typically 3–4 months), because long-term use is unproven and may damage the kidneys. Creatine is not needed during the off-season when the sense of competition is reduced. Christine can continue endurance training during the off-season.
c. product administration procedures	
d. expected time to onset of relief	Strength gains from creatine supplementation are subjectively felt within 1–2 days.
e. degree of relief that can be reasonably expected	The degree of performance enhancement is difficult to measure. Soccer matches involve repeated, short bursts of anaerobic activity lasting 10–15 seconds. Around 40 minutes into a match, Christine would experience an attenuation of this sprint ability as either a decrease in top end speed, or a decrease in the time that speed was available. Creatine supplementation should delay this attenuation for 10–15 minutes later into the match.
f. most common side effects	Side effects of creatine are not commonly reported by clinical research. Heat illness, muscle cramping, and GI intolerance have been reported. Adequate hydration should be part of the athlete's plan regardless of the use of creatine.
g. side effects that warrant medical intervention should they occur	N/A
h. patient options in the event that condition worsens or persists	N/A
i. product storage requirements	Creatine is available in tablets that can be stored at room temperature and as powdered drinks that can be stored at room temperature until mixed with water. Mixed powders should be consumed within 2 hours or refrigerated immediately.
j. specific nondrug measures	N/A

Key: ADP, adenosine diphosphate; ATP, adenosine triphosphate; GI, gastrointestinal; N/A, not applicable; NKA, no known allergies; VO$_{2max}$, maximum volume of oxygen consumed in liters per minute.

Patient Counseling for Performance-Enhancing Nutrients

The quest for enhanced physical performance has resulted in serious health consequences for some athletes. Clinical studies of some of the botanical and hormonal dietary supplements touted as performance enhancers reveal significant adverse effects and little or no enhancement in physical performance. Practitioners should be prepared to steer patients asking for advice on these products to the safest and most appropriate product. The box

Patient Education for Performance–Enhancing Nutrients lists specific information to provide patients.

Key Points for Sports Nutrition and Performance-Enhancing Nutrients

➤ Despite marketing claims, most performance-enhancing nutritional products and ergogenic aids are unproven, and several may be unsafe. By comparison, training regularly

---

PATIENT EDUCATION FOR
Performance-Enhancing Nutrients

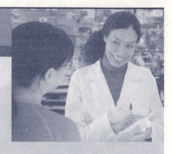

The objective in selecting a performance enhancer is to choose a product that is safe and appropriate for the type, intensity, and duration of the physical activity. Following the recommendations of a primary care provider (PCP) and other clinicians as well as carefully following product instructions and the self-care measures listed here will help ensure optimal therapeutic outcomes.

Muscle Glycogen Preservation

■ High-glycemic-index products, including most carbohydrate-containing sports drinks, contain sucrose and sodium. They are optimal for intermediate sprint activities, such as soccer and football, and for endurance events that last longer than 60 minutes. Small doses repeated every 15–20 minutes may be necessary for sustained energy over longer events, because the insulin effect will outlast a single dose of sucrose.

■ Moderate-glycemic-index products contain maltodextrin, galactose, and fructose. They are optimal for athletic events that last longer than 4 hours.

■ Diabetic athletes should seek the advice of a PCP before beginning an exercise program, and they should be prepared to address the symptoms of hypoglycemia while exercising.

■ Note that sports bars often contain other macronutrients such as fats and proteins. Many of these bars are more appropriate for after-exercise recovery than for use during athletic events. If a well-balanced meal is unavailable within 2 hours of exercise, many of these bars may be an appropriate after-exercise fuel replenishment source. (See Table 25-1 for specific products.)

■ Long-chain triglycerides can cause discomfort and bloating during intense exercise; therefore, consume meals containing large amounts of fat 2 hours before exercise.

Enhancement of Muscle Mass

■ Athletes should not exceed the American Dietetic Association's recommended daily intake of 1.5 grams of protein per kilogram of body weight to increase body mass. Available data do not show that higher intakes produce more muscle mass or additional strength.

■ Athletes who ingest high amounts of protein either through their foods or protein supplements should discuss this practice with their PCP. The PCP may elect to monitor blood urea nitrogen and serum creatinine levels to monitor the effects of high protein intake on kidney function.

■ Little clinical evidence is available to support the claims that arginine and beta-hydroxy-beta-methylbutrate help to increase muscle mass.

Hydration and Electrolytes

■ Athletes exercising for less than 60 minutes usually can complete their exercise with water alone, although the addition

of small amounts of carbohydrates and/or electrolytes may enhance performance.

■ Athletes exercising for longer than 60 minutes should incorporate a carbohydrate- and electrolyte-containing sports drink into the exercise program for optimal performance.

■ Endurance athletes exercising for 4 hours and longer are discouraged from drinking free (regular) water owing to the risk of dilutional hyponatremia. Exercise of this duration (e.g., marathon running and long-distance triathlons) will require electrolyte and carbohydrate replacement for optimal performance.

■ Athletes should consume 400–800 mL of water per hour during exercise. Slower runners/walkers exercising in cool conditions can consume water at the lower rate, whereas faster/heavier athletes and those exercising in heat and humidity should target the higher end for their goal consumption.

■ Athletes should consume 6–12 ounces of plain water if exercising less than 60 minutes. If exercising longer than 60 minutes, consider a carbohydrate- and electrolyte-containing sports drink. (See Fluid Tips for Training and Competition, available at cals.arizona.edu/pubs/health/az1387.pdf; and Food Tips for Training & Competition, available at cals.arizona.edu/pubs/health/az1386.pdf.)

■ Carbonated water may cause gastrointestinal distress and bloating; avoid drinking carbonated water before or during an athletic event.

Ergogenic Supplements

■ Little clinical evidence is available to support the performance-enhancing claims for most herbal supplements.

■ Evidence does not support a performance benefit for antioxidants, arginine, chromium, citrulline, conjugated linoleic acid, ginseng, glycerol, lecithin, or tyrosine.

■ Evidence does not consistently support a performance benefit for branch-chain amino acids, caffeine, carnitine, *Cordyceps sinensis*, hydroxy-beta-methylbutrate, phosphatidylserine, and *Rhodiola*.

■ Creatine may increase muscle strength while it is being used, but gastrointestinal discomfort may occur. Take the loading dose (20 mg) in four separate doses to avoid this problem. Maintain proper hydration to assist in the elimination of metabolic waste. There is no known benefit to long-term use of creatine.

and eating a well-balanced diet have consistently been shown to benefit sports and activities.

➤ Most sports nutrition drinks, gels, and bars are significant sources of carbohydrate calories, and should be avoided unless their use is indicated by the duration of physical activity lasting greater than 60 minutes and by a risk of glycogen depletion.

➤ Dehydration can significantly affect performance. However, there is no evidence that sports nutrition drinks are beneficial when used during events lasting 60 minutes or less.

➤ Sports nutrition drinks that contain electrolytes and carbohydrates can prolong the time until glycogen depletion in events lasting 60 minutes or longer and therefore may improve performance.

➤ Average athletes exercising for very long periods of time should use a sports drink that contains electrolytes and carbohydrates as an alternative to plain water to minimize the risk of hyponatremia caused by the intake of salt-free fluids. An example would be a recreational runner completing a marathon slowly over 5 to 6 hours.

➤ All athletes should be encouraged to continue moving or walking for several minutes at the completion of a race, because the continued muscle contraction of the legs may reduce the risk of orthostasis. Athletes who stop moving or lie down in a prone position immediately after crossing the finish line are at risk of orthostatic hypotension caused by blood pooling in their legs.

➤ Creatine supplementation can increase muscle phosphocreatine concentrations, thus increasing the amount of stored energy in the muscle. Phosphocreatine can lend its high-energy phosphate bond to ADP to rapidly restore ATP, allowing for increased strength and power for single and repeated activities for 30 seconds or less.

➤ Athletes engaging in intense weight training and activities requiring repeated sprints with short recovery times may benefit from creatine supplementation; however, the strength benefits associated with creatine "wash out" when the supplementation stops.

➤ Pseudoephedrine is banned by the U.S. Anti-Doping Agency, and athletes subject to testing for banned substances should be warned of any product containing pseudoephedrine. A similar warning should be given for any cough and cold product that includes a sympathomimetic amine as a decongestant, such as oxymetazoline nasal spray.

REFERENCES

1. Manore MM, Barr SI, Butterfield GE. Position of the American Dietetic Association, Dieticians of Canada, and the American College of Sports Medicine: Nutrition and athletic performance. *J Am Diet Assoc.* 2000;100: 1543–56.

2. National College Athletic Association. NCAA Study of Substance Use Habits of College Student-Athletes. June 2001. Available at: http://www.ncaa.org/library/research/substance_use_habits/2001/substance_use_habits.pdf. Last accessed September 16, 2008.

3. Hoffman JR, Faigenbaum AD, Ratamess NA, et al. Nutritional supplementation and anabolic steroid use in adolescents. *Med Sci Sport Exerc.* 2008;40:15–24.

4. Coyle EF. Physical activity as a metabolic stressor. *Am J Clin Nutr.* 2000; 72(suppl):512S–20S.

5. Spencer MR, Gastin PB. Energy system contribution during 200–1500 meter running in highly trained athletes. *Med Sci Sport Exerc.* 2001;33: 157–62.

6. Achten J, Jeukendrup AE. Optimizing fat oxidation through exercise and diet. *Nutrition.* 2004;20:716–727.

7. Vistisen B, Nybo L, Xu X, et al. Minor amounts of plasma medium-chain fatty acids and no improved time trial performance after consuming lipids. *J Appl Physiol.* 2003;95:2434–43.

8. Wolfe RR. Protein supplements and exercise. *Am J Clin Nutr.* 2000; 72(suppl):551S–7S.

9. Koopman R, Saris WH, Wagenmakers AJ, et al. Nutritional interventions to promote post-exercise muscle protein synthesis. *Sports Med.* 2007; 37:895–906.

10. Tarnopolsky MA, Atkinson SA, MacDougal JD, et al. Evaluation of protein requirements for trained strength athletes. *J Appl Physiol.* 1992;73:1986–95.

11. Brandle E, Sieberth HG, Hautmann RE. Effect of chronic dietary protein intake on the renal function of healthy subjects. *Eur J Clin Nutr.* 1996; 50:734–40.

12. Poortmans JR, Dellalieux O. Do regular high protein diets have potential health risks on kidney function in athletes? *Int J Sport Nutr Exerc Metab.* 2000;10:28–38.

13. Murray D. Exercise and fluid replacement: the American College of Sports Medicine position stand. *Med Sci Sport Exerc.* 2007;39:377–90.

14. Almond CS, Shin AY, Fortescue EB, et al. Hyponatremia among runners in the Boston marathon. *N Engl J Med.* 2005;325:1550–6.

15. Hew-Butler T, Verbalis JG, Noakes TD. Updated fluid recommendation: position statement from the International Marathon Medical Directors Association (IMMDA). *Clin J Sport Med.* 2006;16:283–92.

16. Hampson NB, Pollock NW, Piantadosi CA. Oxygenated water and athletic performance. *JAMA.* 2003;290;2408–9.

17. Saunders MJ, Kane MD, Todd, MK. Effects of a carbohydrate-protein beverage on cycling endurance and muscle damage. *Med Sci Sport Exerc.* 2004;36:1233–8.

18. Ivy JL, Res PT, Sprague RC, et al. Effects of a carbohydrate-protein beverage on endurance performance during exercise of varying intensity. *Int J Sport Nutr Exerc Metab.* 2003;382–95.

19. Romano-Ely BC, Todd MK, Saunders MJ, et al. Effect of an isocaloric carbohydrate-protein-antioxidant drink on cycling performance. *Med Sci Sport Exerc.* 2006;38:1608–16.

20. Van Essen M, Gibala MJ. Failure of protein to improve time trial performance when added to a sports drink. *Med Sci Sport Exerc.* 2006;38: 1476–83.

21. Williams MB, Raven PB, Fogt DL, et al. Effects of recovery beverages on glycogen restoration and endurance exercise performance. *J Strength Cond Res.* 2003;17:12–9.

22. Carrithers JA, Williamson JA, Gallagher PM, et al. Effects of postexercise carbohydrate-protein feedings on muscle glycogen restoration. *J Appl Physiol.* 2000;88:1976–82.

23. Jentjens RL, Addition of protein and amino acids to carbohydrates does not enhance postexercise muscle glycogen synthesis. *J Appl Physiol.* 2001;91:839–46.

24. Shirreffs SM, Watson P, Maughan RJ. Milk as an effective post-exercise rehydration drink. *Br J Nutrition.* 2007;98:173–80.

25. Graham TE. Caffeine and exercise: metabolism, endurance and performance. *Sports Med.* 2001;31:785–807.

26. Bell DG, McLellan TM. Exercise endurance 1, 3, and 6h after caffeine ingestion in caffeine users and non-users. *J Appl Physiol.* 2002;93:1227–34.

27. Bemben MG, Lamont HS. Creatine supplementation and exercise performance. *Sports Med.* 2005;35:107–25.

28. Greenwood M, Kreider RB, Greenwood L, et al. Cramping and injury incidence in collegiate football players are reduced by creatine supplementation. *J Athlet Train.* 2004;38:216–9.

29. Greenwood M, Kreider RB, Melton C, et al. Creatine supplementation during college football training does not increase the incidence of cramping or injury. *Mol Cell Biochem.* 2003;244:83–8.

30. Centers for Disease Control and Prevention. Adverse events associated with ephedrine containing products–Texas, December 1993-September 1995. *MMWR Morb Mortal Wkly Rep.* 1996;45:689–93.

31. Haller CA, Benowitz NL. Adverse cardiovascular and central nervous system events associated with dietary supplements containing ephedra alkaloids. *N Engl J Med.* 2000;343:1833–8.

32. Shekelle PG, Hardy ML, Morton SC, et al. Efficacy and safety of ephedra and ephedrine for weight loss and athletic performance: a meta analysis. *JAMA.* 2003;289:1537–45.

33. Hodges K, Hancock S, Currell K, et al. Pseudoephedrine enhances performance in 1500m runners. *Med SCi Sports Exerc*. 2006;38:329–33.

34. Brown Ga, Vokovich M, King DS. Testosterone prohormone supplements. *Med Sci Sport Exerc*. 2006;38:1451–61.

35. Powers SK, Hamilton K. Antioxidants and exercise. *Clin Sports Med*. 1999;18:525–35.

36. Flakoll P, Sharp R, Levenhagen D, et al. Effect of beta-hydroxy-beta-methylbutyrate, arginine and lysine supplementation on strength, functionality, body composition, and protein metabolism in elderly women. *Nutrition*. 2004;20:455–51.

37. Cheuvront SN, Carter R, Kolka MA, et al. Branched-chain amino acid supplementation and human performance when hypohydrated in the heat. *J Appl Physiol*. 2004;97:1275–82.

38. Davis JM, Welsh RS, De Volve KL, et al. Effects of branched-chain amino acids and carbohydrate on fatigue during intermittent, high-intensity running. *Int J Sports Med*. 1999;20:309–14.

39. Karlic H, Lohninger A. Supplementation of L-carnitine in athletes: does it make sense? *Nutrition*. 2004;20:709–15.

40. Vincent JB. The potential value and toxicity of chromium picolinate as a nutritional supplement, weight loss agent and muscle development agent. *Sports Med*. 2003;33:213–30.

41. Hickner RC, Tanner CJ, Evans CA, et al. L–Citrulline reduces time to exhaustion and insulin response to a graded exercise test. *Med Sci Sports Exerc*. 2006;38:660–6.

42. Kreider RB, Ferreira MP, Greenwood M, et al. Effects of conjugated linoleic acid supplementation during resistance training on body composition, bone density, strength, and selected hematological markers. *J Strength Cond Res*. 2002;16:325–34.

43. Parcell AC, Smith JM, Schulthies SS, et al. Cordyceps sinensis (CordyMax Cs-4) supplementation does not improve endurance exercise performance. *Int J Sport Nutr Exerc Metab*. 2004;14:236–42.

44. Colson SN, Wyatt FB, Johnston DL, et al. Cordyceps sinensis- and rhodiola rosea-based supplementation in male cyclists and its effect on muscle tissue oxygen saturation. *J Strength Cond Res*. 2005;19:358–63.

45. Goulet ED, Dionne IJ. Assessment of the effects of Eleutherococcus senticosus on endurance performance. *Int J Sport Nutr Exerc Metab*. 2005;15:75–83.

46. Engels H, Fahlman MM, Wirth JC. Effects of ginseng on secretory IgA, performance and recovery from interval exercise. *Med Sci Sports Exerc*. 2003;35:690–6.

47. Nelson JL, Robergs RA. Exploring the potential ergogenic effects of glycerol hyperhydration. *Sports Med*. 2007;37:981–1000.

48. Buchman AL, Awal MA, Jenden D, et al. The effect of lecithin supplementation on plasma choline concentrations during a marathon. *J Am Coll Nutr*. 2000;19:768–70.

49. Kinglsey M. Effects of phosphatidylserine supplementation on exercising humans. *Sports Med*. 2006;36:657–69.

50. De Bock K, Eijnde BO, Ramaekers M, et al. Acute Rhodiola rosea intake can improve endurance exercise performance. *Int J Sport Nutr Exerc Metab*. 2004;14:298–307.

51. Earnest CP, Morss GM. Effects of a commercial herbal-based formula on exercise performance in cyclists. *Med Sci Sports Exerc*. 2004;36:504–9.

52. Chinevere TD, Sawer RD, Creer AR, et al. Effects of l-tyrosine and carbohydrate ingestion on endurance performance. *J Appl Physiol*. 2002;93:1590–7.

Infant Nutrition and Special Nutritional Needs of Children

Katherine H. Chessman

Human milk is most physiologically suited to infants and is the optimal milk source for feeding infants until 12 months of age. The American Academy of Pediatrics (AAP) recommends that human milk be used as the sole source of nutrition for infants during the first 6 months of life. For infants whose mothers cannot or will not breast-feed, the nutritional quality, safety, and convenience of infant formulas make them an appropriate alternative. Variations among formulas allow for product selection that will meet a specific infant's nutritional needs while offering differences in palatability, digestibility, nutrient sources, convenience, and cost.

A health care practitioner should be able to provide information to parents or other caregivers to encourage successful breast-feeding. In addition, in consultation with the child's parents and primary care provider, the clinician should be able to evaluate indications, advise on formula selection, and help ensure its appropriate use. This service requires knowledge of infant and child nutrition needs, breast-feeding, and commercially prepared infant and pediatric formulas, including differences in formula composition and specific uses for therapeutic formulas.

Some children will require enteral formulas after the age of 1 year because of various disease states and conditions. The clinician needs to be knowledgeable of these products and their appropriate use to be able to answer caregiver questions about them, facilitate their procurement, and successfully triage complications associated with these products.

Organ Maturation and Infant Growth

Knowledge of the development of the gastrointestinal (GI) tract and the kidney is crucial to understanding infant nutrition. Comparison of an individual infant's or child's growth with his or her previous growth rate and plotting their growth on the Centers for Disease Control and Prevention (CDC) age- and gender-specific standardized growth charts for infants and children is the best method for confirming that nutritional needs are being met.

Gastrointestinal Maturation

By the end of the second trimester of pregnancy, all segments of the fetus' GI tract are formed and display some physiologic function. The third trimester, however, is the period of maximal GI tract growth and differentiation. Therefore, premature infants (those born before 38 weeks gestation) often have reduced GI

tract function, especially those born prior to 32 weeks gestation. Transition from intrauterine nutrition through the maternal–fetal unit (i.e., the placenta) to extrauterine nutrition through milk requires the maturation of many physiologic processes. These processes include effective sucking, swallowing, gastric emptying, intestinal peristalsis, and defecation; salivary, gastric, pancreatic, and hepatobiliary secretions; and, intestinal brush border enzymes and transport systems (Table 26-1).[1]

Nutritive sucking develops at approximately 33 to 34 weeks gestation. In term infants, a mature, efficient pattern of sucking is seen within a few days after birth. In premature infants, an immature, inefficient pattern may persist for a month or more. Infants born before 34 weeks gestation cannot coordinate sucking, swallowing, and breathing; therefore, they may require tube feedings for several weeks to months until these reflexes mature. Liquid nutrition is appropriate for all infants until complex tongue movements and swallowing reflexes mature. Maturation of these reflexes typically occurs at 4 to 6 months of age, and it is at this time that solid foods can be safely added to an infant's diet.[1]

Early in life, frequent feedings (every 2–3 hours) are necessary, because the stomach capacity of a term newborn with a birth weight greater than 2500 grams (5 pounds 8 ounces) is only 20 to 90 mL. Gastric capacity increases to 90 to 150 mL by 1 month of age, at which time longer periods between feedings are possible. Human milk empties more rapidly from the stomach than infant formula does; therefore human milk–fed infants will typically eat more often than their formula-fed peers.

In term infants, gastric acid and pepsin secretion peak in the first 10 days of life, decrease between days 10 and 30 of life, and then increase to adult levels by 3 months of age. In premature infants, basal acid output is lower than that of a term infant but increases with postnatal age. Milk in the infant's stomach causes a sharp increase in the pH of the gastric contents and a slower return to lower pH values than in older children and adults. Gastric acidity in the newborn is unsuitable for optimal pepsin action. Therefore, little protein digestion occurs in the stomach because of low pepsin activity. The extent of protein absorption, however, is similar to that seen in children and adults. Amino acids and peptides produced by protein digestion are absorbed passively or by active transport mechanisms that reach adult capacity by the age of 14 weeks.

Premature and full-term infants can digest most carbohydrates, because the production of intestinal enzymes such as sucrase, maltase, isomaltase, and glucoamylase is sufficiently

TABLE 26-1 Gastrointestinal Maturation

Function	Weeks Gestation When First Detectable	Comments
Sucking and swallowing	16	16 weeks: swallowing of amniotic fluid 26 weeks: sucking 33–35 weeks: mature, coordinated sucking, swallowing, and breathing
Gastric motility and secretion	20	Gastric emptying delayed in first few days of life; affected by caloric density, carbohydrate concentration, pathologic conditions
Intestinal motility	20	26–30 weeks: disorganized contractile activity 30–34 weeks: repetitive groups of contractions 34–35 weeks: more mature migrating motor complexes

Digestion and Absorption

Examples of Factors Important in Digestion and Absorption	Weeks of Gestation When First Detectable	Proportion of Adult Values
Protein		
Enterokinase	24–26	20% at 30 weeks 10%–25% at term
Hydrochloric acid	At birth	<20% at 30 weeks <30% at term 50% for first 3 months
Peptidases	<12	15% at 30 weeks Nearly 100% at term
Trypsinogen/chymotrypsinogen	20	10%–60% at term
Amino acid transport	ND	Nearly 100% at term
Macromolecule absorption	ND	Nearly 100% at term
Fat		
Lingual lipase	30	Nearly 100% at term
Pancreatic lipase	16–20	5%–10% at term
Bile acids	22	25% at 32 weeks 50% at term
Medium-chain triglyceride uptake	ND	100% (absorption occurs in the stomach)
Long-chain triglyceride uptake	ND	10%–90% at term
Carbohydrate		
Pancreatic alpha-amylase	22–30	0% at term Secretion begins at 6 months of age
Salivary alpha-amylase	16	0% at 30 weeks 10%–20% at term
Lactase	10	30% at 28–34 weeks Near 100% at term
Monosaccharide absorption	11–19	Glucose absorption: 50%–60% at term

Key: ND, not determined.

Source: References 1, 2, and Kleinman RE, Kamin DS. Gastrointestinal development. In: Baker SS, Baker RD, Davis AM, eds. *Pediatric Nutrition Support.* Sudbury, Mass: Jones and Bartlett Publishers; 2007:15–27.

mature at birth. Lactase activity increases relatively late in fetal life and begins to decline after the age of 3 years, especially in African American and Asian children. By adulthood, approximately 15% of Caucasians, 40% of Asians, and 85% of African Americans are deficient in intestinal lactase.[2] Pancreatic amylase secretion does not reach adult levels until approximately 1 year of age. Salivary amylase may help compensate for this relative lactase and amylase deficiency in early infancy. Despite this relative lactase deficiency, most term and preterm infants tolerate lactose-containing formulas with negligible unabsorbed carbohydrate output in their stools. Unabsorbed lactose that enters the colon undergoes bacterial fermentation (colonic salvage) to short-chain fatty acids, which creates an acidic environment favoring growth of acidophilic bacterial flora (lactobacilli) and suppressing growth of more pathogenic organisms. This acidity also promotes water absorption and prevents osmotic diarrhea. Because of the relative abundance of glucoamylase, compared with lactase, in the premature infant's intestine, glucose polymers are digested and absorbed better than lactose.[1]

Newborns exhibit low pancreatic lipase concentrations and slow rates of bile acid synthesis, both of which are important for fat absorption. The rate of bile acid synthesis increases throughout gestation and with increasing postnatal age. The bile acid pool in a premature infant is one-fourth that of an adult, whereas a term infant's is one-half that of an adult. However, fat malabsorption is not a major problem in preterm or term infants, given that lingual and gastric lipases are present. Infants born earlier than 34 weeks gestation, however, may exhibit steatorrhea.

Intestinal length may also affect nutrient absorption. At birth, a term infant's small intestine is approximately 270 cm long. During the third trimester, the intestinal length approximately doubles. Therefore, infants born prematurely will have less small intestine and, subsequently, decreased surface area for absorption. Adult intestinal length of 4 to 5 meters is reached by about 4 years of age.

Kidney Maturation

Maturation of the kidney is also important in nutrition, because it determines the ability of the kidney to excrete a solute load. Glomerular filtration begins around the ninth week of fetal life; however, kidney function does not appear to be necessary for normal intrauterine homeostasis, given that the placenta serves as the major excretory organ. After birth, the rate of glomerular filtration increases until growth stops, toward the end of the second decade of life. Even after correction for body surface area, the glomerular filtration rate of a child does not approximate adult values until the third year of life.

Growth

Birth weight is determined primarily by maternal pre-pregnancy weight and pregnancy weight changes. The average birth weight of a term infant is approximately 3500 grams (7 pounds 8 ounces). Premature infants are categorized on the basis of birth weight: low-birth-weight (LBW) infants weigh less than 2500 grams (5 pounds 8 ounces); very-low-birth-weight infants weigh less than 1500 grams (3 pounds 4 ounces); extremely low-birth-weight infants weigh less than 1000 grams (2 pounds 3 ounces); and micropremies weigh less than 750 grams (1 pounds 10 ounces).

Water weight loss (6%–10% of body weight) occurs immediately after birth over a period of 1 to 2 weeks and is followed by an average weight gain of 1% to 2% of birth weight daily (25–35 g/day in term infants) during the first 4 months, and 15 g/day over the next 8 months. Most term infants double their birth weight by 4 months of age and triple it by 12 months. Premature infants may reach these milestones sooner. From 2 years to approximately 10 years of age, the growth rate is fairly constant at about 2.3 kg (5 pounds) each year. Growth velocity increases and a major growth spurt occurs during adolescence. Height shows a growth pattern similar to that of weight; most infants increase their length by 50% in the first year, 100% in the first 4 years, and 300% by 13 years of age. Changes in body

composition accompany height and weight changes. Most notably, total body water decreases as adipose tissue increases. Total body water accounts for approximately 90% of total body weight at 24 weeks gestation, 70% at term, and 60% by 1 year of age.

Normal values of weight, length/height, and head circumference (until 3 years of age) for infants and children are generally expressed in terms of percentile-for-age; the reference standards most commonly used are the CDC growth charts developed by the National Center for Health Statistics (NCHS). The 1977 growth charts were significantly revised in 2000 using an expanded data set that is more representative of the diverse ethnicity and combined breast- and bottle-feeding of infants in the United States.[3] Twenty age-, and gender-specific charts can be downloaded free of charge at www.cdc.gov/growthcharts. The infant charts are intended for use in term infants. Once premature infants reach 40 weeks gestational age, their growth parameters can be plotted on these charts, but their age must be corrected for gestational age (i.e., chronological age in weeks minus number of weeks premature) until 24 months of age for weight and 36 months for length/height and head circumference. Charts for premature infants less than 40 weeks gestation and children with specific conditions (e.g., Down syndrome, cerebral palsy, or Turner syndrome) are available and should be used when appropriate. These specialized growth charts can be found on various Web sites including those of the National Down Syndrome Society (www1.ndss.org), the Kennedy Krieger Institute for children with disorders of the brain and spinal cord such as cerebral palsy (www.kennedykrieger.org), and the Turner Syndrome Society of the United States (www.turnersyndrome.org) The most commonly used charts for premature infants are the Babson and Benda charts, which can be accessed at www.biomedcentral.com/1471-2431/3/13. Most infants' growth parameters will fall between the 3rd and 97th percentiles on the gender-specific weight-for-age, length/height-for-age, weight-for-length, and head circumference-for-age charts. Most children grow along a percentile established shortly after birth, but spurts and plateaus are common. Failure to thrive is defined as a fall of two or more growth percentiles from a previously established percentile in 6 months or less. If growth is not progressing as expected, particularly in the first year of life when growth should be rapid, the infant's diet and other potential contributory factors (e.g., environment, diseases, or syndromes) should be evaluated. Satisfactory growth is the most sensitive indicator of meeting nutritional needs.

For children older than 2 years, body mass index (BMI)-for-age charts can be useful in assessing obesity risk. BMI, a measure of body weight adjusted for height, is a useful tool to assess body fat and is calculated as weight in kilograms divided by height in meters squared. According to current CDC guidelines, a child with a BMI at or above the 85th percentile on the gender-specific, BMI-for-age NCHS chart is considered "at risk of overweight," and a child with a BMI at or above the 95th percentile is "overweight." However, in 2005, the American Medical Association in collaboration with the Health Resources and Service Administration and the CDC convened an expert committee that was charged with revising these recommendations. The committee's nomenclature changes were intended to make it easier to discuss these issues with parents and children and to transition to adult assessments. These new recommendations state that a child whose BMI is at or above the 85th percentile but below the 95th percentile or 30 kg/m², whichever is smaller, should be classified as "overweight." A child whose BMI is at or above the 95th percentile or 30 kg/m², whichever is smaller, should be classified as "obese."[4] In 2003–2004, 18.2% of children and adolescents 2 to 19 years of age were classified as overweight according to the earlier CDC guidelines.[5] A BMI below the 5th percentile is indicative of underweight. The clinician should realize that, because of the way the growth charts were developed, 5% of normally growing and healthy children will fall below the 5th and 5% will fall above the 95th percentile on the weight-for-age or height-for-age charts. These children should not be branded as "malnourished" or "obese."

Infant Nutritional Standards

Acceptable growth is achievable only with adequate intake; absorption; and utilization of energy, protein, carbohydrates, minerals, and vitamins. The Food and Nutrition Board of the National Research Council has established dietary reference intakes (DRIs) as reference values for nutrient intake sufficiency and safety. The DRIs for micronutrients are discussed in detail in Chapter 23, and tables in that chapter list the current established recommended dietary allowances (RDAs) and adequate intakes (AIs) for healthy infants and children. Table 26-2 provides the DRIs of macronutrients for healthy infants and children.[5] Children with various diseases and syndromes may have different needs. One example is the need for "catch-up" calories in infants and children recovering from failure to thrive. Calorie requirements for catch-up growth are often 1.5 times or more

those of age-matched peers, depending on the degree of catch-up growth needed.

An amendment to the Federal Food, Drug, and Cosmetic Act (Infant Formula Act of 1980; amended 1986) gives the Food and Drug Administration (FDA) the authority to revise nutrient levels for infant formulas, establish quality control, and require adequate labeling. FDA sets specifications for minimum amounts of 29 nutrients and maximum amounts of nine of those nutrients. All formulas marketed in the United States must meet these requirements. Parents should be cautioned against using any infant formula not manufactured in the United States. FDA alerts have warned of the dangers of using infant formulas from China whose contents fall well below FDA standards. Formulas granted exemption from FDA-established nutrient specifications must be labeled for use by infants who have inborn errors of metabolism, had a low birth weight, or otherwise have unusual medical problems or dietary needs. A list of exempt formulas can be obtained at the FDA's Center for Food Safety and Applied Nutrition Web site (www.cfsan.fda.gov).

Energy requirements vary with age and clinical condition. Total energy expenditure is a combination of basal energy needs, the energy required to digest food (thermic effect of feeding, also called "specific dynamic action of food"), thermoregulation, and activity. Estimates of energy requirements for infants and children are based on meeting total energy expenditure plus promoting growth. An infant's energy requirement is higher in relation to body mass than that of an adult or older child because of the rapid growth experienced during infancy. Estimated energy requirements for term infants and children are shown in

TABLE 26-2 Dietary Reference Intakes of Macronutrients for Full-Term Infants and Children[a,b]

Nutrient	0–6 Months	7–12 Months	1–3 Years	4–8 Years	9–13 Years
Energy[c] (kcal/day)	M: 570 F: 520	M: 743 F: 676	M: 1046 F: 992	M: 1742 F: 1642	M: 2279 F: 2071
Protein[c] (g/kg/day)	1.52	1.2[d]	1.05[d]	0.95[d]	0.95[d]
(g/day)	9.1	13.5[d]	13[d]	19[d]	34[d]
Carbohydrate (g/day)	60	95	130[d]	130[d]	130[d]
Water (L/day)[e]	0.7	0.8	1.3	1.7	M: 2.4 F: 2.1
Fat (g/day)	31	30	ND	ND	ND
Alpha-linolenic acid (g/day)	0.5	0.5	0.7	0.9	M: 1.2 F: 1.0
Linoleic acid (g/day)	4.4	4.6	7	10	M: 12 F: 10
Fiber (g/day)	ND	ND	19	25	M: 31 F: 26

Key: AI, adequate intake; DRI, dietary reference intake; F, female; M, male; ND, not determined; RDA, recommended dietary intake.

[a] Expressed as AIs unless noted otherwise.

[b] DRIs have not been established for premature infants.

[c] Estimated requirements; include needs associated with growth (i.e., energy expenditure plus energy deposition). The assumed normal body weight and length used for the DRIs are 0–6 months: 6 kg, 62 cm; 7–12 months: 9 kg, 71 cm; 1–3 years: 12 kg, 86 cm; 4–8 years: 20 kg, 115 cm; and 9–13 years: 36 kg, 144 cm for males, 37 kg, 144 cm for females.

[d] Expressed as RDA.

[e] Water from all sources including formula, human milk, foods, beverages, and drinking water.

Source: Reference 5.

Table 26-2. Although no RDA has been established, premature infants require as much as 120 to 150 kcal/kg/day or more for adequate growth.

Components of a Healthy Diet

Infants require the same dietary components as adults: fluid, carbohydrates, proteins, fats, and micronutrients. However, the desired proportion of these components in the infant diet differs.

Fluid

Water is an important part of an infant's diet, given that it makes up a larger proportion of the infant's body weight than in older children or adults. The Holliday-Segar method is most often used to estimate maintenance water needs: 100 mL/kg/day for the first 10 kg of body weight, plus 50 mL/kg/day for each kilogram between 10 and 20 kg, and 20 mL/kg/day for each kilogram over 20 kg. Body surface area may also be used to estimate daily fluid requirements; fluid requirements are approximately 1500 mL/m²/day. These methods will underestimate the needs of premature infants whose requirements are, in general, much higher (i.e., 120–170 mL/kg/day or more). Adequate water intake in the first 6 months of life can be derived from human milk or formula. Both contain sufficient amounts of water, so the normal, healthy infant does not need supplemental water. From 6 to 12 months of age, when solid foods are introduced, water intake remains high, because most infant foods contain at least 60% to 70% more water than other foods, and formula or human milk intake should still be high.

Renal excretion, evaporation from the skin and lungs, and, to a lesser extent, feces are the major routes of fluid loss. Increased water loss caused by diarrhea, fever, or unusually rapid breathing, particularly in concert with decreased water intake, may result in significant dehydration and electrolyte imbalance, and must be offset by fluid intake in excess of maintenance needs.

Carbohydrates

An AI for carbohydrates has been established for infants (Table 26-2).[6] Under normal circumstances, an infant can efficiently use a diet with 40% to 50% of total calories from a carbohydrate source. Carbohydrate intake should be balanced with adequate fat intake to allow proper neurologic development. A carbohydrate-free diet is generally undesirable, because it may lead to metabolic modifications favoring fatty acid breakdown, dehydration, and tissue protein and cation loss. However, children with seizures may receive an essentially carbohydrate-free diet, the ketogenic diet, because these metabolic effects may facilitate seizure control. Use of a ketogenic diet should be under the direct/strict supervision of a physician along with a registered dietitian or other qualified practitioner. Lactose, the primary carbohydrate source in human milk and most milk-based formulas, is hydrolyzed to its monosaccharide components, glucose and galactose, by gastric acid and lactase. Congenital lactase deficiency is a rare type of lactose intolerance that results from an inborn error of metabolism. Infants born prematurely, prior to the maturation of significant lactase activity (before approximately 36 weeks gestation), are relatively lactase deficient. Secondary lactase deficiency is a temporary reduction in intes-

tinal lactase caused by gastroenteritis or significant malnutrition. Because of low lactase activity, infants with congenital lactase deficiency, premature infants, and infants recovering from diarrhea or severe malnutrition may be unable to completely metabolize the quantity of lactose found in human milk or milk-based infant formulas, and may develop lactose intolerance resulting in diarrhea, abdominal pain or distention, bloating, gas, and cramping.

Fiber intake is of considerable interest because, in adults, high-fiber diets have been associated with the prevention of diverticular disease, colon cancer, and coronary heart disease. (See Chapter 24 for further discussion of fiber.) The American Health Foundation has recommended a daily fiber intake calculated by using the equation: fiber (grams/day) = age (in years) plus 5. Age plus 10 g/day is also felt to be a safe intake.[7] An AI for fiber for infants 0 to 12 months of age has not been established. Infants rarely require fiber to maintain normal bowel function. However, from age 6 to 12 months, whole cereals, green vegetables, and legumes provide a source of fiber in the infant's diet. The fiber AI for older children is shown in Table 26-2. Adult values are reached by the teens.

Protein and Amino Acids

The most recent revision of the DRIs established new AIs for protein in term infants and children (Table 26-2).[6] Total body protein increases by an average of 3.5 g/day in the first 4 months of life and by 3.1 g/day over the next 8 months, representing an overall increase in body protein composition from 11% to 15% of total body weight.

The protein's amino acid composition (i.e., chemical value) is also important. Amino acids are classified as essential (or indispensable), nonessential, or conditionally essential. Cysteine, histidine, isoleucine, leucine, lysine, methionine, phenylalanine, threonine, tryptophan, tyrosine, and valine are considered essential amino acids for infants, because the human body cannot synthesize them from other amino acid and carbohydrate precursors. In the neonate and young infant, immature biochemical pathways for synthesis or conversion of amino acids may prevent adequate synthesis for normal growth and development.

Taurine is an especially important amino acid in infancy. Quantities in human milk are high, and all infant formulas are supplemented during the manufacturing process to provide the same margin of physiologic safety as that provided by human milk.[8] Taurine is not an energy source nor is it used for protein synthesis, but it serves as a cell membrane protector by attenuating toxic substances (e.g., oxidants, secondary bile acids, and excess retinoids) and acting as an osmoregulator. Taurine deficiency can result in retinal dysfunction, slow development of auditory brain stem–evoked response in preterm infants, and poor fat absorption in preterm infants and children with cystic fibrosis. These conditions can be improved with taurine supplements.

Despite similar amino acid densities and milk intakes, serum concentrations of some amino acids measured in formula-fed infants tend to exceed those measured in human milk–fed infants. The clinical significance of this difference is unknown, however, because the growth of these infants is equivalent. The protein content of human milk adjusts to a growing infant's needs, but the high protein needs of preterm infants are not completely met by early human milk. Fortification with commercially available powders is required to achieve reasonable amino acid profiles and for the preterm infant to meet expected growth rates. In evaluating the adequacy of an infant's protein intake, one must consider not only the absolute amount of protein ingested but also the growth rate, the quantity of nonprotein calories and other nutrients necessary for protein synthesis, and the quality of the protein itself.

Fat and Essential Fatty Acids

Fat is the most calorically dense component in the diet, providing 9 kcal/g compared with 4 kcal/g for both protein and carbohydrates. Fat accounts for approximately 50% of the nonprotein energy in both human milk and infant formula. Infant feeding practices, especially fat and calorie intake, are increasingly being linked to obesity and other diseases (e.g., diabetes and cardiovascular disease) in adulthood. Despite these concerns, children younger than 2 years (the time of most rapid growth and development requiring high-energy intakes) should not receive a fat- or cholesterol-restricted diet unless medically prescribed. AAP supports this position because of the need for adequate fatty acid intake for normal neurologic development and adequate calories for growth.[9] Between 2 and 5 years of age, children should be encouraged to adopt a diet that contains 20% to 30% of total calories from fat with less than 10% of calories from saturated fats.[9]

The diet must also contain small amounts of the essential polyunsaturated fatty acids (PUFAs): linoleic (n-6) and linolenic acid (n-3). These fatty acids are precursors for the n-3 and n-6 long-chain PUFAs (LCPUFAS): docosohexanoic acid (DHA) and arachidonic acid (ARA). Essential fatty acid deficiency, rarely seen in the United States, can manifest as increased metabolic rate, failure to thrive, hair loss, dry flaky skin, thrombocytopenia, and impaired wound healing. Because of substantial fat stores, clinical manifestations of essential fatty acid deficiency are generally delayed for months in older children and adults; however, rapid onset (within days to weeks) may occur in premature infants with inadequate linoleic acid in their diets. Linoleic acid represents the bulk of PUFAs in infant formulas. Generally, an intake of linoleic acid equal to 1% to 2% of total dietary calories is adequate to prevent essential fatty acid deficiency; 3% to 7% is the amount found in human milk. The AI for the essential PUFAs is shown in Table 26-2.

Historically, infant formulas contained only the precursor PUFAs: linoleic and linolenic acid. Now, most infant formulas are supplemented during manufacturing with the LCPUFAs: DHA and ARA. In fact, more than 60 countries permit the addition of these fatty acids to infant formulas. AAP has not taken an official stand on whether infant formulas should be supplemented with DHA and ARA. These LCPUFAs, which are abundant in human milk but not in cow milk, are not considered essential but thought to provide extra benefits. DHA is important in both brain and eye development; the direct role of ARA is less clear. However, supplementation of DHA without ARA may lead to ARA deficiency and possible growth suppression.

Whether the addition of DHA and ARA to infant formulas improves visual and cognitive function remains controversial. Some studies have shown benefits to an infant's visual function, cognitive and behavioral development, and growth with DHA and ARA supplementation; other studies have shown no differences in supplemented versus control infants.[10–13] No adverse effects have been noted in infants receiving DHA- and ARA-supplemented formulas; however, two studies in which the formula was supplemented with only DHA reported growth suppression, stressing the importance of supplementation with both DHA and ARA.[13] FDA has issued a "generally recognized as safe" (GRAS) notification to Martek Biosciences Corporation for its patented plant-based fatty acid blends DHASCO and ARASCO, which are currently used to supplement infant formulas only during manufacturing. There is also evidence that maternal diet can affect fatty acid concentrations in the infant both in utero and during lactation for human milk–fed infants.[14] Expecta LIPIL DHA Supplement, softgel capsules that contain 200 mg DHA, is marketed as a non–fish-based supplement for pregnant and lactating women to increase maternal dietary DHA, and potentially increase DHA concentrations in their infants. These capsules may be associated with less aftertaste than are other sources of DHA and ARA. Routine supplementation during pregnancy and lactation remains controversial, and should be discussed with a health care provider.

Micronutrients

DRIs for term infants (given as AIs, if defined, or as RDAs, if AIs are not defined) for vitamins and minerals, including trace elements, are shown in Tables 23-3 and 23-4 in Chapter 23. Precise needs are difficult to define and depend on energy, protein, and fat intakes as well as absorption and nutrient stores. Infant formulas are supplemented with adequate amounts of vitamins and minerals to meet the needs of most term and premature infants when the appropriate formula is chosen. As with protein, human milk must be fortified to meet the micronutrient needs of most premature infants. Appropriate supplementation is included in the discussion of specific milks and formulas.

Infant Food Sources

Human– and cow milk–based formulas are the primary food sources for most infants in the United States. Soy protein–based formulas and goat milk are alternatives. A variety of formulas are available to feed infants with special nutritional needs, including those unable to consume a regular oral diet, those with inborn errors of metabolism, and those with various malabsorptive conditions. Most infants and children receive either human milk or an enteral formula orally; however, some children will receive these through feeding tubes such as naso- or orogastric, gastrostomy, or jejunostomy tubes. A discussion of these feeding techniques is beyond the scope of this chapter.

Human Milk

Both the World Health Organization and AAP recommend infants be breast-fed without supplemental foods or liquids for approximately the first 6 months (i.e., exclusive breast-feeding.)[15,16] Breast-feeding initiation rates have increased steadily since 1990, with the rate at hospital discharge increasing from a low of 24.7% in 1971 to 74% in 2004. At 6 and 12 months of age, however, the rate of any breast-feeding is only 42% and 21%, respectively. Sociodemographic factors affect breast-feeding rates. Black women are less likely than white, Hispanic, and Asian women to breast-feed. For infants born in 2003, approximately 59% of black women were breast-feeding at hospital discharge and 27% when their infants were 6 months of age compared with 76% and 42% for white women, 80% and 42% for Hispanic women, and 79% and 47% for Asian women, respectively. At 1 year of age, rates continue to differ, although less so, with 21% to 25% of white, Hispanic, and Asian women compared with 12% of black women still breast-feeding at that time.[17,18] Poor, unmarried, and poorly educated women are also less likely to breast-feed their infants.

Because breast-feeding is a major public health concern, breast-feeding goals were included in *Healthy People 2000: National Health Promotion and Disease Prevention Objectives,* the national plan to improve the health of the American people.[19] One objective of *Healthy People 2000* was to have 75% of all infants in the United States breast-fed at birth, with 50% receiving human milk at 6 months of age. This objective was not reached by 2000; therefore it was included, along with the objective of having 25% of infants breast-fed at 1 year of age, in *Healthy People 2010.*[20] In 2006, *Healthy People* 2010 expanded its breast-feeding objective to include targets for breast-feeding exclusivity: exclusive breast-feeding through 3 months, 60%; and through 6 months, 25%.[21] AAP recommends support for breast-feeding through the first year of life. The AAP policy statement on breast-feeding has been updated to include recommendations to increase breast-feeding and to address reasons why women are not breast-feeding (e.g., insufficient prenatal breast-feeding education; hospital policies disruptive to breast-feeding; early hospital discharge; physician apathy and misinformation; lack of broad societal support; media portrayal of bottle-feeding as the norm; and promotion of formula through hospital discharge packs, coupons, and television and magazine advertising).[22]

Breast-feeding not only offers an optimal source of nutrition for the infant, it provides other benefits, such as improved mother–child bonding. There are advantages to the infant's general health, growth, and development. Strong evidence indicates that human milk decreases the incidence and/or severity of various infections (e.g., diarrhea, respiratory tract infections, otitis media, bacteremia, bacterial meningitis) in infants, and necrotizing enterocolitis, urinary tract infections, and late-onset sepsis in premature infants.[22] Other proposed benefits of human milk include decreased rates of sudden infant death syndrome, types 1 and 2 diabetes mellitus, lymphoma, leukemia, Hodgkin's disease, overweight, obesity, hypercholesterolemia, and asthma. Breast-feeding has also been associated with slightly enhanced performance on tests of cognitive development; however, the effect of genetic and socioenvironmental factors on intelligence is difficult to measure separately from breast-feeding.[22]

Besides enhanced mother–child bonding, maternal benefits of breast-feeding include decreased postpartum bleeding, more rapid uterine involution, decreased menstrual blood loss, increased spacing between children, earlier return to pre-pregnancy weight, decreased risk of breast and ovarian cancer, and decreased hip fracture and osteoporosis in the postmenopausal period.

At least $3.6 billion in annual health care costs could be saved with improved rates of breast-feeding.[22] An economic analysis of estimated direct health care costs for diarrhea, lower respiratory tract infections, and otitis media in the first year of life found that costs for infants never breast-fed were $300 more than for infants exclusively breast-fed for at least 3 months.[23]

Questions remain about the protective effects of breast-feeding. What is the duration of protection after breast-feeding is discontinued? What influence does maternal age have on the protective effect? How great is the interactive effect of social and demographic variables? How does the addition of solid foods (complementary feeding) to the diet of a human milk–fed infant influence the protective effect? What consequence does partial formula-feeding have on the protective effect? Well-designed studies are needed to answer these questions.

There are very few contraindications to human milk. In developed countries, such as the United States, one reason for women not breast-feeding is the maternal diagnosis of human immunodeficiency virus (HIV) infection, which can be transmitted through human milk. Women with HIV in underdeveloped countries, however, are encouraged to breast-feed, because the risk of infant morbidity and mortality with formula use (from inadequate sanitation, refrigeration, and illiteracy) is greater than the risk of HIV transmission.[22] Other reasons women in developed countries may not be able to breast-feed either temporarily or permanently are classic galactosemia; active, untreated tuberculosis; human T-cell lymphotropic virus types I or II; herpes simplex lesion on the breast (may use other breast); and the use of contraindicated drugs (Table 26-3). Several excellent texts provide information regarding the use of drugs during lactation and pregnancy.[24,25] In addition, a comprehensive database of available information regarding drugs in lactation (LactMed) is maintained by the National Library of Medicine (toxnet.nlm.nih.gov), or questions can be directed to the poison control center or to the National Breastfeeding Helpline at 1-800-994-9662. The overall risk of a drug to a breast-fed infant depends on the concentration in the infant's blood and the effects of the drug on the infant. Feeding immediately before the mother's dose may help minimize exposure, because the concentration in milk is likely to be lowest toward the end of the dosing interval. This may not be true for lipid-soluble drugs. Alternating breast- and bottle-feeds or pumping and discarding breast milk is an option, if the need for a particular drug is short-term.

In the United States and other countries, human milk donor banks have been established. In 2005, approximately 745,329 ounces of human milk (a 45% increase over 5 years) were processed and distributed by the 11 member banks of the Human Milk Banking Association of North America (HMBANA).[26] This milk was sent to hospitals in more than 80 cities located in 29 states and three Canadian provinces. Human milk donations are taken from carefully screened, unpaid donors; then the milk undergoes Holder pasteurization to eliminate potential viral and bacterial contaminants while maintaining most of the milk's unique immunologic factors.[27] It is estimated that about 50% of the immunoglobulin A (IgA) is lost in processing; however, because cow milk contains no IgA, infants who receive donor human milk still benefit from its presence. Donor human milk has been used for many sick and premature infants in neonatal intensive care units (NICUs) across the United States and Canada. It has also been used for older children and adults with a variety of conditions including short-bowel syndrome, metabolic disorders, severe food allergies, cancer, and immune deficiency disorders. Adopted infants with no medical problems have also received donor human milk. The cost is approximately $3 per ounce plus shipping and handling. More information about donor milk banks, including how to be a donor or receive donor milk, can be obtained at HMBANA's Web site (www.hmbana.org).

Cow Milk

Cow milk is the primary nutrient source for commercially prepared milk-based infant formulas. Both human and cow milk contain more than 200 ingredients in the fat- and water-soluble fractions. Estimates of the major nutrients contained

TABLE 26-3   Selected Drugs Contraindicated or to Be Used Cautiously While Breast-Feeding

Prescription Drugs	Drugs of Abuse	Radiopharmaceuticals (Time to Wait after Exposure)
Contraindicated Drugs		
Ciprofloxacin	Amphetamine	Copper 64 (50 hours)
Cyclophosphamide	Cocaine	Gallium 67 (2 weeks)
Cyclosporine	Heroin	Indium 111 (20 hours)
Doxepin	Marijuana	Iodine 123 (36 hours)
Doxorubicin	Phencyclidine	Iodine 125 (12 days)
Ergotamine		Iodine 131 (2–14 days)
Leflunomide		Radioactive sodium (96 hours)
Methotrexate		Technetium 99m (15 hours to 3 days)
Drugs to Be Used Cautiously Owing to Significant Potential Adverse Effects		
Acebutolol	Clemastine	Primidone
Amiodarone	Chloramphenicol	Sulfasalazine
5-Aminosalicylic acid	Gold salts	Tetracyclines (long-term)
Atenolol	Lithium	Vitamin D (high-dose)
Aspirin	Phenobarbital	
Bromocriptine	Phenytoin	

Source: American Academy of Pediatrics, Committee on Drugs. Transfer of drugs and other chemicals into human milk. *Pediatrics.* 2001;108:776–89; manufacturer's prescribing information; and UK Drugs in Lactation Advisory Service at www.ukmicentral.nhs.uk/drugpreg/guide.htm. Last accessed September 3, 2008.

in pooled mature human milk and whole cow milk are listed in Table 26-4.

Whole Cow Milk

Whole cow milk is not suitable for providing nutrition to infants younger than 1 year. Because of the low concentration and poor bioavailability of iron, whole cow milk has been associated with iron-deficiency anemia.[28,29] Sensitivity to dietary proteins, most commonly cow or soy milk proteins, can manifest as occult GI bleeding, further increasing the risk of anemia. In the past decade, convincing evidence has accumulated to indicate that iron deficiency impairs psychomotor development and cognitive function in infants, even with relatively mild anemia. Milk-protein intolerance and/or allergy can also result in rash, wheezing, diarrhea, vomiting, colic, and anaphylaxis when whole cow milk is used. When whole cow milk is fed with solid food, infants receive unnecessarily high intakes of protein and electrolytes, resulting in a high renal solute load (RSL; Table 26-5). The implications of a high RSL will be discussed later in this chapter. The current position of AAP's Committee on Nutrition (CON) is that iron-fortified infant formula is the only acceptable alternative to human milk. The use of cow milk is not recommended during the first year of life.[28]

Reduced-Fat Cow Milk

Reduced-fat cow milk, such as skim milk (0.1% fat), low-fat milk (1% fat), and reduced-fat milk (2% fat), has been advocated to prevent obesity and atherosclerosis as part of a "healthy diet." However, when the low-fat diet recommended for adults is imposed on children younger than 2 years, it puts them at risk for failure to thrive and impaired neurologic development. Infants who receive a major percentage of their caloric intake from reduced-fat milk may receive an exceedingly high protein intake and an inadequate intake of essential fatty acids. The maximum protein concentration allowed by FDA in infant for-

mulas is 4.5 g/100 kcal, but skim milk and 2% milk provide approximately 8 to 10 g/100 kcal and 7 to 10 g/100 kcal, respectively. Therefore, using reduced-fat milk for infant nutrition provides an unbalanced percentage of calories supplied from protein, fat, and carbohydrates.

Per unit volume, skim milk has a slightly higher potential RSL (PRSL) than does whole cow milk (Table 26-5). The solute concentration is further increased by water loss during processing. Reduced-fat milk is not recommended during episodes of diarrhea because of the possibility of hypertonic dehydration. As stated previously, AAP does not recommend the use of low-fat diets during the first 2 years of life.

Evaporated Milk

Between 1930 and 1960, evaporated milk was frequently used in preparing infant formula, but by 1978 few infants received evaporated milk formulas. Evaporated milk is a sterile, convenient source of cow milk that has standardized concentrations of protein, fat, and carbohydrate. When ingested, evaporated milk produces a smaller, softer curd than that formed from boiled whole cow milk. Vitamin D is typically added to evaporated milk during processing, but evaporated milk fails to meet vitamin E recommendations for premature infants, as well as ascorbic acid and essential fatty acid requirements for full-term infants. Therefore, evaporated milk is not recommended for infant feeding.

Goat Milk

Although goat milk is the primary milk source for more than 50% of the world's population, it is used rarely in the United States for infants intolerant to cow milk. Goat milk is commercially available in powdered and evaporated forms. It contains primarily medium- and short-chain fatty acids; therefore, the fat is more readily digested than the fat in cow milk. Unfortified goat milk is not recommended during infancy because it is deficient in folate and low in iron and vitamin D. The evaporated

TABLE 26-4 Average Composition of Mature Human Milk and Whole Cow Milk

Component	Mature Human Milk[a]	Whole Cow Milk	Component	Mature Human Milk[a]	Whole Cow Milk
Water (mL/100 mL)	87.1	87.2	**Vitamins**		
Energy			Vitamin A (IU/L)	2000	1000
(kcal/100 mL)	65–70	66–68	Thiamin (mcg/L)	200	300
(kcal/oz)	19.5–21	19–20	Riboflavin (mcg/L)	400–600	1750
Protein (g/100 mL)	0.9–1.3	3.3–3.4	Niacin (mg/L)	1.8–6	0.8
Whey:casein ratio	72:28	18:82	Pyridoxine (mg/L)	0.1–0.3	0.5
Alpha-lactalbumin (g/100 mL)	0.3	0.1	Pantothenate (mg/L)	2–2.5	3.6
Alpha-lactoglobulin (g/100 mL)	—	0.4	Folic acid (mcg/L)	80–140	50
Lactoferrin (g/100 mL)	0.2	Trace	Biotin (mcg/L)	5–9	35
Secretory IgA (g/100 mL)	0.1	Trace	Vitamin B_{12} (mcg/L)	0.5–1	4
Albumin (g/100 mL)	0.04	0.04	Vitamin C (mg/L)	80–100	17
Fat (g/100 mL)	3.9	3.4–3.8	Vitamin D (IU/L)	22	24
Carbohydrate (g/100 mL)	6.7–7.2[b]	4.7–4.8[c]	Vitamin E (IU/L)	2–8	0.4–0.9
			Vitamin K (mcg/L)	2–3	5
Minerals					
Calcium (mg/L)	200–280	1200	**Trace Minerals**		
Phosphorus (mg/L)	120–140	960	Chromium (mcg/L)	45–55	20
Calcium:phosphorus ratio	2:1	1.3:1	Manganese (mcg/L)	3	20–40
Sodium (mg/L)	120–250	500	Copper (mg/L)	0.2–0.4	100
Potassium (mg/L)	400–550	1560	Zinc (mg/L)	1–3	3.5
Chloride (mg/L)	400–450	1020	Iodine (mcg/L)	150	80
Magnesium (mg/L)	30–35	120	Selenium (mcg/L)	7–33	5–50
			Iron (mcg/L)	400	460
			Fluoride (mcg/L)	4–15	—

[a] ≥28 days postpartum.

[b] As lactose, glucose, and oligosaccharides.

[c] As lactose.

Source: Picciano MF. Representative values for constituents of human milk. In: Schanler RJ, ed. Breastfeeding 2001, part 1: the evidence for breastfeeding. *Ped Clin N Am.* 2001;48:263–4; American Academy of Pediatrics, Committee on Nutrition. Appendix A and Appendix E. In: Kleinman RE, ed. *Pediatric Nutrition Handbook.* 5th ed. Elk Grove Village, Ill: American Academy of Pediatrics; 2004:880–3 and 938; and American Academy of Pediatrics, Committee on Nutrition. Appendix A. In: Kleinman RE, ed. *Pediatric Nutrition Handbook.* 4th ed. Elk Grove Village, Ill: American Academy of Pediatrics; 1998:631–2.

TABLE 26-5 Potential Renal Solute Load of Selected Milks and Infant Formulas

	PRSL	
	mOsm/L	mOsm/100 kcal
Human milk	93	14
Milk-based formula	135–260	20–39
Soy protein–based formula	160	24
Whole cow milk	308	46
Skim cow milk	326	93
FDA upper limit	277	41
Beikost[a]	153	23

Key: FDA, Food and Drug Administration; PRSL, potential renal solute load.

[a] Beikost is foods other than milk or formula.

Source: References 32 and 33.

form of Meyenberg goat milk, however, is supplemented with vitamin D and folic acid. Powdered Meyenberg goat milk is supplemented with only folic acid; therefore, it is recommended only for children older than 1 year. Because the powder formulation is not a complete formula, vitamin supplementation is required if it is used for infant nutrition.

Commercial Infant Formulas

When provision of human milk to an infant is not possible or not desired by the mother, then commercially supplied infant formulas are an acceptable alternative (Table 26-6). Differences in palatability, digestibility, sources of nutrients, convenience of administration, and cost among these formulas allow for individualization to the infant's special nutrient needs and the family's resources.

Formula Properties

The Infant Formula Council (a voluntary, nonprofit trade association composed of the four companies that manufacture and

TABLE 26-6 Selected Formulas for Infants and Children

Trade Name [Form] (Mfr)	Kilocalories[a] (per ounce)	Protein[a] (g/L) (C:W ratio)	Carbohydrate[a] (g/L)	Fat[a] (g/L)	MCTs (% fat kcal)	Iron[a,b] (mg/L)
Infant Formulas						
Milk-Based Formulas						
Enfamil LIPIL [C,P,R] (MJ)	20	14 (40:60)	72.7	35.3	—	12.2
Enfamil Gentlease LIPIL [P] (MJ)	20	15.3 (60:40)	72	35.3	—	12.2
Enfamil 24 [R] (MJ)	24	17.4 (40:60)	88	43	—	14.6
Good Start Supreme/Good Start Supreme DHA&ARA [C,P,R] (Nes)	20	14.7 (0:100)	75	34.2	—	10.1
Good Start Natural Cultures[c] [P] (Nes)	20	14.7 (0:100)	75	34.2	—	10.1
Similac Advance [C,P,R] (A)	20	14 (52:48)	73	36.5	—	12
Similac Organic [P,R] (A)	20	14 (82:18)	71.4	37.1	—	12.2
Store Brand Milk-based Formula [C,P,R] (Wy)	20	15 (40:60)	72	36	—	12
Soy Protein–Based Therapeutic Formulas						
Good Start Supreme Soy DHA&ARA [C,P,R] (Nes)	20	16.8	75	34.2	—	10.1
Similac Isomil Advance [C,P,R] (A)	20	16.6	69.7	36.9	—	12.2
Similac Isomil DF [R] (A)	20	18	68.3 (6 g fiber)	36.9	—	12.2
Enfamil ProSobee LIPIL [C,P,R] (MJ)	20	16.7	70.7	35.3	—	12.2
Store Brand Soy Infant Formula [C,P,R] (Wy)	20	18	69	36	—	12
Other Therapeutic Infant Formulas						
Enfamil A.R. LIPIL [P,R] (MJ)	20	16.7 (80:20)	73.3	34	—	12.2
Similac Sensitive [C,P,R]/Similac Sensitive R.S. [P,R] (A)	20	14.5 (82:18)	72.4	36.5	—	12.2
Enfamil LactoFree LIPIL [C,P,R] (MJ)	20	14 (80:20)	72.7	35.3	—	12.2
Similac PM 60/40 [P] (A)	20	15 (40:60)	69	37.9	—	4.7
Nutramigen LIPIL [C,P,R]/Nutramigen AA LIPIL [P] (MJ)	20	18.7	68.7	35.3	—	12.2
Enfamil Pregestimil [R]/Pregestimil LIPIL [P,R] (MJ)	20	18.7	68	37.3	55	12.5
Enfamil Pregestimil [R]/Pregestimil LIPIL [P,R] (MJ)	24	22.2	81	44.4	55	14.9
Similac Alimentum [R,P] (A)	20	18.6	69	37.5	33	12.2
Neocate Infant [P]/Neocate Infant with DHA&ARA [P] (Nut)	20	20.7	78	30	5	12.3
Portagen [P] (MJ)	20	25.2	65.9	34	87	13.3
RCF[d] [C] (A)	20	20.3	68.2	35.8	—	12.2
3232A [P] (MJ)	12.7	18.9	91	28	85	12.5
3232A[d] [P] (MJ)	20	18.9	91	28	85	12.5
Formulas for Premature Infants: Initial Feeding						
Enfamil Premature LIPIL Iron Fortified/ Enfamil Premature LIPIL Low Iron [R] (MJ)	20	20 (40:60)	73.3	34	40	12.2 (3.4)
Similac Special Care 20 with Iron/ Similac Special Care 20 Low Iron [R] (A)	20	20.3 (40:60)	69.7	36.7	50	12.2 (2.5)
Enfamil Premature LIPIL Iron Fortified/ Enfamil Premature LIPIL Low Iron [R] (MJ)	24	24 (40:60)	88	40.8	40	14.6 (4.1)
Good Start Premature 24 [R] (Nes)	24	24 (0:100)	84	41.6	40	14.4
Similac Special Care 24 with Iron/ Similac Special Care 24 Low Iron [R] (A)	24	24.3 (40:60)	83.6	44.1	50	14.6 (3)
Similac Special Care 30 with Iron [R] (A)	30	30.4 (50:50)	78.4	67.1	50	18.3
Formulas for Premature Infants: Transition or Postdischarge						
Similac NeoSure [P,R] (A)	22	20.8 (50:50)	75.1	40.9	25.3	13.4
Enfamil EnfaCare LIPIL [P,R] (MJ)	22	20.5 (40:60)	76.3	38.9	20	13.3
Infant/Toddler or Children's Formulas						
Good Start 2 Supreme DHA&ARA [C,P,R] (Nes)	20	14.7 (0:100)	75	34.2	—	13.4
Similac Go & Grow Milk-based Formula [P] (A)	20	14 (52:48)	71.7	37.1	—	12.2

TABLE 26-6 Selected Formulas for Infants and Children (continued)

Trade Name [Form] (Mfr)	Kilocalories[a] (per ounce)	Protein[a] (g/L) (C:W ratio)	Carbohydrate[a] (g/L)	Fat[a] (g/L)	MCTs (% fat kcal)	Iron[a,b] (mg/L)
Store Brand Formula for Older Infants [P] (Wy)	20	18 (50:50)	69	36	—	12
Enfamil Next Step LIPIL [P,R] (MJ)	20	17.3 (82:18)	70	35.3	—	13.3
Enfamil Kindercal Beverage/Enfamil Kindercal TF [R] (MJ)	31.8	30	135	44	20	10.6
Enfamil Kindercal Beverage with Fiber/Enfamil Kindercal TF with Fiber [R] (MJ)	31.8	30	138 (6.3 g fiber)	44	20	10.6
PediaSure/PediaSure Enteral Formula[e] [R] (A)	30	30	132.5	39.7	16	14
PediaSure With Fiber and scFOS/ PediaSure Enteral Formula With Fiber and scFOS[§] [R] (A)	30	30	138 (5g/8 g fiber)	39.7	16	14
Nutren Junior/Nutren Junior With Fiber [R] (Nes)	30	30	110 (6 g fiber; PreBio[1])[f]	49.6	22	14
Resource Just For Kids/RESOURCE Just For Kids with Fiber [R] (Nes)	30	30	110 (6 g fiber)	50	20	14
Resource Just For Kids 1.5 CAL/ Resource Just For Kids 1.5 CAL with Fiber [R] (Nes)	45	42	165 (9 g fiber)	75	20	14
Compleat Pediatric [R] (Nes)	30	38	130 (6.8 g fiber)	39	20	13
Carnation Instant Breakfast Junior [R] (Nes)	30	32	108 (7.2 g fiber as Prebio[1])[f]	48	—	14

Therapeutic Infant/Toddler or Children's Formulas

Soy-Based Products

Nestlé Good Start 2 Supreme Soy DHA&ARA [P] (Nes)	20	20.8	80.4	29.5	—	12.1
Enfamil Next Step ProSobee LIPIL [P] (MJ)	20	22	78.7	29.3	—	13.3
Similac Go & Grow Soy-based Formula [P] (A)	20	16.6	69.7	36.9	—	12.2

Other Therapeutic Formulas

E028 Splash [R] (Nut), flavored	30	25	146	35	35	7.7
EleCare [P] (A), flavored or unflavored	20	20.9	72.3	32.4	33	10.1
	30	31	107	48	33	15
Modulen IBD [P] (Nes)	30	36	110	47	26	11
Neocate Junior [P] (Nut), unflavored	30	33	104	50	35	15
Neocate Junior [P] (Nut), flavored	30	35	110	47	35	16
Neocate One + Powder [P] (Nut)	30	25	146	35	35	7.7
Pediatric Peptinex DT/Pediatric Peptinex DT with Fiber [R] (Nes)	30	30	138 (6 g fiber)	39	50	14
Pepdite Junior [P] (Nut), flavored or unflavored	30	31	106	50	35	14
Peptamen Junior [P,R] (Nes)	30	30 (0:100)	132 (R) / 138 (P)	40 (R) / 38 (P)	60	11 (R) / 10 (P)
Peptamen Junior Fiber [R] (Nes)	30	30 (0:100)	137 (7.2 g fiber)	38.4	60	14
Peptamen Junior with PreBio [R] (NES)	30	30 (0:100)	137 (3.6 g fiber)	38.4	60	14
Vivonex Pediatric [P] (Nes)	24	24	130	24	69	10

Key: A, Abbott Nutrition (formerly Ross Nutritionals); C, concentrate; MCTs, medium-chain triglycerides; MJ, Mead Johnson Nutritionals; Nes, Nestlé (includes former Novartis Nutritionals); Nut, Nutricia North America (formerly SHS North America); P, powder; R, ready-to-feed; scFOS, short-chain fructooligosaccharides; Wy, Wyeth Nutritionals.

Note: Federal regulations require nutrient values be reported as intakes per 100 kcal. These intakes can be found on the manufacturers' Web sites. Values per liter of formula are provided for ease of calculation.

[a] When powder is prepared to the stated caloric density.

[b] Values in parentheses pertain to low-iron version of formula.

[c] Contains Bifidus BL, *Bifidobacterium lactis*, which is similar to probiotics found in human milk.

[d] When carbohydrate is added as directed to make a 20 kcal/oz concentration.

[e] Enteral formula contains less sucrose and has a lower osmolality.

[f] Prebio[1] is a unique blend of fructooligosaccharides and inulin. These compounds may increase colonic mucosal integrity and permeability, promote potentially beneficial bacteria, and improve colonic absorption of water and electrolytes.

Source: Abbott Nutrition at www.abbottnutrition.com; Mead Johnson Nutritionals at www.meadjohnson.com; Nestlé Infant and Clinical Nutrition at www.nestle-nutrition.com; and Nutricia North America at www.nutricia-na.com. Last accessed October 11, 2008.

market infant formulas: Abbott Nutrition; Mead Johnson Nutritionals, Nestlé Nutrition, and Wyeth Nutrition) has established guidelines requiring liquid formulations to be free of all viable pathogens, their spores, and other organisms that may cause product degradation. In addition, infant formula constituents must meet certain concentrations to ensure optimum nutrition. Guidelines have been established to ensure safety and efficacy of infant formulas.

MICROBIOLOGIC SAFETY

Manufacturers sterilize liquid formulas using heat treatment. Samples of the sterilized formulas are incubated and analyzed for guideline compliance. Quality control measures help to ensure the production of a sterile product that is free of microbes as long as the container remains intact. Powdered formulas, however, are not required or guaranteed to be sterile, given that heat sterilization of the powder would destroy some of the nutrients. Manufacturers culture powdered formulas to ensure that coliforms and other pathogens are absent, and that contamination with other microorganisms is below acceptable government standards. If clinically significant microbiologic contamination occurs, an infant ingesting the formula could develop diarrhea with subsequent fluid and electrolyte losses. In 2002, FDA issued an alert after the death of an infant in a NICU because of contamination of powdered formula with *Enterobacter sakazakii* at the manufacturing site.[30]

Risk for infection after exposure to contaminated formula likely depends on a number of factors including immune status. For this reason, to minimize risk for premature infants, ready-to-feed or liquid concentrates are recommended unless there is no suitable alternative to a powdered formula. The initial FDA response to the *Enterobacter* contamination incident recommended reconstituting powdered formulas with boiling water; however, this recommendation was withdrawn. Use of boiling water to reconstitute powdered formula results in loss of some nutrients, including vitamins and protein, and clumping of formula. In addition, although the use of boiling water may not kill bacteria that are present, it is potentially dangerous for those preparing the formula and for the infant if the formula is not allowed to cool to a proper temperature before feeding.[31] It is best to avoid using powdered formulas for feeding premature or immunocompromised infants if at all possible; however, there is currently no alternative to the powdered, human milk fortifiers that are used for supplementation in premature infants. These products will be discussed later in this chapter.

PHYSICAL CHARACTERISTICS

Infant formulas are emulsions of edible oils in aqueous solutions, but fat separation rarely occurs. If it does, shaking the container will usually redisperse the fat. Redispersion may not happen if stabilizers are lacking or if the formula was stored beyond its shelf life. Liquid infant formulas may contain thickening agents, stabilizers, and emulsifiers to provide uniform consistency and prolong stability. Protein agglomeration may occur, however, if storage time is excessive. This agglomeration ranges from a slight, grainy development through increased viscosity and gel formation to eventual protein precipitation. Agglomeration and separation do not affect a formula's safety or nutritional value; however, the formula's appearance may deter caregivers from using it.

CALORIC DENSITY

The standard caloric density for infant formulas is 20 kcal/oz or approximately 67 kcal/100 mL, which mimics the average caloric density of human milk. A healthy, term infant should have no difficulty consuming enough formula to meet both calorie and fluid needs with this caloric density. Premature, malnourished, volume-restricted (i.e., cardiac or liver disease, or poor oral feeding), or severely ill infants may require more calories (130–150 kcal/kg/day or higher) or formulas with higher caloric densities (e.g., 22, 24, or 27 kcal/oz) to meet their calorie needs. Infant formulas with caloric densities significantly lower or higher than 20 kcal/oz are regarded as therapeutic formulas to be used in managing special clinical conditions (Tables 26-6 and 26-7). Concentrated formulas should be used only under close medical supervision, especially with monitoring for dehydration due to the reduction in free water consumed.

OSMOLARITY AND OSMOLALITY

Osmolality is the preferred term for reporting the osmotic activities of infant formulas. Osmolality represents the number of osmoles of solute per kilogram of solvent (Osm/kg). Any dietary component soluble in water contributes to osmolality. Osmolality is directly related to the concentration of molecular or ionic particles in the solution (i.e., amino acids, small peptides, electrolytes, and simple sugars) and inversely proportional to the concentration of water in the formula. The osmolality of human milk is approximately 295 mOsm/kg; osmolality of standard caloric density formulas is 200 to 300 mOsm/kg.

The osmolarity of an infant formula may be expressed as the concentration of solute per unit of total volume of solution or as the number of osmoles of solute per liter of solution (Osm/L). The osmolarity of human milk is approximately 273 mOsm/L. Formulas for infants should have osmolarities no higher than 400 mOsm/L. Unless the formula is very concentrated, there is no meaningful difference between osmolality and osmolarity of infant formulas.

The osmolality of a formula increases with increasing caloric density. The relationship between osmolality and caloric density is reasonably linear within the range of caloric concentrations usually fed to infants. Therefore, if the osmolality of a 20 kcal/oz formula is known, that of the same formula with any other caloric density can be calculated, assuming a direct proportion between osmolality and caloric density. For example, if a 20 kcal/oz formula has an osmolality of 283 mOsm/kg, then the same formula concentrated to 24 kcal/oz would have an osmolality of approximately 340 mOsm/kg.

No clinically meaningful difference exists in the osmolalities of the commonly used 20 kcal/oz, ready-to-use formulas. In addition, when concentrated products are diluted to provide a formula with 20 kcal/oz, there are no meaningful differences in osmolalities compared with the similar ready-to-use product. However, directions for diluting concentrated and powdered formulas must be followed exactly. Soy protein–based formulas have somewhat lower osmolalities than milk-based formulas because of the difference in carbohydrate source.

POTENTIAL RENAL SOLUTE LOAD

The PRSL is the solute load derived from the diet requiring excretion by the kidney if the amino acids from protein digestion are not used for growth or eliminated by nonrenal routes. The PRSL of an infant formula can be calculated with the following equation: PRSL (mOsm) = N/28 + sodium + chloride + potassium + phosphorus$_{(available)}$, where N is the total nitrogen in milligrams, and sodium, chloride, potassium, and phosphorus$_{(available)}$ (P_a) are expressed as millimoles (or milliosmoles). The P_a is assumed to be the total phosphorus content except in soy-based formulas, in which it is only two-thirds of the total phosphorus. Table 26-5 lists PRSLs for various milks

TABLE 26-7 Indications for Therapeutic Infant Formulas[a]

Problem	Suggested Therapeutic Formula	Comments
Allergy or sensitivity to cow milk or soy protein	Nutramigen LIPIL, Nutramigen AA LIPIL, Similac Alimentum, Enfamil Pregestimil LIPIL, Neocate Infant, EleCare	Protein hydrolysate or free amino acid formula is best. Up to 50% cross-sensitivity between cow milk and soy protein allergies.
Biliary atresia, cholestatic liver disease	Enfamil Pregestimil LIPIL, Similac Alimentum, EleCare, Portagen	Impaired digestion and absorption of long-chain fats; higher percentage of MCTs may improve absorption. Monitor for linoleic acid deficiency, especially if Portagen used.
Carbohydrate intolerance (severe)	RCF, 3232A	Carbohydrate-free; a patient-tolerated carbohydrate source is added gradually (e.g., sucrose, fructose).
Cardiac disease	No therapeutic formula generally necessary	Low electrolyte content (Similac PM 60/40), if renal insufficiency. Electrolyte supplementation may be needed in patients receiving diuretics. Calorically dense, standard formulas often used owing to failure to thrive and volume restriction.
Celiac disease	Enfamil Pregestimil LIPIL, Nutramigen LIPIL, Nutramigen AA LIPIL, Enfamil LactoFree LIPIL, EleCare, Neocate Infant, Similac Isomil DF	Advance to standard formulas as intestinal epithelium returns to normal; diet must be gluten-free.
Chylothorax or chylous ascites	Portagen	High MCT intake decreases flow through the lymphatic system.
Constipation	No therapeutic formula necessary	Continue routine formula; increase water; refer severe constipation.
Cystic fibrosis	Enfamil Pregestimil LIPIL, Similac Alimentum, EleCare	Impaired digestion and absorption of long-chain fats; cow milk–based formula or human milk may be used with appropriate pancreatic enzyme supplementation. Enzyme supplementation may be required even with predigested therapeutic formulas; soy protein–based formulas contraindicated.
Diarrhea		
Chronic nonspecific	Enfamil Lactofree LIPIL, Similac Sensitive (Lactose Free), Enfamil ProSobee LIPIL, Similac Isomil Advance, Nutramigen LIPIL	Trial of lactose-free cow milk or soy protein–based formula may be needed; avoid fruit juices.
Intractable	Enfamil Pregestimil LIPIL, Similac Alimentum, EleCare, RCF, 3232A, Nutramigen AA LIPIL	Hydrolyzed protein needed owing to impaired digestion of intact protein, long-chain fats, and disaccharides. Similac Alimentum contains sucrose and may not be appropriate for all cases.
Failure to thrive	No therapeutic formula generally necessary; Enfamil Pregestimil LIPIL, Similac Alimentum, EleCare	Most cases related to inadequate intake. Start with standard formula, may need more calorically dense formula for catch-up growth; change to predigested formula only if malabsorption present.
Galactosemia	Similac Isomil, Enfamil ProSobee LIPIL	Soy protein–based formula is given initially; cow and human milk contraindicated.
Gastroesophageal reflux	Enfamil A.R. LIPIL, Similac Sensitive R.S.	In otherwise healthy children, may start with standard formula thickened with rice cereal. (Start with 1–2 teaspoons per ounce of formula and increase to a maximum of 1 tbsp/oz as tolerated.)

TABLE 26-7 Indications for Therapeutic Infant Formulas[a] (continued)

Problem	Suggested Therapeutic Formula	Comments
		Thickening formula with rice cereal increases the caloric density, may cause constipation, results in delivery of less volume, and usually requires enlarging the nipple.
		Some infants may have an allergic-type reaction to rice cereal; oatmeal may be used in these cases.
		Attempt small, frequent feedings; avoid using products like Thick-It and Simply-Thick to thicken formula (products are intended for patients with dysphagia or swallowing difficulties); use more calorically dense formula if decreased volume or catch-up growth needed.
Hepatitis		
Without liver failure	No therapeutic formula necessary	Impaired digestion or absorption of long-chain fats is uncommon.
With liver failure	Enfamil Pregestimil LIPIL, EleCare, Similac Alimentum, Portagen	Impaired digestion or absorption of long-chain fats may occur.
Lactose intolerance (primary or secondary)	Enfamil Lactofree LIPIL, Similac Sensitive (Lactose Free), Enfamil ProSobee LIPIL, Similac Isomil	Remove lactose from diet; use lactose-free formula.
Necrotizing enterocolitis (during recovery or postresection)	Enfamil Pregestimil LIPIL, Similac Alimentum, Neocate Infant, EleCare	Impaired digestion or absorption requires a hydrolysate or free amino acid formula.
Prematurity	Fortified human milk, preferred; Similac Special Care, Enfamil Premature LIPIL, Good Start Premature 24 or transition infant formula (Similac NeoSure, Enfamil EnfaCare LIPIL)	Human milk fortifier needed; transition formula (Enfamil EnfaCare LIPIL, Similac NeoSure) can be added to human milk to increase caloric density after discharge (1 tsp/90 mL milk makes 24 kcal/oz).
Renal insufficiency	Similac PM 60/40	Formula is low-phosphate, low-PRSL.

Key: MCT, medium-chain triglyceride; PRSL, potential renal solute load.

[a] List is not all-inclusive; other products may be acceptable.

Source: Abbott Nutrition at www.abbottnutrition.com; Mead Johnson Nutritionals at www.meadjohnson.com; Nestlé Nutrition at www.nestle-nutrition.com; and, Nutricia North America at www.nutricia-na.com. Last accessed October 11, 2008.

and infant formulas compared with the FDA-recommended upper PRSL limit.[32,33] Excretion of 1 mOsm of ingested solute requires 1 mL of water intake. Standard 20 kcal/oz infant formulas supply approximately 1.5 mL of water per kilocalorie ingested, an adequate amount of water to provide usual needs. Therefore, during health the PRSL is generally not a factor; however, during illnesses associated with water loss such as vomiting, diarrhea, and fever, or in infants with compromised renal function or diabetes insipidus, the PRSL of the infant's formula becomes a factor in maintaining fluid balance. Feeding a formula with a high PRSL (i.e., high protein content or concentrated to more than 24 kcal/oz) may produce a hypertonic urine, leading to increased renal water losses and dehydration.

Types, Uses, and Selection of Commercial Infant Formulas

Standard formulas for term infants are milk-based or milk-based with added whey protein (whey-predominant). Other formulas are available for infants and children with specific dietary needs and should be used only under medical supervision.

MILK-BASED FORMULAS

Milk-based formulas (Table 26-6) are prepared from nonfat cow milk, vegetable oils, and added carbohydrate (lactose). The added carbohydrate is necessary, because the ratio of carbohydrate to protein in nonfat cow milk solids is less than desirable for infant formulas. Protein provides approximately 9% to 11% of calories, and fat provides 48% to 50% of calories. The most widely used vegetable oils are corn, coconut, safflower, sunflower, palm olein, and soy. Replacement of the butterfat with vegetable oils allows for better fat absorption. Vitamins and minerals are added to meet FDA guidelines. Most standard formulas contain iron. There are no known contraindications to the use of iron-fortified formulas; concerns that iron-fortified formulas contribute to colic, constipation, fussiness, cramping, and gastroesophageal reflux have not been proven.[28,29] Therefore, most low-iron formulas except those intended for use in NICUs have been removed from the market in the United States. Although Enfamil Lactofree LIPIL and Similac Sensitive (Lactose Free) are milk-based formulas, they contain corn syrup solids or corn syrup solids with sucrose, rather than lactose, as the carbohydrate source and may be used for infants with lactose intolerance.

THERAPEUTIC FORMULAS

Therapeutic infant formulas are used for infants with conditions that require dietary adjustment and should be used with medical supervision, rather than being self-selected by parents. Table 26-7 lists indications for various therapeutic formulas including soy protein–based, casein-based, casein hydrolysate–based or whey hydrolysate–based, and low-electrolyte and low-mineral formulas. Formulas intended for use by premature infants and those formulated specifically for children from 1 to 10 years of age are also considered therapeutic formulas.

Prethickened Milk-Based Formulas
Enfamil A.R. LIPIL with Iron was developed specifically for infants with gastroesophageal reflux. This iron-fortified formula contains a carbohydrate blend of lactose (57%), rice starch (30%), and maltodextrin (13%), as well as a high amylopectin rice starch for thickening. Before ingestion, Enfamil A.R. LIPIL with Iron has a viscosity 10 times that of ready-to-use Enfamil LIPIL with Iron. In contrast, Enfamil LIPIL with Iron thickened with rice cereal (1 tbsp/oz) has a viscosity 30 times that of Enfamil LIPIL with Iron. Therefore, Enfamil A.R. LIPIL with Iron flows better through a nipple than standard infant formula thickened with rice cereal. Once ingested, however, the viscosity increases dramatically in the stomach's acidic pH, reaching a viscosity equal to the Enfamil LIPIL with Iron plus rice cereal combination. This effect may be minimized in infants receiving a histamine$_2$-receptor antagonist (e.g., ranitidine or famotidine) or proton pump inhibitor (e.g., omeprazole, lansoprazole, or esomeprazole) for treatment of their gastroesophageal reflux, if the gastric pH is greater than 5.4. Similac Sensitive R.S. is a milk-based, lactose-free formula with added rice starch intended to help reduce spitting up. Neither Enfamil A.R. LIPIL with Iron nor Similac Sensitive R.S. is recommended for use in premature infants, because neither will adequately meet their needs, especially protein, calcium, and phosphorus.

Soy Protein–Based Formulas
Despite relatively few true indications for soy protein–based formulas, approximately 25% of formulas sold in the United States are soy protein–based, suggesting that these formulas are being selected by parents rather than being prescribed by health care practitioners.[28,34] Soy protein–based formulas (Table 26-6) contain a soy isolate fortified with L-methionine. Vegetable oils, including palm olein, soy, coconut, high-oleic safflower, and sunflower, provide the fat content. Corn maltodextrin, corn syrup solids, and sucrose supply the carbohydrate in these formulas; none contains lactose. Soy formulas are a safe and nutritionally sound alternative for normal growth and development in infants who are not fed human milk, do not tolerate cow milk–based formula, or whose parents choose them for other reasons. Soy protein–based formulas provide an alternative nutritional source for infants whose parents are vegetarians and do not wish to use animal protein–based formulas.

Food allergy occurs in infants because the immature digestive and metabolic processes may not be completely effective in converting dietary proteins into nonallergenic amino acids. Cow milk protein allergy occurs in 2% to 3% of infants and is defined as symptomatology involving the respiratory tract (wheezing), skin (rash), or GI tract (diarrhea and bloody stools) that disappears when cow milk is removed from the diet and reappears on two separate challenges when cow milk is reintroduced during a symptom-free period. Symptoms of cow milk protein intolerance generally regress within 3 to 4 years in most children.

Soy protein–based formulas are appropriate for infants with lactose intolerance because of lactase deficiency and with documented IgE-mediated allergy to cow milk protein. However, infants with cow milk protein–induced enteropathy or enterocolitis are also frequently sensitive to soy protein (up to 50% cross-sensitivity); therefore, AAP/CON recommends protein hydrolysate formulas for these infants.[34] Most infants suspected of having adverse reactions to milk-based formulas have not experienced life-threatening manifestations. These infants appear to tolerate soy protein–based formulas that are less expensive and better tasting than the protein hydrolysate formulas. Routine use of soy protein–based formulas has no proven value in prevention of atopic disease.[35] Some infants with moderate-to-severe gastroenteritis develop intolerance to lactose and sucrose because of a temporary lactase and sucrase deficiency. However, after rehydration most infants with diarrhea can be managed by continuing their usual nutrition regimen whether milk-based or soy protein–based.

The high protein and manganese content of soy protein–based formulas is a concern because PRSL is increased. In addition, manganese absorption is enhanced in children who are iron-deficient, which may result in manganese accumulation and neurologic symptoms in children whose biliary manganese excretion is compromised (e.g., those with biliary atresia or cholestasis). On the positive side, exposure to phytoestrogens early in life may have long-term health benefits for hormone-dependent diseases.[36]

RCF is a soy protein–based formula that contains no carbohydrates. This formula is used in the dietary management of only infants unable to tolerate the type or amount of carbohydrates in human milk or infant formulas. A carbohydrate source (sucrose, dextrose, fructose, or glucose polymers) is added gradually in increasing amounts to slowly improve carbohydrate tolerance.

Similac Isomil DF contains added dietary fiber from soy and was specifically formulated for infants with diarrhea secondary to antibiotics. It is best used short term until diarrhea resolves. It may also help increase the consistency of ileostomy or colostomy output in those term infants without malabsorption who require these devices for conditions such as Hirschsprung's disease, imperforate anus, necrotizing enterocolitis, or intestinal atresias.

Soy protein–based formulas are not recommended for the routine feeding of preterm infants because of reduced calcium, phosphorus, and vitamin D bioavailability, which predisposes these infants, especially those weighing less than 1500 grams, to developing rickets.[34] In addition, soy protein–based formulas are not recommended for infants with cystic fibrosis, because these children do not use soy protein adequately, will lose substantial nitrogen in their stools, and develop hypoproteinemia or even anasarca (generalized infiltration of fluid into subcutaneous connective tissue). Formula-fed infants with cystic fibrosis do well nutritionally when given an easily digested formula that contains elemental protein and medium-chain triglycerides (MCTs) (e.g., a casein hydrolysate–based formula). However, recent studies have shown that infants with cystic fibrosis grow equally well on a regular cow milk–based formula or human milk as long as adequate pancreatic enzyme supplementation is given.[37]

Casein Hydrolysate–Based Formulas
Protein is supplied by enzymatically hydrolyzed, charcoal-treated casein rather than by whole protein in casein hydrolysate–based formulas, which include Enfamil Pregestimil LIPIL, Nutramigen LIPIL, and Similac Alimentum (Table 26-6). These formulas are classified as semi-elemental and contain nonantigenic polypeptides with

molecular weights less than 1200 daltons; therefore, they can be fed to infants who are sensitive to intact milk protein. Casein hydrolysate formulas are supplemented with L-cysteine, L-tyrosine, and L-tryptophan (Similac Alimentum also contains L-methionine), because the concentrations of these amino acids are reduced during the charcoal treatment.

Carbohydrate sources in casein hydrolysate–based formulas vary and include corn syrup solids, modified corn and tapioca starch, sucrose, and dextrose (Table 26–8). Glucose polymers found in corn syrup solids or modified corn starch are particularly useful in infants who have malabsorption disorders and are frequently intolerant to high concentrations of lactose, sucrose, and glucose. In addition, glucose polymers contribute little to the total osmolar load. Low osmolality is an advantage in intestinal disorders in which the osmolar load of disaccharide- or glucose-containing elemental diets may not be tolerated. 3232-A is an extensively hydrolyzed casein-based formula with added amino acids that is intended, like RCF, to be used with small amounts of carbohydrate to gradually improve tolerance. This product contains modified tapioca starch and fat, 85% of which is MCTs.

Hydrolysate formulas usually contain modified fat sources: MCTs from fractionated coconut and palm olein oils and corn, soy, and high-oleic safflower oils. MCTs do not require emulsification with bile and are more easily digested and absorbed than long-chain fats. Shorter-chain fatty acids and MCTs are directly absorbed into the portal system, not into the lacteals of the lymphatic system. In addition, MCTs enhance the absorption of long-chain triglycerides and do not require carnitine for transport into the mitochondria, where oxidation and energy production occur. However, MCTs cannot be the sole source of dietary fat, given that they do not provide essential fatty acids, increasing the risk of essential fatty acid deficiency. Diarrhea can result from MCT malabsorption caused by overfeeding or intestinal mucosal disease.

Enfamil Pregestimil LIPIL is often used for infants with massive small bowel resection (short-bowel syndrome), severe

TABLE 26-8　Composition of Selected Hydrolysate and Amino Acid–Based Formulas

Formula	Carbohydrate	Protein	Fat
Enfamil Pregestimil LIPIL/ Pregestimil LIPIL	Corn syrup solids, tapioca starch	Casein hydrolysates	MCT 55%; corn oil
Similac Alimentum	Sucrose; tapioca starch	Casein hydrolysates, L-cystine, L-tyrosine, L-tryptophan, L-methionine	MCT 33%; safflower and soy oils
Nutramigen LIPIL	Corn syrup solids, modified corn starch	Casein hydrolysates	MCT 0%; corn oil
Nutramigen AA LIPIL	Corn syrup solids, modified tapioca starch	Free amino acids	MCT 0%; palm olein, soy, coconut, and high-oleic sunflower oils
3232A	Modified tapioca starch	Casein hydrolysates, L-cystine, L-tyrosine, L-tryptophan	MCT 85%; corn oil
Pepdite Junior	Corn syrup solids	Hydrolyzed pork and soy proteins	MCT 35%; fractionated coconut, canola and high-oleic safflower oils
Neocate Infant	Corn syrup solids	Free amino acids	MCT 5%; safflower, coconut, and soy oils
Neocate One + Powder	Corn syrup solids	Free amino acids	MCT 35%; fractionated coconut, canola, and high-oleic safflower oils
E028 Splash	Maltodextrin, sucrose	Free amino acids	MCT 35%; fractionated coconut, canola, and high-oleic safflower oils
Neocate Junior	Corn syrup solids	Free amino acids	MCT 35%; fractionated coconut, canola, and high-oleic safflower oils
EleCare	Corn syrup solids	Free amino acids	MCT 33%; high-oleic safflower, fractionated coconut, and soy oils
Peptamen Junior	Maltodextrin, corn starch	Hydrolyzed whey protein	MCT 60%; fractionated coconut and palm kernel, soybean, and canola oils
Peptamen Junior with Prebio[1]	Maltodextrin, corn starch, sucrose (flavored)	Hydrolyzed whey protein	MCT 60%; fractionated coconut and palm kernel, soybean, and canola oils

Key: MCT, medium-chain triglycerides.

Source: Abbott Nutrition at www.abbottnutrition.com; Mead Johnson Nutritionals at www.meadjohnson.com; Nestlé Infant and Clinical Nutrition at www.nestleusa.com; Nutricia North America at www.nutricia.na.com. Last accessed October 11, 2008.

intractable diarrhea, steatorrhea, protein-calorie malnutrition, or cystic fibrosis. Nutramigen LIPIL and Nutramigen AA LIPIL can be used for infants with severe diarrhea or GI disturbances and for infants with severe or multiple food allergies but not for infants with fat malabsorption disorders. In cases of galactosemia, a relatively rare disorder resulting from a deficiency of galactose-1-phosphate uridyltransferase (type 1), galactokinase (type II), or galactose epimerase (type III), dietary lactose must be eliminated; the body converts glucose to the amount of galactose it requires. Infants with galactosemia must be fed formulas without lactose or sucrose (Enfamil Nutramigen LIPIL, Enfamil Nutramigen AA LIPIL, Enfamil Pregestimil LIPIL, or Enfamil ProSobee LIPIL). Similac Alimentum contains sucrose and modified tapioca starch. These carbohydrates are digested and absorbed by separate mechanisms (principally glucoamylase and sucrase-alpha-dextrinase). This formula can be used for infants with protein sensitivity, pancreatic insufficiency (e.g., cystic fibrosis), or intractable diarrhea.

Use of casein hydrolysate–based formulas for allergy prophylaxis is controversial. AAP's policy statement on hypoallergenic formulas states that infants with a high risk for developing allergy identified by a strong family history (both parents or one parent and a sibling) may benefit from a hypoallergenic formula, but studies are not conclusive.[34] Currently, no evidence exists to support the use of hydrolysate formulas for treating colic, irritability, or gastroesophageal reflux. Although these symptoms are common in infants, they are rarely a result of an IgE-mediated allergic reaction to cow milk protein.

Extensively hydrolyzed casein formulas are less palatable than standard formulas. If the formula is rejected by the infant when first offered, it should be tried again after a few hours. These products are designed to provide a sole source of nutrition for infants up to 4 to 6 months of age and a primary source of nutrition through 12 months of age, when indicated. Extended use of hydrolysate formulas as a sole source of nutrition in children older than 6 months requires close medical supervision and monitoring.

Whey Hydrolysate–Based Formula   Enzymatically hydrolyzed whey protein is another protein source used in infant formulas (Good Start Supreme). Infants who have GI intolerance to cow milk but are not allergic to it often tolerate whey hydrolysate-based formula. This product is promoted as having a pleasant taste, smell, and appearance. It may be better accepted than casein hydrolysate–based formulas, which parents and infants find differ noticeably from cow milk– and soy protein–based formulas in both appearance and taste. There are no specific indications for these products, so they may be chosen according to parent/patient or program preference.

Amino Acid–Based Formulas   Occasionally, infants are intolerant to even hydrolyzed casein and require a free amino acid–based formula. Neocate Infant, EleCare, and Nutramigen AA LIPIL contain 100% free amino acids and are considered hypoallergenic. They are used for infants with cow milk–protein allergy, multiple food protein allergies, or intolerance to casein hydrolysate formulas.

High MCT Formula   Portagen is a unique formula because of its high MCT content (i.e., 87% of the fat). It also contains higher concentrations of both lipid- and water-soluble vitamins than are found in casein hydrolysate–based formulas. The higher concentrations of MCTs and vitamins in Portagen help compensate for the impaired digestion and absorption of long-chain fats in patients with pancreatic insufficiency (e.g., cystic fibrosis), bile acid deficiency (e.g., biliary atresia or cholestatic jaundice), and intestinal resection. Another use for Portagen is to decrease lymphatic flow in patients with lymphatic anomalies such as chylothorax and chylous ascites. It can be used as the sole dietary source for infants, children, and adults or as a beverage to be consumed with each meal as a supplement. Mead Johnson Nutritionals does not market Portagen as an infant formula because of concerns with bacterial contamination of powdered formulas, leading to a recall of one batch in March 2002. Because there is no good alternative for infants, including premature infants, with certain medical conditions such as chylothorax and chylous ascites, such infants will require Portagen. These infants should be monitored carefully for signs of GI infection such as diarrhea and abdominal distention. Infants and children with fat malabsorption who receive Portagen can develop essential fatty acid deficiency. Linoleic acid (e.g., corn or safflower oil, or Microlipid) can be given in the diet, either by mixing with the formula or by syringe through a feeding tube, to prevent essential fatty acid deficiency.

Low PRSL Formula   Similac PM 60/40 is an infant formula with lower mineral (potassium and phosphorus) and protein (1.5 g/100 mL) content, and therefore lower PRSL than standard infant formulas. It is most appropriately used for infants with renal insufficiency. Similac PM 60/40 also contains less calcium and iron than standard infant formulas; supplementation of these minerals may be necessary.

Premature Infant Formulas   Inadequate nutrient intake can occur in human milk–fed premature infants because human milk does not meet the needs of this population. Because of their increased nutrient needs and somewhat decreased ability to consume an adequate volume, premature infants (especially those less than 34 weeks gestation) often need formulas that provide a higher caloric density, as well as increased protein, calcium, phosphorus, and other nutrients. The nutritional goal for a preterm infant is to achieve a postnatal growth rate that approximates the intrauterine growth rate of a normal fetus of the same postconceptional age.

No commercially available formula is completely satisfactory for premature infants. Formulas for premature infants (Table 26-6) share features, such as whey-predominant proteins, carbohydrate mixtures of lactose and corn syrup solids, and fat mixtures containing both medium- and long-chain triglycerides. They differ in electrolyte, vitamin, mineral, protein, and caloric content. When given in sufficient volume, these formulas promote adequate growth in preterm infants. An isotonic osmolality (approximately 300 mOsm/kg of water) is maintained at a caloric density of 24 kcal/oz or 80 kcal/100 mL.

Calcium and phosphorus are crucial to the development and maintenance of the human skeleton. In addition, calcium and phosphorus are integral components of many biochemical reactions. Calcium requirements are affected by protein and phosphorus intake in that these nutrients interact with the renal tubular reabsorption of calcium. Calcium-to-phosphorus weight ratios vary significantly for human milk (2:1) and cow milk (1.2:1). This ratio also varies in commercial infant formulas. Formulas designed for term infants will not meet the calcium and phosphorus needs of premature infants. For these infants, the additional calcium and phosphorus found in premature infant formulas is necessary for normal bone growth and mineralization. Typical amounts of calcium and phosphorus found in 20 kcal/oz preterm and term infant formulas are 112 to 120 mg calcium and 56 to 68 mg phosphorus/100 mL versus 53 to 73 mg calcium and 28 to 36 mg phosphorus/100 mL). Human milk fed to premature infants requires calcium and phosphorus fortification with either a human milk fortifier or a transitional premature formula, which is discussed later in this chapter.

Nutrient-enriched transition or postdischarge formulas are designed specifically to provide for continued catch-up growth in premature infants after hospital discharge. Similac NeoSure and Enfamil EnfaCare LIPIL (both milk-based formulas) contain MCTs as part of the fat source. The caloric (22 kcal/oz), protein, vitamin, and mineral content of these formulas exceeds that of standard term formulas but is less than that of 24 kcal/oz premature infant formulas. Use of these formulas in preterm infants until 9 months postnatal age results in greater linear growth, weight gain, and bone mineral content than is seen with the use of standard, term infant formulas.[38]

Human Milk Fortifiers Mothers who deliver prematurely produce milk that is higher in protein, sodium, potassium, and possibly other nutrients than the milk of mothers who deliver at full term. However, these nutrients decline to the amounts found in mature human milk by 4 to 8 weeks after delivery. During the third trimester, the fetus receives 125 to 150 mg of calcium and 65 to 80 mg of phosphorus daily, most of which is deposited in bone. Human milk, whether preterm or mature, cannot supply this amount of calcium and phosphorus, which is needed to prevent osteopenia of prematurity.

Commercial products have been developed to supplement the nutrient content of human milk so that it meets the needs of most preterm infants. Enfamil Human Milk Fortifier and Similac Human Milk Fortifier are powders that add nutrients to human milk without displacing a significant amount of volume. Both products are made from cow milk supplemented with whey protein to provide a whey:casein ratio of 60:40 and a fat mixture that provides MCTs. When added to human milk, fortifiers increase the osmolality by only 10 to 35 mOsm/kg. Table 26-9 lists the composition of the human milk fortifiers. Studies support adequate weight gain and nutrient retention in infants when either fortified human milk or commercial preterm formulas are ingested. Although both groups gained weight at rates equivalent to intrauterine growth rates (15 g/kg/day), as recommended by AAP, time to reach a weight of 1800 grams was reduced by 7 days in a group of premature infants receiving Similac Human Milk Fortifier compared with those receiving Enfamil Human Milk Fortifier.[39,40] This improved weight gain has the potential to shorten length of hospital stay, but this outcome has not been evaluated. Linear growth was also consistent with goals (1 cm/week) in both groups but higher in the Similac Human Milk Fortifier group, an effect likely resulting from the increased calcium and phosphorus found in the Similac product. The use of either product will result in weight gain that is equivalent to intrauterine growth rates in most premature infants. Product selection will, therefore, be dictated by cost and clinical preference. These products are expensive, costing as much as $1.50 per packet, and one packet is generally added to each 25 mL of human milk to yield a 24 kcal/oz concentration. Once the infant is ready for discharge from the hospital or has reached a weight of 2.5 kg, one of the transition or postdischarge formulas can be added to human milk to increase the caloric density (1 teaspoon powder added to 90 mL formula yields 24 kcal/oz) and delivery of other nutrients.

TABLE 26-9 Human Milk Fortifiers

Component	Similac Human Milk Fortifier[a]	Enfamil Human Milk Fortifier[a]
Calories	14	14
Protein (g)	1	1.1
Fat (g)	0.36	1
Carbohydrates (g)	1.8	<0.4
Vitamin A (IU)	620	950
Vitamin D (IU)	120	150
Vitamin E (IU)	3.2	4.6
Vitamin K (mcg)	8.3	4.4
Thiamin (mcg)	233	150
Riboflavin (mcg)	417	220
Vitamin B$_6$ (mcg)	211	115
Vitamin B$_{12}$ (mcg)	0.64	0.18
Niacin (mg)	3.57	3
Folic acid (mcg)	23	25
Pantothenic acid (mg)	1.5	0.73
Biotin (mcg)	26	2.7
Vitamin C (mg)	25	12
Calcium (mg)	117	90
Phosphorus (mg)	67	50
Magnesium (mg)	7	1
Iron (mg)	0.35	1.44
Zinc (mg)	1	0.72
Manganese (mcg)	7.2	10
Copper (mcg)	170	44
Selenium (mcg)	0.5	—
Sodium (mg)	15	16
Potassium (mg)	63	29
Chloride (mg)	38	13

[a] Amount per 4 packets; generally mixed with 100 mL human milk to yield 120 mL with a caloric density of 24 kcal/oz.

Source: Abbott Nutrition at www.abbottnutrition.com, and Mead Johnson Nutritionals at www.meadjohnson.com. Last accessed October 11, 2008.

Metabolic Formulas Infants with various inherited inborn errors of metabolism require specific formulas tailored to their particular condition and must be under the care of a specialist, usually a pediatric endocrinologist or geneticist. Information about these formulas is available on the various manufacturers' Web sites. These formulas, as well as formulas intended for use in LBW infants or in patients with specific medical conditions or dietary needs, are classified by FDA as "exempt formulas," which means they are exempt from FDA nutrient content and labeling requirements.[41]

Concentrated Formulas A child with caloric needs exceeding normal requirements may be given concentrated formula under medical supervision. A few ready-to-use formulas made from cow milk are available in a caloric density of 22 or 24 kcal/oz (Table 26-6). Various concentrations can be prepared from liquid concentrates or powders by varying the amount of water added (Tables 26-10 and 26-11). Increasing caloric density by adding

TABLE 26-10	Dilution of Concentrated Liquid Infant Formulas[a]	

Caloric Concentration Desired (kcal/oz)	Liquid Formula Concentrate (oz)	Added Water (oz)
20	1	1
22 (actual 21.8)	3	2.5
24	3	2
26–27 (actual 26.7)	3	1.5
28–29 (actual 28.6)	5	2

[a] Commercial concentrates of infant formula contain 40 kcal/oz before dilution with water.

TABLE 26-11	Dilution of Powdered Term Infant Formulas[a]	

Caloric Concentration Desired (kcal/oz)	Formula Powder (scoop)[b]	Added Water (oz)
20	1	2
24	3	5
28	4	5.5
28	7	10

[a] Powdered infant formulas generally contain 44 kcal per level, packed scoop before dilution. If a large volume of formula is to be prepared, add powder necessary to supply desired calories; then add water to the final volume desired. Directions for preparation may vary; check manufacturer's information.

[b] Historically, the conversion 1 scoop = 1 tablespoon of powder has been used. However, this measurement varies between powders. For improved accuracy, parents and caregivers should be instructed to use the manufacturer's provided scoop for all measurements.

less water also increases delivery of all nutrients, including protein and electrolytes, and decreases free water delivery. Increased concentration of protein and electrolytes (i.e., PRSL) in conjunction with decreased fluid intake may result in dehydration and electrolyte imbalances. Careful monitoring of the infant's fluid intake and output, weight, serum electrolytes, blood urea nitrogen, serum creatinine, and urine specific gravity and osmolality is recommended, especially on initiation of the concentrated formula.

Modular macronutrient components (Table 26-12) that can be added to either human milk or infant formula are available as alternatives to concentrating formulas. Adding carbohydrates as glucose can result in diarrhea. Protein supplementation may increase the PRSL. Fat may be added as MCTs (MCT Oil) or Microlipid for infants with fat malabsorption or intolerance. Microlipid is an emulsion made from safflower oil that provides long-chain fatty acids and mixes well with formula. Addition of fat can lead to diarrhea, steatorrhea, delayed gastric emptying, vomiting, and gastroesophageal reflux. Adding modular components is more expensive and time-consuming than simply concentrating the formula; these components should be reserved for situations in which a single nutrient is needed or concentrating the formula further is not appropriate.

Follow-Up Formulas   "Follow-up," "follow-on," or toddler formulas (Table 26-6) are designed for infants 4 to 12 months

of age. AAP/CON, however, has stated that these formulas offer no nutritional advantages; standard formulas are appropriate for infants up to 12 months of age.[28]

Formulas for Children 1 to 10 Years of Age   Nutritionally complete, isotonic, virtually lactose-free enteral formulas designed for young children who cannot tolerate a normal diet or eat solid food are available (Table 26-6). Flavored products contain sucrose, have a pleasant taste, and can be used as oral supplements. These formulas are also appropriate to use as tube feedings regardless of tube tip placement. They contain adequate amounts of calcium, phosphorus, iron, and vitamin D for this age group; the amounts contained in adult enteral products are typically inadequate.

Several therapeutic formulas have also been developed for children 1 to 10 years of age (Table 26-6). Peptamen Junior and Pepdite One+ are peptide-based, semi-elemental formulas. Vivonex Pediatric, Neocate One+, Neocate Junior, E028 Splash (a liquid, flavored version of Neocate One+), and EleCare are amino acid–based elemental formulas. These products

TABLE 26-12	Modular Additives		

Additive[a] (Mfr)	Nutrient(s) Provided	Amount of Nutrient(s)	Calories
Resource Beneprotein (Nes)	Whey protein (milk)	Per 7 g scoop or packet: protein 6 g	25 kcal/scoop
Polycose (A)	Carbohydrate	Per tbsp: carbohydrate 6 g	23 kcal/tbsp
Microlipid (Nes)	Long-chain fats (safflower oil)	Per mL: fat 0.5 g	4.5 kcal/mL
MCT Oil (Nes)	MCTs	Per mL: fat 0.93 g	7.7 kcal/mL
Super Soluble Duocal (Nut)	Carbohydrate, fat (MCT 35%)	Per tbsp: carbohydrate 6 g; fat 2 g	25 kcal/scoop 42 kcal/tbsp
Resource Benecalorie (Nes) (liquid)	Protein, fat	Per 1.5 oz: protein 7 g; fat 33 g	7 kcal/mL

Key: A, Abbott Nutrition; MCT, medium-chain triglycerides; Nes, Nestlé Infant and Clinical Nutrition; Nut, Nutricia North America.

[a] Products listed are powders unless specified otherwise.

are intended for use in children with altered digestion and/ or absorptive capabilities caused by a number of conditions (Table 26-7).

Potential Problems with Infant Formulas

As with any food, GI problems, especially diarrhea, can occur with the use of infant formulas as well as human milk. Tooth decay and nutritional deficiencies are other potential problems.

DIARRHEA

Diarrhea can lead to failure to thrive (chronic) and dehydration (acute). Infants are particularly susceptible to dehydration because of their high metabolic rate and ratio of surface area to weight and height. Fluid depletion by diarrhea or vomiting may quickly (within 24 hours) produce severe dehydration with fluid and electrolyte imbalances, shock, and possible death. A potential formula-related cause of diarrhea and vomiting is the improper dilution of a concentrated liquid or powdered formula or the incorrect addition of a modular product.

If diarrhea develops, the clinician should ascertain the severity and duration of the diarrhea, stool frequency, and formula preparation method. If the diarrhea appears severe (i.e., many more stools per day than normal) or has continued for more than 72 hours, or if the infant is clinically ill (fever, lethargy, anorexia, irritability, dry mucous membranes, or decreased urine output), the infant should be referred for medical attention. (Diarrhea is discussed in Chapter 17.)

Mild diarrhea will usually resolve without the need for medical intervention, but the infant should be observed closely for signs of dehydration. Temporarily discontinuing usual dietary intake is not recommended except during a 4- to 6-hour period of oral rehydration if the infant is dehydrated. Oral electrolyte replacement solutions manufactured especially for infants (e.g., Pedialyte) may be used for short-term replacement of fluid and electrolyte losses in mild-to-moderate dehydration to augment fluid intake, but these solutions should not replace formula or human milk intake.[42] Prevention of dehydration by replacement of ongoing losses with a glucose/electrolyte solution in liquid or frozen form is the best intervention for diarrhea in infants and children.

Lactose-free formulas or a lactose-free diet may be considered for those infants and children with moderate-to-severe diarrheal illness, but full-strength lactose-containing formulas, human milk, or a regular diet can be used in most infants. Parents should be advised that diarrhea is likely to continue for 3 to 7 days regardless of type of formula, and seeking medical consultation is advised if a sudden increase in stool output occurs with resumption of feeding.[42]

OTHER GI ISSUES

Adverse GI effects of formula include mechanical obstruction (inspissated milk curds) and hypersensitivity to specific milk protein. Cow milk intolerance is associated most often with an inability to digest lactose or milk proteins. Hyperosmolar formulas may adversely affect premature infants during the early neonatal period and may be a contributing factor to the development of necrotizing enterocolitis, a severe inflammation of the intestinal mucous membranes. For this reason, initiation of feedings in these infants is most often done with unfortified human milk or a 20 kcal/oz premature infant formula. Only after the infant has reached 100 to 150 mL/kg/day of enteral feedings is the caloric density advanced.

TOOTH DECAY

Baby bottle tooth decay can occur in children who are bottle-fed beyond the typical weaning period (1 year) and who go to sleep with their bottles. It can also occur if the infant is allowed to sip on a bottle or training cup frequently during the day. Caries can be seen in children younger than 2 years and may involve the maxillary incisors, maxillary and mandibular first molars, or maxillary and mandibular canines. Restorative dentistry is often required, leading to the potential for difficulty in speech development. Methods for prevention once teeth start to erupt include substituting plain water for carbohydrate-containing formula or other drinks given in a bottle until the infant is weaned from the bottle, ensuring adequate fluoride intake, cleaning the baby's mouth at least once daily, and weaning from breast or bottle by 10 to 12 months of age.[43] Going to sleep with a bottle should be actively discouraged for all infants.

NUTRITIONAL DEFICIENCIES OR TOXICITIES

Generally, age- and condition-appropriate commercial infant formulas are nutritionally adequate and safe for most infants and children. Nutritional deficiencies reported historically with commercial infant formulas are unlikely today with appropriate supplementation procedures and technologic advances in processing.

Because of concern about possible aluminum contamination of infant formulas, the Food and Agricultural Organization of the United Nations has set a provisional tolerable aluminum intake of 1 mg/kg per day. Aluminum toxicity can interfere with cellular and metabolic processes in the nervous system as well as negatively affect bone and liver tissues.[44] Aluminum toxicity is primarily a concern in patients with decreased or immature renal function, such as premature infants. If an infant were to ingest as much as 200 mL/kg per day of a formula known to have the highest aluminum content, the amount of aluminum received per day would still be less than 0.5 mg/kg per day. The highest aluminum concentrations in infant formulas (500–2400 mg/L) have been reported in soy protein–based formulas, because plants readily absorb aluminum from soil.

Infant Formula Preparation

Most formulas are available as a ready-to-use liquid or as a liquid concentrate or powder for reconstitution that is mixed with water. Ready-to-use formulas are convenient but usually more expensive. These formulas should never be diluted. Concentrated liquids typically require the mixing of equal amounts of water and concentrated liquid (e.g., 13-ounce can of formula with 13-ounce can of water) to prepare a 20 kcal/oz formula (Table 26-10). These formulas should never be given undiluted. Powdered term and preterm transition or postdischarge formulas provide a measuring scoop in the can and require addition of 1 packed level scoop of powder to each 2 ounces of water for a 20 kcal/oz formula and 22 kcal/oz formula, respectively. Directions for preparation may vary and should always be compared with the manufacturer's or health care professional's directions. For example, mixing directions for Neocate Infant vary substantially from those for other formulas. In addition, if the family is given alternative directions from those printed on the can, these should be given in writing and explained thoroughly to the caregiver. Directions should be provided in the appropriate language for non–English-speaking patients. Before use, infant formula containers should be inspected for the expiration date and damage. Unopened formula containers, cans, or bottles can be stored at room temperature but must not be subjected to extreme temperature changes.

PREPARATION TECHNIQUES

Each infant formula has specific instructions for preparation, and most formulas have symbols on the containers that can be used as guidelines in preparing formula. Because infants may be more susceptible to infection, various sterilization methods have been recommended for infant formula preparation. Table 26-13 reviews sterilization methods for different types of formulas. Studies have shown that the clean method of preparing formula (i.e., not boiling the water) is as safe as terminal sterilization (i.e., boiling the water); therefore, some practitioners do not recommend boiling water. AAP currently recommends that all water for formula preparation be boiled because of reports of municipal water supply contamination in some areas. If well or pond water is used or if the area is prone to flooding, the water must be boiled. If tap water is used, cold water should be run for at least 2 minutes before use to decrease lead expo-

sure by clearing any lead that might be in the pipes. For the same reason, water from the hot water tap should never be used for formula preparation or for drinking. Tap water should not be boiled for more than 5 minutes, given that excessive boiling may concentrate lead and other impurities in the water. If bottled water is used in infant formula preparation, it should be treated the same as tap or well water (i.e., boil and cool it prior to use) unless the water is labeled as sterile.

Using a microwave oven to warm infant formula or expressed human milk, or to thaw frozen human milk can cause scald injuries, palatal burns, and exploding containers. In addition, glass bottles can get hotter than plastic bottles, and the temperature of the milk may not be evenly distributed. Patient Counseling for Infant Nutrition provides specific guidelines on using a microwave oven for formula preparation.

Table 26-13 provides handling instructions and recommendations for storage of infant formulas once the original container has been opened. Expressed human milk should be stored in glass or plastic airtight containers, refrigerated, and used within 24 to 48 hours. Human milk can be frozen, preferably in the

---

TABLE 26-13 Sterilization Method for Infant Formula Preparation

General Preparation

- Always wash hands before preparing formula or handling bottles and nipples; repeat washing if interrupted.
- Sterilize bottles and other equipment (e.g., glass measuring cup, spoons, nipples, rings, and disks) separately from the formula.[a]
- Using tongs, place all equipment in a deep pan or sterilizer, cover all equipment with cold tap water, bring to a boil, and continue boiling for 5 minutes.
- Tap and bottled water should be heated until it reaches a rolling boil, allowed to continue to boil for 1 to 2 minutes, and then allowed to cool to room temperature. Boiling for a longer period of time may concentrate impurities (e.g., lead) in the water.
- Using tongs, remove all items from the pan or sterilizer and place on a clean towel. Place bottles and nipples on the towel with their open ends facing down.

Concentrated Liquid Formula

- Wash top of can with hot water and detergent, rinse in hot running water, and dry.
- Shake can well and open it with a clean punch-type can opener.
- Mix appropriate amounts of concentrated liquid and sterilized water (according to product label or health care practitioner instructions). For accuracy, use a measuring cup for all measurements of formula and water.
- Pour formula into sterilized bottles; place nipples, rings, and disks on bottles.
- Tightly cover any unused formula and store in refrigerator. Use formula within 48 hours of preparation or discard.

Powdered Formula

- Wash top of can with hot water and detergent, rinse in hot running water, and dry.
- Open can and mix appropriate amounts of powder and sterilized water (according to product label or health care practitioner instructions). For accuracy, use the scoop provided or a dry measuring cup for all measurements.

- Pour formula into sterilized bottles; place nipples, rings, and disks on the bottles.
- Tightly cover any unused formula and store in the refrigerator. Use formula within 48 hours of preparation.
- Cover any formula remaining in the can with the plastic top. Write the date on the opened can. Store in a cool, dry place for up to 1 month.

Ready-to-Use Formula

Ready-to-Use Cans

- Wash top of can with hot water and detergent, rinse in hot running water, and dry.
- Shake can well, and open it with a clean punch-type can opener.
- Add the amount of formula needed for a single feeding to one sterilized bottle or to the number of bottles needed for a full day's feedings.
- *Do not add water.*
- Prepared bottles and any formula left in the can should be tightly covered and refrigerated for up to 48 hours after the can was opened.

Ready-to-Use Bottles

- The protective cap must be removed, and a sterile nipple screwed onto the bottle before feeding.
- Shake each bottle well to ensure mixing of formula.

All Types of Formulas

- Warm bottle to desired temperature by immersing in hot water bath or running under hot water.
- Heating bottles in the microwave is not recommended.
- Never boil or overheat formula.
- Shake each bottle well before feeding infant.
- Test formula temperature before feeding infant.
- After feeding, discard any formula left in bottle, and immediately rinse bottle and nipple in cool water.

---

[a] If disposable bottle liners are used, only nipples, rings, and screw tops of bottles need to be sterilized; the manufacturer has sterilized the bottle liners.

rear of the freezer compartment, for up to 2 weeks if the freezer compartment is inside the refrigerator, 3 to 4 months when the freezer has a separate door from the refrigerator, and up to 6 months if in a 0°F freezer. Frozen milk should be rapidly thawed by holding the container under tepid running water or placing it in a tepid water bath. Thawed human milk should always be used within 24 hours of thawing and never refrozen.

ADVERSE EFFECTS OF IMPROPERLY PREPARED AND/OR ADMINISTERED FORMULAS

As stated previously, the failure to properly dilute a concentrated infant formula can result in a hypertonic solution that could result in diarrhea and dehydration. In extreme cases, the ingestion of an overly concentrated formula can lead to hypernatremic dehydration (induced by water deficit), metabolic acidosis, and renal failure. Excessive formula dilution can lead to water intoxication that can result in irritability, hyponatremia, coma, brain damage, or death. Such a situation may occur when a caregiver misunderstands the instructions for preparing a concentrated formula, dilutes a ready-to-use formula, or tries to make the baby's formula last longer by diluting it.

Parents or other caregivers may have questions about how much infant formula their child should receive. Typically, a health care provider at the hospital will have given parents feeding instructions prior to discharge. However, when a formula change is made after hospital discharge, adequate information may not be provided in some health settings. Generally, the required daily formula intake depends on an infant's age, weight, and individual considerations such as the need for catch-up growth (Table 26-14). During the first year of life, a normal healthy formula-fed term infant usually eats every 3 to 5 hours (average of 4 hours). Small or weak infants may eat every 2 to 3 hours, because they have smaller stomach capacities or shorter gastric emptying times, or tire easily during feedings. Breast-fed infants or those receiving human milk from a bottle also will nurse or eat more often, given that human milk empties from the stomach more rapidly than formula. Most term infants will lengthen the interval between feedings to 4 hours by the age of 3 to 4 weeks. Premature infants may continue to require frequent feedings past 6 to 8 weeks of age, depending on the infant's birth weight and growth. Typically, infants begin to stop nighttime feedings after 1 to 2 months of age or when they reach 8 to 10 pounds (3.5–4.5 kg).

The amount of formula offered to a bottle-fed infant should be consistent with the DRI for energy according to age and weight (Table 26-2). Table 26-14 lists typical quantities of feedings for various age groups. The infant should be fed on demand

and not forced to take more formula than is desired at any one feeding. If the infant finishes a bottle and still seems hungry, more formula should be offered. Parents should also be aware that an infant typically loses weight (mostly water) during the first week of life, but by 2 weeks of age, the child should be gaining weight. Appropriate weight gain usually indicates that an infant is receiving an appropriate amount of formula. The NCHS standardized growth curves are used to determine whether an infant is growing appropriately. Weight, length/height, and head circumference should be plotted at each medical visit.

Both underfeeding and overfeeding are potential problems. Breast-fed infants who like to "graze" all day can take in too much milk and gain too much weight. Other problems associated with overfeeding are regurgitation, gastroesophageal reflux, vomiting, loose stools, constipation, and colic. Spitting up a small amount of formula, even if it is after every feeding, is usually not a cause for concern. If an infant is regurgitating or vomiting significant amounts, a primary care provider should be consulted. Bilious (green) emesis is always a reason to consult immediately the child's primary care practitioner.

Loose stools are normal for some infants, especially those receiving human milk or hydrolyzed formulas. They may also be caused by an improperly concentrated formula, overfeeding, or administration of contaminated formula. Human milk–fed infants may have only 1 stool every 1 to 3 days; however, some infants will have 10 to 12 stools each day. Formula-fed infants usually have 1 to 3 stools per day. Diarrhea, defined as increased stool volume and frequency that differ from the usual volume and frequency, warrants medical attention when it persists for more than 3 days or when the infant appears dehydrated. Constipation is rare in human milk- or formula-fed infants; it most often results from inadequate formula intake. Severe or prolonged constipation with straining and blood streaks on the stool warrant a visit to the primary care provider.

PRODUCT SELECTION GUIDELINES

For healthy, term infants who do not need a therapeutic formula, a milk-based formula with or without added whey protein is indicated. When recommending a formula, the clinician should consider preparation methods, the caregiver's ability to follow directions, the parents' attitudes and preferences, sanitary conditions and refrigeration facilities available, and cost. Before assisting parents in selecting a therapeutic formula, the clinician should determine whether a primary care provider recommended the formula.

For many parents, cost may be a critical factor in formula selection. Concentrated liquids and powders are typically less expensive than ready-to-use products. Convenience is also a consideration. The preparation of powdered and concentrated liquid formulas requires more manipulative functions and more attention to clean technique. The formula selected should be one that is well tolerated by the infant, convenient for the parents, and priced to fit the family's budget. To simplify formula preparation away from home, parents can select products that are available in unit-of-use packaging for ready-to-use liquids, or powder packets or powder can be placed in an empty bottle and water added whenever needed.

The federal grant program Special Supplemental Nutrition Program for Women, Infants, and Children (WIC) helps ensure that all infants, children (up to 5 years of age), and pregnant, postpartum, and breast-feeding women have access to adequate nutrition. State health departments and other agencies regulate and allocate funds in the federal grant program (i.e., $6.1 billion in

TABLE 26-14 Average Age-Appropriate Number of Daily Feedings and Volume per Feeding		
Age	Average Number of Daily Feedings	Average Volume per Feeding (oz)
Birth–2 weeks	6–10	2–3
2 weeks–1 month	6–8	4–5
1–3 months	5–6	5–6
3–4 months	4–5	6–7
4–12 months	3–4	7–8

2008). Formula and other preventive services are free to eligible participants. More than 8.3 million people received WIC benefits each month in 2007, most of them infants and children.[45]

Vitamin and Mineral Supplementation

Routine multivitamin and mineral supplementation is generally unnecessary for most formula- or human milk–fed term infants. However, some infants may be at risk for deficiency and require supplementation. Cases of vitamin D–deficiency rickets continue to be reported in the United States, and the prevalence of iron-deficiency anemia in children 1 to 2 years of age (7%) is still above 5%, the goal set by *Healthy People 2010,* despite routine use of iron-fortified formulas and infant foods. Therefore, particular care should be given to ensure that children in this age group get adequate dietary iron. AAP does not, however, endorse routine iron supplementation in this age group.

Vitamin and mineral supplementation may be needed for preterm and human milk–fed infants whose mothers are inadequately nourished (Table 26-15).[46] These infants and those with other nutritional deficiencies, malabsorptive and other chronic diseases, rare vitamin-dependent conditions, inborn errors of vitamin or mineral metabolism, or deficiencies related to the intake of certain medications will need medically supervised vitamin and mineral supplementation.

Human Milk–Fed, Full-Term Infants

The healthy, full-term human milk–fed infant requires little to no special supplementation for the first 4 to 6 months of life except for vitamin D and iron. AAP recommends vitamin D supple-

mentation (200 IU/day; cholecalciferol 5 mg/day) for all human milk–fed infants unless they are weaned to at least 500 mL/day of vitamin D–fortified formula. Risk factors for vitamin D deficiency include increased birth order (third child or later), dark skin, cultural factors that minimize maternal skin exposure to sunlight, and delayed intake of dairy products in the infant or mother because of intolerance or other factors.[47] Mothers should be encouraged to maintain a balanced diet and to drink three to five 8-ounce glasses of milk each day while breast-feeding. If the mother cannot tolerate milk because of lactose intolerance, lactose digestion aids (e.g., Lactaid, Dairy Aid, Lactogest, and Dairy Ease) or lactose-free milk are available. Mothers who do not drink milk should be encouraged to increase vitamin D and calcium intake through other dietary sources or by taking supplements.

Human milk–fed infants rarely develop iron-deficiency anemia before 4 to 6 months of age. Although the iron concentration in human milk averages only 0.3 to 0.5 mg/L, the form of iron is well absorbed. At 4 to 6 months of age and beyond, the iron stores in infants exclusively human milk–fed may become exhausted, requiring a supplemental source. The addition of iron-enriched foods such as fortified infant cereals will usually meet needs, or alternatively, an iron supplement (elemental iron 2 mg/kg/day) can be given. Term infants who are small-for-gestational age are likely to have higher requirements, but the necessity of supplementation in this population is unclear.[48]

The first iron-enriched food introduced into the infant's diet is typically infant cereal. Bioavailability of the large-particle, electrolytic iron powder used to fortify dry infant cereals is substantially less than that of the ferrous sulfate iron used in milk- or soy protein–based formulas. Cereals also contain potent inhibitors of iron absorption and are unreliable in preventing iron deficiency

TABLE 26-15 Guidelines for Use of Vitamin and Mineral Supplements in Healthy Infants[a]

	Multivitamin/Mineral	Vitamin D[b]	Vitamin E	Folate	Iron[c]
Full-Term Infants					
Human milk–fed	0	+	0	0	±
Formula-fed	0	±[d]	0	0	0
Preterm Infants					
Human milk–fed[e]	+	+	0	0	+
Formula-fed[e]	+	+	0	0	+
Older Infants (>6 Months)					
Normal	0	0	0	0	±
High-risk[f]	+	0	0	0	±

Key: +, supplement usually indicated; ±, supplement sometimes indicated; 0, supplement not usually indicated.

[a] Not shown is vitamin K for newborn infants and fluoride in areas where there is insufficient fluoride in the water (see Table 26-16).

[b] All infants should have a minimal intake of 200 IU vitamin D per day beginning during the first 2 months of life; this intake should be continued throughout childhood and adolescence.

[c] Iron-fortified formula and infant cereals are more convenient and reliable sources of iron than a supplement.

[d] Supplement indicated if receiving less than 500 mL/day of infant formula.

[e] Multivitamin supplements (plus added folate) are needed primarily when calorie intake is below approximately 300 kcal/day or when the infant weighs less than 2.5 kg; vitamin D should be supplied at least until 6 months of age in human milk–fed infants. Iron should be started by 2 months of age.

[f] Multivitamin/mineral preparations including iron are preferred to supplements containing iron alone.

Source: References 6 and 46.

when infants receive minimal iron from other sources. Iron-fortified, wet-packed cereal and fruit combinations marketed in jars offer no exposure of the iron sulfate to oxygen until the jar is opened; therefore, iron absorption is improved. Consuming fruit juices and other products containing ascorbic acid along with iron-fortified cereals has been shown to enhance iron absorption.[49]

Formula-Fed, Full-Term Infants

Full-term infants who consume adequate amounts of an iron-fortified, milk-based formula do not need vitamin and mineral supplementation in the first 6 months of life. An iron-fortified formula is preferred to ensure adequate iron stores for growing infants. Infants fed iron-fortified formulas do not demonstrate a difference in stool consistency, fussiness, colic, or regurgitation compared with infants fed low-iron formulas. Vitamin and mineral supplements are not needed for infants older than 6 months who receive a diet consisting of formula and increasing amounts of infant and table foods. A multivitamin with minerals may be needed, however, if the infant is at special nutritional risk.

Preterm Infants

Preterm infants, either human milk- or formula-fed, need vitamin and mineral supplementation. Their nutrient needs are greater than those of full-term infants because of their more rapid growth rate, inability to ingest an adequate volume of formula or human milk, decreased intestinal absorption, and decreased body stores. Until these infants can consume about 300 kcal/day or until they reach a body weight of 2.5 kg, a multivitamin supplement should be administered to provide the equivalent of the recommended intakes for full-term infants.

Premature infants are especially susceptible to iron-deficiency anemia because of marginal iron stores at birth. Without supplementation (e.g., blood transfusions), iron stores will be depleted by 2 months of age, in contrast to depletion at 4 to 6 months of age in full-term infants. AAP/CON recommends iron supplementation at a dosage of 2 mg elemental iron per kilogram daily for premature infants with birth weights between 1500 and 2500 grams once they are 2 months old or have doubled their birth weight.[29,38] Preterm infants weighing less than 1500 grams should receive 4 mg of elemental iron per kilogram daily, and those receiving erythropoietin should receive 6 mg of elemental iron per kilogram daily. To minimize the possibility of hemolytic anemia in infants with insufficient vitamin E absorption, iron supplements should be withheld until the preterm infant is several weeks old. However, with adequate vitamin E supplementation in the formula, the risk of hemolytic anemia is minimal.

Supplementation of calcium, phosphorus, and vitamin D in preterm infant formulas is necessary to ensure adequate bone mineralization and to prevent osteopenia and rickets. The prevention of severe bone disease in preterm infants appears to depend on both high oral intakes of calcium and phosphorus and the intake of at least 400 IU (12.5 mg) vitamin D per day.[38] Therefore, preterm infants should receive a special preterm infant formula containing appropriate amounts of calcium, phosphorus, and vitamin D. Depending on the volume of formula consumed, vitamin D supplementation may be necessary along with a premature formula to provide 400 to 800 IU per day.

Fluoride Supplementation

When used appropriately, fluoride is both safe and effective in preventing and controlling dental caries. Fluoride reduces dental decay by reducing the solubility of enamel, reducing the ability of bacteria to produce acid, and promoting remineralization. Systemic fluoride, such as that obtained from fluoridated water, primarily provides a topical benefit to teeth, given that fluoride is secreted from the salivary glands. Slightly less than two-thirds of the municipalities in the United States optimally fluoridate water at a cost of $0.50 per person per year.[50]

Fluoride supplementation is currently not recommended from birth to 6 months of age. Furthermore, the recommended supplementation for children 6 months to 6 years of age whose drinking water is inadequately fluoridated and who do not receive adequate fluoride from other sources has been decreased from previous recommendations because of an increased incidence of fluorosis.[51] Fluorosis, which affects approximately 22% of children, is a cosmetic change in the appearance of the teeth ranging from minor white lines running across the teeth to a very chalky appearance resulting from too much fluoride. If a powdered or concentrated formula is used, fluoride supplements should be administered only if the community's drinking water contains less than 0.3 ppm of fluoride. Table 26-16 can be used to determine the proper fluoride supplementation for a child, depending on the fluoride level in the drinking water. Ready-to-use formulas are manufactured with defluoridated water and contain less than 0.3 ppm of fluoride. The primary care provider may recommend a fluoride supplement for infants not receiving adequate fluoride.

Assessment of Infant Nutrition: A Case-Based Approach

Body weight and length, and head circumference are the growth standards for determining whether infants are receiving the appropriate nutrients, are properly using ingested nutrients, or both. If an infant appears to be underweight or underdeveloped, the clinician should advise the parent to take the infant to a primary care provider for evaluation.

The clinician's primary role is to provide information about breast-feeding and infant formula products, including assistance with product selection and preparation instructions.

Cases 26-1 and 26-2 are examples of assessment of infant nutrition.

TABLE 26-16 Recommended Fluoride Supplementation (mg/day)[a]

Age	Fluoride Concentration of Drinking Water (ppm)		
	<0.3	0.3–0.6	>0.6
Birth–6 months	0	0	0
6 months–3 years	0.25	0	0
3–6 years	0.50	0.25	0
6–16 years	1.00	0.50	0

[a] Sodium fluoride 2.2 mg contains fluoride 1 mg.

Source: References 50 and 51.

CASE 26-1

Relevant Evaluation Criteria	Scenario/Model Outcome
Information Gathering	
1. Gather essential information about the patient's symptoms, including:	
a. description of symptom(s) (i.e., nature, onset, duration, severity, associated symptoms)	Infant has been spitting up formula after every feeding, almost always with a little force. Although some emesis has occurred since birth, the amount and frequency has increased over the last week. The infant also appears to have more gas, often crying from "gas pains." The infant girl appears well hydrated.
b. description of any factors that seem to precipitate, exacerbate, and/or relieve the patient's symptom(s)	Emesis occurs only after feedings. The infant appears to be more comfortable after each episode of emesis. Irritability associated with gas pains appears to be relieved by simethicone.
c. description of the parent's efforts to relieve the symptoms	Simethicone has been given for gas. Nothing specific has been done for the emesis.
2. Gather essential patient history information:	
a. patient's identity	Lauren Smith
b. patient's age, sex, height, and weight	6-week-old girl; 22 inches; 8 lb 5 oz (3.8 kg)
c. parents' occupation	Father is a mechanic; mother is a receptionist at an insurance agency.
d. patient's dietary habits	Lauren was receiving breast milk plus Enfamil LIPIL 20 kcal/oz, if desired, until 1 week ago when her mother stopped breast-feeding. The infant was changed to Enfamil LIPIL. Per the mother's report, the formula is being mixed to a 24 kcal/oz concentration on the advice of her PCP. The infant takes approximately 120 mL (4 oz) every 3 hours. No extra water or juice is given during the day.
e. patient's sleep habits	Lauren has not started sleeping through the night.
f. concurrent medical conditions, prescription and nonprescription medications, and dietary supplements	Lauren is a healthy, term infant.
g. allergies	NKA
h. history of other adverse reactions to medications	None
Assessment and Triage	
3. Differentiate the patient's signs/symptoms and correctly identify the patient's primary problem(s).	Primary problem: emesis with feedings Secondary problem: increased intestinal gas
4. Identify exclusions for self-treatment.	Bloody or bilious emesis Signs of dehydration: sunken fontanelle, dry mucous membranes, decreased wet diapers, dark urine, decreased oral intake
5. Formulate a comprehensive list of therapeutic alternatives for the primary problem to determine if triage to a medical practitioner is required, and share this information with the parents.	Options include: (1) Call Lauren's PCP to verify the caloric density and volume of feedings desired. Give Lauren's parents instructions on the proper feeding of the infant. (2) Refer Lauren's parents to the PCP. (3) Take no action.
Plan	
6. Select an optimal therapeutic alternative to address the patient's problem, taking into account patient preferences.	Lauren's current feeding schedule, 120 mL every 3 hours of 24 kcal/oz formula, provides 252 mL/kg/day and 202 kcal/kg/day. Both significantly exceed the usual recommended intakes for a healthy, term infant (see Tables 26-2 and 26-14). The most appropriate plan would be to decrease the overall intake. The PCP should be contacted to verify the caloric density of the formula. The family should then be instructed to feed Lauren approximately 2.5 ounces every 3 hours or 3–3.5 ounces every 4 hours. This decreased intake of formula should decrease the episodes of emesis, and decrease fussiness and irritability caused by overfeeding.

Relevant Evaluation Criteria	Scenario/Model Outcome
7. Describe the recommended therapeutic approach to the parents.	The primary care practitioner should be contacted to verify the desired concentration of Enfamil LIPIL. The volume of the feedings should be reduced to the volumes listed in step 6. If the symptoms persist after these interventions, Lauren should be taken to the PCP.
8. Explain to the parents the rationale for selecting the recommended therapeutic approach from the considered therapeutic alternatives.	Because the symptoms started (or acutely worsened) with the change from breast milk to infant formula, and both the caloric density and the volume of the infant formula exceed the usual needs of a healthy term infant, overfeeding is the most likely cause of Lauren's emesis and irritability. If overfeeding is the major issue, decreasing the caloric density and volume of feedings will have almost immediate results.

Patient Education

9. When recommending self-care with non-prescription medications and/or nondrug therapy, convey accurate information to the parents:	
a. appropriate dose and frequency of administration	New feeding regimen: Enfamil LIPIL 2.5 ounces every 3 hours or 3–3.5 ounces every 4 hours. Watch for cues to the baby's hunger and satiety patterns to avoid under- or overfeeding.
b. maximum number of days the therapy should be employed	If no improvement is seen in 2–3 days, then the primary care provider should be contacted for a possible change in the formula (see Table 26-6).
c. product administration procedures	The formula should be mixed per product instruction (e.g., 1 scoop in 2 ounces of water to make 20 kcal/oz formula) per the information given in the box Patient Education for Infant Nutrition.
d. expected time to onset of relief	Several days
e. degree of relief that can be reasonably expected	Emesis likely will not be eliminated. All infants have some gastroesophageal reflux and spit or vomit from time to time. Forceful emesis and emesis with every feeding as well as irritability from gas pains should improve.
f. most common side effects	None
g. side effects that warrant medical intervention should they occur	Persistent vomiting, especially if severe, bilious, or bloody; weight loss; dehydration
h. patient options in the event that condition worsens or persists	Contact primary care provider to evaluate for other causes such as cow-milk intolerance, gastroesophageal reflux, or other conditions.
i. product storage requirements	Infant formula should be used soon after mixing or kept tightly covered in the refrigerator and used within 24 hours of preparation. See product information for any specific storage requirements.
10. Solicit follow-up questions from parents.	What if Lauren doesn't appear to be satisfied with the smaller volume of feedings?
11. Answer parents' questions.	From the history, it sounds like Lauren's stomach is too full after each feeding, resulting in a forceful emesis to remove the extra volume. If she receives only the amount needed, she should feel satisfied, without an episode of emesis. If she takes the smaller amount and still appears to be hungry, then an additional 0.5 ounces can be given.

Key: PCP, primary care provider.

Patient Counseling for Infant Nutrition

The number and variety of infant formulas available may bewilder some parents. Once the formula type recommended or prescribed by the baby's primary care provider is known, the clinician can direct parents to the appropriate product. If parents need further assistance with product selection, the practitioner can recommend a product to match the parents' preferences. At these encounters, the parents should be questioned to make sure they know how to properly prepare their baby's formula and how much formula to give at each feeding. The box Patient Education for Infant Nutrition lists specific information to provide parents. In addition, families who may qualify for WIC but are not enrolled can be advised of its availability and benefits.

CASE 26-2

Relevant Evaluation Criteria	Scenario/Model Outcome
Information Gathering	
1. Gather essential information about the patient's symptoms, including:	
a. description of symptom(s) (i.e., nature, onset, duration, severity, associated symptoms)	Infant has cried constantly since coming home from the hospital. The parents think that this is his "hungry cry" and feed him almost every 1–2 hours. He rarely goes 2 hours between feedings. Despite these frequent feedings, he never seems satisfied and is very irritable. He appears to have lost weight since coming home from the hospital 4 weeks ago. He has very frequent bowel movements but no emesis. The parents also report a significant diaper rash and streaks of blood in the diaper. The boy appears to be somewhat lethargic.
b. description of any factors that seem to precipitate, exacerbate, and/or relieve the patient's symptom(s)	Crying is relieved briefly by feeding.
c. description of the parent's efforts to relieve the symptoms	The parents' efforts to relieve the crying have just been to feed him more.
2. Gather essential patient history information:	
a. patient's identity	Miquel Alvarez-Lopez
b. patient's age, sex, height, and weight	Hispanic, 4-week-old boy born at 38 weeks gestational age; birth weight 7 lb 11 oz (3.5 kg)
c. parents' occupation	Mother works at a local hospital on the housekeeping staff; father works at the shipping port.
d. patient's dietary habits	Miquel is receiving a standard, term infant formula, Good Start Supreme (see Table 26-6). The parents cannot verbalize the exact amount he is taking because they cannot keep up with it.
e. patient's sleep habits	Rarely sleeps more than 2 hours at a time
f. concurrent medical conditions, prescription and nonprescription medications, and dietary supplements	Term infant with no preexisting medical conditions
g. allergies	NKA
h. history of other adverse reactions to medications	None
Assessment and Triage	
3. Differentiate the patient's signs/symptoms and correctly identify the patient's primary problem(s).	Primary problem: dehydration Secondary problems: malabsorption of feedings and failure to thrive
4. Identify exclusions for self-treatment.	Dehydration and failure to thrive are exclusions for self-care.
5. Formulate a comprehensive list of therapeutic alternatives for the primary problem to determine if triage to a medical practitioner is required, and share this information with the parents.	Options include: (1) Refer to the PCP. (2) Refer to the pediatric emergency department. (3) Recommend a formula change. (4) Take no action.
Plan	
6. Select an optimal therapeutic alternative to address the patient's problem, taking into account patient preferences.	Depending on the time of day and availability of the PCP, the parents should be instructed to take Miquel either to the PCP or to the emergency department. This decision should be made prior to allowing the family to leave, if possible. Discussion with the PCP would also be prudent.
7. Describe the recommended therapeutic approach to the parents.	Miquel appears to be suffering from dehydration and needs to see a doctor right away. You should take Miquel to see his primary care provider [or go to the emergency department, depending on what was decided] right away. [Be sure Miquel's family understands the directions and the directions to the facility; use an interpreter, if necessary.]

CASE 26-2 *(continued)*

Relevant Evaluation Criteria	Scenario/Model Outcome
8. Explain to the parents the rationale for selecting the recommended therapeutic approach from the considered therapeutic alternatives.	Miquel does not appear to be tolerating his formula well. He is hungry all the time, because he is not absorbing the nutrients in the formula. Currently, he needs immediate medical attention to correct his dehydration. After that problem is corrected, the doctors will evaluate him to determine the cause of his malabsorption and failure to thrive.

Patient Education

9. When recommending self-care with non-prescription medications and/or nondrug therapy, convey accurate information to the parents.	Criterion does not apply in this case.
10. Solicit follow-up questions from parents.	Why can't we just change formulas and see if he does better?
11. Answer parents' questions.	Dehydration can quickly lead to serious problems in small infants including seizures and other complications. He should be evaluated by a medical professional prior to making any interventions related to his feedings.

Key: PCP, primary care provider.

PATIENT EDUCATION FOR
Infant Nutrition

Optimal nutrition is critical in infants and children to ensure normal growth and development. Parents who carefully follow product instructions and the measures listed here will help ensure optimal nutrition-related outcomes.

- Check unopened formula containers for damage. Do not use products if they are significantly dented or if the expiration date has passed.
- When preparing formula from powder or liquid concentrate, carefully follow instructions for diluting the formula to the desired caloric density (see Tables 26-10 and 26-11). If the formula is too concentrated, the baby may have diarrhea or become dehydrated. If it is too dilute, the baby can become water intoxicated, which might lead to irritability, seizures, coma, or brain damage.
- When preparing formula from powder or liquid concentrate, follow the technique for aseptic sterilization. Be sure to sterilize the bottles (or use sterile liners) and other equipment, and boil the water used to make the formula (see Table 26-13).
- When preparing ready-to-use formulas, do not add water to the formula. Follow the instructions in Table 26-13. Be sure to sterilize the bottles (or use sterile liners) and other equipment.
- Use prepared or opened ready-to-use formula within 48 hours. Keep refrigerated.
- Feed your baby according to the frequency and quantities listed in Table 26-14 unless instructed otherwise by the baby's primary care provider. Paying careful attention to your infant's hunger and fullness cues is important to avoid over- and underfeeding. Discuss any concerns with your infant's primary care provider.
- Heating formula in a microwave is not recommended. However, if formula or human milk is warmed in a microwave, follow the

instructions below to prevent exploding containers, scalds, or burns to the baby's mouth:

—Remove the bottle's lid to allow heat to escape.
—Heat only 4 ounces or more of refrigerated milk; do not thaw frozen human milk in a microwave. Place frozen human milk in a tepid water bath to thaw.
—Heat 4 ounces of refrigerated formula on full power for no longer than 30 seconds; heat 8 ounces of refrigerated formula for 45 seconds.
—After heating the formula, replace the nipple assembly and invert the bottle a minimum of 10 times.
—Test the formula's temperature by putting a few drops on your tongue or the top part of your hand or the back of the wrist. Do not feed the baby the formula unless it feels cool to the touch.

⚠️ Seek medical attention if:
—Your baby is regurgitating or vomiting significant amounts of formula. A small amount of spitting up is normal. Projectile vomiting or bilious vomiting (i.e., green) always requires immediate medical attention.
—Your baby has severe diarrhea or diarrhea that persists for more than 3 days.
—Your baby appears dehydrated (e.g., decreased number of wet diapers, dark urine, limp, no tears, or lethargic).
—Your baby's bowel movements have blood in them.

Key Points for Infant Nutrition and Special Nutritional Needs of Children

➤ Human milk is the optimal food for infants under 12 months of age, and its use should be encouraged for nearly all infants. When breast-feeding or provision of human milk is not possible or desired, commercial infant formulas provide a safe, nutritionally adequate substitute.

➤ Commercial formulas are available in a variety of types to meet the needs of most infants and children with special nutritional needs, including premature infants and those with alterations in requirements caused by disease or other conditions. Therapeutic formulas vary in content and are not generically equivalent.

➤ Accurate preparation of formula is critical to ensure optimal nutrition outcomes. Patients should be counseled on proper preparation techniques.

➤ Some infants will require vitamin and/or mineral supplementation when their needs are not adequately met by their formula intake.

➤ Parents should be referred to their child's primary care provider if their infant or child has persistent vomiting or at any time the emesis is bilious (green).

➤ Parents should be referred to their child's primary care provider if their infant or child has diarrhea lasting more than 3 days, especially if dehydration develops, if the child looks clinically ill, or if there is blood in the bowel movements.

REFERENCES

1. Committee on Nutrition, American Academy of Pediatrics. Infant nutrition and the development of gastrointestinal function. In: Kleinman RE, ed. *Pediatric Nutrition Handbook*. 5th ed. Elk Grove Village, Ill: American Academy of Pediatrics; 2004:3–22.

2. Garcia-Careagg M, Kerner JA. Malabsorptive disorders. In: Behrman RE, Kliegman RM, Jenson HB, eds. *Nelson Textbook of Pediatrics*. 17th ed. Philadelphia: Elsevier Science; 2004:1258–72.

3. Kuczmarski RJ, Ogden CL, Grummer-Strawn LM, et al. *CDC Growth Charts: United States*. Hyattsville, Md: National Center for Health Statistics; 2000. *Advance Data from Vital and Health Statistics, No. 314*. DHHS Pub No. PHS 2000–1250. Available at: http://www.cdc.gov/growthcharts. Last accessed October 11, 2008.

4. Krebs NF, Himes JH, Jacobson D, et al. Assessment of child and adolescent overweight and obesity. *Pediatrics*. 2007;120(suppl)4:S193–S228.

5. Ogden CL, Carroll MD, Curtin LR, et al. Prevalence of overweight and obesity in the United States, 1999–2004. *JAMA*. 2006;13:1549–55.

6. Institute of Medicine, Food and Nutrition Board, Standing Committee on the Scientific Evaluation of Dietary Reference Intakes. *Reference Intakes for Energy, Carbohydrate, Fiber, Fat, Fatty Acids, Cholesterol, Protein, and Amino Acids*. Washington, DC: National Academy Press; 2002. Available at: http//www.nal.usda.gov/fnic/etext/ 000105.html. Last accessed October 11, 2008.

7. Committee on Nutrition, American Academy of Pediatrics. Carbohydrate and dietary fiber. In: Kleinman RE, ed. *Pediatric Nutrition Handbook*. 5th ed. Elk Grove Village, Ill: American Academy of Pediatrics; 2004:247–59.

8. Heird WC. Taurine in neonatal nutrition—revisited. *Arch Dis Child Fetal Neonatal*. 2004;89:473–4.

9. Committee on Nutrition, American Academy of Pediatrics. Cholesterol in childhood. *Pediatrics*. 1998:101:141–7. [Guideline reaffirmed by AAP in April 2001.]

10. Koletzko B, Lien E, Agostoni C, et al. The roles of long-chain polyunsaturated fatty acids in pregnancy, lactation and infancy: review of current knowledge and consensus recommendations. *J Perinat Med*. 2008;36:5–14.

11. Smithers LG, Gibson RA, McPhee A, et al. Effect of long-chain polyunsaturated fatty acid supplementation of preterm infants on disease risk and neurodevelopment: a systematic review of randomized controlled trials. *Am J Clin Nutr*. 2008;87:912–20.

12. Simmer K, Patole SK, Rao SC. Longchain polyunsaturated fatty acid supplementation in infants born at term. *Cochrane Database Syst Rev*. 2008;1:CD000376.

13. Simmer K, Schulzke SM, Patole S. Longchain polyunsaturated fatty acid supplementation in preterm infants. *Cochrane Database Syst Rev*. 2008;1: CD000375.

14. Hadders-Algra M. Prenatal long-chain polyunsaturated fatty acid status: the importance of a balanced intake of docosahexaenoic acid and arachidonic acid. *J Perinat Med*. 2008;36:101–9.

15. World Health Organization. *Global Strategy for Infant and Young Child Feeding*. Geneva, Switzerland: World Health Organization; 2003. Available at: http://www.who.int/nutrition/publications/gs_infant_feeding_text_eng.pdf. Last accessed October 11, 2008.

16. Committee on Nutrition, American Academy of Pediatrics. Complementary Feeding. In: Kleinman RE, ed. *Pediatric Nutrition Handbook*. 5th ed. Elk Grove Village, Ill: American Academy of Pediatrics; 2004:103–15.

17. McDowell MM, Wang C-Y, Kennedy-Stephensen J. Breastfeeding in the United States: findings from the National Health and Nutrition Examination Surveys, 1999–2006. Hyattsville, MD: National Center for Healthy Statistics; 2008. NCHS Data Brief, No 5. Available at: http://www.cdc.gov/nchs/data/databriefs/db05.pdf. Last accessed October 11, 2008.

18. Centers for Disease Control and Prevention. Breastfeeding Practices—Results from the National Immunization Survey. Available at: http://www.cdc.gov/breastfeeding/data/NIS_data/index.htm. Last accessed October 11, 2008.

19. U.S. Department of Health and Human Services. *Healthy People 2000: National Health Promotion and Disease Prevention Objectives*. Washington, DC: US Government Printing Office; 1990. Publication No. PHS 9450212.

20. US Department of Health and Human Services. *Healthy People 2010*. Washington, DC: US Government Printing Office; 2000.

21. US Department of Health and Human Services. *Healthy People 2010: Midcourse Review*. Washington, DC: US Government Printing Office; 2006. Available at: http://www.healthypeople.gov/data/midcourse/pdf/FA16.pdf. Last accessed October 11, 2008.

22. Section on Breastfeeding, American Academy of Pediatrics. Breastfeeding and the use of human milk. *Pediatrics*. 2005;115:496–506. Available at: http://www.pediatrics.org/cgi/content/ full/115/2/496. Last accessed October 11, 2008.

23. Ball TM, Bennett DM. The economic impact of breastfeeding. *Pediatr Clin North Am*. 2001;48:253–62.

24. Briggs GG, Freeman RK, Yaffee SJ, ed. *Drugs in Pregnancy and Lactation*. 7th ed. Philadelphia: Lippincott Williams & Wilkins; 2005.

25. Hale TW. *Medications & Mothers' Milk 2004*. 11th ed. Amarillo, Tex: Pharmasoft Publishing; 2004.

26. Human Milk Banking Association of North America. Available at: http://www.hmbana.org. Last accessed October 11, 2008.

27. Jones F. History of North American donor milk banking: one hundred years of progress. *J Hum Lact*. 2003;19:313–8. Available at http://jhl.sagepub.com/cgi/content/abstract/19/3/313. Last accessed September 3, 2008.

28. Committee on Nutrition, American Academy of Pediatrics. Formula feeding of term infants. In: Kleinman RE, ed. *Pediatric Nutrition Handbook*. 5th ed. Elk Grove Village, Ill: American Academy of Pediatrics; 2004:87–97.

29. Committee on Nutrition, American Academy of Pediatrics. Iron fortification of infant formulas. *Pediatrics*. 1999;104:119–23. [Guideline reaffirmed by AAP in November 2002.]

30. Centers for Disease Control and Prevention. Enterobacter sakazakii infections associated with the use of powdered infant formula—Tennessee, 2001. *MMWR Morb Mortal Wkly Rep*. 2002;51(RR–15):297–300.

31. Baker RD. Infant formula safety. *Pediatrics*. 2002;110:833–5.

32. Fomon SJ, Ziegler EE. Renal solute load and potential renal solute load in infancy. *J Pediatr*. 1999;134:11–4.

33. Fomon SJ. Potential renal solute load: considerations related to complementary feedings of breastfed infants. *Pediatrics*. 2000;106 (5 suppl):1284.

34. Committee on Nutrition, American Academy of Pediatrics. Soy protein-based formulas: recommendations for use in infant feeding. *Pediatrics*. 1998;101:148–53. [Guideline reaffirmed by AAP in April 2001.]

35. Committee on Nutrition, American Academy of Pediatrics. Hypoallergenic infant formulas. *Pediatrics*. 2000;106:346–9.

36. Setchell KD, Zimmer-Nechemias L, Cai J, et al. Isoflavone content of infant formula and the metabolic fate of these phytoestrogens in early life. *Am J Clin Nutr*. 1998;68(6 suppl):1453–61S.

37. Ellis L, Kalnias D, Corey M, et al. Do infants with cystic fibrosis need a protein hydrolysate formula? A prospective, randomized, comparative study. *J Pediatr*. 1998;132:270–6.

38. Committee on Nutrition, American Academy of Pediatrics. Nutritional needs of preterm infants. In: Kleinman RE, ed. *Pediatric Nutrition Handbook*. 5th ed. Elk Grove Village, Ill: American Academy of Pediatrics; 2004:23–54.

39. Reis BB, Hall RT, Schanler RJ, et al. Enhanced growth of preterm infants fed a new powdered human milk fortifier: a randomized, controlled trial. *Pediatrics*. 2000;106:581–8.

40. Porcelli P, Schanler R, Greer F, et al. Growth in human milk-fed very low birth weight infants receiving a new human milk fortifier. *Ann Nutr Metab*. 2000;44:2–10.

41. US Food and Drug Administration. Center for Food Safety and Applied Nutrition. Exempt Infant Formulas Marketed in the United States by Manufacturer and Category. Available at: http://www.cfsan.fda.gov/~dms/inf-exmp.html. Last accessed October 11, 2008.

42. Centers for Disease Control and Prevention. Managing acute gastroenteritis among children: oral rehydration, maintenance, and nutritional therapy. *MMWR Morb Mortal Wkly Rep*. 2003;52 (RR-16):1–20. Available at: http://www.cdc.gov/mmwr/PDF/rr/rr5216.pdf. Last accessed October 11, 2008.

43. Caufield PW, Griffen AL. Dental caries: an infectious and transmissible disease. *Pediatr Clin North Am*. 2000;47:1001–20.

44. Committee on Nutrition, American Academy of Pediatrics. Aluminum toxicity in infants and children. *Pediatrics*. 1996;97:413–6. [Guideline reaffirmed by AAP in April 1999.]

45. US Department of Agriculture, Food and Nutrition Service. WIC: the special supplemental nutrition program for women, infants and children. Available at: http://www.fns.usda.gov/wic. Last accessed October 11, 2008.

46. Committee on Nutrition, American Academy of Pediatrics. Vitamins. In: Kleinman RE, ed. *Pediatric Nutrition Handbook*. 5th ed. Elk Grove Village, Ill: American Academy of Pediatrics; 2004:339–65.

47. Gartner LM, Greer FR, Section on Breastfeeding and Committee on Nutrition, American Academy of Pediatrics. Clinical report: prevention of rickets and vitamin D deficiency: new guidelines for vitamin D intake. *Pediatrics*. 2003;111:908–10.

48. Griffin IJ, Abrams SA. Iron and breastfeeding. *Pediatr Clin North Am*. 2001;48:401–13.

49. Lynch SR, Stoltzfus RJ. Iron and ascorbic acid: proposed fortification levels and recommended iron compounds. *J Nutr*. 2003;133:2978S–84S.

50. Committee on Nutrition, American Academy of Pediatrics. Nutrition and oral health. In: Kleinman RE, ed. *Pediatric Nutrition Handbook*. 5th ed. Elk Grove Village, Ill: American Academy of Pediatrics; 2004:789–800.

51. Centers for Disease Control and Prevention. Recommendations for using fluoride to prevent and control dental caries in the United States. *MMWR Morb Mortal Wkly Rep*. 2001;50 (RR-14):1–59. Available at: http://www.cdc.gov/mmwr/PDF/rr/rr5014.pdf. Last accessed October 11, 2008.

Overweight and Obesity 27

Sarah J. Miller and Cathy L. Bartels

Overweight and obesity have increased in recent decades in both the United States and worldwide. In the United States, increasing concern centers on the developing epidemic of overweight and obesity in children and adolescents. Overweight and obesity are conditions of considerable significance, because they are associated with increased morbidity from various conditions, including cardiovascular diseases, type 2 diabetes mellitus (DM), gallbladder disease, osteoarthritis, respiratory problems, and several cancers.[1]

The National Health and Nutrition Examination Surveys (NHANES) of the U.S. population have tracked prevalence of overweight and obesity in adults from 1960 to the present. These surveys have demonstrated a marked increase in obesity in both men and women across all age and ethnic groups. More than one-third of U.S. adults are currently obese (Figure 27-1).[2] It is encouraging that changes in obesity prevalence for either males or females between 2003–2004 and 2005–2006 were not significant.[3] Large disparities in obesity prevalence exist in non-Hispanic black and Mexican American women compared with white women; these disparities are not currently seen in men.[2] *Healthy People 2010* set an objective for obesity prevalence less than 15%; with current trends, achievement of this objective is unlikely.[3] Figure 27-1 also illustrates the changes in prevalence of overweight across the various NHANES surveys. These have remained fairly stable at 32% to 34%.[2]

Prevalence of overweight and obesity during childhood and adolescence, as tracked by the NHANES data, has risen considerably, as shown in Figure 27-1.[2] Overweight children often become overweight adults. The increases in overweight children have been particularly striking in non-Hispanic black and Mexican American adolescents.

The economic impact of overweight and obesity is substantial. For 2003, the estimated direct cost of obesity in the United States was $75 billion; this value does not include indirect costs associated with lost productivity and mortality.[4] Quantitation of indirect costs is difficult given that many of the comorbidities of obesity may have etiologies other than obesity. Patients with obesity may experience more hospitalizations, take more prescription drugs, make more professional health care claims, and make more outpatient visits than patients who are not obese.

Americans spend tens of billions of dollars on weight control products and services annually. A 2007 survey indicated that about 15% of U.S. adults admitted to having used a nonprescription or dietary supplement weight-loss product, and 9% indicated use within the last year.[5] This survey was completed

before ephedra was removed from the market and before orlistat received approval for nonprescription sale. Because of the dearth of proven, available nonprescription products for weight loss, the practitioner should be knowledgeable in discussing the limitations and potential harm of weight-loss products and gimmicks, as well as comfortable in recommending nonpharmacologic therapies including diet and exercise. In addition, because evidence for available prescription drug therapies exists, the practitioner may also refer patients who fail nonpharmacologic therapies for medical evaluation and consideration for prescription weight-loss therapies.

Clinical Indicators of Overweight and Obesity

The 1998 National Heart, Lung, and Blood Institute (NHLBI) expert report, *Clinical Guidelines on the Identification, Evaluation, and Treatment of Overweight and Obesity in Adults,* defines overweight and obesity in adults in terms of the body mass index (BMI), a reliable parameter that takes into account both height and weight.[1] Table 27-1 illustrates BMI values for persons of various heights and weights and gives equations for calculation of the BMI value; BMI calculators are also available online. Overweight is defined in adults as a BMI of 25 to 29.9 and obesity as a BMI of 30 or greater. The World Health Organization has adopted the same BMI cutoffs as an international standard. Persons who are very muscular may be classified by BMI as overweight or obese when in fact they are not carrying excessive adipose tissue. The NHLBI report and subsequent reports also address the possible importance of the distribution of body fat to risk of morbidity and mortality from various diseases. Abdominal fat is associated with greater health risk than fat in the buttock or thigh region. The NHLBI classifies men with waist circumference greater than 40 inches and women with waist circumference greater than 35 inches as being at increased relative risk of type 2 DM and cardiovascular disease. In children and adolescents, the Centers for Disease Control and Prevention discourage the use of the term *obesity* because of its negative connotations. They define a BMI percentile for age between the 85th and 95th percentiles as "at risk for overweight" and a BMI percentile of 95 or greater as "overweight."[6] However, a 2005 report from the Institute of Medicine did use the term *obesity* in describing children and adolescents with BMI greater than the 95th percentile. Measurement of height and weight to

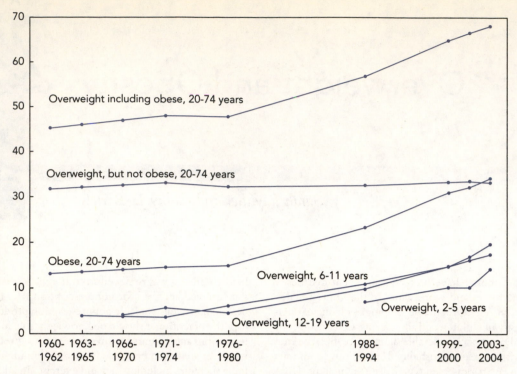

Notes: Estimates for adults are age-adjusted. For adults: overweight including obese is defined as a body mass index (BMI) greater than or equal to 25; overweight but not obese as a BMI greater than or equal to 25 but less than 30; and obese as a BMI greater than or equal to 30. For children: overweight is defined as a BMI at or above the sex- and age-specific 95th percentile BMI cut points from the 2000 CDC Growth Charts: United States. Obese is not defined for children.

FIGURE 27-1 Age-adjusted prevalence of overweight (BMI 25–29.9) and obesity (BMI > 30). Key: BMI, body mass index; NHES, National Health Examination Survey; NHANES, National Health and Nutrition Examination Survey. (*Source:* Reference 2.)

calculate BMI and measurement of waist circumference are physical assessment techniques easily accomplished even in a busy clinical setting.

A syndrome characterized by the presence of certain metabolic risk factors has been associated with increased risk of coronary artery disease, other vascular diseases, and diabetes. Patients with three or more of the following are said to have the metabolic syndrome:

■ Waist circumference greater than 40 inches in men or 35 inches in women
■ Serum triglycerides 150 mg/dL or greater
■ High-density lipoprotein (HDL) cholesterol less than 40 mg/dL in men or less than 50 mg/dL in women
■ Blood pressure level 130/85 mm Hg or higher
■ Fasting serum glucose of 100 mg/dL or greater

Individuals with metabolic syndrome are likely to demonstrate insulin resistance and may benefit more from weight loss in terms of reduced morbidity and mortality compared with overweight or obese persons who are not insulin-resistant. Persons with metabolic syndrome are at especially high risk of morbidity and mortality from cardiovascular disease.

Some studies have challenged the concept that persons with a BMI of 25 to 29.9 have an increased risk of mortality compared with those with a BMI less than 25. Both underweight (BMI

< 18.5) and obesity have been associated with higher mortality rates than either normal weight or overweight categories. There is also some evidence that the association between obesity and cardiovascular disease (CVD) mortality has decreased over time, perhaps because of improvements in medical care for CVD and its risk factors. However, the reduction in obesity-related CVD mortality has been accompanied by an increase in obesity-associated disability, perhaps related to the population becoming overweight or obese at earlier ages; overweight and obesity may contribute to disability, and these developments may contribute to disability in a cumulative fashion over time.[7] There is some evidence to support cardiorespiratory fitness as an independent determinant of mortality in overweight and obese persons (i.e., the concept that being fat but fit carries significantly lower risk than being fat and unfit), although fitness probably only partially offsets the mortality risks associated with obesity.[8]

Pathophysiology of Overweight and Obesity

Contributing Factors

Simply put, weight gain is a reflection of energy intake exceeding energy expenditure. A pound of adipose tissue represents about 3500 calories (kcal) of energy. An excessive intake of only

TABLE 27-1 BMI Corresponding to Height and Body Weight[a]

	BMI (kg/m²)[b]													
	19	20	21	22	23	24	25	26	27	28	29	30	35	40
Height (inches)	**Body Weight (pounds)**													
58	91	96	100	105	110	115	119	124	129	134	138	143	167	191
59	94	99	104	109	114	119	124	128	133	138	143	148	173	198
60	97	102	107	112	118	123	128	133	138	143	148	153	179	204
61	100	106	111	116	122	127	132	137	143	148	153	158	185	211
62	104	109	115	120	126	131	136	142	147	153	158	164	191	218
63	107	113	118	124	130	135	141	146	152	158	163	169	197	225
64	110	116	122	128	134	140	145	151	157	163	169	174	204	232
65	114	120	126	132	138	144	150	156	162	168	174	180	210	240
66	118	124	130	136	142	148	155	161	167	173	179	186	216	247
67	121	127	134	140	146	153	159	166	172	178	185	191	223	255
68	125	131	138	144	151	158	164	171	177	184	190	197	230	262
69	128	135	142	149	155	162	169	176	182	189	196	203	236	270
70	132	139	146	153	160	167	172	181	188	195	202	207	243	278
71	136	143	150	157	165	172	179	186	193	200	208	215	250	286
72	140	147	154	162	169	177	184	191	199	206	213	221	258	294
73	144	151	159	166	174	182	189	197	204	212	219	227	265	302
74	148	155	163	171	179	186	194	202	210	218	225	233	272	311
75	152	160	168	176	184	192	200	208	216	224	232	240	279	319
76	156	164	172	180	189	197	205	213	221	230	238	246	287	328

[a] To determine BMI, find the height in the left-hand column; then move across the row to a given weight. The number above the weight column is the BMI for that height and weight.

[b] BMI calculations: weight (kg)/height (m²) or (weight [lb]/height [in²]) × 703.

Source: Reprinted with permission from reference 1.

10 kcal per day over the level of energy expenditure could result in a gain of approximately 1 pound of fat in a year's time. The physiology of energy intake and expenditure is complex and involves numerous body systems, including the hypothalamic-pituitary axis, the autonomic nervous system, the central nervous system, the endocrine system, the gastrointestinal (GI) tract, and adipose tissue.

Both genetic and environmental factors are important in the etiology of overweight and obesity, and there is a complex interplay between these factors. The rapid increase in overweight individuals over the past few decades argues for a strong environmental role, given that the genetic makeup of our race would not be expected to change dramatically over a short period of time. It is likely that our current environment is facilitating the genetic expression of the propensity to store body fat in many individuals.

A multitude of genes are involved in human obesity, and these factors may make some individuals more likely to become obese when exposed to certain environmental factors. For many obese persons, a complex interplay between genetics and environment contributes to weight gain. The discovery of leptin, a hormone secreted by adipocytes that signals the hypothalamus regarding the amount of energy reserves in the body, generated excitement that a cure for human weight control problems might be imminent. Although the administration of leptin to certain strains of obese mice led to dramatic weight loss, most obese humans are not leptin-deficient but rather have increased leptin levels and are thus believed to be leptin-resistant. However, discovery of the gene for leptin and other genes is increasing our understanding of weight regulation. Ghrelin, a hormone produced by the stomach, has been shown to increase food intake. Ghrelin levels have been shown to rise in persons following diet-induced weight loss. Increased ghrelin levels, along with reductions in resting energy expenditure with weight loss, could help explain the difficulty in trying to keep from regaining weight. Peptide YY_{3-36} and alpha-melanocyte–stimulating hormone are other endogenous compounds whose roles in the etiology of obesity are being studied.

Environmental factors fueling the recent increase in overweight and obesity in the United States, as well as many other parts of the world, include decreases in physical activity coupled with increases in food availability, especially calorie-dense foods. Fewer than half of Americans meet guidelines for regular moderate physical activity.[2] Significant increases in portion sizes of food and increased working hours, which lead to less time to prepare food at home, may be other environmental factors contributing to excessive energy intake relative to energy expenditure. Average caloric intakes for U.S. males increased by about 250 kcal per day from 1971–1974 to 2001–2004; the comparable increase for females was about 350 kcal per day.[2] The *Surgeon General's 2001 Call to Action to Prevent and Decrease Overweight and Obesity* emphasizes that efforts must be made at multiple levels (i.e., individual, family, community, state, and nation) and across multiple sectors (i.e., schools, government, and business) to effectively tackle this complex problem.[9] (See Chapter 23 for a discussion of a healthy diet and the Food Guide Pyramid.)

Another factor that is receiving increasing attention as a possible etiology of overweight and obesity is sleep duration. Several epidemiologic studies have associated high BMI values with shorter sleep duration, although the optimal number of hours of sleep nightly in terms of BMI has varied between studies. Decreased leptin and increased ghrelin levels with shorter sleep duration may explain this association. The percentage of adults sleeping no more than 6 hours per day has increased markedly over the past 2 decades.

A provocative new concept in the etiology of obesity relates to gut flora.[10] Obese persons have been found to have a lower proportion of Bacteroidetes bacteria and relatively more Firmicutes bacteria compared with lean persons. Furthermore, the number of Bacterioidetes bacteria increased with weight loss in obese persons. Perhaps the greater degree of diversity within the Firmicutes bacteria leads to more efficient extraction of calories from foodstuffs (i.e., metabolism and subsequent absorption of foodstuffs generally considered indigestible). These interesting findings may lead to further investigation of prebiotics, probiotics, and antibiotics as tools for weight maintenance and weight loss.

Medications are a potential etiology of weight gain.[11] Many of the newer atypical antipsychotics, especially clozapine, olanzapine, and risperidone, can contribute to significant (sometimes massive) weight gains. Older antidepressants (tricyclics and monoamine oxidase inhibitors) are associated with weight gain, although the amount of gain is usually modest. Although some of the selective serotonin reuptake inhibitor antidepressants have actually been touted as producing weight loss, this loss is usually short lived and weight gain can occur. Other important groups of medications that may contribute to significant weight gain are hormonal contraceptives, corticosteroids, certain anticonvulsants, certain sulfonylureas, thiazolidinediones, and insulins. The latter three groups are particularly noteworthy, because type 2 DM patients placed on these medications frequently are already overweight, a condition that may contribute to poor blood glucose control.

Complications of Obesity

Overweight and obesity are associated with a myriad of chronic health problems.[1] Many of these conditions improve with weight loss. Obese persons have been shown to be more likely to experience difficulties in performing activities of daily living such as walking several flights of stairs or bending and kneeling.

Obesity is associated with coronary heart disease (CHD) through its impact on risk factors such as hypertension, dyslipidemia, and type 2 DM. Overweight and obesity have been linked to increased risk for congestive heart failure (CHF), arrhythmias, and stroke. Prevalence of hypertension begins to increase at relatively low levels of overweight. Patients with a BMI of 30 and higher are more than twice as likely to have hypertension than those with a BMI of 25 or lower.[12] The pathophysiology of obesity-related hypertension is multifactorial. Weight loss in obese persons is associated with significant reductions in blood pressure.[12]

The relationship between CHD and obesity is confounded by other risk factors such as blood lipid levels, blood pressure, DM, and smoking. Several studies that have carefully controlled for confounders have shown BMI and abdominal fat to be sig-

nificantly associated with the risk of CHD in both men and women.[12] There appears to be an association between BMI in childhood and risk of CHD in adulthood, with risk increasing across the entire BMI spectrum.[12]

Overweight and obesity predispose patients to CHF by promoting CHD, hypertension, and DM.[12] However, once CHF is present, obesity may not adversely affect outcome.[12] There is an increased risk of atrial fibrillation associated with obesity, an effect that appears to be mediated by enlargement of the left atrium.[12] Many obese subjects have prolonged QT intervals on electrocardiogram. There is an increased risk of arrhythmias and sudden cardiac death in obese persons, regardless of whether they have diagnosed cardiac dysfunction.

Data from the Physicians' Health Study showed approximately a twofold increase in risk of either ischemic or hemorrhagic stroke in subjects with a BMI of 30 and higher compared with those with a BMI of 23 or less.[12] This effect was apparently independent of the presence of hypertension, DM, or dyslipidemia. BMI may affect stroke risk through an increase in prothrombotic and proinflammatory factors found in obese persons. Venous thromboembolism risk is also increased in obese persons.[12]

There is a strong correlation between BMI and triglyceride levels in both men and women in all adult age groups.[1] Beneficial HDL cholesterol levels are lower in both men and women with higher BMI values.[1] Low-density lipoprotein (LDL) cholesterol tends to increase as BMI increases.[1] The beneficial impact of even modest weight loss on blood lipid levels has been well documented.[1]

The relationship between overweight and obesity and DM is well documented (see Chapter 47). Data from NHANES III indicate that 67% of patients with type 2 DM have a BMI of at least 27.[13] Data from the Behavioral Risk Factor Surveillance System in 2001 indicated approximately a 1.6-fold increase in DM in patients with a BMI of 25 to 29.9 compared with those with a BMI of 18.5 to 24.9.[14] The corresponding number for patients with a BMI of 30 to 39.9 was a 3.4-fold increase, and there was a 7.4-fold increase in DM for those with a BMI of 40 or greater. Modest weight gains after 18 years of age, as well as visceral adiposity (high waist circumference), have been shown to be risk factors for development of type 2 DM.[13] Persons who are initially insulin-resistant, typically evidenced by high plasma triglycerides and low HDL cholesterol, are most likely to benefit from weight loss in terms of reduced morbidity and mortality. Modest weight loss has been shown to be effective in improving blood glucose control in patients with type 2 DM and preventing development of type 2 DM in those at risk.

Negative attitudes toward obese people, leading to social stigmatization and discrimination, have been reported, particularly among Caucasians.[1] Studies relating to whether obesity has significant psychological and emotional impacts have yielded disparate results.[1] Obese patients who seek treatment in clinic settings demonstrate more psychopathology than obese patients who do not seek treatment.[1] Overweight children may develop psychosocial difficulties stemming from compromised peer relationships. These difficulties can lead to poor self-esteem, depression, and poor school functioning in these children, in addition to physical complications such as an increased risk of diabetes.

Obesity appears to increase the risk for a number of other diseases, including gallbladder disease, osteoarthritis, sleep apnea, certain types of cancer, disorders of female reproduction, end-stage renal disease (ESRD), and psoriasis.[13,15] For some of these conditions, weight gain during adulthood has also been shown to be a risk factor. The risk for gallstones and cholecystectomy increases with obesity; rapid weight loss may precipitate gallstones. Osteoarthritis and pain in weight-bearing joints is increased in obese patients. Obesity is also a risk factor for hyperuricemia and gout. The risk of sleep apnea increases with upper body obesity and is the most important modifiable risk factor for this condition.[12]

Obesity may contribute to 14% to 20% of cancer deaths in the United States.[15] Of particular concern are cancers with a hormonal basis such as cancers of the breast, prostate, endometrium, colon, and gallbladder. In addition, female reproduction disorders are associated with obesity, including menstrual irregularities and infertility. Polycystic ovary syndrome is associated with abdominal obesity. Hypertension and gestational diabetes are more likely to develop in obese women who become pregnant, and labor and delivery complications are more common. Babies of obese women may be more likely to have a neural tube defect.

Obesity has recently been shown to be associated with development of ESRD and may be related to renal hyperperfusion and glomerular hyperfiltration.[16] The link between obesity and psoriasis may be explained by overproduction of inflammatory cytokines with adiposity.[17]

Management of Overweight and Obesity

Management Goals and General Management Approach

For many individuals, losing weight or maintaining a weight loss is a lifelong challenge. Lifestyle changes, dietary modification, and increased exercise are the cornerstones of management. Successful weight loss and especially maintenance of weight loss typically require significant behavioral modification. Pharmacologic therapy using nonprescription agents should be only a short-term measure unless a primary care provider supervises the therapy. Long-term use of prescription therapies under the care of a primary care provider is emerging as an option for patients with a BMI of 30 or higher, or a BMI of 27 or higher with comorbid conditions.[1] However, pharmacologic interventions are not a panacea for weight loss and often result in only modest loss of weight that tends to be regained after discontinuation of the drug. Bariatric surgery should be considered for only patients with a BMI of 40 or higher, or a BMI of 35 or higher with comorbid conditions.[1] This surgery is very effective for achieving weight loss for many patients.

Many chronic diseases and conditions improve with weight loss. However, weight-loss goals set by many individuals are unrealistic and are based more on cosmetic effect than on health benefit. Weight loss (and maintenance of that loss) of 5% to 10% of initial weight has been shown to have positive benefits in individuals with hypertension and DM. The NHLBI guidelines state that the initial goal of weight loss is to reduce body weight by about 10% over 6 months.[1] If this goal is achieved and further weight loss is indicated, it can be attempted. However, the first 10% loss probably carries the most health benefit and is also easiest to attain, given that weight often plateaus after 6 months because of decreased basal metabolic rate at the lower weight. It is probably more important to maintain the 10% weight loss than to pursue further weight loss in many patients. An often overlooked approach may be to simply prevent further weight gain in persons who have been slowly but steadily gaining

weight over a period of years or decades; this approach would be particularly appropriate for persons who are still in the overweight (not yet obese) category. Figure 27-2 is a guide for the practitioner in recommending weight-loss measures.

Weight loss is indicated for individuals with health problems (e.g., sleep apnea, hypertension, osteoarthritis, or type 2 DM) that can be lessened by weight loss. Unsupervised weight loss should be discouraged in individuals, as outlined in Figure 27-2.

Nonpharmacologic Therapy (Lifestyle Modification)

Dietary modification or restriction is the mainstay of weight-loss therapy. Although physical activity alone produces less weight loss than caloric restriction, such activity is an important component of maintaining weight loss and improving overall fitness. The term *lifestyle modification* is increasingly being used to describe a structured strategy of dietary change, physical activity, and behavior therapy for management of overweight and obesity.[8] Results from studies utilizing comprehensive lifestyle modification have generally become more impressive over the past several decades in terms of weight loss, because the duration of treatment has increased and behavioral strategies have evolved. Data are also accumulating as to how pharmaceutical care services can emerge as an integral component of lifestyle modification programs.[18,19]

Dietary Change

Dietary change is the most commonly used weight-loss strategy. Diet strategies include caloric restriction; changes in dietary proportions of fat, protein, and carbohydrate; use of macronutrient substitutes (i.e., sugar and fat substitutes); and changes in timing or frequency of meals. Short-term success for many of these methods has been documented; however, information on effectiveness and safety in the longer term is limited. Weight loss at the end of relatively short-term programs can exceed 10% of initial body weight. However, there is a strong tendency to regain weight, in part due to decreases in basal metabolic rate as a person loses weight. Nonetheless, a small percentage of participants do maintain weight loss over more extended periods. The National Weight Control Registry tracks individuals who have maintained a weight loss of at least 30 pounds for at least 1 year.[20] To initially lose weight, persons in this registry used a variety of methods, from self-directed diet programs to liquid formula diets. Most of these individuals reported maintaining weight loss through a combination of a low-calorie, low-fat diet and exercise. This group generally reported that weight maintenance became easier the further out in time from their initial weight loss, perhaps as a result of ingrained behavioral changes. Persistent changes in both eating habits and activity levels should help guard against weight regain.

Even small changes in dietary patterns can have a positive effect. Cutting portion sizes (e.g., two pieces of pizza instead of the usual three), eating fast food one fewer time per week, switching to water or diet soda rather than soda sweetened with sugar, using smaller plates for meals, and keeping healthy snacks such as fruits and vegetables on hand are useful, sustainable strategies for decreasing calories. Trying to emphasize foods in the diet with low energy density (i.e., low calories per weight of food), for example, fruits and vegetables, may be helpful as these foods tend to promote satiation. Again, the reader is referred to Chapter 23 for more details regarding healthy diets.

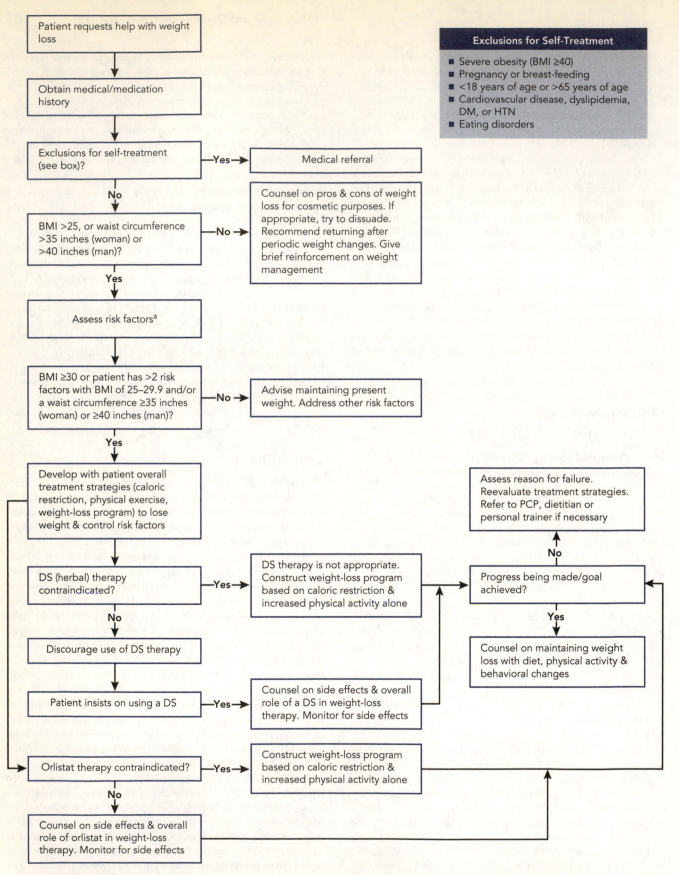

Patient requests help with weight loss

Obtain medical/medication history

Exclusions for self-treatment (see box)? — Yes → Medical referral

No

BMI >25, or waist circumference >35 inches (woman) or >40 inches (man)? — No → Counsel on pros & cons of weight loss for cosmetic purposes. If appropriate, try to dissuade. Recommend returning after periodic weight changes. Give brief reinforcement on weight management

Yes

Assess risk factors[a]

BMI ≥30 or patient has >2 risk factors with BMI of 25–29.9 and/or a waist circumference ≥35 inches (woman) or ≥40 inches (man)? — No → Advise maintaining present weight. Address other risk factors

Yes

Develop with patient overall treatment strategies (caloric restriction, physical exercise, weight-loss program) to lose weight & control risk factors

DS (herbal) therapy contraindicated? — Yes → DS therapy is not appropriate. Construct weight-loss program based on caloric restriction & increased physical activity alone

No

Discourage use of DS therapy

Patient insists on using a DS — Yes → Counsel on side effects & overall role of a DS in weight-loss therapy. Monitor for side effects

Orlistat therapy contraindicated? — Yes → Construct weight-loss program based on caloric restriction & increased physical activity alone

No

Counsel on side effects & overall role of orlistat in weight-loss therapy. Monitor for side effects

Assess reason for failure. Reevaluate treatment strategies. Refer to PCP, dietitian or personal trainer if necessary

No

Progress being made/goal achieved?

Yes

Counsel on maintaining weight loss with diet, physical activity & behavioral changes

[a] Risk factors as defined by the NHLBI include established coronary heart disease, presence of other atherosclerotic disease, type 2 DM, cigarette smoking, hpyertension, low-density lipoprotein cholesterol > 160 mg/dL, high-density lipoprotein cholesterol < 35 mg/dL, impaired fasting glucose, family history of premature coronary heart disease, age (male > 45 years; female > 55 years), physical inactivity, and high triglycerides.

FIGURE 27-2 Self-care of overweight and obesity. Key: BMI, body mass index; DM, diabetes mellitus; DS, dietary supplement; HTN, hypertension; NHLBI, National Heart, Lung, and Blood Institute; PCP, primary care provider.

Caloric Restriction

Daily caloric allowances for moderately active individuals vary with age, gender, and body weight. The U.S. population as a whole seems to suffer from "portion distortion" and needs to relearn the appropriate food portion sizes based on age and activity levels. Daily caloric intake allowances for an average 30-year-old man (BMI, 18.5–25; height, 5 ft 11 in) in a temperate climate range from 2200 to 3000 kcal/day, depending on activity level. Corresponding figures for an average 30-year-old woman (BMI, 18.5–25; height, 5 ft 5 in) are 1800 to 2800 kcal/day.[21] These figures are lower for older persons, whereas they are higher for younger adults. Caloric requirements for women increase during pregnancy and lactation (see Chapter 23).[21] Self-initiated weight loss during pregnancy is not recommended and should be discussed with a primary care provider, even for severely overweight women, because of possible risk to the developing baby.

A diet that is individually planned and takes into account the patient's overweight status to create a deficit of 300 to 1000 kcal/day should be an integral part of any weight-loss program.[1] Two levels of caloric restriction are commonly used. A low-calorie diet (LCD) of about 800 to 1500 kcal/day may involve a structured commercial program with formulated and calorically defined food products, or it may involve guidelines for selecting conventional foods, including careful attention to portion sizes. Weight loss on an LCD is typically 1 to 2 pounds per week. A very-low-calorie diet (VLCD) of 800 or fewer calories per day should be conducted under the supervision and monitoring of a primary care provider, and it should be restricted to patients with a BMI higher than 30. A VLCD should contain at least 1 g/kg of ideal body weight per day of protein. VLCDs are frequently administered as liquid formulas given several times a day. Although weight loss with VLCDs over 12 to 16 weeks is typically double that of LCDs, long-term results are generally no better. A multivitamin/multimineral preparation should be recommended to patients consuming fewer than 1200 kcal/day for prolonged periods.

VLCDs and fasting are associated with numerous short-term adverse effects. Rapid weight loss is frequently associated with fatigue, hair loss, dizziness, diarrhea or constipation, dry skin, irregular menses in females, and other symptoms, some of which are transient. More serious is the increased risk for gallstones and acute gallbladder disease.

Total fasting or semistarvation is sometimes proposed as a means of weight reduction in severely obese persons. However, starvation depletes the body of some lean tissue (protein) and essential electrolytes in addition to fat. The ketosis and ketoacidosis that result from fasting represent a significant metabolic alteration. If total fasting is used to treat obesity, hospitalization and intensive medical supervision are recommended.

Altered Proportions of Food Groups

The most commonly recommended diets for weight loss are reduced-calorie diets that emphasize decreased fat intake, particularly decreased saturated fat. NHLBI recommends a diet that supplies no more than 30% of total calories from fat, of which 8% to 10% of total calories come from saturated fat, and at least 55% from carbohydrates.[1] Future guidelines will probably follow the lead of the *Dietary Guidelines for Americans, 2005,* placing less emphasis on restricting fat calories and more on inclusion of monounsaturated and polyunsaturated fat while minimizing saturated fat.[22] NHLBI guidelines emphasize that a low-fat diet alone is inadequate for weight loss; the diet must also reduce total calories, not simply replace fat with carbohydrate or protein.

Very-low-fat vegetarian diets in the context of other lifestyle changes have been advocated. Although such programs have actually resulted in regression of coronary atherosclerosis in some patients with moderate-to-severe CHD, their applicability to larger populations remains questionable in terms of compliance with strict dietary and lifestyle modifications. Dietary fat must be carefully chosen when consuming a very-low-fat diet to prevent essential fatty acid deficiency. These diets increase triglyceride levels and lower HDL cholesterol in the short term because of high carbohydrate content.

There is a spectrum of currently popular high-protein, higher-fat, low-carbohydrate diets. Some contain very low amounts of carbohydrates (about 5%–15% of total calories; e.g., Atkins diet) and are ketogenic, whereas others are considered moderate carbohydrate diets (about 35%–50% of calories from carbohydrate; e.g., Zone diet). People often start out on the ultralow form of the diet and transition to a more moderate form; despite the initial impression that eating high-protein and high-fat foods will be enjoyable, many persons get tired of a regimen in which consumption of items such as bread, pasta, fruits, and vegetables is severely curtailed. Nevertheless, part of the success of low-carbohydrate diets in terms of weight loss may lie in the fact that they simplify food choices, thus facilitating dietary adherence.

The theory behind very-low-carbohydrate diets is that they prevent the elevated insulin levels that promote storage of body fat seen with higher-carbohydrate diets. In reality, much of the weight loss seen with these diets is a result of decreased caloric intake from avoidance of high-carbohydrate foods. Initial weight loss results partially from a diuretic effect and glycogen depletion. Ketosis accompanying these diets may also result in decreased appetite.

Low-carbohydrate diets result in significant weight loss over the short term (6–12 months). Many concerns regarding long-term safety of these diets still exist. Most of these studies have indicated that serum lipid levels, overall, are not affected deleteriously over the short term in most dieters, mainly because of the weight loss achieved. Triglycerides and HDL cholesterol levels are generally affected more favorably with low-carbohydrate diets, whereas low-fat diets have more favorable effects on LDL and total cholesterol.[23] Effects on lipids still need to be studied for longer periods of time in people maintained on these diets, which typically contain more fat (more than 30%–35% of total calories) than currently recommended by most dietary authorities. Other potential adverse effects associated with these diets include lack of essential nutrients such as potassium, calcium, and magnesium that are important for blood pressure regulation. High-protein foods consumed in large quantities on these diets are high in purines, which could increase uric acid levels and precipitate gout, although this has not been a common problem in studies with up to a year of follow-up. High animal protein content promotes calcium excretion in the urine that could be deleterious to bone health. Restriction of fruits, vegetables, whole grains, and milk products could, according to standard current nutritional thinking, increase a person's risk of various cancers by depleting essential vitamins, minerals, and fiber and could also lead to constipation. The diets' high protein content may predispose the dieter to dehydration and hyperfiltration by the kidneys, leading to eventual kidney damage that could be particularly deleterious in diabetic patients. Headache, muscle weakness, and fatigue are other adverse events reported by some persons on low-carbohydrate diets. Several published randomized trials of these diets demonstrated relative safety of the low-carbohydrate, higher-fat, high-protein diets for 6 to 12 months, with greatest weight loss seen in the first 6 months.[23] A recent study of the Atkins, Zone, Ornish (very-low-fat), and a traditional low-fat diet showed weight loss with the Atkins diet that was equal to or greater than the other diets at 1 year.[24]

A controversial but provocative line of reasoning regarding support for low-carbohydrate diets for prevention of cardiovascular disease is supported by some data. In the Women's Health Initiative trial, reduction of total fat intake for 8 years did not reduce risk for CVD.[25] This finding may be related to the observation that carbohydrate-restricted diets have more favorable effects, when compared with fat-restricted diets, not only on triglyceride and HDL cholesterol levels, but also on small dense LDL cholesterol mass, a factor that is only recently beginning to receive attention as a marker of cardiovascular risk.

The concept of high- versus low-glycemic-index foods in weight-loss diets is gaining notoriety, with low-glycemic-index food products being promoted commercially. The glycemic index of a food refers to the amount of blood glucose rise seen after ingestion of a standardized amount of the food. Many high-carbohydrate, low-fat diets exhibit a high glycemic index. By choosing carbohydrate choices carefully, a lower glycemic response can be obtained. Proponents of low-glycemic-index diets believe that they prevent carbohydrate oxidation from predominating over fat oxidation, a situation that may occur in the setting of hyperinsulinemia following a high-glycemic-index meal. Low-glycemic-index diets would thus promote satiety and prevent large fluctuations in insulin concentrations and might help maintain insulin sensitivity. Studies have not consistently supported the usefulness of low-glycemic diets in weight control, although this topic deserves further research attention, especially in light of the suggestion that such diets may result in reduction of cardiovascular risk even in the absence of weight loss.[8]

Use of Food Additives

Some patients may use food additives such as artificial sweeteners and fat substitutes as adjunctive measures to reduce caloric intake. Although theoretically their use should help decrease caloric intake, data showing that use of these substances is associated with significant weight loss or better weight maintenance are conflicting. Table 27-2 outlines pertinent information related to sugar and fat substitutes.

Meal Replacement Therapy

These commercial products are typically geared toward replacing up to two meals a day with a liquid drink, a snack bar, or a measured frozen meal, with the dieter encouraged to eat a "reasonable" third meal each day. The main advantage to this approach is portion control. These products might typically contain about 200 kcal per serving, consisting of 50% to 60% carbohydrate, up

---

TABLE 27-2 Sugar and Fat Substitutes

Substitute (Sample Trade Name)	Comments
Sugar Substitutes	
Saccharin (Sweet 'n Low)	Has bitter taste; has been replaced largely by newer sweeteners
Aspartame (Nutra Sweet)	Contains phenylalanine, therefore, contraindicated in patients with phenylketonuria; not for use in cooking or baking as heat breaks it down into free amino acids, which impart a bitter taste
Fructose	Nutritive sweetener and should not be viewed as "sugar-free"; insulin not required for fructose utilization in the body
Sorbitol	Nutritive sweetener and should not be viewed as sugar-free; does not cause tooth decay, but can cause osmotic diarrhea when ingested in large quantities
Xylitol	Nutritive sweetener and should not be viewed as sugar-free; does not cause tooth decay
Acesulfame-potassium (Sunette, Sweet One)	May be substituted for sucrose in cooking; may be combined with aspartame, because some people detect a metallic aftertaste with acesulfame-potassium alone
Sucralose (Splenda)	May be used in cooking
Neotame	May be used in cooking
Cyclamates	Banned by FDA in 1969 because of association with cancer in animals; applicability of this finding to humans has been challenged, but petition before FDA for reapproval is pending
Stevia	Approved in United States as a dietary supplement but cannot be added to foods; has shown carcinogenic and infertility effects in vitro and in animal studies
Fat Substitutes	
Microparticulated protein (Simplesse)	Used in frozen desserts
Soluble fiber (Oatrim)	Derived from oats and designed to replace fat in meats, cheeses, baked goods, and frozen desserts
Sucrose polyester (Olean)	Also known as olestra; is not absorbed; can cause malabsorption of fat-soluble vitamins; manufacturers must supply specified amounts of fat-soluble vitamins A, D, E, and K to foods containing olestra; GI side effects can be seen with ingestion of large quantities; can be used for cooking and frying

to 30% protein, and 10% fat. Early weight loss with these products, part of which may be a result of low sodium content that leads to water loss, can give a psychological boost to the dieter to adhere to the program. Implementation of a meal replacement regimen overseen by community pharmacists has been reported as an effective strategy for shorter-term weight loss and weight maintenance.[26] Meal replacement products are discussed further in Chapter 24.

Commercial Weight-Loss Programs

Structured commercial weight-loss programs such as Weight Watchers, Jenny Craig, and Take Off Pounds Sensibly (TOPS) are very popular in the United States. Women tend to gravitate to these programs more than men do. A systematic review of commercial weight-loss programs concluded that data supporting the use of these programs are suboptimal, and that controlled trials are necessary before their efficacy and cost-effectiveness can be touted.[27]

Participation in some of the structured commercial programs may be expensive, because participants are required to purchase specially packaged meals available only from the company. A large component of the success of these programs is likely the social support aspect that develops with periodic meetings of groups of dieters. Online tools such as diet and exercise diaries and support groups are also available; these resources may be less expensive than community-based structured commercial programs.

Physical Activity

Encouragement of physical activity as a method for preventing overweight and obesity is an important public health strategy for all age groups, including children. The *Dietary Guidelines for Americans, 2005* outline physical activity recommendations as shown in Table 27-3.[22] For older adults, participation in regular exercise can help reduce functional declines of aging.

Increased physical activity is an important component of weight-loss therapy and, perhaps, is even more important in weight maintenance after weight loss.[8] Patients who regularly exercise may, in general, be more committed to a healthy lifestyle. Exercise may also build muscle that has a higher metabolic rate than a corresponding amount of fat. The amount of weight loss that can be achieved by an exercise program is modest; combining a reduced-calorie diet with increased physical activity produces greater weight loss and reduction in abdominal fat than either approach alone. Some patients may have underlying medical conditions that make some types of exercise ill advised. These patients are advised to have a medical evaluation before starting an exercise regimen. Regardless of concomitant disease states, current recommendations call for all men older than 40 years and women older than 50 years to undergo a medical evaluation before starting an exercise program.

For sedentary patients, a walking program is often a good place to begin exercise. Patients can start by walking 30 minutes each day for 3 days a week, building up to at least 60 minutes of moderate intensity physical activity on most days of the week.[21] The 60-minute activity periods can be accrued in multiple smaller increments throughout the day with similar benefit.[8] Table 27-3 lists the calories expended during 1 hour of various types of exercise for an average-size male. These values vary with gender, weight, and body composition. Patients should be encouraged to participate in activities that they enjoy and are thus more likely to continue.

TABLE 27-3 Physical Activity Recommendations[a] and Caloric Expenditure Rates

Children and Adolescents

- 60 minutes most days of week

Adults

For reduction of chronic disease:
- 30 minutes of moderate intensity exercise (e.g., brisk walking) most days of week

For prevention of body weight gain over time
- 60 minutes of moderate-to-vigorous activities most days of week

For sustaining weight loss:
- 60 to 90 minutes of moderate intensity exercise daily

Activity (1 hour)	Calories Expended
Bicycling (6 mph)	240
Bicycling (12 mph)	410
Cross-country skiing	700
Jogging (5.5 mph)	740
Jogging (7 mph)	920
Jumping rope	720
Running in place	650
Swimming (50 yards/minute)	500
Tennis (singles)	400
Walking (2 mph)	240
Walking (3 mph)	320
Walking (4.5 mph)	440

[a] As proposed by the *Dietary Guidelines for Americans, 2005.*[22]

Nonexercise energy thermogenesis (NEAT) has received increasing attention over the past several years. NEAT is all energy expenditure beyond that of sleeping, eating, and formal exercise. Modern conveniences have decreased NEAT for the population as a whole. People who engage in more spontaneous activities such as fidgeting and standing rather than sitting have an advantage in maintaining lower body weights.

Behavioral Therapy

Behavioral therapy can improve the outcome of weight-loss programs when used in combination with other strategies such as diet, exercise, and medications. The benefit of behavioral therapy is most evident during the active stage of treatment. Behavioral therapy may be administered in either an individual or group setting by professionals or lay leaders. Emerging data indicate that group treatment may be as beneficial or even more beneficial than individual treatment for weight loss, whereas individual treatment may be superior during maintenance following weight loss.[8] Telephone, Internet, or e-mail contact with a therapist or support group is probably not as effective as face-to-face contact for weight loss and weight maintenance, but the former approaches are less expensive and may prove to be beneficial for some patients.[8]

Behavioral techniques include the following[28]:

- *Environmental modification:* Do not have high-calorie foods readily available, thus avoiding problem foods altogether.

- *Modifying thinking patterns:* Set reasonable, specific, proximate goals; identify and plan for potential obstacles to the goals.
- *Self-efficacy:* Maintain an optimistic and positive approach.
- *Social support:* Rely on family, friends, and health care practitioners.

Pharmacologic Therapy

Pharmacologic therapy is generally not recommended for most individuals seeking to lose weight, as exemplified by the fact that more weight-loss products have been removed from the market than approved in recent years because of safety concerns. The ideal drug, which would provide fast and permanent weight loss with no adverse effects, simply does not exist despite the billions of dollars spent on these products by consumers.

The most current federal guidelines for treatment of overweight and obesity recommend that prescription weight-loss medications approved by the Food and Drug Administration (FDA) for long-term use be reserved as an adjunct to diet and physical activity for patients with BMI of 30 or higher, or for patients with BMI of 27 or higher with concomitant diseases or risk factors. They recommend these drugs be used singly (not in combination) and at the lowest effective dose to reduce the likelihood of adverse events.[1] The same guidelines should apply to all weight-loss products, whether prescription or nonprescription drugs or dietary supplements, although nonprescription orlistat is recommended for BMI greater than 25 as outlined below. Any of these medications or supplements should be used with concomitant lifestyle modification and continuous assessment for efficacy, safety, and tolerance. In only situations in which the drug is efficacious in weight loss and maintenance, and has minimal adverse effects should pharmacotherapy be continued.

Status of Nonprescription Weight-Loss Products

Because of the lack of safety and efficacy data, FDA banned 111 weight-control ingredients in nonprescription drug products in 1991.[29] In 2000, FDA requested that all drug companies discontinue marketing phenylpropanolamine-containing products because of safety issues.[30] In addition, nonprescription drugs containing ephedrine and related alkaloids in combination with a stimulant or analgesic could no longer be marketed as of 2001,[31] and the stimulant laxative ingredients aloe and cascara sagrada were banned as ingredients in nonprescription drugs in 2002.[32] However, many of these ingredients may still be marketed in dietary supplements and are often found as components of weight-loss products.

Dietary supplements are distinct entities from nonprescription drugs. They include herbal and other products meant to supplement the diet, and are regulated under the Dietary Supplement Health and Education Act of 1994 (see Chapter 54). They are generally recognized as safe unless FDA proves otherwise. Nonprescription drugs, conversely, are regulated as drugs by FDA and must adhere to more stringent regulations of safety, efficacy, and quality.

The majority of drugs currently considered safe and efficacious for weight loss are restricted to prescription-only status and include benzphetamine (Didrex), diethylpropion (Tenuate), mazindol (Sanorex), methamphetamine (Desoxyn), orlistat (Xenical), phendimetrazine (Bontril), phentermine (Ionamin), and sibutramine (Meridia). The reader is directed to standard references for more information about these drugs.

Orlistat was approved by FDA as a prescription weight-loss medication (Xenical) in 1999 and as a nonprescription weight-loss medication (alli) in 2007.[33] The prescription strength of orlistat is approved for use in patients 12 years of age and older, whereas the nonprescription medication is approved for those 18 years and older.

GlaxoSmithKline Consumer Healthcare provides free support to those using alli through an individually tailored online plan called myalliplan (www.myalli.com). The alli Starter Pack provides reference guides to help patients follow the program as well as information for joining the online plan.

Orlistat aids in weight loss by decreasing absorption of dietary fats. It inhibits gastric and pancreatic lipases, and specifically reduces absorption of fat by inhibiting hydrolysis of triglycerides.[34]

The drug is recommended for use along with a reduced-calorie, low-fat diet, and exercise program. The product labeling for the prescription product states that the drug is indicated for obese patients with a BMI of 30 kg/m² or higher, or for patients with a BMI of 27 kg/m² or higher who also demonstrate risk factors such as diabetes, hypertension, or dyslipidemia. Interestingly, the labeling for the nonprescription product simply states that the drug is for use in overweight adults, which by the standard definition would be persons with a BMI of 25 kg/m² or higher.[34]

Prescription strength orlistat is recommended at a dosage of 120 mg 3 times a day before meals containing fat; at this dosage it inhibits dietary fat absorption by about 30% through inhibition of gastric and pancreatic lipase.[34] The nonprescription form of the drug is recommended at a dosage of 60 mg 3 times a day before meals containing fat; therefore, its inhibition of fat absorption may be less. Because of its mechanism of action, there is no need to give the drug with a fat-free meal.

Most studies have used the 120 mg dosage in combination with a reduced-calorie diet and have reported modest weight losses, especially during the first 6 months of therapy. This dosage may also be useful for weight-loss maintenance following initial weight loss. In one of the few full-text studies published with the 60 mg nonprescription dose, weight loss after 16 weeks in the active drug group was significantly greater than in patients receiving placebo (3.05 kg vs. 1.90 kg; $P < 0.001$).[35] The nonprescription product labeling notes that most patients lost 5 to 10 pounds (about 2–5 kg) over 6 months in clinical trials. Patients receiving orlistat have had significantly greater reductions in LDL cholesterol and blood pressure compared with placebo. Effects on lipid levels may be independent of weight loss, whereas the changes in blood pressure are probably largely due to weight loss. One-year data, published to date in only abstract form, showed persistent beneficial effects of the 60 mg dosage on weight loss and LDL cholesterol outcomes.[36] Orlistat in the 120 mg dosage has been shown to be effective in preventing and delaying development of type 2 diabetes over a 4-year period in patients with impaired glucose tolerance.[37]

Orlistat may decrease absorption of fat-soluble vitamins. It is recommended that patients taking this medication take a multivitamin once daily at bedtime or separated by at least 2 hours from an orlistat dose. Orlistat is minimally absorbed and therefore exhibits little systemic toxicity. Common GI side effects include flatulence with oily spotting, loose and frequent stools, fatty stools, and fecal urgency and incontinence. Decreasing the amount of ingested fat can minimize these effects. These side effects are expected to be less common with the nonprescription dosage compared with the prescription dosage, and they generally resolve within a few weeks of initiating therapy.

Drug interactions with orlistat are unlikely because of the drug's limited absorption. A theoretical concern exists when a patient is taking both orlistat and warfarin because of the potential for orlistat to decrease vitamin K absorption; close monitoring of the international normalized ratio would be recommended with concomitant use of these medications. Orlistat should be avoided in patients receiving cyclosporine; reductions in cyclosporine plasma concentrations have been noted. Patients with malabsorption disorders should avoid taking orlistat, and patients with a history of thyroid disease, cholelithiasis, nephrolithiasis, or pancreatitis should consult their primary care provider before taking orlistat. In addition, the package label advises patients taking medication to treat diabetes to consult a doctor or pharmacist before using orlistat.

There has been concern regarding potential associations between orlistat and development of breast cancer and colon cancer. A petition from Public Citizen in 2006 asked FDA to remove prescription orlistat from the market or to at least consider these associations when deliberating approval of nonprescription orlistat. After consideration of the data, FDA ruled that the preponderance of evidence favored the beneficial effects of orlistat over the potential harm.[38] FDA concluded that there was not a causal relationship between orlistat and cancer, and no compelling mechanism for orlistat as a cause for cancer has been presented.

Nonprescription orlistat may be useful as an adjunct to lifestyle changes in helping patients lose modest amounts of weight. Results will be more favorable when this agent is combined with a reduced-calorie, low-fat diet and increased physical activity. Patients should also be aware that the GI side effects of the medication are likely to be exacerbated by concomitant ingestion of a low-carbohydrate, high-fat diet.

There is also some concern that this nonprescription agent may be misused, particularly by adolescents; it would be prudent for clinicians to watch for adolescents purchasing this medication.

Benzocaine

Benzocaine is thought to produce appetite suppression and weight loss by local anesthetic effects on the oral cavity and GI mucosa, altering the taste of food. It is currently undergoing review by the FDA Advisory Panel on OTC Miscellaneous Internal Drug Products as an anorectic. A final rulemaking will address the adequacy of available efficacy data for benzocaine as an anorectic.[39] Certain nonprescription products continue to include benzocaine as the active ingredient (e.g., ZoCal lozenges).

Use of Inappropriate Medications for Weight Loss

Individuals seeking to lose weight will sometimes turn to inappropriate, potentially dangerous methods to induce weight loss, such as laxatives or diuretics. The risks associated with laxatives and diuretics are discussed in Chapters 16 and 9, respectively.

Complementary Therapies

A recent survey conducted in the United States has shown that roughly 15% of adults attempting weight loss reported using a dietary supplement for weight loss. The majority of these individuals were women aged 18 to 34 years, and the majority used a supplement containing a stimulant such as caffeine and/or bitter orange. Approximately 10% of users reported use of these products for 12 months or longer.[5]

The Ephedra Debate

Until recently, ephedra, or ma huang, was the most widely used weight-loss dietary supplement in the United States. Ephedrine alkaloids are the active ingredients in ephedra; these compounds have nervous and cardiovascular system stimulant activity.[40] Although some studies suggest that synthetic ephedrine, previously found in many nonprescription allergy and cold preparations, may be beneficial for weight loss when used alone or in combination with caffeine, it is not approved as a nonprescription weight-loss ingredient. Many manufacturers of dietary supplement products incorporated the natural product ma huang, as a source of ephedra, and guarana or cola nut, as sources of caffeine. Although a limited number of clinical studies report modest weight losses with these products, safety issues are of concern, especially when the products are used together.

The results of a RAND Corporation study commissioned by the National Institutes of Health provided evidence of health risks associated with ephedra together with limited evidence of a beneficial effect on weight loss. The RAND study reviewed over 16,000 adverse events reported after ephedra use and found approximately 20 "sentinel events," including heart attack, stroke, and death, that occurred in the absence of other contributing factors.[41] On the basis of this and other evidence, FDA published the final rule on dietary supplements containing ephedrine alkaloids on February 11, 2004, declaring these supplements adulterated because they present an unreasonable risk of illness or injury. Common names used for the various botanicals that contain the ephedrine alkaloids include sea grape, yellow horse, joint fir, popotillo, ma huang, and country mallow.[42] The rule went into effect on April 12, 2004. On April 15, 2005, a federal judge in Utah limited the scope of this ban, stating that FDA's methods in banning ephedra violated DSHEA (see Chapter 53) by shifting the burden of proof of safety from FDA to the manufacturers. This ruling applied to only products containing a maximum of 10 mg of ephedrine alkaloids per daily serving, and it had no effect on those states that already banned all sales of dietary supplements containing ephedrine alkaloids.[43] An appeal by FDA to the U.S. District Court of Utah led to reinstatement of the ban in 2006.[44]

Reformulated Weight-Loss Products

Since the FDA ruling on ephedra-containing dietary supplements, many manufacturers are including bitter orange (*Citrus aurantium*) in weight-loss medications, often in combination with sources of caffeine such as cola nut (*Cola acuminata* or *Cola nitida*), guarana (*Paullinia cupana* or *Paullinia sorbilis*), or maté (*Ilex paraguariensis*). Bitter orange contains synephrine, which is structurally similar to epinephrine, and octopamine, which is similar to norepinephrine. Bitter orange is being touted as a safe alternative to ephedra in many herbal weight-loss products. Although adrenergic effects of synephrine and octopamine have the potential for appetite suppression and lipolysis, these products also carry the same potential health risks as ephedra. A recent randomized, double-blind, placebo-controlled study of single doses of *C. aurantium* in healthy adults reported significant increases in heart rate and blood pressure, compared with placebo. The authors state that the effects likely are due to a combination of *C. aurantium*, caffeine, and other stimulants contained in the multicomponent preparation.[45] Clinical trials of *C. aurantium* for weight loss have failed to support efficacy for this indication.

Many nonprescription weight-loss products list multiple ingredients, many of which are herbal extracts with varying active ingredients, together with vitamins and minerals. Many of these ingredients lack any scientific evidence for usefulness in weight loss. To confuse matters even more, many of the herbal extracts are listed by their common or not-so-common names (e.g., bitter orange, Seville orange, and sour orange are all common names for *C. aurantium*), and many do not list the botanical name, making it difficult to determine exactly what the herbal product contains. The majority of these products have not been clearly demonstrated to be effective or safe, and many have been associated with serious adverse effects. Practitioners are advised to carefully review the labels of all dietary supplement weight-loss products to determine the risk for adverse reactions and drug–herb interactions.

Herbal Products

A summary of botanicals commonly used in weight-loss supplements is provided in Table 27-4.[40,45,46–49] Many of these supplements also contain vitamins and minerals, presumably to ensure adequate intake of these essential nutrients by patients on low-caloric diets. In addition, the majority of these supplements contain multiple ingredients with several purported actions, although the advertising claims frequently focus on one solitary ingredient and/or action. To further complicate the problem, many of the supplements contain "proprietary blends." Ingredients of proprietary blends must be listed, but the amounts of the ingredients do not have to be specified. It is important to note, however, that none of these ingredients have sufficient scientific evidence to support their usefulness in weight loss. Broadly speaking, the ingredients of weight-loss supplements can be categorized as follows:

- *Stimulants and energy boosters and thermogenic aids* claim to increase basal metabolism, increase energy, and counteract fatigue (e.g., caffeine and bitter orange).
- *Fat and carbohydrate modulators* claim to alter fat and/or carbohydrate metabolism, resulting in decreased body fat mass and increased lean muscle mass (e.g., green tea, chromium, and garcinia).
- *Appetite suppressants and satiety promoters* claim to decrease caloric intake by suppressing appetite or promoting satiety (e.g., guar gum, glucomannan, and psyllium)
- *Fat absorption blockers* claim to block intestinal absorption of dietary fat (e.g., chitosan, derived from exoskeletons of marine organisms).
- *Carbohydrate absorption blockers* claim to block intestinal absorption of dietary carbohydrates (e.g., kidney bean extract and mung bean extract).
- *Cortisol blockers* claim to block stress-induced release of cortisol, which is claimed to cause increased appetite and fat storage (e.g., beta-sitosterol, phosphatidylserine, and theanine).
- *Laxatives* (e.g., cascara sagrada and psyllium).
- *Diuretics* (e.g., dandelion and caffeine).

Herbal laxatives and diuretics are often included in multiple-ingredient dietary supplements marketed for weight loss. For example, "dieter's" or "slimming" teas contain a variety of botanical laxatives and diuretics. Diuretics, whether herbal or drug, may result in an initial transient weight loss, but this effect lasts only a few days. Herbal or drug laxatives typically act in the colon and, therefore, will not decrease caloric absorption in the small intestine, which is the primary site of food absorption. Many of these botanicals are stimulant laxatives that should be used for only 1 to 2 weeks at a time. Prolonged use may lead to electrolyte imbalances and dependence on the laxative for regular bowel movements (cathartic colon), as discussed in Chapter 16.

Herbal sources of caffeine have often been used in combination with ephedra and willow bark (as a source of salicin) for weight loss because of purported synergistic effects. This combination is often referred to as a "fat-burning stack" or "ECA" (ephedrine-caffeine-aspirin), with claims of additive thermogenic or heat-producing effects.[40] However, adverse reactions to these products, either alone or in combination, range from relatively mild symptoms, such as headache, nervousness, and hypertension, to more severe reactions, such as stroke, myocardial infarction, and sudden death. In several cases, significant adverse events occurred in otherwise healthy young or middle-aged adults, and many occurred following consumption of relatively low doses for short periods.[47,48]

Calcium

Some evidence suggests that increasing calcium intake from dairy products results in increased weight loss in patients on a calorie-restricted diet. Data suggest that an increased calcium intake of approximately two dairy servings per day is associated with a weight loss ranging from 0.11 to 4.9 kg/year.[49] However, a similar effect was not demonstrated using calcium supplementation with 1000 mg/day in conjunction with moderate dietary restriction.[49]

Chromium

Chromium is an essential nutrient with adequate intake set at 20 to 35 mcg/day. It is promoted for weight loss either alone or as a component of multi-ingredient weight-loss supplements. There is some evidence that chromium picolinate can increase lean body mass and decrease fat mass, although this finding remains controversial and some studies have shown no benefit.[47,48] Chromium is known to increase insulin sensitivity and is often referred to as a glucose tolerance factor. The picolinate salt of chromium is a naturally occurring derivative of the amino acid tryptophan and may be responsible for the changes in mood and sleep, headaches, and cognitive and perception dysfunction that have been reported with chromium picolinate. Perhaps of even greater concern are several recent cases of rhabdomyolysis and/or renal failure in patients taking megadoses of chromium.[47,48]

Glucomannan

Glucomannan is composed of a polysaccharide chain of glucose and mannose, and it is derived from the konjac root (*Amorphophallus kopnjac* C. Koch). Four randomized controlled trials suggest modest weight loss with glucomannan dosages of 3 to 4 grams daily. However, these trials were small and lacked design robustness.[48]

Hoodia

Hoodia (*Hoodia gordonii*) is a succulent native to the Kalahari Desert. Although the manufacturer, Phytopharm, cites a clinical

TABLE 27-4 Complementary Therapies Commonly Used for Weight Loss

Agent	Risks
Stimulants, Energy Boosters, and Thermogenic Aids	
Bitter orange (*Citrus aurantium*)	Synephrine may cause hypertension, cardiovascular toxicity, myocardial infarction, stroke, and seizure.
Caffeine: Cola nut (*Cola acuminata, Cola nitida*), green tea (*Camellia sinensis*), guarana (*Paullinia cupana, Paullinia sorbilis*), Maté (*Ilex paraguariensis*)	Caffeine may cause GI distress, nausea, dehydration, headaches, insomnia, nervousness, anxiety, muscle tension, heart palpitations, hypertension, addiction, and possible genetic damage; avoid in patients with gastric ulcers.
Fat and Carbohydrate Modulators	
Chromium	Chromium is generally well tolerated at low doses.
Conjugated linoleic acid (CLA)	CLA causes GI upset.
Garcinia or brindleberry (*Garcinia cambogia*)	Hydroxycitric acid may cause GI distress with high doses; not recommended in patients with diabetes mellitus or dementia.
Green tea (*Camellia sinensis*)	Caffeine and catechin components may cause decreased appetite, hyperactivity, increased heart rate, and gastric irritation; high doses are associated with headache, heart palpitations, and vertigo.
	Use with caution in patients with renal disease, panic disorder, hyperthyroidism, anxiety, or susceptibility to spasm; use only under medical supervision in patients with peptic ulcers, cardiovascular disease, or blood-clotting abnormalities; discontinue use at least 24 hours before surgery; may alter effects of anticoagulant medications.
Licorice (*Glycyrrhiza glabra*)	Pseudoaldosteronism, hypertension, and hypokalemia may occur.
Pyruvate	GI upset may occur.
Appetite Suppressants and Satiety Promoters	
Glucomannan (*Amorphophallus konjac*)	Risks are similar to those of plantain.
Guar gum (*Cyamopsis tetragonolobus*)	Risks are similar to those of plantain.
Hoodia (*Hoodia gordonii*)	No risks are reported.
Plantain or psyllium (*Plantago lanceolata, Plantago major, Plantago psyllium, Plantago arenatia*)	Flatulence, GI distress, nausea, and vomiting may occur; plantain may interact with lithium or carbamazepine.
Fat Absorption Blockers	
Chitosan	Chitosan is generally well tolerated; may cause GI upset, flatulence, nausea, increased stool bulk, constipation; may exhibit cross-sensitivity in patients with shellfish allergies.
Carbohydrate Absorption Blockers	
Ginseng (*Panax* sp.)	Ginseng may cause nervousness, excitation, inability to concentrate, estrogenic effects, Stevens-Johnson syndrome, allergy, and hypoglycemic effects; may interact with several drugs including warfarin, digoxin, alcohol, and phenelzine.
Laxatives and Diuretics	
Cascara sagrada (*Rhamnus purshiana*)	Abdominal pain, cramps, and diarrhea may occur; chronic use can lead to potassium depletion, disturbed heart function, and muscle weakness; avoid in patients taking digoxin or potassium-depleting diuretics.
Dandelion (*Taraxacum officinale*)	Avoid use in patients with allergies to ragweed, marigolds, etc. (Asteraceae/Compositae family); contraindicated in patients with gallbladder or bile duct obstruction, or with bowel obstruction or pus in the pleural cavity.
Miscellaneous	
Calcium	Constipation, nausea, and vomiting may occur; possibly effective when ingested as naturally occurring calcium in foods.
Chromium	Rhabdomyolysis and renal failure with large doses may occur.
Guggul (*Commiphora mukul*)	GI distress, diarrhea, nausea, and skin rash may occur; use only under medical supervision in patients with hyperthyroidism; may alter effects of thyroid medications, cholesterol-lowering medications, anticoagulants, antiplatelet medications, propranolol, and diltiazem.
Pyruvate	No risks are reported.
Willow bark (*Salix alba*)	Willow bark is a salicin source; no risks reported when taken orally.

Key: GI, gastrointestinal.
Source: References 40, 45, and 46–49.

trial in 18 human subjects wherein hoodia consumption reduced caloric intake compared with placebo, this study was not published nor subjected to peer review. Another study reported modest weight loss in 7 overweight patients given 1000 mg hoodia capsules daily; again, this study was not published nor subjected to the peer-review process.[50]

Assessment of Overweight and Obesity: A Case-Based Approach

When practitioners are asked to recommend a weight-loss method or product, they should find out why the patient wants to lose weight. The reason may be immediately obvious for some patients; others may want to lose a few pounds to improve appearance or to enhance their perception of good health. The practitioner should calculate the BMI to determine whether the patient is, in fact, overweight or obese. The practitioner should also review the current prescription and nonprescription drugs, and ask about use of herbal products and other dietary supplements. Anyone with significant diseases superimposed on obesity should be discouraged from using dietary supplements. The

practitioner should find out what type of weight-loss methods were used previously and whether the attempts were successful so that other methods or adjunctive products may be considered, if needed. Whether the patient received dietary counseling or was seeing a registered dietitian should be determined.

A dieter needs support from family and friends to succeed at losing weight. It may be difficult to change eating and other behavioral habits if family members are not willing to support the dieter. Cultural differences and food preferences in different parts of the country may complicate weight-loss efforts. The practitioner must explore the family dynamic before recommending weight-loss measures. Still, such factors should not be seen as insurmountable obstacles.

Individuals within the normal height/weight range who want to lose weight for other reasons (e.g., improved appearance or sense of well-being) should be advised about the difficulty of the task and the potential adverse physical and psychological effects.

Using all information obtained during the assessment, the practitioner can decide whether weight loss is appropriate and, if warranted, can help select the type, intensity, and length of a weight-loss program. Cases 27-1 and 27-2 illustrate assessment of patients who seek assistance with weight control.

CASE 27-1

Relevant Evaluation Criteria	Scenario/Model Outcome
Information Gathering	
1. Gather essential information about the patient's symptoms, including:	
a. description of symptom(s) (i.e., nature, onset, duration, severity, associated symptoms)	Patient has battled overweight and obesity his entire adult life. He has never been severely obese but tends to gain 10 to 15 pounds per decade. His obesity does not affect his ability to perform activities of daily living.
b. description of any factors that seem to precipitate, exacerbate, and/or relieve the patient's symptom(s)	Patient is a stress eater; he tends to snack on unhealthy foods at work and late at night.
c. description of the patient's efforts to relieve the symptoms	Various diets and exercise programs have been tried over the past 2 decades. Patient is usually able to lose a few pounds but gains it back when stresses of life contribute to declining compliance with diet and exercise regimens.
2. Gather essential patient history information:	
a. patient's identity	John Coughlin
b. patient's age, sex, height, and weight	45-year-old male, 5 ft 10 in, 220 lb
c. patient's occupation	Computer software engineer
d. patient's dietary habits	Typically skips breakfast and eats a sweet roll with his coffee mid-morning on workdays. Eats healthy lunch in workplace cafeteria. Wife fixes large dinner in evenings. He often gets pretzels and chips from snack machine at work and likes to eat candy and popcorn when working on home computer late at night.
e. patient's sleep habits	Goes to bed late, gets up early in morning; averages about 6 hours of sleep per night
f. concurrent medical conditions, prescription and nonprescription medications, and dietary supplements	Simvastatin 20 mg daily for hyperlipidemia; lisinopril 10 mg daily for hypertension
g. allergies	NKA
h. history of other adverse reactions to medications	None
i. other (describe) _____	N/A

CASE 27-1 (continued)

Relevant Evaluation Criteria	Scenario/Model Outcome
Assessment and Triage	
3. Differentiate the patient's signs/symptoms and correctly identify the patient's primary problem(s).	Patient's BMI is 32, placing him in the obese category (see Table 27-1). Lack of exercise and poor dietary habits are probably contributory.
4. Identify exclusions for self-treatment (see Figure 27-2).	On the basis of the patient's age and weight, he should see a primary care provider for medical clearance before beginning an exercise program.
5. Formulate a comprehensive list of therapeutic alternatives for the primary problem to determine if triage to a medical practitioner is required, and share this information with the patient.	Options include: (1) Refer John to a dietitian and/or personal trainer for diet and exercise advice, respectively. (2) Refer John to a primary care provider for prescription medication for obesity. (3) Counsel John on diet and exercise. (4) Recommend nonprescription orlistat. (5) Recommend a dietary supplement for weight loss. (6) Take no action.
Plan	
6. Select an optimal therapeutic alternative to address the patient's problem, taking into account patient preferences.	Because of previous failures with diet and exercise alone, the patient chooses to try orlistat while again trying to diet.
7. Describe the recommended therapeutic approach to the patient.	Take orlistat up to 3 times a day before meals that contain fat, as described in the text.
8. Explain to the patient the rationale for selecting the recommended therapeutic approach from the considered therapeutic alternatives.	You can anticipate that weight loss may be slightly easier to achieve when combining orlistat with diet and exercise, compared with diet and exercise alone.
Patient Education	
9. When recommending self-care with non-prescription medications and/or nondrug therapy, convey accurate information to the patient:	
a. appropriate dose and frequency of administration	60 mg up to 3 times a day
b. maximum number of days the therapy should be employed	Greatest benefit is usually seen within first 6 months of therapy.
c. product administration procedures	Take before meals containing fat. Minimizing dietary fat and spreading it out between all meals should help to minimize the gastrointestinal side effects such as flatus and oily discharge associated with orlistat. Taking a multivitamin supplement at bedtime is wise in case fat-soluble vitamin malabsorption occurs with orlistat.
d. expected time to onset of relief	Weight loss should be detected with the first 2 weeks of initiating orlistat therapy along with diet and exercise regimen.
e. degree of relief that can be reasonably expected	Many patients lose 5 to 10 pounds during the first 6 months of therapy.
f. most common side effects	Flatulence, oily spotting, loose and frequent stools, fatty stools, fecal urgency, fecal incontinence
g. side effects that warrant medical intervention should they occur	None
h. patient options in the event that condition worsens or persists	Consult a dietitian or personal trainer for diet and exercise advice, respectively, or see a primary care provider for prescription medication for weight loss.
i. product storage requirements	No special requirements
j. specific nondrug measures	Continue diet and exercise measures. Find exercise that is enjoyable and thus sustainable. Attempt to reduce stress and thus stress eating. Too little sleep has been associated with increased body weight, so sleep hygiene measures may be helpful.
10. Solicit follow-up questions from patient.	Can I double the dose of medication if weight loss slows?
11. Answer patient's questions.	Dosage above 60 mg up to 3 times a day should be attempted only under the supervision of a primary care provider.

Key: BMI, body mass index; N/A, not applicable; NKA, no known allergies.

Relevant Evaluation Criteria	Scenario/Model Outcome
Information Gathering	
1. Gather essential information about the patient's symptoms, including:	
a. description of symptom(s) (i.e., nature, onset, duration, severity, associated symptoms)	Patient is concerned about her weight and overall appearance. She has never been obese, but she is slightly overweight and wants to lose approximately 15 pounds over the next month or two.
b. description of any factors that seem to precipitate, exacerbate, and/or relieve the patient's symptom(s)	Patient tends to snack on sweets, particularly in the afternoon and when she studies at night.
c. description of the patient's efforts to relieve the symptoms	Patient has tried several diets over the past 6 months, but she has not been successful in losing weight.
2. Gather essential patient history information:	
a. patient's identity	Heidi McMaster
b. patient's age, sex, height, and weight	15-year-old female, 5 ft 5 in, 165 lb
c. patient's occupation	High-school sophomore
d. patient's dietary habits	She typically skips breakfast because she "doesn't have time." Usually eats lunch at the salad bar at school. Often gets candy bar from snack machine in the afternoon. She has a big dinner every night with her family, often including dessert.
e. patient's sleep habits	Averages about 7–8 hours per night
f. concurrent medical conditions, prescription and nonprescription medications, and dietary supplements	Ortho Tri-Cyclen 1 tablet once daily beginning on day 1 of menstrual cycle
g. allergies	NKA
h. history of other adverse reactions to medications	None
i. other (describe) _____	Patient participates in physical education classes at school twice a week. She has no other regular exercise activity. Both of her parents are also overweight.
Assessment and Triage	
3. Differentiate the patient's signs/symptoms and correctly identify the patient's primary problem(s).	Patient's BMI is 27.5, placing her in the overweight category (see Table 27-1). This places her at increased risk for type 2 DM, high cholesterol, hypertension, sleep apnea, and orthopedic problems during both adolescence and adulthood if her weight is not normalized. Her skipping breakfast, regularly consuming sweets, and eating heavy dinners, together with minimal physical activity, are contributing to her weight problem.
4. Identify exclusions for self-treatment (see Figure 27-2).	Age less than 18 years is an exclusion for self-treatment.
5. Formulate a comprehensive list of therapeutic alternatives for the primary problem to determine if triage to a medical practitioner is required, and share this information with the patient.	Options include: (1) Refer Heidi to a primary care provider for a health screen. (2) Refer to dietitian and/or personal trainer for diet and exercise advice, respectively. (3) Recommend nonprescription orlistat. (4) Recommend a dietary supplement weight-loss product. (5) Take no action.
Plan	
6. Select an optimal therapeutic alternative to address the patient's problem, taking into account patient preferences.	Refer the patient to a primary care provider for a health screen.
7. Describe the recommended therapeutic approach to the patient.	N/A
8. Explain to the patient the rationale for selecting the recommended therapeutic approach from the considered therapeutic alternatives.	You need to see a primary care provider to determine if a diet and exercise program is appropriate. Healthy eating habits and exercise are the mainstays of successful weight loss, and these should be a lifelong goal.

C A S E   2 7 - 2 (continued)

Relevant Evaluation Criteria	Scenario/Model Outcome
Patient Education	
9. When recommending self-care with non-prescription medications and/or nondrug therapy, convey accurate information to the patient.	Criterion does not apply in this case.
10. Solicit follow-up questions from patient.	Is there an OTC medication that might work?
11. Answer patient's questions.	No OTC medications are approved and/or appropriate to recommend without referral from a primary care provider.

Key: BMI, body mass index; DM, diabetes mellitus; N/A, not applicable; NKA, no known allergies; OTC, over-the-counter.

Patient Counseling for Overweight and Obesity

The objectives for counseling patients who want to lose weight are to foster realistic goals for weight loss together with a healthy restricted-calorie diet and increased physical activity. The ultimate goal is to achieve a healthy weight and maintain that weight over the long term. For those patients unable to lose weight, the objective is to prevent further weight gain.

Evaluation of Patient Outcomes for Overweight and Obesity

Successful weight loss generally requires a lifelong approach that combines healthy eating and exercise patterns. Realistic weight-loss goals of 10% of the initial weight over 6 months, or 1 to 2 pounds per week, should be encouraged. During any weight-loss program, the patient should be monitored for healthy eating and exercise patterns, and, at a minimum, blood pressure

---

PATIENT EDUCATION FOR
Overweight and Obesity

The objectives of self-treatment are to (1) foster realistic weight-loss and exercise goals, (2) maintain a healthy weight, and (3) prevent further weight gain. For most patients, carefully following the self-care measures listed here, together with continued adherence to a safe and effective weight-loss program, will help ensure optimal therapeutic outcomes.

Health Risks of Obesity
- Health risks related to overweight and obesity include the following:
  —Coronary heart disease
  —Type 2 diabetes mellitus
  —Sleep apnea
  —Elevated serum triglycerides and dyslipidemia
  —Hypertension
  —Stroke
  —Gallbladder disease
  —Osteoarthritis
  —Certain types of cancers

Nondrug Treatment Guidelines
- Focus on small, gradual changes in eating and exercise patterns.
- Maintain realistic goals for weight loss and increased activity levels.
- Eat a low-calorie balanced diet.
- Eat meals at the table, and do nothing else while eating (no television, etc.).
- Set a regular eating schedule, and avoid skipping meals.
- Eat slowly and enjoy the food.

- Put your fork or spoon down between bites.
- Try to leave some food on your plate each time you eat.
- Wait 5 minutes before going back for extra helpings of food.
- Remove serving dishes from the table after the first servings have been made.
- Leave the table after eating.
- Use smaller plates so moderate servings do not appear too small.
- Start a meal with a broth-based soup (low-salt) to help you feel fuller.
- Strive to consume at least five servings a day of fruits and vegetables.
- Keep on hand healthful snacks such as fruits and vegetables, low-fat cheese and yogurt, and frozen fruit juice bars.
- Drink at least eight glasses of noncaloric beverages each day to help you feel full.
- When you experience a craving, try doing something else, such as going for a walk; cravings generally pass within minutes.
- Shop for food immediately after a meal, and use a prepared list.
- Gradually increase your activity level, with the goal of engaging in 60 minutes of moderate-intensity physical activity most days of the week.
- Increase your lifestyle activity: Walk more, climb stairs, and park farther from destination.
- Limit the amount of time spent watching television, playing video games, or surfing the Internet.

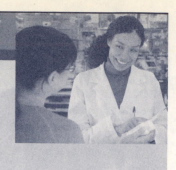

PATIENT EDUCATION FOR
Overweight and Obesity (continued)

■ Keep a diary of your weight, physical activity, and caloric intake so you can see your progress and success.

Drug Management Guidelines

■ Avoid taking OTC drugs and supplements marketed for weight loss, with the exception of orlistat. They are not proven to work, and they can cause significant side effects.

■ If you do decide to take one of these products, make sure to notify your primary care provider and pharmacist so you can be adequately followed for potential side effects and interactions with drugs.

---

should be routinely measured. More extensive physical examinations and laboratory measures may be indicated, particularly in those patients with comorbid conditions such as hypertension or DM. Follow-up with patients attempting weight loss should be encouraged, preferably on a monthly basis. In addition to measuring weight at monthly follow-ups, the practitioner should explore eating habits and exercise patterns with the patient, especially if weight loss is not being achieved. Referral to a dietitian or personal trainer may be helpful in such cases. Referral to a primary care provider for pharmacologic therapy may be an option for patients with more significant obesity who fail to lose weight through lifestyle modifications.

Key Points for Overweight and Obesity

➤ A reasonable goal for weight loss in most overweight and obese subjects is a 10% loss over 6 months.

➤ Even though this amount of weight loss may not result in the cosmetic effect desired by the dieter, it is associated with a reduction in risk for chronic disease.

➤ The safest approach to losing weight entails combining a reduced-calorie diet with increased physical activity.

➤ Physical activity typically needs to be something the person enjoys if it is to be sustained over long periods of time.

➤ A key to sustained weight loss is modification of behavior related to eating and exercise.

➤ If nonprescription or dietary supplement products for weight loss are used, they should be continuously assessed for efficacy, safety, and tolerance.

➤ Labels of nonprescription or dietary supplement weight-loss products should be carefully reviewed to determine the risk for adverse reactions and drug–herb interactions.

REFERENCES

1. National Institutes of Health, National Heart, Lung, and Blood Institute. Clinical guidelines on the identification, evaluation, and treatment of overweight and obesity in adults: the evidence report. 1998. Available at: http://www.nhlbi.nih.gov/guidelines/obesity/ob_gdlns.htm. Last accessed October 5, 2008.

2. National Center for Health Statistics. *Health, United States, 2007*. Washington, DC: US Government Printing Office; 2007. Publication No. (PHS) 2007-1232. Available at: http://www.cdc.gov/nchs/hus.htm. Last accessed October 5, 2008.

3. Ogden CL, Carroll MD, McDowell MA, et al. Obesity among Adults in the United States—No Statistically Significant Change since 2003–2004. National Center for Health Statistics. NCH Data Brief. November 2007. Available at: http://www.cdc.gov/nchs/data/databriefs/db01.pdf. Last accessed October 5, 2008.

4. Finkelstein EA, Fiebelkorn IC, Wang G. State-level estimates of annual medical expenditures attributable to obesity. *Obes Res.* 2004;12:18–24.

5. Blanck HM, Serdula MK, Gillespie C, et al. Use of nonprescription dietary supplements for weight loss is common among Americans. *J Am Diet Assoc.* 2007;107:441–7.

6. National Center for Health Statistics. Centers for Disease Control and Prevention Growth Charts: United States. 2000. Available at: http://www.cdc.gov/growthcharts. Last accessed October 5, 2008.

7. Alley DE, Chang VW. The changing relationship of obesity and disability, 1988–2004. *JAMA.* 2007;298:2020–7.

8. Wadden TA, Butryn ML, Wilson C. Lifestyle modification for the management of obesity. *Gastroenterology.* 2007;132:2226–38.

9. US Department of Health and Human Services. *The Surgeon General's Call to Action to Prevent and Decrease Overweight and Obesity*. Rockville, Md: U.S. Department of Health and Human Services, Public Health Service, Office of the Surgeon General; 2001. Available at: http://www.surgeongeneral.gov/topics/obesity. Last accessed October 5, 2008.

10. Ley RE, Turnbaugh PJ, Klein S, et al. Microbial ecology: human gut microbes associated with obesity. *Nature.* 2006;444:1022–3.

11. Malone M. Medications associated with weight gain. *Ann Pharmacother.* 2005;39:2046–55.

12. Poirier P, Giles TD, Bray GA, et al. Obesity and cardiovascular disease: pathophysiology, evaluation, and effect of weight loss. *Circulation* 2006; 113:898–918.

13. Overweight, obesity, and health risk. National Task Force on the Prevention and Treatment of Obesity. *Arch Intern Med.* 2000;160: 898–904.

14. Mokdad AH, Ford ES, Bowman BA, et al. Prevalence of obesity, diabetes, and obesity-related health risk factors, 2001. *JAMA.* 2003;289:76–79.

15. Calle EE, Rodriguez C, Walker-Thurmond K, et al. Overweight, obesity, and mortality from cancer in a prospectively studied cohort of U.S. adults. *New Engl J Med.* 2003;348:1625–38.

16. Hsu CY, McCulloch CD, Iribarren C, et al. Body mass index and risk for end-stage renal disease. *Ann Intern Med.* 2006;144:21–8.

17. Setty AR, Curhan G, Choi HK. Obesity, waist circumference, weight change, and the risk of psoriasis in women: Nurses' Health Study II. *Arch Intern Med.* 2007;167:1670–5.

18. Malone M, Alger-Mayer SA, Anderson DA. The lifestyle challenge program: a multidisciplinary approach to weight management. *Ann Pharmacother.* 2005;39:2015–20.

19. Lloyd KB, Thrower MR, Walters NB, et al. Implementation of a weight management pharmaceutical care service. *Ann Pharmacother.* 2007;41: 185–92.

20. The National Weight Control Registry. Available at: http://www.nwcr.ws. Last accessed October 5, 2008.

21. Food and Nutrition Board, Institute of Medicine. *Dietary Reference Intakes for Energy, Carbohydrate, Fiber, Fat, Fatty Acids, Cholesterol, Protein, and Amino Acids (Macronutrients)*. Washington, DC: National Academies Press; 2002. Available at: http://www.nap.edu/books/0309085373/html. Last accessed October 5, 2008.

22. US Department of Health and Human Services, US Department of Agriculture. *Dietary Guidelines for Americans, 2005*. 6th ed. Washington, DC: US Government Printing Office; January 2005. Available at: http://www.healthierus.gov/dietaryguidelines. Last accessed October 5, 2008.

23. Nordmann AJ, Nordmann A, Briel M, et al. Effects of low-carbohydrate vs. low-fat diets on weight loss and cardiovascular risk factors: a meta-analysis of randomized controlled trials. *Arch Intern Med.* 2006;166:285–93.

24. Gardner CD, Kiazand A, Alhassan S, et al. Comparison of the Atkins, Zone, Ornish, and LEARN diets for change in weight and related risk factors among overweight premenopausal women: the A to Z weight loss study: a randomized trial. *JAMA.* 2007;297:969–77.

25. Wood RJ. Effect of dietary carbohydrate restriction with and without weight loss on atherogenic dyslipidemia. *Nutr Rev.* 2006;64:539–45.

26. Ahrens RA, Hower M, Best AIM. Effects of weight reduction interventions by community pharmacists. *J Am Pharm Assoc.* 2003;43:583–90.

27. Tsai AG, Wadden TA. Systematic review: an evaluation of major commercial weight loss programs in the United States. *Ann Intern Med.* 2005; 143:56–66.

28. Thompson WG, Cook DA, Clark MM, et al. Treatment of obesity. *Mayo Clin Proc.* 2007;82:93–101.

29. Aikman B. FDA to ban 111 Diet Product Ingredients. October 29, 1990. Available at: http://www.fda.gov/bbs/topics/NEWS/NEW00035.html. Last accessed October 5, 2008.

30. Woodcock J. Phenylpropanolamine (PPA) information page. November 23, 2005. Available at: http://www.fda.gov/cder/drug/infopage/ppa/default.htm. Last accessed October 5, 2008.

31. Dotzel MM. Cold, cough, allergy, bronchodilator, and antiasthmatic drug products for over-the-counter human use; partial final rule for combination drug products containing a bronchodilator. Department of Health and Human Services, Food and Drug Administration. 21 CFR Part 341 [Docket No. 76N-052G] RIN 0910-AA01. September 20, 2001. Available at: http://www.epa.gov/fedrgstr/EPA-IMPACT/2001/September/Day-27/i24127.htm. Last accessed October 5, 2008.

32. Dotzel MM. Status of certain additional over-the-counter drug category II and III active ingredients. Department of Health and Human Services. Food and Drug Administration. 21 CFR Part 310 [Docket No. 78N-0366] RIN 0910-AA01. April 29, 2002. Available at: http://www.fda.gov/OHRMS/DOCKETS/98fr/050902a.htm. Last accessed October 5, 2008.

33. Food and Drug Administration. FDA Approves Orlistat for Over-the-Counter Use [news release]. February 7, 2008. Available at: http://www.fda.gov/bbs/topics/NEWS/2007/new01557.html. Last accessed October 5, 2008.

34. GlaxoSmithKline. alli healthcare professionals. 2008. Available at: http://www.allihcp.com. Last accessed October 5, 2008.

35. Anderson JW, Schwartz SM, Hauptman J, et al. Low-dose orlistat effects on body weight of mildly to moderately overweight individuals: a 16-week, double-blind, placebo-controlled trial. *Ann Pharmacother.* 2006;40:1717–23.

36. GlaxoSmithKline. Study Results Found Low-Dose Orlistat (60 mg) Demonstrates Significant Reduction in LDL Cholesterol While Providing Weight Loss for Up to 2 Years. Available at: http://www.pslgroup.com/dg/2034FA.htm. Last accessed October 5, 2008.

37. Torgerson JS, Hauptman J, Boldrin MN, et al. XENical in the prevention of diabetes in obese subjects (XENDOS) study: a randomized study of orlistat as an adjunct to lifestyle changes for the prevention of type 2 diabetes in obese patients. *Diabetes Care.* 2004;27:155–61.

38. US Food and Drug Administration. Remove from the Market, the Prescription Version of Xenical (Orlistat, Roche Pharmaceuticals). Available at: http://www.fda.gov/ohrms/dockets/dockets/06p0154/06p0154.htm. Last accessed October 5, 2008.

39. US Food and Drug Administration. OTC Ingredient List. Updated August 2006. Available at: http://www.fda.gov/cder/Offices/OTC/Ingredient_List_D-O.pdf. Last accessed October 5, 2008.

40. Shekelle PG, Hardy ML, Morton SC, et al. Efficacy and safety of ephedra and ephedrine for weight loss and athletic performance: a meta-analysis. *JAMA.* 2003;289:1537–45.

41. US Food and Drug Administration. HHS Acts to Reduce Potential Risks of Dietary Supplements Containing Ephedra. February 28, 2003. Available at: http://www.fda.gov/bbs/topics/NEWS/2003/NEW00875.html. Last accessed October 5, 2008.

42. McClellan MB. Final rule declaring dietary supplements containing ephedrine alkaloids adulterated because they present an unreasonable risk. Department of Health and Human Services. Food and Drug Administration. 21 CFR Part 119 [Docket No. 1995N-0304] RIN 0910-AA59. February 11, 2004. Available at: http://www.cfsan.fda.gov/~lrd/fr040211.html. Last accessed October 5, 2008.

43. Amin RM, Blumenthal M. Federal court overturns FDA ban on ephedra at low doses. *HerbalGram.* 2005;64:52–3.

44. US Food and Drug Administration. FDA statement on tenth circuit's ruling to uphold FDA decision banning dietary supplements containing ephedrine alkaloids (8-31-06). Available at: http://www.fda.gov/bbs/topics/NEWS/2006/NEW01434.html. Last accessed October 5, 2008.

45. Haller CA, Benowitz NF, Jacob P III. Hemodynamic effects of ephedra-free weight-loss supplements in humans. *Am J Med.* 2005;118:998–1003.

46. Blumenthal M, Busse WR, Goldberg A, et al., eds. *The Complete German Commission E Monographs. Therapeutic Guide to Herbal Medicines.* Austin, Tex: American Botanical Council; 1998.

47. Pittler MH, Ernst E. Dietary supplements for body-weight reduction: a systematic review. *Am J Clin Nutr.* 2004;79:529–36.

48. Saper RB, Eisenberg DM, Phillips RS. Common dietary supplements for weight loss. *Am Fam Physician.* 2004;70:1731–8.

49. Heaney RP, Davies M, Barger-Lux J. Calcium and weight: clinical studies. *J Am Coll Nutr.* 2002;21:152S–5S.

50. Doheny K. Hoodia: lots of hoopla, little science. Available at: http://www.webmd.com/diet/guide/hoodia-lots-of-hoopla-little-science. Last accessed October 5, 2008.

Ophthalmic, Otic, and Oral Disorders

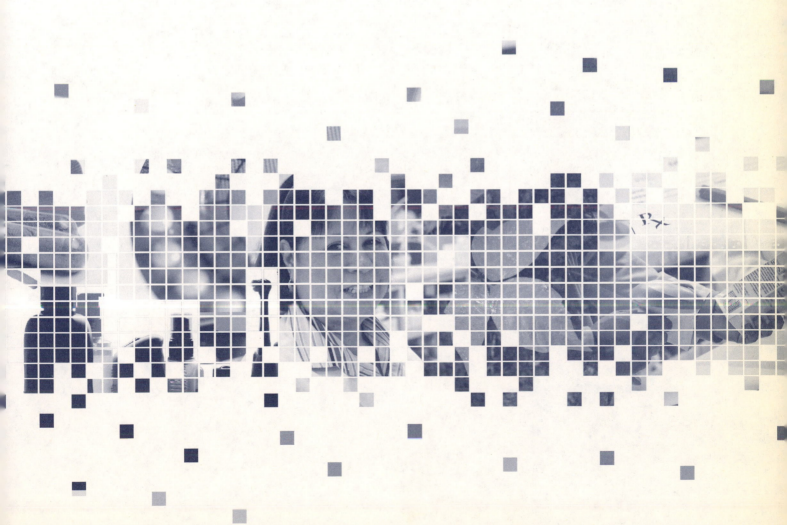

Ophthalmic Disorders

Richard G. Fiscella and Michael Kirk Jensen

The nonprescription ophthalmic market consists of products that treat a wide range of disorders. Little population-based data are available on the epidemiology of these disorders. People with ocular conditions are commonly seen in the primary care provider's office, the emergency department, the eye care practitioner's office, or the pharmacy. Ocular discomfort associated with dry eye may be the most common condition for which nonprescription ophthalmic products can be used. It may affect as many as 4.3 million people in the United States and 20% of persons of advanced age.[1]

Many common conditions causing ocular discomfort are minor and self-limiting. In some instances, however, relatively minor symptoms may be associated with severe, potentially vision-threatening conditions. Practitioners should be well versed in eye anatomy and physiology, as well as in common ocular conditions, so they can provide the best possible guidance for patients who want help in choosing between self-treatment and professional medical care.

Self-treatable ophthalmic disorders occur primarily on the eyelids; however, a few disorders of the eye surface may be responsive to self-treatment. The latter include dry eyes, allergic conjunctivitis, diagnosed viral conjunctivitis and corneal edema, presence of loose foreign debris, minor ocular irritation, diagnosed age-related macular degeneration, and the cleaning or lubricating of artificial eyes. Disorders of the eyelid and adjacent areas that are amenable to self-care include contact dermatitis, hordeolum, chalazion, and blepharitis. Careful assessment is important, especially with ongoing symptoms, to rule out more complicated manifestations that may require referral to an eye care specialist.

ROLE OF EYE ANATOMY IN OCULAR DRUG PHARMACOKINETICS

The external location and exposure of the eye make it susceptible to environmental and microbiologic contamination. However, the eye has many natural defense mechanisms to protect it against contamination, and the eyelid is one of its major protective elements (Figure 28-1).

The eyelids are a multilayer tissue covered externally by the skin and internally by a thin, mucocutaneous epithelial layer called the palpebral conjunctiva. The middle portion of the eyelid contains glandular tissue and muscles for lid movement. The five main types of glandular tissue found within the eyelid, along with conjunctival goblet cells, secrete the bulk of nonstimulated tears.

The eyelids primarily protect the anterior surface of the eye and spread the tears produced by the glandular tissue over the ocular surface. The lids force the flow of tears toward the nose and into the drainage canals located in the upper and lower eyelids. The drainage canals converge, forming the lacrimal sac between the inner eyelid and nose. The lacrimal sac is drained by a canal opening just below the inferior turbinate of the nasal cavity. A highly vascularized epithelium lines the lacrimal drainage system, and absorption into the systemic circulation along this pathway gives rise to potential systemic effects of topically administered eye medications.[2]

The tear layer keeps the ocular surface lubricated, provides a mechanism for removing debris that touches the ocular surface, and has potent antimicrobial action provided by specific enzymes and a number of immunoglobulins, most notably immunoglobulin A. The tear layer is a complex multilayer film. The outer lipid layer maintains the eyes' optical properties and reduces evaporation. The middle aqueous layer is largely responsible for the wetting properties of the tear film. The inner mucinous layer allows the aqueous and lipid layers to maintain constant adhesion across the cornea and conjunctiva. Abnormalities within any one of the tear layers can result in ocular discomfort.

Tears are produced at a rate of 1 to 2 μL per minute, with a turnover of approximately 16% of the total volume per minute.[3,4] As much as 25% of the total tear volume is lost to evaporation.[3] An ambient tear volume of approximately 7 to 10 μL is found on the ocular surface at any point in time.[3] During episodes of ocular irritation, reflex tearing is stimulated by the lacrimal gland found underneath the outer portion of the upper eyelid, and tear production increases to greater than 300% of the nonstimulated production rate.[5] Reflex tearing occurs immediately on instillation of a drug into the eye, diluting the drug's concentration. Drug penetration into the eye is reduced because of increased lacrimal drainage and tearing that falls down the cheek. Studies have shown that as much as 90% of an instilled dose of a drug administered to the eye may be lost.[6]

The visible external portion of the eye is composed of the cornea and sclera; the former is innervated, whereas the latter is not. The sclera is a tough, collagenous layer that gives the eye

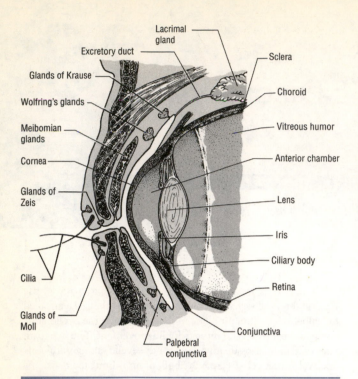

FIGURE 28-1   Anatomy of the eyelid and eye surface.

rigidity and encases the internal eye structures. The visible sclera is covered by two epithelial layers: the episclera and the bulbar conjunctiva. The bulbar conjunctiva is contiguous with the palpebral conjunctiva at the junction between the eyelid and the ocular surface (the fornix). The episcleral and bulbar conjunctival layers contain the vascular and lymphatic systems of the anterior eye surface, and are the sources of visible eye redness in ocular irritation or inflammation.

The cornea is an aspherical, avascular tissue that is the principal refractive element of the eye. It is approximately 12 mm wide and 0.5 mm thick, and consists of five distinct layers. Of the five corneal layers, the outermost epithelium layer, the middle and most abundant stromal layer, and the innermost endothelial layer affect the pharmacokinetics of ocularly administered drugs. The corneal epithelium is lipophilic and facilitates the passage of fat-soluble drugs. However, if a drug is too lipophilic, it may become trapped in the corneal epithelium. The epithelium is often the rate-limiting step in absorption of medication into the anterior chamber. The corneal stroma is hydrophilic and allows the passage of water-soluble drugs. Damage to the corneal epithelium may often increase drug absorption rates. Comparative studies with intact and compromised epithelium have shown that drug penetration into the aqueous humor may be increased by as much as threefold in corneas with compromised epithelium.[7] Corneal epithelium can be compromised by trauma, routine contact lens wear, topical ocular anesthetics, and thermal or ultraviolet (UV) light exposure.

Directly behind the cornea is the anterior chamber, a cavity filled with aqueous humor. The aqueous humor maintains the normal intraocular pressure (IOP) and provides nutritional support for the cornea and crystalline lens. It is produced by the ciliary body and drained from the anterior chamber through the uveoscleral tract and the trabecular meshwork. The trabecular

meshwork, which is located at the junction of the cornea and iris, accounts for approximately 80% to 90% of aqueous drainage from the anterior chamber. The uveoscleral tract, located posteriorly to the iris and comprising the sclera, ciliary body, and choroid areas, accounts for approximately 10% to 20% of aqueous drainage, although this percentage may vary with age and disease state. During episodes of internal eye inflammation, inflammatory cells may block the drainage system, causing the IOP to rise. Increased IOP is one of the most significant risk factors for primary open-angle glaucoma. Similarly, during episodes of closed-angle glaucoma, the iris physically blocks the trabecular meshwork, thereby also resulting in an increase in IOP. Dilating the pupil with mydriatic drugs may precipitate an angle-closure attack. Such attacks often occur as the pupil is returning to its normal state several hours after the mydriatic drug has been instilled. Any agent with anticholinergic or dilating effect has the potential to cause angle closure. The most common symptoms are brow ache or headache, often accompanied by nausea and vomiting. These symptoms are severe enough to cause an individual to visit an eye care practitioner.

The visible, colored portion of the eye, the iris, is located in the anterior segment of the eye, behind the cornea. It functions in much the same way as an aperture on a camera by regulating the amount of light striking the retina. The central opening in the iris is the pupil. The pupillary diameter is controlled by two opposing muscles within the iris: the sphincter and the dilator. Sphincter muscles are circular at the pupillary border and cause a miotic (closing) effect through parasympathetic stimulation. Dilator muscles are radial from the pupillary border and cause a mydriatic (opening) effect through sympathetic stimulation. Prostaglandins released by the iris during episodes of inflammation may affect the sphincter muscle, resulting in constriction of the pupil.

The ciliary body is bordered anteriorly by the iris and is continuous posteriorly with the choroid. Besides aqueous humor production, it participates in focusing the optical mechanism (lens) for near viewing, a process known as accommodation. During episodes of ocular inflammation, the ciliary muscle may go into spasm, resulting in fluctuating vision and pain. Therefore, inhibition of the ciliary muscle (cycloplegia) with anticholinergic agents is a frequent treatment for internal ocular inflammation.

The vitreous cavity, located in the posterior segment of the eye, is the largest portion of the eye and is filled with vitreous humor. Floating spots in the visual field ("floaters") are related to this area. Floaters are deposits in the vitreous humor of various shapes, sizes, and motility; they may be related to degenerative changes in gel that is normally transparent. Problems in this area are not amenable to self-treatment and require professional evaluation because of the possibility of concurrent retinal problems.

The retina is responsible for the initial processing and transmission of light signals. A number of inflammatory conditions of the retina can occur, and most have prominent symptoms. Some, however, have relatively mild symptoms, mimicking common irritative conditions. Trauma, even minor, may cause the retina to separate from its underlying layer (the pigment epithelium), resulting in retinal detachment. The retinal pigment epithelium provides vital "electrical" support to the retina. Macular degeneration, the leading cause of blindness in the United States, is directly related to atrophy in the pigment epithelium. Diabetic retinopathy is also a major cause of vision loss.

DRY EYE

Pathophysiology and Clinical Presentation of Dry Eye

Dry eye is among the most common disorders affecting the anterior eye.[1] Most often associated with the aging process (especially with postmenopausal women), dry eye can also be caused by lid defects, corneal defects, loss of lid tissue turgor, Sjögren's syndrome, Bell's palsy, thyroid eye disease, various collagen diseases such as rheumatoid arthritis, and systemic medications. Refractive surgery patients may complain of transient dry eyes for weeks to months after the procedure. This effect is usually mild if it does occur but can be more pronounced in some patients. Drugs with anticholinergic properties (e.g., antihistamines and antidepressants), decongestants, diuretics, and beta-blockers are some of the more common pharmacologic causes of dry eye. The condition may be exacerbated by allergens or other environmental conditions such as dry, dusty working situations, or by heating and air conditioning systems that reduce relative humidity, thereby increasing the evaporation of tears.

Dry eye is characterized by a white or mildly red eye, and patients may complain of a sandy, gritty feeling or a sensation that something is in the eye. Contrary to what the name suggests, dry eye may often initially present with excessive tearing. Abnormalities in the tear layer cause less-than-optimal lubrication of the ocular surface, thus producing more inadequate tears and beginning a vicious cycle. Failure to properly diagnose and treat dry eye syndromes can result in severe damage to eye tissue, particularly to the corneal surface (see Color Plates, photograph 3). Recent evidence demonstrates that dry eye disease can be linked to a T-cell–mediated inflammatory process, which can respond to immunomodulatory agents such as cyclosporine.[8]

Treatment of Dry Eye

Treatment Goals

The goal in treating dry eye is to alleviate and control the dryness of the ocular surface, thereby relieving the symptoms of irritation and preventing possible tissue and corneal damage.

General Treatment Approach

The primary self-treatment for dry eye is the use of ocular lubricants. The availability of synthetic chemicals suitable for topical application to the eye has resulted in the development of various solutions (artificial tears) to help alleviate dryness of the ocular surface. Artificial tear products vary by viscosity according to the ingredients used in their preparation. Increasing the viscosity of the product results in a more prolonged ocular contact time and greater resistance to tear dilution. Mild cases of dry eye may be treated with less viscous products, whereas more severe cases may require more viscous products. Bland (nonmedicated; e.g., petrolatum) ophthalmic ointment is another type of ocular lubricant. Ointment preparations are typically reserved for use at bedtime or for severe cases of dry eye because of their tendency to cause blurred vision. As with ointments, as the viscosity of tear drops increases, the blurring effect is greater. Vitamin A preparations are also available for treating dry eye. Nonpharmacologic measures, such as lid scrubs with warm compresses, may also increase eye comfort for patients with this disorder. Recommending the use of omega-3 oils or flax seed oil in the normal doses recommended per manufacturer is thought to improve lid function that is possibly related to some anti-inflammatory properties.

Eye care practitioners treat the most severe cases of dry eye with punctual plugs that provide occlusion of the lacrimal drainage system to increase the available tear pool. As mentioned previously, recent advances in the underlying pathophysiology of dry eye suggest that patients may benefit from treatment with topical cyclosporine.[8] However, minor dry eye disease may require relief of only ocular surface dryness, whereas more moderate-to-severe dry eye disease may benefit from a combined approach of immunomodulating agents, such as topical cyclosporine, in conjunction with ocular surface lubrication.

Nonpharmacologic Therapy

The primary nondrug measure is avoiding environments that increase evaporation of the tear film. If possible, the patient should avoid dry or dusty places. Using humidifiers or repositioning workstations away from heating and air conditioning vents may help alleviate dry eyes. Also, avoiding prolonged viewing of computer screens and wearing eye protection in windy, outdoor environments without eye protection (e.g., sunglasses or goggles) may further help alleviate dry eye problems.

Pharmacologic Therapy

Nonmedicated ointments are a mainstay of treating minor ophthalmic disorders, including dry eye. Because ointments can cause blurred vision, resulting in severe vision limitations, combination therapy using artificial tears and nonmedicated ointments is usually recommended. Gels offer some advantage to patients in that they do not disturb vision as much as ointments do and are better tolerated. The effectiveness of retinol solutions for treating dry eye is still speculative.

Artificial Tear Solutions

Although many advances have been made in understanding the mechanisms involved in tear film formation, the role of tears in maintaining a normal conjunctival and corneal surface is still not completely understood. Lubricants that are formulated as artificial tear solutions consist of preservatives, inorganic electrolytes to achieve tonicity and maintain pH, and water-soluble polymeric systems. The lubricating agents in artificial tear products are similar, but buffering agents, preservatives, pH, and other formulation components may vary (Table 28-1).

One class of ophthalmic vehicles or ocular lubricants is the substituted cellulose ethers, which include hydroxypropyl methylcellulose (HPMC), hydroxyethylcellulose, hydroxypropylcellulose, methylcellulose, and carboxymethylcellulose (CMC). These solutions are colorless and vary in viscosity, depending on the grade and concentration of cellulose ether. Polyvinyl alcohol (PVA) and povidone are two other vehicles commonly used as ocular lubricants. The section Formulation Considerations for Ocular Lubricants and Other Ophthalmic Products discusses ophthalmic vehicles, preservatives, and excipients in greater detail.

Perhaps the most important property of the cellulose ethers in artificial tear formulations is their ability to stabilize the tear film, which retards tear evaporation. Both effects are beneficial for patients with dry eye.[9] Combining drugs with these vehicles

TABLE 28-1 More Commonly Used Ophthalmic Lubricants

Artificial Tear Solutions

Bion Tears[a]	Hydroxypropyl methylcellulose 0.3%; dextran 70, 0.1%
Celluvisc[a]	CMC sodium 1%
Clear Eyes Contact Lens Relief Drops	Sorbic acid 0.25%; EDTA 0.1%; NaCl; hypromellose, glycerin
Dry Eyes	PVA 1.4%; sodium phosphate; NaCl; BAK 0.01%; EDTA
Dry Eye Therapy	Glycerin 0.3%, NaCl; KCl; sodium citrate; sodium phosphate
Eye-Lube-A	Glycerin 0.25%; EDTA; NaCl; BAK
GenTeal Tears, Mild and Moderate Formulations	Hydroxypropyl methylcellulose; boric acid; phosphonic acid; NaCl; sodium perborate
HypoTears[b]	PVA 1%; PEG 400; BAK 0.01%
Isopto Plain	Hydroxypropyl methylcellulose 2910, 0.5%; BAK 0.01%; NaCl; sodium citrate; sodium phosphate
Isopto Tears	
LubriTears	Hydroxypropyl methylcellulose 2906, 0.3%; dextran 70, 0.1%; EDTA; KCl; NaCl; BAK 0.01%
Moisture Eyes[b]	Propylene glycol 1%; glycerin 0.3%; BAK 0.01%
Murine Tears Lubricant	Povidone 0.6%; PVA 0.5%; BAK
Nature's Tears	Hydroxypropyl methylcellulose 2906, 0.4%; potassium chloride; NaCl; sodium phosphate; BAK 0.01%; EDTA
Nature's Tears Spray	Pure water mist
Nu-Tears	PVA 1.4%; EDTA; NaCl; BAK; potassium chloride
Nu-Tears II	PVA 1.4%; PEG-400; EDTA; BAK
Ocucoat Lubricating[b]	Hydroxypropyl methylcellulose 0.8%; dextran 70, 0.1%; BAK 0.01%
Optive	CMC 0.5%; glycerin 0.9%; Purite[c]; boric acid; calcium chloride; magnesium chloride; KCl; levocarnitine; erythritol
OptiZen	Polysorbent 80, 0.5%; EDTA; NaCl; sodium phosphate; sorbic acid
Preservative Free Moisture Eyes[a]	Propylene glycol 0.95%; boric acid; NaCl; KCl; sodium borate; EDTA
Refresh	PVA 1.4%; povidone 0.6%
Refresh Dry Eye Therapy	Glycerin 1.0%; polysorbate 80, 1.0% (polymer matrix; emulsifying agent; carbomer; castor oil)
Refresh Liquigel	CMC sodium 1%; Purite[c]
Refresh Plus[a]	CMC sodium 0.5%
Refresh Tears	CMC sodium 0.5%; Purite[c]
Soothe	Restoryl (Drakeol-15 1.0% and Drakeol-35 4.5%); polysorbate 80, 0.4%; octoxynol 40; NaCl; sodium phosphate; EDTA; polyhexamethylene biguanide preservative
Systane	PEG-400, 0.4%; propylene glycol 0.3%; boric acid; calcium chloride; hydroxypropyl guar; magnesium chloride; polyquaternium preservative; potassium chloride; NaCl; zinc chloride; water
Teargen	BAK 0.01%; EDTA; NaCl; PVA
Teargen II	Hydroxypropyl methylcellulose 2910, 4 mg; dextran 70, 0.1%; NaCl; potassium chloride; sodium borate
Tears Naturale	Hydroxypropyl methylcellulose 0.3%; dextran 70, 0.1%; BAK 0.01%
Tears Naturale Forte	Dextran 70, 0.1%; hydroxypropyl methylcellulose 0.3%; glycerin 0.2%; polyquaternium 1, 0.001%; NaCl; KCl; sodium borate
Tears Naturale Free[a]	Hydroxypropyl methylcellulose 0.3%; dextran 70, 0.1%
Tears Naturale II	Hydroxypropyl methylcellulose 0.3%; dextran 70, 0.1%; Polyquad 0.001%
Tears Plus	PVA 1.4%; povidone 0.6%; chlorobutanol 0.5%
Tears Renewed	BAK 0.01%; EDTA; dextran 70, 0.1%; NaCl; hydroxypropyl methylcellulose 2906, 0.3%
Theratears PF[a]	Carboxymethylcellulose 0.25%
Visine Pure Tears Drops[b]	Glycerin 0.2%, hypromellose 0.2%; PEG 400, 1%

Nonmedicated Ointments

Artificial Tears PF[a]	White petrolatum; anhydrous liquid lanolin; mineral oil
Dry Eyes	White petrolatum; mineral oil, lanolin
DuraTears Naturale[a]	Petrolatum; mineral oil; lanolin
HypoTears	White petrolatum; light mineral oil
Lacri-Lube N.P.[a]	White petrolatum 57.3%; mineral oil 42.5%; lanolin alcohols
Lacri-Lube S.O.P.	White petrolatum 56.8%; mineral oil 42.5%; lanolin alcohols; chlorobutanol 0.5%
LubriFresh PM	White petrolatum 83%, 15% mineral oil
Moisture Eyes PM[a]	White petrolatum 80%; mineral oil 20%
Preservative Free Moisture Eyes PM	White petrolatum 80%, mineral oil 20%
Refresh P.M.[a]	White petrolatum 56.8%; mineral oil 41.5%; lanolin alcohols
Tears Renewed[a]	White petrolatum; light mineral oil

TABLE 28-1 More Commonly Used Ophthalmic Lubricants (continued)	
Nonmedicated Gels	
GenTeal Lubricant Eye Gel	Hydroxypropyl methylcellulose 0.3%; sodium perborate 0.028%; carbopol 980; phosphoric acid; sorbitol
Tears Again Gel	CMC[d] 1.5%
Theratears Gel	Carboxymethylcellulose 1%; KCl; sodium bicarbonate; NaCl; sodium phosphate

Key: BAK, benzalkonium chloride; CMC, carboxymethylcellulose; EDTA, ethylenediamine tetraacetic acid; PEG, polyethylene glycol; PVA, polyvinyl alcohol.

[a] Preservative-free product.

[b] Preservative-free formulation available.

[c] Stabilized oxychloro complex.

[d] Stabilized oxyborate complex.

increases the vehicles' viscosity, thereby enhancing the drug's action. The increased viscosity retards drainage of the active ingredient from the eye, thus increasing the retention time of the active drug and enhancing bioavailability at the external ocular tissues. These effects generally occur without irritation or toxicity to the ocular tissues. Similar to the cellulose ethers, PVA also enhances stability of the tear film without causing ocular irritation or toxicity.

Povidone has surface-active properties similar to those of cellulose ethers. This compound is believed to form a hydrophilic layer on the corneal surface, mimicking natural conjunctival mucin. This mucomimetic property has firmly established the role of povidone as an artificial tear formulation. Because this agent promotes wetting of the ocular surface, both mucin- and aqueous-deficient dry eyes appear to benefit from its use.

A few examples of the most commonly recommended and newer products on the market include Refresh Dry Eye Therapy, which contains glycerin (1%), polysorbate 80 (1%), and castor oil. This product is an oil-in-water emulsion that is believed to supplement the lipid component of the tear film. It provides lubrication for a more prolonged period (it is dosed two or three times daily) and may be supplemented with aqueous artificial tears. It is the vehicle of the prescription product Restasis (cyclosporine 0.05%). Soothe is an artificial tear that contains a lipid restorative layer, which provides a barrier to prevent loss of the aqueous component of the tears.

Systane is a lubricant eyedrop that contains a gelling and polymer system. Hydroxypropyl guar binds to the hydrophobic corneal surface forming a glycocalyx, or gel-like, environment that keeps the demulcent system in contact with the ocular surface for a longer period of time. Systane is said to create an ocular shield, allowing for epithelial repair that promotes patient comfort and relief of symptoms. Optive is a combination of CMC and glycerin, which is believed to help protect the corneal epithelium through an osmotic protective effect.

Studies have shown that formulations of artificial tears without preservatives are less likely than those with preservatives to irritate the ocular surface.[10] Practitioners and patients should be aware, however, that nonpreserved products are recommended to be discarded after being opened.

Most patients with mild cases of dry eye instill drops of artificial tears once or twice per day, typically on arising in the morning and/or before bedtime (Table 28-2).[11] Recommending drops at least twice per day is a good starting point. The viscosity of the drops and amount used can then be adjusted according to the

TABLE 28-2   Administration Guidelines for Eyedrops
1. If you have difficulty telling whether eyedrops have touched your eye surface, refrigerate the solution before instilling it. Do not refrigerate suspensions. Always check the expiration date.
2. Wash hands thoroughly. Wash areas of the face around the eyes. Contact lenses should be removed unless the product is designed specifically for use with contact lenses.
3. Tilt head back.
4. Gently grasp lower outer eyelid below lashes, and pull eyelid away from eye to create a pouch.
5. Place dropper over eye by looking directly at it, as shown in the drawing.

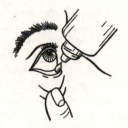

6. Just before applying a single drop, look up.
7. As soon as the drop is applied, release the eyelid slowly. Close eyes gently for 3 minutes by placing your head down as though looking at the floor (using gravity to pull the drop onto the cornea). Minimize blinking or squeezing of the eyelid.
8. Use a finger to put gentle pressure over the opening of the tear duct.
9. Blot excessive solution from around the eye.
10. If multiple medications are indicated, wait at least 5 minutes before instilling the next drop. This pause helps ensure that the first drop is not flushed away by the second, or that the second drop is not diluted by the first.
11. If using a suspension, shake well before instilling. If using the suspension with another dosage form, place the suspension drop last, because it has prolonged retention time in the tear film.
12. If both drop and ointment therapy are indicated, instill the drops at least 10 minutes before the ointment so that the ointment does not become a barrier to the drops' penetrating the tear film or cornea.

patient's response. For more severe cases, the dosage can be increased to three to four times daily. If the patient's clinical needs and response to therapy indicate more frequent use, these solutions may be given as often as hourly. Preservative-free products or those with less-toxic preservatives (e.g., Purite or sodium perborate; see Ophthalmic Preservatives) are preferred in patients with moderate-to-severe dry eye disease.

Use of ocular lubricants requires balancing the number of drops per day, the viscosity of the recommended solution, and the presence of a preservative. As the number of drops per day increases, toxicity from preservatives becomes more likely.[12]

Although PVA is compatible with many commonly used drugs and preservatives, certain compounds (including sodium bicarbonate, sodium borate, the sulfates of sodium, potassium, and zinc) can thicken or gel solutions. For example, sodium borate is found in some extraocular irrigating solutions or irrigants and may react with contact lens wetting solutions containing PVA.[13] Therefore, it is important to be cautious when using solutions that contain PVA.

Nonmedicated Ophthalmic Ointments

The primary ingredients in commercial nonprescription ophthalmic ointments (Table 28-1) are white petrolatum (a lubricant and ointment base), mineral oil (which helps the ointment melt at body temperature), and lanolin (which facilitates incorporation of water-soluble medications and also prevents evaporation).

The principal advantage of nonmedicated (bland) ointments is their enhanced retention time in the eye, which appears to enhance the integrity of the tear film. Therefore, both mucin- and aqueous- deficient eyes can benefit from the application of lubricating ointments.

Ointment formulations are usually administered twice daily (Table 28-3). However, depending on the patient's clinical needs and therapeutic response, ointments may be administered as often as every few hours, or only occasionally as needed. Many patients prefer to instill the ointment at bedtime to keep the eyes moist during sleep and improve morning symptoms of dry eye.

Because of the viscosity of the melted ointment base in the tear film, many patients complain of blurred vision when using ointments. This problem can usually be managed by decreasing the amount of ointment instilled or by administering the ointment at bedtime. The practitioner should routinely counsel the patient about the blurred vision associated with eye ointments.

Ointment preparations are generally nonirritating, but preservatives can be toxic to ocular tissues. Some patients develop hypersensitivity reactions, which may prompt them to discontinue therapy. Changing to preservative-free formulations (e.g., Duratears Naturale, HypoTears, Lacri-Lube N.P., or Refresh PM) can often eliminate symptoms associated with ointment products containing preservatives; preservative-free products are particularly helpful in long-term treatment. As a rule, it is better to recommend nonmedicated ointments without preservatives for the treatment of dry eye to avoid the potential problems associated with preservatives.

Formulation Considerations for Ocular Lubricants and Other Ophthalmic Products

Ocular lubricants and other nonprescription ophthalmic drugs are formulated to reduce the stinging, burning, and other side effects common with some ophthalmic drugs. Carefully controlling the pH, as well as the use of buffers, tonicity adjusters, and

TABLE 28-3   Administration Guidelines for Eye Ointments

1. Wash hands thoroughly. Wash areas of the face around the eyes.
2. If both drop and ointment therapy are indicated, instill the drops at least 10 minutes before the ointment so that the ointment does not become a barrier to the drops' penetrating the tear film or cornea.
3. Tilt head back.
4. Gently grasp lower outer eyelid below lashes, and pull eyelid away from eye as shown in the drawing.

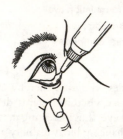

5. Place ointment tube over eye by looking directly at it.
6. With a sweeping motion, place one-fourth to one-half inch of ointment inside the lower eyelid by gently squeezing the tube, but avoid touching the tube tip to any tissue surface.
7. Release the eyelid slowly.
8. Close eyes gently for 1–2 minutes.
9. Blot excessive ointment from around the eye.
10. Vision may be temporarily blurred. Avoid activities that require good visual ability until vision clears.

preservative systems produces a product that is comfortable to use and, therefore, encourages patients to adhere to self-treatment. Drug vehicle and preservative systems are among the most important inactive ingredients of these products. Various other ingredients are often included as excipients.

OPHTHALMIC VEHICLES/OCULAR LUBRICANTS

Ophthalmic vehicles enhance drug action by providing increased viscosity. The greater viscosity of ophthalmic vehicles, compared with aqueous solution vehicles, increases the retention time of the active drug, thereby enhancing its bioavailability at the external ocular tissues. These polymers are generally of high molecular weight. Some of the molecules can even bind to the corneal surface to increase drug retention and stabilize the tear film.

The most commonly used ophthalmic vehicles are CMC, povidone, PVA, HPMC, and poloxamer 407.[14–17] Ointments are also used as vehicles. PVA is a water-soluble viscosity enhancer commonly used in a concentration of 1.4%.[14] HPMC is available in several molecular weights; however, HPMC 0.5% has been shown to exhibit twice the ocular retention time of PVA 1.4%.[16] CMC in concentrations of 0.5% and 1% is also frequently used. The most common complaint associated with these ocular lubricants are caking on the eyelids, and minor ocular irritation and stinging.

Ophthalmic ointments, which are semisolids at room temperature, are produced by mixing white petrolatum and mineral oil with or without a water-miscible agent such as lanolin. The mineral oil in the vehicle allows the ointment to melt at body temperature, whereas the lanolin absorbs water. This formulation allows for the incorporation of water and water-soluble drugs into the delivery system. Commercial ophthalmic ointments are generally derivatives of a mixture of petrolatum 60% USP and mineral oil 40% USP. In general, ointments are well tolerated by the ocular tissues. The primary clinical purpose for an ophthalmic ointment is to increase the ocular contact time of the instilled product. The ocular contact time of an ointment vehicle is about twice as long in the blinking eye and four times as long in the nonblinking or patched eye as that of a saline vehicle. Other commonly used vehicles are dextran 70, gelatin, glycerin, hydroxyethylcellulose, methylcellulose, polyethylene glycol, and propylene glycol.

OPHTHALMIC PRESERVATIVES

Preservatives are incorporated into multidose ophthalmic products. These components are intended to destroy or limit the growth of microorganisms inadvertently introduced into the product. Surfactants, one of two distinct groups of preservatives, are usually bactericidal. These molecules disrupt the bacterial plasma membrane. The other group includes the metals mercury and iodine, their derivatives, and alcohols. Of the quaternary surfactants, benzalkonium chloride (BAK) and benzethonium chloride are preferred by many manufacturers because of their stability, excellent antimicrobial activity, and long shelf life. Unfortunately, these agents have toxic effects on both the tear film and the corneal epithelium.[18,19] Long-term use of topical products containing BAK can damage conjunctival and corneal epithelial cells. Complications associated with BAK include allergy, fibrosis, dry eye syndrome, and increased risk of glaucoma surgery failure.[20] These complications may become problematic for only those using multiple doses per day. Polyquad, a large-molecular-weight quaternary compound, does not bind to contact lenses and is less toxic than BAK.

Chlorhexidine is useful as an antimicrobial agent in the same range of concentrations as BAK, yet it is used at lower concentrations in commercial ophthalmic formulations. Because it does not alter corneal permeability to the same extent as BAK, chlorhexidine is not as toxic to the eye.

Of the mercurial preservatives, patients who become sensitized to thimerosal develop contact blepharitis or conjunctivitis after several weeks of exposure and must discontinue the use of products that contain it. These products are rapidly disappearing from the marketplace.

Chlorobutanol is less effective than BAK as an antimicrobial preservative and, in fact, tends to disappear from bottles during prolonged storage.[14] However, prolonged use of chlorobutanol does not appear to produce allergic reactions. Chlorobutanol is often used in 0.5% concentrations and has both antifungal and antibacterial properties.

Methylparaben and propylparaben, both p-hydroxybenzoic acid derivatives, have a long history of use in some ophthalmic medications, especially artificial tears and nonmedicated ointments. However, these preservatives are unstable at high pH and can sometimes induce allergic reactions.

Ethylenediamine tetraacetic acid (EDTA) is a chelating agent that preferentially binds and sequesters divalent cations. EDTA assists the action of thimerosal, BAK, and other agents. EDTA can sometimes induce contact allergic reactions.[21]

Sodium perborate, which has been used extensively as a tooth-bleaching agent, has found a new use as an ophthalmic preservative. One of two so-called disappearing preservatives, sodium perborate dissociates on contact with the eye to form hydrogen peroxide, which in turn rapidly dissociates to oxygen and water. The amount of hydrogen peroxide formed is so small

that it does not produce eye irritation. Purite (oxychloro complex) is also designed to dissociate on contact with the eye. After exposure to long-wavelength UV light, Purite breaks down quickly to water and sodium chloride. The disappearing preservatives have the advantage of microbial protection while potentially limiting preservative toxicity.

Other, less common ophthalmic preservatives include cetylpyridinium chloride, phenylethyl alcohol, sodium propionate, and sorbic acid.

OPHTHALMIC EXCIPIENTS

Other useful excipients are antioxidants, wetting agents, buffers, and tonicity adjusters. Antioxidants prevent or delay deterioration of products that are exposed to oxygen. Wetting agents reduce surface tension, allowing the drug solution to spread more easily over the ocular surface. Buffers are added to help maintain a pH range of 6.0 to 8.0, thereby preventing ocular discomfort on product instillation. Tonicity adjusters allow the medication to be isotonic with the physiologic tear film. Products in the sodium chloride equivalence range of 0.9% to 1.2% are considered isotonic; they help reduce ocular irritation and tissue damage. Solutions in the tonicity range of 0.6% to 1.8% are usually comfortable when placed on the human eye. Hypertonic solutions used for corneal edema are not well tolerated.

Product Selection Guidelines

In recent years, artificial tear preparations have been introduced in preservative-free formulations and, more recently, in so-called disappearing preservative formulations. These preparations are beneficial for patients who are sensitive to preservatives such as BAK and thimerosal, those who use drops frequently, and/or those with compromised corneas. Three solution products, Genteal (mild-moderate-severe), Refresh Liquigel, and Refresh Tears, and two lubricant gels, Genteal Lubricant Eye Gel (mild-moderate-severe) and Tears Again Gel, are uniquely formulated to allow the preservative to rapidly dissociate into nontoxic components on the ocular surface. True preservative-free artificial tear preparations (e.g., Bion Tears, Celluvisc, HypoTears, and Refresh Plus) are available in a variety of unit-dose dispensers, and some of these products are formulated to provide electrolyte support to the damaged surface epithelium of the eye. Preservative-free formulations are not only more expensive than preserved artificial tear solutions, they are easily contaminated by the patient during use. Therefore, patients must follow strict hygienic procedures for self-administration and should discard any unused solution according to the manufacturer's guidelines.

Although a benefit of ophthalmic lubricant therapy is to increase the viscosity of existing tears, high viscosity alone does not necessarily provide relief for all dry eye conditions. Methylcellulose, in a concentration of 0.25% to 1.0%, was the primary cellulose ether in the first artificial tear solutions. Most contemporary artificial tear solutions incorporate other less viscous substituted cellulose ethers, especially CMC, hydroxyethylcellulose, and hydroxypropylcellulose. The latter ethers, which have emollient properties equal or superior to those of methylcellulose, can also be combined with other polymers such as PVA or povidone for use as artificial tears. PVA is generally used in a 1.4% concentration and is considerably less viscous than methylcellulose.

Clinical results and patient acceptance remain the final criteria for determining a product's efficacy in the treatment of patients with dry eye. Importantly, no single formulation has yet been identified that will universally improve clinical signs and symptoms while maintaining patient comfort and acceptance.[12,13] If there is no response after use of multiple artificial tear products, the patient should be encouraged to seek professional assessment and care from an ophthalmic practitioner.

ALLERGIC CONJUNCTIVITIS

Pathophysiology and Clinical Presentation of Allergic Conjunctivitis

The list of antigens that can cause ocular allergy is virtually endless, but the most common allergens include pollen, animal dander, and topical eye preparations. Patients with ocular allergy will often report seasonal allergic rhinitis as well. Allergic conjunctivitis is characterized by a red eye with watery discharge (see Color Plates, photograph 4). The hallmark symptom accompanying ocular allergy is itching. Vision is usually not impaired but may be blurred because of excessive tearing. Contact lenses should not be used until the condition resolves.[22]

Treatment of Allergic Conjunctivitis

Treatment Goals

The goals in treating allergic conjunctivitis are to (1) remove or avoid the allergen, (2) limit or reduce the severity of the allergic reaction, (3) provide symptomatic relief, and (4) protect the ocular surface.

General Treatment Approach

Questioning the patient about exposure to allergens may help identify the offending substance. Removal or avoidance of the responsible allergen is the best treatment, but nonprescription ocular lubricants, ocular decongestants, ocular decongestant/ antihistamine preparations, ocular antihistamines/mast cell stabilizers, and oral antihistamines, and cold compresses will help relieve symptoms.

Nonpharmacologic Therapy

In addition to removing and/or avoiding exposure to the offending allergen, applying cold compresses to the eyes three to four times per day will help reduce redness and itching. Avoidance of allergic response is also important such as checking the pollen count, keeping doors and windows closed, running air conditioning, using air filters, and so on.

Pharmacologic Therapy

The first-line treatment of allergic conjunctivitis is to instill artificial tears as needed (see Treatment of Dry Eye). If symptoms persist, the patient should switch to an ophthalmic antihistamine/ mast cell stabilizer product. Approval of reclassification of the prescription product to nonprescription status has been a very favorable improvement for the treatment of allergic conjunctivitis. Ketotifen fumarate 0.025% (Zaditor, Alaway) is very safe and can be used in persons 3 years and older; it is dosed twice daily and is very effective in relieving the signs and symptoms of allergic conjunctivitis. An oral antihistamine can still be added to the

second regimen if needed. Medical referral is indicated if symptoms do not resolve.

Nonprescription ophthalmic products designated specifically for treatment of allergic conjunctivitis include decongestants, antihistamines, combinations of the two agents, and more recently the antihistamine/mast cell stabilizer combination. (See Chapter 11 for discussion of systemic nonprescription antihistamines.)

Ophthalmic Decongestants/ Alpha-Adrenergic Agonists

Four decongestants are available in nonprescription strength for topical application to the eye: phenylephrine, naphazoline, tetrahydrozoline, and oxymetazoline (Table 28-4). In nonprescription ophthalmic products, phenylephrine is available in a concentration of 0.12% or less. Higher concentrations of phenylephrine (2.5% and 10%) are prescription products and are used for pupillary dilation. Naphazoline, tetrahydrozoline, and oxymetazoline are chemically classified as imidazoles. As Table 28-4 shows, these agents are available as solutions in a variety of concentrations.

Phenylephrine acts primarily on alpha-adrenergic receptors of the ophthalmic vasculature to constrict conjunctival vessels, thereby reducing eye redness. The higher-concentration, prescription-only products that contain this agent are generally reserved for the short-term dilation needed for eye examinations. Similar to phenylephrine, the imidazoles have greater alpha- than beta-receptor activity and are, therefore, clinically useful in constricting conjunctival blood vessels. These agents have only minimal effect on the underlying vessels of the episclera and sclera. Naphazoline has been shown to be effective in constricting conjunctival vessels as well as in reducing tearing and pain associated with superficial ocular inflammation.[23] Satisfactory results have also been obtained with tetrahydrozoline in most patients with allergic or chronic conjunctivitis. Topical treatment with oxymetazoline will improve most symptoms associated with allergic or noninfectious conjunctivitis, including burning, itching, tearing, and foreign body sensation.

See Table 28-5 for dosages of ophthalmic decongestants.

When used as directed, ocular decongestants generally do not induce ocular or systemic side effects. However, their availability to and use in children should be carefully monitored. Ingestion of these products can result in coronary emergencies and death. Ocular decongestants have the potential for producing rebound conjunctival hyperemia, allergic conjunctivitis, and allergic blepharitis when used excessively or long term.[24] Rebound congestion appears to be less likely with topical ocular use of naphazoline or tetrahydrozoline than with oxymetazoline or phenylephrine. Rebound congestion may be experienced within a few days of initiating treatment, although a case was reported within 8 hours.[24] Patients with apparent rebound congestion should be referred to an eye care practitioner for differential diagnosis and management.

Indiscriminate use of decongestants in an irritated eye can induce papillary dilation and precipitate angle-closure glaucoma in eyes that have narrow anterior chamber angles. Use of these products in angle-closure glaucoma is contraindicated, and practitioners should counsel patients with angle-closure glaucoma against using these products in treating allergic conjunctivitis.

Some patients may experience epithelial xerosis (abnormal dryness) from prolonged topical instillation of ocular decongestants, which may exacerbate the symptoms of irritation, pain, and dryness associated with allergic conjunctivitis.

Ocular decongestants should be used cautiously by patients with systemic hypertension, arteriosclerosis, other cardiovascular

TABLE 28-4 More Commonly Used Ophthalmic Products Containing Decongestants, Antihistamines, and/or Astringents

Trade Name	Primary Ingredients
Decongestant Eyedrop Products	
All Clear	Naphazoline 0.012%; PEG 300, 0.2%; BAK 0.01%; EDTA
All Clear AR	Naphazoline 0.03%; BAK 0.01%; hydroxypropyl methylcellulose 0.5%; EDTA
Allerest	Naphazoline 0.012%; BAK; EDTA
Clear Eyes	Naphazoline HCl 0.012%; glycerin 0.2%; BAK
Clear Eyes ACR	Naphazoline 0.012%; BAK; EDTA; zinc sulfate 0.25%; glycerin 0.2%
Murine Tears Plus	Tetrahydrozoline HCl 0.05%; povidone 0.6%; PVA 0.5%; BAK
Naphcon	Naphazoline HCl 0.012%; BAK 0.01%
Opti-Clear	Tetrahydrozoline 0.05%; BAK 0.01%; boric acid; EDTA; sodium borate; NaCl
Relief[a]	Phenylephrine; PVA 1.4%; EDTA
Tetrasine Extra	Tetrahydrozoline 0.05%; PEG 1.0%, 400; EDTA; BAK
Visine Advanced Relief	Tetrahydrozoline HCl 0.05%; PEG 400, 1.0%; povidone 1.0%; BAK 0.01%; dextran 70, 1.0%
Visine L.R.	Oxymetazoline HCl 0.025%; BAK 0.01%
Visine Moisturizing	Tetrahydrozoline HCl 0.05%; BAK 0.01%; EDTA; hydroxypropyl methylcellulose 0.5%
Visine Original	Tetrahydrozoline HCl 0.05%; BAK 0.01%
Vision Clear	Tetrahydrozoline 0.05%; BAK 0.01%; boric acid; EDTA; sodium borate; NaCl
Antihistamine/Mast Cell Stabilizer Eyedrop Products	
Zaditor and Alaway	Ketotifen 0.025%; BAK 0.01%; glycerol; sodium hydroxide and/or hydrochloric acid; purified water
Antihistamine/Decongestant Eyedrop Products	
Naphcon A	Pheniramine maleate 0.3%; naphazoline HCl 0.025%; BAK 0.01%
Opcon-A	Pheniramine maleate 0.315%; naphazoline HCl 0.02675%; hydroxypropyl methylcellulose 0.5%; BAK 0.01%
Vasocon A	Antazoline phosphate 0.5%; naphazoline HCl 0.05%; BAK 0.01%
Visine-A	Pheniramine maleate 0.3%; naphazoline HCl 0.025%; BAK 0.01%
Decongestant/Astringent Eyedrop Products	
Clear Eyes ACR	Naphazoline HCl 0.012%; zinc sulfate 0.25%; glycerin 0.2%; BAK
Visine Allergy Relief	Tetrahydrozoline HCl 0.05%; zinc sulfate 0.25%; BAK 0.01%
Zincfrin	Phenylephrine HCl 0.12%; zinc sulfate 0.25%; BAK 0.01%

Key: BAK, benzalkonium chloride; EDTA, ethylenediamine tetraacetic acid; PEG, polyethylene glycol; PVA, polyvinyl alcohol.
[a] Preservative-free formulation.

TABLE 28-5 Dosage Guidelines for Ophthalmic Decongestants and Antihistamines

Agent	Nonprescription Concentration (%)	Dosage	Duration of Action (hours)	Duration of Use
Decongestant Products				
Phenylephrine	0.12	1–2 drops up to 4 times/day	0.5–1.5	72 hours
Naphazoline	0.1, 0.12, 0.02, 0.03	1–2 drops up to 4 times/day	3–4	72 hours
Oxymetazoline	0.025	1–2 drops every 6 hours	4–6	72 hours
Tetrahydrozoline	0.05	1–2 drops every 4 hours	1–4	72 hours
Antihistamine/Mast Cell Stabilizer				
Ketotifen	0.025	1 drop every 8–12 hours	8–12	>72 hours
Decongestant/Antihistamine Products				
Naphazoline/pheniramine	0.025 (naphazoline) 0.3 (pheniramine)	1–2 drops 3–4 times/day	3–4	72 hours
Naphazoline/antazoline	0.05 (naphazoline) 0.5 (antazoline)	1–2 drops 3–4 times/day		72 hours

diseases, or diabetes. Adverse cardiovascular events are also possible when these agents are used in patients with hyperthyroidism.[25] Because of these possible adverse reactions, patients should not use phenylephrine and other ocular decongestants as ocular irrigants. Women should use ocular decongestants sparingly, if at all, during pregnancy. Storage of solutions at high temperatures may cause ocular reactions and severe mydriatic responses to instillation. If offending ophthalmic signs or symptoms do not resolve within 72 hours, the patient should see an eye care practitioner.

Ophthalmic Antihistamines and Ophthalmologic Antihistamines/Mast Cell Stabilizers

Two nonprescription antihistamines are available for topical ophthalmic use: pheniramine maleate and antazoline phosphate. Although these antihistamines are effective by themselves, nonprescription products containing them also contain a decongestant. The two combinations are pheniramine/naphazoline and antazoline/naphazoline (Table 28-4).

Pheniramine and antazoline are in different antihistamine classes, but both act as specific histamine₁-receptor antagonists.[26,27] Topical antihistamines are used for rapid relief of symptoms associated with seasonal or atopic conjunctivitis. Using a decongestant with the topical antihistamines has been shown to be more effective than using either agent alone.[23,28] The Food and Drug Administration (FDA) has classified topical antihistamines as less than effective, primarily because clinical trial data on effectiveness are lacking.

Ketotifen fumarate is an ophthalmic antihistamine and mast cell stabilizer. It produces very potent H₁-receptor-antagonist activity, thereby preventing acute histamine-mediated allergy symptoms. The mast cell stabilization activity inhibits mast cell degranulation, preventing the release of inflammatory mediators including histamine. Ketotifen also inhibits eosinophils, thereby inhibiting the release of late phase mediators. The advantages of these products are that they provide relief within minutes, the effects may last up to 12 hours from a single dose, and they do not contain a vasoconstrictor. Therefore, they are very safe product with no concerns for vasoconstrictor overuse.

See Table 28-5 for dosages of the antihistamine combination products.

Burning, stinging, and discomfort on instillation are the most common side effects of ophthalmic antihistamines.[29–33]

Ophthalmic antihistamines have anticholinergic properties and may cause pupil dilation. This effect is most commonly seen in people with light-colored irides or compromised corneas, such as contact lens wearers.[34] In susceptible patients, pupil dilation can lead to angle-closure glaucoma. Therefore, these drugs are contraindicated in people with a known risk of angle-closure glaucoma.[35] Sensitivity to one of the components is another contraindication to the use of products containing topical antihistamines.

Product Selection Guidelines

Ketotifen is the safest and most effective product for the treatment of allergic conjunctivitis. It is the largest improvement in the nonprescription market place for allergic eye disease in many years. The twice-daily dosing and the safety of this product for children ages 3 years and older make it the primary therapy for patients with signs and symptoms of allergic conjunctivitis.

Although decongestant and antihistamine ophthalmic products have product-to-product comparisons available, it is difficult

to reach definitive conclusions regarding clinical comparisons of the available nonprescription ocular decongestants. The concentration 0.02% is an excellent choice for nonprescription therapy of mild-to-moderate conjunctivitis of environmental, viral, or noninfectious origin.

Because rebound congestion appears to be less likely following topical ocular use of naphazoline or tetrahydrozoline, these agents should generally be recommended over phenylephrine or oxymetazoline.

Complementary Therapies

The homeopathic product known as Similasan Eye Drops #2 is indicated for relief from itching and burning caused by allergic reactions. The active homeopathic ingredients are Apis, Euphrasia, and Sabadilla. The efficacy of this formulation has not been established in controlled clinical trials.

VIRAL CONJUNCTIVITIS

Pathophysiology and Clinical Presentation of Viral Conjunctivitis

Viral conjunctivitis ("pink eye") is the most common form of conjunctivitis. This condition is highly contagious and poses a significant health problem in schools and workplaces where touch contamination from contaminated fingers, medical instruments, and so on is poorly controlled. A recent cold, sore throat, or exposure to someone with viral conjunctivitis is a common precursor of this condition. Patients with viral conjunctivitis will usually have a pink eye with a copious amount of watery discharge (see Color Plates, photograph 5). Symptoms include an acute red eye, watery discharge, and conjunctival swelling. Less common symptoms include nonspecific ocular discomfort and a mild-to-moderate sensation of a foreign object in the eye, photophobia, and blurred vision. It may be contagious for about 1 week. Low-grade fever may be present, and swollen preauricular or submandibular lymph nodes may be found. If the etiology of the conjunctivitis is not clear, the patient should be referred to an eye care practitioner. Intense eye pain probably indicates trauma to the cornea and requires immediate referral to an eye care practitioner to rule out a corneal abrasion.

Treatment of Viral Conjunctivitis

Treatment Goals

The goal in treating viral conjunctivitis is to relieve symptoms while the infection runs its course.

General Treatment Approach

Viral conjunctivitis is usually self-limiting, with symptoms resolving within 1 to 3 weeks. Artificial tear preparations and ocular decongestants may be used for symptomatic relief for blurred vision.[36] Because certain forms of viral conjunctivitis can be extremely contagious, strict adherence to proper hygienic measures is also important. Cold compresses may be helpful in providing symptomatic relief.

Nonpharmacologic Therapy

Patients with viral conjunctivitis should wash their hands after touching an infected eye and properly dispose of tissues used to blot an infected eye. They should also avoid sharing towels or other objects that might come in contact with the infected eye. Patients should avoid wearing contact lenses or possibly replace them after having viral conjunctivitis.

Pharmacologic Therapy

See Treatment of Dry Eye, Pharmacologic Therapy section for discussion of artificial tear preparations and ocular decongestants.

CORNEAL EDEMA

Pathophysiology and Clinical Presentation of Corneal Edema

Corneal edema may occur from a variety of conditions, including overwear of contact lenses, surgical damage to the cornea, and inherited corneal dystrophies. The edematous area of the cornea is often confined to the epithelium. Because fluid accumulation distorts the optical properties of the cornea, halos or starbursts around lights (with or without reduced vision) are a hallmark symptom of corneal edema. An eye care practitioner must diagnose this disorder.

Treatment of Corneal Edema

Treatment Goals

The goal in treating corneal edema is to draw fluid from the cornea, thereby relieving the associated symptoms.

General Treatment Approach

Once the initial diagnosis is established, patients can use topical hyperosmotic formulations to treat corneal edema. Of the topical ophthalmic hyperosmotic agents available, only sodium chloride can be obtained without a prescription in both solution and ointment formulations (Table 28-6). Sodium chloride is available as a 2% or 5% solution, and as a 5% ointment. First-line treatment is instillation of a 2% solution four times per day. If symptoms persist, nighttime use of a 5% hyperosmotic ointment should be added to the regimen. If symptoms do not respond to the augmented treatment, the patient should switch to a 5% hyperosmotic solution and continue nighttime use of the ointment. If symptoms still persist, medical referral is necessary.

Pharmacologic Therapy

Hyperosmotics

Hyperosmotic agents increase the tonicity of the tear film, promoting movement of fluid from the cornea to the more highly osmotic tear film. Normal tear flow mechanisms then eliminate the excessive fluid. Many patients with mild-to-moderate corneal epithelial edema may experience improved subjective comfort and vision following appropriate use of these medications.

Usually, the patient instills one or two drops of the solution every 3 to 4 hours (Table 28-2). The ointment formulation, however, requires less frequent instillation and is usually reserved for use at bedtime to minimize symptoms of blurred vision (Table 28-3). Because vision associated with edematous corneas is often worse on awakening, several instillations of the solution during the first few waking hours may be helpful.

In general, sodium chloride 5% in ointment form is the most effective in reducing corneal edema and improving vision, but it tends to cause stinging and burning. For that reason, patients often prefer the 2% solution for long-term therapy. Hypertonic saline is nontoxic to the external ocular tissues, and allergic reactions are rare.

The most important contraindication to topical hyperosmotic sodium chloride is its use to clear edematous corneas with traumatized epithelium. The intact corneal epithelium permits only limited permeability to inorganic ions; therefore, an absent or compromised corneal epithelium will result in increased corneal penetration of the hyperosmotic product, reducing its osmotic effect. Consequently, the management of corneal edema associated with traumatized epithelium requires the use of organic hyperosmotic agents that are available by prescription only.[37] Patients whose history or physical appearance suggests a damaged corneal epithelium should be referred to an eye care practitioner immediately. Patients must be informed never to prepare homemade saline solutions for use in the eye because of the risk of infection.

LOOSE FOREIGN SUBSTANCES IN THE EYE

Pathophysiology and Clinical Presentation of Loose Foreign Substances in the Eye

Despite the protective effect of the lids, foreign substances often contact the ocular surface. The immediate response of the eye is watering (tearing). If the substance causes only minor irritation and does not abrade the eye surface, self-treatment is appropriate.

Treatment of Loose Foreign Substances in the Eye

Treatment Goals

The goal in treating loose foreign substances in the eye is to remove the irritant by irrigating the eye. Known foreign substances from wood or metal fragments should be treated promptly by an eye care practitioner owing to the potential for penetrating injuries.

General Treatment Approach

If reflex tearing does not remove the foreign substance, the eye may need to be flushed. Lint, dust, and similar materials can usually be removed by rinsing the eye with sterile saline or specific eyewash preparations (irrigants).[38] Outside of a medical setting, in the case of loose particles and chemical exposures to the eyes, the eyes should be flushed with copious amounts of water from a sink faucet or a garden hose.

TABLE 28-6 More Commonly Used Miscellaneous Ophthalmic Products

Trade Name	Primary Ingredients
Irrigant Solutions	
Blinx	NaCl; KCl; sodium phosphate; BAK 0.005%; EDTA 0.02%
Collyrium for Fresh Eyes	Boric acid; sodium borate; BAK
Bausch and Lomb Eye Wash	Sodium borate; boric acid; NaCl; sorbic acid 0.1%; EDTA 0.025%
Eye Stream	Sodium acetate 0.39%; sodium citrate 0.17%; sodium hydroxide and/or hydrochloric acid; BAK
Eye Wash	NaCl; sodium phosphate dibasic; sodium phosphate monobasic; EDTA; preserved with benzalkonium chloride in purified water
Irrigate Eye Wash	NaCl; mono- and dibasic sodium phosphate; EDTA; BAK
Optigene	NaCl; mono- and dibasic sodium phosphate; EDTA; BAK
Visual-Eyes	NaCl; mono- and dibasic sodium phosphate; BAK; EDTA
Hyperosmotics	
AK-NaCl Solution	NaCl 5%; methylparaben 0.023%; propylparaben 0.017%
AK-NaCl Ointment[a]	NaCl 5%; lanolin oil; mineral oil; white petrolatum
Muro 128 Solution 2%	NaCl 2%; hydroxypropyl methylcellulose 2906; methylparaben 0.046%; propylparaben 0.02%; propylene glycol; boric acid
Muro 128 Solution 5%	NaCl 5%; boric acid; hydroxypropyl methylcellulose 2910; propylene glycol; methylparaben 0.023%; propylparaben 0.01%
Muro 128 Ointment[a]	Mineral oil; white petrolatum; lanolin
Eyelid Scrubs	
Eye Scrub Solution	Polyethylene glycol 200 glyceryl monotallowate; disodium laureth sulfosuccinate; cocoamido-propylamine oxide; polyethylene glycol 78 glyceryl monococoate; benzyl alcohol; EDTA
Lid Wipes-SPF Pads	Polyethylene glycol 200 glyceryl monotallowate; polyethylene glycol 80 glyceryl cocoate; laureth-23; cocoamidopropylamine oxide; NaCl; glycerin
OcuSoft Solution and Pads	Polyethylene glycol 80 sorbitan laureth; sodium trideceth sulfate; cocoamidopropyl hydroxysulftaine; polyethylene glycol 150 distearate; lauroamphocarboxyglycinate; sodium laureth-13 carboxylate; polyethylene glycol 15 tallow polyamine; quaternium-15
Prosthesis Lubricant/Cleaner	
Enuclene Solution	Tyloxapol 0.25%; hydroxypropyl methylcellulose 0.85%; BAK 0.02%
SteriLid Eyelid Cleanser	Water; PEG-80; sorbitan laurate; sodium trideceth sulfate

Key: BAK, benzalkonium chloride; EDTA, ethylenediamine tetraacetic acid; PEG, polyethylene glycol.

[a] Preservative-free formulation.

Pharmacologic Therapy

Ocular Irrigants

An ocular irrigant is used to cleanse ocular tissues while maintaining their moisture; these solutions must be physiologically balanced with respect to pH and osmolality. Because the tissues that the irrigant contacts obtain nutrients elsewhere, the role of irrigants is primarily to clear away unwanted materials or debris from the ocular surface. Patients should use ocular irrigants on only a short-term basis to reduce risk of contamination and should be sure that no other ocular pathology is being missed. All ophthalmic irrigating solutions are available without a prescription (Table 28-6).

In the ophthalmic practitioner's office, irrigating solutions come in handy following certain clinical procedures, and they are often used to wash away mucous or purulent exudates from the eye. They are also administered in the hospital to clean out eyes between changes of ocular dressings.

Ocular irrigants should not be used for open wounds in or near the eyes. Although irrigating solutions may be used to wash out the eyes after contact lens wear, they have no particular value as contact lens wetting, cleansing, or cushioning solutions.

If the patient experiences continuous eye pain, changes in vision, or continued redness or irritation of the eye, or the ocular condition persists or worsens, evaluation by an eye care practitioner should be strongly encouraged. Irrigants may be packaged with an eyecup. Because contamination of the eyecup is possible, it should not be used to rinse the eye.

MINOR EYE IRRITATION

Pathophysiology and Clinical Presentation of Minor Eye Irritation

Nonallergic, minor eye irritation can be caused by a loose foreign substance in the eye; contact lens wear; or exposure of the eye to wind, sun (e.g., snow skiing without protective eye goggles), smog, chemical fumes, or chlorine. Redness of the eye is a common sign of minor irritation. In cases of snow blindness, other burns from UV light, or arc welder's burns, pain and the feeling of "sand in the eyes" are additional common symptoms.

Treatment of Minor Eye Irritation

Minor irritation often responds well to artificial tear solutions or nonmedicated ointments (see Treatment of Dry Eye).

Zinc sulfate, a mild astringent, may be recommended for temporary relief of minor ocular irritation. The dosage is one to two drops up to four times daily.

The homeopathic product known as Similasan Eye Drops #1 is marketed to relieve dryness and redness caused by smog, contact lenses, and other causes. The active homeopathic ingredients are Belladonna, Euphrasia, and Mercurius sublimatus. Controlled clinical trials have not demonstrated the efficacy of this formulation in the treatment of this condition.

CHEMICAL BURN

Pathophysiology and Clinical Presentation of Chemical Burn

Chemical burns may occur from exposure to alkali (e.g., oven cleaners, cement, or lye), acids (e.g., battery acid or vinegar), detergents, and various solvents and irritants (e.g., tear gas or mace). Burns may range from mild to severe depending on the inciting agent and/or exposure time. Patients complain of pain, irritation, photophobia, and tearing. Signs vary depending on the severity. Less severe signs include superficial punctate keratitis (small pinpoint loss of epithelial cells in the cornea), perilimbal ischemia, chemosis, hyperemia, eyelid edema, hemorrhages, and first- or second-degree burns of the lid and outer skin. More severe signs include corneal edema and opacification, anterior chamber inflammation, increased IOP, and retinal toxicity from scleral penetration. Alkali burns are more penetrating and potentially more damaging to eye tissues than acid burns. Alkali burns are often more resistant to irrigation and have greater tissue destruction when they penetrate into the deeper (stromal) layers of the cornea. If the burns are more superficial and just several layers of the corneal epithelium are affected, the cells should be replenished within approximately 24 hours.

Treatment of Chemical Burn

Emergent treatment includes immediate copious irrigation with sterile saline (Table 28-6) or even tap water if nothing else is available. It cannot be stressed enough that irrigation must be continued until an eye care practitioner can be seen. If irrigation is stopped prematurely, the pH of the tear film may revert back to either acidic or alkaline because of residual material that may still be under the lid or in the inferior cul-de-sac. Further treatment after irrigation may include the use of cycloplegic agents, topical antibiotics, and analgesics. In more severe cases, topical steroids are sometimes used if significant inflammation of the anterior chamber or cornea is present. Antiglaucoma medications are also used if the IOP is elevated. Follow-up by the eye care practitioner is required to prevent conjunctival adhesions and corneal complications. Chemical burns are considered ophthalmic emergencies and should be immediately referred to an eye care practitioner or emergency department.

ARTIFICIAL EYES

Besides the obvious esthetic benefits, clearing dried mucus or fluid secretions from the surfaces of artificial eyes eliminates a potential medium for bacterial growth. A sterile isotonic buffered solution containing tyloxapol 0.25% and BAK 0.02% is available especially for cleaning and lubricating ophthalmic prostheses. The primary method of preventing bacterial growth is routine hygiene with mild, nonallergenic soap and water.

Tyloxapol is a surfactant that softens solid matter on the prosthesis, and BAK aids tyloxapol in wetting the artificial eye. The solution is used in the same manner as ordinary artificial tears. With the artificial eye in place, one or two drops of solution should be applied three or four times daily. In addition, the solution can be used as a cleaner to remove oily or mucous deposits; in this case, the artificial eye is then rubbed between the fingers and rinsed with tap water before reinsertion.

MACULAR DEGENERATION

Age-related macular degeneration (AMD) is the leading cause of blindness in the United States. It takes two forms: neovascular (wet or bleeding) and atrophic (dry). Presently, there is no definitive "cure" for AMD, and research into the etiology and possible cure of the disease is being pursued vigorously. Until a cure is found, the treatments used are aimed at slowing the rate of progression and extent of visual loss.

Treatment of the neovascular form is limited by side effects and a substantial risk for the development of hemorrhagic macular degeneration, requiring continual follow-up care and medical treatment by an ophthalmologist. Currently, it is believed that antioxidants plus zinc therapy may provide some benefit in the dry or atrophic form of the disease. It is not well-known if the antioxidants would have a benefit in wet macular degeneration. Animal models have shown that oxidative mechanisms play a role in the development of both forms of this disorder. Human studies have indicated a general inverse association with antioxidant levels.[39]

Beta-carotene (a specific vitamin A analogue), ascorbic acid (vitamin C), and tocopherol (vitamin E), as well as the trace elements zinc and selenium, have been implicated as possibly helpful in reducing progression of the disorder.[39,40] The most definitive results on antioxidant therapy to date came from the Age-Related Eye Disease Study (AREDS) report of 2001. These researchers concluded that patients older than 55 years with moderate or advanced AMD, or vision loss caused by AMD in one eye, and without contraindications (e.g., smoking history) would benefit from taking antioxidants plus zinc. The recommended doses of these antioxidants are vitamin C 500 mg, vitamin E 400 IU, beta-carotene 15 mg, zinc oxide 80 mg, and cupric oxide 2 mg.[41] In addition, dietary factors lutein and zeaxanthin (related to beta-carotene) are factors that may potentially be associated with a reduced risk of advanced AMD.[42] These two factors were not part of the original AREDS study. The AREDS II study is underway to evaluate the effects of high supplemental doses of dietary xanthophylls (lutein and zeaxanthin) and omega-3 long-chain polyunsaturated fatty acids such as DHA (docosahexaenoic acid) and EPA (eicosapentaenoic acid) on the development of advanced AMD. The study will also investigate the effects of these supplements on cataract and moderate vision loss, and whether reducing zinc in the original AREDS formulation will have an effect on development and progression of AMD.

The possible benefit of antioxidants in treating this disorder has led to the development of numerous nonprescription oral ophthalmic preparations containing these vitamins. However, only one product containing these ingredients is recommended by the AREDS study (Ocuvite PreserVision). Because other treatment options are limited and side effects are rare, eye care practitioners frequently recommend these products to their patients diagnosed with AMD.

These products are generally taken twice daily and are usually well tolerated, with gastrointestinal side effects rarely reported (see Chapter 23). Practitioners should make sure that ophthalmic vitamin products are not taken in conjunction with other multivitamin supplements, which could possibly lead to hypervitaminosis.

CONTACT DERMATITIS

Pathophysiology and Clinical Presentation of Contact Dermatitis

Contact dermatitis of the eyelid can be a reaction to either an allergen or an irritant. Causes of contact dermatitis include a change in cosmetics or soap, exposure to eye medications, or contact with other foreign substances. The involvement of both eyelids suggests allergy because both eyes are often exposed. Common symptoms include swelling, scaling, or redness of the eyelid along with profuse itching. Sunburns of the eyelids and ultraviolet burns to the cornea (e.g., recent sun exposure without eye protection from beach or ski outings) should be ruled out.

Treatment of Contact Dermatitis

Questioning the patient about use of eye medications or new products (e.g., eyeliner or eye shadow) may quickly identify the offending substance. Discontinuing use of the suspected products is the best treatment. If swelling of the eyelid is marked, nonprescription oral antihistamines along with cold compresses applied three to four times per day will help reduce the inflammation and itching.

LICE INFESTATION OF THE EYELID

Pathophysiology and Clinical Presentation of Lice Infestation of the Eyelid

Infestation of the eyelids with the organisms *Phthirus pubis* (crab louse) or *Pediculus humanus capitis* (head louse) may cause symptoms similar to blepharitis (i.e., red, scaly, thickened eyelids). These organisms are also responsible for sexually transmitted lice infestation. Children are rarely affected by the crab louse but are commonly affected by the head louse. Ocular disease is often treated by eye care physicians.

Treatment of Lice Infestation of the Eyelid

Frequent (four to five times daily) cleaning with a mild soap and water and the use of a bland (nonmedicated) ophthalmic ointment (e.g., petrolatum) for 10 days are the recommended self-treatment. The ointment suffocates the louse and deprives its eggs of adequate oxygen to hatch. Practitioners should carefully instruct patients about the need to take appropriate hygienic measures, such as washing clothing and bedding that may contain unhatched eggs. Lice shampoo products cannot be used on the eyelids.

BLEPHARITIS

Pathophysiology and Clinical Presentation of Blepharitis

Blepharitis is an external common inflammatory condition with an accumulation of debris along the eyelid margins. The most commonly associated factors are *Staphylococcus epidermidis, Staphylococcus aureus,* and seborrheic dermatitis or a combination of these.[43] Red, scaly, thickened eyelids (often with loss of the eyelashes), mild foreign body sensation, and crusting of the eye upon waking are typical signs of blepharitis. Itching and burning are the most common complaints. All forms of blepharitis tend to be chronic, and onset can occur in childhood with periods of exacerbation and remission; therefore, individuals are often aware of their diagnosis.

Treatment of Blepharitis

Treatment Goals

The goals in treating blepharitis are to (1) control the disorder with good eyelid hygiene and (2) provide symptomatic relief.

General Treatment Approach

Careful and diligent eyelid hygiene is the mainstay of therapy for the many forms of blepharitis. The chronic nature of blepharitis makes the use of careful eyelid hygiene preferable to the long-term use of topical antibiotics. Ocular lubricants can be used if eye irritation is also present (see Treatment of Dry Eye). Some clinicians are recommending the use of oral omega-3 oils to help restore normal lid Meibomian gland function.

Good eyelid hygiene involves the use of warm compresses for 15 to 20 minutes, two to four times daily. Each application of a compress should be followed by lid scrubs, using a mild detergent cleanser compatible with the ocular tissues, which helps loosen crusts in the eyelids.

Pharmacologic Therapy

Lid Scrubs

Lid scrub procedures are usually effective and well tolerated. Table 28-7 provides instructions on how to perform lid scrubs. This procedure can also be used for hygienic eyelid cleansing in

TABLE 28-7 Administration Guidelines for Eyelid Scrubs

1. Wash hands thoroughly.
2. Apply 3–4 drops of baby shampoo or eyelid cleanser to cotton-tipped applicator or gauze pad.
3. Close one eye. Clean the upper eyelid and eyelashes using side-to-side strokes, being careful not to touch the eyeball with applicator or fingers.
4. Open eye, look up, and clean lower eyelid and eyelashes using side-to-side strokes.
5. Repeat the procedures on the other eye using a clean applicator or gauze pad.
6. Rinse eyelids and eyelashes with clean, warm water.

people who wear contact lenses. Eyelid cleansers are commercially available. However, cleansers for lid scrubs can be made from various brands of "no more tears" baby shampoos (e.g., Johnson and Johnson's) by mixing one-fourth teaspoonful of shampoo in 1 cup of tepid warm water, mixing the solution to a bubbly froth, and scrubbing the lids with a clean, cotton-tipped applicator. Lids should be rinsed thoroughly after each cleaning. Although this approach is acceptable, the commercially available cleansers are equally effective, and patients may experience less ocular stinging and burning with their use.[44]

Commercial lid scrub products are specifically intended for the removal of oils, debris, or desquamated skin associated with the inflamed eyelid (Table 28-6). Some commercial products are packaged with gauze pads, which provide an abrasive action to augment the cleansing properties of the detergent solution.

Eyelid scrubs using commercially available detergents are most effective in patients with noninfectious blepharitis. If the patient's signs or symptoms fail to improve, the patient should be referred to an eye care practitioner.

HORDEOLUM AND CHALAZION

Pathophysiology and Clinical Presentation of Hordeolum and Chalazion

By definition, a hordeolum (stye) is an infection of one of the glands of the eyelid. An internal hordeolum is an infection of the Meibomian glands, whereas an external hordeolum is an infection of the glands of Zeis and Moll (Figure 28-1). There is often lid margin redness and some minor pain associated with styes. A palpable, tender nodule is always present. Swelling of the eyelid, almost to the point of closure, can occur with a severe internal hordeolum. The cause is invariably one of the staphylococcal species associated with blepharitis.

By definition, a chalazion is not infectious and may involve one of the lid glands or may be located near (but not on) the eyelid (see Color Plates, photograph 6). A chalazion, which is a sterile granuloma, is very similar in appearance to an internal hordeolum. However, a chalazion is not tender to gentle touching, whereas a hordeolum is typically quite tender.

It is important to be aware that basal cell carcinoma on the eyelid may present as a nodule with a white, pearl-like appearance, and carcinoma of a sebaceous gland may be black in appearance, with loss of cilia (eyelashes), neovascularization, and/or bleeding. Patients who have an ocular nodule with these symptoms should see an eye care practitioner for evaluation.

Treatment of Hordeolum and Chalazion

A hordeolum typically responds well to warm compresses applied three to four times daily for 5 to 10 minutes. Gentle pressure, applied by rolling the compress gently around the affected area, is recommended. A fresh, clean compress should be used with each treatment. Clearing usually occurs within 1 week. An external hordeolum may be treated with a topical antibiotic; however, an internal hordeolum does not respond well to such treatment and is best treated with a course of oral antibiotics. Surgical drainage may be required in recalcitrant cases. The nonprescription homeopathic product Stye may offer some relief for pain, swelling, and redness, although there is little clinical evidence to support these effects.

Warm compresses applied in the same manner are usually sufficient to drain a chalazion. If either type of nodule does not drain within 1 week or has been present chronically, medical referral is appropriate. Periodic use of lid scrubs may reduce the recurrences of chalazion and hordeolum (Table 28-7). Chalazia may or may not resolve and are often a cosmetic problem, but they have been associated with changes in visual acuity when they occur on the eyelid margin.

ASSESSMENT OF OPHTHALMIC DISORDERS: A CASE-BASED APPROACH

For patients who have not seen an eye care practitioner, the pharmacist or primary care practitioner must determine whether the ophthalmic disorder is self-treatable or requires medical referral. The practitioner must also take great care in assessing a patient with a new, acute problem. Ocular inflammation and irritation can be caused by many conditions, some of which can be treated safely and effectively with nonprescription ophthalmic products. These products are used primarily to relieve minor symptoms of burning, stinging, itching, and watering. FDA has suggested that self-treatment may be indicated for tear insufficiency, corneal edema, and external inflammation or irritation. Self-treatment may also be effective in managing hordeolum (stye), blepharitis, and allergic and viral conjunctivitis.

Cases 28-1 and 28-2 are examples of the assessment of patients with ophthalmic disorders.

Table 28-8 describes the major features of disorders that require medical referral. Any self-treated condition that does not resolve within a reasonably short time should be referred to an eye care practitioner for care.

PATIENT COUNSELING FOR OPHTHALMIC DISORDERS

Before counseling a patient, the practitioner should carefully consider the nature and extent of ocular involvement. It is important that patients with acute ocular disease receive a prompt, definitive

Relevant Evaluation Criteria	Scenario/Model Outcome
Information Gathering	
1. Gather essential information about the patient's symptoms, including:	
a. description of symptom(s) (i.e., nature, onset, duration, severity, associated symptoms)	Patient has suffered from allergies over the past couple of weeks this spring. She currently is taking a systemic nonsedating OTC antihistamine, loratadine 10 mg, but is still having ocular symptoms. Her ocular irritation and dry eye symptoms are definitely affecting her day-to-day activities. She is willing to do anything to cure the problem.
b. description of any factors that seem to precipitate, exacerbate, and/or relieve the patient's symptom(s)	Symptoms appeared about the same time as last year, at the start of spring. Patient started her loratadine last year and did fine. This year, however, her eyes are itchy, red, and dry, and her eyelids are swollen, even though her systemic complaints seem under control. The dryness and ocular irritation began prior to the allergy season.
c. description of the patient's efforts to relieve the symptoms	The decongestant eyedrops to get the "red out" do not appear to give her any relief from her ocular symptoms.
2. Gather essential patient history information:	
a. patient's identity	May Wong
b. patient's age, sex, height, and weight	49-year-old female; 5 ft 6 in, 125 lb
c. patient's occupation	Full-time employee, mother of two
d. patient's dietary habits	Normal healthy diet with occasional social drinking; works out on tread mill 4 times weekly
e. patient's sleep habits	Stays up late and sleeps in as allotted by her schedule
f. concurrent medical conditions, prescription and nonprescription medications, and dietary supplements	Loratadine 10 mg once daily for seasonal allergies (spring and fall), glucosamine capsules 2 times daily, aspirin 75 mg daily, tetrahydrozoline eyedrops 3–4 times daily in both eyes
g. allergies	Pollen and some plants, otherwise NKA
h. history of other adverse reactions to medications	None
i. other (describe) _____	N/A
Assessment and Triage	
3. Differentiate the patient's signs/symptoms and correctly identify the patient's primary problem(s).	Patient is experiencing exacerbation of seasonal allergy. This is the first year she has complaints of ocular irritation and dryness; some complaints have occurred a little earlier than expected.
4. Identify exclusions for self-treatment (see Table 28-8 and Figure 28-2).	None
5. Formulate a comprehensive list of therapeutic alternatives for the primary problem to determine if triage to a medical practitioner is required, and share this information with the patient.	Options include: (1) Refer Mrs. Wong to an eye care specialist (optometrist or ophthalmologist). (2) Suggest that Mrs. Wong discontinue her topical decongestant eyedrops and switch to ketotifen topical drops twice daily. (3) Recommend an OTC artificial tear. (4) Take no action.
Plan	
6. Select an optimal therapeutic alternative to address the patient's problem, taking into account patient preferences.	The patient prefers to discontinue her decongestant drops, and start the artificial tear product and the new ocular antihistamine.
7. Describe the recommended therapeutic approach to the patient.	Instill 1 drop of the ketotifen eyedrops twice daily in both eyes, as described in Table 28-2. Supplement throughout the day with the artificial tear product as much as you desire; however, wait at least 5 minutes after instilling the ketotifen eyedrops.
8. Explain to the patient the rationale for selecting the recommended therapeutic approach from the considered therapeutic alternatives.	Seeing an eye care physician may not be necessary if you follow the administration guidelines in Table 28-2.

CASE 28-1 (continued)

Relevant Evaluation Criteria	Scenario/Model Outcome
Patient Education	
9. When recommending self-care with nonprescription medications and/or nondrug therapy, convey accurate information to the patient:	
a. appropriate dose and frequency of administration	See Tables 28-4 and 28-5.
b. maximum number of days the therapy should be employed	See Table 28-5.
c. product administration procedures	See Table 28-2.
d. expected time to onset of relief	See Table 28-5.
e. degree of relief that can be reasonably expected	Complete symptom control should be possible. It is likely that some minor symptoms may occasionally appear.
f. most common side effects	Burning, stinging, and discomfort on instillation
g. side effects that warrant medical intervention should they occur	Worsening eye pain and continued redness
h. patient options in the event that condition worsens or persists	An eye doctor should be consulted if the condition does not improve or if irritation and pain become intolerable.
i. product storage requirements	Store under room temperature and away from heat and light. Observe product expiration date.
j. specific nondrug measures	Remove and/or avoid exposure to the offending allergen, for example check the pollen count, keep doors and windows closed, run air conditioning, use air filters, and so on.
	Applying cold compresses to the eyes 3–4 times per day to help reduce redness and itching.
10. Solicit follow-up questions from patient.	(1) May I use the drops that I was using previously to get the red out if my eyes still bother me?
	(2) Also, my spouse has eyedrops (Tobradex) that he used previously, and they seemed to help him very quickly. May I try his eyedrops?
11. Answer patient's questions.	(1) No. The get-the-red-out eyedrops actually can cause more ocular redness (rebound) and eye dryness.
	(2) The Tobradex drops (steroid and antibiotic) can cause significant eye complications such as secondary infection, glaucoma, and cataract.

Key: N/A, not applicable; NKA, no known allergies; OTC, over-the-counter.

CASE 28-2

Relevant Evaluation Criteria	Scenario/Model Outcome
Information Gathering	
1. Gather essential information about the patient's symptoms, including:	
a. description of symptom(s) (i.e., nature, onset, duration, severity, associated symptoms)	Patient has suffered from allergies for years. The allergies flare up every spring and fall. She does occasionally have trouble wearing her contact lenses during this time period because of ocular irritation and dryness. Once in while, she will stop wearing her lenses if the eye irritation is bothersome, but that doe not occur often. Usually she gets pretty good relief by just taking OTC Zyrtec.

Relevant Evaluation Criteria	Scenario/Model Outcome
	Although her eyes occasionally get a little dry, just using the contact lens rewetting solution usually does the trick. However, she fell asleep with her contacts in and had a little too much to drink at dinner. She remembers her eyes were irritating her and she rubbed them quite a bit before she fell asleep. She woke up with red irritated eyes, especially the right eye. She is experiencing some distorted vision and a little sensitivity to light in that right eye.
b. description of any factors that seem to precipitate, exacerbate, and/or relieve the patient's symptom(s)	This time of the year, around spring, her symptoms seem to get worse.
c. description of the patient's efforts to relieve the symptoms	Taking the OTC antihistamine seems to help, as does the rewetting solution.
2. Gather essential patient history information:	
a. patient's identity	Sofia Castillo
b. patient's age, sex, height, and weight	24-year-old female, 5 ft 6 in, 135 lb
c. patient's occupation	Sales representative
d. patient's dietary habits	Balanced diet, with occasional junk food and alcohol
e. patient's sleep habits	Averages 6 hours per night
f. concurrent medical conditions, prescription and nonprescription medications, and dietary supplements	Zyrtec 1 tablet every 24 hours as needed for allergy symptoms, omega-3 capsules 2 times daily
g. allergies	NKA
h. history of other adverse reactions to medications	None
i. other (describe) _____	Ms. Costillo has had only minor problems with her contacts over the years, even with her allergies. She usually receives good response to the rewetting drops for occasional dry eye.
	She wants to try some OTC drops to get the red out, because she is not getting any relief, and now the eye pain and ocular discomfort are getting worse. She is complaining of more redness and pain in the right eye. She also has trouble trying to open that eye because of the sensitivity to light and tearing.

Assessment and Triage

3. Differentiate the patient's signs/symptoms and correctly identify the patient's primary problem(s).	The symptoms in the right eye differ from those she has experienced in the past with her allergies, contact lenses, and use of rewetting solution. It seems the symptoms, especially the increased tearing and sensitivity to light, are getting worse.
4. Identify exclusions for self-treatment (see Table 28-8 and Figure 28-2).	When a patient complains of sensitivity to light and/or blurry vision, especially with pain, they must be referred to an eye care practitioner.
5. Formulate a comprehensive list of therapeutic alternatives for the primary problem to determine if triage to a medical practitioner is required, and share this information with the patient.	Options include: (1) Immediately refer patient to an eye care practitioner (optometrist or ophthalmologist) for a differential diagnosis. (2) Recommend an OTC decongestant eyedrop or the new antihistamine/mast cell stabilizer eyedrop ketotifen, and tell patient to remove her contact lenses for a few hours. (3) Take no action.

Plan

6. Select an optimal therapeutic alternative to address the patient's problem, taking into account patient preferences.	Refer the patient to an eye care specialist immediately for a differential diagnosis.
7. Describe the recommended therapeutic approach to the patient.	N/A
8. Explain to the patient the rationale for selecting the recommended therapeutic approach from the considered therapeutic alternatives.	You need to see an eye doctor, because OTC eyedrops are not appropriate to treat a potentially blinding infection.

CASE 28-2 (continued)

Relevant Evaluation Criteria	Scenario/Model Outcome
Patient Education	
9. When recommending self-care with nonprescription medications and/or nondrug therapy, convey accurate information to the patient.	Criterion does not apply in this case.
10. Solicit follow-up questions from patient.	Eye doctors are expensive. Is there an OTC eye medication that might work?
11. Answer patient's questions.	No OTC eye medications are approved and/or appropriate to recommend for your problem. You may have a corneal ulcer and that would require aggressive topical prescription antibiotic eyedrops—and maybe even hospitalization. Corneal ulcers left untreated may cause ocular complications, including corneal scarring, perforations, and even eye transplant.

Key: N/A, not applicable; NKA, no known allergies; OTC, over-the-counter.

TABLE 28-8 Differentiation of Ophthalmic Disorders That Require Medical Referral

Disorder	Potential Signs/Symptoms	Complications	Treatment Approach
Blunt trauma	Ruptured blood vessels, bleeding into eyelid tissue space, swelling, ocular discomfort, facial drooping	Internal eye bleeding, secondary glaucoma, detached retina, periorbital bone fracture (blowout fracture)	Medical referral is appropriate.
Foreign particles trapped/embedded in the eye	Reddened eyes, profuse tearing, ocular discomfort	Corneal abrasions/scarring, chronic red eye, interocular penetration from metal striking metal at high speeds	Medical referral for removal of particles is appropriate.
Ocular abrasions	Partial/total loss of corneal epithelium, blurred vision, profuse tearing, difficulty opening the eye	Risk of bacterial/fungal infection if eye exposed to organic material, corneal scarring, anterior chamber rupture	Medical referral is appropriate.
Infections of eyelid/eye surface	Red, thickened lids; scaling	Scarring of lids, dry eye, corneal abrasion or scarring, loss of vision	Medical referral is appropriate.
Eye exposure to chemical splash, solid chemical, or chemical fumes	Reddened eyes, watering, difficulty opening eye	Scarring of eyelids and eye surface, loss of vision	To prevent/reduce scarring of eyelids from chemical burns, flush eye immediately for at least 10 minutes, preferably with sterile saline/water. If neither is available, flush with tap water. After flushing eye, arrange immediate transportation to an emergency facility. No recommendation is noted for chemical neutralization.
Thermal injury to eye (welder's arc)	Reddened eyes, pain, sensitivity to light	Corneal scarring, secondary infection	Medical referral for definitive care, including possible eye patching, is appropriate.
Bacterial conjunctivitis	Reddened eyes with purulent (mucous) discharge, ocular discomfort, eyelids stuck together on awakening	Typically self-limiting in 2 weeks	Medical referral for treatment with topical antibiotics to clear infection more quickly; some infections require systemic antibiotic treatment.
Chlamydial conjunctivitis	Watery or mucous discharge, ocular discomfort, low-grade fever, possible blurred vision	Scarring	If infection with *Chlamydia* sp. is known or suspected, or if symptoms are too vague to rule in viral or allergic conjunctivitis, medical referral is mandatory.

diagnosis, including baseline visual acuity, before the practitioner considers the appropriateness of nonprescription therapy. Some acute conditions, which may or may not involve ocular pain or blurred vision, can be appropriately treated with nonprescription agents, but a recent diagnosis from an ophthalmic practitioner can give additional reassurance and confidence in recommending such treatment. Although the cost-effectiveness of ophthalmic care can be greatly improved through the use of nonprescription agents, severe visual impairment, including blindness, can be a serious clinical and medicolegal complication if the practitioner delays referral for definitive diagnosis and treatment. After careful consideration of the history, the practitioner should always counsel patients on the indications for and limitations of self-treatment. The algorithms in Figures 28-2 and 28-3 can assist the practitioner in recommending the appropriate treatment for disorders of the eye surface and eyelid, respectively.

Numerous nonprescription ophthalmic products for treating minor ocular irritations are available for self-administration by the patient with minimal or no supervision. Such products are also adequate for treating certain clinical conditions diagnosed by primary care providers or eye care practitioners. First-line therapy should always include counseling on nonpharmacologic treatment. These treatments alone are frequently sufficient to relieve the ocular symptoms or are necessary as an adjunct to the ophthalmic drug therapy. Proper drug instillation technique is critical if the target tissue (the eye) is to receive the maximum benefit from the medication. Ophthalmic solutions and ointments, as well as eyelid scrubs, are often used incorrectly. By carefully instructing patients in the proper self-administration procedures, the practitioner can help ensure maximum safety and effectiveness of these agents. Appropriate patient education and counseling must accompany dispensing of any ophthalmic product.

Although drug side effects and interactions are rare with topically applied ophthalmic products, the potential for such effects does exist. Therefore, the practitioner should advise the patient of possible adverse effects, including the clinical signs of drug toxicity or allergy.

The practitioner must actively assist patients in selecting the appropriate product that will enhance compliance, minimize or avoid side effects, and reduce the attendant costs of therapy. The other major considerations in making therapeutic recommendations are whether the person has a sensitivity to one of the product constituents, the product can be used with contact lenses, and the product has the potential to wash out prescription ophthalmic drugs the patient may be using. With the exception of ophthalmic antihistamines and decongestants, little product-to-product comparative research has been done for nonprescription ophthalmic preparations. The practitioner must, therefore, make therapy recommendations based on the patient's diagnosis and the products the patient is currently using. The box Patient Education for Ophthalmic Disorders lists specific information to provide patients.

EVALUATION OF PATIENT OUTCOMES FOR OPHTHALMIC DISORDERS

Patients who self-treat allergic conjunctivitis, loose foreign substances in the eye, or minor eye irritation should see an eye care practitioner if the symptoms persist after 24 hours of treatment. Those who are self-treating viral conjunctivitis should seek med-

ical care if vision loss occurs or symptoms persist after 96 hours of treatment. Dry eye is often a chronic disorder, requiring continuous treatment with ophthalmic lubricants. Patients with this disorder should be advised to seek medical care if the symptoms worsen despite diligent self-treatment. Patients with corneal edema should consult an eye care practitioner if the symptoms persist or worsen despite adherence to the instructions for treating the disorder.

The treatment period for eyelid disorders differs considerably. Patients with lice infestation of the eyelids should see an eye care practitioner if symptoms persist after 10 days of treatment. If the nodule of a hordeolum/chalazion is not drained after 1 week of treatment, the patient should seek medical care. Recurrent episodes of hordeolum/chalazion in the same area or gland require evaluation by an eye care practitioner. Symptoms of contact dermatitis should resolve quickly once the offending substance is removed. If symptoms persist after 72 hours of antihistamine use, the patient should see an eye care practitioner. Blepharitis usually requires chronic treatment. Patients with diagnosed blepharitis should self-treat the disorder daily as described in Treatment of Blepharitis but seek medical care if symptoms worsen.

KEY POINTS FOR OPHTHALMIC DISORDERS

➤ The pharmacist is positioned in the community to treat patients with ophthalmic pathology or to recommend self-management with one or more nonprescription drugs.

➤ Many ophthalmic products are available to manage the symptoms of minor acute or chronic conditions of the eye and eyelid.

➤ By understanding the pathophysiology of certain ocular conditions and knowing how to assess patients who present with such conditions, a pharmacist should be able to optimize the safe, appropriate, effective, and economical use of nonprescription drugs to manage selected conditions of the eye and eyelid.

➤ Nonprescription ophthalmic products should be used in only cases of minor pain or discomfort. If doubt exists concerning the nature of the problem, the practitioner should refer the patient for professional care.

➤ Nonprescription ocular medications should not be recommended to patients who have demonstrated an allergy to any of the active ingredients, preservatives, or other excipients in the product.

➤ Patients who already are using a prescription ophthalmic product should use nonprescription products only after consulting with an ophthalmic practitioner or pharmacist.

➤ Patients with narrow anterior chamber angles or narrow-angle glaucoma should not use topical ocular decongestants because of the risk of angle-closure glaucoma.

➤ Drug administration should be conservative in patients with hyperemic conjunctiva because of the potential for increased systemic drug absorption and the risk of adverse effects.

➤ The lowest concentration and conservative dosage frequencies should be used, especially for ocular decongestants, and overuse should be avoided.

➤ Ophthalmic products frequently are used incorrectly; therefore, counseling on appropriate application of products is crucial.

Patient with reddening of eye surface

↓

Determine signs & symptoms or events that preceded/accompany the disorder

---

Exclusions for Self-Treatment

- Eye pain
- Blurred vision not associated with use of ophthalmic ointments
- Sensitivity to light
- History of contact lens wear
- Blunt trauma to eye
- Chemical exposure to eye
- Eye exposure to heat, excluding sun exposure
- Symptoms that have persisted for >72 hours

Exclusions for self-treatment (see box)? —**Yes**→ Immediate referral to eye care practitioner (see Table 28-8 for first-aid measures for chemical exposure)

↓ **No**

Eyes burn, sting, itch & water? Gritty sensation, but no foreign material present? —**Yes**→ Dry eye suspected. Avoidance of situations that cause tear evaporation. Use of OTC agents determined by degree of discomfort

↓ **No**

Mild discomfort → Low-viscosity artificial tears 1-2x/day. Follow up in 1 week

Moderate discomfort → Low-viscosity artifical tears 3-4x/day, or switch to high-viscosity solution. Follow up in 1 week

Severe discomfort → Nonpreserved artifical tears used every hour if needed + nighttime use of ophthalmic ointment. Follow up in 1 week

↓

Symptoms worsen despite diligent treatment? —**Yes**→ Refer to eye care practitioner

↓ **No**

Continue therapy as needed

Eyes burn, sting, itch & water? Patient history of "pink eye" exposure, cold, or flu? —**Yes**→ Viral conjunctivitis suspected. Hygienic measures (see box Patient Education for Ophthlamic Disorders) + as-needed use of artificial tears. If needed, ophthalmic decongestant + nighttime use of ointment. Follow up in 96 hours → Symptoms persist or vision loss has occurred? —**Yes**→ (to Refer to eye care practitioner)

↓ **No**

Go to next page

Symptoms persist or vision loss has occurred? ↓ **No** → D/C therapy

---

FIGURE 28-2 Self-care of eye surface disorders. Key: AH, antihistamine; D/C, discontinue; MSC, mast cell stabilizer; OTC, over-the-counter. *(continued on next page)*

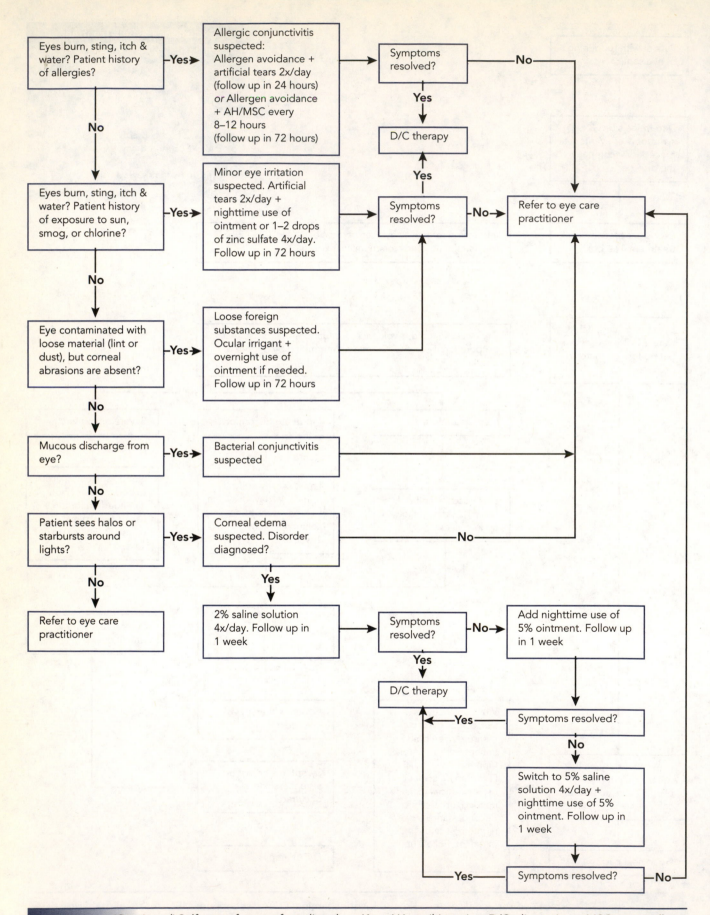

FIGURE 28-2 *(Continued)* Self-care of eye surface disorders. Key: AH, antihistamine; D/C, discontinue; MSC, mast cell stabilizer; OTC, over-the-counter.

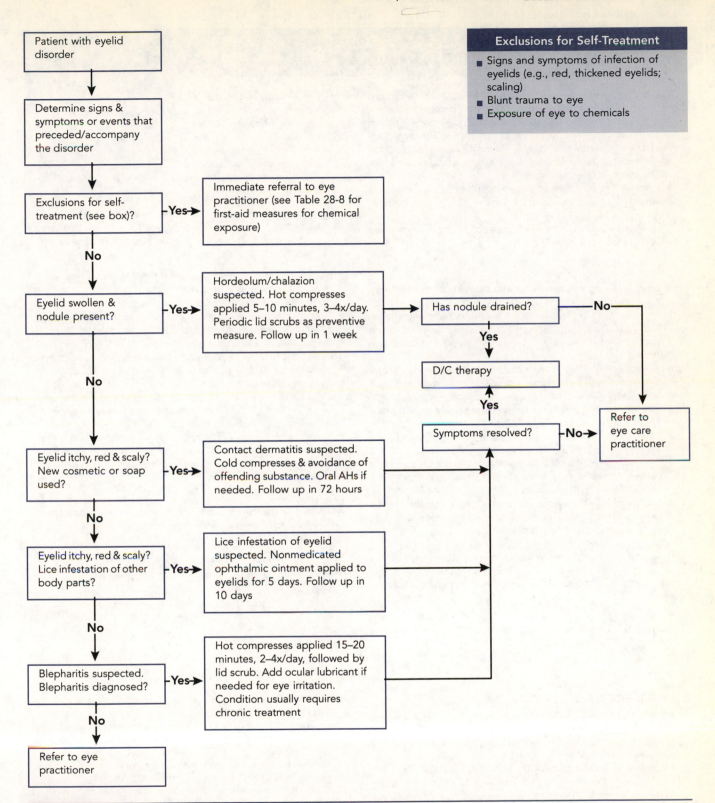

FIGURE 28-3 Self-care of eyelid disorders. Key: AH, antihistamine; D/C, discontinue.

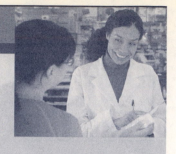

PATIENT EDUCATION FOR
Ophthalmic Disorders

The objectives of self-treatment are to (1) relieve the symptoms of minor ophthalmic disorders using the appropriate nonprescription products or nondrug measures and (2) use nonprescription products as adjunctive treatment of ophthalmic disorders diagnosed by an eye care practitioner. For most patients, carefully following product instructions and the self-care measures listed here will help ensure good outcomes.

■ Remove the causative ocular agent/irritant that predisposes you to your ocular condition or disease.

 If *blunt trauma* to the eye occurs, obtain an eye examination as soon as possible.

■ If you have *dry eye syndrome* and the first ophthalmic lubricants used to treat it are not effective, ask your eye care practitioner or a pharmacist about the following treatment options: increasing the dosage, switching to a product with increased viscosity, and/or switching to a preservative-free product (see Table 28-1).

■ When treating *allergic conjunctivitis,* do not exceed the recommended dosages of ophthalmic antihistamine/mast cell stabilizer, decongestant, or antihistamine/decongestant products (see Tables 28-4 and 28-5). Consult an eye care practitioner if symptoms persist after 72 hours of treatment.

■ When treating *viral conjunctivitis,* wash your hands after touching the infected eye and properly dispose of tissues used to blot the infected eye. Do not share towels or other objects that might come in contact with the infected eye. Consult an eye care practitioner if symptoms persist after 72 hours of treatment.

■ Discard or replace eyedrop bottles 30 days after the sterility safety seal is opened. The manufacturer's expiration date does not apply once the seal is broken.

 If *eye exposure to chemicals* occurs, irrigate the eye continuously for 10 minutes with copious amounts of water or eye irrigants (see Table 28-6) and seek immediate eye care.

■ If *loose foreign substances* such as lint, dust, or pollen enter the eye, flush the substance from the eye using an eye irrigant or water (see Tables 28-6).

 If a *foreign substance* becomes embedded in the eye or trapped under the eyelid, see an eye care practitioner. Failure to remove the substance could cause an eye infection or tissue damage.

 Consult an eye care practitioner before treating *corneal edema.* If hyperosmotic solutions (see Table 28-6) are recommended, follow the recommended dosages even though the product may sting.

■ Note that taking ophthalmic vitamin supplements for macular degeneration along with general multivitamins may result in gastrointestinal upset or vitamin toxicity.

■ For the treatment of *chronic blepharitis,* maintain lid hygiene with the regular use of lid scrubs (see Tables 28-6 and 28-7).

■ Do not *treat lice infestations of the eyelids* with pediculicides (lice products); use regular lid hygiene and a nonmedicated ointment for 10 days instead (see Tables 28-1 and 28-3).

■ If *contact dermatitis of the eyelid* occurs, wash the affected areas, identify the cause of the reaction, and try to avoid future contact with the substance. Consult an eye care practitioner if symptoms persist after 72 hours of use of oral antihistamines.

■ To clear a *hordeolum* or *chalazion,* apply hot compresses three to four times daily for 5 to 10 minutes at each session. Consult an eye care provider if the disorder persists after 1 week of treatment.

 Pearl-like or black nodules with loss of eyelashes and bleeding require immediate evaluation by an eye care specialist to rule out carcinoma (cancer).

 If the disorder persists or worsens after the recommended length of therapy, consult an eye care provider.

REFERENCES

1. Schein OD, Munoz B, Tielsch JM, et al. Prevalence of dry eye among the elderly. *Am J Ophthalmol.* 1997;124:723–8.
2. Warwick R. In: *Anatomy of the Eye and Orbit.* 7th ed. Philadelphia: WB Saunders; 1975:195–219.
3. Milder B. The lacrimal apparatus. In: Moses RA, Hart WM, eds. *Adler's Physiology of the Eye.* 8th ed. St Louis: Mosby; 1987:15–35.
4. Mishima S, Gasset A, Klyce SO, et al. Determination of tear volume and tear flow. *Invest Ophthalmol.* 1966;3:264–76.
5. Jordan A, Baum J. Basic tear flow. Does it exist? *Ophthalmology.* 1980;9:920–30.
6. Harris LS, Galin MA. Dose response analysis of pilocarpine–induced ocular hypotension. *Arch Ophthalmol.* 1970;1:605–8.
7. Pfister RR, Burstein N. The effects of ophthalmic drugs, vehicles, and preservatives on corneal epithelium; a scanning electron microscope study. *Invest Ophthalmol.* 1976;15:246–59.
8. Stern ME, Beurman RW, Fox RI, et al. The pathology of dry eye: the interaction between the ocular surface and lacrimal glands. *Cornea.* 1998; 17:584–9.

9. Norn MS. Desiccation of the precorneal film, I: corneal wetting time. *Acta Ophthalmol.* 1969;47:865–80.
10. Lopez–Bernal D, Ubels JL. Quantitative evaluation of the corneal epithelial barrier effect: effect of artificial tears and preservatives. *Curr Eye Res.* 1991;7:645–66.
11. Swanson M. Compliance with and typical usage of artificial tears in dry eye conditions. *J Am Optom Assoc.* 1998;69:649–55.
12. Berdy GJ, Abelson MB, Smith LM, et al. Preservative free artificial tear solutions. *Arch Ophthalmol.* 1992;110:528–32.
13. Pensyl CD. Lubricants and other preparations for ocular surface disease. In: Bartlett JD, Jaanus SD, eds. *Clinical Ocular Pharmacology.* 4th ed. Boston: Butterworth-Heinemann; 2001:315–32.
14. Schilling H, Koch JM, Waubke TN, et al. Treatment of dry eye with vitamin A acid: an impression cytology controlled study. *Fortschr Ophthalmol.* 1989;5:530–4.
15. Mullen W, Sheppard W, Leibowitz J. Ophthalmic preservatives and vehicles. *Surv Ophthalmol.* 1973;17:469–83.
16. Sabiston DW. The dry eye. *Trans Ophthalmol Soc N Z.* 1969;21:96–100.
17. Linn ML, Jones LT. Rate of lacrimal excretion of ophthalmic vehicles. *Am J Ophthalmol.* 1968;65:76–8.

18. Fiscella R, Burstein NL. Ophthalmic drug formulations. In: Bartlett JD, Jaanus SD, eds. *Clinical Ocular Pharmacology*. Boston: Butterworth-Heinemann; 2001:19–40.

19. Burstein NL. Preservative cytotoxic threshold for benzalkonium chloride and chlorhexidine digluconate in cat and rabbit corneas. *Invest Ophthalmol Vis Sci*. 1980;19:308–13.

20. Debbasch C, Brignole F, Pisella P-J, et al. Quarternary ammoniums and other preservatives, contribution in oxidative stress and apoptosis on chang conjunctival cells. *Invest Ophthalmol Vis Sci*. 2001;42:642–52.

21. Wilson WS, Duncan AJ, Jay JL. Effect of benzalkonium chloride on the stability of the precorneal tear film in rabbit and man. *Br J Ophthalmol*. 1975;59:667–9.

22. Mondino BJ, Salamon SM, Zaidman GW. Allergic and toxic reactions in soft contact lens wearers. *Surv Ophthalmol*. 1982;26:337–44.

23. Miller J, Wolf EM. Antazoline phosphate and naphazoline hydrochloride, singly and in combination for the treatment of allergic conjunctivitis—a controlled double-blind clinical trial. *Ann Allergy*. 1975;35:81–6.

24. Soparkar CN, Wilhelmus KR, Koch DD, et al. Acute and chronic conjunctivitis due to over-the-counter ophthalmic decongestants. *Arch Ophthalmol*. 1997;115:34–8.

25. Portello JK, Jaanus SD. Mydriatics and mydriolytics. In: Bartlett JD, Jaanus SD, eds. *Clinical Ocular Pharmacology*. 4th ed. Boston: Butterworth-Heinemann; 2001:135–48.

26. Jaanus SD. Antiallergy drugs and decongestants. In: Bartlett JD, Jaanus SD, eds. *Clinical Ocular Pharmacology*. 4th ed. Boston: Butterworth-Heinemann; 2001:299–314.

27. Krupin T, Silverstein B, Faitt M, et al. The effect of H1 blocking antihistamines on intraocular pressure in rabbits. *Ophthalmology*. 1980;87:1167–72.

28. Abelson MB, Allansmith MR, Freidlaender MH. Effects of topically applied ocular decongestant and antihistamine. *Am J Ophthalmol*. 1980;90:254–7.

29. Petrusewicz J, Kalizan R. Blood platelet adrenoreceptor: aggregatory and antiaggregatory activity of imidazole drugs. *Pharmacology*. 1986;33:249–55.

30. Pahissa A, Guardia J, Botil JM, et al. Antazoline induced allergic pneumonitis. *BMJ*. 1979;2:1328.

31. Bengtsson U, Larsson O, Lindstedt G, et al. Antazoline induced immune hemolytic anemia, hemoglobulinuria, and acute renal failure. *Acta Med Scand*. 1975;198:223–7.

32. Neilsen JL, Dahl R, Kissmeyer-Neilsen F. Immune thrombocytopenia due to antazoline. *Allergy*. 1981;36:517–9.

33. Ogbuihi S, Audick W, Bohn G. Sudden infant death-fatal intoxication with pheniramine. *Z Rechtsmed*. 1990;103:221–5.

34. Berdy GJ, Abelson MB, George MA, et al. Allergic conjunctivitis—a survey of new antihistamines. *J Ocul Pharmacol*. 1991;7:313–24.

35. Gelmi C, Occuzzi R. Mydriatic effect of ocular decongestants studied by pupillography. *Ophthalmologica*. 1994;208:243–6.

36. Abelson MB, Yamamoto GK, Allansmith MR. Effects of ocular decongestants. *Arch Ophthalmol*. 1980;98:856–8.

37. Lamberts DW. Topical hyperosmotic agents and secretory stimulants. *Int Ophthalmol Clin*. 1980;20:163–9.

38. Hales RH. Contact lens solutions. In: *Contact Lenses: A Clinical Approach to Fitting*. Baltimore: Williams & Wilkins; 1978:32–50.

39. Christen WG. Antioxidant vitamins and age-related eye disease. *Proc Assoc Am Phys*. 1999;111:16–21.

40. Sperduto RD, Ferris FL, Kurinij N. Do we have a nutritional treatment for age-related cataract or macular degeneration? *Arch Ophthalmol*. 1990;108:1403–5.

41. Age-Related Eye Disease Study Research Group. A randomized, placebo-controlled, clinical trial of high-dose supplementation with vitamins C and E, beta carotene, and zinc for age-related macular degeneration and vision loss. *Arch Ophthalmol*. 2001;119:1417–36.

42. Marse-Perlman JA, Fisher AI, Klein R, et al. Lutein and zeaxanthin in the diet and serum and their relation to age-related maculopathy in the Third National Health and Nutrition Examination Survey. *Am J Epidem*. 2001;153:424–32.

43. Jones DB, Liesegang TJ, Robinson NM. Laboratory diagnosis of ocular infections. Paper presented at the Annual Meeting of the American Society for Microbiology, Washington, DC; May 26–30, 1981.

44. Polack FM, Goodman DF. Experience with a new detergent lid scrub in the management of chronic blepharitis. *Arch Ophthalmol*. 1988;106:719–20.

Prevention of Contact Lens–Related Disorders

Janet P. Engle

The greatly enhanced comfort of soft contact lenses over hard lenses, introduced in the 1970s, led to a significant expansion of the contact lens market. Rigid gas permeable (RGP) lenses provide improved comfort and safety in comparison with older polymethylmethacrylate (PMMA)-based hard lenses. Continuous-wear lenses, toric lenses for astigmatism, tinted lenses, bifocal contact lenses, and disposable lenses have also greatly expanded the patient population who can successfully wear contact lenses.

Although much of the motivation to wear contact lenses may be cosmetic, properly fitted lenses can provide significant vision advantages over eyeglasses. Of the more than 36 million Americans currently wearing contact lenses, nearly 90% use the lenses to correct the vision of an otherwise healthy eye. Contact lenses reduce size distortion and prismatic effects, improve peripheral vision, and can enable improved acuity in patients with irregular acuity. Elimination of spectacle fogging, dirt accumulation, and frame distraction are also significant advantages to many users. Most patients who wear soft contact lenses say their lenses are more comfortable than eyeglasses. Of the almost 3 million patients who stop wearing their lenses every year, the most commonly cited reason is lens discomfort. Proper care and fitting of lenses can help eliminate discomfort and encourage patients to continue wearing their lenses.

It has been well established that contact lenses, even when expertly fitted, somewhat alter ocular tissues and change the corneal metabolism. Therefore, it is imperative that both the user and the health care professional understand the proper care, maintenance, and safe use of these products. Failure to do so can greatly increase the chance of corneal infection, corneal ulcers, and other ocular conditions that may result in permanent eye damage and blindness. Fortunately, most complications from contact lens wear are reversible if attended to promptly.

More than 100 nonprescription contact lens care products are available, and consumers are likely to be overwhelmed by the variety. Other than the lens prescriber, pharmacists are the most accessible health care professionals to counsel contact lens wearers which products to choose. Selection depends on the product compatibility with each other as well as with the specific contact lens. Therefore, the pharmacist's responsibility is to understand this area of professional practice and provide effective, up-to-date information when consulting with the contact lens wearer.

Use of Contact Lenses

Most people can wear one or more types of contact lenses without problems if certain precautions are taken. In a few cases, use of contact lenses is contraindicated.

Indications for Contact Lenses

The decision to wear contact lenses rather than eyeglasses is sometimes based on therapeutic necessity. For example, in patients with keratoconus, a corneal dystrophy causing a gradual protrusion of the central cornea, satisfactory vision is usually unattainable with ordinary eyeglasses but can be enabled with use of rigid contact lenses. Other examples of therapeutic necessity are collagen lenses used to provide a "bandage" effect and soft contact lenses saturated with antibiotic agents for sustained release.

Aphakic patients, patients who do not have an intraocular lens, characteristically see better with contact lenses than with spectacles. Continuous-wear contacts are particularly beneficial for such patients, because their poor near vision makes it difficult for them to insert and remove lenses. However, this patient population may not have the necessary mental and physical faculties to safely use contact lenses as seen in certain geriatric patients who have undergone glaucoma corrective surgeries and cataract extraction procedures.

Visual aberrations caused by corneal scarring are also often better corrected with rigid contact lenses. Whereas eyeglasses simply correct refractive error by changing the focus of light incident on the cornea, the proximity of the rigid contact lens actually masks irregularities in corneal topography. Prosthetic lenses may also improve cosmetic appearance by rendering corneal scarring virtually unnoticeable. However, surface aberrations on the cornea carry greater risk for corneal ulcers, given that bacteria and other pathogens may sequester there.

Other indications for the use of contacts include correction of refractive errors such as myopia (nearsightedness), hyperopia (farsightedness), astigmatism, and presbyopia.

Astigmatism occurs when unequal curvatures of the refractive surface of the eye results in a blurred image. RGP lenses, hard lenses, and toric soft lenses can be used to correct astigmatism.

Presbyopia (old vision) is a condition caused by aging, in which the eye muscles of the crystalline lens have deteriorated to the point that one cannot properly focus on near objects. More than 50% of visually corrected patients are presbyopic. Contact lens correction of presbyopia using bifocal contact lenses has proven difficult, with a success rate of only 60% to 70%. Because vision correction is needed for both near vision and far vision, two optical corrections are required in each bifocal contact lens. Presbyopia is not to be confused with cataracts, another common cause of visual loss due to loss of clarity in the crystalline lens, which is usually attributable to long-term oxidation and genetic predisposition.

If patients are properly identified and indoctrinated, 60% to 70% can achieve adequate vision with bifocal contact lenses. "Monovision" is one method of presbyopic contact lens correction that has been successful in many cases; the dominant eye is fitted with a lens for far vision, and the other eye is fitted with a lens that corrects for close-up objects and reading. In most individuals, the eyes adjust in a relatively short time.

Perhaps the main reason for choosing contact lenses is the perceived improvement in personal appearance. Other strongly influencing factors include (1) no obstruction of vision from eyeglass frames, (2) greater clarity in peripheral vision, (3) no fogging of lenses caused by sudden temperature changes, and (4) more freedom of motion during vigorous activity (e.g., sports). A number of factors, such as increased sensitivity to light and improved quality of the retinal image, contribute to the subjective perception of vision improvement by the contact lens wearer. With eyeglasses, the myopic individual sees a smaller-than-normal image and the hyperopic individual sees a larger-than-normal image. With contacts, both myopic and hyperopic individuals see objects in nearly their true sizes; for highly myopic persons, the increase in image size with contact lenses is significant and decidedly beneficial.

Contraindications and Warnings for Contact Lenses

Some individuals who require vision correction cannot or should not wear contact lenses. Contraindications are often based on lifestyle as well as on medical history.

Occupational conditions that may prohibit the wearing of contact lenses include exposure to wind, glare, molten metals, irritants, dust and particulate matter, tobacco smoke, chemicals, and chemical fumes. Certain chemical fumes may be particularly hazardous because of the potential concentration of irritants under a hard lens or inside a soft lens. The lens theoretically prolongs contact of such substances with the cornea and can lead to corneal toxicity. However, these theoretical occupational contraindications have not been proven.

Contact lenses should not be used if a patient has active pathologic intraocular or corneal/conjunctival conditions. Medical contraindications to wearing contact lenses include (1) dry eye syndrome, (2) blepharitis, (3) patients who must dose eye medications frequently such as glaucoma patients, and (4) poor blink rate or incomplete blink. Patients who have insufficient tear production, a deficiency or excess of mucin, excessive lipid production, or need to spend time in excessively dry environments may also be unable to use contact lenses successfully.

Diabetic patients are often advised against continuous-wear contact lenses because of retarded healing processes and the tendency toward prolonged corneal abrasion with such use. This precaution is probably unnecessary for daily wear of lenses unless problems occur.

Chronic common colds or allergic conditions such as hay fever and asthma may also make contact lens wear extremely uncomfortable or impossible.

In women, the corneal topography may be altered by pregnancy or the use of oral contraceptives. The fluid-retaining properties of estrogen may lead to edema of the cornea and eyelids as well as to decreased tear production. Keratitis sicca or dry eye syndrome, often found in postmenopausal women, may also preclude successful contact lens wear.

Contact lenses can be used with care by persons of advanced age; care is needed because of possible lacrimal insufficiency and loose lid tissues. Contact lenses should be used with caution by patients with severe arthritis. Individuals with arthritis (as well as other conditions such as stroke) may lack the dexterity needed to insert and remove lenses.

Lens wearers moving from a low to a high altitude may encounter hypoxia (causing edema of the cornea) or metabolic deficiency, resulting in irritation and corneal abrasions.

During the period needed for adapting to rigid contact lenses, the eyelids may become hyperemic (congested with excessive blood). Short pseudoblinks, by new wearers of hard lenses, may irritate the conjunctiva of the upper eyelid. Chin elevation and squinting may result from the patient's efforts to minimize the irritation.

Characteristics of Contact Lenses

Contact lenses are often broadly classified into three distinct groups, soft contact lenses, rigid gas permeable lenses, and hard lenses, on the basis of their chemical makeup and physical properties (Table 29-1). Lenses that are relatively inflexible, do not appreciably absorb water (less than 10%), and retain their shape when removed from the eye are commonly called rigid lenses. Rigid lenses made of PMMA are not permeable to oxygen and are called hard contact lenses. Rigid lenses made of more flexible polymers are permeable to oxygen and therefore are called rigid gas permeable (RGP) lenses. Hard lenses are now seldom pre-

TABLE 29-1 Comparison of Contact Lens Characteristics

	Hard Lenses	Soft Lenses	RGP Lenses
Lens Characteristics			
Rigidity	+++	0	+++
Durability	+++	+	++
Oxygen transmission	0	++	+++
Chemical adsorption	0	+++	0
Optical Quality			
Visual acuity	+++	+	+++
Correction of astigmatism	Yes	Toric	Yes
Photophobia	++	+	++
Spectacle blur	+++	0	++
Convenience			
Comfort	+	+++	++
Adaptation period	Weeks	Days	Weeks
Continuous wear	No	Yes	Yes
Intermittent wear	No	Yes	No

Key: + indicates the degree to which the characteristic is present; 0 means the characteristic is not present.

scribed but may be replaced for individuals who successfully wore them before the advent of RGP lenses. Contact lenses that are moderately to highly flexible, absorb a high percentage of water (greater than 10%), and conform to the shape of a supporting structure are commonly called soft lenses.

Subgroups of contact lenses are classified according to wear (daily-wear or continuous-wear) or replacement schedule (conventional, planned-replacement, and disposable lenses). Continuous-wear lenses can be either soft or, occasionally, RGP lenses that are designed to be worn for an extended time, including while sleeping, before removal. Planned replacement lenses are worn from 1 to 3 months and then discarded. Disposable lenses are designed to be worn for 1 to 14 days and then discarded.

Contact lenses are manufactured from polymers that vary widely in their chemical and physical properties. Each material has physical and surface characteristics that correlate with the specific problems that the patient may encounter.

Physical characteristics of contact lenses include size, dimensional stability, strength or resistance to breakage, and polymer stability. Generally, hard lenses are dimensionally stable and tend to hold their parameters with little change. Soft lenses, however, are much less stable physically; water content, to a large extent, dictates their physical strength. RGP lenses are thicker and larger than hard lenses and generally have a high degree of dimensional stability. As they dehydrate, however, curvature of the plastic surfaces may be altered slightly. Even though RGP lenses have clear advantages over other lenses in terms of clarity and durability, they tend to cause more discomfort and can be less desirable to patients.

Physical characteristics of the different contact lenses account for most of the problems that patients encounter. Unfortunately, many patients do not know which type of lens they are wearing. This problem underscores the importance of the pharmacist establishing an excellent relationship with eye care practitioners in the area.

To maintain a healthy cornea, an adequate amount of oxygen is needed. As the oxygen that passes through the contact lens increases, the corneal metabolism can be better maintained. Oxygen permeability describes the ability of a specific material to permit the passage of oxygen. Oxygen permeability is expressed as the Dk value of the material, where D is the diffusion coefficient, and k is the solubility coefficient. A higher Dk value indicates higher oxygen permeability. Oxygen transmission is represented by Dk/L, in which L corresponds to the thickness of a specific lens, and is the value to which most practitioners and manufacturers refer. Because the lens thickness varies depending on the power of the lens, many manufacturers report the Dk/L value for a lens with a −3.00D (diopter) prescription. For example, a lens that corrects myopia (minus lens) will be thinner in the center than a lens that corrects hyperopia (plus lens), which will be thicker in the center than in the periphery.

In non–silicone-based soft lenses, oxygen transmission depends primarily on the water content of the soft lens. With higher water content, more oxygen is transmitted through the lens. However, as water content increases, durability decreases and the lens must be made thicker, which in turn hinders oxygen permeability. Therefore, a thick lens with high water content may transmit the same amount of oxygen as a thin lens with lower water content.[1] In addition, as water content increases, the lenses tend to attract tear deposits such as lipids, proteins, and polysaccharides. Compared with lenses having a lower water content, lenses with a high water content tend to be more susceptible to the growth of bacteria and fungi on the surface, especially if

large pores or many pores are present.[2] Regardless of the lens type, insoluble deposits can occur as soon as in the first hour of wear. This problem is especially of concern in people who are exposed to tobacco smoke and other environmental pollutants.

The majority (87%) of patients who wear contact lenses are fitted with soft (hydrophilic) lenses. Rigid (primarily RGP) lenses are prescribed for 13% of patients. Continuous-wear lenses (soft or RGP) are worn by 25% of patients wearing contact lenses. Approximately 76% of patients wearing contact lenses wear some type of disposable or planned replacement lenses.[3]

Formulation Considerations for Lens Care Products

Lens care products include surface-active cleaners, enzymatic cleaners, disinfecting solutions, wetting and rewetting solutions, and multipurpose solutions that combine several steps into one. Each type of contact lens has specific care procedures.

The manufacturing and marketing of contact lenses are regulated by the ophthalmic devices division of the Food and Drug Administration (FDA). Even though contact lens solutions are not considered drug products, formulation considerations are still applicable. Patients who wear contact lenses should use only lens care products that have been approved by FDA for use with their specific contact lenses.

The basic considerations for a well-formulated contact lens solution include pH, viscosity, isotonicity with tears, stability, sterility, and provision for maintenance of sterility (bactericidal action). The pH range of comfort is not well defined because, although normal tear pH is 7.4, tear pH varies among individuals. It is best to have a weakly buffered solution that can readily adjust to any tear pH, given that highly buffered solutions can cause significant discomfort, even ocular damage, when they are instilled. However, as with therapeutic ophthalmic solutions, the stability of the solution takes precedence over comfort. For this reason, many contact lens solutions are formulated with pH values above or below 7.4. These systems are weakly buffered and are usually well tolerated by the eye.

Solutions from different manufacturers should not be mixed because a precipitate may form. For instance, a product containing alkaline borate buffers forms a gummy, gel-like precipitate on lenses if mixed with a wetting solution containing polyvinyl alcohol. Furthermore, solutions containing a cationic preservative, such as chlorhexidine, polyquaternium-1, or polyaminopropyl biguanide, should not be mixed with solutions containing an anionic preservative such as sorbic acid; this combination, too, will cause a precipitate to form.[4]

Preservatives

Daily use of the same bottle of any contact lens solution over a long period of time increases the risk of bacterial contamination. Depending on specific lens care procedures, a single container may last for a month or more. The solution must therefore contain a bactericidal agent that is both effective over the long term and nonirritating to the eye with daily use. Few preservatives fulfill these criteria.

Several preservatives are used in contact lens products. Older types of preservatives include benzalkonium chloride, thimerosal, sorbic acid, chlorhexidine, and ethylenediaminetetraacetic acid (EDTA) (see Chapter 28). Polyquaternium-1 and polyaminopropyl biguanide are more commonly used. These preservatives are believed to cause fewer adverse effects than some of the older preservatives.

Polyquaternium-1

Polyquaternium-1 (Polyquad) is a quaternary ammonium preservative shown to be effective against certain bacteria, fungi, and yeast. To date, few toxicity or sensitivity problems have been noted with this preservative. When it was introduced to the market, formulations containing polyquaternium-1 were not compatible with lenses that had a high water content, because the methacrylic acid component of the lens had the ability to adsorb the preservative in toxic levels. However, recent formulations do not seem to have this problem.

Polyhexamethylene Biguanide

Polyhexamethylene biguanide, also known as polyaminopropyl biguanide, Dymed, or polyhexanide, is a cationic polymeric biguanide that is effective against certain bacteria and yeast, although its activity against *Acanthamoeba* and fungi is limited. No significant adverse effects to polyaminopropyl biguanide have been reported in lens wearers.

Hard Contact Lenses

Hard contact lenses were the first lenses to be used in the United States. Hard lenses are polymerized products of esters of acrylic acid or methacrylic acid. The most common plastic found in hard lenses is PMMA, known commercially as Lucite or Plexiglas. Although these lenses are rarely prescribed, some patients still wear this type of lens.

Care of Hard Lenses

Hard contact lens care products help minimize stress on the eye and prevent infection. These products aid the wearer, providing comfort and safety. Hard lens care involves three important steps: cleaning, soaking/disinfecting, and wetting (Figure 29-1). For optimal lens care, all three steps should be performed each time the lenses are removed from the eye. Fortunately, modern care solutions enable disinfection/soaking and wetting in the same step.

Cleaning Solutions

Normal tears are composed of secretions from many specialized glands lining the lacrimal apparatus, conjunctiva, and lids. Many components are somewhat hydrophobic and tend to adhere to the surface of a hard lens during normal daily wear. This residue, primarily proteinaceous debris and oils, acts as a growth medium for bacteria. If it is not routinely removed by daily cleaning, the residue may harden to form coatings or tenacious deposits that create an irregular surface on the lens. This residue will eventually irritate the eyelids and corneal epithelium, and it may progress to infection. Decreased visual acuity and shorter toleration time are likely consequences of a cloudy lens or allergenic reactions to the residue.

Contact lens cleaning solutions typically contain nonionic or amphoteric surfactants that emulsify oils and aid in solubilizing other debris. Proteins and lipids are soluble in highly alkaline media, but high pH can cause lens decomposition. Weak alkaline solutions may dislodge deposits from the lens in conjunction with the surface tension–lowering properties of the surfactants. Home-

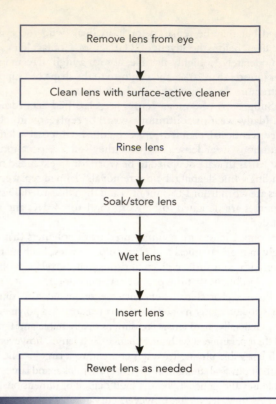

made cleaning solutions such as baking soda mixed with distilled water or cleaning solution may scratch lenses and may not rinse off easily.[5] Use of household cleansers and homemade solutions (including salt tablet solutions) of any kind should be strongly discouraged to prevent lens damage, contamination leading to infection, and ocular irritation. Tables 29-2 and 29-3 provide instructions for properly cleaning hard lenses.

FIGURE 29-1   Self-care of hard lenses.

[Figure content:]
- Remove lens from eye
- Clean lens with surface-active cleaner
- Rinse lens
- Soak/store lens
- Wet lens
- Insert lens
- Rewet lens as needed

TABLE 29-2   General Cleaning Procedures for All Lens Types

- Wash hands with noncosmetic soap and rinse thoroughly before handling lenses.
- Clean contact lenses with only commercially manufactured products made specifically for that type of lens. Homemade cleansers can scratch the lenses or cause eye irritation or injury.
- Do not mix contact lens care products from different manufacturers unless an eye care practitioner says they are compatible.
- When handling lenses over a sink, cover or close the drain to prevent loss of a lens.
- During cleaning, check lenses for scratches, chips, or tears, and the presence of foreign particles, warping, or discoloration. Also, check that lenses are clean and thoroughly rinsed of cleaner. These factors could cause eye discomfort.
- When cleaning a lens, rub it in a back-and-forth, rather than a circular, direction.
- Clean the second lens as thoroughly as the first to prevent "left lens syndrome," in which the left lens has more deposits than the right lens, because the right lens is often removed first and cleaned more thoroughly.
- Discard cleansers and other lens care products if the labeled expiration date has passed.

TABLE 29-3 Specific Cleaning Procedures for Hard Lenses

- Apply appropriate cleaning solution to both surfaces of the lenses; rub the lens between thumb and forefinger or between forefinger and palm of opposite hand for approximately 20 seconds.
- Do not wipe lenses dry with tissue; the tissue may scratch the lenses.
- Avoid overly vigorous cleaning of lenses, which may cause scratches or warping.
- Always clean hard lenses before storing them.

Soaking Solutions

A soaking solution is used to store hard contact lenses whenever they are removed from the eyes. The solution maintains the lens in a constant state of hydration for maximum comfort and visual acuity when inserted in the eye. It also aids in removing deposits that accumulate on the lens during wear.

If lenses are allowed to dry out during overnight storage, accumulated deposits are more difficult to remove by normal cleaning. Storage in a soaking solution reduces the likelihood of deposits forming.

To maintain sterility, storage solutions use essentially the same preservatives as wetting solutions. The main difference is that the concentration can be somewhat higher in a soaking solution, given that the solution is rinsed from the lens before insertion. However, preservative levels are carefully selected, because higher levels do not necessarily result in increased effectiveness and may lead to impaired wetting or corneal irritation because of the adsorption of preservatives onto the lens.

Wetting Solutions

An ideal wetting solution performs the following functions: (1) converts the hydrophobic lens surface to a hydrophilic surface by means of a uniform film that does not easily wash away; (2) increases comfort by providing cushioning and lubrication between the contacting surfaces; (3) places a viscous coating on the lens to protect it from oil on the fingers during insertion; and (4) stabilizes the lens on the fingertip to ease insertion, particularly for individuals with poor manual dexterity or unsteady hands.

If the lens is thoroughly cleaned before insertion, lacrimal fluid can adequately wet the lens. Indeed, the wetting action of popular wetting solutions is sometimes not significantly better than that of saline. Furthermore, patients whose tears are capable of wetting a lens almost immediately upon insertion often do not use these solutions.

The cushioning effect of a wetting solution is achieved by hydrophilic polymers that lubricate the interface between the lens and the surfaces of the cornea and eyelid. Cellulose gum derivatives are often used. Although compounds such as methylcellulose possess a degree of surfactant activity, they do not promote uniform wetting of a rigid lens. For this reason, polyvinyl alcohol is also often used to decrease surface tension.

Saliva should never be used to wet contact lenses; it can lead to infection by *Acanthamoeba*, *Pseudomonas aeruginosa*, or other pathogens.

Rewetting Solutions

Rewetting solutions are intended to clean and rewet the contact lens while it is in the eye. These solutions depend on the use of surfactants to loosen deposits; removal is assisted by the natural cleaning action of blinking. Although these products function well to recondition the lens, the cornea benefits more if the lens is actually removed, cleaned, and rewetted. Removing the lens for even a brief time allows the cornea to be resurfaced with a new proteinaceous or mucinaceous layer.

Other Products

Other ophthalmic products are available to the hard lens wearer for occasional use. Some, such as artificial tears and ocular decongestants, are not recommended for use with the lenses in place. Because of their emollient and lubricating effect, artificial tears can be used to soothe the eye, but the hard contact lens must be removed prior to use. Ocular decongestants reduce mild conjunctival hyperemia associated with prolonged lens wear. However, these topical decongestants can induce a rebound hyperemia if used for more than 72 hours with cessation of the drug. Therefore, routine use of these products should be avoided. If symptoms requiring their use persist, a visit to an eye care practitioner is advised.

Product Selection Guidelines

Several lens care solutions are available to hard lens wearers. These products are also labeled for certain RGP lenses as well (Table 29-4). Product selection is an area in which pharmacists can perform a much-needed role as a consultant. A surfactant cleaner, a soaking solution, a wetting solution, and a rewetting solution should be recommended.

TABLE 29-4 Selected Hard Contact Lens Products	
Trade Name	**Primary Ingredients**
Cleaning Solutions	
Bausch and Lomb Concentrated Cleaner	Alkyl ether sulfate; triquaternary cocoa-based phospholipid; silica gel; ethoxylated alkyl phenol
Wetting Solutions	
Liquifilm	Hydroxypropyl methylcellulose; polyvinyl alcohol; benzalkonium chloride 0.004%; EDTA; NaCl; KCl
Wetting/Soaking Solutions	
Bausch and Lomb Wetting/Soaking Solution	Cationic cellulose derivative polymer; edentate calcium disodium 0.05%; chlorhexidine gluconate 0.006%
Rewetting/Lubricating Solutions	
Clerz 2	Hydroxyethyl cellulose; sorbic acid 0.1%; EDTA 0.1%; NaCl; KCl; sodium borate; boric acid

Key: EDTA, ethylenediamine tetraacetic acid; KCl, potassium chloride; NaCl, sodium chloride.

Insertion and Removal

Tables 29-5 and 29-6 provide instructions for inserting and removing hard lenses.

RGP Contact Lenses

The new generation of RGP lenses combines the optical qualities of PMMA and the oxygen permeability of soft lenses. Generally, RGP lenses can deliver two to three times more oxygen to the cornea than non–silicone-based soft lenses of the same thickness. However, to maintain rigidity (which is important for the proper lens fit and correction of astigmatism), RGP lenses are generally thicker than soft lenses. Newer RGP lenses still transmit much more oxygen to the cornea than do most soft lenses, while covering only the central 75% of the cornea. RGP lenses, unlike soft lenses, enable exchange up to 20% of the post-lens tear volume per blink.

RGP lenses have been investigated for continuous-wear use, and some have been approved for 1 to 30 days of extended wear. The use of continuous-wear lenses is somewhat controversial. These lenses have been implicated in causing corneal ulcers (epithelial erosion with inflammation or infection), which, in rare instances, can lead to partial or complete blindness.

RGP lenses are available in several types of materials. The earliest types of RGP lens were composed of silicone acrylates that combine silicone with methyl methacrylate and methacrylic acid and/or hydroxyethyl methacrylate (HEMA) in varying amounts. These materials are relatively stable and fairly inflexible. Examples of lenses made with this type of material include Polycon II and Paraperm O_2.

TABLE 29-5 Insertion of Hard and RGP Lenses

- After washing hands, remove one lens from the lens storage case, rinse it with fresh conditioning/soaking solution, and inspect it for cleanliness and signs of damage (cracks or chips).
- If a wetting or conditioning solution is being used, place a few drops on the lens.
- Place the lens on the top of the index finger, as shown in drawing A.
- Place the middle finger of the same hand on the lower lid and pull it down. (See drawing B.)
- With the other hand, use a finger to lift the upper lid and then place the lens on the eye. (See drawing C.)
- Release the lids and blink.
- Check vision immediately to see if the lens is in the proper position.
- If vision is blurred, blink three to four times. If vision is still blurred, the lens may be off center, on the wrong eye, or dirty.
  —Instill one to three drops of rewetting or reconditioning drops into the eye.
  —If vision is not improved, remove the lens, place several drops of wetting/conditioning solution onto both surfaces, and reinsert.
- Repeat all steps with the other lens.

A

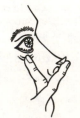

B

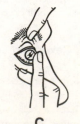

C

TABLE 29-6 Removal of Hard and RGP Lenses

- Before removing the lens, fill the storage cases with soaking/conditioning solution.
- Remove the top from the cleaning solution.
- Place a hand (or a towel) under the eye.
- Use one of the following methods to remove the lens from the eye.

Two-Finger Method of Removing Lenses

- Place the tip of the forefinger of one hand on the middle of the upper eyelid by the lashes, as shown in drawing A.
- Place the forefinger of the other hand on the middle lower lid margin. (See drawing A.)
- Push the lids inward and then together, as shown in drawing B. The lens should pop out.
- If the lens becomes decentered onto only the white part of the eye, recenter the lens and try again.

Temporal Pull/Blink Method of Removing Lenses

- Place an index finger on the temporal edge of the lower and upper lids. Initially, widen the eyelids a little. (See drawing C.)
- Stretch the skin outward and slightly upward without allowing the lid to slide over the lens. Blink briskly, as shown in drawing D. The lens will pop out because of the pressure of the eyelids at the top and bottom of the lens. Blinking facilitates removal after the lids have been tightened around the lens.

A

B

C

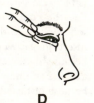

D

Fluorine is a newer component of RGP materials, and in combination with older materials, forms either fluorosilicone acrylate or fluoropolymer lenses. Examples of lenses made with this type of material are Boston EO/XO and Fluoroperm. Of all RGP materials available, the fluorosilicone acrylates or modified fluorosilicone acrylates are the most commonly used.[6]

Advantages of RGP lenses vary depending on the type of materials used. Fluorinated lenses offer the advantages of increased oxygen transmissibility and reduced lipophilicity problems. These lenses also have less surface reactivity, thereby decreasing tear film deposits.

As with hard lenses, the main drawback of RGPs is discomfort and long adaptation time. Material disadvantages of RGP lenses also vary with the type of materials used. Silicone acrylate lenses have less surface wettability than PMMA because silicone is more hydrophobic. Silicone acrylates also tend to have a negative surface charge, which can attract lysozymes and other positively charged deposits. Fluorinated lenses have the disadvantage of greater mass, which can affect RGP lens fit. These lenses also tend not to be highly wettable.

Care of RGP Lenses

Lens wearers should be advised by their eye care practitioners about the products and regimens recommended for their particular lenses. The labeling on contact lens products also indicates the lenses for which they are approved; however, patients must know what type of lens they are wearing to be able to use this information.

The care of an RGP lens is similar to that of a hard contact lens (Figure 29-2). (See Tables 29-2 and 29-7 for the proper cleaning procedures.)

Some RGP lenses have a high silicone content and therefore have decreased surface wettability. As previously noted, the lens surface tends to have a negative charge, which promotes the binding of positively charged tear constituents. Cleaners designed for conventional hard or RGP lenses may not effectively remove the more tenacious deposits. Other cleaners formulated for this type of lens (e.g., Boston Advance Cleaner and Original Formula Boston Cleaner) contain silica gel, which acts to mechanically break the adhesive bonds that have formed between the lens and the deposits. Patients should be counseled to discard these solutions 90 days after opening the product. There is a space on the label to record the date that the product is opened.

Because high silicone–containing RGP lenses have decreased surface wettability, conditioning solutions are generally used instead of soaking solutions to aid the formation of a cushioning tear layer. A conditioning solution is essentially a specially formulated wetting solution. The conditioner system enhances wettability of the lens, increases comfort, and disinfects the lens. The lenses must be soaked at least 4 hours in this solution before they are reinserted into the eyes. It is important to counsel the patient that the Boston Advance Conditioning solution must be discarded 90 days after opening. There is a space on the label to record the date that the product is opened.

Reconditioning and rewetting drops may also be used while the lens is on the eye to rewet the lens as necessary. Boston Rewetting Drops must be discarded 90 days after opening. Heat disinfection cannot be used with RGP lenses.

TABLE 29-7	Specific Cleaning Procedures for RGP Lenses

- Use the cleansing, soaking, and conditioning products recommended by your eye care practitioner to clean your lenses.
- Upon removal, apply an appropriate cleaning solution to both surfaces of the lens. Then rub the lens between forefinger and palm of opposite hand to avoid chipping an edge, which may occur if the lens is cleaned between the fingers.
- When cleaning the lens, do not apply too much pressure. If debris is still on the lens, soak a cotton swab in the surfactant cleaner, and use the swab to clean the lens.
- If unsure of lens type, ask the eye practitioner about proper cleaning procedures.
- After cleaning RGP lenses, soak them in a soaking or conditioning solution recommended by the eye practitioner for the specified amount of time. Rewet lenses before inserting them in the eyes.

As the silicone content of RGP lenses increases, so does the amount of protein adherence. Silicone acrylate lenses have an active surface that promotes the binding of tear constituents. Protein deposits on a lens will decrease the oxygen permeability, and the patient may experience discomfort. If daily cleaning is not sufficient, lenses of this type should be cleaned with an enzymatic product once weekly.[7] Failure to comply with this cleaning step may result in the need for professional polishing or replacement of the lens.

Fluorosilicone acrylate lenses should not be cleaned more than one time with MiraFlow. Cracking, changes in parameters, and brittleness have been noted when this type of lens is cleaned repeatedly with alcohol-based cleaners like MiraFlow.

Product Selection Guidelines

The appropriate lens care regimen for RGP lenses is fairly straightforward with the abundance of combination wetting/disinfection solutions now on the market. Lens wearers should be advised against substituting other products for those specifically recommended by their eye care practitioner. Patients wearing RGP lenses should be advised to purchase a surface-active cleaning product, an enzymatic product, and a conditioning or soaking solution, depending on the type of lens worn. A rewetting or reconditioning product should also be recommended. Table 29-8 lists examples of products for RGP lenses.

Insertion and Removal

Wearers of RGP lenses should be counseled to follow the same insertion and removal procedures as hard lenses (Tables 29-5 and 29-6).

Soft Contact Lenses

The main chemical difference between the hydrophobic rigid lens and the hydrophilic soft lens is that the soft lens contains hydroxyl or hydroxyl and lactam groups, which allow it to absorb and hold water. Table 29-9 classifies the different types of soft contact lenses into four groups, according to water content and

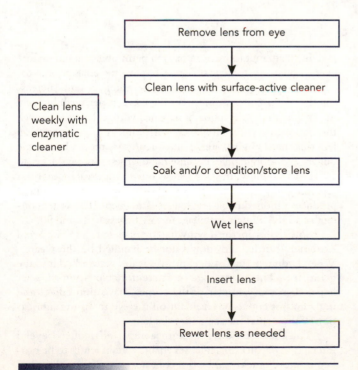

FIGURE 29-2 Self-care of RGP lenses.

TABLE 29-8 Selected Products for RGP Lenses	
Trade Name	**Primary Ingredients**
Cleaning Solutions	
Boston Advance Cleaner[a]	Silica gel; alkyl ether sulfate; ethoxylated alkyl phenol; triquaternary cocoa-based phospholipid
Boston Cleaner	Silica gel; alkyl ether sulfate; titanium dioxide; NaCl
Opti-Clean II Daily Cleaner	Cleaning agent; polysorbate 21; hydroxyethyl cellulose; EDTA 0.1%; polyquaternium-1, 0.001%, boric acid; sodium borate; NaCl; sodium hydroxide
Opti-Free Daily Cleaner	Nylon 11; polysorbate 21; hydroxyethyl cellulose; polyquaternium-1; EDTA; boric acid; sodium borate; hydrochloric acid and/or sodium hydroxide
Enzymatic Cleaning Products	
Boston One Step Liquid Enzymatic Cleaner	Subtilisin; glycerol
Wetting/Soaking/Disinfecting Solutions	
Boston Advance Comfort Formula Conditioning Solution	Cellulosic viscosifier; polyvinyl alcohol; cationic cellulose derivative polymer; derivatized PEG; chlorhexidine gluconate 0.003%; polyaminopropyl biguanide 0.0005%; EDTA 0.05%
Boston Conditioning Solution	Hydroxyethyl cellulose; polyvinyl alcohol; cationic cellulose derivatives; poloxamer 407; chlorhexidine gluconate 0.006%; EDTA 0.05%
Rewetting/Lubricating Solutions	
Boston Rewetting Drops	Hydroxyethyl cellulose; polyvinyl alcohol; cationic cellulose derivatives; poloxamer 407; chlorhexidine gluconate 0.006%; EDTA 0.05%
Multipurpose Solutions	
Boston Simplus	Poloxamine; hydroxyalkylphosphonate; boric acid; sodium borate; sodium chloride; hydroxypropylmethyl cellulose; Glucam; chlorhexidine gluconate (0.003%); polyaminopropyl biguanide (0.0005%)

Key: EDTA, ethylenediamine tetraacetic acid; NaCl, sodium chloride; PEG, polyethylene glycol.

[a] Preservative-free formulation.

ionic charge based on 1986 FDA recommendations. Soft lenses are composed of hydrophilic groups, including hydroxyl, amide, lactam, and carboxyl, with small amounts of cross-linking agents that form a hydrophilic gel (hydrogel) network. The degree of cross-linking determines lens hydrophilicity and water content. Greater cross-linking means that fewer hydrophilic groups are available to interact with water, which in turn produces a less flexible, less hydrated lens than those originally available.

Ionic lenses have a negative surface charge, which tends to attract more protein deposits than nonionic lenses. Soaking ionic lenses in sorbate-preserved saline yellows the lenses prematurely. Nonionic lenses are electrically neutral and tend to be less reactive with the tear film, resulting in a more deposit-resistant lens. High-water-content lenses (greater than 50%), which tend to attract tear film deposits into their matrix, usually cannot withstand daily heat disinfection. If soaked in enzymes for a prolonged period, these lenses may also cause sensitivity reactions. Silicone hydrogel lenses (e.g., Night and Day, Pure-Vision, and Acuvue Oasys) have recently gained popularity. These lenses are highly permeable to oxygen, are durable, and have less protein deposition but more lipid deposition. Currently, only four lens care products (Clear Care, Aquify, Opti-Free Replenish, and Opti-Free Express) have received FDA approval for use with silicone hydrogel lenses.

In an attempt to increase oxygen permeability and therefore safety profiles, the trend in designing soft lens materials prior to the "silicone-age" was to gradually increase water content. Increasing the water content improves the oxygen permeability of a material, with the exception of silicone hydrogel lenses for which the opposite is true. However, permeability also depends on lens thickness. High-water-content lenses are more physiologic but are also more fragile. Because these lenses must be thicker to offset their fragility, the two factors often cancel each other out regarding oxygen transmissibility. Lowering the water content produces a more durable and longer-lasting lens. The water content of a HEMA-type material can vary between 5% and 90%.

Soft lenses in the nonhydrated (dry) state are rigid and extremely brittle, and should not be handled by the wearer. When hydrated, the lenses expand as water is absorbed into the gel matrix. These lenses are most comfortable when they are larger than the diameter of the cornea, have thin edges, and undergo just enough movement on the eye to ensure lubrication of the ocular surface under the lens.

The increased oxygen permeability and reduced eyelid interaction of soft contact lenses enable certain lenses to be broken in more quickly and worn continuously. Table 29-10 lists examples of some of the soft contact lenses approved for wear in the United States.

TABLE 29-9 Soft Contact Lens Classification	
Classification	**Water Content (%)**
Group I: Low Water, Nonionic	
Hefilcon A and B	45%
Polymacon	38%
Senofilcon A	38%
Tefilcon	38%
Tetrafilcon A	43%
Group II: High Water, Nonionic	
Lidofilcon A	70%
Lidofilcon B	79%
Nelfilcon A	69%
Group III: Low Water, Ionic	
Bufilcon A	45%
Deltafilcon A	43%
Phemfilcon	38%
Group IV: High Water, Ionic	
Bufilcon A	55%
Etafilcon	58%
Perfilcon A	71%
Phemfilcon A	55%
Vilfilcon A	55%

TABLE 29-10 Examples of Soft Contact Lenses		
Trade Name (Manufacturer)	**Water/Saline Content (%)**	**Group Classification[a]**
Daily-Wear Soft Lenses		
Cibasoft Visitint (CIBA Vision)	37.5	I
Hydrasoft Sphere (Coopervision)	55.0	IV
Satureyes (Metro)	59.0	II
Soft Mate B (CIBA Vision)	45.0	III
Continuous-Wear Soft Lenses		
DuraSoft 3 (CIBA Vision)	55.0	IV
Focus Night and Day (CIBA Vision)	24.0	I
LL-70 (Unilens Corporation)	70.0	II
Permalens (Coopervision)	71.0	IV
Disposable Soft Lenses		
Focus Dailies (CIBA Vision)	69.0	II
1 Day Acuvue (Vistakon)	58.0	IV
Soflens one day (Bausch and Lomb)	70.0	II
Silicone Hydrogels		
Night and Day (CibaVision)	24%	I
PureVision (Bausch and Lomb)	36%	III
Soft Toric Lenses		
Frequency 55 Toric (Coopervision)	55.0	IV
Optima Toric (Bausch & Lomb Optics)	45.0	I
Soft Bifocal Lenses		
Acuvue Bifocal (Vistakon)	58.0	IV
Hydrocurve II Bifocal (Ciba-Vision)	45.0	III

[a] See Table 29-9 for group classifications.

Continuous-Wear Lenses

In 1981, cosmetic, soft continuous–wear lenses were originally approved by FDA to be worn for 30 days. However, as with RGP continuous-wear lenses, problems with contamination, infection, and ulceration suggested that they should not be worn for more than 7 days and, in 1989, FDA rescinded its approval of 30-day continuous wear.[8] However, FDA has since approved certain contact lenses for up to 30 nights of continuous wear. Even though the lenses are approved for 30 nights of continuous wear, some patients, depending on tear flow rate, sleep pattern, and ocular anatomy, may not be able to tolerate wearing them for this length of time.

Disposable and Planned Replacement Lenses

Disposable lenses represent the fastest-growing segment of the soft lens market. Depending on the lens, there are several approved wearing schedules. Some lenses are worn for 1 day and then discarded; others are worn daily for up to 2 weeks and then discarded; and others can be worn as continuous–wear lenses for up to 2 weeks, with the patient wearing them on various schedules (e.g., wearing them for 6 nights and then removing them for 1 night). Planned replacement lenses are discarded and replaced usually after 1 to 3 months of wear, depending on how quickly the lenses build up deposits and how well the patient complies with proper lens care. Planned replacement lenses and disposable lenses other than the daily disposables are cared for in a manner similar to other soft contact lenses. In most patients, an enzymatic cleaner is generally not necessary for disposable lenses that will be discarded after a few weeks of wear.

Daily disposable lenses have the following advantages: (1) each lens is sterile prior to removal from its package for immediate insertion into the eye; (2) no cleaning regimen is necessary because the lens is discarded after wear; (3) deposit formation is minimal; and (4) lens–related problems, such as giant papillary conjunctivitis or allergic reactions to lens care solutions, occur less frequently. At a cost of $1 to $2 per day for daily disposable lenses to correct both eyes, they are sometimes considered to be too expensive by patients. However, if the cost of solutions is factored into the use of frequent replacement lenses, daily disposable lenses can actually be less expensive overall.

Specialty Lenses

Some soft contacts are classified as specialty lenses. These include toric, bifocal, and tinted lenses. Toric soft lenses have been developed specifically to correct astigmatism (improper focusing attributed to an irregularly shaped cornea). Traditional soft lenses do not correct astigmatism, because they conform to the corneal surface rather than retain their original shape, as do rigid lenses. Toric soft lenses are fabricated with both spherical and cylindrical optical corrections, and remain on axis because of design features such as weighting on the bottom edge of the lens. Spherical soft lenses can be fitted to eyes with an upper limit of astigmatism of about 1.00 diopters.

Bifocal or multifocal lenses, which can be weighted in a fashion similar to that of toric lenses, are prescribed to correct presbyopia.

Tinted lenses are available to facilitate handling and for cosmetic purposes (i.e., to change eye color) as well as for corrective purposes. Three types of tinted lenses are available: translucent lenses, opaque lenses, and lenses that absorb ultraviolet radiation. Translucent lenses can be tinted in varying degrees to facilitate handling and increase the visibility of the lens or to enhance eye color. Opaque lenses cover the iris and hide its natural color. These lenses may also be used as a prosthetic to mask corneal scarring or to cover an amblyopic (lazy) eye. Some lenses incorporate designs such as football team logos and come in plano (no correction) and various corrections (e.g., WildEyes). Finally, some lenses have material incorporated into them that absorbs ultraviolet radiation.

Advantages

Soft lenses are easier to remove and are considerably more comfortable than rigid lenses. This effect is most apparent during the initial break-in period. Photophobia is not likely to occur with soft lenses, and glare is significantly reduced. As with rigid lenses, however, flare around the periphery may be noticed at night, particularly in individuals who have large pupils. This flare is caused by refracted light entering the eye through the edge of the corrective area or optic zone of the contact lens.

The typical patient wearing soft contact lenses does not usually experience the spectacle blur common among hard lens wearers and even occasionally experienced by RGP wearers.

Soft lenses are less likely than rigid lenses to trap dust particles, eyelashes, or other foreign material under the lens. They are also less likely to become dislodged or fall out. Therefore, soft lenses are often better suited for occasional wear and for use during participation in sports, including contact sports.

Disadvantages

Although many people prefer the comfort of soft lenses, not all soft lens wearers can achieve excellent visual acuity. The hydration of the lens may change either in or out of the eye, particularly with extreme temperatures and low relative humidity. This change can decrease the quality of the visual image. Because a soft lens conforms in large part to the corneal shape, it is difficult to project the degree of vision improvement before the lens is actually placed on the eye. Furthermore, because soft lenses cannot be as precisely tailored to the specific requirements of an individual cornea, the fitting process is less exact than it is with rigid lenses. As a result, the overall quality of vision with soft contact lenses does not usually equal that of a properly fitted pair of rigid lenses. Fortunately, these differences are often small and are not clinically significant for most wearers.

Unlike rigid lenses, soft lenses can absorb chemical compounds from topically administered ophthalmic products.[9] As previously discussed, ocular irritation may result, and the lens may be damaged. With the exception of specially formulated rewetting solutions, no solution should be instilled into the eye with the soft lens in place. If a drug solution is instilled into the eye prior to lens insertion, the wearer must wait to insert a lens until the solution has cleared from the lower eyelid's precorneal (conjunctival) pocket (about 5 minutes). A nonprescription ophthalmic product not specifically designed for use with contact lenses should not be used when lenses are in the eye. When topical ophthalmic ointments, gels, or suspensions are being used, the lenses should not be worn at all.

Unlike rigid lenses, soft lenses cannot be easily marked to identify the left and the right lens. A soft lens wearer who is uncertain of the identity of the lenses may have to see an eye care practitioner.

The care given to contact lenses varies considerably with each wearer. Soft lenses rapidly degenerate to useless pieces of plastic if they are neglected. However, when used with a fastidious care and cleaning program, conventional soft lenses can have an average life of 12 to 18 months, compared with 18 to 36 months for RGP lenses.

Care of Soft Lenses

Conventional hard and RGP lens solutions should never be used with soft lenses unless the label is specifically labeled for soft lens products; absorption of the ingredients can damage the lenses. Because soft lenses contain a high percentage of water, they are most prone to bacterial contamination. Lens disinfection is crucial to prevent ocular infection and damage to the lens by bacteria and fungi. Wearers of soft hydrophilic contact lenses should also be particularly cautious in exposing their lenses to chemicals. These chemicals, many of which penetrate and bind with the lens material, can come from cosmetics, environmental pollutants, and ophthalmic and systemic products.

The basic care regimen for soft lenses (Figure 29-3) differs from that for hard and RGP lenses. All steps must be completed to avoid ocular complications. The only exception is with daily-wear frequent replacement soft lenses. Because these lenses are disposed of within 2 weeks, enzymatic cleaners are usually not necessary. Frequent replacement lenses should, however, be cleaned and disinfected after each wearing until disposal.

Cleaning Products

A troublesome aspect of soft lens wear is the accumulation of deposits on the lens. The nature of these deposits varies, but generally they consist of proteins and lipids from the wearer's lacrimal secretions. Deposits are a greater problem with the more highly hydrated lenses, but the rate at which these deposits accumulate depends on the lens and the tears. Some wearers experience little difficulty and wear soft lenses for long periods without significant buildup; others may show deposits in as little as 2 or 3 days. Whatever the cause or accumulation rate, the result is an uncomfortable lens of poor optical quality.

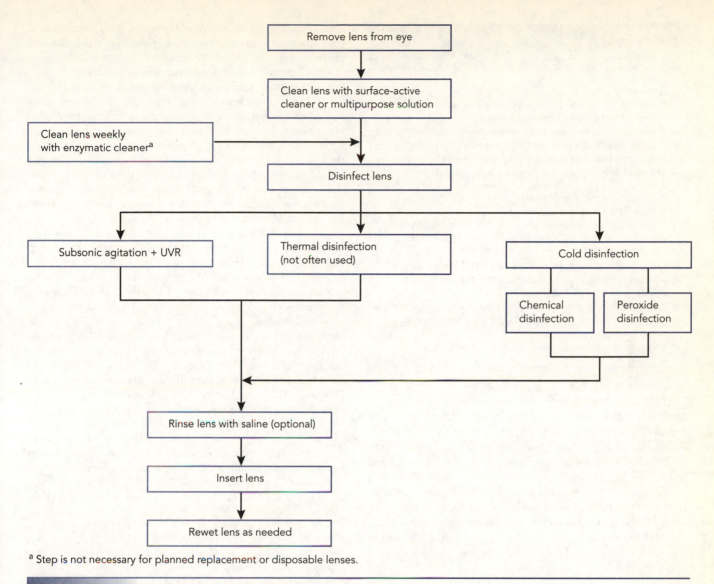

ᵃ Step is not necessary for planned replacement or disposable lenses.

FIGURE 29-3 Self-care of soft lenses. Key: UVR, ultraviolet radiation.

Daily-wear soft contact lenses require two cleaning steps to rid them of debris (Tables 29-2 and 29-11). Cleaning with a surface-active cleaner must be done daily or, in the case of continuous-wear lenses, each time they are removed from the eyes. Cleaning with an enzymatic cleaner should be done daily (e.g., Supraclens) or weekly (e.g., Ultrazyme). Soft lens cleaning solutions generally contain a nonionic detergent, a wetting agent, a chelating agent, buffers, preservatives, and, in some cases, polymeric cleaning beads.

Although the surface-active cleaners are generally quite effective in removing lipid deposits, they remove tenacious protein debris less successfully. Enzymatic cleaners are an additional cleaning aid that can help solve this problem. These enzymes hydrolyze polypeptide bonds of protein and dissolve the protein deposits. For the enzyme solution to work properly, however, the lens must be cleaned with a surface-active cleaner first; enzymes are ineffective on debris that covers or is mixed with protein.

Enzymatic regimens were developed to be used simultaneously with chemical or hydrogen peroxide disinfection on either a daily or a weekly basis. Products that combine enzymatic cleaning and disinfecting steps tend to increase compli-ance by decreasing the number of lens care steps a patient must perform. Table 29-12 lists characteristics of various enzymatic products.

Disinfecting Methods

FDA recommends disinfecting soft contact lenses before each reinsertion. Disinfection is performed after the lens is cleaned. Two methods of cold disinfection are currently approved: chemical and hydrogen peroxide. Thermal disinfection has also been used, but this method has largely been replaced by cold disinfection systems. Studies have shown that microorganisms do not actually enter the matrix of soft lenses, but surface contamination can lead to ocular infection. Chemical disinfection with hydrogen peroxide has increased in popularity with certain types of lenses over earlier chemical disinfectants because of decreased ocular allergenicity and toxicity. A system that uses subsonic agitation and high-intensity ultraviolet light is available (Purilens). LensComfort Ultrasonic Cleaning and Disinfecting system utilizes ultrasound for cleaning and an antimicrobial multipurpose solution to disinfect.

TABLE 29-11 Specific Cleaning Procedures for Soft Lenses

- Clean regular soft lenses daily with a surface-active cleaner. Clean continuous-wear and disposable soft lenses with a surface-active cleaner after each wearing.
- Wash hands before handling your lenses.
- Place several drops of a cleaning product (if not using a no-rub product) on the lens; gently rub the lens between the thumb and forefinger, or between the fingertip of the forefinger and the palm of the opposite hand for 20–30 seconds.
- Avoid cutting the lens with a fingernail or scratching the lens surface with grit or dirt on the hands.
- Rinse lenses with a sterile isotonic buffered solution. Never use tap water: It is not isotonic and contains harmful microorganisms.
- Clean lenses at least weekly (or every day if using a daily product) with enzymatic cleaners, either separately from disinfection or as part of the disinfecting process.
- When combining enzyme cleaning and disinfecting of the lenses as one step, see Table 29-12 for the appropriate combinations of products.
- Discard any enzyme cleaner that is discolored.

CHEMICAL DISINFECTION

In chemical disinfection, the lenses are stored for a prescribed period of time (usually 4–6 hours) in a solution containing bactericidal agents that are compatible with soft lens materials. Two basic chemical disinfection methods are available in the United States. The first is based on the original chemical disinfecting solutions, which consisted of antimicrobial preservatives of sufficient concentration in storage solutions primarily composed of saline. These initial disinfecting solutions contained chlorhexidine and thimerosal, both of which induce sensitivity reactions in many soft lens wearers. To avoid this problem, solutions with less sensitizing disinfecting preservatives are currently being marketed for soft contact lens care. Some of these preservatives are sorbic acid, polyquaternium-1, polyaminopropyl biguanide, and amidoamine, which are touted as much less toxic or allergenic than their predecessors. However, some of these agents may also be less effective, especially against fungi and protozoans.

The second chemical method uses hydrogen peroxide as the antimicrobial agent (Table 29-13). Soft lenses are placed in purified hydrogen peroxide and disinfected by the liberation of oxygen from peroxide. Household hydrogen peroxide solution should not be used; its pH is too low and it may discolor

lenses.[10] Following disinfection, the peroxide is neutralized to trace levels by a neutralizing tablet or the catalytic action of a platinum disk.

One potential disadvantage of hydrogen peroxide disinfection is that patients may mistakenly insert the lens directly from the peroxide solution without neutralization. A peroxide-soaked lens placed on the eye will cause great pain, photophobia, redness, and, perhaps, corneal epithelial damage. If this occurs, the patient should immediately remove the lens from the eye and flush the eye with sterile saline solution. The pain should subside within a few hours. If it does not, the patient should consult an eye care practitioner. If the patient has any doubt as to whether the peroxide was neutralized, the entire disinfection cycle should be started over again.

Several hydrogen peroxide products help the patient avoid the possibility of forgetting to perform the neutralization step: AO Sept, AO Sept Clear Care, and Oxysept UltraCare.

Patients who use the AO Sept platinum disk for neutralization should replace the disk after 100 uses or 3 months, whichever comes first. Failure to comply with these instructions may result in disk failure, and the patient may sustain a peroxide burn on the cornea. Although the catalytic disk systems require only one step, that step takes 6 hours for disinfection and neutralization, which decreases the system's flexibility and rules out morning use. Suboptimal disinfection is another concern with AO Sept. The catalytic disk will neutralize the surrounding peroxide quickly, and there may not be adequate time for disinfection. Once the catalytic disk neutralizes the peroxide, a nonpreserved solution remains. If the lenses are left in the case for long periods of time, bacterial contamination may occur. Patients should not store their lenses in neutralized AO Sept Clear Care for more than 7 days or neutralized AO Sept for more than 24 hours unless they once again disinfect the lenses prior to insertion.

It should be noted that AO Sept Clear Care contains a built-in cleaner and is approved as a "no-rub" product. AO Sept Clear Care can also be used for cleaning, disinfection, and storage of RGP lenses.

With Oxysept UltraCare, the user adds a delayed-release neutralizing tablet at the beginning of the 6-hour disinfecting cycle. Disinfection and neutralization then occur at the appropriate time intervals. This tablet contains catalase and cyanocobalamin; the latter ingredient turns the solution pink, reminding the user that the tablet has been added. The tablet is coated with hydroxypropyl methylcellulose, which helps lubricate the eye if the lens is not re-rinsed between disinfection and insertion. Exposure of the lenses to the disinfecting effects of hydrogen peroxide before neutralization allows optimal activity against

TABLE 29-12 Enzymatic Cleaners

Trade Name	Active Ingredient	Concurrent Use with Chemical Preservative Disinfection	Concurrent Use with Hydrogen Peroxide Disinfection
Opti-Free SupraClens (used daily)	Liquid pancreatin	Yes, with Opti-Free Express	No
ReNu 1-Step Liquid (daily use)	Subtilisin	Yes, with ReNu Multi-purpose Solution	No
Ultrazyme/Unizyme	Subtilisin	No	Yes, with any hydrogen peroxide 3% disinfecting solution

TABLE 29-13	Guidelines for Disinfecting RGP and Soft Lenses

Chemical Disinfection with Hydrogen Peroxide

- Using the cup provided with the hydrogen peroxide product, soak lenses for the length of time specified by the manufacturer. Do not use lens cups or cases that came with other products.
- To disinfect and neutralize in one step, place platinum catalytic disk in lens case and leave the disk there until time to replace it. Add hydrogen peroxide, insert lenses, and leave for at least 6 hours.
- Never place neutralizing solution in lens case with a catalytic disk. An unwanted chemical reaction may occur, or a gummy residue may form on the disk.
- Make sure hydrogen peroxide is completely neutralized by carefully following product instructions before inserting lenses in the eyes.
- Rinse lenses thoroughly with saline before inserting them.

Combination Enzyme Cleaning and Disinfection

- When combining enzyme cleaning and disinfecting of the lenses as one step, select products compatible with your disinfecting system (Table 29-12).
- Add appropriate solution (hydrogen peroxide or chemical disinfecting product) to storage case of disinfecting system.
- Add lenses, and then add appropriate enzymatic cleaner.
- Follow directions above for appropriate disinfecting system.
- Rinse lenses thoroughly with saline to remove residual enzymes

Chemical Preservative Disinfection

- Store lenses for prescribed period of time (usually a minimum of 4 hours) in a preservative disinfecting solution appropriate for the lenses.
- Rinse lenses thoroughly with saline to remove disinfecting solution if you experience irritation.

Acanthamoeba. Patients using Oxysept UltraCare should know the following:

- This product requires a minimum of 6 hours to complete disinfection and neutralization of the peroxide.
- The neutralizing tablet should not be crushed or used if there are cracks in the coating, or the tablet will start neutralizing the peroxide before adequate disinfection occurs.
- MiraFlow and Pliagel, which are used for surface-active cleaning, can leave a film on the lenses and lens cup if they are not carefully rinsed off the lens. This film may result in foaming and overflow of the peroxide-neutralizer solution.[11] If this occurs, lenses should be rinsed more carefully or another surface-active cleaner should be used.
- Before lenses are removed from the eye, the lens container should be filled with fresh Oxysept UltraCare disinfection solution, the neutralization tablet added, and the cap tightened; the cup is turned upside down and then right side up three times to allow the solution to bathe the upper portion of the cup and the top.
- When lenses are to be inserted, the cup should be turned upside down to ensure full neutralization of all residual disinfecting solution in the lens case; then the lenses are removed from the case and inserted.

- Oxysept UltraCare should not be used with Illusions soft contact lenses. Lens damage may result.
- If the lenses are not going to be worn for a while, they can be stored unopened in the neutralized solution. However, they should be disinfected once weekly and just before wear.

Multipurpose Products

Initially, manufacturers recommended three different products for the cleaning, protein removal, and disinfection of soft contact lenses. However, there has been a trend toward using multipurpose solutions for these functions; some single solutions claim to be effective for all three procedures.

The major problem with a multipurpose solution is that ingredients required in its formulation perform different and somewhat incompatible functions. For example, high concentrations of preservatives are necessary to kill bacteria; however, these same concentrations can cause ocular irritation when placed directly on the eye with a contact lens. If lenses are stored overnight in a cleaning solution containing an anionic surfactant, the detergent may eventually build up on the lens and cause irritation.

Some cold disinfection systems are considered multipurpose solutions, including ReNu MultiPlus MultiPurpose Solution, ReNu Multipurpose Disinfecting Solution, OptiFree Express, and SOLO-care 10 minute. All these solutions are indicated for surface-active cleaning of the lens as well as disinfection. Some of the products also perform protein removal. Some have also met FDA requirements to be labeled as "no rub required," meaning that no rubbing is needed during the cleaning step.[12] Examples include OptiFree Express, ReNu Multi-Plus, and AO Sept Clear Care. It should be noted that all of the no-rub products require thorough rinsing of the lenses, not just soaking without rinsing first.

These products are useful for patients with planned replacement lenses, because these lenses are usually discarded before a significant amount of protein or lipid builds up on the lens. Patients who wear traditional soft contact lenses usually benefit from using separate solutions for cleaning, protein removal, and disinfection rather than multipurpose solutions.

Recently, ReNu Multiplus has been implicated in causing corneal staining in some patients when used to clean and disinfect PureVision silicone hydrogel contact lenses. This combination should be avoided.

In recent years, several cold disinfection products have been recalled from the market amid reports of serious eye infections involving *Fusarium*, a fungus, and *Acanthamoeba*, a parasite. These recalls have underscored the importance of compliance with a good contact lens care regimen, given that poor compliance with lens care was a factor in these reports. The FDA has recommended that patients consider performing a "rub and rinse" lens cleaning method rather than a no-rub method to decrease the chances of infection.

Saline Solutions

The hydrophilic soft contact lens must be maintained in a constant state of hydration. Furthermore, the hydrated lens must be isotonic with tears, because changes in tonicity can alter the conformation and optical properties of the lens. Isotonic normal saline is the basic solution used for rinsing, thermally disinfecting, and storing soft contact lenses.

Prepared saline is available in either preserved or preservative-free forms. Because thimerosal and chlorhexidine can cause sensitivity reactions or irritation in many patients, sorbic acid–preserved products are commonly promoted for sensitive eyes and appear to be acceptable to most wearers.

Several preservative-free saline solutions are also available. Preservative-free buffered saline is available in multiuse bottles (which must be discarded 30 days after opening) and as aerosol sprays.

Patients using nonpreserved saline should be counseled that only aerosolized solutions can be used to rinse lenses just before insertion into the eye. Multipurpose nonpreserved saline (e.g., Unisol 4) should never be used to rinse lenses just before insertion, unless the bottle is new and has not been opened. Once these products have been opened, they should be used only if a disinfection step will be performed before insertion.

Patients should avoid using other forms of saline such as intravenous normal saline or saline squirts; these products are usually too acidic for use with soft contact lenses.

Some patients prepare their own preservative-free saline using salt tablets and USP purified water. Using salt tablets is inexpensive, but the clear superiority of commercial saline solutions argues strongly against use of homemade saline. This practice and the application of improper lens care are the greatest predisposing factors to *Acanthamoeba* keratitis and many anterior eye infections contracted by hydrophilic lens wearers. When contact lens patients started using homemade salt tablet solutions, there was a resurgence of *Acanthamoeba* infections. Usually nonpathogenic, *Acanthamoeba* has been isolated from airborne dust, soils, surface water, tap water, and even distilled water. In unfavorable environments, it forms a very resistant cyst that can survive many antimicrobial agents, even though its vegetative form (trophozoite) may be susceptible. Viable cysts have been found in swimming pools and hot tubs that are adequately chlorinated to kill trophozoites. *Acanthamoeba* infection was very rare until contact lenses became popular. Most victims of *Acanthamoeba* keratitis have used improper lens hygiene, gone swimming without removing their contact lenses, used nonsterile saline solution made from salt tablets and distilled water, or used tap water in the maintenance of their soft contact lenses. Because they are very resistant, *Acanthamoeba* cysts often can survive attempts to eradicate them from the eye with antimicrobial agents. Multiple antibiotic regimens have been applied with variable or poor therapeutic response. Many cases of *Acanthamoeba* keratitis are severe enough to require keratoplasty (a partial or complete cornea transplant) in an attempt to save the eye. Unfortunately, the persistent presence of cysts gives this eye infection a poor prognosis and in many cases, ultimately leads to enucleation—the partial or total removal of the affected eye. For these reasons, FDA no longer condones the use of salt tablets, and neither should a concerned practitioner.

Rewetting Solutions

Accessory solutions for use with soft lenses permit lubricating and rewetting (and, in some cases, cleaning) of the lens in the eye. These solutions typically contain a low concentration of a nonionic surfactant to promote cleaning and a polymer to lubricate the lens surface, along with buffering agents. Clerz Plus Lens Drops contains Clens 100, a patented surfactant that acts on protein, lipid, and calcium deposits. Besides rewetting activity, this product provides some on-the-eye cleaning, which can help improve lens comfort.[12] Other rewetting products, blink Contacts and AQuify, contain sodium hyaluronate, which strongly adheres to the mucin layer of the tear film. This property allows for a water-retaining layer that resists evaporation.

Rewetting solutions are particularly useful to patients with highly hydrated lenses, such as the continuous-wear type. Exposing lenses to wind and high temperature causes some dehydration, even with the lens in the eye. The resultant discomfort is sometimes relieved by one or two drops of rewetting solution. To minimize contamination, the tip of the applicator bottle should not touch the eye, eyelid, or any other surface. (See chapter 28 for a discussion of administration of eye drops.)

Product Selection Guidelines

Many problems associated with soft lens wear arise from the way people handle their lenses; unsatisfactory results may stem from improper procedures rather than inadequate products. It should be noted, however, that patients who choose to buy generic (e.g., mass merchandiser labeled) multipurpose lens solutions may be purchasing older, potentially obsolete formulas. Mass merchandisers generally purchase older formulations of nationally known brands of multipurpose solutions and then market them under their private label. In addition, the composition of a particular generic formulation can vary, because the stores bid from manufacturers two to three times per year. Generally, it is preferable that patients not use generic brands unless they carefully read the label and compare all of the ingredients to the product that was recommended by their eye care professional or pharmacist. It is important to note that manufacturers are not required to use the same name for generic and brand-name ingredients, so it may be difficult to compare formulations.

Table 29-14 lists examples of products designed specifically for soft contact lenses. Specific questions about the care and maintenance regimen a wearer uses can often bring these problems to light.

SURFACE-ACTIVE CLEANERS

Some surface-active cleaners (e.g., Bausch & Lomb Sensitive Eyes Daily Cleaner) have a lower viscosity and may be easier to rinse off the lens. These products are good choices for patients who have difficulty completely rinsing the cleaner off their lens.

In addition to surfactants, some products (e.g., Opti-Clean II) contain mild abrasives that aid in the removal of lens deposits. Patients who have difficulty removing deposits from their lenses will benefit from this type of cleaner. These products should be shaken before use. Some patients may have difficulty rinsing these cleaners off their lenses. Care should be taken to be sure that no residue from the cleaning solution remains on the lens prior to insertion.

Finally, one surfactant cleaner (MiraFlow) contains isopropyl alcohol. This product is useful for patients who discover heavy lipid deposits on their lenses.

ENZYMATIC CLEANERS

Enzymatic cleaners can be recommended according to the disinfection system used by the patient. Ultrazyme and Unizyme are good choices for the patient using a hydrogen peroxide cleaning system. These products can be placed in the peroxide solution, thereby cleaning and disinfecting at the same time. If the patient uses Opti-Free disinfecting solution, Supra-Clens or Opti-Free Enzymatic Cleaner would be a good choice, because they can be placed directly in the Opti-Free solution during the disinfection cycle. If the patient uses ReNu Multipurpose

TABLE 29-14 Selected Products for Soft Lenses

Trade Name	Primary Ingredients
Surface-Active Cleaning Solutions	
Bausch & Lomb Sensitive Eyes Daily Cleaner	Hydroxypropyl methylcellulose; sorbic acid 0.25%; EDTA 0.5%; NaCl; borate buffer; poloxamine
MiraFlow Extra Strength	Isopropyl alcohol 20%; poloxamer 407; amphoteric 10
Opti-Clean II Daily Cleaner	Nylon 11; polysorbate 21; hydroxyethyl cellulose; polyquaternium-1; EDTA; boric acid; sodium borate; NaCl
Opti-Free Daily Cleaner	Nylon 11; polysorbate 21; hydroxyethyl cellulose; polyquaternium-1, 0.001%; EDTA; boric acid; sodium borate; hydrochloric acid and/or sodium hydroxide
Pliagel	Sorbic acid 0.25%; EDTA 0.5%; poloxamer 407; KCl; NaCl
Enzymatic Cleaning Products	
Opti-Free SupraClens Daily Protein Remover Solution[a]	Highly purified porcine pancreatin enzymes; PEG; sodium borate
ReNu 1 Step Daily Protein Remover Liquid	Subtilisin; glycerin; borate buffers
Ultrazyme Enzymatic Cleaner Tablet	Subtilisin A; effervescing agents; buffers
Unizyme Tablet	Subtilisin
Chemical Disinfecting Solutions	
ReNu Multipurpose Solution	Poloxamine; polyaminopropyl biguanide; boric acid; edetate disodium
Hydrogen Peroxide Disinfecting Solutions and Rinsing/Neutralizing Products	
AO Sept	Disinfecting solution: hydrogen peroxide 3%; NaCl 0.85%; phosphate buffers; phosphoric acid Neutralizer: platinum disk
AO Sept Clear Care	Hydrogen peroxide 3%; pluronic; platinum disk
Oxysept UltraCare	Disinfecting solution: hydrogen peroxide 3%; sodium stannate; sodium nitrate; phosphates Neutralizer: catalase tablet; cyanocobalamin (color indicator)
Preserved Saline Solutions	
Bausch & Lomb Sensitive Eyes Saline	Sorbic acid 0.1%; NaCl; borate buffer; EDTA
Preservative-Free Saline Products	
AMO Lens Plus	NaCl; boric acid
Unisol 4 Saline Solution	NaCl; sodium borate; boric acid
Rewetting/Lubricating Solutions	
Clerz Plus	Clens 100; Tetronic 1304
Clerz 2	Hydroxyethyl cellulose; sorbic acid 0.1%; EDTA 0.1%; NaCl; KCl; sodium borate
Opti-Free Rewetting Drops	Polyquaternium-1, 0.001%; citric acid; sodium citrate; NaCl
ReNu Rewetting Drops	Sorbic acid 0.15%; EDTA; borate buffer; poloxamine; NaCl
Multipurpose Solutions	
AQuify	Sorbitol; dexpanthenol; pluronic F127; tromethamine; polyhexanide; EDTA
Opti-Free Express Multipurpose Solution Opti-Free Replenish	Polyquaternium-1, 0.001%; EDTA; sodium citrate; NaCl; citric acid; myristamidopropyl demethylamine; citrate buffer; C9-ED3A; Tetronic 1304
ReNu MultiPlus Solution	Polyaminopropyl biguanide; EDTA; NaCl; sodium borate; boric acid; poloxamine
ReNu Multi-Purpose Solution	Polyaminopropyl biguanide; EDTA; NaCl; sodium borate; boric acid; poloxamine

Key: EDTA, ethylenediamine tetraacetic acid; KCl, potassium chloride; NaCl, sodium chloride; PEG, polyethylene glycol.
[a] Preservative-free formulation.

Disinfecting solution, then ReNu 1 Step liquid (daily use) would be a good choice. If the patient uses another chemical disinfection system, product comparisons are very idiosyncratic unless the patient is allergic to one of the components.

DISINFECTING METHODS

When counseling a patient about the best disinfecting method to use, compliance and convenience should be considered. Ultra-Care (2-hour exposure to hydrogen peroxide) is a good choice; it is the only method that eradicates *Acanthamoeba* besides heat disinfection, which is no longer commonly used. If a patient does not want to use a hydrogen peroxide system, a second-generation chemical system (i.e., Opti-Free Express or ReNu Multipurpose) can be recommended.

When choosing a chemical disinfection product, several factors should be considered. If the patient has a history of sensitivity reactions to lens solutions or is unsure if sensitivity exists, it is best to recommend a product containing one of the nonsensitizing preservatives. A recommendation can be made on the basis of the brand and type of enzymatic cleaner the patient is using. For example, if the patient is using Supra-Clens Enzymatic cleaner, then Opti-Free or Opti-Free Express should be recommended as the disinfecting agent. If a patient has no preference for a particular enzymatic product, then any of the chemical disinfection solutions that can be used concurrently with an enzymatic product are appropriate.

PRODUCT INCOMPATIBILITY

Several incompatibilities may occur when mixing soft lens products. Most manufacturers test for compatibility within their own product lines; however, compatibility with other manufacturers' products is usually not determined. Generally, chemical disinfecting solutions should not be interchanged or used concurrently. If a patient mixes a disinfecting solution containing chlorhexidine and thimerosal with a product containing a quaternary ammonium compound, a toxic keratopathy known as mixed solution syndrome may occur. Patients should be counseled not to switch from a chlorhexidine-containing chemical disinfection system to a hydrogen peroxide system, unless they procure new lenses. A fine black precipitate may form on the lenses if chlorhexidine is still present in the lens matrix. Other chemical disinfection system residue on soft lenses may cause the lens to turn pink, yellow, brown, black, or purple if the lens is exposed to a hydrogen peroxide system.[4]

Insertion and Removal

Table 29-15 provides instructions for inserting and removing soft lenses.

Lens Storage Case

Choice of a lens storage case is important. The case should have left and right clearly identified on the caps and in the lens wells. The lens wells should have ridges or flutes so the RGP lens does not adhere to the case, an occurrence that is common in smooth cases and can cause warping of the lens or inversion on removal.

The proper care and cleaning of the contact lens storage case are as important as lens care itself. A storage case should be able to hold at least 2.5 mL of the storage solution.[13] This volume minimizes the chance that the soaking solution will be overwhelmed by an inoculum of bacteria. The lens case should be cleaned thoroughly on a routine basis and replaced at least

---

TABLE 29-15 Insertion and Removal of Soft Lenses

Insertion

- Wash the hands with noncosmetic soap and rinse thoroughly; dry the hands with a lint-free towel.
- Remove the lens for the right eye from its storage container.
- (Optional) Rinse the lens with saline solution to dilute any preservatives left from disinfection.
- Place the lens on the top of a finger, and examine it to be sure it is not inside out. This determination can be done by using the "taco test." Gently fold the lens at the apex (not the edges) between the thumb and forefinger. The edges should look like a taco shell with the edges pointed inward. If the edges roll out, the lens is inverted and must be reversed.
- Examine the lens for cleanliness. If necessary, clean it and rinse again.
- Insert the lens on the right eye using the same procedure as for hard and RGP lenses (see Table 29-5).
- Repeat the process for the left eye.

Removal

- Before removing the lenses, wash hands with a noncosmetic soap; rinse the hands thoroughly and dry them with a lint-free towel.
- Using the right middle finger, pull down the lower lid of the right eye. Touch the right index finger to the lens and slide the lens off the cornea, as shown in drawing A.
- Using the index finger and thumb, grasp the lens and remove it (see drawing B).
- Repeat the procedure for the left eye.

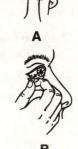

A

B

---

every 3 months.[14] Routine cleaning entails air drying the case between periods of use and scrubbing it weekly. Air-drying should be done daily to discourage biofilm formation. Some manufacturers recommend cleaning the case twice weekly using a few drops of lens cleaner and hot water. If the case can withstand routine boiling (such as those cases made of polycarbonate or noryl plastic), it can be boiled in a pot of water for 10 minutes weekly. Examine the case for cracks and replace it periodically. Lens cases can be contaminated with a biofilm that will attract pathogens and increase the risk of infection.

Assessment of Contact Lens–Related Problems: A Case-Based Approach

Although contact lenses are usually safe, lens wearers can experience a variety of problems. During the patient interview, the practitioner should first determine what type of eye problems exist and how long the patient has been experiencing them. Asking the patient whether a history of eye problems exists and what medications are currently being taken will give a general sense of the etiology and urgency of the current eye problem. The answers will also help the practitioner determine whether the problem is related to noncompliance with care regimens or to drug–lens interactions.

Determining which type of contact lenses a patient is wearing and for how long is crucial in assessing problems related to improper lens care or deteriorated lenses. Each type of lens has unique physical characteristics that, in turn, dictate which methods and products for cleaning and disinfecting lenses are appropriate. Patients should be asked to describe how they care for their lenses, which lens care products they use, and whether they have recently changed products. Many lens care–related problems are minor and can be easily solved by a knowledgeable practitioner.

The individual sections on types of contact lenses discuss problems related to lens care. The following sections discuss other types of lens–related problems and their symptoms, as well as problems that require medical referral.

Precautions for Contact Lenses

Contact lenses generally can match or exceed the vision obtained with spectacles. However, depending on the type of lens, vision may become worse in certain situations. Some patients wearing lenses with high water content may experience hazy vision around the edges of objects. In some cases, patients wearing hard lenses experience nighttime ghosting, which occurs when the patient's pupil dilates enough to see the edges of the lens. This can sometimes be corrected with larger-diameter lenses. Other patients complain of spiderweb vision, usually at night; this problem can be due to crazing (i.e., the development of fine cracks) and is usually experienced with RGP lenses.

Potential Transmission of Viral Infections

The human immunodeficiency virus (HIV) has been isolated from the tears of infected individuals as well as from the contact lenses worn by infected individuals. This contamination seemingly becomes an issue in the case of trial contact lenses, which may be reused by different patients in the lens–fitter's office. Use of disposable contact lenses is advisable in this situation. Generally, trial lenses are not dispensed to a patient except as loaner lenses (i.e., to a patient waiting for new replacement lenses). Even in this scenario, after the lenses have been used in any patient, they are disinfected with heat or chemicals before being dispensed to another patient. Studies have shown that heat and the routinely available hydrogen peroxide products are effective in inactivating HIV.

Adverse Effects of Drugs

Many undesired effects have been reported when a patient who wears contact lenses ingests, applies, or encounters certain drugs (Table 29-16). The practitioner must understand these drug-induced problems to counsel patients effectively.

Topical Drugs

In general, patients should be counseled not to place any ophthalmic solution, suspension, gel, or ointment into the eye when contact lenses are in place. The only exceptions to this rule are products specifically formulated to be used with contact lenses, such as rewetting drops, or those products that an eye care practitioner has specifically recommended for use with contact lenses.

Topical administration of ophthalmic drugs may have physiologic consequences or may modify pharmacologic responses to drugs. The use of solutions that may be considered benign, such as artificial tears, may reduce tear breakup time and alter the distribution of the mucoid, aqueous, and lipid components of tears, perhaps causing initial discomfort on instillation of the drops.[4] The pharmacologic effect of a topically administered drug while soft lenses are in place may be exaggerated. The soft lens may absorb the drug and either release it over time, creating a sustained-release dosage form, or bind it tightly so that none of it is released into the eye. Furthermore, the presence of any kind of contact lens may increase the amount of time the medication is in contact with the eye. Finally, increased drug absorption may occur secondary to a compromised corneal epithelium during contact lens wear.[4]

In certain cases, patients will be treated with topical ophthalmic medications while wearing contact lenses. For example, these medications are used in conjunction with disposable soft contact lenses as an alternative to bandage contact lenses in the treatment of persistent epithelial corneal defects. Yet, an opaque precipitate has been noted in case reports of some patients who used SeeQuence disposable contact lenses and were treated with topical ciprofloxacin and topical prednisolone acetate concurrently.[15] When studied in the laboratory, neither drug alone produced precipitates in the contact lens; white crystalline deposits were noted only when the two topical agents were used in combination. In another study, the combination of topical gentamicin and methylprednisolone produced precipitates.[16] Therefore, if a patient who wears contact lenses is treated with a topical antibiotic and steroid combination, the eye care practitioner must carefully monitor for deposits in the lenses. If deposits are noted, the lenses should be removed and replaced with a new pair.

In addition, the preservatives, vehicles, tonicity, and pH of the solution instilled into the eye may alter the properties of the lenses. For instance, instillation of hypertonic solutions such as sodium sulfacetamide 10% or pilocarpine 8% may cause soft lens dehydration and lens disfigurement. Topical medications with an acidic pH promote lens dehydration and steepening; alkaline medications promote hydration and flattening.[17] Topical suspensions may lead to lens intolerance, because particulate matter builds up and causes discomfort. Gel and oil formulations may alter the surface relationship between the contact lens and the cornea.[9] Finally, the active ingredient of certain topical products may discolor lenses. For example, exposure to light and air causes epinephrine to form adrenochrome deposits, which range in color from pink to brown.

Airborne Drugs and Particulate Matter

Some drugs present in indoor air may damage lenses. For example, nurses who care for patients receiving ribavirin have reportedly experienced cloudy lenses after repeated exposure to the drug.[18,19] Similarly, contact lens wearers who have been exposed to a large amount of cigarette smoke have discovered a brown discoloration and nicotine deposits on their lenses. This problem is especially true for those who smoke and have nicotine-stained fingers.[20]

Systemic Medications

Some systemic medications are secreted into tears and may interact with (primarily soft) contact lenses. For example, rifampin will stain both lenses and tears orange. Drugs and dietary supplements such as gold salts and garlic are secreted into the tears and may cause ocular irritation. Other drugs may affect tear production, the refractive properties of the eye, the shape of the cornea, or the actual lens (Table 29-16).[21] Some medications

TABLE 29-16 Drug–Contact Lens Interactions

Changes in Tear Film and/or Production

Decreased Tear Volume

Anticholinergic agents

Antihistamines

Beta-blockers

Benzodiazepines

Botulinum toxin type A (Botox)

Conjugated estrogens

Diuretics

Oral contraceptives

Phenothiazines

Serotonin reuptake inhibitors

Sildenafil citrate

Statins

Timolol (topical)

Tricyclic antidepressants

Vardenafil HCl

Increased Tear Volume

Cholinergic agents

Garlic (dietary supplement)

Reserpine

Changes in Lens Color (Primarily Soft Lenses)

Diagnostic dyes (i.e., fluorescein)

Epinephrine (topical)

Fluorescein (topical)

Nicotine

Nitrofurantoin

Phenazopyridine

Phenolphthalein

Phenothiazines

Phenylephrine

Rifampin

Sulfasalazine

Tetracycline

Tetrahydrozoline (topical)

Changes in Tonicity

Pilocarpine (8%)

Sodium sulfacetamide (10%)

Lid/Corneal Edema

Chlorthalidone

Clomiphene

Conjugated estrogens

Oral contraceptives

Primidone

Ocular Inflammation/Irritation

Diclofenac (topical ophthalmic)

Garlic (dietary supplement)

Salicylates

Gold salts

Isotretinoin

Changes in Refractivity (Induction of Myopia)

Acetazolamide

Sulfadiazine

Sulfamethizole

Sulfamethoxazole

Sulfisoxazole

Changes in Pupil Size

Pupillary Dilation

Anticholinergic agents

Antidepressants

Antihistamines

CNS stimulants

Kava

Phenothiazines

Pupillary Miosis

Opiates

Miscellaneous Agents (Effects)

Digoxin (increased glare)

Ribavirin (cloudy lenses)

Topical ciprofloxacin/prednisolone acetate (precipitate)

Hypnotics/sedatives/muscle relaxants (decreased blink rate)

Key: CNS, central nervous system.

Source: Adapted with permission from Engle JP. Contact lens care. *Am Druggist.* 1990;201:5465.

may influence the size of the pupil, causing complaints of glare or flare when lenses are in place. Visual performance may be diminished, especially in patients who wear multifocal lenses or gas permeable lenses for which pupil size may determine placement of the reading segment or the optic zone of the lens, respectively.[22]

Use of Cosmetics

Patients who wear contact lenses should choose—and use—cosmetics with care. Individuals should insert lenses before applying makeup and should avoid touching the lens with eyeliner or mascara. Cosmetics, moisturizers, and makeup removers with an aqueous base should be used, because oil-based products may cause blurred vision and irritation if they are deposited on the lens. Cream eye shadows are preferable to powder shadows. Water-resistant (as opposed to waterproof) mascara (which requires an oil-based remover) should be applied to only the very tips of the lashes. Eyeliners should never be applied inside the eyelid margin; the liner can clog glands in the eyelid and contaminate the contact lens. Aerosol products, in particular, must be used with caution. Irritation may occur if some of the spray particles are trapped in the tear layer beneath the lens, and some sprays may actually damage the lens. One way to avoid this problem is to insert the lenses, go into another room, cover the eyes with a cloth, use the spray, and then leave the area with the eyes still closed.

Nail polish, hand creams, and perfumes should also be applied only after the lenses have been inserted. Nail polish and remover can destroy a lens. Men often contaminate their lenses with hair preparations and spray deodorants; they should take special care to clean their hands thoroughly before handling their lenses. Soaps that contain cold cream or deodorants should be avoided; they can leave a film on the fingers after rinsing. This residue readily transfers to a lens and can cause blurred vision. Moreover, if a lens comes in contact with residual petrolatum-based lotion on the patient's fingers, the lens's surface can be modified. This modification cannot be detected by inspection; it will be noted, however, once the lens is worn. The surface-wetting properties of the lens are disrupted approximately 20 to 30 minutes after insertion of the lens.

Corneal Hypoxia and Edema

An adequate supply of oxygen exists only if the cornea is continuously bathed with oxygenated tears. During blinking, metabolic byproducts from the surface epithelium are flushed from under the contact lenses, and oxygen is brought in as the lenses move toward and away from the cornea. Even when properly fitted, however, both rigid and soft lenses can produce a progressive hypoxia of the cornea while the lenses are in place, especially in persons who have low blink frequency or incomplete blinks.

One major effect of this hypoxia is edema of the corneal tissues. It has been demonstrated that corneal thickness is increased by hard (PMMA) lenses. After approximately 16 hours of continuous wear, hard and, to a lesser extent, soft lenses cause the glycogen content of the cornea to fall to a level that is accompanied by significant edema. Symptoms associated with corneal edema include photophobia; rainbows around a light; sensations of hotness, grittiness, and itchiness; fogging of vision; and blurred vision. Although it is not usually necessary, a patient experiencing corneal edema from overuse of contact lenses can be treated with one to two drops of a sodium chloride (2% or 5%) ophthalmic solution every 3 to 4 hours after the lenses have been removed. The patient should be counseled that transient stinging or burning may occur on instilling the drops. Furthermore, the patient should be counseled not to overuse the lenses.

Another effect of corneal hypoxia is neovascularization (the development of new vessels), which is potentially irreversible. Routine follow-up visits to the eye care practitioner are important to monitor this effect of contact lens wear.

Corneal Abrasions

Corneal abrasions are surface defects in the epithelial layer of the cornea. The causes of these abrasions range from poorly fitted lenses or simple overwear to the entrapment of foreign bodies under the lens. The cornea is sensitive to abrasion, so blepharospasm (reflex lid closure), tearing, and rubbing the affected eye occur immediately. However, rubbing the eye can cause more extensive damage while the lens remains in the eye and must be avoided.

Fortunately, the pain associated with corneal abrasion is usually of greater magnitude than the damage. The epithelium regenerates quickly; most minor epithelial defects (i.e., those 22 mm in diameter or less) generally heal within 12 to 24 hours. The lens should be left out for 2 to 7 days. The wearer may then proceed using a modified break-in schedule suggested by the eye care practitioner. More extensive abrasions require the attention of an eye care practitioner.

Symptoms of Lens Problems

Patients may initially encounter various problems in adapting to contact lenses, particularly RGP lenses; even longtime wearers occasionally experience difficulty. Many of these problems arise from different causative factors, and identifying and solving a specific problem may require an eye care practitioner. The following list provides a perspective for counseling a lens wearer who seeks advice. Most of this information is particularly applicable to rigid lens wear.

- *Deep aching of eye:* This pain persists even after the lens is removed, and it may be caused by poorly fitted lenses. The eye care practitioner must be consulted.
- *Blurred vision:* This effect may be produced by improper refractive power, lenses switched right for left, lenses placed on the eye inside out, tear film buildup, cosmetic film buildup, corneal edema, or the use of oral contraceptives.
- *Excessive tearing:* Tearing is normal when lenses are first worn; however, poorly fitted lenses or chipped, rough edges on the lenses may also cause tearing.
- *Fogging:* Misty or smoky vision can be caused by corneal edema, overwearing of contact lenses, coatings or deposits on lens surfaces, or poor wetting of the lens while on the eye.
- *Flare:* Point sources of light having a sunburst or streaming quality can be caused by inadequate optic zone size or decentration of a poorly fitting lens.
- *Itching:* This symptom may be caused by allergic conjunctivitis and may be treated with short-term use of topical steroids (with the lenses out of the eyes).
- *Lens falling out of eye:* Poorly fitted lenses could be the cause. However, even properly fitted rigid lenses may occasionally slide off the cornea or be blinked out of the eye.
- *Inability to wear lenses in the morning:* This problem may be caused by corneal edema or mild conjunctivitis. The most likely cause is that the patient's eyes dry out overnight because of incomplete eyelid closure.
- *Pain after removal of lens:* This problem is usually caused by corneal abrasion. The presence of the lens anesthetizes the cornea owing to hypoxia; sensation returns after 4 to 6 hours and pain develops.
- *Sudden pain in the eye:* A foreign body or a chipped or folded lens may be the problem.
- *Squinting:* This effect is caused by excessive movement of a lens or by a poorly fitted lens. The wearer will squint to center the optical portion of the lens over the pupil.

Exclusions for Self-Care

When lens care is appropriate but the lenses are old or, in the case of hard lenses, chipped or scratched, the patient should see an eye care practitioner for replacement lenses. Other situations that require referral are suspected vision changes, deep aching of the eyes, last eye examination occurring more than 1 year ago, and a suspected interaction between the lenses and oral contraceptives or other systemic medications. Patients experiencing lens problems related to the medical conditions or other factors discussed in Contraindications for Contact Lenses should also be referred for further evaluation.

Cases 29-1 and 29-2 illustrate the assessment of patients with contact lens–related problems.

Patient Counseling for Prevention of Contact Lens–Related Disorders

The box Patient Education for Preventing Contact Lens–Related Disorders outlines the care regimen for each type of contact lens.

CASE 29-1

Relevant Evaluation Criteria	Scenario/Model Outcome

Information Gathering

1. Gather essential information about the patient's symptoms, including:

   a. description of symptom(s) (i.e., nature, onset, duration, severity, associated symptoms)

   Patient complains of eye discomfort associated with soft contact lenses. Patient began wearing this particular pair of lenses 4 months ago. She did not experience discomfort when she first began wearing the lenses; however, during the past 2–3 weeks, she has noticed discomfort and some irritation that occurs only when she wears the lenses. The patient does not complain of other symptoms such as discharge from the eye. Her last visit to the lens prescriber was 4 months ago when she received her lenses.

   b. description of any factors that seem to precipitate, exacerbate, and/or relieve the patient's symptom(s)

   None

   c. description of the patent's efforts to relieve the symptoms

   The patient's lens care regimen includes cleaning the lenses with Sensitive Eyes Daily Cleaner each time she removes them. She then soaks the lenses in Oxysept Ultra-Care with a neutralization tablet (hydrogen peroxide disinfection system) for 6 hours. She cleans her storage container once per week according to the manufacturer's recommendations.

2. Gather essential patient history information:

   a. patient's identity

   Elizabeth Gallagher

   b. age, weight, sex, and height

   18-year-old female

   c. patient's occupation

   College student

   d. patient's dietary habits

   N/A

   e. patient's sleep habits

   Stays up late most nights; tries to get at least 7 hours of sleep each night; removes contacts before going to bed

   f. concurrent medications and medical conditions

   Famotidine as needed for occasional heartburn

   g. allergies

   Penicillin

   h. history of other adverse reactions to medications

   None

   i. other (describe) _____

   Does not smoke; drinks 1–2 martinis per week

Assessment and Triage

3. Correctly identify the patient's primary problem(s).

   Lens discomfort secondary to protein buildup on the lens

4. Identify exclusions for self-care.

   None

5. Formulate a comprehensive list of therapeutic alternatives to address the primary problem and share this information with the patient.

   Options include:
   (1) Refer Elizabeth to her eye care practitioner.
   (2) Recommend a change in her lens care routine.
   (3) Take no action.

Plan

6. Select an optimal therapeutic alternative to address the patient's problem.

   Add an enzymatic product to the lens care regimen.

CASE 29-1 (continued)

Relevant Evaluation Criteria	Scenario/Model Outcome
7. Describe the recommended therapeutic approach to the patient.	Add Ultrazyme to the lens care regimen. Place one enzyme tablet in the Oxysept Ultracare solution once weekly. See Table 29-13 for more details.
8. Explain to the patient the rationale for selecting the recommended therapeutic approach from the considered therapeutic alternatives.	There are no symptoms of infection or of a poor-fitting lens. Because you were not doing the enzymatic step to clean your lenses, it is appropriate to recommend the addition of an enzymatic product. Ultrazyme was chosen because you use Oxysept Ultracare disinfection. The Ultrazyme tablet can be placed directly in the Oxysept Ultracare weekly to perform the enzymatic and disinfection step concurrently, which enhances compliance.

Patient Education

9. When recommending self-care with non-prescription medications, convey accurate information to the patient:	
a. appropriate dose and frequency of administration	Use the Ultrazyme once weekly. If the lenses seem to get uncomfortable before the week is finished, the Ultrazyme can be used more frequently.
b. maximum number of days the therapy should be employed	N/A
c. product administration procedures	N/A
d. expected time to onset of relief	After 1 or 2 weekly uses of the enzymatic cleaner, the lenses should feel more comfortable.
e. degree of relief that can be reasonably expected	The lenses should feel as comfortable as when you first received them.
f. most common side effects	Stinging, burning, itching (uncommon for most people)
g. side effects that warrant medical intervention should they occur	Continued feelings of irritation and discomfort after two to three enzymatic cleanings
h. patient options in the event that condition worsens or persists	The lens prescriber should be consulted if the discomfort or irritation persists or worsens, or if symptoms of infection appear, such as a thick discharge from either eye or eyelids glued together when you awake.
i. product storage requirements	Store at room temperature in a dry place.
j. specific nondrug measures	N/A
10. Solicit follow-up questions from patient.	May I use any other enzyme product to clean my lenses?
11. Answer patient's questions.	Two products can be used with hydrogen peroxide disinfection. You can also try Unizyme if you prefer.

Key: N/A, not applicable.

CASE 29-2

Relevant Evaluation Criteria	Scenario/Model Outcome
Information Gathering	
1. Gather essential information about the patient's symptoms, including:	
a. description of symptom(s) (i.e., nature, onset, duration, severity, associated symptoms).	Patient began wearing 2-week frequent replacement soft contact lenses 3 weeks ago. She is looking for information about the proper care of her lenses.

CASE 29-2 (continued)

Relevant Evaluation Criteria	Scenario/Model Outcome
b. description of any factors that seem to precipitate, exacerbate, and/or relieve the patient's symptom(s).	The patient has never worn contact lenses before, and she is not sure of the proper care and wearing regimen for her lenses.
c. description of the patent's efforts to relieve the symptoms.	N/A
2. Gather essential patient history information:	
a. patient's identity	Debra Walsh
b. age, weight, sex, and height	32-year-old female
c. patient's occupation	Engineer
d. patient's dietary habits	N/A
e. patient's sleep habits	Has a regular sleep schedule
f. concurrent medications and medical conditions	Acetaminophen as needed for occasional headaches and pseudoephedrine for occasional nasal congestion
g. allergies	NKA
h. history of other adverse reactions to medications	None
i. other (describe)_____	She does not smoke and is a social drinker (an occasional glass of wine or a beer).

Assessment and Triage

3. Correctly identify the patient's primary problem(s).	Debra is wearing frequent replacement lenses and needs help with her lens care regimen. She is also not replacing her lenses as prescribed.
4. Identify exclusions for self-care.	None
5. Formulate a comprehensive list of therapeutic alternatives to address the primary problem and share this information with the patient.	Options include: (1) Refer Debra to her eye care practitioner. (2) Recommend a lens care routine and reinforce replacement schedule. (3) Take no action.

Plan

6. Select an optimal therapeutic alternative to address the patient's problem.	Recommend a multipurpose chemical disinfection product such as Opti-Free Express.
7. Describe the recommended therapeutic approach to the patient.	Because you are wearing frequent replacement lenses, you can try a one-bottle simplified regimen such as Opti-Free Express. Remove the lens from your eye. Apply a few drops of solution to the lens and rub the lens. Fill the lens case with enough fresh Opti-Free Express to cover the lenses. Store lenses in the closed lens case overnight or at least 6 hours. After soaking, lenses are ready to wear. The lenses may be left in the unopened lenses case for up to 30 days prior to wear. Fill your case with fresh solution every time you store your lenses. Never reuse solution. Be sure to replace your lenses every 2 weeks. Do not wear them for a longer period of time.
8. Explain to the patient the rationale for selecting the recommended therapeutic approach from the considered therapeutic alternatives.	Many options are appropriate to care for your lenses. Because you will be replacing them every 2 weeks, you can start out with a product such as Opti-Free Express. Some other options include multipurpose solutions such as Opti-Free Replenish, ReNu Multiplus, or Aquify.

Patient Education

9. When recommending self-care with non-prescription medications, convey accurate information to the patient:	
a. appropriate dose and frequency of administration	Use this product every time you remove your contact lenses.
b. maximum number of days the therapy should be employed	N/A
c. product administration procedures	N/A

Relevant Evaluation Criteria	Scenario/Model Outcome
d. expected time to onset of relief	N/A
e. degree of relief that can be reasonably expected	N/A
f. most common side effects	Stinging, burning, itching (uncommon for most people)
g. side effects that warrant medical intervention should they occur	If the lenses stop feeling comfortable or visual acuity is lessened, a different lens care regimen may be necessary. Some patients experience deposits on their lenses. Using cleaning products such as Mira Flow or Opti-Clean II and digital cleaning of the lenses will help in removing the deposits.
h. patient options in the event that condition worsens or persists	The lens prescriber should be consulted if the patient does not get good results from the recommended lens care regimen.
i. product storage requirements	Store at room temperature.
j. specific nondrug measures	N/A
10. Solicit follow-up questions from patient.	Are there other products that I could use?
11. Answer patient's questions.	There are many other soft contact lens products that could be used. However, because you have frequent replacement lenses, you can start out with one of the simpler regimens (one-bottle, multipurpose) to see if it is adequate for your needs.

Key: N/A, not applicable; NKA, no known allergies.

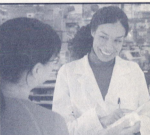

The objective of contact lens care is to prevent lens–related problems such as abrasions or infections of the cornea. For most patients, following the prescribed lens care regimen, product instructions, and self-care measures listed here will help ensure trouble-free use of contact lenses.

General Instructions for All Contact Lens Types

- Wash hands with noncosmetic soap and rinse thoroughly before touching contact lenses.
- Avoid wearing oily cosmetics while wearing lenses. Bath oils or soaps with an oil or a cream base may leave an oil film on the hands that will be transferred to the lenses.
- To avoid mixing up the lenses, always work with the same lens first. Check hard lenses for a dot in the lens periphery to avoid confusing lenses.
- If the lenses are not comfortable after insertion or vision is blurred, check to see if they are on the wrong eyes or are inside out.
- To avoid damaging lenses, apply aerosol cosmetics and deodorants either before lens insertion or with eyes closed until the air is clear of spray particles.
- Except for prescription continuous-wear lenses, do not wear lenses while sleeping.
- To avoid excessive dryness of the eyes, do not wear lenses while sitting under a hair dryer, overhead fans, or air ducts.
- When lenses are worn outside on windy days, protect the eyes from soot and other particles that may become trapped under the lens and scratch the cornea.
- Use eye protection in industry, sports, or any other occupation or hobby that has the potential for eye damage.
- Store contact lenses in a proper lens case when not in use.

- Never reuse contact lens solutions.
- Replace soaking/disinfecting solutions in lens case after each use. Do not top off the storage solution in the case after it has been used.
- Never store lenses in tap water.
- Do not wear contact lenses in swimming pools, hot tubs, or natural bodies of water without using external eye protection such as goggles.
- To prevent contamination, do not touch dropper tips or the tips of lens care product containers.
- While wearing lenses, apply to the eyes only ophthalmic solutions specifically formulated for contact lens use.
- Never use saliva to wet contact lenses. This practice can result in eye infections.
- Do not insert lenses in red or irritated eyes. If the eyes become irritated while lenses are being worn, remove the lenses until the irritation subsides. If irritation or redness does not subside, consult an eye care practitioner.
- If an eye infection is suspected, see an eye care practitioner immediately.

Instructions for Hard Lenses

- Do not store lenses dry.
- Clean lenses every time they are removed from the eyes. See Tables 29-2 and 29-3 for cleaning procedures.
- Inspect lenses regularly for chips and scratches.
- Do not rub eyes while lenses are in place.

- Do not rinse contact lenses with very hot or very cold water, because temperature extremes may warp the lenses.
- Do not get oils or lanolin on the lens.

Instructions for RGP Lenses

- See Tables 29-2 and 29-7 for guidelines on cleaning RGP lenses.
- Do not use tap water to rinse off cleaner or to rewet lenses. If tap water is used, disinfect lenses before inserting them in the eyes.[23]
- Do not disinfect these lenses with thermal disinfecting systems.
- See Table 29-13 for guidelines on using other types of disinfecting systems.

Instructions for Soft Lenses

- See Tables 29-2, 29-11, and 29-13 for guidelines on cleaning and disinfecting these lenses.
- Handle soft lenses carefully because they are very fragile and can easily be torn.
- Remove these lenses before instilling any ophthalmic preparation not specifically intended for concurrent use with soft contact lenses. Wait at least 20 to 30 minutes before reinserting the lenses, unless directed otherwise by an eye care practitioner.

- Do not wear lenses when a topical ophthalmic ointment is being used.
- Do not wear soft contact lenses in the presence of irritating fumes or chemicals.

Instructions for Continuous-Wear Lenses (RGP or Soft)

- Remove mascara before sleeping, because mascara can flake off during sleep and become trapped underneath the lens.[24]
- If lenses appear to be lost on awakening, check eyes to see if the lenses were displaced. Soft lenses can fold over on themselves and get lodged underneath the top or bottom eyelid.
- Each morning, check eyes carefully for unusual, persistent redness, discharge, or pain. If redness does not abate within 45 minutes or discharge or pain is present, remove the lens and call the lens care practitioner.
- Check vision after inserting lenses. (Some hazy vision is normal on awakening because of corneal hypoxia, which develops overnight.) Apply a few drops of rewetting solution to improve hydration of the lens and help resolve hypoxia. If the problem is not resolved, remove lenses, clean them, and reinsert. If vision is not improved within an hour, remove lenses and call your lens prescriber.

Key Points for Prevention of Contact Lens–Related Disorders

➤ Following the prescribed lens care program is the best strategy for avoiding lens wear–related problems.

➤ The practitioner should explain the care regimen for the patient's particular lens type and stress that the patient should use only the products recommended for his or her lenses.

➤ Instructions on avoiding practices or situations that can cause eye irritation or lens damage are also important in educating the patient about successful wearing of contact lenses. The patient should also be advised of signs and symptoms that indicate medical care is needed.

REFERENCES

1. Weisbarth RE, McCartnery DL. In: Kastl PR, ed. *Contact Lenses, The CLAO Guide to Basic Science and Clinical Practice.* 3rd ed. Dubuque, Iowa: Kendall/Hunt Publishing; 1995:II113–29.
2. Yamaguchi T, Hubbard A, Fukushima A, et al. Fungus growth on soft contact lenses with different water contents. *CLAO J.* 1984;10:166–71.
3. Contact Lens Council. Available at: http://www. contactlenscouncil.org/stats.htm. Last accessed September 2, 2008.
4. Rakow PL. Mixing contact lens solutions. *J Ophthalmic Nurs Technol.* 1989;8:67–8.
5. Diefenbach CB, Seibert CK, Davis LJ. Analysis of two home remedy contact lens cleaners. *J Am Optom Assoc.* 1988;59:518–21.
6. Bartlett JD. In: *Ophthalmic Drug Facts.* St Louis: Wolters Klewer Health; 2007:289–314.
7. Key JE, Bennett ES. In: Kastl PR, ed. *Contact Lenses, The CLAO Guide to Basic Science and Clinical Practice.* 3rd ed. Dubuque, Iowa: Kendall/Hunt Publishing; 1995:II51–74.
8. Nichols JJ. The controversy of contact lens convenience. *Contact Lens Spectrum.* January 2000;32–5.
9. Krezanoski JZ. Topical medications. *Int Ophthalmol Clin.* 1981;21:173–6.
10. Harris MG. Practical considerations in the use of hydrogen peroxide disinfection systems. *CLAO J.* 1990;16(suppl 1):S53–S60.
11. Wittman G. Personal communication of data on file at company. Irvine, Calif: Allergan; January 17, 1995.
12. Barr JT. Contact lens solutions and lens care update. *Contact Lens Spectrum.* June 2001;26–33.
13. Krezanoski JZ, Dabezies OH. In: Dabezies OH, ed. *Contact Lenses, The CLAO Guide to Basic Science and Clinical Practice.* 2nd ed. Boston: Little, Brown and Company; 1992:31.1–31.17.
14. Driebe WT. In: Kastl PR, ed. *Contact Lenses, The CLAO Guide to Basic Science and Clinical Practice.* 3rd ed. Dubuque, Iowa: Kendall/Hunt Publishing; 1995:II237–62.
15. Macsai MS, Goel AK, Michael MM, et al. Deposition of ciprofloxacin, prednisolone phosphate, and prednisolone acetate in SeeQuence disposable contact lenses. *CLAO J.* 1993;19:166–8.
16. Lee BL, Matoba AY, Osato MS, et al. The solubility of antibiotic and corticosteroid combinations. *Am J Ophthalmol.* 1992;114:212–5.
17. Plotnik RD, Mannis MJ, Schwab IR. Therapeutic contact lenses. *Int Ophthalmol Clin.* 1991;31:35–52.
18. Diamond SA, Dupuis LL. Contact lens damage due to ribavirin exposure. *DICP Ann Pharmacother.* 1989;23:428–9.
19. Rodriguez WJ, Bui RH, Connon JD, et al. Environmental exposure of primary care personnel to ribavirin aerosol when supervising treatment of infants with respiratory syncytial virus infections. *Antimicrob Agents Chemother.* 1987;31:1143–6.
20. Broich J, Weiss L, Rapp J. Isolation and identification of biologically active contaminants from soft contact lenses. *Invest Ophthalmol Vis Sci.* 1980;19:1328–35.
21. Miller D. Systemic medications. *Int Ophthalmol Clin.* 1981;21:177–83.
22. Schornack JA. Drugs and pupillary interaction in contact lens practice. *Contact Lens Spectr.* May 2003;46.
23. Campbell RC, Caroline PJ. RGPs and tap water. *Contact Lens Forum.* 1990;15:64.
24. Key JE, Bennett ES. In: Kastl PR, ed. *Contact Lenses, The CLAO Guide to Basic Science and Clinical Practice.* 3rd ed. Dubuque, Iowa: Kendall/Hunt Publishing; 1995:II:51–74.

Otic Disorders

Linda Krypel

Ear complaints are common and vary from simple complaints of excessive earwax (cerumen) or itching to painful ear infections. Ear disorders affect all ages, with younger patients and patients of advanced age being the most prone. Otic disorders account for 1.5% of ambulatory care visits per year.[1] Cerumen impaction can affect up to 10% of children and more than 50% of the elderly nursing home population; it is the most common cause of hearing loss in all ages.[2-5] Approximately 4% of patients will visit their primary care physician because of cerumen impaction.[3]

Self-treatment with nonprescription medications and complementary therapies should be restricted to external ear disorders, which include disorders of the auricle and the external auditory canal (EAC). Excessive cerumen and water-clogged ears are self-treatable EAC disorders for which the Food and Drug Administration (FDA) has approved nonprescription otic medications. Other self-treatable disorders of the auricle include allergic and contact dermatitis, seborrhea, and psoriasis. Nonprescription medications used to treat the latter disorders when they appear on other parts of the body are also appropriate for treating the auricle. If improvement does not occur within 7 days, the patient should be referred to the primary care provider.

Diseases of the head and neck can cause referred pain, which the patient often perceives as pain originating from the ear. The clinician must attempt to determine the cause of pain prior to recommending self-treatment or medical referral. The assessment of self-treatable otic disorders and discussions for patient counseling and evaluation for patient outcomes are presented later in the chapter. This chapter will briefly examine the anatomy and pathophysiology of the ear, as well as the three most common otic disorders, the pathophysiology for each, and associated nonprescription therapies.

The external ear consists of the auricle (also called the pinna) and the EAC (Figure 30-1), and is closed by the tympanic membrane (eardrum), which separates the external ear from the middle ear.[6] The auricle is composed of a thin layer of highly vascular skin that is tightly bound to cartilage. Adipose or subcutaneous tissue, which would insulate blood vessels, is absent except in the lobe. The lobe has fewer blood vessels and is composed primarily of fatty tissue. The triangular piece of cartilage in front of the ear canal adjacent to the cheek is called the tragus.

The EAC consists of an outer cartilaginous portion, which comprises one-third to one-half of its length, plus an inner body or osseous portion.[6] The canal forms a blind cul-de-sac. Chil-dren have a shorter, straighter, and flatter EAC than that of adults, whose canals tend to lengthen and form an "S" shape.[6] At the same time, an adult's eustachian tube (part of the inner ear) lengthens downward as it enters the nasal cavity. This shape helps to promote drainage, and inhibits aspiration of pharyngeal and nasal contents into the middle ear, which may help to explain why children suffer from more middle ear infections than do adults.[6,7]

The skin that covers the auricle is especially susceptible to bleeding when scratched because of the lack of flexibility usually afforded by a subcutaneous layer of fat and the large blood supply to the area.[6] The skin is highly innervated, causing a disproportionate otalgia (ear pain) when inflammation is present. Skin farther into the EAC is thicker, and contains apocrine and exocrine glands as well as hair follicles.[8] The skin in the canal is continuous with the outer layer of the tympanic membrane.

Oily secretions from the exocrine glands mix with the milky, fatty fluid from the apocrine glands to form cerumen, which appears on the surface of the skin on the outer half of the EAC. Cerumen lubricates the canal, traps dust and foreign materials, and provides a waxy, waterproof barrier to the entry of pathogens.[8,9] It also contains various antimicrobial substances such as lysozymes, and it has an acidic pH, which aids in the inhibition of bacterial and fungal growth.[8,10]

The canal skin is shed continuously and mixes with cerumen. The debris-laden cerumen slowly migrates outward with jaw movements (such as chewing and talking). This migration serves as a process of self-cleaning.[9] Cerumen may appear dry and flaky or oily and paste-like. Color varies from light gray to orange or brown and may darken on exposure to air.[11]

The normal tympanic membrane or eardrum is smooth, translucent, and pearl gray. It is concave and oval, with an average thickness of 0.074 mm, and is composed of three layers. The continuous skin layer of the EAC forms the outer tympanic membrane layer. The middle layer is fibrous tissue, and the internal layer is a mucous membrane continuous with the lining of the middle ear.[6] The tympanic membrane transmits sound waves and acts as a protective barrier to the middle ear.[9]

The natural defenses of the ear canal include the skin layer with its protective coating of cerumen, an acidic pH, and hairs that line the outer half of the canal. Together, they protect against injury from foreign material and infection. It is important for the clinician to explain the normal role and function of cerumen when educating patients.

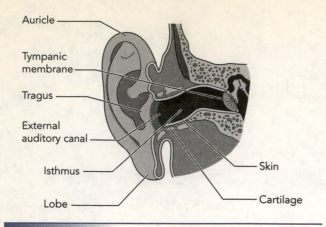

Auricle

Tympanic membrane

Tragus

External auditory canal

Isthmus

Lobe

Skin

Cartilage

FIGURE 30-1 Anatomy of the auricle and external ear.

PATHOPHYSIOLOGY OF OTIC DISORDERS

Because the EAC forms a blind cul-de-sac, it is especially prone to collecting moisture. Its dark, warm, moist environment is ideal for fungal and bacterial growth. In the preinflammatory stage, moisture, local trauma, or both remove the lipid layer covering the skin. Local trauma from fingernails, cotton-tipped swabs, or other items inserted into the canal can abrade the skin and allow pathogens to enter. Because a normal, healthy ear canal is impervious to potentially pathogenic organisms, skin integrity generally must be interrupted before an organism can produce an infection. Trauma to the ear from thermal injuries, sports injuries, ear piercing, and poorly fitting or improperly cleaned ear molds or hearing aids can contribute to the breakdown of the EAC's natural defenses.[12] Dermatologic skin disorders, such as contact dermatitis, seborrhea, psoriasis, and malignancies, also compromise these defenses.[8]

Viral illnesses, such as colds and upper respiratory infections, can contribute to the breakdown of natural defenses of the middle and inner ear, especially in children, who are very susceptible to middle ear infections following such illnesses. Because a child's eustachian tube is shorter and angled flatter than that of an adult, it is commonly believed that nasopharyngeal secretions can easily be aspirated and accumulate in the middle ear, leading to proliferation of bacteria.[7] Holding back or trying to stifle a sneeze can force secretions into the middle ear and therefore should be strongly discouraged, even in adults.

EXCESSIVE/IMPACTED CERUMEN

Cerumen can be considered an undervalued defense system. Widespread misinformation has often led the public to believe that cerumen production is a pathologic condition and that cerumen must be continually removed. In fact, improper or excessive attempts to remove cerumen can actually damage the EAC.[10]

Pathophysiology of Excessive/Impacted Cerumen

Individuals with abnormally narrow or misshapen EACs and/or excessive hair growth in the canal are predisposed to impacted cerumen. These physiologic anomalies disrupt the normal migration of cerumen to the outer EAC. Individuals who have overactive ceruminous glands or who wear hearing aids, earplugs, and sound attenuators often suffer from impacted cerumen. Such devices worn in the ear can inhibit the migration of cerumen, causing wax buildup.[3,10]

Older adults often experience impacted cerumen resulting from atrophy of ceruminous glands.[9] This population secretes drier cerumen, which is more difficult to expel from the ear.

Clinical Presentation of Excessive/Impacted Cerumen

The most common symptoms of impacted cerumen are a sense of fullness or pressure in the ear and a gradual hearing loss, which can lead to a decrease in cognition in the elderly.[13] A dull pain is sometimes associated with this disorder, along with vertigo (a sensation of spinning or whirling), tinnitus, chronic cough, or pain.[3] Attempting to remove cerumen by means of cotton-tipped applicators, bobby pins, toothpicks, fingernails, or other such objects can force the cerumen into the inner half of the EAC, where it becomes hardened and compacted over time.[9] Hardened cerumen generally does not cling to cotton-tipped applicators, and using them may serve only to remove the protective waxy layer and force the cerumen plug further into the canal. The delicate skin of the auditory canal can also be scratched or damaged, providing an entry point for water and pathogens.[9,10] Cerumen whose migration to the outer EAC is blocked by devices in the ear will also harden and become compacted. Frequent removal and proper cleaning of ear devices may help prevent wax buildup.

Treatment of Excessive/Impacted Cerumen

Treatment Goals

The goal of treating excessive/impacted cerumen is to soften and remove it using proper methods and safe, effective agents. Proper treatment should eliminate temporary hearing loss and other symptoms.

General Treatment Approach

The initial step in removing impacted cerumen is the use of a safe and effective agent to soften cerumen. Gently irrigating the ear, using an otic bulb syringe filled with warm water, is often recommended. Caution must be used to ensure complete removal of water and avoid a possible infection attributable to water-clogged ears. Cotton-tipped swabs or other foreign objects should not be used to remove cerumen or water. The algorithm in Figure 30-2 outlines the appropriate self-treatment of excessive/impacted cerumen and lists exclusions for self-treatment.

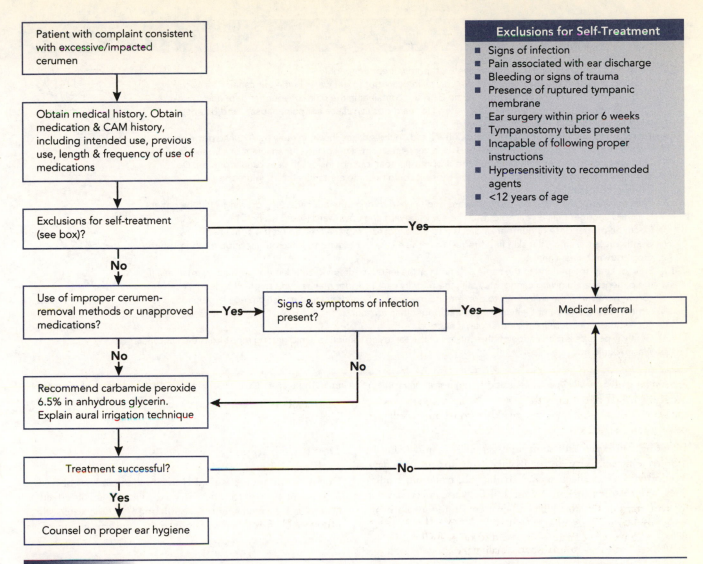

The flowchart contains the following text:

- Patient with complaint consistent with excessive/impacted cerumen
- Obtain medical history. Obtain medication & CAM history, including intended use, previous use, length & frequency of use of medications
- Exclusions for self-treatment (see box)?
- Use of improper cerumen-removal methods or unapproved medications?
- Signs & symptoms of infection present?
- Medical referral
- Recommend carbamide peroxide 6.5% in anhydrous glycerin. Explain aural irrigation technique
- Treatment successful?
- Counsel on proper ear hygiene

Exclusions for Self-Treatment

- Signs of infection
- Pain associated with ear discharge
- Bleeding or signs of trauma
- Presence of ruptured tympanic membrane
- Ear surgery within prior 6 weeks
- Tympanostomy tubes present
- Incapable of following proper instructions
- Hypersensitivity to recommended agents
- <12 years of age

FIGURE 30-2 Self-care of excessive/impacted cerumen. Key: CAM, complementary and alternative medicine.

Nonpharmacologic Therapy

Earwax should be removed only when it has migrated to the outermost portion of the EAC. The only recommended non-pharmacologic method of removing cerumen is to use a wet, wrung-out washcloth draped over a finger. Making this procedure part of daily aural hygiene can prevent impacted cerumen if physiologic abnormalities or physical devices are not the cause of the impaction. This method is not effective once cerumen becomes impacted.

Pharmacologic Therapy

Carbamide peroxide 6.5% in anhydrous glycerin is currently the only FDA-approved nonprescription cerumen-softening agent.[14] Other agents such as mineral oil, olive oil (sweet oil), glycerin, docusate sodium, and dilute hydrogen peroxide have been used by primary care providers and patients as inexpensive home remedies to soften cerumen. There are no data, however, to support these remedies as being more effective than carbamide peroxide in anhydrous glycerin.

Carbamide Peroxide

Carbamide peroxide 6.5% in anhydrous glycerin is approved as safe and effective in softening, loosening, and removing excessive earwax in adults and children 12 years and older.[14] (See Table 30-1 for the proper instillation of eardrops.) Carbamide peroxide is prepared from hydrogen peroxide and urea. When carbamide peroxide is exposed to moisture, nascent oxygen is released slowly and acts as a weak antibacterial. The effervescence that occurs during this process, along with the effect of urea on tissue debridement, helps to mechanically break down and loosen cerumen that has been softened by anhydrous glycerin.[15]

Any cerumen remaining after treatment may be removed with gentle, warm-water irrigation administered with a rubber otic bulb syringe (Table 30-2). Caution is important in that improper use of an otic syringe or using an oral jet irrigator to remove cerumen can leave excess moisture in the canal or further compress cerumen. These actions can also cause otitis externa, perforated tympanic membrane, pain, vertigo, otitis media, tinnitus (ringing, hissing, or buzzing noises in the ear), and even cardiac arrest.[3,16]

TABLE 30-1 Guidelines for Administering Eardrops

1. Wash your hands with soap and warm water; then dry them thoroughly.
2. Carefully wash and dry the outside of the ear, taking care not to get water in the ear canal.
3. Warm eardrops to body temperature by holding the container in the palm of your hand for a few minutes. Do not warm the container in hot water. Hot eardrops can cause ear pain, nausea, and dizziness.
4. If the label indicates, shake the container.
5. Tilt your head (or have the patient tilt his or her head) to the side, as shown in drawing A. Or lie down with the affected ear up, as shown in drawing B. Use gentle restraint, if necessary, for an infant or a young child.
6. Open the container carefully. Position the dropper tip near, but not inside, the ear canal opening. Do not allow the dropper to touch the ear, because it could become contaminated or injure the ear. Eardrop bottles must be kept clean.
7. Pull your ear (or the patient's ear) backward and upward to open the ear canal (see drawing A). If the patient is a child younger than 3 years old, pull the ear backward and downward (see drawing B).
8. Place the proper dose or number of drops into the ear canal. Replace the cap on the container.
9. Gently press the small, flat skin flap (tragus) over the ear canal opening to force out air bubbles and push the drops down the ear canal.
10. Stay (or keep the patient) in the same position for the length of time indicated in the product instructions. If the patient is a child who cannot stay still, the primary care provider may tell you to place a clean piece of cotton gently into the child's ear to prevent the medication from draining out. Use a piece large enough to remove easily, and do not leave it in the ear longer than an hour.
11. Repeat the procedure for the other ear, if needed.
12. Gently wipe excess medication off the outside of the ear, using caution to avoid getting moisture in the ear canal.
13. Wash your hands.

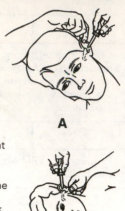

Source: APhA Special Report: Medication Administration Problem Solving in Ambulatory Care. Washington, DC: American Pharmaceutical Association; 1994:9.

Carbamide peroxide solution is generally considered to be nonirritating and may be used twice daily for up to 4 days. Reported adverse effects include pain, rash, irritation, tenderness, redness, discharge, or dizziness.[17] If adverse effects develop or symptoms persist after 4 days, the patient should see a primary care provider for evaluation.[18]

Docusate Sodium

Docusate sodium is classified as an emollient and has been used by some physicians to soften earwax. Evidence for its effectiveness over approved agents is conflicting.[19–21] Docusate sodium is more expensive, has varying results, and causes superficial

TABLE 30-2 Guidelines for Removing Excessive/Impacted Cerumen

1. Place 5–10 drops of the cerumen-softening solution into the ear canal, and allow it to remain for at least 15 minutes, as described in Table 30-1.
2. Do this procedure twice daily for no longer than 4 consecutive days.
   Optional treatment: If cerumen remains in the ear canal, the following irrigation technique may be tried as outlined below, with special attention paid to cautionary instructions.
3. Prepare a warm (not hot) solution of plain water or other solution as directed by your primary care provider. Eight ounces of solution should be sufficient to clean out the ear canal.
4. To catch the returning solution, hold a container under the ear being cleaned. An emesis basin is ideal because it fits the contour of the neck. Tilt the head down slightly on the side where the ear is being cleaned.
5. Gently pull the earlobe down and back to expose the ear canal, as shown in the drawing.
6. Place the open end of the syringe into the ear canal with the tip pointed slightly upward toward the side of the ear canal (see drawing). Do not aim the syringe into the back of the ear canal. Use caution and make sure the syringe does not obstruct the outflow of solution.
7. Squeeze the bulb gently—not forcefully—to introduce the solution into the ear canal and to avoid rupturing the eardrum. (*Note:* Only health professionals trained in aural hygiene should use forced water sprays [e.g., Water Pik] to remove cerumen.)
8. Do not let the returning solution come into contact with the eyes.
9. If pain or dizziness occurs, remove the syringe and do not resume irrigation until a clinician is consulted.
10. Make sure all water is drained from the ear to avoid predisposing to infection from water-clogged ears.
11. Rinse the syringe thoroughly before and after each use, and let it dry.
12. Store the syringe in a cool, dry place (preferably, in its original container) away from hot surfaces and sharp instruments
13. If cerumen still remains, consult a clinician.

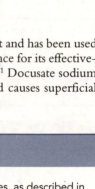

Source: Adapted with permission from *Ohio Clinician.* 1996;14(5):10.

erythema in some cases; therefore, it should not be recommended over FDA–approved agents.[20]

Glycerin

Glycerin has emollient and humectant properties, and is widely used as a solvent and vehicle.[15] It is safe and nonsensitizing when applied to abraded skin. It has been used to soften earwax, although FDA does not recognize this use.

Hydrogen Peroxide

Hydrogen peroxide releases nascent oxygen when exposed to moisture and acts as a weak antibacterial.[15] A 1:1 solution of warm water and hydrogen peroxide 3% can be used to flush the ear canal when softening or removing earwax.[3] This solution, however, is not an effective ear-drying agent. Overuse of 1:1 aqueous hydrogen peroxide solutions may predispose the ear to infection from tissue maceration caused by excessive water left in the canal.

Olive Oil (Sweet Oil)

Olive oil is used as an emollient and has been used to soften earwax.[18] It has also been used in the ear canal to alleviate itching and pain.[3] Using olive oil to treat ear pain can delay seeking proper treatment and should not be recommended.

Product Selection Guidelines

Table 30-3 lists examples of cerumen-softening and other otic products.

Complementary Therapies

Although major herbal references do not list herbal remedies for self-treatable otic disorders,[22,23] some folk remedies remain popular in many regions. One of the more interesting—and dangerous—is the use of ear candles to remove cerumen. A hollow candle is burned with one end inserted in the ear canal. The intent is to create negative pressure and draw cerumen from the ear. Studies have shown that this method does not aid in removing cerumen but has caused serious ear injuries.[24] Candle wax was deposited in the ear canal in some patients, and severe blockages and burns have occurred. FDA issued an alert warning against the import and sale of these devices.[25]

The herb yerba santa is listed as an ingredient in two available products. It contains flavonoids such as eriodictyol and tannins. Eriodictyol is reported to exert an expectorant effect when taken orally. Although the manufacturer lists yerba santa as a "dermprotective" factor, there is no evidence for safety and effectiveness of yerba santa used topically.[22] A product advertised for ear pain in children contains olive oil, garlic oil, and willow bark; the latter is a form of salicylate.[22] Although garlic oil claims to have some antibacterial properties, self-treating ear pain can delay seeking an appropriate diagnosis. Another available

---

TABLE 30-3 Selected Products for Otic Disorders

Trade Name	Primary Ingredients
Cerumen-Softening Products	
Auro Ear Drops	Carbamide peroxide 6.5%; anhydrous glycerin
Debrox	Carbamide peroxide (non-USP) 6.5%; glycerin; propylene glycol; sodium stannate
Murine Earwax Removal System	Carbamide peroxide 6.5%; glycerin; alcohol 6.3%; polysorbate 20; packaged with syringe
Murine Earigate Ear Cleaning System	Isotonic, desalinated sea water; packaged with syringe
OTIX drops	Carbamide peroxide 6.5%; anhydrous glycerin; propylene glycol; water; trolamine triethanolamine; sodium citrate
Physician's Choice	Carbamide peroxide 6.5%; anhydrous glycerin; sodium lauryl sarcosinate
Ear-Drying Products	
Auro-Dri Drops	Isopropyl alcohol 95%; anhydrous glycerin
Star Otic	Isopropyl alcohol; anhydrous glycerin
Swim Ear Drops	Isopropyl alcohol 95%; anhydrous glycerin
Botanical and Homeopathic Products	
Earsol-HC Drops	Alcohol 44%; hydrocortisone 1%; propylene glycol; yerba santa; benzyl benzoate
Herbs for Kids Willow/Garlic Ear Oil	Extra virgin olive oil; garlic, calendula; willow bark; usnea; Vitamin E oil
Murine Earache Relief	Chamomilla HPUS 10X; mercurius solubus HPUS 15X; sulfur HPUS 12X; Lycopodium clavatum HPUS 8x
Similasan Healthy Relief Homeopathic Ear Drops	Chamomilla HPUS 10X; mercurius solubus HPUS 15X; sulfur HPUS 12X; glycerin

Key: *HPUS, Homeopathic Pharmacopoeia of the United States.*

herb is chamomilla, which is believed to help with ear inflammation. Although these herbal and homeopathic products are available, no published studies document safety and effectiveness (Table 30-3).

WATER-CLOGGED EARS

Water-clogged ears is a separate disorder from swimmer's ear (external otitis). FDA has not approved any nonprescription products for preventing or treating external otitis. Manufacturers have argued that removing moisture from a water-clogged ears with an approved agent may prevent tissue maceration, a process that can lead to inflammation and infection of the EAC (commonly referred to as swimmer's ear). FDA, however, prohibits this extrapolation and manufacturers may no longer label their products as preventing swimmer's ear.[26,27] Most available nonprescription products for water-clogged ears have been reformulated to contain only FDA-approved ingredients.

Pathophysiology of Water-Clogged Ears

Some patients are more prone to retaining water because of the shape of their ear canals or the presence of excessive cerumen.[8] The cerumen can swell, thereby trapping water. Excessive moisture in the ears can result from hot, humid climates, sweating, swimming, bathing, or improper use of aqueous solutions to cleanse the ear. Therefore, simple attempts to remove water by mechanical manipulation may be insufficient. In addition, the use of cotton-tipped applicators has been linked to otitis externa.[28]

Clinical Presentation of Water-Clogged Ears

A feeling of wetness or fullness in the ear, accompanied by gradual hearing loss, can occur after exposure to any of the etiologic factors. The trapped moisture can compromise the natural defenses of the EAC, causing tissue maceration that, in turn, can lead to itching, pain, inflammation, or infection.[10]

Treatment of Water-Clogged Ears

Treatment Goals

The goals of treating a water-clogged ear are to dry it using a safe and effective agent, and to prevent recurrences in persons who are prone to retaining moisture in the ears.

General Treatment Approach

Before recommending an agent to treat water-clogged ears, the clinician should determine whether a patient has a ruptured tympanic membrane or has a tympanostomy tube in place. Ear-drying agents are very painful if instilled in either of these situations. Figure 30-2 lists additional exclusions for self-treatment.

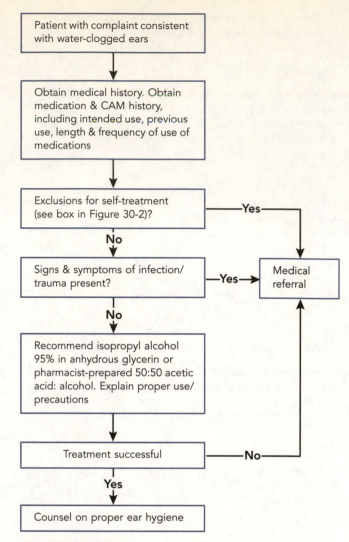

FIGURE 30-3 Self-care of water-clogged ears. Key: CAM, complementary and alternative medicine.

The algorithm in Figure 30-3 outlines the appropriate treatment of water-clogged ears. The clinician should recommend a product containing isopropyl alcohol 95% in anhydrous glycerin 5%.[26,27]

Nonpharmacologic Therapy

Tilting the affected ear downward and gently manipulating the auricle can expel excessive water from the ear. This procedure should be performed after swimming or bathing, or during periods of excessive sweating, especially by persons who are prone to developing this disorder. Using a blow-dryer on a low setting around (not directly into) the ear immediately after swimming or bathing may help dry the ear canal.

Pharmacologic Therapy

FDA has approved only isopropyl alcohol 95% in anhydrous glycerin 5% as a safe and effective "ear-drying aid."[26,27] (See Table 30-3 for examples of products containing these agents.)

In addition, a 50:50 mixture of acetic acid 5% (white household vinegar) and isopropyl alcohol 95% has also commonly been recommended to help dry water-clogged ears.[5,8]

Ear-drying agents, which are recommended for use in adults and children ages 12 years and older, may be used whenever ears are exposed to water. Table 30-1 presents guidelines for administering these agents. Medical referral is necessary if symptoms persist after several days of simultaneous use of ear-drying agents and prevention of exposure of ears to water. Symptoms of infection also require medical referral.

Isopropyl Alcohol in Anhydrous Glycerin

Alcohol is highly miscible with water and acts as a drying agent. In concentrations greater than 70%, it is also an effective skin disinfectant.[15] Glycerin has been used in pharmaceutical preparations for its solvent, emollient, or hygroscopic properties. It is safe and nonsensitizing when applied to open wounds or abraded skin. Combined with alcohol, glycerin provides a product that reduces moisture in the ear without overdrying.

Acetic Acid

The acetic acid in a 50:50 mixture of acetic acid 5% and isopropyl alcohol 95% has bactericidal and antifungal properties.[15] Species of *Pseudomonas, Candida,* and *Aspergillus* are particularly sensitive to this agent. As discussed previously, alcohol has anti-infective properties as well, is highly miscible with water, and helps remove water from the ear. Repeated use can cause overdrying of the canal. Care must be taken to advise patients against using cider vinegar instead of white vinegar. Cider vinegar is produced from fruit and contains impurities that could hinder antibacterial activity.

A 50:50 mixture of white vinegar 5% and isopropyl alcohol 95% provides an acetic acid 2.5% solution. Concentrations of acetic acid between 2% and 3% may lower the pH of the ear canal below the optimal pH of 6.5 to 7.5 needed for bacterial growth.[15] The solution is well tolerated and nonsensitizing, and does not induce resistant organisms. It may sting or burn slightly, especially if the skin is abraded. The clinician should provide an accurately compounded solution in an appropriately sized and labeled dropper bottle.

CONTACT DERMATITIS, SEBORRHEA, AND PSORIASIS OF THE EAR

Pathophysiology of Contact Dermatitis

Contact dermatitis is categorized as either allergic contact dermatitis or irritant contact dermatitis. The external ear is susceptible to both types of this dermatitis.

Topical neomycin, nickel in earrings, poison ivy, and the chemicals used to process the rubber or plastic of hearing aid molds or earphones typically cause allergic reactions of the external ear.[9,10] Soaps and detergents are mild irritants, which generally require repeated or extended contact to cause a significant inflammatory response. However, such substances have been shown to cause reactions similar to allergic contact dermatitis.[9,10] (See Chapter 35 for a detailed discussion of the etiology and treatment of these disorders.)

Clinical Presentation of Contact Dermatitis

Allergic dermatitis is associated with various skin manifestations, including maculopapular rash and formation of vesicles. The rash, in turn, causes pruritus, erythema, and edema, and may encourage placing objects in the ear to decrease pruritus.

Treatment of Contact Dermatitis

Dermatitis of the external ear frequently is treated with an astringent such as 1:40 aluminum acetate (Burow's solution). Solutions of aluminum acetate have antipruritic, antiinflammatory, and limited antibacterial properties. They are useful for treating itchy, weeping, swollen conditions of the external ear when diluted to concentrations of 1:10 to 1:40.[9] Astringents precipitate proteins and dry the affected area by reducing the secretory function of skin glands.[15] The dilute solution has an acidic pH that inhibits bacterial and fungal growth. A wet compress of diluted aluminum acetate solution applied several times per day is useful for acute contact dermatitis.

Seborrhea and Psoriasis

Seborrhea and psoriasis are chronic dermatologic disorders usually associated with the scalp, face, and trunk. Seborrhea can usually be managed with nonprescription medications. Psoriasis that involves mild inflammation is sometimes responsive to nonprescription medications. However, a primary care provider or dermatologist should make the initial diagnosis of psoriasis. (See Chapter 34 for a detailed discussion of these disorders.)

ASSESSMENT OF OTIC DISORDERS: A CASE-BASED APPROACH

The most common complaints of ear disorders are otalgia, pruritus (itching), and hearing loss. Evaluating the characteristics of particular symptoms, such as pain and hearing loss, and the specific combination of symptoms is the key to assessing otic disorders. To that end, the following discussion of common otic symptoms describes their possible causes. Furthermore, Table 30-4 compares the signs and symptoms and other features of common otic disorders, and Table 30-5[29-32] describes the common etiologies and treatments for otalgia, otic pruritus, hearing loss, dizziness, and tinnitus. A verbal 5-minute hearing loss test is available at the American Academy of Otolaryngology Head and Neck Surgery, Inc. Web site (www.entnet.org/healthinformation/hearing-loss.cfm). Finally, Case 30-1 gives an example of the assessment of patients with otic disorders.

TABLE 30-4 Differentiation of Common Otic Disorders

Disorder	Etiology	Pain	Itching
Ruptured tympanic membrane	Otitis media or trauma to ear such as sharp blows, diving into water, forceful irrigation of ear	Brief, severe	No
External otitis (swimmer's ear)	Local trauma to EAC caused by excessive moisture or abrasions; subsequent fungal/bacterial infections	Acute onset, varies from mild to severe, increases with movement of tragus or auricle	Yes
Otitis media	Bacterial infection of middle ear, usually following upper respiratory tract infections	Sharp, steady, frequently unilateral; does not increase with movement of tragus or auricle	No
Foreign object in ear	Insects, insertion of objects by children, hearing aids, sound attenuators	Dull-to-severe pain with sense of fullness or pressure while chewing	Yes
Trauma to ear	Burns from curling iron, frostbite, hematomas/injuries from contact sports or ill-fitting helmets, ear piercing, improper cerumen removal techniques, abrasions of EAC, rapid changes in air pressure	Varies from sharp and steady to brief and severe	Rare
Tinnitus	Hearing disorders, blockage of EAC, exposure to high noise levels, acoustic trauma, systemic diseases, drug toxicities (salicylate, quinidine, aminoglycosides, and other antibiotics)	Possible	No
Excessive/impacted cerumen	Overactive ceruminous glands, obstructed migration of cerumen	Rare, dull pain if present	No
Water-clogged ears	Excessive moisture in EAC	None	No

Key: EAC, external auditory canal.
Source: References 29–32.

TABLE 30-5 Treatment of Common Otic Disorders

Disorder	Etiology	Treatment
Otalgia	Intrinsic: infection, trauma, foreign objects, perichondritis Extrinsic: dental or jaw problems, nasopharyngeal infections, tumors, cysts, migraine headaches, neuralgias, cervical arthritis	Medical referral unless cause is clearly obvious, self-limiting, and self-treatable; always refer infections; self-care may delay seeking proper treatment
Otic pruritus	Contact dermatitis, seborrhea, psoriasis, infection (external otitis), excessive dryness related to decreased sebum production	Excessive dryness: 1–2 drops of mineral oil; avoid application of alcohol, insertion of foreign objects; medical referral if severe; see also Chapters 34 and 35.
Hearing loss	Foreign objects, water trapped in canal, infection, upper respiratory tract congestion, neoplasms, tympanic membrane perforation (abrupt), excessive pressure in ear canal, excessive cerumen, excessive noise, medications	Medical referral unless hearing loss is related to excessive water or impacted cerumen
Dizziness	Inner ear lesions, otitis media, rapid change in pressure on the tympanic membrane, migraine headache, ototoxic drugs, postural hypotension, cardiac disease, neoplasms, irrigation of ear canal with very hot or cold water, motion sickness	Medical referral unless related to motion sickness
Tinnitus	Hearing disorders, blockage of EAC, exposure to high noise levels, acoustic trauma, systemic diseases, drug toxicities (salicylate, quinidine, aminoglycosides, and other antibiotics)	Check for impacted cerumen; discontinuation of offending drug; medical referral for all other causes (OTC medications are ineffective)
Foreign body	Insects, beads, seeds, small batteries, or other objects	Medical referral; mineral oil can quickly suffocate the insect until removed by a clinician; moisture causes seeds to swell, making removal more difficult

Source: References 29–32.

Loss of Hearing	Discharge	Other Features
Abrupt	If associated with otitis media	May be associated with otitis media (see subsequent text)
Occasional	Occasionally, clear discharge changing to seropurulent	Swollen ear canal, stuffiness, discharge, swollen lymph nodes, fever, usually occurring in summer or in warm, humid climates
Is sometimes decreased	Possible exudate through perforated eardrum	Perforated or bulging eardrum, lymph nodes sometimes swollen, fever, dizziness, usually occurring in winter
Yes	Possible exudate from secondary bacterial infection	If obstruction not removed promptly, acute otitis externa and tinnitus may develop
Varies, can be abrupt to seldom	Seldom	Untreated hematomas may cause swelling/scarring; ear piercing may cause metal sensitivies, keloids, perichondritis, toxic shock syndrome, hepatitis B
Sometimes	None	Continuous or intermittent alien noises in ear such as ringing, roaring, or humming
Often	None	Sense of fullness or pressure in the ears
Often	None	Sense of fullness or wetness

PATIENT COUNSELING FOR OTIC DISORDERS

Patients who self-treat otic disorders must understand how easily the EAC can be injured. The clinician should discourage common harmful practices of relieving itching of the ear, and instruct patients on the proper methods of removing excessive cerumen and moisture from the ears. Patients who are susceptible to these disorders should be advised to incorporate the removal methods as part of their aural hygiene. The clinician should explain the proper use and possible adverse effects of all recommended medications. The box Patient Education for Self-Treatable Otic Disorders lists specific information to provide patients.

A WORD ABOUT **Fluid Monitors**

In 1997, a medical device that detects the presence of fluid in the middle ear was approved for marketing and for use by patients ages 6 months to adult.[33] It is marketed as an aid to monitoring fluid resolution in the middle ear following middle ear infections.

The device uses sonar-like technology to detect the presence of fluid by measuring reflected sound. An acoustic transducer emits a soft, complex series of sound waves into the ear canal. In a normal ear, the tympanic membrane is flexible and vibrates when sound waves reach it. When fluid is in the middle ear, the tympanic membrane is not as mobile and reflects sound waves differently from that of the normal ear. The intensity of the reflected sound is measured by the device, using a microphone and microprocessor.[34] Three color levels are coded according to the probability of fluid being present.

Users of the device should be reminded that the presence of fluid in the middle ear does not always indicate an infection. The device will not work if a tympanostomy tube, a ruptured eardrum, or impacted cerumen is present. Normal amounts of cerumen in the canal do not appear to affect the results. Precautions for use of the device include not reusing the disposable tips and not forcing the tip far into the ear.

Although used primarily by clinicians, this device is available to the public; however, expense limits its public use.

CASE 30-1

Relevant Evaluation Criteria	Scenario/Model Outcome
Information Gathering	
1. Gather essential information about the patient's symptoms, including:	
a. description of symptom(s) (i.e., nature, onset, duration, severity, associated symptoms)	Patient reports a gradual hearing loss over the past few weeks in left ear that has become painful and swollen after itching started 2 days ago.
b. description of any factors that seem to precipitate, exacerbate, and/or relieve the patient's symptom(s)	Pain and itching started several days after the patient attempted to remove wax in his ear using a bulb syringe and warm water along with a toothpick. Removal was unsuccessful. Pain is preventing use of his earpiece.
c. description of the patient's efforts to relieve the symptoms	Patient used a cotton-tipped applicator to relieve the itching with poor results.
2. Gather essential patient history information:	
a. patient's identity	Charles Smith
b. patient's age, sex, height, and weight	62-year-old male, 5 ft 9 in, 150 lb
c. patient's occupation	Realtor
d. patient's dietary habits	Balanced diet; occasional alcohol
e. patient's sleep habits	Averages 6–7 hours per night
f. concurrent medical conditions, prescription and nonprescription medications, and dietary supplements	Hypertension; losartan 50 mg daily, aspirin 81 mg daily
g. allergies	NKA
h. history of other adverse reactions to medications	Penicillin
i. other (describe) _____	Patient recently started using an earpiece when speaking on his cell phone.
Assessment and Triage	
3. Differentiate the patient's signs/symptoms and correctly identify the patient's primary problem(s) (see Table 30-4).	Improper removal of excessive cerumen has resulted in a probable infection (pruritus followed by pain and swelling).
4. Identify exclusions for self-treatment treatment (see Figure 30-2).	Signs of infection
5. Formulate a comprehensive list of therapeutic alternatives for the primary problem to determine if triage to a medical practitioner is required, and share this information with the patient.	Options include: (1) Refer patient to a PCP for a differential diagnosis. (2) Recommend OTC cerumen-softening agent with proper ear hygiene. (See Table 30-3.) (3) Recommend OTC ear-drying agent. (See Table 30-3.) (4) Take no action.
Plan	
6. Select an optimal therapeutic alternative to address the patient's problem, taking into account patient preferences.	Refer the patient to a PCP for a differential diagnosis.
7. Describe the recommended therapeutic approach to the patient.	N/A
8. Explain to the patient the rationale for selecting the recommended therapeutic approach from the considered therapeutic alternatives.	Seeing a PCP is necessary because of the signs and symptoms of a possible infection. Water remaining in the ear, along with possible toothpick abrasions, is likely to cause an infection.

CASE 30-1 (continued)

Relevant Evaluation Criteria	Scenario/Model Outcome
Patient Education	
9. When recommending self-care with non-prescription medications and/or nondrug therapy, convey accurate information to the patient.	For future prevention of excessive cerumen, use proper ear hygiene along with regular breaks from using an earphone. See the box Patient Education for Self-Treatable Otic Disorders.
10. Solicit follow-up questions from patient.	Is there an OTC product to help loosen cerumen I can use in the future that might work?
11. Answer patient's questions.	Yes. Refer to Figure 30-2 and Tables 30-2 and 30-3.

Key: N/A, not applicable; NKA, no known allergies; OTC, over-the-counter; PCP, primary care provider.

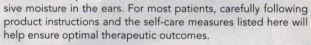

PATIENT EDUCATION FOR
Self-Treatable Otic Disorders

Excessive/Impacted Cerumen

The objective of self-treatment is to soften and remove excessive or impacted cerumen (earwax) that is already present, or to prevent the disorder from recurring in susceptible patients. For most patients, carefully following product instructions and the self-care measures listed here will help ensure optimal therapeutic outcomes.

Nondrug Measures for Excessive/Impacted Cerumen

- Use a washcloth draped over a finger to remove earwax from the outer canal.
- Do not insert objects in the ear to remove earwax. Such attempts may injure the ear canal or push the wax further into the canal.
- Never use the hollow candle method to remove earwax; it can cause serious ear injury.

Nonprescription Medications for Excessive/Impacted Cerumen

- Cerumen is necessary to lubricate the canal, trap dust and foreign materials, and provide a waxy, waterproof barrier to the entry of pathogens.
- Carbamide peroxide in anhydrous glycerin work together to soften and mechanically break down excessive/impacted cerumen.
- See Tables 30-1 and 30-2 for guidelines on using carbamide peroxide to remove excessive or impacted earwax.
- Do not let the medication come into contact with the eyes.
- Do not use this medication if you have a fever, ear drainage, pain more severe than a dull pain, dizziness, or a ruptured eardrum, or if you had ear surgery within the past 6 weeks.
- Do not use this medication to treat inflamed ear tissue, swimmer's ear, or itching of the ear canal.
- Prolonged contact between carbamide peroxide solution and skin of the ear canal can cause dermatitis. Discontinue treatment if irritation or a rash appears.
- Monitor for changes in your hearing and symptoms of infection such as pain and itching. If severe pain occurs or your hearing worsens, see a primary care provider immediately. Severe pain may indicate a ruptured eardrum.
- Store product in a cool, dry area and check expiration date before using.

Water-Clogged Ears

The objective of self-treatment is to remove water from ears already clogged with water or to prevent the disorder in persons who are susceptible to excessive moisture in the ears. For most patients, carefully following product instructions and the self-care measures listed here will help ensure optimal therapeutic outcomes.

Nondrug Measures for Water-Clogged Ears

- Tilt the affected ear down, and gently manipulate it to help drain water from the ear. Immediately after swimming or bathing, use a blow-dryer on a low setting to help dry the ear canal. Do not blow air directly into the ear canal.

Nonprescription Medications for Water-Clogged Ears

- Water can become trapped in the ear causing a sense of fullness or wetness.
- Use a product that reduces moisture content in the ear without overdrying. Isopropyl alcohol 95% in anhydrous glycerin 5% is the only FDA-approved formula.
- Do not use the medications if you have a ruptured eardrum or have tympanostomy tubes in place.
- Place 5–10 drops of the solution in the ear canal, and allow the solution to remain for 1–2 minutes.
- See Table 30-1 for instructions on instilling the medication.
- Do not let the medication come into contact with the eyes.
- Discontinue the medication if stinging or burning occurs.
- If pain, fever, or discharge develops, see a primary care provider immediately.
- Store product in a cool, dry area and check expiration date before using.

Dermatologic Disorders of the Ear

The objective of self-treatment is to relieve the symptoms. For most patients, carefully following product instructions and the self-care measures listed in Chapters 34 and 35 will help ensure optimal therapeutic outcomes.

EVALUATION OF PATIENT OUTCOMES FOR OTIC DISORDERS

If the symptoms of excessive/impacted cerumen, water-clogged ears, or self-treatable dermatologic disorders of the ear persist or worsen after 4 days of proper treatment, the patient should consult a primary care provider. The patient should also consult a primary care provider if ear pain or discharge develops during treatment. The clinician can follow up by phone in 4 days to determine whether the therapy is successful.

KEY POINTS FOR OTIC DISORDERS

➤ Limit the self-treatment of otic disorders to minor symptoms such as a sense of fullness, pressure, or wetness in the ears.
➤ Refer patients with acute onset of hearing loss, dizziness, pain, discharge, or other symptoms associated with infection, tympanostomy tubes, or ear surgery within the past 6 weeks for further evaluation.
➤ Instruct patients on how to use specific otic products that have been proven safe and effective (Tables 30-1 and 30-2).
➤ Advise patients with self-treatable symptoms to contact a primary care provider if symptoms worsen or do not improve after 4 days.
➤ Advise patients about proper ear hygiene and the importance of cerumen to prevent further problems or complaints.

REFERENCES

1. Woodwell DA, Cherry DK. *National Ambulatory Medical Care Survey: 2002 Summary.* Hyattsville, Md: National Center for Health Statistics; 2004:21. Advance Data from Vital and Health Statistics, No. 346.
2. Roland PS, Eaton D, Meyerhoff WL. Aging in the auditory and vestibular system. In: Bailey BJ, Calhoun KH, Healy GB, et al., eds. *Head and Neck Surgery—Otolaryngology.* 3rd ed. Philadelphia: Lippincott Williams & Wilkins; 2001:1941–7.
3. McCarter DF, Courtney AU, Pollart SM. Cerumen impaction. *Am Fam Phys.* 2007;75:1523–8, 1530.
4. Aung T, Mulley GP. Removal of earwax. *BMJ.* 2002;325:27.
5. Ears, nose and throat. In: Litin SC, ed. *Mayo Clinic Family Health Book.* 3rd ed. New York: Harper Resource; 2003:661–96.
6. Bluestone CD. Anatomy and physiology of the eustachian tube system. In: Bailey BJ, Calhoun KH, Healy GB, et al., eds. *Head and Neck Surgery—Otolaryngology.* 3rd ed. Philadelphia: Lippincott Williams & Wilkins; 2001:1059–69.
7. Northern JL, Downs MP. *Hearing in Children.* 5th ed. Philadelphia: Lippincott Williams & Wilkins; 2002:65–89.
8. Kryzer TC, Lambert PR. Diseases of the external auditory canal. In: Canalis RF, Lambert PR, eds. *The Ear: Comprehensive Otology.* Philadelphia: Lippincott Williams & Wilkins; 2000:341–57.
9. Linstrom CJ, Lucente FE, Joseph EM. Infections of the external ear. In: Bailey BJ, Calhoun KH, Healy GB, et al., eds. *Head and Neck Surgery—Otolaryngology.* 3rd ed. Philadelphia: Lippincott Williams & Wilkins; 2001:1711–24.
10. Hughes E, Lee JH. Otitis externa. *Pediatr Rev.* 2001;22:191–7.
11. Hawke M. Update on cerumen and ceruminolytics. *Ear Nose Throat J.* 2002;81(suppl):23–4.
12. Holten KB, Gick J. Management of the patient with otitis externa. *J Fam Prac.* 2001;50:353.
13. Moore AM. Cerumen, hearing, and cognition in the elderly. *J Am Med Dir Assoc.* 2002;3:136–9.
14. *Fed Regist.* 1986;51:28656–61.
15. Beringer P, Gupta PK, DerMarderosian A, et al., eds. *Remington: The Science and Practice of Pharmacy.* 21st ed. Philadelphia: Lippincott Williams & Wilkins; 2006:1081–4, 1628.
16. Folmer RL. Chronic tinnitus resulting from cerumen removal procedures. *Int Tinnitus J.* 2004;10(1):42–6.
17. Eye, ear, nose and throat (EENT) preparations: carbamide peroxide. *AHFS Drug Information.* Bethesda, Md: American Society of Health System Pharmacists; 2005:2666–7.
18. Borgsdorf LP, Selevan JR, Cada DJ, et al., eds. *Drug Facts and Comparison.* St Louis: Facts and Comparisons; 2007:1803–5.
19. Burton MJ, Doree CJ. Ear drops for the removal of ear wax. *Cochrane Database Syst Rev.* 2003;3:CD004326.
20. Whatley VN, Dodds CL, Paul RI. Randomized clinical trial of docusate, triethanolamine polypeptide, and irrigation in cerumen removal in children. *Arch Pediatr Adolesc Med.* 2003;157:1177–83.
21. Singer AJ, Sauris E, Viccellio AW. Ceruminolytic effects of docusate sodium: a randomized, controlled trial. *Ann Emerg Med.* 2000;36:228–32.
22. Jellin JM, Gregory PJ, Batz F, et al., eds. *Pharmacist Letter/Prescriber Letter Natural Medicines Comprehensive Database.* 4th ed. Stockton, Calif; 2002:1367.
23. Office of Dietary Supplements International Bibliographic Information on Dietary Supplements. Available at: http://dietary-supplements.info.nih.gov/Health_Information/IBIDS.aspx. Last accessed September 16, 2008.
24. Ernst E. Ear candles: a triumph of ignorance over science. *J Laryngol Otol.* 2004;118:1–2.
25. US Food and Drug Administration. *Detention without Physical Examination of Ear Candles.* Important Alert #77-01. 2007. Available at: http://www.fda.gov/ora/fiars/ora_import_ia7701.html. Last accessed September 5, 2008.
26. US Food and Drug Administration. Topical otic drug products for over-the-counter human use; products for drying water-clogged ears; proposed amendment of monograph. *Fed Regist.* 1999;64:44671.
27. US Food and Drug Administration. Topical otic drug products for over-the-counter human use; products for drying water-clogged ears; amendment of monograph; lift of partial stay of effective date. *Fed Regist.* 2000;65:48902.
28. Nussinocitch M, Rimon A, Volovitz B, et al. Cotton-tipped applicators as a leading cause of otitis externa. *Int J Pediatr Otohinolaryngol.* 2004;68:433–5.
29. Beers MH, Porter RS, Jones TV, et al., eds. *The Merck Manual of Diagnosis and Therapy.* 18th ed. Whitehouse Station, NJ: Merck Research Laboratories; 2006:776–95, 797–805.
30. Brockenbrough JM, Rybak LP, Matz GJ. Ototoxicity. In: Bailey BJ, Calhoun KH, Healy GB, et al., eds. *Head and Neck Surgery—Otolaryngology.* 3rd ed. Philadelphia: Lippincott Williams & Wilkins; 2001:1893–8.
31. Hashisaki GT. Sudden sensory hearing loss. In: Bailey BJ, Calhoun KH, Healy GB, et al., eds. *Head and Neck Surgery—Otolaryngology.* 3rd ed. Philadelphia: Lippincott Williams & Wilkins; 2001:1919–24.
32. Schleuning AJ, Martin WH. Tinnitus. In: Bailey BJ, Calhoun KH, Healy GB, et al., eds. *Head and Neck Surgery—Otolaryngology.* 3rd ed. Philadelphia: Lippincott Williams & Wilkins; 2001:1925–32.
33. US Food and Drug Administration. Premarket Notification Database. [Search for 510K numbers 070312 and 971859.] Available at: http://www.accessdata.fda.gov/scripts/cdrh/cfdocs/cfPMN/pmn.cfm. Last accessed September 5, 2008.
34. How EarCheck® Works [product information]. Available at: http://www.earcheck.com/Consumer/ProductInfo/About/Index.htm. Last accessed September 5, 2008.

Prevention of Hygiene-Related Oral Disorders

Amy L. Whitaker

Dental diseases are the most prevalent chronic diseases in American society. Each year, dental conditions cause 7.05 million days of work loss. Among all Americans, 50% need dental treatment, and nearly 80% have some form of periodontal disease. Of all 12- to 17-year-olds, 68% have experienced tooth decay, and the average adult has 21.5 decayed or filled tooth surfaces. Only 42% of adults 65 years and older visit a dentist during a given year. Furthermore, nearly 44% of Americans 75 years and older have lost all their natural teeth, but that percentage is declining. The increasing number of persons of advanced age with natural teeth has many dental implications.[1]

Improper oral hygiene is a direct cause of dental caries (decay), periodontal disease (gingivitis and periodontitis), halitosis, and some cases of denture-related discomfort. Nonprescription products for prevention of oral disease are widely available in pharmacies, food stores, and other retail stores; therefore, educating the public about proper use of these products is the key to preventing dental diseases.

The teeth and supporting structures are necessary for normal mastication and articulation as well as for appearance. The primary (deciduous) dentition first appears at approximately age 6 months, when the mandibular (lower jaw) central incisors erupt; the process is usually complete with the eruption of the upper second molars at approximately age 24 months. There are 20 deciduous (baby) teeth, 10 in each arch. Generally, the permanent dentition first appears when the mandibular first molar erupts behind the deciduous second molar at approximately age 6 years, and the process continues in a regular pattern, usually replacing shedding deciduous teeth. All 32 permanent teeth are present by age 14, except third molars (wisdom teeth), which may appear between the ages of 17 and 21 years.

Anatomically, the teeth are grossly viewed as having two parts, the roots and the crown (Figure 31-1). The roots are normally below the gingival (gum) line or margin, and are essential in supporting and attaching the tooth to the surrounding tissues. The crown is above the gingival margin and is responsible for mastication. Each tooth has four basic components: enamel, dentin, pulp, and periodontium.

Enamel is composed of very hard, crystalline calcium phosphate salts (hydroxyapatite). It is 1.5 to 2 mm thick at its thickest part and protects the underlying tooth structure. It covers the crown of the tooth, ending around the gum line at the cemento-enamel junction. Its hardness enables the crown to withstand the wear of mastication. Dentin, which is softer, lies beneath the enamel and makes up the largest part of the tooth structure. It is transected by microscopic tubules that transport nutrients from the dental pulp. Dentin protects the dental pulp from mechanical, thermal, and chemical irritation.

The pulp occupies the pulp chamber and is continuous with the tissues surrounding the tooth by an opening at the apex of the root (apical foramen). The pulp consists primarily of vascular and neural tissues. The only nerve endings in the pulp are free nerve endings; therefore, any type of stimulus to the pulp is interpreted as pain.

The periodontium comprises the tissues that support the teeth, including the cementum, the periodontal ligament, the encompassing alveolar bone, and the gingiva. The bone-like cementum is softer than dentin and covers the root of the tooth, extending apically from the cementoenamel junction. Therefore, the tooth is suspended in bone but is not continuous with it. The cementum's major function is to attach the tooth to the periodontal ligament by periodontal fibers. The periodontal ligament is connective tissue that attaches the tooth to the surrounding alveolar bone and gingival tissue. The four functions of the periodontal ligament are supportive, formative, sensory, and nutritive. The alveolar bone forms the sockets of the teeth. Alveolar bone is thin and spongy, and it attaches to the principal fibers of the periodontal ligament, as well as to the gingiva. The gingiva is the soft tissue surrounding the teeth. It is normally pink, stippled (looking like an orange peel) and keratinized, and it is attached to the cementum by the gingival group of periodontal ligament fibers.

The major salivary glands (parotid, submandibular, and sublingual) are responsible for secreting saliva, an alkaline, slightly viscous, clear secretion that contains enzymes (lysozymes and ptyalin), albumin, epithelial mucin (a mucopolysaccharide), immunoglobulin, leukocytes, and minerals. Normal salivary gland function promotes good oral health in several ways. Saliva lubricates and facilitates the removal of carbohydrates and microorganisms from the oral cavity. Saliva also buffers the decline in pH caused by the acid formed by carbohydrate fermentation. Its mineral components have a protective role in the demineralization and remineralization of tooth enamel.

Editor's Note: This chapter is based on the 15th edition chapter with the same title, written by Gary D. Klasser and Michael Colvard.

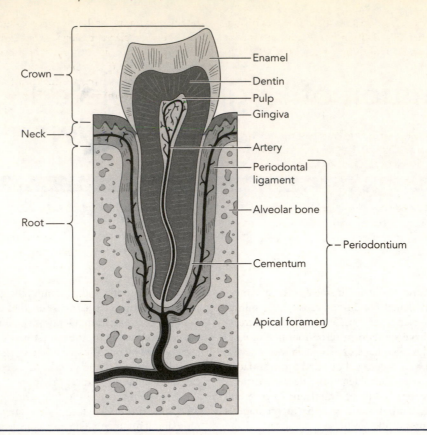

Crown

Neck

Root

Enamel
Dentin
Pulp
Gingiva
Artery
Periodontal ligament
Alveolar bone
Cementum
Apical foramen
Periodontium

FIGURE 31-1 Anatomy of the tooth.

CARIES

The number of individuals who experience dental caries remains high, with approximately 20% of the population being affected.[2] Although the incidence of dental caries in children has declined over the past several decades, this reduction in caries most likely results from the presence of fluoride in public water supplies and toothpastes, not improved oral hygiene.[3] Nevertheless, dental caries remains a public health problem, and the importance of prevention should not be ignored.

Patients with poor oral hygiene are at greatest risk for developing caries. Patients at increased risk for caries include those with orthodontic appliances, xerostomia (dry mouth), and gum tissue recession that exposes root surfaces. Certain prescription medications may cause xerostomia (see Chapter 32). Patients who received head and neck radiation therapy may also be more likely to manifest xerostomia.

Evidence also supports the association of use of tobacco products with increased dental caries attributable to worsening deposition of plaque and difficulty in appropriately removing plaque because of tar buildup on the teeth.[4] Because alcohol consumption can cause xerostomia, individuals who consume alcohol may also have a higher risk of caries.

Pathophysiology of Caries

Dental caries is now considered to be an infectious disease that affects the calcified tissues of the teeth. Certain plaque bacteria generate acid from dietary carbohydrates; the acid demineralizes tooth enamel, leading to the formation of carious lesions (pits or

perforations), which, if left untreated, will eventually destroy the tooth. Formation of dental caries requires growth and attachment of many cariogenic microorganisms (e.g., *Streptococcus mutans, Lactobacillus casei,* and *Actinomyces viscosus*) to exposed surfaces. *S. mutans* is the primary organism to initiate the carious process. Lactobacilli continue the process after entering established pits and fissures in biting surfaces of teeth, whereas *A. viscosus* is associated with root caries. These organisms are spread by saliva and can be spread from direct contact via kissing, sharing a spoon, blowing on food, or other shared activities. If oral hygiene is neglected, dental plaque containing these organisms remains on the tooth surfaces and, in time, attracts more bacteria, thereby promoting decay.

The carious process is characterized by alternating periods of destruction (demineralization) and repair (remineralization). Demineralization is caused by organic acids, such as lactic and formic acids, which are produced (usually anaerobically) by microbial metabolism of low-molecular-weight carbohydrates (sugars) that readily diffuse into plaque. The resultant reduction in pH on the tooth surface causes demineralization of dental enamel. Saliva, rich in calcium and phosphate ions, is crucial in remineralizing early carious lesions. The presence of fluoride ions in the mouth also promotes remineralization and slows demineralization, thereby retarding enamel dissolution.

A carious lesion starts slowly on the enamel surface and initially produces no clinical symptoms. Once demineralization progresses through the enamel to the softer dentin, the destruction proceeds much more rapidly, becoming clinically or radiographically evident as a carious lesion. At this point, the patient can become aware of the process by either observing it or experiencing symptoms of sensitivity to stimuli (such as heat, cold, or sweet foods) or chewing. If untreated, the carious lesion can result in damage to the dental pulp itself (with continuous pain as a common symptom) and, eventually, in necrosis of vital pulp tissue.

Clinical Presentation of Caries

Plaque is commonly recognized as the source of microbes that cause caries and periodontal disease; therefore, plaque buildup is directly related to the incidence of oral disease. Plaque begins with the formation of acquired pellicle on a clean tooth surface. Pellicle appears to be a thin, acellular, glycoprotein/mucoprotein coating that adheres to the enamel within minutes after a tooth is cleaned. Its source is believed to be saliva. The pellicle seems to serve as an attachment for cariogenic bacteria that, along with acids, produces long-chain polymers such as dextrans and levans that adhere to the pellicle and tooth surface. The resultant sticky, adherent mass is soft and readily disrupted by toothbrushing or flossing.

After meals, food residue may be incorporated into plaque by bacterial degradation. Left undisturbed, plaque thickens and bacteria proliferate. Plaque growth begins in protected cracks and fissures, and along the gingival margin. If not removed within 24 hours, dental plaque (especially in areas opposite the salivary glands) begins to calcify by calcium salt precipitation from the saliva, forming calculus, or tartar. This hardened, adherent deposit is removable by only professional dental cleaning.

Calculus is generally considered to be a substrate on which additional plaque can develop and is not considered the primary cause in periodontal disease. However, most periodontists agree that supragingival (above) and subgingival (below the gingival margin) calculus can promote the progression of periodontal disease by accumulating new bacterial plaque in contact with sensitive tissue sites and by interfering with local self-cleaning efforts to remove plaque. Subgingival calculus may also intensify the inflammatory process. Thorough removal of subgingival calculus in periodontal therapy is an important step in delaying the reestablishment of periodontal pathogens and resolution of inflammation.

Prevention of Caries

General Approach

The key to preventing caries is controlling dental plaque. Because a combination of diet (carbohydrate substrate), oral bacteria, and host resistance is involved in developing caries, prevention should be aimed at modifying these factors. The frequency of refined carbohydrate intake should be reduced; plaque, which supports cariogenic bacterial growth, should be removed, usually by mechanical means (brushing and flossing); and host resistance should be increased through appropriate exposure to fluoride ion. Antiplaque products aid in mechanical removal of plaque or retard its buildup. The declining prevalence of dental caries in children may be attributed to a combination of these interventions (e.g., increased exposure to fluoride in drinking water, dentifrices, and mouth rinses; changed patterns of diet; and overall improved oral hygiene).

Two methods are used to manage plaque: The first is mechanical removal (i.e., brushing with a dentifrice and flossing) and the second is chemical management (i.e., using specific products to prevent plaque accumulation or aid in its removal). The best way to ensure healthy teeth and gingival tissues is to mechanically remove plaque buildup by brushing at least twice daily and flossing at least once a day. Toothbrushing removes plaque from the lingual (tongue) side, buccal (cheek) side, and occlusal (biting) surfaces of the teeth. Plaque found on interproximal (between the teeth) surfaces can be removed efficiently with only dental floss and other interdental cleaning aids (e.g., interproximal brush, dental tape, or tapered picks).

Nonpharmacologic Therapy

Dietary Measures

Cariogenic foods should be avoided in favor of less cariogenic foods. A food is considered highly cariogenic if it contains more than 15% sugar, clings to the teeth, and remains in the mouth after it is chewed. Conversely, foods are less cariogenic if they have a high water content (e.g., fresh fruit); stimulate the flow of saliva (i.e., fibrous foods that require lots of chewing); or are high in protein (e.g., dairy products). Both the water content of fresh fruit and the flow of saliva tend to wash the sugar away and neutralize the acid it creates. Milk protein also raises pH and tends to inhibit binding of bacteria.

Oral hygiene products such as mouth rinses and dentifrices may contain a low concentration of saccharin, which is a potent noncariogenic sugar substitute that appears to present no caries hazard. The Food and Drug Administration's (FDA) limit on saccharin is 1.0 g/day for adults; ingestion from normal use of both mouth rinse and dentifrice would result in a total saccharin exposure of only about 20 to 40 mg/day. Other noncariogenic sugar substitutes such as sugar alcohols (sorbitol, xylitol) and aspartame (amino acid methyl ester) are currently used as sweetening agents.

Plaque Removal Devices

Toothbrushes, dental floss, oral irrigating devices, and specialty aids (e.g., interproximal dental brushes) are the primary devices used in facilitating plaque removal.

TOOTHBRUSHES

The toothbrush is the most universally accepted device available for removing dental plaque and maintaining good oral hygiene.

The proper frequency and method of brushing will vary from patient to patient. Thoroughness of plaque removal without gingival trauma is more important than the method used. Table 31-1 describes the proper method of brushing teeth

Manual toothbrushes vary in size, shape, texture, and design, with new product designs proliferating rapidly. These toothbrushes have either nylon or natural bristles. The firmness of the bristles is usually rated as soft, medium, or firm.

Electric toothbrushes, of which there are many on the market, are either battery operated or have a rechargeable battery system. The battery-operated variety, such as the Crest Spinbrush or Colgate 360 Sonic Power Toothbrush, use a rotary and/or vibratory motion, and are less expensive, but the efficiency of their actions deteriorates as a result of the inherent properties of the disposable battery. Rechargeable battery toothbrushes use a rotary and/or vibrating motion (Oral B Braun) or high-frequency sound (Sonicare) to remove plaque. These power brushes tend to be more expensive, but they maintain constant efficiency because of their rechargeability. Dental professionals consider the power toothbrush to have a positive effect on the

---

TABLE 31-1 Guidelines for Brushing Teeth

- Brush teeth after each meal or at least twice a day.
- If using a toothpaste, apply a small amount of paste to the toothbrush.
- If using a powder, apply the powder to a wet toothbrush, completely covering all bristles.
- Use a gentle scrubbing motion with the bristle tips at a 45-degree angle against the gumline so that the tips of the brush do the cleaning.
- Do not use excessive force, because it may result in bristle damage, cervical abrasion, irritation of delicate gingival tissue, and gingival recession with associated hypersensitivity.
- Brush for at least 30 seconds, cleaning all tooth surfaces systematically.
- Gently brush the upper surface of the tongue to reduce debris, plaque, and bacteria that can cause oral hygiene problems.
- If using a powder, reapply powder as described previously and brush again. (Two applications of powder are needed to deliver an amount of sodium fluoride comparable to one application of a paste formulation.)
- Rinse the mouth, and spit out all the water.

---

oral health of 80.5% of their patients.[5] Electric toothbrushes may also benefit certain patients, such as those who are disabled or of advanced age, patients with orthodontic devices; and those who may have difficulty mastering manual brushing techniques.

Best results can be expected if a patient uses a brush carrying the American Dental Association's (ADA's) seal of acceptance and follows a dental professional's specific directions for use. ADA's criteria for acceptance are based on safety and efficacy concerns. Advertisements may mention plaque reduction but may not claim to improve any existing oral disease.[1] Positive results (i.e., significant reductions in dental plaque accumulation) depend, to some extent, on the proper use of the device, implying a need for patient education.

There is no definite guideline as to how often a patient should buy a new toothbrush, although 3 months has been suggested as the average toothbrush life expectancy. Marketing data suggest that consumers, on average, replace their toothbrushes only 1.7 times per year. Two major reasons exist for replacing toothbrushes frequently: wear and bacterial accumulation. Different methods of brushing cause bristles to wear differently. Worn, bent, or matted bristles do not remove plaque effectively. Therefore, patients should replace toothbrushes at the first sign of bristle wear, rather than after a defined period of use. Ideally, they should rotate two or three toothbrushes to allow each to dry completely between uses, thereby decreasing bristle wear and matting. Some brands of toothbrushes have color-impregnated bristles that indicate the need for replacement when the color disappears halfway down the brush.

Product Selection Guidelines　Dental professionals recommend toothbrushes according to the individual patient's manual dexterity, oral anatomy, and periodontal health. The toothbrush should be of a size and shape to allow the patient to reach every tooth in the mouth. Many dentists and dental hygienists prefer soft, rounded, multitufted, nylon bristle brushes, because nylon bristles are more durable and easier to clean than natural bristles, and because soft, rounded bristle tips are also more effective in removing plaque below the gingival margin and on proximal

tooth surfaces. Unfortunately, toothbrush firmness is not standardized; toothbrushes designated as soft, medium, or hard may not be comparable across manufacturers. Most dental professionals recommend a soft brush, even though many individuals may believe that a firm brush will do a better job of cleaning. Use of medium- or hard-bristled toothbrushes may result in damage to the tooth enamel and gingival tissue. The softer bristles are more effective at working themselves into crevices and spaces between the teeth, and are less abrasive on teeth with exposed recession. Innovations in head shapes and bristle configurations continue to be introduced in an attempt to improve cleaning contact with tooth and gumline surfaces.

The handle size and shape of a toothbrush should allow the individual to maneuver the brush easily while maintaining a firm grasp. Many modifications (e.g., angle bends or flexible areas in the handle) that may improve contact between the bristles and some less-accessible tooth surfaces have been introduced. The dentist can fabricate customized handles for physically impaired individuals by adding moldable acrylic to the handles.

Soft bristles are recommended for children's toothbrushes. Children's toothbrushes are smaller than an adult's and are available in baby (for children up to age 6 or 7 years) and junior (ages 7 years to teens) sizes. Toothbrush size and shape should be individualized according to the size of the child's mouth. Children can usually remove plaque more easily with a brush that has short and narrow bristles.

DENTAL FLOSS

Plaque accumulation in the interdental spaces contributes to proximal caries and periodontal pocketing. Interdental plaque removal has been reported to reduce gingival inflammation and prevent periodontal disease and dental caries. Dental flossing is the most widely recommended method of removing dental plaque from proximal tooth surfaces that are not adequately cleaned by toothbrushing alone. Besides removing plaque and debris interproximally, proper flossing also polishes the tooth surfaces, massages interdental papillae, and reduces gingival inflammation. Proper flossing technique requires some finger dexterity and practice. If performed improperly, flossing can injure gingival tissue and cause cervical wear on proximal root surfaces.[1] Table 31-2 describes the proper use of dental floss.

Most floss is a multifilament nylon yarn that is available in waxed or unwaxed form and in varying widths, from thin

---

TABLE 31-2 Guidelines for Using Dental Floss

- Pull out approximately 18 inches of floss, and wrap most of it around the middle finger.
- Wrap the remaining floss around the same finger of the opposite hand. About an inch of floss should be held between the thumbs and forefingers.
- Do not snap the floss between the teeth; instead, use a gentle, sawing motion to guide the floss to the gumline.
- When the gumline is reached, curve the floss into a C-shape against one tooth, and gently slide the floss into the space between the gum and tooth until you feel resistance
- Hold the floss tightly against the tooth, and gently scrape the side of the tooth while moving the floss away from the gums.
- Curve the floss around the adjoining tooth, and repeat the procedure.

---

thread to thick tape. Many brands feature product lines of flosses that are impregnated or coated with additives, such as flavoring, baking soda, and fluoride. In addition, several manufacturers are marketing floss made of materials with superior antishredding properties (e.g., Glide, Reach Tight Teeth Floss, and Oral B Essential). ADA has recognized nearly 35 brands of dental floss and tape as safe and effective.[6]

Product Selection Guidelines   Because no particular product has been proven to be superior, patient factors (e.g., tightness of tooth contacts, tooth roughness, manual dexterity, and personal preference) should be considered in product selection. Similarly, clinical studies show no difference between waxed and unwaxed floss in terms of removing plaque and preventing gingivitis.[7] Evidence does not support concern about waxed floss leaving a residual wax film on tooth surfaces.

Waxed floss may pass interproximally between tight-fitting teeth without shredding more easily than unwaxed floss can. Teflon floss, such as Glide, also resists shredding and slips easily between tight teeth. If contacts at the crowns of teeth are too tight to force floss interdentally, floss threaders can be used to pass floss between the teeth and under the replacement teeth (pontics) of fixed bridges. Floss threaders, which are available in reusable and disposable forms, are usually thin plastic loops or soft plastic, needle-like appliances. Patients who also have braces may find that the use of threaders aids in the flossing process. Electrically powered (flossing) interdental cleaning devices may be used to remove interproximal debris. However, electrically powered interdental devices or floss threaders should be used cautiously to avoid physical trauma of the gingiva.[8] Floss holders have one or two forks rigid enough to keep floss taut and a mounting mechanism that allows quick rethreading of floss. Both floss and electrically powered interdental cleaning devices may improve compliance among some people, and are recommended for patients who lack manual dexterity and for caregivers who assist disabled or hospitalized patients.

SPECIALTY AIDS

Cleaning devices that adapt to irregular tooth surfaces better than dental floss are recommended for interproximal cleaning of teeth with large interdental spaces, such as is found in patients with periodontal disease. The Flossbrush is such a device; it features woven dental floss with a time-release fluoride system that is molded into a plastic handle for interdental cleaning. The most common aids are tapered triangular wooden toothpicks (Stim-U-Dent), holders for round toothpicks (Perio-Aid), miniature bottle brushes (Proxabrush), rubber stimulator tips, denture brushes, and denture clasp brushes.

The evidence for plaque-removal efficacy among these interproximal cleaning devices is conflicting. Differences in methodology and patient populations prevent generalizations from being made, whereas individual patient motivation and dexterity may also influence results. The dental professional considers the patient's oral anatomy, the presence of periodontal disease, the size of the interproximal spaces, and the patient's dexterity when recommending an interdental cleaning aid.

ORAL IRRIGATING DEVICES

Oral irrigators work by directing a high-pressure stream of water through a nozzle to the tooth surfaces. These devices can remove only a minimal amount of plaque from tooth surfaces. Therefore, oral irrigators cannot be viewed as substitutes for a toothbrush, dental floss, or other plaque-removal devices but should be con-

sidered as adjuncts in maintaining good oral hygiene. These devices are useful for removing loose debris from those areas that cannot be cleaned with the toothbrush (e.g., around orthodontic bands and fixed bridges). Several brands on the market carry the ADA seal of acceptance.[7]

Oral irrigators have also been valuable as vehicles for administering chemotherapeutic agents that inhibit microbial growth in inaccessible regions of the mouth. Patients with advanced periodontal disease should use these devices only under professional supervision, because it is possible for transient bacteremia to occur after manipulative procedures with the oral irrigator. Oral irrigation devices are also contraindicated in patients who are predisposed to bacterial endocarditis.

Pharmacologic Therapy

Chemical Management of Plaque

Chemical management of plaque and calculus can enhance mechanical removal either by acting directly on the plaque bacteria or by disrupting components of plaque to aid in its removal during routine oral hygiene. The use of chemical agents in plaque control may be particularly appropriate for selected patients who may be unable to brush and floss effectively. Physically or mentally disabled individuals (who may not be able to master the necessary manual techniques) and orthodontia patients (i.e., those with fixed prostheses) may benefit from adding antiplaque agents to their oral hygiene regimen.

Desirable characteristics for antiplaque agents include the following:

- Selective antibacterial activity, interference with the rate of accumulation, or metabolism of supragingival plaque
- Substantivity (sustained retention of the agent in the mouth)
- Compatibility with dentifrice ingredients
- Lack of undesirable side effects for the user
- Noninterference with the natural ecology of the normal oral microflora

Use of Fluoride

Fluoride is believed to help prevent dental caries through a combination of effects. When it is incorporated into developing teeth, fluoride systemically reduces the solubility of dental enamel by enhancing the development of a fluoridated hydroxyapatite (which is more resistant to demineralizing acids) at the enamel surface. The topical effect facilitates remineralization of early carious lesions during repeated cycles of demineralization and remineralization. Some evidence exists that fluoride interferes with the bacterial cariogenic process. Fluoride that is chemically bound to organic constituents of plaque may interfere with plaque adherence and inhibit glycolysis, the process by which sugar is metabolized to produce acid.[1]

Fluoridation of the public water supply is an effective and economically sound public health measure that has played a major role in decreasing the incidence of caries.[9] More than one-half of the U.S. population resides in communities in which the public water supply contains either naturally occurring or added fluoride at optimal levels for decay prevention (e.g., 1 ppm, or 1 mg/L). Besides reducing dental caries in children, fluoridation has benefits that extend through adulthood, resulting in (1) fewer decayed, missing, or filled teeth; (2) greater tooth retention; and (3) a lower incidence of root caries. Systemic fluoride supplementation in children is based on the preventive mechanism of fluoride when incorporated into developing enamel. Current concepts of the action of fluoride relative to its presence in saliva and plaque provide a rationale for its topical application to prevent caries in all age groups. It must be noted, however, that any decision to supplement fluoride intake must consider the concentration of fluoride present in the drinking water.[1] Bottled water does not contain fluoride.

Mouth rinses and gels that contain sodium fluoride are therapeutic topical applications of fluoride for prevention of dental caries (Table 31-3). Fluoride mouth rinsing enables patients to apply fluoride interproximally.

Examples of patients who may benefit from fluoride rinsing are those with orthodontic appliances, those with decreased salivary flow, those at risk for developing root caries, and anyone with difficulty maintaining good oral hygiene. Orthodontic patients are at risk of developing decalcified areas while under treatment, and their ability to thoroughly clean interdental spaces may be inhibited.

Because fluoride rinses and gels provide a therapeutic fluoride treatment, package directions should be followed closely to maximize the safe and effective use of these products. Table 31-4 describes the proper method of applying fluoride rinses and gels.[10] When recommending a nonprescription fluoride mouth rinse, the practitioner should stress that children younger than 12 years should be supervised as necessary until they are capable of using the product correctly. Furthermore, children younger than 6 years should use these products only as directed by a dentist or primary care provider. Concern has been raised about whether unsupervised home use of fluoride gels is justified.

Dental fluorosis, a mottled appearance of the surface enamel of the tooth, may develop in certain children. Fluorosis develops during time of tooth formation and in children who live in a community with an optimally fluoridated water supply; long-term ingestion of drinking water containing fluoride along with use of fluoride dentifrices places them at risk for mild form of dental fluorosis. Although a mild degree of fluorosis is an esthetic concern, more severe cases can result in pitting and surface defects (see Color Plates, photograph 7).

Related to this concern, FDA considered comments regarding formulation of a reduced-strength fluoride dentifrice during the anticaries final rule process. It was determined that, unlike dental caries, mild dental fluorosis does not compromise oral health or tooth function. Therefore, the risk of dental caries from inadequate fluoride protection is a greater health hazard than the cosmetic effect of fluorosis.

Because of the concerns about dental fluorosis in children, FDA required that dentifrice products with sodium monofluorophosphate containing 1500 ppm of theoretical total fluorine carry the following label: "Keep out of the reach of children under 6 years of age."

TABLE 31-4 Guidelines for Using Topical Fluoride Treatments

- Use topical fluoride treatments no more than once a day.
- Brush teeth with a fluoride dentifrice before using a fluoride treatment.
- If using a fluoride rinse, measure the recommended dose (most commonly 10 mL), and vigorously swish it between the teeth for 1 minute.
- If using a fluoride gel, brush the gel on the teeth. Allow the gel to remain for 1 minute.
- After 1 minute, spit out the fluoride product. Do not swallow it.
- Do not eat or drink for 30 minutes after the treatment.
- Supervise children as necessary until they can use the product without supervision.
- Instruct children younger than 12 years in good rinsing habits to minimize swallowing of the product.
- Consult a dentist or primary care provider before using fluoride products in children younger than 6 years.

Source: Reference 11.

The ADA revised its recommendations for fluoride supplement dosing in children. The new schedule slightly lowers the dose amounts, recommends beginning treatment not earlier than age 6 months, and extends the age limit from 13 to 16 years. Evaluation of studies reporting on the intake of fluoride among children prompted the revision.

Studies of dentifrice ingestion by children show great variation in the amount of dentifrice retained and consistently show that younger children are more likely than older ones to swallow some dentifrice. Limiting ingestion of fluoride dentifrice is advised.

Fluoride rinsing presents a similar problem for children (ages 3–5 years) who may swallow significant amounts of rinse each time they swish. A usual dose of fluoride 0.05% rinse contains 2 mg of fluoride ion and may contribute to mild fluorosis in the presence of a fluoridated public water supply. Fluoride rinses should be used by only children 6 years and older who have mastered the swallowing reflex. These products should be kept out of children's reach, and children younger than 12 years should be supervised during fluoride rinsing. High-dose ingestion requires prompt medical care. Toxicity is related to both the fluoride and the alcohol content. Parents should be able to identify the product and to estimate the amount ingested.

Dentifrices

Dentifrices are used with a toothbrush for cleaning accessible tooth surfaces. Use of a dentifrice enhances removal of dental plaque and stain, resulting in a decreased incidence of dental caries and gum disease, reduced mouth odors, and enhanced personal appearance.

Dentifrices are available as powders, pastes, or gels (Table 31-5). The powder forms commonly contain abrasive and flavoring agents and, sometimes, a surfactant (foaming agent). Dentifrice powders are either moistened to form a slurry and applied with a dry brush, or used dry with a brush moistened with water. The powder is more abrasive when it is used dry. The gels and pastes commonly contain an abrasive, a surfactant, a humectant (moistening agent), a binder/thickener, a sweetener, flavoring

TABLE 31-3 Selected Topical Fluoride Products

Trade Name	Primary Ingredients
ACT for Kids	Sodium fluoride 0.05%; cetylpyridinium chloride
GelKam Gel	Stannous fluoride 0.4%
Oral-B Anti-Cavity Rinse	Sodium fluoride 0.05%
Phos-Flur Fluoride Rinse	Sodium fluoride 0.044%

TABLE 31-5	Selected Dentifrices

Trade Name	Primary Ingredients
Fluoride Toothpastes	
Aquafresh Extra Fresh Toothpaste	Calcium carbonate; hydrated silica; sodium monofluorophosphate (fluoride 0.15%)
Colgate Toothpaste	Dicalcium phosphate dihydrate; sodium monofluorophosphate (fluoride 0.15%)
Crest Cavity Protection Gel	Hydrated silica; sodium fluoride (fluoride 0.15%)
Tartar-Control Toothpastes	
Colgate Baking Soda and Peroxide Tartar Control Toothpaste	Hydrated silica; sodium monofluorophosphate (fluoride 0.15%); pentasodium triphosphate; tetrasodium pyrophosphate
Crest Tartar Protection Gel/Toothpaste	Silica; sodium fluoride (fluoride 0.15%); tetrapotassium pyrophosphate; disodium pyrophosphate; tetrasodium pyrophosphate
Viadent Advanced Care	Hydrated silica; sodium monofluorophosphate (fluoride 0.13%); zinc citrate trihydrate
Antiplaque/Antigingivitis Toothpastes	
Colgate Total Toothpaste	Hydrated silica; sodium bicarbonate; sodium fluoride (fluoride 0.14%); triclosan 0.3%
Crest Multicare Toothpaste	Hydrated silica; sodium fluoride (fluoride 0.15%); sodium bicarbonate; tetrasodium pyrophosphate
Whitening Toothpastes	
Aquafresh Whitening Gel/Toothpaste	Hydrated silica; sodium fluoride; titanium dioxide
Mentadent Advanced Whitening Gel/Toothpaste	Hydrated silica; sodium bicarbonate; sodium fluoride (fluoride 0.24%); titanium dioxide
Ultrabrite Toothpaste	Hydrated silica; alumina; sodium monofluorophosphate (fluoride 0.14%); titanium dioxide
Sodium Lauryl Sulfate–Free Toothpastes	
Biotène Dry Mouth Toothpaste	Lactoperoxidase; glucose oxidase; lysozyme; sodium monofluoro-phosphate 0.15%
Oral B Rembrandt Whitening Natural Toothpaste	Dicalcium phosphate; silica; sodium monofluorophosphate; papain
Sensodyne Original Flavor Toothpaste	Potassium nitrate 5%; sodium fluoride (fluoride 0.13%)
Botanical-Based Toothpastes	
Dr. Burt's	Peppermint; coconut oil; lavender oil; rosemary; eucalyptus; comfrey
Tom's of Maine	Peppermint; spearmint; orange; mango; fennel; carrageenan; propolis; cassia; myrrh; cinnamon
Viadent Original	Sanguinaria

agents, and a therapeutic agent such as fluoride for anticaries activity.

Dentifrice abrasives are pharmacologically inactive and insoluble compounds. Common abrasives include silicates, dicalcium phosphate, alumina trihydrate, calcium pyrophosphate, calcium carbonate, and sodium metaphosphate. Although dentifrices vary in their degree of abrasiveness, abrasion is an essential property for removing stained pellicle from teeth.[1] The ideal abrasive would maximally aid in cleaning while causing minimal damage to tooth surfaces. Unfortunately, because of the variability in patients' brushing techniques and oral conditions, the ideal dentifrice abrasive does not exist. Low-abrasive dentifrices, which include most dentifrice formulations currently marketed in the United States, usually have a low concentration (10%–25%) of silica abrasives, whereas high-abrasive dentifrices typically have higher concentrations (40%–50%) of the inorganic calcium or aluminum salts mentioned previously. Baking soda, a mild abrasive, is found in a number of dentifrices. Although they are safe to use, toothpastes with baking soda have not been shown to clean teeth better than toothpastes without this substance.

FLUORIDE DENTIFRICES

Fluoride dentifrices are indicated for both preventing and treating carious lesions. Use of fluoride-containing dentifrices is the one method of caries prevention that is common to all countries that show a reduction in caries. ADA accepts as safe and effective fluoride-containing toothpaste and fluoride-containing gel dentifrice formulations with compatible abrasives. FDA promulgated a final rule for nonprescription anticaries drug products in 1995; the ingredients that meet the monograph conditions are outlined in Table 31-6. Although a theoretical total fluorine concentration of sodium monofluorophosphate 1500 ppm was

TABLE 31-6	FDA-Approved Active Ingredients for Anticaries Dentifrices

Ingredient	Concentration (ppm) (Dosage Form)
Sodium fluoride	850–1150 (paste)
	850–1150 (powder)
Sodium monofluorophosphate	850–1150 (paste)
Stannous fluoride	850–1150 (paste)

previously recognized as safe, clinical data submitted in the final rulemaking process also established that this ingredient had efficacy for enhanced anticaries benefit.

The possibility of staining exists with the use of stannous fluoride. About 10% to 20% of patients experience slight, but noticeable, tooth discoloration after 2 to 3 months of continuous use. The discoloration is not permanent and is readily removed at the next professional dental cleaning. This product is for use by adults and children ages 12 years and older.

TARTAR-CONTROL DENTIFRICES

A number of fluoride dentifrices contain anticalculus, or tartar-control, compounds. Although plaque—not supragingival calculus—is the primary etiologic factor in marginal periodontal disease, reducing calculus formation is still a goal of good oral hygiene. The ingredients that prevent or retard new calculus formation are zinc chloride, zinc citrate, and soluble pyrophosphates (which act to inhibit crystal growth). Placebo-controlled clinical studies have reported a significant reduction in calculus occurrence and severity.[11]

ADA regards the inhibition of supragingival calculus as a nontherapeutic use and, therefore, does not evaluate anticalculus claims. However, all advertising claims made for accepted products are reviewed for accuracy. ADA has directed that the following additional statement appear on all package and container labeling for accepted fluoride dentifrice products with calculus-control activity: "[Product name] has been shown to reduce the formation of tartar above the gumline, but has not been shown to have a therapeutic effect on periodontal diseases."[12]

The use of tartar-control toothpastes has been associated with a type of contact dermatitis in the perioral region. Adding pyrophosphate compounds to these products increases alkalinity and requires increased concentrations of other components, such as flavorings and surfactants, for solubilizing. It is hypothesized that the pyrophosphates, either alone or combined with the higher concentrations of inactive ingredients, are implicated as the cause of irritant contact dermatitis. Patients experiencing such a reaction should be advised to discontinue the tartar-control dentifrice and should switch to a non–tartar control fluoride product.

ANTIPLAQUE/ANTIGINGIVITIS DENTIFRICES

Colgate Total contains triclosan, an antibacterial agent and promoter of substantivity that has antigingivitis and antiplaque activity. The product also contains fluoride for caries protection and a copolymer delivery system for the triclosan. It is also the only toothpaste currently accepted by ADA for this indication (see the box American Dental Association Seal of Acceptance).[6,12]

Approval was based on clinical data for safety and efficacy. The product is not intended for use in children younger than 6 years.

WHITENING/ANTISTAIN DENTIFRICES

Cosmetic dentifrices make no therapeutic claims and are usually chosen by patients because of taste, whitening ability, or antistain properties. Some dentifrices claiming to remove stubborn coffee or tobacco stains may contain higher concentrations of abrasives. High-abrasive formulations are not advised for long-term use or for use by patients with exposed root surfaces. Plain baking soda, which is a water-soluble mild abrasive, or toothpastes containing baking soda have limited polishing and stain-removal capacity. Other products may contain a pigment (e.g., titanium dioxide) that produces a temporary brightening effect. Rembrandt Whitening Toothpaste contains a chemical complex of aluminum oxide, a citrate salt, and papain. Whitening dentifrices that contain oxygenating agents rely on a debriding action to remove stained pellicle. Numerous products offer a combination of baking soda and peroxide with fluoride. Whitening dentifrices should not be confused with tooth-bleaching products (see the box A Word about Tooth-Bleaching Products).

ADMINISTRATION GUIDELINES

Table 31-1 describes the proper method for brushing teeth using a fluoride dentifrice. Children are usually unable to brush by themselves until they are 4 or 5 years of age, and they may require supervision until age 8 or 9 years to clean teeth effectively. FDA recommends that parents instruct children ages 6

A WORD ABOUT Tooth-Bleaching Products

The popularity of tooth bleaching has increased in the United States in recent years. Three methods are currently in use: (1) in-office dental bleaching, (2) dental office–supported home bleaching, and (3) nonprescription home bleaching. All three methods use basically the same chemical agents: carbamide peroxide or hydrogen peroxide in various strengths. The in-office method has the advantage of a one-time treatment, but the stronger bleach and the accelerator light are not necessary to obtain the same result with the dental office–supported home-bleaching process. The latter method involves the use of custom trays. With this process, patients can fine-tune the extent of lightening to their own preferences.

The following two nonprescription products (among the many) may aid in lightening:

- Rembrandt Professional Bleaching System includes a lower concentration of the company's professional product, which contains carbamide peroxide gel and fluoride. The kit contains a mouth guard that is boiled to form a one-size-fits-all tray similar to nonprescription athletic mouth guards. Because the tray cannot be trimmed exactly to the gumline, there is no way to keep the bleaching gel away from the gingival tissue (gums), and a large quantity of product is required to fill the tray. A kit contains enough product for 30 doses.
- Crest WhiteStrips Classic provides translucent film strips impregnated with hydrogen peroxide and other ingredients. The strips are peeled away from a protective backing and folded over the six upper or lower front teeth (different strips are provided for upper and lower teeth). The teeth will look as though they are covered with small pieces of transparent food wrap. The strips are applied twice a day and left in place for 30 minutes. A kit contains enough strips for 14 days. A stronger version of the same system is available over the counter and is used for a shorter period of time.

to 12 years about good brushing and rinsing habits to minimize swallowing of fluoride. Parents should apply the toothpaste (only a pea-sized amount) to a child-sized toothbrush and should brush the teeth of preschoolers until the children can manage it properly by themselves. Children should be taught to rinse thoroughly and expectorate after brushing. Only regular-strength fluoride toothpaste is recommended for use in children from 2 to 6 years of age. Use in children younger than 2 years should be under the direction of a dentist or primary care provider.

All fluoride dentifrice products must contain the following warning on the labeling: "Warning: Keep out of the reach of children under 6 years of age. If you accidentally swallow more than used for brushing, seek professional assistance or contact a Poison Control Center immediately."

PRODUCT SELECTION GUIDELINES

Unless advised otherwise by their dentists, patients—especially those with periodontal disease, significant gum recession, and/or exposed root surfaces—should choose the least abrasive dentifrice that effectively removes stained pellicle. Although dentifrice abrasives do not pose a risk to dental enamel, toothbrushing action and excessive abrasiveness, which may lead to tooth hypersensitivity, can damage the softer material of exposed root surfaces (cementum) and dentin.

Children younger than 6 years should not use a fluoride dentifrice. Extra-strength fluoride dentifrices, however, may be beneficial to patients who have a greater tendency to develop cavities or who reside in an area with nonfluoridated water.

Popular gel dentifrices are flavored and disperse rapidly in the mouth. Manufacturers of gel dentifrices have advertised that children brush longer and more thoroughly because of the gel's consistency, translucence, dispersibility, and flavor. This claim has not been substantiated, but many dentifrices marketed for children are of the gel type. The children's products usually have fruit flavors, rather than the breath-freshening minty or cinnamon flavors that adults prefer.

Mouth Rinses and Gels

A mouth rinse with plaque or calculus-control properties is indicated as an adjunct to proper flossing and toothbrushing with a fluoride toothpaste. Further research is necessary to determine the efficacy of the antiplaque activity of these products.

Mouth rinse and dentifrice formulations are very similar. As with dentifrices, mouth rinses may be cosmetic or therapeutic (Table 31-7). Both may contain surfactants, humectants, flavor, coloring, water, and therapeutic ingredients.

A mouth rinse approximates a diluted liquid dentifrice that contains alcohol but no abrasive. Alcohol adds bite and freshness, enhances flavor, solubilizes other ingredients, and contributes to the mouth rinse's cleansing action and antibacterial activity. Flavor contributes to pleasant taste and breath freshening. Surfactants are foaming agents that aid in the removal of debris. Other active ingredients may include astringents, demulcents (soothing agents), antibacterial agents, and fluoride.

Cosmetic mouth rinses freshen the breath and clean some debris from the mouth. Mouth rinses can be classified by appearance, alcohol content, and active ingredients. In general, mouth rinses are minty or spicy, medicinal or alcoholic, and contain various miscellaneous ingredients such as (1) glycerin, a topical protectant that tastes sweet and is soothing to oral mucosa; (2) benzoic acid, an antimicrobial agent; or (3) zinc chloride/citrate, an astringent that neutralizes odoriferous sulfur compounds produced in the oral cavity. The most popular cosmetic mouth rinses are medicinal and mint flavored. It is normal for healthy individuals to have some degree of oral malodor (e.g., morning breath). This malodor results from reduced activity of tongue, cheeks, and salivary flow, which enhances bacterial activity and production

TABLE 31-7 Selected Mouth Rinses

Trade Name	Primary Ingredients
Cosmetic Mouth Rinses	
Bioténe	Lysosyme; lactoferrin; glucose oxidase; lactoperoxidase
Lavoris	Zantate; clove oil; zinc chloride
Targon	Polyethylene glycol 40; hydrogenated castor oil
Therapeutic Mouth Rinses	
Crest Pro-Health Rinse	Cetylpyridinium chloride 0.07%
Listerine Tartar Control Antiseptic	Sodium lauryl sulfate; tetrasodium pyrophosphate
Scope	Cetylpyridinium chloride; domiphen
Botanical-Based Mouthwashes	
Glyoxide	Carbamide peroxide
Listerine	Thymol; eucalyptol; methyl salicylate; menthol
Tom's of Maine	Peppermint; spearmint; cinnamon; fennel; aloe vera; witch hazel

of odoriferous sulfur compounds. Therefore, products that are intended to eliminate or suppress mouth odor of local origin in healthy people with healthy mouths are considered by the FDA Advisory Review Panel on Over-the-Counter Oral Health Care Products to be cosmetics, unless they contain antimicrobial or other therapeutic agents. ADA's acceptance program does not evaluate mouth rinses labeled and advertised as only cosmetic agents.

An important consideration is the potential for breath-freshening mouth rinses to disguise or delay treatment of pathologic conditions that may contribute to lingering oral malodor (e.g., periodontal disease, purulent oral infections, and respiratory infections). If marked breath odor persists after proper toothbrushing, the cause should be investigated and not masked with mouth rinse.

Since the 1990s, nonprescription mouth rinses promoted for antiplaque or tartar-control activity have proliferated. Ingredients added to mouth rinses for plaque control include (1) aromatic oils (thymol, eucalyptol, menthol, and methyl salicylate), which are antibacterial and have some local anesthetic activity; and (2) agents with antimicrobial activity (e.g., quaternary ammonium compounds). Of the latter, cetylpyridinium chloride is a cationic surfactant capable of bactericidal activity, although it does not penetrate plaque well. Domiphen bromide is a bactericidal agent similar to cetylpyridinium. Another ingredient, phenol, is a local anesthetic, antiseptic, and bactericidal agent that penetrates plaque better than either cetylpyridinium or domiphen.

Listerine, containing the active ingredients thymol, eucalyptol, methyl salicylate, and menthol, was the first mouth rinse to be accepted by ADA as a nonprescription antiplaque/antigingivitis mouth rinse. The phenol oils (active ingredients) control plaque by destroying bacterial cell walls, inhibiting bacterial enzymes, and extracting bacterial lipopolysaccharides. ADA has since added Cool Mint, FreshBurst Listerine, and more than 100 similarly formulated private-label antiseptic mouth rinses to the antiplaque/antigingivitis category of accepted therapeutic products.[6]

Many practitioners have found anecdotally that use of rinses containing phenol oils, methyl salicylate, and alcohol often brings about a sloughing of the oral epithelium, which subsides when the rinse is discontinued. A similar event seems to occur with the use of lozenges or candies containing cinnamon or other common flavoring substances.

Advanced Formula Plax, intended for use as a prebrushing rinse, contains an enhanced level of detergent (sodium lauryl sulfate) and the addition of detergent builders, tetrasodium pyrophosphate, and sodium benzoate. Approximately 1 to 2 tablespoons of the product is vigorously swished between the teeth and then expectorated. Patients should refrain from eating, drinking, or smoking for 30 minutes after use. The FDA Dental Plaque Subcommittee concluded that insufficient data are available to classify sodium lauryl sulfate as an effective antigingivitis/antiplaque agent.[13]

With the exception of Advanced Formula Plax, plaque- or calculus-control mouth rinses are intended for use twice daily after brushing. In general, an amount equal to 1 to 2 tablespoons of rinse should be swished vigorously in the mouth and between the teeth for about 30 seconds and then expectorated; the rinse should not be swallowed. Patients should be advised to refrain from smoking, eating, or drinking for 30 minutes following use. Children younger than 12 years should be instructed to develop good rinsing habits (to minimize swallowing) until they are capable of using mouth rinses without supervision.

Mouth rinses and gels are generally safe when used as directed, but occasional adverse reactions (e.g., burning sensation or irritation) have been reported. Overuse should be discouraged. Consultation with a health professional is indicated if irritation occurs and persists after the patient discontinues use of the product. The detergent sodium lauryl sulfate is also present in nearly all toothpastes and has been implicated as a cause of aphthous ulcers (canker sores).[14] Some dentifrices that do not contain sodium lauryl sulfate are listed in Table 31-5. Aphthous ulcers are discussed in Chapter 32.

Unsupervised use is contraindicated in patients with mouth irritation or ulceration. These products should be kept out of children's reach. In case of accidental ingestion, the caregiver should seek professional assistance or contact a poison control center.

The alcohol content in mouth rinses ranges from 0% to 27%; the most popular adult mouth rinses contain between 14%

and 27%. Ingestion of alcohol-containing products poses a danger for children, who may be attracted by bright colors and pleasant flavors. Toxicity data concerning a child's ingestion of an alcohol-containing mouth rinse demonstrate that the amount of alcohol in available mouth rinse preparations is sufficient to cause serious illness and injury. Acute alcoholic intoxication and death resulting from high-dose ingestion are possible. For a child weighing 26 pounds, 5 to 10 ounces of a mouth rinse containing alcohol can be lethal.[1] Responding to concern over the potential danger to children, the Consumer Products Safety Commission issued a final rule that required child-resistant packaging for mouth rinses containing 3 grams or more of absolute alcohol per package—the amount that is present in a small quantity (approximately 2.6 ounces) of a mouth rinse with alcohol 5%: "For the purposes of this final rule, the term *mouthwash* includes liquid products that are variously called mouthwashes, mouth rinses, oral antiseptics, gargles, fluoride rinses, antiplaque rinses, and breath fresheners. It does not include throat sprays or aerosol breath fresheners." These products should be kept out of children's reach and should not be administered to children younger than 12 years. Labeling includes a warning not to swallow the product but to seek professional assistance or contact a poison control center immediately in case of accidental ingestion.

Plaque-Control Chewing Gum and Lozenges

Additions to the plaque-control market include baking soda chewing gum (e.g., Between Dental Gum) for plaque reduction. Gum chewing contributes to increased saliva flow that apparently produces a beneficial buffering effect against acids in the oral cavity. Therefore, especially for patients with xerostomia, these products may have some value as an adjunct to their oral hygiene. In addition, the chewing gums are sugar-free and sweetened with sugar alcohols (e.g., xylitol and sorbitol) that do not promote caries and may reduce the risk of caries formation. The patient is directed to chew two pieces of gum daily after eating. These products are not regulated for their antiplaque claims by FDA, and should not be substituted for a regular program of brushing, flossing, and rinsing to remove plaque.

Special Population Considerations for Plaque Removal

At birth, the 20 primary teeth that will erupt are present but not visible. It is important to start oral hygiene early in life. Accordingly, the practitioner should recommend removal of plaque and milk residue by wiping the baby's gums with a wet gauze pad after each feeding. The deciduous teeth will usually start to erupt at about age 6 months and can decay at any time. "Baby bottle caries" results when an infant is allowed to nurse continuously from a bottle of juice, milk, or sugar water. The prolonged contact of teeth with the cariogenic liquid promotes caries. When the teeth have erupted, a soft, child-sized toothbrush can be used for cleaning. Parents must do the brushing and should take care to use only a very small amount of fluoride toothpaste or none at all. Children at this age will swallow the toothpaste, which will contribute to overall systemic fluoride ingestion. Therefore, younger children need to be taught the proper brushing technique or be supervised while brushing.

In patients with fixed orthodontia, very careful attention to oral hygiene to prevent gingivitis and caries is required because of the ease with which plaque accumulates along the orthodontic brackets. Patients with these appliances require a combination of toothbrush types to clean all surfaces effectively. Use of power toothbrushes or oral irrigating devices may help remove plaque and debris around orthodontic bands. It may be advisable for orthodontic patients to use a nonprescription fluoride mouth rinse while undergoing treatment.

Patients with removable orthodontic appliances should consult their orthodontist about using a denture cleanser. Some dental practitioners have recommended, in addition to brushing, a denture cleanser to remove plaque, tartar, odor-causing bacteria, and stain that accumulate on orthodontic appliances.

In patients of advanced age who have natural dentition, topical fluoride application in the form of a dentifrice, rinse, or gel is indicated to prevent coronal and root caries. Practitioners should continue to recommend fluoride anticaries products to their older adult patients. When a practitioner counsels these patients on oral health care, it becomes very important to consider the patients' medication use. Because this population is more likely to be taking multiple medications, the incidence of drug-induced or disease-related changes in oral physiology is increased.

Assessment of Caries: A Case-Based Approach

When asked to recommend plaque-control products, the practitioner should determine what dental care measures the patient is taking, whether these measures meet recommended oral hygiene standards, and how often the patient sees a dentist. The patient's concern about caries should alert the practitioner to ask whether the patient has a history of caries or suspects a new carious lesion has developed.

Case 31-1 illustrates the assessment of patients with caries.

Patient Counseling for Caries

The practitioner should tailor all explanations of the purpose of various oral hygiene products and the methods for using them to the patient's level of knowledge. Patients with a history of caries should be encouraged to brush after meals and to consult with a dentist regarding the use of topical fluoride products. If caries recur or are widespread, the patient should be encouraged to visit a dentist for treatment. The practitioner may recommend products with anticaries agents (e.g., chlorhexidine, povidone iodine, or xylitol). The practitioner should explain the precautions for these products as well as the possible adverse effects of some therapeutic ingredients in other products. Patients should be advised of signs and symptoms that indicate a dental evaluation is necessary. The box Patient Education for Prevention of Caries, Gingivitis, and Halitosis lists specific information to provide patients about plaque-induced oral disorders.

Because dental disease is a commonly encountered health problem, the practitioner needs a well-developed knowledge of oral health care products and their use. Useful resources, references, and information related to ongoing FDA and ADA evaluations of nonprescription dental products are easily available on the Internet. Sites maintained by government agencies, industry, and professional associations provide valuable professional and patient education material. Table 31-8 lists some of these organizations.

Relevant Evaluation Criteria	Scenario/Model Outcome

Information Gathering

1. Gather essential information about the patient's symptoms, including:

   a. description of symptom(s) (i.e., nature, onset, duration, severity, associated symptoms)

   Patient has experienced mild pain in the right lower jaw for the past several days. The pain is occurring occasionally, especially after she eats something sweet.

   b. description of any factors that seem to precipitate, exacerbate, and/or relieve the patient's symptom(s)

   Symptoms began when the patient was eating salt water taffy but improved after she brushed her teeth and rinsed her mouth.

   c. description of the patient's efforts to relieve the symptoms

   She used Orajel (benzocaine) to relieve pain but has not seen an improvement in symptoms.

2. Gather essential patient history information:

   a. patient's identity

   Irene Rudenko

   b. patient's age, sex, height, and weight

   52-year-old female, 5 ft 3 in, 125 lb

   c. patient's occupation

   Paralegal

   d. patient's dietary habits

   Normal healthy diet but has a sweet tooth

   e. patient's sleep habits

   Normal

   f. concurrent medical conditions, prescription and nonprescription medications, and dietary supplements

   Lipitor 10 mg every day

   g. allergies

   NKA

   h. history of other adverse reactions to medications

   None

   i. other (describe) _____

   N/A

Assessment and Triage

3. Differentiate the patient's signs/symptoms and correctly identify the patient's primary problem(s).

   Patient would appear to have either dental caries or a cracked tooth possibly related to poor oral hygiene.

4. Identify exclusions for self-treatment.

   None

5. Formulate a comprehensive list of therapeutic alternatives for the primary problem to determine if triage to a medical practitioner is required, and share this information with the patient.

   Options include:
   (1) Refer Irene to a dentist.
   (2) Recommend appropriate OTC products along with education about proper oral care and referral to a dentist.
   (3) Take no action.

Plan

6. Select an optimal therapeutic alternative to address the patient's problem, taking into account patient preferences.

   OTC analgesics such as an NSAID can be used temporarily to relieve the dental pain the patient is experiencing. Practice appropriate oral hygiene using a fluoride-containing toothpaste and floss. Reduce consumption of sugary foods.

7. Describe the recommended therapeutic approach to the patient.

   NSAIDs such as ibuprofen, naproxen, or aspirin will reduce the inflammation and pain that you are experiencing in your tooth. The amount of sugary foods that you eat should be limited in quantity as well as frequency of consumption.

8. Explain to the patient the rationale for selecting the recommended therapeutic approach from the considered therapeutic alternatives.

   Only a dentist will be able to identify the tooth decay and correct the problem so that you do not continue to have tooth-related pain. The recommendation of an analgesic is temporary and will help to relieve the pain. Appropriate oral hygiene will help to prevent the development of tooth decay in the future.

CASE 31-1 *(continued)*

Relevant Evaluation Criteria	Scenario/Model Outcome
Patient Education	
9. When recommending self-care with nonprescription medications and/or nondrug therapy, convey accurate information to the patient:	
a. appropriate dose and frequency of administration	One of the following: ibuprofen 400 mg every 4–6 hours; aspirin 650 mg every 4 hours; naproxen 220 mg every 8–12 hours
b. maximum number of days the therapy should be employed	This is temporary treatment to reduce pain only. Use for the shortest amount of time possible until you can be seen by a dentist.
c. product administration procedures	Take NSAID with food.
d. expected time to onset of relief	Approximately 1 hour
e. degree of relief that can be reasonably expected	Total pain relief will not occur until decay has been removed and tooth appropriately restored.
f. most common side effects	GI upset including nausea, heartburn, dyspepsia
g. side effects that warrant medical intervention should they occur	GI bleeding; severe nausea, heartburn, or dyspepsia
h. patient options in the event that condition worsens or persists	If some pain relief does not occur within 1 hour, seek immediate dental treatment.
i. product storage requirements	Keep medication in original packaging, tightly closed and at room temperature.
j. specific nondrug measures	Avoid sweet foods and foods that are hard.
10. Solicit follow-up questions from patient.	Can I double the dose of any of these products to get better more quickly?
11. Answer patient's questions.	No. Doubling the dose of any of these products will only increase your risk of suffering unwanted adverse effects.

Key: GI, gastrointestinal; N/A, not applicable; NKA, no known allergies; NSAID, nonsteroidal anti-inflammatory drug; OTC, over-the-counter.

TABLE 31-8 Internet Oral Health Care Resources for the Pharmacist

Agency/Organization/Publication	Web Site	Available Resources/Services
American Dental Association	www.ada.org	Patient education, product news, research, publications, references, accepted products
Federal Register	www.access.gpo.gov	OTC advisory committee actions and recommendations; proposed and final rules, etc.
National Institute of Dental and Craniofacial Research	www.nidcr.nih.gov (site maintained by National Institutes of Health)	Health care and patient information, *NIDCR Research Digest,* and links to oral health resources
Academy of General Dentistry	www.agd.org	Reliable source for consumer dental health information
American Dental Hygienists' Association	www.adha.org	Consumer oral health information and related links
American Association of Public Health Dentistry	http://www.aaphd.org	Databases and links to Internet resources on oral health
Various manufacturers of oral health care products	Search for home pages on the Internet	Product information and links to related dental sites

Key: OTC, over-the-counter.

GINGIVITIS

Periodontal disease, the prevalence and severity of which are related primarily to the degree and quality of oral health care, remains the principal cause of tooth loss in adults older than 45 years.[11] Controlling buildup of plaque and calculus can prevent or control this common and significant public health problem. All forms of periodontal disease are associated with oral hygiene status, not with age. However, as life spans increase and people retain more teeth later in life, both the number of teeth at risk and the time for risk of periodontal disease increase.[1]

Gingivitis, the mildest form of periodontal disease, is reversible and affects nearly everyone. Gingivitis may progress to more severe periodontal diseases, such as acute necrotizing ulcerative gingivitis and periodontitis. The latter can cause significant, irreversible alveolar bone loss.

Periodontitis and gingivitis can be distinguished in the following way. Whereas gingivitis is the inflammation of the gingiva without loss or migration of epithelial attachment to the tooth, periodontitis occurs when the periodontal ligament attachment and alveolar bone support of the tooth have been compromised or lost. This process involves apical migration of the epithelial attachment from the enamel to the root surface (see Color Plates, photographs 8 and 9).

Because caries and gingivitis can result from buildup of plaque, the epidemiology of caries can be extended to that of gingivitis. In addition, hormonal changes influence gingivitis, accounting for its increased frequency during puberty and pregnancy.

Pregnant patients are more susceptible to both dental caries and gingivitis. An inflammatory condition so common that it is called "pregnancy gingivitis" is characterized by red, swollen gingival tissue that bleeds easily. Local factors cause this gingivitis, as in any patient. Pregnancy modifies the host's response, however, making gingival tissue more sensitive to bacterial dental plaque. Hormone level and increased production of prostaglandins have been implicated in the heightened inflammatory response.[1] Pregnancy gingivitis can be prevented or resolved with thorough plaque control. The severity of the inflammatory response and the resultant gingivitis decrease postpartum and return to pre-pregnancy levels after approximately 1 year.

Pathophysiology of Gingivitis

Gingivitis results from the accumulation of supragingival bacterial plaque. If this accumulation is not controlled, the plaque proliferates and invades subgingival spaces. At the same time, specific types of bacteria are associated with plaque at different stages of accumulation; the composition of the bacterial flora changes to a more complex mix of organisms. Although not all gingivitis progresses to periodontitis, the progression from supragingival plaque to gingivitis to periodontitis is relatively common; therefore, controlling gingivitis is a reasonable approach to limiting periodontitis.[1]

Gingivitis also may manifest as a result of (1) blood dyscrasias such as leukemia, (2) mucocutaneous diseases such as lichen planus, and (3) viral infections such as acute herpetic gingivostomatitis. Most importantly, disturbances of the immune system (e.g., acquired immunodeficiency syndrome) can lead to a severe form of this disease.[15]

Other possible etiologies include medications such as calcium channel blockers, cyclosporine, and phenytoin. Anticholinergics and antidepressants may cause gingivitis by reducing the flow of saliva. The use of tobacco (both smokeless and smoked) has also been linked to periodontal disease.

Clinical Presentation of Gingivitis

The marginal gingiva (the border of the gingiva surrounding the neck of the tooth) is held firmly to the tooth by a network of collagen fibers. Microorganisms present in the plaque in the gingival sulcus (the space between the gingiva and the tooth) are capable of producing harmful products, such as acids, toxins, and enzymes that damage cellular and intercellular tissue. Dilation and proliferation of gingival capillaries, increased flow of gingival fluid, and increased blood flow with resultant erythema of the gingiva are found in early stages. The gingiva may also enlarge, change contour, and appear puffy or swollen as a result of the inflammation (see Color Plates, photograph 8). In the early stage of gingivitis, the inflammatory process is reversible with effective oral hygiene.

In time and with neglect, the condition becomes chronic as capillaries become engorged, venous return is slowed, and localized anoxemia results in a bluish hue to areas of the reddened gingiva. Chronic gingivitis may be localized to the area around one or several teeth, or it may be generalized, involving the gingiva around all the teeth. The inflammation may involve just the marginal gingiva or it may be more diffuse, involving all the gingival tissue surrounding the tooth. Changes in gingival color, size, and shape, as well as the ease with which gingival bleeding occurs, are common indications of chronic gingivitis that both the patient and the practitioner can recognize. The flat knife-edge appearance of healthy gingiva is replaced by a ragged or rounded edge. The presence of red cells in extravascular tissue and the breakdown of hemoglobin also deepen the color of gingival tissue. Progression of these conditions is usually slow and insidious—and often painless.

Left untreated, chronic gingivitis may advance to the inflammatory condition of chronic destructive periodontal disease, or periodontitis (see Color Plates, photograph 9). Bacterial species that predominate in periodontitis, but are not present in healthy periodontium, have been found in low proportions in gingivitis. Progression of gingivitis may parallel the increasing proportions of bacterial species implicated in the genesis of periodontitis.

Prevention of Gingivitis

Because prevention of gingivitis and caries depends on calculus prevention and plaque control, the same measures described in Prevention of Caries pertain to gingivitis. The active antigingivitis ingredients in dentifrices, mouth rinses, and other plaque removal and antiplaque products are triclosan, cetylpyridinium chloride, and stabilized stannous fluoride.[16]

Brushing and flossing can cure early gingivitis that arises from irritating food debris and plaque. Adequate removal and control of supragingival plaque are the most important factors in reversing gingivitis, and in preventing and controlling periodontal disease. Gum massage is also recommended, with such devices as soft brushes, special rubber cup massagers, a Stim-U-Dent, or toothpicks. Practitioners should immediately refer for dental care any patient who describes bleeding during brushing or shows signs of early gingivitis.

Assessment of Gingivitis: A Case-Based Approach

Before recommending oral hygiene products, the practitioner should evaluate the patient's oral hygiene regimen. At a minimum, the practitioner should find out whether the patient has a history of gingivitis, whether signs and symptoms of gingivitis are currently present, and what preventive measures the patient has tried or is using. Checking the patient's medical and medication history will identify asymptomatic patients who are at risk for gingivitis.

The practitioner is quite often alerted to pregnancy gingivitis during counseling on prescription prenatal vitamins. Besides monitoring the pregnant patient's medications for safety, the practitioner has an opportunity to encourage the patient to have a dental checkup and to stress the importance of careful attention to brushing and flossing to avoid oral health complications.

Case 31-2 is an example of the assessment of patients with gingivitis.

Patient Counseling for Gingivitis

Because gingivitis is usually not associated with pain, patients are unlikely to seek a practitioner's advice for this problem alone. More likely, patients will ask for oral hygiene information and product recommendations. The practitioner may have to suggest

---

CASE 31-2

Relevant Evaluation Criteria	Scenario/Model Outcome
Information Gathering	
1. Gather essential information about the patient's symptoms, including:	
a. description of symptom(s) (i.e., nature, onset, duration, severity, associated symptoms)	Patient has been experiencing sore, swollen gums for the past several months.
b. description of any factors that seem to precipitate, exacerbate, and/or relieve the patient's symptom(s)	Gum tissue bleeds freely during toothbrushing. Bleeding increases with use of dental floss.
c. description of the patient's efforts to relieve the symptoms	He has decreased the frequency of toothbrushing to a couple times a week and avoids using floss.
2. Gather essential patient history information:	
a. patient's identity	William Fisher
b. patient's age, sex, height, and weight	31-year-old male, 5 ft 11 in, 185 lb
c. patient's occupation	Police officer
d. patient's dietary habits	Eats meals on the go, frequently fast food
e. patient's sleep habits	Varies depending on which shift he is working
f. concurrent medical conditions, prescription and nonprescription medications, and dietary supplements	None
g. allergies	None
h. history of other adverse reactions to medications	Codeine caused vomiting.
i. other (describe) _____	N/A
Assessment and Triage	
3. Differentiate the patient's signs/symptoms and correctly identify the patient's primary problem(s).	William appears to have gingivitis and signs of possible periodontal disease.
4. Identify exclusions for self-treatment.	None
5. Formulate a comprehensive list of therapeutic alternatives for the primary problem to determine if triage to a medical practitioner is required, and share this information with the patient.	Options include: (1) Refer William to a dentist. (2) Recommend appropriate OTC products along with education about proper oral care and referral to a dentist. (3) Take no action.

CASE 31-2 *(continued)*

Relevant Evaluation Criteria	Scenario/Model Outcome
Plan	
6. Select an optimal therapeutic alternative to address the patient's problem, taking into account patient preferences.	Refer patient to the dentist.
7. Describe the recommended therapeutic approach to the patient.	N/A
8. Explain to the patient the rationale for selecting the recommended therapeutic approach from the considered therapeutic alternatives.	You need to see a dentist because you have signs of periodontal disease. Although there are steps you can take to improve your oral hygiene, a dentist will need to evaluate your condition and develop a treatment plan.
Patient Education	
9. When recommending self-care with non-prescription medications and/or nondrug therapy, convey accurate information to the patient.	Criterion does not apply in this case.
10. Solicit follow-up questions from patient.	Is there an OTC medication that might work?
11. Answer patient's questions.	OTC medications do not treat gingivitis and periodontal disease. They may reduce the symptoms, but ultimately your dental care professional will need to develop a treatment strategy. Once you have been diagnosed, there are OTC products you may use as part of your oral care regimen. Gingivitis and periodontal disease, if left untreated, may result in tooth loss.

Key: N/A, not applicable; OTC, over-the-counter.

oral hygiene methods and alert the patient to the possible adverse effects of certain products. The box Patient Education for Prevention of Caries, Gingivitis, and Halitosis lists specific information to provide patients.

The practitioner should also use this opportunity to warn patients with suspected gingivitis (bleeding, swollen gums) that this disease is a serious problem warranting professional attention. The practitioner should stress, especially to pregnant patients and teenagers, that adherence to an oral hygiene program is vital to preventing gingivitis.

HALITOSIS

Halitosis, oral malodor usually known as bad breath, may be a symptom of oral pathology. However, in 90% of cases, poor oral hygiene is the cause.

Pathophysiology of Halitosis

Common oral causes related to poor oral hygiene include malodorous decaying food particles, tonsillar crypt debris, plaque on the dorsum of the tongue (particularly the posterior third), caries, and periodontal disease.[17] Xerostomia can also cause mouth odor. Medications that have anticholinergic properties often cause xerostomia. Garlic, tobacco, onions, alcohol, and other substances commonly placed into the mouth have their own odors that are not always appreciated by others.

Pulmonary diseases such as purulent lung infections, tuberculosis, bronchiectasis, sinusitis, tonsillitis, and rhinitis are responsible for a small percentage of mouth odors. Renal failure, carcinoma, hepatic failure, and hyperglycemic acetone breath (ketosis) are also examples of nonoral causes.[18]

Most foul breath odors occur because of a breakdown of sulfur-containing proteins into volatile sulfur compounds (VSCs) including hydrogen sulfide, methylmercaptan, and dimethyl sulfide.[19]

Prevention of Halitosis

Prevention of halitosis relies on the removal of plaque and the prevention of calculus formation as described in Prevention of Caries. One of the primary sites for the formation of VSCs is the back of the tongue. Plaque and VSCs in this area of the mouth can seed the tonsillar crypts with malodorous debris. Brushing the teeth and tongue are helpful, but some dentists have found that the use of a tongue-cleaning device such as a tongue blade may be the best way to clean the circumvallate papillae area of the tongue. Cleaning this posterior dorsal area will not only remove the fetid VSCs but also prevent them from spreading to the tonsils.

Zinc salts and chlorine dioxide are most effective in the chemical prevention of oral malodor. The two are combined in two-part rinses such as Smart-Mouth (Triumph Pharmaceuticals). Zinc chloride, citrate, and acetate reduce the receptor binding necessary for VSC production. Chlorine dioxide breaks disulfide bonds and oxidizes the precursors of VSCs. The zinc salts also kill gram–negative bacteria.

Any patient who complains of severe or lingering halitosis without a readily identifiable cause (e.g., smoking) should be advised to see a dentist for a thorough evaluation. Masking foul taste and odor with cosmetic mouth rinses may delay necessary dental or medical assessment and any needed treatment.

Assessment of Halitosis

When assessing a patient for halitosis, the practitioner should evaluate the patient's dental hygiene. Ideally, the practitioner should obtain a medication and medical history to determine whether the halitosis might arise from one of the illnesses discussed in Pathophysiology of Halitosis (see also Xerostomia in Chapter 32.)

Patient Counseling for Halitosis

For patients with mouth odor related to poor dental hygiene, the practitioner should recommend the appropriate products and explain their use. Nonpharmacologic measures should also be explained. The practitioner should stress to patients whose mouth odor is related to medical conditions that proper oral hygiene is still necessary to prevent tooth and gum problems. The box Patient Education for Prevention of Caries, Gingivitis, and Halitosis lists specific information to provide patients.

PATIENT EDUCATION FOR Prevention of Caries, Gingivitis and Halitosis

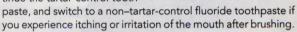

The primary objective of self-care is the removal of plaque to prevent caries, gingivitis, and halitosis. For most patients, carefully following product instructions and the self-care measures listed here will help ensure good oral hygiene.

Nondrug Measures and Other Considerations

- Avoid cariogenic foods, such as foods that contain more than 15% sugar, that cling to the teeth, and that remain in the mouth after they are chewed.
- Eat low-cariogenic foods, such as foods that have a high water content (e.g., fresh fruit); that stimulate the flow of saliva (e.g., fibrous foods that require lots of chewing); or that are high in protein (e.g., dairy products).
- To help prevent mouth odor, drink at least eight 8-ounce glasses of water a day, if possible. Also, if you wear dentures, do not wear them while sleeping.
- Note that use of alcohol and tobacco can cause caries, gingivitis, and halitosis.
- Note that hormonal changes during pregnancy increase the risk of gingivitis.
- Consider incorporating gum massage as an antigingivitis measure, using such devices as soft brushes, special rubber cup massagers, a Stim-U-Dent, or toothpicks.

Plaque Removal
Brushing Teeth
- Mechanically remove plaque buildup by brushing teeth at least twice daily with a fluoride dentifrice. (See Table 31-1 for proper brushing technique.)
- Use a brush with soft nylon bristles.
- Replace the brush when the bristles show signs of wear.
- For children younger than 2 years, clean the teeth with a soft cloth, and massage the gums.
- For preschool children, apply a pea-sized amount of toothpaste to a child-sized toothbrush, and brush the child's teeth until the child can brush properly.
- Use only regular-strength fluoride toothpaste for children ages 2–6 years. Consult a dentist before using fluoride toothpastes in children younger than 2 years.
- Teach children how to rinse the mouth and spit out the toothpaste to avoid swallowing fluoride.

- Note that tartar-control toothpastes have been related to a type of contact dermatitis in the perioral region. Discontinue the tartar-control toothpaste, and switch to a non–tartar-control fluoride toothpaste if you experience itching or irritation of the mouth after brushing.
- If you are prone to developing caries or gingivitis, consider using a toothpaste classified as having antiplaque/antigingivitis activity. Such toothpastes contain stannous fluoride.
- If you are prone to developing aphthous ulcers, consider using a toothpaste that does not contain sodium lauryl sulfate.

Flossing Teeth
- Floss your teeth at least once a day. (See Table 31-2 for proper flossing technique.)
- Use a waxed or Teflon-coated floss for teeth with tight contacts.

Using Plaque-Disclosing Products
- For maximum plaque removal, use a plaque-disclosing product to see whether toothbrushing and flossing have removed all the plaque.
- Rinse the mouth with water.
- Chew a disclosing tablet, or apply a solution to the teeth with a cotton-tipped applicator.
- Swish the product around the mouth for 30 seconds, and then spit out the product.
- Rinse the mouth with water, and spit out the solution. Look for red areas on the teeth that indicate areas of plaque accumulation. If teeth are red, brush and floss again.

Using Mouth Rinses and Gels
- To freshen breath, use a mouth rinse that contains zinc chloride (Viadent) and zinc citrate. Zinc chloride and chlorine dioxide are found in Smart-MouthTri-Oral two-part rinse. These ingredients eliminate odoriferous volatile sulfur compounds.
- If you are prone to developing caries or gingivitis, consider using a mouth rinse classified as having antiplaque/antigingivitis activity. Such mouthwashes contain cetylpyridinium chloride or a combination of thymol, eucalyptol, methyl salicylate, and menthol.

HYGIENE-RELATED DENTURE PROBLEMS

Pain along the gingival ridge under a denture prosthesis suggests conditions such as denture stomatitis (an inflammation of the oral tissue in contact with a removable denture), inflammatory papillary hyperplasia, and chronic candidiasis. Denture stomatitis, which results from poor cleaning of dentures, can lead to chronic candidiasis (fungal infection).

Pathophysiology of Hygiene-Related Denture Problems

Dentures accumulate plaque, stain, and calculus by a process very similar to that occurring on natural teeth. The denture plaque mass that is in contact with oral tissues produces predictable toxic results. Poor denture hygiene contributes to fungal and bacterial growth that not only affects the patient esthetically (unpleasant odors and staining), but also seriously affects the patient's oral health (inflammation and mucosal disease) and ability to successfully wear the dentures.

Chronic atrophic candidiasis, sometimes referred to as denture stomatitis or denture sore mouth, is common in patients with full or partial dentures. This condition may be attributed to infection with *Candida albicans*, which can be found resident on the denture base.[20] Symptomatically, the inflamed denture-bearing area may appear granular or erythematous and edematous with soreness or a burning sensation (see Color Plates, photograph 10). Inflammation secondary to *Candida* organisms is generalized to the entire denture-bearing tissue area, whereas inflammation secondary to the trauma of ill-fitting dentures is usually localized to the specific area of the trauma. It appears that *Candida* organisms either adhere to the denture material or reside in pores of the denture material and can reinfect the mouth. Failure to remove the denture at bedtime and clean it regularly worsens this condition. Angular cheilitis (soreness and cracking at corners of the mouth) is commonly associated with

chronic atrophic candidiasis and other forms of oral candidiasis. The corners of the mouth can often be effectively treated with terbinafine cream. If a staphylococcal organism is also involved, a prescription will be needed.

Prevention of Hygiene-Related Denture Problems

Removing plaque from dentures helps prevent gum infections, staining of dentures, and mouth odor. Specialty brushes and aids are available to remove plaque from hard-to-clean areas (e.g., spaces around a fixed bridge, implants, or orthodontic bands) and dentures. Dentures should be cleaned thoroughly at least once daily to remove unsightly stain, debris, and plaque. Abrasive and chemical cleansers formulated specifically for dentures are available (Table 31-9). A combination regimen of brushing dentures with an abrasive cleaner and soaking them in a chemical cleanser is recommended.

Denture (paste or powder) cleansers containing mild abrasives (e.g., calcium carbonate) must be applied properly with

TABLE 31-9 Selected Denture Cleaners

Trade Name	Primary Ingredients
Ban-A-Stain Liquid	Phosphoric acid 25%
Dentu-Cream Paste	Dicalcium phosphate dihydrate; calcium carbonate; aluminum silicate
Efferdent Plus Tablets	Sodium bicarbonate; sodium perborate; potassium monopersulfate; detergents
Polident Tablets	Potassium monopersulfate; sodium perborate monohydrate; sodium carbonate; sodium bicarbonate; citric acid; surfactant; chelating agents

specialty brushes adapted to the denture's contour to remove stains, plaque, and calculus. Overly vigorous scrubbing can abrade the acrylic materials of dentures and bend the metal clasps. To prevent irritation of oral tissues, the patient should thoroughly rinse the abrasive cleaner from the denture.

The brushing routine can be followed by soaking the denture in an alkaline peroxide cleansing solution to help remove remaining plaque and bacteria. Plaque removal is then enhanced by brushing the denture after it has soaked; instructions for this procedure are included on some products.

The other method of cleaning is to use a soaking solution containing one of the three chemical cleansers: hypochlorite, alkaline peroxide, or dilute acids.

Alkaline peroxide cleaners are the most commonly used chemical denture cleansers. These powders or tablets become alkaline solutions of hydrogen peroxide when dissolved. The ingredients are alkaline detergents and perborates; the latter cause oxygen release for a mechanical cleaning effect. These products are most effective on new plaque and stains that are soaked for 4 to 8 hours. The alkaline peroxides have few serious disadvantages and do not damage the surface of acrylic resins.

Hypochlorites (bleach) remove stains, dissolve mucin, and are both bactericidal and fungicidal. Denture plaque consists of cells embedded in a matrix that serves as a surface on which calculus may develop. Hypochlorite cleansers act directly on the organic plaque matrix to dissolve its structure, but they cannot dissolve calculus once it has formed. The most serious disadvantage of hypochlorite is that it corrodes metal denture components such as the framework and clasps of removable partial dentures, solder joints, and possibly the pins holding the teeth. The addition of anticorrosive phosphate compounds has greatly reduced this problem, but these products should be used for only 15-minute soaks to limit exposure and not more often than once a week.

Acid-containing soaking solutions can also be corrosive to metals, and short soaking times in these solutions are recommended. A sonic or ultrasonic cleaning device, when used with a commercially prepared solution, is easier to use and cleans more effectively than soaking alone. However, some hand brushing may still be required.

All denture-cleansing products should be completely rinsed off the denture before it is inserted into the mouth. Abrasive cleansers coming in contact with oral or other mucous membranes may cause tissue irritation. Chemical cleansers may cause tissue irritation or possibly severe chemical burns. All denture cleansers should be kept out of children's reach owing to the potential for eye or skin irritation, or for toxicity from accidental ingestion. A dentist should evaluate stains that are resistant to proper denture brushing and soaking in available solutions.

Only products that are specifically formulated for denture cleansing should be used. Household cleansers (used for soaking) are not appropriate and may either be ineffective or damage the denture material. The use of whitening toothpastes, which are formulated for use with natural dentition, should be discouraged; they are too abrasive to be used safely on denture material.

Patients should not soak or clean dentures in hot water or hot soaking solutions because distortion or warping may occur.

Patients of advanced age or disabled patients may prefer an alkaline peroxide soak solution for daily, overnight cleaning. Unlike alkaline hypochlorite and acid cleansers, alkaline peroxide cleansers do not corrode metal components of dentures.

Assessment of Hygiene-Related Denture Problems

Before recommending any type of oral hygiene product, the practitioner should determine what denture care measures the patient is taking and whether those measures are adequate. At a minimum, the practitioner should determine whether the patient suffers from denture stomatitis or inflammation secondary to ill-fitting dentures.

Patient Counseling for Hygiene-Related Denture Problems

Denture wearers may tend to blame any oral discomfort on the appliances rather than their hygiene regimen. The practitioner should stress that diligent plaque removal from dentures is the key to preventing denture stomatitis. The methods of cleaning dentures, including their advantages and disadvantages, should be explained. Using the patient's preferences, the practitioner should recommend a denture cleanser and reinforce the methods of use. The box Patient Education for Hygiene-Related Denture Problems lists specific information to provide patients.

PATIENT EDUCATION FOR
Hygiene-Related Denture Problems

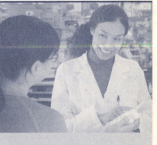

The objective of self-care is to prevent bacterial or fungal infections of the mouth by removing plaque from the dentures. For most patients, carefully following product instructions and the self-care measures listed here will help ensure good denture hygiene.

- Clean dentures thoroughly at least once daily to remove unsightly stain, debris, and potentially harmful plaque.
- Preferably, brush dentures with an abrasive cleaner, and then soak them in a chemical cleanser. This combination regimen is more effective in removing plaque and bacteria.
- Apply the abrasive cleaner to the denture, using a brush designed to adapt to the denture's contour.

- Do not scrub the denture surface vigorously; such action can abrade the acrylic materials and bend the metal clasps.
- To prevent irritation of oral tissues, rinse the abrasive cleaner thoroughly from the denture.
- After brushing the dentures, soak them in an alkaline peroxide cleansing solution for 4–8 hours. Rinse the dentures thoroughly to avoid chemical burns of the mouth.
- If possible, brush the dentures again, and rinse them thoroughly.

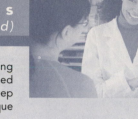

PATIENT EDUCATION FOR
Hygiene-Related Denture Problems
(continued)

- Note that alkaline peroxide cleansers cannot damage the denture, but hypochlorite or dilute acid (phosphoric acid) cleansers can.
- If using an alkaline peroxide or acid cleanser, soak the dentures for only 15 minutes to avoid corrosion of metal denture components.
- Keep all denture cleansers out of children's reach. These agents can cause eye or skin irritation or toxicity if accidentally ingested.
- Do not use household cleansers or whitening toothpastes to clean dentures. These agents may damage denture material.
- Do not soak or clean dentures in hot water or hot soaking solutions. Distortion or warping of the denture may occur.

- Do not sleep while wearing your dentures. Decreased levels of saliva during sleep may contribute to plaque buildup on the denture.

 If your mouth becomes sore or shows sign of infection, see a dentist.

Key Points for Prevention of Hygiene-Related Oral Disorders

➤ Removing plaque and modifying diet are the main goals of self-care to prevent caries, gingivitis, and halitosis.

➤ Mechanical removal of plaque by brushing and flossing is essential for good oral health.

➤ Mouth rinses may augment brushing and flossing procedures and may be used to freshen breath and/or as antiplaque/antigingivitis adjuncts.

➤ Topical fluorides may be used in individuals with high caries activity.

➤ Supervision of children younger than 12 years or until they are capable of using the products correctly must be enforced.

➤ Denture cleaners may be used, in addition to physical removal of debris, to prevent bacterial and/or fungal infections.

➤ If individuals have specific problems related to the purpose or use of these products, consultation with a dentist should be recommended.

REFERENCES

1. Harris NO, Garcia-Godoy F. *Primary Preventive Dentistry*. 6th ed. Stamford, Conn: Appleton & Lange; 2004:76–85, 96–102, 124–5, 128–30, 165–6, 242–7, 249–53, 419, 440, 471, 489–90, 655–9.
2. ten Cate JM. Fluorides in caries prevention and control: empiricism or science. *Caries Res*. 2004;38:254.
3. Davies RM. The rational use of oral care products in the elderly. *Clin Oral Invest*. 2004;8:2.
4. Taybos G. Oral changes associated with tobacco use. *Am J Med Sci*. 2003;326:179.
5. Warren PR, Ray TS, Cugini M, et al. A practice-based study of a power toothbrush: assessment of effectiveness and acceptance. *J Am Dent Assoc*. 2000;131:389.
6. Council on Scientific Affairs. *Products of Excellence ADA Seal Program*. Chicago: American Dental Association; 2007.
7. Carr MP, Rice GL, Horton JE. Evaluation of floss types for interproximal plaque removal. *Am J Dent*. 2000;13:212–4.
8. Rawal SY, Claman LJ, Kalmar JR, et al. Traumatic lesions of the gingiva: a case series. *J Periodontol*. 2004;75:762–9.
9. Petersen PE, Lennon MA. Effective use of fluorides for the prevention of dental caries in the 21st century: the WHO approach. *Community Dent Oral Epidemiol*. 2004;32:319–21.
10. Gluck GM, Morganstein WM, eds. *Jong's Community Dental Health*. 4th ed. St Louis: Mosby-Year Book; 1998:127–33.
11. Fairbrother KJ, Heasman PA. Anticalculus agents. *J Clin Periodontol*. 2000;27:285–301.
12. Council on Scientific Affairs. *Guidelines for Acceptance of Chemotherapeutic Products for the Control of Gingivitis*. Chicago: American Dental Association; 1997.
13. US Food and Drug Administration. Oral health care drug products for over-the-counter human use; antigingivitis/antiplaque drug products; establishment of a monograph. *Fed Regist*. 2003;68:32235, 32263, 32285–6.
14. Herlofson BB, Barkvoll P. The effect of two toothpaste detergents on the frequency of recurrent aphthous ulcers. *Acta Odontol Scand*. 1996;54:150–3.
15. Eisen DE, Lynch DP. *The Mouth: Diagnosis and Treatment*. St Louis: Mosby; 1998.
16. US Food and Drug Administration. Oral health care drug products for over-the-counter human use; antigingivitis/antiplaque drug products; establishment of a monograph. *Fed Regist*. 2003;68:32232.
17. Sanz M, Roldan S, Herrera D. Fundamentals of breath malodor. *J Contemp Dent Pract*. 2001;2:1–17.
18. Tangerman A. Halitosis in medicine: a review. *Int Dent J*. 2002;52 (suppl 3):201–6.
19. ADA Council on Scientific Affairs. Oral malodor. *J Am Dent Assoc*. 2003;134:209.
20. Kulak-Ozkan Y, Kazazoglu E, Arikan A. Oral hygiene habits, denture cleanliness, presence of yeasts and stomatitis in elderly people. *J Oral Rehabil*. 2002;29:300.

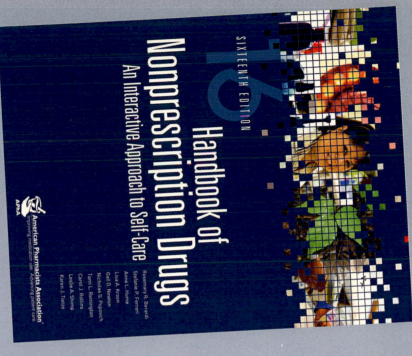

Handbook of Nonprescription Drugs eBook

Welcome!

As a free bonus, purchasers of the 16th edition of the *Handbook of Nonprescription Drugs* get

- ONE free download to ONE computer
- Fast access to the complete contents of the book from your laptop or desktop computer. It is completely searchable and can be annotated with your comments.
- Technical support information is available by clicking on *http://www.OTCHandbook.com/faq.aspx*

How to Get Started

1. Open your browser and visit *http://www.OTCHandbook.com.*
2. Click on "Download eBook."
3. Fill out ALL required fields on the registration form.
4. Enter the unique download code on this card. (You must do this *before* clicking "Submit")
5. Click "Submit" only once.

eBook Download Code:

3363e36e

Oral Pain and Discomfort

Macary Weck Marciniak

Oral pain and discomfort are common ailments affecting persons in the United States.[1–3] Many children experience irritation and soreness during the teething process. As adults, oral pain may be associated with sudden exposure of or damage to nerves in a tooth or to the unexpected cracking or breaking of teeth, fillings, or crowns (caps). Similarly, pain in the mucosa of the oral cavity and lips can be generated by injury to the mouth, recurrent aphthous stomatitis (canker sores), or herpes simplex labialis (cold sores). Some adults experience xerostomia (dry mouth) that is significant enough to require treatment with nonprescription medications. Oral pain and discomfort can interfere with daily activities such as drinking, eating, and working; cause mental anxiety and distress; and result in economic costs from visits to health care providers.[1–3] By distinguishing the patient's self-treatable problems from those potentially requiring professional dental or medical care, the health care practitioner plays an important advisory role in oral health care.

TOOTH HYPERSENSITIVITY

Tooth hypersensitivity, or dentin hypersensitivity, is characterized by a short, sharp pain arising from exposed dentin (i.e., mineralized tissue of teeth internal to crown enamel and root cementum) in response to a stimulus (thermal, chemical, or physical) that cannot be ascribed to any other form of dental defect or disease.[4] Tooth hypersensitivity affects approximately 40 million people in the United States each year and up to 30% of adults at some point during their lifetime.[5] For many patients, tooth hypersensitivity is not perceived as a severe oral health problem; in fact, dentists believe it is a serious problem for only 1% of their diagnosed patients.[6] Whitening dentifrices may contribute to tooth sensitivity and are discussed in Chapter 31.

Pathophysiology of Tooth Hypersensitivity

Two processes are essential for the development of dentin hypersensitivity: Dentin must become exposed (lesion localization) through loss of enamel or gingival recession, and the dentin

tubules must be open to both the oral cavity and the pulp (lesion initiation).[4,6] The roots of teeth are usually covered by gum tissues (gingiva) but, with infection (periodontal disease) or injury (traumatic brushing), the gums recede. The cementum covering affected root surfaces may be reduced by further injury (attrition, abrasion, or erosion), eventually exposing the underlying porous dentin. When stimuli such as heat, cold, pressure, or acid touch exposed dentin or reach an open tubule, fluid flow in the dentinal tubule is increased and the underlying nerves are stimulated, resulting in pain.[4,6]

Enamel, which covers the anatomic crowns of the teeth and is the most mineralized body tissue, is resistant to abrasion by normal toothbrushing, but excessive brushing with an abrasive dentifrice or a medium- or hard-bristled toothbrush can be problematic. The etiology of dental erosion is primarily attributed to the presence of extrinsic or intrinsic acid.[7,8] Extrinsic sources of acid include frequent consumption of acidic medications, foods, or drinks. Persons who regularly consume citrus juices and fruits, carbonated drinks, wines, and ciders may be at risk for tooth hypersensitivity. The most common source of intrinsic acid is regurgitation of gastric contents into the mouth, which occurs with disorders such as gastroesophageal reflux disease or bulimia nervosa.[7] Erosion of tooth enamel and dentin by acidic vomitus is the most notable oral consequence of frequent purging in patients suffering from bulimia; according to one report, one-third of patients will exhibit erosion of the anterior teeth (primarily the lingual or tongue surfaces of the upper incisors).[8] Brushing of acid-softened (eroded) enamel has a marked abrasive effect.[4]

Tooth hypersensitivity is more common in persons with periodontitis or after procedures such as deep scaling, root planing, orthodontic tooth movement, or periodontal (gum) surgery.[9,10] Sensitivity to hot and cold for several weeks following dental therapy is normal. Hypersensitivity can also occur as a result of clenching or grinding teeth (bruxism) and from gumline grooves (abfraction lesions or toothbrush abrasions) formed by abrasive or inappropriate toothbrushing technique. Over the past several years, patients have become increasingly interested in the esthetic benefits of whitening systems that can be used at home.[11] Tooth-whitening procedures may adversely affect both hard and soft tissues in the oral cavity, as well as the dental pulp.[11] A recent study showed that mild tooth sensitivity can be expected

Editor's Note: This chapter is based on the 15th edition chapter with the same title, written by Gary D. Klasser and Charles S. Greene.

in approximately half of patients who undergo home whitening treatment; approximately 10% experience moderate sensitivity and 4% experience severe sensitivity.[11] This hypersensitivity is transient, occurs early in treatment, decreases as treatment continues, and subsides once treatment is completed.[11-13] The hypersensitivity is rarely severe enough to prevent the patient from finishing the full course of treatment.[11] Tooth-whitening products are discussed in Chapter 31.

Clinical Presentation of Tooth Hypersensitivity

A patient with tooth hypersensitivity experiences pain from hot/cold and sweet/sour solutions, as well as when hot/cold air touches the teeth. As individual pain thresholds vary, so does the pain experienced from tooth hypersensitivity. Pain varies from mild discomfort to sharp, excruciating pain. If the pain from tooth hypersensitivity is intense, the patient may limit oral hygiene, which in turn contributes to plaque accumulation and the progression of oral plaque diseases. Although tooth hypersensitivity is self-treatable, toothache is not; therefore, it is critical for the practitioner to differentiate between these two conditions (Table 32-1). Resolution of pain associated with toothache, fractured dentition, ill-fitting dentures or suspected infection (abscess) requires professional dental care. Only a dental/medical provider can adequately evaluate and treat these conditions; therefore, the practitioner should advise the patient to see a dentist without delay.

Treatment of Tooth Hypersensitivity

Treatment Goals

The goals of self-treating tooth hypersensitivity are to (1) alter the damaged tooth surface using the appropriate toothpaste and (2) stop abrasive toothbrushing practices. When these goals have been achieved, tooth hypersensitivity may be eliminated.

General Treatment Approach

Most patients seek care early in the course of their symptoms.[3] Patients frequently report an inability to cope with toothache and often consult non–dental health care professionals, such as physicians or pharmacists.[14] Before recommending self-treatment of tooth pain, the practitioner should determine whether the patient has a history of dental problems (caries, periodontal, or endodontic problems), whether the patient regularly cares for his or her teeth, and whether the patient receives regular professional dental care. This information will help determine the patient's level of care and risk for a toothache versus tooth hypersensitivity. Figure 32-1 outlines the self-treatment of tooth hypersensitivity and lists exclusions for self-care. A patient presenting with a possible toothache should be advised to seek professional dental assistance as soon as possible.

Nonpharmacologic Therapy

Treatment plans for tooth hypersensitivity should include identification and elimination of predisposing factors such as extrinsic and intrinsic acid and improper (harsh) toothbrushing technique. Tooth hypersensitivity can be prevented by brushing less vigorously with standard fluoride dentifrice (toothpaste) and a soft-bristled toothbrush. Fluoride dentifrices and oral fluoride supplementation can help limit sensitivity issues. Fluoride is discussed in more detail in Chapter 31.

Pharmacologic Therapy (Desensitizing Dentifrices)

Pharmacologic treatment of tooth hypersensitivity involves the use of desensitizing dentifrices that contain a potassium salt. Potassium diffuses along the dentinal tubules to decrease the excitability of intradental nerves and alter their membrane potential. A tooth desensitizer acts on the dentin to block the perception of stimuli that patients with normal teeth usually do not perceive. Because the most common cause of tooth sensitivity is exposed dentin, a desensitizing dentifrice must inhibit

---

TABLE 32-1 Differentiation of Tooth Hypersensitivity and Toothache

	Tooth Hypersensitivity	Toothache
Etiology	Exposed and open dentin tubules	Bacterial invasion to the pulp
Pathophysiology	Stimuli (heat, cold, pressure, acid) cause fluid in the dentinal tubules to expand and shrink stimulating pulp nerve fibers, resulting in pain	Inflammatory response to invading bacteria stimulates free nerve endings in the pulp
Causes	Attrition, abrasion, erosion, tooth/restoration fracture, faulty restoration, or gingival recession	Cavitation/decay present in tooth/teeth under existing restoration, tooth/restoration fracture, or trauma to the dentition
Symptoms	A quick, fleeting, sharp, or stabbing pain on stimulation by thermal, chemical, or physical stimuli, which stops after stimuli are no longer present	Intermittent, short, and sharp pain on stimulation may indicate reversible damage; continuous, dull, and throbbing pain without stimulation usually indicates irreversible damage
Assessment	Hypersensitivity due to attrition, abrasion, or erosion is not serious and self-treatable; sensitivity due to fracture, faulty restoration or gingival recession should be referred to a dentist	Requires dental/medical care for resolution

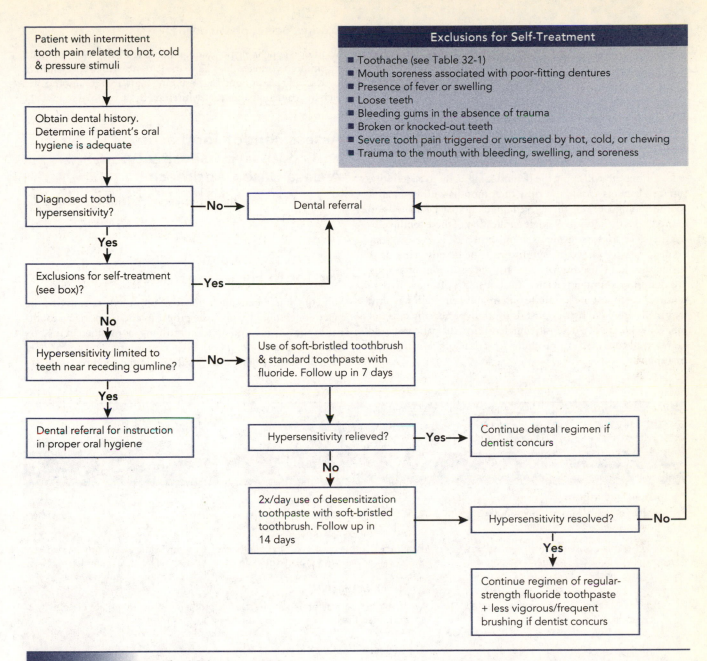

FIGURE 32-1 Self-care of tooth hypersensitivity.

sensitization while also being nonabrasive. Table 32-2 lists selected desensitizing toothpastes and their active ingredients.

Two well-controlled clinical studies and three supportive studies provided sufficient data to the Food and Drug Administration (FDA) to establish the effectiveness of potassium nitrate 5% for protection against painful sensitivity of the teeth caused by cold, heat, acids, sweets, or contact. As a tooth desensitizer, potassium nitrate 5% is classified as a Category I agent (safe and effective).[15] Combination products containing potassium nitrate 5% and fluoride are available. When used as directed, these products can relieve tooth hypersensitivity and prevent dental caries. Two studies demonstrated that the dentifrice containing potassium nitrate 5% and stannous fluoride 0.454% (Colgate Sensitive Maximum Strength) is superior to products containing potassium nitrate 5% and sodium monofluorophosphate 0.76% (Fresh Mint

TABLE 32-2 Selected Desensitizing Toothpastes

Trade Name	Primary Ingredients
Colgate Sensitive Maximum Strength Whitening	Potassium nitrate 5%; sodium fluoride 0.24%
Crest Maximum Strength Sensitivity Protection Extra Whitening	Potassium nitrate 5%; sodium fluoride 0.243%
Sensodyne Maximum Strength with Fluoride	Potassium nitrate 5%; sodium fluoride 0.15%
Orajel Sensitive Pain-Relieving	Potassium nitrate 5%; sodium monofluorophosphate 0.20%

Sensodyne).[16,17] New combination dentifrices in development that contain potassium nitrate, stannous fluoride, and sodium fluoride have demonstrated significantly better reduction in dentin hypersensitivity compared with dentifrices containing sodium fluoride or potassium chloride, triclosan, and sodium fluoride (Sensodyne F).[18] Other studies have demonstrated benefit in combining potassium nitrate with dimethyl isosorbide.[19]

For optimum effectiveness, patients should apply at least a 1-inch strip of the desensitizing dentifrice to a soft-bristled toothbrush and use the product twice daily. Brushing thoroughly for at least 1 minute will apply the desensitizing agent to all sensitive surfaces. Patients should not rinse their mouths with water after toothbrushing, because the active ingredient may be diluted and cleared from the mouth. A single application of these toothpastes has no effect; for some patients, long-term use (2–4 weeks) may be necessary to relieve the symptoms. The desensitizing dentifrice should be used until the sensitivity subsides or as long as a dentist recommends its use. In about 25% of adults, hypersensitive teeth are a chronic problem and require long-term treatment provided by a dentist. If tooth hypersensitivity is not relieved with use of a desensitizing dentifrice, the patient should be referred to a medical provider for an in-office method of treatment.

Product Selection Guidelines

Dentifrices containing potassium nitrate 5% are not recommended for children younger than 12 years. Patients with hypersensitive teeth should be cautioned against using high-abrasion toothpastes such as cosmetic pastes that whiten teeth or remove stains.

Assessment of Toothache and Tooth Hypersensitivity: A Case-Based Approach

Case 32-1 illustrates the assessment of patients with toothache or tooth hypersensitivity.

Patient Counseling for Tooth Hypersensitivity

Subsequent to a definite diagnosis of tooth hypersensitivity, the practitioner should explain the proper use of desensitizing toothpastes and safe methods of toothbrushing, as outlined in the box Patient Education for Tooth Hypersensitivity. The practitioner should also explain precautions for using the toothpastes.

CASE 32-1

Relevant Evaluation Criteria	Scenario/Model Outcome
Information Gathering	
1. Gather essential information about the patient's symptoms, including:	
a. description of symptom(s) (i.e., nature, onset, duration, severity, associated symptoms)	Patient is complaining of tooth pain for the last 4 days. It is a continuous, dull pain in an upper right molar. The pain came on somewhat slowly and has not improved over the last few days. The pain is bothersome enough that it is interfering with his life.
b. description of any factors that seem to precipitate, exacerbate, and/or relieve the patient's symptom(s)	When asked, the patient denies any specific problems when eating hot or cold foods; rather, the pain seems to be constant.
c. description of the patient's efforts to relieve the symptoms	The patient has not tried anything yet.
2. Gather essential patient history information:	
a. patient's identity	Jordan Wiseman
b. patient's age, sex, height, and weight	21-year-old male, 5 ft 9 in, 195 lb
c. patient's occupation	College student
d. patient's dietary habits	N/A
e. patient's sleep habits	The pain is making it difficult to fall asleep at night.
f. concurrent medical conditions, prescription and nonprescription medications, and dietary supplements	Loratidine 10 mg 1 tablet by mouth every day for allergies
g. allergies	NKA
h. history of other adverse reactions to medications	None
i. other (describe) _____	The patient brushes his teeth at least once a day and flosses once a month. Life on campus is busy, and the patient now indicates that he is not sure exactly when the pain started. In fact, it might have been around for longer than 4 days. The semester is coming to a close, and final exams are coming up in the next week.

Relevant Evaluation Criteria	Scenario/Model Outcome

Assessment and Triage

3. Differentiate the patient's signs/symptoms and correctly identify the patient's primary problem(s) (see Table 32-1).

The pain is continuous in nature and is not brought on by stimulation with heat or cold. Based on the information available, it is likely that the pain is related to a toothache, rather than tooth hypersensitivity.

4. Identify exclusions for self-treatment (see Figure 32-1).

Toothache is not a self-treatable condition.

5. Formulate a comprehensive list of therapeutic alternatives for the primary problem to determine if triage to a medical practitioner is required, and share this information with the patient.

Options include:
(1) Refer Jordan to a dentist.
(2) Take no action.

Plan

6. Select an optimal therapeutic alternative to address the patient's problem, taking into account patient preferences.

Refer the patient to a dentist for evaluation.

7. Describe the recommended therapeutic approach to the patient.

N/A

8. Explain to the patient the rationale for selecting the recommended therapeutic approach from the considered therapeutic alternatives.

You need to see a dentist because your pain appears to be related to a toothache, which is not a self-treatable condition. You will likely require prescription medications or medical intervention for resolution of your problem.

Patient Education

9. When recommending self-care with nonprescription medications and/or nondrug therapy, convey accurate information to the patient.

Criterion does not apply in this case.

10. Solicit follow-up questions from patient.

I would like to wait and see my dentist at home. May I use a nonprescription medication to "get me through" the end of the semester?

11. Answer patient's questions.

Evaluation by a dentist should occur as soon as possible. Short-term use of oral analgesics can help control the pain so that studying for final exams can be continued in comfort; however, an appointment should be made as soon as possible. Waiting to make the appointment until after final exams are finished will likely delay treatment, and the condition could worsen and become more serious.

Key: N/A, not applicable; NKA, no known allergies

PATIENT EDUCATION FOR
Tooth Hypersensitivity

The objectives for self-care of tooth hypersensitivity are to (1) repair the damaged tooth surface using the appropriate toothpaste and (2) stop abrasive toothbrushing practices. For most patients, carefully following product instructions, the dentist's recommendations, and the self-care measures listed here will help ensure optimal therapeutic outcomes.

- Use a soft-bristled toothbrush, and brush with light pressure with a fluoride toothpaste for sensitive teeth at or near a receding gumline.
- If correct brushing techniques with a fluoride toothpaste are ineffective, a desensitizing toothpaste should be used.
- If a desensitizing toothpaste is needed, apply a 1-inch strip of toothpaste to a soft-bristled toothbrush. Brush for at least 1 minute twice daily.
- Note that relief of the sensitivity may take several days to several weeks. The better the patient is at removing bacterial plaque, the quicker the sensitivity will resolve.

- Use the toothpaste as long as the dentist recommends, and then switch to a low-abrasion (nonwhitening) fluoride dentifrice.
- Note that some cases of hypersensitive teeth require long-term treatment or several repeated treatments.
- Do not use desensitizing toothpastes in children younger than 12 years.
- Do not use high-abrasion toothpastes such as cosmetic pastes that whiten or remove stains.

 See a dentist if the pain worsens during treatment or if new symptoms develop.

Evaluation of Patient Outcomes for Tooth Hypersensitivity

The patient with hypersensitive teeth should use a desensitizing dentifrice for a maximum of 4 weeks. If the pain is resolved, the patient should continue treatment as recommended by a dentist. The patient should be advised to continue the recommended dental hygiene measures. If the pain persists or worsens or if new symptoms develop, the patient should see a dentist for further evaluation.

TEETHING DISCOMFORT

Not all babies suffer discomfort during teething. For those who do, nonprescription products can provide symptomatic relief.

Pathophysiology of Teething Discomfort

Teething is the eruption of the deciduous (primary or baby) teeth through the gingival tissues. Usually, this normal physiologic process is uneventful. However, it can cause pain, sleep disturbances, or irritability in some individuals.

Clinical Presentation of Teething Discomfort

Mild pain, irritation, reddening, excessive drooling, or slight swelling of the gums may precede or accompany sleep disturbances or irritability. Teething is not associated with vomiting, diarrhea, nasal congestion, malaise, fever, or rashes, but these symptoms may be a sign of ear or stomach infection. Bluish, soft, and round swellings (called eruption cysts) sometimes form over emerging incisors and molars. Eruption cysts are not the result of infection and will disappear if left alone. In addition, three bumps (called mamelons) may be present on the biting surfaces (incisal edges) of emerging incisors. The mamelons will wear away as the teeth begin to occlude against the opposing dentition. If the underside of the tongue becomes irritated, a dentist may try to smooth the edges of the mamelons to prevent further irritation.

Treatment of Teething Discomfort

Treatment Goals

The goal of self-care of teething discomfort is to relieve gum pain and irritation, thereby reducing the child's irritability and sleep disturbances.

General Treatment Approach

Parents/caregivers should be cautioned to exercise restraint in treating a child's teething discomfort. Eruption cysts are a part of the normal physiologic process and should be left alone to resolve spontaneously. If cut or punctured, the cysts will leave scars that may delay the tooth's eruption. Parents/caregivers should also exercise restraint in the use of nonprescription teething products. Various nonpharmacologic measures are recommended for alleviating teething discomfort. Parents should try all measures to determine which are helpful. If additional treatment is needed, topical analgesics that are approved specifically for teething discomfort or pediatric doses of systemic analgesics can be used.

Nonpharmacologic Therapy

If the baby cooperates, massaging the gum around the erupting tooth may provide relief. Babies may be made more comfortable by giving them a frozen pacifier (teething ring) or a cold wet cloth, or if they are at an age to tolerate food (such as dry toast), they may be given such food to chew.

Pharmacologic Therapy

Pharmacologic management of teething discomfort is limited to topical analgesics that are approved for use in infants and pediatric doses of systemic analgesics.

Topical Oral Analgesics

FDA review of nonprescription drug products for relief of oral discomfort has classified benzocaine 5% to 20% and phenol 0.5% preparations as Category I (safe and effective) topical anesthetics/analgesics for teething pain. In the highest concentration (20%) that is approved for nonprescription use, benzocaine is too potent for infants and can even cause death from drug overdose. The risk of hypersensitivity to local anesthetics also exists. Currently, no phenol 0.5% products are marketed for teething pain, although phenol products are marketed for other types of oral pain. Parents/caregivers should be careful to select only products that are labeled for teething. Table 32–3 lists selected products that are marketed for teething pain.

Systemic Analgesics

Pediatric doses of systemic nonprescription analgesics (e.g., acetaminophen) may be used to relieve teething discomfort. (See Chapter 5 for discussion of these agents and their recommended dosages.)

Product Selection Guidelines

Teething products are labeled, "For the temporary relief of sore gums due to teething in infants and children 4 months of age and older."[15] A product containing benzocaine 10% might be preferable for nighttime use to help babies sleep. For ease of application, gels are the best choice; unlike liquids, they do not drip when applied. Products containing benzocaine in solution or suspension should be rubbed onto the gums not more than four

---

TABLE 32-3 Selected Teething Products

Benzocaine 7.5% Products
Baby Anbesol Gel
Baby Orajel Teething Pain Medicine Gel/Liquid/Swabs

Benzocaine 10% Products
Baby Orajel Teething Nighttime Formula

PATIENT EDUCATION FOR
Teething Discomfort

The objective of self-care for teething discomfort is to relieve gum pain and irritation, thereby reducing the child's irritability and sleep disturbances. For most patients, the parent's or caregiver's careful following of product instructions and the self-care measures listed here will help ensure optimal therapeutic outcomes.

Nondrug Measures

- If possible, massage the gum around the erupting tooth to provide relief.
- Give the baby a frozen pacifier (teething ring), a cold wet cloth, or food (such as dry toast) to chew.

Nonprescription Medications
Topical Analgesics

- Use only products that are labeled for teething.
- Rub commercial teething products containing benzocaine onto the gums not more than four times daily.
- Do not use teething preparations containing benzocaine 20%, because this concentration is too potent for infants and can even cause death from drug overdose.

- Benzocaine can cause hypersensitivity. If redness or irritation of the gum increases after use of this medication, stop using it.
- Use alcohol- and sucrose-free products that carry the American Dental Association's acceptance seal.

Systemic Analgesics

- If desired, use pediatric formulations of oral nonprescription analgesics such as acetaminophen to relieve teething discomfort.
- Read the label carefully, and do not exceed recommended doses or frequency of use.

 If the baby is vomiting or has diarrhea, fever, nasal congestion, malaise, pain, or other symptoms not typical of teething discomfort, take the baby to a primary care provider or pediatrician.

---

times daily. The American Dental Association (ADA) recommends using an alcohol-free product. Parents/caregivers should check the ingredients of teething products for the presence of alcohol.

Assessment of Teething Discomfort: A Case-Based Approach

In most cases, the practitioner must assess teething discomfort based on the parent's description of the child's symptoms. If the child cooperates, visual inspection of the gums may confirm that the child is teething. Nonetheless, the practitioner must distinguish the signs and symptoms of teething from those of an infection.

Patient Counseling for Teething Discomfort

The practitioner should be prepared to suggest both nonpharmacologic and pharmacologic remedies for teething discomfort, as outlined in the box Patient Education for Teething Discomfort. Parents should be urged to contact a primary care provider when symptoms uncharacteristic of teething discomfort are present.

Evaluation of Patient Outcomes for Teething Discomfort

The practitioner should ask the parent to call back after 3 to 5 days of treatment. If neither nonpharmacologic therapy nor nonprescription medications are relieving the symptoms, the parent should be advised to take the baby to a primary care provider, pediatrician, or pediatric dentist. Furthermore, if symptoms

uncharacteristic of teething discomfort have developed, the baby should be evaluated by a primary care provider or pediatrician.

RECURRENT APHTHOUS STOMATITIS

Recurrent aphthous stomatitis (RAS), also known as canker sore or aphthous ulcer, affects approximately 25% of Americans and has a recurrence rate of 50% within 3 months.[20] RAS occurs more commonly during the second and third decades of life. There may be a female predominance in some adult and child patient groups, and children of higher socioeconomic status may be more commonly affected than those from lower socioeconomic groups.[21] Also, the incidence is slightly higher in stressed than in nonstressed populations. Minor RAS is the most common form of RAS, representing 80% to 90% of all cases.[22] The disease usually begins in childhood or early adolescence. In patients older than 50 years, RAS declines in both frequency and severity.

Pathophysiology of Recurrent Aphthous Stomatitis

The cause of RAS is unknown in most patients. The most likely precipitating factors are stress and local trauma. Trauma (e.g., chemical irritation, biting the inside of cheeks or lips, or injury caused by toothbrushing or braces) has been implicated as a leading cause of lesions.[20] A genetic component to the disease is possible, given that more than 42% of patients with RAS have first-degree relatives with RAS.[23] Additional precipitating or contributing factors may include food allergy and hormonal changes. Patients suffering from RAS are usually nonsmokers.[23] Many smokers have reported RAS following smoking cessation, which may be a result of the stress of cessation or the changes that occur to the oral mucosa after cessation. Smoking is an irritant to the oral mucosa that results in a thickening process that may protect the oral mucosa from traumatic injury. Ex-smokers need reassurance during this time period to be successful in giving up this habit. Systemic conditions associated with RAS include Behçet's disease; systemic lupus erythematosus; neutrophil dysfunction; allergy; nutritional deficiencies of vitamins B_1, B_2, B_6, B_{12}, and folic acid, or iron; inflammatory bowel disease; and human immunodeficiency virus/acquired immunodeficiency syndrome.[20,23,24]

Clinical Presentation of Recurrent Aphthous Stomatitis

RAS appears as an epithelial ulceration on nonkeratinized mucosal surfaces of movable mouth parts, such as the tongue, floor of the mouth, soft palate, or the inside lining of the lips and cheeks. Rarely, ulcerations affect keratinized tissue such as the gingiva or the external lips (vermillion). Individual ulcers are usually (1) round or oval, (2) flat or crater-like in appearance, and (3) gray to grayish yellow with an erythematous halo of inflamed tissue surrounding the ulcer (see Color Plates, photograph 11).

RAS occurs in three clinical forms: minor, major, and herpetiform. The RAS form can be distinguished primarily on the number of lesions, the size of the ulcer, and the number of days that the lesion persists. Table 32-4 compares the features of these three forms. Some patients may experience a pricking or burning sensation (prodrome) about 24–48 hours before the lesion actually appears. The lesions can be very painful—with the pain increasing on eating and drinking—and may inhibit normal eating, drinking, swallowing, and talking, as well as routine oral

hygiene. Although many patients have recurrent episodes of oral lesions with periods of remission, some patients chronically experience one or more lesions in the mouth for very long periods without the knowledge of their presence. Usually, fever or lymphadenopathy does not accompany RAS; however, such symptoms may arise if a secondary bacterial infection is present.

Treatment of Recurrent Aphthous Stomatitis

RAS cannot be cured; however, nonprescription medications can provide symptomatic relief.

Treatment Goals

The goals in treating RAS are to (1) control pain of the ulcer, (2) promote ulcer healing, (3) prevent recurrence, and (4) prevent complications such as secondary infection.[22]

General Treatment Approach

If possible, the lesion(s) should be inspected to determine whether their appearance and location are characteristic of RAS. The practitioner should try to identify what factors may have led to development of the ulcer. If possible, precipitating or contributing factors should be removed. For example, if trauma is suspected, perhaps a gentler toothbrush and gentler brushing technique could be suggested. It is also helpful to determine whether the patient has a history of RAS. The practitioner should ask about previous self-treatments and their effectiveness. If the treatments used are appropriate and have been successful for the patient, then they should be continued. Treatment should focus on protecting the ulcerations from irritating stimuli and reduc-

TABLE 32-4 Differentiation of RAS and HSL

| | RAS (Canker Sores) | | | |
	Minor	Major	Herpetiform	HSL (Cold Sores)
Manifestation	Oval, flat ulcer; erythematous tissue around ulcer	Oval, ragged, gray/yellow ulcers; crater form	Small ulcers in crops, similar to minor RAS	Red, fluid-filled vesicles; lesions may coalesce; crusted when mature
Location	All areas except gingiva, hard palate, vermilion (border of the oral mucosa and external skin)	All areas except gingiva, hard palate, vermilion (border of the oral mucosa and external skin)	Any intraoral area	Junction of oral mucosa and skin of lip and nose
Incidence	85%	10%	5%	
Number of lesions	Usually one	Several (1–10)	Multiple (crops)	Several
Size of lesion	<1 cm	0.5–2 cm	1–4 cm	1–3 mm
Duration (days)	5–7	>14 days	10–14	10–14
Pain	None-to-moderate	None-to-moderate	Moderate-to-severe	None-to-moderate
Scarring	None	Common	None	Rare
Comments	Immunologic defect	Immunologic defect	Immunologic defect	Induced by HSV-1

Key: HSL, herpes simplex labialis; HSV-1, herpes simplex virus-1; RAS, recurrent aphthous stomatitis.

ing the severity of pain and irritation. Figure 32-2 outlines the self-treatment of RAS and lists exclusions for self-care.

Nonpharmacologic Therapy

If a nutritional deficiency (e.g., iron, folate, or vitamin B$_{12}$) is suspected as a contributing factor, the patient should increase consumption of foods high in these nutrients or take nutritional supplements. For patients in whom a food allergy is thought to be a contributing factor, elimination of the offending agent from the diet may help to improve or resolve RAS. Spicy foods, acidic foods, and foods that have the potential to cause local

injury should be avoided until ulcerations improve. Ice applied in 10-minute increments directly to the lesions can give temporary relief. However, heat may cause the spread of infection (if present) and should not be used. As stress may play a role in the development of RAS, relaxation and imagery training may be useful and has shown reductions in ulcer frequency.

Pharmacologic Therapy

Several types of nonprescription medications (oral debriding and wound cleansing agents, topical oral anesthetics, topical oral protectants, oral rinses, and systemic analgesics) provide symptomatic

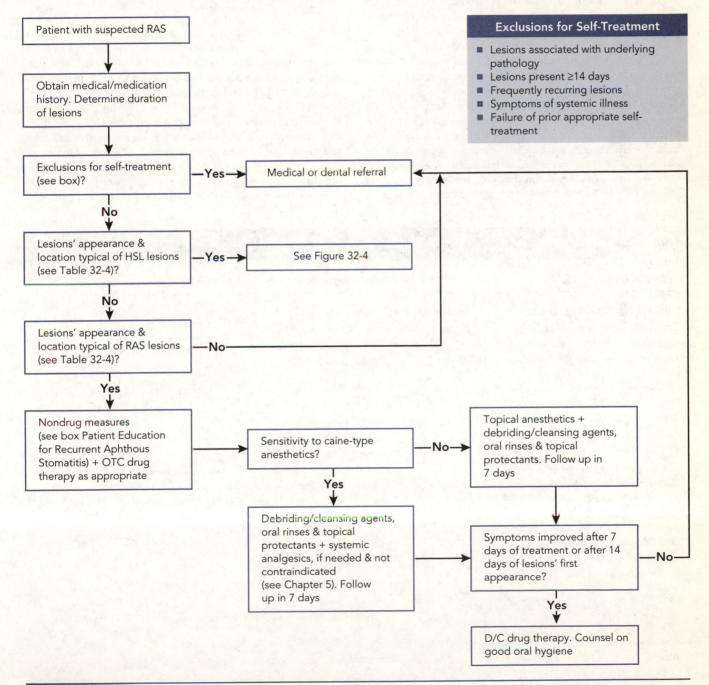

FIGURE 32-2 Self-care of recurrent aphthous stomatitis; Key: D/C, discontinue; HSL, herpes simplex labialis; OTC, over-the-counter; RAS, recurrent aphthous stomatitis.

relief of RAS, but they do not prevent its recurrence. Table 32-5 lists a variety of commercial products containing these agents.

Oral Debriding and Wound Cleansing Agents

Debriding agents/oral wound cleansers may be used to (1) aid in the removal of debris or phlegm, mucus, or other secretions associated with sore mouth; (2) cleanse minor wounds or minor gum inflammation; and (3) cleanse recurrent aphthous ulcers. Products that release nascent oxygen can be used as debriding and cleansing agents to provide temporary relief of RAS discomfort. After a thorough review process, FDA has determined that carbamide peroxide 10% to 15% in anhydrous glycerin, hydrogen peroxide 3%, and sodium bicarbonate are Category I (safe and effective) for use as nonprescription debriding agents or oral wound cleansers for oral health care.[25] FDA has determined that no ingredient is generally recognized as safe and effective for use as a nonprescription healing agent for oral wounds. Hydrogen peroxide and carbamide peroxide release oxygen immediately on contact with tissue enzymes (catalase and peroxidase), but tissue and bacterial exposure to the oxygen is very brief.[26] The foaming of the liberated oxygen has a mechanical effect, which loosens particulate matter and cleanses debris from wounds. The efficacy of oxidizing products in killing anaerobic bacteria when treating infections and periodontitis has not been established.

For direct application, a few drops of carbamide peroxide or hydrogen peroxide are applied to the affected area and allowed to remain in place for 1 minute. As a rinse, carbamide peroxide drops are placed on the tongue, mixed with saliva, and swished in the mouth for 1 minute. An aqueous solution of hydrogen peroxide 3% should be mixed with an equal amount of water before rinsing the mouth. Some products (e.g., Peroxyl Rinse) are a solution of hydrogen peroxide 1.5% and should be used without dilution. These products can be used up to four times daily (after meals) for no longer than 7 days. Prolonged rinsing with oxidizing products can lead to soft-tissue irritation, transient tooth sensitivity from decalcification of enamel, cellular changes, and overgrowth of undesirable organisms that will possibly lead to a black hairy tongue.[27,28]

Topical Oral Anesthetics

FDA has classified topical oral anesthetic/analgesic products that contain benzocaine 5% to 20%, dyclonine 0.05% to 0.1%, hexylresorcinol 0.05% to 0.1%, menthol 0.04% to 2.0%, phenol 0.5% to 1.5%, phenolate sodium 0.5% to 1.5%, benzyl alcohol 0.05% to 0.1%, and salicylic alcohol 1% to 6% as Category I (safe and effective) for temporary relief of pain associated with RAS.[29] Benzocaine is the most commonly used local anesthetic in nonprescription products. It is a known sensitizer (allergen) and should not be used by patients with a history of hypersensitivity to other common local anesthetic products. The patient should avoid using potentially inflammatory products containing counterirritants (e.g., menthol, phenol, and camphor)

TABLE 32-5 Selected Nonprescription Medications for RAS and HSL

Trade Name	Primary Ingredients
Debriding/Cleansing Agents[a]	
Gly-Oxide Oral Cleanser Liquid	Carbamide peroxide 10%
Orajel Antiseptic Mouth Sore Rinse	Hydrogen peroxide 1.5%
Peroxyl Hygienic Dental Rinse Liquid/Gel	Hydrogen peroxide 1.5%
Topical Anesthetics	
Anbesol Regular Strength Gel/Liquid	Benzocaine 10%
Zilactin-B Gel	Benzocaine 10%
Kank-A Liquid	Benzocaine 20%
Orabase Maximum Strength Paste/Gel	Benzocaine 20%
Orajel Mouth Sore Medicine Gel	Benzocaine 20%; benzalkonium chloride 0.02%; zinc chloride 0.1%
Campho-Phenique Gel/Liquid	Camphor 10.8%; phenol 4.7%
Blistex Lip Medex Ointment	Camphor 1%; menthol 1%; phenol 0.5%
Carmex Lip Balm Ointment	Menthol 0.7%; camphor 1.7%; phenol 0.4%; salicylic acid
Oral Mucosal Protectants[a]	
Canker Cover	Menthol 2.5 mg; carbomer
Orabase Soothe-N-Seal	Cyanoacrylate
Oral Rinses	
Listerine Antiseptic	Eucalyptol 0.92%; menthol 0.042%; methyl salicylate 0.060%; thymol 0.064%
Topical Treatments[b]	
Abreva	Docosanol 10%

[a] Use limited to RAS.
[b] Use limited to HSL.
Key: HSL, herpes simplex labialis; RAS, recurrent aphthous stomatitis.

in concentrations that exceed those approved as Category I (safe and effective) as anesthetic, counterirritant, or antiseptic treatments for RAS. These agents may cause tissue irritation and damage, which may prevent spontaneous healing or cause systemic toxicity, especially if overused. To reduce the incidence irritation of RAS, patients should also be advised to avoid the use of dentifrices containing sodium lauryl sulfate.[26]

Topical Oral Protectants

Oral mucosal protectants are pharmacologically inert substances that coat and protect the area. Coating the ulcer with a topical oral protectant can be effective in protecting ulcerations, decreasing friction, and affording temporary symptomatic relief.[26] The products available in this category create a barrier by using a paste, an adhering film, or a dissolvable patch to cover the lesion. Some products are available in combination with an oral anesthetic. Products available as a patch or dissolving disc must be placed against the sore for 10 to 20 seconds. Once the disc adheres to the lesion, the barrier is formed and the disc will stay in place until dissolved. These products can be applied as needed for pain relief, often three to four times daily.[30]

Oral Rinses

Rinsing the mouth with Listerine Antiseptic will hasten the healing of the lesions. Saline rinses (1–3 teaspoons of salt in 4–8 ounces of warm tap water) may soothe ulcers and can be used before topical application of a medication. Similarly, a paste of baking soda applied to the lesions for a few minutes may soothe irritation.

Systemic Analgesics

Systemic nonprescription analgesics (e.g., aspirin, nonsteroidal anti-inflammatory drugs, and acetaminophen) afford additional relief of mouth discomfort. (See Chapter 5 for discussion of these agents and their recommended dosages.) Aspirin should not be retained in the mouth before swallowing or placed in the area of the oral lesions. The acid can cause a chemical burn with subsequent tissue damage (see Color Plates, photograph 12).

Product Selection Guidelines

Patients with known hypersensitivity to common local anesthetics should not use a product containing a local anesthetic. Patients with known sensitivity to aspirin should avoid salicylic acid. Only products containing menthol, phenol, and/or camphor in the concentrations approved as Category I (safe and effective) should be used for RAS. Higher concentrations are potentially inflammatory. Various dosage forms exist (e.g. liquid, gel, rinse, dissolvable patch) for symptomatic treatment of RAS; therefore, the practitioner's recommendation should take into account the patient's preference for a particular dosage form.

Assessment of Recurrent Aphthous Stomatitis: A Case-Based Approach

Case 32-2 illustrates the assessment of patients with RAS.

Patient Counseling for Recurrent Aphthous Stomatitis

The practitioner should explain all nonpharmacologic and pharmacologic measures for treating RAS, as outlined in the box Patient Education for Recurrent Aphthous Stomatitis. The patient should be cautioned about using ineffective or harmful therapies. Possible adverse effects, contraindications, and precautions should be explained for all nonprescription agents. In addition, the practitioner must alert patients to the conditions that warrant dental or medical evaluation.

C A S E   3 2 - 2

Relevant Evaluation Criteria	Scenario/Model Outcome
Information Gathering	
1. Gather essential information about the patient's symptoms, including:	
a. description of symptom(s) (i.e., nature, onset, duration, severity, associated symptoms)	Patient is complaining of an uncomfortable sore on the inside of her mouth. She noticed the sore about 2 days ago and does not recall having anything like it before. When you ask the patient if she can show you the sore, she pulls down her lower lip to reveal one flat, gray sore surrounded by an erythematous halo of inflamed tissue in nonkeratinized, movable mucosa.
b. description of any factors that seem to precipitate, exacerbate, and/or relieve the patient's symptom(s)	The pain gets worse when she eats and drinks, and it is pretty hard to ignore throughout the day.
c. description of the patient's efforts to relieve the symptoms	She has sucked on ice chips to relieve/numb the pain with some success.
2. Gather essential patient history information:	
a. patient's identity	Jennifer Fuller
b. patient's age, sex, height, and weight	32-year-old female, 5 ft 4 in, 125 lb

CASE 32-2 (continued)

Relevant Evaluation Criteria	Scenario/Model Outcome
c. patient's occupation	She is an elementary school teacher. Talking aggravates the sore, and it is causing her to lose her patience more often with the children.
d. patient's dietary habits	Normal healthy diet with occasional junk food
e. patient's sleep habits	Gets up early and works long hours
f. concurrent medical conditions, prescription and nonprescription medications, and dietary supplements	Yaz 1 tablet by mouth every day for 28 days
g. allergies	NKA
h. history of other adverse reactions to medications	None
i. other (describe) _____	She recently quit using tobacco after smoking about 1 pack per day for 12 years. The pain from this sore is so unbearable that she is frustrated and really wants a cigarette to "relieve the stress."

Assessment and Triage

3. Differentiate the patient's signs/symptoms and correctly identify the patient's primary problem(s) (see Table 32-4).	Patient's signs and symptoms appear consistent with minor recurrent aphthous stomatitis (RAS). It is likely that the stress from her job or from recently quitting smoking (or perhaps mucosal changes after the quit attempt) have precipitated this event.
4. Identify exclusions for self-treatment (see Figure 32-2).	None
5. Formulate a comprehensive list of therapeutic alternatives for the primary problem to determine if triage to a medical practitioner is required, and share this information with the patient.	Options include: (1) Refer Jennifer to a dentist or primary care provider. (2) Recommend a nonprescription oral debriding/wound cleansing agent. (3) Recommend a nonprescription oral anesthetic. (4) Recommend a nonprescription oral protectant. (5) Recommend a nonprescription oral rinse. (6) Take no action.

Plan

6. Select an optimal therapeutic alternative to address the patient's problem, taking into account patient preferences.	The patient prefers a product that is more potent than ice chips and would be easier to use throughout her busy day.
7. Describe the recommended therapeutic approach to the patient.	Orabase Maximum Strength Gel
8. Explain to the patient the rationale for selecting the recommended therapeutic approach from the considered therapeutic alternatives.	This product contains an anesthetic (benzocaine), which should help to relieve the pain and discomfort.

Patient Education

9. When recommending self-care with nonprescription medications and/or nondrug therapy, convey accurate information to the patient:	
a. appropriate dose and frequency of administration	Apply a small amount of medicine to the painful areas up to 4 times a day.
b. maximum number of days the therapy should be employed	7 days
c. product administration procedures	Apply the medicine to the sore places with a clean finger, a cotton-tipped applicator, or a piece of gauze.
d. expected time to onset of relief	Quickly, within 5 minutes, you should begin to feel relief.
e. degree of relief that can be reasonably expected	You should feel more comfortable, although 100% relief may not be achieved.

C A S E   3 2 - 2   (continued)

Relevant Evaluation Criteria	Scenario/Model Outcome
f. most common side effects	None
g. side effects that warrant medical intervention should they occur	If rash or fever develops, contact your dentist or primary care provider.
h. patient options in the event that condition worsens or persists	A dentist or primary care provider should be consulted if the condition does not improve with 7 days of treatment or 14 days after the lesion first appeared.
i. product storage requirements	Store product in a cool, dry place.
j. specific nondrug measures	Avoid spicy and acidic foods or any substances that could irritate the ulcer. Your recent quit attempt was a healthy move; try to resist the urge to start smoking again during this stressful time. Relaxing as much as possible may help to heal the ulcer and to avoid a smoking relapse.

Key: NKA, no known allergies.

PATIENT EDUCATION FOR
Recurrent Aphthous Stomatitis

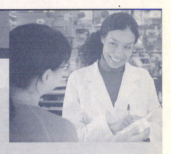

The primary objective of self-treatment for RAS is to relieve pain and irritation so the lesions can heal, and the patient can eat, drink, and perform routine oral hygiene. The secondary objective is to prevent complications, such as secondary infection. For most patients, carefully following product instructions and self-care measures will help ensure optimal therapeutic outcomes.

Nondrug Measures

- If a deficiency of iron, folate, or vitamin B_{12} is suspected as a contributing factor, increase consumption of foods high in these nutrients, or take nutritional supplements.
- Avoid spicy or acidic foods until the lesions heal.
- Avoid sharp foods that may cause increased trauma to the lesion.
- If desired, apply ice in 10-minute increments directly to the lesions.
- Do not use heat. If infection is present, heat may spread the infection.

Nonprescription Medications

- If longer-lasting relief is desired, ask your pharmacist to recommend one or more of the following types of nonprescription medications: debriding and cleansing agents, topical oral anesthetics, topical oral protectants, oral rinses, and systemic analgesics.
- Do not cauterize lesions with silver nitrate. This treatment is not effective and may stain teeth and damage healthy tissue.

Debriding and Cleansing Agents

- Use a product containing one of the following ingredients: carbamide peroxide 10%-15%, hydrogen peroxide 1.5%, or perborates. Apply after meals up to four times daily.
- Do not use these medications longer than 7 days. Chronic use can cause tissue irritation, decalcification of enamel, and black hairy tongue.
- Do not swallow these medications.

Topical Oral Anesthetics

- Ask your pharmacist to recommend a product containing one of the following medications: benzocaine 5%–20%, benzyl alcohol 0.05%–0.1%, butacaine sulfate 0.05%–0.1%, dyclonine 0.05%–0.1%, hexyl-resorcinol 0.05%–0.1%, or salicylic alcohol 1%–6%.
- Do not use benzocaine if you have a history of hypersensitivity to other benzocaine-containing products.
- Avoid using potentially inflammatory products containing menthol, phenol, or camphor in concentrations that exceed those approved as Category I (safe and effective). These agents may cause tissue irritation and damage or systemic toxicity.

Topical Oral Protectants

- Use topical oral protectants or denture adhesives to coat and protect the lesions. These agents will also provide temporary relief of discomfort.
- Apply these products as needed.

Oral Rinses

- Rinse the mouth with Listerine Antiseptic to hasten healing of the lesions.
- Rinse the mouth with a saline solution to soothe discomfort or to prepare the lesion for application of a topical medication. For saline solution, add 1–3 teaspoons of salt to 4–8 ounces of warm tap water.

Systemic Analgesics

- If desired, take an oral analgesic (e.g., aspirin, ibuprofen, or acetaminophen) for additional relief of mouth discomfort.
- Do not hold aspirin in the mouth or place it on oral lesions. The acid can cause a chemical burn with tissue damage.

⚠️ See a primary care provider if any of the following occur:
- —Symptoms do not improve after 7 days of treatment with debriding/wound cleansing agents.
- —The lesions do not heal in 14 days.
- —Symptoms worsen during self-treatment.
- —Symptoms of systemic infection such as fever, rash, or swelling develop.

Evaluation of Patient Outcomes for Recurrent Aphthous Stomatitis

RAS lesions are typically self-limiting and resolve within 14 days. Oral debriding and wound cleansing agents are labeled for use for up to 7 days. If the symptoms have improved, the patient should discontinue treatment but continue other dental hygienic measures. Symptoms that are unimproved or that have worsened during treatment require medical evaluation.

MINOR ORAL MUCOSAL INJURY OR IRRITATION

Pathophysiology of Minor Oral Mucosal Injury or Irritation

Minor wounds or inflammation resulting from minor dental procedures, accidental injury (e.g., biting of the cheek or abrasion from sharp, crisp foods), or other irritations of the mouth, gums, or palate may be treated with various nonprescription medications.

Treatment of Minor Oral Mucosal Injury or Irritation

Treatment of mouth injury (traumatic laceration or ulcer) and irritation is similar to that for RAS. Mouth injury and irritation differ from RAS, however, with regard to etiology and certain treatment considerations.

Treatment Goals

The goals of treating minor mucosal injury and irritation are to (1) control discomfort and pain, (2) aid healing with the appropriate use of nonpharmacologic and pharmacologic measures, and (3) prevent secondary bacterial infection.

General Treatment Approach

Treatment should focus first on relieving discomfort. Application of ice can relieve discomfort. Local anesthetics, oral analgesics, and saline rinses are safe and effective choices. Once the discomfort has resolved, patients should focus on healing the affected area. Homemade sodium bicarbonate rinses and oral debriding/wound cleansing agents can help achieve this objective. Finally, concomitant use of oral protectants can relieve discomfort and aid healing by protecting the area from further irritation. Figure 32-3 outlines this approach and lists exclusions for self-care.

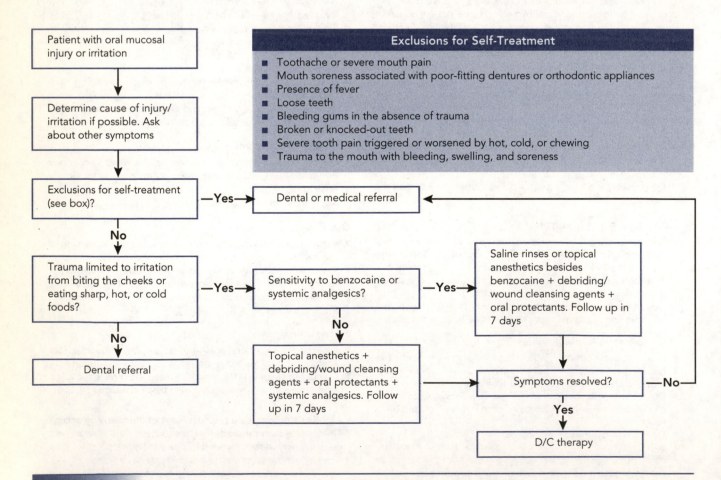

FIGURE 32-3   Self-care of minor oral mucosal injury or irritation. Key: D/C, discontinue.

Nonpharmacologic Therapy

When tissues of the lips, cheeks, or palate are bruised, direct application of ice may reduce the swelling. Ice should be applied in 10-minute increments. Longer application times may cause local tissue damage. Sodium bicarbonate solutions (household baking soda one-half to 1 teaspoon in 4 ounces of water) can act as an oral debriding agent/wound cleanser. The solution is swished in the mouth over the affected area for at least 1 minute and then expectorated. Sodium bicarbonate's mucolytic action is related to its alkalinity. Saline rinses (1–3 teaspoons of salt in 4–8 ounces of warm tap water) can cleanse and soothe the affected area.

Pharmacologic Therapy

As with RAS, topical analgesics/anesthetics, oral protectants, and oral debriding/wound cleansing agents are the mainstay of pharmacologic therapy. The Pharmacologic Therapy section for RAS discusses these agents in further detail.

In addition, astringents may be used. Astringents cause tissues to contract or arrest secretions by causing proteins to coagulate on a cell surface. Dentists may suggest that their patients use oxidizing mouth rinses or topically applied steroids (which are available only by prescription) as an adjunctive treatment of specific conditions or a postoperative aid to cleaning the affected area, relieving discomfort, and assisting the healing process. FDA review of oral antiseptic products found insufficient data to support efficacy for oral antiseptic use (i.e., to decrease the chance of infection in minor oral irritation).[25] Patients who

dislike complicated regimens may want to use a combination preparation (Table 32-5). These preparations may contain (1) a single anesthetic/analgesic combined with a single astringent, an oral mucosal protectant, or a denture adhesive or (2) benzocaine combined with menthol or phenol.

Assessment of Minor Oral Mucosal Injury or Irritation: A Case-Based Approach

The cause and nature of the injury or irritation are the primary considerations in patient assessment. If the disorder is self-treatable, the practitioner should determine whether the patient has had previous episodes, how they were treated, and whether the patient has known contraindications to the nonprescription medications used to treat these disorders.

Patient Counseling for Minor Oral Mucosal Injury or Irritation

Once the problem is determined to be minor irritation or injury of the mouth, the practitioner should explain (1) the steps in the treatment regimen, (2) the purpose of each agent, and (3) the length of time the products can be used safely. Signs and symptoms that indicate infection should also be explained. (See the box Patient Education for Minor Oral Mucosal Injury or Irritation.)

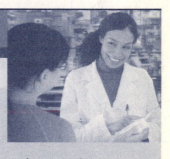

PATIENT EDUCATION FOR
Minor Oral Mucosal Injury or Irritation

The objectives of self-treatment for minor oral mucosal injury or irritation are to (1) control discomfort and pain, (2) aid healing with the appropriate use of drug and nondrug measures, and (3) prevent secondary bacterial infection. For most patients, carefully following product instructions and the self-care measures listed here will help ensure optimal therapeutic outcomes.

Nondrug Measures

- Rinse with a sodium bicarbonate solution to remove injured tissue and cleanse the affected area. Add one-half to 1 teaspoon of sodium bicarbonate to 4 ounces of water. Swish the solution in the mouth over the affected area for 1 minute; then spit out the solution.
- Use saline rinses to cleanse and soothe the affected area. Add 1–3 teaspoons of salt to 4–8 ounces of warm tap water.
- For bruised lips or cheeks, apply ice in 10-minute increments to reduce swelling. Do not apply ice longer than 20 minutes in a given hour.

Nonprescription Medications

- If longer-lasting relief is desired, ask your pharmacist to recommend one or more of the following types of nonprescription medications: debriding and cleansing agents, topical oral anesthetics, topical oral protectants, and systemic analgesics.

Debriding and Cleansing Agents

- Use a product containing one of the following ingredients: carbamide peroxide 10%-15%, hydrogen peroxide 1.5%, or perborates. Apply after meals up to four times daily.
- Do not use these medications longer than 7 days. Chronic use can cause tissue irritation, decalcification of enamel, and black hairy tongue.
- Do not swallow these medications.

Topical Oral Anesthetics

- Ask your pharmacist to recommend a product containing one of the following medications: benzocaine 5%–20%, benzyl alcohol 0.05%–0.1%, butacaine sulfate 0.05%–0.1%, dyclonine 0.05%–0.1%, hexylresorcinol 0.05%–0.1%, or salicylic alcohol 1%–6%.
- Do not use benzocaine if you have a history of hypersensitivity to other benzocaine-containing products.
- Avoid potentially inflammatory products containing substantial amounts of menthol, phenol, or camphor. These agents may cause tissue irritation and damage or systemic toxicity.

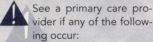

PATIENT EDUCATION FOR
Minor Oral Mucosal Injury or Irritation
(continued)

Topical Oral Protectants

- Use topical oral protectants or denture adhesives to coat and protect the lesions.
- Apply these products as needed.

Systemic Analgesics

- If desired, take an oral analgesic (e.g., aspirin, ibuprofen, acetaminophen) for additional relief of mouth discomfort.
- Do not hold aspirin in the mouth or place it on oral lesions. The acid can cause a chemical burn and tissue damage.

⚠ See a primary care provider if any of the following occur:
—Symptoms persist after 7 days of treatment.
—Symptoms worsen during self-treatment.
—Symptoms of systemic infection such as fever, redness, or swelling develop.

Evaluation of Patient Outcomes for Minor Oral Mucosal Injury or Irritation

Minor injury or irritation should resolve within 7 days of treatment and within 10 days of the initial insult or injury. If the symptoms are resolved, no further treatment is necessary. If symptoms persist or worsen, or swelling, rash, or fever develops, the patient should be evaluated by a medical provider.

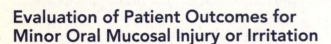

HERPES SIMPLEX LABIALIS

Herpes simplex labialis (HSL), also known as cold sores or fever blisters, is a disorder caused by a virus of the family Herpesviridae. Herpes simplex virus 1 (HSV-1) is primarily associated with oral and labial lesions, whereas herpes simplex virus 2 (HSV-2) is usually involved in producing genital sores. However, preference of a specific HSV type for an anatomic site is changing, in part owing to varying sexual practices.[31] Any of the human herpes viruses (cytomegalovirus, Epstein–Barr virus, and others), not just HSV-1 and 2, can cause oral lesions. Anyone who comes in contact with the herpes virus can potentially become infected. Most often, exposure to HSV occurs in childhood and adolescence, and 99% of exposed individuals have subclinical cases on primary exposures; only 1% of exposed patients present with primary manifestations of the infection.[31] By the age of 40 years, 84% of the population has positive antibodies for HSV-1.[31] Approximately 30%–40% of persons exposed to HSV will develop recurrent infections (reactivation of HSV infection, not reinfection).[31]

Pathophysiology of Herpes Simplex Labialis

HSV is contagious and is believed to be transmitted by direct contact. Fluid from herpes vesicles contains live virus and may serve to transmit the virus from patient to patient. Because the virus remains viable on surfaces for several hours, contaminated objects may also be a source of infection. HSL enters the host through a break in the skin or intact mucous membranes. Once the virus has infected a host, it remains in a latent state in the trigeminal ganglia. The virus can be reactivated upon exposure to a trigger such as ultraviolet radiation, stress, fatigue, cold, and windburn. Other possible triggers include fever, injury, menstruation, dental work, infectious diseases, and factors that depress the immune system (e.g., chemotherapy or radiation therapy).[31,32] Although the virus can go through periods of dormancy and reactivation, the person is infected for life. Upon reactivation, the lesions often arise repeatedly in the same location.

Clinical Presentation of Herpes Simplex Labialis

HSL is so named because it commonly occurs on the lip or on areas bordering the lips; the usual site is at the junction of mucous membrane and skin of the lips or nose. However, these lesions may also occur intraorally (primarily involving keratinized mucosa such as hard palate or gingiva). The lesions are recurrent, painful, and cosmetically objectionable; these symptoms often prompt patients to seek the advice of a practitioner. HSL lesions are often preceded by a prodrome in which the patient notices burning, itching, tingling, or numbness in the area of the forthcoming lesion. Other symptoms include pain, fever, bleeding, swollen lymph nodes, and malaise.[32] The lesion first becomes visible as small, red papules of fluid-containing vesicles 1 to 3 mm in diameter. Often, many lesions coalesce to form a larger area of involvement. An erythematous, inflamed border around the fluid-filled vesicles may be present. A mature lesion often has a crust over the top of many coalesced, burst vesicles; its base is erythematous (see Color Plates, photograph 13). Pustules or pus present under the crust of a herpes virus lesion may indicate a secondary bacterial infection; prompt evaluation and treatment with an appropriate antibiotic, if indicated, are appropriate. Table 32–4 further describes the clinical presentation of HSL and compares its features with that of RAS.

Patients may relate a history of primary herpetic stomatitis (viral-induced inflammation of the mouth), which usually manifests itself as vesicles (blisters) in the mouth. However, most primary oral infections of herpes virus seem to be subclinical, and most patients are unaware of their previous primary exposure. The recurrence rate and extent of lesions vary greatly among patients. Some patients may experience several large lesions every few weeks; other patients may have only a single small lesion at infrequent intervals.

A related disease, acute (primary) herpetic gingivostomatitis, is seen mainly in children but can occur in adults, especially those who are immunocompromised. Although the oral lesions of this disease can develop anywhere on the oral mucosal surface, they commonly occur on the lips, areas bordering the lips, or the gums. Herpetic gingivostomatitis is distinguished from RAS gingivostomatitis by infected gums that are very red and covered by a pseudomembrane or are studded with ulcerations.

The appearance of HSL and RAS should easily be distinguished from oral candidiasis, which develops as part of yeast infections. In the mouth, candidiasis is often referred to as thrush, and is characterized by white plaques with a milk curd appearance. Such plaques, which are attached to the oral mucosa, can usually be detached easily, displaying erythematous, bleeding, sore areas beneath (see Color Plates, photograph 10).

Treatment of Herpes Simplex Labialis

Although the etiologies of HSL and RAS differ, global treatment of these disorders is similar. The patient should be instructed to avoid circumstances that induce more lesions (e.g., stress), keep the lesions free of counterirritants, and keep existing lesions as clean as possible, thereby avoiding secondary infections. Table 32-5 lists common classes of nonprescription medications used to treat RAS and HSL. (*Note:* Of the products listed in Table 32-5, debriding/cleansing agents and oral mucosal protectants are not used to treat HSL.)

Treatment Goals

The goals of treating HSL are to (1) relieve the discomfort of the lesions, (2) prevent secondary bacterial infection, and (3) prevent autoinoculation or spread of the virus to others.

General Treatment Approach

The lesion(s) should be inspected to determine whether their appearance and location are characteristic of HSL. The practitioner should try to identify what factors may have led to development of the lesion. If possible, precipitating or contributing factors should be removed. For example, if trauma is suspected, perhaps a gentler toothbrush and gentler brushing technique could be suggested. It is also helpful to determine whether the patient has a history of HSL. The practitioner should obtain the patient's medical history to determine whether an underlying pathology predisposes the patient to recurrent HSL or could complicate treatment. The practitioner should ask about previous self-treatments and their effectiveness; if treatments used are appropriate and have been successful for the patient, then they should be continued. Treatment should focus on cleansing the affected area, protecting the lesions from infection, and relieving the discomfort of burning, itching, and pain. Figure 32-4 outlines the self-treatment of HSL and lists exclusions for self-care.

Nonpharmacologic Therapy

Lesions should be kept clean by gently washing with mild soap solutions. Handwashing is important in preventing lesion contamination and minimizing autoinoculation of herpes virus. The lesion should be kept moist to prevent drying and fissuring. Cracking of the lesions may render them more susceptible to secondary bacterial infection, may delay healing, and usually increases discomfort. Factors that delay healing (e.g., stress, local trauma, wind, excessive sun exposure, and fatigue) should be avoided. Patients who identify sun exposure as a precipitating event should be advised to routinely use a lip and face sunscreen product (with a minimum sun protection factor [SPF] of 15).

Pharmacologic Therapy

Topically applied skin protectants are effective nonprescription medications for relieving the discomfort of HSL, but not for reducing the duration of symptoms.[33] Topical skin protectants help to protect the lesions from infection, relieve dryness, and keep the lesions soft.

Externally applied analgesics/anesthetics, in bland, emollient vehicles, also relieve the discomfort of burning, itching, and pain, but they do not reduce the duration of symptoms. Ingredients that are generally recognized as safe and effective include benzocaine 5% to 20%, dibucaine 0.25% to 1%, dyclonine hydrochloride 0.5% to 1%, benzyl alcohol 10% to 33%, camphor 0.1% to 3%, and menthol 0.1% to 1%.[34] Higher concentrations of certain ingredients (i.e., camphor > 3% and menthol > 1%) that stimulate cutaneous sensory receptors and produce a counterirritant effect are contraindicated.[35]

Docosanol 10% (Abreva) is the only FDA-approved nonprescription product proven to reduce the duration and severity of symptoms. The agent inhibits direct fusion between the herpes virus and the human cell plasma membrane, thereby preventing viral replication.[36] Docosanol should be applied at the first sign of an outbreak (prodromal stage), five times a day until the lesion is healed. Treatment with docosanol reduces the median time to healing by approximately 1 day (18 hours) compared with placebo.[37] Docosanol-treated patients also note a significant reduction in the duration of symptoms, including pain and/or burning, itching, or tingling, compared with placebo (20% reduction in the median time to complete cessation of these symptoms).[37]

If evidence of secondary bacterial infection (e.g., failure of crusting to occur or persistence of erythematous border) is seen, topical application of a thin layer of triple-antibiotic ointment three to four times daily is recommended. (See Chapter 42 for more information about these agents.) Systemic nonprescription analgesics may provide additional pain relief.

Studies suggest that patients suffering from sideropenia, a condition resulting from a deficiency of iron in the body, who have recurrent HSL may experience fewer episodes following treatment with iron replacement therapy.[38]

HSL is not considered to be a steroid-responsive dermatosis; therefore, the use of topical steroids is contraindicated. Products that are highly astringent should be avoided. Tannic acid and zinc sulfate are Category II agents for topical management of HSL, because their frequent application to the lip and oral cavity could cause oral mucosal absorption and toxicity.[35]

Complementary Therapies

The essential oil of *Melaleuca alternifolia,* or tea tree oil, has activity against HSV in vitro. Studies have shown healing time with tea tree oil is reduced versus placebo and similar to topical acyclovir 5%.[39,40] Lysine has preventive effects and has been shown to decrease the frequency of outbreaks when taken daily.[41] LongoVital is a dietary supplement that includes vitamins A, B_1, B_2, B_3, B_5, B_6, C, D, and E, as well as paprika, rosemary, peppermint, hawthorn, pumpkin seeds, and yarrow flowers. After 2 months of therapy, LongoVital decreased the number, duration, and size of lesions. In addition, patients perceived the number and duration of recurrences to be decreased after the trial.[42] Extracts of the leaves of *Melissa officinalis,* or lemon balm, have also been used in patients with HSL. Studies comparing lemon balm with placebo have shown a reduction in symptoms, shortened healing time, prevention of infection spread, and patient preference for lemon balm.[43]

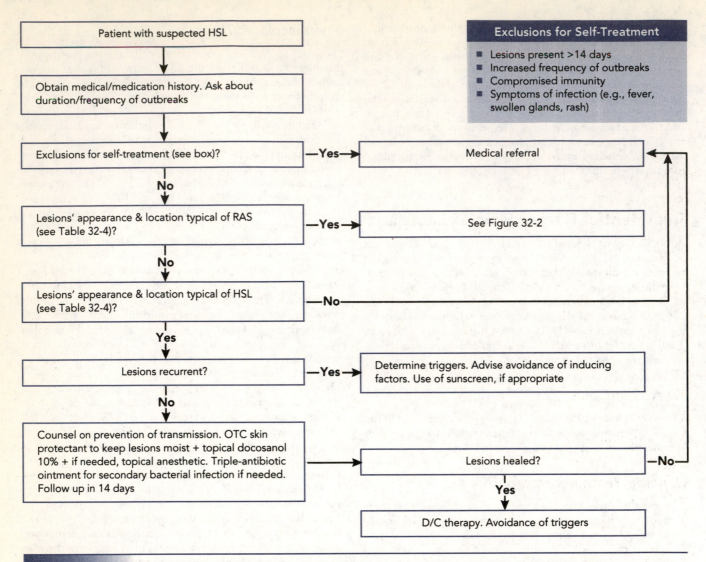

FIGURE 32-4 Self-care of herpes simplex labialis. Key: D/C, discontinue; HSL, herpes simplex labialis; OTC, over-the-counter; RAS, recurrent aphthous stomatitis.

Assessment of Herpes Simplex Labialis: A Case-Based Approach

Although many of the same nonprescription medications are indicated for RAS and HSL, the practitioner still needs to differentiate the disorders. Because herpes simplex lesions are contagious, additional measures are necessary to prevent transmission of the virus. The practitioner should obtain the patient's medical history to determine whether an underlying pathology predisposes the patient to recurrent HSL or could complicate treatment.

Patient Counseling for Herpes Simplex Labialis

The practitioner should stress that HSL lesions are contagious and should explain to the patient appropriate measures to prevent

transmission of the virus, as outlined in the box Patient Education for Herpes Simplex Labialis. Patients should be advised that the disorder is self-limiting, and that pharmacologic therapy can keep the lesions moist and supple, decrease the itch and pain, protect the lesions from secondary bacterial infection, and help reduce the duration of active infection. The practitioner should explain the action of each recommended product, its proper use, and possible adverse effects.

Evaluation of Patient Outcomes for Herpes Simplex Labialis

HSL typically resolves within 10 to 14 days. If the symptoms have resolved, no further treatment is necessary. However, if the condition worsens (pain and itching persist, redness increases, or signs of secondary infection are apparent), the patient should be referred to a medical provider for evaluation.

PATIENT EDUCATION FOR
Herpes Simplex Labialis

The objectives of self-treatment for herpes simplex labialis (cold sores) are to (1) relieve pain and irritation while the sores are healing, (2) prevent secondary infection, and (3) prevent spread of the lesions. For most patients, carefully following product instructions and the self-care measures listed here will help ensure optimal therapeutic outcomes.

Nondrug Measures

- Keep labial or extraoral lesions clean by gently washing them with mild soap solutions.
- Wash hands frequently to prevent contaminating the lesions and to avoid spreading the virus.
- Avoid factors believed to delay healing such as stress, injury to the lesions, wind, excessive sun exposure, and fatigue.
- If outbreaks are related to sun exposure, use a lip and face sunscreen routinely.

Nonprescription Medications

- Use skin protectants such as allantoin, petrolatum, and cocoa butter to keep lesions moist and to prevent cracking of the lesions. (See Chapter 41 for discussion of these agents.) These measures help prevent secondary bacterial infection.
- Use topical anesthetics such as benzocaine or dibucaine to relieve burning, itching, and pain. Do not use benzocaine if you have a history of hypersensitivity to other benzocaine-containing products.

- If using products containing camphor and menthol, make sure the concentration of camphor does not exceed 3% and the concentration of menthol does not exceed 1%.
- Do not apply hydrocortisone to the lesions.
- If evidence of secondary bacterial infection is seen, apply a thin layer of triple-antibiotic ointment three to four times daily.
- Apply topical agent docosanol 10% (Abreva) to limit the burning, tingling, and itching sensations. Docosanol 10% can also speed up the healing process, thus reducing the duration of the symptoms.
- If desired, take oral nonprescription analgesics (e.g., aspirin, ibuprofen, acetaminophen) for additional pain relief.
- Do not hold aspirin in the mouth or place it on oral lesions. The acid can cause a chemical burn and tissue damage.

⚠ See a primary care provider if any of the following occurs:
  —The lesions do not heal in 14 days.
  —The self-treatment measures do not relieve discomfort.
  —Symptoms of systemic illness such as fever, malaise, rash, or swollen lymph glands occur.

XEROSTOMIA

Xerostomia, commonly referred to as dry mouth, is a disorder in which salivary flow is limited or completely arrested. A person with normal salivary flow reportedly produces up to 1.5 liters of saliva every 24 hours.[44] About 20% of older adult patients are affected with xerostomia.

Pathophysiology of Xerostomia

Patients with certain disease states, including Sjögren's syndrome (an autoimmune condition in which the salivary glands become partly or completely dysfunctional and patients typically present with dry mouth and/or dry eyes), diabetes mellitus, depression, and Crohn's disease, are prone to xerostomia. Estimates of the total number of U.S. cases of Sjögren's syndrome range from 1 to 4 million.[45] Radiation therapy of the head and neck can cause atrophy of the salivary glands. Following treatment, the vast majority of patients have compromised salivary function for the rest of their lives. Medications with anticholinergic activity or that cause depletion of salivary flow volume (e.g., antihistamines, decongestants, antihypertensives, diuretics, antidepressants, antipsychotics, sedatives) can cause xerostomia.[46,47] Older patients who are more likely to be taking multiple medications for chronic diseases may be more greatly affected.[47] However, if xerostomia is drug-induced and the medication can be discontinued, the condition may be reversed in some cases.[48] Nonpharmacologic causes of xerostomia include use of alcohol, tobacco, or caffeine; salivary gland stones (sialolithiasis); and mouth-breathing.

Clinical Presentation of Xerostomia

Xerostomia can result in difficulty talking and swallowing, stomatitis, burning tongue, and halitosis. Unmoistened food cannot be tasted; therefore, xerostomia can cause loss of appetite and eventual decline in nutritional status. Patients' teeth can become hypersensitive, which can be related to a decrease in salivary flow and the lack of buffering capacity that saliva provides.[49] Xerostomia can also result in a higher-than-normal incidence of cervical caries (decay around the root surfaces of teeth) despite excellent oral hygiene.[50] Depending on the status of a patient's dentition, this disorder also can increase the incidence of caries, gingivitis, and more severe periodontal disease, or reduce denture-wearing time. Furthermore, reduced flow of saliva can disturb the balance of microflora in the oral cavity and predispose it to candidiasis. The absence of lubrication and buffering can lead to tooth erosion, decalcification, and decay.[51]

Treatment of Xerostomia

Dry mouth should never be discounted as inconsequential. Failure to treat it can result in serious complications for some patients.

Treatment Goals

The goals in treating dry mouth are to (1) relieve discomfort, (2) prevent and treat oral infections and periodontal disease, and (3) reduce the risk of dental caries by either replacing lost saliva with exogenous sources, or stimulating the remaining functional gland tissue to produce saliva.[52]

General Treatment Approach

The patient should discontinue using substances that dry the mouth or erode tooth enamel. If possible, medications that are known to cause xerostomia should be discontinued. To reduce the risk of caries, the patient must maintain good oral hygiene, and use sugarless sweets and chewing gums to stimulate residual salivary flow.[52] Commercial artificial saliva products can be used as needed to relieve soft-tissue discomfort. Figure 32-5 outlines the self-treatment of xerostomia and lists exclusions for self-care.

Nonpharmacologic Therapy

The patient should avoid substances that reduce salivation, including tobacco (smoked and smokeless) and products that contain alcohol (including mouth rinses). Modification of medication schedules, in consultation with the treating medical provider, to coincide with periods of natural stimulation should be considered. For example, patients could take medications that cause dry mouth 1 hour prior to meals, because eating naturally stimulates an increase in salivary flow. Consequently, the duration of dry mouth would be reduced.

To prevent tooth decay, the xerostomic patient should limit intake of sugary and acidic foods that may have been tolerated before, but now pose significant danger to the patient's oral health. The sugar promotes bacterial growth, whereas the acid creates caries and increases tooth erosion. Similarly, the patient should avoid sucking on hard candy or lozenges sweetened with sugar because of their cariogenic potential. Chewing gum sweetened with sugar alcohols (e.g., xylitol), however, may be beneficial. Chewing gum increases salivary flow, and xylitol has not been shown to be cariogenic.[27] Increasing water intake, especially if it is fluoridated, would also be of benefit. Finally, the use of very soft toothbrushes will help prevent decay by minimizing tissue abrasion.

Pharmacologic Therapy (Artificial Saliva Products)

Artificial saliva products are the primary agents for relieving the discomfort of dry mouth. They are designed to mimic natural saliva both chemically and physically. However, they do not contain the many naturally occurring protective components that are present in innate saliva. Because they do not stimulate natural salivary gland production, however, they must be considered replacement therapy, not a cure for xerostomia. Closely resembling natural saliva, artificial saliva is formulated with the following properties:

- *Viscosity:* Carboxymethylcellulose and glycerin are used to mimic natural saliva viscosity.
- *Mineral content:* All products contain calcium and phosphate ions, and some also contain fluoride. With normal use, no product has demonstrated the ability to remineralize enamel. Therefore, the ADA does not recognize any such claims made by the manufacturers.
- *Palatability:* Flavorings (e.g., mint and lemon) and sweeteners (e.g., sorbitol and xylitol) are commonly used.

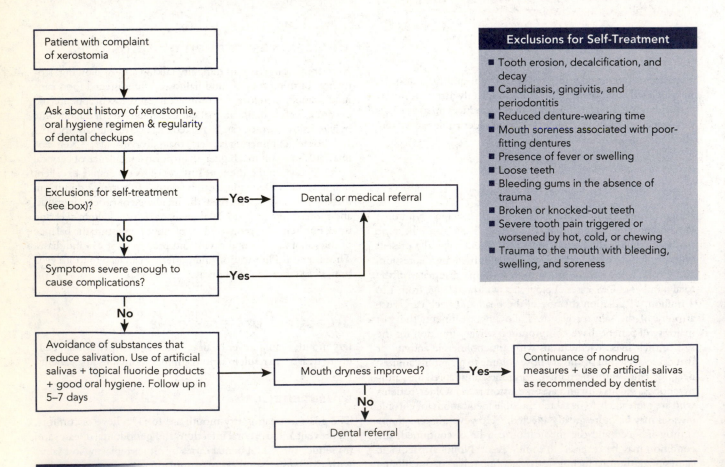

FIGURE 32-5 Self-care of xerostomia.

Artificial salivas are of value and can be used on an as-needed basis in patients with little or no saliva flow. Table 32-6 lists selected nonprescription saliva substitutes.

Product Selection Guidelines

The majority of artificial saliva products are available as a spray. Oral Balance is also available as a gel; its proper use involves placing approximately a half-inch length of gel onto the tongue and spreading thoroughly in the mouth. These products can be used at any time; a minimum suggested use is after meals and before going to bed. Salivart does not contain preservatives because it is packaged as a sterile aerosol. Other products containing preservatives, such as methyl- or propylparaben, may cause hypersensitivity reactions in certain patients. Patients on low-sodium diets should avoid artificial salivas that contain sodium.

Assessment of Xerostomia: A Case-Based Approach

The practitioner should inquire about the patient's history of xerostomia, oral hygiene practices, and regularity of dental visits. The practitioner should then evaluate the patient's symptoms to determine whether the symptoms have progressed to the point that complications are likely. A review of the patient's medical and medication history can identify medical conditions and/ or medications known to reduce salivation. Furthermore, the practitioner should determine whether lifestyle or other practices could be contributing to the condition. The patient should be questioned as to whether he or she has concurrent dry eyes or joint symptoms to assess any risk for Sjögren's syndrome. Similarly, the patient should be questioned as to whether any salivary gland pain or swelling occurs with meals to assess the risk for salivary gland stones.

TABLE 32-6 Selected Nonprescription Saliva Substitutes	
Trade Name	**Primary Ingredients**
Biotene Oral Balance Dry Mouth Relief Moisturizing Gel/Spray	Hydroxyethylcellulose; hydrogenated starch; glyceryli polymethacrylate; potassium thiocyanate; glucose oxidase; lactoperoxidase; lysozyme; lactoferrin; aloe vera; xylitol
Salivart Synthetic Saliva Spray	Sodium carboxymethylcellulose; dibasic potassium phosphate; calcium; magnesium and potassium chlorides; sorbitol
Entertainer's Secret Spray	Sodium carboxymethylcellulose; dibasic sodium phosphate; potassium chloride; parabens; aloe vera gel; glycerin

Patient Counseling for Xerostomia

It is generally necessary for xerostomic patients to have professional dental management of their condition as well as the self-care methods discussed above and outlined in the box Patient Education for Xerostomia. Patients should be encouraged to practice good oral hygiene measures and to see their dentist regularly. In addition, the practitioner should advise patients about what they need to know regarding which nonpharmacologic and pharmacologic measures will keep the oral cavity moist, and can be used to treat dry mouth to minimize the increased risk for tooth decay associated with xerostomia. Finally, the practitioner must alert patients to signs and symptoms that indicate complications from dry mouth.

PATIENT EDUCATION FOR Xerostomia

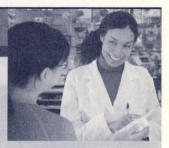

The objectives of self-treatment for xerostomia (dry mouth) are to (1) relieve the discomfort of dry mouth, (2) reduce the risk of dental decay, and (3) prevent and treat infections and periodontal disease. For most patients, carefully following product instructions and the self-care measures listed here will help ensure optimal therapeutic outcomes.

Nondrug Measures
- To prevent reduced levels of saliva, avoid use of cigarettes and smokeless tobacco.
- Do not use products that contain alcohol (including mouth rinses) or medications that cause depletion of salivary flow.
- Avoid food or drinks that contain caffeine.
- To prevent tooth decay, limit consumption of sugary and acidic foods. Do not suck on hard candy or lozenges sweetened with sugar.
- If desired, chew gum sweetened with sugar alcohols such as xylitol to help increase flow of saliva.
- If possible, take medications 1 hour before meals so that the natural saliva flow caused by food can counteract any mouth dryness.

- To help prevent tooth decay, use a very soft toothbrush to reduce abrasion of the teeth.

Nonprescription Medications
- Use artificial saliva products that contain fluoride to relieve the discomfort of dry mouth and prevent tooth decay.
- If you are on a low-sodium diet, avoid artificial salivas that contain sodium.
- Brush and floss your teeth at least twice daily using a regular toothpaste with fluoride, and see your dentist regularly.

⚠️ If your symptoms do not improve or if they worsen, see a dentist.

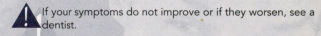

Evaluation of Patient Outcomes for Xerostomia

The patient with xerostomia should return for evaluation after 5 to 7 days of self-treatment. If the mouth dryness is improved, the patient should continue using artificial saliva and fluoride products as recommended by a medical provider. The patient should also be advised to continue the nonpharmacologic measures. If the dryness becomes worse or symptoms of complications develop, the patient should return to a dental/medical provider for further evaluation.

KEY POINTS FOR ORAL PAIN AND DISCOMFORT

➤ Tooth hypersensitivity and teething are nonserious and self-treatable problems.

➤ Self-treatment of toothache should be limited to the temporary relief of pain, because professional treatment is required for complete resolution of pain.

➤ RAS is amenable to self-treatment for the relief of pain and irritation so the lesions can heal, thereby allowing the patient the ability to eat, drink, and perform routine oral hygiene while preventing further complications.

➤ Minor oral mucosal injury or irritation may be self-treated by controlling discomfort and pain, by using drug and non-drug measures appropriately to aid healing, and by preventing secondary bacterial infection.

➤ The goals of self-treatment for HSL (cold sores) are to relieve pain and irritation while the sores are healing, prevent secondary infection, and prevent spread of the lesions to other areas of the body and other individuals.

➤ Self-treatment of xerostomia (dry mouth) can relieve discomfort from dry mouth, thereby reducing the risk of dental decay as well as preventing and, at times, treating infections.

➤ It is critical for practitioners to recognize and understand that, in the event conditions worsen or persist after self-treatment and nonprescription measures, it is imperative to strongly advise the individual to seek professional assistance form a dentist or primary care provider.

REFERENCES

1. US Department of Health and Human Services Centers for Disease Control and Prevention. Oral Health: Preventing Cavities, Gum Disease, and Tooth Loss 2008. Available at: http://www.cdc.gov/nccdphp/publications/aag/pdf/doh.pdf. Last accessed September 25, 2008.
2. US Department of Health and Human Services. *Healthy People 2010*. Vol 2. 2nd ed. Washington, DC: US Government Printing Office; November 2000. Available at: http://www.healthypeople.gov/Document/HTML/Volume2/21oral.htm. Last accessed September 25, 2008.
3. Riley JL III, Gilbert GH, Heft MW. Race/ethnic differences in health care use for orofacial pain among older adults. *Pain*. 2002; 100:119–30.
4. Canadian Advisory Board on Dentin Hypersensitivity. Consensus-based recommendations for the diagnosis and management of dentin hypersensitivity. *J Can Dent Assoc*. 2003;69:221–6.
5. Walters PA. Dentinal hypersensitivity: a review. *J Contemp Dent Pract*. 2005;6:107–17.
6. Orchardson R, Gillam DG. Managing dentin hypersensitivity. *J Am Dent Assoc*. 2006;137:990–8.
7. Linnett V, Seow WK. Dental erosion in children: a literature review. *Pediatr Dent*. 2001;23:37–43.
8. Woodmansey KF. Recognition of bulimia nervosa in dental patients: implications for dental care providers. *Gen Dent*. 2000; 48:48–52.
9. Leavitt AH, King GJ, Ramsay DS, et al. A longitudinal evaluation of pulpal pain during orthodontic tooth movement. *Orthod Craniofacial Res*. 2002;5:29–37.
10. Simon J. Biomechanically-induced dental disease. *Gen Dent*. 2000;48: 598–605.
11. Jorgensen MG, Carroll WB. Incidence of tooth sensitivity after home whitening treatment. *J Am Dent Assoc*. 2002;133:1076–82.
12. Hasson H, Ismail AI, Neiva G. Home-based chemically-induced whitening of teeth in adults. *Cochrane Database Syst Rev*. 2006;4: CD006202.
13. American Dental Association. *ADA Statement on the Safety and Effectiveness of Tooth Whitening Products*. Chicago: American Dental Association; 2008.
14. Pau AKH, Croucher R, Marcenes W. Perceived inability to cope and care seeking in patients with toothache: a qualitative study. *Br Dent J*. 2000: 189:500–2.
15. *Fed Regist*. 1991;56:48308–10, 48315–6, 48325, 48335–46.
16. Sowinski JA, Bonta Y, Battista GW, et al. Desensitizing efficacy of Colgate Sensitive Maximum Strength and Fresh Mint Sensodyne dentifrices. *Am J Dent*. 2000;13:116–20.
17. Schiff T, Bonta Y, Proskin HM, et al. Desensitizing efficacy of a new dentifrice containing 5.0% potassium nitrate and 0.454% stannous fluoride. *Am J Dent*. 2000;13:111–5.
18. Sowinski J, Ayad F, Petrone M, et al. Comparative investigations of the desensitizing efficacy of a new dentifrice. *J Clin Periodontol*. 2001;28: 1032–6.
19. Hodosh M. Potentiating potassium nitrate's desensitization with dimethyl isosorbide. *Gen Dent*. 2001;49:531–6.
20. Barrons RW. Treatment strategies for recurrent aphthous ulcers. *Am J Health Syst Pharm*. 2001;58:41–53.
21. Porter SR, Hegarty A, Kaliakatsou F, et al. Recurrent aphthous stomatitis. *Clin Dermatol*. 2000;18:569–78.
22. Shashy RG, Ridley MB. Aphthous ulcers: a difficult clinical entity. *Am J Otolaryngol*. 2000;21:389–93.
23. Scully C, Gorsky M, Lozada-Nur F. The diagnosis and management of recurrent aphthous stomatitis: a consensus approach. *J Am Dent Assoc*. 2003;134:200–7.
24. Casiglia JM. Recurrent aphthous stomatitis: etiology, diagnosis, and treatment. *Gen Dent*. 2002;50:157–66.
25. *Fed Regist*. 1994;59:6084.
26. Greenberg MS. Drug use for connective tissue disorders and oral mucosal diseases. In: Ciancio SG, ed. *ADA Guide to Dental Therapeutics*. 2nd ed. Chicago: ADA Business Enterprises; 2000:450–1.
27. Harris NO, Garcia-Godoy F. *Primary Preventive Dentistry*. 6th ed. Stamford, Conn: Appleton & Lange; 2004:76–85, 96–102, 124–5, 128–30, 165–6, 242–7, 249–53, 419, 440, 471, 489–90, 655–9.
28. American Dental Association. *ADA Statement on the Safety of Hydrogen-Peroxide-Containing Dental Products Intended for Home Use*. Chicago: American Dental Association; 1997.
29. *Fed Regist*. 1988;53:2436.
30. Burgess J, van der Ven P, Martin M, et al. Review of over-the-counter treatments for aphthous ulceration and results from use of a dissolving oral patch containing glycyrrhiza complex herbal extract. *J Contemp Dent Pract*. 2008;9:88–98.
31. Siegel MA. Diagnosis and management of recurrent herpes simplex infections. *J Am Dent Assoc*. 2002;133:1245–9.
32. Gonsalves WC, Chi AC, Neville BW. Common oral lesions, part I: superficial mucosal lesions. *Am Fam Physician*. 2007;75:501–7.
33. *Fed Regist*. 1992;57:29173.
34. *Fed Regist*. 1990;55:3372,3379.
35. *Fed Regist*. 1993;58:27638.

36. ADA news: FDA approves OTC cold sore medication. *J Am Dent Assoc.* 2000;131:1256–60.

37. Sacks SL, Thisted RA, Jones TM, et al. Clinical efficacy of topical docosanol 10% cream for herpes simplex labialis: a multicenter, randomized, placebo-controlled trial. *J Am Acad Dermatol.* 2001;45:222–30.

38. Wilis A, Hyland P, Lamey P-J. Response to replacement iron therapy in sideropenic individuals with recrudescent herpes labialis. *Eur J Clin Microbiol Infect Dis.* 2000;19:355–7.

39. Carson CF, Ashton L, Dry L, et al. Melaleuca alternifolia (tea tree) oil gel (6%) for the treatment of recurrent herpes labialis. *J Antimicrob Chemother.* 2001;48:450–1.

40. Allen P. Tea tree oil: the science behind the antimicrobial hype. *Lancet.* 2001;13:1245.

41. Tomblin FA, Lucas KH. Lysine for management of herpes labialis. *Am J Health Syst Pharm.* 2001;58:298–304.

42. Pederson A. LongoVital and herpes labialis: a randomised, double-blind, placebo-controlled study. *Oral Dis.* 2001;7:221–5.

43. Gaby AR. Natural remedies for herpes simplex. *Altern Med Rev.* 2006; 11:93–101.

44. Guyton AC. *Textbook of Medical Physiology.* 8th ed. Philadelphia: WB Saunders; 1991:711–2.

45. Fox PC. Management of dry mouth. *Dent Clin North Am.* 1997; 41:863–75.

46. Ciancio SG. Medications' impact on oral health. *J Am Dent Assoc.* 2004; 135;1440–48.

47. Guggenheimer J, Moore PA. Xerostomia: etiology, recognition and treatment. *J Am Dent Assoc.* 2003;134:61–9.

48. Wynn RL, Meiller TF, Crossly HL. *Drug Information Handbook for Dentistry.* 9th ed. Hudson, Ohio: Lexi-Comp; 2003:1553–61.

49. Garg AK, Malo M. Manifestations and treatment of xerostomia and associated oral effect secondary to head and neck radiation therapy. *J Am Dent Assoc.* 1997;128:1128–33.

50. Atkinson JC, Wu AJ. Salivary gland dysfunction: causes, symptoms, treatment. *J Am Dent Assoc.* 1994;125:409–16.

51. Yagiela JA. Agents affecting salivation. In: Ciancio SG, ed. *ADA Guide to Dental Therapeutics.* 2nd ed. Chicago: ADA Business Enterprises; 2000: 198–210.

52. Jonsson R, Moen K, Vestrheim D, et al. Current issues in Sjögren's syndrome. *Oral Dis.* 2002;8:130–40.

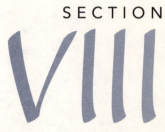

SECTION VIII

Dermatologic Disorders

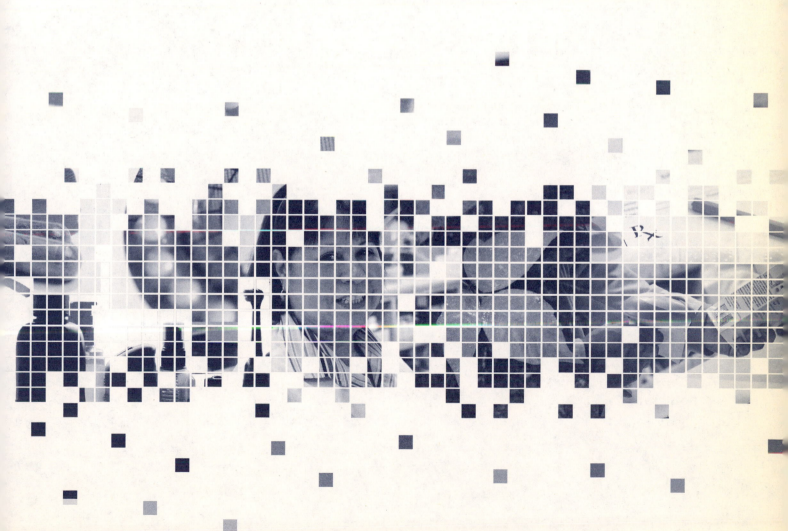

Atopic Dermatitis and Dry Skin

Steven A. Scott

An estimated 5% of the population suffer from a chronic skin, hair, or nail condition, and many others experience acute or seasonal disorders. Numerous skin disorders present as early as infancy and continue to appear throughout childhood and adulthood.[1] Patients with skin disorders typically present with some type of rash and/or itching (pruritus), which may indicate dermatitis. It is essential for clinicians to be able to recognize, differentiate, and suggest appropriate treatment for common skin conditions, and to know when to refer patients to a primary care provider or dermatologist for severe skin disorders.

Dermatitis is a nonspecific term describing numerous dermatologic conditions that are generally characterized by erythema (redness). The terms *eczema* and *dermatitis* are used interchangeably to describe a group of inflammatory skin disorders of unknown etiology. When the cause of a particular skin condition is elucidated, the disorder is given a specific name. Known causes of dermatitis include allergens, irritants, and infections; however, several distinct forms of dermatitis exist for which the causes remain unclear.

This chapter discusses atopic dermatitis, a common form of dermatitis, and dry skin, another frequent dermatologic complaint. Almost everyone will experience dry or chapped skin (xerosis) at some point, and the incidence increases with age. Although dry skin is often not severe, it may be annoying and uncomfortable for patients with mild-to-moderate dryness because of the attendant pruritus and, in some cases, infection, pain, and inflammation occur.

ROLE OF SKIN IN DRUG ABSORPTION

The skin is involved in numerous physical and biochemical processes.[2] Skin thickness is variable but averages about 1 to 2 mm, with the thickest skin on the palms and soles, and the thinnest skin on the scrotum. Thinner areas are more permeable, allowing substances to be absorbed more easily than through thicker skin. Although skin is exposed to a variety of chemical and environmental insults, it demonstrates remarkable resiliency and recuperative ability.

Human skin has three functionally distinct regions: epidermis, dermis, and hypodermis (Figure 33-1). The epidermis, the outermost thin layer of the skin, regulates the water content of

the skin and controls drug transport into the lower layers and systemic circulation. The dermis is 40 times thicker than the epidermis and contains nerve endings, vasculature, and hair follicles. The hypodermis primarily provides nourishment and cushioning for the upper two layers.

The most important function of skin and its appendages (hair and nails) is to protect the body from external harmful agents, such as pathogenic organisms and chemicals. The skin's ability to do this depends on age, immunologic status, underlying disease states of the individual, concurrent medications, and preservation of an intact stratum corneum.[3]

Normal skin flora also acts as a defense mechanism by controlling the growth of potential pathogenic organisms, and preventing their possible invasion of the skin and body. The skin also contributes to sensory experiences, and is involved in temperature control, pigment development, and synthesis of some vitamins. It is important in hydroregulation as well, controlling moisture loss from the body and moisture penetration into the body. If the stratum corneum becomes dehydrated, it loses elasticity and its permeation characteristics are altered. Aging skin becomes more fragile, requiring a longer recovery time after injury.

A drug must be released from its vehicle if it is to exert an effect at the desired site of activity (skin surface, epidermis, or dermis). Release occurs at the interface between the skin surface and the applied layer of product. The physical–chemical relationship between the drug and the vehicle determines the rate and amount of drug released. Considerations such as the drug's solubility and diffusion coefficient in the vehicle, and its partition coefficient into the sebum and stratum corneum are significant to its efficacy.[3] A drug with a strong affinity for the vehicle has a lower rate and extent of percutaneous absorption than drugs with weaker affinity for the vehicle. Therefore, a drug with an approximately equal balance of polar and hydrocarbon moieties (i.e., a partition coefficient) penetrates the stratum corneum more readily than one that is either highly polar or highly lipoidal.

Other factors influencing drug release include degree of hydration of the stratum corneum, pK_a of the drug, pH of the drug vehicle and the skin surface, drug concentration, thickness of the applied layer, and temperature. As temperature increases at the site of application, blood flow in the area also increases, as does the rate of percutaneous absorption.

Oily hydrocarbon bases such as petrolatum are transiently occlusive, promote hydration, and generally enhance the transport of agents through the skin layers. Hydrous emulsion bases are less occlusive. Water-soluble bases (polyethylene glycols)

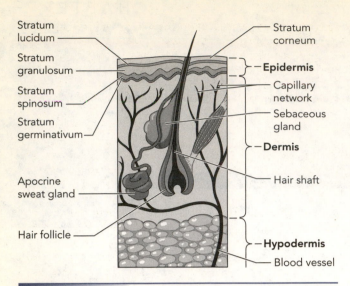

FIGURE 33-1 Cross-section of human skin.

are minimally occlusive, may attract water from the stratum corneum, and may decrease drug transport. Powders with hydrophilic ingredients presumably decrease hydration, because they promote evaporation from the skin by absorbing available water.

Substances are transported from the skin surface to the general circulation through percutaneous absorption. The routes of such transport are presumed to involve passages through skin between the keratinized units of the stratum corneum and through skin appendages (e.g., hair follicles, sweat glands, and sebaceous glands). The major mechanism of drug absorption is passive diffusion through the stratum corneum, followed by transport through the deeper epidermal regions and then the dermis.

Drug movement into and through the skin is enhanced or inhibited to varying degrees, depending on the physical–chemical properties of a drug, the sebum, and area of skin. The stratum corneum provides the greatest resistance and is often a rate-limiting barrier to percutaneous absorption. Because it is nonliving tissue, the stratum corneum may be viewed as having the general characteristics of an artificial and semipermeable membrane. Once a molecule has crossed this layer, there is much less resistance to its transport through the rest of the epidermis and into the dermis. When the stratum corneum is hydrated, drug diffusion is sometimes accelerated. Occlusion also increases hydration of the stratum corneum, which enhances the transfer of most drugs. The increased amount of water present in the skin under such conditions probably further enhances the transfer of polar molecules.

Wounds, burns, chafed areas, and dermatitis can alter the integrity of the stratum corneum, and can result in artificial shunts of the percutaneous absorption process. Inflammation can also enhance percutaneous absorption of topically applied medications, which may result in dangerous systemic drug levels. Therefore, caution should be used in applying topical medication to compromised skin, particularly if large surface areas are involved.

Topical medications should not be used on children ages 2 years or younger, except under the advice and supervision of a primary care provider. Infants have a reduced capability to biotransform drugs absorbed by the cutaneous route, and they have immature hepatic enzyme systems. In addition, because the ratio of surface area to body weight in a newborn is approx-imately two to three times that of an adult, the proportion of drug absorbed per kilogram of body weight is greater in a newborn.[4] Infants are, therefore, at increased risk for systemic effects from topically applied drugs.

ATOPIC DERMATITIS

Atopy is a genetically predisposed tendency to exaggerated skin and mucosal reactivity in response to environmental stimuli. The atopic triad is asthma, allergic rhinitis (hay fever), and atopic dermatitis (AD). AD is a chronic, relapsing skin disorder that typically begins during infancy or early childhood and often lasts into adulthood. Over time it moves through three age-related phases (infancy, childhood, and adult).[5] The incidence of AD may be increasing (from 3% of children after World War II to 10%–15% today) possibly, in part, from increased exposure to pollutants, irritants, indoor allergens (particularly house dust mites), and a decline in breast-feeding.[6]

The estimated worldwide incidence of AD is 5% to 10% of the children under the age of 14 years and 2% to 5% of adults.[6] It is considered the most common dermatologic condition of children, with more than 5% of children affected by age 6 months. AD persists or recurs in about 60% of affected individuals and is more common in boys, whites, higher socioeconomic classes, and urban areas.[6] Allergic rhinitis (hay fever) and asthma occur in 30% to 80% of cases of AD. Areas commonly affected (e.g., face, flexural areas on the inside of the knees and elbows, and collar area of the neck) depend on the patient's age. Two-thirds to three-quarters of patients with AD do not seek medical care and therefore are likely to look for advice regarding self-care of this condition.[6]

Pathophysiology of Atopic Dermatitis

AD has a genetic basis, but its expression is modified by a broad spectrum of exogenous manifestations.[7] Seventy percent of cases have an atopic family history. For example, if one parent (especially the father) has an atopic disorder, there is a 60% chance of the child being atopic. If both parents are affected, the likelihood is 80%. In families without atopia, the likelihood of having an atopic child is roughly 20%.

AD is diagnosed according to clinical criteria (Table 33-1). No established laboratory tests exist, although many patients have shown an elevated immunoglobulin E level and peripheral blood eosinophilia. AD may be accompanied by allergic respiratory

---

TABLE 33-1 Diagnostic Criteria for Atopic Dermatitis

An itchy skin condition, plus three or more of the following criteria:

- Onset at <2 years of age
- History of skin crease involvement (including cheeks in children < 10 years of age)
- History of generally dry skin
- Personal history of other atopic disease (or history of any atopic disease in first-degree relative in children < 4 years of age)
- Visible flexural dermatitis (or dermatitis of cheeks/forehead and other outer limbs in children < 4 years of age)

disease but often is the initial clinical manifestation of an allergic disease.

Common exacerbating factors include foods, soaps, detergents, fragrances, chemicals, temperature changes, dust, pollens, certain bacteria, and emotional changes. Clinically relevant food allergy in AD is estimated to range up to 33% to the age of 24 months. Patients with AD may be more sensitive to irritants than the general population; therefore, it is important for affected patients to minimize exposure to known irritants, allergens, plus any other factor known to exacerbate the condition.[8]

Irritants (e.g., solvents, industrial chemicals, fragrances, soaps, fumes, paints, bleach, wool, and astringents) may cause burning, itching, or redness. Patients with AD may be especially sensitive to low concentrations of irritants that would not generally cause a reaction on normal skin.[9]

Allergens—typically, plant or animal proteins from food, pollens, or pets—may aggravate AD. However, the role of food allergies in exacerbating AD is unclear. It is claimed that up to 20% of children younger than 2 years with AD are affected by allergic reactions to foods through either ingestion or skin contact, and specific hypersensitivities to milk products and eggs have been identified. Restricting offending foods, especially in children, creates overwhelming compliance problems. Moreover, although dietary restriction may produce some improvement in the condition initially, complete resolution is unlikely to occur. Therefore, it is probably best to reserve dietary management for patients who have severe symptoms and are unresponsive to other treatments.[10]

Patients with AD are often intolerant of sudden and extreme changes in temperature and humidity. High temperature may enhance perspiration, leading to increased itching. Low humidity, often found in heated buildings during the winter, dries the skin and increases itching. Use of humidifiers in dry environments will provide some benefit. As with asthma, emotional stress is an exacerbating factor in some patients.

Clinical Presentation of Atopic Dermatitis

Although AD is often first manifested in infancy, it is rarely present at birth. If it does develop early in life, it typically occurs within the first year (often beginning at age 2–3 months) in approximately 80% of the cases. It initially appears as redness and chapping of the infant's cheeks, which may continue to affect the face, neck, and trunk (Table 33-2). At times, this dermatitis

may progress to become more generalized, with crusting developing on the forehead and cheeks.[10] Crusts consist of dried exudate containing proteinaceous and cellular debris from erosion or ulceration of primary skin lesions. Remission usually occurs between the ages of 2 and 4 years, with recurrences often diminishing in intensity or even disappearing as the child approaches adulthood.

A classic case of infantile or childhood AD involves the cheeks and extensor surfaces of the forearms and legs (see Color Plates, photographs 14A, B, and C). Later manifestations of AD typically present on flexor surfaces. Lesions are typically symmetric in patients with AD.

The primary sign of AD is intense pruritic papules (solid, circumscribed, elevated lesions less than 1 cm in diameter) and vesicles (sharply circumscribed, elevated lesions containing fluid). Pruritus is common and causes significant morbidity in AD. Patients with AD react more readily and more persistently to pruritic-inducing stimuli. Scratching and lichenification (increased epidermal markings) can produce a vicious cycle and lead to excoriation (abrasion of the epidermis by trauma).[11]

AD has three clinical forms. Acute AD is characterized by intensely pruritic, erythematous papules or vesicles over erythematous skin, and is often associated with excoriation and serous exudate. Subacute AD is characterized by erythematous, excoriated, scaling papules. Chronic AD is characterized by thickened plaques of skin and accentuated skin markings (lichenification). In chronic AD, all three stages of skin reactions frequently coexist in the same individual.

Secondary or associated cutaneous infections, especially bacterial, can be common, difficult to prevent, and typically aggravate AD. More than 90% of the skin lesions in patients with AD (in contrast to 5% of unaffected individuals) harbor *Staphylococcus aureus*.[6] Although *S. aureus* is the most common cause, streptococci may also be found alone or in association with *S. aureus*. Infections present as yellowish crusting of the eczematous lesions. Patients should be counseled to seek medical attention promptly when signs of bacterial or viral skin infection such as pustules (circumscribed, elevated lesions less than 1 cm in diameter containing pus), vesicles (especially exudate or pus-filled), and crusting (dried exudate) are noticed.

Treatment of Atopic Dermatitis

Treatment Goals

The goals of self-treatment of AD are to (1) stop the itch–scratch cycle, (2) maintain skin hydration, (3) avoid or minimize factors that trigger or aggravate the disorder, and (4) prevent secondary infections.

General Treatment Approach

To prevent unrealistic expectations, clinicians should stress to patients that AD cannot be cured but that most patients' symptoms can be managed satisfactorily. The condition should be explained as a multifactorial disorder, and it must be appreciated that just as there is no "cure," there is no single "cause." Often no explanation can be found for a particular flare-up of the condition, and many factors are probably working in combination at all times.

Regardless of a patient's age, the stratum corneum in patients with AD contains less moisture than that of normal skin. Enhancing skin hydration can be achieved through nonpharmacologic

TABLE 33-2 Characteristics of Atopic Dermatitis by Age

Age	Location	Signs
2 months	Chest, face	Red, raised vesicles; dry skin; oozing
2 years	Scalp, neck, and extensor surface of extremities	Less acute lesions; edema; erythema
2–4 years	Neck, wrist, elbow, knee	Dry, thickened plaques; hyperpigmentation
12–20 years	Flexors, hands	Dry, thickened plaques; hyperpigmentation

measures, as well as through the use of emollients and moisturizers. Hydrocortisone relieves itching and inflammation, and cool water compresses relieve weeping vesicles. An effective preventive measure is to minimize exposure to factors known to trigger AD. The algorithm in Figure 33-2 outlines the self-treatment of this disorder and lists exclusions for self-treatment.

Nonpharmacologic Therapy

The variability in severity and age of onset requires tailoring treatment to an individual's needs, bearing in mind their age, gender, and social conditions, and the site(s) and severity of the lesions.[11] Extensive patient education about the skin disorder is

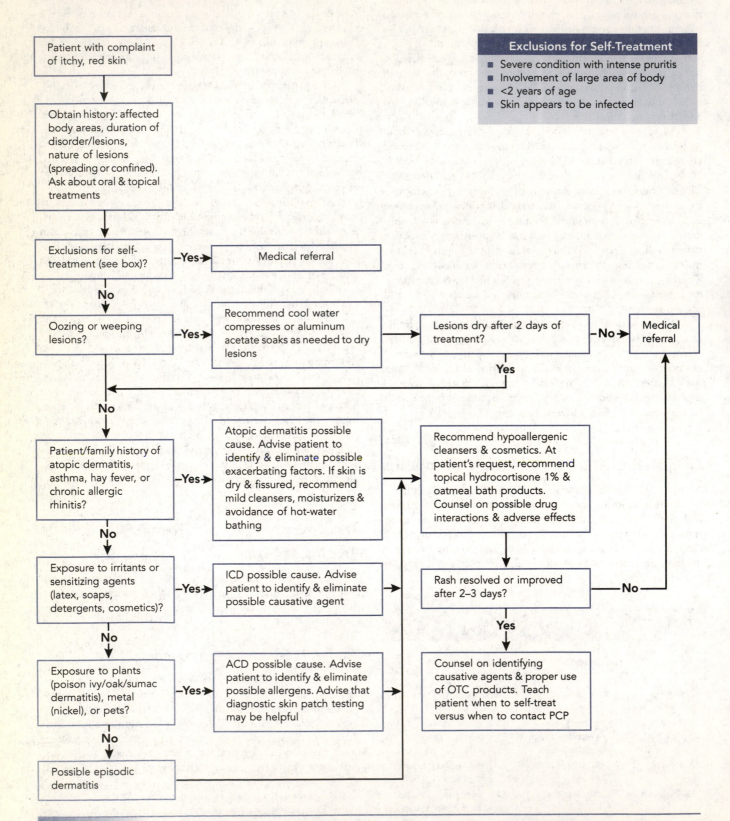

FIGURE 33-2 Self-care of dermatitis. Key: ACD, allergic contact dermatitis; ICD, irritant contact dermatitis; OTC, over-the-counter; PCP, primary care provider.

paramount at the onset. Successful treatment of AD requires a systematic, multipronged approach that incorporates (1) skin hydration; (2) the identification and elimination of flare factors such as irritants, allergens, infectious agents, and emotional stressors; and (3) the use of topical and sometimes systemic therapy.

Patients with AD may be more susceptible to irritants than normal individuals are. Reducing or eliminating exposure to or contact with trigger factors (soaps, cigarette smoke, animal dander, molds, pollens, etc.) is crucial. Laundering and thoroughly rinsing new clothing, wearing nonirritating fabrics such as cotton, and avoiding sunburn by using nonirritating sunscreens are all encouraged practices.

Errors in bathing and moisturizing are by far the most common factors in persistent AD. Some dermatologists oppose daily bathing because it dries the skin, causing microfissures and cracks that serve as portals of entry for skin pathogens, irritants, and allergens. In contrast, other dermatologists claim that "appropriate" bathing in AD sufferers hydrates the stratum corneum, removes allergens and irritants, cleanses and debrides crusts, and enhances the effects of moisturizers and topical steroids.[12] The answer to the apparent paradox is that bathing hydrates the skin as long as an effective moisturizer is applied within 3 minutes to prevent evaporation from the stratum corneum. When evaporation occurs, this barrier dries and cracks. Patients should bathe for only 3 to 5 minutes using fragrance-free bath oils to soothe the skin, or dehydration of the skin occurs. Common bar soaps are often too drying and irritating for some AD patients.[13] Preferred frequency of bathing is every other day (to minimize removal of natural oils), with tepid rather than hot water. Because of the significant drying effect of most soaps, mild nonsoap cleansers (e.g., Cetaphil) are often recommended. After bathing, moisturizers can be applied and excessively dry areas of skin covered with a lubricating ointment.

Treatment of acute weeping or oozing lesions is directed toward drying the lesions. Wet compresses using tap water should be applied for 20 minutes, four to six times daily. Bathing with tepid water containing colloidal oatmeal may also be soothing.

For itching, simply telling a patient not to scratch is generally ineffective. Therefore, adjunctive measures may be used to minimize scratching and the damage it produces. Fingernails should be kept short, smooth, and clean. Because scratching may increase at night, even while the patient is sleeping, wearing cotton gloves or socks on the hands at night may lessen scratching. Excessive scratching can result in open sores that may need to be treated with a topical antibiotic preparation. Use of bacitracin/polymyxin B ointment (Polysporin) may be preferred over bacitracin/polymyxin B/neomycin ointment, given that some patients may be sensitized to neomycin. Patients should avoid occlusive, tight clothing. If possible, patients should remain in moderate temperature settings and moderate relative humidity conditions.

Treatment of chronic lesions focuses on measures to maintain skin hydration and decrease itching. A water-miscible bath oil may be added to the water near the end of the bath. The skin should be patted dry gently; vigorous rubbing produces irritation. An emollient should be applied within 3 minutes while the skin is still damp. Although ointments with a petrolatum or water-in-oil base maintain hydration best, sweating after the application of heavy ointments may add to the propensity for itching. Patients should be instructed to rub a very small amount of ointment into the affected area very well. Oil-in-water preparations (creams and lotions) are often more cosmetically acceptable, but they need to be applied more frequently than ointments because their ability to maintain moisture in the skin is often

more short lived. If applied correctly, they should have a good emollient effect and not produce dryness.

Few alternative and complementary remedies exist to treat atopic dermatitis. Oral preparations containing bifidobacteria or lactobacillus and topical application of rice bran are considered possibly effective at decreasing the severity of AD in some patients. Insufficient evidence exists to determine whether products containing the following ingredients provide any benefit to patients with AD: grapefruit seed extract, licorice, puncture vine, schizonepeta, and vitamin B_{12}. The use of products containing evening primrose oil, borage, gamma linolenic acid, zinc, and tea tree oil have all failed to demonstrate any benefit in the treatment of atopic dermatitis to date.

Pharmacologic Therapy

Hydrocortisone in an oil-in-water base is the primary pharmacologic nonprescription agent used to treat AD. These preparations are primarily used to decrease inflammation and relieve itching.

Magnesium ions inhibit the antigen-presenting function of skin cells and thereby may decrease cutaneous irritation and inflammation.[14] Topical magnesium salts (chloride and sulfate) are, therefore, used as nonprescription products to provide antiinflammatory benefit in dermatoses that include psoriasis and AD. Several products (shampoo and topical cream as well as bathing salts) that contain salt from the Dead Sea (46% magnesium chloride) have been used to manage these dermatoses, although there is little evidence to support their use.

DRY SKIN (XEROSIS)

Xerosis, or dry skin, is the result of decreased water content of the skin with resultant abnormal loss of cells from the stratum corneum. Environmental dry skin is often associated with the patient's taking long, hot showers or not consuming enough water. The prevention and care of dry skin may become a major focus for practitioners as the population of persons of advanced age continues to increase. There is a heightened awareness among those caring for persons of advanced age that prophylactic dry skin care can reduce morbidity by minimizing the risk of skin breakdown and, therefore, can ultimately reduce the cost of dermatologic health care.[15]

Xerosis is a common problem, affecting more than 50% of older adults, and is the most common cause of pruritus.[6] It is a frequent cause of pruritus in cooler climates during the winter season (i.e., "winter itch"). Individuals who live or work in arid, windy, or cold environments also have an increased risk for dry skin. Most cases of xerosis are either undertreated or ignored as a cause of the patients' problem.

Pathophysiology of Dry Skin

Dry skin can result from various etiologies. It can be caused by disruption of keratinization and impairment of water-binding properties.[16] Dry skin may also occur secondary to prolonged detergent use, malnutrition, or physical damage to the stratum corneum. It may also signal a systemic disorder such as hypothyroidism or dehydration.

Dry skin is related to decreased water retention in the stratum corneum, not a lack of natural skin oils. Dry skin pathophysiology, therefore, can be described by examining the factors involved in skin hydration. One major factor is frequent or prolonged bathing or showering with hot water, as well as excessive use of soap, both of which increase dryness of the skin. Soap removes the skin's natural oils, and the short duration of contact with water is usually insufficient to hydrate dry skin. A second factor relates to environmental conditions, such as low relative humidity. Dry air allows the outer skin layer to lose moisture, become less flexible, and crack when flexed, leading to an increased rate of moisture loss. High wind velocity also causes moisture loss in skin. A third factor is physical damage to the stratum corneum, such as a leg ulcer, which dramatically increases transepidermal water loss. However, after the insult is removed, partial recovery occurs within 1 or 2 days with the formation of a temporary barrier consisting of incompletely keratinized cells. The maximum barrier effect is restored in 2 to 3 weeks if the skin barrier is not severely disrupted.

With advancing age, the epidermis changes because of abnormal maturation or adhesion of the keratinocytes, resulting in a superficial, irregular layer of corneocytes. This condition may be described as a thinning of the entire epidermis, which produces a roughened skin surface. The skin's hygroscopic substances also decrease in quantity with advancing age. Hormonal changes that accompany aging result in lowered sebum output. Older patients also typically have inadequate water intake, which contributes to this condition.

Clinical Presentation of Dry Skin

Xerosis is characterized by one or more of the following signs and symptoms: roughness, scaling, loss of flexibility, fissures, inflammation, and pruritus. Clinically, fine plate-like scaling particularly on the arms and legs that may be associated with a "cracked" appearance (eczema craquelé) or fish scaling (ichthyosis) appearance of the skin is common.

Treatment of Dry Skin

Treatment Goals

The goals of self-treatment of dry skin are to (1) restore skin hydration, (2) restore the skin's barrier function, and (3) educate the patient about this chronic condition

General Treatment Approach

Treatment involves recognizing the problem as well as modifying the environment (humidity) and bathing habits to maintain skin hydration. Nonprescription products such as bath oils, emollients/moisturizers, humectants, and keratolytic agents also aid in restoring and maintaining barrier function. If needed, topical hydrocortisone can be used to reduce pruritus and erythema.

Nonpharmacologic Therapy

The most important aspects of care are the proper use of emollients and modifications to bathing practices. Products such as oilated oatmeal or bath oil added near the end of the bath may be used to enhance skin hydration. The patient should apply oil-based emollients immediately after bathing while the skin is damp and should reapply them frequently. The room humidity should be increased with a humidifier or even a vaporizer. Care should

---

TABLE 33-3 Dry Skin Therapy

- Take tub baths two to three times per week, using bath oil, for brief periods (3–5 minutes). Take sponge baths on other days.
- The water should be tepid, not more than 3°F above body temperature.
- Stay in the bath water only 3–5 minutes.
- Within 3 minutes of getting out of the tub, pat the body dry, leaving beads of moisture, and generously apply body lotion to trap the moisture.
- Apply the body lotion at least three more times during the day to (preferably) the whole body or at least the most affected areas.
- Additional measures include:
  —Use corticosteroid ointments rather than creams.
  —Keep room humidity higher.

---

be taken to clean humidifiers per manufacturers' instructions to prevent mold or mildew that may grow in the device if not cleaned properly. The patient, if medical conditions allow, should be encouraged to drink at least eight 8-ounce glasses of water daily. Table 33-3 reviews nonpharmacologic therapy of dry skin.

Pharmacologic Therapy

More severe cases of dry skin may require a product containing urea or lactic acid to enhance hydration. The patient may apply topical hydrocortisone ointment on a short-term basis (no longer than 7 days) to reduce inflammation and itching. Dry skin responds minimally to topical corticosteroid therapy, although short-term use of topical corticosteroids may reduce symptoms of erythema and pruritus.[17,18] If resolution does not occur within 1 or 2 weeks, a primary care provider should be consulted, because higher potency corticosteroid products (e.g., betamethasone or halobetasol) or one of the immunomodulatory agents (e.g., pimecrolimus or tacrolimus) may be required to control the skin disorder.[5] Dry skin is more prone to itching, inflammation, and development of secondary infections. Most moisturizers are mixtures of oils and water. Moisturizers containing ammonium lactate 12% have improved the appearance of skin covered with cracks and fissures.[19] Alpha-hydroxy acids and related compounds have been shown to normalize keratinization and to result in more normal stratum corneum.[16] Indications for using alpha-hydroxy acid products include treatment of xerosis (dry skin), acne, and photoaging. The emergence of such products allows the practitioner to choose from a vast array of nonprescription products.

TREATMENT OF ATOPIC DERMATITIS AND DRY SKIN

Nonprescription products for dermatitis and dry skin that restore skin hydration include bath products, emollients, hydrating agents, and keratin-softening agents (Table 33-4). Astringents, antipruritics, protectants, and hydrocortisone are used to relieve weeping and/or itching of lesions and to protect the affected area.

TABLE 33-4 Selected Dry Skin Products

Trade Name	Primary Ingredients
Absorbase Ointment[a]	Petrolatum; mineral oil; ceresin wax; wool wax alcohol; potassium sorbate
AmLactin Cream/Lotion	Ammonium lactate 12%
Aquaphor Ointment	Petrolatum 41%; water
Aveeno Cleansing Bar[a]	Disodium lauryl sulfosuccinate; cetyl alcohol; wheat starch; paraffin
Aveeno Daily Moisturizing Lotion[a]	Dimethicone 1.25%; cetyl alcohol; oat kernel flour; glycerin
Aveeno Moisturizing Bath Treatment Formula[a]	Mineral oil; colloidal oatmeal 43%
Aveeno Moisturizing Cream/Lotion[a]	Petrolatum; dimethicone; isopropyl palmitate; cetyl alcohol; colloidal oatmeal 1%; glycerin
Aveeno Skin Relief Moisturizing Lotion[a]	Dimethicone 1.25%; menthol 0.1%; oat kernel flour
Aveeno Soothing Bath Treatment Formula[a]	Colloidal oatmeal 100%
Carmol 10 Lotion	Urea 10%
Carmol 20 Cream	Urea 20%
Cetaphil Gentle Cleansing Bar[a]	Sodium cocoyl isethionate; stearic acid; sodium tallousate; PEG-20; petrolatum
Cetaphil Gentle Skin Cleanser Liquid[a]	Cetyl alcohol; stearyl alcohol; PEG
Corn Huskers Lotion	Glycerin 6.7%; SD alcohol 40, 5.7%; algin; guar gum
Eucerin Cream[a]	Petrolatum; mineral oil; mineral wax; wool wax alcohol
Jergens Advanced Therapy Ultra Healing Lotion	Petrolatum; mineral oil; dimethicone; cetearyl alcohol; cetyl alcohol; glycerin; allantoin
Keri Original Formula Therapeutic Dry Skin Lotion	Mineral oil; lanolin oil; glyceryl stearate; propylene glycol
Lac-Hydrin Five Lotion	Urea 5%
Lubriderm Advanced Therapy Lotion	Cetyl alcohol; glycerin; mineral oil; PEG-40; emulsifying wax; vitamin E
Lubriderm Bath and Shower Oil	Mineral oil
Lubriderm Daily Moisturizing Lotion	Mineral oil; petrolatum; sorbitol; lanolin; lanolin alcohol; triethanolamine
Moisturel Cream/Lotion[a]	Petrolatum; dimethicone; cetyl alcohol; glycerin
Neutrogena Body Oil	Isopropyl myristate; sesame oil
Neutrogena Norwegian Formula Body Moisturizing Lotion[a]	Glycerin; distearyldimonium chloride; petrolatum; cetyl alcohol; dimethicone; colloidal oatmeal
Neutrogena Soap	TEA-stearate; triethanolamine; glycerin
Nivea Body Lotion	Mineral oil; glycerin isopropyl palmitate; vitamin E; lanolin alcohol
Purpose Gentle Cleansing Bar	Sodium tallowate; sodium cocoate; glycerin; BHT
Sarna Anti-Itch Lotion	Camphor 0.5%; menthol 0.5%; carbomer 940; cetyl alcohol; DMDM hydantoin, glyceryl stearate; petrolatum
Vaseline Dermatology Formula Lotion	White petrolatum 5%; mineral oil 4%; dimethicone 1%; glyceryl stearate; cetyl alcohol; glycerin

Key: BHT, butylhydroxytoluene; DMDM, dimethylol dimethyl; PEG, polyethylene glycol; TEA, triethanolamine.

[a] Fragrance-free formulation.

Bath Products

Bath Oils

Bath oils generally consist of a mineral or vegetable oil, plus a sur-factant. Mineral oil products are adsorbed better than vegetable oil products. Adsorption onto and absorption into the skin increase as temperature and oil concentration increase. Bath oils are minimally effective in improving a dry skin condition because they are greatly diluted in water. Their major effect is the slip or lubricity they impart to the skin, which may be important to the patient. When applied as wet compresses, however, bath oils (1 teaspoon in one-fourth cup of warm water) help lubricate dry skin and may allow a decrease in the frequency of full-body bathing.[5,18] Bath oils make the tub and floor slippery, creating a safety hazard, especially for patients of advanced age or children. They also make cleansing the skin with soaps more difficult.

Oatmeal Products

Colloidal oatmeal bath products contain starch, protein, and a small amount of oil. Although these products combine the effect of oatmeal and a bath oil, they are less effective than bath oils. Evidence-based efficacy is minimal; however, colloidal oatmeal is claimed to be soothing and antipruritic, and it does have a lubricating effect.

Cleansers

Typical bath soaps generally contain salts of long-chain fatty acids (commonly oleic, palmitic, or stearic acid) and alkali metals (e.g., sodium or potassium). Combined with water, such products act as surfactants that will remove many substances from the skin, including the lipids that normally keep the skin soft and pliable. Some authorities recommend special soaps that contain extra oils to minimize the drying effect of washing. However, these soaps usually lather and clean poorly.

Glycerin soaps, which are transparent and more water soluble, have a higher oil content than standard toilet soaps because of the addition of castor oil. They are closer to a neutral pH and are, therefore, regarded as less drying than soaps, which are alkaline. Although little objective proof exists to prove their superiority, glycerin soaps are advertised for, and well accepted by, people with skin conditions.

Clinicians may choose to recommend mild cleansers such as Cetaphil or pHisoDerm, if soap is to be avoided. Most of these products consist primarily of surfactants and may contain oil. Although these products claim to have a low potential for irritation, clear evidence of their superiority over soaps is lacking. On application, they foam mildly, and on gentle wiping, they leave a thin layer of lipid material on the skin, which helps retain water in the stratum corneum. Leave-on, no-rinse skin cleansers are a useful tool to minimize the skin barrier disruption seen with traditional soaps and body bathing.

Emollients and Moisturizers

Emollients function by filling the spaces between the desquamating skin scales with oil droplets, but their effect is only temporary. Many terms are used to describe the effects of creams and lotions such as lubricants (i.e., products that increase skin slip in dry skin), moisturizers (i.e., products that impart moisture to the skin, increasing skin flexibility), repair or replenishing products (i.e., intended to reverse the appearance of aging skin), emollients, and so forth.

Most moisturizers consist of the following:

- Water (60%–80%), which functions as a diluent and evaporates, leaving behind the active agents
- Lipids (essential fatty acids)
- Emulsifiers, which keep water and lipids in one continuous phase
- Humectants, which help skin retain water
- Preservatives
- Fragrance (or may be fragrance-free)
- Color
- Specialty additives, such as (1) vitamins (vitamins A, C, D, and B complex), which have no effect, and (2) natural moisturizing factors, a group of substances (e.g., lactate, urea, ammonia, uric acid, and glucosamine) reported to regulate the moisture content of the stratum corneum.

Facial moisturizers are either oil-in-water emulsions or water-in-oil emulsions. The differences between moisturizer products are caused by the addition of fragrances, exotic oils, vitamins, protein or amino acid products, and other minor moisturizing aids. The selection of an appropriate facial moisturizer depends on skin type. Oily complexion products are oil-free or contain small amounts of light oils (mineral oil) with silicone derivatives and talc, clay, starch, or synthetic polymers (oil control). Normal skin products contain predominantly water, mineral oil, and propylene glycol with very small amounts of petrolatum or lanolin. These products leave an oilier residue on the face than oil-free formulations. Dry skin products contain water, mineral oil, propylene glycol, and larger amounts of petrolatum or lanolin.[20]

Body moisturizers come in lotion, cream, and ointment. Lotions are the most popular. Creams and ointments are more difficult to spread, especially in hair-bearing areas. Body lotions are generally oil-in-water emulsions containing 10% to 15% oil phase, 5% to 10% humectant, and 75% to 85% water phase.

Hand moisturizers are much heavier than body or facial emollients. The simplest and most economical hand ointment is petroleum jelly. Although it is greasy, which leads to poor compliance, petroleum jelly is effective when applied correctly. Hand creams are nongreasy oil-in-water emulsions with 15% to 40% oil phase, 5% to 15% humectant, and 45% to 80% water phase. Adding silicone derivatives renders hand cream water-resistant through four to six washings.

Because sebum and skin surface lipids contain a relatively high concentration of fatty acid glycerides, vegetable and animal oils derived from avocado, cucumber, mink, peanut, safflower, sesame, turtle, and shark liver are included in dry skin products, presumably because of their unsaturated fatty acid content. However, although use of such oils contributes to skin flexibility and lubricity, their occlusive effect is less than that of white petrolatum.

Emollients are occlusive agents and moisturizers that are used to prevent or relieve the signs and symptoms of dry skin. Such products act primarily by leaving an oily film on the skin surface through which moisture cannot readily escape. Cosmetically, emollients make the skin feel soft and smooth by helping to reestablish the integrity of the stratum corneum. Lipid components make the scales on the skin translucent and flatten them against the underlying skin. This flattening eliminates air between the scales and the skin surface, which is partly responsible for a white, scaly appearance.[15]

Frequency of application depends on the severity of the dry skin condition, as well as the hydration efficiency of the occlusive agent. Generally, moisturizers must be applied three to four times daily to achieve maximum benefit. For dry hands, the patient may need to apply the occlusive agent after each hand washing, as well as at numerous other times during the day.

Emollient products are available as petrolatum-containing ointments that are typically very greasy and generally lack consumer appeal because of their texture, difficulty of spreading and removing, and staining properties. To avoid a greasy feel, patients should be advised to gently warm the product in the hands, apply a very thin layer, and massage it gently, but thoroughly, into the skin. Ointments are inappropriate for an oozing AD, because they do not allow the lesions to dry and ultimately heal.

Lotions and creams are either water-in-oil or oil-in-water emulsions. As the lipid content of the moisturizer increases, the occlusive effect increases. In most cases, patients prefer the less effective but more esthetic oil-in-water emulsions for their cosmetic acceptability. Such agents help alleviate the pruritus associated with dry skin by virtue of their cooling effect as water evaporates from the skin surface. Moreover, enough oil exists in most oil-in-water emulsions to form a continuous occlusive film.[5,15]

Lanolin, a natural product derived from sheep wool, is found in many nonprescription moisturizing products. Patients rarely develop an allergic reaction to this substance, presumably because its wool wax fraction is recognized as antigenic. Patients with a previous history of allergic reactions to lanolin should generally avoid lanolin-containing products. However, products containing refined lanolin are generally less likely to be sensitizing and may even be tolerated by those with a history of allergic contact reactions to unrefined lanolin.

Although most commercial formulations generally are bland, contact with the eye or with broken or abraded skin should be avoided, because formulation ingredients may cause irritation. This irritation is especially true with emulsion systems, given that the surfactants in them denature protein and therefore may produce further irritation.

Petrolatum should not be applied over puncture wounds, infections, or lacerations, because its high occlusive ability may lead to maceration and further inflammation. Application of petrolatum to intertriginous areas, mucous membranes, and acne-prone areas should be minimized; only a preparation with a low concentration of petrolatum is tolerated in these areas.

Humectants

Humectants or hydrating agents are hygroscopic materials that may be added to an emollient base. Commonly used hydrating agents are glycerin, propylene glycol, and phospholipids.

Humectants draw water into the stratum corneum to hydrate the skin. Water may come from the dermis or from the atmosphere. However, high relative humidity (80% or greater) is necessary for the latter to occur. Humectants are distinct from emollients, which serve to retain water already present.

Because of glycerin's hygroscopic properties, high concentrations may actually increase water loss by drawing water from the skin rather than from the atmosphere. At lower concentrations (i.e., 5%), however, humectants such as glycerin help decrease water loss by keeping water in close contact with skin and accelerating moisture diffusion from the dermis to the epidermis. In addition, glycerin lubricates the skin surface.

Propylene glycol is a viscous, colorless, odorless solvent with hygroscopic properties. It is less viscous than glycerin and is included in many skin care formulations for its humectant action. However, it can cause skin irritation, usually on a concentration-dependent basis. Phospholipid products contain lecithin, a water-binding compound normally present in the skin. Each phospholipid molecule can complex with up to 15 molecules of water.

Urea

Urea in concentrations of 10% to 30% is mildly keratolytic and increases water uptake in the stratum corneum, giving it a high water-binding capacity. Urea has a direct effect on stratum corneum elasticity because of its ability to bind to skin protein. It is considered safe and has been recommended for use on crusted, necrotic tissue. Concentrations of 10% have been used on simple dry skin; 20% to 30% formulations have been used for treating more resistant dry skin conditions. Lotion and cream formulations containing urea may better at helping to remove scales and crusts, whereas urea in emollient ointments (e.g., urea in a hydrophilic ointment base) may be better at rehydrating the skin. However, urea preparations can cause stinging, burning, and irritation, particularly on broken skin.[19]

Alpha-Hydroxy Acid

Lactic acid is an alpha–hydroxy acid that has been useful in concentrations of 2% to 5% for treating dry skin conditions. Lactic acid increases the hydration of human skin and may act as a modulator of epidermal keratinization, rather than a keratolytic agent at low concentrations. Lactic acid may be added to urea preparations for both its stabilizing and its hydrating effects.

Other alpha-hydroxy acids, derived from fruits, are used for a number of common skin conditions such as dry skin, acne, and photoaging (see Chapter 40). Such acids include malic acid (in apples), citric acid (in oranges and lemons), tartaric acid (in grapes), and glycolic and gluconic acids (in sugar cane).[21]

Allantoin

Allantoin and allantoin complexes soften keratin by disrupting its structure. A product of purine metabolism, allantoin is considered to be a relatively safe compound. However, it is less effective than urea. The Food and Drug Administration (FDA) classifies allantoin as a Category I (safe and effective for nonprescription use) skin protectant for adults, children, and infants when applied in concentrations of 0.5% to 2.0%.[19]

Astringents

Astringents retard oozing, discharge, or bleeding of dermatitis when applied to unhealthy serous skin or mucous membranes. When applied as a wet dressing or compress, astringents cool and dry the skin through evaporation. They cause vasoconstriction and reduce blood flow in inflamed tissue. They also cleanse the skin of exudates, crust, and debris. Because astringents generally have low cell penetrability, their activity is limited to the cell surface and interstitial spaces. The protein precipitate that forms may serve as a protective coat, allowing new tissues to grow underneath.[19]

FDA has identified two astringent solutions as Category 1: aluminum acetate (Burow's solution) and witch hazel (hamamelis water). Aluminum acetate solution USP contains approximately 5% aluminum acetate. The solution must be diluted 1:10 to 1:40 with water before use.

The patient may soak the affected area two to four times daily for 15 to 30 minutes. Alternatively, the patient may loosely apply a compress of washcloths, cheesecloth, or small towels soaked in the solution, and then wring them gently so they are wet but not dripping. The dressings should be rewetted and applied every few minutes for 20 to 30 minutes, four to six times daily. Less expensive alternatives to aluminum acetate include isotonic saline solution (1 teaspoon salt in 2 cups of water), tap water, diluted white vinegar (one-fourth cup per pint of water), and plain water.

Topical Hydrocortisone

Hydrocortisone is currently the only corticosteroid available without a prescription for the topical treatment of dermatitis. Although its exact mechanism is unknown, hydrocortisone most likely suppresses cytokines associated with the development of inflammation and itching associated with various dermatoses. FDA monograph indications for its use include temporary relief of itching associated with minor skin irritations, inflammation, and rashes caused by dermatitis, seborrheic dermatitis, insect bites, poison ivy/oak/sumac dermatitis, soaps, detergents, cosmetics, and jewelry. Concentrations of 0.5% to 1% are regarded as appropriate for treating localized dermatitis (Table 33-5).

Hydrocortisone should be applied sparingly to the affected area three or four times a day. An ointment formulation generally provides the best results for chronic, non-oozing dermatoses. The drug should not be applied to infected skin; it may mask the symptoms of dermatologic infections and allow the infection to progress. Topical hydrocortisone rarely produces systemic complications, because its systemic absorption is relatively minimal (approximately 1%). Absorption increases in the presence of

TABLE 33-5 Selected Dermatitis Products

Trade Name	Primary Ingredients
Cortaid Maximum Strength Ointment/Cream	Hydrocortisone 1%
Cortizone-5 Cream	Hydrocortisone 0.5%; aluminum sulfate; calcium acetate
Lanacort-5 Cream/Ointment	Hydrocortisone 0.5%; aloe

skin inflammation, when occlusive dressings are used, or when the temperature of the skin is elevated. Certain local adverse effects such as skin atrophy rarely occurs with nonprescription concentrations; it is more common with the more potent prescription products. Because response to topical corticosteroids may decrease with continued use owing to tachyphylaxis, intermittent courses of therapy are advised when possible.[5]

Antipruritics

The itching associated with dermatitis may be mediated through several mechanisms, which may explain how three major classes of pharmacologic agents—local anesthetics, antihistamines, and corticosteroids (discussed previously)—are useful as antipruritics. Cooling the area through application of a soothing, bland lotion may reduce the extent of the pruritus, but this effect is only transitory.

The itching sensation is mediated by the same nerve fibers that carry pain impulses. Local anesthetics block conduction along axonal membranes, thereby relieving itching as well as pain. However, because local anesthetics may cause systemic side effects, they should not be used in large quantities or over long periods of time, particularly if the skin is raw or blistered. Nonprescription topical anesthetics that appear to be safe and effective are pramoxine, lidocaine, and benzocaine. Topical anesthetics may be applied to affected areas three or four times daily, but caution should be used because these agents may have a sensitizing effect in a small number of people. Counterirritants such as camphor and menthol, in concentrations of 0.5% to 1%, are available in or can also be added to lotions and creams to serve as an inexpensive antipruritic.[19]

Itching may also be mediated by various endogenous substances, including histamine. Accordingly, topical antihistamines such as diphenhydramine are effective in alleviating this symptom. Their activity stems from an ability to compete with histamine at H_1-receptor sites and to exert a topical anesthetic effect. Local anesthesia may be the more important mechanism of action, given that the cause of itching in many conditions (e.g., atopic dermatitis) is most likely due to cytokine release and may not be related to histamine release at all. Antihistamines are considered safe and effective for use as nonprescription external analgesics. However, because of their significant sensitizing potential, FDA does not recommend the topical use of such agents for more than 7 consecutive days, except under the advice and supervision of a primary care provider.[22]

Oral antihistamines have been used to treat the itching of dermatologic disorders with variable results. Some researchers claim that the antipruritic effect is a result of the sedative side effect; others claim the efficacy is caused by antihistaminic activity, although with a delayed onset of several days. If histamine is involved, it has already reached and stimulated the receptor sites to produce itching, and the antihistamine requires a finite amount of time to displace it. In either case, central nervous system depression may be a problem, as may the anticholinergic side effects in patients with conditions such as prostatic hypertrophy or closed-angle glaucoma.[10]

Product Selection Guidelines

When deciding which product to recommend for dermatitis or dry skin, the clinician must evaluate the active ingredients and the vehicle. Primary active ingredients contained in nonprescription skin products are water and oil. However, a variety of secondary ingredients are added to enhance product elegance and stability, and many of them have the potential to produce contact dermatitis through either an irritant or a sensitizing effect. These agents may include the following:

- *Emulsifiers:* cholesterol, magnesium aluminum silicate, polyoxyethylene lauryl ether, polyoxyethylene monostearate, polyoxyethylene sorbitan monolaurate (Tween), propylene glycol monostearate, sodium borate plus fatty acid, sodium lauryl sulfate, sorbitan monopalmitate (Span), or triethanolamine plus fatty acid
- *Emulsion stabilizers (thickening agents):* carbomer, cetyl alcohol, glyceryl monostearate, methylcellulose, spermaceti, or stearyl alcohol
- *Preservatives*

The type of vehicle (e.g., ointment, cream, lotion, gel, solution, or aerosol) may have a significant effect on dermatitis. The following guidelines may be used to choose an appropriate vehicle:

1. "*If it's wet, dry it.*" If a drying effect is desired, the practitioner may recommend solutions, gels, and occasionally creams. However, components of these systems may quickly diffuse into the underlying tissue and possibly cause irritation.
2. "*If it's dry, wet it.*" If slight lubrication is needed, creams and lotions are preferable. If the lesion is very dry and fissured, an ointment is the vehicle of choice. However, avoid use in intertriginous areas because of the potential for maceration. Also, in an acute process, the occlusive effects of an ointment may cause further irritation.

In recommending aerosols, gels, or lotions for dermatitis affecting a hair-covered area of the body, the practitioner must keep in mind that gels can be very drying when used for prolonged periods of time.

Numerous cosmetic dry skin formulations are available; they may contain natural oils, vitamins, or fragrances that have psychological appeal. However, the fragrances found in many formulations may be allergenic to sensitive, dry skin and should be avoided. Efficacy of any skin care product may need to be sacrificed or compromised somewhat to achieve patient acceptance. The practitioner should recommend the most efficacious product that the patient will accept.

Topical nonprescription products come in varying package sizes and strengths. Table 33-6 lists the amount of drug needed to cover a given area of the body three times daily over a 1-week

TABLE 33-6 Amount of Topical Medication Needed for Three Times Daily Application for 1 Week

Part of Body	Cream or Ointment (g)	Lotion, Solution, or Gel (mL)
Face	5–10	100–120
Both hands	25–50	200–240
Scalp	50–100	200–240
Both arms or both legs	100–200	240–360
Trunk	200	360–480
Groin and genitalia	15–25	120–180

Source: Adapted from Bingham EA. Topical dermatologic therapy. In: Rook A, Parish LC, Beare JM, eds. *Practical Management of the Dermatologic Patient.* Philadelphia: JB Lippincott; 1986: 2278.

period. By being aware of such details, the practitioner can serve the patient economically as well as therapeutically.

ASSESSMENT OF ATOPIC DERMATITIS AND DRY SKIN: A CASE-BASED APPROACH

Initially, the signs and symptoms are similar for most forms of dermatitis. A diagnosis of atopic dermatitis is often made after excluding other dermatologic conditions such as contact dermatitis (see Chapter 35) or scaly dermatoses (see Chapter 34). Because AD is primarily a disease of the young, patient age is important in assessment. The practitioner should determine whether the patient (or patient's family) has a history of atopic disorders. Inquiries should be made regarding onset and duration of the eruption, anatomic location, and distribution of the lesions (Table 33-1).

When recommending the use of an appropriate nonprescription product or referring the patient to a primary care provider, the practitioner must consider the cosmetic, psychological, and work- or recreation-related aspects of a dermatologic disorder, in addition to the underlying pathology

Dry skin is typically visible, with roughness and scaling. Practitioners can question patients about their bathing habits, the soaps and detergents used, and any other medical condition that may predispose them to excessive dryness. Patients should note that changes in climate can also affect their skin, such as winter air drying the skin, even though it may be raining.

Cases 33-1 and 33-2 are examples of the assessment of patients with AD or dry skin.

PATIENT COUNSELING FOR ATOPIC DERMATITIS AND DRY SKIN

Patients with atopic dermatitis should be educated on achieving control of their disease with proper information on the chronic nature of the disease, exacerbating factors, and appropriate treatment options.

CASE 33-1

Relevant Evaluation Criteria	Scenario/Model Outcome
Information Gathering	
1. Gather essential information about the patient's symptoms, including:	
a. description of symptom(s) (i.e., nature, onset, duration, severity, associated symptoms)	Patient has persistent itching on the neck and wrist areas, which has intensified during the past 6–9 months. The skin is dry and thickened, and plaques with slight hyperpigmentation are present in both locations.
b. description of any factors that seem to precipitate, exacerbate, and/or relieve the patient's symptom(s)	Symptoms seem to worsen during the winter months.
c. description of the patient's efforts to relieve the symptoms	Once daily use of Vaseline Intensive Care Lotion has not helped to date.
2. Gather essential patient history information:	
a. patient's identity	Anne Parker
b. patient's age, sex, height, and weight	3 1/2-year-old female, 41 inches
c. patient's occupation	None
d. patient's dietary habits	Normal childhood diet
e. patient's sleep habits	9–11 hours per night

CASE 33-1 *(continued)*

Relevant Evaluation Criteria	Scenario/Model Outcome
f. concurrent medical conditions, prescription and nonprescription medications, and dietary supplements	Singulair 5 mg once daily for mild chronic asthma
g. allergies	House dust
h. history of other adverse reactions to medications	None
i. other (describe) _____	The child's mother notes that Anne's skin has always seemed sensitive.

Assessment and Triage

3. Differentiate the patient's signs/symptoms and correctly identify the patient's primary problem(s).	Lesions associated with atopic dermatitis may vary with time and are likely to worsen with continued irritation from scratching.
4. Identify exclusions for self-treatment (see Figure 33-2).	If this child were younger than 2 years of age, any form of self-treatment would be avoided. Further evaluation should take place prior to using any pharmacologic agent on a chronic basis.
5. Formulate a comprehensive list of therapeutic alternatives for the primary problem to determine if triage to a medical practitioner is required, and share this information with the patient.	Options include: (1) Refer Anne to a PCP or dermatologist for a differential diagnosis. (2) Recommend an appropriate OTC product with nondrug measures. (3) Recommend an appropriate OTC product until Anne can be seen by a PCP or dermatologist. (4) Take no action.

Plan

6. Select an optimal therapeutic alternative to address the patient's problem, taking into account patient preferences.	See Figure 33-2. A topical emollient would be appropriate to recommend and should be applied 3–4 times daily to the lesions until Anne can be seen by her primary care provider or a dermatologist. An ointment would be ideal to use because the skin is especially dry, but a cream-based product may be preferred by the parent. The frequency of bathing should be minimized (no more than once daily) and moisturizer should be applied frequently.
7. Describe the recommended therapeutic approach to the patient.	N/A
8. Explain to the patient the rationale for selecting the recommended therapeutic approach from the considered therapeutic alternatives.	Because Anne is a child, it is important to have a definitive diagnosis prior to recommending any chronic treatment with any pharmacologic agent, such as hydrocortisone.

Patient Education

9. When recommending self-care with nonprescription medications and/or nondrug therapy, convey accurate information to the patient.	Encourage Anne not to scratch the lesions. See the box Patient Education for Atopic Dermatitis and Dry Skin for additional information that you can discuss with Anne's primary care provider or a dermatologist.
10. Solicit follow-up questions from parent.	Is there an OTC medication that might work?
11. Answer parent's questions.	No OTC medication is appropriate to recommend without a definite diagnosis from a primary care provider or dermatologist.

Key: N/A, not applicable; OTC, over-the-counter; PCP, primary care provider.

CASE 33-2

Relevant Evaluation Criteria	Scenario/Model Outcome

Information Gathering

1. Gather essential information about the patient's symptoms, including:

   a. description of symptom(s) (i.e., nature, onset, duration, severity, associated symptoms)

   Patient has pruritic, fine, scaly skin on the exterior surfaces of his lower legs. Significant flaking is observed when he removes his socks. Physical observation reveals no evidence of weeping, vesicles, or crusting.

   b. description of any factors that seem to precipitate, exacerbate, and/or relieve the patient's symptom(s)

   Symptoms are more bothersome in the winter months and have worsened as he has aged.

   c. description of the patient's efforts to relieve the symptoms

   Use of a store-brand lotion for dry skin on a sporadic basis has proven minimally effective.

2. Gather essential patient history information:

   a. patient's identity

   James Thayer

   b. patient's age, sex, height, and weight

   70-year-old male, 5 ft 10 in, 185 lb

   c. patient's occupation

   Retired postal worker

   d. patient's dietary habits

   Normal diet

   e. patient's sleep habits

   6–7 hours of sleep per night

   f. concurrent medical conditions, prescription and nonprescription medications, and dietary supplements

   Hydrochlorothiazide 25 mg once daily, diltiazem-CR 360 mg once daily for hypertension

   g. allergies

   None

   h. history of other adverse reactions to medications

   None

   i. other (describe) _____

   James takes daily, long hot showers. He lives in Minneapolis, Minnesota, and says that he does not have a humidifier in his house.

Assessment and Triage

3. Differentiate the patient's signs/symptoms and correctly identify the patient's primary problem(s).

   James has dry skin that is most likely due to environmental factors in combination with his advancing age.

4. Identify exclusions for self-treatment (see Figure 33-2).

   None

5. Formulate a comprehensive list of therapeutic alternatives for the primary problem to determine if triage to a medical practitioner is required, and share this information with the patient.

   Options include:
   (1) Refer James to a PCP or dermatologist.
   (2) Recommend appropriate OTC product(s) and nondrug measures.
   (3) Recommend appropriate OTC product(s) for use until James can be seen by a PCP.
   (4) Take no action.

Plan

6. Select an optimal therapeutic alternative to address the patient's problem, taking into account patient preferences.

   OTC treatment with a moisturizing cream will be appropriate for this patient. Use of a store-brand product is preferred by the patient owing to limited resources. If intense itching is troublesome, hydrocortisone 1% cream or ointment may be applied to the affected area 2–4 times daily in addition to emollients.
   See Table 33-3 for other information on dry skin therapy.

7. Describe the recommended therapeutic approach to the patient.

   See Table 33-3 and the box Patient Education for Atopic Dermatitis and Dry Skin.

8. Explain to the patient the rationale for selecting the recommended therapeutic approach from the considered therapeutic alternatives.

   Your condition should be easily managed with nonprescription topical therapy plus modification of your bathing habits.

C A S E   3 3 - 2   *(continued)*

Relevant Evaluation Criteria	Scenario/Model Outcome
Patient Education	
9. When recommending self-care with non-prescription medications and/or nondrug therapy, convey accurate information to the patient:	
a. appropriate dose and frequency of administration	See the box Patient Education for Atopic Dermatitis and Dry Skin.
b. maximum number of days the therapy should be employed	It is likely the emollient will need to be used chronically. Avoid daily prolonged use (>7 days) of topical hydrocortisone, if possible.
	See the box Patient Education for Atopic Dermatitis and Dry Skin.
c. product administration procedures	See the box Patient Education for Atopic Dermatitis and Dry Skin.
d. expected time to onset of relief	See the box Patient Education for Atopic Dermatitis and Dry Skin.
e. degree of relief that can be reasonably expected	See the box Patient Education for Atopic Dermatitis and Dry Skin.
f. most common side effects	See the box Patient Education for Atopic Dermatitis and Dry Skin.
g. side effects that warrant medical intervention should they occur	See the box Patient Education for Atopic Dermatitis and Dry Skin.
h. patient options in the event that condition worsens or persists	See the box Patient Education for Atopic Dermatitis and Dry Skin.
i. product storage requirements	See the box Patient Education for Atopic Dermatitis and Dry Skin.
j. specific nondrug measures	See the box Patient Education for Atopic Dermatitis and Dry Skin.
10. Solicit follow-up questions from patient.	Will putting Vaseline on my legs at bedtime produce better results than using a cream?
11. Answer patient's questions.	Yes, most likely. Ointments, such as Vaseline, do a better job of holding moisture in the skin than do creams or lotions. You may wish to wear high cotton stockings to prevent staining of your bed linens.

Key: OTC, over-the-counter; PCP, primary care provider.

Patients with dry skin should be informed that they have more control over mild-to-moderate forms of this disorder than most other types of dermatologic disorders. The practitioner should also explain factors that cause dry skin and the appropriate measures for restoring barrier function. The box Patient Education for Atopic Dermatitis and Dry Skin lists specific information to provide patients.

worsened (continued or additional itching, redness, scaling, lesions, or tissue breakdown), the patient should see a primary care provider.

EVALUATION OF PATIENT OUTCOMES FOR ATOPIC DERMATITIS AND DRY SKIN

The practitioner should reevaluate a patient with atopic dermatitis within 2 to 3 days of the patient's initial visit. A patient with dry skin should be reevaluated in 7 days.

Visual assessment is the best method of determining treatment response. Therefore, a scheduled visit is the preferred follow-up method. If the symptoms have not improved or have

KEY POINTS FOR ATOPIC DERMATITIS AND DRY SKIN

➤ Note that most patients with mild-to-moderate atopic dermatitis or dry skin are candidates for self-treatment with a combination of nonprescription and nonpharmacologic therapies.

➤ Refer patients with yellow, crusting, eczematous atopic dermatitis lesions and all children younger than 2 years with atopic dermatitis to a primary care provider or dermatologist for evaluation and treatment.

➤ Question patients presenting with dry or eczematous skin lesions about exposure to soaps, detergents, fragrances, chemicals, irritants, changes in temperature, allergens, and bathing.

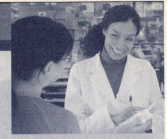

PATIENT EDUCATION FOR
Atopic Dermatitis and Dry Skin

The primary objectives of self-treating atopic dermatitis are to (1) relieve symptoms of itching and weeping and (2) avoid or minimize exposure to factors that trigger or aggravate the disorders. The primary objective in self-treating dry skin—restoring skin moisture and the skin's barrier function—can also help relieve the discomfort of atopic dermatitis. For most patients, carefully following product instructions and the self-care measures listed here will help ensure optimal therapeutic outcomes.

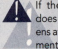 If the atopic dermatitis does not improve or worsens after 2–3 days of treatment, consult a primary care provider.

Atopic Dermatitis

Nondrug Measures

- Avoid factors that trigger allergic reactions. Do not wear occlusive, tight clothing. Remain in areas with a moderate temperature and low humidity.
- Bathe or shower every other day, if possible. Take short showers or baths, using warm (tepid) water and a nonsoap cleanser.
- If possible, substitute sponge baths with tepid water for full-body bathing.
- To dry weeping lesions, apply cool tap water compresses for 5–20 minutes, four to six times daily.
- To prevent injury to the affected area caused by scratching, keep your fingernails short, smooth, and clean. At night, wear cotton gloves or socks on your hands to lessen scratching.

Nonprescription Medications

- To decrease itching, bathe in tepid water that contains colloidal oatmeal, or add a water-miscible bath oil to the water near the end of the bath.
- Gently wash the affected areas with a nonsoap cleanser prior to applying any emollient or medication. Gently pat your skin dry, and apply an emollient within 3 minutes after washing while your skin is still damp.
- Wash hands before and after applying any medication.
- Apply a thin layer of medication over the affected areas.
- Apply hydrocortisone three to four times daily to dry weeping lesions and relieve itching. Do not use this medication for longer than 7 days.
- With proper use of medications and nondrug measures, noticeable improvement can be observed in 24–48 hours.
- Although complete eradication of the rash and itching is possible, it is likely that exacerbation may occasionally recur, especially during the winter and summer months.
- Atrophy of the skin while using hydrocortisone should be reported to a primary care provider.

Dry Skin

Nondrug Measures

- Avoid excessive bathing; take brief (3- to 5-minute) full-body baths two to three times per week, using bath oil and tepid, not hot, water.
- If possible, take sponge baths on other nights, using warm water to maintain skin hydration.
- Drink plenty of water daily. Do not substitute sodas, coffee, or tea for water.
- Copious quantities of moisturizer should be applied three to four times daily and continued as long as dry skin persists.
- Moisturizers should be applied within 3 minutes after bathing, plus an additional three times per day.
- Complete eradication of dry skin is unlikely, but significant symptomatic improvement should start to be observed within 24 hours.
- Avoid caffeine, spices, and alcohol as these can contribute to dehydration.
- Keep the room humidity higher than normal to minimize evaporation from the skin.

Nonprescription Medications

- Add products such as oilated oatmeal or bath oil near the end of your bath to enhance skin hydration. Colloidal oatmeal products, if used on a regular basis, may clog plumbing pipes and can leave the tub slick.
- Apply an oil-based emollient immediately after bathing while your skin is damp. Reapply the emollient frequently.
- For more severe cases of dry skin, use a product that contains urea or lactic acid.
- Apply topical hydrocortisone ointment to reduce inflammation and itching. Do not use this medication for longer than 7 days.

 If skin dryness worsens after 7 days of treatment, consult a primary care provider.

- ➤ Counsel patients with dry skin conditions to take brief baths, using tepid water, and apply moisturizers within 3 minutes of completing the bath or shower.
- ➤ Advise patients to use mild skin cleansers, to avoid products with fragrances or other potential irritants, and to apply copious quantities of moisturizers three to four times daily.
- ➤ Educate the patient with chronic dry skin conditions about the importance of stopping the itch–scratch cycle, maintaining adequate hydration, and avoiding triggers of the condition.
- ➤ Advise patients to use cream-based products, whenever possible, to maximize the hydrating properties of the product and compliance. Ointment-based products should be

recommended for patients not responding adequately to creams.
- ➤ Instruct patients how to properly apply topical emollients, and anti-inflammatory and antipruritic agents.
- ➤ Advise patients with self-treatable symptoms to contact their primary care provider if symptoms worsen or do not improve within 7 days.

REFERENCES

1. Kligman AM, Koblenzer C. Demographics and psychological implications for the aging population. *Dermatol Clin.* 1997;15:549–53.
2. MacKie RM. *Clinical Dermatology.* 4th ed. Oxford: Oxford University Press; 1997:3–4.

3. Micali G, Lacarrubba F, Bongu A, et al. The skin barrier. In: Freinkel R, Woodely D, eds. *The Biology of the Skin*. New York: Parthenon; 2001:227.

4. Micali G, West D. Poisoning and paediatric skin. In: Harper J, Oranje A, Prose N, eds. *Textbook of Pediatric Dermatology*. Oxford: Blackwell Scientific; 2000:1753–4.

5. Leung DY, Tharp M, Boguniewicz M. Atopic dermatitis. In: Freedberg IM, Eisen AZ, Wolff K, eds. *Fitzpatrick's Dermatology in General Medicine*. 7th ed. New York: McGraw-Hill, Inc; 2008:1464–80.

6. Thompson J, Avery M, Honeywell M, et al. Atopic dermatitis: a review of clinical management. *US Pharm*. April 2006: 89–96.

7. Abramovits WA. A clinician's paradigm in the treatment of atopic dermatitis. *J Am Acad Dermatol*. 2005; 53: S70–S77.

8. Leung DY, Hanifin JM, Charlesworth EN, et al. Disease management of atopic dermatitis: a practice parameter. Joint Task Force on Practice Parameters, representing the American Academy of Allergy, Asthma and Immunology, the American College of Allergy, Asthma and Immunology, and the Joint Council of Allergy, Asthma and Immunology, Work Group on Atopic Dermatitis. *Ann Allergy Asthma Immunol*. 1997;79:197–209.

9. Zhai H, Maibach HI. *Dermatoxicology*. 6th ed. Boca Raton, Fla: CRC Press; 2004:795–800.

10. Greaves MW. Antihistamines. In: Wolverton SE, ed. *Comprehensive Dermatologic Drug Therapy*. Philadelphia: WB Saunders; 2001:360–72.

11. Holden CA, Parish WE. In: Champion RH, Burton JL, Burns DA, et al., eds. *Textbook of Dermatology*. 6th ed. Oxford: Blackwell Scientific; 1998: 681–708.

12. Hanifin JM, Cooper KC, Ho CV, et al. Guidelines of care for atopic dermatitis. *J Am Acad Dermatol*. 2004;50:391–404.

13. White MI, McElwan-Jenkinson D, Lloyd DH. The effect of washing on the thickness of the stratum corneum in normal and atopic individuals. *Br J Dermatol*. 1987;116:525–30.

14. Schempp CM, Dittmar HC, Hummler D, et al. Magnesium ions inhibit the antigen-presenting function of human epidermal Langerhans cells in vivo and in vitro: involvement of ATPase, HLA-DR, B7 molecules, and cytokines. *J Invest Dermatol*. 2000;115:680–6.

15. Lazar AP, Lazar P. Dry skin, water, and lubrication. *Dermatol Clin*. 1991;9:45–51.

16. Kempers S, Katz HI, Wildnauer R, et al. An evaluation of the effect of an alpha-hydroxy acid-blend skin cream in the cosmetic improvement of symptoms of moderate to severe xerosis, epidermolytic hyperkeratosis, and ichthyosis. *Cutis*. 1998;61:347–50.

17. Shwayder T, Ott F. All about ichthyosis. *Pediatr Clin North Am*. 1991;38:835–57.

18. Draelos ZK. *Cosmetics in Dermatology*. 2nd ed. New York: Churchill-Livingstone; 1995.

19. Knutson K, Pershing LK. Topical drugs. In: Hendrickson, R, Beringer, P, Der Marderosian AH, et al., eds. *Remington: The Science and Practice of Pharmacy*. 21st ed. Philadelphia: Lippincott Williams & Wilkins; 2005: 1277–93.

20. Loden M, Maiback HI. *Dry Skin and Moisturizers: Chemistry and Function*. Boca Raton, Fla: CRC Press; 2006:323–8.

21. Jackson EM. AHA-type products proliferate in 1993. *Cosmet Dermatol*. 1993;6:22–4.

22. Gebhardt M, Elsner P, Marks JG. *Handbook of Contact Dermatitis*. Boca Raton, Fla: CRC Press; 2004:125–30.

Scaly Dermatoses

Steven A. Scott

Dandruff, seborrheic dermatitis (seborrhea), and psoriasis are chronic, scaly dermatoses. They may be placed on a spectrum ranging from dandruff (a less inflammatory form of seborrheic dermatosis with relatively fine scaling confined to the scalp), to seborrhea (inflammatory seborrheic dermatitis involving scalp, face, and trunk), to psoriasis (an inflammatory clinical condition with plaques and relatively adherent thick scales that can have profound physical, psychological, and economic consequences). These conditions involve the uppermost layer of skin, the epidermis.[1]

Nonprescription products are appropriate treatment for most cases of dandruff and seborrheic dermatitis. Mild psoriasis may be responsive to nonprescription treatment, but the initial diagnosis of psoriasis and the management of acute flare-ups require the attention of a primary care provider.[1]

DANDRUFF

Dandruff is a chronic, noninflammatory scalp condition that results in excessive scaling of the scalp. It is a substantial cosmetic concern and is associated with social stigma. This disorder represents the less inflammatory end of the seborrheic dermatitis spectrum. Authorities disagree over whether inadequate shampooing exacerbates dandruff; however, they agree that a consistent washing routine is important in managing the condition.[1,2]

Dandruff occurs in approximately 1% to 3% of the population.[3] Dandruff is uncommon in children and generally appears at puberty, reaches a peak in early adulthood, levels off in middle age, and is less prominent after 75 years of age.[1] There is no gender preference, and bald spots on males are typically dandruff-free. Dandruff is less severe during the summer.[1,2] The specific cause of accelerated cell growth seen in dandruff is unknown. Debate continues as to whether dandruff is a result of accelerated cell turnover or of elevated microorganism levels—particularly of *Pityrosporum* (a yeast-like fungus that is normal flora of the scalp).[4]

Pathophysiology of Dandruff

Dandruff is a hyperproliferative epidermal condition, characterized by an accelerated epidermal cell turnover (twice that of normal scalp[5]) and an irregular keratin breakup pattern, resulting in the shedding of large, nonadherent white scales. The horny layer of the scalp normally consists of 25 to 35 fully keratinized, closely coherent cells per square millimeter arranged in an orderly fashion. However, in dandruff, the intact horny layer has fewer than 10 normal cells per square millimeter, and nonkeratinized cells are common. With dandruff, crevices occur deep in the stratum corneum, resulting in cracking, which generates relatively large scales.[1] If the large scales are broken down to smaller units, the dandruff becomes less visible.

Clinical Presentation of Dandruff

Dandruff is diffuse rather than patchy and is minimally inflammatory. Scaling, the only visible manifestation of dandruff, is the result of an increased rate of horny substance production on the scalp and the sloughing of large white or gray scales. Pruritus, although not universal in all patients, is common. The crown of the head is often a prime location for formation of dandruff flakes.

Treatment of Dandruff
Treatment Goals

The goals of self-treating dandruff are to (1) reduce the epidermal turnover rate of the scalp skin, (2) minimize the cosmetic embarrassment of visible scaling, and (3) minimize itch.

General Treatment Approach

Washing the hair and scalp with a general-purpose nonmedicated shampoo every other day or daily is often sufficient to control mild-to-moderate dandruff. If it is not, the clinician may recommend medicated nonprescription antidandruff products.

With medicated shampoos, contact time is the key to effectiveness. The patient should massage the shampoo into the scalp

Editor's Note: This chapter is based on the 15th edition chapter with the same title, written by Robert W. Martin III and Steven A. Scott.

with a scalp scrubber, and leave the medicated shampoo on the hair for 5 minutes before rinsing and repeating. Medicated shampoos need to be used only two to three times weekly for 2 to 3 weeks, and then once weekly or every other week to control the condition. Thorough rinsing is important in the use of all shampoo products. It is the scalp, not the hair, that is being treated; therefore, use of a scalp scrubber will help ensure adequate contact of the medicated shampoo with the scalp.

A cytostatic agent (e.g., pyrithione zinc, selenium sulfide, or coal tar) is generally recommended initially. Such agents reduce scaling by decreasing the epidermal turnover rate. However, shampoos containing coal tar may tend to discolor light hair as well as clothing and jewelry, and may not appeal to some patients. A keratolytic shampoo, containing salicylic acid or sulfur, or a ketoconazole shampoo may also be used (see Treatment of Scaly Dermatoses). If dandruff proves resistant to these agents after 4 to 8 weeks of use, the patient should be referred to a primary care provider for treatment with products containing a higher concentration of selenium sulfide, ketoconazole, or coal tar.[1]

SEBORRHEIC DERMATITIS

Seborrheic dermatitis is a subacute or chronic inflammatory disorder that occurs predominantly in the areas of greatest sebaceous gland activity (e.g., scalp, face, and trunk).[6] Seborrheic dermatitis is a common chronic red, scaly, itchy rash with two age peaks of occurrence, one within the first 3 months of life and the second around the fourth to the seventh decade of life. Seborrheic dermatitis is common in infants and affects 2% to 5% of adults, more commonly men. There is no ethnic predilection. Seborrheic dermatitis is more severe in winter and is commonly found in people with parkinsonism, zinc deficiency, endocrine states associated with obesity, and human immunodeficiency virus (HIV) infection.

The cause of seborrheic dermatitis is unknown, although the lipophilic, pleomorphic fungus *Pityrosporon* has been proposed as contributing to seborrheic dermatitis. Emotional stress may serve as an aggravating factor.

Pathophysiology of Seborrheic Dermatitis

Seborrheic dermatitis is more inflammatory than dandruff and is marked by accelerated epidermal proliferation in areas with dense distribution of sebaceous glands.[7] Cell turnover rate for seborrheic dermatitis is 9 to 10 days compared with 13 to 15 days for dandruff.[1] The characteristic accelerated cell turnover and enhanced sebaceous gland activity give rise to the prominent scale displayed in the condition.

Clinical Presentation of Seborrheic Dermatitis

Seborrheic dermatitis occurs in the scalp, eyebrows, glabella, eyelid margins (often with conjunctivitis), cheeks, paranasal areas, nasolabial folds, beard area, presternal area, central back, retroauricular (behind the ear) creases, and in and about the external ear canal. The disorder typically presents as dull, yellowish, oily, scaly areas on red skin that are fairly well-demarcated. Pruritus is common.[8] In the axillae, inframammary, umbilicus, groin, and intergluteal cleft (i.e., intertriginous) areas, the lesions consist of bright erythema with or without fissures but are usually devoid of scale.

The infantile form occurs in the first months of life as greasy scales and scale crusts on a bright erythematous base, and affect the scalp (cradle cap), retroauricular creases, lateral neck, and intertriginous folds. Cradle cap usually clears without treatment by age 8 to 12 months (because of the gradual disappearance of hormones passed from the mother to the child before birth), after which the disease is rare until puberty.

The most common form in adults is seborrhea of the scalp, characterized by greasy scales on the scalp that often extend to the middle third of the face with subsequent eye involvement (see Color Plates, photograph 15). Asymptomatic, fluffy white dandruff of the scalp represents the mild end of the spectrum of seborrheic dermatitis. An oily type, at times accompanied by erythema and an accumulation of thick crusts, is also encountered. Other types of seborrheic dermatitis on the scalp are more severe and are manifested by greasy, scaling patches or plaques, exudation, and thick crusting.

On the face, flaky scales or yellowish scaling patches on red, itchy skin are seen in the eyebrows and glabella. The eyelid edges may be erythematous and granular (marginal blepharitis) with injected conjunctivae. In the nasolabial creases, there may be yellowish or reddish-yellow, scaling macules, sometimes with fissures. In men, folliculitis of the upper lip may occur. Red scaling, fissures, and swelling may be present in the ear canals, around the auditory meatus, in the postauricular region, or under the earlobe.

V-shaped areas of the chest and back and, less frequently, intertriginous areas such as the side of the neck, axillae, submammary region, umbilicus, and genitocrural folds may also be involved. In adults, the disease lasts for years to decades with periods of improvement in warmer seasons and periods of exacerbation in the colder months.

Treatment of Seborrheic Dermatitis

Treatment Goals

The goals of self-treatment of seborrheic dermatitis are to (1) reduce inflammation and the epidermal turnover rate of the scalp skin and (2) minimize or eliminate visible erythema and scaling.

General Treatment Approach

The treatment of seborrheic dermatitis is similar to that of dandruff. There is no way to cure seborrheic dermatitis. Patients should be informed about the chronic nature of the disease and understand that therapy works by controlling the disease rather than curing it. Therapy is directed toward loosening and removal of scales and crusts, inhibiting yeast colonization, controlling secondary infection, and reducing erythema and itching. When a medicated shampoo is used for treatment, patients should be instructed to work the shampoo into the scalp, and then leave the lather on the hair and affected areas for 3 to 5 minutes. Initially, the shampoo should be used two times per week for 4 weeks and then applied once a week when the condition is controlled. A double application of medicated shampoos and use of a scalp scrubber ensure penetration to the scalp.

In infants, seborrheic dermatitis is usually self-limited and treated primarily by gently massaging the scalp with baby oil, followed by the use of a nonmedicated shampoo to remove scales.[1,6,8] For more severe cases, crusts can be removed with salicylic acid 3% to 5% in olive oil or a water-soluble base and warm olive oil compresses, followed by gentle shampooing with a mild shampoo or a shampoo containing salicylic acid. Following shampooing, a low-potency nonprescription glucocorticoid (e.g., hydrocortisone 1%) in a cream or lotion may be tried for a few days in children 2 years of age and older. When the face is involved in infants, gentle washing with mild soap and application of a facial emollient are all that is necessary. The application of corticosteroids to an infant's face is to be avoided, unless its use is directed by a dermatologist, to avoid adverse reactions.

In adults, shampooing is the foundation of treatment. The scalp should be shampooed several times per week with shampoos containing pyrithione zinc, selenium sulfide, sulfur, ketoconazole, salicylic acid, or coal tar. If the odor of a medicated shampoo is objectionable, it can be followed by a more cosmetically acceptable shampoo/conditioner. A regular nonmedicated shampoo or liquid dishwashing soap (e.g., Dawn) can be used to soften and remove crusts or scales.[9]

Seborrheic dermatitis involving the ears can be treated with a medicated shampoo during a bath or shower followed by application of an emollient and hydrocortisone 0.5% to 1.0% cream. Adult patients should avoid greasy ointments and pre- or aftershave lotions containing alcohol, and reduce the use of soaps.

The primary difference between the treatment of dandruff and that of seborrheic dermatitis is the frequency of topical corticosteroid use. Such products may be used to manage seborrheic dermatitis whenever erythema is persistent after therapy with medicated shampoos or creams. Hydrocortisone should be applied two to three times a day until symptoms subside, and then intermittently to control acute exacerbations. Lotions are preferred for hairy areas, and care should be taken to prevent any corticosteroid from being used on eyelids or entering the eyes. The hair should be parted, and the product applied directly to the scalp and massaged in thoroughly. The patient should repeat this process until desired coverage of the affected area is achieved. The absorption of medication into the scalp is enhanced by applying the lotion after shampooing; skin hydration promotes drug absorption. Shampooing removes natural body oils, which also allows for better medication penetration.

Use of nonprescription hydrocortisone should not exceed 7 days. If the condition worsens or symptoms persist longer than 7 days, a primary care provider should be consulted. A more potent topical corticosteroid may be indicated.[5]

PSORIASIS

Psoriasis is a chronic inflammatory disease estimated to afflict 1% to 3% of Americans.[10] Lesions are often localized, but they may become generalized over much of the body surface, resulting in disability caused by deformities that impair use of the hands and feet.[11] Remissions and exacerbations are unpredictable. Approximately 30% of people with psoriasis find that lesion involvement clears spontaneously.[10] Unrelenting generalized psoriasis may cause enough psychological distress to adversely affect the patient's quality of life. Psoriatic arthritis may result in joint deformity and, in some cases, disability.[12] Treatment of severe psoriasis can also produce a significant physical and economic burden.[13]

The incidence of psoriasis is distributed almost equally among men and women. Psoriasis is seen in all races and geographic regions, but the incidence is lower among people living in countries close to the equator and among blacks, Native Americans, and Asians.[10,13,14]

Psoriasis may be categorized into two types. Patients with type I disease typically present at an early age, have a strong family history of the disorder (36% of patients have relatives with psoriasis, but the mode of inheritance is not clear), and have a higher frequency of human lymphocyte antigen. In contrast, type II psoriasis develops in the later decades of life and does not show a high incidence of family history.

The cause of psoriasis is unknown. However, the onset of psoriasis can be triggered by:

- Environmental factors such as physical, ultraviolet (UV), and chemical injury.
- Various infections (streptococcal infections, but also acute viral infections and HIV infections).
- Prescription drug use (e.g., beta-blockers, lithium, antimalarials, indomethacin, and quinidine) and withdrawal of systemic corticosteroids.
- Psychological stress.
- Endocrine/hormonal changes.
- Obesity.
- Use of alcohol and tobacco.

There is a distinct tendency for improvement or even temporary disappearance during pregnancy. After childbirth, there is a tendency for exacerbation of lesions. During menopause, lesions may change for better or worse, with no set pattern of behavior. Hot weather and sunlight exposure improve the lesions in many patients.[13]

Pathophysiology of Psoriasis

Accelerated epidermal proliferation leading to excessive scaling is one hallmark symptom of psoriasis. Normal epidermal cell turnover is 25 to 30 days, whereas it is approximately 4 days in a psoriatic plaque. The duration of psoriasis is variable, and lesions may last a lifetime or disappear quickly. When lesions disappear, they may leave the skin either hypopigmented or hyperpigmented. The disease course is marked by spontaneous exacerbations and remissions, and it tends to be chronic and relapsing.[13]

Clinical Presentation of Psoriasis

There are several clinical forms of psoriasis including plaque, inverse, guttate, pustular, and erythrodermic. Regardless of the clinical form, psoriasis is usually symmetrical, with minimal itching.

Plaque psoriasis is by far the most common form, occurring in about 90% of patients. Lesions start as small papules that grow and unite to form plaques. These lesions are well-circumscribed, sharply demarcated, light pink to bright red or maroon plaques, with overlying opaque, thick, adherent, white scale that can be pulled off in layers (see Color Plates, photographs 16A, B, and C). This typical feature has been likened to the mineral mica and descriptively termed *micaceous scale*. When scale is lifted from the base of the plaque, punctate bleeding points sometimes occur at the sites of scale removal (Auspitz sign). The most common locations are the extensor surfaces of the elbow and knees, the lumbar region of the back, the scalp, the posterior auricular area, the external auditory canal, and the glans penis.

Inverse or flexural psoriasis involves folds, recesses, and flexor surfaces: ears, axillae, groin, inframammary folds, navel, intergluteal crease, glans penis, lips and, above all, the palms, soles, and nails.

Guttate (drop-like) psoriasis is characterized by the rapid onset of "crops" of uniformly sized, scattered papules with light pink, flaking scale on the trunk and proximal extremities. This form of psoriasis is often seen in adolescents. In patients with chronic, persistent plaque-type psoriasis, guttate psoriasis is a sign of an acute exacerbation. Guttate psoriasis arises very rapidly but responds to antibiotic treatment and ultraviolet light therapies better than psoriatic lesions that have a longer onset.[13,15] Pustular psoriasis is either localized to hands or widespread over the entire body.

Treatment of Psoriasis

Treatment Goals

The goals of self-treatment of psoriasis are to (1) control or eliminate the signs and symptoms (inflammation, scaling, and itching) and (2) prevent or minimize the likelihood of flares.

General Treatment Approach

The Food and Drug Administration (FDA) recommends that only mild cases of psoriasis be self-treated. Individuals with moderate-to-severe cases, involving more than 10% of body surface area, should be treated by a primary care provider.[2] Furthermore, recalcitrant cases (cases not responding to emollients and nonprescription strengths of hydrocortisone) or cases in children younger than 2 years should be referred to a primary care provider for evaluation.

Numerous nondrug measures can be used by patients in the treatment of psoriasis. However, it is unlikely that these measures alone will control the signs and symptoms of the disorder. Patients should avoid psychological stress, as well as physical, UV, and chemical injury of the skin. Overweight patients should be encouraged to lose weight, smoking should be stopped, and alcohol consumption should be discouraged. Patients with psoriasis should be encouraged to bathe with lubricating bath products two to three times per week using tepid water. Scales can be removed by gently rubbing with a soft cloth. Emollients should be applied to the lesions within 3 minutes of bathing.

The selection of the most effective but appropriate therapy depends on the site, severity, duration, previous treatment, and age of the patient. Treatment may be topical, systemic, or a combination of both. The treatment selected will be more accepted if the patient and/or the parent/guardian are educated about the nature of psoriasis and the alternatives available for treatment.

Factors in determining appropriate therapy include the morphologic type of psoriasis, extent, age, cost, and ability of the patient to comply with the regimen. Topical treatment of psoriasis is usually the first line of therapy. Pruritic dry skin is common in psoriasis, and emollients and lubricating bath products often provide relief for these symptoms (see Chapter 33). Daily lubrication of the skin after a bath or shower is an essential part of therapy. Emollients moisturize, lubricate, and soothe dry and flaky skin, as well as reduce fissure formation within plaques and help maintain flexibility of the surrounding skin. To be effective, they need to be applied liberally, four to six times daily. Gentle rubbing of affected areas with a soft cloth following the bath helps to mechanically remove scales. Depending on the anatomic site, self-treatment may progress to the use of topical hydrocortisone, coal tar products, and/or keratolytic agents such as salicylic acid.[2] The patient should avoid vigorous rubbing, which can aggravate the lesions.

Acute localized flares, characterized by bright red lesions, call for soothing local therapy with emollients and hydrocortisone. Tars, salicylic acid, and aggressive UV radiation therapy at this stage may exacerbate the disease. After the flare has subsided and the usual thick-scaled plaques appear, the patient may use agents such as keratolytics. Many patients respond well to simple measures, whereas others have disease that is refractory even to aggressive treatments.[5]

In many cases, psoriasis will not be controlled by nonprescription treatment, and a dermatologic referral from the clinician will be necessary. Prescription topical agents such as calcipotriol, topical retinoids (tazarotene), and anthralin are effective. For severe or recalcitrant psoriasis, systemic agents may be necessary. These include oral retinoids (acitretin), methotrexate, cyclosporine, and the newer biologicals (alefacept, efalizumab, etanercept, and infliximab). Phototherapy with narrow-band ultraviolet B radiation or PUVA, ultraviolet A (UVA) radiation in combination with methoxsalen (a chemical photosensitizing psoralen [P]) is also a treatment option available in many dermatologists' offices.

Scalp psoriasis can be treated with tar-based and salicylic acid–based nonprescription shampoos. Again, sufficient contact time is the key to successful therapy, the goal of which is scale removal. In addition, although hydrocortisone 1% products may be used for scalp itching and mild lesional skin involvement, widespread involvement and involvement of the face dictate that the patient be treated by a dermatologist for more effective prescription medications. If a nonprescription product is used, the clinician should counsel the patient to consult a primary care provider if the condition does not improve in 7 days, or if it worsens.

Agents such as coal tar and salicylic acid should be used with extreme caution, if at all, to treat psoriasis in intertriginous areas (e.g., armpits and genital/anal region). Instead, hydrocortisone cream may be applied sparingly two or three times a day for up to 2 weeks and should be used less often as improvement occurs.

Salicylic acid products, which are most useful if thick scales are present, may be more cosmetically acceptable than coal tar products to some patients and may encourage compliance. Soaking the affected area in warm (not hot) water for 10 to 20 minutes before applying a salicylic acid product enhances keratolytic activity.

Coal tar products may be applied to the body, arms, and legs, preferably at bedtime. Because coal tar stains most materials, the patient should be advised to use bed linen and clothing for which staining would not present a problem. Overnight application is followed by a bath in the morning to remove residual coal tar and loosen psoriatic scales. Patients using coal tar preparations should avoid sun exposure for 24 hours after application. Topical hydrocortisone 1% ointment for the body may be applied sparingly to lesions and massaged into the skin thoroughly but gently (see Treatment of Scaly Dermatoses).

Psoriasis cannot be cured, but signs and symptoms can usually be controlled adequately with appropriate patient education and treatment, and remissions do occur. The patient should be reassured that, in most cases, control is possible. Such reassurance increases compliance with burdensome and prolonged treatment regimens. Also, if the practitioner can help the patient gain some understanding and acceptance of the condition, that knowledge may reduce the patient's emotional stress and psychogenic exacerbations. Prevention of flares, which can be achieved by minimizing identified precipitating factors such as emotional stress, skin irritation, and physical trauma, should be emphasized.

TREATMENT OF SCALY DERMATOSES

Cytostatic agents and keratolytic agents, usually in the form of medicated shampoos, are used to reduce epidermal turnover rate. Ketoconazole, an antifungal agent, is used in self-treatment of seborrheic dermatitis and dandruff. Hydrocortisone controls the inflammation associated with seborrheic dermatitis and psoriasis. Table 34-1 summarizes the concentrations and indications of currently approved agents, and the algorithm in Figure 34-1 outlines self-treatment with these agents.

Patients should shampoo with a nonmedicated, nonresidue shampoo to remove scalp and hair dirt, oil, and scale before using a medicated shampoo. Many shampoos leave a residue on the hair shaft and scalp that may aggravate scaly dermatoses of the scalp. Nonresidue shampoos (e.g., Prell or Johnson's Baby Shampoo) do not interfere with these scalp conditions, but rather leave the scalp clean and receptive to optimal effects from medicated shampoos. A nonresidue shampoo application and rinse may be followed by a medicated shampoo left on the scalp for the labeled length of time. The patient can use this treatment as often as daily until symptoms are relieved, then two to three times weekly or as needed.[5]

TABLE 34-1 Concentrations of Approved Nonprescription Ingredients for Products Used to Treat Scaly Dermatoses

	Concentration (%)		
Ingredient	**Dandruff**	**Seborrheic Dermatitis**	**Psoriasis**
Coal tar	0.5–5.0	0.5–5.0	0.5–5.0
Ketoconazole	1	1	1
Pyrithione zinc (brief exposure)	0.3–2.0	0.95–2.0	2.0
Pyrithione zinc (residual)	0.1–0.25	0.1–0.25	0.25
Salicylic acid	1.8–3	1.8–3.0	1.8–3.0
Selenium sulfide	1	1	1
Sulfur	2–5	2–5	
Hydrocortisone		0.5–1.0	0.5–1.0

Source: Reference 11.

Cytostatic Agents

Although their mechanism of action is not completely understood, topical cytostatic agents are known to decrease the rate of epidermal cell replication. This action increases the time required for epidermal cell turnover, which, in turn, allows the possibility of normalizing epidermal differentiation, resulting in a dramatic decline in visible scales. Therefore, use of products containing cytostatic agents (Table 34-2) represents a direct approach to controlling dandruff and seborrheic dermatitis.

Pyrithione Zinc

Pyrithione zinc's mechanism of action is likely caused by a nonspecific toxicity for epidermal cells. The pyrithione moiety is apparently the active part of the molecule. Product effectiveness is influenced by several factors. Pyrithione zinc is strongly bound to both hair and the external skin layers, and the extent of binding correlates with clinical performance. The drug's absorption increases with contact time, temperature, concentration, and frequency of application. Some researchers consider pyrithione zinc to be slower acting than selenium sulfide.[2]

For pyrithione zinc products intended to be applied and washed off within minutes, FDA allows concentrations of 0.3% to 2.0% for treating dandruff and 0.95% to 2.0% for treating seborrheic dermatitis. Concentrations for products intended to be applied and then left on the skin or scalp are 0.1% to 0.25% for treating both dandruff and seborrheic dermatitis.[7] Shampoos and soaps are currently available in 1% and 2% concentrations. Long-term use of pyrithione zinc 1% to 2% rinse-away products has rarely been associated with toxicity. Rare cases of contact dermatitis have been reported with use of this agent on broken or abraded skin.[4]

Selenium Sulfide

Selenium sulfide is believed to have a direct antimitotic effect on epidermal cells.[4] Like pyrithione zinc, it is more effective with longer contact time and therefore should be applied in a similar manner.[4] The product must be rinsed from the hair thoroughly or discoloration may result, especially in blond, gray, or dyed hair. Frequent use of selenium sulfide tends to leave a residual odor and an oily scalp.

Selenium sulfide has been approved in a 1% concentration as an active ingredient in nonprescription products to treat dandruff and seborrhea.[16] A higher concentration is available by prescription for use in resistant cases.

Irritation from selenium sulfide is minimal. Contact with the eyelids should be avoided because of the potential for eye irritation. If such contact does occur, the patient should flush the eyes with copious amounts of water. Selenium sulfide is toxic if ingested. Because of the risk of systemic toxicity, it should be applied to only intact skin.

Coal Tar

Coal tar products have long been popular for treating dandruff, seborrheic dermatitis, and psoriasis. Many nonprescription products are available.

Crude coal tar 1% to 5% and UV radiation therapy have been used to treat psoriasis since 1925 in a method known as the Goeckerman treatment. A therapeutic benefit has been

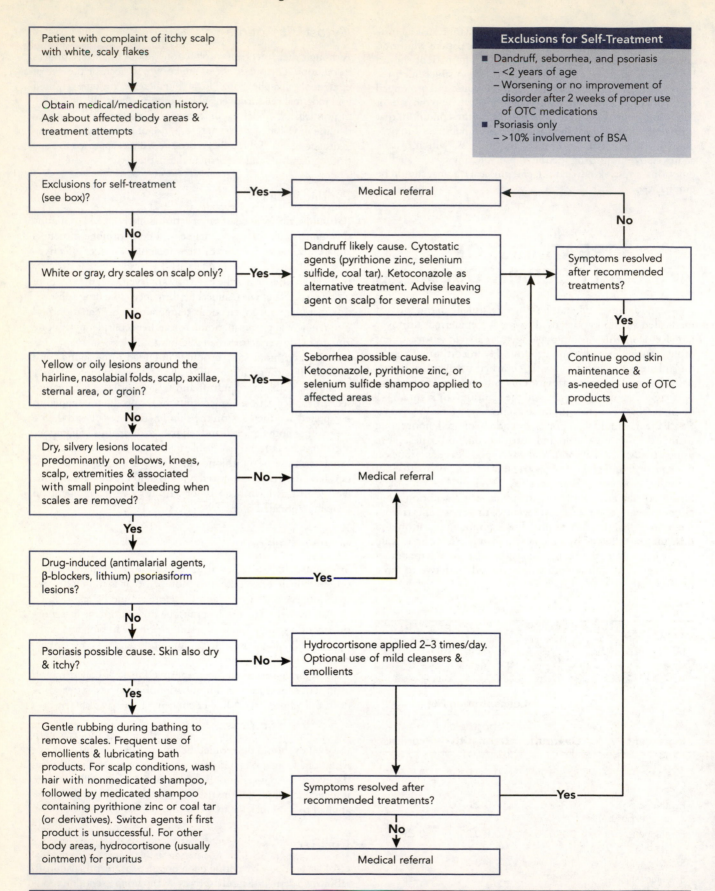

FIGURE 34-1 Self-care of scaly dermatoses. Key: BSA, body surface area; OTC, over-the-counter.

TABLE 34-2 Cytostatic Products for Scaly Dermatoses

Trade Name	Primary Ingredients
Balnetar Bath Oil	Coal tar 2.5% in mineral oil
Denorex Everyday Shampoo	Pyrithione zinc 2%
DHS Tar Shampoo	Coal tar 0.5%
DHS Tar Gel Shampoo	Coal tar 0.5%
DHS Zinc Shampoo	Pyrithione zinc 2%
Head & Shoulders Dandruff Shampoo	Pyrithione zinc 1%
Head & Shoulders Intensive Treatment Shampoo	Selenium sulfide 1%
Ionil T Plus Shampoo	Coal tar 2%
MG217 Medicated Tar Lotion	Coal tar solution 5%
MG217 Medicated Tar Ointment	Coal tar solution 10%
MG217 Medicated Tar Shampoo	Coal tar solution 15%
Neutrogena T/Derm Body Oil	Tar 5% (equivalent to coal tar 1.2%)
Neutrogena T/Gel Extra Strength Therapeutic Shampoo	Tar 4% (equivalent to coal tar 1%)
Neutrogena T/Gel Shampoo	Tar 2% (equivalent to coal tar 0.5%)
Nizoral AD Shampoo	Ketoconazole 1%
Pentrax Shampoo	Coal tar extract 5%
Polytar Shampoo	Tar 4.5% (equivalent to coal tar 0.5%)
Polytar Cleansing Bar	Tar 2.5% (equivalent to coal tar 0.5%)
P&S Plus Gel	Coal tar solution 8%; salicylic acid 2%
Sebulon Shampoo	Pyrithione zinc 2%
Sebutone Shampoo	Coal tar 0.5%; sulfur 2%; salicylic acid 2%
Selsun Blue Medicated Treatment Shampoo	Selenium sulfide 1%
X-Seb Plus Shampoo	Pyrithione zinc 1%; salicylic acid 2%
X-Seb T Shampoo	Coal tar solution 10%; salicylic acid 4%
X-Seb T Plus Shampoo	Coal tar solution 10%; salicylic acid 3%; menthol 1%
Zincon Shampoo	Pyrithione zinc 1%
ZNP Cleansing Bar	Pyrithione zinc 2%

demonstrated for both the tar alone and the irradiation alone, but the combination is more effective than either agent by itself. Rare remissions lasting up to 12 months have been reported after 2 to 4 weeks of therapy.

For many years, the therapeutic response to this form of therapy was believed to be caused solely by its phototoxicity. Now it is believed that the beneficial effect of coal tar lies primarily in its ability to cross-link with DNA.[4]

Coal tar is available in creams, ointments, pastes, lotions, bath oils, shampoos, soaps, and gels. This variety of dosage forms is partly a result of an attempt to develop a cosmetically acceptable product, one that masks the odor, color, and staining properties of crude coal tar that most patients find esthetically unappealing. Liquor carbonis detergens is a tincture of coal tar 20% that has been useful in developing acceptable tar products. It is used in concentrations of 3% to 15%.

Tar gels represent a special product that appears to deliver the beneficial elements of crude coal tar in a form both convenient to apply and cosmetically acceptable. These gels are nongreasy, nonstaining, and nearly colorless. Many of these gels may have a drying effect on the skin, however, necessitating the use of an emollient.

Side effects are associated with the use of coal tar, including folliculitis (particularly of the axilla and groins); stains to the skin and hair (particularly blond, gray, and dyed hair); photosensitization; and irritant contact dermatitis.[2] Rarely, the disorder may worsen on exposure to coal tar products. This situation is of particular concern in the acute phase of psoriasis, when topical corticosteroids are recommended to reduce inflammation before coal tar preparations are used.

Coal tar contains known human carcinogens. However, because of the relatively short contact time and therefore the low lifetime exposure, FDA considers the benefits of coal tar to outweigh the risks for use in topical formulations. Therefore, coal tar is available in concentrations of 0.5% to 5% for the self-treatment of scalp conditions such as dandruff, seborrheic dermatitis, and psoriasis.[16]

Keratolytic Agents

The keratolytic agents salicylic acid and sulfur are used in dandruff and seborrheic dermatitis products to loosen and lyse keratin aggregates, thereby facilitating their removal from the scalp in smaller particles. These agents act by dissolving the "cement" that holds epidermal cells together. Vehicle composition, contact time, and concentration are important factors in the success of a keratolytic agent. The keratolytic concentrations in nonprescription scalp products (Table 34–3) are not sufficient

TABLE 34-3 Selected Keratolytic Products for Scaly Dermatoses	
Trade Name	**Primary Ingredients**
MG217 Medicated Tar-Free Shampoo	Salicylic acid 3%; sulfur 5%
Neutrogena Healthy Scalp Anti-Dandruff Shampoo	Salicylic acid 1.8%
Neutrogena T/Sal Maximum Strength Therapeutic Shampoo	Salicylic acid 3%, coal tar extract 2%
Scalpicin Maximum Strength Foam/Solution	Salicylic acid 3%; menthol
Sebucare Lotion	Salicylic acid 1.8%
Sebulex Conditioning Shampoo with Protein	Salicylic acid 2%; sulfur 2%
Sulfoam Medicated Antidandruff Shampoo	Sulfur 2%
Sulray Cleansing Bar	Sulfur 5%
Sulray Dandruff Shampoo	Sulfur 2%
X-Seb Shampoo	Salicylic acid 4%

to impair the normal skin barrier, but do affect the abnormal, incompletely keratinized stratum corneum.

Keratolytic agents may produce several adverse effects, and patients should be counseled accordingly. These agents have a primary, concentration-dependent irritant effect, particularly on mucous membranes and the conjunctiva of the eye. They also have the potential of acting on hair and skin keratin; therefore, extended use may alter hair appearance. The directions and precautions for the use of keratolytic shampoos are similar to those for shampoos containing cytostatic agents.

Salicylic Acid

Salicylic acid decreases skin pH, which causes increased hydration of keratin and therefore facilitates its loosening and removal. Because contact time is minimal for a shampoo, percutaneous absorption of the agent is minimal.[4]

Topical salicylic acid is useful for psoriasis when thick scales are present. However, application over extensive areas should be avoided because of the potential for percutaneous absorption and systemic toxicity, as evidenced by symptoms of salicylism such as tinnitus.

Salicylic acid has been approved in concentrations of 1.8% to 3% for the self-treatment of dandruff, seborrheic dermatitis, and psoriasis.[16] At these concentrations, the keratolytic effect typically takes 7 to 10 days. In higher concentrations for other uses, the keratolytic effect may be evident in 2 to 3 days.

Sulfur

Sulfur is believed to cause increased sloughing of cells and to reduce corneocyte counts. Sulfur has been approved in concentrations of 2% to 5% for the self-treatment of dandruff only. Although it is approved as a single-entity active ingredient, sulfur is often combined with salicylic acid.[16] Although not an FDA-

approved indication, this combination has been commonly used for the self-treatment of seborrheic dermatitis.[6]

Topical Hydrocortisone

Topical hydrocortisone 0.5% and 1% is available without a prescription and is FDA-approved for the temporary relief of itching associated with minor skin irritations, inflammation, and rashes caused by eczema, psoriasis, seborrheic dermatitis, poison ivy/oak/sumac dermatitis, insect bites, soaps, detergents, cosmetics, and jewelry, and for external feminine and anal itching. It is not indicated, nor is evidence available that it is effective in treating dandruff. However, it may be useful for seborrhea accompanied by inflammation that is unresponsive to medicated shampoos.[6]

Nonprescription hydrocortisone products can play a role in managing mild psoriasis. Relapse occurs more quickly after use of topical corticosteroids than after use of tar therapy. Nevertheless, corticosteroids are more appealing to patients on cosmetic grounds, which is a consideration in long-term therapy.[13]

Topical corticosteroids have several effects (e.g., anti-inflammatory, antimitotic/antisynthetic, antipruritic, vasoconstrictive, and immunosuppressive) on cellular activity. Efficacy may be enhanced by using the ointment dosage form and an occlusive dressing (cover with plastic wrap for 12–24 hours). If the patient does not respond adequately to hydrocortisone, referral to a primary care provider is appropriate; the use of more potent corticosteroids may be in order.

Adverse effects associated with the use of topical corticosteroids include local atrophy after prolonged use, as well as the aggravation of certain cutaneous infections. The possibility of systemic sequelae exists and is enhanced by the use of the more potent compounds, by occlusive dressings, or by application to large areas of the body. Because children have a greater ratio of surface area to body mass, they are at greater risk for developing systemic complications. In general, however, the concentrations of hydrocortisone available in nonprescription preparations are highly unlikely to cause systemic sequelae.

Other Agents

Ketoconazole

Ketoconazole, a synthetic azole antifungal agent, is available as a nonprescription shampoo formulation. Nizoral AD (ketoconazole 1%) is active against most pathogenic fungi but is indicated specifically for *Pityrosporon yeast*. Therefore, it is used to treat dandruff and seborrheic dermatitis of the scalp. Although the fungal etiology of dandruff and seborrhea has been debated in the past, the efficacy of newer antifungal agents against these conditions has resulted in an FDA OTC review panel endorsing these agents for treatment of these two common skin disorders. In addition to ketoconazole shampoo, other antifungals such as miconazole (cream or solution) have been used to treat seborrheic dermatitis of areas other than the scalp.

As with other medicated shampoos, contact time is crucial. The scalp and hair should be wet; then the shampoo should be massaged well into the scalp and left on for 3 to 5 minutes. The scalp and hair should be thoroughly rinsed and the process repeated. The patient should use ketoconazole shampoo twice a week for 4 weeks, with at least 3 days between each treat-

TABLE 34-4 Distinguishing Features of Scaly Dermatoses

	Dandruff	Seborrheic Dermatitis	Psoriasis
Location	Scalp	Adults and children: head and trunk; children only: back, intertriginous areas	Scalp, elbows, knees, trunk, lower extremities
Exacerbating factors	Generally a stable condition, exacerbated by dry climate	Exacerbated by many external factors, notably stress	Exacerbated by irritation, stress, climate, medications, infection, endocrine factors
Appearance	Thin, white, or grayish flakes; even distribution on scalp	Macules, patches, and thin plaques of discrete yellow, oily scales on red skin	Discreet symmetrical, red plaques with sharp border; silvery white scale; small bleeding points when removed; difficult to distinguish from seborrhea in early stages or in intertriginous zones
Inflammation	Absent	Present	Present
Epidermal hyperplasia	Absent	Present	Present
Epidermal kinetics	Turnover rate 2 times faster than normal	Turnover rate about 3 times faster than normal	Turnover rate about 5–6 times faster than normal
Percentage of incompletely keratinized cells	Rarely exceeds 5% of total corneocyte count	Commonly makes up 15%–25% of corneocyte count	Commonly makes up 40%–60% of corneocyte count

Source: Adapted from reference 3 and McGinley KJ, Marples RR, Plewig G, et al. A method for visualizing and quantitating the desquamating portion of the human stratum corneum. *J Invest Dermatol.* 1969;53:107.

ment. Once the condition is controlled, the shampoo can be applied once weekly or once every other week. Adverse effects associated with ketoconazole are minimal, but hair loss, skin irritation, abnormal hair texture, and dry skin have been reported.

other symptoms or the location of the dermatitis provides additional important clues to its assessment. Factors that precipitate or exacerbate the disorder are also helpful in defining the disorder. Table 34-4 describes the distinguishing features of these three dermatoses.

Cases 34-1 and 34-2 illustrate the assessment of patients with scaly dermatoses.

ASSESSMENT OF SCALY DERMATOSES: A CASE-BASED APPROACH

Differentiation of the scaly dermatoses involves several factors. The appearance of the scales in the early stages of a disorder is not always definitive. In these cases, the presence and nature of

PATIENT COUNSELING FOR SCALY DERMATOSES

Patients need to know that scaly dermatoses are rarely cured by pharmacotherapy; rather, nonprescription agents help control

C A S E   3 4 - 1

Relevant Evaluation Criteria	Scenario/Model Outcome
Information Gathering	
1. Gather essential information about the patient's symptoms, including:	
a. description of symptom(s) (i.e., nature, onset, duration, severity, associated symptoms)	Patient has had mild dandruff since adolescence but now complains of yellow, oily scales along his hairline and around his nose and mouth. Some minor erythema is also present in these areas.

Relevant Evaluation Criteria	Scenario/Model Outcome
b. description of any factors that seem to precipitate, exacerbate, and/or relieve the patient's symptom(s)	The condition has grown worse since he moved from Houston to Chicago 6 months ago.
c. description of the patient's efforts to relieve the symptoms	Routine facial hygiene with hand soap has not proven beneficial. Dandruff is generally controlled with Head and Shoulders shampoo.
2. Gather essential patient history information:	
a. patient's identity	Aaron Smith
b. patient's age, sex, height, and weight	27-year-old male, 5 ft 11 in, 175 lb
c. patient's occupation	Commodities trader
d. patient's dietary habits	Normal healthy diet with occasional junk food
e. patient's sleep habits	6–7 hours per night (more on the weekend)
f. concurrent medical conditions, prescription and nonprescription medications, and dietary supplements	He takes a vitamin pack from the health food store on a daily basis.
g. allergies	NKA
h. history of other adverse reactions to medications	None
i. other (describe) _____	N/A

Assessment and Triage

3. Differentiate the patient's signs/symptoms and correctly identify the patient's primary problem(s) (see Table 34-4).	Aaron appears to have seborrheic dermatitis on his face. His scalp should be examined closely to differentiate dandruff (dry flakes) from seborrheic dermatitis (oily flakes).
4. Identify exclusions for self-treatment (see Figure 34-1).	None
5. Formulate a comprehensive list of therapeutic alternatives for the primary problem to determine if triage to a medical practitioner is required, and share this information with the patient.	Options include: (1) Recommend self-care with an appropriate OTC product and nondrug measures. (2) Recommend self-care with an appropriate OTC product and nondrug measures until a PCP or dermatologist can be consulted. (3) Refer Aaron to a PCP or dermatologist. (4) Take no action.

Plan

6. Select an optimal therapeutic alternative to address the patient's problem, taking into account patient preferences.	OTC treatment with Head and Shoulders shampoo (pyrithione zinc) can be used initially, if the patient would like to use a product on hand or if cost is a factor. Use of Nizoral AD (ketoconazole) is a good alternative agent to recommend if the patient would prefer to use an alternative product. A mild, fragrance-free soap should be used on the face. Hydrocortisone cream 1% should be applied to affected areas of the face and scalp if the redness does not respond to the medicated shampoo.
7. Describe the recommended therapeutic approach to the patient.	Apply the medicated shampoo to the scalp and affected areas of the face twice a week (at least 3 days between applications) for the next 4 weeks. Once the condition is controlled, the shampoo can be applied once a week. If hydrocortisone cream is applied to the face, it should be applied 2–3 times daily for 7 days.
8. Explain to the patient the rationale for selecting the recommended therapeutic approach from the considered therapeutic alternatives.	You may use the Head and Shoulders shampoo or the Nizoral AD shampoo according to personal preference and cost. Because pyrithione zinc has worked for you in the past, it may prove useful in this case as well. Avoid selenium products; they can increase oiliness of the scalp and face. We will not consider a coal tar shampoo because you find the odor objectionable.

C A S E   3 4 - 1   (continued)

Relevant Evaluation Criteria	Scenario/Model Outcome
Patient Education	
9. When recommending self-care with non-prescription medications and/or nondrug therapy, convey accurate information to the patient:	
a. appropriate dose and frequency of administration	See the box Patient Education for Scaly Dermatoses.
b. maximum number of days the therapy should be employed	See the box Patient Education for Scaly Dermatoses.
c. product administration procedures	See the box Patient Education for Scaly Dermatoses.
d. expected time to onset of relief	See the box Patient Education for Scaly Dermatoses.
e. degree of relief that can be reasonably expected	Control of the condition can be expected in most cases with the use of a medicated shampoo every week or every other week. The condition will not be cured.
f. most common side effects	See the box Patient Education for Scaly Dermatoses.
g. side effects that warrant medical intervention should they occur	See the box Patient Education for Scaly Dermatoses.
h. patient options in the event that condition worsens or persists	See the box Patient Education for Scaly Dermatoses.
i. product storage requirements	See the box Patient Education for Scaly Dermatoses.
j. specific nondrug measures	See the box Patient Education for Scaly Dermatoses.
10. Solicit follow-up questions from patient.	May I use my regular shampoo after using my medicated shampoo?
11. Answer patient's questions.	Yes, but the effectiveness of the medicated shampoo is related to contact time with the face and scalp. Therefore, be sure to leave it on for at least 3–5 minutes prior to rinsing and then using your regular shampoo.

Key: N/A, not applicable; NKA, no known allergies; OTC, over-the-counter; PCP, primary care provider.

C A S E   3 4 - 2

Relevant Evaluation Criteria	Scenario/Model Outcome
Information Gathering	
1. Gather essential information about the patient's symptoms, including:	
a. description of symptom(s) (i.e., nature, onset, duration, severity, associated symptoms)	The patient has had shiny scales bilaterally on her knees, legs, and elbows for greater than 6 months. Some minor bleeding occurs when the scales are removed. She now complains of worsening lesions and the development of similar lesions on her back.
b. description of any factors that seem to precipitate, exacerbate, and/or relieve the patient's symptom(s)	The lesions appeared to worsen following a recent respiratory infection. Being out in the sun appears to be somewhat beneficial.
c. description of the patient's efforts to relieve the symptoms	Use of Eucerin Cream once daily is somewhat soothing but has not resolved the lesions. The patient has not sought medical attention for this condition in the past.
2. Gather essential patient history information:	
a. patient's identity	Agnes Morehead
b. patient's age, sex, height, and weight	46-year-old female, 5 ft 4 in, 155 lb
c. patient's occupation	Secretary

CASE 34-2 *(continued)*

Relevant Evaluation Criteria	Scenario/Model Outcome
d. patient's dietary habits	Normal diet
e. patient's sleep habits	Averages 6–7 hours per night
f. concurrent medical conditions, prescription and nonprescription medications, and dietary supplements	Depression × 10 years, well controlled with sertraline 50 mg daily
g. allergies	Penicillin (rash)
h. history of other adverse reactions to medications	None
i. other (describe) _____	Agnes likes to soak in her tub to relax.

Assessment and Triage

3. Differentiate the patient's signs/symptoms and correctly identify the patient's primary problem(s) (see Table 34-4).	Agnes has dry scaly skin most likely caused by psoriasis. The bilateral appearance supports this assessment.
4. Identify exclusions for self-treatment (see Figure 34-1).	The worsening symptoms and spread of the lesions to the patient's back indicate a worsening condition that requires more than self-care. The condition was likely exacerbated by the stress associated with her recent infection.
5. Formulate a comprehensive list of therapeutic alternatives for the primary problem to determine if triage to a medical practitioner is required, and share this information with the patient.	Options include: (1) Refer Agnes to a PCP or dermatologist for a differential diagnosis. (2) Recommend an OTC product (hydrocortisone) with bathing modifications. (3) Recommend self-care until a PCP or dermatologist can be consulted. (4) Take no action.

Plan

6. Select an optimal therapeutic alternative to address the patient's problem, taking into account patient preferences.	Refer the patient to a PCP or dermatologist for a differential diagnosis and treatment.
7. Describe the recommended therapeutic approach to the patient.	Contact your primary care provider or a dermatologist to diagnose your condition. Until the time of your appointment, avoid prolonged baths and apply an emollient to the affected areas 3–4 times daily.
8. Explain to the patient the rationale for selecting the recommended therapeutic approach from the considered therapeutic alternatives.	You need to see a PCP or dermatologist, because OTC therapy may not be appropriate for extensive disease.

Patient Education

9. When recommending self-care with non-prescription medications and/or nondrug therapy, convey accurate information to the patient.	See the box Patient Education for Scaly Dermatoses.
10. Solicit follow-up questions from patient.	Is there an OTC medication that might work?
11. Answer patient's questions.	Hydrocortisone ointment may be useful for patients with mild cases of psoriasis, but your worsening condition and larger affected area will likely require more aggressive treatment with one or more products requiring a prescription and monitoring by your clinician. The use of emollients will continue to play a major role in the treatment of your condition.

Key: OTC, over-the-counter; PCP, primary care provider.

the signs and symptoms of the disorders. The practitioner should also explain that fluctuation in severity of seborrhea and psoriasis may be related to emotional, physical, or environmental factors.

Explanations of the proper use of cytostatic and keratolytic agents should include information about the length of time to leave the agent on the affected area. The practitioner should also explain possible adverse effects and drug interactions with recommended agents. Finally, the practitioner should advise the patient what signs and symptoms indicate that medical attention is needed. The box Patient Education for Scaly Dermatoses lists specific information to provide patients.

PATIENT EDUCATION FOR
Scaly Dermatoses

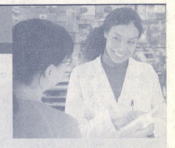

The primary objective for self-treating dandruff, seborrhea, and psoriasis is to reduce the turnover rate of skin cells, which is responsible for the scaly lesions. Controlling inflammation and itching of the affected areas is another treatment objective for seborrhea and psoriasis. Although these disorders are chronic and incurable, carefully following product instructions and the self-care measures can help ensure optimal therapeutic outcomes for many patients.

General Measures

- Shampoo the hair with the medicated shampoo three times per week initially, leaving the shampoo on the hair for 3–5 minutes. Work the shampoo into the scalp and affected area of the face. Use a scalp scrubber to ensure penetration to the scalp. Repeat application.
- If used, apply a thin layer of the hydrocortisone cream 2–3 times daily. Wash the affected areas before use.
- Use the shampoo for a minimum of 2 weeks to determine effectiveness and then on a weekly or biweekly basis to control the condition.
- With usage of medication and proper nondrug therapy, noticeable improvement could be observed within 7–14 days. Complete control of the condition is possible with periodic use of the medicated shampoo. It is likely that exacerbations may occasionally appear, especially during the winter months.
- Stinging or burning may occur if medicated shampoo enters the eyes.
- Use of coal tar products can stain light-colored hair and sensitize patients to the sun.

Dandruff

- Use a medicated shampoo containing ketoconazole, pyrithione zinc, selenium sulfide, or coal tar. If these agents are ineffective, use a medicated shampoo containing sulfur or salicylic acid.
- Coal tar can stain light hair and cause folliculitis (inflammation of hair follicles), dermatitis, and photosensitization (sensitivity of the skin to sunlight).
- Shampoo the hair with the medicated shampoo, and leave it on the hair for several minutes. Rinse the hair thoroughly and repeat.

Seborrhea

- Use a medicated shampoo containing ketoconazole, pyrithione zinc, or selenium sulfide. Note that selenium sulfide may increase scalp oiliness or worsen seborrhea in some individuals.
- If redness persists after therapy with medicated shampoos, apply hydrocortisone 2–3 times a day until symptoms subside and then intermittently to control acute exacerbations. Do not use this agent longer than 7 days. Prolonged use can cause rebound flare-ups when the hydrocortisone is discontinued.

- After shampooing, part the hair, apply the product directly to the scalp, and massage it in thoroughly. Repeat this process until the affected area is covered.

Psoriasis

- For itchy, dry skin, use emollients and lubricating bath products (see Chapter 33, Table 33-4). Remove scales by gently rubbing them with a soft cloth following the bath. Do not rub vigorously.
- Avoid alcohol and smoking. Obese patients should lose weight.
- For scalp psoriasis, use medicated shampoos containing coal tar or salicylic acid.
- For daytime treatment of itchiness, apply hydrocortisone 1% cream three to four times daily. Reduce frequency of application as the condition improves. Do not use this agent longer than 7 days.
- To help loosen and remove scales during the day, soak the affected body area in warm (not hot) water for 10–20 minutes; then apply a salicylic acid product. Do not apply salicylic acid to extensive areas of the body; the agent may be absorbed into the bloodstream.
- For more effective removal of scales, apply coal tar products to lesions on the body, arms, and legs at bedtime. Note that this agent stains bed linen and clothing. Bathe in the morning to remove residual coal tar and to also loosen psoriatic scales. If preferred, apply salicylic acid at bedtime.
- For psoriasis of the armpits, genital areas, and anus, use hydrocortisone instead of coal tar or salicylic acid.
- When bright red lesions are present, use only emollients and hydrocortisone until the flare-up has subsided. Resume therapy with coal tar and salicylic acid when the thick-scaled plaques appear.
- Prevent flare-ups by minimizing factors such as emotional stress, skin irritation, and physical trauma that you know will exacerbate the disorder.
- Consult a primary care provider before treating psoriasis with sun exposure.
- Take a nonsteroidal anti-inflammatory drug (e.g., aspirin, ibuprofen, or naproxen) for swelling of joints associated with psoriatic arthritis (see Chapter 7).

 Consult a primary care provider if the condition does not improve or if it worsens after 1–2 weeks of treatment with nonprescription medications.

EVALUATION OF PATIENT OUTCOMES FOR SCALY DERMATOSES

Follow-up on the patient's progress should occur after 1 week of self-treatment. A scheduled visit to the practitioner is preferable if the lesions are on a part of the body that can be inspected. If the symptoms persist or have worsened after 1 week of treatment, the patient should consult a primary care provider. If the disorder has not worsened, the practitioner should ask the patient to return after a second week of treatment. If the symptoms persist or have worsened after this period, the patient should consult a primary care provider.

KEY POINTS FOR SCALY DERMATOSES

➤ Mild-to-moderate scaly dermatoses can often be effectively managed with topical nonprescription products.

➤ Products should be selected on the basis of the patient's history and prior response to treatment, as well as on the basis of a careful evaluation of the risks and benefits of using the nonprescription products.

➤ The practitioner should be sure to educate patients about the proper application of topical therapy, which greatly impacts the efficacy of therapy.

REFERENCES

1. Odom RB, James WD, Berger T. *Andrews Diseases of the Skin: Clinical Dermatology*. 9th ed. Philadelphia: WB Saunders; 2000.
2. Hay RJ, Graham-Brown RAC. Dandruff and seborrheic dermatitis: causes and management. *Clin Exp Dermatol*. 1997;22:3–6.
3. Johnson M-LT, Roberts J. *Prevalence, Disability, and Health Care for Psoriasis among Persons 1–74 Years of Age*. Hyattsville, Md: National Center for Health Statistics; 1978. Advance Data from National Center for Health Statistics, No. 47.
4. Brodell RT, Cooper KD. Therapeutic shampoo. In: Wolverton SE, ed. *Comprehensive Dermatologic Drug Therapy*. Philadelphia: WB Saunders; 2001:647–58.
5. Han NH, West DP. Scaly dermatoses. In: Berardi RR, DeSimone EM, Newton GD, et al., eds. *Handbook of Nonprescription Drugs*. 12th ed. Washington, DC: American Pharmaceutical Association; 2000:633–45.
6. Wright, AL. Seborrheic eczema. In: Lebwohl MG, Heymann WR, Berth-Jones J, et al., eds. *Treatment of Skin Disease: Comphrehensive Therapeutic Strategies*. London: Mosby; 2002:582–4.
7. Rudikoff D. Atopic dermatitis. In: Lebwohl MG, Heymann WR, Berth-Jones J, et al., eds. *Treatment of Skin Disease: Comphrehensive Therapeutic Strategies*. London: Mosby; 2002:58–64.
8. Plewig G, Jansen T. Seborrheic dermatitis. In: Freedberg IM, Eisen AZ, Wolff K, et al., eds. *Fitzpatrick's Dermatology in General Medicine*. 6th ed. New York: McGraw-Hill, Inc; 2003:1482–3.
9. Holden CA, Berth-Jones J. Eczema, lichenification, prurigo and erythroderma. In: Burns T, Breathnach S, Cox N, et al., eds. *Rook's Textbook of Dermatology*. 7th ed. Malden, Mass: Blackwell Publishing; 2004:17: 10–17.15.
10. Griffiths CEM, Camp RDR, Barker JNWN. Psoriasis. In: Burns T, Breathnach S, Cox N, et al., eds. *Rook's Textbook of Dermatology*. 7th ed. Malden, Mass: Blackwell Publishing; 2004:35.1–35.51.
11. Christophers E, Mrowietz U. Psoriasis. In: Freedberg IM, Eisen AZ, Wolff K, et al., eds. *Fitzpatrick's Dermatology in General Medicine*. 6th ed. New York: McGraw-Hill, Inc; 2003:495–521.
12. Sege-Peterson K, Winchester RJ. Psoriatic arthritis. In: Freedberg IM, Eisen AZ, Wolff K, et al., eds. *Fitzpatrick's Dermatology in General Medicine*. 6th ed. New York: McGraw-Hill, Inc; 2003:522–33.
13. Lebwohl MG. Psoriasis. In: Lebwohl MG, Heymann WR, Berth-Jones J, et al., eds. *Treatment of Skin Disease: Comprehensive Therapeutic Strategies*. London: Mosby; 2002:533–43.
14. MacKie RM. Psoriasis, papulosquamous diseases, and disorders of keratinization. In: *Clinical Dermatology*. 5th ed. Oxford: Oxford University Press; 2003:44–62.
15. Camp RD. Psoriasis. In: Champion RH, Burton JL, Burns DA, et al., eds. *Textbook of Dermatology*. 6th ed. Oxford: Blackwell Science; 1998:1595–6.
16. *Fed Regist*. 1991;56:63554–69.

Contact Dermatitis

Kimberly S. Plake and Patricia L. Darbishire

Contact dermatitis accounts for 5.7 million primary care provider (PCP) visits per year, not including the number of requests for the clinician to evaluate and help relieve this condition. Contact dermatitis is defined as an inflammatory skin condition characterized by inflammation, redness, itching, burning, stinging, and vesicle and pustule formation on dermal areas exposed to irritant or allergenic agents.[1-3] Irritant contact dermatitis (ICD) is an inflammatory reaction of the skin caused by exposure to an irritant. Allergic contact dermatitis (ACD) is an inflammatory reaction of the skin caused by exposure to an allergen.[3] In industrial societies, ICD and ACD commonly occur in 1% to 10% of the population.

IRRITANT CONTACT DERMATITIS

The majority of ICD cases are related to occupation, particularly jobs that involve wet work or exposure to irritant chemicals. Although contact dermatitis may be caused by chemical exposure in the home, available statistics include only those associated with occupations and job tasks. According to the most recent statistics, work-related skin disorders comprise 15% of the total workplace injuries.[4] Overall, persons employed in forestry, agriculture, and fishing industries have the greatest incidence at 155 per 100,000 workers. Workers in the manufacturing and service sectors follow with 110 and 50 incidents per 100,000 workers, respectively.[5,6]

Contact dermatitis is commonly seen in health care professionals and individuals in personal service occupations (e.g., hair stylists). The Bureau of Labor Statistics (BLS) annual survey of occupational illnesses reveals that occupational contact dermatitis accounts for 90% to 95% of all occupational skin diseases, with 80% of the cases of contact dermatitis related to ICD. The BLS identified that 12% of all occupational illnesses reported are skin diseases/disorders and make up the highest percentage of nontraumatic work-related illness. The number of cases is estimated to be 10 to 50 times greater than actually reported because of changes in industry procedure, underreporting of incidents, and limitations in data collection for the BLS survey. It has been estimated that the national medical costs for treating occupational skin diseases is $4.7 million annually.[5]

Pathophysiology of Irritant Contact Dermatitis

Approximately 80% to 90% of the cases of contact dermatitis are caused by exposure to chemicals, solvents, and detergents (Table 35-1).[7-9]

Most instances of ICD occur on exposed or unprotected skin surfaces, especially the face and dorsal surfaces of the hands and arms. Approximately 80% of the cases of ICD involve the hands and 10% involve facial dermatitis.[6] Contact dermatitis may appear after a single exposure or following multiple exposures to the same agent. Several mechanisms may be responsible for causing ICD. First, the chemical may directly damage the dermal cells by direct absorption through the cell membrane, destroying cell systems. A second mechanism may be through mediators released by naive T cells.[10] The reaction does not require previous exposure to an irritant for the dermatitis to appear.

Several factors may affect the magnitude of the skin response. The presence of existing skin diseases or conditions can result in a more profound dermatitis by allowing the irritant to easily enter the dermis. The quantity and concentration of chemical exposure also impact the severity. Chemical irritants, acids, and alkalis are more likely to produce immediate and severe inflammatory reactions. Mild irritants, such as detergents, soaps, and solvents, may require successive exposures before the dermatitis appears. Occlusive clothing can harbor irritants, leading to a more severe reaction. This reaction develops simply through normal skin respiration and humidification; the occluded skin allows greater skin penetrability of the irritant. In addition, environmental factors, such as warmer ambient temperature and higher humidity, or wet work, may contribute to more severe dermatologic conditions.[1,8]

Clinical Presentation of Irritant Contact Dermatitis

On exposure to an irritant, the skin becomes inflamed and swollen, turns red, and may develop small vesicles or papules that ooze fluid when opened. Itching, stinging, and burning commonly occur with the rash. The inflammatory reaction varies, ranging from these initial symptoms to ulcer formation and localized necrotic areas of skin. Within several days, the dermatitis

Editor's Note: This chapter is based on the 15th edition chapter with the same title, written by Kenneth R. Keefner.

TABLE 35-1 Selected Common Irritants Associated with Contact Dermatitis

Strong acids (hydrochloric, nitric, sulfuric, hydrofluoric)

Strong alkalis (sodium, potassium, calcium hydroxides)

Detergents

Epoxy resins

Ethylene oxide

Fiberglass

Leather tanning agents

Oils (cutting, lubricating, etc.)

Solvents

Oxidizing agents

Reducing agents

Oxidants, plasticizers, and activators in athletic shoes

Wood dust and products

Source: Adapted from references 7–9.

may crust. If the patient remains free of the irritant, the dermatitis will resolve in several days. In patients chronically exposed to an irritant, the affected areas of skin will remain inflamed, begin to furrow and scale, and may become hyper- or hypopigmented.[1,8,10,11] A portion of patients chronically exposed to irritants recover completely, whereas many improve but continue to have recurrences. Some patients continue to have an inflammatory process comparable to or worse than the original insult.[12]

Treatment of Irritant Contact Dermatitis

Treatment Goals

The goals in self-treating ICD are to (1) relieve the inflammation, dermal tenderness, and irritation; (2) prevent continued exposure to the irritant substance; and (3) educate the patient on self-management to prevent and treat recurrences.

General Treatment Approach

Regardless of the severity, the area of initial exposure to the irritant substance should be washed with copious amounts of water and cleansed with a mild or hypoallergenic soap. Application of wet compresses of the astringent aluminum acetate soothes and dries weeping lesions. Hydrocortisone, calamine lotion, and colloidal oatmeal baths are helpful in relieving associated itching. The use of topical caine-type anesthetics should be avoided because of their ability to sensitize the skin to a contact dermatitis. Avoidance of the irritant is a hallmark of treatment and patient education. Figure 35-1 outlines self-treatment of ICD and lists exclusions for self-treatment.

Nonpharmacologic Therapy

Immediately washing exposed areas will reduce the contact time of the offending substance and, if a dermal response occurs, help prevent the spread of the dermatitis. (See Hygienic Measures for specific bathing/showering information.) Educating the patient in techniques to reduce risk of exposure is fundamental. Using protective clothing, gloves, and other protective equipment, and limiting the time skin areas are occluded through frequent changes in coverings will aid in reducing irritant exposure. Emollients, moisturizers, and barrier creams also can be used in the treatment and prevention of ICD. Hydropel and Hollister Moisture Barrier Cream claim to prevent ICD if applied before contact with an irritant.[13]

Pharmacologic Therapy

The same pharmacologic treatment is used for ICD and ACD. (See Treatment of Allergic Contact Dermatitis for a detailed discussion of the appropriate pharmacologic agents.)

ALLERGIC CONTACT DERMATITIS

Although ACD accounts for a small percentage of contact dermatitis cases, poison ivy/oak/sumac dermatitis is responsible for a large number of field occupational injuries and is the primary cause of ACD. For these reasons, poison ivy/oak/sumac dermatitis is discussed in more detail than other ACDs.

Allergen exposure is the cause of 10% to 20% of contact dermatitis cases. Poison ivy/oak/sumac (*Toxicodendron* genus) dermatitis is the principal cause of ACD in the United States and exceeds the incidence of all other causes of ACD combined. Several million cases of poison ivy are reported each year in the United States, and they account for the largest number of worker's compensation claims.[14] After poison ivy/oak/sumac, metal allergy, most often caused by nickel, is the most common form of ACD. In fact, approximately 16.7% of all patients patch tested for allergies are allergic to nickel.[15] Fragrances, cosmetics, and skin care products also can cause ACD.[16]

As much as 80% of the U.S. population is estimated to be sensitive to poison ivy's urushiol, the oleoresin that causes the dermatitis. Poison ivy/oak/sumac dermatitis can present in patients as young as 3 years old. Sensitivity to urushiol increases as individuals age, with adult sensitization patterns occurring after 10 years of age. Patients of advanced age, in contrast, appear to have a declining sensitivity because of reduced response, but they have a prolonged duration of symptoms. Itching in patients of advanced age has been observed to be greater than in younger adults. Presentation of symptoms in the older patient may be explained, in part, by a general decline in immune competence that occurs with age and a reduced ability to be sensitized to a new antigen.[11,17]

Various occupations are linked to *Toxicodendron* exposure in the daily work environment, as shown in Table 35-2.[18,19]

Pathophysiology of Allergic Contact Dermatitis

Numerous environmental substances may act as an antigen. Urushiol (from poison ivy/oak/sumac plants), nickel salts (in jewelry, clothing, and cell phones), and fragrances (in cosmetics) are examples of allergens capable of producing ACD. Table 35-3 lists *selected* allergenic substances and is not comprehensive.[15,20]

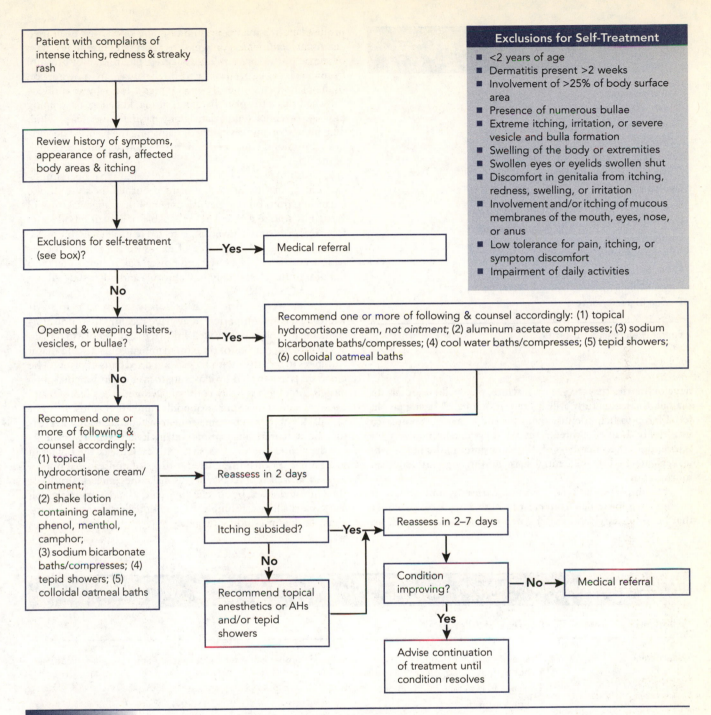

FIGURE 35-1 Self-care of contact dermatitis. Key: AH, antihistamine.

Urushiol-Induced ACD

In the United States, five species of *Toxicodendron* plants, which belong to the family Anacardiaceae, are primarily responsible for dermatoses associated with exposure to plants[21] (Table 35-4).[17,18,22] Many of these plants were previously considered to belong to the genus *Rhus*, but the term *Toxicodendron* is now the accepted genus for this group of antigenic plants. This genus is used throughout the chapter to appropriately refer to these plants. The change in genus and the difficulty in classifying these plants are the result of the variability in the morphology of the plants. Botanists claim that such variability is based on the effects associated with geographic

location, soil, water, and climatic conditions. The plants were reclassified into the genus *Toxicodendron*, but terms such as *Rhus radicans*, *Rhus rash*, and *Rhus dermatitis* are still used, especially in early literature and reference works.

If patients have sensitivity to any one *Toxicodendron* species, they are usually allergic to all members of the genus. Although all five species are common to the United States, they are somewhat indigenous to specific regions of the country. These species are most easily identified as having three leaves emanating from a central stem, with the middle leaflet appearing at the terminal end of the stem. The plants flower in the spring and produce small, waxy, white five-petaled flowers. In the late fall, the plants

TABLE 35-2 Occupations That Pose Risk for Poison Ivy/Oak/Sumac Dermatitis

Civil engineers
Construction workers
Farm and agricultural workers
Firefighters
Forestry personnel and conservationists
Gardeners and groundskeepers
Geologists
Highway and road construction crews
Land surveyors
Loggers
Park maintenance personnel
Police officers
Power utilities and maintenance personnel
Truck and tractor drivers

Source: References 18 and 19.

develop berries that are greenish white, pale yellow, or tan. In the fall, the leaves turn brilliant red or orange. A saying taught to children to help identify the plant and to avoid exposure to urushiol is "Leaves of three; let it be!" In general, this statement is true, but other members of the genus differ in the number of leaflets attached to the central stalk, and in the berry and leaf morphology.[17,18]

Urushiol is quite sensitive to oxidation by ambient air. It changes in appearance from clear fluid to a black inky lacquer that becomes tarry and may harden on the damaged portion of the plant in a matter of minutes. This oddity has been used as a visual identifier to confirm the existence of poison ivy, oak, or sumac in the surrounding foliage.[23] The release of urushiol from the plant can occur only through damage to some portion of the plant itself, either through direct damage by an individual who bruises the plant by lying, sitting, kneeling, or stepping on it, or by contact after damage by natural causes (e.g., wind, rain, insects, or animals eating or damaging the plant). The antigenic urushiol is contained and carried only within resin canals of the plant.[17,18]

Urushiol is not a volatile substance, but it has been implicated in dermatitis when the plant is burned, because smoke emanating from burned plants contained the antigen. Urushiol carried by smoke particulates is capable of affecting body surface areas ordinarily viewed as protected (e.g., genitals, buttocks, anus, and lungs). This source of exposure is a primary occupational cause of poison ivy and poison oak in personnel who fight forest fires, especially in California and other states along the West Coast.[17,18]

Patients presenting with poison ivy dermatitis in mid-winter or off-season periods may have recently used urushiol-contaminated objects. It is well-known that urushiol can remain active for long periods of time on inanimate objects, and that it continues to be active within dead and dried parts of plants. The oleoresin is inactivated by exposure to wet environmental conditions. An object is easily contaminated with the oleoresin and becomes a common source of oddly timed dermatitis. It is not unusual for objects to become contaminated in one growing season; the contaminating urushiol retains its antigenicity throughout the winter and causes rashes with each use of the object in succeeding seasons. Implicated sources of nonseasonal poison ivy rash, as well as of recurrent seasonal rashes, include urushiol-contaminated shoes, boots, clothing, garden and work tools, golf clubs, baseball bats, fishing rods, and other recreational equipment, or the fur of domestic pets.[17,18]

TABLE 35-3 Selected Common Allergens Associated with Allergic Contact Dermatitis

Allergen	Sources of Allergen
Benzocaine	The caine-type anesthetics have crossover allergy to other caine-type local anesthetics, topical medications (for skin, eye, ear), other oral medications
Bacitracin	Topical and injectable medications
Balsam of Peru	Cough syrups, flavors
Chromium salts	Potassium dichromate electroplating, cement, leather tanning agents, detergents, dyes
Cobalt chloride	Cement, metal plating, pigments in paints
Colophony (rosin)	Rosin cake for string instrument bows, sport rosin bags, cosmetics, adhesives
Epoxy resins	Constituents prior to mixing and hardening
Formaldehyde	Germicides, plastics, clothing, glue, adhesives
Fragrances	Cosmetics, household products, eugenol, cinnamic acid, geraniol, oak moss absolute
Lanolin	Lotions, moisturizers, cosmetics, soaps
Latex	Gloves, syringes, vial closures
Nickel sulfate	In jewelry, blue jean studs, utensils, pigments, coins, tools, many metal alloys encountered daily
Neomycin sulfate	Medications, antibiotic ointments, other aminoglycosides
Plants	*Toxicodendron* species (poison ivy, oak, sumac), primrose (*Primula obonica*), tulips, others
Rubber (carba mix)	Added ingredients, accelerators, activators, other processing chemicals
Thiomersal	Preservative in many medications, injectables, cosmetics

Source: References 15 and 20.

TABLE 35-4 Toxicodendron Plants Indigenous to North America		
Plant	**Other Common Names**	**Common Geographic Location**
Poison ivy	Poison vine, mark weed, three-leaved ivy, poor man's liquid amber	Exists throughout North America, ranging throughout the United States (central, midwest, south central, southeastern, lower Mississippi Valley regions); Canada (Ontario, Nova Scotia); and Mexico
Poison sumac	Poison elder, poison ash	Exists from Quebec to Florida in primarily the eastern third of the U.S. coast
Western poison oak		Exists throughout Pacific Coast
Eastern poison oak		Exists widely in the southeastern United States

Source: Adapted from references 17, 18, and 22.

Poison Ivy

The most common *Toxicodendron* plant found throughout the United States is poison ivy (*Toxicodendron radicans* and *Toxicodendron rydbergii*). Poison ivy is quite common throughout central and northeastern United States and Canada. It has been described as a climbing shrub or hairy vine that commonly grows up poles, trees, and building walls (see Color Plates, photograph 17A). It also grows along roads, hiking trails, streams, dry rocky canyons, and embankment slopes. *T. radicans* is composed of nine subspecies that can exist as a shrub or a climbing vine, whereas *T. rydbergii* is a dwarf shrub that has large, broad, spoon-shaped leaves with a hairy underside. *T. rydbergii* is the principal variety of poison ivy that grows in the northern United States and southern Canada. *T. radicans* grows over much of the United States as a climbing vine with aerial rootlets.[17,18,22]

Poison Oak

Poison oak has two species indigenous to the United States: *Toxicodendron diversilobum,* which inhabits the West Coast, and *Toxicodendron toxicarium,* which inhabits the East Coast. Both species possess leaves similar to those of oak trees; most have an unlobed leaf edge and commonly display three leaflets per stem (see Color Plates, photograph 17B). The leaves and berries of eastern poison oak (*T. toxicarium*) are covered with fine hairs. The plant ordinarily exists as a nonclimbing shrub. Western poison oak (*T. diversilobum*) differs by usually possessing between three and 11 leaflets per stem; its leaves are quite similar to California live oak. Poison oak bears fruit covered with numerous fine hairs. It exists as a shrub capable of climbing to distances as high as 131 feet (40 meters). Poison oak grows along streams, in thickets, on wooded slopes, and in dry woodlands. As a rule, poison oak grows well at altitudes below 4000 to 5000 feet.[17,18,22]

Poison Sumac

Poison sumac (*Toxicodendron vernix*) grows in remote areas of the eastern third of the United States in peat bogs and swampy areas. It appears as a shrub or small tree, attains a height of roughly 9.8 feet (3 meters), and may resemble, to some extent, either elder or ash trees. Therefore, it has been given the names "poison elder" or "poison ash." Its leaves are pinnate and may be almost 16 inches (40 cm) in length; they are odd numbered, ranging between 7 and 13 leaflets. The edges of the leaves are smooth and come to a tip (see Color Plates, photograph 17C).[17,18,22]

Other Causative Plants

In addition to the genus *Toxicodendron*, several other plants are known to have cross-sensitivity with urushiol, causing a poison ivy–like dermatitis in individuals who have been previously sensitized to urushiol. Although this discussion is not all–inclusive, several plants deserve specific mention. The cashew nut tree (*Anacardium occidentale* L.) bears an edible nut, the shells of which contain oils that share a cross-sensitivity to urushiol and produce a similar rash. The peel of the mango fruit (*Magnifera indica* L., Indian mango, king of the fruits, apples of the tropics)[22] contains an antigenic substance that has been responsible for facial, oral, and lip dermatitis and cheilosis. The mango allergen is found in the stems, leaves, and peel, but not in the edible fruit of the mango itself. Such rashes are commonly encountered in Malaysia and Hawaii when urushiol-sensitive visitors to these locations are exposed to the peels of fresh mangoes.

Lacquer from the Japanese lacquer tree (*Toxicodendron vernicifluum*) is used as an ingredient in the finish of varnished boxes, rifle stocks, floors, bar rails, teapots, canes, and toilet seats. Urushiol-sensitive individuals who are exposed and reexposed to these lacquered products may have recurrent episodes of ACD. In Korea, the sap of the Japanese lacquer tree is used as an herbal medicament, and in basting and boiling chicken. Currently, there are two Korean reports of patients developing generalized dermal reactions to ingestion of the lacquer.[24,25] The fruit of the ginkgo tree (*Ginkgo biloba* L.) contains a cross-sensitive resin that leads to rashes on the lower extremities (caused by walking through an area with fallen fruit) and to dermatitis of the mucous membranes, cheilitis, stomatitis, or proctitis associated with consumption of the fruit.

ACD is an inflammatory dermal reaction related to exposure to an allergen that activates sensitized T cells, which migrate to the site of contact and release their inflammatory mediators. ACD ordinarily does not appear on first contact, because allergens responsible for ACD are immunologically connected, and several steps must occur before the dermatitis is manifested. An initial exposure to the antigen must take place to sensitize the immune system. This process is known as the induction phase. With the immune system now sensitized, the next contact with the allergen induces a type IV delayed hypersensitivity reaction, which is a cell-mediated (allergen-sensitized T cells) allergic reaction that can take 24 to 48 hours or longer to develop. This reaction results in the symptoms and dermatitis associated with ACD.[26–28]

Most clinicians think that the initial exposure is not ordinarily associated with dermal symptoms, although some reports suggest that the initial exposure in very sensitive patients may not only sensitize the patient to urushiol, but also lead to dermatitis as much as 2 to 10 days later.[29] The first sensitizing dose may not produce a rash until as long as 3 weeks after the initial exposure. Other reports suggest that numerous, recurrent exposures may be needed to develop the clinical dermatitis in highly resistant or tolerant patients. In people previously sensitized, the rash and related symptoms may appear at any time between 2 and 48 hours after the second exposure.

The allergic response appears to be a two-step process: initial sensitization (step one), followed by a delayed hypersensitivity reaction (step two) in the dermal layers of the skin. Some clinicians think the urushiol rapidly (10 minutes) enters the skin and attaches to protein molecules found on the surface of Langerhans cells (specialized white blood cells) in the epidermis and to macrophages in the dermis. The Langerhans cells communicate the antigen information to lymphocytes (inducer cells); these cells, in turn, proliferate into circulating T-effector and T-memory lymphocytes. This process allows the immune lymphocytes to become sensitized to future entry of urushiol into the skin layers.[18] With succeeding urushiol exposure, the patient has a delayed hypersensitive reaction that allows T cells to invade the skin area containing the newly deposited urushiol. It has been reported that as little as 2 to 2.5 mg or less of urushiol is enough to stimulate the typical dermal rash in sensitive patients.[30] In patients who are tolerant or show subclinical reactions to the same level of urushiol, as much as 5, 10, or 50 mg may be necessary to elicit an allergic response. Symptoms of pruritus, erythema, vesiculation, and local edema are the result of this cytotoxic immune response.[31,32]

Clinical Presentation of Allergic Contact Dermatitis

General Presentation

Signs and symptoms of ACD vary depending on the allergen, site, and duration of exposure and host factors. Typically, the skin appears red and swollen. Blisters may also appear and form crusts or scales when they break open. Itching, burning, and pain are common symptoms of ACD. A more detailed discussion of the signs and symptoms of the primary plant-induced dermatitis follows.

Presentation of Urushiol-Induced Dermatitis

The initial dermal reaction to urushiol is an intense itching of the skin's surface areas exposed to the antigen, followed by erythema. Scratching the area may spread the urushiol to other unexposed skin surfaces if it has not been previously washed from the skin. As the dermatitis progresses, vesicles (blisters) or bullae form, depending on an individual's sensitivity. The vesicles/bullae may break open, releasing their fluid (see Color Plates, photograph 18A). Vesicular fluid does not contain any antigenic material to further spread the dermatitis. A common patient description that highly suggests poison ivy or oak exposure is streaks of vesicles that correspond to the points of urushiol contact from the damaged plant (see Color Plates, photograph 18C). In fact, specks of black oxidized urushiol may form on the skin and clothing after contamination.

Patients may continue to scratch for several days after exposure and excoriate the surface dermal layer, leading to open lesions and the potential for secondary wound infections. Common microbes found in infected poison ivy dermatitis consist of *Staphylococcus aureus,* group A *Streptococcus,* and *Escherichia coli.*[33] In addition to these microbes, other organisms may be identified depending on where the infection arose on the skin. Oozing and weeping of the vesicular fluid continues to occur for several days, until the affected area develops crusts and begins to dry (see Color Plates, photograph 18B).

Lesions may develop on skin that is ordinarily considered protected (e.g., the genitals, anus, buttocks, or other covered body surfaces), which occurs primarily through contact with urushiol-contaminated fingers and hands. Unwashed, contaminated hands and fingernails are the primary sources of rash on protected areas of the body. Numerous reports describe the dermatitis on the face and around the eyes, and on lips, underarms, buttocks, and the anus, as well as the genitalia of the affected patient and his or her sexual partner.

Severity of Poison Ivy/Oak/Sumac Dermatitis

Mild dermatitis is characteristically seen in a linear streaking arrangement. Marked swelling of the eyelids without associated swelling of other parts of the face may occur[22] and is caused by rubbing the eyelids with urushiol-contaminated fingers and hands. Clinically, the dermatitis is localized in distinct patches on the unprotected lower and upper extremities.

Signs and symptoms of moderate dermatitis include the appearance of bullae and edematous swellings of various body parts, in addition to the pruritus, erythema, papules, and vesicles of mild dermatitis.

Severe dermatitis is distinguished by extensive involvement and edema of the extremities and the face. Often the eyelids are swollen closed. Extreme itching, irritation, and formation of severe vesicles, blisters, and bullae may also be present. Furthermore, daily activities may be hampered in some patients. Dermatitis or edema affecting large areas of the face, eyes, or genitalia requires immediate medical referral for systemic or parenteral therapy. Dark-skinned patients may experience a permanent discoloration in areas of dermatitis where severe inflammatory changes and blistering have occurred.

Complications of Poison Ivy/Oak/Sumac Dermatitis

On rare occasions, various other diseases have been associated with exposure to *Toxicodendron* plants and the development of ACD. Such diseases have included eosinophilia (ordinarily seen with exposure to poison ivy), secondary mania,[34] erythema multiforme,[35] acute respiratory distress syndrome (caused by inhaling urushiol particles carried in smoke),[36] renal failure, dyshydrosis of the hands and feet,[29] and urethritis.

Treatment of Allergic Contact Dermatitis

Treatment Goals

The goals of self-treating ACD are to (1) protect the area affected during the acute phase of the rash, (2) prevent itching and excessive scratching that may lead to open lesions and potential secondary skin infections, and (3) prevent the accumulation of debris that arises from oozing, crusting, and scaling of the vesicle fluids.

Customarily, the first several days following the initial appearance of ACD are usually the most uncomfortable for the patient. Treated or untreated dermatitis will naturally resolve in approximately 10 to 21 days as a result of the patient's own immune system. Topical nonprescription products may be used for symptomatic relief. Patients will seek the practitioner's counsel principally because of the intensity of itching and pain associated with a mild localized rash, or because of the widespread nature of the dermatitis and the magnitude of symptoms.

The following discussion deals primarily with treatment of poison ivy dermatitis, but the same therapeutic approaches apply to ICDs and other ACDs. Therapy is indicated primarily to relieve symptoms associated with the dermatitis and to prevent secondary infection of excoriated portions of the skin caused by excessive scratching.

General Treatment Approach

Removing the known allergen from the skin as soon as possible may reduce the chance and/or severity of the immune response. In the case of poison ivy/oak/sumac dermatitis, cleansing the affected area within the first 10 minutes of exposure reduces the immune response.

The aggressiveness of and type of treatment for the allergic reaction depend on the severity of the allergic reaction: mild, moderate-to-severe, or severe. (See the algorithm in Figure 35-1 for a summary of appropriate treatments and exclusions for self-treatment.) If, at the time of presentation, the patient exhibits mild dermatitis (only localized patches of rash with intense pruritus and erythema), the practitioner may initially recommend treatment that includes the topical application of an antipruritic (shake) lotion containing calamine, menthol, phenol, camphor, and antipruritic agents, or the application of a hydrocortisone cream or ointment. As long as the rash does not begin to weep and remains dry, the patient may use shake lotions and ointments. If the rash spreads to larger areas but does not affect the eyes or genitals and does not cover the body (moderate-to-severe reaction), the patient may use astringent compresses and baths to treat the rash.

Mild Poison Ivy/Oak/Sumac Dermatitis

Initial treatment recommendations may consist of several options to relieve pruritic symptoms. One option is the use of a shake lotion consisting of calamine lotion with the addition of phenol (1%) and/or menthol (0.25%). The lotion should be shaken well and then applied topically to the itchy or erythematous areas every 4 hours as needed for relief of pruritus. The lotion should not be applied if open lesions are present. Calamine leaves a light pink film in the application area, and the patient may find it cosmetically distasteful, especially when applied to the face. Instead, the patient may find a hydrocortisone cream or ointment more esthetically acceptable.

Alternatively, patients may use sodium bicarbonate (baking soda) as either a paste or a cool compress to relieve itching and irritation. For paste application, cool tap water is added to sodium bicarbonate powder in sufficient quantity to prepare a paste for direct application to the vesicles. In addition, 1 or 2 cups of sodium bicarbonate powder may be added to a warm bath. The affected areas should be soaked for 15 to 30 minutes and then the paste applied. The skin should be dried by patting rather than wiping so that a film of baking soda remains on the skin. For very localized dermatitis, baking soda compresses may be applied for 15 to 30 minutes and repeated as needed. Patients should be warned not to use baking soda near the eyes and to consult a primary care provider (PCP) if relief is not obtained within 7 days of treatment. Baking soda should not be applied to patients younger than 2 years.

Topical ointments and creams containing anesthetics (benzocaine), antihistamines (diphenhydramine), or antibiotics (neomycin) should not be used. These agents are known sensitizers and can cause a drug-induced dermatitis along with the existing dermatitis.[17,18]

Moderate-to-Severe Poison Ivy/Oak/Sumac Dermatitis

Treatment of numerous large, coalesced bullae should be referred to a PCP. An initial recommendation is the application of a cool water compress to the affected area for as long and as often as needed. Mild edema or swelling of the eyelids should be treated with only cold water dressings. Cool compresses of aluminum acetate solution (Burow's) may be applied to other affected areas.

A 1:40 dilution of Burow's solution may be prepared from prepackaged tablets or powder by adding 1 tablet or package to 1 pint of cool tap water. Clean white compresses are soaked in the solution and then applied to the affected areas for 15 to 30 minutes, three times a day (soak) or as often as needed (compress). Any remaining solution should be discarded and a fresh solution prepared for each application. Burow's solution provides an astringent action on the papulovesicular lesions of the dermatitis that dries the weeping vesicles.[37] In addition, Burow's solution is useful in softening and removing crusting. A cream or lotion can be applied to provide an emollient effect following the use of the Burow's solution.

Colloidal oatmeal baths can cleanse and soothe the lesions, and reduce itching. One packet (30 grams) of colloidal oatmeal per tub of water is sprinkled into warm, running water to allow for good mixing of the milled oatmeal. Stirring the bath water occasionally will help prevent lumps from developing. Colloidal oatmeal makes the bathtub extremely slippery. Placing a rubber mat in the tub and a dry rug or towel on the floor will help prevent falling. Soaking for 15 or 20 minutes one to two times each day is recommended. The skin should be patted dry (not wiped) to leave a film of colloidal oatmeal on the skin.

Severe Poison Ivy/Oak/Sumac Dermatitis

Symptomatic topical treatment of severe dermatitis is similar to that used in moderately severe cases; however, the PCP will likely prescribe an anti-inflammatory glucocorticoid. The prescriber should ensure a good treatment outcome by recommending a systemic glucocorticoid that consists of a tapering dosage of not fewer than 12 days to as long as 21 days of therapy. On average, about 1 mg/kg body weight per day (approximately 40–100 mg) of prednisone is used when initiating therapy and is tapered over the next 2 to 3 weeks. The use of prepackaged dosage packs of glucocorticoid (tapered over 6 days) in numerous instances has led to the use of a second or third dose pack, or may even lead to rebound dermatologic symptoms if this shorter therapy period is selected.[38]

Nonpharmacologic Therapy

Hygienic Measures

The primary nondrug measure to relieve symptoms of contact dermatitis is to take cold or tepid soapless showers to temporarily relieve the pruritus. A tepid shower is approximately 90° (32.2°C) or cooler. The clinician should recommend that a patient be cautious about taking a hot shower (temperatures greater than 105°F [40.5°C]), because it may cause scalding or thermal skin injuries (second-degree burns) as well as intensifies the pruritus. The clinician may recommend that patients bathe or shower using hypoallergenic face soap to maintain cleanliness; they should never use harsh soaps. Furthermore, when a rash is present, affected areas should not be vigorously scrubbed. Along with applying topical treatment, all patients, both adults and children, should trim their fingernails to help reduce the degree of scratching injury.

Preventive/Protective Measures

In the case of *Toxicodendron* plants, recreational or work-related outdoor activities should include a survey of the surrounding vegetation to determine the potential risk of exposure. In addition, clinicians can educate patients by providing descriptions and photographs of the plants. Table 35-5 describes preventive and protective measures for avoiding poison ivy/oak/sumac dermatitis.

USE OF PROTECTIVE CLOTHING
Individuals should wear additional protective clothing that can be removed and immediately washed after exposure. They should use ordinary laundry detergent to wash clothes contaminated with urushiol separately from noncontaminated clothing.

REMOVAL OF URUSHIOL OR OTHER ALLERGENS FROM SKIN
To reduce the contact and spread of the dermatitis, the individual should immediately wash the area that was exposed to poison ivy plants or other allergens. Even though urushiol is a water-insoluble compound, clinicians have shown that immediate and early washing of urushiol-exposed areas with soap and water may avoid or reduce the severity of the rash. Researchers have shown[39] that washing the contaminated area must take place within 10 minutes of exposure to significantly reduce the risk of dermatitis. Studies have also revealed that, for up to 30 minutes after exposure, washing will remove unreacted oleoresin. Therefore, washing after the initial 10-minute period is still useful in removing any oleoresin that remains on the skin's surface and has not entered the dermal layers. Once urushiol has entered the skin and attached to tissue proteins, it can no longer be removed.

"In the field" washing is difficult, but simply using large volumes of water will rinse away much of the surface irritant and oleoresin. Historically, PCPs and many home remedies recommended vigorous scrubbing of contaminated skin surfaces with a harsh soap (e.g., Fels Naphtha or homemade lye soap). Instead, the current recommendation is to use a mild face soap and water to wash all body areas believed to have been exposed to urushiol. In lieu of this approach, copious amounts of plain water may be sufficient to reduce the chance of dermatitis. In addition, it is crucial that at-risk patients practice good hand-washing, including meticulous cleansing under the fingernails, to avoid contaminating other clean skin surfaces with allergen trapped under the fingernails.

Other cleansers and organic solvents have been used to rinse off skin surface urushiol, including isopropyl alcohol. However, general thought holds that although urushiol is soluble in alcohol, its use should be followed immediately by washing with a mild soap and water to remove any remaining surface oleoresin. Alcohol may dissolve and transport the surface oleoresin to clean

TABLE 35-5 Preventive and Protective Measures for Poison Ivy/Oak/Sumac Dermatitis

Preventive Measures

- Learn the physical characteristics and usual habitat of *Toxicodendron* plants.
- Eradicate *Toxicodendron* plants near your residence either by mechanically removing the plant and its roots, or by applying an herbicide recommended by the state farm bureau or the USDA extension services.
- Apply bentoquatam on exposed areas of body to reduce the risk of contamination before visiting an outdoor site. Repeat application every 4 hours until your potential exposure has ended. This application should be followed by flushing the area with water to remove bentoquatam and any urushiol deposited on the skin surface.
- Survey the area of an outdoor visit, identify surrounding plants, and assess potential risk for exposure to *Toxicodendron* plants.
- Take the protective measures listed here for suspected exposure.

Protective Measures

- Wear protective clothing to cover exposed areas.
- Cover the nose and mouth with a protective mask when removing or eradicating *Toxicodendron* plants.
- Remove all clothing worn during exposure, and place the clothing directly into a washing machine.
- Wash the suspected area as soon as possible with soap and water as well as with other suggested removal products.
- If thorough washing is not possible, rinse with water as soon as possible.
- At the earliest convenience, take a complete shower instead of a bath, using soap and water. Avoid tub baths right after exposure, because oleoresin may remain in the tub and potentially affect other unexposed areas.
- Meticulously clean under the fingernails to avoid transferring trapped urushiol to clean skin surfaces.
- Wash all clothing exposed to urushiol separately from other clothes in a washing machine using ordinary detergent. If clothes are dry cleaned to remove urushiol, warn cleaning personnel of the possible contamination. Put contaminated clothing in a plastic bag for transport.
- As soon after use as possible, thoroughly wash with soap and water—or with water alone—any shoes, gloves, jackets, or other protective garments; sports equipment; garden and work tools; and any equipment that is capable of carrying urushiol. Wear vinyl gloves for washing contaminated objects.
- Cleanse the fur of pets after known or suspected exposures to poison ivy plants.

Key: USDA, U.S. Department of Agriculture.

skin surfaces, generating additional areas of dermatitis. Alcohol may also remove natural protective oils from the skin and can be a source of irritation.

One product used as a cleanser for urushiol is Tecnu Outdoor Skin Cleanser, whose constituents include mineral spirits, water, soap, and a surface-active agent. The cleanser was originally developed as an agent to wash away radioactive matter from the skin surface of exposed individuals. This product is recommended for use after exposure and should be rubbed into the affected area as soon after exposure as possible, but it can be used up to 8 hours after exposure. The patient should cleanse the contaminated area for a minimum of 2 minutes. No water is required for the initial cleansing application, but the cleanser may be wiped away with a cloth or rinsed with cool water. The manufacturer recommends using the product before eating, smoking, or using the bathroom in an effort to minimize spreading urushiol to uncontaminated skin. In a study comparing untreated urushiol exposures with those cleansed with Tecnu, Dial Ultra dishwashing soap, and Goop grease remover, it was found that any of the three provided good protection against poison ivy rash when used to cleanse skin exposed to urushiol.[40] The difference in protective ability among the products was not significant.

USE OF BARRIER PRODUCTS

Several studies have evaluated the use of barrier creams and lotions as agents to prevent urushiol from entering the skin. A comprehensive study[13] identified three products that had notable protective qualities when used in subjects who were experimentally challenged with *Toxicodendron* extract. The three products (Hydropel, Hollister Moisture Barrier, and Stokogard Outdoor Cream) reduced dermatitis severity by 48%, 52%, and 59%, respectively. At the present time, Stokogard is not available. The remaining two products (Hydropel and Hollister Moisture Barrier Cream) do not claim protection from poison ivy dermatitis; instead they claim prevention of ICD or diaper rash.

IvyBlock Lotion is the only barrier product approved by the Food and Drug Administration (FDA) to provide protection against exposure to poison ivy, oak, and sumac. This product's active ingredient is an organoclay known as quaternium-18 bentonite (bentoquatam).[41,42] The product contains 5% bentoquatam in a lotion containing alcohol. Bentoquatam is a nonsensitizing and nonirritating organoclay that appears to possess little antigenicity or toxicity when applied topically. The mechanism by which this ingredient works is not presently known, but it is believed to physically block urushiol from being absorbed into the skin. It is effective in protecting patients from exposure to the urushiol common to all *Toxicodendron* plants, as well as urushiol that adheres to smoke particles from burned plants.

This barrier lotion claims protection when it is topically applied at least 15 minutes before exposure to *Toxicodendron*. It should be reapplied once every 4 hours or as needed after the initial application to maintain effective protection. The lotion should be shaken vigorously before application to skin likely to be exposed to poison ivy, oak, or sumac. The individual must apply the lotion generously to clean dry skin, leaving a smooth wet film of lotion where it is applied. One may determine skin coverage by looking for the faint white coating that appears when the lotion has dried. After the period of exposure has ended, the patient may remove the lotion by washing with soap and water.[43] This product is flammable and should not be used around the eyes or applied to an existing poison ivy rash. In addition, its use is not recommended in children younger than 6 years.

ERADICATION OF TOXICODENDRON PLANTS

The eradication of Toxicodendron plants has been suggested in situations in which extremely sensitive individuals are affected by close proximity to the plant and its oleoresin. Two methods of eradication have been recommended: either mechanically removing (hand grubbing of plants and the root system) or applying an appropriate herbicide. When considering the use of herbicides, patients should contact the U.S. Department of Agriculture Extension Service (www.csrees.usda.gov/Extension/index.html) or the appropriate state or county agency to determine the recommended herbicide and prescribed methods of application to *Toxicodendron* species indigenous to the area.

HYPOSENSITIZATION TO TOXICODENDRON PLANTS

History and scientific literature are replete with folklore and stories of Native Americans who ate poison ivy to desensitize themselves. Beginning in the early 1940s, numerous oral and injectable forms of poison ivy extract products were available for use. Their purpose was to desensitize patients to urushiol. From the numerous studies published since these products were introduced, clinicians have learned that such desensitization methods are incapable of adequately desensitizing the patient to poison ivy. Although hyposensitization was possible, it could be maintained only with consistent maintenance doses of injectable extracts. Any protection provided through hyposensitization was lost within 3 months of discontinuing maintenance doses. Several hundred milligrams of urushiol was required to provide clinical hyposensitization. Injectable products could be given in only small doses because of the development of poison ivy symptoms and the side effects associated with administering higher doses. PCPs have long doubted the potency of such commercial products. However, some clinicians prepared their own injectables, which then led to overall claims that were confusing and did not convincingly support the hyposensitization process. FDA took actions in 1994 and 1995 to remove injectable *Toxicodendron* oleoresin extracts (poison ivy or poison oak) from the marketplace.[44,45] No products can currently be recommended as hyposensitization programs for human use (P. M. Scott, Bayer Allergy Products, Miles, Inc., Spokane, Wash; personal communication; March 1999).

Pharmacologic Therapy

Because treatment is primarily aimed at relieving itching, patients should use topical hydrocortisone, oral antihistamines, and other antipruritic agents. Oral antihistamines have the additional benefit of producing sedation for nighttime relief. Patients can use astringents to promote drying of the moist, wet, oozing lesions and to provide a protective covering for the inflamed, tender skin beneath the affected areas. Combination products that contain one or more of these ingredients are available for use. Many dosage forms are available for use on the dermatitis, according to the skin condition and patient-specific preferences. In addition, antiseptics can be included in the formulation, theoretically to provide antimicrobial protection. FDA recently provided final monograph approval for the antipruritic and astringent ingredients discussed in this section.[46,47]

Hydrocortisone

Hydrocortisone is the most effective form of topical therapy for treating symptoms of mild-to-moderate ICD or ACD that does not involve edema and extensive areas of the skin. Hydrocortisone is a low-potency, naturally occurring corticosteroid capable of relieving pruritus and reducing inflammation associated with dermatitis (see Chapter 34). FDA's advisory panel and dermatologists believe that hydrocortisone is safe to apply to all parts of the body except the eyes and eyelids. Generally, topical hydrocortisone is free from systemic absorption when used according to manufacturer's recommendations. Systemic absorption can occur with use over large surface areas, with prolonged use, or with use of occlusive dressings. Hydrocortisone may be applied up to three or four times a day and is available without a prescription in concentrations from 0.50% to 1%. Topical hydrocortisone should not be used for children younger than 2 years, except on a PCP's advice. Practitioners should advise patients that hydrocortisone dosage forms should not be used if the dermatitis persists for longer than 7 days, or if symptoms clear and then reappear in a few days, unless patients have consulted with a PCP.

Other Topical Antipruritics

Several longstanding topical analgesics have been used for their local antipruritic and anesthetic properties, and are incorporated into nonprescription products to relieve the pruritus of ICD or ACD (see Chapter 7). Phenol, camphor, and menthol appear in numerous products at various low concentrations. All three are capable of depressing the skin's sensory receptors, which contributes to their topical analgesic effectiveness. Using such products on open lesions and tender, inflamed tissues may cause local burning and irritation at the application site.

Astringents

Astringents are pharmacologic entities that are known protein precipitants used to stop or reduce the oozing of capillaries or the fluid release from blisters or inflamed tissues. These substances promote drying of wet dermatitis and, in turn, promote reduced inflammation and improved healing. FDA-approved astringents include aluminum acetate (Burow's solution), zinc oxide, zinc acetate, sodium bicarbonate, calamine, and witch hazel (hamamelis water).[46] They are often used as soaks or in wet compresses applied to the affected area several times a day. This type of application aids in cleansing and removing crusting or surface debris that arises from the natural progression of poison ivy or poison oak dermatitis. Therapy may be continued for approximately 5 to 7 days, when the dermatitis is moist and oozing.

After the use of astringents, patients may notice drying, tightening, and contracting of the skin. As a note of caution, prolonged use of calamine lotion or zinc oxide lotion/paste may lead to a buildup of debris and caked material on the skin, which will lead to further irritation and discomfort. Regular cleansing of the affected area to avoid buildup is recommended. The clinician may recommend the use of colloidal oatmeal baths to help provide skin hydration, to aid in cleansing or removing skin debris, and to allay the drying and tightening symptoms noted after frequent use. Also available is an oilated form of colloidal oatmeal, which contains mineral oil to provide an emollient action on the skin.

Antihistamines

Although antihistamines block the histamine₁ (H₁) receptor, such receptors do not play a significant role in type IV cell-mediated responses. Antihistamines have been included in topical formulations for anesthetic action, but they should be avoided in poison ivy/oak/sumac. Topical antihistamines can act as dermatologic sensitizers, which can cause secondary inflammatory dermatologic conditions. Oral antihistamines can be used to assist with itching and sedation at night.

Product Selection Guidelines

Numerous dosage forms are available for nonprescription recommendation by the clinician. The choice of dosage form depends on several factors, especially the severity of the dermatitis and the

presence of vesicles (dry or weeping). Ointments hold moisture within the skin and act as a reservoir for the active ingredient, keeping it on the affected site. Ointments are effective agents when they are applied before the lesions open and begin oozing fluid. Ointments should not be applied to open lesions for several reasons: Removal of ointments from the skin is more difficult, and they may trap bacteria beneath the oleaginous film, leading to secondary infections.

Applying a cream base allows vesicle fluid to flow freely from the blisters and does not trap bacteria, because the medication is quickly absorbed into the skin. Gels offer ease of application and a rapid absorption of active ingredients into the skin. Some gels may contain alcohol or similar organic solvents that may cause irritation or burning when applied to open lesions.

Spray products provide the easiest form of drug application. They allow even distribution to relatively larger areas and are convenient to use, but they are somewhat more expensive. One advantage of a spray product is that touching the area of dermatitis is not necessary, which may curtail additional scratching. Aerosol sprays may contain propellants that cause additional inflammation. Table 35-6 lists selected products containing primarily colloidal oatmeal, astringents, or bentoquatam. (See Chapter 37 for products that contain local anesthetics, hydrocortisone, or topical antihistamines.)

Complementary Therapies

Jewelweed (*Impatiens biflora*, *Impatiens pallida*) is a well-known natural product and folk remedy used by Native Americans to treat a vast array of dermal conditions, including the prevention of poison ivy/oak/sumac dermatitis. Studies have shown that this therapy does not reduce or prevent poison ivy dermatitis in humans.[48,49]

TABLE 35-6 Selected Products for Poison Ivy/Oak/ Sumac Dermatitis

Trade Name	Primary Ingredients
Aveeno Bath Treatment Moisturizing Formula Powder	Colloidal oatmeal 43%
Aveeno Bath Treatment Soothing Formula Powder	Colloidal oatmeal 100%
Cortaid	Hydrocortisone 1%
Domeboro Powder	Aluminum sulfate 1191 mg
Ivy Dry Cream	Benzyl alcohol 10 mg/g; camphor 6 mg/g; menthol 4 mg/g; zinc acetate 20 mg/g
Ivy Dry Liquid	Isopropyl alcohol 12.5%; zinc acetate 20 mg/mL
Ivy Super Dry Liquid	Benzyl alcohol 0.1 mg/g; camphor 4 mg/g; menthol 2 mg/g; isopropyl alcohol 35%; zinc acetate 20 mg/mL
IvyBlock Lotion	Benzyl alcohol; SDA alcohol 40, 25%; bentoquatam (quaternium-18 bentonite) 5%

TABLE 35-7 Differentiation of Irritant and Allergic Contact Dermatitis

Symptom or Characteristic	Irritant Contact Dermatitis	Allergic Contact Dermatitis
Itching	Yes, later	Yes, early
Stinging, burning	Early	Late or not at all
Erythema	Yes	Yes
Vesicles	Yes, minimal	Yes, early
Pustules	Yes	Yes, minimal
Dermal edema	Yes	Yes
Delayed reaction to exposure	Minutes to hours	Days, slower reaction
Appearance of symptoms in relation to exposures	Single or multiple exposures	Delayed
Causative chemical substances	Alkalis, acids, solvents, salts, surfactants, oxidizers	Low-molecular-weight and lipid-soluble substances, fragrances, metals
Substance concentration at exposure	Very important	Less important
Mechanism of reaction	Direct tissue damage	Immunologic reaction

Source: Adapted from references 1, 11, and 12.

ASSESSMENT OF CONTACT DERMATITIS: A CASE-BASED APPROACH

Diagnostically, ICD and ACD are difficult to differentiate from each other (Table 35-7). Circumstances surrounding the occurrence of the dermatitis help the clinician determine the type of dermatitis; these factors include the time relationship to irritant or allergen exposure (at home, work, or recreation); the distribution of the dermatitis on exposed skin areas; symptomatology; and whether dermatitis improves with avoidance of potential antigens.[3]

Assessment of a suspected irritant, allergic, or plant-induced dermatitis is based on characteristic symptoms, history of sensitivity, and activities that indicate exposure to causative substances. Determining the type and success of previous treatments of such rashes will aid in recommending the appropriate nonprescription medications. Cases 35–1 and 35–2 illustrate the assessment of patients with contact dermatitis.

PATIENT COUNSELING FOR CONTACT DERMATITIS

When approached by a patient with ICD or ACD, the practitioner should take the opportunity to explain preventive and protective measures, as well as treatment measures. If the

---

C A S E   3 5 - 1

Relevant Evaluation Criteria	Scenario/Model Outcome
Information Gathering	
1. Gather essential information about the patient's symptoms, including:	
a. description of symptom(s) (i.e., nature, onset, duration, severity, associated symptoms)	Patient has irritated hands and wishes to treat condition. She works in a salon as a stylist. Her job consists of washing, cutting, and dying hair for most of the day. She uses gloves only when mixing and handling dye. She noticed her hands becoming more irritated as her client load has increased over the last 2 months.
	Patients' hands appear dry, red, and cracked. She complains of itching, pain and tenderness. There appears to be no vesicles or infection present. Irritation is confined to hands.
b. description of any factors that seem to precipitate, exacerbate, and/or relieve the patient's symptom(s)	Symptoms worsened when her client load increased at the salon. Dryness and itching progressively increased over last 2 months.
c. description of the patient's efforts to relieve the symptoms	She has used hand lotion periodically to help with the dryness.

Relevant Evaluation Criteria	Scenario/Model Outcome
2. Gather essential patient history information:	
a. patient's identity	Lily Baldwin
b. patient's age, sex, height, and weight	27-year-old female, 5 ft 1 in, 145 lb
c. patient's occupation	Hair stylist
d. patient's dietary habits	Balanced diet; occasional junk food and alcohol
e. patient's sleep habits	Averages 5 hours per night
f. concurrent medical conditions, prescription and nonprescription medications, and dietary supplements	Ortho Tri-Cyclen 1 tablet once daily beginning on day 1 of menstrual cycle
g. allergies	NKA
h. history of other adverse reactions to medications	None
i. other (describe) _____	N/A

Assessment and Triage

3. Differentiate the patient's signs/symptoms and correctly identify the patient's primary problem(s) (see Table 35-7).	Lily is suffering from irritant contact dermatitis. The likely sources are detergents, shampoos, bleach, and general wet work.
4. Identify exclusions for self-treatment (see Figure 35-1).	None
5. Formulate a comprehensive list of therapeutic alternatives for the primary problem to determine if triage to a medical practitioner is required, and share this information with the patient.	Options include: (1) Refer Lily to the appropriate health care professional. (2) Recommend self-care with a nonprescription product and/or nondrug measures. (3) Recommend self-care until Lily can see an appropriate health care professional. (4) Take no action.

Plan

6. Select an optimal therapeutic alternative to address the patient's problem, taking into account patient preferences.	Lily should continue to use gloves when handling chemicals. She should increase her use of gloves when performing any wet work, and change gloves periodically to prevent irritant exposure of chemicals and other liquids. She should continue to use hand lotion but increase frequency of application. In addition, she can use a nonprescription antipruritic product.
7. Describe the recommended therapeutic approach to the patient.	While working, use protective gloves that have high sleeves and are impermeable. Regularly wash and completely dry hands throughout the day, and use a hypoallergenic hand lotion. Apply hydrocortisone cream (1%) 3–4 times a day to the affected area. Apply moisturizer at night using cotton gloves.
8. Explain to the patient the rationale for selecting the recommended therapeutic approach from the considered therapeutic alternatives.	Protective gloves will reduce irritation to your hands from wet work by reducing contact time with the irritant. Washing and drying hands will cleanse hands of irritants. The hypoallergenic hand lotion will relieve dryness. The hydrocortisone cream will relieve itching. The addition of cotton gloves will increase the moisture retained in skin.

Patient Education

9. When recommending self-care with nonprescription medications and/or nondrug therapy, convey accurate information to the patient:	
a. appropriate dose and frequency of administration	See the box Patient Education for Contact Dermatitis.
b. maximum number of days the therapy should be employed	See the box Patient Education for Contact Dermatitis.
c. product administration procedures	See the box Patient Education for Contact Dermatitis.
d. expected time to onset of relief	See the box Patient Education for Contact Dermatitis.

C A S E   3 5 - 1   *(continued)*

Relevant Evaluation Criteria	Scenario/Model Outcome
e. degree of relief that can be reasonably expected	Complete symptomatic relief is likely.
f. most common side effects	See the box Patient Education for Contact Dermatitis.
g. side effects that warrant medical intervention should they occur	See the box Patient Education for Contact Dermatitis.
h. patient options in the event that condition worsens or persists	A PCP should be consulted if the condition does not improve or if irritation is intolerable.
i. product storage requirements	See the box Patient Education for Contact Dermatitis.
j. specific nondrug measures	See the box Patient Education for Contact Dermatitis.
10. Solicit follow-up questions from patient.	(1) How long should I use the hydrocortisone cream? (2) When should the irritation get better?
11. Answer patient's questions.	(1) You may continue to use the cream for up to 7 days. (2) You should see a difference in 1 week. If you do not see improvement, contact your PCP.

Key: N/A, not applicable; NKA, no known allergies; PCP, primary care provider.

C A S E   3 5 - 2

Relevant Evaluation Criteria	Scenario/Model Outcome
Information Gathering	
1. Gather essential information about the patient's symptoms, including:	
a. description of symptom(s) (i.e., nature, onset, duration, severity, associated symptoms)	Patient complains of intense itching, redness, and streaking on face (with eye involvement), arms, and hands. Symptoms have developed within the last 24 hours.
b. description of any factors that seem to precipitate, exacerbate, and/or relieve the patient's symptom(s)	A hot shower this morning intensified the itching.
c. description of the patient's efforts to relieve the symptoms	Patient has not tried anything yet.
2. Gather essential patient history information:	
a. patient's identity	William Dell
b. patient's age, sex, height, and weight	35-year-old male, 6 ft 1 in, 220 lb
c. patient's occupation	Construction worker
d. patient's dietary habits	Normal diet with junk food
e. patient's sleep habits	7 hours a night; awake by 5 am
f. concurrent medical conditions, prescription and nonprescription medications, and dietary supplements	No current medications
g. allergies	None
h. history of other adverse reactions to medications	None
i. other (describe) _____	Patient is unsure of contact with any allergens. He works outdoors and is clearing trees for a new subdivision.

CASE 35-2   (continued)

Relevant Evaluation Criteria	Scenario/Model Outcome
Assessment and Triage	
3. Differentiate the patient's signs/symptoms and correctly identify the patient's primary problem(s) (see Table 35-7).	William is suffering from poison ivy resulting from his workplace. His symptomatology (e.g., weeping vesicles, linear rash, intense itching), delayed onset, and the clearing of trees at work are indicative of this problem.
4. Identify exclusions for self-treatment (see Figure 35-1).	Eye involvement
5. Formulate a comprehensive list of therapeutic alternatives for the primary problem to determine if triage to a medical practitioner is required, and share this information with the patient.	Options include: (1) Refer William to the appropriate health care professional. (2) Recommend self-care with a nonprescription product and/or nondrug measures. (3) Recommend self-care until William can see an appropriate health care professional. (4) Take no action.
Plan	
6. Select an optimal therapeutic alternative to address the patient's problem, taking into account patient preferences.	William should be referred to his PCP because the rash involves his eyes. Advise patient to trim and wash underneath fingernails to ensure oleoresin is gone. Cool water compresses/dressings on affected areas can be used to ease discomfort until PCP is seen.
7. Describe the recommended therapeutic approach to the patient.	
8. Explain to the patient the rationale for selecting the recommended therapeutic approach from the considered therapeutic alternatives.	The only effective treatments to resolve poison ivy rash with eye involvement require prescription medications.
Patient Education	
9. When recommending self-care with nonprescription medications and/or nondrug therapy, convey accurate information to the patient.	The rash will resolve in 10–21 days depending on its severity. Contact your primary care provider if the rash worsens or persists.
10. Solicit follow-up questions from patient.	(1) Is this rash going to spread if I scratch and touch other parts of my body? (2) Will the doctor give me something to make it go away?
11. Answer patient's questions.	(1) No. The rash will occur only where the plant or its resin touched the body. This resin is not in the fluid from the blisters. Be sure to clean your hands and underneath your fingernails so that any remaining resin is removed. (2) The medication the doctor will prescribe helps with the symptoms. The rash will still run its course, which can take approximately 21 days.

Key: PCP, primary care provider.

patient cannot identify contact with irritant chemicals, allergens, or *Toxicodendron* plants, the practitioner should review chemicals or allergens likely to cause dermatitis, show illustrations of *Toxicodendron* plants, if possible, or refer the patient to an appropriate reference. The practitioner should also explain the purpose and appropriate use of nonprescription agents, their possible adverse effects, and signs and symptoms that indicate one should see a clinician. The box Patient Education for Contact Dermatitis lists specific information to provide patients.

EVALUATION OF PATIENT OUTCOMES FOR CONTACT DERMATITIS

After recommending treatment for a contact dermatitis, the practitioner may choose to follow up with the patient after several days of treatment, or may instead encourage the patient to call for additional advice if the itching has not subsided significantly within 5 to 7 days. If, at follow-up, the rash has signif-

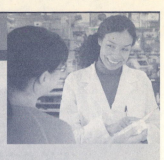

PATIENT EDUCATION FOR
Contact Dermatitis

Irritant Contact Dermatitis

The goals in self-treating irritant contact dermatitis are to (1) relieve the inflammation, dermal tenderness, and irritation; (2) prevent continued exposure to the irritant substance; and (3) educate the patient on self-management to prevent and treat recurrences. For most patients, carefully following product instructions and the self-care measures listed here will help ensure optimal therapeutic outcomes.

Nondrug Measures

- Decrease exposure to common skin irritants such as detergents, soaps, and solvents.
- Avoid occlusion of the skin by changing gloves (especially latex gloves used for cleaning chores), diapers, and clothing more frequently.
- Wash the affected area gently to remove traces of the offending agent.

Nonprescription Medications

- To help the lesions dry, apply compresses of cool tap water or aluminum acetate for 20 minutes, four to six times daily.
- Apply calamine lotion between compress applications, and take colloidal oatmeal baths to soothe and help relieve itching.
- Apply a thin layer of hydrocortisone cream/ointment to the affected area three or four times daily for up to 7 days to relieve itching and/or inflammation.
- If itching keeps you awake at night, take an oral antihistamine that has a sedative effect, such as diphenhydramine or doxylamine, and follow the labeled instructions. Be aware that such medications can cause drowsiness the next morning.
- Store nonprescription medications in a cool, dry place out of the reach of children.
- If the contact dermatitis does not begin to improve in 2–3 days or if it worsens, consult a primary care provider.

Allergic Contact Dermatitis

The goals of self-treating allergic contact dermatitis are to (1) protect the area affected during the acute phase of the rash, (2) prevent itching and excessive scratching that may lead to open lesions and potential secondary skin infections, and (3) prevent the accumulation of debris that arises from the oozing, crusting, and scaling of vesicle fluids. For most patients, carefully following product instructions and the self-care measures listed here will help ensure optimal therapeutic outcomes.

Nondrug Measures

- Apply the preventive measures outlined in Table 35-5 to prevent poison ivy/oak/sumac dermatitis.
- If exposure is suspected and if preventive measures were not taken, implement the protective measures outlined in Table 35-5.
- Take tepid, soapless showers to relieve itching.
- When cleansing the affected areas, do not use harsh cleansers or scrub vigorously.
- To avoid potential allergic reactions, use hypoallergenic cosmetics and soapless cleansers.

Nonprescription Medications

- Note that the dermatitis will subside with or without treatment in 14–21 days.
- If treatment is desired, consult a clinician about the use of one or more of the following nonprescription medications to relieve the intense itching, inflammation, weeping, and crusting that may accompany this dermatitis.
- If desired, use sodium bicarbonate paste or compresses as follows to relieve itching:
  —Apply paste directly to the rash.
  —Use clean white cloths to apply cool water compresses; apply for 20–30 minutes as often as needed or desired. Use a fresh solution with each new application.
- If desired, apply topical hydrocortisone cream or ointment as follows to reduce the itching and dissipate the dermal inflammation and erythema:
  —Apply sparingly to affected areas four times a day.
  —Avoid direct application around the eyes or eyelids.
  —Note that ointment dosage forms appear to maintain hydrocortisone application for longer periods of time than cream forms.
- To avoid potential dermal infections, do not apply ointments to open or excoriated pustules or lesions.
- Use aluminum acetate (Burow's solution) compresses as follows to dry open and weeping pustules or lesions:
  —Mix a prepackaged tablet or packet of aluminum acetate with a pint of cool tap water, wet a cloth with the solution, and apply the compress to rash areas.
  —Apply compresses for 30 minutes at least four times a day or as needed.
  —Prepare fresh Burow's solution for each application period.
- Use colloidal oatmeal baths or soaks as follows to soothe and cleanse areas of rash, as well as reduce pruritus:
  —Sprinkle a 30 gram packet or a cup full of milled oatmeal into fast-running bath water, and mix water periodically to avoid lumping of the oatmeal.
  —Soak for 15–20 minutes in the oatmeal bath at least twice a day. Pat skin dry rather than wiping it.
  —Be cautious on entry and exit from the bathtub, because oatmeal baths are quite slippery.
- Store nonprescription medications in a cool, dry place out of the reach of children.

! Contact a primary care provider for systemic and topical treatment in the following situations:
  —Symptoms become worse.
  —The rash becomes more widespread on the body.
  —The rash covers large areas of the face or causes swelling of the eyelids.
  —The rash involves the genitalia.

icantly increased in size, affects the eyes or genitals, or covers extensive areas of the face, the practitioner must reassess the patient for further therapy or referral to a PCP. Overall, complete remission of the dermatitis may take up to 3 weeks. However, the patient should see slow but steady reduction in itching, weeping, and dermatitis after 5 to 7 days of therapy.

KEY POINTS FOR CONTACT DERMATITIS

➤ The leading cause of irritant contact dermatitis is exposure to a chemical irritant, primarily related to occupation. Irritants include such agents as acids, alkalis, solvents, and numerous other harsh chemicals.

➤ Allergic contact dermatitis, the next largest segment of contact dermatitis, is produced through sensitization to an antigenic substance.

➤ Many substances are antigenic, such as fragrances, metals, medications, plants, and chemicals. Urushiol from poison ivy/oak/sumac is the best-known allergen.

➤ Patients who are sensitive to irritants, allergens, or urushiol may take precautions to eliminate unnecessary exposure by avoiding these agents, limiting exposure time, and wearing protective clothing and equipment.

➤ In the case of poison ivy, avoiding geographic areas endemic with *Toxicodendron* plants is helpful. In addition, patients sensitive to urushiol should make liberal and timely applications of bentoquatam barrier lotion every 4 hours until the exposure period is over to reduce the risk of dermatitis.

➤ Once exposed to an irritant or allergen, the patient can take protective measures that include bathing with mild soap and water or using large volumes of cool water immediately after exposure to reduce the risk of dermatitis.

➤ Dermatitis may begin as localized streaks or patches of highly pruritic rash that proceed to larger areas on exposed dermal areas. The rash may affect the eyelids or face and, in some cases, areas ordinarily considered to be protected.

➤ The practitioner should refer patients to a PCP if the rash causes edema of the eyelids, closes the eyelids, affects the external genitalia or anus, or produces massive areas of body rash or edema.

➤ Treatment of localized, pruritic rash consists of a topical application of hydrocortisone cream or ointment, sodium bicarbonate paste, compresses, or baths. Weeping of vesicles or bullae, which is caused by the patient's scratching, may be treated with aluminum acetate compresses as an astringent to soothe and dry the weeping. Colloidal oatmeal baths may be used to treat the pruritic rash, to soothe, and to provide an emollient action on dry skin.

➤ Irritant, allergic, and poison ivy/oak/ sumac dermatitis will resolve in approximately 7 to 21 days with or without topical therapy. Nonprescription medication recommendations serve in part to relieve the intense itching, inflammation, weeping, and crusting that may accompany these dermatoses.

REFERENCES

1. Wigger-Alberti W, Iliev D, Elsner P. Contact dermatitis due to irritation. In: Adams RM, ed. *Occupational Skin Disease*. 3rd ed. Philadelphia: WB Saunders; 1999:1–22.

2. Cohen DE, Heidary N. Treatment of irritant and allergic contact dermatitis. *Dermatol Ther*. 2004;17:334–40.

3. Wolff K, Johnson RA, Suurmond D. Contact dermatitis. In: *Color Atlas and Synopsis of Clinical Dermatology*. 5th ed. New York: McGraw-Hill, Inc; 2005:18–32.

4. McCall BP, Horwitz IB, Feldman SR, et al. Incidence rates, costs, severity, and work-related factors of occupational dermatitis. *Arch Dermatol*. 2005;141:713–8.

5. Centers for Disease Control and Prevention. Occupational dermatoses: a program for physicians. Available at: http://www.cdc.gov/niosh/ocderm1. html. Last accessed September 12, 2008.

6. Lushniak BD. Occupational skin diseases. Occupational and environmental medicine. *Prim Care*. 2000;27:895–915.

7. Koch P Occupational contact dermatitis, recognition and management. *Am J Dermatol*. 2001;2:353–65.

8. Belisto DV. Allergic contact dermatitis. In: Freedberg IM, Eisen AZ, Wolff K, et al., eds. *Fitzpatrick's Dermatology in General Medicine*. 5th ed. New York: McGraw-Hill Inc; 1999:1447–61.

9. Belisto DV. The diagnostic evaluation, treatment, and prevention of allergic contact dermatitis in the new millennium. *J Allergy Clin Immunol*. 2000;105:409–20.

10. Slodownik D, Lee A, Nixon R. Irritant contact dermatitis: a review. *Australas J Dermatol*. 2008;49:1–11.

11. Talor JS, Sood A. Occupational skin disease. In: Freedberg IM, Eisen AZ, Wolff K, et al., eds. *Fitzpatrick's Dermatology in General Medicine*. 5th ed. New York: McGraw-Hill Inc; 1999:1609–31.

12. Aajjachareonpong P, Cahill J, Keegel T, et al. Persistent post-occupational dermatitis. *Contact Dermat*. 2004;51:278–81.

13. Grevelink SA, Murrell DF, Olsen EA. Effectiveness of various barrier preparations in preventing and/or ameliorating experimentally produced *Toxicodendron* dermatitis. *J Am Acad Dermatol*. 1992;27(2 pt 1):182–8.

14. Klingman DL, Davis DE, Knake ED, et al. *Poison Ivy, Poison Oak, Poison Sumac*. Washington, DC: US Department of Agriculture Extension Service; 1983.

15. Pratt MD, Belsito DV, DeLeo VA, et al. North American Contact Dermatitis Group patch-test results, 2001–2002 study period. *Dermatitis*. 2004;15:176–83.

16. Cosmeceuticals facts & your skin. Available at: http://www.aad.org/public/ publications/pamphlets/general_cosmeceutical.html. Last accessed September 22, 2008.

17. Allen PLJ. Leaves of three, let them be: if it were only that easy. *Dermatol Nurs*. 2006;18:236–42.

18. Gladman AC. Toxicodendron dermatitis: poison ivy, oak, and sumac. *Wilderness Environ Med*. 2006;17:120–8.

19. Peate WF. Occupational skin disease. *Am Fam Physician*. 2002;66:1025–32.

20. Scheman A, Jacob S, Zirwas M, et al. Contact allergy: alternatives for the 2007 North American Contact Dermatitis Group (NACDG) standard screening tray. *Disease-a-Month*. 2008;54:7–156.

21. Botanical Dermatology Database. Anacardiaceae. Available at: http:// bodd.cf.ac.uk/BotDermFolder/BotDermA/ANAC-1.html. Last accessed September 22, 2008.

22. Reitschel RL, Fowler JF, eds. *Fisher's Contact Dermatitis: Toxicodendron Plants and Spices*. 4th ed. Baltimore: Williams & Wilkins; 1995:461–74.

23. Guin JD. The black spot test for recognizing poison ivy and related species. *J Am Acad Dermatol*. 1980;2:332–3.

24. Park YM, Park JG, Kang H, et al. Acute generalized exanthematous pustulosis induced by ingestion of lacquer chicken. *Br J Derm*. 2000; 143:230–3.

25. Park SD, Lee S-W, Chun JH, et al. Clinical features of 31 patients with systemic contact dermatitis due to the ingestion of Rhus (lacquer). *Br J Derm*. 2000;142:937–42.

26. Funk JO, Maibach HI. Horizons in pharmacologic intervention in allergic contact dermatitis. *J Am Acad Derm*. 1994;31:999–1014.

27. Gayer KD, Burnett JW. Toxicodendron dermatitis. *Cutis*. 1988;42:99–100.

28. Epstein WL. Plant-induced dermatitis. *Ann Emerg Med*. 1987;16:950–5.

29. Klingman AM. Poison ivy (Rhus) dermatitis: an experimental study. *Arch Dermatol*. 1958;77:149–80.

Color Plates

Color Illustration Contributors

Allergan, Inc.

Lawrence R. Ash

Umberto Benelli (eyeatlas.com)

Jean A. Borger

Richard C. Childers

Stanley Cullen

emedicine.com, Inc.

Jeffery A. Goad

Alfred C. Griffin (deceased)

Harold L. Hammond

Hollister Incorporated

Christopher Huerter

Thomas C. Orihel

Joan Lerner Selekof

R. Gary Sibbald

George Yatskievych

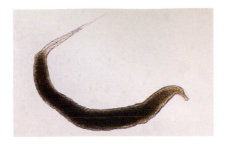

1A

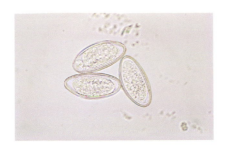

1B

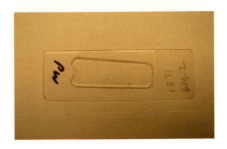

1C

1A, B, and C **Pinworm infection,** the most common worm infestation in the United States, is caused by ingestion of pinworm eggs from fecally contaminated hands, food, clothing, or bedding. **A,** The adult pinworm is a small (1-cm long), white, thread-like worm with a pin-shaped, pointed tail. **B,** The mature female stores approximately 11,000 eggs in her body, which she deposits in the perianal region of the host, usually at night. Reinfection occurs when the hatched larvae return to the large intestine or when eggs are transferred from the anus to the mouth and swallowed. **C,** Commercial pinworm detection kits use a sticky paddle, instead of tape, to affix the adult pinworm to a slide, which is then examined microscopically (see Chapter 19). (Photographs 1A and B courtesy of Lawrence R. Ash, PhD, and Thomas C. Orihel, PhD, © 1997, *Atlas of Human Parasitology.* 4th ed. Chicago: ASCP Press; 1997. Photograph 1C courtesy of Jeffery A. Goad, PharmD, University of Southern California, School of Pharmacy, Los Angeles, © 2003.)

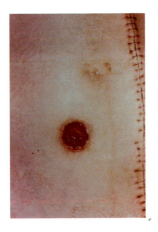

2A

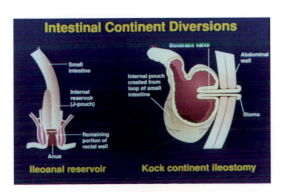

2B

2A–B There are three major types of ostomies: ileostomy, colostomy, or urinary diversion. **A,** In an ileostomy, a portion of the ileum is brought through the abdominal wall. **B,** The two most common types of continent ileostomies are the ileoanal reservoir and the Kock continent ileostomy. The ileoanal reservoir is created by stripping diseased mucosa from the rectum, creating an internal pouch from the ileum, and pulling the distal end of the pouch through the rectum and attaching it. In the Kock continent ileostomy, an internal pouch is created from the ileum and an intussusception of the bowel is used to create a "nipple."

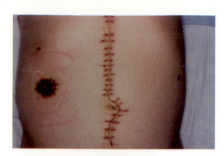

2C

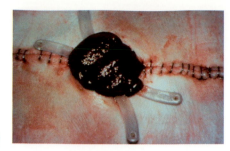

2D

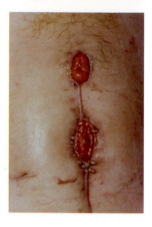

2E

2C–F Colostomies are located on the ascending, transverse, or descending/sigmoid colon. **C,** Ascending colostomies are uncommon. The ascending colon is retained, but the rest of the large bowel is removed or bypassed. The stoma is usually on the right side of the abdomen. The transverse colon is the site of most temporary colostomies. A loop of the transverse colon is lifted through the abdominal incision, and a rod or bridge is placed under the loop to give it support. **D,** Loop colostomies have one large opening, but two tracts. The proximal tract discharges fecal material; the distal tract secretes small amounts of mucus. **E,** In a double-barrel transverse colostomy, the bowel is completely divided by bringing both the proximal end and the distal end through the abdominal wall and suturing it to the skin. **F,** Descending and sigmoid colostomies are fairly common and generally are on the left side of the abdomen.

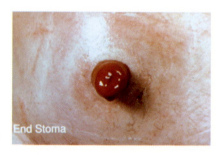

End Stoma

2F

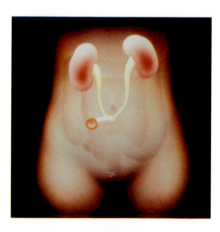

2G

2G–I Urinary diversion surgery diverts the urinary stream through an opening in the abdominal wall. **G,** In the ileal conduit, the most common type of urinary diversion, ileal and colon conduits are created after removal of the bladder by implanting the ureters into an isolated loop of bowel, the distal end of which is brought to the surface of the abdomen. **H,** Mucous shreds will be present if the bowel is used to create the diversion. **I,** In an ureterostomy, one or both ureters are detached from the bladder and brought to the outside of the abdominal wall, where a stoma is created. This procedure is used less frequently because the ureters tend to narrow unless they have been dilated permanently by previous disease (see Chapter 22). (Copyrighted photographs 2B, D, and G courtesy of Hollister Incorporated, Libertyville, Illinois. Copyrighted photographs 2A, C, E, F, H, and I courtesy of Joan Lerner Selekof, BSN, CWOCN, University of Maryland Medical Center, Baltimore, Maryland.)

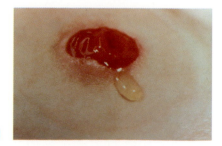

2H

2I

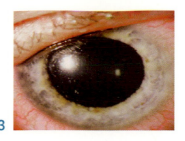

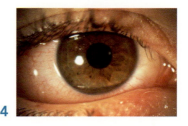

3 **Severe dry eye** can result from failure to properly diagnose and treat dry eye syndromes. Severe damage to eye tissue, particularly the corneal surface, can occur (see Chapter 28). (Photograph courtesy of Allergan, Inc., Irvine, California.)

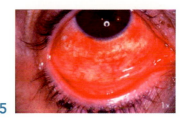

4 **Allergic conjunctivitis** is characterized by itchy, red eyes with a watery discharge. Vision is usually not impaired, but it may be blurred because of excessive tearing (see Chapter 28).

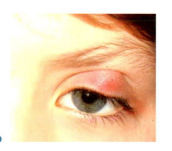

5 **Viral conjunctivitis,** the most common form of conjunctivitis, is usually characterized by a "pink eye" with a copious amount of watery discharge. A recent cold, sore throat, or exposure to someone with viral conjunctivitis is a common precursor of this condition (see Chapter 28). (Copyrighted photograph courtesy of Umberto Benelli, MD, eyeatlas.com.)

6 **Chalazion** is a sterile granuloma that may involve one of the lid glands or may be located near (but not on) the eyelid. Unlike a hordeolum, a chalazion is neither infectious nor tender to gentle touching (see Chapter 28). (Copyrighted photograph courtesy of Umberto Benelli, MD, eyeatlas.com.)

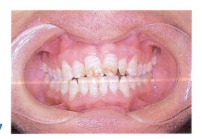

7 **Dental fluorosis (mottled enamel)** occurs during the time of tooth formation and is caused by the long-term ingestion of drinking water containing fluoride at concentrations greater than 1 ppm. Discoloration of the teeth varies, depending on the level of fluoride in the water, and ranges from white flecks or spots to brownish stains, small pits, or deep irregular pits that are dark brown in color (see Chapter 31).

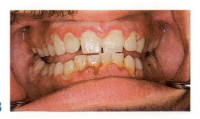

8 **Chronic gingivitis,** an asymptomatic inflammation of the gingivae (gums) at the necks of the teeth, is an early stage of periodontitis and is usually caused by poor oral hygiene. The gingivae are erythematous (red) and may have areas that appear swollen and glossy. In addition, mild hemorrhage may occur during toothbrushing (see Chapter 31).

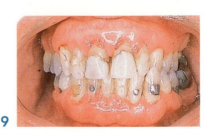

9 Chronic periodontitis (pyorrhea), an inflammation of the tissues surrounding the teeth, including the gingivae, periodontal ligaments, alveolar bone, and the cementum (bony material covering the root of a tooth), is caused by plaque accumulation resulting from poor oral hygiene. The gingivae may be erythematous and swollen, and may recede from the necks of the teeth. The condition is not painful and usually is accompanied by halitosis, loosening of the teeth, and mild hemorrhage during toothbrushing (see Chapter 31).

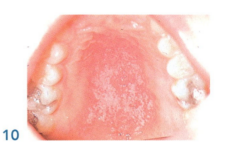

10 Candidiasis (candidosis, moniliasis, thrush), an infection caused by overgrowth of *Candida albicans,* tends to occur in people with debilitating or chronic systemic disease or those on long-term antibiotic therapy. Candidiasis commonly presents as a whitish-gray to yellowish, soft, slightly elevated pseudomembrane-like plaque on the oral mucosa; the plaque is often described as having a milk curd appearance. If the membrane is stripped away, a raw bleeding surface remains. A dull, burning pain is often present (see Chapters 31 and 32).

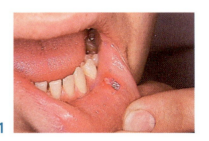

11 Recurrent aphthous ulcers (canker sores) are recurrent, painful, single, or multiple ulcerations of bacterial origin. The central ulceration is sharply demarcated, often has a yellow to white surface of necrotic debris, and is surrounded by an erythematous margin (see Chapter 32).

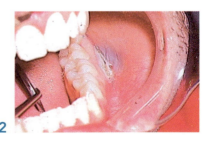

12 Aspirin burn results from the topical use of aspirin to relieve toothache. An aspirin tablet is placed against the tooth, where it is held in place by pressure from the buccal (cheek) mucosa. The mucosa becomes necrotic and is characterized by a white slough that rubs away, revealing a painful ulceration (see Chapter 32).

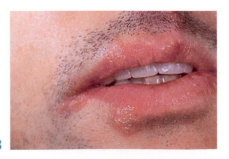

13 Herpes simplex lesions of the mouth and the eye usually start as a small cluster of vesicles (tiny blisters) that subsequently heal over with a serosanguineous (blood-tinged) crust. Local stinging, burning, and pain often herald the onset of lesions. Eye involvement should always be referred to an ophthalmologist (see Chapter 32).

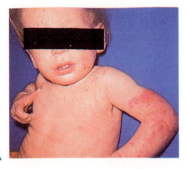

14A

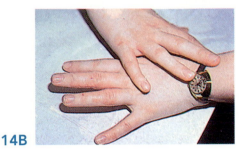

14B

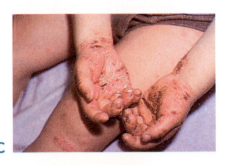

14C

14A, B, and C **Atopic dermatitis (eczema)** is an inflammatory condition that occurs **(A)** on the extensor surface of the elbows and knees during the first year of life and then **(B)** involves predominantly the flexors. **C,** The hands, feet, and face are often involved as well. The dermatitis is characterized by erythema, scale, increased skin surface markings, and crusting; secondary infection is common (see Chapter 33).

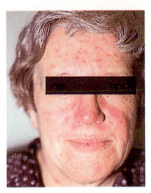

15

15 **Seborrheic dermatitis** is a red scaling condition of the scalp, midface, and upper midchest of adults. This dermatitis is marked by characteristic greasy, yellowish scaling and is associated with erythema (see Chapter 34).

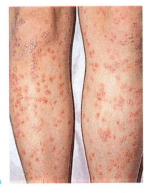

16A

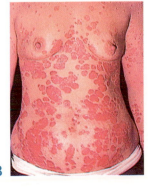

16B

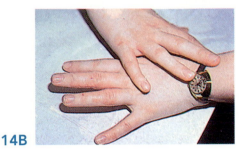

16C

16A, B, and C **Psoriasis** is a scaling condition in which erythematous plaques (red raised areas) are covered by a thick adherent scale. The borders of the lesions are well developed and vary from guttate (very small drop-shaped plaques) to much larger plaques: **(A)** guttate, **(B)** medium-size plaques, **(C)** large plaques (see Chapter 34).

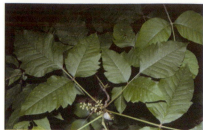

17A

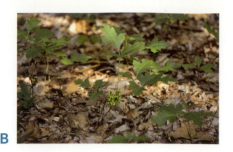

17B

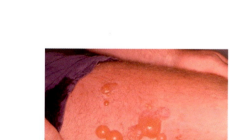

17C

17A, B, and C **Poison ivy, oak, and sumac** account for the majority of plant-induced allergic contact dermatitis. **A,** In the United States, poison ivy is the most common of the three plants. It usually grows as a scrambling shrub or a climbing hairy vine that often grows up poles, trees, and building walls. Its leaves are usually large, broad, and spoon-shaped. **B,** Two species of poison oak are indigenous to the United States; both possess leaves with unlobed edges that look similar to those of oak trees. Eastern poison oak (*Toxicodendron toxicarium*) commonly displays three leaflets, whereas Western poison oak (*Toxicodendron diversilobum*) has between 3 and 11 leaflets per stem. Poison oak usually grows as a shrub capable of reaching heights of 131 feet (40 meters). **C,** Poison sumac (*Toxicodendron vernix*) grows in remote areas of the eastern one third of the United States in peat bogs and swampy areas. It grows as a shrub or small tree and attains a height of about 9.8 feet (3 meters). Its pinnate leaves have smooth edges that come to a tip and may be almost 16 inches (40 cm) in length. The leaves are odd numbered, ranging between 7 and 13 leaflets (see Chapter 35). (Photographs courtesy of George Yatskievych, PhD, Missouri Botanical Garden, St. Louis, © 2000.)

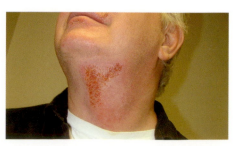

18A

18A, B, and C **Poison ivy** dermatitis is often associated with **(A)** fluid-filled vesicles (blisters) or bullae, depending on a person's sensitivity. **B,** Oozing and weeping of the vesicular fluid occur for several days, until the affected area develops crusts and begins to dry. **C,** Streaks of vesicles that correspond to the points of urushiol contact from the damaged plant are highly suggestive of poison ivy exposure. Similar reactions can also be caused by poison oak and poison sumac (see Chapter 35). (Photographs courtesy of Christopher Huerter, MD, Creighton University Medical Center, Omaha, Nebraska, © 2002.)

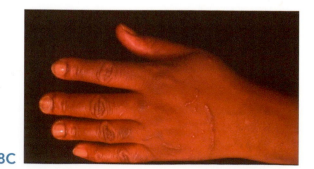

18B

18C

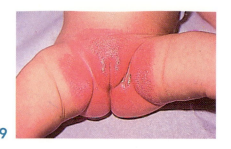

19 **Diaper dermatitis** presents as erythema of the groin (crease area around the genitals) and is common in infants. The case shown here was caused by a contact allergen. Contact irritants, such as urine and feces, and secondary bacterial and yeast infections may also cause problems in this area (see Chapter 36). (Photograph reprinted with permission from emedicine.com, Inc., © 2003.)

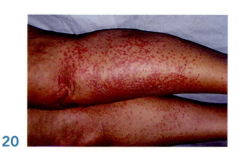

20 **Miliaria rubra (heat rash)** is an obstruction of sweat glands. Superficial involvement results in only tiny vesicles (blisters) appearing on the skin surface (miliaria crystallina). When deeper inflammation is present, the surrounding erythema is characteristic of miliaria rubra (see Chapter 36). (Photograph reprinted with permission from emedicine.com, Inc., © 2003.)

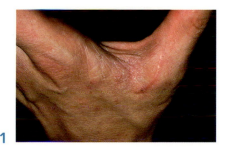

21 **Scabies** is caused by a small mite that burrows under the superficial skin layers. Small linear blisters that cause intense itching can be seen between the finger webs, on the inner wrists, in the axilla, around the areola (nipple) of the breast, and on the genitalia (see Chapter 37). (Photograph reprinted with permission from emedicine.com, Inc., © 2003.)

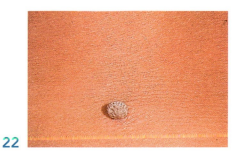

22 **Ticks** can attach to human skin and burrow into superficial skin layers. With careful examination, the back of the organism is usually visible on the skin surface. Ticks are vectors of several systemic diseases (see Chapter 37).

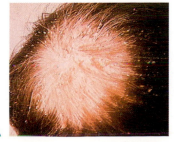

23A and B **Pediculosis humanus capitis** is a louse infestation of the scalp. **A,** Examination of the scalp hair in this infestation shows tiny nits (eggs) attached to the hair shaft. **B,** The organism shown is only occasionally seen (see Chapter 37).

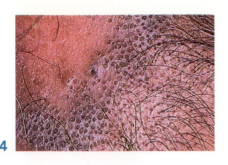

24 **Comedonic acne (noninflammatory)** occurs when follicles become plugged with sebum, forming a comedone on the surface. The black color is caused by oxidation of lipid and melanin, not dirt as is commonly believed (see Chapter 38).

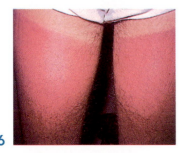

25 **Pustular acne (inflammatory)** presents as inflamed papules that are formed when superficial hair follicles become plugged and rupture at a deeper level. Superficial inflammation results in pustules; deep lesions cause large cysts to form with possible resultant scarring (see Chapter 38).

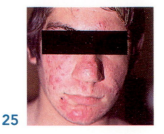

26 **Sunburn** presents as an erythema that occurs after excessive sun exposure; severe burns can result in large blister formation. Proper sunscreen application can provide photoprotection for susceptible patients (see Chapters 39 and 41).

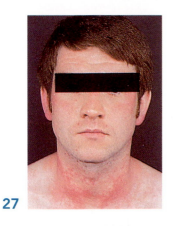

27 **Drug-induced photosensitivity** is a reaction that occurs on sun-exposed surfaces of the head, neck, and dorsum (back) of the hands. The erythema does not occur on photoprotected areas, such as under the nose and chin, behind the ears, and between the fingers (see Chapters 39 and 41).

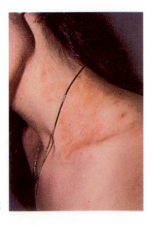

28 **Cosmetic-induced photosensitivity** can be caused by ingredients in certain topical colognes and perfumes. This immunologic reaction produces a local erythema that leaves characteristic post-inflammatory pigmentation (see Chapters 39 and 41).

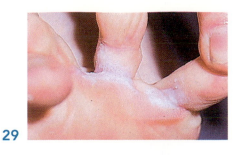

29 **Tinea pedis** infection of the toes characteristically starts between the fourth and fifth web space and spreads proximally. Scaling can progress to maceration with resultant small fissures (see Chapter 43).

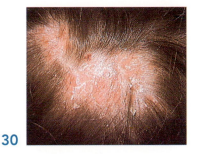

30 **Tinea capitis,** a fungal infection of the scalp, is marked by scale on the scalp with local breaking or loss of hair; erythema (redness) is usually not observed (see Chapter 43).

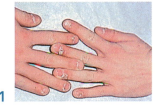

31 **Common warts** are viral-induced lesions that present as localized rough accumulations of keratin (hyperkeratosis) containing many tiny furrows. If the wart's surface is pared, small bleeding points can be seen (see Chapter 44).

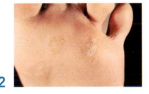

32 **Plantar warts,** caused by a viral infection, are often found on the plantar surface of the foot and present with hard, localized accumulations of keratin. The punctate bleeding points seen when the lesions are pared distinguish plantar warts from calluses (see Chapter 44). (Photograph reprinted with permission from emedicine.com, Inc., © 2003.)

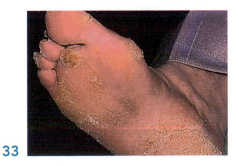

33 **Calluses** are thickened scales that often form on joints and weight-bearing areas. A callus on the plantar surface of the foot is shown here (see Chapter 45).

30. Epstein WL, Epstein JH. Plant induced dermatitis. In: Auerbach PL, ed. *Wilderness Medicine Management of Wilderness and Environmental Emergencies.* 3rd ed. St Louis: Mosby-Yearbook; 1995:843–61.

31. Gayer KD, Burnett JW. Toxicodendron dermatitis. *Cutis.* 1988;42:99–100.

32. Epstein WL. Plant-induced dermatitis. *Ann Emerg Med.* 1987;16: 950–5.

33. Brook I. Secondary bacterial infections complicating skin lesions. *J Med Microbiol.* 2002;51:808–12.

34. D'Mello DA, MacAuley L. Poison ivy dermatitis and secondary mania. *J Nerv Ment Dis.* 1994;182:116–7.

35. Werchniak AE, Schwarzenberger K. Poison ivy: an underreported cause of erythema multiforme. *J Am Acad Dermatol.* 2004:51:S87–8.

36. Gealt L, Osterhoudt KC. Adult respiratory distress syndrome after smoke inhalation from burning poison ivy. *JAMA.* 1995;274: 358–9.

37. Williford PM, Sheretz EF. Poison ivy dermatitis: nuances in treatment. *Arch Fam Med.* 1994;3:184–8.

38. Ives TJ, Tepper RS. Failure of a tapering dose of oral methylprednisolone to treat reactions to poison ivy. *JAMA.* 1991;266:1362.

39. Fisher AA. Poison ivy/oak dermatitis, part 1: prevention soap and water, topical barriers, and hyposensitization. *Cutis.* 1996;57:384–6.

40. Stibach AS, Yagan M, Sharma V, et al. Cost-effective post-exposure prevention of poison ivy dermatitis. *Int J Dermatol.* 2000;39:515–8.

41. Epstein WL. Topical prevention of poison ivy/oak dermatitis. *Arch Dermatol.* 1989;125:499–501.

42. Marks JG Jr, Fowler JG Jr, Sheretz EF, et al. Prevention of poison ivy and poison oak allergic contact dermatitis by quaternium-18 bentonite. *J Am Acad Dermatol.* 1995;33(2 pt 1):212–6.

43. IvyBlock Lotion [package insert]. Plymouth, Mass: EnviroDerm Pharmaceuticals; 1998.

44. Biological products; allergenic extracts; implementation of efficacy review. *Fed Regist.* 1985;50:3082–288.

45. Biological products; allergenic extracts classified in category IIIB; final order; revocation of licenses. *Fed Regist.* 1994;59:59228–37.

46. Skin protectant drug products for over-the-counter human use; final monograph. *Fed Regist.* 2003;68:33362–81.

47. Skin protectant drug products for over-the-counter human use; final monograph; technical amendment. *Fed Regist.* 2004;69:51362.

48. Zink BJ, Otten EJ, Rosenthal M, et al. The effect of jewel weed in preventing poison ivy dermatitis. *J Wilderness Med.* 1991;2:178–82.

49. Long D, Ballentine NH, Marks JG Jr. Treatment of poison ivy/oak allergenic contact dermatitis with an extract of jewelweed. *Am J Contact Dermat.* 1997;8:150–3.

Diaper Dermatitis and Prickly Heat

Nicholas E. Hagemeier

"Diaper rash" is the common name for diaper dermatitis, an acute dermatitis of the skin occurring in the region of the perineum, buttocks, lower abdomen, and inner thighs. By definition, diaper rash cannot occur without the presence of a diaper. Diaper rash can appear in adults or children on any skin surface area enclosed by a diaper or brief. This chapter will focus on infant diaper dermatitis. However, information presented in this chapter is generalizable to the adult population. Specific information about treatment of adult incontinence and its signs and symptoms can be found in Chapter 52.

Prickly heat (miliaria or miliaria rubra) is a transient inflammation of the skin that appears as a very fine, usually red, rash. It can appear on any part of the body that has sweat glands (e.g., groin, chest, and axilla regions).

In most circumstances, neither diaper rash nor prickly heat causes serious illness. These conditions typically produce discomfort, irritation, or itching. They may lead to fussiness, agitation, and irritability, especially in the infant population. Diaper dermatitis and prickly heat can also be devoid of any discomfort or may be only a minor annoyance in both adults and infants.

DIAPER DERMATITIS

Diaper dermatitis is the most common dermatologic disorder of infancy, resulting in more than 1 million physician office visits per year.[1] The majority of diaper dermatitis cases appear in diapered infants younger than 20 months of age. Approximately 70% of infants exhibit some features of diaper-induced skin compromise as early as 7 days after birth.[2] Two-thirds of all infants have overt symptoms of diaper rash at some time in their infancy. There are no known racial, gender, or socioeconomic status differences that influence the incidence of diaper rash. The steady decline in the number of cases of diaper rash in infants since the 1970s is attributed to the increased use of disposable diapers. The decline was accelerated in the 1980s and 1990s with improvements in diaper technology, and the rise of super-absorbent core materials and breathable coverings.[3,4]

Pathophysiology of Diaper Dermatitis

Diaper dermatitis can be caused by a combination of factors. Occlusion, moisture, bacteria, a shift away from the normal acidic skin pH (pH 4.0–5.5) to a more alkaline pH, mechanical chafing and friction, and proteolytic enzymes and bile salts from the gastrointestinal tract can all combine in additive or synergistic ways to cause diaper rash.[5–9]

The skin of the infant perineal region is about one-half to one-third of the thickness of adult skin. Because the perineal region is typically enclosed by a diaper and has little exposure to the outside environment, this area tends to hold moisture and wetness, predisposing it to irritation and infection. This environment has been described as "tropical."[8] Infrequent changing of the diaper contributes to increased skin moisture. Skin left in contact with wetness for long periods becomes waterlogged or hyperhydrated, which plugs sweat glands, increases susceptibility to abrasion and frictional harm, and diminishes the barrier function of the stratum corneum in the infant diaper area. Diminished barrier capabilities in turn make the skin more susceptible to irritation, absorption of chemicals, and opportunistic microbials.

A majority of infants are exceptionally gifted in production of moisture in the diaper area. The typical infant begins to urinate within 24 hours after birth. Urination occurs in infants up to 20 times a day until they are approximately 2 months old; the frequency falls to about 8 times a day until age 8 months. Defecation occurs from 3 to 6 times a day up to about age 8 months. As the infant's autonomic and muscular control develops, defecation gradually declines to 1 to 3 times a day. In the first months of life, it is common for infants to need in excess of six diaper changes per day.

Urine and fecal bacteria can contribute to skin breakdown; urea-splitting bacteria from the colon are believed to convert urine contents into ammonia. Ammonia can raise the pH of the skin, making it more susceptible to damage or infection; ammonia from urine can also rapidly produce a serious chemical burn. This etiologic factor has been diminished by the use of absorbent disposable diapers, which prevent mixing of urine and feces in the diaper area.

Mechanical irritation of the skin can also be the initial insult that breaks down the epidermis, allowing other irritants to harm the skin. Tight-fitting, stiff, or rough diapers and the

Editor's Note: This chapter is based on the 15th edition chapter with the same title, written by Victor A. Padrón.

use of occlusive plastic or rubberized covers or pants over the diaper can contribute to occlusion and mechanical friction of the skin.

Reusable cloth diapers can contribute to diaper rash and skin irritation if the diapers are not adequately washed and rinsed. Harsh chemicals used to clean and sanitize the diapers may leave chemical residues on the diaper that then come into contact with the skin.

Medications and foods that affect the motility and microbial flora of the GI tract, and that hinder autonomic control of urination and defecation may contribute to diaper rash. Foods high in hexitols, sorbitol, sucrose, and fructose may induce diarrhea and predispose to diaper rash. Dairy products can also induce diarrhea, especially in the presence of lactose intolerance. Infant feeding preferences can also influence prevalence of diaper dermatitis. Breast-fed infants have decreased incidences of diaper rash compared with bottle-fed infants.[10] The feces of breast-fed infants are less copious, less alkaline, and less caustic to the skin. Studies have shown that starting a child on solid food early, of itself, has no effect on the incidence of diaper rash in infants, but foods that increase the urinary and fecal pH, such as high-protein diets, may contribute to diaper rash.

Some products (e.g., antioxidants, detergent or soap residues, household cleaning products, lotions, sunscreens, insect repellents), and plant materials (e.g., ragweed and thistle) can produce a contact dermatitis that resembles diaper rash or predispose infants to diaper rash. Although many of these agents commonly are not used in the diaper region, they may have an unexpected effect on skin under a diaper should they be placed in the diaper region through accident or ignorance.

Clinical Presentation of Diaper Dermatitis

Diaper rash usually presents as red to bright red (erythematous), sometimes shiny, wet-looking patches and lesions on the skin (see Color Plates, photograph 19). They may appear dusky maroon or purplish on darker skin. Generally, diaper rash occurs on the skin spaces covered by the diaper, but severe cases can spread outside the diaper area, moving up the abdomen or onto the upper buttocks and lower back. If the infant lies primarily on his or her abdomen, the rash may appear more anterior to the perineum. If the infant lies primarily on his or her back, the rash may appear more posterior to the perineum.

A very disconcerting feature of diaper rash is that it can present in a matter of hours and take days or weeks to completely resolve. The onset of observable diaper rash can occur in the time between two diaper changes. Most likely, the process of skin breakdown is not pronounced or observable initially, and the breakdown goes from unobservable to observable in a matter of hours. The entire process from normal to noticeably inflamed skin takes longer than the time between normal diaper changes.

Severe diaper rash can progress to maceration, papule formation, the presence of vesicles or bullae, oozing, erosion of the skin, or ulceration. Diaper rash can also predispose infants to secondary infection and genital damage. As skin pH changes, it can foster the growth of opportunistic infections that can be bacterial (e.g., streptococci or staphylococci), fungal (e.g., yeasts), and even viral (e.g., herpes simplex). Untreated or infected diaper rash can progress to skin ulceration, infections of the penis or vulva, and/or urinary tract infections. Such developments require medical referral.

Diaper rash can also be a manifestation of other diseases such as Kawasaki's syndrome, granuloma gluteale infantum, cytomegalovirus infection, and nutritional deficiencies. Infants born to immunocompromised mothers (e.g., HIV-positive for human immunodeficiency virus; genital herpes; other chronic, congenital, or sexually transmitted infections) should be considered at increased risk for unusual manifestations of diaper rash or diaper rash–like presentations. Primary infections of the skin by yeasts may initially resemble diaper rash and be misdiagnosed. Inguinal swelling, fever, chills, tachycardia, blisters, vesicles, and irregular borders bounded by bumps or vesicles are indicators of infections that require medical referral.[11,12]

It is important to note that diaper rash can exist concurrent with other skin conditions such as psoriasis and seborrhea. Skin conditions that can occur on other parts of the body can exist in the diaper region and may be misdiagnosed as diaper rash.

Treatment of Diaper Dermatitis

Treatment Goals

The goals of diaper rash treatment are to (1) relieve the symptoms, (2) rid the patient of the rash, and (3) prevent recurrences.

General Treatment Approach

The general treatment approach for diaper rash is the use of nondrug therapy or a combination of drug and nondrug therapy as outlined in Figure 36-1.

The best treatment for diaper rash is prevention. The ideal preventive therapy would be to change the diaper each time the infant defecates or urinates. This treatment is impractical, because it would require a 24-hour vigil and a way to know immediately when the infant has defecated or urinated. Electronic devices (moisture alarms) for constant monitoring of when individuals urinate are available. However, these devices are better used for bed-wetting and potty training in the older child. In infants it is more realistic to use standard prevention and treatment of diaper rash.

Self-treatment should be limited to diaper rash that is uncomplicated and mild-to-moderate in presentation. Self-treatment will most often involve increased vigilance in keeping the infant dry and use of barrier creams to protect the skin in the diaper area. These areas will be covered in more detail in the following nonpharmacologic and pharmacologic sections. Medical referral should occur when diaper rash manifests one or more of the exclusions listed in Figure 36-1.

Nonpharmacologic Therapy

The goals of nonpharmacologic therapy are to (1) reduce occlusion, (2) reduce contact time of urine and feces with skin, (3) reduce mechanical irritation and trauma to the inguinal and perineal skin, (4) protect the skin from further irritation, (5) encourage healing, and (6) discourage the onset of secondary infection.

Treatment of uncomplicated diaper rash should be initiated with nondrug therapy. Increasing the frequency of diaper changes to a minimum of six per day may be a good starting place. If feasible, more than six changes a day combined with careful diaper change procedures may alleviate mild symptoms. During each diaper change, careful flushing of the skin with plain water

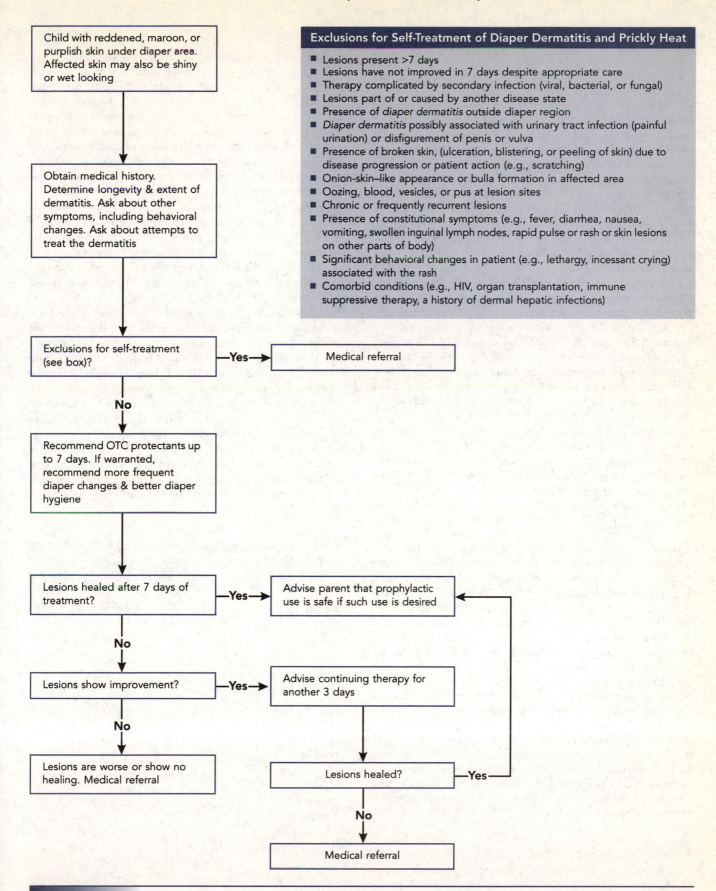

FIGURE 36-1 Self-care of diaper dermatitis. Key: HIV, human immunodeficiency virus; OTC, over-the-counter.

followed by gentle nonfriction drying is to be encouraged. Should wiping be needed, gentle rubbing with a bland soft cloth or wipe is appropriate. Importantly, the unsoiled part of a diaper should not be used to clean or wipe the infant because it may harbor unseen fecal bacteria.

Anecdotally, both professional and nonprofessional caregivers have suggested using a shower sprayer on a low power setting to rinse the child, because a sprayer head is maneuverable and can flush skin folds and natural skin creases without directly touching the area. Another method is holding the infant in a sitting position in a basin of lukewarm water and gently washing the area; however, this method may spread fecal contamination to other parts of the body. Holding the child over a basin or sink as the infant is washed is better, but holding a wiggling wet infant may not be as simple as it sounds and may require more than one set of hands. Some caregivers will let the child air dry and run naked for a short time, but there is the risk that the infant has more urine or bowel contents ready to evacuate. Regardless, thorough drying before re-diapering is essential to good diaper-changing procedures.

The use of commercial baby wipes is no longer controversial. Most wipes are now low in abrasives and chemically bland for use on diaper rash. Used with finesse and gentle wiping, infant wipes are as mild as or milder than washcloths.[13] Few baby wipes still contain alcohol, perfumes, soap, or other ingredients that can cause contact dermatitis or actually burn or sting the infant. Those that do should be avoided.

In the past two decades, the trend toward the use of disposable diapers has been overwhelming, driven by convenience to the caregiver, advertising, and a quelling of environmental issues by the advent of biodegradable disposable diapers. As the technology of disposable diapers has improved, the disposable diaper has become a critical component of nondrug therapy for diaper rash.[14] Disposable diapers are available in various absorbencies to match the waste output of the infant. Some disposable diapers have absorptive materials that pull moisture away from direct contact with the skin to reduce skin hyperhydration and mixing of urine with feces. Some disposable diapers have a protectant (e.g., petrolatum) already in the diaper. These innovations in diaper technology favor the disposable diaper. Studies have shown that use of disposable diapers versus cloth diapers decreases the incidence of severe diaper dermatitis.[3]

Using detergents or lye-based soaps to launder cloth diapers may cause irritation and aggravate diaper rash or cause contact dermatitis. Starched or very stiff diapers can cause mechanical irritation and trauma to the skin. If cloth diapers are used, the following guidelines should be observed:

- Wash with mild detergent.
- Avoid harsh detergents and water softeners.
- If bleach or other sanitizing agents are used, conduct additional rinses to remove chlorine or chemical residues; boiling the diapers for 10 to 15 minutes after washing will also sterilize the diapers.

Pharmacologic Therapy

The goals involved in initiating pharmacologic therapy are to (1) clean and dry the skin, (2) protect the skin from further contact with urine and feces, (3) soothe any discomfort caused by the lesion(s), (4) encourage healing, and (5) discourage the onset of secondary infection.

Skin Protectants

Protectants are the only products considered safe and effective for use in diaper rash without supervision by a medical practitioner. Seventeen ingredients, all skin protectants, have been approved for treatment of diaper rash (Table 36-1). It is common for two or more of the approved ingredients to be combined in commercial products for treating diaper rash. Some products contain an approved ingredient in combination with other ingredients that are unsafe or of dubious value for treating diaper rash. The other ingredient(s) may be unsuitable or even toxic when applied to skin compromised by diaper rash. Therefore, practitioners should suggest only those products that are labeled for diaper rash or contain only 1 or more of the 17 approved ingredients. By law, products that contain antimicrobials, external analgesics, and antifungals cannot claim they are for treatment of diaper rash. Ingredients included in skin protectant formulations but not approved for treatment of diaper rash are provided in Table 36-2.[15]

Of the 17 skin protectants listed in Table 36-1, a select few are commonly incorporated into trade-name skin protectant products. Zinc oxide is an excellent protectant commonly used in products that treat diaper rash. It is typically formulated as a semisolid. Zinc oxide paste USP is a classic example of the protectant group of products; it contains zinc oxide 25%, cornstarch 25%, and white petrolatum 60%. The paste's major drawback is that it is thick and tacky to the touch. Removal from the skin requires wiping with mineral oil. Some zinc oxide preparations are formulated to be less difficult to use, more washable, more cream-like, and easier to apply and remove. Zinc oxide is often combined with other ingredients that may or may not have Food and Drug Administration (FDA) approval (Table 36-2).

TABLE 36-1 Skin Protectants Approved to Treat Diaper Rash

Agent	Concentration (%)
Allantoin	0.5–2
Calamine	1–25
Cocoa butter	50–100
Cod liver oil (in combination)	5.0–13.56
Colloidal oatmeal	≤0.007
Dimethicone	1–30
Glycerin	20–45
Hard fat	50–100
Kaolin	4–20
Lanolin	12.5–50
Mineral oil	50–100
Petrolatum	30–100
Topical starch	10–98
White petrolatum	30–100
Zinc acetate	0.1–2
Zinc carbonate	0.2–2
Zinc oxide	1–25

Source: Reference 15.

TABLE 36-2	Selected Nonmonograph Ingredients Found in Diaper Rash Products

Aloe vera sp. (aloe)	Poplar bud
Aluminum acetate or hydroxide	Shepherd's purse
Arnica (flower)	Silicone
Bovine collagen	Sodium bicarbonate
Castor oil	Sweet clover
Comfrey (herb)	St. John's wort
Emu oil	Tea tree oil
Goldenseal	Vitamins A and D
Jambolan bark	Vitamin E
Melissa (lemon balm)	Walnut leaf
Peruvian balsam	Witch hazel
Plantain	

Use of plain approved ingredients avoids irritation and possible allergic responses from additive ingredients. Few useful comparative studies of the skin protectants are available.

Calamine is a mixture of zinc and ferrous oxides. It has absorptive, antiseptic, and antipruritic properties and is available in numerous dosage forms. Mineral oil coats the skin with a water-impenetrable film that must be washed off with each diaper change to avoid buildup in pores and subsequent folliculitis. Mineral oil is often used in small quantities in skin protectant products. It is often listed as an inactive ingredient in formulations.

Petrolatum is a yellow oleaginous hydrocarbon that, when decolorized, becomes white petrolatum. In either form, it is an excellent protectant and a ubiquitous ointment base. Similar to mineral oil, petrolatum may be listed as an active ingredient (e.g., in Eucerin cream) or as an inactive ingredient (e.g., in Boudreaux's Butt Paste) in skin protectant formulations. Lanolin is a bacteriostatic, hypoallergenic product obtained from wool-bearing animals. It can be used alone or in combination with other skin protectants. Dimethicone is a silicone-based oil that repels water, and soothes and counteracts inflammation. It is used in combination with other skin protectants such as petrolatum.

Topical cornstarch is used almost exclusively as a loose powder. Cornstarch carries a warning against inhalation of the powder because of a history of injury and fatality from improper use around infants. The warning states "Do not use on broken skin. Keep powder away from child's face to avoid inhalation, which can cause breathing problems." Powders should be carefully applied with as little aerosolization as possible. Concerns about inhalation of powders have caused some practitioners to suggest pouring the powder into the hands away from the infant and gently rubbing it onto the perineal area, whereas others recommend avoiding any use of powders around infants.

Skin protectants serve as physical barriers between the skin and external irritants. By preventing further insult or aggravation, they protect surfaces that are healing. Protectants serve as lubricants in areas in which skin-to-skin or skin-to-diaper friction could aggravate diaper rash or predispose the area to dia-

per rash. Protectants absorb moisture or prevent moisture from coming into direct contact with skin. Protective effects of these products allow the body's normal healing processes to work. Because skin protectants are remarkably safe, their use either as treatment or prophylaxis is acceptable. Research suggests that applying a skin protectant regularly with each diaper change is one element of preventing diaper dermatitis.[5]

When diaper rash is present and pharmacologic therapy is indicated, the practitioner should inform caregivers about their choices between semisolid and powdered protectants. Caregivers may be more comfortable with a semisolid product if they are anxious about the inhalation warning on powders, or when hands-on application is not painful or uncomfortable to the patient. Fortunately, the products in this category are relatively inexpensive, and socioeconomic status tends not to be a major issue in treating diaper rash. Table 36-3 lists selected tradename products and their ingredients.

Skin protectant dosing and application are straightforward. The protectant is applied liberally to the skin in the diaper area. Special attention should be paid to completely cover erythematous areas with the protectant if diaper rash is already present. Overapplication (overdosage) of approved skin protectants should not be a concern. Underapplication, however, can reduce the protective effectiveness of the product. The protectant should be reapplied as needed and with every diaper change. Most protective barriers are developed as water-in-oil emulsions (ointments). Therefore, removal of the protectant from the skin will require mild soap and water. Powder preparations of skin protectants, however, are also available.

Contraindicated Agents

Topical nonprescription antibiotic and antifungal agents are not appropriate to use in the self-treatment of diaper rash. The general public is not considered adequately educated to diagnose and treat infectious diseases in the infant's inguinal area. Topical analgesics are not recommended, because they can alter sensory perception in a population that cannot communicate perceptual changes. These agents may also excoriate macerated skin, be painful, retard healing, and further complicate diaper rash.

Hydrocortisone is indicated for minor skin irritation, but it should not be used in diaper rash without supervision by a medical practitioner. This contraindication is especially true in infants. First, hydrocortisone may suppress local immune response, an action that may be undesirable when secondary infection is possible. Second, the diaper area is a significant portion of the infant's body surface area. Hydrocortisone absorption into the skin is enhanced under occlusive conditions. When applied to macerated skin or a large surface area, absorption of hydrocortisone may lead to blood levels that interfere with the infant's pituitary-adrenal axis. Nonprescription hydrocortisone is labeled not to be used in patients younger than 2 years (see Chapter 33).

Product Selection Guidelines

Product selection for treatment of diaper dermatitis focuses mainly on product formulation. Patient preference for ointment or powder formulations will determine which type of product caregivers choose. Comparative studies of skin protectants are lacking in the literature. Whereas no particular product among

TABLE 36-3 Selected Products for Diaper Dermatitis

Trade Name	Primary Ingredients
A + D Ointment with Zinc Oxide	Zinc oxide 10%; dimethicone 1%
Aveeno Bath Treatment Soothing Formula Powder	Colloidal oatmeal 100%
Balmex Diaper Rash Ointment	Zinc oxide; aloe vera; vitamin E[a]
Boudreaux's Butt Paste	Zinc oxide 16%; Peruvian balsam[a]; boric acid[a]; castor oil; mineral oil; white wax; petrolatum
Desitin Diaper Rash Ointment	Zinc oxide 40%; cod liver oil; petrolatum; lanolin; talc
Desitin with Zinc Oxide Powder	Cornstarch 88.2%; zinc oxide 10%
Desitin Creamy Ointment	Zinc oxide 10%; parabens; petrolatum; mineral oil
Diaper Guard Ointment	Dimethicone 1%; white petrolatum 66%; cocoa butter; parabens; vitamins A, D, and E[a]; zinc oxide
Diaparene Cornstarch Baby Powder	Corn starch; aloe[a]
Eucerin Cream	Petrolatum; mineral oil; mineral wax
Johnson & Johnson No More Rash Cream with Zinc Oxide	Zinc oxide 13%; water; mineral oil; dimethicone; glycerin; lanolin; petrolatum
Mexsana Medicated Powder	Kaolin; eucalyptus oil; camphor; corn starch; lemon oil; zinc oxide
Vaseline Pure Petroleum Jelly	White petrolatum 100%

[a] Nonmonograph ingredients.

the approved products has more advantages, personal preferences for particular product characteristics will likely determine which product(s) caregivers use to treat the diaper rash.

As previously mentioned, some commonly used products contain nonapproved (nonmonograph) ingredients. These products may be used for formulation purposes, or they may be unregulated nutraceuticals listed as inactive or active ingredients. Unapproved ingredients could also be included in preparations to support marketing claims. For example, camphor may be present to provide a "medicated" fragrance; aloe may be present to appeal to the public perception that aloe is a wound healer; or vitamins may be present to sound "natural." To make the claim to treat diaper rash, the product must, however, meet the FDA-published guidelines for active ingredients. Although the products used in diaper dermatitis generally have a wide margin of safety, the practitioner should not recommend them indiscriminately.

Complementary Therapies

Products containing complementary therapies are not recommended for use on newborn and infant skin for several reasons. Not enough is known about their effects on infant skin. The amount and effect of systemic absorption are unknown. Appropriateness of product strength to use is unknown. Although some of these agents have been used without incidence in adults, there are no credible data on their safety or efficacy in infants. Infants and children should be treated with the mildest and blandest effective products available.

Assessment of Diaper Dermatitis: A Case-Based Approach

When a caregiver consults a practitioner about a suspected diaper rash, the practitioner should find out whether factors con-

ducive to diaper dermatitis are present. Specifically, the caregiver should be asked what type of diaper is being used and how frequently diapers are changed. Drawing on that response, the practitioner must consider whether increasing the frequency of diaper changes would reduce the diaper rash problem or whether medication is warranted.

If cloth diapers are used, the practitioner should find out how they are laundered and should determine whether the laundering method is adequate to remove chemical residues or fecal bacteria. The practitioner should also ask how the infant is cleaned during diaper changes. The caregiver's response may indicate a cleaning method that does not remove all fecal bacteria or the use of a disposable wipe that may cause skin irritation. To find out whether occlusion of the diaper area is a problem, the practitioner should find out whether plastic pants are being used over the diaper or whether high-absorbency diapers are being used. The practitioner should ask questions to determine whether self-care is appropriate.

Case 36-1 illustrates assessment of patients with diaper dermatitis.

Patient Counseling for Diaper Dermatitis

The practitioner should review with the caregiver proper cleaning of the diaper area, and caution the caregiver to avoid occlusion of the area and to prevent prolonged contact of urine or feces with the infant's skin. The practitioner should explain the proper methods of applying nonprescription skin protectants, and should warn the caregiver of signs and symptoms that indicate the dermatitis has worsened and needs medical attention. The box Patient Education for Diaper Dermatitis lists specific information to provide patients.

CASE 36-1

Relevant Evaluation Criteria	Scenario/Model Outcome
Information Gathering	
1. Gather essential information about the patient's symptoms, including:	
a. description of symptom(s) (i.e., nature, onset, duration, severity, associated symptoms)	Ms. Rose indicates that her daughter is very fussy and thinks it may be because of a rash on her "bottom." The rash has progressively worsened over the past 7 days. Mr. Rose describes the rash as "very red and wet." She also says, "It looks like some of the blisters are oozing a little pus."
b. description of any factors that seem to precipitate, exacerbate, and/or relieve the patient's symptom(s)	Ms. Rose says that her daughter has had "looser stools than normal" over the past week. Her daughter recently finished a course of antibiotics, but the mother does not know if the medication had anything to do with the rash.
c. description of the patient's efforts to relieve the symptoms	The mother has been putting baby powder on the rash for the last 4 days. She does not think it is helping the rash. She has not tried any additional OTC products. She has been changing Clara's diaper more often in an effort to keep her bottom dry.
	She has not contacted her daughter's pediatrician, because she was "just at the doctor a little more than a week ago for an ear infection."
2. Gather essential patient history information:	
a. patient's identity	Clara Rose
b. patient's age, sex, height, and weight	4-month-old female, 25 inches, 14 lb
c. patient's occupation	N/A
d. patient's dietary habits	Breast-fed; normal eating habits
e. patient's sleep habits	Normal for age
f. concurrent medical conditions, prescription and nonprescription medications, and dietary supplements	None; recently finished course of amoxicillin/clavulanic acid for treatment of ear infection
g. allergies	NKA
h. history of other adverse reactions to medications	None
i. other (describe) _____	N/A
Assessment and Triage	
3. Differentiate the patient's signs/symptoms and correctly identify the patient's primary problem(s).	Symptoms similar to moderate-to-severe diaper rash in the inguinal area. The condition was likely precipitated by the antibiotic therapy (change in intestinal flora), which consequently caused loose stools in the infant.
4. Identify exclusions for self-treatment (see Figure 36-1).	Presence of blistered skin in the inguinal area; presence of the condition for about 7 days with no improvement; presence of constitutional symptoms (i.e., loose stools)
5. Formulate a comprehensive list of therapeutic alternatives for the primary problem to determine if triage to a medical practitioner is required, and share this information with the caregiver.	Options include: (1) Refer Clara immediately to her pediatrician or other PCP. (2) Recommend self-care until an appropriate PCP can be consulted. (3) Recommend self-care with an OTC product. (4) Recommend self-care with nonpharmacologic methods. (5) Take no action.
Plan	
6. Select an optimal therapeutic alternative to address the patient's problem, taking into account patient preferences.	Recommend that Ms. Rose contact Clara's pediatrician for a workup of the condition
7. Describe the recommended therapeutic approach to the caregiver.	Because the condition has worsened in the last week and Clara has had loose stools during this time, it is important to rule out other conditions, prevent secondary infection, and keep the condition from worsening.
8. Explain to the caregiver the rationale for selecting the recommended therapeutic approach from the considered therapeutic alternatives.	Clara meets multiple exclusion criteria (see Figure 36-1). Although appropriate self-care may improve the condition in this situation, it is in Clara's best interests to be evaluated by a primary care provider.

CASE 36-1 *(continued)*

Relevant Evaluation Criteria	Scenario/Model Outcome
Patient Education	
9. When recommending self-care with non-prescription medications and/or nondrug therapy, convey accurate information to the caregiver.	See Nondrug Measures in the box Patient Education for Diaper Dermatitis.
10. Solicit follow-up questions from caregiver.	I have some aloe vera gel at home. Would it help if I put some on Clara's bottom to take away some of the pain?
11. Answer caregiver's questions.	No. Aloe vera is not an appropriate product to use in this situation. It would be best to discuss with Clara's pediatrician appropriate treatment options for this condition.

Key: N/A, not applicable; NKA, no known allergies; PCP, primary care provider.

Evaluation of Patient Outcomes for Diaper Dermatitis

Treatment of diaper dermatitis should be relatively short, approximately 1 week. If 7 days have elapsed and the condition is improved but not healed, therapy should be continued for another 3 days or until complete healing has occurred. If the condition has not improved or has worsened after 7 days of treatment, medical referral should occur. At each diaper change, the parent should inspect the lesions for signs of improvement. At the conclusion of therapy, the skin should have returned to pre–diaper rash condition.

PATIENT EDUCATION FOR Diaper Dermatitis

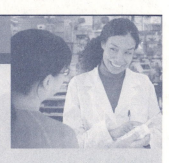

The objectives of self-treatment are to (1) eliminate the rash, (2) relieve the symptoms, and (3) prevent recurrent rashes. For most patients, carefully following product instructions and the self-care measures listed here will help ensure optimal therapeutic outcomes.

Nondrug Measures

- Change diapers frequently, at least six times a day, to prevent prolonged exposure of the infant's skin to moisture and feces.
- To prevent occlusion of skin in the diaper area, avoid putting rubber pants over cloth diapers. Tightly covering the skin causes it to break down.
- During every diaper change, flush the infant's skin with plain water, and gently pat it dry or allow it to air dry.
- Do not wipe the infant with any part of the diaper. Even areas that appear unsoiled may be contaminated with fecal bacteria.
- To prevent irritating the infant's skin, do not use harsh detergent or ordinary lye-based soaps to launder cloth diapers; avoid starched or very stiff diapers; and avoid commercial baby wipes that contain alcohol, perfumes, and soap, which may burn or sting the skin.
- If feasible, allow the infant to go without a diaper, even for short instances, in an effort to dry the rash.

Nonprescription Medications

- To treat diaper rash, use a product containing one or more of the skin protectants listed in Table 36-1. The product can be used even after the rash clears to prevent recurrences.

- Do not use products that contain ingredients listed in Table 36-3 if they are combined with benzocaine or an antibacterial such as benzethonium chloride. Benzocaine can cause an allergic reaction; antibacterials are not suitable for use on diaper rash.
- Do not use hydrocortisone.
- Do not use external analgesics such as phenol, menthol, methyl salicylate, or capsaicin to treat diaper rash. These medications are inappropriate for use on infant skin and may cause harm.
- Powders for children or infants should be gently poured into the hands then rubbed onto the skin, using a sufficient amount to cover the affected area. Do not vigorously shake powders near infants. Avoid infant inhalation of powders.
- Apply sufficient cream or ointment, by hand or with a disposable or washable spatula, to cover the affected area.
- If using mineral oil, wash it off at every diaper change to avoid clogging skin pores, which may lead to prickly heat and folliculitis.
- Discard products that are discolored or whose expiration date has passed. (The practitioner should point out expiration dates on the products.)
- Consult a primary care provider if any of the exclusions in Figure 36-1 apply.

PRICKLY HEAT

Prickly heat (also called heat rash or miliaria) can occur at any age in anyone who has active sweat glands. It probably is significantly underreported, because it is less troublesome than diaper rash and clears up very rapidly if left alone and/or if its cause is removed. Because persons of advanced age are less tolerant to heat, sweat less, are less physically active, and spend more time indoors and in controlled environments than younger people, they may have less opportunity to develop prickly heat.

Pathophysiology of Prickly Heat

Prickly heat results from blocked or plugged sweat glands. Prickly heat can arise from normal skin with little or no anatomic prodrome. The condition is most often associated with very hot, humid weather or can occur during illnesses that cause significant or profuse sweating. It also results from inability of the skin to "breathe" (interact with air) because of excessive clothing; very tight clothing; or clothing that is occlusive, such as leather and polyester, or athletic protective or safety garments and devices.

The pores that house the sweat glands are obstructed in prickly heat. The inability of sweat to be secreted and escape the pores causes dilation and rupture of epidermal sweat pores. This situation causes an acute inflammation of the dermis that may manifest as stinging, burning, or itching.

Clinical Presentation of Prickly Heat

The pinpoint-size lesions that are the hallmark of prickly heat are raised and red or maroon, forming erythematous papules (see Color Plates, photograph 20). The pinhead-size lesions may appear in small numbers clustered together or spread out over the occluded area on a pink to red field ("miliaria rubra"). Common sites for prickly heat dermatitis include the axillae (armpits), chest, upper back, back of the neck, abdomen, and inguinal area (groin). The lesions usually trace the pattern of the occlusion and, in uncomplicated cases, do not extend beyond the occluded area. Lesions can occur on the body wherever occlusion occurs and active sweat glands are present. If lesions are not resolved in a reasonable length of time (approximately 3–10 days), they can evolve into the same kinds of complications seen in diaper rash (e.g., infection, pustule formation, or generalized dermatitis). Complications are extremely rare.

Treatment of Prickly Heat

Treatment Goals

The primary goal in treatment of prickly heat is removal of the causative agent. Lesions associated with prickly heat usually resolve without pharmacologic treatment if the cause is removed. A secondary goal in the treatment of prickly heat is alleviation of symptoms associated with prickly heat.

General Treatment Approach

The goals in nonpharmacologic therapy of prickly heat include (1) eliminating occlusion of skin, (2) protecting skin from fur-

ther irritation, (3) promoting healing of skin, and (4) discouraging onset of secondary infection.

Pharmacologic therapy and nondrug therapy have the same goals. The pharmacologic products help to (1) keep skin dry, (2) promote healing, (3) soothe any discomfort caused by lesion(s), and (4) discourage onset of secondary infection. The algorithm in Figure 36-2 outlines the self-treatment of prickly heat.

Nonpharmacologic Therapy

Nondrug therapy for prickly heat consists of taking measures to decrease sweating. If the sweating is caused by a fever, the use of internal antipyretics, if not contraindicated, is appropriate. Wearing loose, light-colored, and lightweight clothing is palliative in prickly heat and is also good prevention in that it allows airflow to the skin. In infants, frequent diaper changes and sparing use of soap or chemical irritants can reduce discomfort of existing prickly heat. Practitioners should warn patients not to apply oleaginous or oily substances to prickly heat lesions, because these substances plug pores that need to be patent.

Pharmacologic Therapy

Nonprescription treatment of prickly heat should be limited to mild-to-moderate, uncomplicated cases. Prickly heat should not be occluded during therapy. This disorder can be ameliorated in less time and with less total drug exposure than diaper rash.

Emollients, Skin Protectants, and Antipruritics

For prickly heat, washing the skin with bland soap and soaking in colloidal oatmeal may be all that is needed. The choice of a drug product should be limited to one product that relieves burning and itching but does not block skin exposure to the air. Water-washable antipruritic products as well as bland emollients and protectants that soothe the skin and maintain skin moisture and texture can be used to treat the symptoms of prickly heat while they resolve. Powders should be used only prophylactically to absorb moisture and keep skin dry, rather than as treatment of active prickly heat. Powders can actually clog pores and complicate therapy. (See Table 36-4 for selected trade-name products and Chapter 33 for a discussion of skin emollients.)

Other Pharmacologic Agents

As in diaper rash, hydrocortisone is contraindicated in infants. In adults, hydrocortisone may be useful if the surface area involved is equal to or less than approximately 10% of body surface area. (See Figure 41-3 for information on calculating body surface area.) Because prickly heat rapidly clears without drug therapy, the only real use for hydrocortisone is to relieve itching.

Topical antihistamines and local anesthetics (see Chapter 37) carry the risk of sensitization.

Product Selection Guidelines

Petrolatum and other oil-in-water emulsions are not desirable in prickly heat, given that they trap moisture beneath them and keep the area hydrated. In prickly heat, the skin needs to dry and dissipate moisture. Only water-washable, cream-based products should be applied to prickly heat to relieve symptoms. For moisture absorption and prevention of wetness, powders are a reasonable choice. However, prolonged use or overuse of

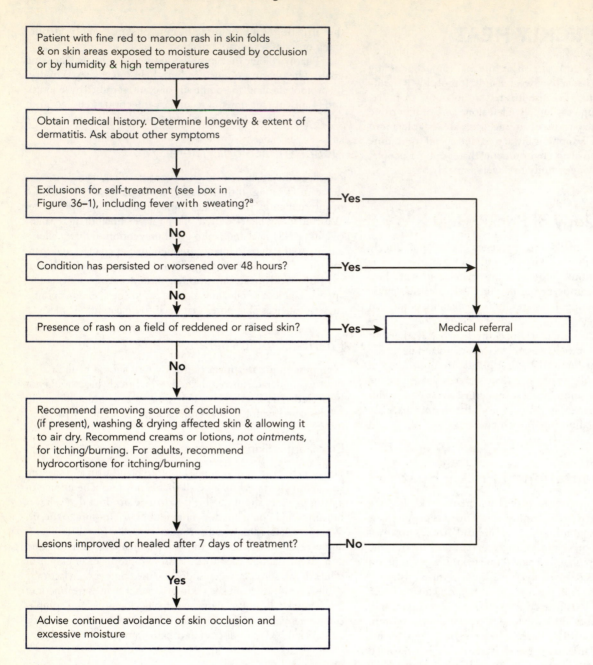

Patient with fine red to maroon rash in skin folds & on skin areas exposed to moisture caused by occlusion or by humidity & high temperatures

↓

Obtain medical history. Determine longevity & extent of dermatitis. Ask about other symptoms

↓

Exclusions for self-treatment (see box in Figure 36–1), including fever with sweating?[a] —**Yes**——→ Medical referral

No ↓

Condition has persisted or worsened over 48 hours? —**Yes**——→

No ↓

Presence of rash on a field of reddened or raised skin? —**Yes**—→ Medical referral

No ↓

Recommend removing source of occlusion (if present), washing & drying affected skin & allowing it to air dry. Recommend creams or lotions, *not ointments*, for itching/burning. For adults, recommend hydrocortisone for itching/burning

↓

Lesions improved or healed after 7 days of treatment? —**No**——→ Medical referral

Yes ↓

Advise continued avoidance of skin occlusion and excessive moisture

[a] High fever without sweating, high pulse rate, possible increased respiration, or hot, flushed dry skin (patient seems to be "burning up") may indicate hyperpyrexia ("heatstroke" or "sunstroke"). Refer the patient immediately to a PCP and/or transport patient to an emergency facility. Slow or weak pulse, lethargy, cold, pale clammy skin, absence of fever, or disorientation may indicate heat exhaustion. Move patient to a cool environment, and have the patient recline and take regular sips of water or slightly salty liquids or electrolyte solutions every few minutes.

FIGURE 36-2 Self-care of prickly heat. Key: PCP, primary care provider.

powders can lead to clogged pores and actually can precipitate prickly heat. When applied to the chest or neck, cornstarch or talc powder should be placed in the hand and applied manually to the skin with light friction. Practitioners should be very careful not to recommend any product for an infant that has an ingredient (e.g., phenols or boric acid) that could be toxic if absorbed through thin, compromised skin. Bathing children and infants with prickly heat in colloidal oatmeal or lukewarm water may be recommended as a first option.

Assessment of Prickly Heat: A Case-Based Approach

Patient assessment for prickly heat involves identifying the site of lesions and having patients reconstruct their activities and attire over the past 24 hours. If the patient is an infant, the practitioner should ask whether the infant sleeps in a warm or humid environment and whether additional clothing or occlusive coverings are used at night or when the infant is asleep.

TABLE 36-4 Selected Products for Prickly Heat

Trade Name	Primary Ingredients
Aveeno Moisturizing Cream	Colloidal oatmeal 1%; glycerin; petrolatum; dimethicone
Band-Aid Itch Relief Gel Spritz	Camphor 0.5%
Benadryl Maximum Strength Itch Relief Cream	Diphenhydramine HCl 2%; zinc acetate 0.1%; parabens; aloe vera
Cortizone-5, Cortizone-10 Cream	Hydrocortisone 0.5% or 1.0%
Curel Moisturizing Cream	Glycerin; petrolatum; dimethicone; parabens
Eucerin Moisturizing Lotion	Mineral oil; PEG-40 sorbitan peroleate; lanolin acid glycerin ester; sorbitol; lanolin alcohol
Lubriderm Cream	Mineral oil; petrolatum; lanolin; lanolin alcohol; lanolin oil; glycerin

Case 36-2 is an example of assessment of patients with prickly heat.

Patient Counseling for Prickly Heat

The practitioner should stress to the patient that prickly heat is easily prevented by removing factors that clog skin pores, while also explaining appropriate nondrug and drug measures for healing/alleviating symptoms of prickly heat. The practitioner should explain that excessive use of skin protectants can exac-erbate the disorder. The box Patient Education for Prickly Heat lists specific information to provide patients.

Evaluation of Patient Outcomes for Prickly Heat

Treatment of prickly heat should be relatively short. If the condition is improved but not completely resolved after 7 to 10 days of treatment, therapy can be continued another 3 to 4 days until complete healing has occurred. If the condition has not improved

CASE 36-2

Relevant Evaluation Criteria	Scenario/Model Outcome
Information Gathering	
1. Gather essential information about the patient's symptoms, including:	
a. description of symptom(s) (i.e., nature, onset, duration, severity, associated symptoms)	Patient has a fine, pinpoint-sized rash around his groin, thigh, and gluteal area. The rash has been present since he woke up this morning. Although the rash is not painful, the patient indicates that it does itch.
b. description of any factors that seem to precipitate, exacerbate, and/or relieve the patient's symptom(s)	Patient has had previous rashes. He tends to get the rash more often in the summer, but he sometimes has it in the winter months as well. He tends to get the rash more often when he is riding his bicycle. He did go for a 15-mile ride yesterday afternoon.
c. description of the patient's efforts to relieve the symptoms	Patient tries to prevent rash through good personal hygiene techniques; however, these measures do not always keep him from getting the rash. He has not tried any OTC products to treat the rash.
2. Gather essential patient history information:	
a. patient's identity	William Edwards
b. patient's age, sex, height, and weight	23-year-old male, 5 ft 11 in, 178 lb
c. patient's occupation	Meteorologist
d. patient's dietary habits	Normal healthy diet with occasional junk food; occasional alcohol
e. patient's sleep habits	Gets up early for occupation; averages 5–7 hours of sleep nightly
f. concurrent medical conditions, prescription and nonprescription medications, and dietary supplements	Hyperlipidemia well controlled by diet, exercise, and simvastatin 40 mg daily

Relevant Evaluation Criteria	Scenario/Model Outcome
g. allergies	NKA
h. history of other adverse reactions to medications	None
i. other (describe) _____	William is an avid cyclist, often logging 75–100 miles each week when the weather is fit. He wears tight-fitting cycling clothing when he rides.

Assessment and Triage

3. Differentiate the patient's signs/symptoms and correctly identify the patient's primary problem(s).	Prickly heat secondary to sweating and occlusive clothing
4. Identify exclusions for self-treatment (see Figure 36-1).	None
5. Formulate a comprehensive list of therapeutic alternatives for the primary problem to determine if triage to a medical practitioner is required, and share this information with the patient.	Options include: (1) Refer William to a dermatologist or his PCP. (2) Recommend self-care until an appropriate PCP can be consulted. (3) Recommend self-care with OTC products. (4) Recommend self-care with nonpharmacologic methods. (5) Take no action.

Plan

6. Select an optimal therapeutic alternative to address the patient's problem, taking into account patient preferences.	A moisturizing cream will likely relieve the itching associated with the prickly heat. Appropriate creams listed in Table 36-4 are Aveeno Moisturizing Cream, Curel Moisturizing Cream, and Lubriderm Cream. Patient education about the cause of prickly heat is important in prevention of future occurrences.
7. Describe the recommended therapeutic approach to the patient.	Apply moisturizing cream 2 times daily and as needed until the rash subsides.
8. Explain to the patient the rationale for selecting the recommended therapeutic approach from the considered therapeutic alternatives.	With mild symptoms such as itching, a moisturizer will likely minimize discomfort. Removing sweaty clothing and taking a shower as soon as possible after cycling will help prevent future occurrences of prickly heat rash.

Patient Education

9. When recommending self-care with nonprescription medications and/or nondrug therapy, convey accurate information to the patient:	
a. appropriate dose and frequency of administration	See the box Patient Education for Prickly Heat.
b. maximum number of days the therapy should be employed	N/A
c. product administration procedures	See the box Patient Education for Prickly Heat.
d. expected time to onset of relief	See the box Patient Education for Prickly Heat.
e. degree of relief that can be reasonably expected	See the box Patient Education for Prickly Heat.
f. most common side effects	Side effects are not common with moisturizing creams.
g. side effects that warrant medical intervention should they occur	See the box Patient Education for Prickly Heat.
h. patient options in the event that condition worsens or persists	See the box Patient Education for Prickly Heat.
i. product storage requirements	Store the product in its original container in a location near the showering area.
j. specific nondrug measures	See the box Patient Education for Prickly Heat.
10. Solicit follow-up questions from patient.	Can I get this rash on other parts of my body?
11. Answer patient's questions.	Yes. Prickly heat can occur in any location where sweat glands are present.

Key: N/A, not applicable; NKA, no known allergies; OTC, over-the-counter; PCP, primary care provider.

PATIENT EDUCATION FOR
Prickly Heat

The objectives of self-treatment are to (1) relieve the discomfort of prickly heat and (2) eliminate its cause. For most patients, following product instructions and the self-care measures listed here will help ensure optimal therapeutic outcomes.

Nondrug Measures

- To prevent clogging skin pores, avoid excessive sweating by resting, cooling off, or going to a cool environment.
- Wear loose, light-colored, porous, and/or lightweight clothing to allow airflow to the skin.
- Decrease the discomfort of prickly heat in infants by changing diapers frequently and by using soaps or possible chemical irritants (e.g., baby wipes) sparingly.
- Shower, bathe, or change clothes immediately after heavy sweating, and wear loose-fitting clothes when such activity is anticipated. Remember to drink plenty of fluids and allow the body to cool down after any strenuous activity.

Nonprescription Medications

- Unless a primary care provider advises otherwise, use internal analgesics (e.g., aspirin, acetaminophen, ibuprofen) to reduce a fever and the sweating it can cause.
- Do not apply oleaginous or oily substances to prickly heat lesions because they clog skin pores.
- Use powdered skin protectants to absorb moisture and help prevent wetness (see Table 36-3). Place cornstarch or talc powder in the hand, and apply to the skin with light friction. Note that prolonged use or overuse of powders can lead to clogged pores and can precipitate prickly heat.
- Do not use hydrocortisone on infants. However, it may be used to relieve itching in adult cases of prickly heat if no more than 10% of the body surface area is involved.
- Water washable emollients applied in a thin film twice a day can help the skin return to normal.
- If redness, burning, itching, peeling, or swelling develops after a product is applied, rinse any remaining product off the skin and avoid further use.
- For older children and adults, consider using oral antihistamines for relief of itching. Note that topical antihistamines can cause allergic reactions (see Chapter 11).
- To soothe discomfort in adults or infants, wash the affected skin with bland soap or soak the skin in a colloidal oatmeal solution.
- The condition should show observable improvement in 24 hours.

⚠️ If the condition has not improved or has worsened after 7 days of treatment, consult a primary care provider.

---

or has worsened after 7 days, the patient should be referred for further evaluation. Monitoring of treatment success involves simple observation of lesions. At the end of therapy, skin should have returned to normal.

KEY POINTS
FOR DIAPER DERMATITIS
AND PRICKLY HEAT

- ➤ Diaper rash is caused by moisture and occlusion.
- ➤ The frequency of diaper changes (at least six per day) is a major factor in the prevalence of diaper rash.
- ➤ Pharmacologic treatment should be limed to the mildest, blandest products with the fewest ingredients; exotic additives should be avoided.
- ➤ Apply skin protectants liberally to diaper rash areas; over-application should not be a concern.
- ➤ Products containing petrolatum and zinc oxide are the favored semisolid dosage forms; cornstarch and zinc oxide are the favored powders.
- ➤ Do not use hydrocortisone on diaper rash.
- ➤ Caution should be used to prevent infant inhalation of powders used for both diaper dermatitis and prickly heat.
- ➤ The majority of diaper rash cases will resolve when occlusion and wetness are adequately suppressed.
- ➤ Help the patient to distinguish between ordinary diaper rash and complicated cases that warrant medical referral.

- ➤ Cases that do not resolve in 10 days should be referred for further evaluation.
- ➤ Prickly heat is caused by occluded sweat glands.
- ➤ By removing the occlusion, prickly heat will generally heal itself.
- ➤ Pharmacologic treatment is directed to providing relief from itching or burning.
- ➤ Products containing emollients and/or anti-itch ingredients in water-washable dosage forms are favored; powders may be used to help dry the skin, but they must be used judiciously to prevent clogged pores.
- ➤ Help the patient to distinguish between ordinary prickly heat and complicated cases that warrant medical referral.

REFERENCES

1. Ward DB, Fleischer, AB, Feldman, SR, et al. Characterization of diaper dermatitis in the United States. *Arch Pediatr Adolesc Med.* 2000;154:943–6.
2. Visscher MO, Chatterjee R, Munson KA, et al. Development of diaper rash in the newborn. *Pediatr Dermatol.* 2000;17:52–7.
3. Akin F, Spraker M, Aly R, et al. Effects of breathable disposable diapers: reduced prevalence of Candida and common diaper dermatitis. *Pediatr Dermatol.* 2001;18:282–90.
4. Odio MR, O'Connor RJ, Sarbaugh F, et al. Continuous topical administration of a petrolatum formulation by a novel disposable diaper. *Dermatology.* 2000;200:238–43.
5. Atherton DJ. A review of the pathophysiology, prevention and treatment of irritant diaper dermatitis. *Curr Med Res Opin.* 2004;20:645–9.
6. Shin HT. Diaper dermatitis that does not quit. *Dermatol Ther.* 2005;18:124–35.
7. Scheinfeld N. Diaper dermatitis: a review and brief survey of eruptions of the diaper area. *Am J Clin Dermatol.* 2005;6:273–81.

8. Wolf R, Wolf D, Tuzun B, et al. Diaper dermatitis. *Clin Dermatol.* 2000; 18:657–60.

9. Berg RW. Etiologic factor in diaper dermatitis: a model for development of improved diapers. *Pediatrician.* 1986;14(suppl 1):27–33.

10. Benjamin, L. Clinical correlates with diaper dermatitis. *Pediatrician.* 1987; 14:21–6.

11. Nield LS, Kamat D. Prevention, diagnosis, and management of diaper dermatitis. *Clin Pediatr.* 2007;46:480–86.

12. Gupta AK, Skinner AR. Management of diaper dermatitis. *Int J Dermatol.* 2004;43:830–4.

13. Odio M, Streicher-Scott J, Hansen RC. Disposable baby wipes: efficacy and skin mildness. *Dermatol Nurs.* 2001;13:107–13.

14. Odio M, Friedlander SF. Diaper dermatitis and advances in diaper technology. *Curr Opin Pediatr.* 2000;12:342–6.

15. US Food and Drug Administration. Skin protectant drug products for over-the-counter human use: final monograph. *Fed Regist.* 2003;68:33362–81.

Insect Bites and Stings and Pediculosis

Wayne Buff and Cliff Fuhrman

Insect bites and stings are common, and anyone who spends time outdoors, whether for work or recreation, is at risk. These injuries usually cause only a local reaction, but they can produce a mild allergic reaction or life-threatening anaphylaxis in patients who are sensitive. About 0.5% of the population may show signs of systemic allergic reactions to insect stings, and simultaneous multiple insect stings of 500 or more may cause death from toxicity. In the United States, more people die of insect stings than of bites from all poisonous animals combined. The exact number of people who experience systemic allergic reactions to insect bites is unknown.

Despite the potentially fatal consequences, encounters with biting and stinging insects are typically brief. Pediculosis (lice infestation) and scabies, by contrast, are parasitic infections, and the arachnids remain on the host until eradicated. Approximately 10 to 12 million people in the United States are affected by pediculosis each year, most of them children ages 3 to 12 years.

Although the public usually refers to all biting and stinging invertebrate animals as "insects," these animals are members of the phylum Arthropoda, which includes insects, arachnids, and crustaceans. This chapter covers the stings of insects only, but discusses the bites of both insects and arachnids (e.g., ticks, mites, spiders, and lice). The term *insect* is used to cover general statements about these invertebrates.

INSECT BITES

Pathophysiology and Clinical Presentation of Insect Bites

Bites from insects (e.g., mosquitoes, fleas, and bedbugs) and from arachnids (e.g., ticks and chiggers) are nonvenomous. Each biting arthropod has distinctive biting organs and salivary secretions that contribute to the characteristic signs and symptoms for each type of bite.

Mosquitoes

Mosquitoes are found in abundance worldwide, particularly in humid, warm climates. After landing on the skin, mosquitoes inject an anticoagulant saliva into the victim. The antigenic components of this secretion cause the characteristic welt and itching. Bites are most common on exposed skin, but mosquitoes can also bite through thin clothing.

Malaria and West Nile virus are serious systemic infections that are transmitted by mosquitoes. West Nile virus was first diagnosed in the United States in New York in 1999 and has since been found in 47 states.[1] The most common symptoms are flu-like with fever and fatigue, but they can progress to muscle weakness, encephalitis, or meningitis. Although research is underway to develop a vaccine, the only currently available treatments are supportive care. Controlling mosquito populations is particularly important in preventing the spread of this disease.[2,3]

Fleas

Fleas are tiny bloodsucking insects that can be found worldwide but breed best in a humid climate. It is believed that fleas are attracted to their bird or mammalian host by body warmth or exhaled carbon dioxide. Although they are parasites, fleas may survive and multiply without food for several weeks. Humans are often bitten after moving into a vacant flea-infested habitat or when living with infested pets. Fleabites are usually multiple and grouped and, in humans, occur primarily on legs and ankles. Each lesion is characterized by an erythematous region around the puncture and intense itching. In addition to being annoying, fleas can transmit diseases such as bubonic plague and endemic typhus.

Sarcoptes scabiei

Scabies, commonly called "the itch," is a contagious parasitic skin infection caused by *Sarcoptes scabiei,* a very small and rarely seen arachnid mite. The mites burrow up to 1 cm into the stratum corneum, and the females deposit eggs in their "tunnels." Common infestation sites are interdigital spaces of fingers, flexor surfaces of the wrists, external male genitalia, buttocks, and anterior axillary folds (see Color Plates, photograph 21). Scabies infection is characterized by inflammation and intense itching secondary to an immunologic response. Mites are transmitted from an infected individual to others through physical contact. The mite that causes scabies should not be confused with lice or chiggers; a scabies infection requires prescription therapy rather than nonprescription treatment.

Bedbugs

Bedbugs usually hide and deposit their eggs in crevices of walls, floors, picture frames, bedding, and furniture during the day; they bite their victims at night. People may also be bitten in subdued light while sitting in theaters or other public places.

The increased mobility of society worldwide has heightened concern for an increased incidence of bedbug infestations in the United States in places frequented by travelers, such as hotels.[4] The reaction to a bedbug bite can range from irritation at the site to a small dermal hemorrhage, depending on the sensitivity of the individual. Hepatitis B may be transferred through bedbug bites, but this type of transmission has not yet been confirmed.[5]

Ticks

Ticks feed on the blood of humans and both wild and domesticated animals. During feeding, the tick's mouthparts are introduced into the skin, enabling it to hold firmly (see Color Plates, photograph 22). If the tick is removed but the mouthparts are left behind, intense itching and nodules requiring surgical excision may develop. If left attached, the tick becomes fully engorged with blood and remains for up to 10 days before dropping off. Ticks should be removed intact with fine tweezers. If fingers are used instead, protect with gloves and wash afterward. Matches or petrolatum should not be applied to the tick to aid removal because they may damage the patient's skin or induce salivation by the tick and possibly contribute to infection in the bite area.[6,7]

The local reaction to tick bites consists of itching papules that disappear within 1 week. Certain species of ticks, however, can transmit systemic diseases such as Rocky Mountain spotted fever and Lyme disease. Rocky Mountain spotted fever is transmitted by wood ticks or dog ticks, and is characterized by severe headache, rash, high fever, and extreme exhaustion. Symptoms appear 3 to 12 days after the bite occurs and must be treated with antibiotics.[6] Lyme disease is an inflammatory infection that affects the joints, heart, and nervous system. It is caused by a spirochete found in deer ticks that is transmitted into the victim after a tick bite.[8] Deer ticks are also referred to as black-legged ticks; these ticks are smaller than wood ticks or dog ticks and, therefore, may sometimes be overlooked by patients performing skin inspections.[6] Lyme disease has been identified in 49 states, but the highest percentage of cases occur in the northeastern, upper midwestern, and Pacific coast states.[6] Most acute stages of Lyme disease are heralded by skin rash and flu-like symptoms. The rash appears first as a papule at the bite site and may become an enlarged circle with a clear center called a "bull's-eye." Tender urticarial lesions appear 3 to 32 days after the bite and disappear spontaneously within 3 to 4 weeks. If left untreated, neurologic symptoms ranging from headache and stiff neck to partial paralysis or aseptic meningitis may occur. Cardiac disturbances and musculoskeletal symptoms may develop and last up to several months. Finally, the patient may experience arthritis and a red discoloration of the skin on hands, wrists, feet, or ankles. Early diagnosis and prompt treatment with antibiotics are essential to prevent development of serious neurologic, cardiac, and rheumatologic manifestations.

Chiggers

Chiggers, or red bugs, live in shrubbery, trees, and grass. After attaching to the skin, the larvae secrete a digestive fluid that causes cellular disintegration of the affected area, a red papule, and intense itching. This fluid also causes the skin to harden and form a tiny tube where the chigger lies and continues to feed until engorged. It then drops off and changes into an adult.

Spiders

Although all species of spiders are poisonous, most are unable to penetrate the skin because their fangs are too short or too fragile.

The black widow and brown recluse are two major exceptions. Bites from these species may not be noticed initially, but symptoms develop shortly. Deaths from bites of either species are rare, but symptoms can be serious. Reaction to black widow bites includes delayed intense pain, stiffness and joint pain, abdominal disturbances, fever, chills, and dyspnea. Brown recluse bites can cause these symptoms as well as a spreading ulcerated wound at the bite site.[6] If a spider bite is suspected but cannot be confirmed, the wound area should be monitored for these symptoms.

Complications of Insect Bites

Secondary bacterial infection of insect bites can occur if skin of the affected area is abraded from scratching. Skin infections such as impetigo may be a complication of insect bites; these infections may appear as yellow crusting, purulent drainage, and/or significant redness and swelling of the skin around the bite.

Treatment of Insect Bites

Specific nonprescription external analgesics are labeled for use in treating minor insect bites. These agents are not, however, effective for treating scabies.

Treatment Goals

The goals of self-treating insect bites are to relieve symptoms and prevent secondary bacterial infections.

General Treatment Approach

Application of an ice pack may provide sufficient relief of pain and irritation of bites from mosquitoes, chiggers, bedbugs, or fleas. If this treatment does not work, applying an external analgesic to the site should relieve symptoms. Patients should be advised to avoid scratching the bite. For children, trimming their fingernails may prevent further injury from scratching. Prevention of future insect bites is also important.

Self-treatment of insect bites with a nonprescription product is appropriate if the reaction is confined to the site and the patient is older than 2 years; parents should seek a primary care provider's advice for treatment of children younger than 2 years. No effective nonprescription product is available to treat scabies. Because of possible systemic effects, a primary care provider should evaluate and treat bites from ticks and spiders. There are no nonprescription drug treatments for Lyme disease; the disease is treated with prescription antibiotics such as tetracycline, doxycycline, amoxicillin, and cephalosporins.[6] If a black widow or brown recluse spider bite is suspected, immediate medical attention should be sought. Figure 37-1 outlines treatment of insect bites and lists exclusions for self-treatment.

Nonpharmacologic Therapy

Nondrug measures include the two methods of preventing insect bites: avoiding insects and using repellents. Specific measures are discussed in the box Patient Education for Insect Bites.

Avoidance of Insects

Measures to avoid insect bites include covering skin as much as possible with clothing, hats, and shoes; cuffing clothing around

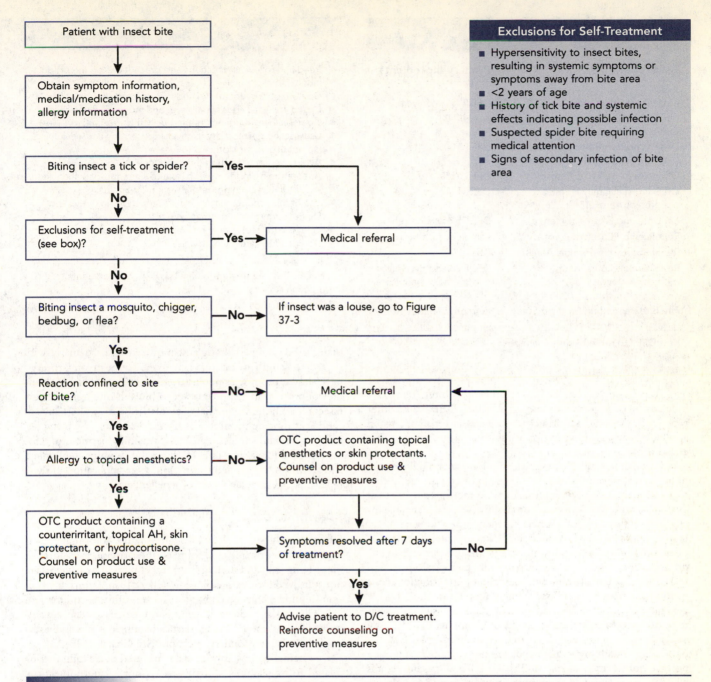

Exclusions for Self-Treatment

- Hypersensitivity to insect bites, resulting in systemic symptoms or symptoms away from bite area
- <2 years of age
- History of tick bite and systemic effects indicating possible infection
- Suspected spider bite requiring medical attention
- Signs of secondary infection of bite area

FIGURE 37-1 Self-care of insect bites. Key: AH, antihistamine; D/C, discontinue; OTC, over-the-counter.

ankles, wrists, and neck; avoiding swamps, dense woods, and brush that harbors ticks, mosquitoes, and chiggers; keeping pets free of pests; and removing standing water from around he home to reduce breeding areas for mosquitoes. It should be noted that scabies is transmitted by close, prolonged personal contact with an infected individual.[6]

Use of Insect Repellents

Insect repellents are useful in preventing bites from insects such as mosquitoes, fleas, and ticks, but these products are not effective in repelling stinging insects, such as wasps, hornets, bees, or yellow jackets. An insect repellent should have an inoffensive odor, protect for several hours, be effective against as many insects as possible, be relatively safe, withstand all weather conditions, and have an esthetic feel and appearance. Selection of an insect repellent should be based on product ingredients, concentration, and the anticipated type and length of exposure. Most commercial products contain n,n-diethyl-m-toluamide, commonly called DEET, in concentrations ranging from 7% to 40%, which are effective concentrations for routine insect exposure situations. Products containing up to 100% DEET are also available. Other ingredients that may be combined with DEET include ethylbutylacetylaminopropionate and dimethylpthalate (Table 37-1).

N,N-DIETHYL-M-TOLUAMIDE
The best all-purpose repellent is n,n-diethyl-m-toluamide, or DEET.

TABLE 37-1   Selected Insect Repellents

Trade Name	Primary Ingredients
Cutter Skinsations Pump	DEET 7%; aloe vera; vitamin E
Cutter Advanced Pump	Picaridin 7%
Deep Woods Off! For Sportsmen Insect Repellent I Pump Spray	DEET 100%
Off Insect Repellent II Aerosol	DEET 15%
Off Skintastic Family Formula Pump or Aerosol	DEET 7%
Off Light and Fresh Towelettes	DEET 5.6%; aloe vera
Repel Lemon Eucalyptus Lotion	Lemon eucalyptus oil
Repel Sportsman Formula Aerosol	DEET 29%
Repel Sun and Bug Lotion	DEET 20%; ethyl hexyl-p-methoxy-cinnamate 7.5%; oxybenzone 5%
Fite Bite Permethrin Clothing Spray	Permethrin 0.5%

Key: DEET, n,n-diethyl-m-toluamide.

TABLE 37-2   EPA Guidelines for Safe Use of DEET

- Read and follow all directions and precautions on the product label.
- Do not apply over cuts, wounds, or irritated skin.
- Do not apply to hands or near eyes and mouth of young children.
- Do not allow young children to apply this product.
- Use just enough repellent to cover exposed skin and/or clothing.
- Do not use under clothing.
- Avoid overapplication of this product.
- After returning indoors, wash treated skin with soap and water.
- Wash treated clothing before wearing it again.
- Use of this product may cause skin reactions in rare cases.
- Do not spray in enclosed areas.
- To apply to face, spray on hands first, and then rub on face.
- Do not spray directly onto face.

Key: DEET, n,n-diethyl-m-toluamide; EPA, Environmental Protection Agency.
Source: Reference 12.

Repellents protect the skin against insect bites. The exact mechanism of action is not known fully, but DEET, like other repellents, does not kill insects. The volatile repellent, when applied to skin or clothing, releases vapors that tend to discourage the approach of insects.

Repellents, available in sprays, solutions, creams, wipes, and other forms, are applied as needed to skin or clothing according to package directions, which usually is no more frequently than every 4 to 8 hours. Concentrations below 30% are preferable for children, but use of DEET insect repellents on children younger than 2 months should be discouraged[9]; appropriate clothing may offer some protection against insect bites in these younger children. Products with DEET concentrations ranging from 10% to 40% provide adequate effect and sufficient protection for adults in routine situations. Products containing 50% to 100% DEET generally are promoted for adults with high exposure to insects for long periods, and when high heat and humidity may decrease adherence of the product; higher concentrations of DEET may be associated with higher incidence of skin reactions.[10] A unique polymer formulation of 25% or 33% DEET is also available; it is promoted as an extended duration product offering 8 to 12 hours of protection.[11] Table 37-2 provides a summary from the Environmental Protection Agency regarding the application and safe use of DEET products.[12]

Skin irritation is the most frequent DEET-related problem, with occlusion of the application area possibly contributing to skin rashes or eruptions.[11,12] Central nervous system reactions, including seizures, ataxia, hypotension, encephalopathy, and angioedema, have been reported in association with improper use or ingestion.[11,13,14] These products are considered safe if used appropriately, even in women who are pregnant or breastfeeding.[11,13,14] Table 37-2 lists warnings and precautions for use of DEET.

OTHER INSECT REPELLENTS

Alternative products include citronella, lemon eucalyptus oil, soybean oil, cedar oil, lavender oil, tea tree oil, garlic, thiamin, and scented moisturizers in mineral oil, such as Skin So Soft. These products generally have been found to be less effective than DEET as repellents against mosquitoes, particularly with regard to length of action; however, soybean oil products have shown promise as potential repellents, providing 90 minutes of protection against mosquito bites in one test.[10] A new insect repellent, picaridin, has been marketed as an alternative to DEET; it is being promoted as having less odor and being less irritating to skin.[11] Insect repellents containing permethrin 0.5% are designed for use on only clothing and camping equipment, and are not to be applied to the skin. One application of these repellents may provide weeks of repellent activity.

Pharmacologic Therapy

External analgesics such as local anesthetics, topical antihistamines, hydrocortisone, and some counterirritants are approved for treating pain and itching from insect bites. These agents are not approved for use in children younger than 2 years; a physician should be consulted about treatment of these children.

Topical skin protectant agents may be used to reduce inflammation and promote healing. First-aid antiseptics and antibiotics can help prevent secondary infections (see Chapter 42).

Systemic antihistamines often are used in treating itching related to insect bites, but this use is not a label indication. Chapter 11 discusses systemic antihistamines in detail.

Local Anesthetics

Local anesthetics such as benzocaine, pramoxine, benzyl alcohol, lidocaine, dibucaine, and phenol are used in topical preparations for relief of itching and irritation caused by insect bites.

Local anesthetics cause a reversible blockade of conduction of nerve impulses at the site of application, thereby producing loss of sensation. Phenol exerts topical anesthetic action by depressing cutaneous sensory receptors.

Local anesthetics are approved for use on burns, sunburns, minor cuts, insect bites, and minor skin irritation to relieve pain and itching.[15]

Topical preparations containing local anesthetics are applied in the form of creams, ointments, aerosols, or lotions. These products are generally applied to the bite area up to three to four times daily for no longer than 7 days.

Even though local anesthetics, including benzocaine, are relatively nontoxic when applied topically, allergic contact dermatitis may occur. Pramoxine and benzyl alcohol do not commonly cause adverse effects and exhibit less cross-sensitivity than other local anesthetics. Dibucaine, a common allergen, may cause systemic toxicity if there is excessive absorption. Phenol solutions of greater than 2% are irritating, and may cause sloughing and necrosis of skin, but the concentration of phenol in nonprescription products ranges from 0.5% to 1.5%.

Local anesthetics should not be used longer than 7 days. Some individual agents have specific precautions or warnings.

Preparations containing benzocaine should not be applied to skin of individuals with confirmed or suspected hypersensitivity (typically allergic contact dermatitis) to benzocaine or other ester-type local anesthetics.

Although in the same class as benzocaine, dibucaine products carry additional labeling warning against use of large quantities, especially over raw surfaces or blistered areas.[16] Convulsions, myocardial depression, and death have been reported from systemic absorption.

Nonprescription products containing phenol should not be applied to extensive areas of the body, especially under compresses or bandages, because of risk of skin damage and systemic absorption[16]; systemic toxicities of phenol include convulsions and cardiac failure. Products containing phenol should be avoided in pregnant patients and children.

Topical Antihistamines

Diphenhydramine hydrochloride in concentrations of 0.5% to 2% is the agent used in most products that contain a topical antihistamine.

Topical antihistamines exert an anesthetic effect by depressing cutaneous receptors, thereby relieving pain and itching.

Topical antihistamines are approved for temporary relief of pain and itching related to minor burns, sunburns, insect bites, poison oak/ivy/sumac dermatitis, and minor skin irritation.[17] Products are available in several topical dosage forms; they are generally applied to the bite area up to three to four times daily for no longer than 7 days.

Although absorption occurs through skin, topical antihistamines generally are not absorbed in sufficient quantities to cause systemic side effects, even when applied to damaged skin. Systemic absorption is of more concern when these products are used over large body areas, especially in young children. Topical antihistamines are capable of producing hypersensitivity reactions, specifically allergic and photoallergic contact dermatitis; continued use of these agents for 3 to 4 weeks increases the possibility of contact dermatitis.

Topical antihistamines should not be used longer than 7 days, except as advised by a primary care provider.

Counterirritants

Low concentrations of the counterirritants camphor and menthol are used in some external analgesic products. Chapter 7 discusses these agents in more detail. These products generally are applied to the bite area three or four times daily for up to 7 days.

CAMPHOR

At concentrations of 0.1% to 3%, camphor depresses cutaneous receptors, thereby relieving itching and irritation by exerting an anesthetic effect. However, camphor-containing products can be very dangerous if ingested. Patients should be warned to keep these products out of children's reach.

MENTHOL

In concentrations of less than 1%, menthol depresses cutaneous receptors and exerts an analgesic effect. Menthol is considered a safe and effective antipruritic when applied to the affected area in concentrations of 0.1% to 1%.

Hydrocortisone

The Food and Drug Administration (FDA) has approved topical preparations containing hydrocortisone in concentrations up to 1% for nonprescription use.

Topically applied, hydrocortisone is an antipruritic and anti-inflammatory agent capable of preventing or suppressing development of edema, capillary dilation, swelling, and tenderness that accompany inflammation. Reduction in inflammation results in relief of pain and itching.

Topical absorption of hydrocortisone is increased after prolonged use of occlusive dressings. After application, a minimal amount of hydrocortisone may enter circulation; however, this penetration increases if skin is broken or inflamed.

Hydrocortisone topical preparations are indicated for temporary relief of minor skin irritations, itching, and rashes caused by dermatitis, insect bites, poison ivy/oak/sumac, soaps, cosmetics, and jewelry.

A wide variety of topical hydrocortisone dosage forms are available and should be applied as directed to the bite area three or four times daily for up to 7 days.

Prolonged administration of hydrocortisone may cause epidermal atrophy, acneiform eruptions, irritation, folliculitis, and tightening and cracking of the skin.

Patients who suffer from scabies, fungal or bacterial infections, or candidiasis should be warned against using topical hydrocortisone. Not only may the underlying conditions be worsened, but hydrocortisone may also mask these disorders, thereby making accurate diagnosis difficult. Chapter 35 provides more information about topical hydrocortisone.

Skin Protectants

Medications such as zinc oxide, calamine, and titanium dioxide are applied to insect bites mainly in the form of lotions, ointments, and creams. These agents act as protectants and tend to reduce inflammation and irritation. Zinc oxide works as a mild astringent with weak antiseptic properties.[18] Zinc oxide and calamine also absorb fluids from weeping lesions.

FDA considers preparations with zinc oxide and calamine to be safe and effective in concentrations from 1% to 25% as nonprescription drugs. Although its mechanism of action is similar to that of zinc oxide, titanium dioxide's safety and effectiveness has not been determined by FDA. These preparations should be applied to the affected area as needed. They have minimal adverse effects and are recommended for adults, children, and infants.

Product Selection Guidelines

Sensitization, specifically contact dermatitis, can occur with local anesthetics. If these agents are preferred, pramoxine and benzyl alcohol have a low incidence of adverse effects. Dibucaine and phenol have the most potential for adverse effects, especially if systemic absorption occurs from improper application.

Adverse effects and systemic absorption generally are not a concern with short-term use of the topical antihistamine diphenhydramine hydrochloride. However, its prolonged use can cause

TABLE 37-3 Selected External Analgesic Products for Insect Bites and Stings

Trade Name	Primary Ingredients
Local Anesthetics	
Itch-X Gel/Pump Spray	Pramoxine HCl 1%; benzyl alcohol 10%
Lanacane Aerosol Spray	Benzocaine 20%
Nupercainal Ointment	Dibucaine 1%
Solarcaine Medicated First Aid Aerosol Spray	Benzocaine 20%; triclosan 0.13%
Unguentine Maximum Strength Cream	Benzocaine 5%; resorcinol 2%
Topical Antihistamines	
Dermarest Gel	Diphenhydramine HCl 2%; resorcinol 2%; menthol
Di-Delamine Gel/Spray	Diphenhydramine HCl 1%; tripelennamine 0.5%; benzalkonium chloride 0.15%; menthol
Maximum Strength Benadryl Cream/Spray	Diphenhydramine HCl 2%
Counterirritants	
Blue Star Ointment	Camphor 1.2%
Sarna Lotion	Camphor 0.5%; menthol 0.5%
Corticosteroids	
Cortaid with Aloe Cream/Ointment	Hydrocortisone 0.5%; aloe vera
Cortizone-5 Cream	Hydrocortisone 0.5%
Maximum Strength Cortaid Cream/Ointment	Hydrocortisone 1%
Combination Products	
Aveeno Anti-Itch Cream/Lotion	Pramoxine HCl 1%; calamine 3%; camphor 0.3%
Benadryl Itch Stopping Maximum Strength Gel	Diphenhydramine HCl 2%; zinc acetate 1%; camphor
Caladryl Clear Lotion	Diphenhydramine HCl 1%; zinc oxide 2%; camphor
Campho-Phenique Gel	Camphor 11%; phenol 5%; eucalyptus oil
Chigarid	Camphor 2.8%; phenol 2%; eucalyptus oil 0.5% in collodion
Medi-Quik Spray	Lidocaine 2%; benzalkonium chloride 0.2%; camphor
Sting-Kill Swabs	Benzocaine 19%; menthol 0.9%

allergic or photoallergic contact dermatitis. Similarly, short-term use of hydrocortisone usually does not cause adverse effects or clinically significant systemic absorption, but patients with scabies, bacterial infections, or fungal infections should not use this agent without medical supervision. Hydrocortisone can worsen or mask these disorders, making accurate diagnosis difficult. Camphor-containing products can be very dangerous if ingested, making them an inappropriate choice for use in children. Topical diphenhydramine's side effect profile makes it a suitable topical antipruritic to recommend. However, patients must understand that topical antipruritics and anesthetics should not be used longer than 7 days.

The patient's preference of dosage forms should also guide product recommendations. Creams, lotions, and sprays are the most commonly used dosage forms. Table 37–3 lists selected trade-name products in various dosage forms.

Assessment of Insect Bites: A Case-Based Approach

The practitioner should first determine what type of insect inflicted the patient's injury. A primary care provider or dermatologist should evaluate bites from ticks and spiders because of

the serious diseases or adverse effects associated with these bites. For other insect bites, the practitioner should evaluate the seriousness of the reaction before recommending a nonprescription product or nondrug measure. If a nonallergic reaction is present, the appropriate external analgesic for symptomatic relief should be recommended. The practitioner should explain proper use of the selected product as well as its possible adverse effects. If the patient is a child, recommendation of a skin protectant to prevent secondary bacterial infection is appropriate.

Patient Counseling for Insect Bites

Counseling for insect bites includes an explanation of how to treat the injury as well as how to prevent recurrences. The practitioner should explain nondrug measures and/or proper use of recommended nonprescription products. The explanation should include potential adverse effects of these agents plus signs and symptoms that indicate the injury needs medical attention. Appropriate use of insect repellents to prevent further bites should also be discussed. The box Patient Education for Insect Bites lists specific information to provide patients.

The objectives of self-treatment for insect bites are to (1) relieve swelling, pain, and itching; (2) prevent scratching that may lead to secondary bacterial infection; (3) monitor for infections transmitted by ticks; and (4) prevent future insect bites. For most patients, carefully following product instructions and the self-care measures listed here will help ensure optimal therapeutic outcomes.

Nondrug Measures

- Apply ice pack promptly to bite area to reduce swelling, itching, and pain.
- Avoid scratching affected area; keep fingernails trimmed.
- Remove ticks with tweezers by grasping the tick's head and gently pulling; the head should be removed. Keep the removed tick in a sealed container for future identification in case of systemic symptoms.
- Do not wear rough, irritating clothing over bite area.

Preventive Measures

- To prevent exposure, cover skin as much as possible with clothing and socks.
- Avoid swamps, dense woods, and dense brush that harbor mosquitoes, ticks, and chiggers.
- Keep pets free of pests.
- Apply insect repellent according to package recommendations to repel biting insects (see Table 37-2); these repellents do not deter stinging insects.
- To prevent transmission of scabies, avoid close, physical contact with infected individuals.

Nonprescription Medications

Topical Analgesics

- Use an external analgesic to relieve pain and itching of insect bites. Choice of medications includes local anesthetics, topical antihistamines, counterirritants, and hydrocortisone.
- These products can be applied to the bite area three or four times daily. Do not use on children younger than 2 years. Do not use longer than 7 days.

- Note that local anesthetics can cause sensitization. If these agents are preferred, pramoxine and benzyl alcohol are less likely to cause adverse effects.
- Do not use dibucaine in large quantities, particularly over raw surfaces or blistered areas. Such use could cause myocardial depression, convulsions, or death.
- Do not apply phenol to extensive areas of the body or under compresses/bandages. Such application increases the possibility of skin damage or systemic absorption.
- Do not use topical diphenhydramine longer than the recommended 7 days. Prolonged use can cause hypersensitivity reactions or systemic effects.
- Do not use hydrocortisone on scabies, bacterial infections, or fungal infections without medical recommendation. Hydrocortisone can mask or worsen these disorders.
- Do not allow children to ingest camphor-containing products. Camphor is toxic when ingested.

Skin Protectants

- If needed to reduce irritation or inflammation, use a skin protectant such as zinc oxide or calamine.
- Apply protectant to affected area as needed up to four times daily.
- Protectants can be applied to skin of children younger than 2 years.
- Some insect bite products contain external analgesics and skin protectants.

Seek medical attention if the condition worsens during treatment or symptoms persist after 7 days of topical treatment.

Evaluation of Patient Outcomes for Insect Bites

Follow-up should occur after 7 days of self-treatment. The patient should be advised to seek medical attention if symptoms such as redness, itching, and localized swelling worsen during treatment, or if patient develops secondary infection, fever, joint pain, or lymph node enlargement. Medical attention is also necessary if symptoms persist after 7 days of treatment.

INSECT STINGS

Pathophysiology and Clinical Presentation of Insect Stings

Venomous insects such as bees, wasps, hornets, yellow jackets, and fire ants belong to the order Hymenoptera. They attack their victims to defend themselves or to kill other insects. The injected venom contains allergenic proteins and pharmacologically active molecules. Because venom contents vary within the Hymenoptera order, venom is discussed in general terms.

Most people will complain of pain, itching, and irritation at the site following an insect sting, but they will have no systemic symptoms. People who are allergic to insect stings may experience hives, itching, swelling, and burning sensations of the skin. Although anaphylaxis is rare, those with severe allergies may experience a fall in blood pressure, light-headedness, chest tightness, dyspnea, and even loss of consciousness. Nausea, vomiting, abdominal cramps, and diarrhea may also occur.

Wild Honeybees, Wasps, Hornets, Yellow Jackets, and Africanized Bees

Wild honeybees are most commonly found in the western and midwestern United States; they usually nest in hollow tree trunks. Because the honeybee stinger is barbed, it remains embedded in the skin, even after the bee pulls away or is brushed off, and continues to inject venom. Paper wasps, hornets, and yellow jackets are found more commonly in the southern, central, and southwestern United States. Paper wasps tend to nest in high places, under eaves of houses, or on branches of high trees, whereas hornets prefer to nest in hollow spaces, especially hollow trees. Yellow jackets, considered the most common stinging culprits, usually nest in low places, such as burrows in the ground, cracks in sidewalks, or small shrubs. The stinging mechanism of wasps, hornets, and yellow jackets resembles that of the honeybee, except their stingers are not barbed. Their stingers can be withdrawn easily after venom is injected, enabling them to sting repeatedly. A species of "killer bees" or Africanized bees may be found in certain areas of the southwestern United States. These bees are known for their aggressive, swarming behavior and large number of stings.[19] Their venom is similar in potency to that of honeybees, but the large number of stings per individual causes an increased risk of severe allergic reaction. Deaths have been reported as the result of venom toxicity from massive numbers of stings.

Fire Ants

Fire ants, imported from South America early in the 20th century, are now found in the southern and western United States, live in underground colonies, and form large raised mounds. Some ants only bite, while others bite and sting simultaneously, but it is often believe that it is the bite that causes the reactions. Fire ants are considered a health hazard because of the severity of reactions to their bite. Fire ant stings cause intense itching, burning, vesiculations, tissue necrosis, and anaphylactic reactions in hypersensitive persons. It appears that very limited or no cross-sensitivity exists between venom of fire ants and that of bees, wasps, hornets, and yellow jackets.

Treatment of Insect Stings

Although labeling of nonprescription products for insect-related injuries mentions only "insect bites" as an indication, it is generally accepted that FDA had intended the term to also cover insect stings.

Treatment Goals

The goal of self-treating insect stings is to relieve the itching and pain of cutaneous nonallergic reactions. Allergic reactions require evaluation and treatment by a primary care provider.

General Treatment Approach

Removal of the stinger and application of an ice pack in 10-minute intervals[6] are the first steps in treating insect stings. Application of a local anesthetic, skin protectant, antiseptic, or counterirritant to the sting site is appropriate if the reaction is confined to the site and if none of the exclusions for self-treatment listed in Figure 37-2 applies. Nonprescription systemic antihistamines can also be taken to alleviate itching. Figure 37-2 outlines the treatment of insect stings.

Avoiding future insect stings can prevent an individual from developing allergic reactions to stings. If symptoms of an allergic reaction develop, emergency treatment should be administered, and the patient should seek medical attention. Patients with severe allergic reactions might want to consider prophylactic treatment such as hyposensitization therapy. Such patients should be advised to wear a bracelet or carry a card identifying the nature of the allergy. They should also contact their primary care provider about carrying an injectable form of epinephrine.

Nonpharmacologic Therapy

Prompt application of cold packs to the sting site in 10-minute intervals helps to slow absorption and reduce itching, swelling, and pain. It is important to remove the honeybee's stinger and venom sac, which are usually left in the skin. The patient should remove the stinger before all venom is injected; it takes approximately 2 to 3 minutes to empty all contents from the honeybee's venom sac. Current recommendations suggest immediate removal of the stinger by any means.[6] Ideally, the patient should not squeeze the sac because rubbing, scratching, or grasping it releases more venom. Scraping away the stinger with a fingernail or edge of a credit card minimizes the venom flow. After the stinger is removed, an antiseptic, such as hydrogen peroxide or alcohol, should be applied.

To avoid attracting stinging insects, the patient should adhere to the following measures: avoid wearing perfume, scented lotions, and brightly colored clothes; control odors in picnic and garbage areas; change children's clothing if it becomes contaminated with summer foods such as fruits; wear shoes when outdoors; and destroy nests of stinging insects near homes.

Pharmacologic Therapy

The section Treatment of Insect Bites discusses the following external analgesics approved for treatment of insect bites and, by inference, insect stings: local anesthetics, topical antihistamines, counterirritants, hydrocortisone, and skin protectants.

Product labels for systemic antihistamines do not include treatment of itching associated with insect stings as an indication even though these products are often used in this way.

Complementary Therapies

Meat tenderizer has been used on insect stings to "break down" proteins in venom. Ammonia and baking soda have been used to "neutralize" venom in insect bites. These products may affect itching, but most reports of success are anecdotal and currently their effectiveness has not been determined.

Emergency Treatment of Allergic Reactions

Epinephrine is the initial drug of choice for combating anaphylactic reactions precipitated by insect stings. Antihistamines often are used in conjunction with epinephrine hydrochloride and are given either orally or parenterally to relieve itching. Antihistamines alone are insufficient in life-threatening anaphylactic reactions.

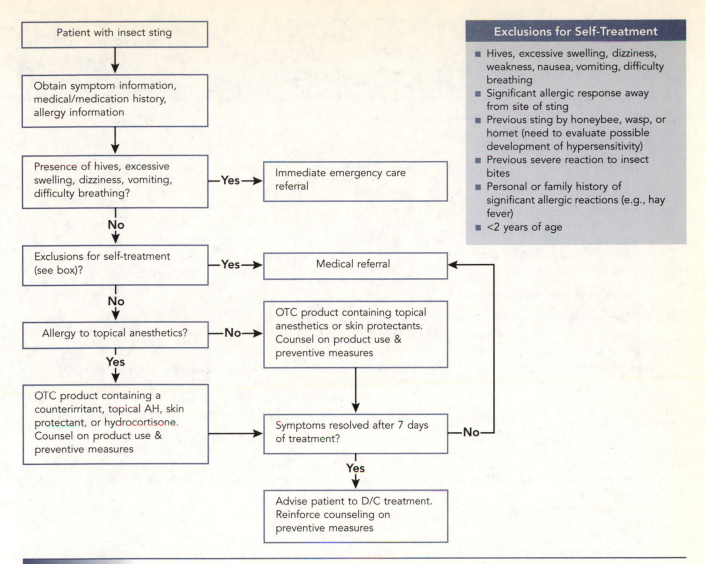

FIGURE 37-2 Self-care of insect stings. Key: AH, antihistamine; D/C, discontinue; OTC, over-the-counter.

Epinephrine is an alpha$_1$-agonist, and a beta$_1$- and beta$_2$-agonist. Activation of alpha$_1$-receptors, which constrict blood vessels in internal organs, mucosa surface, and skin, results in a systemic increase in blood pressure. Because beta–receptors control the bronchial tree, activation of these receptors results in bronchial dilation, thereby relieving chest tightness, dyspnea, and wheezing. Patients who are allergic to insect stings should carry an injectable form of epinephrine with them to use only when stung; epinephrine is not used as a maintenance therapy. A prescription–only product such as the EpiPen Auto-Injector is available; it contains a 0.3 mg intramuscular dose of 1:1000 epinephrine in a 2 mL disposable single–dose syringe designed for self-injection in the thigh. Because of infrequent use and product stability, patients should observe the product for discoloration and regularly monitor the expiration date.

Prophylactic Treatment of Insect Stings

Hymenoptera venom is used prophylactically to treat patients who had reactions to stings. Venom immunotherapy is accomplished by subcutaneous injection of small amounts of venom at regularly scheduled intervals. The dose of the venom is gradually increased over many weeks until a predetermined maintenance dose is reached. The length of treatment is usually 3 to 5 years.[19] Benefits of immunotherapy appear to be greater the younger the age of the patient at the beginning of therapy, and include a decreased risk of reaction for up to 10 to 20 years after treatments are stopped.[20]

Assessment of Insect Stings: A Case-Based Approach

The critical determination in assessing a patient with an insect sting is whether the patient is allergic to the venom. Patients experiencing allergic reactions should be referred immediately for emergency medical attention.

Case 37-1 illustrates assessment of a patient who has been stung by an insect.

CASE 37-1

Relevant Evaluation Criteria	Scenario/Model Outcome
Information Gathering	
1. Gather essential information about the patient's symptoms, including:	
a. description of symptom(s) (i.e., nature, onset, duration, severity, associated symptoms)	Patient comes into the pharmacy and says he was stung by a honeybee 20 minutes ago while working in his yard. Although he is not having difficulty breathing, the area is still very red and the pain is not subsiding.
b. description of any factors that seem to precipitate, exacerbate, and/or relieve the patient's symptom(s)	None
c. description of the patient's efforts to relieve the symptoms	Patient applied ice to the affected area for about 5 minutes and took ibuprofen 200 mg in an attempt to relieve pain.
2. Gather essential patient history information:	
a. patient's identity	Michael Jones
b. patient's age, sex, height, and weight	32-year-old male, 6 ft 2 in, 180 lb
c. patient's occupation	Self-employed
d. patient's dietary habits	Patient says that he eats fast food for lunch about 3 times a week but tries to eat a balanced diet the rest of the time.
e. patient's sleep habits	6–7 hours per night
f. concurrent medical conditions, prescription and nonprescription medications, and dietary supplements	Cetirizine 10 mg daily as needed for seasonal allergies
g. allergies	Seasonal allergies, PCN
h. history of other adverse reactions to medications	Patient states he gets a rash all over his body when he takes PCN.
i. other (describe) _____	N/A
Assessment and Triage	
3. Differentiate the patient's signs/symptoms and correctly identify the patient's primary problem(s).	Patient presents with typical response to honeybee sting. Unremitting pain could be from injected honeybee venom, or it could be due to stinger still embedded in skin
4. Identify exclusions for self-treatment (see Figure 37-2).	None
5. Formulate a comprehensive list of therapeutic alternatives for the primary problem to determine if triage to a medical practitioner is required, and share this information with the patient.	Options include: (1) Recommend self-care with nonprescription insect sting products. (2) Refer Michael to a PCP. (3) Recommend self-care until a PCP can be consulted. (4) Take no action.
Plan	
6. Select an optimal therapeutic alternative to address the patient's problem, taking into account patient preferences.	Because the patient is not presenting with any symptoms of anaphylaxis, self-care is appropriate in this case. Removing the embedded stinger is the most important step, followed by self-care with appropriate nonprescription insect sting products
7. Describe the recommended therapeutic approach to the patient.	Remove stinger immediately by scraping it off with a credit card or fingernail. Be careful not to squeeze stinger, which may force more venom into the skin. Disinfect the site with hydrogen peroxide or alcohol, and apply a topical antihistamine or hydrocortisone to the area to reduce redness and itching.
8. Explain to the patient the rationale for selecting the recommended therapeutic approach from the considered therapeutic alternatives.	Honeybees embed their stinger in the victim, and it can continue injecting venom into skin for several minutes after the bee is gone.

CASE 37-1 *(continued)*

Relevant Evaluation Criteria	Scenario/Model Outcome
Patient Education	
9. When recommending self-care with nonprescription medications and/or nondrug therapy, convey accurate information to the patient.	Apply diphenhydramine or hydrocortisone to sting site as directed on package for no more than 7 days. If you begin to exhibit signs of anaphylaxis, seek emergency medical treatment immediately.
10. Solicit follow-up questions from patient.	What can I do to prevent future bee stings?
11. Answer patient's questions.	The best way to prevent insect stings is to avoid wearing brightly colored clothing or perfume, destroying any nests or hives outside, and always wearing shoes when outdoors. Insect repellents are most effective at preventing insect bites, not insect stings.

Key: N/A, not applicable; PCN, penicillin; PCP, primary care provider.

Patient Counseling for Insect Stings

The practitioner should advise the patient that local reactions to insect stings usually are transient and are experienced by the vast majority of the population, but that severe reactions to insect stings can occur if sensitization to the insect venom develops with repeated exposure. The symptoms of allergic reactions should be explained. The importance of consulting a primary care provider if such symptoms occur should also be emphasized. Patients who have a known hypersensitivity to insect stings should have epinephrine injection available at all times for emergency self-treatment.

For nonallergic reactions to stings, the practitioner should recommend one or more topical medications to manage immediate symptoms. The patient should be advised about adverse effects and any contraindications. The box Patient Education for Insect Stings lists specific information that should be provided.

PATIENT EDUCATION FOR
Insect Stings

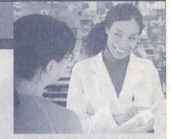

The objectives of self-treatment for insect stings are to (1) relieve swelling, pain, and itching of insect stings; (2) monitor any reaction to the sting to determine whether an allergic reaction is developing; and (3) prevent future insect stings. For most patients, carefully following product instructions and the self-care measures listed here will help ensure optimal therapeutic outcomes.

Nondrug Measures

■ For honeybee stings, it is important to remove the honeybee stinger immediately. Scraping the stinger away with the edge of a credit card is effective. Try not to squeeze or rub the stinger; these actions will actually release more venom.

■ Apply an ice pack or a cold compress promptly to the sting site to help slow absorption of the venom. This action will reduce itching, swelling, and pain.

■ Avoid scratching the affected area; keep fingernails trimmed. Gloves or mittens may be used on small children during sleep to avoid unconscious scratching.

■ To prevent stings, avoid wearing brightly colored clothing, as well as scented lotions or perfume/cologne, which attract stinging insects.

■ If you are hypersensitive to stings, wear a bracelet or carry a card showing the nature of the allergy.

Nonprescription Medications

■ For nonallergic stings, apply a topical nonprescription external analgesic such as a local anesthetic, topical antihistamine,

counterirritant, or hydrocortisone to the affected site to relieve pain and itching.

■ These products can be applied three to four times daily for up to 7 days.

 If you have experienced previous severe reactions to insect stings, seek emergency medical care immediately. If a primary care provider has prescribed epinephrine and/or an oral antihistamine and you have it on your person, administer it according to the primary care provider's instructions.

 Seek medical attention if you develop symptoms of an allergic reaction, such as hives, excessive swelling, dizziness, vomiting, or difficulty breathing.

 Seek medical attention if the pain and itching worsen during treatment or if they do not improve after 7 days of topical treatment.

Evaluation of Patient Outcomes for Insect Stings

Follow-up for nonallergic reactions to insect stings should occur within 7 days. The patient should be advised to seek medical attention if symptoms of pain, itching, and localized swelling worsen during the treatment period or persist after 7 days of treatment. Symptoms of secondary infection or fever also warrant medical attention. Follow-up for patients who have allergic reactions should occur the same day, if possible. The need to have emergency epinephrine injection available for future situations should be emphasized.

PEDICULOSIS

Pathophysiology and Clinical Presentation of Pediculosis

Lice are irritating pests, and lice infestations in the United States are common. Three types of lice that infest humans are head lice (*Pediculus humanus capitis*), body lice (*Pediculus humanus corporis*), and pubic lice (*Phthirus pubis*).

Head Lice

Head lice are the most common cause of lice infestation, affecting 10 to 12 million Americans annually, with most cases involving children ages 3 to 12 years.[21] Outbreaks of lice infestation are common in places such as schools and day care centers. Infestations are spread through close personal contact or sharing personal items such as caps, hairbrushes, combs, and so forth. Head lice are not spread by way of toilet seats, and they do not live on pets. Outbreaks usually peak after the opening of schools each year, between August and November.[21] All socioeconomic groups are affected, but the slightly lower incidence in the African American population probably is due to the unique oval structure of their hair shafts that make it more difficult for lice to attach to the hair.[21,22] Head lice create problem infestations, but they generally do not contribute to the spread of other diseases in the United States.[22]

Head lice usually infest the head and live on the scalp (see Color Plates, photographs 23A and B). A lice egg or nit is about 1 mm in diameter and is yellowish or grayish-white. Once hatched, the louse must begin feeding within 24 hours or it dies. The nymph, or newly hatched, immature louse resembles an adult and matures within 8 to 9 days. The nymph is active and tends to move about the head, whereas adults are less active. Without treatment, this cycle may repeat every 3 weeks.[22] The bite of a louse causes an immediate wheal to develop around the bite, with a local papule appearing within 24 hours. Itching and subsequent scratching may result in secondary infection. Adult lice, which are about the size of a sesame seed, are often difficult to locate because they move, but nits and nit casings generally can be spotted at the base of hair shafts when hair is parted for physical inspection. Hair inspections should focus on the crown of the head, near ears, and at the base of the neck. The grayish nits blend in well with the hair, but nit casings (hatched nits) are a lighter color and more easily located. Nits and nit casings may be differentiated from dandruff, dirt, and so forth because of their firm attachment to the hair shaft. A lice comb may be beneficial in removing some nits and nit casings as part of the inspection. The presence of black powdery specks, lice feces, is also evidence of an infestation.

Body Lice

Body lice (or "cooties") live, hide, and lay their eggs in clothing, particularly in seams and folds of underclothes. They periodically attack body areas for blood feedings and can transmit infections such as typhus and trench fever.[6] Body lice are controlled easily by appropriate hygiene; therefore, infestations generally are hygiene related, occurring in individuals who do not shower or change clothing frequently, such as the homeless.[6]

Pubic Lice

Pubic lice or "crabs," referring to their crab-like appearance, are generally transmitted through high-risk sexual contact, but may also spread by way of toilet seats, shared undergarments, or bedding. The lice usually are found in the pubic area but may infest armpits, eyelashes, mustaches, beards, and eyebrows.[6]

Treatment of Pediculosis

Nonprescription pediculicide agents, appropriate hair combing for nit removal, and home vacuuming/cleaning of personal items are primary treatments for lice infestation.[22] Awareness of the problem and appropriate actions by parents, as well as health and school officials, are also essential.

Treatment Goals

The goal of treating pediculosis is to rid the infested patient of lice by killing adult and nymph lice, and by removing nits from the patient's hair.

General Treatment Approach

A pediculicide is applied to the infested body area for the designated amount of time to rid the patient of lice. The hair is then combed with a lice/nit comb to remove nits from the hair shaft; combing will also remove dead lice.

Products containing formic acid or enzymes, used as secondary treatments, are purported to break down the substance cementing nits and eggs to hair shafts. These products may be used on the hair, before combing, to loosen lice eggs and facilitate their removal. Once rid of lice, patients should be instructed on how to avoid future infestations. Figure 37-3 outlines treatment of lice infestations and lists exclusions for self-treatment.

Nonpharmacologic Therapy

Because none of the pediculicides kills 100% of lice eggs, careful visual inspection of the hair for nits and combing with a nit comb, such as the LiceMeister comb, to remove nits are helpful in treating and controlling head lice.[22,23] It should be noted that some schools have "no nit" policies that do not allow students to attend school until they have been treated for the lice infestation and nits are not visible on inspection. Direct physical contact with an infested individual should be avoided, and articles such as combs, brushes, towels, caps, and hats should not be shared. Clothing and bedding should be washed in hot water and dried in a clothes

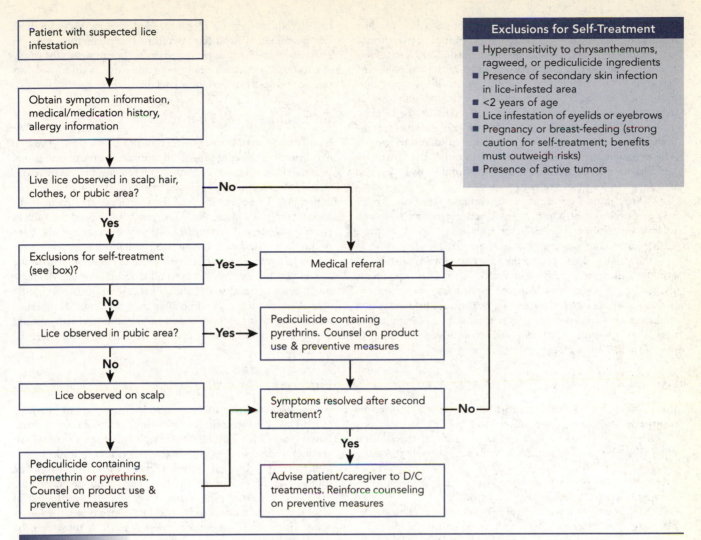

Exclusions for Self-Treatment

- Hypersensitivity to chrysanthemums, ragweed, or pediculicide ingredients
- Presence of secondary skin infection in lice-infested area
- <2 years of age
- Lice infestation of eyelids or eyebrows
- Pregnancy or breast-feeding (strong caution for self-treatment; benefits must outweigh risks)
- Presence of active tumors

FIGURE 37-3 Self-care of pediculosis. Key: D/C, discontinue.

dryer to kill lice and their nits; an alternative to washing would be to seal contaminated items in a plastic bag for 2 weeks. Hairbrushes and combs should be washed in very hot water. Carpets, rugs, and furniture should be vacuumed thoroughly and regularly.[22] Insecticidal sprays should be used on these items sparingly, if at all, because of the difficulty in controlling human exposure through possible absorption or inhalation, and because lice generally survive for less than 48 hours when not in contact with a host.[22] Given the increasing resistance to pediculicides, some patients are choosing to use nondrug therapy exclusively; these nondrug methods, specifically combing and vacuuming, can be effective but are labor intensive and tedious.[24] Complete head shaving has also been used as a lice treatment, but the social stigma involved makes this a questionable option. Body lice are controlled by appropriate body hygiene and frequent changing and appropriate laundering of clothing and bed linens.[6]

Pharmacologic Therapy

Two nonprescription pediculicide agents are available for treating pediculosis: permethrins and synergized pyrethrins. Patients should be warned about overusing these agents because of an apparent increasing trend of lice resistance to pediculicides,

including the nonprescription products; the resistance may be due to overuse, improper use, or insufficient contact time.[21,25] Resistance is contributing to increased use of nonpharmacologic treatments.[23,24] A prescription-only therapy, 0.5% malathion, was found to be significantly more pediculicidal and ovicidal than 1% permethrin. This product is also advantageous because the application time is only 20 minutes.[26]

The oral antibiotic sulfamethoxazole/trimethoprim has demonstrated effectiveness against head lice when used in conjunction with permethrin; the mechanism of action is not clearly defined, but it may be due to direct toxicity of the antibiotic ingredients or possibly death of symbiotic bacteria in the gut of lice.[22,27]

Synergized Pyrethrins

Pyrethrins, oleoresins obtained from chrysanthemum flowers, are synergized by addition of piperonyl butoxide, a petroleum derivative. Pyrethrins are approved for treating head and pubic lice.

Pyrethrins block nerve impulse transmission, causing the insect's paralysis and death. Addition of piperonyl butoxide to pyrethrins synergizes their insecticidal effect through inhibition of pyrethrin breakdown, increasing insecticide levels within the louse.[21,28]

Excessive contact time or occlusion of scalp after product application may increase skin absorption of topical pyrethrins.

Pyrethrins, in concentrations ranging from 0.17% to 0.33%, generally are used in combination with 2% to 4% piperonyl butoxide. This combination is considered an effective pediculicide when applied topically as shampoos, foams, solutions, or gels. The medication is applied to the affected area for 10 minutes, and then the treated area is rinsed or shampooed as recommended. Combing with a lice comb should follow treatment. The treatment is repeated in 7 to 10 days to kill any remaining nits that have since hatched. The drug should not be applied more than twice in 24 hours.

When applied according to directions, pyrethrins have a low order of toxicity. Most adverse reactions are cutaneous and include irritation, erythema, itching, and swelling.[22,29] Contact with eyes and mucous membranes should be avoided.

Individuals allergic to pyrethrins or chrysanthemums should not use this agent; ragweed-sensitive individuals risk cross-sensitivity. This agent should not be applied to eyelashes or eyebrows; upon recommendation of a health care professional, a nonmedicated ointment such as petrolatum can be applied to these areas to smother lice. (See discussion of lice infestation of the eyelid in Chapter 28.)

Permethrin

Permethrin is a synthetic pyrethroid available as a nonprescription cream rinse for treating head lice. Permethrin acts on the nerve cell membrane of lice. It disrupts the sodium channel, delaying repolarization and causing paralysis of the parasite.

When permethrin is applied, an estimated less than 2% is absorbed, after which the agent is metabolized.

Nonprescription permethrin is indicated for treating head lice only; prescription versions are used in treating scabies.

The 1% cream rinse is applied in sufficient quantities to cover or saturate washed hair and scalp. It is left on the hair for 10 minutes before rinsing; the hair is then combed with a lice comb. The rinse has residual effects for up to 10 days; therefore, re-treatment in 7 to 10 days is not required unless active lice are detected.

Primary adverse effects include transient pruritus, burning, stinging, and irritation of the scalp. Contact with eyes and mucous membranes should be avoided.

Permethrin is contraindicated in patients who are sensitive to pyrethrins or chrysanthemums. Permethrin should not be used on infants younger than 2 years.

Pharmacotherapeutic Comparison

When treatment involves a single application of a pediculicide, permethrin is more effective than the pyrethrin and piperonyl butoxide combination. However, no significant difference exists in effectiveness of these agents when treatment consists of two applications.[23] Recent studies indicate a possible decline in effectiveness of both products related to increasing resistance.[29]

Product Selection Guidelines

Preparations that contain pyrethrins may be used on infants and young children, but they should be used in pregnancy and lactation only if prescribed by a physician.

Pyrethrins may be recommended for treating pubic lice. For treatment of head lice, pyrethrins or permethrin may be selected on the basis of preferred dosage form, desire for single application, or patient allergies/sensitivities. Table 37-4 lists selected trade-name products containing these agents.

Complementary Therapies

Lice enzyme shampoos, which claim to break down the lice exoskeleton, are being promoted as an alternative to traditional pediculicides. Products containing ingredients such as olive oil, eucalyptus oil, rosemary oil, and pennyroyal oil are being used as pesticide-free alternatives to traditional lice treatments with anecdotal reports of success.[21] Other oil-based products such as petroleum jelly and mayonnaise are also being used on the basis of the theory that they impair lice respiration; however, these products are not very effective and most likely only slow the movement of lice.[22,29] Tea tree oil, another alternative treatment, must be used with caution because of potential significant allergic reactions and possible liver toxicity.[30] Dangerous alternative treatments such as gasoline and kerosene should always be avoided because of their flammability and potential for toxicity.[24]

Emerging Therapies

A new potential treatment under study is a class of products called DSP (Dry-on, Suffocation-based Pediculicide) lotions. Nuvo lotion, also marketed as Cetaphil cleanser, the first DSP product to be tested, is a nontoxic lotion that "shrink wraps" lice. It is applied to hair and dried with a hairdryer to form a shrink-wrap film over hair and lice. The lotion covers breathing holes, suffocating the louse. Nuvo Lotion must be left in place for at least 8 hours to be effective. Once dried, the lotion is not visible and hair can be styled as usual. It must then be reapplied 7 to 10 days later to kill lice that may have hatched since the first treatment.[29]

Dimeticone 4% lotion has also been shown to cure pediculosis while causing less irritation than traditional therapy. Dimeticone may also be advantageous in that it is not absorbed transdermally. Furthermore, dimeticone works by coating the lice and irreversibly immobilizing them within 5 minutes of application, which causes disruption of water balance. Because dimeticone is not a neurotoxin like most commonly used pediculicides, resistance to this product is unlikely.[31]

TABLE 37-4 Selected Pediculicides

Trade Name	Primary Ingredients
A-200 Lice Killing Shampoo	Pyrethrins 0.33%; piperonyl butoxide 3%
RID Lice Killing Shampoo, Maximum Strength	Pyrethrins 0.33%; piperonyl butoxide 4%
RID Mousse Foam, Maximum Strength	Pyrethrins 0.33%; piperonyl butoxide 4%
Nix Cream Rinse Lice Treatment	Permethrin 1%
Pronto Lice Killing Shampoo	Pyrethrins 0.33%; piperonyl butoxide 4%

Assessment of Pediculosis: A Case-Based Approach

In many cases of pediculosis, visual inspection of the scalp will verify presence or absence of head lice or nits. Similarly, presence of body lice can be determined by identifying adult lice and nits in seams of clothing. If a patient does not want such inspection or if lice have not been confirmed by another health care professional, the practitioner should not recommend a pediculicide. When the disorder is confirmed, the practitioner should recommend the appropriate pediculicide according to the type of pediculosis and the patient's allergic history to chrysanthemums or ragweed.

Case 37–2 illustrates assessment of a patient with pediculosis.

CASE 37-2

Relevant Evaluation Criteria	Scenario/Model Outcome
Information Gathering	
1. Gather essential information about the patient's symptoms, including:	
a. description of symptom(s) (i.e., nature, onset, duration, severity, associated symptoms)	Patient complains of intense itching of her scalp that has caused minor irritation and redness from scratching. The discomfort has kept her awake at night and distracts her during school hours. These symptoms began shortly after the start of the school year.
b. description of any factors that seem to precipitate, exacerbate, and/or relieve the patient's symptom(s)	The mother says that regular shampooing has not relieved the symptoms.
c. description of the patient's efforts to relieve the symptoms	The mother was aware of many reports of lice infestation among Brittney's classmates. She recognized nits after examining the patient's scalp and has tried regular shampooing with store-brand permethrin shampoo every night this week.
2. Gather essential patient history information:	
a. patient's identity	Brittney Smith
b. patient's age, sex, height, and weight	5-year-old female, 40 inches, 38 lb
c. patient's occupation	Kindergartner
d. patient's dietary habits	Mother says Brittney usually eats a well-balanced diet.
e. patient's sleep habits	9 hours per night
f. concurrent medical conditions, prescription and nonprescription medications, and dietary supplements	Multivitamin chewables
g. allergies	Nuts
h. history of other adverse reactions to medications	None
i. other (describe) _____	Mother bathes Brittney each night and washes her hair.
Assessment and Triage	
3. Differentiate the patient's signs/symptoms and correctly identify the patient's primary problem(s).	After examination of the patient, you find no evidence of a current lice infestation. The scalp is red and irritated owing to overuse of permethrin.
4. Identify exclusions for self-treatment (see Figure 37-3).	None
5. Formulate a comprehensive list of therapeutic alternatives for the primary problem to determine if triage to a medical practitioner is required, and share this information with the patient.	Options include: (1) Recommend that patient discontinue permethrin shampoo and monitor scalp improvement. (2) Refer Brittney to a PCP. (3) Recommend self-care until a PCP can be consulted. (4) Take no action.
Plan	
6. Select an optimal therapeutic alternative to address the patient's problem, taking into account patient preferences.	The mother and patient should discontinue permethrin shampoo, because there is no longer evidence of pediculosis.

CASE 37-2 *(continued)*

Relevant Evaluation Criteria	Scenario/Model Outcome
7. Describe the recommended therapeutic approach to the patient.	Irritation of the patient's scalp has occurred from inappropriate use of permethrin. Discontinuing the shampoo will allow the scalp to heal. If no improvement is seen over several days, Brittney should see her PCP.
8. Explain to the patient the rationale for selecting the recommended therapeutic approach from the considered therapeutic alternatives.	Explain to Brittney and her mother that package instructions for permethrin shampoo should be followed to ensure effectiveness and safety. Resistance of the lice and toxicity to the patient can result from inappropriate use of these products.

Patient Education

9. When recommending self-care with non-prescription medications and/or nondrug therapy, convey accurate information to the patient:	
a. appropriate dose and frequency of administration	See the box Patient Education for Pediculosis.
b. maximum number of days the therapy should be employed	See the box Patient Education for Pediculosis.
c. product administration procedures	See the box Patient Education for Pediculosis.
d. expected time to onset of relief	See the box Patient Education for Pediculosis.
e. degree of relief that can be reasonably expected	See the box Patient Education for Pediculosis.
f. most common side effects	See the box Patient Education for Pediculosis.
g. side effects that warrant medical intervention should they occur	See the box Patient Education for Pediculosis.
h. patient options in the event that condition worsens or persists	See the box Patient Education for Pediculosis.
i. product storage requirements	See the box Patient Education for Pediculosis.
j. specific nondrug measures	See the box Patient Education for Pediculosis.
10. Solicit follow-up questions from parent.	If a lice infestation occurs again in the future, should everyone in the household be treated?
11. Answer parent's questions.	No. Only those in the household with evidence of a lice infestation should be treated. However, you can prevent the spread of lice by thoroughly washing bed sheets and clothes on the hottest settings, and by reminding household members not to share brushes or hats with the affected person.

Key: PCP, primary care provider.

Patient Counseling for Pediculosis

Control of pediculosis requires both pharmacologic and non-pharmacologic intervention, as well as the patient's understanding of lice control. The practitioner should reassure parents of children with head lice that the condition is not the result of poor hygiene. Patients with confirmed head or pubic lice infestations should be counseled on which product is best for the situation and how to use the product properly; preventive measures should also be discussed.

PATIENT EDUCATION FOR
Pediculosis

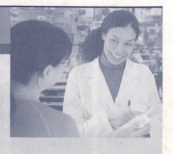

The objectives for self-treatment of pediculosis are to (1) rid the body of lice and nits and (2) implement measures to prevent future infestations. For most patients, carefully following product instructions and the self-care measures listed here will help ensure optimal therapeutic outcomes.

Nondrug Measures
- Wash hairbrushes, combs, and toys of infested patients in water at a temperature of 130°F (39.4°C) or greater for 10 minutes.[22]

PATIENT EDUCATION FOR
Pediculosis (continued)

- Use water at a temperature of 130°F (39.4°C) or greater to wash the clothes, bedding, and towels of infested patients. Dry the items on the hottest dryer setting the fabric permits.[22]
- Objects or clothing that cannot be washed should be sealed in plastic bags for the length of the louse's life cycle (2 weeks) so that it is unable to feed on a host.
- Avoid close, physical contact with an infested patient; do not share articles such as combs, brushes, towels, caps, and hats.
- Vacuum living areas thoroughly and regularly during treatment period.
- Visually inspect the hair and scalp before, during, and after treatment for evidence of lice or nits:
  —Use a nit comb diligently to remove nits.
  —Comb the hair in segments. (Individual hairs can be trimmed if nit removal proves difficult.)

Nonprescription Medications

- Treatment of other family members should be determined on the basis of presence of lice or nits and the family members' level of contact with the infested individual; unnecessary treatment should be avoided.
- Application steps for a pyrethrin shampoo include:
  —Apply sufficient quantity to wet the dry hair and scalp. (Foams should also be applied to dry hair.)
  —Allow the treatment to remain for 10 minutes.
  —Work the shampoo into a lather and then rinse thoroughly. (Remove foams with shampoo or soap and water.)
  —Use a nit comb to remove dead lice and eggs as described previously.
- Application steps for a permethrin cream rinse include:
  —Shampoo with regular shampoo, rinse, and towel dry hair.
  —Apply sufficient cream rinse to wet hair and scalp.

  —Allow the treatment to remain for 10 minutes; then rinse and towel dry.
  —Use a nit comb as described previously.
- Avoid contact of the pediculicide with eyes and mucous membranes.
- The pediculicide can cause temporary irritation, erythema, itching, swelling, and numbness of the scalp; itching should be relieved in a few days.
- For pyrethrin products, repeat entire process in 7–10 days; permethrin products can be used again in 7–10 days if lice or nits are detected. Because of resistance, proper use of these products is required and overuse must be avoided.
- If desired, contact the National Pediculosis Association at www.headlice.org or 1-781-449-6487 for information about treatment of lice infestations.

⚠ Significant skin irritation or excessive exposure of eyes or mucous membranes to pediculicides warrants medical intervention.

⚠ Seek medical attention if symptoms of lice infestation persist after the second treatment.

Evaluation of Patient Outcomes for Pediculosis

Follow-up of lice infestations should occur within 10 days. The practitioner should advise the patient to seek medical attention if signs of lice infestation persist after a second application of a pediculicide. Overuse of these products should be discouraged and nonpharmacologic control measures emphasized.[24]

Key Points for Insect Bites and Stings and Pediculosis

➤ In people who are not hypersensitive, insect stings and bites cause local irritation, inflammation, swelling, and itching that provoke rubbing and scratching; a cold pack may be applied promptly to the bite area to reduce local symptoms.

➤ For relief of the itching and pain resulting from insect bites, typical nonprescription preparations that contain local anesthetics, antihistamines, hydrocortisone, or counterirritants are considered safe and effective in adults and children 2 years and older. Oral antihistamines may also aid in the relief of local symptoms.

➤ In hypersensitive people, anaphylactic reactions may pose serious emergency problems; immediate, active treatment such as administration of epinephrine hydrochloride is required. Nonprescription products are of minimal value to hypersensitive patients.

➤ Suspected spider bites should be referred; nonprescription treatments are not appropriate.

➤ A tick should be removed by grasping it near the head with tweezers and gently pulling to cause the tick to release from the skin; the tick should then be maintained in a sealed container for identification. The patient should be monitored for systemic effects such as Lyme disease and Rocky Mountain spotted fever.

➤ Prevention of bites from mosquitoes, ticks, and chiggers is an important component of self-care; appropriate use of insect repellents containing DEET will help to prevent insect bites.

➤ Exposure to mosquito bites warrants monitoring the patient for symptoms of West Nile virus.

➤ Lice infestation, especially in school-age children, continues to be a significant problem; nondrug measures are an important component in treatment of lice infestation.

➤ Available nonprescription pediculicides contain either synergized pyrethrins or permethrin. Both agents are effective in treatment of head lice infestations, but only synergized pyrethrins are effective in treatment of pubic lice.

➤ Pediculicides, available in shampoo, cream rinse, and mousse formulations, are designed for initial treatment and re-treatment in 7 to 10 days; hair combing with a nit comb after treatment is recommended. Overuse should be avoided because resistance to pediculicides is a growing problem and impacts the products' effectiveness.

REFERENCES

1. Centers for Disease Control and Prevention. Statistics, Surveillance, and Control of West Nile Virus. Available at: http://www.cdc.gov/ncidod/dvbid/westnile/surv&controlCaseCount04_detailed.htm. Last accessed September 15, 2008.
2. Petersen L, Marfin A. West Nile virus: a primer for the clinician. *Ann Intern Med.* 2002;137:173–9.
3. Nash D, Mostashari F, Fine A, et al. The outbreak of West Nile virus infection in the New York City area in 1999. *N Engl J Med.* 2001;344:1807–14.
4. Paul J, Bates J. Is infestation with the common bedbug increasing? *BMJ.* 2000;320:1141.
5. Silverman A, Qu L, Low J, et al. Assessment of hepatitis B virus DNA and hepatitis C virus RNA in the common bedbug and kissing bug. *Am J Gastroenterol.* 2001;96:2194–8.
6. Beers MH, Berkow R. *The Merck Manual.* 18th ed. West Point, Pa: Merck & Co; 2006:994–7, 1478–81, 1492–3, 2638–40, 2650.
7. Gammons M, Salam G. Tick removal. *Am Fam Physician.* 2002;66:643–4.
8. Steere AC. Lyme disease. *New Engl J Med.* 2001;345:115–25.
9. Hayes E, O'Leary D. West Nile virus infection: a pediatric perspective. *Pediatrics.* 2004;113:1375–81.
10. Fradin M, Day J. Comparative efficacy of insect repellents against mosquito bites. *N Engl J Med.* 2002;347:13–8.
11. Abramowicz M. Insect repellants. *Med Lett Drugs Ther.* 2003;45:41–2.
12. US Environmental Protection Agency. The Insect Repellent DEET. March 2007. Available at: http://www.epa.gov/pesticides/factsheets/chemicals/deet.htm. Last accessed September 15, 2008.
13. Koren G, Matsui D, Bailey B. DEET-based insect repellants: safety implications for children and pregnant and lactating women. *CMAJ.* 2003;169:209–11.
14. Sudakin D, Trevathan W. DEET: a review and update of safety and risk in the general population. *J Toxicol.* 2003;42:831–9.
15. Gennaro A. *Remington: The Science and Practice of Pharmacy.* 20th ed. Baltimore: Lippincott Williams & Wilkins; 2000:1045–6.
16. McEvoy G. *AHFS Drug Information.* Bethesda, Md: American Society of Health-System Pharmacists; 2002:3444–5.
17. Wickersham, R. *Drug Facts and Comparisons.* St Louis: Facts and Comparisons; 2008:1599.
18. Zinc oxide. Lexi-Drugs Online. Available at: http://www.crlonline.com. Last accessed February 26, 2008.
19. Morrit J, Golden D, Reisman R, et al. Stinging insect hypersensitivity: a practice parameter update. *J Allergy Clin Immunol.* 2004;114:869–86.
20. Golden D, Kagey-Sobotka A, Norman P, et al. Outcomes of allergy to insect stings in children, with and without venom immunotherapy. *N Engl J Med.* 2004;351:668–74.
21. Stephens MB. Controlling head lice. *Patient Care.* September 15, 2000:99–107.
22. Frankowski B, Weiner L, Clinical report: head lice, guidance for the clinician in rendering pediatric care. *Pediatrics.* 2002;110:638–43.
23. Meinking T, Serrano L, Hard B, et al. Comparative in vitro pediculicidal efficacy of treatments in a resistant head lice population in the United States. *Arch Dermatol.* 2002;138:220–4.
24. Pray S. Pediculicide resistance in head lice: a survey. *Hosp Pharm.* 2003;38:241–6.
25. Meinking T, Entzel P, Villar M, et al. Comparative efficacy of treatments for pediculosis capitis infestations. *Arch Dermatol.* 2001;137:287–91.
26. Meinking T, Vicaria M, Eyerdam D, et al. Efficacy of a reduced application time of Ovide lotion (0.5% malathion) compared to Nix crème rinse (1% permethrin) for the treatment of head lice. *Pediatr Dermatol.* 2004;21:670–4.
27. Meinking T, Clineschmidt C, Chen C, et al. An observer-blinded study of 1% permethrin cream rinse with and without adjunctive combing in patients with head lice. *J Pediatr.* 2002;141:665–70.
28. Burkhart C. Relationship of treatment-resistant head lice to the safety and efficacy of pediculicides. *Mayo Clin Proc.* 2004;79:661–6.
29. Pearlman D. A simple treatment for head lice: dry-on, suffocation based pediculicide. *Pediatrics.* 2004;114:275–9.
30. Alternative Treatments: What the NPA Is Saying About Mayonnaise, Vaseline, and Tea Tree Oil. Available at: http://www.headlice.org/faq/treatments/alternatives.htm. Last accessed September 15, 2008.
31. Burgess I, Brown C, Lee P. Treatment of head louse infestation with 4% dimeticone lotion: randomized controlled equivalence trial. *Br Med J.* 2005:330;1423–5.

Acne

Kristi Quairoli and Karla T. Foster

Acne vulgaris is a common skin condition that affects approximately 15% of the U.S. population[1] and accounts for over 20% of all visits to a dermatology practice.[2] An estimated 90% of the world's population will experience acne to some extent during their lifetime.[3] Acne is likely to be more severe in young men but more persistent in women. Although roughly 85% of those who suffer from acne are adolescents, it can occur at any time, with upwards of 40% of men and women older than 25 having the diagnosis.[1]

Although many adolescents will achieve spontaneous remission of their acne, some patients will experience acne into adulthood and may already have scarring by age 18.[1] Although patients tend to overestimate the severity of their acne, physicians tend to underestimate the impact of the disease on patients. The effect of acne on patients should not be overlooked: Whether or not physical scarring exists, the potential for psychological scarring exists. Associations have been shown between acne and lower self-esteem, reduced employability as adults,[4] and a negative impact on quality of life to a degree comparable to that of asthma, epilepsy, diabetes, and arthritis.[1]

A wide variety of nonprescription treatment options are available for acne vulgaris. Sales of nonprescription drugs for acne are $100 million annually.[2] Practitioners can be instrumental in helping patients make informed choices about their selection of acne products. This interaction also represents an opportunity for clinicians to introduce a new group of consumers to the value of pharmaceutical care.

Pathophysiology of Acne

Acne is the result of several pathologic processes that occur within the pilosebaceous unit located in the dermis, or middle layer of the skin (Figure 38-1A). These units, consisting of a hair follicle and associated sebaceous glands, are connected to the skin surface by a duct (infundibulum) lined with epithelial cells through which the hair shaft passes. The sebaceous glands produce sebum, which passes to the skin surface through the duct, and then spreads over the skin to retard water loss and maintain proper 10% hydration of the skin and hair.

The exact cause of acne has not yet been determined; however, what is known is that the causes are multifactorial and largely influenced by both genetic and hormonal factors. Although there is no direct correlation to severity, a patient's likelihood of developing acne is increased if it was experienced by one or both of the patient's parents.[3,5] The inhabitation of the skin by *Propionibacterium acnes* (*P. acnes*) and the occurrence of follicular plugging to some extent are normal processes for everyone. The development of clinical lesions is determined by the level of immune response (hypersensitivity) that occurs; this response is already genetically determined.[4] The pathologic factors involved in the development of acne are (1) androgenic hormonal triggers, (2) excessive sebum production, (3) abnormal follicular desquamation, (4) proliferation of *P. acnes,* and (5) resultant inflammatory responses.[1]

The timing of the start of puberty and the appearance of acne is not a coincidence. The rise in androgenic hormones triggers these processes. The conversion of testosterone to dihydrotestosterone stimulates an increase in the size and metabolic activity of sebaceous glands. The excessive sebum serves as a breeding ground for *P. acnes* as the comedo develops.[5]

Increases in androgen levels are also partly responsible for abnormal follicular desquamation within the infundibulum. Some evidence exists for the role of sebum lipid abnormalities, such as deficiencies of linoleic acid and excesses of free fatty acids, in hyperkeratinization. In addition, there is evidence that follicular keratinocytes release interleukin 1, which may stimulate comedone formation. Regardless of the cause, hyperproliferation of these keratinocytes results in cell cohesion and formation of a plug that blocks the follicular orifice. This plug distends the follicle to form a microcomedo, the initial pathologic lesion of acne (Figure 38-1B). As more cells and sebum accumulate, the microcomedo enlarges and becomes visible as a closed comedo, or whitehead, a small, pale nodule just beneath the skin surface (Figure 38-1C). If the contents of the plug cause distension of the pore's orifice, the plug will protrude from the pore, causing an open comedo or blackhead (Figure 38-1D; see also Color Plates, photograph 24). The lesion is so named because of the presence of melanin and oxidization of lipids upon exposure to air. Comedones are the precursor of other acne lesions.[1]

Behind the plug, the buildup of sebum is an ideal habitat for proliferation of *P. acnes*. This bacterium breaks down sebum into highly irritating free fatty acids through production of lipases and is also responsible for the production of proinflammatory

Editor's Note: This chapter is based on the 15th edition chapter with the same title, written by Karla T. Foster and Cynthia W. Coffey.

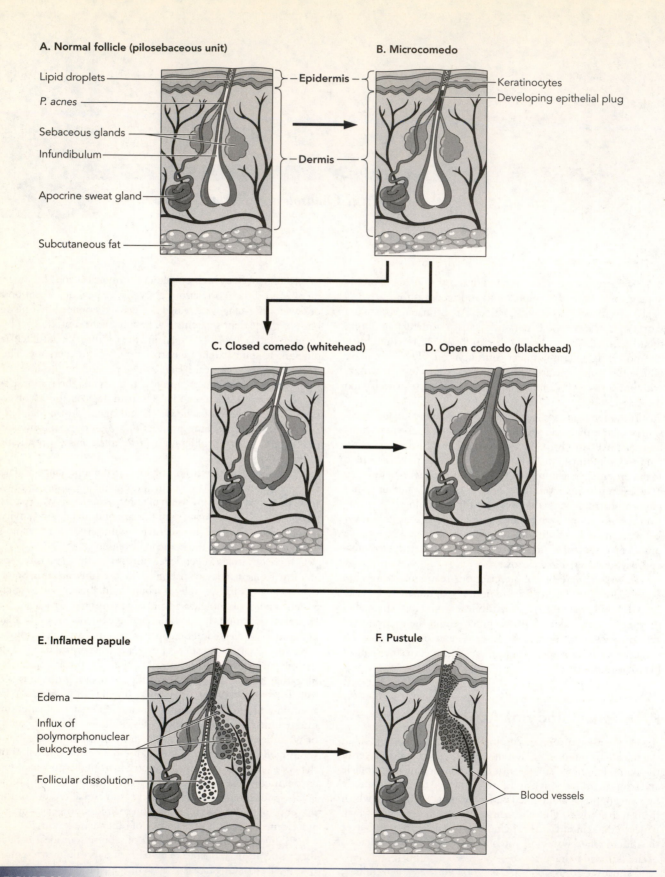

A. Normal follicle (pilosebaceous unit)

Lipid droplets

P. acnes

Sebaceous glands

Infundibulum

Apocrine sweat gland

Subcutaneous fat

– Epidermis –

– Dermis –

B. Microcomedo

Keratinocytes

Developing epithelial plug

C. Closed comedo (whitehead)

D. Open comedo (blackhead)

E. Inflamed papule

Edema

Influx of polymorphonuclear leukocytes

Follicular dissolution

F. Pustule

Blood vessels

FIGURE 38-1 Pathogenesis of acne. (Adapted with permission from Fulton JE, Bradley S. *Cutis*. 1976;7:560.)

TABLE 38-1 Exacerbating Factors in Acne

Factor	Description of Factor
Acne mechanica	Local irritation or friction from occlusive clothing, headbands, helmets, or other friction-producing devices
	Excessive contact between face and hands, such as resting the chin or cheek on the hand
Acne cosmetica	Noninflammatory comedones on the face, chin, and cheek due to occlusion of the pilosebaceous unit by oil-based cosmetics, moisturizers, pomades, or other health and beauty products
Occupational acne	Exposure to dirt, vaporized cooking oils, or certain industrial chemicals, such as coal tar and petroleum derivatives
Medications	Some drugs known to exacerbate acne: phenytoin, isoniazid, moisturizers, phenobarbital, lithium, ethionamide, steroids (helpful mnemonic: P.I.M.P.L.E.S)[8]
	Implicated drugs: azathioprine, rifampin, quinine[9]
Stress and emotional extremes	May induce expression of neuroendocrine modulators, which play a role in centrally and topically induced stress of the sebaceous glands, and possibly progression of acne[10]
High-humidity environments and prolonged sweating	Hydration-induced decrease in size of pilosebaceous duct orifice and prevention of loosening of comedone
Hormonal alterations	Increased androgen levels induced by medical conditions, pregnancy, or medications[11]

Source: References 8–11.

mediators that induce neutrophil chemotaxis and activate complement.[1] As a result of the irritation and inflammation, localized tissue destruction occurs.[6] Redness and inflammation in and around the follicular canal constitute a papule (Figure 38-1E). A pustule (Figure 38-1F; see also Color Plates, photograph 25) possesses the same qualities of a papule but has visible purulence in the center of the lesion. Nodules result from disruption of the follicular wall and release of its contents into the surrounding dermis.[7]

Several factors contribute to the exacerbation of existing acne and cause periodic flare-ups of acne in some patients (Table 38-1).[8-11] Other factors widely assumed to cause acne, including hygiene and diet, have not been directly proven as etiologic factors. Patients may falsely believe that they have acne as a result of dirty skin or not cleansing their skin thoroughly. No research supports this belief. In addition, most studies that looked at the correlation between acne and the consumption of certain foods, such as chocolate or greasy foods, have shown no relationship between the two. However, some patients are insistent that certain foods worsen their acne. In this case, it is best to recommend avoidance of the particular food. Recently, some evidence has suggested that acne may be influenced by consuming diets rich in high-glycemic foods (a typical Western culture diet). This theory rose from a study that observed no cases of acne between two populations (Kativan Islanders of Papua New Guinea and the Ache hunter-gatherers of Paraguay) whose diets consist of fruits, fish and wild game, and locally cultivated grains.[12]

Clinical Presentation of Acne

Acne lesions can generally be classified as noninflammatory or inflammatory. Noninflammatory lesions consist of either open or closed comedones. These lesions are often the first to manifest in the early stages of puberty and often appear initially on the forehead. With the progression of puberty and with age, especially in women, lesions tend to appear on areas of the body below

the neck, such as the chest and back.[13] It is not uncommon for women in their 30s and 40s to have acne that is concentrated on the chin and along the jaw line. Inflammatory lesions are further characterized as papules, pustules, or nodules. On presentation to the practitioner, the patient may exhibit one or more types of lesion.

If acne lesions persist beyond the mid-20s or develop in the mid-20s or later, the symptoms may signal rosacea rather than acne vulgaris. A differential diagnosis is necessary because the treatment of rosacea, although similar to that for acne, has unique elements.[4]

Complications associated with acne include scarring and negative psychosocial impact. An acute complication of acne is postinflammatory erythema or hyperpigmentation.[1] This complication is often mistaken for scarring, but in fact it is a remnant of the inflammatory process that fades with time. To minimize this discoloration, patients should use a sunscreen to prohibit pigmentation of the area. True scars are a chronic complication of severe or poorly managed acne. Risk of scarring is higher with more severe acne and is also increased by picking and squeezing acne lesions. More aggressive treatment strategies are warranted if complications, either physical or psychological, are present.

Treatment of Acne

In most cases, acne is self-limiting and can be controlled to varying degrees. Adherence to therapeutic regimens will reduce symptoms and minimize scarring. Because acne persists for long periods, treatment must be long term, continuous, and consistent.

Treatment Goals

Patients and practitioners should identify any exacerbating factors of acne (Table 38-1). It is also imperative that patients and practitioners classify the patient's acne (Table 38-2) to allow selection of the most appropriate therapeutic options.[14] Once the classification of acne has been determined, the primary goals are

TABLE 38-2 Assessment of Acne Severity

Grade of Acne	Qualitative Description	Quantitative Description
Comedonal		
I	Comedonal acne	Comedones only, <10 on face, none on trunk, no scars; noninflammatory lesions only
	Blackheads	Open comedo; dilated hair follicle with open orifice to skin
		Dark color may be caused by oxidation of melanin or compacted epithelial cells; presence of lipids may contribute
	Whiteheads	Closed comedo; dilated hair follicle filled with keratin, sebum, and bacteria with obstructed opening to the skin
Papulopustular		
II	Papular acne	10–25 papules on face and trunk, mild scarring; inflammatory lesions < 5 mm in diameter
III[a]	Pustular acne	More than 25 pustules, moderate scarring; size similar to papules but with visible, purulent core
IV[a]	Severe/persistent pustulocystic acne	Nodules or cysts, extensive scarring; inflammatory lesions > 5 mm in diameter
	Recalcitrant severe cystic acne	Extensive nodules/cysts

[a] Some overlap with previous grade of acne.

Source: Reference 2 and Baldwin HE. The interaction between acne vulgaris and the psyche. *Cutis.* 2002;70:133–9.

to prevent new lesions, prevent scarring, and decrease morbidity associated with the psychological implications of acne.[15]

General Treatment Approach

Zaenglien and Thilboutot[16] recommend that one or more acne treatments, either topical or topical and systemic, be combined to target a greater number of pathogenic factors. The treatment of acne depends on the severity of the disease[6] (Table 38-2). Only patients with type I acne should self-treat with nonprescription products. Patients under the care of a practitioner should be instructed to avoid use of nonprescription products unless the practitioner recommends their use. Combining some non-prescription products with prescription acne drugs may decrease a patient's ability to tolerate prescribed topical drugs.

Nonpharmacologic Therapy

Patients with acne should eliminate exacerbating factors of acne (Table 38-1). This measure should promote understanding and prevention of the disease as well as adherence to therapy. Patients seeking self-care options should cleanse the skin with a mild soap or non–soap cleanser twice daily. The use of abrasive products and over cleansing may worsen the acne.[6] Self-care options should also include staying well hydrated. Dehydration may increase the inflammatory chemicals in the cell and may cause dysfunction in the natural desquamation process of the stratum corneum.[17]

Physical Treatments

Physical treatments have increased in popularity. There is a wide range of self-applied, acrylate glue–based material strips that aid in the extraction of impacted comedones. These products are a better alternative to picking the acne, which ultimately results

in scarring.[18] Professional comedo extraction is a useful adjunct to the overall acne regimen and often results in immediate improvement. Patients should be aware that the risks include tissue damage or scarring if these procedures are not done correctly.

Pharmacologic Therapy

Topical therapy is the standard of care in acne treatment.[19] The cornerstone of all acne treatment is topical retinoids.[11] Because topical retinoids are available by prescription only, it is recommended that most patients seek medical referral for treatment of moderate-to-severe acne. Most of these patients will benefit from a therapeutic regimen that contains a combination of medications including, but not limited to, topical retinoids. Topical retinoids inhibit microcomedone formation and prevent the formation of new lesions.

Many are familiar with benzoyl peroxide, the most common topical antibiotic acne product available both with and without a prescription. It has been the mainstay of treatment for type I acne since the 1950s.[20] Benzoyl peroxide is currently classified by the Food and Drug Administration (FDA) as Category III (i.e., more data needed to determine safety and use for "non-monograph conditions") because of concern about its tumorigenic potential.[21]

Category I (generally recognized as safe and effective) topical antiacne ingredients include salicylic acid 0.5% to 2%, sulfur 3% to 10% (in single-ingredient products), and a combination of sulfur 3% to 8%, with either resorcinol 2% or resorcinol monoacetate 3%.[21,22]

In addition, after reviewing a time-and-extent application for triclosan as an active, topical acne agent, FDA determined that this antibacterial agent is eligible for inclusion in the OTC topical acne drug products monograph. The agency announced December 5, 2005, that it is seeking safety and effectiveness information to determine whether the concentrations 0.2% to 0.5% and 0.3% to 1.0% are safe and effective in leave-on and rinse-off dosages, respectively.[22]

Benzoyl Peroxide

Benzoyl peroxide has the ability to prevent or eliminate the development of *P. acnes* resistance,[11,19] which has increased with the use of conventional antibiotics (macrolides and tetracyclines) over the last three decades. Resistant strains have been found in 50% of close contacts of acne patients with a resistant organism.[11] The use of benzoyl peroxide in combination with antibiotics has been recommended to minimize *P. acnes* resistance.[11] Benzoyl peroxide reduces inflammatory and noninflammatory lesions by generating free radicals that oxidize protein in the cell membranes.[21] It is also characterized as a keratolytic because of its ability to reduce follicular hyperkeratosis. Benzoyl peroxide is often used in combination with other oral or topical antibiotics. In a recent literature review, benzoyl peroxide was more effective than topical antibiotics such as clindamycin and erythromycin. In addition, benzoyl peroxide in combination with either of these antibiotics was more effective and better tolerated than either of the antibiotics alone.[11]

Nonprescription formulations of benzoyl peroxide are available in concentrations from 2.5% to 10%. Prescription concentrations are available up to 20%. The higher strengths of benzoyl peroxide have the same antibacterial effects as the lower strengths.[2] Some minor improvement may occur with daily application of benzoyl peroxide; the number of applications can be increased or decreased until a mild peeling occurs. Many patients may experience mild erythema and scaling during the first few days, which usually subside within 1 or 2 weeks. Allergic reactions, which may occur in 2% of patients, are characterized by a sudden onset of erythema and vesiculation.[5] The product should be discontinued when contact allergy is suspected. Patients may be advised to test the product in the antecubital area before use.[20] Avoidance of contact with clothes or hair is advised because this product may cause bleaching. In addition, avoidance of excessive sun exposure and use of a sunscreen product are recommended.

Salicylic Acid

Salicylic acid is a mild comedolytic and keratolytic agent available in various nonprescription acne products in concentrations of 0.5% to 2%. It provides a milder, less effective alternative to the prescription agent tretinoin.[21] In cleansing preparations, salicylic acid is considered adjunctive treatment.

Alpha- and Beta-Hydroxy Acids

Keratolytic agents such as alpha- and beta-hydroxy acids are also common nonprescription acne products. Hydroxy acids are considered less potent and are often used when patients cannot tolerate other topical acne products.[19] Hydroxy acids have comedolytic properties and are weakly effective in the treatment of acne.[11]

Beta-hydroxy acids, such as salicylic acid, are indicated for hyperkeratotic skin disorders and have been used for many years in the treatment of acne. These products are contraindicated in diabetic patients or patients with poor blood circulation.[22] Use of this product should be limited to the affected area. Use of the product over a large area for prolonged periods of time could result in toxicity. Signs of salicylate toxicity include nausea, vomiting, dizziness, loss of hearing, tinnitus, lethargy, hyperpnea, diarrhea, and psychic disturbances.[22] It is available in 0.5% to 5% formulations for both nonprescription and prescription drugs for acne.

Alpha-hydroxy acids (AHAs) are natural exfoliating acids that occur in sugar cane, milk products, and fruits.[18] The most common acids are glycolic, lactic, and citric acids, respectively. AHAs are available in several nonprescription formulations in concentrations from 4% to 10% or through dermatologists at higher concentrations. In a study comparing AHAs with benzoyl peroxide, benzoyl peroxide was superior to the AHAs at 8 weeks. Currently, there is not enough evidence to support the use of these agents in the treatment of acne.[2] However, once acne is controlled, a light chemical peel with AHAs may be useful to help correct scarring and hyperpigmentation.[11]

Sulfur

Sulfur has met the criteria of FDA's Advisory Review Panel for Over-the-Counter Topical Acne Products, although the claim for its antibacterial effects was disallowed.[21] Sulfur, precipitated or colloidal, is included in acne products as a keratolytic and antibacterial in concentrations of 3% to 10%. It is generally accepted as effective in promoting the resolution of existing comedones but, on continued use, may have a comedogenic effect. Alternative forms of sulfur, such as sodium thiosulfate, zinc sulfate, and zinc sulfide, are not recognized as safe and effective.

Sulfur-containing products are applied in a thin film to the affected area one to three times daily.[21] An esthetic consideration is the noticeable color and odor of these products.

Sulfur/Resorcinol

Combinations of sulfur 3% to 8% with resorcinol 2% to 3%, which enhances the effect of the sulfur, are available in nonprescription acne products. The products function primarily as keratolytics, fostering cell turnover and desquamation. Resorcinol produces a reversible, dark brown scale on some darker-skinned individuals.[21]

Sulfur/Sodium Sulfacetamide

Sodium sulfacetamide is combined with sulfur in acne preparations. This combination has been said to destroy para-aminobenzoic acid, an essential component for bacterial cellular growth. Sulfur has been postulated to inhibit the growth of *P. acnes* and the development of free fatty acids.[6]

Pharmacotherapeutic Comparison

Table 38-3 provides a comparison of the therapeutic properties of the major acne products.

Product Selection Guidelines

Skin cleansers and topical acne products are available in a variety of vehicles and strengths. Medicated cleansing products (bars and liquids) are not of much value; they leave little active ingredient residue on the skin. Generally, gels are the most effective formulations, because they are astringents and remain on the skin the longest. Gels and solutions have a drying effect that may sometimes cause contact dermatitis. However, gels and solutions are nongreasy and may be more beneficial in patients with oily skin.[2] Creams and lotions are generally less irritating to the skin than gels and solutions. Lotions and creams with a low fat content are intended to counteract drying (astringent effect) and peeling (keratolytic effect).[10] They are an acceptable alternative to the

TABLE 38-3 Comparison of Nonprescription Topical Acne Agents

	Benzoyl Peroxide	Salicylic Acid	Sulfur
Bactericidal	Yes		Yes
Keratolytic	Slight	Yes	Yes
Comedolytic		Yes	Yes
Concentration	2.5%–10%	0.5%–2%	3%–10%
Frequency of use	1–2 times daily	Used mainly as cleanser, then rinsed off	1–3 times daily
Adverse effects	Bleached hair and clothing	Potent keratolytic at high concentration	Color, unpleasant odor

Source: Adapted with permission from reference 2.

TABLE 38-4 Selected Acne Products

Benzoyl Peroxide Products

Stridex Power Pads	Benzoyl peroxide 2.5%
Clean & Clear Gel	Benzoyl Peroxide 10%
Oxy Maximum Strength Acne Wash	Benzoyl Peroxide 10%

Salicylic Acid Products

Neutrogena Rapid Defense	Salicylic acid 2%
Nature's Cure Body Acne Spray	Salicylic acid 2%

Benzoyl Peroxide/Salicylic Acid Products

University Medical AcneFree Spot Treatment	Salicylic acid 1.5%; benzoyl peroxide 1.5%

Alpha-Hydroxy Acid Products

Gly Derm	Glycolic acid
Total Skin Care	Glycolic acid
M.D. Forte	Glycolic acid

Alpha/Beta-Hydroxy Acid Products

Neutrogena Pore Refining Lotion	Glycolic and salicylic acids

Sulfur Product

Bye Bye Blemish	Sulfur 10%

Triclosan Product

Clearasil Daily Face Wash	Triclosan 0.3%

Combination Product

Clearasil Acne Control	Resorcinol 2%; sulfur 8%

Physical Treatments

Biore Ultra Deep Cleansing Pore Strips
Clean & Clear Oil Absorbing Sheets

more effective gels, and are recommended for dry or sensitive skin and for use during dry winter weather. Ointment vehicles are not used because they are occlusive and tend to worsen acne. Patients should start with the lowest strength available and gradually increase the concentration to minimize the irritating effects of the product. Table 38-4 lists selected trade-name acne products in these and other formulations.

Many patients will use nonprescription medications in combination with prescription products to manage acne. Product selection is important for the successful treatment and management of acne. It is important that patients seek medical referral for proper diagnosis and grading of acne. For example, women who experience acne related to hormonal imbalance may benefit more from correction of hormone imbalances with the use of hormone replacement such as oral contraceptives, whereas a peripubertal teenager or young adult may benefit more from consultation on avoidance of comedogenic products and adherence with nonprescription products such as benzoyl peroxide.[18]

SPECIAL POPULATIONS

Pregnant women may have problems with acne owing to hormonal imbalances. In most cases, if women become pregnant while taking any acne medication, they should stop taking the acne medication and advise their obstetrician of current or previous product use because of the potential for teratogenic effects. Topical benzoyl peroxide is a Pregnancy Category C medication. It may be necessary for pregnant women to begin or discontinue treatment depending on the severity of the acne. This decision will be considered if the practitioner deems it is necessary.

Neonatal acne, which is caused by the mother's hormones, affects 20% of newborns. It is more common in males, and usually begins at 6 weeks and clears at 4 to 6 months of age.[6] It is advised that caregivers use clean fingertips or a soft washcloth to wash the baby's skin with mild soap and water twice a day.

Complementary Medicine

Tea tree oil, widely known for its antibacterial properties, has been postulated to work by disturbing cytoplasmic membranes of *Staphylococcus aureus* and weakening the cells' ability to fight off other cytocidal agents.[23] Guyette and Rygwelski[23] conducted an investigator-blind, comparative, randomized controlled trial in 124 patients with mild-to-moderate acne. Tea tree oil 5% water-based gel was used for 3 months compared with benzoyl peroxide 5% water-based lotion for 3 months. The results showed that both treatments are effective in reducing lesions; however, tea tree oil has a slower onset of action.

Oral zinc may be considered an alternative to tetracyclines.[11,24] Zinc inhibits chemotaxis and shows effectiveness against noninflammatory lesions (not including comedones). One study found that zinc was 17% less effective than minocycline; however, zinc may be used as an alternative to tetracycline therapy, especially in the summer, because it does not cause phototoxicity. Nausea and gastralgia are adverse effects.

Few data support the use of nicotinamide for the use of inflammatory acne. The product is occasionally used in Europe and has some anti-inflammatory properties.

Assessment of Acne: A Case-Based Approach

Patient assessment begins with asking questions to define the condition. Physical assessment, which involves observing the affected area and questioning the patient further, is the next

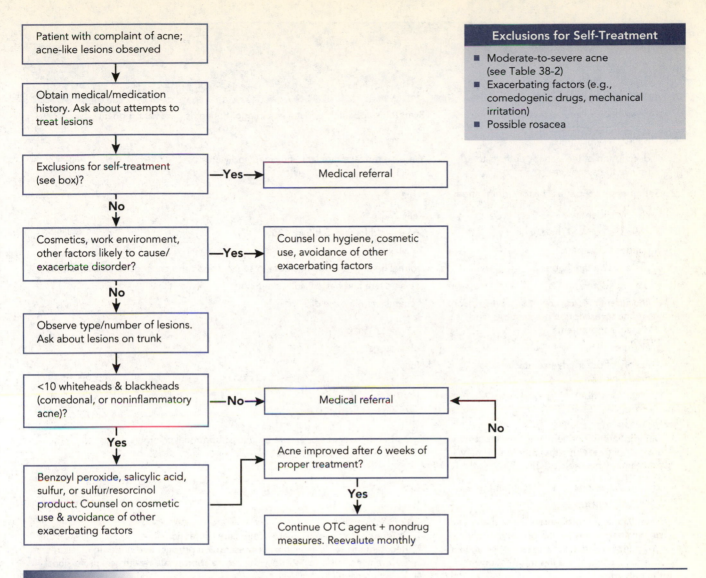

Exclusions for Self-Treatment

- Moderate-to-severe acne (see Table 38-2)
- Exacerbating factors (e.g., comedogenic drugs, mechanical irritation)
- Possible rosacea

Patient with complaint of acne; acne-like lesions observed

↓

Obtain medical/medication history. Ask about attempts to treat lesions

↓

Exclusions for self-treatment (see box)? —Yes→ Medical referral

No ↓

Cosmetics, work environment, other factors likely to cause/exacerbate disorder? —Yes→ Counsel on hygiene, cosmetic use, avoidance of other exacerbating factors

No ↓

Observe type/number of lesions. Ask about lesions on trunk

↓

<10 whiteheads & blackheads (comedonal, or noninflammatory acne)? —No→ Medical referral

Yes ↓

Benzoyl peroxide, salicylic acid, sulfur, or sulfur/resorcinol product. Counsel on cosmetic use & avoidance of other exacerbating factors → Acne improved after 6 weeks of proper treatment? —No→ Medical referral

Yes ↓

Continue OTC agent + nondrug measures. Reevalute monthly

FIGURE 38-2 Self-care of acne. Key: OTC, over-the-counter.

step in evaluating the disorder. This evaluation helps determine whether the condition is acne vulgaris or another dermatologic condition with similar signs and symptoms. Physical assessment also determines whether the severity of the condition precludes self-treatment (Figure 38-2). Before self-care is rec-

ommended, an assessment of current medication use (prescription and nonprescription) is necessary to reveal prescribed treatments for the disorder or use of medications known to cause acne (Table 38-1).

Case 38-1 is an example of assessment of patients with acne.

CASE 38-1

Relevant Evaluation Criteria	Scenario/Model Outcome
Information Gathering	
1. Gather essential information about the patient's symptoms, including:	
a. description of symptom(s) (i.e., nature, onset, duration, severity, associated symptoms)	Patient has come into the pharmacy to get advice on a recent outbreak along her jaw line.

C A S E   3 8 - 1   *(continued)*

Relevant Evaluation Criteria	Scenario/Model Outcome
b. description of any factors that seem to precipitate, exacerbate, and/or relieve the patient's symptom(s)	Symptoms appeared about 4 weeks ago. Patient is 8 weeks pregnant.
c. description of the patient's efforts to relieve the symptoms	Washing the face regularly with soap and water
2. Gather essential patient history information:	
a. patient's identity	Kelly Wade
b. patient's age, sex, height, and weight	30-year-old female, 5 ft 5 in, 136 lb
c. patient's occupation	Retail associate
d. patient's dietary habits	Normal healthy diet with increase in sugary foods and cravings for Mexican food
e. patient's sleep habits	Stays up late and has difficulty sleeping
f. concurrent medical conditions, prescription and nonprescription medications, and dietary supplements	Prenatal vitamin once daily
g. allergies	Sulfur drugs
h. history of other adverse reactions to medications	None
i. other (describe) _____	N/A

Assessment and Triage

3. Differentiate the patient's signs/symptoms and correctly identify the patient's primary problem(s) (see Table 38-1).	Exacerbation of acne appears to be due to hormonal changes.
4. Identify exclusions for self-treatment (see Figure 38-2).	None
5. Formulate a comprehensive list of therapeutic alternatives for the primary problem to determine if triage to a medical practitioner is required, and share this information with the patient.	Options include: (1) Refer Kelly to an appropriate health care professional. (2) Recommend self-care with a nonprescription product and nondrug measures. (3) Recommend self-care until Kelly can see an appropriate health care professional. (4) Take no action.

Plan

6. Select an optimal therapeutic alternative to address the patient's problem, taking into account patient preferences.	Kelly should use nondrug and preventive measures.
7. Describe the recommended therapeutic approach to the patient.	You should use nondrug and preventive measures.
8. Explain to the patient the rationale for selecting the recommended therapeutic approach from the considered therapeutic alternatives.	The outbreaks have probably peaked due to pregnancy and may normalize during the third trimester.

Patient Education

9. When recommending self-care with nonprescription medications and/or nondrug therapy, convey accurate information to the patient:	
a. appropriate dose and frequency of administration	See the box Patient Education for Acne.
b. maximum number of days the therapy should be employed	See the box Patient Education for Acne.

CASE 38-1 *(continued)*

Relevant Evaluation Criteria	Scenario/Model Outcome
c. product administration procedures	See the box Patient Education for Acne.
d. expected time to onset of relief	See the box Patient Education for Acne.
e. degree of relief that can be reasonably expected	
f. most common side effects	See the box Patient Education for Acne.
g. side effects that warrant medical intervention should they occur	
h. patient options in the event that condition worsens or persists	Medical referral
i. product storage requirements	See the box Patient Education for Acne.
j. specific nondrug measures	See the box Patient Education for Acne.
10. Solicit follow-up questions from patient.	May I try benzoyl peroxide temporarily until I can see a practitioner?
11. Answer patient's questions.	Some clinical studies have shown that benzoyl peroxide promotes growth of tumors in animals. Because you are in your first trimester, the risks of using this medication outweigh the benefits.

Key: N/A, not applicable.

Patient Counseling for Acne

The success of the treatment regimen depends largely on the patient. Therefore, it is crucial that the practitioner educate the patient on the causes of acne, correct any misconceptions, and clearly explain the rationale for treatment. Patient buy-in will facilitate adherence and increase the likelihood of a successful outcome. The practitioner must also evaluate the patient's maturity and willingness to comply with a skin care program that involves a continued daily regimen of washing affected areas and applying medication. Because acne cannot be cured but only controlled, reassurance and emotional support are often necessary to reduce patient concern.

The box Patient Education for Acne lists specific information to provide patients.

PATIENT EDUCATION FOR Acne

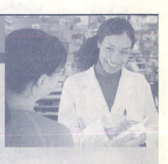

The goal of self-treatment is to control mild acne, therefore, preventing more serious forms from developing. Acne usually goes away without treatment. Symptoms can usually be managed with diligent and long-term treatment. The best approaches to controlling acne are using cleansers and medications to keep the pores open, and avoiding situations that worsen acne. For most patients, carefully following product instructions and the self-care measures listed here will help ensure optimal therapeutic outcomes.

Disease Information
- Acne is a common skin condition caused by clogging of the pores by sebum (oil) and dead skin cells; inflammation can occur when normal skin bacteria get trapped behind the oil and skin plug.
- Acne is not caused by poor hygiene or eating greasy or sugary foods.
- Acne can be controlled by using certain medications, but it cannot be cured.

Nondrug and Preventive Measures
- Cleanse skin thoroughly but gently twice daily to produce a mild drying effect that loosens comedones. Use a mild, oil-free cleanser and warm water.
- To prevent or minimize acne flare-ups, avoid or reduce exposure to environmental factors such as dirt, dust, petroleum products, cooking oils, or chemical irritants.
- To prevent friction or irritation that may cause acne flare-ups, do not wear tight-fitting clothes, headbands, or helmets; avoid resting the chin on the hand. To minimize acne related to cosmetic use, do not use oil-based cosmetics and shampoos.
- To prevent excessive hydration of the skin, which can cause flare-ups, avoid areas of high humidity and do not wear tight-fitting clothes that restrict air movement.
- Avoid stressful situations when possible and practice stress-management techniques. Stress can worsen existing acne.

- Do not pick or squeeze pimples, which can further irritate skin and possibly lead to worsening of acne and scarring.
- Note that sexual activity plays no role in the occurrence or worsening of acne, although the onset of sexual activity and occurrence of acne may be simultaneous or occur within the same time span.

Nonprescription Medications

- Most common available nonprescription products contain benzoyl peroxide, salicylic acid, or sulfur and come in a variety of formulations (cleansers, creams, gels, astringents).
- Benzoyl peroxide is the most effective and widely used nonprescription medication for treating acne.

Benzoyl Peroxide

- Benzoyl peroxide inhibits the growth of *P. acnes*, the bacteria involved in acne development; it also helps unclog pores by causing a mild peeling effect.
- Apply a thin layer to the entire affected area, not just on visible blemishes.
- Some mild stinging or peeling is normal and should diminish with continued use. To minimize irritation, the product should not be applied for 15–20 minutes after washing the affected area with a mild cleanser.
- Begin with one application daily or every other day for the first few weeks using the 2.5% strength. This approach will aid in determining sensitivity to the product.
- Leave initial application on the skin for only 15 minutes; then wash off.
- If no discomfort occurs, increase the time the product is left on the skin in 15-minute increments as tolerance allows.
- Once the product is tolerated for 2 hours, leave it on overnight. Once-daily application may be all that is needed.
- After the initial 1–2 weeks of treatment, applications can be increased up to two to three times per day over a period of 2–3 days, as tolerated
- For fair-skinned individuals, initiate therapy at the 2.5% strength and apply only once daily during the first few weeks of therapy.
- Slight improvement may be noticed in as little as a few days, but maximum effectiveness may take up to 4–6 weeks of continued use
- If treatment is tolerated, but the problem persists, the strength may be increased to 5% after 1 week and to 10% after 2 weeks, if necessary.

- Continue the treatment regimen even after lesions have cleared to prevent the formation of new ones.
- If improvement has not occurred after 6 weeks of treatment, or if the adverse effects cause discontinuation of therapy, seek medical evaluation.
- Use carefully near the eyes, mouth, lips, and nose, as well as near cuts, scrapes, and other abrasions, because excessive irritation may occur.
- Use of other acne medications with this product may cause excessive dryness and peeling. Do so only as directed by a medical practitioner.
- This product may cause increased sensitivity to the sun. Avoid direct sun exposure or use of sunlamps, and apply a non-comedogenic sunscreen with a sun protection factor (SPF) of 15 or higher when going outdoors.
- Product may bleach clothing, hair, and bed linens.

Salicylic Acid

- Salicylic acid helps unclog pores by causing slight peeling.
- This medication is less effective than benzoyl peroxide.
- Salicylic acid can be used once or twice daily as a cleanser or as a topical gel.
- Gel formulations should be applied to only the affected area.
- If excessive peeling occurs, limit use to once daily or every other day.
- Salicylic acid may cause sun sensitivity, so use a sunscreen (see Benzoyl Peroxide).
- Maximum effectiveness and duration of use are similar to those of benzoyl peroxide.
- Lack of response after 6 weeks is an indication of need for medical referral.

Sulfur

- Sulfur is believed to work by inhibiting the growth of *P. acnes*.
- This medication can be applied one to three times daily, but its use is limited by its chalky yellow color and characteristic unpleasant odor.
- Use of sulfur is mostly adjunctive; it is not as effective as benzoyl peroxide.

The Internet lists supplemental information about acne in lay language, including discussions of acne, nonprescription drugs used to treat it, and treatment expectations. Selected sites that appear to provide accurate information are listed in Table 38-5. If not copyrighted, these materials can be printed and given to the patient during the consultation. If the material is copyrighted, the practitioner should instead give the patient the Web site address.

Evaluation of Patient Outcomes for Acne

Although the patient may expect complete resolution of the acne, an improvement in the disorder, as defined by a decrease in both the number and severity of lesions, is a more realistic expectation for effective self-treatment. The practitioner should determine

TABLE 38-5 Selected Web Sites for Acne Information

Web Site

www.aad.org

www.acne.org

www.derm-infonet.com/acnenet

www.fda.gov

www.nlm.nih.gov/medlineplus/acne.html

www.skincarephysicians.com/acnenet

www.holisticonline.com/Remedies/Acne.htm

whether patients whose acne shows no improvement after 6 weeks of self-treatment are following the recommended regimen. If they have been adherent, medical referral is appropriate. Patients who have not diligently followed the regimen should be encouraged to do so. The practitioner should again explain the expected results and the rigor with which treatment must be pursued. If some improvement is evident, the practitioner may suggest monthly follow-up to check for improvement in the condition and potential adjustment of the maintenance regimen.

Key Points for Acne

➤ Acne cannot be cured, but it may be controlled enough to improve cosmetic appearance and prevent development of severe acne with resultant scarring.

➤ Adherence to any regimen to treat acne is a crucial factor in achieving a successful outcome.

➤ Minimizing environmental and physical factors that exacerbate acne can help limit the extent of the condition.

➤ Pharmacologic and nonpharmacologic therapies should be tailored to the patient.

➤ According to current guidelines, medical referral is the preferred initial step before implementing nonprescription therapy.

➤ Some people have chronic acne into adulthood and must care for their skin for a long time before improvement will occur.

➤ If given proper counseling, including empathy and reassurance, patients with acne may understand that the condition may not exist forever.

REFERENCES

1. Yan AC. Current concepts in acne management. *Adolesc Med.* 2006; 17;613–37

2. Federman DG, Kirsner RS. Acne vulgaris: pathogenesis and therapeutic approach. *Am J Manage Care.* 2000;6:78–87.

3. Rodan K, Fields K. *Unblemished.* New York: Atria Books; 2004:12–20.

4. Webster GF. Acne and rosacea. In: Rakel RE, Bope ET, eds. *Conn's Current Therapy 2007.* 59th ed. Philadelphia: Saunders; 2007. Available to subscribers at: http://www.mdconsult.com/das/book/body/89163103-2/0/1444/449.html?tocnode=53006947&fromURL=449.html#4-u1.0-B978-1-4160-3281-6.X5001-4—section13_3048. Last accessed January 4, 2008.

5. Habif TP. *Clinical Dermatology.* 4th ed. Edinburgh: Mosby; 2004. Available to subscribers at http://www.mdconsult.com/das/book/body/89193507-2/0/1195/43.html?tocnode=51440414&fromURL=43.html#4-u1.0-B0-323-01319-8.50009-1_567. Last accessed January 3, 2008.

6. Rudy SJ. Overview of the evaluation and management of acne vulgaris. *Pediatr Nurs.* 2003;29:287–93.

7. Farrar MD, Ingham E. Acne: inflammation. *Clin Dermatol.* 2004;22: 380–4.

8. Burrall BA. Clinical Pearls from the Literature and Experience. Presented at the 59th Annual Meeting of the American Academy of Dermatology, Washington, DC, March 2–7, 2001.

9. Allen LV. Secundum Artem. Available at: http://www.paddocklabs.com/forms/secundum/Vol.%2011.1.pdf. Last accessed September 28, 2008.

10. Zouboulis CC, Bohm. Neuroendocrine regulation of sebocytes a pathogenic link between stress and acne. *Exp Dermatol.* 2004;13(suppl 4):31–5.

11. Gollnick H, Cunliffe W, Berson D. Management of acne: a report from a global alliance to improve outcomes in acne. *J Am Acad Dermatol.* 2003; 49:S1–S38.

12. Wolf R, Matz H, Orion E. Acne and diet. *Clin Dermatol.* 2004;22: 387–93.

13. Presentations at different stages (defining characteristics of acne). *J Drugs Dermatol.* 2004;3(4 suppl):S7–S9.

14. Van de Kerkhof PC, Kleinpenning MM, De Jong EM, et al. Current and future treatment options for acne. *J Dermatol Treat.* 2006;17:198–204.

15. Feldman S, Careccia R. Diagnosis and treatment of acne. *Am Fam Physician.* 2004;69:2123–30.

16. Zaenglein AL, Thilboutot DM. Expert committee recommendation for acne management. *Pediatrics.* 2006:118:1188–99.

17. Perricone N. *The Clear Skin Prescription: The Perricone Program to Eliminate Problem Skin.* New York: Harper Collins; 2003:28–30.

18. Brown SK, Shalita AR. Acne vulgaris. *Lancet.* 1998; 351:1871–6.

19. Strauss JS, Krowchuk DP, Leyden JJ. Guidelines of care for acne vulgaris management. *J Am Acad Dermatol.* 2007;56:651–3.

20. Russell JJ. Topical therapy for acne. *Am Fam Physician.* 2000;61:357–66.

21. Knox-Koh CP, Scott SA, Popovich NG. Therapy and topical treatment of acne vulgaris. *US Pharm.* 2002;22:4. Available at: http://www.uspharmacist.com. Last accessed September 22, 2008.

22. efacts [subscription resource]. Salicylic Acid. Available at: http://online.factsandcomparisons.com/MonoDisp.aspx?monoID=fandc-hcp11854&inProdGen=true&quick=Salicylic%20Acid&search=Salicylic%20Acid. Last accessed October 9, 2008.

23. Guyette JR, Rygwelski JM. Complementary or alternative medicine: therapies for common dermatologic conditions. *Clin Pharm Pract.* 2002; 4:947–66.

24. Goodman G. Managing acne vulgaris effectively. *Am Fam Physician.* 2006; 35:705–8.

Prevention of Sun-Induced Skin Disorders

Kimberly M. Crosby

Current research has demonstrated that exposure to ultraviolet radiation (UVR) is cumulative and can produce serious, long-term problems such as premature skin aging. In addition, cumulative exposure from childhood to adulthood, even without a serious sunburn, may predispose a person to develop precancerous and cancerous skin conditions. This fact is clear: Avoiding excessive exposure to UVR will reduce the incidence of premature aging of the skin, skin cancer, and other long-term dermatologic effects.

The most common skin problem caused by UVR is sunburn. However, other conditions are either directly caused or exacerbated by UVR. These conditions include both drug and nondrug photosensitivity. Photodermatoses are idiopathic (self-originated) or exacerbated (photoaggravated) by radiation of varying wavelengths, including ultraviolet A (UVA) and some visible light. Ultraviolet B (UVB), however, is most often responsible for the reactions. More than 20 disorders are classified as photodermatoses (Table 39-1).[1,2]

Along with the heightened awareness of the dangers of UVR has come a multitude of sunscreen (rather than *suntan*) products intended not only to help darken but also to protect the skin from the harmful effects of exposure to the sun. Applied properly, these products can block most of the sun's harmful UV rays. Unfortunately, the average consumer lacks sufficient understanding of both the process of tanning and the necessity of using sunscreens properly. There is a public health need for education about the safe and effective use of sunscreen and suntan products. To perform this function, health professionals should be aware of the hazards of UVR, as well as the criteria for selecting and properly using sunscreen products. Practitioners are encouraged to become involved in educational efforts to help minimize the morbidity and mortality associated with UVR exposure.

In 2000, the market for sun care products was $853 million, with sunscreen/sunblock products representing 65% of the total.[3] Although spending on sun care products continues to rise, there has been a slow but steady shift in sales from pharmacies to mass merchandisers.

Pathophysiology of Sun-Induced Skin Disorders

Each of the more than 20 photodermatoses presents with a unique morphology. The common factor in the development of each of these disorders is the onset or exacerbation of signs and symptoms after exposure to UVR. Other UVR-induced disorders include neoplastic disorders such as premalignant actinic keratosis (which usually develops into squamous cell carcinoma if left untreated), keratoacanthoma, Kaposi's sarcoma, and malignant melanoma.

In addition to the idiopathic photodermatoses, UVR can precipitate or exacerbate many photoaggravated dermatologic conditions, including herpes simplex labialis (cold sores), systemic lupus erythematosus (SLE) and associated skin lesions, and chloasma, which may affect pregnant women and women taking oral contraceptives.

One of the other long-term hazards of UVR is premature photoaging of the skin. It is now believed that 50% to 80% of all photodamage to the skin occurs by 20 years of age.[4]

Epidemiologic studies conducted since the 1950s demonstrate a strong relationship between chronic, excessive, and unprotected sun exposure and human skin cancer. Skin cancer is the most common type of cancer, accounting for approximately 50% of all malignancies. The majority of nonmelanoma skin cancers (NMSCs) occur on the most exposed areas of the body, such as the face, head, neck, and back of the hands. An estimated more than 1 million people are diagnosed with NMSC each year in the United States.[5] The two most common types of NMSC are basal cell carcinoma (BCC) and squamous cell carcinoma (SCC). Most of these cases of NMSC are curable with early detection and treatment. In contrast, an estimated 62,480 new cases of malignant melanoma were expected to be diagnosed in 2008. Of the estimated 11,200 deaths from skin cancer, 8420 are from melanoma.[6] Some of the risk factors for skin cancer include fair skin (difficulty tanning/burning easily), large numbers of melanocytic nevi (moles), large-sized moles, a family history of melanoma, previous history of SCC or BCC, severe sunburns as a child, and excessive sun exposure or visits to a tanning salon.[5,6]

Research has shown that the type of skin cancer varies significantly according to the causes and contributing factors. For example, studies have shown conclusively that skin cancer occurs more often in light-skinned as opposed to dark-skinned individuals. This is believed to occur because individuals with darker pigmentation have more melanin. Melanin absorbs UVR, thereby preventing the radiation from penetrating into the tissue.[7] Although follow-up studies need to be performed before a definitive relationship can be made between the type of sun exposure and the type of skin cancer, there is no question that skin cancer is linked to sun exposure.

TABLE 39-1 Common Photodermatoses

Idiopathic Disorders

Actinic prurigo
Chronic actinic dermatitis
Hydroa vacciniforme
Polymorphous light eruption
Solar urticaria

Photoaggravated Dermatoses

Atopic dermatitis	Lichen planus actinicus
Chronic actinic dermatitis	Pellagra
Cutaneous T-cell lymphoma	Pemphigus
Dermatomyositis	Porphyrias
Disseminated superficial actinic porokeratosis	Psoriasis
Drug-induced photosensitivity	Reticular erythematous mucinosis
Erythema multiforme	Rosacea
Herpes simplex labialis	Systemic lupus erythematosus
	Transient acantholytic dermatosis

Source: References 1 and 2.

Another factor affecting skin cancer has been generally accepted—its relationship to latitude. The incidence of skin cancer increases steadily in populations closer to the equator. The quantity of harmful UVR increases as the angle of the sun to the Earth approaches 90 degrees and as the distance of the sun to Earth decreases.[8] People in the southern part of the United States are at greater risk from the harmful effects of UVR than are those in northern areas. A constant rate of increase in the incidence of skin cancer is found as one approaches the equator from north to south; the incidence approximately doubles for every 3° 48′ decrease in latitude. Also, the irradiance of UVB increases by 4% for every 1000-foot increase in altitude. This increase may be of particular concern to skiers and to people who live and work in higher elevations.[9,10]

Various bands of UVR cause or exacerbate sun-induced skin disorders. UVR is commonly referred to as UV light. However, *light* technically refers to only the visible spectrum; therefore, the correct terminology in this context is *radiation*.

Bands of UVR

The UV spectrum is divided into three major bands: ultraviolet C (UVC), UVB, and UVA. The wavelength of UVC, also known as germicidal radiation, is within the 200 to 290 nm band. Little UVC radiation from the sun reaches Earth, because it is screened out by the ozone layer of the upper atmosphere. However, UVC is emitted by some artificial sources of UVR, and most of the UVC that strikes the skin is absorbed by the dead cell layer of the stratum corneum.

The wavelength of the UVB band is between 290 and 320 nm. This is the most active UVR wavelength for producing erythema, which is why it is called sunburn radiation. The irradiance (i.e., intensity of the radiation reaching Earth) of UVB is most intense from 10 am to 4 pm.

The only true therapeutic effect of UVB exposure is vitamin D_3 synthesis in the skin. Vitamin D deficiency does not seem to be a problem for infants who receive vitamin D–fortified milk.[11] Vitamin D deficiency can be avoided in most individuals by 5 to 20 minutes of exposure to sunlight two to three times per week most months of the year.[12] Its therapeutic benefit notwithstanding, UVB is considered to be primarily responsible for inducing skin cancer, and its carcinogenic effects are believed to be augmented by UVA.[13,14] UVB is also primarily responsible for wrinkling, epidermal hyperplasia, elastosis, and collagen damage. However, UVA also contributes to premature aging of the skin.[15]

The wavelength of UVA radiation ranges from 320 to 400 nm. Although most concerns regarding the hazards of sun exposure to date have focused specifically on UVB, concern about the adverse effects of UVA has been slowly developing since the early 1980s. UVA radiation penetrates deeper into the skin than UVB; therefore, it has a greater effect on the dermis than on the epidermis. This deeper penetration can cause both histologic and vascular damage. Evidence suggests that subsequent UVA exposure may cause further and more serious acute and chronic damage to the underlying tissue than that of UVB exposure.[16] It was believed previously that only UVB produced premature aging effects on the skin. Now UVA is believed to be involved in suppression of the immune system as well as in damage to DNA.[3] UVA radiation can trigger herpes simplex labialis. In addition, it can produce a photosensitivity reaction in patients who have ingested or applied photosensitizing agents. Although approximately 20 times more UVA than UVB reaches Earth at noon (30 times more in winter), erythemogenic activity is relatively weak in the UVA band.[17]

Most tanning beds or devices use UVR sources comprising more than 96% UVA and less than 4% UVB, a different mix of UVR than that obtained from natural sunlight. Tanning bed use has been associated with an increased risk of skin cancers.[18,19]

The Food and Drug Administration (FDA) sets standards for sunlamp products and UV lamps.[20] These regulations deal with issues such as timers, exposure time, and device labeling, as well as the use of goggles with specified transmittance limits. Despite all FDA precautions and warnings, however, its regulations do not include any specified limits on the amount of UVA and UVB emitted from tanning devices. The only requirement is that the ratio of UVB to UVA shall not exceed 0.05 (5%). Health care practitioners should advise patients that the long-term hazards related to tanning devices have begun to surface and that these devices currently provide no accepted health benefits.

Transmission/Reflection of UVR

Contrary to popular opinion, cloud cover filters very little UVR; 70% to 90% of UVR will penetrate clouds, depending on their density. Clouds tend to filter out the infrared radiation that contributes to the sensation of heat, creating a false sense of security against a burn.[21] Fresh snow reflects 85% to 100% of the light and radiation that strikes it, creating the need for sunglasses when skiing on a sunny day. This reflected radiation can also cause significant sunburn in skiers, even on a cloudy day; therefore, skiers should use a sunscreen. Similarly, sand and white-painted surfaces, although not as reflective as snow, reflect 10% to 15% of the radiation striking them.[13] A person sitting in the shade of a beach umbrella may still be bombarded by UVR reflecting off the sand. This reflection contributes to the overall radiation received, and severe sunburn may result.

Water reflects no more than 5% of UVR, allowing the remaining 95% to penetrate and burn the swimmer. Therefore, time in the water, even if the swimmer is completely submerged, should be considered part of the total time spent in the sun. In addition, although dry clothes reflect almost all UVR, wet clothes allow transmission of approximately 50% of UVR. However, if light passes through dry clothing when held up to the sun, UVR will also penetrate that clothing. Tightly woven material offers the greatest protection.[4,10]

Although UVB does not penetrate window glass, UVA does. Most automobile windshields are made from laminated glass that filters most of the UVA. However side windows are not made from laminated glass; therefore, a significant amount of UVA may pass through to persons in the vehicle. Patients sensitive to UVA (e.g., those with photodermatoses or those taking photosensitizing drugs) should use appropriate sunscreens even when driving with the window closed.[22]

The Environmental Protection Agency has developed a UV index that uses a scale to rate the amount of skin-damaging UV radiation that reaches the earth's surface at any instance in time (Table 39-2). As the rating increases, the risk of exposure increases. When a UV index is given in the United States, it typically is given for noon, but it is important to remember that the UV index changes throughout the day. Factors that influence the UV index are time of day (midday has greater UVR exposure than early morning or late afternoon), ozone (limited amounts of ozone increase the amount of UVR exposure), altitude (higher altitudes receive greater UVR exposure), season of year (spring and summer have greater UVR exposure), surface (reflective surfaces increase UVR exposure), latitude (closer to equator increase UVR exposure), and land cover (less tree cover increases UVR exposure).[23]

Sunburn and Suntan

The degree to which a person will develop a sunburn or a tan depends on several factors, including type and amount of radiation received, thickness of the epidermis and stratum corneum, skin pigmentation, skin hydration, and distribution and concentration of peripheral blood vessels. Most UVR that strikes the skin is absorbed by the epidermis.

A sunburn involves a number of mediators, including histamine, lysosomal enzymes, kinins, and at least one prostaglandin. These mediators produce peripheral vasodilatation as the UVR penetrates the epidermis; then, an inflammatory reaction involving a lymphocytic infiltrate develops. Swelling of the endothelium and leakage of red blood cells from capillaries will also occur. Although the exact mechanism is not fully understood, it is believed that UVB radiation produces erythema by first causing

damage to cellular DNA. The intensity of the UVB-induced erythema peaks at 12 to 24 hours after exposure.[21]

A tan is produced when UVR stimulates the melanocytes in the germinating skin layer to generate more melanin, and when UVR oxidizes the melanin already in the epidermis. Both processes serve as protective mechanisms by diffusing and absorbing additional UVR. Although UVB and UVA contribute to the tanning process, they induce pigmentation by different mechanisms. UVB acts by stimulating epidermal hyperplasia as well as by shifting of melanin up through the skin. UVA acts by increasing the total amount of melanin in the basal layer. Because of the location of melanin in each case, greater photoprotection from UVB-induced pigmentation is available than from UVA-induced pigmentation. UVA produces a tan through two processes. The first process is known as immediate pigment darkening, which involves photooxidation of existing melanin. It begins to be visible from 5 to 10 minutes after exposure and reaches its maximum effect in 60 to 90 minutes. The effects of immediate pigment darkening begin to fade quickly and may be gone within 24 hours. The second process is delayed tanning, or melanogenesis, which involves an increase in the number and size of melanocytes, as well as in the number of melanosomes or pigment granules produced by melanocytes. This delayed tanning contributes to the development of a slow natural tan.[21]

Drug Photosensitivity

Photosensitivity encompasses two types of conditions: photoallergy and phototoxicity. Drug photoallergy, a relatively uncommon immunologic response, involves an increased, chemically induced reactivity of the skin to UVR and/or visible light. UVR (primarily UVA) triggers an antigenic reaction in the skin. This reaction, which is not dose-related, is usually seen after at least one prior exposure to the involved chemical agent or drug.

Phototoxicity is an increased, chemically induced reactivity of the skin to UVR and/or visible light. However, this reaction is not immunologic. It is often seen on first exposure to a chemical agent or drug, is dose-related, and usually exhibits no drug cross-sensitivity. Some drugs associated with phototoxicity are listed in Table 39-3. This type of reaction is not limited to drugs; it is also associated with plants, cosmetics, and soaps.[2]

Premature Aging

Premature skin aging is genetically influenced. For example, whites are more susceptible than blacks. It is called *premature* photoaging because the obvious physical findings are similar to those seen in natural aging, although there are significant histologic and biochemical differences.

Skin Cancer

BCC is often an aggressive, invasive disorder of the epidermis and dermis, which can cause serious damage to the skin and underlying tissue. However, it rarely metastasizes. SCC is found in epithelial keratinocytes and grows very slowly. The pathophysiology of melanoma differs from that of the NMSCs. Although most melanomas come from normal skin, about 30% arise from existing nevi. The role that exposure to sunlight plays in the development of all types of skin cancers is continually being investigated. However, a growing amount of evidence supports the supposition that sun exposure plays a role in the development of all types of skin cancers.[24]

TABLE 39-2 Global Solar UV Index	
Rating Number	**Interpretation of UVR Exposure Risk**
1–2	Low
3–5	Moderate
6–7	High
8–10	Very high
11+	Extreme

Source: Reference 23.

TABLE 39-3 Selected Medications (by Drug Category) Associated with Photosensitivity Reactions

Anticancer Drugs

Dacarbazine
Daunorubicin
Fluorouracil
Methotrexate
Vinblastine

Anticonvulsants

Carbamazepine
Gabapentin
Lamotrigine
Phenytoin

Antidepressants

Bupropion
Selective serotonin reuptake inhibitors
Trazodone
Venlafaxine

Antihistamines

Cetirizine
Diphenhydramine

Antihypertensives

Angiotensin-converting enzyme inhibitors
Calcium channel blockers
Hydralazine
Labetalol
Methyldopa
Minoxidil
Sotalol

Anti-Infectives

Azithromycin
Ceftazidime

Dapsone
Gentamicin
Griseofulvin
Itraconazole
Ketoconazole
Metronidazole
Pyrazinamide
Quinolones
Ritonavir
Saquinavir
Sulfonamides
Tetracyclines
Trimethoprim
Trovafloxacin
Zalcitabine

Antimalarials

Chloroquine
Quinine

Antipsychotics/Phenothiazines

Haloperidol
Olanzapine
Ziprasidone

Coal Tar and Derivatives

DHS Tar Gel Shampoo
Ionil T Plus Shampoo
Neutrogena T/Derm Body Oil
Neutrogena T/Gel Extra Strength

Diuretics

Acetazolamide
Amiloride
Furosemide

Metolazone
Triamterene
Thiazide diuretics

Nonsteroidal Anti-Inflammatory Drugs

Celecoxib
Ibuprofen
Indomethacin
Naproxen
Psoralens
Methoxsalen
Trioxsalen

Sunscreens

Aminobenzoic acid
Aminobenzoic acid esters
Benzophenones
Cinnamates
Homosalate
Menthyl anthranilate
Oxybenzone

Miscellaneous

Amiodarone (antiarrhythmic)
Benzoyl peroxide
Gold salts (antiarthritic)
Isotretinoin (antiacne)
Quinidine sulfate (antiarrhythmic)
Retinoids
Statins

Source: Stein KR, Scheinfeld NS. Drug-induced photoallergic and phototoxic reactions. Expert Opin Drug Saf. 2007;6:431–43; and Moore DE. Drug-induced cutaneous photosensitivity. *Drug Saf.* 2002;25:45–372.

Clinical Presentation of Sun-Induced Skin Disorders

Sunburn

Sunburn is, in fact, a burn. It is most often seen as a first-degree (superficial) burn, with a reaction ranging from mild erythema to tenderness, pain, and edema (see Color Plates, photograph 26). Severe reactions to excessive UVR exposure can sometimes produce a second-degree burn, with the development of vesicles (blisters) or bullae (many large blisters), as well as fever, chills, weakness, and shock. Shock caused by heat prostration or hyperpyrexia can lead to death. (See Chapter 41 for treatment of sunburn.)

Drug Photosensitivity

Drug photoallergy presents similar to allergic contact dermatitis (e.g., poison ivy) and is characterized by pruritus with erythematous papules, vesicles, bullae, and/or urticaria (see Color Plates, photograph 27). Phototoxicity is most likely to appear as

exaggerated sunburn with pruritis.[1] Urticaria may also occur (see Color Plates, photograph 28).

Photodermatoses

Each photodermatosis has a unique morphology. Polymorphous light eruption alone can have multiple morphologic presentations of pruritus with papules, vesicles, plaques, and/or urticaria.

Premature Aging

This condition is characterized by wrinkling and yellowing of the skin. Conclusive evidence reveals that prolonged exposure to UVR results in elastosis (degeneration of the skin due to a breakdown of the skin's elastic fibers). Pronounced drying, thickening, and wrinkling of the skin may also result.[4] Other physical changes include cracking, telangiectasia (spider vessels), solar keratoses (growths), and ecchymoses (subcutaneous hemorrhagic lesions).[2] (See Chapter 40 for measures for reversing photoaging.)

Skin Cancer

BCC is a translucent nodule with a smooth surface. It is usually firm to the touch and may be ulcerated or crusted. It is generally found as an isolated lesion on the nose or other parts of the face, although multiple lesions are sometimes found. SCC, on the other hand, is a slow-growing, isolated papule or plaque on sun-exposed areas of the body.

Self-examination for melanoma uses four factors (A–B–C–D) for evaluation: *A*symmetric shape, *B*order irregularity or poorly defined border, *C*olor variation within the same mole or a change in color, and *D*iameter larger than 6 mm. A mole with these characteristics and any new growth or change in appearance of the skin (including the lips) should be evaluated by a dermatologist.[25]

Prevention of Sun-Induced Skin Disorders

The short-term goals in preventing sun-induced skin disorders are relatively simple: avoiding or minimizing sunburn, photosensitivity reactions, and UVR-induced or exacerbated photodermatoses. The expected long-term outcomes are prevention of skin cancer and avoidance of premature aging of the skin.

UVR-induced skin disorders can be prevented by minimizing exposure to UVR and using sunscreen agents. The selection of a sunscreen product and the degree of protection vary, depending on the patient's intended use for the product, as well as the conditions under which the product will be used (Figure 39-1).

The greater the risk a patient has of developing a UVR-induced skin disorder, the greater is the need to avoid sun exposure. However, most people do not spend warm, sunny July afternoons sitting inside, nor do they go to the beach or pool wearing lots of clothing. Practitioners can assist the patient in striking a balance between completely avoiding sun exposure, wearing protective clothing, and using sunscreen products. If, however, the patient suffers from a UVR-induced skin disorder, such as SLE, few options are available. With regard to preventing sunburn, the patient's natural skin type will be the primary factor in deciding the potency of the sunscreen product to be used. The lighter the natural skin color is (and the more *quickly* a burn develops), the higher is the required potency of the sunscreen product.

Avoidance of Sun Exposure

Complete avoidance of UVR, although unrealistic, is often the best approach for patients who have the physical characteristics or history listed in Table 39-4. For people who refuse to stay indoors or who must be outdoors for extended periods, the use of protective clothing such as a hat with a 4-inch brim, long pants, and a long-sleeved shirt should be recommended. In situations in which the patient is unwilling or unable to avoid the sun or to wear protective clothing, the next best choice is to use a sunscreen product.[26]

Use of Sunscreens

The final monograph (FM) for sunscreen products was published in 1999, with the new rules initially scheduled to become effective May 21, 2000, and May 21, 2001.[27] However, several key issues such as UVA protection factors and professional labeling were not addressed, because they remained under review by the

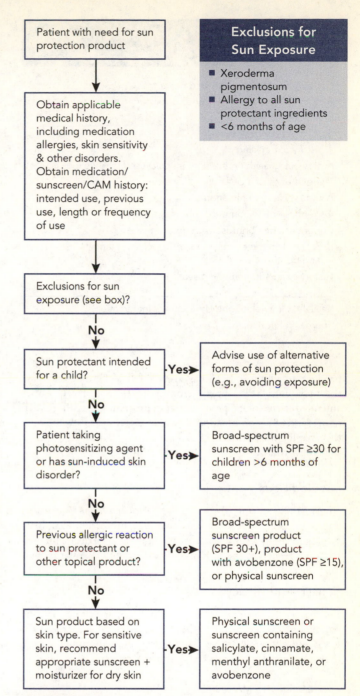

FIGURE 39-1 Self-care for sun protection. Key: CAM, complementary and alternative medicine; SPF, sun protection factor.

agency. On December 31, 2001, FDA delayed the effective implementation date of the sunscreen FM until they could address key issues such as formulation, labeling, and testing for sunscreens providing UVA protection. In August 2007, FDA issued new proposed regulation for the sunscreen drug products FM. These proposed changes included a new "four star" rating system for UVA protection of sunscreen products to be included with the sun protection factor (SPF) labeling for the product. Ratings would be derived from two tests that FDA has proposed to assess the effectiveness of UVA protection in the sunscreen

TABLE 39-4   Patient Risk Factors for the Development of UVR-Induced Problems

Fair skin that always burns and never tans

A history of one or more serious or blistering sunburns

Blonde or red hair

Blue, green, or gray eyes

A history of freckling

A previous growth on the skin or lips caused by UV exposure

The existence of a UV-induced disorder

A family history of melanoma

Current use of an immunosuppressive drug

Current use of a photosensitizing drug

Excessive lifetime exposure to UVR, including tanning beds and booths

History of an autoimmune disease

Key: UV, ultraviolet light; UVR, ultraviolet radiation.
Source: Reference 25.

product. In addition, FDA has amended its 1999 rule to increase the maximum SPF labeling from SPF30+ to SPF50+. Other amended items include a new testing procedure for SPF (UVB) ratings and new combinations of active ingredients.[28] At the time this chapter was written, FDA had not issued a final notice for these new rules.

Labeled Uses

The FM allows only the term *uses*—not *indications*—on sunscreen labels and approves only two uses: protection (minimal/moderate/high) against sunburn and tanning. The degree of protection is related to the SPF of a sunscreen and UVA star ratings.

Sunscreen Efficacy

Purchasers of sunscreens are usually familiar with SPF, one parameter for determining the effectiveness of sunscreens for UVB protection. Another parameter, minimal erythema dose (MED), is used to calculate the SPF of a sunscreen.

MINIMAL ERYTHEMA DOSE

The MED is defined as the "minimum UVR dose that produces clearly marginated erythema in the irradiated site, given as a single exposure."[24,26] It is a dose of radiation and not a grade of erythema. Generally, two MEDs will produce a bright erythema; four MEDs, a painful sunburn; and eight MEDs, a blistering burn. However, because of variations in thickness of the stratum corneum, different parts of the body may respond differently to the same MED. Furthermore, the MED for heavily pigmented blacks is estimated to be 33 times higher than that for lightly pigmented whites.

SUN PROTECTION FACTOR

The important measure for sunscreens is the SPF, derived by dividing the MED on protected skin by the MED on unprotected skin. For example, if a person requires 25 mJ/cm² of UVB radiation to experience 1 MED on unprotected skin and requires 250 mJ/cm² of radiation to produce 1 MED after applying a

TABLE 39-5   Proposed Product Category Designations

SPF	Category Designation
2–<12	Low sunburn protection
12–<30	Medium sunburn protection
30–>50	High sunburn protection
50+	Highest sunburn protection

Source: Adapted from references 27 and 28.

given sunscreen, the product would be given an SPF rating of 10. The higher the SPF, the more effective the agent is in preventing sunburn. If it normally takes 60 minutes for someone to experience two MEDs (a bright erythematous sunburn), a sunscreen with an SPF of 6 will allow that person to stay in the sun six times longer (or 6 hours) before receiving the same degree of sunburn (assuming the sunscreen is reapplied at the recommended intervals). The SPF is product-specific, given that it is calculated on the basis of the final formulation of the product and cannot be determined on the basis of the active ingredient alone.[26,28]

FDA reduced the original five SPF categories to three (Table 39-5) and eliminated designation of a skin type for each category. Manufacturers use the classification system in Table 39-6 to select test subjects for general testing procedures for sunscreens. However, this system is not allowed on product labeling.

A product with an SPF of 15 blocks 93% of UVB. Raising the SPF to 30 increases UVB protection to only 96.7%, and an SPF of 40 blocks 97.5%.[27] A hypothetical SPF of 70 would increase UVB protection to only 98.6%.[26,27] The small gain in protection made when SPF is increased from 30 to 40 may require up to 25% more sunscreen ingredients, which could increase the possibility of systemic and local adverse effects, as well as significantly increase product cost.

MEASURES OF UVA PROTECTION

With concern growing about the long-term adverse effects of UVA, the utility of the SPF value has been questioned. SPF provides a measure of a patient's erythemogenic response to UVB when using a sunscreen. However, UVA is at least 200 times less potent than UVB in producing erythema, and UVA's effects on

TABLE 39-6   Sunburn and Tanning History[a]

Skin Type	Sunburn/Tanning History
I	Always burns easily; never tans (sensitive)
II	Always burns easily; tans minimally (sensitive)
III	Burns moderately; tans gradually (normal)
IV	Burns minimally; always tans well (normal)
V	Rarely burns; tans profusely (insensitive)
VI	Never burns; deeply pigmented (insensitive)

[a] Used for selection of test subjects for general testing procedures and is not to be used as part of any sunscreen label.
Source: Adapted from references 27 and 28.

the skin differ somewhat from those produced by UVB.[17] Investigations have shown that sunscreens with similar SPFs demonstrate significant differences in their abilities to protect against UVR-induced immunologic injury to the skin.[17,26] Data suggest that high-SPF products block significant amounts of UVA. However, among products of equal SPF, UVA blockage may vary considerably. SPF is not a reliable measure of UVA protection.[28,29]

SUBSTANTIVITY

The efficacy of a sunscreen is also related to its substantivity—that is, its ability to remain effective during prolonged exercising, sweating, and swimming. This property can be a function of the active sunscreen, the vehicle, or both. Generally speaking, products with cream-based (water-in-oil) vehicles appear more resistant to removal by water than those with alcohol bases, and will reduce desquamation of the skin. In addition, part of a sunscreen's effectiveness may relate to the ability of the active agent to bind with constituents of the skin. This binding characteristic may be independent of the vehicle. Oil-based products have traditionally been the most popular and are easiest to apply; however, they tend to have lower SPF values.

The FM requirements for sunscreen product substantivity according to sweating, perspiring, or participating in water activities are as follows:

- *Water resistant:* Product retains its SPF for at least 40 minutes.
- *Very water resistant:* Product retains its sun protection for at least 80 minutes.

The category of *very water resistant* is intended to replace *waterproof*. This terminology is one of the areas in which manufacturers do not agree with FDA (they prefer *waterproof*). The FM does not allow for the use of labeling that claims a specific number of hours of protection or "all-day protection." The only allowed labeling will be "higher SPF gives more sunburn protection."

The mechanism of action of sunscreens is related to the definitions for the two therapeutic sunscreen types[27,28]:

1. *Sunscreen active ingredient:* An active ingredient absorbs at least 85% of the radiation in the UV range at wavelengths from 290 to 320 nm but may or may not allow transmission of radiation to the skin at wavelengths longer than 320 nm.
2. *Sunscreen opaque sunblock:* An opaque sunscreen active ingredient reflects or scatters all light in the UV and visible range at wavelengths from 290 to 777 nm, and the sunscreen thereby prevents or minimizes suntan and sunburn.

Types of Sunscreens

According to the therapeutic definitions, topical sunscreens can be divided into two major subgroups: chemical and physical sunscreens. Chemical sunscreens work by absorbing and thus blocking the transmission of UVR to the epidermis. Physical sunscreens are generally opaque, and act by reflecting and scattering UVR, rather than absorbing it.

The FM lists 14 chemical agents and 2 physical agents as safe and effective for use as sunscreens. Table 39-7 lists these agents, their UVR absorbance range, and their maximum concentrations. Because the SPF is product-specific and does not depend on the sunscreen's active agent alone, the FM has eliminated a required minimum strength for sunscreens that contain a single active ingredient. At the time of this publication, a new ingredient for sunscreens, octyl triazone, has not been approved by FDA for use in the United States, although it is being used in other countries. Octyl triazone is a polymer designed to enhance the capacity of other sunscreen active ingredients to protect against UVA and UVB radiation. Some studies have shown increases in SPFs by up to 70% when octyl triazone is added to other chemical sunscreen agents.[30]

AMINOBENZOIC ACID AND DERIVATIVES

Aminobenzoic acid (formerly para-aminobenzoic acid [PABA]), once the most widely used sunscreen agent, has been replaced by other agents, because it has been shown to be a major sensitizer. Because of the continuing confusion about the name of this sunscreen, the FM requires that product labels list it as "aminobenzoic acid" and that each time this name appears on product labeling, it shall be followed by "(PABA)" so consumers know which chemical entity they are using.

Aminobenzoic acid is an effective UVB sunscreen, especially when formulated in a hydroalcoholic base (maximum of 50%–60% alcohol). The SPF of such formulations increases proportionally as the concentration of aminobenzoic acid increases from 2% to 5%. One advantage of this agent is its ability to penetrate into the horny layer of the skin and provide lasting protection. Its substantivity on sweating skin is significant but is reduced on skin that is immersed in water. The primary advantage of aminobenzoic acid derivatives over aminobenzoic acid is that the derivatives do not stain clothing. The only Category I derivative is padimate O.

The disadvantages of alcoholic solutions of aminobenzoic acid include contact dermatitis, photosensitivity, stinging and drying of the skin, and yellow staining of clothes on exposure to the sun. Patients who have experienced a photosensitivity reaction to a sunscreen product containing aminobenzoic acid or any of its derivatives should avoid using these products.[17,26,28]

ANTHRANILATES

The anthranilates are ortho-aminobenzoic acid derivatives. Menthyl anthranilate, the menthyl ester of anthranilic acid, is a weak UV sunscreen with maximal absorbance in the UVA range. It is usually found in combination with other sunscreen agents to provide broader UV coverage.[17,26,28]

BENZOPHENONES

Three agents are in the benzophenone group: dioxybenzone, oxybenzone (benzophenone-3), and sulisobenzone (benzophenone-4). As a group, these agents are primarily UVB absorbers, with maximum absorbance between 282 and 290 nm. However, their absorbance extends well into the UVA range, with oxybenzone up to 350 nm and dioxybenzone up to 380 nm. Because of the possibility of allergic reactions to aminobenzoic acid and its derivatives, many sunscreen products now contain benzophenones in their formulations because of the broader spectrum of action. Oxybenzone, also found in some cosmetic formulations, is a significant sensitizing agent among sunscreens. There has been a rise in reports of sensitivity to the benzophenones as the use of these agents has increased.[17,26,28,31,32]

CINNAMATES

Cinnamates include cinoxate, octyl methoxycinnamate, and octocrylene. As shown in Table 39-7, cinoxate and octyl methoxycinnamate have similar absorbance ranges and maximum absorbances. Octocrylene, however, has an absorbance range of 250 to 360 nm, well into the UVA range. Octocrylene is currently found in more commercial sunscreen preparations than

TABLE 39-7 Sunscreens Considered to Be Safe and Effective

Sunscreen Agent	Absorbance Range (nm)	Maximum Range (nm)	Approved Maximum Concentration (%)
ABA and Derivatives			
Aminobenzoic acid (PABA)	260–313	288.5	15
Padimate O	290–315	310	8
Anthranilates			
Menthyl anthranilate (meradimate)	260–380[a]	340[a]	5
Benzophenones			
Dioxybenzone	260–380[b]	282[c]	3
Oxybenzone	270–350	290[d]	6
Sulisobenzone	260–375	285[e]	10
Cinnamates			
Cinoxate	270–328	310	3
Octocrylene	250–360	303	10
Octyl methoxycinnamate (octinoxate)	290–320	308–310	7.5
Dibenzoylmethane Derivatives			
Avobenzone[f]	320–400	360	3
Salicylates			
Homosalate	295–315	306	15
Octyl salicylate (octisalate)	280–320	305	5
Trolamine salicylate	260–320	298	12
Miscellaneous			
Phenyl benzimidazole sulfonic acid (ensulizole)	290–320	302	4
Terephthalyidene dicamphor sulfonic acid (ecamsule)	290–390	345	2
Titanium dioxide[g]	290–770	—	25
Zinc oxide[g]	290–770	—	25

[a] Values are for concentrations higher than those normally found in nonprescription drugs.

[b] Values are achieved when used in combination with other sunscreen agents.

[c] Second peak occurs at 217 nm.

[d] Second peak occurs at 329 nm.

[e] Second peak occurs at 324 nm.

[f] Agent is currently marketed through a new drug application.

[g] Agent scatters, rather than absorbs, radiation in the 290–770 nm range.

Source: References 17, 26–28, 30, and Shaath NA. Encyclopedia of UV absorbers for sunscreen products. *Cosmet Toiletries.* 1987;102:21–36.

it was in the past, possibly reflecting its broader spectrum of absorbance.

Unfortunately, cinnamates do not adhere well to the skin and must rely on the vehicle in a given formulation for their substantivity.[17,26,28]

DIBENZOYLMETHANE DERIVATIVES

Avobenzone (butyl methoxydibenzoylmethane, originally known as Parsol 1789) is the first of a new class of sunscreen agents effective throughout the entire UVA range (320–400 nm; full spectrum). It has a maximum absorbance at approximately 360 nm. This agent entered the market through a new drug application and was officially approved in the published FM. Although avobenzone absorbs UVR throughout the UVA spectrum, its absorbance falls off sharply at 370 nm. Therefore, reactions from photosensitive drugs and chemicals that are highly reactive in the 370 to 400 nm range could still occur. Avobenzone, however, offers the best protection in the UVA range compared with the other chemical sunscreens on the market. It is commonly included in sunscreen products to increase UVA coverage. Avobenzone is easily degraded by exposure to sunlight. It is found in newer sunscreen products combined with octocrylene, salicylates, methybenzylidene camphor, and micronized zinc oxide and/or titanium dioxide to enhance stability of the product, as well as extend the spectrum of coverage of the product through the UVA and UVB spectrum.[17,26,28]

SALICYLATES

Salicylic acid derivatives are weak sunscreens and must be used in high concentrations. They do not adhere well to the skin and are easily removed by perspiration or swimming.[17,26,28]

OTHER CHEMICAL SUNSCREENS

Phenylbenzimidazole sulfonic acid does not fit into any of the above classes. It is a pure UVB sunscreen with an absorbance range of 290 to 320 nm. Terephthalylidene dicamphor sulfonic acid (ecamsule) is a new molecule that FDA approved in 2006. It is a water-resistant broad-spectrum sunscreen. Octocrylene is often combined with this product to increase stability to light.[17]

PHYSICAL SUNSCREENS

Physical sunscreens scatter rather than absorb UVR and visible radiation (290–777 nm). They are most often used on small and prominently exposed areas by patients who cannot limit or control their exposure to the sun (e.g., lifeguards). A white or colored substance containing zinc oxide or titanium dioxide is often used to coat the nose and top of the ears. Manufacturers have also developed a way to make titanium dioxide transparent while maintaining efficacy as a sunscreen. Disadvantages of physical sunscreens are that they can discolor clothing, and they may occlude the skin to produce miliaria (prickly heat) and folliculitis. Because titanium dioxide increases the effective SPF of a product and extends the spectrum of protection well into the UVA range, the number of commercial products containing this agent has increased. The FM allows zinc oxide to be used alone or combined with any of the other sunscreen agents except avobenzone; the exception is due to a lack of data on effectiveness.[17,26,28]

Combination Products

FDA has not recommended limits on the number of sunscreen agents that may be used together. However, each sunscreen agent must contribute to the efficacy of a product and must not be included merely for marketing promotion purposes. Therefore, the FM requires that each active ingredient contribute a minimum SPF of not less than 2, and that the finished product must have a minimum SPF of not less than the number of sunscreen active ingredients used in the combination multiplied by 2.

Dosage and Administration Guidelines

The two major causes of poor sun protection with sunscreen use are application of inadequate amounts and infrequent reapplication. In a report on sunscreen application to eight areas of the face, the degree of complete coverage ranged from 8% periorbital and 18% ears, to 80% forehead and 94% cheeks.[33] Although many sunscreen products that prevent burning of the lips (or nose) are available, the lips are often neglected. Although they differ in ingredients and in the UVA and UVB spectrum, products for the lips carry most of the same labeling, including the SPF, used on sunscreen lotions. The SPF of products for lips is usually at least 15. Studies have shown that lip protection not only helps prevent drying and burning of the lips, but it also helps prevent the development of cold sores or fever blisters triggered by the herpes simplex virus in patients who are susceptible to recurrent outbreaks.

Sunscreens must be liberally applied to all exposed areas of the body and reapplied at least as often as the label recommends for maximum effectiveness. One recent study suggested that sunscreens be applied 15 to 30 minutes before UV exposure and every 15 to 30 minutes thereafter. The study also suggested reapplication after every episode of swimming, toweling dry, or excessive sweating.[34] Although these two factors drive up the cost of sunscreen use, the long-term benefits of proper sunscreen use outweigh the costs.

The FDA standard for application of sunscreens is 2 mg/cm^2 of body surface area. This standard means that, for sufficient protection, the average adult in a bathing suit should apply nine portions of sunscreen of approximately one-half teaspoon each, or approximately 4 and one-half teaspoons (22.5 mL) total. The sunscreen should be distributed as follows:

- *Face and neck:* one-half teaspoon
- *Arms and shoulders:* one-half teaspoon to each side of body
- *Torso:* one-half teaspoon each to front and back.
- *Legs and top of feet:* 1 teaspoon to each side of body

Because of the cost of sunscreen products and the need to apply them often and in sufficient amounts, people may use far less sunscreen than is necessary to provide adequate protection. A study on sunscreen failure reported that men were significantly less likely to use sunscreens than were women.[35] In addition, when men used sunscreens, they applied less to exposed skin than did women.

Outdoor exposure to UVR should be within the limits of the SPF value of the sunscreen. Another factor to consider is the time that it takes the sunscreen to bind to the various skin constituents and to become fully effective. For most sunscreen products, the interval is 15 to 30 minutes, although at least one product claims immediate effectiveness. Because this lag time varies from product to product, the FM allows each product to include its individual lag time on the label. Sunscreens should be reapplied as often as label instructions direct. Water-resistant products are reapplied every 40 minutes, whereas very-water-resistant products are reapplied after every 80 minutes of water exposure.

If properly applied, products with an SPF of 15 to 30 allow an individual to stay out in the sun for long periods and to slowly develop a tan over several days to weeks. As an individual tans, a natural protection against burning also develops. Therefore, an individual who insists on tanning should begin the summer using a product with an SPF of at least 15 to 30 (depending on skin type and tanning history) and should switch to a product with a lower SPF (e.g., 12, then 10, then 8, etc.) as the natural tan progresses. This change will allow a more rapid deepening of the tan while helping to build up natural protection in the skin. The individual can, however, continue to use the product with the higher SPF; it will simply take longer to achieve the desired tan.

Patients should be advised that, although tanning and thickening of the skin serve as protective mechanisms against future injury, peeling of the skin removes part of this protection. The amount of exposure to the sun as well as the SPF of the product being used must be reevaluated as tanning and peeling occur.

Safety Considerations

The development of a rash, vesicles (blisters), hives, or an exaggerated sunburn is most likely a sign of either a photosensitivity or allergic reaction. Product labels must state the following: "Stop use if skin rash occurs." The patient should be referred to a primary care provider for evaluation of the situation. The degree of the reaction will determine what type of medical intervention (if any) is necessary.

If a patient has had a prior reaction to a sunscreen product, the name of the product and the ingredients it contained should be identified, if possible. This action may be difficult because product formulations change frequently. Photosensitivity and contact dermatitis are more likely to occur with aminobenzoic acid and its esters, although the benzophenones, cinnamates, homosalate, avobenzone, and menthyl anthranilate have also been reported to produce both conditions. In a French study of contact dermatitis, 15.4% of patients were found to have an allergy to sunscreens with almost one-half attributed to oxybenzone.[36] In addition, patients who are allergy prone and have allergies to various drugs (e.g., benzocaine, thiazides, or sulfonamides) may also develop an allergic reaction to either aminobenzoic acid or its esters.

Although no evidence exists of significant effects from eye contact, FDA requires the warning label: "Keep out of eyes."

Additional Product Considerations

SUNSCREENS IN COSMETIC PRODUCTS

The FM addresses a gray area that has allowed the proliferation of cosmetics claiming to offer sun protection. It stipulates that sunscreen products will be classified as drugs rather than cosmetics, because consumers expect that sunscreens will protect them from some of the sun's damaging effects. However, cosmetics that contain sunscreen agents will be classified as cosmetics as long as no therapeutic claims are made, and the sunscreen is intended for a nontherapeutic, nonphysiologic purpose. In addition, if the term *sunscreen* appears on the product labeling, a statement must appear that describes the cosmetic purpose of the sunscreen (e.g., "contains a sunscreen—to protect product color").

SUNTAN PRODUCTS

Two types of products fall under the general heading of suntan products: those that contain a pigmenting agent and those that do not. Products that do not contain a pigmenting agent are formulated with oily vehicles (e.g., mineral oil) that tend to concentrate UVR onto the skin. Although they are also formulated with emollients, these products provide no protection whatsoever against the short- and long-term hazards of UVR exposure. The other type of suntan product contains the pigmenting agent dihydroxyacetone (DHA). This agent may be formulated with or without an oily vehicle. DHA has been the major ingredient in products that claim to tan without the sun. It produces a reddish-brown color by binding with specific amino acids in the stratum corneum. The intensity of the tan is related to the thickness of the skin. If the product is not washed off the hands immediately after application, however, the palms may also develop this tan (turn orange). In addition, dry areas, such as elbows and kneecaps, will absorb the DHA more readily, resulting in uneven coloration. The color fades after 5 to 7 days with desquamation of the stratum corneum.

One new requirement from the final monograph did go into effect in 2000. All suntan products that do not contain a sunscreen must carry the following labeling: "Warning—This product does not contain a sunscreen and protect against sunburn. Repeated exposure of unprotected skin while tanning may increase the risk of skin aging, skin cancer, and other harmful effects to the skin even if you do not burn."[25,27]

ORAL PIGMENTING AGENTS

A number of products have claimed to be effective oral tanning compounds. Their active ingredients are the dyes canthaxanthin and beta-carotene, which are chemically similar. Beta-carotene and canthaxanthin are both approved by FDA as color additives in foods and drugs, and beta-carotene is also approved for use in cosmetics. Canthaxanthin is a synthetic dye that is similar to dyes found naturally in fruits, vegetables, and flowers. Both agents are used to enhance the appearance of foods such as pizza, barbecue and spaghetti sauces, soups, salad dressings, fruit drinks, baked goods, pudding, cheese, ketchup, and margarine.[37] However, the concentrations of these agents in food are lower (1/20 to 1/40) than those found in oral products that claim to produce tanning.

The dyes alter skin tone by coloring the fat cells under the epidermal layer. Because of variations in fat cells and epidermal thickness, the extent of the tan varies from person to person. Canthaxanthin is dosed by body weight. The promotional literature cautions the user that if the palms turn orange, too much of the product is being consumed.

According to the 1960 Color Additive Amendment, any new use of a color additive must be submitted to FDA for approval. FDA has not yet approved either beta-carotene or canthaxanthin for artificial tanning. One major concern with these additives is the discoloration of the feces to brick red, which could mask gastrointestinal bleeding. A second concern is the long-term adverse effects that may be associated with the large doses recommended. Although beta-carotene is used on a prescription basis to help prevent photosensitivity in patients with erythropoietic protoporphyria, no evidence documents the safety of canthaxanthin at the high doses found in oral tanning products. In fact, a case has been reported of fatal aplastic anemia associated with canthaxanthin ingestion from an oral tanning product. Reported cases of retinopathy as well as other medical problems associated with the use of oral tanning agents have prompted FDA to issue further warnings on such products.[27] Canada, which previously allowed the nonprescription sale of canthaxanthin for tanning purposes, has decided that there is insufficient evidence of its safety and no longer allows such sales.

TAN ACCELERATORS

Tan accelerators are cosmetic products that claim to stimulate a faster and deeper tan. Their major ingredient is tyrosine, an amino acid necessary to produce melanin. Product literature recommends application of these products once daily for at least 3 days before sun exposure. However, there is currently no evidence that tan accelerators work. FDA recognizes this fact and has stated that "any product containing tyrosine or its derivatives and claiming to accelerate the tanning process is an unapproved new drug."[27]

MELANOTROPINS AND MELANIN PRODUCTS

A hormone known as alpha-melanotropin or alpha-melanocyte–stimulating hormone (alpha-MSH) has been located within the human central nervous system. The role of alpha-MSH in humans, if any, has not yet been fully identified. However, this hormone is produced by the pituitary gland of numerous vertebrates and has been shown to affect skin color through its action on melanocytes.[38] Alpha-melanotropin is currently under investigation to determine whether it can affect skin tanning. Also, the FM states that melanin and artificial melanin ingredients are not recognized sunscreens, and that any products containing these agents and making sunscreen claims are new drugs and must be under a new drug application.

Product Selection Guidelines

Two primary factors will determine the best product for a given patient: the intended use of the product and specific patient characteristics. The decision on which sunscreen product to use must be based on the information obtained from both categories.

INTENDED USE

Some patients may want to use sunscreens to prevent sunburn or the photoaging effects of UVR, or to protect themselves from skin cancer. Others may need protection from sun exposure, because they are taking photosensitive drugs or they suffer from a photodermatosis.

The higher the SPF of the sunscreen product, the greater the protection it provides against sunburn and tanning. Studies have shown that sunscreens can protect against the long-term hazards of skin cancer.[37] Considerable research is currently being conducted on all aspects of UVR and its effects. However, experts are debating whether low-SPF products protect individuals from UV skin damage or allow them to receive dangerously high levels of UVR over extended periods of time. Because of the known hazards associated with UVR, FDA and other organizations such as the American Academy of Dermatology recommend the use of sunscreen products of at least SPF 15. Compared with lower-SPF products, any product in the SPF range of 15 to 30+ will significantly reduce the total amount of both UVB and some UVA radiation received. Generally, if a product is to be used to prevent skin cancer, reduce the chances of a photosensitivity reaction, or reduce the risk of triggering a skin disorder induced or aggravated by UVR, a broad-spectrum 30+ SPF is best.

A number of commercial products claim to be broad spectrum; FDA allows such claims if the product contains ingredients that absorb or reflect UVB (290–320 nm) *and* absorb UVA up to 360 nm.[27] Products with equal SPFs may still differ significantly in total UVR protection, depending on the absorbances of the various sunscreens they contain. Most currently available broad-spectrum products have a minimum of two sunscreen ingredients, whereas many incorporate three or even four sunscreens.

No one generally accepted measure exists to evaluate the actual efficacy of a product that claims to provide UVA protection. The best recommendation would be to select a product that contains a combination of sunscreen agents that protect throughout the entire UVB range and across the widest possible UVA range. A product labeled as broad spectrum that contains avobenzone and has an SPF of at least 15 is an excellent choice for patients who have UVR-induced disorders or who are taking photosensitizing drugs. If the sunscreen product does not contain avobenzone, then a broad-spectrum sunscreen with an SPF of 30+ is recommended. A very broad spectrum of coverage can be obtained by using a sunscreen product containing padimate O with one of the benzophenones, octocrylene, or menthyl anthranilate. An increasing number of products have added micronized titanium dioxide to increase the SPF and to provide a broad spectrum of coverage.

PATIENT FACTORS

For patients not concerned with photosensitivity, photodermatoses, or prevention of skin cancer, product selection is much simpler. The following factors can serve as a guide in selecting products with the appropriate properties for a patient's particular situation.

Skin Type and Tanning History The most important factors in product selection are the individual's natural skin type and tanning history. An SPF product of 30+ should be used by people who always burn easily and tan minimally at best. The average person who uses sunscreen products does so to avoid getting burned while still obtaining a tan. For that individual, a product with an SPF of 12 to 30 is recommended, with the lower end for people who always tan well and the higher end for those who tan gradually. An SPF from 2 to 12 is recommended for people who are deeply pigmented or who tan easily. A higher-SPF product can always be recommended, although tanning will occur at a slower than normal rate.

Physical Activity If the individual plans to swim, participate in vigorous activity (e.g., sand volleyball), or work outdoors, the sunscreen product must be able to adhere to the skin more substantially than if the individual just lies on the beach. The expected duration of the physical activity can also help to determine which sunscreen to use. Water-resistant products are usually effective for at least 40 minutes when used during the above activities, whereas very-water-resistant products are labeled as effective for at least 80 minutes.

Cosmetic Considerations At least one-third of the current commercial products are labeled noncomedogenic, fragrance-free, and hypoallergenic. Noncomedogenic products do not plug the pores and, therefore, do not exacerbate acne. This property is especially important for teenagers, who usually spend more time outdoors than other age groups and would generally prefer not to use comedogenic sunscreens. Regarding fragrance-free and hypoallergenic properties, many patients are sensitive to various ingredients, including fragrances, emulsifiers, and preservatives. In a randomized, placebo-controlled study of adverse reactions to sunscreens, 16% of subjects developed a local reaction to the topically applied product.[39] Of these subjects, 53% agreed to be patch-tested and photopatch-tested. None of this subset showed an allergic sensitivity to the sunscreen agents. Instead, all the reactions were found to be caused by formulation ingredients such as fragrances and preservatives. This finding reinforces the belief that most sensitivity may be caused by ingredients other than sunscreens. Although it may not be possible to figure out what specific ingredient a patient is sensitive to, patients who have a history of sensitivity to certain types of ingredients would do well to use a fragrance-free, hypoallergenic product.

Some patients have normally dry skin. Sunbathing can further exacerbate this problem. These patients should avoid ethyl and isopropyl alcohols, which are included in a number of commercial sunscreen products and can further dry the skin.

Use in Special Populations Absorptive characteristics of human skin in children younger than 6 months differ from those of adult skin. The metabolic and excretory systems of infants are not fully developed to handle any sunscreen agent absorbed through the skin. Therefore, only patients older than 6 months are considered to have skin with adult characteristics. FDA requires that sunscreen products be labeled with the statement "children under 6 months of age: ask a doctor." Caregivers should be extremely wary regarding sun exposure in children, especially infants. Although the evidence is not yet conclusive, researchers and clinicians agree that use of an SPF-15 product starting after age 6 months and continuing throughout one's lifetime can reduce the incidence of long-term skin damage due to UVR. A product with an SPF of 30+ may result in even higher reductions in sunburn, premature skin aging, skin cancer, and other skin problems. No special consideration is needed for the use of sunscreen-containing products in the elderly or in pregnant or lactating women.

Assessment of Sun-Induced Skin Disorders: A Case-Based Approach

The approach to UVR-induced skin disorders differs from that used in most self-care situations. Such disorders are addressed from a preventive, rather than a treatment, standpoint. According to FDA, the primary indication for sunscreen products is to protect against sunburn. A voluntary labeling "sun alert" may also advise that such products "may reduce the risks of skin aging, skin cancer, and other harmful effects of the sun."[40]

Consequently, assessment of the patient should focus on the *intended use* of the product. Two primary situations exist in which clinical practitioners' interventions with patients occur. The first situation involves a request by the patient for the practitioner to recommend a sunscreen product to prevent a burn and/or to allow development of a tan. The second situation is initiated by the practitioner when a patient is placed on a drug that can produce a photosensitivity reaction. In this second scenario, no real patient assessment is needed because prevention of exposure to UVR is the standard approach.

Case 39-1 illustrates the assessment of patients with sun-induced skin disorders.

C A S E   3 9 - 1

Relevant Evaluation Criteria	Scenario/Model Outcome
Information Gathering	
1. Gather essential information about the patient's symptoms, including:	
a. description of symptom(s) (i.e., nature, onset, duration, severity, associated symptoms)	The patient is light-skinned with blonde hair. She has experienced multiple sunburns in the past and would like some help choosing a sunscreen product.
b. description of any factors that seem to precipitate, exacerbate, and/or relieve the patient's symptom(s)	The patient has noticed that since she started using tazarotene and tetracycline for her acne, her face tends to get sunburned more quickly and more severely than other parts of her body.
c. description of the patient's efforts to relieve the symptoms	The patient does not normally wear any type of daily sunscreen product.
2. Gather essential patient history information:	
a. patient's identity	Daisy Mitchell
b. patient's age, sex, height, and weight	20-year-old female, 5 ft 3 in, 145 lb
c. patient's occupation	College student
d. patient's dietary habits	Diet consists of mainly "fast food"
e. patient's sleep habits	She stays up late and sleeps in as allotted by her schedule.
f. concurrent medical conditions, prescription and nonprescription medications, and dietary supplements	Ortho-Novum 7/7/7, tetracycline 500 mg by mouth three times daily for acne, tazarotene applied to face in the morning
g. allergies	NKA
h. history of other adverse reactions to medications	None
i. other (describe) _____	N/A
Assessment and Triage	
3. Differentiate the patient's signs/symptoms and correctly identify the patient's primary problem(s) (see Table 39-3).	The patient appears to have phototoxicity related to the use of her acne medications, specifically the tetracycline.
4. Identify exclusions for self-treatment (see Figure 39-1).	None
5. Formulate a comprehensive list of therapeutic alternatives for the primary problem to determine if triage to a medical practitioner is required, and share this information with the patient.	Options include: (1) Suggest that Daisy see her dermatologist to change acne regimen. (2) Recommend use of a regular OTC sunscreen. (3) Take no action.

CASE 39-1 *(continued)*

Relevant Evaluation Criteria	Scenario/Model Outcome
Plan	
6. Select an optimal therapeutic alternative to address the patient's problem, taking into account patient preferences.	The patient prefers to stay on the medications for her acne and would like to try to prevent the phototoxicity from occurring with the use of a sunscreen-containing product.
7. Describe the recommended therapeutic approach to the patient.	Use a sunscreen product that is at least 30 SPF and provides both UVA and UVB coverage. Apply the product liberally to all areas of the body exposed to the sun.
8. Explain to the patient the rationale for selecting the recommended therapeutic approach from the considered therapeutic alternatives.	Seeing a primary care provider may not be necessary if you use a sunscreen product.
Patient Education	
9. When recommending self-care with nonprescription medications and/or nondrug therapy, convey accurate information to the patient:	
a. appropriate dose and frequency of administration	Apply the sunscreen product 10–30 minutes prior to going out into the sun. Reapply the sunscreen as directed on the product or at least every 30 minutes.
b. maximum number of days the therapy should be employed	Apply sunscreen every day when exposed to the sun.
c. product administration procedures	Apply one-half teaspoon of sunscreen to face, one-half teaspoon to arms and shoulders, one-half teaspoon to torso, and 1 teaspoon to legs and feet.
d. expected time to onset of relief	
e. degree of relief that can be reasonably expected	Proper application of sunscreen should prevent sun damage.
f. most common side effects	If you develop a rash, hives, or skin irritation with application of the sunscreen, try another product that contains a different sunscreen.
g. side effects that warrant medical intervention should they occur	Severe allergy or rash requires medical attention.
h. patient options in the event that condition worsens or persists	If regular use of sunscreen does not prevent sunburn, you should see your primary care provider regarding use of alternative agents for treatment of your acne.
i. product storage requirements	Sunscreen-containing products should be stored at normal room temperature.
j. specific nondrug measures	Try to wear a large-brimmed hat and cover sun-exposed areas of skin when you are in the sun for extended periods of time.
10. Solicit follow-up questions from patient.	Is there anything I can apply one time a day?
11. Answer patient's questions.	No sunscreen products will provide all-day coverage. All products should be reapplied regularly with continued sun exposure.

Key: N/A, not applicable; NKA, no known allergies; OTC, over-the-counter; SPF, sun protection factor; UVA, ultraviolet A; UVB, ultraviolet B.

Patient Counseling for Sun-Induced Skin Disorders

Health care practitioners can provide a great service by counseling consumers about the suntanning process, and about properly selecting and using sunscreens. One study of Italian teenagers reported that "young people are aware of the risks associated with sunbathing, but they continue to expose themselves without taking precautions."[41] An American study reported that among the participants, 13% of children and 9% of adults had a sunburn during the previous week, and there was a relationship between sunburn and a parental attitude that tanning is healthy.[36]

One simple way to find out if a patient is using a sunscreen properly is to ask how long the current bottle has lasted. When applied properly, according to the suggested dosing guidelines and in accordance with the appropriate substantivity of the product, a sunbather could easily use about 1 ounce every 80 to 90 minutes. This use would amount to several ounces a day and several bottles per week. Incredibly, many frequent sunbathers use only one bottle in an entire season. This diminished usage demonstrates the importance of individuals receiving adequate counseling to get the protection they desire. The box Patient Education for Protection from Sun Exposure lists specific information to provide patients.

PATIENT EDUCATION FOR
Protection from Sun Exposure

The objectives of self-care depend on a patient's specific goal or health status. Protection from sun exposure can prevent sunburn or tanning, photosensitivity reactions in susceptible persons, or exacerbation of sun-induced photodermatoses. The primary long-term benefits are to prevent skin cancer and premature aging of the skin. For most patients, carefully following product instructions and the self-care measures listed here will help ensure optimal therapeutic outcomes.

Avoiding/Minimizing Sun Exposure

- Avoid exposure to the sun and other sources of ultraviolet radiation (UVR) such as tanning beds/booths and sunlamps.
- The rays of the sun are the most direct and damaging between 10 am and 4 pm. Avoid sun exposure during this time of day as much as possible.
- Sunburn can occur on a cloudy or overcast day; 70%–90% of UVR penetrates clouds.
- Wear protective clothing such as long pants, a long-sleeved shirt, and a hat with a brim. Tightly woven fabrics that do not allow light to pass through will provide the most protection.
- Use a beach umbrella or other protection to reduce UVR.
- Wet clothing and water allow significant transmission of UVR. Consider time in the water, even if the body is completely submerged, as part of the total time spent in the sun.

Use of Sunscreens

- An SPF of 30+ provides the greatest protection against sunburn and other UVB-induced skin problems.
- A broad-spectrum sunscreen product (e.g., avobenzone used in combination with padimate O and/or octocrylene, menthyl anthranilate, titanium dioxide, or one of the benzophenones) provides optimal protection against UVA and UVB sun exposure. This type of sunscreen is especially recommended if you have a sun-induced disorder or are taking photosensitizing drugs, or if you just want to reduce sun exposure as much as possible to prevent long-term effects.

- Apply first dose 15–30 minutes before exposure.
- Apply approximately 1 ounce of sunscreen to each exposed area of the body. Avoid contact with the eyes.
- Use the most substantive sunscreen available (very-water-resistant).
- Reapply the sunscreen according to the label instructions, usually every 40 minutes for water-resistant sunscreens or 80 minutes for very-water-resistant sunscreens.
- Higher altitudes and lower latitudes increase the amount of UVR to which an individual is exposed. Take proper precautions, including use of a sunscreen with a high SPF, to protect skin from UVR.
- Snow and sand reflect UVR. Take proper precautions, such as wearing sunglasses and using high SPF sunscreens, to protect exposed skin.
- Keep sunscreen out of direct sun to avoid reduction in potency.
- Continue to use a sunscreen as long you are taking a photosensitizing drug or exhibit signs and symptoms of photodermatitis.
- Avoid sunscreens containing aminobenzoic acid esters, benzophenones, cinnamates, or menthyl anthranilate if you have had a prior allergic reaction to a sunscreen product.

 Stop using the sunscreen if redness, itching, rash, or exaggerated sunburn occurs.

A WORD ABOUT — Sun-Induced Ocular Damage

Recent studies have demonstrated a relationship between both UVA and UVB in cataract formation.[42] UVR has been shown to cause temporary injuries such as photokeratitis (a painful type of snow blindness associated with highly reflective surfaces). Another concern involves an increase in the incidence of uveal (iris plus ciliary body) melanoma.[43,44] These concerns are even more serious because of the erroneous belief that all sunglasses screen out UVR. In response, the Sunglass Association of America, working with FDA, has developed a voluntary labeling program. Abbreviated information concerning the UVR-screening properties is directly attached to each pair of sunglasses, and brochures describing the appropriate use of each type of lens are available at outlets selling the sunglasses.

According to its UVR filtration properties, each pair of sunglasses is placed in one of the following three categories[45]:

1. *Cosmetic sunglasses* block at least 70% UVB and 20% UVA. They are recommended for activities in nonharsh sunlight, such as shopping.
2. *General-purpose sunglasses* block at least 95% UVB and 60% UVA. With shades that range from medium to dark, they are recommended for most activities in sunny environments, such as boating, driving, flying, or hiking.
3. *Special-purpose sunglasses* block at least 99% UVB and 60% UVA. They are recommended for activities in very bright environments, such as ski slopes and tropical beaches.

Evaluation of Patient Outcomes for Sun-Induced Skin Disorders

The short-term outcomes for sunscreen use are readily apparent. Twenty-four hours after use, there will be no obvious sunburn, photosensitivity reaction, or eruption of photodermatosis. This success indicates that the appropriate sunscreen agents and/or SPF were used. However, the long-term effects of UVR (e.g., skin cancer or premature aging of the skin) may take up to 20 to 30 years to become evident.

Key Points for Sun-Induced Skin Disorders

Current research in the area of UVR, its effects on the body, and prevention of its damaging effects has clearly delineated the following:

➤ UVR (UVA and UVB) triggers a variety of photodermatoses, and causes sunburn, photosensitivity, skin cancer, premature aging of the skin, cataracts, and a variety of other medical problems.

➤ The effects of ultraviolet radiation are cumulative over one's lifetime.

➤ The best protection against ultraviolet radiation is avoidance. The next best approach is to wear a hat, long sleeves, pants, and UV-protective sunglasses.

➤ Maximum protection is provided by using a sunscreen of SPF 30+.

➤ A broad-spectrum sunscreen, because of its added UVA protection, is the best type to prevent long-term effects regardless of the patient's history.

Practitioners need to appreciate sunscreen products as therapeutic agents rather than cosmetics. Unfortunately, most people have the latter view. This perception makes good patient counseling even more important. It is important to identify the patient's skin type as well as understand the intended use of the product when recommending a sunscreen product.

REFERENCES

1. Roelandts R. The diagnosis of photosensitivity. *Arch Dermatol.* 2000;136:1152–7.
2. Hawk JLM, Norris PG, Hönigsmann H. Abnormal responses to ultraviolet radiation: idiopathic, probably immunologic, and photoexacerbated. In: Freedberg IM, Eisen AZ, Wolff K, et al., eds. *Fitzpatrick's Dermatology in General Medicine.* 6th ed. New York: McGraw-Hill, Inc; 2003:1283–98.
3. MarketResearch.com. The U.S. Market for Suncare and Lipcare Products. March 1, 2001. Available at: http://www.marketresearch.com/map/prod/222308.html. Last accessed September 14, 2008.
4. Kim HJ. Photoprotection in adolescents. *Adolesc Med.* 2001;12:181–93.
5. *Skin Cancer Facts.* American Cancer Society. August 2007. Available at: http://www.cancer.org/docroot/PED/content/ped_7_1_What_You_Need_To_Know_About_Skin_Cancer.asp?sitearea=&level=. Last accessed September 14, 2008.
6. American Cancer Society. Cancer Facts & Figures 2008. Available at: http://www.cancer.org/docroot/STT/content/STT_1x_Cancer_Facts_and_Figures_2008.asp?from=fast. Last accessed September 14, 2008.
7. Armstrong BK, Kricker A. The epidemiology of UV-induced skin cancer. *J Photochem Photobiol B.* 2001;63:8–18.
8. Urbach F, O'Beirn S, Judge P, et al. The influence of environment and genetic factors on cancer of the skin in man [abstract]. *Tenth International Cancer Congress.* Philadelphia: JB Lippincott; 1970:109–10.
9. Averbach H. Geographic variation in incidence of skin cancer in the United States. *Public Health Rep.* 1961;76:345–8.
10. *Skin Cancer Prevention and Early Detection.* American Cancer Society. June 2007. Available at: http://www.cancer.org/docroot/PED/content/ped_7_1_Skin_Cancer_Detection_What_You_Can_Do.asp?sitearea=&level=. Last accessed September 14, 2008.
11. Moloney FJ, Collins S, Murphy GM. Sunscreens: safety, efficacy and appropriate use. *Am J Clin Dermatol.* 2002;3:185–91.
12. Holick MF. Sunlight "D"elimma: risk of skin cancer, bone disease and muscle weakness. *Lancet.* 2001;357:4–6.
13. US Environmental Protection Agency. *The Burning Facts.* Washington, DC: US Environmental Protection Agency; September 2006. Publication No. EPA430-F-060-013.
14. Moyal DD, Fourtanier AM. Effects of UVA radiation on an established immune response in humans and sunscreen efficacy. *Exp Dermatol.* 2002;11(suppl 1):28–32.
15. Brenneisen P, Sies H, Scharffetter-Kochanek K. Ultraviolet-B irradiation and matrix metalloproteinases: from induction via signaling to initial events. *Ann N Y Acad Sci.* 2002;973:31–43.
16. Gasparro FP. Sunscreens, skin photobiology, and skin cancer: the need for UVA protection and evaluation of efficacy. *Environ Health Perspect.* 2000;108(suppl 1):71–8.
17. Palm MD, O'Donoghue MN. Update on photoprotection. *Dermatol Ther.* 2007;20:360–76.
18. O'Riordan DL, Field AE, Geller AC, et al. Frequent tanning bed use, weight concerns, and other health risk behaviors in adolescent females (United States). *Cancer Causes Control.* 2006;17:679–86.
19. Karagas MR, Stannard VA, Mott LA, et al. Use of tanning devices and risk of basal cell and squamous cell skin cancers. *J Natl Cancer Inst.* 2002;94:224–6.
20. Sunlamp products and ultraviolet lamps intended for use in sunlamp products. 21 CFR 1040. 20 (1992):519–22.
21. Walker SL, Hawk JL, Young AR. Acute and chronic effects of ultraviolet radiation on the skin. In: Freedberg IM, Eisen AZ, Wolff K, et al., eds. *Fitzpatrick's Dermatology in General Medicine.* 6th ed. New York: McGraw-Hill, Inc; 2003:1275–81.
22. Tuchinda C, Srivannaboon S, Lim HW. Photoprotection by window glass, automobile glass, and sunglasses. *J Am Acad Dermatol.* 2006;54:845–54.
23. US Environmental Protection Agency. *A Guide to the UV Index.* Washington, DC: US Environmental Protection Agency; May 2004. Publication No. EPA30-F-04-020. Available at: http://www.epa.gov/sunwise/publications.html. Last accessed October 4, 2008.
24. Kripke ML, Honnavara N, Ananthaswamy HN. Carcinogenesis: ultraviolet radiation. In: Freedberg IM, Eisen AZ, Wolff K, et al., eds. *Fitzpatrick's Dermatology in General Medicine.* 6th ed. New York: McGraw-Hill, Inc; 2003:371–7.
25. American Cancer Society. Skin Cancer Prevention and Early Detection. June 2007. Available at: http://www.cancer.org/docroot/PED/content/ped_7_1_Skin_Cancer_Detection_What_You_Can_Do.asp?sitearea=&level=. Last accessed September 14, 2008.
26. Kullavanijaya P, Lim HW. Photoprotection. *J Am Acad Dermatol.* 2005;52:937–58.
27. US Food and Drug Administration. Sunscreen drug products for over-the-counter human use; final monograph. *Fed Regist.* 1999;64:27666–93.
28. US Food and Drug Administration. Over-the-counter human drugs; labeling requirements; delay of implementation date. Final rule: delay of implementation date of certain provisions. *Fed Regist.* 2004;69:53801–04.
29. Fourtanier A, Gueniche A, Compan D, et al. Improved protection against solar-simulated radiation-induced immunosuppression by a sunscreen with enhanced ultraviolet A protection. *J Invest Dermatol.* 2000;114:620–7.
30. Tuchinda C, Lim HW, Osterwalder U, et al. Novel emerging sunscreen technologies. *Dermatol Clin.* 2006;24:105–17.
31. Berne N, Ros AM. 7 years experience of photopatch testing with sunscreen allergens in Sweden. *Contact Dermat.* 1998;38(2):6–14.
32. Journe F, Marguery MC, Rakotondrazafy J, et al. Sunscreen sensitization: a 5-year study. *Acta Derm Venereol.* 1999;79:211–3.
33. Loesch H, Kaplan DL. Pitfalls in sunscreen application. *Arch Dermatol.* 1994;130:665–6.

34. Diffey BL. When should sunscreens be reapplied? *J Am Acad Dermatol.* 2001;45:882–5.

35. Wright MW, Wright ST, Wagner, RF. Mechanisms of sunscreen failure. *J Am Acad Dermatol.* 2001;44:781–4.

36. Journe F, Marguery MC, Rakotondrazafy J, et al. Sunscreen sensitization: a 5-year study. *Acta Derm Venereol.* 1999;79:211–3.

37. US Food and Drug Administration. *Tanning Pills.* Rockville, Md: Center for Food Safety and Applied Nutrition, Office of Cosmetics and Colors Fact Sheet. October 18, 2000; revised June 14, 2001. Available at: http://www.cfsan.fda.gov/~dms/cos-tan2.html. Last accessed October 4, 2008.

38. Brown DA. Skin pigmentation enhancers. *J Photochem Photobiol B.* 2001; 63:148–61.

39. Foley P, Nixon R, Marks R, et al. The frequency of reactions to sunscreens: results of a longitudinal population-based study on the regular use of sunscreens in Australia. *Br J Dermatol.* 1993;128:512–8.

40. Monfrecola G, Fabbrocini G, Posteraro G, et al. What do young people think about the dangers of sunbathing, skin cancer and sunbeds? A questionnaire survey among Italians. *Photodermatol Photoimmunol Photomed.* 2000;16:15–8.

41. Dummer R, Maier T. UV protection and skin cancer. *Recent Results Cancer Res.* 2002;160:7–12.

42. Hayashi LC, Hayashi S, Yamaoka K, et al. Ultraviolet B exposure and type of lens opacity in ophthalmic patients in Japan. *Sci Total Environ.* 200320;302:53–62.

43. Zigman S. Lens UVA photobiology. *J Ocul Pharmacol Ther.* 2000; 16:161–5.

44. Guenel P, Laforest L, Cyr D, et al. Occupational risk factors, ultraviolet radiation, and ocular melanoma: a case-control study in France. *Cancer Causes Control.* 2001;12:451–9.

45. Sunglass Association of America. *SAA UV Labeling Program.* Norwalk, Conn: Sunglass Association of America; 1997.

Skin Hyperpigmentation and Photoaging

Kimberly M. Crosby

Photoaging of the skin is related directly to exposure to ultra-violet (UV) radiation. Although sun exposure often is not the cause of hyperpigmentation, such exposure during or after treatment may negate the therapeutic effects. This chapter focuses on the treatment of hyperpigmentation and photoaging once they have occurred. Nonprescription products used to minimize sun exposure are discussed in Chapter 39.

Alpha-hydroxy acids (AHAs) play a role in treating both disorders. Hydroquinone, a skin-bleaching agent (fading cream), can be used alone or in combination with an AHA for self-treatment of hyperpigmentation. AHAs, beta-hydroxy acids (BHAs), and *N*-furfuryladenine are promoted as nonprescription treatments for photoaging.

SKIN HYPERPIGMENTATION

Hyperpigmentation, manifested as increased or more intense skin color, is usually a benign phenomenon, but may occasionally represent a sign of systemic disease. Hyperpigmentation may be perceived by the patient as disfigurement, especially when it occurs on the face and neck. Therefore, agents that can reduce pigmentation when applied topically are used worldwide, especially when hyperpigmented skin is in noticeable contrast to surrounding normal skin color. Although these products serve a cosmetic function, it is important to emphasize that they are drugs with potential toxicity and side effects.

Systemic as well as localized skin diseases may cause pigment cells to become overactive (resulting in skin darkening) or to become underactive (resulting in skin lightening). Endocrine imbalances caused by Addison's disease, Cushing's disease, hyperthyroidism, and pregnancy are capable of altering skin pigmentation. Metabolic alterations affecting the liver and certain nutritional deficiencies can be associated with diffuse melanosis. Inflammatory dermatoses (e.g., contact dermatitis from poison ivy or acne lesions) or physical trauma to the skin (e.g., thermal burn) may cause prolonged postinflammatory hyperpigmentation. In addition, certain drugs (Table 40-1) have an affinity for melanin and may cause hyperpigmentation. Skin hyperpigmentation resulting from these conditions may occur as a result of increased melanin, increased melanocytes, or deposits in the skin of other darkening chemicals.[1–3]

Melanocytes (pigment cells) produce melanosomes, pigment granules that contain a complex protein called melanin, a brown-black pigment. These cells can be viewed as tiny one-celled glands with long projections used to pass pigment particles into the keratinocytes, which migrate upward to the skin surface. Melanocytes are also present in hair bulb cells that pass pigment granules to the hair.

There are about 800 to 1000 melanocytes per square millimeter of human epidermis. The number of melanocytes is the same in equivalent body sites in light and dark skin, but the rate of production of pigment and its distribution are different. It is believed that the function of the melanocyte is to provide protection from ultraviolet radiation (UVR). Dark skin usually has more active melanocytes than light skin, which explains why UVR-induced skin cancers of all types are less common in dark skin than in light skin.[4]

Freckles are spots of uneven skin pigmentation that first appear in childhood and are exacerbated by the sun. Melasma (also called chloasma), a condition in which macular hyperpigmentation appears, usually on the face or neck, is often associated with pregnancy ("the mask of pregnancy") or the use of oral contraceptives, as well as with sun exposure. Lentigines, hyperpigmented macules that may appear at any age anywhere on the skin or mucous membranes, are caused by an increased deposition of melanin and an increased number of melanocytes. These macules are not known to be induced by UVR. However, solar or "senile" lentigines (age spots or liver spots) appear on exposed skin surfaces, particularly in fair-skinned people, and are induced by UVR.

Clinical Presentation of Skin Hyperpigmentation

Depending on the etiology of hyperpigmentation, patients can present with varying signs and symptoms. Most notably, patients complain of persistent macular discoloration on the face or other sun-exposed areas. Discoloration typically consists of a more intense brown coloration than that of surrounding normal skin; the discoloration may range from dark to faint in appearance.[5] As noted earlier, some hyperpigmentation can occur in areas of trauma or inflammation. Clinical evidence of hyperpigmentation and photoaging, as well as response to treatment, is not easily quantifiable by standard light photography or by routine clinical evaluation. Fluorescence photography is used to detect subtle but significant decreases in diffuse and mottled hyperpigmentation after topical treatment to clinically evaluate and effectively assess efficacy of topical products.[6]

TABLE 40-1   Medications That May Cause Hyperpigmentation

- Amiodarone
- Amitriptyline
- Antimalarial agents (chloroquine, hydroxychloroquine)
- Antineoplastic agents (cyclophosphamide, daunorubicin, doxorubicin, fluorouracil, busulfan)
- Clofazimine
- Heavy Metals (gold compounds, arsenic, mercury, silver, bismuth)
- Hormone replacement therapy
- Minocycline
- Oral contraceptives
- Phenothiazines (chlorpromazine, thioridazine, imipramine, clomipramine)
- Phenytoin
- Zidovudine

Adapted from references 1, 2, and Cheigh NH. Dermatologic drug reactions, self-treatable skin disorders and skin cancer. In: Dipiro JT, Talbert RL, Yee GC, et al., eds. *Pharmacotherapy: A Pathophysiologic Approach.* 6th ed. New York: McGraw-Hill, Inc; 2005:1741–53.

Treatment of Skin Hyperpigmentation

Treatment Goals

The goal of treating skin hyperpigmentation is to diminish the degree of pigmentation of affected areas so the skin tone of these areas is consistent with surrounding normal skin.

General Treatment Approach

Several types of hyperpigmentation, including freckles, melasma, and lentigines, are amenable to self-treatment with topical non-prescription skin-bleaching agents.[7] They diminish hyper-pigmentation by inhibiting melanin production within skin.[8] Many treatments are available for melasma, but the combination of a bleaching agent (e.g., hydroquinone) with an exfoliant (e.g., an AHA) is considered efficacious (see Treatment of Photoaging), giving patients acceptable outcomes with minimal adverse effects.[9,10]

To prevent negation of the effects of treatment, patients must avoid even minimal exposure to UVR, and they must use sunscreen agents and protective clothing on an indefinite, ongoing basis, even after discontinuing the bleaching agent. The algorithm in Figure 40-1 outlines the self-treatment of skin hyperpigmentation.

Management of hyperpigmentation directed by a primary care provider may include topical prescription agents composed of ingredients known to cause lightening of the skin, such as tretinoin (retinoic acid), azelaic acid, hydroquinone, and a corticosteroid, or even laser therapy. A combination of ingredients may sometimes be effective for postinflammatory hyperpigmentation that is resistant to nonprescription treatment.[11]

Pharmacologic Therapy

Historically, a number of topical agents have been used in skin-bleaching preparations. These agents have included hydro-

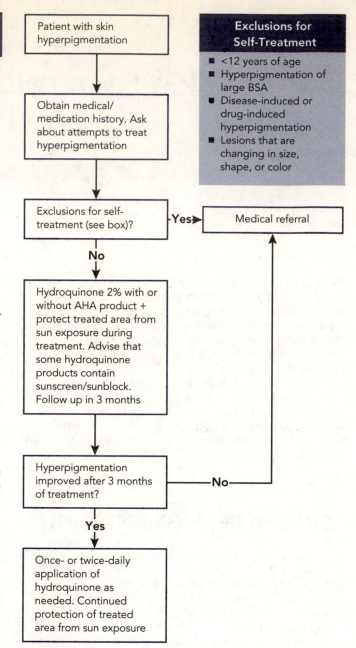

FIGURE 40-1   Self-care of skin hyperpigmentation. Key: AHA, alpha-hydroxy acid; BSA, body surface area.

quinone, monobenzyl and monomethyl ethers of hydroquinone, ammoniated mercury, ascorbic acid, peroxides, and kojic acid. However, only preparations containing hydroquinone were submitted to the Food and Drug Administration's (FDA's) Advisory Review Panel on Over-the-Counter Miscellaneous External Drug Products. Pigment disorders may present with both hypo- and hyperpigmented skin or skin that may appear mottled. Nonprescription skin-staining products such as Dy-O-Derm or Chromelin Complexion Blender, which contain dihydroxy-acetone (the active ingredient in self-tanning products), may be used to adjust color in lightened skin areas to approximate natural darker tones in mixed hypo- and hyperpigmented disorders.[12] Once the desired skin color is attained, applications are decreased from daily to every fourth to seventh day to maintain the desired outcome. Because this product has a higher concentration of active ingredient than that found in self-tanning products, it is not intended for widespread application.

Hydroquinone

Hydroquinone (*p*-dihydroxybenzene) in concentrations of 1.5% to 2.0% is currently available for nonprescription use for the treatment of skin hyperpigmentation.[7] The safety of bleaching creams containing hydroquinone has been separately reviewed in the literature.[13] However, in 2006, FDA proposed withdrawal of the tentative final monograph for skin-bleaching creams. This new proposed final rule states that all drug products (including hydroquinone) used for skin lightening in nonprescription products are no longer considered generally recognized as safe and effective. If this final monograph is published, hydroquinone products will be removed from the nonprescription marketplace.

Table 40-2 lists selected trade-name products.

Hydroquinone and its derivatives act by reducing conversion of tyrosine to dopa and, subsequently, to melanin by inhibiting the enzyme tyrosinase. Other possible mechanisms of action include destruction of the melanocyte or melanosomes.[9,14] Topical preparations of hydroquinone 2% to 5% are effective in producing cutaneous hypopigmentation. The 2% concentration is safer and produces results equivalent to those of higher concentrations.[14] Exfoliants such as topical glycolic acid (an AHA) or topical tretinoin are sometimes combined with hydroquinone to enhance hydroquinone's absorption and effect.[15]

Monobenzone, the monobenzyl ether of hydroquinone, is a prescription medication, whose use usually is restricted to depigmenting remaining areas of normally pigmented skin in patients with extensive vitiligo (a condition resulting in patches of depigmentation, often with hyperpigmented borders).

Hydroquinone is dosed as a thin topical application of a 2% concentration, rubbed gently but thoroughly into affected areas twice daily. The agent should be applied to clean skin before application of moisturizers or other skin care products. It should not be applied to damaged skin or near the eyes. If no improvement is seen within 3 months, its use should be discontinued and a primary care provider should be consulted.[8] Once the desired benefit is achieved, hydroquinone can be applied as often as needed in a once- or twice-daily regimen to maintain lightening of the skin. Because of the lack of safety data, hydroquinone is not recommended for children younger than 12 years. Other contraindications to the use of hydroquinone include hypersensitivity to the product and pregnancy.

Adverse effects, such as tingling or burning on application, are mild with low concentrations of topical hydroquinone.[16] If desired, patients can apply the agent to a small test area and check for signs of irritation after 24 hours. Higher concentrations frequently irritate the skin and, if used for prolonged periods, may cause side effects including epidermal thickening, skin darkening, which may result in pitch-black pigmentation of the treated areas, and colloid milium (yellowish papules associated with colloid degeneration).[17]

The effectiveness of hydroquinone varies among patients, and treatment must usually be maintained on an indefinite basis to retain lightening once it has been achieved. Results are best on lighter skin and lighter lesions. In dark skin, the response to hydroquinone depends on the amount of pigment present. Hyperpigmented areas fade more rapidly and completely than surrounding normal skin. Although treatment may not lead to complete disappearance of hypermelanosis, the results are often satisfactory enough to reduce self-consciousness. A disadvantage of treatment with hydroquinone is that it tends to overshoot the intended degree of hypopigmentation and may produce treated areas that are lighter than the surrounding normal skin color. Therefore, the patient must carefully observe the degree of lightening as the treatment progresses and must subsequently decrease applications when sufficient lightening has occurred.

A decrease in skin color usually becomes noticeable in about 4 weeks; however, the time of onset varies from 3 weeks to 3 months. Hypopigmentation lasts for 2 to 6 months but is reversible upon UVR exposure. Although sunscreens may help to prevent repigmentation, even visible light may cause some darkening. Therefore, a sunscreen containing opaque ingredients, such as zinc oxide or titanium dioxide, is preferable for sun protection.[18] Some nonprescription hydroquinone products are formulated to include a sunscreen.

In some cases, lesions become slightly darker before fading. A transient inflammatory reaction may develop after the first few weeks of treatment. Inflammation makes subsequent lightening more likely, although inflammation can occur without the development of hypopigmentation. Mild inflammation is not an indication to stop therapy except when the reaction increases in intensity, at which point a patch test can be done for allergy to hydroquinone, although most reactions are irritant rather than allergic in nature. Topical hydrocortisone may be used temporarily to alleviate the inflammatory reaction. Contact with eyes should be avoided. Accidental ingestion of hydroquinone seldom produces serious systemic toxicity. However, oral ingestion of 5 to 15 grams has produced tremor, convulsions, and hemolytic anemia.[13] Reversible brown discoloration of nails has been reported occasionally after application of hydroquinone 2% to

TABLE 40-2   Selected Skin-Bleaching/Fading Products

Trade Name	Primary Ingredients
Eldopaque	Hydroquinone 2%
Esoterica Facial	Hydroquinone 2%; octyl dimethyl PABA 3.3%; benzophenone-3, 2.5%
Esoterica Regular	Hydroquinone 2%
NeoStrata Skin Lightening	Hydroquinone 2%
Nadinola Skin Discoloration Fade Cream Deluxe for Oily Skin	2-Ethyl hexyl salicylate 3%; hydroquinone 2%
Porcelana Skin Discoloration Fade Cream Night Time Formula	Hydroquinone 2%; octyl methoxycinnamate 2.5%
Solaquin	Hydroquinone 2%

the back of the hand.[19] Discoloration is probably caused by formation of oxidation products of hydroquinone.

Product Considerations

Hydroquinone is readily oxidized in the presence of light and air. Discoloration or darkening of the cream indicates product deterioration as well as a possible decline in the strength of available hydroquinone. Because hydroquinone is oxidized by contact with air, antioxidants such as sodium bisulfite may be added to the formulation. Hydroquinone is incompatible with alkali or ferric salts.[18] The inclusion of a sunscreen agent is rational and appropriate, provided that combination products are intended primarily as skin-bleaching agents with added sunscreen.

Kojic Acid

Kojic acid, a product derived from certain species of fungus (e.g., *Acetobacter, Aspergillus,* and *Penicillum*), can be found in cosmetic products promoted for the treatment of hyperpigmentation. This product is usually found in combination with AHAs with or without hydroquinone. Kojic acid works by inhibiting the production of tyrosinase. Adverse effects associated with this product include contact dermatitis and erythema. One study comparing the combination of kojic acid and glycolic acid to hydroquinone and glycolic acid demonstrated similar results between the two therapies.[2,9–11,20]

Product Selection Guidelines

Hydroquinone is listed as FDA Pregnancy Category C. Pregnancy is considered a contraindication to the use of hydroquinone. It is unknown how much drug is systemically absorbed or how much is passed into breast milk. Therefore use during pregnancy and during breast-feeding should be avoided. Hydroquinone is indicated for use in adults and children younger than 12 years.[21]

Product selection should be based on a suitable dosage form (i.e., cream, lotion, or gel) for the patient's skin type (dry, normal, or oily) and anatomic site (face or neck). For example, an emollient cream-based product may be more suitable for dry skin, whereas a gel-based preparation may be preferable for an oily skin type.

Assessment of Skin Hyperpigmentation: A Case-Based Approach

The practitioner should evaluate the affected areas to determine whether they are characteristic of freckles, melasma, or lentigines. The patient's medication history and health status are important factors in pinpointing possible causes of the hyperpigmentation.

Case 40-1 is an example of the assessment of patients with skin hyperpigmentation.

CASE 40-1

Relevant Evaluation Criteria	Scenario/Model Outcome
Information Gathering	
1. Gather essential information about the patient's symptoms, including:	
a. description of symptom(s) (i.e., nature, onset, duration, severity, associated symptoms)	The patient is experiencing darkened areas of skin on her upper lip and forehead, which appeared over the last 6 months.
b. description of any factors that seem to precipitate, exacerbate, and/or relieve the patient's symptom(s)	These skin changes began appearing after the patient began taking oral contraceptives. The areas appear darker when the patient spends more time in the sunlight.
c. description of the patient's efforts to relieve the symptoms	The patient has tried topical moisturizing lotions, but she has seen little improvement.
2. Gather essential patient history information:	
a. patient's identity	Diane Kempton
b. patient's age, sex, height, and weight	23-year-old female, 5 ft 6 in, 140 lb
c. patient's occupation	Retail salesperson
d. patient's dietary habits	Diet is well balanced. She drinks wine regularly with dinner.
e. patient's sleep habits	Normal sleep schedule; she averages 6–8 hours per night.
f. concurrent medical conditions, prescription and nonprescription medications, and dietary supplements	LoOvral 1 tablet every day, ibuprofen 200 mg as needed for headaches or menstrual cramps
g. allergies	Sulfonamides
h. history of other adverse reactions to medications	None
i. other (describe) _____	

CASE 40-1 (continued)

Relevant Evaluation Criteria	Scenario/Model Outcome
Assessment and Triage	
3. Differentiate the patient's signs/symptoms and correctly identify the patient's primary problem(s) (see Table 40-1).	The patient has hyperpigmented areas on her upper lip and forehead, which appeared after she began oral contraceptive agents. The areas appear darker when exposed to sunlight, but they have not changed since they appeared.
4. Identify exclusions for self-treatment (see Figure 40-1).	The patient has no exclusions for self-treatment.
5. Formulate a comprehensive list of therapeutic alternatives for the primary problem to determine if triage to a medical practitioner is required, and share this information with the patient.	Options include: (1) Refer Diane to a dermatologist. (2) Recommend a 3-month trial of an OTC 2% hydroquinone product and use of daily sunscreen. (3) Take no action.
Plan	
6. Select an optimal therapeutic alternative to address the patient's problem, taking into account patient preferences.	The patient would prefer to try OTC hydroquinone.
7. Describe the recommended therapeutic approach to the patient.	Apply a thin film of hydroquinone to the affected areas on the lip and forehead twice a day. The product should be applied after cleansing the skin and before applying any moisturizers or creams. It should be rubbed into the skin gently until absorbed.
8. Explain to the patient the rationale for selecting the recommended therapeutic approach from the considered therapeutic alternatives.	Seeing a dermatologist may not be necessary with proper use of the product.
Patient Education	
9. When recommending self-care with non-prescription medications and/or nondrug therapy, convey accurate information to the patient:	
a. appropriate dose and frequency of administration	Hydroquinone-containing products should be applied directly to clean skin as a thin application twice a day.
b. maximum number of days the therapy should be employed	Improvement may be seen in as little as 3 weeks but may take as long as 3 months.
c. product administration procedures	The product should be applied after cleansing the face and rubbed into the affected areas gently until absorbed.
d. expected time to onset of relief	Improvement is usually seen by 1 month.
e. degree of relief that can be reasonably expected	The areas of darkened skin may lighten significantly, although they may not completely disappear.
f. most common side effects	Mild irritation may occur. In addition, the areas being treated may appear lighter than surrounding skin.
g. side effects that warrant medical intervention should they occur	If the treated areas of skin become severely irritated or if they darken significantly, you should see your primary care provider or a dermatologist.
h. patient options in the event that condition worsens or persists	If no improvement is seen after 3 months of use, you should see your primary care provider or a dermatologist.
i. product storage requirements	The product should be kept at normal room temperature and tightly closed when not in use.
j. specific nondrug measures	To prevent worsening of the condition and to protect treated skin areas, daily sunscreen should be used.
10. Solicit follow-up questions from patient.	(1) May I use this product more often than twice a day? (2) Should I always use a sunscreen or only when I am using this product?
11. Answer patient's questions.	(1) No. This product should be used only twice daily. However once the desired lightening of the skin areas has occurred, you may decrease the frequency of applications to maintain results. (2) Sun exposure can result in worsening or reappearance of the darkened areas of skin. Continued sunscreen use is necessary to maintain results even after stopping the hydroquinone product.

Key: OTC, over-the-counter.

PATIENT EDUCATION FOR
Skin Hyperpigmentation

The objective of self-treatment with skin-bleaching products is to diminish the degree of pigmentation in affected areas. For most patients, carefully following product instructions and the self-care measures listed here will help ensure optimal therapeutic outcomes.

- Use hydroquinone to lighten only limited areas of hyperpigmented skin that show brownish discoloration.
- Do not use these products on nevi (moles) or reddish or bluish areas, such as port wine discoloration.
- Time to initial response averages 6–8 weeks, but it may take up to 3 months to see noticeable results.
- Test for possible irritant reactions to the product by applying it to a small test area, and by checking the area for redness, itching, or swelling after 24 hours.
- Do not apply the product near the eyes or to damaged skin.
- Apply a thin layer of the product to clean, dry skin in the affected area only. Rub product into the skin gently but thoroughly.
- If moisturizers or other topical agents are being used at the same time, apply the hydroquinone first.

- When you are outdoors for even a short time, apply an opaque sunblock or broad-spectrum sunscreen (see Chapter 39) to the affected area after applying the hydroquinone, if the product does not already contain a sunscreen in the formulation.
- Once the desired lightening of skin is reached, apply the hydroquinone once or twice daily to prevent hyperpigmentation from recurring. Continue to protect the treated area from sun exposure.

⚠ Consult a primary care provider if:
— No improvement is seen after 3 months of using hydroquinone.
— Skin pigmentation becomes darker during treatment with hydroquinone.

Patient Counseling for Skin Hyperpigmentation

The clinician should explain which types of hyperpigmentation are self-treatable, while stressing the importance of avoidance of sun exposure during and after treatment. To ensure a successful therapeutic outcome, the practitioner should review the product instructions with the patient. The box Patient Education for Skin Hyperpigmentation lists specific information to provide patients.

Evaluation of Patient Outcomes for Skin Hyperpigmentation

The clinician should check on the patient's progress after 3 months of therapy. Follow-up can be achieved through a telephone call or a scheduled visit to the practitioner. If the pigmented area shows no improvement, the patient should consult a primary care provider or a dermatologist. If the desired outcome has been achieved, the patient should continue applying the hydroquinone once or twice daily to maintain lightening of the skin.

PHOTOAGING

Photoaging, or dermatoheliosis, is the pattern of characteristic skin changes associated with sun exposure. Most fair-skinned Americans will have some signs of photodamaged skin by 50 years of age. A variety of therapies are available for treatment of photodamaged skin, which range from procedures such as face-lifts, Botox injections, and laser resurfacing to less invasive topical products and cosmetics. Although some products are available by prescription only, many others are nonprescription, with AHAs being widely used to combat photoaged skin.[22]

Pathophysiology of Photoaging

Aging skin results from a combination of extrinsic and intrinsic factors. Clinical and histologic changes that intrinsically occur include genetically controlled skin and muscle changes, expression lines, sleep lines, and hormonal changes. The second component, extrinsic aging, relates to environmental influences such as UVR, smoking, wind, and chemical exposure.[23,24] Medications known to induce photosensitivity can contribute to photoaging by making the skin sensitive to UVR (see Chapter 39).

Prematurely aged facial skin, with creases and wrinkles, dry texture, and blotchy hyperpigmentation, is largely attributed to cumulative UVR, or photoaging. Exposure to UVB (290–320 nm) is primarily responsible for photoaging, although the longer UVA (320–400 nm) wavelengths also contribute to damage. The amount of UVA present in sunlight is 10-fold greater than that of UVB, which allows for greater amounts of skin exposure. UVA can penetrate into the deeper dermal layer and can work synergistically with UVB to cause photodamage and skin cancers.

Microscopically, sun-damaged skin shows dysplasia (abnormal tissue development), atypical keratinocytes, and occasional cell necrosis. Irregularity of epidermal cell alignment is also common. Deeper in the dermal layer is a loss of collagen and elastin.[24,25]

Clinical Presentation of Photoaging

Clinical signs of photoaging include changes in color, surface texture, and functional capacity (Table 40-3). Photoaged skin may have a sallow yellow color with discoloration and may show telangiectasias (visible distended capillaries). Textural changes include loss of smoothness, loss of subcutaneous tissue around the mouth, and epidermal thinning around the lip. As sebaceous glands hypertrophy, the skin begins to show coarse texture with increased pore size. In addition, fine vellus hairs can develop into unwanted terminal hairs. Other manifestations of photoaged

TABLE 40-3 Classification of Photoaging	
Type I (Mild)	No wrinkles, early photoaging, mild pigment changes 20–30 years of age
Type II (Moderate)	Wrinkles in motion, early-to-moderate photoaging, keratoses palpable 30–40 years of age
Type III (Advanced)	Wrinkles at rest, advanced photoaging, obvious dyschromia and keratoses ≥50 years of age
Type IV (Severe)	Only wrinkles, severe photoaging, yellow-gray skin ≥60 years of age

Source: Glogau RG. Aesthetic and anatomic analysis of the aging skin. *Semin Cutan Med Surg.* 1996;15:134–8.

skin may include development of precancerous (actinic keratosis) and cancerous (basal cell, squamous cell, and melanoma) tumor development.[22,24,25] Cosmetically, patients notice freckling, discolorations, or "crow's feet" (small parallel lines around the eyes). In contrast, postmenopausal skin is susceptible to reduced estrogen receptor stimulation of dermal metabolism and undergoes significant changes in collagen and moisture content. These changes lead to signs of skin aging, as evidenced by diminished elasticity and wrinkles.[26]

Treatment of Photoaging

Treatment Goals

The first goal is to prevent or minimize the likelihood of skin photoaging by appropriate sun protection, including sunscreens.[27] The goals of treating photoaging are to (1) reverse cumulative skin damage with prescription and nonprescription products and (2) maintain the skin and protect it from further extrinsic damage by making lifestyle changes and, most importantly, protecting the skin from further and prolonged sun exposure

General Treatment Approach

The first step in preventing and treating photoaged skin is for the patient to commit to daily sun protection. Broad-spectrum sunscreens (UVA and UVB coverage) with a sun protection factor (SPF) of 15 or greater can minimize further photodamage during UVR exposure (see Chapter 39).[28]

Proper cleansing of the skin removes bacteria, dirt, desquamated keratinocytes, cosmetics, sebum, and perspiration. However, excessive use of soap leads to xerosis, eczematous dermatitis, and other skin conditions.[29] Use of AHAs enhances skin water retention and repairs damaged skin by improving the skin's elasticity.[30,31]

Pharmacologic Therapy

Within the vast array of available nonprescription products for skin care, the division of categories is blurred. Cosmetics and moisturizers are not pharmaceuticals, whereas antiperspirants and sunscreens are considered nonprescription pharmaceuticals.

Although "cosmeceuticals" are an undefined category of products recognized by practitioners and dermatologists, no final regulatory guidance currently is available for these products from FDA. Many cosmeceutical ingredients, such as AHAs, function as active pharmaceuticals that are known to penetrate and alter the stratum corneum.[32]

Various topical products are being used to treat aging skin. Nonprescription products include vitamin C and vitamin K products, N-furfuryladenine (Kinerase), and AHAs and BHAs.

Alpha- and Beta-Hydroxy Acids

AHAs have generated much interest in the treatment of aging skin.[9] The AHAs are used in various concentrations, with a wide array of available products. Most AHAs are sold as cosmeceuticals; however, some are sold as cosmetics, and yet others are sold as pharmaceuticals through a primary care provider. These products range in concentration from 2% to 20% (as nonpeeling AHAs) and act as peeling agents (as used by estheticians or dermatologists) in concentrations above 20%.

Of the available nonprescription products, AHAs currently play a major role in reliably reversing and cosmetically improving aging skin.[9,33] Many types of AHAs are available, with the most common being lactic and glycolic acids (Table 40–4). Other AHAs that are not as widely used include malic acid, citric acid, and tartaric acids. Although termed a *cosmeceutical* by industry, FDA has not yet defined AHAs as either cosmetics or drugs.[34]

The Cosmetic Ingredient Review Expert Panel, the cosmetic industry self-regulatory body, concluded that use of AHAs in cosmetic products is safe if (1) concentrations are less than or equal to 10%, (2) final pH is greater than or equal to 3.5, and (3) the product is formulated with a sunscreen or directions to use a sunscreen are included.[34]

TABLE 40-4 Selected Products for Photoaged Skin	
Trade Name	**Active Ingredients**
Alpha-Hydroxy Acid Products	
Alpha Hydrox Creme Enhanced[a,b]	Glycolic acid 10%
AmLactin 12% Moisturizing Lotion	Lactic acid 12%
Aqua Glycolic Hand & Body Lotion	Glycolic acid 14%
Cetaphil Moisturizing Lotion[a]	Citric acid
Dermal Therapy Body Lotion Extra Strength	Urea 10%; lactic and malic acids 5%
Eucerin Dry Skin Therapy Plus Intensive Repair Lotion With Alpha Hydroxy	Sodium lactate; urea; panthenol
Lac-Hydrin Five Lotion[a]	Lactic acid
Nutraderm 30 Lotion	Lactic acid; malic acid
Olay Age Defying Daily Renewal Cream, Beta Hydroxy Complex	Salicylic acid
WellSkin Body Lotion with SPF 15	Octyl methoxycinnamate 7.5%; octyl salicylate 5%; oxybenzone 3%; glycolic acid

[a] Fragrance-free formulation.

[b] Oil-free formulation.

Of the BHAs, salicylic acid is used widely, even as a chemical peel for resurfacing moderately photodamaged facial skin.[35] Compared with AHA products, BHAs are less soluble and unstable in water, and demonstrate keratolytic effects. Although BHAs are now marketed as cosmetics, they have been used to treat skin conditions such as dermatitis and psoriasis for quite some time. Products containing BHAs as the active ingredients may be beneficial to acne-prone skin.

Used appropriately, AHA products act as exfoliants by causing detachment of keratinocytes, resulting in a smoother, non-scaly skin surface with eventual normalization of keratinization. The product's pH is important, because products with a lower pH produce greater results, but they may carry an increased risk of irritation.[23,28]

By improving skin elasticity, AHAs have been shown to make skin more flexible and less vulnerable to cracking and flaking. Long-term use has led to an increase in skin collagen and elastin.[9,30,31] Regular application of AHAs results in smoother skin texture, lessening of fine lines, and normalization of pigmentation.[36]

Current labeling on AHA cosmetic products includes recommendations for melasma, acne, solar lentigines, and fine wrinkling of photoaging.[9]

Guidelines for treatment with AHAs include identification of patient factors such as medications, prior procedures, and medical history, all of which may affect treatment outcome and realistic patient expectations.[37] Care should be taken to apply AHAs to completely dry skin, with an estimated wait time of 10 to 15 minutes after cleansing the face. It is also prudent to begin application gradually, starting every other night for approximately 1 week and then increasing as tolerated to a maximum of twice-daily application. AHA products may make the skin more sensitive to sun exposure. Patients should be advised to use daily sunscreen or sunblock with an SPF of 15 or greater during use of AHAs and after their discontinuation.[28]

Common adverse effects include mild, transient stinging, burning, pruritus, skin lightening, and dryness. Many of these effects can be ameliorated if products are used with caution and proper counseling. Patients should also note that other topically applied products, both medications and cosmetics, may contain active ingredients (e.g., AHA, BHA, and hydroquinone) capable of exacerbating irritation.

Product Selection Guidelines

Skin type should determine the vehicle chosen. Creams are appropriate for drier skin types, lotions are best for combination or normal skin, and gels or solutions are useful for oilier skin. Use of products with higher concentrations and a lower pH may produce faster results. However, the patient should be warned that these products may also cause greater skin irritation.

There are limited data on the safety of AHAs in special populations such as lactating women, and pediatric and geriatric populations. AHA products appear to be safe when used topically in adults. In addition, AHAs are not contraindicated in pregnancy.[38]

Other Agents

There is little scientific information to support mechanism of action for other agents used in photoaging treatment. However, the indications, dosage, and adverse events are similar to those for AHAs.

Assessment of Photoaging: A Case-Based Approach

If visual inspection of the patient's skin causes the clinician to suspect photoaging, the patient should be questioned about his or her history of UVR (sunlight as well as artificial light) exposure. Knowing whether the patient's current occupational or recreational habits require excessive exposure is useful not only in determining the cause of the skin disorder but also in developing a treatment plan. It is important to assess for a history of diseases or medications that may predispose the patient to premature photodamage or photosensitivity. The patient's health status, lifestyle practices, and daily skin maintenance regimen are other pertinent assessment criteria.[22]

Patient Counseling for Photoaging

The practitioner should advise patients that premature wrinkling, creases, dry texture, and blotchy hyperpigmentation are not inevitable.[24] The practitioner should be proactive in identifying and recommending products that are appropriate for a specific patient.

Evaluation of Patient Outcomes for Photoaging

Patients treated with nonprescription products for photoaging should set a reasonable goal. Obviously, these preparations cannot "erase wrinkles." The practitioner should monitor the progress of the treatment and be sensitive to issues that may require intervention by a primary care provider.

PATIENT EDUCATION FOR
Photoaging

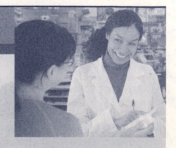

The objectives of self-treatment are to (1) reverse skin damage by using available nonprescription products and (2) protect the skin from further damage by making lifestyle changes and protecting skin from sun exposure. For most patients, carefully following product instructions and the self-care measures listed here will help ensure optimal therapeutic outcomes.

■ Protect the skin from sun exposure by covering the skin with clothing. FDA recommends advising patients to wear long-sleeved clothing and hats with brims of at least

PATIENT EDUCATION FOR
Photoaging (continued)

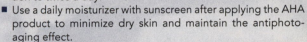

4 inches. Patients should also use a sunblock or sunscreen product with an SPF of 15 or greater during use of alpha-hydroxy acids (AHAs) and regularly in the future to prevent further damage.

■ To prevent dry skin, cleanse the skin with a mild soap or a soap-free liquid cleanser. Do not cleanse skin more often than twice daily. Apply a pea-sized amount of an AHA product to clean, dry skin.

■ To minimize transient mild tingling and stinging, wait 10–15 minutes after cleansing the face to apply an AHA product.

■ Excessive skin dryness or irritation warrants decreased application.

■ Note that AHA products contain an active ingredient and that the use of other products, including cosmetics, could result in skin irritation, including mild stinging, burning, or erythema.

■ Do not apply the product too close to the eyes or mucous membranes.

■ Begin applying this product once at bedtime every other day for approximately 1 week. Gradually increase application to twice a day.

■ Use a daily moisturizer with sunscreen after applying the AHA product to minimize dry skin and maintain the antiphotoaging effect.

■ Store this product in a cool dry place out of the reach of children.

■ Discontinue the AHA product if severe irritation, such as redness or excessive dryness, or a rash occurs.

KEY POINTS FOR SKIN HYPERPIGMENTATION AND PHOTOAGING

➤ Photoaging and hyperpigmentation are cosmetically unacceptable skin conditions. Patients who have reasonable expectations should be able to achieve even skin tone and minimize appearance and occurrence of fine wrinkling with the use of nonprescription products.

➤ Hydroquinone is the only FDA-approved nonprescription skin-bleaching product. Patients should apply a 2% concentration to skin twice daily.

➤ Patients younger than 12 years; those with large areas of hyperpigmentation, or disease- or drug-induced hyperpigmentation; or those with lesions that have changed in size, shape, or color should consult their primary care provider.

➤ Patients should be referred to a primary care provider if no improvement occurs within 3 months or if skin darkens during treatment of hyperpigmentation.

➤ Patients should avoid applying hydroquinone-containing products near the eye area or on damaged skin areas.

➤ Patients using AHAs to reduce photoaging should be advised to apply AHAs up to twice daily to dry skin. Patients who do not see a desired improvement in skin appearance in 2 months, or who experience excessive irritation or drying of the skin should contact their primary care provider.

➤ Patients who use products to prevent photoaging or hyperpigmentation should be instructed to protect their skin from daily sun exposure by using a sunscreen with SPF 15 or greater to maintain results.

REFERENCES

1. Nicolaidou E, Antoniou C, Katsambas A. Origin, clinical presentation and diagnosis of facial hypermelanoses. *Dermatol Clin.* 2007;25:321–6.
2. Stulberg DL, Clark N, Tovey D. Common hyperpigmentation disorders in adults, part 1: diagnostic approach, café au lait macules, diffuse hyperpigmentation, sun exposure and phototoxic reactions. *Am Fam Physician.* 2003;68:1955–60.
3. Lacz NL, Vafaie J, Kihicazak N, et al. Postinflammatory hyperpigmentation: a common but troubling condition. *Int J Dermatol.* 2004;43:362–5.
4. Nordlund JJ, Boissy R. The biology of melanocytes. In: Freinkel R, Woodley D, eds. *The Biology of the Skin.* New York: Parthenon; 2001:117.
5. Habif TP, Campbell JL, Quitadamo MJ, et al. *Skin Disease: Diagnosis and Treatment.* St Louis: Mosby; 2001:318–9.
6. Kollias N, Gillies R, Cohen-Goihman, et al. Fluorescence photography in the evaluation of hyperpigmentation in photodamaged skin. *J Am Acad Dermatol.* 1997;36:226–30.
7. US Food and Drug Administration. Skin bleaching drug products for over-the-counter human use; proposed rule. *Fed Regist.* 2006;71:51146–55.
8. Briganti S, Camera E, Picardo M. Chemical and instrumental approaches to treat hyperpigmentation. *Pigment Cell Res.* 2003;16:101–10.
9. Halder RM, Richards GM. Topical agents used in the management of hyperpigmentation. *Skin Ther Lett.* 2004;9:1–3.
10. Gupta AK, Gover MD, Nouri K, et al. The treatment of melasma: a review of clinical trials. *J Am Acad Dermatol.* 2006;55:1048–65.
11. Picardo M, Carrera M. New and experimental treatments of cloasma and other hypermelanoses. *Dermatol Clin.* 2007;25:353–62.
12. Brown DA. Skin pigmentation enhancers. *J Photochem Photobiol.* 2001;63:148–61.
13. Nordlund JJ, Grimes PE, Ortonne JP. The safety of hydroquinone. *JEAVD.* 2006;20:781–7.
14. Kasraee B, Handjani F, Aslani FS. Enhancement of the depigmenting effect of hydroquinone and 4-hydroxyoxyanisole by all-TRANS-retinoic acid (tretinoin): the impairment of glutathion-dependent cytoprotection? *Dermatology.* 2003; 206:289–91.
15. Draelos ZD. Cosmetic therapy. In: Wolverton SE, ed. *Comprehensive Dermatologic Drug Therapy.* Philadelphia: WB Saunders; 2001:695.
16. Perez-Bernal A, Munoz-Perez MA, Camacho F. Management of facial hyperpigmentation. *Am J Clin Dermatol.* 2000;1:261–8.
17. Levin CY, Maibach H. Exogenous echronosis: an update on clinical features, causative agents and treatment options. *Am J Clin Dermatol.* 2001; 2:213–7.
18. Arndt KA, Bowers KE. *Manual of Dermatologic Therapeutics.* 6th ed. Philadelphia: Lippincott Williams & Wilkins; 2002:118–24.
19. Ozluer SM, Muir J. Nail staining from hydroquinone cream. *Australas J Dermatol.* 2000;41:255–6.
20. Garcia A, Fulton JE. The combination of glycolic acid and hydroquinone or kojic acid for the treatment of melasma and related conditions. *Dermatol Surg* 1999;22:443–7.
21. Micromedex® Healthcare Series [database online]. Greenwood Village, Colo: Thomson Healthcare. Updated periodically.
22. Drake L, Dinehart S, Farmer E, et al. Guidelines of care for photoaging/photodamage. *J Am Acad Dermatol.* 1996;35:462–4.
23. Holck DE. Facial skin rejuvenation. *Curr Opin Opthalmol.* 2003;14:246–52.
24. Yarr M, Gilchrest B. Aging of skin. In: Freedberg IM, Eisen AZ, Wolff K, et al., eds. *Fitzpatrick's Dermatology in General Medicine.* 6th ed. New York: McGraw-Hill, Inc; 2003:1386–98.

25. Hashizume H. Skin aging and dry skin. *J Dermatol.* 2004;31:603–9.

26. Raine-Fenning N, Brincat M, Muscat-Baron Y. Skin aging and menopause: implications for treatment. *Am J Clin Dermatol.* 2003; 4:371–8.

27. Levy SB. Sunscreens. In: Wolverton SE, ed. *Comprehensive Dermatologic Drug Therapy.* Philadelphia: WB Saunders; 2001:632–46.

28. Stern RS. Treatment of photoaging. *N Eng J Med.* 2004;350:1526–34.

29. Engasser PG, Maibach HI. Cosmetics and skin care in dermatologic practice. In: Freedberg IM, Eisen AZ, Wolff K, et al., eds. *Fitzpatrick's Dermatology in General Medicine.* 6th ed. New York: McGraw-Hill, Inc; 2003:2369–79.

30. Stiller MJ, Bartolone J, Stern R, et al. Topical 8% glycolic acid and 8% L-lactic acid creams for the treatment of photodamaged skin. *Arch Dermatol.* 1996;132:631–6.

31. Ditre CM. Griffin TD. Murphy GF et al. Effects of alpha-hydroxy acids on photoaged skin: a pilot clinical, histologic, and ultrastructural study. *J Am Acad Dermatol.* 1996;34:187–95.

32. Draelos ZD, Jegasothy SM. Should cosmeceuticals be regulated by the FDA? *Skin Aging.* 1999;7:52–4.

33. Clark CP 3rd. New directions in skin care. *Clin Plast Surg.* 2001; 28:745–50.

34. US Food and Drug Administration. Guidance for Industry. Labeling for Topically Applied Cosmetic Products Containing Alpha Hydroxy Acids as Ingredients. December 2, 2002. Available at: http://www.cfsan.fda.gov/~dms/ahaguide.html. Last accessed September 11, 2008.

35. Kligman D, Kligman AM. Salicylic acid peels for the treatment of photoaging. *Dermatol Surg.* 1998;24:325–8.

36. Lewis AB. Alpha-hydroxy acids. In: Wolverton SE, ed. *Comprehensive Dermatologic Drug Therapy.* Philadelphia: WB Saunders; 2001:659–70.

37. Tung RC, Bergfeld WF, Vidimos AT, et al. Alpha-hydroxy acid-based cosmetic procedures: guidelines for patient management. *Am J Clin Dermatol.* 2000;1:81–8.

38. Cosmetic ingredient review. Final report on the safety assessment of glycolic acid, ammonium, calcium, potassium, and sodium glycolates, methyl, ethyl, propyl, and butyl glycolates, and lactic acid, ammonium, calcium, potassium, sodium, and TEA-lactates, methyl, ethyl, isopropyl, and butyl lactates, and lauryl, myristyl, and ceryl lactates. *Int J Toxicol.* 1998;17(suppl 1):1–242.

Minor Burns and Sunburn

Valerie T. Prince

More than 500,000 patients per year are estimated to receive burn injuries that require medical treatment.[1] Many of these patients can be managed without hospitalization. Nonprescription products can play an important role in the treatment of minor burns and sunburn. Because deep burn injuries can lead to scarring and nonhealing wounds, it is important to accurately assess the injury and determine whether self-care or referral for further evaluation is appropriate.

Deaths from fires and burns are among the top five most common causes of unintentional deaths in the United States and are one of the top three causes of fatal home injury.[2] Groups at increased risk of fire-related injuries and deaths include children ages 4 years and younger; adults ages 65 and older; African Americans; Native Americans; persons living in rural areas, manufactured homes, or substandard housing; and the poor.[2] Sunburn, in comparison, occurs at all ages. The incidence and significance of sunburn have been underrated, and the injury goes unreported in most burn surveys, because the public often does not consider sunburn in the same context as thermal, electrical, and chemical burns.

Pathophysiology of Minor Burns and Sunburn

The skin is the largest organ of the human body, accounting for approximately 17% of the body weight of an average person. The skin performs a number of vital physiologic functions. It protects the body from injury and serves as a barrier against microorganisms. By synthesizing melanin, the skin protects underlying tissues from certain forms of irradiation. In addition, the skin is a sense organ, receiving sensory input (especially touch and temperature) from the proximal environment. Cholecalciferol (vitamin D_3), which is involved in calcium regulation, is produced in the skin through exposure to ultraviolet radiation (UVR). The skin plays a major role in thermoregulation, because cutaneous blood flow and perspiration are vital in maintaining core body temperature at a normal level and also help maintain body water balance. Sebaceous glands produce oil, which lubricates and prevents excessive drying of the skin.

Figure 41-1 shows a cross-section of the anatomy of the skin and the depths of injury caused by thermal burns. (See Chapter 33 for further discussion of skin anatomy and physiology.)

Burns are tissue injuries caused by thermal, electrical, chemical, or UVR exposure. Excluding sunburns, most burns occur in the home and are usually thermal burns. Thermal burns result from skin contact with flames, scalding liquids, or hot objects (e.g., irons, oven broiler elements, hot pans, curling irons, or radiators) or from the inhalation of smoke or hot vapors. Most fire-related deaths occur in December through February. The increased occurrence of deaths during the winter months reflects the seasonal use of space heaters, portable heaters, fireplaces, and Christmas trees.

Thermal Burns

Thermal damage to the respiratory tract from exposure to steam or hot gases can cause immediate upper airway obstruction, as well as obstruction of the lower bronchioles caused by slowly developing edema. Smoke inhalation produces extensive lung damage because of toxic particles. Resultant injury to small airway alveolar capillaries can cause progressive respiratory failure. If smoke or heated gas inhalation has occurred, emergency services personnel should quickly transport the patient to a hospital emergency room.

There are two types of electrical burns: flash electrical burns, which result from a high-temperature arc of current close to the skin, and contact electrical burns, which are caused by contact with a high-voltage source. Contact electrical burns generally have entry and exit sites, and tissue at every depth along the current's path, including bone, can be injured. Electrical burns result from exposure to heat of up to 9000°F (5000°C). Electrical burns always injure the skin because the electrical energy is dissipated as heat. For the same reason, they can also cause extensive damage to underlying tissues. Progressive necrosis and sloughing are usually greater than the initial lesion indicates. The patient may appear to be healthy despite the presence of unknown internal damage. For this reason, referral of these patients to an emergency department, primary care provider, or burn center is necessary.

Chemical Burns

Chemical burns can result from skin contact with acids or alkalis contained in household products or from substances used in the workplace. These burns can be partial- or full-thickness. Clothing that has been exposed to chemicals should be removed,

Editor's Note: This chapter is based on the 15th edition chapter with the same title, written by John D. Bowman.

Depth of Burn

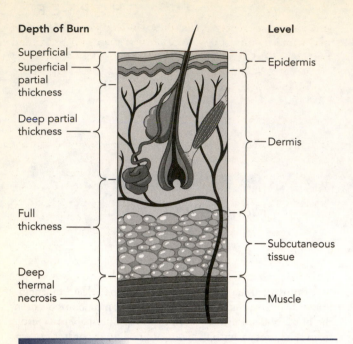

Superficial
Superficial partial thickness
Deep partial thickness
Full thickness
Deep thermal necrosis

Level

Epidermis
Dermis
Subcutaneous tissue
Muscle

FIGURE 41-1 Cross-section of skin showing depth of burns.

if not adherent, to prevent continued burn insult to the affected skin. Adherent clothing can be left for removal during the cleaning phase of treatment.[3] The clinician should refer such patients to the emergency department of a hospital.

Sunburn

Sunburn is caused by acute overexposure of the skin to UVR (see Color Plates, photograph 26). Sunburn can be caused from natural sunlight (primarily ultraviolet band B), tanning beds, and ultraviolet lamps.[4] (See Chapter 39 for a discussion of UVR bands.)

Photosensitive reactions (photoallergy and phototoxicity) are related to the administration of drugs and chemicals. Photoallergy is relatively uncommon, is usually caused by topical agents, and is characterized by an intensely pruritic eczematous dermatitis that may evolve into thickened leathery changes in sun-exposed skin (see Color Plates, photograph 28). The clinical presentation of phototoxicity includes erythema that resembles a sunburn, which desquamates (peeling of the skin) within several days[5]; edema, vesicles (blisters), and bullae (large blisters) may occur. Sun-exposed skin is the only area of involvement (see Color Plates, photograph 27). This reaction occurs more often with systemic rather than topical medications.

Cosmetics that contain fragrances such as musk ambrette, sandalwood oil, and bergamot oil are the most likely to cause a photoallergic reaction. A number of medications may cause photoallergy or phototoxicity reactions (see Chapter 39).

The extent of thermal injury to the skin is a function of the temperature generated and the duration of exposure. The skin can tolerate temperatures up to 104°F (40°C) for relatively long periods of time before injury. Temperatures above this produce a logarithmic increase in tissue destruction. Cell damage occurs as a result of protein denaturation. This damage is reversible unless temperatures exceed 113°F (45°C). At this temperature, protein denaturation exceeds the capacity for cellular repair.

Clinical Presentation of Minor Burns and Sunburn

Classification of Burns

The traditional classification of burns as first, second, or third degree has been replaced by the terms *superficial, superficial partial thickness, deep partial thickness,* and *full thickness,* which are related to the depth of injury to the skin. Sunburn is discussed separately.

Skin burns are classified primarily according to depth of injury (Figure 41-1). This pathophysiologic criterion is used to determine whether a burn patient needs emergency medical care. A second system developed by the American Burn Association (Injury Severity Grading System) classifies burn injuries as minor, moderate, and major.[6] Table 41-1 lists the criteria for these burn injury classifications, which incorporate the percentage of affected body surface area (BSA), depth of injury, location of burn, and cause of burn. This system is used by burn care treatment centers for major burn injuries.

Minor burns can often be managed in an outpatient environment if the eyes, ears, face, or perineum (genitalia) are not involved.[6] Either system can be used to assess a patient's burn; this chapter uses the depth of injury classification.

TABLE 41-1 American Burn Association Injury Severity Grading System

Type of Burn	Criteria
Minor	■ 15% BSA superficial and superficial partial-thickness burn in an adult ■ 10% BSA superficial and superficial partial-thickness burn in a child ■ 2% BSA deep partial-thickness or full-thickness burn in a child or adult not involving the eyes, ears, face, or genitalia
Moderate	■ 15%–25% BSA superficial partial-thickness burn in an adult ■ 10%–20% BSA superficial partial-thickness burn in a child ■ 2%–10% BSA deep partial-thickness or full-thickness burn in a child or adult not involving the eyes, ears, face, or genitalia
Major	■ 25% BSA superficial partial-thickness burn in an adult ■ 20% BSA superficial partial-thickness burn in a child ■ All deep partial-thickness or full-thickness burns greater than 10% BSA ■ All burns involving the eyes, ears, face, or genitalia ■ All inhalation injuries ■ Electrical burns ■ Complicated burn injuries involving fractures or other major trauma ■ All poor-risk patients (preexisting condition such as closed head injury, cerebrovascular accident, psychiatric disability, emphysema or lung disease, cancer, or diabetes)

Key: BSA, body surface area.

Source: Adapted from reference 5.

Superficial Burns

Superficial burns usually result from a brief exposure to low heat, causing a painful area of erythema similar to sunburn but without significant damage to epithelial cells. Superficial burns involve only the epidermis. In most circumstances, no blistering occurs. Redness, warmth, and slight edema are present. The burn may be painful because the sensory nerve endings are intact. Avoidance of additional injury and symptomatic relief of pain and fever are usually the only treatment required. Sunburn is classified most often in this category. The majority of superficial burns can be managed through self-care or ambulatory care centers and will heal within 3 to 6 days.

Superficial Partial-Thickness Burn

Higher levels of heat or longer exposures than those involved in superficial burns will damage the outer epidermal layers and produce painful blistering, causing a superficial partial-thickness burn. If the damage does not involve the deeper proliferating area of the epidermis, rapid regeneration of a normal epidermis usually results. Superficial partial-thickness burns are often moist and weeping, and they blanch with pressure (lighten in color when pressed with a finger). They are painful and sensitive to temperature and air. They often occur from a splash or spill of hot liquid, a brief contact with a hot object, or a flash ignition. Healing is generally spontaneous, occurring within 2 to 3 weeks, with minimal or no scarring. If this type of burn occurs in a child or in a patient with multiple medical problems, or covers more than 10% BSA, fluid restoration may be required. The patient should be transported to a hospital emergency room. Lesser degrees of superficial partial-thickness burn injuries can often be managed in an ambulatory setting; small burns (1%–2% BSA) can usually be managed through self-care. All superficial partial-thickness burns that have failed to heal within 2 weeks should be referred to a burn care specialist. Presence of pain, redness, exudate formation, fever, odor, or malaise that persists days or weeks after the initial injury is an indication for referral.[7]

Deep Partial-Thickness Burns

Deep partial-thickness burns result from more extensive heat exposure than that involved in superficial partial-thickness burns. The heat damages deeper layers of the skin including the dermis, resulting in a blanched rather than moist erythematous wound. Such burns result from a spill of scalding liquid, contact with a hot object, flash ignition, and chemical contact, as well as from flame exposure. Such wounds can resurface because of surviving nests of epithelial cells that line the hair follicles and sweat glands. In this case, healing may be slow and scarring is likely to occur. In addition, these injuries are prone to infection because of the loss of barrier function and the loss of vasculature. Infection will worsen the severity of a burn injury, its depth, or both.

Deep partial-thickness burns involve the entire depth of the epidermis and may extend into the dermis. The appearance may be a patchy white to red area, and large blisters may be present. Blanching indicates loss of blood vessels to the area. Pain may be more intense than in superficial burns because of the irritation to nerve endings, although some areas may lack sensation. More of the dermis is involved than in superficial partial-thickness burns, so these burns take longer to heal (up to 6 weeks) and may cause thick scar formation (hypertrophic scarring or cheloid), as well as contractures of the skin and underlying tissues that can affect use of the affected areas. Itching and hypersensitivity of the scar

often occur when deep partial-thickness wounds are allowed to heal without skin grafting. Patients with deep partial-thickness burns should be examined in a hospital's emergency department. These burn injuries can convert to full-thickness injuries if not properly and promptly managed.

Full-Thickness Burns

Even more extensive heat exposure than that involved in deep partial-thickness burns will cause death of the full thickness of skin in the affected area, resulting in a dry, leathery area that is painless and insensate. These full-thicknesses burns result from immersion in scalding liquid, flame exposure, electricity, and chemical contact, and are considered serious. The body attempts to heal these wounds by sloughing off the dead layer and contracting the wound. If the wounds are not surgically managed, significant scarring may result, as well as failure to completely heal. Full-thickness burns destroy both the dermis and epidermis and may extend into underlying tissues. Initially, the wound may appear red but will fade to white over 24 hours. Healing occurs slowly over months, and grafting is often required to achieve wound closure. Scarring usually results, and severe contractures may occur if physical therapy is not undertaken. Hospitalization is normally required for treatment of full-thickness burns, and patients should seek emergency care as soon as possible.

Sunburn

Sunburn causes a superficial burn injury, characterized by erythema and slight dermal edema resulting from an increase in blood flow to the affected skin. The increased blood flow begins approximately 4 hours after exposure, and peaks between 12 and 24 hours following exposure. Severe sunburn can lead to blistering (partial-thickness injury), fever, vomiting, delirium, and shock. If blisters occur, they will desquamate or "peel" over a period of several days. There is a slight chance of bacterial infection because of the loss of the outer skin barrier (see Color Plates, photograph 26). With mild exposure, erythema with subsequent scaling and exfoliation (peeling) of the skin occurs. Pain and low-grade fever may accompany the erythema. More prolonged exposure causes pain, edema, skin tenderness, and possibly blistering. Systemic symptoms similar to those of thermal burn, such as fever, chills, weakness, and shock, may be seen in patients in whom a large portion of the BSA has been affected. Following exfoliation and for several weeks thereafter, the skin will be more susceptible than normal to sunburn.

Long-Term Effects of Burns

A specialist should promptly examine patients who have received burns to the ear or eye, because loss of function in these structures may be devastating. Facial burns may be associated with respiratory injuries caused by inhalation, and intubation for airway protection may be required. Burns that are deeper than superficial may result in permanent scarring of the face. Hand burns can result in scarring and loss of range of motion, leading to major functional problems. Feet burns are often slow to heal, particularly in adults, and may become infected. Perineal burn victims are often chair-bound patients of advanced age or paraplegic patients who suffer spill scalds. These wounds are difficult to dress and are readily infected by fecal organisms. Patients who are immunocompromised or otherwise at high risk for infection (e.g., advanced age or diabetes) can develop serious infections without specialized care of the burn injuries. These patients should be referred for further evaluation.

Injuries deeper than superficial may require specialized care at a burn center. If treatment is delayed or not performed at all, incomplete wound healing, hypertrophic scarring, or abnormal pigmentation may occur.

Repeated sunburns are a risk factor for melanoma, particularly in children. Excessive unprotected exposure to the sun can also cause photoaging and ocular damage (see Chapter 39).[4]

Treatment of Minor Burns and Sunburn

Superficial and some superficial partial-thickness burn injuries are the only types suitable for self-treatment. Deeper burns are referred for medical or hospital care.

Treatment Goals

The goals in treating superficial and superficial partial-thickness burns are to (1) relieve pain associated with the burn, (2) provide physical protection, and (3) provide a favorable environment for healing that minimizes the chances of infection and scarring.

General Treatment Approach

The treatment of a burn depends on its depth and severity. When a patient with burns presents for treatment, it is critical to assess the extent and depth of the injury, both initially and again in 24 to 48 hours. If first aid is appropriate and the patient has not already done so, the clinician should administer this therapy. If the patient has none of the exclusions for self-treatment listed in Figure 41-2, the clinician should treat the patient (or guide the patient's treatment) using the treatment approach outlined in the algorithm.

Superficial burns are not likely to become infected and do not pose a problem with exudates. Physical protection for comfort can be provided by a number of wound dressings (see Chapter 42) and skin protectants that are currently marketed.

Superficial partial-thickness burns in which the epithelium is lost and the surface is weeping are prone to surface infection. Blisters should not be disturbed because blister fluid protects the skin below. Once debrided (dead skin removed), a blistered area may become infected and should be cleansed periodically. For ambulatory care or self-care, cleansing and/ or the use of first-aid antiseptics or topical antibiotics is sufficient. Dressings and skin protectant agents should be used to protect the injured area.

Most patients with superficial or superficial partial-thickness burns complain of pain. Therapeutic strategies include topical cold compresses, skin protectants, external anesthetics, topical corticosteroids, and oral nonprescription analgesics.

Generally, if the burned area is 2% of BSA or larger and consists of superficial partial-thickness or greater injury, medical attention is needed. The inflammatory response to a burn injury evolves over the first 24 to 48 hours; therefore, the initial appearance of the injury often leads to an underestimation of its actual severity. As a rule, the patient should return after that period for reevaluation of the injury. Figure 41-3 illustrates the rule-of-nine method for estimating the percentage of BSA burned.

Some medications can cause a photosensitivity reaction (see Chapter 39). These reactions require further referral.

Nonpharmacologic Therapy

First-aid measures are described in Figure 41-2. The goals of first aid are to stop the burning process, cool the burn, provide pain relief, and cover the burn. Stop the burning process by removing the source of heat. Active cooling delays progression of the burn and increases wound healing if performed within 20 minutes of the injury.[8,9] The affected area should be immersed or irrigated in tepid tap water for up to 20 minutes. Iced water can cause harmful vasoconstriction and should be avoided. Chemical burns should be irrigated with copious amounts of water. This phase of treatment does not apply when the depth or extent of the burn or both are serious, because such action would delay emergency treatment. Cool immersion decreases cutaneous vasodilation and has been shown to decrease edema, blister formation, and pain. In addition, an internal analgesic drug product such as aspirin, nonsteroidal anti-inflammatory drugs (NSAIDs), or acetaminophen can be given to reduce pain (see Chapter 5).[9]

Patients with moderate-to-severe injuries should be transported to an emergency center promptly. If some delay is anticipated before emergency care can be initiated, the patient should drink water, if possible, to replace vascular losses.

In the case of chemical burns, the patient should immediately remove any clothing on or near the affected area. The affected area should then be washed with tap water for at least 15 minutes or longer until the offending agent has been removed. This treatment, however, should not delay transport to a hospital emergency department.

If the eye is involved, the eyelid should be pulled back and the eye irrigated with tap water for at least 15 to 30 minutes. The irrigation fluid should flow from the nasal side of the eye to the outside corner to prevent washing the contaminant into the other eye. The area poison information center should be contacted immediately for treatment guidelines. Referral for further evaluation is frequently encouraged and should be sought as soon as possible.

No attempt should be made to counteract or neutralize a chemical burn. This action may produce an exothermic (heat-generating) chemical reaction, which can damage the injured area more than the original offending agent. For example, treating a burn caused by an acid by applying a base such as sodium bicarbonate is inappropriate. It should be noted that for certain chemicals, even a small area of contact can produce serious or lethal injury. For example, exposure to hydrofluoric acid, an industrial chemical, can result in life-threatening hypocalcemia.[10]

Initial treatment for minor sunburn is to get out of the sunlight and avoid further exposure. Minor sunburn can be relieved to some extent with cool compresses or a cool bath.

Heat stroke may occur with excessive exposure to sunlight in an environment that is hot or humid, or both. Because of complications from heat stroke, patients exhibiting fever, confusion, weakness, or convulsions should be referred for further evaluation immediately.

Preventive Measures

Preventing or reducing the number of burn injuries is an important public health measure. However, if a burn does occur, nondrug measures such as cleansing and protecting the burned area are important therapeutic modalities.

Several public health strategies are effective in reducing burn injuries. People should install smoke alarms in all homes and periodically test them. Families should develop escape plans; remove fire ignition sources from homes with children; and teach chil-

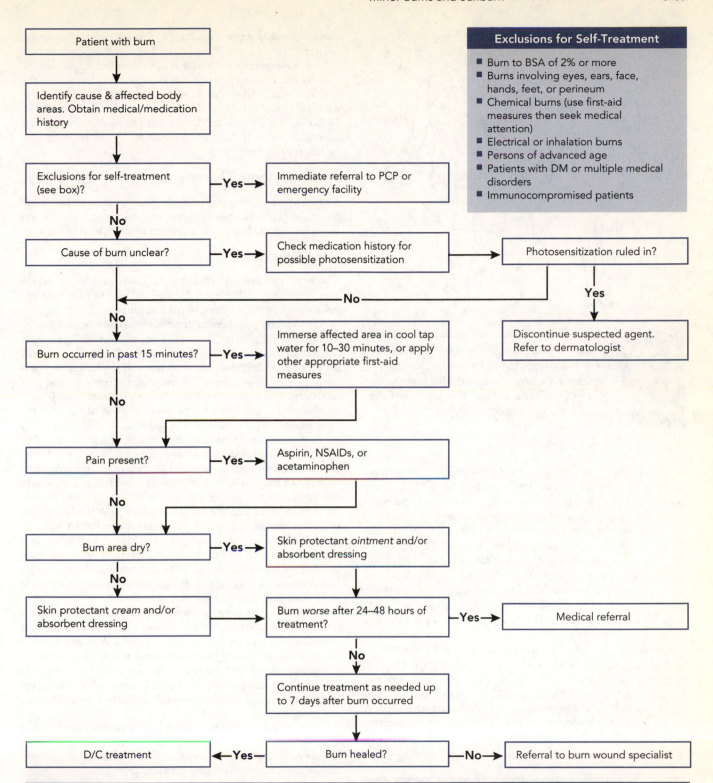

Exclusions for Self-Treatment

- Burn to BSA of 2% or more
- Burns involving eyes, ears, face, hands, feet, or perineum
- Chemical burns (use first-aid measures then seek medical attention)
- Electrical or inhalation burns
- Persons of advanced age
- Patients with DM or multiple medical disorders
- Immunocompromised patients

FIGURE 41-2 Self-care of minor burns and sunburn. Key: BSA, body surface area; D/C, discontinue; DM, diabetes mellitus; NSAID, nonsteroidal anti-inflammatory drug; PCP, primary care provider.

dren not to play with matches or lighters. Food that is being cooked requires constant monitoring. Patients should refrain from smoking in bed or under the influence of alcohol.[2]

Sunburn can be prevented by avoiding overexposure to sunlight and using appropriate sunscreen agents (see Chapter 39).

After applying cool moisture to a burned area to help stop the progression of the burn injury, the patient should gently cleanse

the area with water-based disinfectant.[10] Alcohol-containing preparations should not be used, because they dehydrate the area and cause pain to denuded skin (skin missing the outer protective epithelial layer). Hydrogen peroxide should also be avoided; it will damage healthy tissue. After the burn is cleansed, a nonadherent, hypoallergenic dressing may be applied if the area is small. A skin protectant or lubricant may be applied instead of,

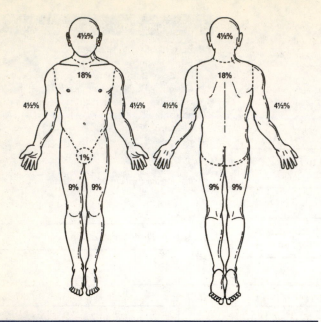

FIGURE 41-3 Rule-of-nine method for quickly establishing the percentage of adult body surface burned. (*Source:* Adapted with permission from *The Guide to Fluid Therapy.* Deerfield, Ill: Baxter Laboratories; 1969:111.)

or in addition to, a dressing, particularly if the burn is extensive or in an area that cannot be dressed easily (Table 41-2). If the burn is weeping, soaking it in cool tap water three to six times a day for 15 to 30 minutes will provide a soothing effect and diminish the weeping. Minor burns usually heal without additional treatment. For blistering burns in which blisters are no longer intact, cleansing once or twice daily to remove dead skin is recommended. Patients should be advised not to pull at loose skin or peel off burned skin, because viable skin may be removed in the process, thereby delaying healing.

All burns appropriate for management in a primary care setting should be covered. Modern wound dressings based on hydrocolloids, hydrofiber, silicones, alginates, and polyurethane provide a moist healing environment for burn injuries.[7] Sterile, nonadherent gauze dressings are the most convenient means of covering a small burn on a body area that is easily bandaged, such as the arm or leg. For superficial burns, films that are self-adhesive, waterproof, and semipermeable provide a protective barrier that is transparent and permits wound inspection without dressing

TABLE 41-2 Skin-Protectant Ingredients Used in Treatment of Minor Burns and Sunburn

Ingredient	Proposed Concentrations (%)
Allantoin	0.5–2
Cocoa butter	50–100
Petrolatum	30–100
Shark liver oil	3
White petrolatum	30–100

Source: Adapted from reference 11.

changes (e.g., OpSite or Tegaderm).[11] Pressure points (the sacrum, heels, and elbows) should be covered with self-adherent hydrocolloid dressings such as DuoDERM or Comfeel.

Newer dressings have been designed to incorporate the desirable characteristics of exudate absorption with occlusiveness (e.g., DuoDERM, Vigilon, and Viasorb; see Chapter 42). Blistering burns should be dressed with these absorbent hydrocolloid dressings. If the dressing remains dry and intact, it may be left in place for 10 days.[7]

Pharmacologic Therapy

Various products are useful in treating minor burns and sunburn. Some agents relieve pain, swelling, and/or inflammation. Others either protect the burn from infection or aid in healing the skin.

Skin Protectants

The Food and Drug Administration (FDA) has recognized the skin protectants in Table 41-2 as safe and effective for the temporary protection of minor burns and sunburn.

Skin protectants benefit patients with minor burns by making the wound area less painful. They protect the burn from mechanical irritation caused by friction and rubbing, and they prevent drying of the stratum corneum. Rehydrating the stratum corneum helps relieve the symptoms of irritation and permits normal healing to continue. Skin protectants provide only symptomatic relief. FDA has proposed revised labeling for the indications of skin protectants as follows: "For the temporary protection of minor cuts, scrapes, burns, and sunburn."[12] In selecting a skin protectant for burns, the clinician should choose products that prevent dryness and provide lubrication. Accordingly, FDA has proposed that bismuth subnitrate and boric acid not be considered safe or effective when used as skin protectants. FDA has also proposed that products with labeling claims of "cures any irritation" or "prevents formation of blisters" should not be generally recognized as safe and effective, and should not be included in the proposed skin protectant monograph. FDA has not accepted claims that certain substances (e.g., live yeast cell derivatives) contained in skin protectants are safe and effective in accelerating wound healing.[13]

Liver oils have been used for many years as folk remedies for wound healing. Shark liver oil contains a high concentration of vitamin A and is proposed as a skin protectant. Vitamin A and D ointment has been used to treat minor skin burns and abrasions. FDA recommends that the restriction preventing the use of skin protectants on children younger than 2 years be waived, except for products containing live yeast cell derivatives, shark liver oil, and zinc acetate.

Generally, the patient with minor burns may apply a skin protectant as often as needed. If the burn has not improved in 7 days or if it worsens during or after treatment, the patient should consult a primary care provider promptly.

Systemic Analgesics

An initial step in treating the patient with a minor burn is to recommend short-term administration of an internal analgesic, preferably one with anti-inflammatory activity, such as the NSAIDs (aspirin, naproxen, or ibuprofen). As prostaglandin inhibitors, NSAIDs may decrease erythema and edema in the burned area. NSAIDs may be especially beneficial in the patient with mild sunburn, especially in the first 24 hours after overexposure to UV radiation. Their use has been shown to decrease inflammation caused by exposure to UV radiation. However, this effect has been found to last only about 24 hours,[14] possibly because the initial inflammation of sunburn is mediated by prostaglandins, whereas the later inflammation is associated primarily with leukocytes. For patients who cannot tolerate NSAIDs, acetaminophen can provide pain relief, although it is a weak prostaglandin inhibitor and is not an anti-inflammatory agent. (See Chapter 5 for discussion of dosages and safety considerations for systemic analgesics.)

Topical Anesthetics

The pain of minor burns and sunburn can be attenuated by the judicious use of topical anesthetics. Agents proposed as safe and effective in providing temporary relief of pain associated with minor burns are listed in Table 41-3.

Topical anesthetics relieve pain by inhibiting the transmission of pain signals from pain receptors. Relief is short lived, lasting only 15 to 45 minutes.

Benzocaine (5%–20%) and lidocaine (0.5%–4%) are the two anesthetics most often used in nonprescription drug preparations. Dibucaine (0.25%–1%), tetracaine (1%–2%), butamben (1%), and pramoxine (0.5%–1%) are also found in external anesthetic preparations. The higher concentrations of the topical anesthetics are appropriate for burns in which the skin is intact. Lower concentrations are preferred when the skin surface is not intact because absorption is enhanced. They should be applied only to small areas to avoid systemic toxicity.

Topical anesthetics should be applied no more than three or four times daily. Because their duration of action is short, continuous pain relief cannot be obtained with these agents. Increasing the number of applications increases the risk of a hypersensitivity reaction and, more importantly, the chance for systemic toxicity.

Benzocaine produces a hypersensitivity reaction in about 1% of patients, a higher incidence than that seen with lidocaine. In a patch test study of 4000 patients with dermatitis, 9% were sensitive to benzocaine, and only neomycin was more sensitizing (10%).[15] In contrast, benzocaine is essentially free of systemic toxicity, whereas the systemic absorption of lidocaine can lead to a

number of side effects. However, systemic toxicities caused by lidocaine are rare if the product is used on intact skin, on localized areas, and for short periods.

Topical Hydrocortisone

Although not FDA-approved for use in treating minor burns, topical hydrocortisone 1% is often used in the first-aid treatment of minor burns covering a small area.

Hydrocortisone, an anti-inflammatory agent, should be used with caution if the skin is broken, because it may allow infections to develop. Topical corticosteroid treatment with high-potency agents has been shown to decrease collagen synthesis and delay reepithelialization in dermal wounds, whereas low-potency hydrocortisone 1% ointment does not interfere with resurfacing of the skin (see Chapter 34).[16]

Antimicrobials

Silver sulfadiazine (SSD) has been the gold standard agent used traditionally for the outpatient management of minor or partial-thickness burns. Recent studies have questioned the appropriateness of this practice owing to a lack of superiority demonstrated in trials comparing SSD to honey and membrane-like dressings.[17] Recent findings also suggest that SSD may delay wound healing and may have cytotoxic activity on host cells.[18] However, for minor burns, nonprescription first-aid antibiotic or antiseptic products are of limited value, especially on burns in which the skin is intact. These preparations may be used on minor burns when the skin has been broken. Chapter 42 discusses preparations that may be used to help prevent infection in minor burns or sunburn. The petrolatum base present in some first-aid products, such as triple-antibiotic ointment, is a skin protectant that can provide symptomatic relief.

Vitamins

Vitamin supplements are commonly used by burn centers for severe burn injuries. Although the benefits of vitamin supplementation for minor burns are not known, a frank deficiency of vitamin C (ascorbic acid) or vitamin A will impair wound healing. No scientific evidence suggests that vitamin dosages beyond the normal daily requirements will accelerate wound healing. However, vitamin C does play a key role in healing wounds, given that it is required for collagen synthesis. Because vitamin C is not stored in the body, it is reasonable to recommend up to 2 grams of vitamin C daily from the time of injury until healing is complete.

Animal studies indicate that vitamin A enhances healing in a variety of wounds. Following serious injury, the patient may have an increased requirement for vitamin A. In addition, deficiency states are associated with increased infections. Because vitamin A is stored in large amounts in the liver, supplemental vitamin A should not be used for long periods. Minor burn injuries will probably not benefit from supplemental oral vitamin A, but topical vitamin A (fish or shark liver oil–based products) may be helpful.

Deficiency of B vitamins may retard wound healing, so B vitamins should be supplemented if nutritional status is poor. Excess vitamin E may delay wound healing and does not play a role in burn injury. Vitamin D is not significantly involved in healing wounds. Administering zinc is beneficial in only people who are zinc-deficient. Iron-deficiency anemia can decrease the oxygen supply to the healing area and should be corrected if present. Copper deficiency may impair healing and can be corrected through normal dietary intake. Topical application of vitamin C and vitamin E, alone or in combination, may have protective

Agent	FDA-Approved Concentrations (%)
TABLE 41-3 Topical Analgesic Ingredients for Treatment of Minor Burns and Sunburn	
Amine and Caine-Type Local Anesthetics	
Benzocaine	5–20
Butamben picrate	1
Dibucaine	0.25–1
Dibucaine hydrochloride	0.25–1
Dimethisoquin hydrochloride	0.3–0.5
Dyclonine hydrochloride	0.5–1
Lidocaine	0.5–4
Lidocaine hydrochloride	0.5–4
Pramoxine hydrochloride	0.5–1
Tetracaine	1–2
Tetracaine hydrochloride	1–2
Antihistamines	
Diphenhydramine hydrochloride	1–2
Tripelennamine hydrochloride	0.5–2

Source: Reference 12.

benefits against sun-induced skin injury.[19,20] Beta-carotene supplementation, however, does not alter sunburn reactions.[21]

In summary, burned patients with good nutritional status may not benefit from vitamin or mineral supplementation. However, patients whose dietary intake is suboptimal will not be harmed by, and could benefit from, temporary supplementation with standard multivitamin or mineral preparations. Assurance of adequate vitamin C intake is recommended during healing from burn injury.

Counterirritants

Although counterirritants such as camphor, menthol, and ichthammol are currently proposed for use in minor burn treatment, FDA is still evaluating them. They generally should not be used for burns. Even though these agents do reduce pain by stimulating sensory nerve fibers, they increase blood flow to the area, causing further development of edema. They also irritate the already sensitized and damaged skin.

Miscellaneous Agents

The ability of topical forms of aloe vera and vitamin E to aid in the healing of minor burns and sunburn has not been substantiated, so FDA has not approved these agents as healing aids. Topical nitrofurantoin and some petrolatum-containing products have been shown to retard epithelial healing, whereas an oil-in-water cream, triple-antibiotic ointment, and benzoyl peroxide lotion 10% and 20% have increased the rate of healing.[16]

Combination Products

Rarely will a product intended to treat minor burns contain only one ingredient. FDA proposed that two or more of the skin protectant ingredients listed in Table 41-2 may be combined, provided that each ingredient in the combination is within the concentration range in the proposed monograph.[12]

Product Selection Guidelines

If a topical anesthetic or hydrocortisone is to be used, the clinician should recommend the most appropriate product formulation. Such products are available as ointments, creams, solutions (lotions), and sprays (aerosols).

Ointments are oleaginous-based preparations. They provide a protective film to impede the evaporation of water from the wound area, which helps keep the skin from drying. However, if the skin is broken, an ointment may not be appropriate because of its impermeability. The presence of excessive moisture trapped beneath the application may promote bacterial growth or maceration of the skin, thereby delaying healing. Ointments are more appropriate for minor burns in which the skin is intact. Creams are emulsions that allow some fluid to pass through the film and are best for broken skin. Generally, creams are easier to apply and remove than are ointments. To prevent contamination of the preparation, the patient should not apply ointments and creams directly onto the burn from the container.

Lotions spread easily and are easier to apply when the burn area is large. However, lotions that produce a powdery cover should not be used on a burn, because they tend to dry the area, are difficult (and possibly painful) to remove, and provide a medium for bacterial growth under the caked particles.

Generally, aerosol and pump sprays are more costly than other topical dosage forms. Sprays offer the advantage of precluding the need to physically touch the injured area, so there is less pain associated with applying the medication. Proper application requires holding the container approximately 6 inches from the burn and spraying for 1 to 3 seconds. This method decreases the chances of chilling the area. However, sprays are not usually protective in that the aerosol is typically water- or alcohol-based and will evaporate.

Table 41-4 lists selected trade-name topical products appropriate for treating minor burns and sunburn.

Complementary Therapies

Therapy for minor burns and sunburn is largely empirical, with little scientific study. The use of complementary preparations such as herbals is also empirical, but in some societies these remedies have been used for many generations. Plants such as *Calendula, Aloe vera, Garcinia morella,* and *Datura metol* are said to have healing properties.[22] (See Chapter 54 for further discussion of these types of remedies.)

Aloe gel has been widely used externally for its wound-healing properties, although the effectiveness of commercial preparations compared with fresh aloe gel is controversial.[23] Differences in the extraction and processing techniques may be related to variable results in artificial cell culture systems for

TABLE 41-4 Selected Topical Products for Minor Burns and Sunburn

Trade Name	Primary Ingredients
Skin Protectants	
A + D Original Ointment	Petrolatum 80.5%; lanolin 15.5%; cod liver oil (contains vitamins A and D)
Zinc oxide, Desitin Ointments	Zinc oxide 20 or 25%; white petrolatum
Local Anesthetics	
Americaine Aerosol, Ointment	Benzocaine 20%
ELA-Max 4%	Lidocaine 4%
Dermoplast Pain-Relieving Spray	Benzocaine 20%; menthol 0.5%
Dibucaine Topical Ointment	Dibucaine 1%
Itch-X Spray, Gel	Pramoxine HCl 1%; benzyl alcohol 10%
Solarcaine Aloe Extra Burn Relief Gel/Spray	Lidocaine 0.5%
Xylocaine Ointment	Lidocaine 2.5%
Local Anesthetics/Antiseptics	
Bactine First Aid Antiseptic Spray	Lidocaine HCl 2.5%; benzalkonium chloride 0.13%
Dermoplast Antibacterial Spray	Benzocaine 20%; benzethonium chloride 0.2%
Lanacane Maximum Strength Anti-Itch Cream	Benzocaine 20%; benzethonium chloride 0.1%
Unguentine Maximum Strength Cream	Benzocaine 5%, resorcinol 2%

TABLE 41-5 Age-Related Changes in Body Surface Area (%)

Surface	Age					
	Birth	**1 Year**	**5 Years**	**10 Years**	**15 Years**	**Adult**
Head	19	17	13	11	9	7
Neck	2	2	2	2	2	2
Trunk (anterior)	13	13	13	13	13	13
Trunk (posterior)	13	13	13	13	13	13
Buttocks	5	5	5	5	5	5
Perineum	1	1	1	1	1	1
Arms	8	8	8	8	8	8
Forearms	6	6	6	6	6	6
Hands	5	5	5	5	5	5
Thighs	11	13	16	17	18	19
Legs	10	10	11	12	13	14
Feet	7	7	7	7	7	7

processed aloe gel. A few small clinical studies suggest the effectiveness of fresh aloe gel and some prepared products in skin ulcers, burn wounds, frostbite injuries, and psoriasis. Aloe gel's effects may result from inhibition of the pain-producing substance bradykinin. Aloe gel may also inhibit thromboxane and prostaglandins, and may have antibacterial and antifungal properties. FDA does not recognize aloe gel as safe and effective for treating any condition because of insufficient evidence. Nonetheless, aloe gel products are widely used for burns and sunburns, and freshly prepared aloe gel may be worth considering for self-care of minor burns when applied externally. Patients should avoid internal use of aloe vera owing to multiple drug interactions and adverse effects associated with internal use. External aloe preparations are contraindicated in patients who have allergies to garlic, onions, tulips, and other plants in the *Liliaceae* family.[24]

The dried flower heads of *Arnica montana* have been prepared as hydroalcoholic extracts and creams.[23] Arnica has been shown to have antimicrobial, antiedema, and anti–inflammatory properties. Although the German Commission E has approved arnica for external application because of its anti–inflammatory, analgesic, and antiseptic properties, FDA has classified arnica as an unsafe herb.[24] Arnica is contraindicated in patients who have demonstrated hypersensitivity reactions to marigolds and other members of the Asteraceae family.[25]

One prospective randomized trial of honey versus SSD for superficial burns demonstrated that honey dressings resulted in faster healing and fewer infections than did the SSD dressings[26]; however, honey dressings are not advocated by burn centers.

Assessment of Minor Burns and Sunburn: A Case-Based Approach

When a patient presents with a burn, the practitioner should immediately assess the severity of the burn by determining the depth of the injury and the percentage of BSA involved. The percentage of the adult body that has been burned can be estimated by the rule-of-nine method (Figure 41-3). The total BSA is divided into 11 areas, each accounting for 9% or a multiple of 9. An easy way to estimate the percentage of burned BSA is to use the back of the hand as 1% of BSA. The rule of nines is reliable for adults but inaccurate for children and patients with small body surfaces. Table 41-5 illustrates how the BSA of the head, extremities, and other parts of the body changes with age.

Cases 41-1 and 41-2 are examples of the assessment of a patient with a minor burn.

CASE 41-1

Relevant Evaluation Criteria	Scenario/Model Outcome
Information Gathering	
1. Gather essential information about the patient's symptoms, including:	
a. description of symptom(s) (i.e., nature, onset, duration, severity, associated symptoms)	Patient burned her hand on a hot pan about an hour ago. She has a reddened area approximately 1 by 0.5 inch on the side of her hand that burns, and the area is painful to touch. There are no blisters or weeping areas.

Relevant Evaluation Criteria	Scenario/Model Outcome
b. description of any factors that seem to precipitate, exacerbate, and/or relieve the patient's symptom(s)	N/A
c. description of the patient's efforts to relieve the symptoms	Patient washed hand in cool water and applied butter to the burn.
2. Gather essential patient history information:	
a. patient's identity	Jennifer Smith
b. age, sex, height, and weight	31-year-old female, 5 ft 4 in, 155 lb
c. patient's occupation	Accountant
d. patient's dietary habits	Normal healthy diet with occasional junk food
e. patient's sleep habits	Bedtime is 10 pm; she rises at 5 am and usually wakes up once each night to check on baby.
f. concurrent medical conditions, prescription and nonprescription medications, and dietary supplements	Ortho-Novum 7/7/7, calcium carbonate 500 mg 3 times daily
g. allergies	NKA
h. history of other adverse reactions to medications	None
i. other (describe) _____	N/A

Assessment and Triage

3. Differentiate patient's signs/symptoms and correctly identify the patient's primary problem(s) (see Table 41-1).	Patient received a minor burn on her hand while cooking.
4. Identify exclusions for self-treatment (see Figure 41-2).	None
5. Formulate a comprehensive list of therapeutic alternatives for the primary problem to determine if triage to a medical practitioner is required, and share this information with the patient.	Options include: (1) Refer Jennifer to a burn specialist. (2) Suggest Jennifer see her PCP to obtain wound care if appropriate. (3) Recommend an OTC skin protectant, wound dressing, and analgesic product. (4) Take no action.

Plan

6. Select an optimal therapeutic alternative to address the patient's problem, taking into account patient preferences.	Patient prefers to use Desitin as a skin protectant because she also uses it for the baby.
7. Describe the recommended therapeutic approach to the patient.	Apply Desitin to burn and cover with occlusive dressing. Dressing may remain in place up to 5 days. Take ibuprofen for pain relief.
8. Explain to the patient the rationale for selecting the recommended therapeutic approach from the considered therapeutic alternatives.	Referral to a burn specialist or your primary care provider for wound care is necessary only with more severe burns.

Patient Education

9. When recommending self-care with nonprescription medications and/or nondrug therapy, convey accurate information to the patient:	
a. appropriate dose and frequency of administration	Desitin can be applied as often as desired. Occlusive dressing can remain in place for up to 5 days.
b. maximum number of days the therapy should be employed	7 days
c. product administration procedures	Wash hands and affected area with mild soap and water prior to application.
d. expected time to onset of relief	Immediate

C A S E   4 1 - 1   (continued)

Relevant Evaluation Criteria	Scenario/Model Outcome
e. degree of relief that can be reasonably expected	Burning sensation will be decreased, but it may not be entirely eliminated.
f. most common side effects	None
g. side effects that warrant medical intervention should they occur	N/A
h. patient options in the event that condition worsens or persists	If symptoms have not resolved or worsen in 7 days, you should see your primary care provider.
i. product storage requirements	Keep at room temperature.
j. specific nondrug measures	Cover the burn with an occlusive dressing.
10. Solicit follow-up questions from patient.	Is there some reason Desitin is better than butter?
11. Answer patient's questions.	Yes. Butter and other oil–based products can cause further damage to the skin and increase the burning sensation in your hand.

Key: N/A, not applicable; NKA, no known allergies; OTC, over-the-counter; PCP, primary care provider.

C A S E   4 1 - 2

Relevant Evaluation Criteria	Scenario/Model Outcome
Information Gathering	
1. Gather essential information about the patient's symptoms, including:	
a. description of symptom(s) (i.e., nature, onset, duration, severity, associated symptoms)	Patient ran into someone carrying a deep fryer full of hot grease an hour ago. Grease spilled over the entire length of the patient's arm and over a small area of her torso. Multiple large blisters are present. The burned area is bright red and blanches to the touch.
b. description of any factors that seem to precipitate, exacerbate, and/or relieve the patient's symptom(s)	N/A
c. description of the patient's efforts to relieve the symptoms	Patient hopped in a cold shower and put ice packs on the burn after getting out of the shower.
2. Gather essential patient history information:	
a. patient's identity	Joshua Smith
b. age, sex, height, and weight	43-year-old male, 5 ft 11 in, 215 lb
c. patient's occupation	Sales
d. patient's dietary habits	High-fat, high-protein diet, junk food, and alcohol
e. patient's sleep habits	Averages 7–8 hours per night
f. concurrent medical conditions, prescription and nonprescription medications, and dietary supplements	Occasional acetaminophen use for headaches, famotidine for occasional reflux symptoms
g. allergies	NKA
h. history of other adverse reactions to medications	None
i. other (describe) _____	N/A
Assessment and Triage	
3. Differentiate patient's signs/symptoms and correctly identify the patient's primary problem(s) (see Table 41-1).	Patient has experienced a superficial partial-thickness thermal burn.

CASE 41-2 (continued)

Relevant Evaluation Criteria	Scenario/Model Outcome
4. Identify exclusions for self-treatment (see Figure 41-2).	According to the rule of nines, the extent of the burn is greater than 4.5%.
5. Formulate a comprehensive list of therapeutic alternatives for the primary problem to determine if triage to a medical practitioner is required, and share this information with the patient.	Options include: (1) Refer Joshua to PCP or burn specialist for evaluation. (2) Recommend referral to the emergency department. (3) Recommend skin protectant and nonocclusive dressing. (4) Take no action.

Plan

6. Select an optimal therapeutic alternative to address the patient's problem, taking into account patient preferences.	Refer the patient to a PCP for evaluation and follow-up.
7. Describe the recommended therapeutic approach to the patient.	N/A
8. Explain to the patient the rationale for selecting the recommended therapeutic approach from the considered therapeutic alternatives.	Evaluation by a primary care provider is necessary because of the size of the lesion and the possibility that prescription products or other interventions might be necessary. You have no comorbid conditions, and the size of the lesion is not greater than 10% of your body surface area, so referral to a burn center or the emergency department is not necessary.

Patient Education

9. When recommending self-care with nonprescription medications and/or nondrug therapy, convey accurate information to the patient.	Criterion does not apply in this case.
10. Solicit follow-up questions from patient.	Is there an OTC medication that might work?
11. Answer patient's questions.	It is not advisable to self-medicate a burn of this size without evaluation and follow-up from your primary care provider. Burns often worsen slightly over a 24–48 hour period, and yours is already severe enough to warrant evaluation by your primary care provider.

Key: N/A, not applicable; NKA, no known allergies; OTC, over-the-counter; PCP, primary care provider.

Patient Counseling for Minor Burns and Sunburn

Once a burn is assessed as self-treatable, the clinician should address the patient's immediate concern: relieving the pain and swelling. Some patients may not realize the potential complications of even minor burns; therefore, advice on how to protect the injury is vital in preventing possible infection and scarring.

After a 24- to 48-hour follow-up evaluation of the burn, the clinician should either recommend continuation of self-treatment or refer the patient for further evaluation. If self-treatment continues, the patient needs to know how long healing of the burn will take, as well as the signs and symptoms that indicate worsening of the injury. The box Patient Education for Minor Burns and Sunburn lists specific advice for successful treatment of these injuries.

PATIENT EDUCATION FOR
Minor Burns and Sunburn

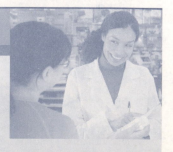

The objectives of self-treatment are to (1) relieve the pain and swelling, (2) protect the burned area from further physical injury, and (3) avoid infection and scarring of the burned area. For most patients, carefully following product instructions and the self-care measures listed here will help ensure optimal therapeutic outcomes.

Nondrug Measures
- Treat superficial burns with no blistering as follows:
  —Immerse the affected area in cool tap water for 10–30 minutes.

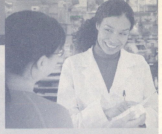

PATIENT EDUCATION FOR
Minor Burns and Sunburn (continued)

—Cleanse the area with water and a mild soap.

—Apply a nonadherent dressing or skin protectant to the burn.

■ For small burns with minor blistering, follow the first two steps above, but use a hydrocolloid dressing to protect the burn.

■ If possible, avoid rupturing blisters.

■ For sunburns, avoid further sun exposure and follow the previous procedures according to whether blistering is present.

Nonprescription Medications

■ For superficial burns (including sunburn) with unbroken skin, treat the affected area with thin applications of skin protectants or topical anesthetics using a tissue to reduce the risk of infection from the fingertips.

■ If the skin is broken, use topical antibiotics to prevent infection.

■ If nutritional status is poor, take supplements for vitamins A, B, and C.

■ Do not apply camphor, menthol, or ichthammol to the burn.

■ For temporary relief of pain, take aspirin, acetaminophen, ibuprofen, or naproxen (see Chapter 5 for dosage guidelines and safety considerations).

 If a skin rash, weight gain, swelling, or blood in the stool occurs while taking pain relievers, report these side effects to a primary care provider.

 Report immediately to a primary care provider any redness, pain, or swelling that extends beyond the boundaries of the original injury.

 If the burn seems to worsen or is not healed significantly in 7 days, see a primary care provider for further treatment.

Evaluation of Patient Outcomes for Minor Burns and Sunburn

Burn wounds should be reassessed after 24 to 48 hours, because the full extent of skin damage may not be initially apparent. If the burn has progressed or worsened, the patient should be referred to an appropriate health care professional for further evaluation.

The burn wound should exhibit decreased redness during healing. Signs of cellulitis or tissue infection, such as increasing redness, pain, and swelling that extend beyond the boundaries of the original wound, or signs of contact dermatitis from topical treatment suggest the need for further evaluation.

Burned skin is more susceptible to sunburn for several weeks after initial injury, so avoiding sun exposure and using sunscreen agents during this period are recommended.

Key Points for Minor Burns and Sunburn

➤ Minor burns and sunburn can often be treated with self-care. However, deeper burn injuries or burns affecting more than 1% to 2% of BSA require medical attention.

➤ Burn injuries may increase in severity over the first 24 to 48 hours, so reassessment is always necessary.

➤ Patient complaints usually focus on pain. Skin protectants and dressings should be recommended, and aspirin or NSAIDs are often helpful. The type of dressing or skin protectant used depends on whether the wound is dry or weeping. Blisters should not be ruptured. Topical hydrocortisone or anesthetics may provide additional relief in some patients but should be used sparingly on broken skin. Counterirritants should be avoided.

➤ Vitamins, whether systemic or topical, are generally of no value unless the patient is malnourished.

➤ Photosensitization reactions can often be assessed by history and must be distinguished from ordinary sunburns.

REFERENCES

1. American Burn Association. Burn Incidence Fact Sheet. Available at: http://www.ameriburn.org. Last accessed September 30, 2008.
2. National Center for Injury Prevention and Control. Fire Deaths and Injuries: Fact Sheet Available at: http://www.cdc.gov/ncipc/factsheets/fire.htm. Last accessed September 25, 2008.
3. Morgan ED, Bledsoe SC, Barker J. Ambulatory management of burns. *Am Fam Physician.* 2000;62:2015–26, 2029–30, 2032.
4. Scarlett WL. Ultraviolet radiation; sun exposure, tanning beds, and vitamin D levels. *J Am Osteopath Assoc.* 2003;:103:371–5.
5. Bickers DR. Photosensitivity and other reactions to light. In: Fauci AS, ed. *Harrison's Principles of Internal Medicine.* 16th ed. New York: McGraw-Hill, Inc; 2005:324–29.
6. Mertens DM, Jenkins ME, Warden GD. Outpatient burn management. *Nurs Clin North Am.* 1997;32:343–64.
7. Alsbjorn B, Gilbert P, Hartmann B, et al. Guidelines for the management of partial-thickness burns in a general hospital or community setting—recommendations of a European working party. *Burns.* 2007;33:155–60.
8. Jandera V, Hudson DA, De Wet PM, et al. Cooling the burn wound: evaluation of different modalities. *Burns.* 2000;2:265–70.
9. Hudspith J, Rayatt S. First aid and treatment of minor burns. *BMJ.* 2004:328; 1487–9.
10. Sheridan RL. Thermal injuries. In: Wolff K, Goldsmith LA., Katz SI et al., eds. *Fitzpatrick's Dermatology in General Medicine.* 7th ed. New York: McGraw-Hill, Inc; 2007.
11. Judson R. Minor burns—modern management techniques. *Aust Fam Physician.* 1997;26:1023–6.
12. *Fed Regist.* 1983;48:6820–33.
13. US Food and Drug Administration. Skin protectant drug products for over-the-counter human use; final monograph. *Fed Regist.* 2003;68:33364.
14. Young AR, Walker SL. Acute and chronic effects of ultraviolet radiation on the skin. In: Wolff K, Goldsmith LA., Katz SI, et al., eds. *Fitzpatrick's Dermatology in General Medicine.* 7th ed. New York: McGraw-Hill, Inc; 2007.
15. Bandmann HJ, Calnan CD, Cronin E, et al. Dermatitis from applied medicaments. *Arch Dermatol.* 1972;106:335–7.
16. Eaglestein WH, Mertz BA, Alvarez OM. Effect of topically applied agents on healing wounds. *Clin Dermatol.* 1984;2:112–5.
17. Chung, JY, Herbert ME. Myth: silver sulfadiazine is the best treatment for minor burns. *West J Med.* 2001;175:205.
18. Atiyeh BS, Costagliola M, Hayek SN, et al. Effect of silver on burn wound infection control and healing: review of the literature. *Burns.* 2007:33;139–48.
19. Krol ES, Kramer-Strickland KA, Lieberler DC. Photoprotective effect of topical vitamin E. *Drug Metab Rev.* 2000;32:413–20.

20. Lin JY, Selim MA, Shea CR, et al. UV photoprotection by combination topical antioxidants vitamin C and vitamin E. *J Am Acad Dermatol.* 2003;48:866–74.

21. Sayre RM, Black HS. Beta-carotene does not act as an optical filter in skin. *J Photchem Photobiol B.* 1992;12:83–90.

22. Sai KP, Babu M. Traditional medicine and practices in burn care: need for newer scientific perspectives. *Burns.* 1998;24:387–8.

23. Robbers JE, Tyler VE. *Tyler's Herbs of Choice.* New York: The Haworth Herbal Press; 1999:215–24.

24. Fetrow CW, Avila JR. *The Professionals Handbook of Complementary and Alternative Medicines.* 3rd ed. Springhouse: Lippincott Williams & Wilkins; 2004:33.

25. Fetrow CW, Avila JR. *The Professionals Handbook of Complementary and Alternative Medicines.* 3rd ed. Springhouse: Lippincott Williams & Wilkins; 2004:53.

26. Subrahmanyam M. A prospective randomised clinical and histological study of superficial burn wound healing with honey and silver sulfadiazine. *Burns.* 1998;24:157–61.

Minor Wounds and Secondary Bacterial Skin Infections

Daphne B. Bernard

Wound care management can be quite resource intensive, with much of the cost related to fees for emergency department visits and the expense of the medications and supplies used for wound healing. In fact, $1 billion are spent worldwide on wound dressings alone.[1] In light of these statistics and the fact that patients commonly use self-care in wound management, a thorough knowledge of wounds and how they heal is essential. Although the skin is well adapted to heal minor wounds over time, proper dressing and the appropriate use of antiseptics and antibiotics will facilitate healing as well as prevent scar formation and secondary bacterial skin infections.

Common concepts of wound care have changed drastically from earlier times and go against conventional wisdom, which encouraged "drying out" a wound and promoting the formation of a scab. Occlusive dressings were expressly avoided, because it was believed that the moist, warm environment they created promoted bacterial colonization. This approach was challenged in the mid-1960s when experiments were conducted to determine the possible benefit of a moist environment in wound healing. Today, there is clear evidence to support the benefits of a moist wound-healing environment. In many circumstances, practitioners should now recommend newer synthetic products that provide a moist environment in place of the traditional gauze dressings that promote dehydration of the wound.

One of the primary goals of this chapter is to provide practitioners with current information to enable them to properly advise consumers on wound care and product selection. Principles of the moist wound-healing method and its proper implementation through the use of selected first-aid products are covered. In addition, the chapter's goals are realized with a thorough review of skin anatomy and function; the physiology of wound healing; the classifications, types, and complications of wounds; wound management through the use of drugs and/or dressings; and a schematic approach to triaging wounds.

Each year millions of individuals are afflicted with various acute and chronic wounds in need of intervention. It is reported that approximately 11 million wounds are evaluated annually in emergency departments in the United States, with the majority of lacerations requiring repair.[2]

The skin is a versatile, multifunctional organ whose intricate workings depend on a delicate balance between structure and function. When a wound alters or disturbs this balance, prompt restoration is required to ensure body homeostasis.

Restoration of homeostasis is accomplished through the process of wound healing, a complex cascade of localized biochemical and cellular events regulated by the immune system and orchestrated by the skin.

The skin is composed of two anatomic layers, the epidermis and the dermis, and supported by a variably thick subcutaneous layer called the hypodermis (see Table 42-1 and Chapter 33, Figure 33-1). The epidermis, the most superficial layer of the skin, is normally in direct contact with the outside environment. Approximately 0.04 mm thick and avascular, it consists of five layers of stratified squamous epithelium (keratinocytes). This keratinized layer provides a tough, resistant, waterproof covering for the skin. Aside from its protective function, the epidermis also serves several other functions, given that it contains the cell types necessary for immune regulation (Langerhans' cells), skin color (melanocytes), and proprioception (Merkel's tactile cells). Skin appendages, including the sweat glands and hair follicles, are also derived from the epidermis.

The dermis is the layer directly below the epidermis. It is approximately 0.5 mm thick and contains a rich vascular supply, multiple nerve endings, lymphatics, collagen proteins, and connective tissue. It also contains two main cell types: fibroblasts and macrophages. The main function of fibroblasts is to produce collagen, a structural support protein necessary for scar formation. Macrophages, however, are multifunctional cells that are vital for wound repair. They serve as both immune regulators and growth regulators; these functions are necessary for the sterilization, debridement (removal of dead, damaged, or infected tissue), and eventual healing of the wound. The dermis also contains the basilar projections of epidermally derived sweat glands and hair follicles.

The subcutaneous tissue contains mostly adipocytes and is the origination site for dermal blood vessels. Its major function is to provide insulation, padding, and protection against mechanical injury. It also stores calories in the form of fat and provides the skin with a moderate degree of mobility, protecting it against friction and shear-related injury.

Physiology of Wound Healing

Wound healing begins immediately after injury and consists of three overlapping stages: inflammatory, proliferative, and maturation (remodeling).[3]

TABLE 42-1 Structure and Function of the Skin

Epidermis
- Thickness of 0.04 mm
- No blood supply
- Composed of epithelium
- Resident flora
- Five layers (two are stratum corneum and stratum germinativum, or basement layer)

Dermis
- Thickness of 0.5 mm
- Main support structure
- Contains nerve endings, lymphatics, vasculature
- Normally moist
- Appendages: hair follicles, sebaceous glands, sweat glands

Subcutaneous Tissue (Hypodermis)
- Variable thickness
- Reservoir for fat storage
- Temperature insulator
- Shock absorber
- Stores calories

Source: Adapted with permission from Bryant R. Wound repair: a review. *J Enterostomal Ther.* 1987;14:262–3.

Inflammatory Phase

The inflammatory phase is the body's immediate response to injury. This phase, which lasts approximately 3 to 4 days, is responsible for preparing the wound for subsequent tissue development and consists of two primary parts: hemostasis and inflammation.

In the initial portion of the inflammatory phase, hemostasis is initiated by the release of thromboplastin from injured cells. Thromboplastin, in turn, activates the body's intrinsic clotting system to form a clot within the first several hours. The newly formed clot stops the bleeding and allows healing to progress with eventual collagen synthesis.

After hemostasis is achieved, an active inflammatory phase begins, cleansing the wound. Polymorphonuclear (PMN) leukocytes are recruited during the first 24 to 48 hours to phagocytize debris and bacteria in the wound.

After the first 24 hours, released chemotactic factors recruit blood monocytes into the wound; the latter become tissue macrophages. Macrophages function as phagocytes and release growth factors that stimulate epithelial mitogenesis and endothelial angiogenesis. They also induce fibroblasts to synthesize collagen, which provides a healthy bed of granulation tissue for future epithelial cells.

The final portion of the inflammatory phase involves epithelial migration into the wound. Epithelial cells from the stratum germinativum migrate from the intact wound edges and epithelial appendages to cover the denuded area of the wound. Once the epithelial cells become established on their granulation bed, they provide the initial (one-cell-thick) layer of new skin for the wound. Epithelial cells can migrate under the clot and eschar (scab) in the wound, but in doing so they delay healing time and promote scar formation.

Proliferative Phase

In the next phase of healing, the proliferative phase, the wound is filled with new connective tissue and covered with new epithelium. This phase starts on about day 3 and continues for about 3 weeks. It involves the formation of granulation tissue, which is a collection of new connective tissue (fibroblasts and newly synthesized collagen), new capillaries, and inflammatory cells.

Maturation Phase

The final phase of healing is known as the maturation or "remodeling" phase. This is the longest phase, beginning at about week 3, when the wound is completely closed by connective tissue and resurfaced by epithelial cells. It involves a continual process of collagen synthesis and breakdown, replacing earlier, weak collagen with high-tensile-strength collagen.

Factors That Affect Wound Healing

Several local and systemic factors can affect how efficiently and to what extent a wound will heal. Local factors include tissue perfusion and oxygenation, infection, and wound characteristics. Only the most important systemic factors that can affect the healing process—nutrition, age and weight, coexisting diabetes mellitus, and medications—are discussed.

Poor vascularization delays wound healing. The resultant poor oxygenation leads to impaired leukocyte activity, decreased production of collagen, decreased epithelialization, and reduced resistance to infection. Common disorders that may cause decreased perfusion include diabetes, severe anemia, hypotension, peripheral vascular disease, and congestive heart failure.

All traumatic wounds are contaminated with bacteria to some degree; this contamination is usually restrained by phagocytic action. However, an infection will develop if the following factors are present: (1) a high level of bacterial contamination (e.g., $>10^5$ bacteria per gram of wound tissue); (2) a compromised tissue microenvironment (e.g., eschar, necrosis); (3) systemic conditions (e.g., age, steroid therapy, and malnutrition); and (4) immunoincompetence.[4]

Localized infection in the wound delays collagen synthesis and epithelialization, and prolongs the inflammatory phase, causing additional tissue destruction. The most common bacteria implicated in community-acquired wound infections include gram-positive *Staphylococcus aureus, Streptococcus pyogenes,* and *Enterococcus faecalis.* Gram-negative *Escherichia coli, Pseudomonas aeruginosa,* and *Klebsiella* species are often associated with hospital-acquired or chronic wounds. Anaerobic organisms, such as *Bacteroides* species, are associated with necrotic or poorly perfused wounds.[4]

The classic signs and symptoms of a local wound infection include erythema, edema, induration, pain, crepitation, and the presence of purulent or odorous exudate in the affected area. Fever, flu-like symptoms, and leukocytosis are frequently associated with systemic infections. Appropriate wound cultures should be taken to identify the infecting organisms when the classic clinical signs of infection are present.[4]

Local features that may impair wound closure include the presence of necrotic tissue, eschar, or foreign bodies (e.g., glass and dirt); the lack of moisture; and the presence of infection.[2,5] Practitioners who are aware of and can recognize problems with such local factors can, through careful counseling, do their part to ensure proper wound healing.

Adequate nutrition provides the building blocks for wound repair. Protein, carbohydrates, vitamins, and trace elements are needed for collagen production and cellular energy.[6,7] Vitamins A and C promote wound integrity. Vitamin A enhances the synthesis of collagen and stimulates epithelialization by causing rapid cell turnover. Vitamin C is necessary to maintain proper cellular membrane integrity and further enhance collagen synthesis and cross-linkage. Zinc may enhance wound healing by promoting cell proliferation. Many practitioners recommend supplements of these and other complementary therapies for promotion of wound healing, despite the lack of substantial clinical evidence of their benefit.

Aging can cause a delayed inflammatory response and is associated with increased capillary fragility, reduced collagen synthesis, and neovascularization. Aging is also associated with slow epithelialization.[8,9] Patients who are obese have problems with poor perfusion (adipose tissue lacks vascular tissue) and tend to have delayed wound healing.[10]

Poorly controlled diabetes is usually associated with reduced collagen synthesis, impaired wound contraction, delayed epidermal migration, and reduced PMN leukocyte chemotaxis and phagocytosis. Strict professional attention should be given to wounds in patients with diabetes because of these inherent difficulties.[11]

Practitioners can play a key role in identifying potential detriments to proper wound closure. Certain medications, for example, can act directly to impede healing through their interaction at various stages of the healing process. Corticosteroids suppress inflammation, resulting in a decrease in angiogenesis, collagen synthesis, and phagocytosis. Antineoplastic drugs and radiation therapy interfere with the cellular division necessary for fibroblast function and reepithelialization. Anticoagulants may interfere early in the inflammatory phase.[12] Patients who are taking these medications should be carefully followed by a wound care specialist to ensure that proper healing occurs.

Classification of Wounds

Classification of wound type is necessary for implementing proper and specific wound therapy; therefore, it is imperative that practitioners who are recommending outpatient first-aid products be aware of these classifications. Wounds can be classified according to their acuity and/or depth.

Using the acuity classification, wounds can be either acute or chronic. Chronic wounds require triage with intense medical treatment and will not be discussed in this chapter.

Acute wounds include abrasions, punctures, lacerations, and burns, and usually result from injury. They take approximately 1 month to heal in healthy individuals. Burns are discussed in Chapter 41. *Abrasions* usually result from a rubbing or friction injury to the epidermal portion of the skin and extend to the uppermost portion of the dermis. *Punctures* usually result from a sharp object that has pierced the epidermis and lodged in the dermis or deeper tissues. *Lacerations* result from sharp objects cutting through the various layers of the skin.[10] Self-treatment of acute wounds such as abrasions and puncture wounds not extending beyond the dermis is generally deemed appropriate.

Wound depth classification (Figure 42-1) is used primarily by health care personnel and is based on the extent or number of skin layers damaged during the wound-initiating process. This classification has been divided, for simplicity's sake, into four descriptive stages. *Stage I* does not involve loss of any skin

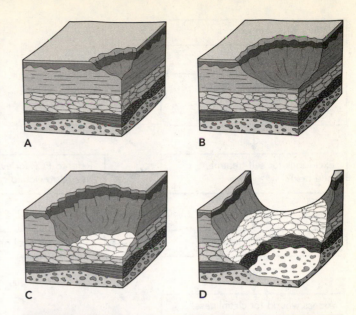

FIGURE 42-1 Stages of wounds. **A: Stage I,** Nonblanchable erythema of intact skin with warmth and redness. **B: Stage II,** Superficial lesions with partial-thickness skin loss involving the epidermis with or without the dermis involved. **C: Stage III,** Full-thickness skin loss with damage to subcutaneous tissue. **D: Stage IV,** Full-thickness skin loss with extensive tissue necrosis and damage to underlying muscle, tendon, and bone.

layers and consists primarily of reddened, nonblanching unbroken skin. *Stage II* includes blister or partial-thickness skin loss involving all the epidermis and part of the dermis. *Stage III,* full-thickness skin loss, includes damage to the entire epidermis, dermis, and dermal appendages, and may involve subcutaneous tissue. *Stage IV* is an extension of stage III but further involves the subcutaneous tissue and underlying muscle, tendon, and bone.[13] Understanding these stages helps in selecting appropriate dressings for proper wound closure.

Treatment of Minor Wounds and Secondary Bacterial Infections

Treatment Goals

The goal in treating wounds is to promote healing by protecting the wound from infection and further trauma, and to minimize scarring. Treatment should include a stepwise approach that involves cleansing the wound, selectively using antiseptics and antibiotics, and creating closure with an appropriate dressing. Figure 42-2 lists exclusions for self-treatment.

General Treatment Approach

Uncontaminated acute wounds at stages I and II (Figure 42-1), such as minor cuts, scrapes, and burns, require only basic supportive measures, including irrigation with saline or bottled water for proper cleansing and using a wound dressing to prevent

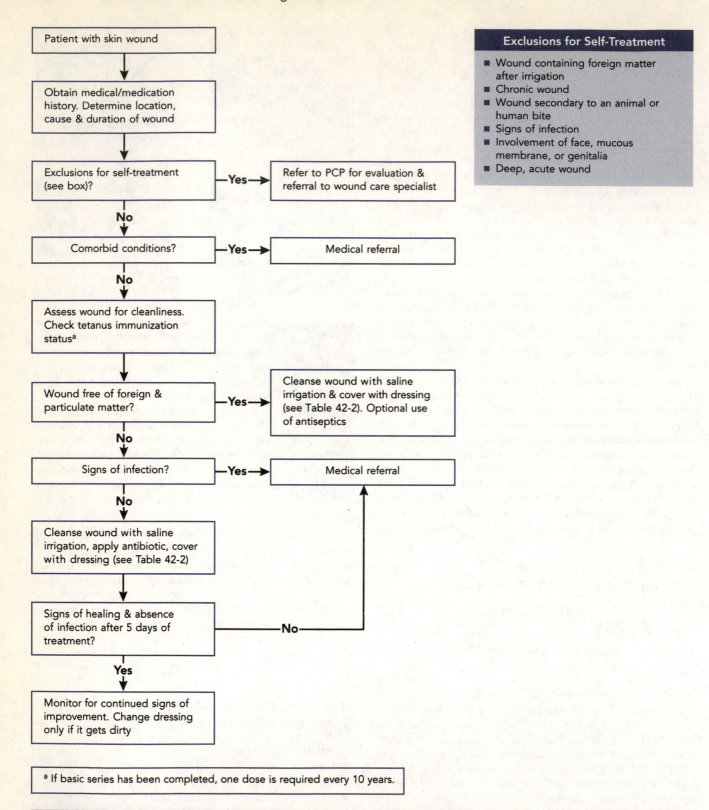

Exclusions for Self-Treatment

- Wound containing foreign matter after irrigation
- Chronic wound
- Wound secondary to an animal or human bite
- Signs of infection
- Involvement of face, mucous membrane, or genitalia
- Deep, acute wound

Patient with skin wound

↓

Obtain medical/medication history. Determine location, cause & duration of wound

↓

Exclusions for self-treatment (see box)? —Yes→ Refer to PCP for evaluation & referral to wound care specialist

No ↓

Comorbid conditions? —Yes→ Medical referral

No ↓

Assess wound for cleanliness. Check tetanus immunization status[a]

↓

Wound free of foreign & particulate matter? —Yes→ Cleanse wound with saline irrigation & cover with dressing (see Table 42-2). Optional use of antiseptics

No ↓

Signs of infection? —Yes→ Medical referral

No ↓

Cleanse wound with saline irrigation, apply antibiotic, cover with dressing (see Table 42-2)

↓

Signs of healing & absence of infection after 5 days of treatment? —No→ Medical referral

Yes ↓

Monitor for continued signs of improvement. Change dressing only if it gets dirty

[a] If basic series has been completed, one dose is required every 10 years.

FIGURE 42-2 Self-care of acute skin wounds. Key: PCP, primary care provider.

entry of bacteria into the affected area. Topical nonprescription antibiotic and antiseptic preparations can also be useful in preventing secondary infection, but these agents should be viewed as extensions of supportive treatment. Figure 42-2 outlines the triage and treatment of acute wounds.

More serious or deeper tissue injury (e.g., animal or human bites, puncture wounds, and severe burns) requires primary care provider consultation to assess the need for systemic or topical prescription antibiotics as well as a tetanus booster.

Nonpharmacologic Therapy (Wound Dressings)

Traditional wound management involves leaving the wound open to air or covering it with a nonocclusive textile dressing (gauze). However, this type of management leads to eschar formation, which impedes reepithelialization of wounds and creates unwanted scars (Figure 42-3A). Wound dehydration with delayed healing and increased risk of bacterial entry into the wound may also occur. Removal of gauze dressings often tears away not only the eschar but also the new tissue under the eschar. These cumulative problems have led primary care providers and nurses to develop new treatment strategies based on creating a moist wound environment (Figure 42-3B). This type of environment prevents eschar development, removes excess exudate without dehydration, and prevents bacterial invasion of the wound.[14] Practitioners should still recommend the use of gauze and gauze-type adhesive dressings; for example, gauze pads may be used with more advanced semiocclusive dressings such as foams for better exudate absorption. They also help in wound debridement with the removal of eschar and necrotic tissue. In addition, gauze-type adhesive bandages may be used for minor cuts and abrasions.

Selection Criteria for Wound Dressings

The primary goal in wound healing is to heal the wound quickly with minimal scarring, deformity, and loss of function. Scarring is closely related to the type of dressing used; occlusive dressings cause less scarring than gauze dressings. The timing of the dressing placement is also important; immediate occlusion leads to resurfacing of epithelium faster than delayed occlusion. The ideal dressing should (1) remove excess exudate, (2) maintain a moist environment, (3) be permeable to oxygen, (4) thermally insulate the wound, (5) protect the wound from infection, (6) be free of particulate or toxic contaminants, and (7) be removable without disrupting delicate new tissue.[15]

Understanding the potential use and function of specific wound dressings should guide the practitioner in proper product selection. It is important to note that wound dressing requirements may change depending on the healing phase. In terms of promoting moist wound healing, the wound dressing may be used to absorb excess moisture, maintain optimal moisture, or provide moisture where it is lacking. Table 42-2 and Figure 42-4 (which provide guidelines for selection of dressings developed by Jeter and Tintle[16]) describe and illustrate the major categories of wound care products available today, as well as provide an overview of their indications, advantages, and disadvantages.

ABRASIONS AND LACERATIONS

Most superficial wounds (minor abrasions and lacerations) that practitioners encounter may simply require the application of adhesive gauze-type bandages such as regular Band-Aid Brand bandages. Recognition of the importance of the moist wound-healing method has led to the development and marketing of more hydrocolloid-based bandages (Band-Aid Brand Advanced Healing Strips and New Skin), which meet the need for moisture retention and control, and may promote faster healing.[17] For individuals with hypersensitive skin, hypoallergenic and latex-free tape (First-Aid Hurt Free Tape) may be less irritating and will not tear the skin or hair on removal. Patients with latex allergies who have generally developed dermatologic problems from synthetic latex exposure may benefit from using dressings containing natural rubber latex (Band-Aid Brand Gentle Care and Curad Sensitive Skin); however, these products may still cause allergic reactions.

Medicated bandages include those with pads containing benzalkonium chloride (Band-Aid Brand Antibacterial), which claim to "kill germs and prevent infection"; benzocaine (Band-Aid Brand Pain & Itch Relief), which claim to decrease wound "pain and itch"; calcium alginate (Band-Aid Brand Quick Stop), which claim to "help blood clot faster"; and ionic silver (Actocoat and Silverderm), which are promoted as having antibacterial properties. In selecting medicated bandages, it is important for a primary care provider to evaluate whether the application of these agents is necessary. Evidence supporting the benefits of these more expensive products compared with more traditional dressings is lacking.

Alternatives to conventional bandages are cyanoacrylate tissue adhesives also known as liquid adhesive bandages (Liquiderm), which are used for small cuts and abrasions. These bandages are preferred for either cosmetic purposes (i.e., when a wound is located on the face) or when a more flexible dressing product is needed (i.e., when a wound is located on the finger or elbow).[18] Cyanoacrylate tissue adhesives offer many advantages: patient comfort, resistance to bacterial growth, and one-time rapid application with no need for removal.

PUNCTURE WOUNDS

It is important for a primary care provider to inspect puncture wounds to ensure that no foreign bodies are retained and to update tetanus prophylaxis, if necessary. If no debris is present, the wound should then be cleansed with either water or sterile saline. The wounds should be left open and soaked with soapy water for 30 minutes, at least four times a day initially, to allow for proper healing.[3,5] Hydrocolloid dressings (i.e., Johnson & Johnson Brand Advanced Healing Pads) are indicated for punctures that produce light exudates, whereas hydrogel dressings (i.e., Biolex Wound Gel) that absorb more exudates may be indicated for punctures extending deeper into the dermis and deeper tissues.

Types of Wound Dressings

Ideal dressings should be able to absorb excess moisture (foams, alginates, etc.); maintain moisture (hydrocolloid and transparent film dressings); or provide moisture where it is lacking (hydrogels).

DRESSINGS THAT ABSORB MOISTURE

Early in the inflammatory phase of healing, the wound tissue may be overly moist as a result of the accumulation of fluid evaporated by exposed damaged tissue, as well as blood and serous drainage. A wound that is "too wet" may result in maceration of the tissue. Exudate contains various components including lysosomal enzymes, white blood cells, and growth cells.[19] A wound that exudes moderate-to-high levels of drainage requires an absorbent dressing (foam, alginates, carbon-impregnated, and composite dressings). These dressings offer the benefit of requiring fewer dressing changes than nonabsorbent dressings, enabling undisturbed wound healing.

Foam dressings usually consist of polyurethane or other polymer material that has been "foamed" by introducing air bubbles to create tiny open pockets capable of filling with and holding fluids to remove drainage from the wound's surface. The "fluid-filled" foam dressing covers the wound to create a humid environment to further promote healing. Care must be taken not to

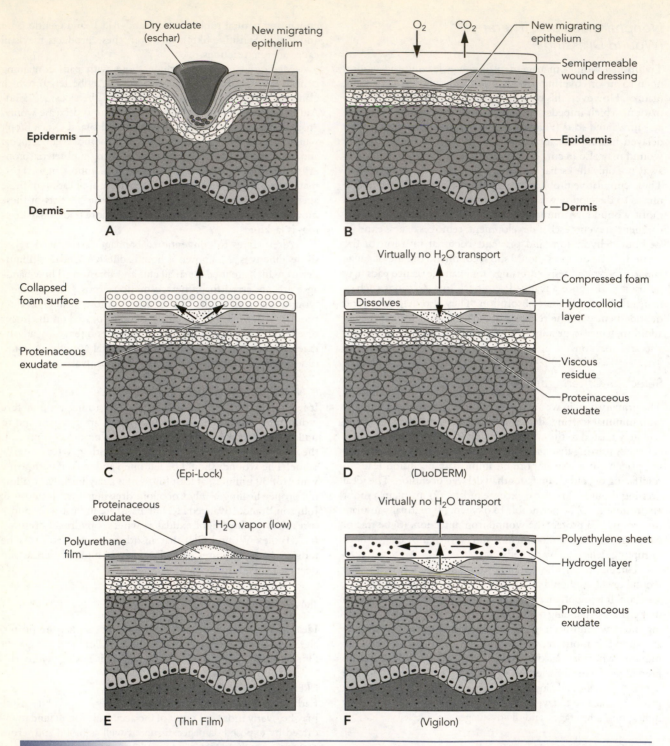

FIGURE 42-3 Mechanisms by which semipermeable wound dressings create a moist environment for wound healing. **A,** Regenerating epidermal cells are forced to "tunnel" below the dry wound eschar to attain wound closure. This tunneling delays wound closure. **B,** Semipermeable wound dressings prevent formation of eschar by maintaining optimal moisture level at the wound bed. Unhindered by the presence of a dry eschar, migrating epithelial cells are able to migrate and close the wound. **C,** Mechanism of action of a hydrophilic polyurethane foam dressing (Epi-Lock). **D,** Mechanisms of action of a hydrocolloid wound dressing (DuoDERM). **E,** Mechanism of water vapor transmission in thin films. **F,** Mechanism of action of a hydrogel wound dressing (Vigilon). (Adapted with permission from Syzcher M, Lee SJ. Modern wound dressings: a systemic approach to wounds. *J Biomater Appl.* 1992;7:142–213.)

TABLE 42-2 Options in Wound Dressing

Description (Trade Name)[a]	Uses/Indications	Advantages	Disadvantages
Gauze Dressings			
Nonocclusive fiber dressing with loose, open weave (Bulky Bandage, Conform, Kerlix Rolls and Sponges, Kling-Fluff)	Stages II-IV Minimal to heavy exuding wounds/topicals Debridement Wound rehydration May use with semiocclusive dressings	Readily available in many sizes Deep wound packing May use with infected wounds/topicals Nonocclusive Conformable	Wound bed may desiccate if dressing is dry Nonselective debridement May cause bleeding/pain on removal Need secondary dressing Frequent dressing changes
Nonadherent (Gauze-Type) Dressings			
Nonadherent, porous dressings. Lightly coated dressings allow exudate to flow through (Adaptic, Nexcare Pads, Release, Telfa, Vaseline Gauze)	Skin donor sites Stage II, shallow stage III Staple/suture lines Abrasions Lacerations Punctures May use with semiocclusive dressings	Readily available Less adherent than plain gauze	Need secondary dressing May cause bleeding/pain on removal Some impregnated dressings may delay healing May require frequent dressing changes Some may cause exudate pooling
Foams			
Semipermeable, nonwoven, absorptive, inert polyurethane foam dressings (Allevyn, EPIGARD, Epi-Lock, Hydrasorb, Lyofoam, VigiFOAM; see Figure 42-3C)	Stage II, shallow-stage III Minimal-to-moderate drainage First- and second-degree burns Contraindicated in third-degree burns	Most are nonadhesive Some can be used with infected wounds/topicals Thermal insulation Reduce pain Nonocclusive Moist environment Conformable Less frequent dressing changes Trauma-free removal Absorbent	Most require secondary dressing May require cutting May cause wound desiccation May be difficult to determine wound contact surface
Alginates			
Hydrophilic, nonwoven dressings composed of calcium-sodium (percentages vary) alginate fibers. Alginates are processed from brown seaweed into pad or twisted fiber form. Exudate transforms fibers to gel at wound interface (AlgiDERM, Algosteril, Band-Aid Brand Quick Stop Adhesive Bandages, Kaltostat, Sorbsan)	Light-to-heavy exuding wounds Stages II, III, IV Skin donor sites	Absorptive Reduce pain Nonocclusive Moist environment Conformable Easy, trauma-free removal Can use on infected wounds Accelerate healing time Less frequent dressing changes Potential to aid in control of minor bleeding	Require secondary dressing Characteristic odor May need wound irrigation May desiccate May promote hypergranulation
Carbon-Impregnated (Odor-Control) Dressings			
Dressings with an outer layer of carbon for odor control (Carboflex, Lyofoam "C")	Malodorous wounds	Control odor	Require appropriate seal or odor may escape Carbon is inactivated when it becomes wet
Composite/Island Dressings			
Nonadherent, absorptive center barrier with adhesive at perimeter (AcryDerm, Allevyn island, Lyofoam "A," Nu-Derm, Viasorb)	Stages II, III Moderate-to-heavy exuding wounds	Nonadherent over wound Semiocclusive Autolysis Suture/staple lines Protective Reduce pain No secondary dressing required Impermeable to fluids/bacteria	May cause periwound trauma on removal

(Continued)

TABLE 42-2 Options in Wound Dressing *(continued)*

Description (Trade Name)[a]	Uses/Indications	Advantages	Disadvantages
Hydrocolloids			
Wafer dressings composed of hydrophilic particles in an adhesive form covered by a water-resistant film or foam (Band-Aid Brand Advanced Healing Strips, Comfeel, Cutinova, DuoDERM CGF Dressing, Tegasorb, ULTEC; see Figure 42-4D)	Stages I, II, shallow stage III Clean, granular wounds Autolysis Minimal-to-moderate exuding wounds Can use with absorption products and alginates	Occlusive Manage exudate by particle swelling Autolysis Long wear time Self-adherent Impermeable to fluids/bacteria Conformable Protective Thermal insulation Reduce pain Moist environment	For uninfected wounds only May cause periwound trauma on removal Difficult wound assessment Characteristic odor Impermeable to gases Some may leave residue on skin or in wound
Transparent Adhesive Films			
Semiocclusive, translucent dressings with partial or continuous adhesive composed of polyurethane or copolyester thin film (ACU-derm, BIOCLUSIVE, Blisterfilm, CarraFilm, OpSite, Tegaderm; see Figure 42-4E)	Stages I, II, shallow stage III Clean granular wounds Minimally exuding wounds Autolysis Can use with absorption products and alginates Can be used in conjunction with some enzymatic debriders	Semiocclusive Gas permeable Easy inspection Autolysis Protection Impermeable to fluids/bacteria Comfortable Self-adherent Reduce pain Moist environment Shear resistant	For uninfected wounds only Not absorptive May cause periwound trauma on removal With continuous adhesive, may reinjure wound on removal With large amounts of exudate, maceration may occur
Hydrogels/Gels			
Nonadherent, nonocclusive dressings with high moisture content that come in the form of sheets and gels (Bioflex Wound Gel, Elasto-Gel, New Skin Burn Relief Dressings, 2nd Skin, Vigilon; see Figure 42-4F)	Stages II, III, some approved for stage IV Granular or necrotic wound beds Autolysis Some used on partial- and full-thickness burns Punctures	Nonadherent Most are nonocclusive Trauma-free removal Varying absorption capabilities Conformable Some can be used in conjunction with topicals Thermal insulation Reduce pain Moist environment	Most require secondary dressings May macerate periwound skin Some products may dehydrate Slow-to-minimal absorption rate in most Most require frequent/daily dressing change

[a] The trade names listed for each type of wound dressing are given as examples of available products; however, these products do not constitute an all-inclusive list of available wound-dressing products.

Source: Adapted with permission from an unpublished document prepared by McIntosh A, Raher E. Silver Cross Hospital, Joliet, Ill; 1991.

dehydrate a wound by using a foam dressing when there is minimal exudate release. Foam dressings vary in thickness, have different absorbance capacities, and may have adhesive borders and/or waterproof coating on one side. A secondary adhesive dressing is required for those that are nonadhesive.

Alginate dressings are made of soft tan fibers derived from a product of brown seaweed (alginic acid) and are considered more conformable than foam dressings. The fibers are compressed in flat sheets and have a high absorbance capacity; the fibers swell and gel on exposure to fluids, creating a moist mass over the top of the wound. A secondary dressing is required to prevent alginate dressings from drying out, and most require an adhesive dressing to hold them in place.

Carbon-impregnated dressings absorb exudates as well as wound odor.

Composite dressings contain several functional layers, including an absorptive layer to absorb heavy wound exudate.[19]

DRESSINGS THAT MAINTAIN MOISTURE

The need for dressings that absorb drainage decreases as healing moves to the proliferative phase with the formation of new connective tissue. Dressings that maintain natural moisture are then preferred.[19]

Hydrocolloid dressings are generally waterproof and have minimal absorption capacity. They also contain adhesive material that covers the entire dressing surface to keep them in place and minimize the need for frequent dressing changes. Hydrocolloid dressings are available in wafer and paste forms.

Transparent film dressings are transparent thin sheets of polymer material that are coated on one side with adhesive. Although

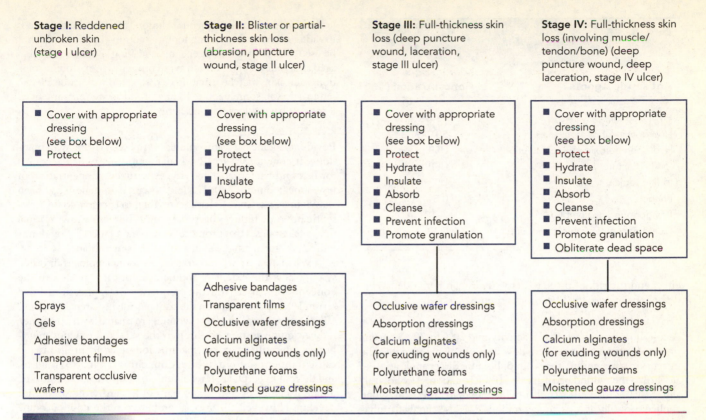

Stage I: Reddened unbroken skin (stage I ulcer)	Stage II: Blister or partial-thickness skin loss (abrasion, puncture wound, stage II ulcer)	Stage III: Full-thickness skin loss (deep puncture wound, laceration, stage III ulcer)	Stage IV: Full-thickness skin loss (involving muscle/tendon/bone) (deep puncture wound, deep laceration, stage IV ulcer)
■ Cover with appropriate dressing (see box below) ■ Protect	■ Cover with appropriate dressing (see box below) ■ Protect ■ Hydrate ■ Insulate ■ Absorb	■ Cover with appropriate dressing (see box below) ■ Protect ■ Hydrate ■ Insulate ■ Absorb ■ Cleanse ■ Prevent infection ■ Promote granulation	■ Cover with appropriate dressing (see box below) ■ Protect ■ Hydrate ■ Insulate ■ Absorb ■ Cleanse ■ Prevent infection ■ Promote granulation ■ Obliterate dead space
Sprays Gels Adhesive bandages Transparent films Transparent occlusive wafers	Adhesive bandages Transparent films Occlusive wafer dressings Calcium alginates (for exuding wounds only) Polyurethane foams Moistened gauze dressings	Occlusive wafer dressings Absorption dressings Calcium alginates (for exuding wounds only) Polyurethane foams Moistened gauze dressings	Occlusive wafer dressings Absorption dressings Calcium alginates (for exuding wounds only) Polyurethane foams Moistened gauze dressings

FIGURE 42-4 Guidelines for product selection on the basis of wound severity. (Adapted with permission from reference 16.)

these film dressings are waterproof, they are capable of allowing adequate gas exchange and maintain a moist wound environment. Transparent film dressings are often used as secondary dressings to both secure and provide a waterproof covering for other dressings.

DRESSINGS THAT PROVIDE MOISTURE

A dry wound that is covered with dead tissue needs to be rehydrated before optimal wound healing can occur. Providing moisture will soften and remove the dead tissue, and promote autolytic debridement, which facilitates the migration of newly formed epithelial tissue to the wound bed. A wound dressing must contain water to effectively add moisture to a wound and promote healing.[19]

Amorphous hydrogels and *hydrogel sheets* are capable of adding moisture to the wound bed and transferring water to tissues. Amorphous hydrogels are clear gels applied directly to the wound surface that release water; hydrogel sheets cover the wound and gradually release water that has been cross-linked in a polymer network to give form. The sheets also provide a cooling effect that soothes the skin and are recommended for painful or inflamed wounds.[20]

Pharmacologic Therapy

Wound Irrigants (Normal Saline)

Wound irrigation is often necessary to clean the wound surface by removing dirt and debris. Normal saline or bottled water is sufficient for irrigation; however, mechanical removal with clean gauze is sometimes appropriate.

First-Aid Antiseptics

Antiseptics are chemical substances designed for application to intact skin up to the edges of a wound, for disinfection purposes. When effective antisepsis is combined with proper wound care technique, including gentle handling of tissue, the infection rate is low. Ideally, antiseptics should exert a sustained effect against all microorganisms without causing tissue damage. However, even therapeutic concentrations of antiseptics can harm tissue. Therefore, antiseptics should be used to disinfect only intact skin after the removal of all organic matter.

Antiseptic active ingredients recognized as safe and effective for use include ethyl alcohol (48%–95%), isopropyl alcohol (50%–91.3%), iodine topical solution USP, iodine tincture USP, povidone/iodine complex (5%–10%), hydrogen peroxide topical solution USP, quaternary ammonium compounds (0.13%), and camphorated phenol (Tables 42-3 and 42-4).

HYDROGEN PEROXIDE

Hydrogen peroxide 3% topical solution USP is a widely used antiseptic. Enzymatic release of oxygen occurs when the hydrogen peroxide comes in contact with the skin, causing an effervescent cleansing action. The duration of action is only as long as the period of active oxygen release. Hydrogen peroxide should be used where released gas can escape; therefore, it should not be used in abscesses, nor should bandages be applied before the compound dries. Using hydrogen peroxide on intact skin is of minimal value, because the release of nascent oxygen is too slow, and the reliance on the effervescent quality of hydrogen peroxide to mechanically debride wounds may come at the expense of tissue toxicity. Because of the limited bactericidal

TABLE 42-3 Nonprescription First-Aid Antiseptic Ingredients	
Antiseptic Agents	**Concentration (%)**
Ethyl alcohol	48–95
Isopropyl alcohol	50.0–91.3
Hydrogen peroxide topical solution	USP
Iodine tincture	USP
Iodine topical solution	USP
Phenol	0.5–1.5
Povidone/iodine complex	5–10
Quaternary ammonium compound	0.13

effect and the risk of tissue toxicity, hydrogen peroxide has little benefit over soapy water for antisepsis.

ETHYL ALCOHOL

Alcohol has good bactericidal activity in a 20% to 70% concentration. Caution must be used, however, when applying it to the intact skin surrounding the wound, because direct application of alcohol to the wound bed can cause tissue irritation. Alcohol usually contains denaturants that will dehydrate the skin when applied topically at high concentrations. It is also highly flammable and must be kept away from fire or flame. Alcohol wash may be used one to three times daily, and the wound may be covered with a sterile bandage after the washed area has dried.

ISOPROPYL ALCOHOL

Isopropyl alcohol 70% aqueous solution, which has somewhat stronger bactericidal activity and lower surface tension than ethyl alcohol, is generally used for its cleansing and antiseptic effects on intact skin. It should not be used to clean open wounds because of possible cytotoxic effects and higher reported infection rates. Isopropyl alcohol has a greater potential for drying the skin (astringent action), because its lipid solvent effects are stronger than those of ethyl alcohol. Similar to ethyl alcohol, it is flammable and must be kept away from fire or flame.

IODINE

Iodine is effective against bacteria, fungi, virus, spores, protozoa, and yeast owing to its ability to oxidize microbial protoplasm.[21] An iodine solution USP of iodine 2% and sodium iodide 2.5% is used as an antiseptic for superficial wounds. An iodine tincture USP of iodine 2%, sodium iodide 2.5, and alcohol about 50% is

TABLE 42-4 Selected Wound Irrigant and Antiseptic Products	
Trade Name	**Primary Ingredients**
Wound Irrigants	
Wound Wash Saline Aerosol	Sodium chloride 0.9%
Antiseptics	
Betadine Skin Cleanser Liquid	Povidone/iodine 7.5%
Campho-Phenique Gel/Liquid	Camphor 10.8%; phenol 4.7%
Unguentine Ointment	Phenol 1%

less preferable than the aqueous solution, because the tincture is irritating to the tissue. Strong iodine solution (Lugol's) must not be used as an antiseptic. In general, bandaging should be discouraged after iodine application to avoid tissue irritation. Iodine solutions stain skin, may be irritating to tissue, and may cause allergic sensitization in some people. Iodine products are recommended if patients have chlorhexidine allergy.[22]

POVIDONE/IODINE

Povidone/iodine is a water-soluble complex of iodine with povidone. It contains 9% to 12% available iodine, which accounts for its rapid bactericidal activity. A reduced concentration of povidone/iodine at 0.001% (e.g., vaginal douches) has been shown to be less toxic to leukocytes than to bacteria, so this antiseptic not only reduces bacterial counts but also allows normal immune responses that promote wound maturation.[21] Povidone/iodine is nonirritating to skin and mucous membranes.

When used as a wound irrigant, povidone/iodine is absorbed systemically; the extent of iodine absorption is related to the concentration used and the frequency of application. Final serum level also depends on the patient's intrinsic renal function. When severe burns and large wounds are treated with povidone/iodine, iodine absorption through the skin and mucous membranes can result in excess systemic iodine concentrations and cause transient thyroid dysfunction, clinical hyperthyroidism, and thyroid hyperplasia. If renal function is normal, the absorbed iodine is rapidly excreted, and signs of hyperthyroidism do not develop. However, the association between the dose of iodine administered and thyroid dysfunction remains controversial. Detergents formed by the combination of surfactants with povidone/iodine have been found to damage wound tissue and potentiate infection. Therefore, these combination products are not recommended for scrubbing wounds.[22]

CAMPHORATED PHENOL

Oily solutions of phenol and camphor are often used as nonprescription first-aid antiseptics. Such products contain relatively high concentrations of phenol (4%) and must be used with caution. If oleaginous phenolic solutions are applied to moist areas, the phenol is partitioned out of the vehicle into water, resulting in caustic concentrations of phenol on the skin. To avoid such damaging effects, these products should be applied to only dry skin. Wounds treated with camphorated phenol should not be bandaged, because the moisture would result in damage.

First-Aid Antibiotics

Topical nonprescription antibiotic agents (e.g., the combination of bacitracin, neomycin, and polymyxin B sulfate) help prevent infection in minor cuts, wounds, scrapes, and burns. When applied within 4 hours of insult, topical antibiotics can reduce the likelihood of wound infection and foster the healing process.[23] Topical and, in some cases, oral antibiotics are indicated in contaminated wounds that have a moderately high risk of infection. However, clean wounds have a low infection rate and do not warrant the use of prophylactic antibiotics. A primary care provider should be consulted if questions arise concerning the degree of contamination and the need for oral antibiotics.

Topical antibiotic preparations should be applied to the wound bed after cleansing and before applying a sterile dressing. Special caution should be taken when applying these preparations to large areas of denuded skin, however, because the potential for systemic toxicity can increase. Prolonged use of these agents may result in the development of resistant bacteria and secondary fungal infection. If significant signs of improvement are not seen within 5 days, the patient should consult a primary care provider.

TABLE 42-5 Selected Antibiotic Products

Trade Name	Primary Ingredients
Betadine First Aid Antibiotics + Moisturizer Ointment	Polymyxin B sulfate 10,000 U/g; bacitracin zinc 500 U/g
Q-tips Treat & Go	Cotton swabs containing bacitracin 500 U/g
Gold Bond First Aid Antibiotic Ointment	Bacitracin zinc 500 U/g; polymyxin B sulfate 10,000 U/g; neomycin base 3.5 mg/g; pramoxine HCL 10 mg
Neosporin Ointment	Polymyxin B sulfate 5000 U/g; bacitracin zinc 400 U/g; neomycin base 3.5 mg/g
Neosporin Plus Pain Relief Ointment	Bacitracin zinc 500 U/g; polymyxin B sulfate 10,000 U/g; neomycin base 3.5 mg/g; pramoxine HCL 10 mg
Neosporin Plus Pain Relief Cream	Polymyxin B sulfate 10,000 U/g; neomycin base 3.5 mg/g; pramoxine HCl 10 mg
Polysporin Ointment/Powder	Polymyxin B sulfate 10,000 U/g; bacitracin zinc 500 U/g

First-aid antibiotics available without a prescription in the United States consist of the active ingredients (Category I) bacitracin, neomycin, and polymyxin B sulfate (Table 42-5).

BACITRACIN

Bacitracin is a polypeptide bactericidal antibiotic that inhibits cell wall synthesis in several gram-positive organisms. The development of resistance in previously sensitive organisms is rare. Minimal absorption occurs with topical administration. The frequency of allergic contact dermatitis (erythema, infiltration, papules, edematous, or vesicular reaction) is approximately 2%. Topical nonprescription preparations usually contain 400 to 500 U/g of ointment and are applied one to three times a day.

NEOMYCIN

Neomycin is an aminoglycoside antibiotic; it exerts its bactericidal activity by irreversibly binding to the 30S ribosomal subunit to inhibit protein synthesis in gram-negative organisms and some species of *Staphylococcus*. Neomycin has been demonstrated to decrease the severity of clinical infection 48 hours after treatment in tape-stripped wounds. Resistant organisms may develop. Neomycin applied topically produces a relatively high rate of hypersensitivity; reactions occur in 3.5% to 6% of patients. Some patients with positive results to neomycin on skin tests will also react to bacitracin. Because the two agents are not chemically related, such responses apparently represent independent sensitization rather than cross-reactions. Although neomycin is not absorbed when applied to intact skin, application to large areas of denuded skin may cause systemic toxicity (ototoxicity and nephrotoxicity).

Neomycin is available in cream and ointment forms, alone or in combination. It is most frequently used in combination with polymyxin and bacitracin to prevent the development of neomycin-resistant organisms. Neomycin has been associated with causing contact dermatitis. However, triple-antibiotic ointment preparations containing neomycin are regularly used by consumers without significant complications. The concentration of neomycin commonly used in nonprescription products is 3.5 mg/g. Applications are made one to three times a day.

POLYMYXIN B SULFATE

Polymyxin B sulfate is a polypeptide antibiotic that is effective against several gram-negative organisms, because it alters the bacterial cell wall permeability. However, its effect on healing is unknown; it also is a rare sensitizer. Concentrations of 5000 U/g and 10,000 U/g are available in nonprescription combination preparations. Applications are usually made one to three times a day.[24]

Product Selection Guidelines

Sterile saline is the preferred choice for effective wound irrigation. The issue of which antiseptic solution is best remains unresolved. When choosing an antiseptic product, one must consider tissue toxicity and costs of the different ingredients.

Topical antibiotics, applied one to three times a day, are effective in eradicating bacteria and producing faster wound healing when combined with appropriate cleansing and the use of proper dressings.

Complementary Therapies

The benefits of vitamins and complementary therapies for wound care remain questionable, because little reliable scientific data exist to substantiate their enhancement of healing. Animal studies have provided some insight on the role of complementary therapies in wound healing, but more reliable human studies are needed to support such claims. Vitamins A and C are believed to enhance collagen synthesis, whereas the antioxidant properties of vitamins C and E may decrease cell destruction by oxygen free radicals. Zinc supplements used to speed wound healing may enhance cell proliferation. Honey is believed to have antibacterial properties and improve healing. Aloe vera's watery composition is thought to increase the migration of epithelial cells to improve wound healing. Practitioners should use their clinical judgment when considering recommending these agents.[25]

Assessment of Minor Wounds and Secondary Bacterial Infections: A Case-Based Approach

The pharmacist should assess the type, depth, location, and degree of contamination of a wound. Visual inspection of the affected area usually provides an accurate evaluation of these factors. The wound should also be assessed for signs of infection. Because noninfectious processes, including drug-induced eruptions, could be involved, the patient's health status and current medication use should also be determined. Antimicrobial agents should generally be recommended when secondary infection is present or might occur.

Cases 42-1 and 42-2 are examples of the assessment of patients with minor wounds.

Relevant Evaluation Criteria	Scenario/Model Outcome
Information Gathering	
1. Gather essential information about the patient's symptoms, including:	
a. description of symptom(s) (i.e., nature, onset, duration, severity, associated symptoms)	Patient has had a wound on the right cheek of her face for more than 2 months. It began as a pimple that later grew bigger and has now turned into a red, swollen sore that is painful to the touch.
	Symptoms appeared 2 months ago as a pimple.
b. description of any factors that seem to precipitate, exacerbate, and/or relieve the patient's symptom(s)	
c. description of the patient's efforts to relieve the symptoms	Patient continues to use an acne cream and hydrogen peroxide with no apparent relief.
2. Gather essential patient history information:	
a. patient's identity	Jill Slater
b. patient's age, sex, height, and weight	26-year-old female, 5 ft 4 in, 135 lb
c. patient's occupation	Graduate college student
d. patient's dietary habits	Well-balanced diet with minimal carbohydrates
e. patient's sleep habits	Averages 6–7 hours per night
f. concurrent medical conditions, prescription and nonprescription medications, and dietary supplements	Occasional ibuprofen for minor aches
g. allergies	Codeine
h. history of other adverse reactions to medications	None
Assessment and Triage	
3. Differentiate the patient's signs/symptoms and correctly identify the patient's primary problem(s) (see Figure 42-4).	Stage II laceration with damage to the entire epidermis and part of the dermis. No puncture involvement. Redness, swelling, pain, and enlargement of wound over a 2-month period were noted.
4. Identify exclusions for self-treatment (see Figure 42-2).	Signs of infection; facial involvement
5. Formulate a comprehensive list of therapeutic alternatives for the primary problem to determine if triage to a medical practitioner is required, and share this information with the patient.	Options include: (1) Recommend self-care management (wound irrigant, antiseptic, antibiotic, and wound dressing). (2) Refer to PCP for further evaluation (3) Recommend self-care management until further medical evaluation can be obtained. (4) Take no action.
Plan	
6. Select an optimal therapeutic alternative to address the patient's problem, taking into account patient preferences.	Refer patient to PCP or dermatologist for further evaluation.
7. Describe the recommended therapeutic approach to the patient.	Continue to keep the wound clean with warm soapy water until you are seen by a practitioner for further evaluation. Discontinue use of hydrogen peroxide; it may further damage the sensitive tissue. In addition, topical antiseptics should be applied to only intact skin to decrease harm to tissues. Application of a topical nonprescription antibiotic containing bacitracin, neomycin, or polymyxin may be somewhat beneficial
8. Explain to the patient the rationale for selecting the recommended therapeutic approach from the considered therapeutic alternatives.	Wounds that appear to be infected require further medical evaluation and treatment with prescription topical and, often, systemic antibiotics.

C A S E   4 2 - 1   *(continued)*

Relevant Evaluation Criteria	Scenario/Model Outcome
Patient Education	
9. When recommending self-care with non-prescription medications and/or nondrug therapy, convey accurate information to the patient.	Criterion does not apply in this case.
10. Solicit follow-up questions from patient.	Should I continue using my acne cream on the wound?
11. Answer patient's questions.	No. The acne cream likely contains benzoyl peroxide or salicylic acid. Both can harm exposed tissue, which will worsen the inflammation and delay healing.

Key: PCP, primary care provider.

C A S E   4 2 - 2

Relevant Evaluation Criteria	Scenario/Model Outcome
Information Gathering	
1. Gather essential information about the patient's symptoms, including:	
a. description of symptom(s) (i.e., nature, onset, duration, severity, associated symptoms)	Patient has suffered from a laceration on the right arm after being cut by a piece of metal at a construction site. The wound is 1-inch long with no dirt or contaminants and was covered with a hand towel to help stop bleeding. However, slight bleeding resumes once the covering is removed, and mild redness and swelling are noted. The patient complains of moderate pain, but he has not taken any pain reliever to resolve this symptom.
b. description of any factors that seem to precipitate, exacerbate, and/or relieve the patient's symptom(s)	Symptoms appeared after patient was cut by a piece of metal.
c. description of the patient's efforts to relieve the symptoms	Covered with a hand towel for slight compression
2. Gather essential patient history information:	
a. patient's identity	Joe Assan
b. patient's age, sex, height, and weight	26-year-old male, 5 ft 6 in, 135 lb
c. patient's occupation	Construction worker
d. patient's dietary habits	Well-balanced diet with lots of meat and rice
e. patient's sleep habits	Averages 6–7 hours per night
f. concurrent medical conditions, prescription and nonprescription medications, and dietary supplements	Occasional Tylenol for muscle aches
g. allergies	NKA
h. history of other adverse reactions to medications	None

CASE 42-2 *(continued)*

Relevant Evaluation Criteria	Scenario/Model Outcome
Assessment and Triage	
3. Differentiate the patient's signs/symptoms and correctly identify the patient's primary problem(s) (see Figure 42-4).	Stage II laceration with damage to the entire epidermis and part of the dermis, but no puncture involvement
4. Identify exclusions for self-treatment (see Figure 42-2).	None
5. Formulate a comprehensive list of therapeutic alternatives for the primary problem to determine if triage to a medical practitioner is required, and share this information with the patient.	Options include: (1) Recommend self-care management (wound irrigant, antiseptic, antibiotic, and wound dressing). (2) Refer to PCP for further evaluation. (3) Recommend self-care management until further medical evaluation can be obtained. (4) Take no action.
Plan	
6. Select an optimal therapeutic alternative to address the patient's problem, taking into account patient preferences.	The patient prefers to self-treat the wound with soapy water, a topical antibiotic, and a wound dressing.
7. Describe the recommended therapeutic approach to the patient.	Clean the wound with warm soapy water to remove debris, and let wound air dry. Apply a topical antibiotic combination that contains a pain reliever such as Gold Bond First Aid Antibiotic Ointment (see Table 42-5). Cover with a nonadherent gauze such as Vaseline Gauze followed by a secondary dressing such as Kerlix Bandage Roll to provide more absorption and to maintain moisture; then secure dressings with bandage tape (see Table 42-2). The dressing should be changed regularly according to the amount of drainage. A more absorbent dressing may be necessary if frequent dressing changes are required.
8. Explain to the patient the rationale for selecting the recommended therapeutic approach from the considered therapeutic alternatives.	Minor wounds are generally appropriate for self-treatment, because the deep layers of the skin have not been damaged and there is no indication of puncture or infection.
Patient Education	
9. When recommending self-care with nonprescription medications and/or nondrug therapy, convey accurate information to the patient.	See the box Patient Education for Acute Wounds.
10. Solicit follow-up questions from patient.	What can I take to stop the pain?
11. Answer patient's questions.	In addition to the topical anesthetic in the ointment that you apply, you may take a regular pain reliever such as acetaminophen or ibuprofen for pain relief.

Key: NKA, no known allergies; PCP, primary care provider.

Patient Counseling for Minor Wounds and Secondary Bacterial Infections

When assessing the wound type, the practitioner should remember that minor cuts and abrasions may be self-treated, whereas chronic and more severe acute wounds or those that appear infected should first be evaluated by a primary care provider (see Classification of Wounds and Figure 42-2). Irrigation with soapy water or normal saline is generally recommended if a wound is dirty. Patients should be instructed to change the dressing only when it is dirty or not intact. The practitioner should ensure that the patient understands the basic steps in wound care, especially the selection of appropriate wound dressings. An explanation of basic skin physiology and the wound-healing process will enhance patient compliance. The box Patient Education for Acute Wounds lists specific information to provide patients. The patient should consult a primary care provider if the wound does not show signs of healing after 5 days of self-treatment.

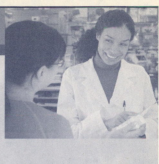

PATIENT EDUCATION FOR
Acute Wounds

The objective of self-treatment is to promote healing by protecting the wound from infection or further trauma. For most patients, carefully following product instructions and the self-care measures listed here will help ensure optimal therapeutic outcomes.

- Position the wound above the level of the heart to slow bleeding and relieve throbbing pain.
- If the wound is dirty, irrigate it with normal saline solution, which is not toxic to cells. Use antiseptic solutions selectively and cautiously. Any inflammation should subside within 12–24 hours.
- When cleansing with soapy water, wash hands, apply mild liquid soap (e.g., Dove soap) to a wet cotton ball, and gently wash the wound area; rinse under running warm water and gently pat the area dry.
- Cover the wound with a dressing that will keep the wound site moist. Make sure the dressing is the appropriate size and contour for the affected body part.
- Continue using a wound dressing until the wound bed has firmly closed and signs of inflammation in surrounding tissue have subsided. This process usually takes 2–3 weeks. Failure to keep the wound covered may delay healing.

- Avoid disrupting the dressing unnecessarily; change it only if it is dirty or is not intact. Most dressings should be changed every 3–5 days. Frequent changes may remove resurfacing layers of epithelium and slow the healing process. Change dressing if excessive fluid is released.
- Use a mild analgesic to control pain.
- All wound dressings should be kept in their original packaging and stored away from moisture.
- Observe the wound for signs of infection. Redness, swelling, and exudate are a normal part of healing; foul odor is not.

 Consult a primary care provider if infection is suspected or the wound does not show signs of healing after 5 days of self-treatment.

Evaluation of Patient Outcomes for Minor Wounds and Secondary Bacterial Infections

The practitioner should check the patient's progress after 5 days. Visual inspection, if possible, is the best method of assessing the healing process; therefore, a scheduled visit to see the practitioner is preferable. If the wound shows no signs of healing or has worsened (i.e., foul odor, worsened inflammation, etc.), the patient should see a primary care provider for more aggressive therapy.

Key Points for Minor Wounds and Secondary Bacterial Infections

➤ Self-treatment of minor acute wounds is appropriate.
➤ First-aid antibiotics are used to prevent infection.
➤ Moist wound healing is now considered the standard of care.
➤ Proper selection of first-aid products, including appropriate wound dressing, is key.

REFERENCES

1. *F-D-C-Reports—The Tan Sheet*. 2001;9(6):12.
2. Capellan O, Hollander JE. Management of lacerations in the emergency department. *Emerg Med Clin North Am*. 2003;21:205.
3. Hunt TK, Hopf H, Hussain Z. Physiology of wound healing. *Adv Skin Wound Care*. 2000;13(suppl 2):6–11.
4. Parker L. Applying the principles of infection control to wound care. *Br J Nurs*. 2000;9:394–6, 398, 400.
5. Pearson AS, Wolford RW. Management of skin trauma. *Dermatology*. 2000;27:475–91.
6. Dabrowski GP, Rombeau JL. Practical nutritional management in the trauma intensive care unit. *Surg Clin North Am*. 2000;8:921–32.
7. Green S, McLaren S. Nutrition and wound healing. *Commun Nurse*. 1998;4:29–32.
8. Partridge C. Influential factors in surgical wound healing. *J Wound Care*. 1998;7:350–3.
9. Lenhardt R, Hopf HW, Marker E, et al. Perioperative collagen deposition in elderly and young men and women. *Arch Surg*. 2000;135:71–4.
10. Wilson JA, Clark JJ. Obesity: impediment to wound healing. *Crit Care Nurs Q*. 2003 April–June;26:119–32.
11. Velander P, Theopod C, Hirsch T, et al. Impaired wound healing in an acute diabetic pig model and the affects of hyperglycemia. *Wound Repair Regen*. 2008 March–April; 16:288–93.
12. Phillips SJ. Physiology of wound healing and surgical wound care. *ASAIO J*. 2000:46(suppl 6):S2–S5.
13. Lindsay-Garvey J. Wound Management: A Long Road to Wound Management. Nurseweek. 2005. Available at: http://www.nurseweek.com/news/Features/05-05/Clinical_WoundHealing.asp. Last accessed September 30, 2008.
14. Wiechula R. The use of moist healing dressings in the management of split-thickness skin graft donor sites: a systemic review. *Int J Nurs Pract*. 2003;9(suppl 2):S9–S17.
15. Mionelli GT, Lawrence WT. *Surg Clin North Am*. 2003;83:617.
16. Jeter KF, Tintle TE. Wound dressings of the nineties: indications and contraindications. *Clin Podiatr Med Surg*. 1991;8:799–816.
17. *F-D-C-Reports—The Gray Sheet*. 2001;27(12):22.
18. *F-D-C-Reports—The Tan Sheet*. 2001;27(23):25.
19. Thompson G, Stephen-Hayes J. An overview of wound healing and exudates management. *Br J Community Nurs*. 2007;12(12):S22, S24–6, S28–S30.
20. Lay-Flurrie K. The properties of hydrogel dressings and their impact on wound healing. *Prof Nurse*. 2004;19:269–73
21. Pearson AS, Wolford RW. Dermatology: management of skin trauma. *Prim Care*. 27:475, 2000.
22. Gouin S, Patel H. Office management of minor wounds. *Can Fam Physician*. 2001;47:769–74.
23. Fletcher J. Choosing an appropriate antibacterial dressing. *Nurs Times*. 2006;102(44):46, 48–9.
24. Sanford JP. *Guide to Antimicrobial Therapy*. Dallas: Antimicrobial Therapy; 2001.
25. MacKay D, Miller AL. Nutritional support for wound healing. *Altern Med Rev*. 2003;8: 359–77.

Fungal Skin Infections

Gail D. Newton and Nicholas G. Popovich

Fungal skin infections, or dermatomycoses, are among the most common cutaneous disorders.[1] They are often referred to as ringworm, because their characteristic lesions are ring-shaped with clear centers and red, scaly borders. However, these lesions can vary from the ring form and may present as single or multiple lesions ranging from mild scaling to deep granulomas (inflamed, nodular-size lesions).

Fungal infections are usually superficial and can involve the hair, nails, and skin. The term *tinea* refers exclusively to dermatophyte infections. Most often, tinea infections are named according to the area of the body that is affected (i.e., scalp [tinea capitis], groin [tinea cruris], body [tinea corporis], feet [tinea pedis], and nails [tinea unguium]). These infections are generally caused by three genera of fungi: *Trichophyton, Microsporum,* and *Epidermophyton.* Species of *Candida* and other yeasts may also be involved[2]; however, currently available nonprescription antifungals are not indicated for self-management of cutaneous infections secondary to the latter microorganisms.[3]

Although many pathogenic fungi exist in the environment, the overall prevalence of actual superficial fungal infections is remarkably low. An estimated 10% to 20% of the U.S. population suffer from a tinea infection at any one time.[4,5] Many degrees of susceptibility, from instantaneous "takes" by a single spore to severe trauma with massive exposure, produce a clinical infection. It appears, however, that trauma to the skin, especially that which produces blisters (e.g., from wearing ill-fitting footwear), may be significantly more important to the occurrence of human fungal infections than is simple exposure to the offending pathogens.[5] Other predisposing factors for the development of tinea infections include diabetes mellitus and other debilitating diseases associated with immune system depression, use of immunosuppressive drugs, impaired circulation, poor nutrition and hygiene, trauma, occlusion of the skin, and warm, humid climates.[5,6]

The most prevalent cutaneous fungal infection in humans is tinea pedis (dermatophytosis of the foot, or athlete's foot). Tinea pedis afflicts approximately 26.5 million people in the United States every year—of every 10 sufferers, 7 are male. Tinea pedis is rare among blacks but common in whites, particularly those who live in urban tropical areas.[7] An estimated 70% of people will be afflicted with athlete's foot in their lifetime. Approximately 45% will suffer with it episodically for more than 10 years. When exposure to infectious environments is equal, the incidence of tinea infections in women approaches that in men.[4,5,8,9] Although tinea pedis may occur at all ages, it is more common in adults, presumably because of their increased opportunities for exposure to pathogens.[5]

Individuals who use public pools or bathing facilities are at greater risk for the development of tinea pedis than the general population. However, tinea pedis may be acquired in the home if one or more members of the household are already infected. High-impact sports that cause chronic trauma to the feet, such as long-distance running, also predispose athletes to tinea pedis.[10–12] This trauma affords infecting fungi the opportunity to invade the outer layers of the skin. In addition, wearing socks and shoes exacerbates the problem by impeding the dispersion of heat and the evaporation of moisture, both of which facilitate fungal growth. In contrast, individuals who most often wear footwear that allows the feet to remain cool and dry (e.g., sandals) are less likely to develop tinea pedis.

Tinea unguium, also called ringworm of the nails or onychomycosis, is sometimes associated with tinea pedis. More than 2.5 million Americans are treated annually for tinea unguium. However, because many cases go untreated, the actual incidence of this infection is probably much higher.[13] Onychomycosis cannot be managed with topical nonprescription antifungals. Rather, the affected nail must be treated with systemic drug therapy (e.g., terbinafine or itraconazole) or removed surgically to rid the area of the offending fungus.

The next two most common infections are tinea corporis and tinea cruris. Tinea corporis, also called ringworm of the body, is most common in prepubescent individuals. It is frequently transmitted among children in day care centers. However, it is also more common in adults and children who live in hot, humid climates. Individuals who are under stress or overweight are also at increased risk for the development of tinea corporis.[14,15]

Tinea cruris, or jock itch, is most common during warm weather, but it can occur at any time of the year when the skin in the groin area is kept warm and moist for long periods of time. For example, sweating or prolonged contact with wet clothing provides an ideal environment for the growth of fungi. Tinea cruris occurs more often in men than in women and rarely affects children. Several reasons exist for more frequent infections in males than in females: (1) males wear more occlusive clothing, (2) scrotal skin may increase occlusion of the groin area, (3) males generally are more active than females, and (4) males have a greater incidence of other tinea infections that may serve as a reservoir for generating new cases of tinea cruris.[14] Close indirect or direct physical contact between infected males and noninfected females does not mitigate the higher prevalence of tinea cruris in males.[5] For example, females who live in the same household with infected males do not develop infections at the same rate as non-infected males in the same household.

Although its true incidence is unknown, tinea capitis, or ringworm of the scalp, occurs most often in children, because they are more likely to have contact with infected individuals and because they are less attentive to personal hygiene than adults. Black female children are infected more often than black males and white children, possibly because of the hair care products and practices (e.g., occlusive hair dressings and tight braiding) that are unique to this population.[5,14]

Tinea capitis can be spread by direct contact with an infected person, but it is often spread by contact with infected fomites (e.g., using infected combs, hats, toys or telephones; wearing infected clothing; using infected towels; or sleeping on infected linens). In some instances, tinea capitis is spread through contact with other infected individuals or with infected cats or dogs.[16]

Pathophysiology of Fungal Skin Infections

Tinea infections are caused by three genera of pathogenic fungi: *Trichophyton, Microsporum,* and *Epidermophyton.* Tinea pedis and tinea cruris are caused by species of *Epidermophyton* and *Trichophyton.* Species of *Trichophyton* and *Microsporum* cause ringworm of the scalp. All species of the three genera can cause tinea corporis.[5] Fungal transmission can occur through contact with infected people, animals, soil, or fomites. Dermatophytes are classified on the basis of their habitat: anthropophilic (humans), zoophilic (animals), and geophilic (soil). Most tinea infections are caused by person–to–person contact with individuals infected with anthropophilic dermatophytes.[14]

In addition to specific fungi, other environmental factors contribute to the disease's development, such as climate and social customs. Footwear is a key variable, as illustrated by the incidence of tinea pedis in any population that wears occlusive footwear, especially in the summer and in tropical or subtropical climates. Nonporous shoe material increases temperature and hydration of the skin, which interferes with the barrier function of the stratum corneum. Similarly, sweating or wearing wet clothing for long periods of time can predispose individuals to the development of tinea corporis and tinea cruris.

Chronic health problems and medications that weaken or suppress the immune system can also increase the risk for development of tinea infections. For example, patients with diabetes and persons of advanced age taking medications such as glucocorticoids should be instructed to monitor themselves for the signs and symptoms of tinea infections. They should also be instructed about the importance of proper hygiene and diet for the prevention of tinea infections as well as other health problems.

After inoculation of a dermatophyte into the skin under suitable conditions, a tinea infection progresses through several stages. These stages include periods of incubation and then enlargement, followed by a refractory period and a stage of involution. During the incubation period, the dermatophyte grows in the stratum corneum, sometimes with minimal signs of infection. After the incubation period and once the infection is established, two factors appear to play a role in determining the size and duration of the lesions: the growth rate of the organism and the epidermal turnover rate.[17] The fungal growth rate must equal or exceed the epidermal turnover rate, or the organism will be quickly shed.

Dermatophytid infestations remain within the stratum corneum. This resistance to the spread of infection seems to involve both immunologic and nonimmunologic mechanisms. For example, the presence of a serum inhibitory factor (SIF) appears to limit the growth of dermatophytes beyond the stratum corneum. SIF is not an antibody but a dialyzable, heat-labile component of fresh sera. It appears that SIF chelates the iron that dermatophytes need for continued growth.[17] Once in the stratum corneum, dermatophytes produce keratinases and other proteolytic enzymes that cause allergic reactions when they reach living epidermis.[5]

The major immunologic defense against fungal skin infections is the type IV delayed–hypersensitivity response. The refractory period precedes complete development of this cell-mediated immunity. The fungal growth rate typically exceeds epidermal turnover, and inflammation and pruritus are at their peak. After development of an adequate immune response, symptoms of superficial fungal infections diminish, and the infection may clear spontaneously during the involution period. Patients with chronic infections typically present with much less inflammation. This presentation may be due to a suppressed hypersensitivity response, which in turn reduces the inflammatory response.[2]

Clinical Presentation of Fungal Skin Infections

The clinical spectrum of tinea infections ranges from mild itching and scaling to a severe, exudative inflammatory process characterized by denudation, fissuring, crusting, and/or discoloration of the affected skin. Individuals experiencing their first tinea infection and patients with infections secondary to zoophilic fungi tend to present with greater inflammation.[14] Table 43–1 summarizes key differences between fungal skin infections, contact dermatitis, and bacterial skin infection.

Tinea Pedis

Clinically, there are four accepted variants of tinea pedis; two or more of these types may overlap. The most common is the chronic, intertriginous type,[5] characterized by fissuring, scaling, or maceration in the interdigital spaces, malodor, pruritus, and/or a stinging sensation on the feet (see Color Plates, photograph 29). Typically, the infection involves the lateral toe webs, usually between either the fourth and fifth, or the third and fourth toes. From these sites, the infection may spread to the sole or instep of the foot but rarely to the dorsum. Warmth and humidity aggravate this condition; consequently, hyperhidrosis (excessive sweating) becomes an underlying problem and must be treated along with the dermatophyte infestation.[5]

Normal resident aerobic diphtheroids may become involved in the athlete's foot process. After initial invasion of the stratum corneum by dermatophytes, enough moisture may accumulate to trigger a bacterial overgrowth. Increased moisture and temperature then lead to the release of metabolic products, which diffuse easily through the underlying horny layer already damaged by fungal invasion. In more severe cases, gram-negative

TABLE 43-1 Differentiation of Fungal Skin Infections and Skin Disorders with Similar Presentation

Criterion	Fungal Skin Infections	Contact Dermatitis	Bacterial Skin Infection
Location	On areas of the body where excess moisture accumulates such as the feet, groin area, scalp, and under the arms	Any area of the body exposed to the allergen/irritant; hands, face, legs, ears, eyes, anogenital area involved most often	Anywhere on the body
Signs	Presents either as soggy malodorous, thickened skin; acute vesicular rash; or fine scaling of affected area with varying degrees of inflammation; cracks and fissures may also be present	Presents as a variety of lesions from raised wheals to fluid-filled vesicles, or both	Presents as a variety of lesions from macules to pustules to ulcers with redness surrounding the lesion, which often are warmer than surrounding, unaffected skin
Symptoms	Itching and pain	Itching and pain	Irritation and pain
Quantity/severity	Usually localized to one region of the body but can spread	Affects all areas of exposed skin but does not spread	Usually localized to one region of the body but can spread
Timing	Variable onset	Variable onset from immediately after exposure to 3 weeks after contact	Variable onset
Cause	Superficial fungal infection	Exposure to skin irritants or allergens	Superficial bacterial infection
Modifying factors	Treated with nonprescription astringents, antifungals, and nondrug measures to keep the area clean and dry	Treated with topical antipruritics, skin protectants, astringents, and nondrug measures to avoid reexposure	Treated with prescription antibiotics

organisms intrude and may exacerbate the condition, causing skin maceration, white hyperkeratosis, or erosions with increased patient symptomatology.[5]

The second variant of athlete's foot is known as the chronic, papulosquamous pattern.[5] It is usually found on both feet and is characterized by mild inflammation and diffuse, moccasin-like scaling on the soles of the feet. Tinea unguium (i.e., ringworm of the nails, or onychomycosis) of one or more toenails may also be present and may continue to fuel the infection. The toenails must first be cured with oral drug therapy, such as itraconazole, ketoconazole, or terbinafine, or must be removed surgically to rid the area of the offending fungus.

The third variant of tinea pedis is the vesicular type, usually caused by *Trichophyton mentagrophytes* var. *interdigitale*.[5] Small vesicles or vesicopustules are observed near the instep and on the mid-anterior plantar surface. Skin scaling is seen on these areas as well as on the toe webs. This variant is symptomatic in the summer and is clinically quiescent during the cooler months.

The acute ulcerative type is the fourth variant of tinea pedis. It is often associated with macerated, denuded, weeping ulcerations on the sole of the foot. Typically, white hyperkeratosis and a pungent odor are present. This type of infection, which is complicated by an overgrowth of opportunistic, gram-negative bacteria such as *Proteus* and *Pseudomonas*, has been called dermatophytosis complex, and it may produce an extremely painful, erosive, purulent interspace that can impede the patient's ability to walk.[5]

Tinea Unguium

Nails affected by tinea unguium gradually lose their normal shiny luster and become opaque. If left untreated, the nails become thick, rough, yellow, opaque, and friable. The nail may separate from the nail bed if the infection progresses secondarily to subungual hyperkeratosis. Ultimately, the nail may be lost altogether. Subungual debris also provides an excellent medium for the growth of opportunistic bacteria and other microorganisms, which can lead to further, infectious complications.[5]

Tinea Corporis

Tinea corporis may have a diverse clinical presentation. Most often, the lesions, which involve glabrous (smooth and bare) skin, begin as small, circular, erythematous, scaly areas. The lesions spread peripherally, and the borders may contain vesicles or pustules. Infected individuals may also complain of pruritus.[18]

Tinea corporis can occur on any part of the body. However, the location of the infection can provide clues to the type of infecting dermatophyte. For example, zoophilic dermatophytes often infect areas of exposed skin such as the neck, face, and arms. In contrast, infections secondary to anthropophilic dermatophytes often occur in occluded areas or in areas of trauma.[5]

Tinea Cruris

Tinea cruris occurs on the medial and upper parts of the thighs and the pubic area, and is more common in males. The lesions have well-demarcated margins that are elevated slightly and are more erythematous than the central area; small vesicles may be seen, especially at the margins. Acute lesions are bright red, and chronic cases tend to have more of a hyperpigmented appearance; fine scaling is usually present. This condition is generally bilateral with significant pruritus; however, the lesions usually spare the penis and scrotum. This characteristic can help to distinguish this infection from candidiasis, which does cause lesions in these areas.[19] Pain may also be present during periods of sweating or when the skin becomes macerated or infected by a secondary microorganism.[4,5]

Tinea Capitis

Clinically, tinea capitis may present as one of four variant patterns, depending on the causative dermatophyte. In noninflammatory tinea capitis, lesions begin as small papules surrounding individual hair shafts. Subsequently, the lesions spread centrifugally to involve all hairs in their path. Although there is some scaling of the scalp, little inflammation is present (see Color Plates, photograph 30). Hairs in the lesions are a dull gray color (because they are coated with arthrospores) and usually break off above scalp level.[5]

The inflammatory type of tinea capitis produces a spectrum of inflammation, ranging from pustules to kerion formation. Kerions are weeping lesions whose exudate forms thick crusts on the scalp.[8] Individuals with this type of tinea capitis also may complain more about pruritus in addition to fever and pain. Regional lymph nodes may also be enlarged.[5]

The black dot variety of tinea capitis was named for the appearance of infected areas of the scalp. The location of arthrospores on the hair shaft causes hairs to break off at the level of the scalp, leaving black dots on the scalp surface. Hair loss, inflammation, and scaling with this type of tinea capitis range from minimal to extensive. Therefore, this variant is especially challenging to diagnose.[5,20,21]

The favus variant of tinea capitis typically presents as patchy areas of hair loss and yellowish crusts and scales known as scutula. Ultimately, these lesions can coalesce to involve a major portion of the scalp. If left untreated, this condition can lead to scalp atrophy, scarring, and permanent hair loss.[5]

Complications ranging from secondary infections to permanent hair loss or scarring may occur if tinea infections are not effectively treated.

Treatment of Fungal Skin Infections

Treatment Goals

The goals of treating fungal skin infections are to (1) provide symptomatic relief, (2) eradicate existing infection, and (3) prevent future infections.

General Treatment Approach

In many instances, patients can effectively self-treat tinea pedis, tinea corporis, and tinea cruris with nonprescription topical antifungals and nonpharmacologic measures. However, individuals with tinea unguium or tinea capitis should be referred to a primary care provider for treatment.

Patients who want to improve the appearance of the nail during prescription treatment can use Fungal Nail Revitalizer to reduce nail discoloration and to smooth out the thick, rough nail. This product contains calcium carbonate (a strong alkali) and urea (a protein denaturant) to debride nail tissue. The patient should apply the cream over the entire surface of the infected nail, scrub this area for at least 1 minute with the provided nailbrush, and then wash and dry the nail completely. For optimum results, this procedure should be performed daily for 3 weeks.

Before recommending therapy, the practitioner must be reasonably sure that the lesions are consistent with a tinea infection. Their appearance should conform to the descriptions provided in Clinical Presentation of Fungal Skin Infections, and photographs 29 and 30 of the tinea lesions (see Color Plates) should be consulted for comparison. Furthermore, the lesions should not resemble any other skin conditions covered in this text. When in doubt about the true cause of a condition, the patient should be advised to consult a primary care provider or dermatologist. Figure 43-1 outlines the appropriate self-treatment options for fungal skin infections as well as exclusions for self-treatment.

A number of topical antifungals are available in a variety of dosage forms for self-treatment of fungal skin infections. The selection of a particular product depends on the type of infection and on individual patient characteristics and preferences. For example, in acute, inflammatory tinea pedis, characterized by reddened, oozing, and vesicular eruptions, the inflammation must be counteracted with solutions of astringent aluminum salts before antifungal therapy can be instituted.

A critical determinant of the outcome of therapy is the patient's ability to comply with the recommended therapy for the appropriate length of time. Compliance may be difficult because these conditions may take between 2 and 4 weeks to resolve. Patients may be tempted to terminate therapy when their symptoms subside but before the infection has been eradicated. Another determinant of therapeutic outcome relates to the patient's compliance with the nonpharmacologic measures intended to complement the effects of nonprescription antifungals and to prevent future infections. These measures include keeping the skin clean and dry, avoiding the sharing of personal articles, and avoiding contact with persons who have a fungal infection or contact with infected fomites.

Nonpharmacologic Therapy

The box Patient Education for Fungal Skin Infections located at the end of the chapter describes nonpharmacologic measures intended to complement the effects of nonprescription antifungals and to prevent future infections. The patient should follow these measures during and after treatment of the infection.

Pharmacologic Therapy

An antifungal ingredient must have at least one well-designed clinical trial demonstrating its effectiveness in treating athlete's foot before the Food and Drug Administration (FDA) will classify it as Category I (Table 43-2).[22] Butenafine hydrochloride, clioquinol, clotrimazole, haloprogin, miconazole nitrate, povidone/iodine, terbinafine hydrochloride, tolnaftate, and various undecylenates are considered safe and effective for nonprescription use in the treatment of fungal skin infections.[3] Except for povidone/iodine, these agents are labeled for treatment of athlete's foot, jock itch, and body ringworm. Although considered safe and effective for treating fungal skin infections, povidone/iodine products do not carry an indication for these infections. Recommended treatment period is a minimum of 2 to 4 weeks.

Clioquinol

Although FDA has approved clioquinol 3% for nonprescription use, no commercially available nonprescription topical antifungals currently contain this agent.

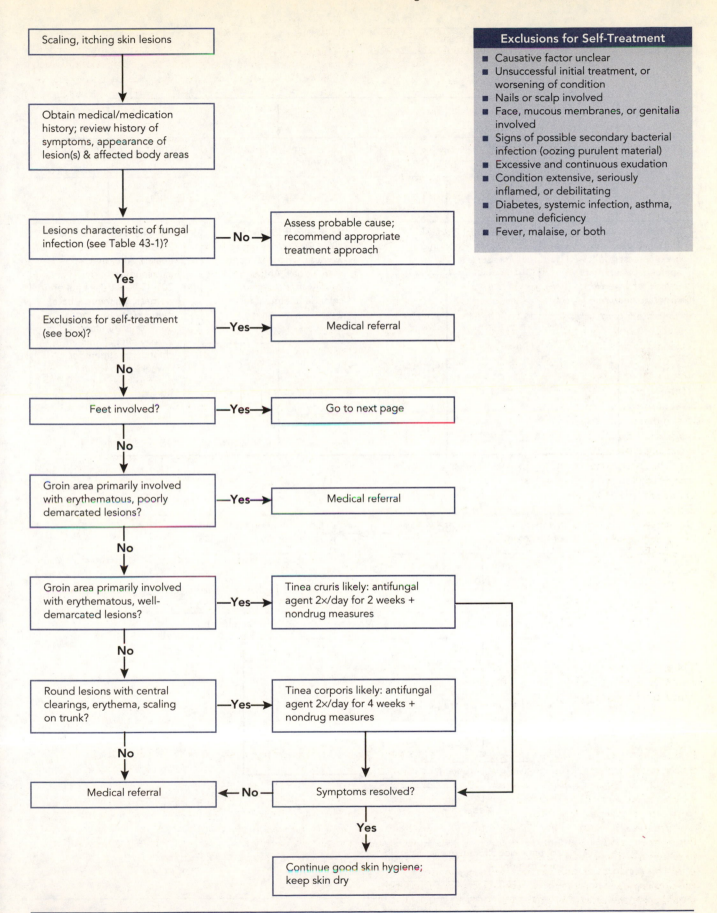

FIGURE 43-1 Self-care of fungal skin infections. *(continued on next page)*

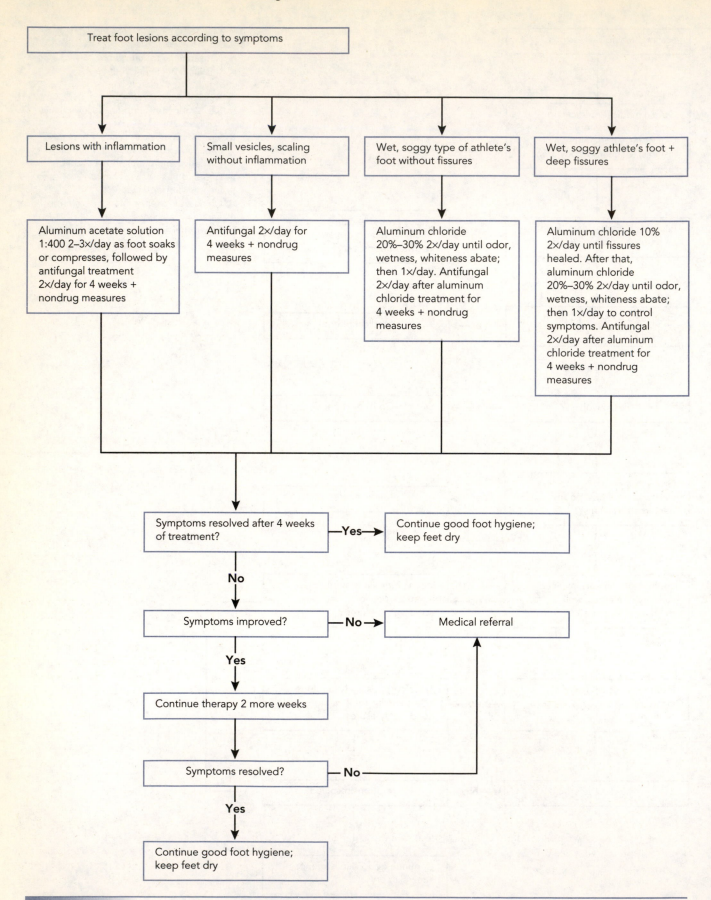

FIGURE 43-1 *(Continued)* Self-care of fungal skin infections.

TABLE 43-2 FDA-Approved Nonprescription Topical Antifungal Drugs

Drug	Concentration (%)
Butenafine hydrochloride	1
Clioquinol	3
Clotrimazole	1
Haloprogin	1
Miconazole nitrate	2
Terbinafine hydrochloride	1
Tolnaftate	1
Povidone/iodine	10
Undecylenic acid and its salts	10–25

Source: Reference 3 and Center for Drug Evaluation Research Approval Package for: Lotrimin Ultra (Butenafine Hydrochloride) Cream. Company: Schering-Plough HealthCare Products Application No.: 21-307 Approval date:12/7/2001. Available at: http://www.fda.gov/cder/foi/nda/2001/21-307_Lotrimin.htm.

Clotrimazole and Miconazole Nitrate

Clotrimazole and miconazole nitrate are imidazole derivatives that demonstrate fungistatic/fungicidal activity (depending on concentration) against *T. mentagrophytes, Trichophyton rubrum, Epidermophyton floccosum,* and *Candida albicans.*

These agents act by inhibiting the biosynthesis of ergosterol and other sterols, and by damaging the fungal cell wall membrane, thereby altering its permeability and resulting in the loss of essential intracellular elements. These drugs have also been shown to inhibit the oxidative and peroxidative enzyme activity that results in intracellular buildup of toxic concentrations of hydrogen peroxide; this toxicity may then contribute to the degradation of subcellular organelles and to cellular necrosis. In *C. albicans,* such drugs have been shown to inhibit the transformation of blastospores into the invasive mycelial form that causes infection.

FDA classified clotrimazole and miconazole nitrate as safe and effective for topical nonprescription use in treating tinea pedis, tinea cruris, and tinea corporis. Clotrimazole and miconazole nitrate are suggested for application twice daily, once in the morning and once in the evening for up to 4 weeks.

Rare cases of mild skin irritation, burning, and stinging have occurred with their use. No drug–drug interactions have been reported with topical use of clotrimazole and miconazole nitrate for up to 4 weeks.

Haloprogin

Although FDA has approved haloprogin 1% for nonprescription use, no commercially available nonprescription topical antifungals currently contain this agent.

Terbinafine Hydrochloride

Topical terbinafine hydrochloride 1% was reclassified as a nonprescription medication in 1999 under the trade name Lamisil AT. This product is available as a cream and a spray.

This antifungal agent inhibits squalene epoxidase, a key enzyme in fungi sterol biosynthesis. This action results in a deficiency in ergosterol and a corresponding accumulation of squalene within the fungal cell, causing fungal cell death.

Terbinafine hydrochloride is indicated for interdigital tinea pedis, tinea cruris, and tinea corporis caused by *E. floccosum, T. mentagrophytes,* and *T. rubrum.* Similar to miconazole and clotrimazole, terbinafine hydrochloride should be applied sparingly to the affected area twice daily.

In clinical trials this drug demonstrated it could cure athlete's foot with 1 week of treatment. However, complete resolution of symptoms may require up to 4 weeks of treatment.

Clinical trials to date have demonstrated a low incidence of side effects for terbinafine hydrochloride. These side effects include irritation (1%), burning (0.8%), and itching/dryness (0.2%).[23,24] No drug–drug interactions have been reported with topical use of terbinafine hydrochloride.

Butenafine Hydrochloride

Topical butenafine hydrochloride 1% was reclassified as a nonprescription medication in 2001 under the trade name Lotrimin Ultra. This product is available as a cream.

Like terbinafine, this antifungal agent is a squalene epoxidase inhibitor. This action results in a deficiency in ergosterol, a corresponding accumulation of squalene within the fungal cell, and cell death.

Butenafine hydrochloride is indicated as a cure for athlete's foot between the toes, jock itch, and ringworm caused by *E. floccosum, T. mentagrophytes,* and *T. rubrum.* Similar to other antifungals, it also relieves the itching, burning, cracking, and scaling that can accompany these conditions. Effectiveness on the bottom or sides of the foot is unknown.

Patients suffering from athlete's foot should be advised to apply a thin film to affected skin between and around toes twice daily for 1 week, once a day for 4 weeks, or as directed by a primary care provider. Patients with jock itch or ringworm should apply a thin film to the affected area once daily for 2 weeks or as directed by a primary care provider.

Effective treatment rates for interdigital tinea pedis with 1-week and 4-week application durations are reported to be approximately 38% and 74%, respectively. In clinical trials, Lotrimin Ultra kept users free of athlete's foot for up to 3 months.[25] To date, clinical trials demonstrate a low incidence of side effects. No drug–drug interactions have been reported with topical use of butenafine hydrochloride.

Tolnaftate

Tolnaftate has demonstrated clinical efficacy since its commercial introduction in the United States in 1965. In addition, it was the standard against which the efficacy of other topical antifungals was compared for many years.

Although tolnaftate's exact mechanism of action has not been reported, it is believed that tolnaftate distorts the hyphae and stunts the mycelial growth of the fungi species. Tolnaftate is the only nonprescription drug approved for both preventing and treating athlete's foot.[3] It acts on fungi typically responsible for tinea infections, including *T. mentagrophytes, T. rubrum,* and *E. floccosum.*

Tolnaftate is valuable primarily in the dry, scaly type of athlete's foot. Superficial fungal infection relapse has occurred after tolnaftate therapy has been discontinued. Relapse may be caused by inadequate duration of treatment, patient nonadherence with the medication, or use of tolnaftate when an oral antifungal should have been used.

As a cream, tolnaftate is formulated in a polyethylene glycol 400/propylene glycol vehicle. The 1% solution is formulated in polyethylene glycol 400 and may be more effective than the cream. The solution solidifies when exposed to cold but liquefies with no loss in potency if allowed to warm. These vehicles are particularly advantageous in superficial antifungal therapy, because they are nonocclusive, nontoxic, nonsensitizing, water miscible, anhydrous, easy to apply, and efficient in delivering the drug to the affected area.

The topical powder formulation of tolnaftate uses cornstarch/talc as the vehicle. Because the two agents absorb water, this vehicle not only is an effective drug delivery system but also offers a therapeutic advantage. The topical aerosol formulation of tolnaftate includes talc, alcohol, and the propellant vehicle.

Tolnaftate (1% solution, cream, gel, powder, spray powder, or spray liquid) is applied sparingly twice daily after the affected area is cleaned thoroughly. Effective therapy usually takes 2 to 4 weeks, although some individuals (patients with lesions between the toes or on pressure areas of the foot) may require treatment lasting 4 to 6 weeks. When medication is applied to pressure areas of the foot, where the horny skin layer is thicker than normal, concomitant use of a keratolytic agent (e.g., Whitfield's ointment) may be advisable. Neither keratolytic agents nor wet compresses, such as aluminum acetate solution (Burow's solution), which promote the healing of oozing lesions, interfere with the efficacy of tolnaftate. If weeping lesions are present, the inflammation should be treated before tolnaftate is applied.

Tolnaftate is well tolerated when applied to intact or broken skin, although it usually stings slightly when applied. Delayed hypersensitivity reactions to tolnaftate are extremely rare. As with all topical medications, however, discontinuation is warranted if irritation, sensitization, or worsening of the skin condition occurs. No drug–drug interactions have been reported with topical use of tolnaftate.

Undecylenic Acid

Combination undecylenic acid and undecylenate salts have been used widely and may be effective for various mild superficial fungal infections, excluding those involving nails or hairy parts of the body. This agent is fungistatic and effective in mild chronic cases of tinea pedis. Compound undecylenic acid ointment (USP XXI) contains 5% undecylenic acid and 20% zinc undecylenate in an ointment base. It is believed that zinc undecylenate liberates undecylenic acid (the active antifungal entity) on contact with perspiration. In addition, zinc undecylenate has astringent properties because of the presence of the zinc ion; this astringent activity can help to decrease the irritation and inflammation of the infection.

FDA approved undecylenic acid and its derivatives (10%–25% total undecylenate content) as Category I for treating athlete's foot.[3] The vehicle in compound undecylenic acid ointment has a water-miscible base, which makes it nonocclusive, removable with water, and easy to apply. The powder uses talc as its vehicle and is absorbent. The aerosol contains menthol, which serves as a counterirritant and an antipruritic. The solution contains 25% undecylenic acid in an isopropyl alcohol vehicle and is available with either an applicator or in

a spray pump container. The foam dosage form contains 10% undecylenic acid.

The product is applied twice daily after the affected area is cleansed. When the solution is sprayed or applied to the affected area, the area should be allowed to air dry; otherwise, water may accumulate and further macerate the tissue. The usual period required for therapeutic results depends on the severity of the infection. However, if improvement does not occur in 2 to 4 weeks, the condition should be reevaluated and an alternative medication used.

Applied to the skin as an ointment, diluted solution, or dusting powder, the combination of undecylenic acid/zinc undecylenate is relatively nonirritating, and hypersensitivity reactions are rare. The relatively high alcohol concentration in undecylenic acid solutions may cause some burning; the strong odor of undecylenic acid can be objectionable to some patients, possibly promoting patient noncompliance. Caution must be exercised to ensure that such ingredients do not come into contact with the eye or that the powder formulation is not inhaled.

Salts of Aluminum

Because these drugs do not have any direct antifungal activity, aluminum salts were not included in the FDA final monograph for topical antifungal drug products. Rather, they are approved for the relief of inflammatory conditions of the skin, such as athlete's foot. However, their effectiveness as astringents and their possible use in treating athlete's foot merit their inclusion in this chapter. Historically, aluminum acetate has been the foremost astringent used for both the acute, inflammatory type and the wet, soggy type of tinea pedis. Aluminum chloride is also used to treat the wet, soggy type of infection.

Aluminum salts do not cure athlete's foot entirely but are useful when combined with other topical antifungal drugs. Application of aluminum salts merely shifts the disease process back to the simple dry type of athlete's foot, which can then be controlled with other agents such as tolnaftate or an azole.

The action and efficacy of aluminum salts appear to be two-pronged. First, these compounds act as astringents. Their drying ability probably involves complexing of the astringent agent with proteins, thereby altering the proteins' ability to swell and hold water. Astringents decrease edema, exudation, and inflammation by reducing cell membrane permeability and by hardening the cement substance of the capillary epithelium. Second, aluminum salts in concentrations greater than 20% possess antibacterial activity. Aluminum chloride solution (20%) may exhibit that activity in two ways: by directly killing bacteria and by drying the interspaces. Solutions of 20% aluminum acetate and 20% aluminum chloride demonstrate equal in vitro antibacterial efficacy.

Aluminum acetate for use in tinea pedis is generally diluted with about 10 to 40 parts of water. Depending on the situation, the patient may immerse the whole foot in the solution for 20 minutes up to three times a day (every 6–8 hours) or may apply the solution to the affected area in the form of a wet dressing.

For patient convenience, aluminum acetate solution (Burow's solution) or modified Burow's solution is available for immediate use in solution or in forms (powder packets, powder, and effervescent tablets) to be dissolved in water.

Aqueous solutions of 20% to 30% aluminum chloride have been the most beneficial for the wet, soggy type of athlete's foot.[7] Twice-daily applications are generally used until the signs and symptoms (odor, wetness, and whiteness) abate. After that, once-daily applications may control the symptoms. In hot, humid weather, the original condition may return within 7 to 10 days after the application is stopped.

Because aluminum salts penetrate the skin poorly, their toxicity, like that of aluminum chloride, is low. However, a few cases of irritation have been reported in patients with deep fissures. Therefore, the use of concentrated aluminum salt solutions is contraindicated on severely eroded or deeply fissured skin. In such a case, the salts must be diluted to a lower concentration (10% aluminum chloride) for initial treatment.

Solutions of aluminum acetate or aluminum chloride have the potential for misuse (accidental childhood poisoning by ingesting the solutions or the solid tablets), and precautions must be taken to prevent this occurrence. Products containing these ingredients are intended for external use only and should not be applied near the eyes. Prolonged or continuous use of aluminum acetate solution may produce tissue necrosis. In the acute inflammatory stage of tinea pedis, this solution should be used for less than 1 week. The practitioner should instruct the patient to discontinue its use if inflammatory lesions appear or worsen.

Pharmacotherapeutic Comparison

All the topical antifungals approved for treating cutaneous fungal infections have been demonstrated to be effective. The allure of butenafine hydrochloride and terbinafine hydrochloride is their demonstrated ability to cure athlete's foot in some patients after 1 week. However, a close analysis of the data demonstrates that the number of patients achieving complete resolution of the problem is low, and that the effectiveness of these agents parallels that of other antifungals (e.g., clotrimazole and miconazole nitrate) previously approved for nonprescription use.[26]

Controlled studies have demonstrated the efficacy of clotrimazole and miconazole nitrate for athlete's foot, as well as for other kinds of fungal skin infections (see Chapter 8). Both would be expected to demonstrate efficacy comparable to that of tolnaftate for tinea infections. If patient factors (e.g., noncompliance or improper foot hygiene) can be ruled out as a cause of treatment failure, both can be suggested as alternative treatment modalities.

Product Selection Guidelines

Cutaneous antifungals are available as ointments, creams, powders, and aerosols (Table 43-3). Creams or solutions are the most efficient and effective dosage forms for delivery of the active ingredient to the epidermis. Sprays and powders are less effective because often they are not rubbed into the skin. They are probably more useful as adjuncts to a cream or a solution or as prophylactic agents in preventing new or recurrent infections.

Patient compliance is influenced by product selection. Therefore, the practitioner should recommend a drug and product form that is likely to cause the least interference with daily habits and activities without sacrificing efficacy. For example, patients of advanced age may require a preparation that is easy to use; obese patients, in whom excessive sweating may contribute to the disease, should use topical talcum powders as adjunctive therapy. Under certain circumstances, it may be necessary for the practitioner to instruct the caregiver rather than the patient in the proper use of foot products.

Before recommending a nonprescription product, the practitioner should review the patient's medical history. For example, patients with diabetes should have their blood glucose levels controlled, because increased glucose in perspiration may promote fungal growth. Patients with allergic dermatitides usually have a history of asthma, hay fever, or atopic dermatitis; therefore, they

TABLE 43-3 Selected Topical Antifungal Products	
Trade Name	**Primary Ingredients**
Cruex Antifungal Spray Powder	Miconazole 2%
Cruex Cream	Total undecylenate 20% (as undecylenic acid and zinc undecylenate)
Cruex Prescription Strength Aerosol Spray Powder	Miconazole nitrate 2%
Cruex Powder	Calcium undecylenate 10%
Desenex Max Antifungal Cream	Terbinafine hydrochloride 1%
Desenex Prescription Strength AF Aerosol Spray Powder/Aerosol Spray Liquid	Miconazole nitrate 2%
Desenex Prescription Strength AF Cream	Clotrimazole 1%
Lamisil AT Cream	Terbinafine HCl 1%
Lamisil AT Gel	Terbinafine HCl 1%
Lotrimin AF Lotion/Solution/Cream	Clotrimazole 1%
Lotrimin AF Aerosol Spray Liquid/Aerosol Spray Powder	Miconazole nitrate 2%
Lotrimin AF Powder	Miconazole Nitrate 20%
Lotrimin Ultra Cream	Butenafine 1%
Micatin Jock Itch Cream	Miconazole nitrate 2%
Micatin Aerosol/Cream/Lotion/Powder/Spray	Miconazole nitrate 2%
Tinactin Aerosol Spray Liquid/Aerosol Spray Powder/Cream	Tolnaftate 1%
Tinactin Jock Itch Cream	Tolnaftate 1%

are extremely sensitive to most oral and topical agents. By acquiring a good medical history, the practitioner may be able to distinguish a tinea infection from atopic dermatitis and avoid recommending a product that may cause further skin irritation.

The practitioner should bear in mind that prescription drugs may sometimes be more beneficial than nonprescription products. If the patient has soggy, macerated athlete's foot complicated by bacterial infection, broad-spectrum antifungal agents (e.g., econazole nitrate) are preferable to both tolnaftate and prescription-strength haloprogin.

The practitioner should also be aware that product line extensions carrying the same brand name do not necessarily have the same active ingredient(s). For example, the cream and solution formulations of Lotrimin AF contain clotrimazole 1%, whereas the topical spray and powder formulations contain miconazole nitrate 2%. Indeed, Lotrimin Ultra, the newest line extension, contains butenafine hydrochloride. It would have been prohibitively expensive for the manufacturer to pursue the new drug application necessary to market these products with clotrimazole 1% or butenafine hydrochloride 1% as their active ingredient. It was more economically prudent to develop them with an active ingredient that had already received FDA approval. Similarly, Desenex spray liquid and spray powder formulations contain miconazole nitrate 2%, whereas these products formerly contained undecylenic acid and zinc undecylenate in a 25% concentration. In addition, Desenex Max Antifungal Cream now contains 1% terbinafine.

Complementary Therapies

Research results suggest that twice-daily application of 100% tea tree oil solution for 6 months can eradicate fungus from infected toenails in about 18% of patients. It also improves nail appearance and symptoms in about 56% of patients after 3 months and 60% of patients after 6 months of treatment. However, lower concentrations of tea tree oil do not seem to be as effective.[27]

Assessment of Fungal Skin Infections: A Case-Based Approach

Fungal skin infections must be differentiated from bacterial infections, as well as from noninfectious dermatitis. If possible, the practitioner should examine the affected area to determine whether the disorder's manifestation is typical of a fungal infection (Table 43-1).[28] The only true determinant of a fungal infection is a clinical laboratory evaluation of tissue scrapings from the affected area. This process involves a potassium hydroxide mount preparation of the scrapings and cuttings on a special growth medium to show the actual presence and specific identity of fungi. The procedure can be ordered and performed only at the direction of a primary care provider, and microscopic confirmation is probably possible only in the dry, scaly type of tinea infections. The recovery of fungi for diagnosis decreases as the infection becomes progressively more severe. In typical cases of dermatophytosis complex, fungus recovery rates are only about 25% to 50%.

The practitioner should question the patient thoroughly regarding the condition and its characteristics to determine symptoms, extent of disease, previous patient compliance with medications, and any compounding disorders (e.g., diabetes or obesity) that might render the patient susceptible. Patients with diabetes, for example, may present with a mixed dermatophytid

and monilial infection. In general, it is appropriate to inspect the area if privacy and sanitary conditions allow, and inspection is especially appropriate for patients with diabetes.

Cases 43-1 and 43-2 are examples of assessment of a patient with a fungal skin infection.

The most common complaint of patients with a cutaneous fungal infection is pruritus. However, if fissures are present, particularly between the toes, painful burning and stinging may also occur. If the area is abraded, denuded, or inflamed, weeping or oozing may be present in addition to pain. Some patients may merely remark on the bothersome scaling of dry skin, particularly if the infection involves the soles of the feet. In other instances, small vesicular lesions may combine to form a larger bullous eruption marked by pain and irritation, or the only symptoms may be brittleness and discoloration of a hypertrophied nail.

The practitioner should seek to distinguish a tinea infection from diseases with similar symptoms, such as bacterial infection, dermatitis, allergic contact dermatitis, and atopic dermatitis. For this reason, the manifestation of these disorders is briefly discussed here. In children, peridigital dermatitis or atopic dermatitis is more common than tinea pedis. Shoe dermatitis is perhaps the most common form of allergic contact dermatitis from clothing. Therefore, the practitioner should inquire about the type of footwear worn by the patient and about recent footwear changes. Since 1950, the increased use of rubber and adhesives in footwear has paralleled the increase in reports of shoe dermatitis in the dermatologic and podiatric literature. Contact allergy to accelerators—the chemical compounds used to speed the processing of rubber used in sponge-rubber insoles for tennis shoes—has also been reported.[29] In addition to accelerators, antioxidants have been implicated as major chemical allergens, and various phenolic resins used in adhesives are also troublesome. The patient is usually unaware that his or her footwear may be causing the problem.

Hyperhidrosis of interdigital spaces and of the sole of the foot is common, as is infection of the toe webs by gram-negative bacteria. In hyperhidrosis, tender vesicles cover the sole of the foot and toes, and may be quite painful. The skin generally turns white, erodes, and becomes macerated. This condition is accompanied by a foul foot odor. A soggy wetness of the toe webs and the immediately adjacent skin characterizes infection by gram-negative bacteria; the affected tissue is damp and softened. The last toe web (adjacent to the little toe) is the most common area of primary or initial involvement, because it is deeper and extends more proximally than the web between the other toes. Furthermore, abundant exocrine sweat glands, a semiocclusive anatomic setting, and the added occlusion provided by footwear enhance development of the disease at this site. The practitioner must be careful not to confuse this condition with soft corns, which also appear between the fourth and fifth toes.

Patient Counseling for Fungal Skin Infections

The practitioner should describe the proper application technique for topical antifungals to the patient to prevent over- or undermedication. The patient should be told the expected duration of therapy and to apply the medication regularly throughout a complete course of therapy. In addition to information about product use, the practitioner may provide information that will help to control or eradicate the infection, and that will minimize the likelihood of recurrent infections. Such information should

Relevant Evaluation Criteria	Scenario/Model Outcome
Information Gathering	
1. Gather essential information about the patient's symptoms, including:	
a. description of symptom(s) (i.e., nature, onset, duration, severity, associated symptoms)	The patient describes intense itching and a red, weeping rash on her right foot, between and atop the fourth and fifth toes. She says that her symptoms have been a problem for the past 2 years. She says that she is embarrassed to wear sandals during warm weather, because the rash and large yellowish toenail on her fifth toe are unsightly.
b. description of any factors that seem to precipitate, exacerbate, and/or relieve the patient's symptom(s)	The patient says that the rash and itching worsen during the summer months.
c. description of the patient's efforts to relieve the symptoms	The patient has tried several nonprescription antifungals over the past 2 years. The problem seems to resolve after about 2 weeks of treatment but recurs within a month of discontinuing treatment.
2. Gather essential patient history information:	
a. patient's identity	Katrina Renner
b. patient's age, sex, height, and weight	48-year-old female, 5 ft 3 in, 115 lb
c. patient's occupation	Administrative professional
d. patient's dietary habits	Eats low-calorie frozen entrees twice daily
e. patient's sleep habits	7 hours nightly
f. concurrent medical conditions, prescription and nonprescription medications, and dietary supplements	Osteoporosis diagnosed at age 46; calcium carbonate 500 mg 3 times/day, Boniva 150 mg monthly
g. allergies	NKA
h. history of other adverse reactions to medications	None
i. other (describe) _____	Patient lives alone. She works out daily at a gym but does not use the public showers.
Assessment and Triage	
3. Differentiate the patient's signs/symptoms and correctly identify the patient's primary problem(s) (see Table 43-1).	Katrina is suffering from recurrent athlete's foot secondary to onychomycosis of the fifth toenail.
4. Identify exclusions for self-treatment (see Figure 43-1).	Nail involvement
5. Formulate a comprehensive list of therapeutic alternatives for the primary problem to determine if triage to a medical practitioner is required, and share this information with the patient.	Options include: (1) Refer Katrina to an appropriate health care professional. (2) Recommend self-care with a nonprescription antifungal and nondrug measures. (3) Recommend self-care until Katrina can see an appropriate health care professional. (4) Take no action.
Plan	
6. Select an optimal therapeutic alternative to address the patient's problem, taking into account patient preferences.	Katrina should consult a health care professional.
7. Describe the recommended therapeutic approach to the patient.	You should consult a health care professional for treatment.
8. Explain to the patient the rationale for selecting the recommended therapeutic approach from the considered therapeutic alternatives.	This option is best because it appears that the toenail on your fifth toe is infected, which is causing the itching and rash. Infected nails cannot be treated with nonprescription products.

CASE 43-1 (continued)

Relevant Evaluation Criteria	Scenario/Model Outcome
Patient Education	
9. When recommending self-care with non-prescription medications and/or nondrug therapy, convey accurate information to the patient.	Criterion does not apply in this case.
10. Solicit follow-up questions from patient.	What about the Dr. Scholl's Fungal Nail Management Kit that I saw in the foot care aisle? Will it work?
11. Answer patient's questions.	This product works only to reduce discoloration and excessive thickening of infected nails. It does not eliminate the underlying infection.

Key: NKA, no known allergies.

CASE 43-2

Relevant Evaluation Criteria	Scenario/Model Outcome
Information Gathering	
1. Gather essential information about the patient's symptoms, including:	
a. description of symptom(s) (i.e., nature, onset, duration, severity, associated symptoms)	The patient describes intense itching and a red rash on the soles of both feet. He says that the symptoms began a week ago not long after he launched his boat at a public dock for the first time this spring.
b. description of any factors that seem to precipitate, exacerbate, and/or relieve the patient's symptom(s)	The patient says the itching is worse when he wears shoes.
c. description of the patient's efforts to relieve the symptoms	The patient has not tried anything other than scratching the affected areas when he removes his shoes after work.
2. Gather essential patient history information:	
a. patient's identity	Mark Somer
b. patient's age, sex, height, and weight	37-year-old male, 6 ft 3 in, 200 lb
c. patient's occupation	Sales representative
d. patient's dietary habits	Skips breakfast and eats out twice daily
e. patient's sleep habits	4–6 hours nightly
f. concurrent medical conditions, prescription and nonprescription medications, and dietary supplements	He uses "Red Bull" energy drink to stay alert while driving.
g. allergies	None
h. history of other adverse reactions to medications	None
i. other (describe) _____	The patient enjoys boating every weekend during the summer. He either goes barefoot or wears boat shoes without socks when doing so.
Assessment and Triage	
3. Differentiate the patient's signs/symptoms and correctly identify the patient's primary problem(s) (see Table 43-1).	Mark is suffering from athlete's foot that he likely contracted at a public dock.
4. Identify exclusions for self-treatment (see Figure 43-1).	None

Relevant Evaluation Criteria	Scenario/Model Outcome
5. Formulate a comprehensive list of therapeutic alternatives for the primary problem to determine if triage to a medical practitioner is required, and share this information with the patient.	Options include: (1) Refer Mark to an appropriate health care professional. (2) Recommend self-care with a nonprescription antifungal and nondrug measures. (3) Recommend self-care until Mark can see an appropriate health care professional. (4) Take no action.
Plan	
6. Select an optimal therapeutic alternative to address the patient's problem, taking into account patient preferences.	Mark should use a nonprescription antifungal and nondrug measures to treat his problem.
7. Describe the recommended therapeutic approach to the patient.	Regular use of any of the commercially available nonprescription antifungals in any dosage form, except a spray or powder, should alleviate the problem. However, to be optimally effective, you will have to take several measures to keep your feet clean and dry.
8. Explain to the patient the rationale for selecting the recommended therapeutic approach from the considered therapeutic alternatives.	Athlete's foot can be effectively managed with nonprescription antifungals and nondrug measures (keeping the feet clean and dry) as long as there is no toenail involvement, evidence of secondary infection, or preexisting medical conditions that would preclude self-treatment, as in your case. Sprays and powders are less effective, because they often are not rubbed into the skin.
Patient Education	
9. When recommending self-care with nonprescription medications and/or nondrug therapy, convey accurate information to the patient:	
a. appropriate dose and frequency of administration	See the box Patient Education for Fungal Skin Infections.
b. maximum number of days the therapy should be employed	See the box Patient Education for Fungal Skin Infections.
c. product administration procedures	See the box Patient Education for Fungal Skin Infections.
d. expected time to onset of relief	Itching may be relieved somewhat within a few days, but eradication of the causative microorganism may take up to 4 weeks.
e. degree of relief that can be reasonably expected	Athlete's foot can be cured if you use the antifungal and nondrug measures properly.
f. most common side effects	See the box Patient Education for Fungal Skin Infections.
g. side effects that warrant medical intervention should they occur	See the box Patient Education for Fungal Skin Infections.
h. patient options in the event that condition worsens or persists	See the box Patient Education for Fungal Skin Infections.
i. product storage requirements	Store in a cool, dry place out of children's reach.
j. specific nondrug measures	See the box Patient Education for Fungal Skin Infections.
10. Solicit follow-up questions from patient.	Why do I have to wear socks even with my boat shoes? I will look stupid.
11. Answer patient's questions.	Socks help to wick moisture away from the foot. Moisture helps the fungus that causes athlete's foot to thrive.

address proper care of the infected skin site, appropriate laundry techniques and products, minimal use of occlusive clothing, and avoidance of habits or behavior that may lead to recurring infections. The patient should also be told which conditions indicate a need to consult a primary care provider (e.g., the development of a secondary bacterial infection). The box Patient Education for Fungal Skin Infections lists specific information to provide patients.

Evaluation of Patient Outcomes for Fungal Skin Infections

In general, the patient should begin to see some relief of the itching, scaling, and/or inflammation within 1 week. If the disorder shows improvement within this time frame, continuing treatment for 1 to 3 more weeks (depending on the type of tinea infection) should be recommended. If the disorder has not improved or has

PATIENT EDUCATION FOR
Fungal Skin Infections

The objectives of self-treatment are to (1) relieve itching, burning, and other discomfort; (2) inhibit the growth of fungi and cure the disorder; and (3) prevent recurrent infections. For most patients, carefully following product instructions and the self-care measures listed here will help ensure optimal therapeutic outcomes.

Nondrug Measures

- To prevent spreading the infection to other parts of the body, either use a separate towel to dry the affected area or dry the affected area last.
- Do not share towels, clothing, or other personal articles with family members, especially when an infection is present.
- Launder contaminated towels and clothing in hot water to prevent spreading the infection.
- Cleanse the skin daily with soap and water, and thoroughly pat dry to remove oils and other substances that promote growth of fungi.
- If possible, do not wear clothing or shoes that cause the skin to stay wet. Wool and synthetic fabrics prevent optimal air circulation.
- If needed, allow shoes to dry thoroughly before wearing them again. Dust shoes with medicated or nonmedicated foot powder to help keep them dry.
- If needed, place odor-controlling insoles (e.g., Odor Attackers, Sneaker Snuffers) in casual or athletic shoes. These insoles also provide some support and cushioning for the feet. Change insoles routinely every 3–4 months or more often if their condition warrants. Take care that the shoe fit is not compromised by the insoles.
- Avoid contact with people who have fungal infections. Wear protective footwear (e.g., rubber or wooden sandals) in areas of family or public use such as home bathrooms or community showers.

Nonprescription Medications

- Ask a practitioner for assistance in picking the appropriate antifungal agent and dosage form for your infection.
- Available agents include butenafine, clioquinol, clotrimazole, miconazole nitrate, terbinafine, tolnaftate, and undecylenic acid/zinc undecylenate.
- It usually takes 2–4 weeks to cure tinea infections. Some cases may require 4–6 weeks of treatment.
- Apply the antifungal to the clean, dry, affected area in the morning and the evening. Massage the medication into the area. Note that creams and solutions are easier to work into the skin and therefore are probably more effective treatment forms.
- Avoid getting the product in your eyes.

- Wash hands thoroughly with soap and water after applying the product.
- Topical antifungals themselves may cause itching, redness, and irritation.
- Clioquinol may interfere with thyroid function tests and also should not be used on children younger than 2 years.
- Note that clioquinol may cause transient stinging or itching, as well as a rash. If these symptoms persist, stop using the product.
- Tolnaftate may sting slightly upon application.
- An undiluted solution of undecylenic acid/zinc undecylenate may cause temporary stinging when applied to broken skin because of its isopropyl alcohol content.
- When medication is applied to pressure areas of the foot, where the horny skin layer is thicker than normal, apply a keratolytic agent (e.g., Whitfield's ointment) initially to the affected area to help the antifungal penetrate the skin.
- If oozing lesions are present, apply aluminum acetate solution (1:40) to the area before applying the antifungal:
  —Soak the area in an aluminum acetate solution for 20 minutes up to three times a day (every 6–8 hours), or apply the solution to the affected area in the form of a wet dressing.
  —Note that aluminum acetate solution (Burow's solution) or modified Burow's solution is available for immediate use in solution or in forms (powder packets, powder, and effervescent tablets) to be dissolved in water.
  —Avoid getting the product in your eyes.
  —To avoid skin damage, use the solution for no more than 1 week. Discontinue use of the solution if inflammatory lesions appear or worsen.
- For the wet, soggy type of athlete's foot, apply to or soak foot in aluminum acetate solution (1:40) before applying the antifungal:
  —Soak feet with aluminum acetate solution (1:40) twice daily until the odor, wetness, and whiteness abate. After that, soak once daily to control the symptoms.
  —If deep fissures are present in the skin, use a more dilute solution of aluminum acetate for initial treatment.

 Discontinue use of the product and contact a primary care provider if itching or swelling occurs, or if the infection worsens.

 Consult a primary care provider if the infection worsens or persists beyond the recommended length of therapy.

---

worsened, referring the patient to a primary care provider for more aggressive therapy is appropriate. Recurrent skin infections may be a sign of undiagnosed diabetes, immunodeficiency, or another organic problem that requires medical evaluation.

Key Points for Fungal Skin Infections

➤ Historically, the nonprescription drug of choice to treat tinea corporis, tinea cruris, and tinea pedis has been tolnaftate. Other agents, such as clioquinol, clotrimazole, miconazole nitrate, terbinafine hydrochloride, butenafine hydrochloride, and undecylenic acid and its derivatives, are also efficacious for this purpose.

➤ The effectiveness of topical antifungals will be limited, however, unless the patient eliminates other predisposing factors to tinea infections.

➤ These drugs are effective in all their delivery vehicles, but the powder forms should be reserved only for extremely mild conditions or as adjunctive therapy.

➤ Because solutions and creams are spreadable, they should be used sparingly.

➤ When recommended for suspected or actual dermatophytosis, these drugs should be used twice daily (morning and night). Treatment should be continued for 2 to 4 weeks, depending on the symptoms. After that time, the patient and practitioner should evaluate the effectiveness of the therapy.

➤ To minimize noncompliance, the practitioner should advise patients that alleviation of symptoms will not occur overnight. Patients should also be cautioned that frequent recurrence of any of these problems is an indication that they should consult a primary care provider.

➤ Immunocompromised patients and those with diabetes or circulatory problems should be treated by a primary health care provider.

REFERENCES

1. Hay RJ, Roberts SOB, MacKenzie DWR. In: Campion RH, Burton JL, Ebling FJG, eds. *Textbook of Dermatology*. 6th ed. Oxford: Blackwell Scientific Publications; 1999:1127–216.

2. Freeberg IM, Eisen AZ, Wolff K, et al., eds. *Dermatology in General Medicine*. 5th ed. New York: McGraw-Hill, Inc; 1999.

3. *Fed Regist*. 1993;58:49890–9.

4. Drake LA, Dinehart SM, Farmer ER, et al. Guidelines for care of superficial mycotic infections of the skin: tinea corporis, tinea cruris, tinea faciei, tinea manuum and tinea pedis. *J Am Acad Dermatol*. 1996; 34(2 pt 1):282–6.

5. Fitzpatrick TB, Eisen AZ, Wolf K, et al., eds. *Dermatology in General Medicine*. 7th ed. New York: McGraw-Hill, Inc; 2007.

6. Lesher J, Levine N, Treadwill P. Fungal skin infections. *Patient Care*. 1994;28:16–44.

7. Shrum JP, Millikan LE, Bataineh O. Superficial fungal infections in the tropics. *Dermatol Clin*. 1994;12:687–93.

8. Bergus GR, Johnson JS. Superficial tinea infections. *Am Fam Physician*. 1993;48:259.

9. Evans EG. Tinea pedis: clinical experience and efficacy of short treatment. *Dermatology*. 1997;194(suppl 1):3–6.

10. Aly R. Ecology and epidemiology of dermatophyte infections. *J Am Acad Dermatol*. 1994;31(3 pt 2):S21.

11. Auger P, Marquis G, Joly J, et al. Epidemiology of tinea pedis in marathon runners: prevalence of occult athlete's foot. *Mycoses*. 1993;36:35–43.

12. Griffin LY. Common sports injuries of the foot and ankle seen in children and adolescents. *Orthop Clin North Am*. 1994;25:83–93.

13. American Pediatric Medical Association. Nail problems. Available at: http://www.apma.org/s_apma/doc.asp?CID=371&DID=9418. Last accessed September 15, 2008.

14. Noble SL, Forbes RC, Stam PL. Diagnosis and management of common tinea infections. *Am Fam Physician*. 1998;58:163–74, 177–8.

15. Odom R. Pathophysiology of dermatophyte infections. *J Am Acad Dermatol*. 1993;28(5 pt 1):S2–S7.

16. Pray SW. *Nonprescription Product Therapeutics*. 2nd ed. Philadelphia: Lippincott Williams & Wilkins; 2006:591.

17. Dahl MV. Dermatophytosis and the immune response. *J Am Acad Dermatol*. 1994;31(3 pt 2):S34–S41.

18. Pray, SW. Ringworm: easy to recognize and treat. Available at: http://www.uspharmacist.com/oldformat.asp?url=newlook/files/cons/acf2f92.htm. Last accessed September 15, 2008.

19. Weinstein A, Berman B. Topical treatment of common superficial tinea infections. *Am Fam Physician*. 2002;65:2095–102.

20. Elewski BE, Silverman RA. Clinical pearl: diagnostic procedures for tinea capitis. *J Am Acad Dermatol*. 1996;34:498–9.

21. Drake LA, Dinehart SM, Farmer ER, et al. Guidelines for care of superficial mycotic infections of the skin: tinea capitis and tinea barbae. *J Am Acad Dermatol*. 1996;34(2 pt 1):290.

22. *Fed Regist*. 1982;47:12480–566.

23. Savin RC. Treatment of chronic tinea pedis (athlete's foot type) with topical terbinafine. *J Am Acad Dermatol*. 1990;23:786–9.

24. Savin RC, Zaias N. Treatment of chronic moccasin-type tinea pedis with terbinafine: a double-blind, placebo-controlled trial. *J Am Acad Dermatol*. 1990;23:804–7.

25. Center for Drug Evaluation and Research Approval Package for: Application Number: 020663, Trade Name: MENTAX CREAM 1%, Generic Name: Butenafine HCl Cream, Sponsor: Penederm, Inc, Approval Date: December 31, 1996. Available at http://www.fda.gov/cder/foi/nda/96/020663ap.pdf. Last accessed September 15, 2008.

26. Gupta AK, Einarson TR, Smmerbell RC, et al. An overview of topical antifungal therapy in dermatomycoses: a North American perspective. *Drugs*. 1998:55;645–74.

27. Buck DS, Nidorf DM, Addino JG. Comparison of two topical preparations for the treatment of onychomycosis: Melaleuca alternifolia (tea tree) oil and clotrimazole. *J Fam Pract*. 1994;38: 601–5.

28. Bruinsma W, ed. *A Guide to Drug Eruptions*. 6th ed. Amsterdam, The Netherlands: Free University Press; 1995.

29. Jung JH, McLaughlin JL, Stannard J, et al. Isolation, via activity-directed fractionation, of mercaptobenzothiazole and dibenzothiazyl disulfide as 2 allergens responsible for tennis shoe dermatitis. *Contact Dermatitis*. 1988;19:254–9.

Warts

44

Nicholas G. Popovich and Gail D. Newton

Warts, or verrucae, are common viral infections of the epithelium of the skin and mucous membranes.[1] Treatments described in this chapter apply to common warts on self-treatable areas of the body.

Approximately 7% to 10% of people have warts, and approximately 24% of the cases involve plantar warts (i.e., warts located on the sole of the foot).[2] Between 4% and 20% of school-age children will have a wart at some time.[3] The peak incidence of warts occurs between the ages of 12 and 16 years. As many as 10% of school-age children younger than 16 years have one or more warts. Warts usually are not permanent; approximately 30% clear spontaneously in 6 months, 65% clear in 2 years, and most warts clear in 5 years.[4] The mechanism of spontaneous resolution is not fully understood.

Pathophysiology of Warts

Warts are caused by human papillomaviruses (HPVs). These are members of the family Papillomavirdidae.[1] HPVs are non-enveloped, measure 50 to 55 nm in diameter, have icosahedral capsids, are composed of 72 capsomeres, and contain a double-stranded circular DNA genome of ~8000 nucleotide base pairs.[1] HPVs differ from one another by the degree of nucleic acid sequence homology, although they share less than 90% of the DNA sequences in the late region of their genomic organization.[1] The late region L1 and L2 genes encode the structured proteins that form the outer protein shell, called the capsid of the viral particle. Each subtype has its own characteristic histopathology and cytopathology. The polymerase chain reaction with its high specificity and sensitivity has made it possible to amplify and sequence any viral isolate. This biotechnology has resulted in HPV types being defined by DNA sequence homology.

HPV infection occurs through person-to-person contact, including sexual inoculation of the virus into viable epidermis through defects in the epithelium. Autoinoculation to another body area is also possible. The individual's immune system must be susceptible to the virus (probably the key reason that certain individuals develop warts and others do not). Indeed, immunodeficient patients (e.g., those maintained on systemic or topical glucocorticoids), once infected, can develop widespread and highly resistant warts.[1] Maceration of the skin is considered a contributing, predisposing factor, as demonstrated by the occurrence of plantar warts in those who frequent public swimming pools. It is conceivable that the heavy traffic area of a pool can be contaminated easily by one person with a plantar wart, making inoculation in that area around the pool likely. Athletes have a high incidence of plantar warts, and those who use communal and public showers are at high risk.[5] The incubation period after inoculation is 1 to 9 months, with an average of 3 to 4 months for a verruca to become clinically apparent.

Studies[6] have shown that common warts are caused by HPV-2, HPV-4, HPV-27, and HPV-29. HPV 1 causes plantar warts, whereas more than 95% of cervical cancers demonstrate HPV DNA of oncogenic (i.e., high-risk types; e.g., HPV 16, HPV 18, HPV 31, HPV 33, HPV 45).[1] Often, flat warts are associated with types HPV-3, HPV-10, HPV-28, and HPV-49. Digital warts often found in butchers display subtype HPV-7. These findings prompted the belief that HPV type dictates the kind of wart and that these viruses are confined to specific body locations. Evidence suggests that HPV types are not restricted to a specific site, but that, for unknown reasons (perhaps epithelial cell receptor specificity), viral particles function in keratinocytes in only specific locations and will induce warts in only these locations.[7] Different types may infect cornified stratified squamous epithelium of the skin or uncornified mucous membranes. Environmental and host factors besides the viral subtype also influence the lesion appearance.[8] (See Chapter 33 for discussion of anatomy and physiology of the skin.)

Papillomavirus particles assemble in the nuclei of upper-layer keratinocytes and are subsequently released into the milieu within the stratum corneum. It has been demonstrated that HPVs do not bud from the cell membrane; therefore, they lack a thermosensitive lipid envelope such as that found in the herpes viruses and the human retroviruses. It is believed that the presence of a heat-stable protein coat allows the HPV to remain infectious outside the host cells for substantial periods of time.[7]

Clinical Presentation of Warts

Common warts are recognized by their rough, cauliflower-like appearance. They are slightly scaly, rough papules or nodules that appear alone or grouped. They can be found on any skin surface although they most often appear on the hands (see Color Plates, photograph 31). Warts begin as minute, smooth-surfaced, skin-colored lesions that enlarge over time. Repeated irritation causes them to continue enlarging. Plantar warts, hyperkeratotic lesions generally associated with pressure, are usually asymptomatic when small and may not be noticed. However, if they are large or occur on the heel or ball of the foot, they may cause severe discomfort and limitation of function as the otherwise raised lesion is pushed inward secondary to pressure caused by walking. The lesion then impinges on the surrounding sensory nerve endings, causing discomfort or pain.

Warts are defined according to their location. Common warts (verruca vulgaris) usually are found on the hands and fingers, but they may also occur on the face. Periungual and subungual warts occur around and underneath the nail beds, especially in nail biters and cuticle pickers. Juvenile, or flat, warts (verruca plana) usually occur on the face, neck, and dorsa of the hands, wrists, and knees of children. Typically, venereal warts (condyloma lata and condyloma acuminata) occur near the genitalia and anus; however, the penile shaft is the most common site of lesions in men. Plantar warts (verruca plantaris) are common on the soles of the feet (see Color Plates, photograph 32).

Plantar warts are more common in older children, adolescents, and adults. They may be confined to the weight-bearing areas of the foot (the sole of the heel, the great toe, the areas below the heads of the metatarsal bones, and the ball of the foot), or they may occur in non–weight-bearing areas of the sole of the foot. Plantar warts, if located on weight-bearing portions of the foot, are under constant pressure and usually are not raised above the skin surface. The wart itself is in the center of the lesion and is roughly circular, with a diameter of 0.5 to 3.0 cm. The surface is usually grayish and friable, and the surrounding skin is thick and heaped. Several warts may coalesce and fuse, giving the appearance of one large wart (mosaic wart).

Calluses are also commonly found on weight-bearing areas of the foot. Because of their smooth keratotic surfaces, calluses may resemble isolated plantar warts. Therefore, the visual distinction between a wart and a callus is sometimes unclear. However, unlike a callus, a plantar wart is tender with pressure and interrupts the footprint pattern. Optimally, a podiatrist or dermatologist will assess the condition and make the differential diagnosis. To make this assessment, the primary care provider may shave away the outer keratinous surface to expose thrombosed capillaries in the papilloma, which appear as black dots or seeds. In instances in which the results of this procedure are inconclusive, a skin sample can be sent to a clinical laboratory to confirm or refute the presence of HPV.

Warts occasionally may be confused with more serious conditions, such as squamous cell carcinoma (SCC) and deep fungal infections. An SCC may develop rapidly, attaining a diameter of 1 cm within 2 weeks. The lesion generally appears as a small, red, conical, hard nodule that quickly ulcerates. Subungual verrucae, which occur under the nail plate, may exist in conjunction with periungual verrucae. A long-standing subungual verruca may be difficult to differentiate from an SCC, especially in patients of advanced age.

Treatment of Warts

No specific effective therapy for curing warts is available, although topical agents and procedures can relieve pain and sometimes help in removing warts. No single treatment is 100% effective, and different types of therapies may be combined.[9] However, self-care therapies should not be combined by the patient or his/her caregiver. Clinical presentation and response to treatment are used to guide therapy. Typically, warts will regress spontaneously in 2 to 3 years, so a valid management option is to do nothing if this approach is acceptable to the patient. However,

the decision to treat is based on the desire for treatment; painful, bleeding, disfiguring, or disabling lesions; prevention of spread; and presence of warts in immunocompromised patients that could develop into SCC.[6]

Treatment Goals

The goals in treating warts are to (1) remove the wart with no recurrence, (2) leave no scars, and (3) prevent autoinoculation or transmission of the HPV to other people.

General Treatment Approach

Many practitioners believe that early and vigorous treatment of warts is best. The urgency for treatment is based on considerations such as the cosmetic effect (facial warts), the number of warts present in an area, the site of the wart (weight-bearing area of the foot), the age of the patient, financial considerations, and available treatment modalities. Prolonged treatment with nonprescription products may increase the chance of autoinoculation. Figure 44-1 outlines the treatment of warts and lists exclusions for self-treatment.

Nonpharmacologic Therapy

To avoid the spread of warts, which are contagious, patients should wash their hands before and after treating or touching wart tissue. A specific towel should be used for drying only the affected area after cleaning. Patients should not probe, poke, or cut the wart tissue. If warts are present on the sole of the foot, patients should not walk in bare feet unless the wart is securely covered.

Pharmacologic Therapy

Salicylic Acid

Topical salicylic acid in three different vehicles has been recognized as the only drug that is safe and effective for self-treatment of common or plantar warts: salicylic acid 12% to 40% in a plaster vehicle, salicylic acid 5% to 17% in a collodion-like vehicle, and salicylic acid 15% in a karaya gum–glycol plaster vehicle (Table 44-1).[10] (See the section Salicylic Acid in Chapter 45 for a discussion of this agent's properties.)

The Food and Drug Administration (FDA) recommends that topical salicylic acid products be labeled for treating only common and plantar warts. The Agency excluded the other wart types from self-therapy because of the difficulty in recognizing and treating them without supervision by a primary care provider.[10] Indeed, painful plantar warts—as well as the other wart types listed in Figure 44-1—should all be treated by a primary care provider.[6,8]

In self-treatment of warts, patients should notice visible improvement within the first or second week of treatment; removal should be complete within 6 to 12 weeks of product use.[1] Therefore, selection of regular and convenient times to apply the product and adherence to the dosage regimen are important. Table 44-2 provides guidelines for using wart removal products that contain salicylic acid.

If the wart remains after a full course of treatment, a primary care provider should be consulted. Because of the latency factor, however, warts may reappear several months after they have been considered "cured."

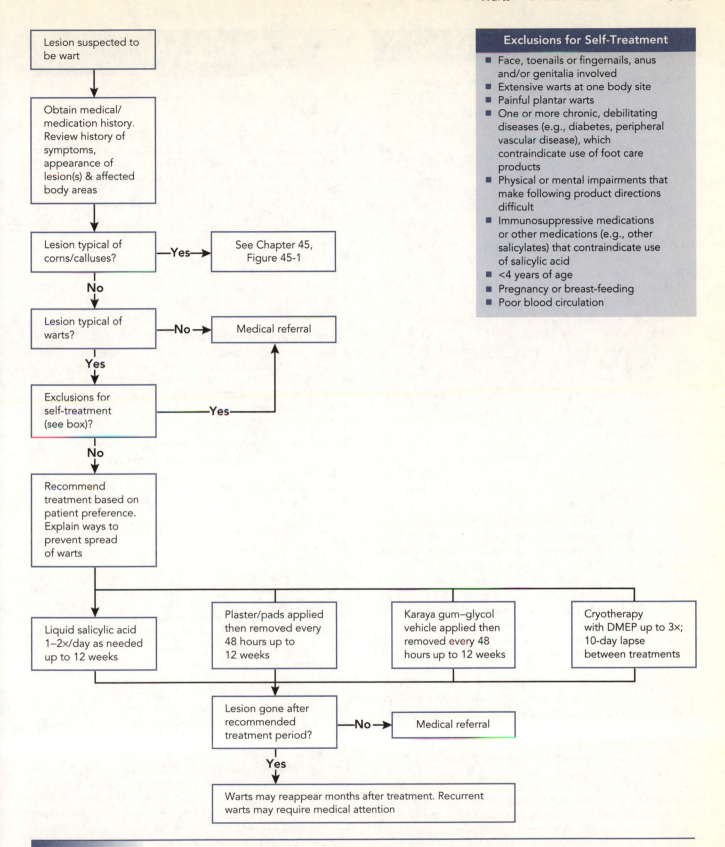

FIGURE 44-1 Self-care of warts. Key: DMEP, dimethyl ether and propane.

TABLE 44-1 Selected Products for Warts	
Trade Name	**Primary Ingredient**
Compound-W for Kids Pad	Salicylic acid 40%
Compound-W Gel, Compound-W Liquid	Salicylic acid 17%
Compound W *Freeze Off*	Dimethyl ether; propane; isobutane
Dr. Scholl's Clear Away Plantar Discs, Dr. Scholl's Clear Away Discs, Dr. Scholl's Clear Away OneStep Invisible Strips	Salicylic acid 40%
Dr. Scholl's Fast Acting Liquid	Salicylic acid 17%
Dr. Scholl's *Freeze Away* Wart Remover	Dimethyl ether; propane
DuoFilm Wart Remover Liquid	Salicylic acid 17%
DuoFilm Wart Remover Patch for Kids	Salicylic acid 40%
OFF-Ezy Wart Remover Kit Liquid	Salicylic acid 17%
Trans-Ver-Sal AdultPatch, Trans-Ver-Sal Pedia Patch	Salicylic acid 15%
Wartner Wart Removal System, Wartner Plantar Wart Removal System, Kids Wartner Wart Removal System	Dimethyl ether; propane

Cryotherapy

Cryotherapy has been standard treatment for wart removal for many years. Although evidence for its efficacy is only equivalent to simpler and safer treatments,[11] cryotherapy is believed to cause irritation and tissue destruction that causes the host to mount an immune response against the causative virus. The most common agent used by dermatologists for this purpose is liquid nitrogen (LN). In 2002, FDA approved a mixture of dimethyl ether and propane (DMEP) that enables patients to treat warts effectively using cryotherapy in the home (Table 44-1).[12] The Wartner Wart Removal System consists of two parts: a pressurized spray can containing the DMEP mixture and a foam applicator that fits into the spray can. Table 44-3 provides guidelines for using the Wartner Wart Removal system. Similar guidelines with minor procedural differences exist for other cryotherapy products. A blister will form under the wart. After about 10 days, the frozen skin and wart fall off and reveal newly formed skin underneath. The patient may repeat the process after 10 days using one of the remaining nine foam applicators. A persistent wart should be treated only three times. The spray can contains enough DMEP for 10 treatments.[13] Studies have shown little difference in treatment effectiveness between LN and DMEP.[14] Because the process involves freezing of skin tissue, the product must be used very carefully to avoid destruction of neighboring healthy tissue.

Other Therapies

Several prescription products (e.g., cantharidin, dichloroacetic acid, trichloroacetic acid, podophyllum, podofilox, and tretinoin) may be used to treat warts. However, the benefits and risks

TABLE 44-2 Guidelines for Treating Warts with Salicylic Acid Product

- Wash and dry affected area before applying the salicylic acid product.

Salicylic Acid 5%–17% in Collodion Vehicle
- Apply product to wart no more than twice daily. Morning and evening are usually the most convenient times.
- Apply solution 1 drop at a time until affected area is covered. Do not overuse the product.
- If the medication touches healthy skin, wash it off immediately with soap and water.
- Allow the solution to harden so that it does not run. Repeat this procedure as needed for up to 12 weeks.
- After use, cap the container tightly to prevent evaporation, which would cause the active ingredient to become more concentrated.
- Store product in an amber or light-resistant container away from direct sunlight or heat.

Salicylic Acid 12%–40% Plaster/Pads
- If using plaster, trim it to follow the contours of the wart. Apply plaster to the skin, and cover it with adhesive occlusive tape.
- If using discs with pads, apply appropriately sized disc directly on the affected area, and cover disc with the pad.
- Apply and remove plasters and pads every 48 hours as needed for up to 12 weeks.

Salicylic Acid 15% in Karaya Gum–Glycol Vehicle
- Apply plaster to wart at bedtime, and leave it on for at least 8 hours.
- Remove and discard plaster in the morning.
- Repeat this procedure every 24 hours as needed for up to 12 weeks.

of other topical interventions (e.g., dinitrochlorobenzene and 5–flurouracil, intralesional bleomycin and interferons, and photodyname therapy) remain unknown.[11] Laser treatments and immunotherapy with or without use of other prescription products are other alternatives. Detailed discussion of these treatments is outside the scope of this chapter. The reader is referred to standard medicine and pharmacotherapy textbooks for such information.[1,15,16]

In recent years, several reports have suggested that occlusion with adhesive tape or duct tape was an effective mode for wart therapy. Results of a prospective, randomized controlled trial suggested that duct tape occlusion therapy was more effective than cryotherapy for treatment of the common wart.[17] Similar to cryotherapy, duct tape is believed to cause irritation. However, whether this irritation leads the host to mount an immune response against the causative virus is unknown. Such speculation is premature; therefore, the exact mechanism remains unknown. In a randomized, double–blind controlled intervention, Wenner et al.[18] studied 90 immunocompetent adult volunteers with at least one wart measuring 2 to 15 mm. Patients were randomized to receive pads consisting of either moleskin with transparent duct tape (i.e., the treatment group) or moleskin alone (i.e., control group). Patients wore the pads for 7 consecutive days and left the pad off on the seventh evening. This process was repeated for 2 months or until the wart resolved. Ultimately, there was no statistically significant difference in

TABLE 44-3 Guidelines for Treating Warts with Wartner Wart Removal System

- Choose the foam applicator that most closely fits the size of the wart. Squeeze the colored end of the foam applicator between the thumb and index finger until a small opening appears.
- Slide the opening on the colored end of the foam applicator over the stick of the applicator holder until the stick is no longer visible. You will find the applicator holder in the bag containing the foam applicators.
- Insert the applicator holder with the attached foam applicator into the opening on the top of the aerosol can so that the foam applicator is no longer visible.
- Place aerosol spray can on a table or sturdy surface. CAUTION! Do not hold the spray can near your face or over parts of your body or clothing!
- Holding can firmly at the bottom, press down valve strongly for 2–3 seconds. You will hear a hissing sound.
- Remove holder with foam applicator from valve. Foam applicator is saturated with cold liquid and condensation will form. This condensation is harmless.
- Leave foam applicator on holder, and then lightly place tip of foam applicator on the wart that is to be frozen. Apply foam applicator to area for no more than 20 seconds. Adjust the exact time depending on size of the wart and thickness of the skin. There will be an aching, stinging sensation. Discard foam applicator after a single use.
- Do not use this system to remove skin growths other than common warts.
- Do not use on genital warts, or warts on mucous membranes, face, nose, lips, ears, or near eyes. Do not use on warts on thin skin such as armpits, breasts, buttocks, or genitals, or on warts in places that you cannot see well, such as your back.
- Do not use on warts in children younger than 4 years, pregnant or breast-feeding women, or patients with diabetes or poor blood circulation.

resolution of the wart between the treatment and control groups. Wenner et al. acknowledged using a transparent duct tape, whereas the Focht study[17] compared acrylic-based adhesive (transparent duct tape) with rubber-based adhesive (standard silver duct tape), which might have been responsible for the difference in efficacy between the two studies. Wenner et al. advocated that further studies are needed to determine whether specific types of adhesive resins are important for efficacy of the duct tape in wart therapy.

The use of oral cimetidine for treatment of warts remains controversial. Randomized, controlled trials have failed to demonstrate a significant effectiveness when cimetidine is compared with placebo or topical agents. Ranitidine has never been evaluated for this therapeutic claim in a randomized controlled trial.[19]

Assessment of Warts: A Case-Based Approach

When assessing a patient with warts, the practitioner should inspect the lesion, if possible, to determine its suitability for self-treatment. The patient's age, health status (especially immunologic status), and use of medications for other disorders should be factored into the choice of treatment. The practitioner should ask whether and how the patient has self-treated the disorder. The answers to these questions will help in evaluating expected compliance with self-treatment of the wart. Other important considerations before initiating treatment are the pain, inconvenience, and risk of scarring from the treatment.

Table 44-4 illustrates differentiation of warts from other disorders with similar presentation. Cases 44-1 and 44-2 provide examples of assessment of patients with warts.

TABLE 44-4 Differentiation of Corns, Calluses, and Warts

Criterion	Corns	Calluses	Warts
Location	Usually over bony prominences of fourth and fifth toes, with hard corns occurring on tops of toes and soft corns in toe webs	Usually over weight-bearing areas of foot	Anywhere virus can gain entry into skin
Signs	Raised, sharply demarcated, hyperkeratotic lesion with central core; hard corns are shiny and soft corns are white	Raised, yellowish lesions with irregular margins and diffuse thickening of skin; may be broad based or have central core; no disruption of normal skin ridges	Slightly scaly, rough papules or nodules, cauliflower-like in appearance; may occur alone or in groups; plantar warts disrupt normal skin ridges
Symptoms	Pain	Pain	Pain if warts appear on weight-bearing areas of foot
Quantity/severity	Can vary from few millimeters to 1 cm	Can vary from few millimeters to several centimeters	Can vary from few millimeters to 3 cm
Timing	Variable onset; lesions may progressively enlarge	Variable onset; lesions may progressively enlarge	1- to 24-month incubation period after inoculation, with average period of 3–4 months
Cause	Friction from tight-fitting hosiery/shoes	Friction from tight-fitting hosiery/shoes; walking barefoot; structural biomechanical problems	Human papilloma viruses
Modifying factors	Well-fitted hosiery/footwear relieve signs and symptoms	Well-fitted hosiery/footwear relieve signs and symptoms	Cryotherapy or salicylic acid; proper hygiene

Relevant Evaluation Criteria	Scenario/Model Outcome
Information Gathering	
1. Gather essential information about the patient's symptoms, including:	
a. description of symptom(s) (i.e., nature, onset, duration, severity, associated symptoms)	A woman points to a growth on her son's finger and asks what she can do to get rid of it. The lesion, located on the left index finger, is a single growth about 0.25 cm in diameter and has a cauliflower-like appearance. The mother says she noticed it about 3 weeks ago. The child says it is not painful. The mother is concerned, because she does not want her other three children to get warts. There is no inflammation, bleeding, or discharge from the growth.
b. description of any factors that seem to precipitate, exacerbate, and/or relieve the patient's symptom(s)	The mother says she is not aware of anything that makes her son's condition better or worse.
c. description of the patient's efforts to relieve the symptoms	No attempts have been made to clear the lesion.
2. Gather essential patient history information:	
a. patient's identity	Jack Wilder
b. patient's age, sex, height, and weight	12-year-old male, approximately 100 lb
c. patient's occupation	Student
d. patient's dietary habits	Generally healthy
e. patient's sleep habits	9–10 hours per night
f. concurrent medical conditions, prescription and nonprescription medications, and dietary supplements	No medical conditions; Flintstones Complete vitamin tablet every morning
g. allergies	Penicillin
h. history of other adverse reactions to medications	None
i. other (describe) _____	Jack is very active in sports and plays on a park-district football team. He has three younger siblings with whom he swims on a regular basis during the summer.
Assessment and Triage	
3. Differentiate the patient's signs/symptoms and correctly identify the patient's primary problem(s) (see Table 44-4).	Jack appears to have an uncomplicated common wart secondary to infection with a human papillomavirus.
4. Identify exclusions for self-treatment (see Figure 44-1).	None
5. Formulate a comprehensive list of therapeutic alternatives for the primary problem to determine if triage to a medical practitioner is required, and share this information with the caregiver.	Options include: (1) Refer Jack to an appropriate health care professional. (2) Recommend self-care with a nonprescription wart removal product and nondrug measures. (3) Recommend self-care until Jack and his mother can consult an appropriate health care professional. (4) Take no action.
Plan	
6. Select an optimal therapeutic alternative to address the patient's problem, taking into account patient preferences.	Because the mother is concerned that Jack will spread his wart to his siblings, Jack should be treated with a nonprescription wart removal product.
7. Describe the recommended therapeutic approach to the caregiver.	Cryotherapy is the best option for treatment of Jack's wart. This method freezes the skin tissue, causing a blister to form underneath the wart. As a result, the frozen skin and wart will fall off, and newly formed skin will be present underneath. Examples of cryotherapy products include Compound-W *Freeze Off*, Dr. Scholl's *Freeze Away* Wart Remover, and Wartner Wart Removal System.

C A S E   4 4 - 1   (continued)

Relevant Evaluation Criteria	Scenario/Model Outcome
8. Explain to the caregiver the rationale for selecting the recommended therapeutic approach from the considered therapeutic alternatives.	Cryotherapy appears optimal for Jack, because the wart can resolve in as little as one treatment at home.
	Salicylic acid liquid products will have to be used twice daily. If a pad containing salicylic acid is used, a new pad will have to be applied every 48 hours and covered with an adhesive occlusive tape. This latter salicylic acid therapy might take between 6–12 weeks for the wart to resolve. Because Jack is very active in sports and swimming, it is unlikely that this type of product would stay in place on his finger.
	Jack's wart is not severe enough to warrant a referral to an appropriate health care professional.

Patient Education

9. When recommending self-care with nonprescription medications and/or nondrug therapy, convey accurate information to the caregiver.	See Table 44-3 and the box Patient Education for Warts for sample patient instructions.
	Be very careful not to touch the applicator to uninfected areas of skin. A blister will form underneath the wart, and within 10 days, the frozen skin and wart should fall off. If after 10 days, the wart is still present, the process may be repeated. The wart can be treated a total of 3 times depending on the product.
	Be sure to read the instructions that come with the product.
10. Solicit follow-up questions from caregiver.	Is the treatment going to hurt? What should I do if the wart is not gone after three treatments?
11. Answer caregiver's questions.	The application of the product will feel very cold and may cause temporary burning/redness. If after three treatments, the wart is still present, Jack should see his primary care provider.

C A S E   4 4 - 2

Relevant Evaluation Criteria	Scenario/Model Outcome
Information Gathering	
1. Gather essential information about the patient's symptoms, including:	
a. description of symptom(s) (i.e., nature, onset, duration, severity, associated symptoms)	Patient asks for something to get rid of a callus on the bottom of his foot that has become increasingly painful. The callus started out about the size of a pencil eraser 6 months ago, but it has enlarged to the size of a quarter.
	The pain has prevented him from participating in pickup basketball games at the gym for the past week. He describes the pain as "constantly walking with a large stone in my shoe."
	The lesion is on the ball of the foot and is flat, whitish, and approximately 1 inch in diameter. It also appears to be a coalescence of four smaller lesions; the normal pattern of skin ridges is interrupted within the lesion. No inflammation, discharge, or bleeding is present.
b. description of any factors that seem to precipitate, exacerbate, and/or relieve the patient's symptom(s)	Patient cannot think of anything that improves or worsens the condition.
c. description of the patient's efforts to relieve the symptoms	Patient attempted to shave off part of the lesion with a razor blade, but that only seemed to cause the lesion to enlarge.
2. Gather essential patient history information:	
a. patient's identity	Bryan Hammond
b. patient's age, sex, height, and weight	37-year-old male
c. patient's occupation	Sales representative

C A S E 4 4 - 2 *(continued)*

Relevant Evaluation Criteria	Scenario/Model Outcome
d. patient's dietary habits	High-carbohydrate diet
e. patient's sleep habits	7 hours per night
f. concurrent medical conditions, prescription and nonprescription medications, and dietary supplements	Dyazide 50 mg once daily for mild hypertension; Imitrex tablets 25 mg as needed for migraine relief
g. allergies	NKA
h. history of other adverse reactions to medications	None
i. other (describe) _____	Recently, Brian was divorced. Until a few months ago, he played basketball at the gym four times each week and used the public shower at the gym afterward.

Assessment and Triage

3. Differentiate the patient's signs/symptoms and correctly identify the patient's primary problem(s) (see Table 44-4).	Brian is suffering from multiple, debilitating plantar warts secondary to infection with human papillomavirus that he likely contracted in the gym shower.
4. Identify exclusions for self-treatment (see Figure 44-1).	None

Plan

5. Formulate a comprehensive list of therapeutic alternatives for the primary problem to determine if triage to a medical practitioner is required, and share this information with the patient.	Options include: (1) Refer Brian to an appropriate health care professional. (2) Recommend self-care with a nonprescription wart removal product and nondrug measures. (3) Recommend self-care until Brian can consult an appropriate health care professional. (4) Take no action.
6. Select an optimal therapeutic alternative to address the patient's problem, taking into account patient preferences.	Brian should consult a health care professional to treat his problem, because the multiple warts seem to have coalesced into one.
7. Describe the recommended therapeutic approach to the patient.	You should consult a health care professional for treatment.
8. Explain to the patient the rationale for selecting the recommended therapeutic approach from the considered therapeutic alternatives.	This option is superior because you have multiple warts that are causing symptoms that interfere with your normal activity.

Patient Education

9. When recommending self-care with nonprescription medications and/or nondrug therapy, convey accurate information to the patient.	Criterion does not apply in this case.
10. Solicit follow-up questions from patient.	Is there anything else I can do to keep from getting this condition?
11. Answer patient's questions.	Yes. See the box Patient Education for Warts.

Key: NKA, no known allergies.

Patient Counseling for Warts

Patients must understand that, unlike corns and calluses, warts are contagious and can spread to other parts of the body unless proper precautions are taken. The practitioner should point out differences in nonprescription salicylic acid products used to treat warts and their proper application. Practitioners should stress contraindications, warnings, and precautions for these products to prevent the wart from progressing to a more serious disorder.

The box Patient Education for Warts lists specific information to provide patients specifically for salicylic acid products.

Evaluation of Patient Outcomes for Warts

Because wart removal using salicylic acid can take from 6 to 12 weeks, the practitioner should schedule the first follow-up on the patient's progress after 6 weeks of treatment. If the wart

PATIENT EDUCATION FOR Warts

The objectives of self-treatment are to (1) remove the wart with no recurrence, (2) leave no scars, (3) induce lifelong immunity, and (4) prevent spread of warts to other parts of the body or other people. For most patients, carefully following product instructions and the self-care measures listed here will help to ensure optimal therapeutic outcomes.

Nondrug Measures

- To avoid spreading warts, wash your hands before and after treating or touching warts.
- Use a specific towel for drying only the affected area after cleansing. Use a separate towel to dry other parts of the body.
- Do not probe, poke, or cut the wart.
- If warts are present on the sole of the foot, do not walk in bare feet unless the wart is securely covered.

Nonprescription Medications

- Be sure to use only topical salicylic products that are labeled for use on warts (see Table 44-1). Table 44-2 describes proper methods for applying the products.
- Treat only common or plantar warts with these agents. Ask your practitioner or primary care provider to identify the type of wart if you are unsure.
- Do not apply the medication to warts on the face, genitals, toenails, or fingernails, or around the anus.
- Do not use this product on irritated skin or on any area that is infected or reddened.
- Do not use this product if you have diabetes or poor circulation.
- Salicylic acid is caustic. Do not allow it to come in contact with the mouth, and keep it out of children's reach.
- Note that the medication sloughs off skin and initially leaves an unsightly pinkish tinge to the skin.
- Expect to see visible improvement within the first or second week of treatment; expect to see complete removal of the wart within 4–12 weeks of product use.

- Note that warts may reappear months after the initial treatment.

Nonprescription Cryotherapy

- Select either the original (for common warts) or the plantar (for plantar warts) product.
- Be sure to read the instructions for the proper use and application of the product.
- Do not use this system to remove skin growths other than either common or plantar warts.
- Do not use this product on genital warts, or warts on mucous membranes, face, nose, lips, ears, or near eyes. Do not use on warts on thin skin such as armpits, breasts, buttocks, or genitals, or on warts in places you cannot see well, such as your back.
- Keep out of children's reach.
- Do not use in children younger than 4 years, pregnant or breast-feeding women, or patients with diabetes or poor blood circulation.
- Expect an aching, stinging sensation after application.
- Expect the frozen skin and wart to fall off after 10 days.
- If necessary, the procedure can be repeated after 10 days using one of the remaining foam applicators.
- A persistent wart can be treated only three times with this product.

 Stop treatment and consult a primary care provider or podiatrist if swelling, reddening, or irritation of the skin occurs, or if pain occurs immediately when applying the product.

 If the wart remains after 12 weeks of treatment, consult a primary care provider.

---

is still present, the patient should be reminded of proper application procedures and advised to continue the treatment. Reevaluation is appropriate for persistent warts. The practitioner should refer the patient to a primary care provider for any warts that persist after 12 weeks of self-treatment.

Cryotherapy can be performed up to three times with a 10-day lapse between each treatment; therefore, medical referral is appropriate if the wart persists after three treatments.

KEY POINTS FOR WARTS

- ➤ Historically, the nonprescription drug of choice to treat common and plantar warts was salicylic acid in a collodion-like vehicle or plaster product form, whichever was more convenient.
- ➤ Plantar warts should be treated with a higher concentration of topical salicylic acid (up to 40%); warts on thin epidermis require a lower concentration (up to 17%).
- ➤ Because warts are usually self-limiting, treatment should be conservative; vigorous therapy with salicylic acid may scar tissue.

- ➤ To minimize noncompliance, the practitioner should advise patients that alleviation of the symptoms should not be expected to occur overnight.
- ➤ Patients should also be cautioned that frequent recurrence of any of these problems indicates they should consult a podiatrist or primary care provider.
- ➤ The introduction of DMEP products enables consumers to treat common and plantar warts effectively using cryotherapy in the home.
- ➤ Consumers should carefully follow directions when using these products, because injury to normal, adjacent skin can occur with product misuse.
- ➤ Patients with diabetes, circulatory problems, immunodeficiencies, and/or arthritis should not self-medicate with any topical nonprescription drug without first checking with their primary care provider, podiatrist, or other health care practitioner.

REFERENCES

1. Reichman RC. Human papillomavirus infections. In: Kasper DL, Fauci AS, Longo DL, et al., eds. *Harrison's Principles of Internal Medicine.* 16th ed. New York: McGraw-Hill, Inc; 2005:1056–8.

2. Wanek EL, Pray WS. Warts: more than a minor nuisance. *US Pharm.* 1996;21:122–7.

3. Williams HC, Pottier A, Strachan D. The descriptive epidemiology of warts in British schoolchildren. *Br J Dermatol.* 1993;128:504–11.

4. Janniger CK. Childhood warts. *Cutis.* 1992;50:15–6.

5. Johnson LW. Communal showers and the risk of plantar warts. *J Fam Pract.* 1995;40:136–8.

6. Berman B, Weinstein A. Treatment of warts. *Dermatol Ther.* 2000; 13:290–304.

7. Bolton RA. Nongenital warts: classification and treatment options. *Am Fam Pract.* 1991;43:2049–56.

8. Sterling JC, Handfield-Jones S, Hudson PM. Guidelines for the management of cutaneous warts. *Br J Dermatol.* 2001;144:4–11.

9. Gibbs S, Harvey I, Sterling J, et al. Local treatments for cutaneous warts: systematic review. *BMJ.* 2002;325:461–9.

10. *Fed Regist.* 1990;55:33246–56.

11. Gibbs S, Harvey I. Topical treatments for cutaneous warts. *Cochrane Database System Rev.* 2006;3:CD001781.

12. Center for Drug Evaluation and Research New Device Clearance for: Application Number: K011708, Trade Name: Wartner Wart Removal System, Sponsor: Wartner Medical Products, Approval Date: February 20, 2002. Available at: http://www.fda.gov/cdrh/pdf/K011708.pdf. Last accessed September 17, 2008.

13. Wartner Medical Products. Available at: http://www.wartner.com. Last accessed September 19, 2008.

14. Caballero MF, Plaza NC, Perez CC, et al. Cutaneous cryosurgery in family medicine: dimethyl ether-propane spray *versus* liquid nitrogen. *Aten Primaria.* 1996;18:211–6.

15. Housman TS, Williford PM. Warts (verrucae). In: Rakel PE, Bope ET, eds. *Conn's Current Therapy 2007.* Philadelphia: Saunders Elsevier; 2007:956–9.

16. DiPiro JT, Talbert RL, Yee GC, eds. *Pharmacotherapy: A Pathophysiologic Approach.* 6th ed. New York: McGraw-Hill, Inc; 2005:2114–6.

17. Focht DR, Spicer C, Fairchiok MP. The efficacy of duct tape vs cryotherapy in the treatment of verruca vulgaris (the common wart). *Arch Pediatr Adolesc Med.* 2002;156:971–4.

18. Wenner R, Askari SK, Cham PM, et al. Duct tape for the treatment of common warts in adults. A double-blind randomized controlled trial. *Arch Derm.* 2007;143:309–13.

19. Fit KE, Williams PC. Use of histamine$_2$-antagonists for the treatment of verruca vulgaris. *Ann Pharmacother.* 2007;41:1222–6.

Minor Foot Disorders

Cynthia W. Coffey and Karla T. Foster

On average, a person walks 115,000 miles in a lifetime, which is equivalent to circling the world nearly four times. Approximately 80% of Americans will have some type of foot disorder during their lifetime.[1] Sales of foot care products in the United States currently exceed $500 million per year. The five most common groups of foot disorders are heel/arch pain; corns, calluses, and plantar warts (see Chapter 44); athlete's foot (see Chapter 43); tired, aching feet; and ingrown toenails. Historically, Americans have used more than just commercially available products for foot disorders, including such harmful self-care practices as scraping or cutting corns and calluses, opening blisters or removing the skin cover, improperly trimming toenails, and inappropriately using hot water to clean and bathe/soak the feet. Therefore, a significant need exists to educate patients about foot care, including appropriate self-treatment measures.

In some instances, foot disorders or inappropriate foot care practices may be life threatening to patients with diabetes, severe arthritis, and impaired circulation (see the box A Word about Chronic Diseases and Foot Disorders).[2-7] Foot disorders may indicate serious underlying conditions. For most patients, however, such problems cause nominal measures of discomfort and impaired mobility.

An estimated 15% to 20% of the 16 million patients with diabetes will be hospitalized with a foot complication during the course of their disease.[3] Foot problems such as ulceration and infection can ultimately lead to gangrene, amputation of the foot/ankle, and even death. These problems are the leading causes of hospitalization for patients with diabetes. Treating a patient with a foot ulcer can cost $28,000 without amputation and up to $34,000 in a patient requiring amputation.[4]

Three distinct groups of patients often encounter foot problems. First are children with a congenital malformation or deformity, or a specific disease that affects the foot (e.g., juvenile arthritis). These patients need special shoes and foot care overseen by an orthopedic surgeon or podiatrist. Second are adolescents who experience rapid growth. Growth plates in their feet may become stressed and irritated. Athletic activity at this age can also contribute to secondary conditions, especially if associated injuries to the feet are not properly treated. Osteoarthritis, for example, can occur secondary to a foot injury. The third group is made up of older patients who encounter foot problems because of aging (e.g., arthritis) and disease (e.g., peripheral vascular disease). In particular, diabetes and arthritis can cause secondary foot problems. Therefore, it is important for patients to check their feet regularly for common foot disorders. These common foot disorders could result in more serious injuries in patients with comorbid disorders such as diabetes.[4]

Individuals who exercise regularly are also at risk for foot disorders. Since the 1980s, society's attitude toward physical fitness and body awareness has changed dramatically. Millions of people exercise every day; jogging, running, and aerobic exercising are methods used most often to remain or get "in shape." Without adequate precautions, however, problems and injuries can arise, particularly involving the feet.[1]

PATHOPHYSIOLOGY OF THE FOOT

At birth, an infant's foot has 33 joints, 19 muscles, 107 ligaments, and cartilage that will develop into 26 bones. These small components continue to develop and mature until age 14 to 16 years for females and age 15 to 21 years for males. Women and men will generally begin to notice changes in their feet in their 40s and 50s, respectively.[8] After years of bearing the body's weight, the feet tend to broaden and flatten, thus stretching ligaments and causing bones to shift positions. These changes subject the feet to stress, which is compounded by prolonged standing. An estimated 40% of the U.S. population spends about 75% of their workday on their feet, increasing the potential for painful foot conditions.

CORNS AND CALLUSES

Although corns and calluses are common foot disorders, they should not be ignored. They may indicate a biomechanical problem in the feet or lead to serious complications in predisposed patients.

Pathophysiology of Corns and Calluses

Under normal conditions, the cells in the skin's basal cell layer undergo mitotic division at a rate equal to the continual surface cellular desquamation, leading to complete replacement of the

Some chronic diseases predispose certain patients to foot complications. Patients who have diabetes often have poor circulation and diminished limb sensitivity, and are especially vulnerable to infectious foot problems. Other susceptible patients include those with peripheral vascular disease or arthritis. The practitioner can identify such patients by asking about daily medication use or reviewing the patient's drug profile. Typical drug use patterns for high-risk patients include insulin, oral antidiabetic drugs (e.g., glipizide, glyburide, metformin, acarbose, and nateglinide), drugs for circulation (e.g., cyclandelate, isoxsuprine, papaverine, and pentoxifylline), drugs used for neuropathic pain (e.g., gabapentin and duloxetine), and drugs for arthritic conditions (e.g., aspirin and other NSAIDs).

Self-treatment with nonprescription products, if not properly supervised in patients with impaired circulation, may induce more inflammation, ulceration, or even gangrene, particularly in cases of vascular insufficiency in the foot. Patients with diabetes and those with peripheral circulatory impairments are particularly susceptible to gangrene. In addition, simple lesions may mask more serious abscesses or ulcerations. If left medically unattended, these lesions may lead to such conditions as osteomyelitis, which may require hospitalization and aggressive parenteral antibiotic therapy.

Diabetes Mellitus[2–6]

Patients who have poorly controlled diabetes are at greater risk for lower extremity complications, which result in increased health care costs as well as decreased quality of life and increased morbidity. Two major causes of foot ulcerations are peripheral neuropathy, which results in loss of injury perception, and excessive plantar pressure, which contributes to decreased mobility and foot deformities. Patients with diabetes also contribute to foot complications by poor foot hygiene such as extreme hot water soaks, inappropriate footwear, and lack of daily foot self-examinations. Patients with diabetes need to be educated on proper foot care such as appropriate toenail trimming, avoidance of creams/lotions between the toes, keeping socks clean and dry, and foot examinations at home and at the health care provider's office. (See Chapter 47 for further discussion of proper foot care and for potentially serious foot disorders in patients with diabetes.)

Peripheral Vascular Disease[4,6]

Patients with peripheral vascular disease often have poor circulation of the feet and legs. Because of decreased blood flow and low oxygen perfusion, ulcerations and decreased wound healing may be problematic. They may complain of persistent and unusual feelings of cold, numbness, tingling, burning, or fatigue. Other symptoms may include discolored skin, dry skin, absence of hair on the feet or legs, or a cramping or tightness in the leg muscles. The clinician should also palpate for pedal pulses. The most discriminating questions that a practitioner can ask this type of patient are (1) Do you experience aching in your calves when you walk? and (2) Do you have to hang your feet over the edge of the bed during sleep to relieve the soreness in your calves? A "yes" response to either question warrants referring the patient to a primary care provider or podiatrist.

Localized redness or unilateral coldness may indicate a possible blockage (a clot) of circulation to the foot. Sometimes the involved foot or lower leg will appear physically larger than the other, may be red or waxy in appearance, may have no hair growth on the toes, and will exhibit thickened nails. If the patient's medication history does not indicate the use of medications intended to relieve such symptoms, the practitioner should advise the patient with suspected circulatory problems to consult a primary care provider or podiatrist for evaluation immediately.

A daily footbath is a simple measure to assist these patients. After the foot is patted dry, an emollient foot cream can be applied to aid in retaining moisture and pliability. The footbath will also soften brittle toenails for clipping and filing. The feet should be kept warm and moderately exercised every day.

Arthritis[6,7]

Osteoarthritis is a noninflammatory, degenerative joint disease that occurs primarily in older people. Degeneration of the articular cartilage and changes in the bone result in a loss of resilience and a decrease in the skeleton's shock-absorption capability. This condition, however, is also experienced by individuals in their late teens and early 20s as a secondary complication of a previous athletic injury. This condition might be evidenced by the development of hallux limitus or rigidus of the big toe (i.e., a stiff toe or painful flexion or extension of the big toe because of stiffness and spur formation in the metatarsophalangeal joint). Subsequently, these patients have a lot of difficulty with their shoes not fitting properly. They may also develop an osteoarthritic condition in the ankle joint. Referral for further evaluation is appropriate. Most patients with rheumatoid arthritis eventually have foot involvement. The major forefoot deformities in these patients are painful metatarsal heads, hallux valgus, and clawfoot. Corrective surgical procedures are often indicated to reduce pain and improve function and mobility. Little evidence exists that conventional nonsurgical therapy (e.g., orthopedic shoes, metatarsal inserts, conventional arch supports, and metatarsal bars) is effective in these cases.

Proper palliative foot care is especially important for arthritic patients. They should wear properly fitted shoes, pad their shoes with insoles to protect their feet from the shock of hard surfaces, and undergo regular podiatric or medical examinations. (See Chapter 5 for use of topical or systemic nonprescription analgesics for osteoarthritis.)

epidermis in approximately 1 month. During corn or callus development, however, friction and pressure increase mitotic activity of the basal cell layer, leading to the migration of maturing cells through the prickle cell (stratum spinosum) and granular (stratum granulosum) skin layers. This migration produces a thicker stratum corneum (hyperkeratosis) as more cells reach the outer skin surface, which is a natural protective mechanism of the skin surface. This process may signal biomechanical problems that cause abnormal weight distribution in a particular area of the foot. In this case, a podiatric examination is warranted to determine whether an imbalance is present. When friction or pressure is relieved, mitotic activity returns to normal, causing remission and disappearance of the lesion.

Clinical Presentation of Corns and Calluses

Corns and calluses are similar in one respect: Both produce a marked hyperkeratosis of the stratum corneum. Besides this one feature, however, there are marked differences. Table 44-4 in Chapter 44 differentiates the signs and symptoms of warts, corns, and calluses.

Corns

A corn (clavus) is a small, raised, sharply demarcated, hyperkeratotic lesion with a central core caused by pressure from underlying bony prominences or joints (Figure 45-1). The central core of the corn differentiates it from a wart (see Chapter 44, Table 44-4). Misidentification of warts and corns is common. A clinician can identify a corn by shaving the central core. A corn has a hard center, and a wart will bleed because of multiple capillary loops.[9] Corns are yellowish gray with diameters ranging from a few millimeters to 1 cm or more. The base of the corn is on the skin surface; its apex points inward and presses on the nerve endings in the dermis, causing pain.

There are two types of corns—hard and soft. Hard corns (heloma durum) are most prevalent; appear shiny, dry, and polished; and usually occur on the bulb of the great toe, the dorsum of the fourth or fifth toe, or tips of the middle toes. Soft corns (heloma molle) are whitish thickenings of the skin and may be extremely painful. Accumulated perspiration macerates

the epidermis, giving the corn a soft appearance. Soft corns may occur between any adjacent toes but are most frequently found between the fourth and fifth toe, because the fifth metatarsal is much shorter than the fourth, and the web between these toes is deeper and extends more proximally than the webs between the other toes.[8,9]

A bony spur, or exostosis (a bony tumor in the form of an ossified muscular or ligamentous attachment to the bone surface) nearly always exists between long-lasting hard and soft corns.[8]

Pressure from inappropriate, tight-fitting shoes is the most frequent cause of pain from corns. As narrow-toed or high-heeled shoes crowd toes into a narrow toe box, the most lateral toe, the fifth, sustains the most pressure and friction and is the usual site of a corn. The resultant pain may be severe and sharp (when downward pressure is applied) or dull and discomforting. Consumer research approximates that 82% of women ages 35 to 54 years suffer moderate-to-intense pain from corns and that 35% are consequently limited or restricted in their activities.

Calluses

A callus has a broad base with relatively even thickening of skin generally found on the bottom of the foot in areas such as the heel, ball of the foot, toes, and sides of the foot (Figure 45-1). It has indefinite borders and ranges from a few millimeters to several centimeters in diameter. The indefinite borders help clinicians differentiate calluses from well-circumscribed margins of corns. A callus is usually raised and yellow, and has a normal pattern of skin ridges on its surface. Calluses form on joints and weight-bearing areas of the hands and feet[9–11] (see Color Plates, photograph 33).

Friction (caused by loose-fitting shoes or tight-fitting hosiery), walking barefoot, and structural biomechanical problems contribute to the development of calluses. Structural problems include improper weight distribution, pressure, and development of bunions with age. Calluses can be symptomatic and protective.

Diffuse-shearing and discrete-nucleated are two types of calluses. The discrete-nucleated callus is smaller and has a localized translucent center; this type of callus is painful with applied pressure. The diffuse-shearing callus covers a larger surface area and does not have a central core.[9,10]

Treatment of Corns and Calluses

Treatment Goals

The goals of self-treatment are to (1) provide symptomatic relief, (2) remove corns and calluses, and (3) prevent their recurrence by correcting underlying causes.

General Treatment Approach

Although effective nonprescription products are available for removing corns and calluses, ultimate success depends on eliminating the causes such as pressure and friction. The algorithm in Figure 45-2 outlines self-treatment of corns and calluses, and lists exclusions for self-treatment.

Nonpharmacologic Therapy

Nondrug adjunctive measures include daily soaking of the affected area throughout treatment for at least 5 minutes in warm (not hot) water to soften dead tissue for removal. Dead tissue should

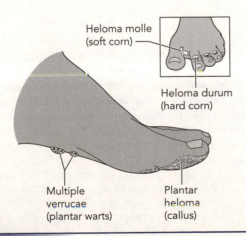

Heloma molle (soft corn)

Heloma durum (hard corn)

Multiple verrucae (plantar warts)

Plantar heloma (callus)

FIGURE 45-1 Disorders affecting top and sole of foot (corns, callus, and plantar warts).

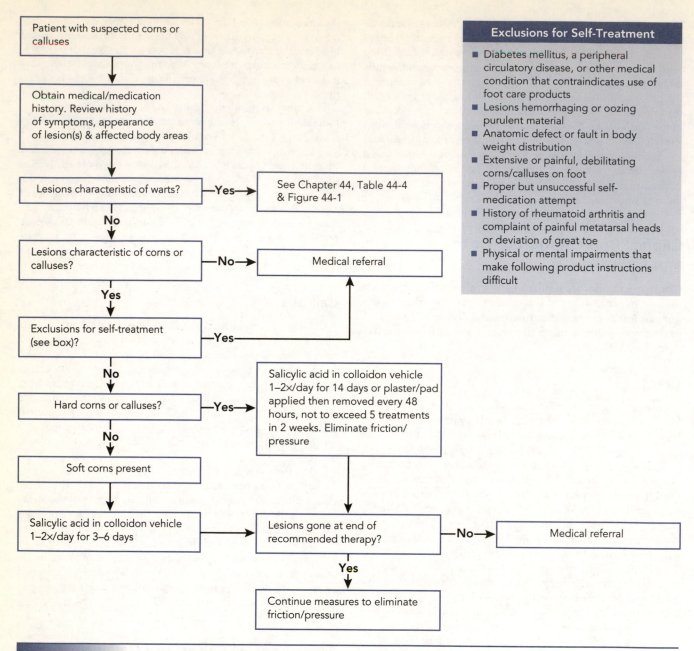

Exclusions for Self-Treatment

- Diabetes mellitus, a peripheral circulatory disease, or other medical condition that contraindicates use of foot care products
- Lesions hemorrhaging or oozing purulent material
- Anatomic defect or fault in body weight distribution
- Extensive or painful, debilitating corns/calluses on foot
- Proper but unsuccessful self-medication attempt
- History of rheumatoid arthritis and complaint of painful metatarsal heads or deviation of great toe
- Physical or mental impairments that make following product instructions difficult

Flowchart:

Patient with suspected corns or calluses → Obtain medical/medication history. Review history of symptoms, appearance of lesion(s) & affected body areas → Lesions characteristic of warts? — Yes → See Chapter 44, Table 44-4 & Figure 44-1

No ↓

Lesions characteristic of corns or calluses? — No → Medical referral

Yes ↓

Exclusions for self-treatment (see box)? — Yes → Medical referral

No ↓

Hard corns or calluses? — Yes → Salicylic acid in colloidon vehicle 1–2×/day for 14 days or plaster/pad applied then removed every 48 hours, not to exceed 5 treatments in 2 weeks. Eliminate friction/pressure

No ↓

Soft corns present ↓

Salicylic acid in colloidon vehicle 1–2×/day for 3–6 days → Lesions gone at end of recommended therapy? — No → Medical referral

Yes ↓

Continue measures to eliminate friction/pressure

FIGURE 45-2 Self-care of corns and calluses.

be removed gently, rather than forcibly, after normal washing to avoid further damage. A callus file or pumice stone effectively accomplishes this purpose. These instruments should be kept clean to avoid autoinoculating other skin areas. Sharp knives or razor blades should not be used; they may lacerate the skin, allowing bacteria to enter the wound, which may result in localized infection.[11]

To relieve painful pressure emanating from inflamed underlying tissue and irritated or hypertrophied bones directly underneath a corn or callus, patients may use a circular foam cushioning pad such as a Dr. Scholl's pad with an aperture for the corn or callus. If the skin can tolerate pads, they may be used for up to 1 week or longer. However, some podiatrists recommend that patients change the pads every day. Concerns stem from the fact that the pad adhesive can macerate the skin, leading to infection. To prevent the pads from adhering to hosiery, patients may cover

the pads with paraffin wax and then powder them daily with a hygienic foot powder or cover with an adhesive bandage. If, despite these measures, friction causes the pads to peel up at the edge and stick to hosiery, the practitioner may recommend that patients cover their toes with the forefoot of an old stocking or panty hose before putting on hosiery.[10]

Many of the disadvantages associated with older pads have been overcome with the introduction of Cushlin, manufactured by Dr. Scholl's. Cushlin is a soft polymer that provides a protective cushion without leaving a sticky residue. When applied to the skin, it molds to the shape of the foot and adheres to the skin without the adhesive properties found in other products. In addition, its smooth outer surface prevents snags and runs in socks and hosiery.[9]

Practitioners should advise patients that if the pad begins to cause itching, burning, or pain at any time, it should be removed immediately and a primary care provider or podiatrist should be consulted. Patients should also be advised that these pads will provide only temporary relief and rarely cure a corn or callus. Practitioners may also recommend silicone toe sleeves for the toes affected by corns. The toe sleeves are lined with silicone, which is impregnated with mineral oil. The mineral oil is slowly released to soften the skin. The sleeves also protect and cushion the corn area. A foam spacer or lamb's wool may be used to provide relief in areas of soft corns. Placement of a metatarsal pad may help relieve pain and pressure from a diffuse-shearing callus.[9]

Eliminating the pressure and friction that induces corns and calluses entails using well-fitting, nonbinding footwear that evenly distributes body weight (Table 45-1). For anatomic foot deformities, orthopedic corrections must be made. These measures relieve pressure and friction, allowing normal mitosis of the basal cell layer to resume and the stratum corneum to normalize after total desquamation of the hyperkeratotic tissue secondary to the use of topical products. Orthotics (i.e., custom-molded arch supports) may have to be used to help compensate for deformities by redistributing the mechanical forces. Ultimately, surgical correction of toe deformities and resection of the underlying bone may be necessary.

Pharmacologic Therapy

Salicylic Acid

Salicylic acid, the oldest of the keratolytic agents, is formulated in many strengths (0.5%–40%), depending on its intended use and dosage form. For the self-treatment of corns and calluses, the approved concentration ranges are 12% to 40% in a plaster vehicle and 12% to 17.6% in a collodion-like vehicle.[9,12]

Salicylic acid is believed to act on hyperplastic keratin in two ways: (1) it decreases keratinocyte adhesion and (2) it increases water binding, which leads to hydration of keratin. Because of the latter effect, the presence of moisture was believed to be an important component of therapeutic efficacy, and soaking the area in a warm water bath for 5 minutes before applying salicylic acid was recommended. However, evidence submitted to the Food and Drug Administration (FDA) indicated that presoaking produced no significant positive effects for any efficacy parameter assessed. In its final rule, FDA proposed allowing manufacturers of these products to state as an optional direction to the consumer: "May soak corn/callus (or wart) in warm water for 5 minutes to assist in removal."[12,13]

The FDA advisory review panel evaluated more than 20 agents for the treatment of corns and calluses. Of these agents, only salicylic acid in plaster, pad, disk, or collodion vehicle is approved as safe and effective for nonprescription marketing for the removal of corns and calluses (Table 45-2). FDA recognized that the term *plaster* includes disks and pads because these dosage forms are similar.[12]

Salicylic acid is usually applied to a corn, callus, or common wart in a collodion or collodion-like vehicle. These vehicles contain pyroxylin and various combinations of volatile solvents such as ether, acetone, or alcohol, or a plasticizer, which is usually castor oil. Pyroxylin is a nitrocellulose derivative that remains on the skin as a water-repellent film after the volatile solvents have evaporated.[12,13]

The advantages of collodions and liquid forms are that they form an adherent flexible or rigid film and prevent moisture evaporation. These qualities aid penetration of the active ingredient into the affected tissue and result in sustained local action of the drug. The systems are largely water insoluble, as are most of their active ingredients such as salicylic acid. They are also less apt to run onto surrounding skin than are other aqueous solutions.[12,13]

Disadvantages of collodions are they are extremely flammable and volatile and, by occluding normal water transport through the skin, they may be mechanically irritating. The collodion's occlusive nature also allows systemic absorption of some drugs. Some patients may abuse these vehicles by sniffing their volatile aromatic solvents.[12,13]

Salicylic acid may also be delivered to the skin through the use of a plaster, disk, or pad. This delivery system provides direct and prolonged contact of the drug with the affected area,

---

TABLE 45-1 Selection of Properly Fitted Footwear

- Buy shoes in the proper size (width and length). To obtain an accurate measurement, ask a trained salesperson to measure your feet. Recheck shoe size every 2 years.
- Base shoe length on the longest toe of your longest foot. There should be approximately one-half inch between the tip of shoe and longest toe.
- For proper arch length, choose a shoe in which the first metatarsal head of the foot fits the metatarsal break of the shoe.
- For proper shoe width, choose a shoe that feels comfortable at the first metatarsal joint (toes do not feel cramped in the toe box).
- Once the shoe size is determined, choose a shoe shaped to match the shape of the foot. For example, choose a shoe shaped inward if the feet are shaped inward like a pigeon's. Choose a shoe shaped outward if the feet are shaped outward like a duck's.
- If you have abnormalities of the toes (e.g., hammer toes) or use orthotics or padding in your shoes, select a shoe with adequate depth (vertical height) of the toe box to prevent friction of the tops of the toes. A wide toe box will help relieve pressure between toes.
- Make sure the heel fits snugly and helps hold the foot straight.
- If you are physically active, make sure the shoe's midsole provides adequate cushioning and support.
- Try on both shoes at the time of purchase, preferably wearing a pair of socks or stockings of the type that will be worn normally with the new pair of shoes.
- If your feet tend to swell, select shoes at the end of the day.

Source: References 1, 8, 9, and 11.

TABLE 45-2 Selected Corn and Callus Products

Trade Name	Primary Ingredients
Curad Mediplast Corn, Callus & Wart Remover	Salicylic acid 40%
Dr. Scholl's Corn/Callus Remover Liquid	Salicylic acid 12.6%
Dr. Scholl's Cushlin Gel Corn/Callus Remover Disk	Salicylic acid 40%
Freezone One Step Corn/Callus Remover Pads	Salicylic acid 40%

resulting in quicker resolution of the condition. Salicylic acid plaster is a uniform solid or semisolid adhesive mixture of salicylic acid in a suitable base, spread on appropriate backing material (e.g., felt, moleskin, cotton, or plastic), which may be applied directly to the affected area. The usual concentration of salicylic acid in the base is 40%. A small piece of a plaster may be cut to the size of the corn or callus and held in place by waterproof tape. More convenient, however, are corn or callus pads that have small salicylic acid disks for direct application to the skin. The patient selects the appropriately sized disk, places it directly on the affected area, and then covers it with the pad.[9,12,13]

Table 45-3 provides instructions for applying salicylic acid products.

Significant percutaneous absorption may occur when salicylic acid is applied over large body areas, for example, during

therapy for extensive psoriasis on the face, trunk, or extremities. Absorbed salicylic acid is largely metabolized in the liver and excreted in the urine. Patients with impaired liver or kidney function are, therefore, predisposed to accumulation and salicylate toxicity. However, although occlusive vehicles can enhance the percutaneous absorption of salicylic acid, it is highly unlikely that salicylate toxicity will result during corn, callus, or wart therapy with recommended dosages.

Because some patients will not use salicylic acid products properly or misapply it, topical salicylic acid therapy is not preferred by some podiatrists (see the box A Word about Chronic Diseases and Foot Disorders). In the past, packaging and labeling for corn and callus products warned patients with diabetes or peripheral vascular disease not to use the products, except under direct supervision of a primary care provider. This warning was included because any acute inflammation or ulcer formation caused by the topical salicylic acid could be dangerous. In its final monograph, FDA determined that the warning should be stronger and should directly caution against using the product under certain conditions, rather than including an "except under" condition for use. Consequently, the revised warning is as follows:

> Do not use this product on irritated skin, any area that is infected or reddened, moles, birthmarks, warts with hair growing from them, genital warts, warts on the face, or warts on the mucous membranes, such as inside the mouth, nose, anus, genitals, or lips. Do not use if you are diabetic, or if you have poor blood circulation.[13]

Petroleum jelly need not be applied to healthy skin surrounding the affected area before corrosive products are applied. However, this precaution should be suggested to patients with poor eyesight or other conditions that increase the likelihood of misapplication or accidental spillage of a salicylic acid product.

TABLE 45-3 Guidelines for Treating Corns and Calluses with Salicylic Acid Products

- Wash and dry the affected area thoroughly before applying any product.

Salicylic Acid 12%–17.6% in Collodion-Like Vehicle

- Apply product no more than twice daily. Morning and evening are usually the most convenient times.
- Do not let adjacent areas of normal healthy skin come in contact with the drug. If they do, wash off the solution immediately with soap and water.
- Apply one drop at a time directly to the corn or callus until the affected area is well covered. Do not overuse the product.
- Allow the drops to dry and harden so the solution does not run.
- For hard corns and calluses, the solution is applied once or twice daily for up to 14 days.
- For soft corns between the toes, hold the toes apart until the solution has dried; then apply a dressing. Treat these corns for 3–6 days.
- After use, cap the container tightly to prevent evaporation and to prevent the active ingredients from assuming a greater concentration.
- Soak the affected foot in warm water for 5 minutes. Then remove the macerated, soft white skin of the corn or callus by scrubbing gently with a rough towel, pumice stone, or callus file. Do not debride the healthy skin.
- Store the product in an amber or light-resistant container away from direct sunlight or heat.

Salicylic Acid 12%–40% Plasters/Pads

- If using plaster, trim the plaster to follow the contours of the corn or callus. Apply the plaster to the affected skin, and cover it with adhesive occlusive tape.
- If using disks with pads, apply the appropriately sized disk directly on the affected area, and then cover it with the pad.
- Remove the plaster/pad and occlusive tape within 48 hours.
- Soak the foot and remove the macerated skin by scrubbing gently with a rough towel, pumice stone, or callus file. Do not debride the healthy skin.
- Reapply the plaster after removing the softened skin.
- Repeat every 8 hours as needed over a 2-week period.

Source: References 12 and 13.

Assessment of Corns and Calluses: A Case-Based Approach

For corns, calluses, and other foot disorders, the practitioner should consider providing a private area where patients can be comfortable removing their shoe(s) to permit direct inspection of the foot. Direct inspection enables the practitioner to accurately assess the nature and extent of the problem.

Before recommending a course of action, the practitioner must identify not only the disorder but also its possible causes. The patient's health status and use of medications should be determined. The patient should be asked whether and how he or she has self-treated the disorder, as well as how successful the attempts were. This information should be recorded and regularly updated in the patient's medication profile.

Patient Counseling for Corns and Calluses

Remission of corns and calluses can take several days to several months. Patients suffering from corns and calluses should understand that effective treatment and maintenance depend on eliminating predisposing factors that contributed to the foot

PATIENT EDUCATION FOR
CORNS AND CALLUSES

The objectives of self-treatment are to (1) provide symptomatic relief, (2) remove corns or calluses, and (3) prevent their recurrence by correcting underlying causes. For most patients, carefully following product instructions and the self-care measures listed here will help ensure optimal therapeutic outcomes.

Nondrug Measures

- To avoid autoinoculating oneself at another body site, keep the instruments used to remove dead skin clean (see Table 45-3).
- Do not use sharp knives or razor blades to remove dead skin of corns and calluses. These instruments may cause bacterial contamination and infection.
- If you have trouble applying the product to only the affected area because of poor eyesight or other conditions, apply petroleum jelly to healthy skin surrounding the affected area before applying the corn and callus remover.
- For temporary relief of painful pressure from the area under a corn or callus, cover the affected area with a pad such as Cushlin. Use the pad for up to 1 week or longer unless it causes itching, burning, or pain.
- Consult a primary care provider or podiatrist if the symptoms described previously occur.

Preventive Measures

- To eliminate the pressure and friction that cause corns and calluses, wear well-fitting, non-binding footwear that evenly distributes body weight (see Table 45-1).
- For anatomic foot deformities, consult a podiatrist about orthopedic corrections.

Nonprescription Medications

- To remove corns and calluses, use a salicylic acid product labeled for use on these types of lesions (see Table 45-2).
- Do not use this product on irritated, infected, or reddened skin.
- Do not use this product if you are diabetic or have poor blood circulation.
- Salicylic acid is poisonous. Do not allow it to come in contact with the mouth, and keep it out of children's reach.
- Note that the medication sloughs off skin and may leave an unsightly pinkish tinge to the skin.

 Stop treatment and consult a primary care provider or podiatrist if swelling, reddening, or irritation of the skin occurs, or if pain occurs immediately with product application.

---

problem in the beginning. It is important to discuss the need for appropriately fitting footwear, which will allow for plenty of width and length. Recommendations also can be made on types of padding to reduce pressure and shearing, which may predispose to corns and calluses.

The practitioner should counsel the patient or caregiver on how to use nonprescription medications that remove corns and calluses. Because many products contain corrosive materials, they must be applied to only the corn or callus. Practitioners should alert patients that products containing collodions are poisonous when taken orally and that these products, as well as all other medications, should be stored out of children's reach. Collodion-containing products are volatile, have an odor similar to that of airplane glue, and may be subject to abuse by inhalation.

Nonprescription products for corns and calluses are not recommended for patients with diabetes or circulatory problems. Practitioners should reinforce contraindications, warnings, and precautions with all patients to avoid the inadvertent use of such products by individuals who have such conditions.

The box Patient Education for Corns and Calluses lists specific information to provide patients.

Evaluation of Patient Outcomes for Corns and Calluses

The progress of patients with hard corns or calluses should be checked after 14 days of treatment. If these conditions are still present, the patient should consult a primary care provider or podiatrist for evaluation.

BUNIONS

An estimated 3% of Americans and 7% of those older than 65 years have bunions. Women are 10 times more likely to develop bunions than men, owing to improperly fitting shoes with narrow toe boxes or too-high heels. Often, several family members suffer from this disorder. However, despite a positive family history, aggravating circumstances (e.g., wearing tight shoes) must also be present for a bunion to actually develop.[8]

Pathophysiology of Bunions

The hallux, or great toe, along with the inner side of the foot, provides the elasticity and mobility needed to walk or run. Thus, the hallux is a dynamic body part. However, this mobility causes several anatomic disorders associated with the foot, such as hallux valgus in which there is a deviation of the great toe, or main axis of the toe, toward the outer toes or lateral side of the foot. Prolonged pressure associated with external shoe irritation over the prominent, angulated metatarsophalangeal joint of the great toe may result in painful inflammation, swelling, and/or exostosis over the involved bony joint structure (Figure 45-3). This process may result in bunion formation, as shown in Figure 45-4.

Bunions can be caused by various conditions. Pressure on the metatarsal head of the great toe may result from the manner in which a person sits, walks, or stands. In women, pressure from high-heeled shoes and/or too-narrow or too-shallow toe boxes force the side of the toe inward and can aggravate the condition.

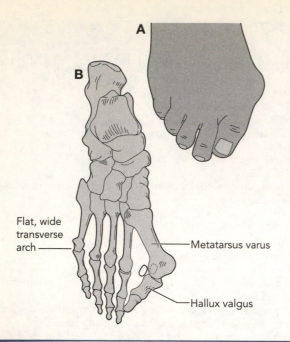

Flat, wide transverse arch

Metatarsus varus

Hallux valgus

FIGURE 45-3 Two views of hallux valgus. **A,** Gross representation of hallux valgus. **B,** Bone structure of hallux valgus.

Friction on the toes from bone malformations (wide heads or lateral bending) is also a major factor in bunion production, as are biomechanical defects. Vigorous exercise such as running can cause bunions or exacerbate existing bunions and increase the severity of a hallux valgus deformity.

Clinical Presentation of Bunions

Bunions are usually asymptomatic but may become quite painful, swollen, red, and tender. Pain is caused by pressure from shoes on the medial aspect of the first metatarsal head. The bunion itself is usually covered by an extensive keratinous overgrowth. Patients may experience increased pain or decreased movement of the great toe.[14–16]

Treatment of Bunions

Corrective steps to alleviate bunions often depend on the degree of discomfort. In some cases, corrective surgery is necessary.

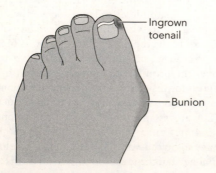

Ingrown toenail

Bunion

FIGURE 45-4 Bunion and ingrown toenail.

Treatment Goals

The self-treatment goals are (1) to decrease irritation of the affected area and (2) prevent worsening of the condition by correcting the cause.

General Treatment Approach

Bunions are not amenable to topical drug therapy, and the chronic use of oral nonprescription analgesics, particularly ibuprofen, is not suggested. Management of the bunion should address the cause, such as tight-fitting or high-heeled shoes, excessive pronation of the foot, or a previous injury. Therefore, self-treatment includes avoiding high-heeled shoes, using protective padding (e.g., bunion pads), and taking oral anti-inflammatory drugs on a short-term basis. Self-treatment relieves only the swelling caused by shoe friction; therefore, well-fitted shoes with a wide toe box should be worn at all times to prevent subsequent flares of inflammation. If shoe adjustments fail to alleviate pain, referral to a properly trained health care professional is indicated. Physical therapy may be beneficial to provide relief from pain and inflammation. Orthotics may help control irregularities of the foot movement.[14] The algorithm in Figure 45-5 outlines self-treatment of bunions and lists exclusions for self-management.

Nonpharmacologic Therapy

Selection of Footwear

Table 45-1 provides guidelines for selecting properly fitted footwear.

Bunion Pads/Cushions

Topical nonprescription padding (e.g., moleskin) can be helpful and may be all that is necessary to decrease the irritation of footwear. Eventually, padding can help to decrease inflammation around the bunion area. Before the protective pad is applied, the foot should be bathed and thoroughly dried. The pad is then cut into a shape that conforms to the bunion. If the intention is to relieve the pressure from the center of the bunion area, the pad should be cut to surround the bunion. Precut pads are available for immediate patient use. To minimize the risk of skin maceration and ulceration, the patient should avoid constant skin contact with adhesive-backed pads, unless their use is recommended by a podiatrist or primary care provider.

For patients who are allergic to adhesives, a nonmedicated, self-adhesive bunion cushion (i.e., Bunion Guard) is commercially available. One advantage of this product is that it protects the bunion and can be easily removed before showering. The cushion, made of a soft polymer gel, can then be reapplied onto the bunion after showering for up to 3 months. Another advantage of Bunion Guard is that it does not contain an adhesive backing, which can be irritating to skin. The outer surface is smooth and not prone to snagging socks or hosiery.

Larger footwear may be necessary to compensate for the space taken up by the pad; in fact, failure to increase shoe size appropriately may cause pressure in other areas. In addition, protective pads should not be used on bunions when the skin is broken or blistered. Abraded skin should receive palliative

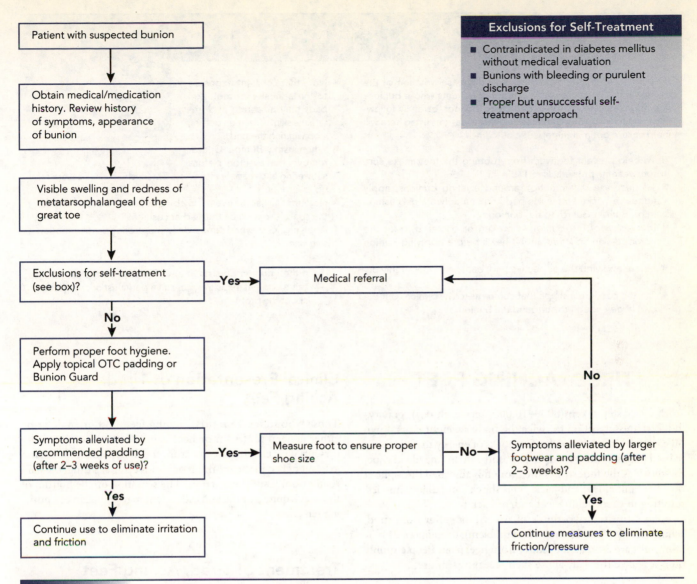

Exclusions for Self-Treatment

- Contraindicated in diabetes mellitus without medical evaluation
- Bunions with bleeding or purulent discharge
- Proper but unsuccessful self-treatment approach

Patient with suspected bunion

↓

Obtain medical/medication history. Review history of symptoms, appearance of bunion

↓

Visible swelling and redness of metatarsophalangeal of the great toe

↓

Exclusions for self-treatment (see box)? —**Yes**→ Medical referral

↓ **No**

Perform proper foot hygiene. Apply topical OTC padding or Bunion Guard

↓

Symptoms alleviated by recommended padding (after 2–3 weeks of use)? —**Yes**→ Measure foot to ensure proper shoe size —**No**→ Symptoms alleviated by larger footwear and padding (after 2–3 weeks)?

↓ **Yes** (from first) — ↓ **Yes** (from last)

Continue use to eliminate irritation and friction — Continue measures to eliminate friction/pressure

No → Medical referral

FIGURE 45-5 Self-care of bunions. Key: OTC, over-the-counter.

treatment before pads are applied. If symptoms persist, these patients should consult a podiatrist or orthopedist.

Assessment of Bunions: A Case-Based Approach

Measures discussed in Assessment of Corns and Calluses: A Case-Based Approach are also appropriate for evaluating bunions. Specific information the practitioner needs to obtain from the patient includes where the lesion is located, how long it has been a problem, whether it occurs with specific footwear, and how painful it is. It is also important to inquire about methods used to relieve symptoms (shoes, pads, and NSAIDs).

Patient Counseling for Bunions

The practitioner should stress to the patient that effective, long-term "treatment" of bunions is to remove the source of irritation.

Patients who do not achieve permanent relief by changing footwear should consult a podiatrist or orthopedist to determine whether anatomic defects are causing bunions. The practitioner should explain the proper short-term use of bunion pads and cushions to patients who want to use them. In addition, non-drug measures such as applying ice to relieve pain and inflammation can be recommended.[17] The box Patient Education for Bunions lists specific information to provide patients.

Evaluation of Patient Outcomes for Bunions

Depending on the severity of the irritation, bunions that are not caused by biomechanical defects of the foot may take a few weeks to resolve. The practitioner should follow up after 2 to 3 weeks to determine whether wearing new shoes and/or using bunion cushions or pads has eliminated the discomfort. If the patient is still experiencing discomfort, medical referral is appropriate.

TIRED, ACHING FEET

With every step taken (8000–10,000 steps each day), gravity-induced pressure of up to twice the body's weight bears down on each foot, releasing powerful shocks of energy that the foot's natural padding must struggle to absorb. In an unpadded shoe, the shock as the foot strikes the ground is absorbed throughout the foot, ankle, leg, and back. This shock can fatigue muscles, resulting in tired, aching feet and/or back pain.[1]

An estimated two-thirds of Americans suffer from tired, aching feet (the most common foot problem). In addition, 21 million adults are estimated to suffer from heel pain. People simply do not realize the daily abuse their feet must endure.

Pathophysiology of Tired, Aching Feet

Aching feet can be caused by increased frequency of standing and/or walking (especially on hard surfaces), age-related erosion of the fat padding on the bottom of the foot, circulatory or neurologic disorders, and poor-fitting/inappropriate footwear.

Because the cause of heel pain is difficult to determine, treatment can often be prolonged and expensive. The two most common types of heel pain are heel spurs (i.e., bony growths on the underside of the heel bone) and plantar fasciitis (strain on the connective tissue that attaches the arch to the front of the heel). Heel spurs are the result of strained foot muscles and the wearing away of the fat tissue surrounding the heel bone. Incorrect walking or running technique, excessive running, poor-fitting shoes, being overweight or experiencing a rapid weight gain, and aging are common contributors to this condition. Heel pain can be an early sign of systemic arthritis.[9,18]

Plantar fasciitis is often caused by high arches, flat feet, repetitive foot stress during athletic activity, pronated feet, or prolonged standing. This disorder can be determined by the patient's description of the pain and its occurrence.[15,18,19]

Clinical Presentation of Tired, Aching Feet

Those who suffer from tired, aching feet most often describe either general foot pain or heel pain. Plantar fasciitis usually presents with pain that occurs from the first moment the person gets out of bed in the morning or stands up after sitting; the pain results from tissue contraction. The sensation on the bottom of the heel is quite painful, and the patient may complain of a burning sensation.[15,19]

Treatment of Tired, Aching Feet

Treatment Goals

The goal in self-treating tired, aching feet is to provide additional support and shock absorbance for the feet to reduce foot pain and fatigue.

General Treatment Approach

The first measure to avoid tired, aching feet is to use well-fitted footwear that has sufficient padding and cushioning (Table 45-1). Wearing sport-specific shoes with good arch support (e.g., running/jogging shoes) is an excellent measure for preventing heel pain. People should purchase shoes carefully to ensure a proper fit.[9]

Active people or those who must stand for prolonged periods during the day may need to take additional measures, such as replacing worn shoes or heel pads, using a night splint, strapping or taping the arch, decreasing the amount of weight-bearing activity, and, if necessary, entering a weight-reduction program.[9,20] Oral anti-inflammatory treatment and topical anti-inflammatory treatments such as ice applications are also appropriate (Table 45-4). Athletes will use Epsom salt soaks to assist with decreasing fatigue and pain in feet and legs caused by

TABLE 45-4 Guidelines for Applying Cold Compresses

Ice Bag Method

- Fill the ice bag one-half to two-thirds of capacity with crushed or shaved ice, if possible. These forms of ice will ensure greater contact with the injured body part.
- If needed, break ice into walnut-sized pieces with no jagged edges. An overfilled bag will be difficult to apply, because it will not rest on the contour of the body area.
- After filling the bag, squeeze out trapped air. Then dry the outside of the bag and check for leaks.
- Bind the injured body part with a wet elastic wrap, and then apply the ice bag. The wet wrap aids transfer of cold to the injured area.
- If the ankle is being treated, keep it in a dorsiflexed position (foot toward the nose) when it is wrapped in the elastic bandage.
- Apply the ice bag to the specific body part.
- To avoid tissue damage, apply the ice bag for 10 minutes and then remove it for 10 minutes. If the bag is not cloth covered, wrap injured area or the ice bag in a thin towel to prevent tissue damage.
- Follow this procedure three to four times a day.
- For most injuries, continue the cryotherapy until swelling decreases or for a maximum of 12–24 hours. Depending on the severity of the injury, application of ice may be necessary for up to 48–72 hours. (For example, the maximum swelling of ankle injuries may occur up to 48 hours after the injury.)
- Before storing the ice bag, drain it and allow it to air dry. If possible, turn it inside out for more efficient drying. Cap the bag, and store it in a cool, dry place.

Cold Wraps

- To activate a single-use cold pack, squeeze the middle of the pack to burst the bubble. This action initiates an endothermic reaction of ammonium nitrate, water, and special additives.
- For a reusable cold wrap (cold pack or gel pack), store it in the freezer for 2 hours. Do not put the cloth cover in the freezer.
- Remove the cold wrap from the freezer, insert it in the cloth cover, and apply it to the injured body part.
- If the cold wrap is uncomfortable, remove it for a minute or 2 and then reapply it.
- Alternate application of the cold wrap (10 minutes on; 10 minutes off) three to four times a day for 24–48 hours.
- After use, store the cold wrap in the freezer.
- Although some gel packs are nontoxic, keep all cold wraps out of children's reach.

inflammation and muscle cramps. Salt baths have historically been used for soothing tired aching muscles, sprains, and bruising, but no scientific evidence supports these claims. Commonly, adding 2 cups of Epsom salt to a warm bathtub and soaking for approximately 12 minutes will prove beneficial. When self-treatment fails, patients should be referred to an appropriate health care professional for evaluation of possible bony malalignments and possible orthotic therapy. Figure 45-6 outlines self-treatment of tired, aching feet.

Nonpharmacologic Therapy

Shoe Inserts, Partial Insoles, and Heel Cups/Cushions

Full-shoe inserts, which can provide cushioning and absorb shock, are available in various sizes and thicknesses to accommodate most individuals. These inserts help decrease the incidence of lower back pain associated with the impact from walking. The patient must select an insert that conforms to the type of shoe worn.[9,11]

Partial insoles are preferred when cushioning or support is desired in a certain portion of the shoe. For example, metatarsal arch supports, which fit into the ball-of-foot region of a woman's shoe, help lift the arch behind the toes to alleviate pain associated with the spreading of the foot, a condition that occurs with increasing age. For women who wear high-heeled shoes, inserts (i.e., Toe Squish Preventer cushions) are available to prevent the toes from becoming cramped in the pointed toe box. Finally, the arch support insert is intended to cushion and support painful longitudinal arches.[9,11]

Depending on the location and extent of the pain, a heel cup or heel cushion may be indicated. For example, a heel cushion might be appropriate when the pain is confined to the bottom of the heel. A heel cushion supports the entire heel as it elevates the sensitive area to prevent further irritation. Alternatively, when the pain is widespread and diffuse, a heel cup might be more appropriate. Heel cups help relieve the pain caused by the breakdown of the heel's natural padding or by intense athletic activity.

Caution should be used when selecting shoe inserts. If an insole affects the patient's gait, referral to a podiatrist or pedorthist (one who specializes in designing, manufacturing, modification, and fit of footwear and orthotics) is recommended. Insoles should be used only to cushion the foot, not to correct malformation, which requires a specialist's attention.

Compression Stockings

Compression stockings are also options to enhance support for those who spend many hours on their feet. Available without a prescription in compressions ranging from 15 to 40 mm Hg, these stockings will decrease inflammation by improving circulation, thereby reducing fatigue of the feet, legs, and back.[21,22]

Assessment of Tired, Aching Feet: A Case-Based Approach

Measures discussed in Assessment of Corns and Calluses: A Case-Based Approach is appropriate for triage of a patient who complains of tired, aching feet. In addition, the practitioner must determine whether the pain affects the soles of the feet, the heels, or the entire foot. The practitioner must also evaluate lifestyle factors (e.g., occupation, daily exercise, and footwear); underlying pathology (e.g., circulatory or neurologic disorders); the possibility of an aggravating event; and the walking/working surface. If underlying pathology is suspected, the practitioner should refer patients to a primary care provider or podiatrist for initial evaluation.

Patient Counseling for Tired, Aching Feet

The practitioner can play an integral role in counseling patients on preventing and treating foot disorders caused by friction and excessive impact. The cornerstone of preventing these disorders

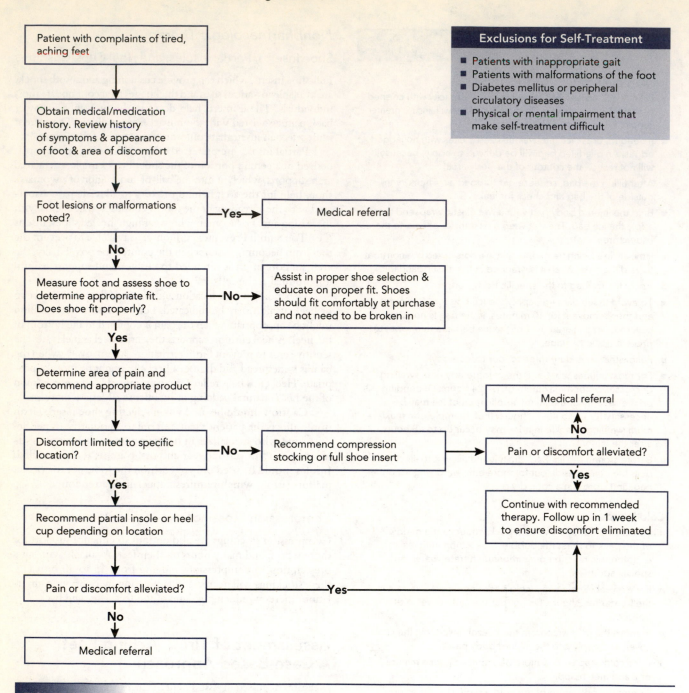

FIGURE 45-6 Self-care of tired, aching feet.

is selecting the appropriate footwear. If the disorder still persists, the practitioner can help patients select in-shoe supports and advise them of other measures to reduce weight-bearing activities. The box Patient Education for Tired, Aching Feet lists specific information to provide patients.

Evaluation of Patient Outcomes for Tired, Aching Feet

Resolution of pain in the soles or heels of the feet depends on the patient and the longevity of the foot problem. The practitioner should follow up after 1 week to determine whether the use of

new shoes and/or in-shoe supports has eliminated the discomfort. If the symptoms persist, the patient should consult a podiatrist for evaluation.

EXERCISE-INDUCED FOOT INJURIES

The practitioner should be aware of possible exercise-induced foot injuries, particularly those caused by running, jogging, or other high-impact physical activities (Figure 45-7) as well as acute injury management techniques (Table 45-5). Often, individuals fail to take certain precautions and dive head first into a strenuous exercise program. People who are typically sedentary, older than 35 years, have hypertension, or a history of heart disease or diabetes should see a clinician before beginning a strenuous exercise program to minimize potential injuries and dangers. Walking may minimize the potential orthopedic problems described here that can result from more strenuous forms of exercise.[23]

Types of Exercise-Induced Injuries

The term *shin splint* is used generically to describe all the pain emanating from below the knee and above the ankle. Shin splints are an overuse phenomenon that occurs in runners or walkers who use hard surfaces. This condition may also occur from not stretching out properly before running, running on a banked track or the sloped shoulder of a road, wearing improper footwear, or overstriding. People who suffer from shin splints experience pain caused by excessive pronation, which causes weakness and strain on the posterior tibialis tendon. This tendon may pull away from the periosteum that lines the shinbone.[16,24]

Exercise-induced stress fractures account for 50% of stress fractures in men and 64% in women.[25] Stress fracture, also known as march, army, or fatigue fracture, may be encountered in runners, especially those who run repetitively on hard, inflexible surfaces. Stress fractures also occur in car salespersons and individuals who climb stairs and/or ladders numerous times during the day. This injury usually involves the long bones of the foot or leg. It is not an overt break of the bone, but rather an alteration in the architecture of the normal bone in which the outer cortex of the bone cracks. Rapid increases in physical activity, running, jumping, nutritional deficiencies, obesity, inappropriate footwear, poor flexibility, and hormone disturbances (i.e., estrogen deficiency) are some of the risk factors for stress fractures.

Achilles tendonitis is a painful inflammation involving the Achilles tendon. Running on hills or on the beach, wearing improper footwear (e.g., running and jogging in shoes designed for racquet sports), and moving with excessive pronation (i.e., rolling in of the feet) are common causes of Achilles tendonitis. However, running by itself does not cause this condition. It may be an early sign of arthritis or rupture of a tendon; the exact cause of the problem is difficult to distinguish. Therefore, patients with Achilles tendonitis should be referred to a primary care provider, podiatrist, or physical therapist.

Blisters occur on the heel or sole of the foot following repeated shearing forces moving across the skin. These forces result in midepidermal cell death between the stratum corneum and stratum lucidum. Heat, sweat, and skin maceration all increase the risk of blistering.[8,26]

Ankle sprains account for 75% of ankle injuries. Approximately 1 million patients seek medical assistance related to acute injuries of the ankle each year.[26] Lateral ligament injury to the ankle is caused by rotation of the body over the fixed foot.

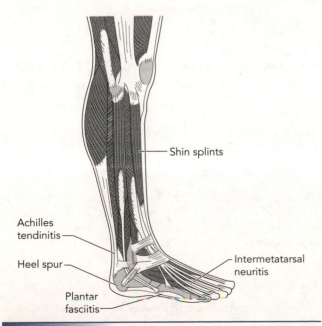

Shin splints

Achilles tendinitis

Heel spur

Plantar fasciitis

Intermetatarsal neuritis

FIGURE 45-7 Selected foot and leg injuries associated with excessive impact shock.

TABLE 45-5 Differentiation of Exercise-Induced Foot Injuries

Type of Injury	Common Causes	Pathophysiology	Signs/Symptoms	Recommendations
Shin splints	Overzealous workout; inappropriate stretching; running/walking on sloped or hard surfaces; wearing ill-fitting footwear; overstriding	Excessive pronation weakens/strains posterior tibialis; anterior tibial muscle stretches away from periosteum that lines shinbone	Pain in medial lower third of shin, or below knee and above ankle; pain worsens with exercise; cramping, burning, and tightness on anterior lateral section of shin	PRICE or RICE therapy; acetaminophen or ibuprofen; shoe orthotic; medical referral
Stress fracture	Running on hard, rigid surfaces; rapid increase in physical activity; jumping; estrogen deficiency; nutritional deficiencies; obesity; ill-fitting footwear	Outer cortex of long bones of leg or foot cracks from alternation in tensile forces sent by ligaments, tendons, and muscles	Deep pain in lower leg; tender to touch; swelling; pain worsens with exercise	Medical referral; complete rest; NSAID therapy
Achilles tendonitis	Running on hills or in sand; ill-fitting footwear; excessive pronation; arthritis	Inflammation of Achilles tendon; rupture of tendon	Posterior heel pain; tenderness; swelling	Medical referral
Blisters	Repetitive movement; ill-fitting footwear; tight hosiery	Continual friction on small surface of foot separates stratum corneum and stratum lucidum skin layers, causing space between layers to fill with fluid	Accumulation of fluid beneath stratum corneum; may be painful	Do not remove blister; protect with topical bandage; medical referral for drainage
Ankle sprains	Ankle rotating outside acceptable range	Lateral ligament damage	Pain; bruising; tenderness; difficulty walking	PRICE or RICE therapy; compression bandage
Intermetatarsal neuritis	Small toe box space	Inflammation of nerves from compression of or entanglement between metatarsal heads and digital bases	Pain and numbness between toes	Proper footwear
Toenail loss	Long, thick toenails in small toe box space; friction and pressure from running in "stop and go" sports, such as tennis	Fluid beneath nail plate pushes toenail from nail bed	Dark discoloration from blood underneath nail plate; pain at toe; nail loss	Referral to podiatrist or PCP

Key: NSAID, nonsteroidal anti-inflammatory drug; PCP, primary care provider; PRICE, protection, rest, ice, compression, elevation; RICE, rest, ice, compression, elevation.

Intermetatarsal neuritis is due to inflamed nerves. These nerves are compressed or caught in the area between the metatarsal heads and digital bases.[27,28]

Toenail loss may be due to blisters under the toenail that occur as a result of the interaction between the toenail and the interior toe box of the shoe. Overgrown, thickened toenails and poorly fitted shoes can produce this problem. Long toenails catch on the sock or inside the shoe toe box, particularly when the individual is running downhill and in "stop and go" sports such as tennis.[29]

Clinical Presentation of Exercise-Induced Foot Injuries

Table 45-5 lists clinical signs and symptoms of the discussed exercised-induced foot injuries.

Treatment of Exercise-Induced Foot Injuries

Treatment Goals

The goals in self-treating exercise-induced foot problems are to (1) relieve pain if present, (2) prevent secondary bacterial infection if the skin is broken, and (3) institute measures to prevent further injury.

General Treatment Approach

Measures to prevent exercise-induced injuries entail using suitable footwear that fits properly (Table 45-1), running on the proper surface, using correct posture (i.e., running erect), and stretching muscles before exercising. Most running injuries can be successfully treated with measures for shoe modifications, inserts, and in-shoe supports as discussed in Treatment of Tired, Aching Feet.

If there is an injury to the leg or foot, activity must usually be interrupted to allow the injured leg or foot to rest. Relative rest (i.e., avoiding activities that produce the symptoms) is often indicated. When an injury occurs, the practitioner should encourage alternative exercise modes, such as swimming, rowing, and/or bicycling (stationary or outdoor).

If the injury warrants it, the practitioner can instruct the patient on selecting and using nonprescription accessories (e.g., cryotherapy, a compression ice wrap, ice bags, compression bandages, arch supports, and heel cushions) that will alleviate injuries or problems. Systemic analgesics can also relieve the pain and inflammation of minor foot injuries (see Chapter 5).

Nonpharmacologic Therapy

Table 45-5 provides specific recommendations for self-treatment of the discussed exercise-induced foot injuries.

Athletic Footwear

Appropriate footwear can be a powerful tool for manipulating human movement and can greatly influence the healing of injured tissues in both positive and negative ways. The importance of appropriate footwear has been reported by Cheung and Ng.[30] These authors demonstrated that the type of footwear chosen by recreational runners is important for injury prevention. Consequently, inappropriate shoes may be problematic, as observed by Burns et al.,[31] who report that an association was found between ill-fitting shoes and self-reported pain. The authors go on to explain that a majority of older people on a rehabilitation ward wore ill-fitting shoes. Table 45-1 provides recommendations for selection of footwear.

Shoe manufacturers offer various types of shoes for different activities (e.g., running, walking, and racquetball sports). Practitioners should advise individuals to use proper sport-specific shoes to prevent exercise-related injuries.[9,18,28]

Shoes are designed to provide stability and cushioning, and decrease friction. Therefore, shoes should be replaced as soon as they become worn. Individuals with a history of stress fractures, osteoarthritis, or rigid high arches should not wait until the outer sole wears through to replace shoes.[9,18]

The Exercise Surface

The exercise surface is another area of consideration with exercise-induced injuries. Because hard surfaces have no give and provide little shock-absorbing capacity, they cause intense shock to the legs, feet, and back. Grassy surfaces, however, are often irregular, which may cause a sprained ankle. Running on a sloping or banked surface may cause the foot to rotate excessively, and place additional stress on the tendons and ligaments of the leg and foot. Uphill training places a strain on the Achilles tendon and muscles of the lower back; downhill running places a lot of impact on the heel. The ideal surface for exercise is relatively smooth, level, and resilient.

Someone who wants to increase energy expenditure may try walking on dirt or sand; these surfaces can boost energy expenditure by as much as one-third. Similarly, walking on a mild, 14-degree slope requires more muscle power than walking on a straight, flat surface.[18]

Compression Bandages

Typically, a compression bandage (e.g., Ace Bandages) is used for an ankle or knee sprain. If a compression bandage is to be used, the width of bandage needed depends on the injury site. For example, a foot or an ankle requires a 2.5- to 3-inch bandage. Table 45-6 describes the proper method of applying this type of bandage.

Cryotherapy

Applying cold compresses to an injury such as a muscle sprain anesthetizes the area and decreases the pain and inflammation. Ice bags or cold wraps are useful for cold application. If an ice bag is used, the English type, which is identified by its commercial cloth material, is preferred, because the patient does not have to wrap a towel around it to protect the skin. Cold packs are available as either single-use (e.g., instant cold pack) or multiple-use products. Another simple, inexpensive method is to prepare ice applications by freezing water in small paper cups, placing ice cubes in a resealable sandwich bag, or using a frozen bag of peas. Table 45-4 describes the proper method of cold application to injuries.

Contrast Bath Soaks

For acute injury, cold application is beneficial in decreasing resultant inflammation. After the acute injury, some podiatrists advocate the use of alternating applications of cold therapy and warm therapy for chronic, nagging pain. Specifically, the cold therapy is intended to decrease inflammation. The warm therapy attempts to bring increased blood flow to the affected area and effect smooth muscle relaxation.

TABLE 45-6 Application Guidelines for Compression Bandages

- Choose the appropriate size of bandage for the injured body part. Purchase a product designed for the appropriate body part if you are unsure of the size.
- Unwind about 12–18 inches of bandage at a time, and allow the bandage to relax.
- If ice is also being applied to the injured area, soak the bandage in water to aid the transfer of cold (see Table 45-4).
- Wrap the injured area by overlapping the previous layer of bandage by about one-third to one-half of its width.
- Tightly wrap the point most distal from the injury. For example, if the ankle is injured, begin wrapping just above the toes.
- Decrease the tightness of the bandage as you continue to wrap. (Follow package directions on how far to extend the bandage past the injury.) If the bandage feels tight or uncomfortable or if circulation is impaired, remove the compression bandage and rewrap. Cold or swollen toes and fingers indicate a bandage is too tight.
- After using the bandage, wash it in lukewarm, soapy water; do not scrub it. Rinse the bandage thoroughly and allow to air-dry on a flat surface.
- Roll up the bandage to prevent wrinkles, and store it in a cool, dry place. Do not iron the bandage to remove wrinkles.

Assessment of Exercise-Induced Injuries: A Case-Based Approach

The practitioner may be called on to play a triage role in treating an exercise-induced injury to the foot. Identifying the location of the pain will help determine the type and extent of the injury. Asking about the nature and duration of the pain will help in determining whether the injury is self-treatable. Figure 45–8 provides therapeutic recommendations for exercise-induced foot injuries.

Patient Counseling for Exercise-Induced Injuries

Although a sports enthusiast may resist such advice, the practitioner should encourage the patient to rest an injured foot or limb, allowing it to heal. The practitioner should also explain measures to prevent recurrences of the patient's particular injury.

When rest alone does not relieve foot discomfort, the proper use of oral analgesics, compression bandages, and cryotherapy should be explained. The practitioner should review with the patient the correct procedure for wrapping, which is also described on the bandage package. If there is reason to believe the patient may cause further injury through inappropriate use of a compression bandage, the practitioner should recommend simply elevating the body part and applying an ice pack or, if warranted by the severity of the injury, consulting a primary care provider. The box Patient Education for Exercise-Induced Injuries lists specific information to provide patients.

Evaluation of Patient Outcomes for Exercise-Induced Injuries

The practitioner should follow up with patients with shin splints or ankle sprains 7 days after the use of compression bandages, cryotherapy, or other anti-inflammatory therapy is begun to find

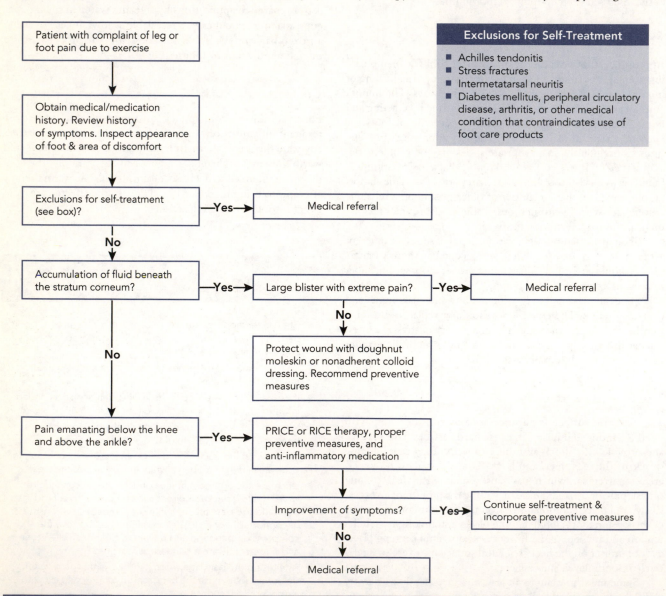

Exclusions for Self-Treatment

- Achilles tendonitis
- Stress fractures
- Intermetatarsal neuritis
- Diabetes mellitus, peripheral circulatory disease, arthritis, or other medical condition that contraindicates use of foot care products

FIGURE 45-8 Self-care of exercise-induced injuries. Key: PRICE, protection, rest, ice, compression, and elevation; RICE, rest, ice, compression, and elevation.

The objectives of self-treatment are to (1) rest the injured foot or limb to allow healing, (2) relieve discomfort, and (3) take measures to prevent further injury. For most patients, carefully following product instructions and the self-care measures listed here will help ensure optimal therapeutic outcomes.

General Measures

■ When a leg or foot injury occurs, rest the injured limb. If desired, perform other types of exercise that do not put a great deal of force on the feet such as swimming or bicycling (stationary or outdoor).

■ Take the following actions to prevent exercise-induced injuries:
—Stretch muscles before exercising.
—Choose sport-specific shoes with good arch support for athletic activities.
—Run or walk on a relatively smooth, level, and resilient surface.
—Keep the back straight when running.

Shin Splints

■ Rest the feet, and apply an ice bag or a cold wrap to the painful area (see Table 45-4).

■ If desired, take aspirin or ibuprofen to relieve pain and reduce tissue inflammation.

■ Do not use analgesics to suppress pain or to increase your endurance during a workout.

■ Seek medical attention if the discomfort becomes a cramping, burning tightness that repeatedly occurs at the same distance or time during a run.

Blisters

■ To prevent blisters during running, wear cotton or woolen socks. If desired, wear two pairs of socks with ordinary talcum powder sprinkled between them. Using an acrylic sock next to the foot will assist in drawing moisture from the foot.

■ Apply compound tincture of benzoin or a flexible collodion product (e.g., New Skin) to the blister before exercise to decrease pain and accelerate healing by promoting reepithelialization.

■ Apply an antiperspirant containing 20% aluminum chloride to decrease incidence of blisters.

■ If blisters break, apply a first-aid antibiotic to the broken skin to prevent secondary bacterial infection.

■ Cover blistered area with moleskin to protect surface.

Ankle Sprains

■ Although maximum swelling will not occur for 48 hours, begin treatment as soon as possible.

■ Stay off the injured foot, wrap a compression bandage around the ankle, apply ice, and elevate the ankle. (See Tables 45-4 and 45-6 for guidelines on applying ice and compression bandages.)

■ Seek medical attention if swelling persists more than 72 hours.

Toenail Blisters/Loss

■ To prevent blisters under the toenail, keep toenails trimmed and run in properly fitted shoes.

■ Should a blister develop, do not disturb or puncture the blister roof.

■ If the toenail separates from the skin or is lost, consult a primary care provider or podiatrist for proper treatment.

out whether the symptoms are resolved. If symptoms of swelling and/or pain persist, referral to a podiatrist or primary care provider is appropriate. Patients with blisters of the feet or under the toenail should also be reevaluated after 7 days of the recommended therapy. If signs of infection are present or if the toenail has separated from the nail bed, medical referral is appropriate.

INGROWN TOENAILS

The most frequent cause of ingrown toenails, or onychocryptosis, is incorrect trimming of the nails. The correct method is to cut the nail straight across without tapering the corners in any way. Wearing pointed-toe or tight shoes or hosiery that is too tight has also been implicated. Other causes are hyperhidrosis, improper-fitting footwear, trauma, obesity, and excessive pressure. In these cases, direct pressure can force the lateral or medial edge of the nail into the soft tissue. The embedded nail may then continue to grow, resulting in swelling and inflammation of the nail fold.[8,11,32]

Bedridden patients may develop ingrown toenails if tight bedcovers press the soft skin tissue against the nails. Nail curling, which can be hereditary or secondary to incorrect nail trimming, onychomycosis, or a systemic, metabolic disease, can also result in ingrown toenails.

Pathophysiology of Ingrown Toenails

An ingrown toenail occurs when a section of nail presses into the soft tissue of the nail groove. The nail curves into the flesh of the toe corners and becomes embedded in the surrounding soft tissue of the toe, causing pain (Figure 45-4). This process results in microtears of the skin that, when coupled with invasion by opportunistic resident foot bacteria, can cause a superficial infection. Swelling, inflammation, and ulceration are secondary complications that can arise from this condition.[31]

Treatment of Ingrown Toenails

Treatment Goals

The goals of self-treating ingrown toenails are to (1) relieve pressure on the toenails, (2) relieve pain, and (3) prevent reoccurrence.

General Treatment Approach

Education is probably the best means of preventing the development of ingrown toenails. In the early stages of development, therapy is directed at providing adequate room for the nail to resume its normal position adjacent to soft tissue. This therapy is accomplished by relieving the external source of pressure. Warm water soaks will help soften the area, and topical antiseptics prescribed by a physician can be applied to prevent possible opportunistic infections. The patient should be referred to a podiatrist or primary care provider if the condition is recurrent or gives rise to an oozing discharge, pain, or severe inflammation. Sometimes surgery is warranted and, even with subsequent systemic antibiotic therapy, the toe may take up to 3 to 4 weeks to heal. Figure 45-9 outlines self-treatment options for ingrown toenails.

Pharmacologic Therapy

In its final rule for ingrown toenail relief products, FDA did not propose any nonprescription active ingredient as safe and effective and not misbranded.[33] Therefore, two previously approved drugs, tannic acid and sodium sulfide,[34] were classified as Category III and withdrawn from the market. Tannic acid was not proven to harden the skin and shrink the soft tissue surrounding the ingrown toenail. Sodium sulfide has considerable adverse reactions such as burning sensations and irritation that made it unacceptable for nonprescription use.[33]

The practitioner, however, must be aware of trade-name product reformulations to accommodate this rule. For example, Outgro Pain-Relieving Formula, which formerly contained tannic acid for treating ingrown toenails, now contains benzocaine 20% to relieve pain associated with ingrown toenails. Patients must be cautious because inappropriate use of this product can result in superficial burns on skin adjacent to the toenail. Furthermore, this product does not treat the underlying problem.

Patients with ingrown toenails often fail to realize they may be helped by oral medication intended to alleviate pain and inflammation. Provided no contraindications exist for use by a particular patient, the practitioner may recommend oral aspirin, ibuprofen, ketoprofen, or naproxen; all four are proven analgesics with anti-inflammatory activity (see Chapter 5).

Assessment of Ingrown Toenail: A Case-Based Approach

The practitioner can play a vital role in prevention and acute pain relief for ingrown toenails. Initial recommendations can be made to offer relief from the ingrown toenail such as warm bath soaks to soften the skin and oral anti-inflammatory therapy for temporary pain relief. If the toenail or nail bed is infected, immediate referral is warranted.

Patient Counseling for Ingrown Toenails

Practitioners should educate patients on proper nail trimming techniques as well as preventive measures to eliminate or avoid future issues with ingrown toenails. They can also offer recommendations on temporary pain relief options. The box Patient Education for Ingrown Toenails lists specific information to provide patients.

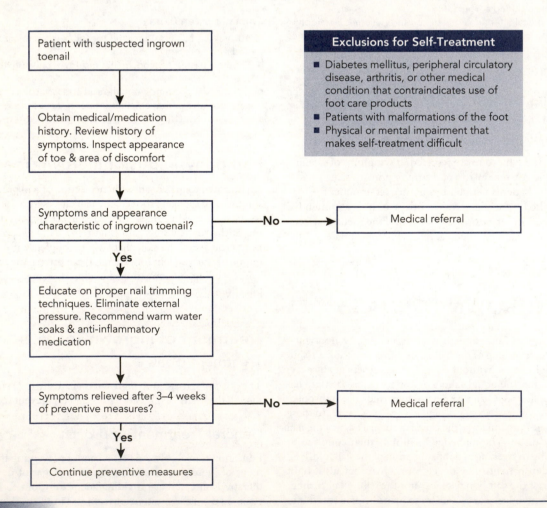

Exclusions for Self-Treatment

- Diabetes mellitus, peripheral circulatory disease, arthritis, or other medical condition that contraindicates use of foot care products
- Patients with malformations of the foot
- Physical or mental impairment that makes self-treatment difficult

Patient with suspected ingrown toenail

↓

Obtain medical/medication history. Review history of symptoms. Inspect appearance of toe & area of discomfort

↓

Symptoms and appearance characteristic of ingrown toenail? —**No**→ Medical referral

↓ **Yes**

Educate on proper nail trimming techniques. Eliminate external pressure. Recommend warm water soaks & anti-inflammatory medication

↓

Symptoms relieved after 3–4 weeks of preventive measures? —**No**→ Medical referral

↓ **Yes**

Continue preventive measures

FIGURE 45-9 Self-care of ingrown toenails.

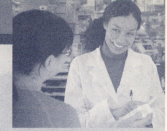

PATIENT EDUCATION FOR
Ingrown Toenails

The ultimate goals for self-treatment of ingrown toenails are to relieve the pain and pressure associated with the condition and to prevent recurrence.

- Ensure proper fit of shoes to eliminate pressure on the toenails.
- Prevent recurrence of ingrown toenails by cutting toenails straight across, rather than at an angle.

- Decrease pain and inflammation of the ingrown toenail by taking a nonsteroidal anti-inflammatory medication such as ibuprofen or naproxen.
- Relieve impingement of the nail by soaking feet in warm water to soften the nail and skin around it.

Evaluation of Patient Outcomes for Ingrown Toenails

Patient evaluations should be made after 3 to 4 weeks to determine whether relief of pressure and preventive measures have been successful. Referrals should be made if there is no improvement, worsening of the condition, or discharge from the site of irritation.

HYPERHIDROSIS

Hyperhidrosis is defined as excessive sweating. The incidence of hyperhidrosis is 2.8% of the population; it occurs in men and women at the same rate.[35,36] It is most prevalent in people ages 25 to 64 years.[35] Hyperhidrosis is a complicated process that involves sympathetic and parasympathetic pathways.[35] There are two types of hyperhidrosis, primary focal hyperhidrosis and secondary hyperhidrosis.

Primary focal hyperhidrosis is defined as visible, excessive sweating of 6 months duration without cause and having two or more of the following characteristics: bilateral and symmetrical presentation, one or more episodes a week, hindrance of social activities, family history of disorder, and absence of sweating during sleep.[35] This disorder seems to begin during childhood. Symptoms of hyperhidrosis usually improve with age. Family history is positive in 30% to 50% of patients.[36] Hyperhidrosis can be embarrassing to individuals and may affect their daily activities, lifestyle, and social interactions. Although its psychological morbidity is prevalent in most patients experiencing hyperhidrosis, few people seek medical attention for the disorder.

Secondary hyperhidrosis can have a focal or generalized presentation affecting the entire body. Secondary hyperhidrosis is usually caused by a variety of medical conditions. Examples of these are endocrine disorders (e.g., hyperthyroidism or diabetes mellitus); pregnancy; neurologic disorders; malignant disorders; cardiovascular disorders; respiratory failure; licit and illicit drugs; and alcohol abuse.[36] This discussion will focus on primary focal hyperhidrosis, because nonprescription medications are available to treat this disorder.

Pathophysiology of Hyperhidrosis

Primary focal hyperhidrosis occurs mainly in the palms, plantar surfaces, and axillae. The more than 4 million sweat glands in the body are classified as either eccrine or apocrine, with eccrine glands making up 75% of the total. Eccrine glands primarily produce colorless, odorless sweat and are located all over the body. They are more concentrated in the soles of the feet, forehead, and palms. The apocrine glands are scented sweat glands located in the axillae and genital areas. The pathophysiology of hyperhidrosis is not fully understood. It may be caused by dysfunction of the autonomic nervous system. It seems that once sweating begins, a vicious cycle predominates, and evaporative cooling of the skin increases a reflex sympathetic outflow, which increases sweating even more.[36]

Clinical Presentation of Hyperhidrosis

The most common sign of hyperhidrosis is profuse sweating. Normal sweating is defined as 1 mL/m^2 per minute by eccrine glands at rest and at room temperature.[36] Excessive sweating is considered any amount of sweat that interferes with daily life and activities. Laboratory diagnosis is not necessary. The starch–iodine test has been used to identify the primary area of sweating. When the starch is applied to the area previously covered by an iodine solution, a purple spot highlights the area of sweating. This process helps direct treatment to the affected areas and allows practitioners to see areas of improvement with treatment as a subsequent decrease in the focal area.[35]

There are no physical complications associated with focal hyperhidrosis. Some patients may experience odor problems from sweaty feet or underarms. There are psychological complications that result from the embarrassment of hyperhidrosis. More than 35% of patients report that they have altered their lifestyle by decreasing leisure activity time owing to hyperhidrosis. Simple social interactions such as shaking hands, holding hands, and hugging may be difficult.

Treatment of Hyperhidrosis
Treatment Goals

The main goal of treatment is to eliminate profuse sweating in a cost-effective, minimally invasive method. Several types of treatments are available.

General Treatment Approach

Patients should consider convenience, ease of administration, side effects, and the financial impact in choosing the best treatment. Figure 45-10 outlines this process.

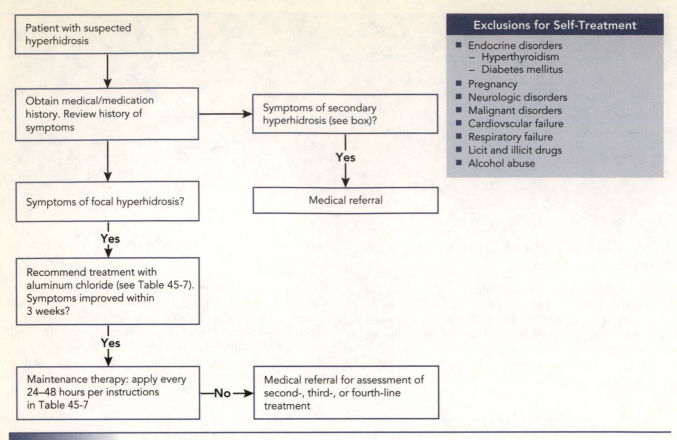

FIGURE 45-10 Self-care of hyperhidrosis.

Nonpharmacologic Therapy

The psychosocial implications of this disorder are one of the primary concerns with the disease. Because the disease mainly involves the autonomic nervous system, few noninvasive methods to treat hyperhidrosis are available. Psychotherapy has been beneficial in a small number of cases.[37] Several surgical and nonsurgical treatments are available. Ionotophoresis is used as a second-line therapy for hyperhidrosis.[35,36,38] This treatment, which involves the passage of a direct electrical current onto the skin, is safe and effective for palm and plantar hyperhidrosis. Its mechanism of action may be related to induction of hyperkeratosis of the sweat pores, which obstructs sweat flow and secretion.[38] Surgical treatment for hyperhidrosis or sympathectomy is recommended as fourth-line treatment for hyperhidrosis.[35,36,38] The treatment involves surgical disruption of second and third thoracic sympathetic ganglia of the palms. Lumbar sympathectomy is used for plantar hyperhidrosis. Patients should pursue surgical treatment cautiously, given that 60% of patients experience compensatory sweating.[38]

Pharmacologic Therapy

Several pharmacologic treatments are available for hyperhidrosis. Aluminum chloride is recommended as first-line treatment in hyperhidrosis, because it is inexpensive and relatively easy to administer.[35,36,38] Drysol is a common prescription drug used to treat hyperhidrosis and contains 20% aluminum chloride hexahydrate in absolute anhydrous ethyl alcohol. The most common nonprescription treatments are topical treatments available as aluminum salts. Aluminum salts, indicated for treatment of excessive perspiration, are commonly found in nonprescription antiperspirants. Their mechanism of action is related to mechanical obstruction of the eccrine gland duct or atrophy of eccrine secretory ducts.[35] Aluminum chloride solutions are available in concentrations of 20% to 25%; nonprescription antiperspirants containing aluminum salts are available in 1% to 2% concentrations. The nonprescription antiperspirant Certain Dri contains 12% aluminum chloride. The products are available in a variety of dosing and delivery formulations to accommodate different application areas.

Patients will need to repeat applications (Table 45-7) often, every 24 to 48 hours; improvement may be seen as early as 3 weeks. The side effects associated with use of aluminum

---

TABLE 45-7 Administration Guidelines for Aluminum Chloride

- Apply product at bedtime and wash off after 6–8 hours. Reapply product every 24–48 hours.
- Apply sparingly by using only a few strokes.
- Do not apply immediately after shaving.
- Do not apply on broken skin.
- Do not apply on irritated skin.
- Do not apply immediately after bathing.
- If desired, apply topical baking soda to reduce skin irritation.

Source: References 35, 36, and 38.

chloride solution include localized burning, stinging, and irritation. These agents may be used on the hands, axillae, or feet. Aluminum chloride in an alcohol–based solution has been shown to be effective in 98% of patients with axillae hyperhidrosis. Aluminum chloride can reduce palmar hyperhidrosis within 48 hours, but reapplication is necessary.

Botulinum toxin A (Botox) is indicated for axillary hyperhidrosis and has shown great promise in the treatment of this disorder. Its mechanism of action is to inhibit the release of acetylcholine at the neuromuscular junction. It also affects the postganglionic sympathetic innervation of sweat glands. Botulinum toxin is safe and effective and is recommended as a third-line treatment.

Assessment of Hyperhidrosis: A Case-Based Approach

For proper assessment of hyperhidrosis, the practitioner should obtain a medical history and medication history related to this disorder. Most often, patients with hyperhidrosis have had symptoms since childhood. A comfortable screening area may allow the practitioner to observe the bilateral excessive sweating. The practitioner should also discuss treatment options and determine the patient's comfort level with the degree of therapies. Case 45-1 illustrates the assessment of patients with hyperhidrosis and other minor foot disorders.

CASE 45-1

Relevant Evaluation Criteria	Scenario/Model Outcome
Information Gathering	
1. Gather essential information about the patient's symptoms, including:	
a. description of symptom(s) (i.e., nature, onset, duration, severity, associated symptoms)	Patient presents with palms and soles of feet that are dripping with sweat. He says that he has had this problem since he was a child. He also says that he especially hates summer and avoids wearing certain shoes, because his feet sweat so much. He often wears thick socks and tennis shoes. He does not like to attend social situations where he will have to hold hands.
b. description of any factors that seem to precipitate, exacerbate, and/or relieve the patient's symptom(s)	Sometimes when he is nervous or uncomfortable, his hands and feet sweat, but they also sweat when watching a scary movie.
c. description of the patient's efforts to relieve the symptoms	He has not tried anything. He makes sure that he has a towel with him to wipe his hands and feet when he can.
2. Gather essential patient history information:	
a. patient's identity	Greg Summer
b. patient's age, sex, height, and weight	25-year-old male, 6 ft 3 in, 210 lb
c. patient's occupation	Student
d. patient's dietary habits	Varies; he eats when he can.
e. patient's sleep habits	Averages 5–6 hours per night
f. concurrent medical conditions, prescription and nonprescription medications, and dietary supplements	None
g. allergies	NKA
h. history of other adverse reactions to medications	None
i. other (describe) _____	Greg will do almost anything to get this problem resolved. He also complains of a painful ingrown toenail that is red with a discharge oozing from the area.
Assessment and Triage	
3. Differentiate the patient's signs/symptoms and correctly identify the patient's primary problem(s).	The patient is experiencing palm and plantar hyperhidrosis. In addition, he has an ingrown toenail.
4. Identify exclusions for self-treatment (see Figures 45-9 and 45-10).	None
5. Formulate a comprehensive list of therapeutic alternatives for the primary problem to determine if triage to a medical practitioner is required, and share this information with the patient.	Options include: (1) Recommend OTC products for focal hyperhidrosis and ingrown toenail. (2) Recommend only a product for hyperhidrosis. Refer patient for ingrown toenail. (3) Take no action.

CASE 45-1 (continued)

Relevant Evaluation Criteria	Scenario/Model Outcome
Plan	
6. Select an optimal therapeutic alternative to address the patient's problem, taking into account patient preferences.	Suggest an OTC product for focal hyperhidrosis, and refer patient to PCP for treatment of ingrown toenail.
7. Describe the recommended therapeutic approach to the patient.	Patient should try a product that contains aluminum chloride (i.e., Certain Dri). If this does not work, he may go to his PCP for a stronger aluminum chloride prescription (i.e., Drysol). Patient must be referred to PCP for the ingrown toenail.
8. Explain to the patient the rationale for selecting the recommended therapeutic approach from the considered therapeutic alternatives.	First-line treatment for focal hyperhidrosis is aluminum chloride. OTC products containing this ingredient are available. You may also obtain a stronger concentration of this ingredient from a medical practitioner.
	If this product does not work, you should consult a medical practitioner for second-line treatment.
	Ingrown toenails are found in patients with hyperhidrosis. The discharge, pain, and possible inflammation may be a sign of infection You should see a medical practitioner for evaluation and treatment.
Patient Education	
9. When recommending self-care with non-prescription medications and/or nondrug therapy, convey accurate information to the patient.	You should try to keep your feet dry throughout the day. You may want to change socks throughout the day or try a powder that will help keep your feet dry.
10. Solicit follow-up questions from patient.	When do I apply the medication to my feet for treatment of hyperhidrosis?
11. Answer patient's questions.	See Table 45-7.

Key: NKA, no known allergies; OTC, over-the-counter; PCP, primary care provider.

Patient Counseling for Hyperhidrosis

The practitioner should discuss the various treatment modalities available for hyperhidrosis. Patients should be made to realize the amount of sweat reduction with the noninvasive therapy of alu-minum hydroxide. Then the patient should also be given details as to the prescription and surgical options to determine if those therapies are worth further exploration. The box Patient Education for Hyperhidrosis and Table 45-7, provide specific information for patients.

PATIENT EDUCATION FOR Hyperhidrosis

The main goal of self-treatment of hyperhidrosis is to eliminate profuse sweating in a cost-effective manner.

- The easiest and most cost-effective therapy would be treatment with aluminum hydroxide. See Table 45-7 for specific administration techniques.
- Use an application modality (e.g., roll-on, aerosol, or cream), which ensures the most beneficial application.
- Use caution with topical treatments; they may result in allergic reaction, burning, stinging, or irritation at the application site.
- Remember to reapply topical product every 24–48 hours to ensure reduction of hyperhidrosis symptoms.

- If satisfactory results are not seen with topical products, consider other therapies such as Botox or surgical procedures.
- There is high patient satisfaction with Botox therapy, but consideration must be given to the level of invasiveness, the pain associated with administration, and the product costs.
- For those who have tried other treatment modalities, surgical treatments may be an option. Compensatory sweating, neuralgia, and sexual dysfunction may result and should be considered before taking this step.

Evaluation of Patient Outcomes for Hyperhidrosis

Patients and practitioners should discuss the expectations of the treatment modalities used. In addition the patient may need to incorporate a routine that will allow continued compliance with treatments that require consistent reapplications. The patients' quality of life should be discussed to determine whether the treatments are effective in improving daily activities.

KEY POINTS FOR MINOR FOOT DISORDERS

➤ The nonprescription drug of choice to treat corns and calluses is salicylic acid in a collodion-like vehicle or plaster product form.

➤ Predisposing factors responsible for corns and calluses must be corrected.

➤ Patients should also be cautioned that frequent recurrence of any of these problems is an indication that they should consult a podiatrist or primary care provider.

➤ Patients with diabetes, circulatory problems, and/or arthritis should be counseled to avoid self-medicating with any topical or oral nonprescription drug without first checking with their primary care provider, podiatrist, or pharmacist.

➤ Nonprescription products are powerful drugs and may exacerbate certain conditions; the practitioner must monitor patient progress carefully and be attuned to patient comments that might indicate the occurrence of drug-related problems.

➤ Be prepared to educate and assist patients who develop exercise-induced injuries.

➤ Most exercise-induced injuries can be treated with shoe modifications, in-shoe supports, modified training methods, ice applications, and stretching exercises.

➤ Maintaining good foot hygiene is an important component of overall health care.

➤ Talking with patients about proper foot hygiene is an important aspect of caring for the patient as a whole.[38]

➤ Patients and practitioners should discuss the expectations of the treatment modalities used in hyperhidrosis.

REFERENCES

1. Georgia Podiatric Medical Association. Available at: http://www.gapma.com/FootFacts.htm. Last accessed October 12, 2008.
2. Plummer ES, Albert SG. Foot care assessment in patients with diabetes: a screening algorithm for patient education and referral. *Diabetes Educ.* 1995;21:47–51.
3. Mayfield J. *The Use of the Semmes-Weinstein Monofilament and Other Threshold Tests for Preventing Foot Ulceration and Amputation in Persons with Diabetes.* Seattle, Wash: School of Public Health and Community Medicine and School of Medicine, University of Washington; Veterans Affairs Puget Sound Health Care System; September 2000.
4. Singh N, Armstrong DG, Lipsky BA. Preventing foot ulcers in patients with diabetes. *JAMA.* 2005;293:217–28.
5. Hunt D. Using evidence in practice foot care in diabetes. *Endocrinol Metab Clin North Am.* 2002;31:306–611.
6. emedicine. Foot infections. Available at: http://www.emedicine.com/orthoped/topic601.htm. Last accessed October 12, 2008.
7. Gorter K, de Poel S, de Melker R, et al. Variation in diagnosis and management of common foot problems by GPs. *Fam Practice* (Oxford). 2001;18(6):569–573.
8. Martin RW, Martin KS, Popovich NG. Podiatry and pharmacy: working together. *Drug Top.* 2001;145(12):43–52.
9. Bedinghaus JM, Niedfeldt MW. Information from your family doctor. Over-the-counter remedies for common foot problems. *Am Fam Physician.* 2001;64:791–804.
10. Freeman DB. Corns and calluses resulting from mechanical hyperkeratosis. *Am Fam Physician.* 2002;65:2277–80.
11. The Children's Hospital—Denver Area, Colorado, Rocky Mountain Region. Blisters, Calluses, and Corns. Available at: http://www.thechildrenshospital.org/wellness/info/kids/22053.aspx. Last accessed October 21, 2008.
12. *Fed Regist.* 1990;55:33258–62.
13. *Fed Regist.* 1990;55:33246–56.
14. American Podiatric Medical Association. Available at: http://www.apma.org/s_apma/doc.asp?TRACKID=&CID=146&DID= 9388. Last accessed October 12, 2008.
15. Are you taking good care of your feet? *Tufts University Health and Nutrition Letter.* Medford, Mass: Tufts University; September 2002:6.
16. American Podiatric Medical Association. [Foot Ailments Table.] Available at: http://www.apma.org/s_apma/doc.asp?TRACKID=&CID=25&DID= 9122. Last accessed October 12, 2008.
17. Bunions: Lifestyle and Home Remedies. Available at: http://www.mayoclinic.com/health/bunions/DS00309/DSECTION=lifestyle-and-home-remedies. Last accessed October 21, 2008.
18. Kennedy JG, Knowles B, Dolan M, et al. Foot and ankle injuries in the adolescent runner. *Curr Opin Pediatr.* 2005;17:34–42.
19. Adams SB, Theodore GH. Extracorporeal shock wave therapy for treatment of plantar fasciitis [serial online]. *OJHMS Online.* Available at: http://orthojournalhms.org/volume5/manuscripts/ms13.htm. Last accessed October 12, 2008.
20. DeLee, Drez. Orthopaedic Sports Medicine. 2nd ed. Philadelphia: Saunders; 2003:chp 30.
21. Ibegbuna V, Delis KT, Nicolaides AN, et al. Effect of elastic compression stockings on venous hemodynamics during walking. *J Vasc Surg.* 2003;37:420–425.
22. Flore R, Gerardino L, Santoliquido A, et al. Reduction of oxidative stress by compression stockings in standing workers. *Occup Med* (Oxford). 2007;57:337–41.
23. McDermott AY, Mernitz H. Exercise and older patients: prescribing guidelines. *Am Fam Physician.* 2006;74:437–44.
24. Goodman A. Foot orthoses in sports medicine. *South Med J.* 2004; 97:867–70.
25. Sanderlin BW, Raspa RF. Common stress fractures. *Am Fam Physician.* 2003;68:1527–32.
26. Freiman A, Barankin B, Elpern DJ. Sports dermatology, part 1: common dermatoses. *CMAJ.* 2004;171:851–3.
27. Childs SG. Interdigital perineural fibroma (a.k.a Morton's neuroma). *Orthopaed Nurs.* 2002;21(6):32–34.
28. Franson J. Intermetatarsal compression neuritis. *J Clin Podiatr Med Surg.* 2006;23:569–578.
29. Mailler-Savage EA, Adams BB. Skin manifestations of running. *J Am Acad Dermatol.* 2006;55:290–301.
30. Cheung RT, Ng G. Influence of different footwear on force of landing during running. *Phys Ther.* 2008 Feb 14 [Epub ahead of print].
31. Burns SL, Leese GP, et al. Older people and ill fitting shoes. *Postgrad Med J.* 2002;78:344–6.
32. Zuber TJ. Ingrown toenail removal. *Am Fam Physician.* 2002;65:2547–50.
33. *Fed Regist.* 1993;58:47602–6.
34. *Fed Regist.* 1982;47:39120–5.
35. Haider A, Solish N. Focal hyperhidrosis: diagnosis and management. *CMAJ.* 2005;172:69–75.
36. Haider A, Solish N. Hyperhidrosis: an approach to diagnosis and management. *Dermatol Nurs.* 2004;16(6):515–23.
37. Connolly M, de Berker D. Management of primary hyperhidrosis: a summary of the different treatment modalities. *Am J Clin Dermatol.* 2003;4:681–97.
38. Thomas I, Brown J, Vafaie J. Palmoplantar hyperhidrosis: a therapeutic challenge. *Am Fam Physician.* 2004;69:1117–20.

Hair Loss

Michael D. Hogue

Significant numbers of both men and women experience either thinning hair or hair loss. Hair loss is most frequently due to hormonal changes, but it may also occur secondary to trauma, medication use, acute or chronic illness, dietary changes, or a combination of these factors. Regardless of the cause, hair loss can have a significant psychological and social impact on individuals' lives. Therefore, patients spend millions of dollars each year on products and procedures both proven and unproven to treat hair loss.

Although only a few causes of hair loss account for the vast majority of cases, many causes and types of baldness exist. Hair loss is broadly categorized as nonscarring or scarring alopecia. Androgenetic alopecia (AGA, or pattern hereditary hair loss), alopecia areata, anagen effluvium (rapid shedding of growing hairs), telogen effluvium (rapid shedding of resting hairs), cosmetic hair damage, and trichotillomania (a compulsive pulling out of one's own hair) are common forms of nonscarring alopecia. With the exception of AGA, other types of nonscarring hair loss should be referred for medical evaluation to determine cause and proper treatment. Types of hair loss secondary to medication use, acute or chronic illness, or dietary changes most typically are also nonscarring; removal of the causative agent or correction of the underlying problem may correct the hair loss. Scarring alopecia may be related to conditions such as discoid lupus erythematosus, syphilis, sarcoidosis, or lichen planus and should also be referred for medical evaluation.[1] Alopecia due to trauma may be either nonscarring or scarring depending on the nature of the trauma. Of all the types of hair loss, the Food and Drug Administration (FDA) has approved nonprescription drug therapy for only AGA; therefore, AGA will be the focus of this chapter.

AGA is the most common form of hair loss, affecting about one-third of the U.S. male population and about one-sixth of the female population. It is characterized by progressive, patterned hair loss from the scalp. By age 30, about 30% of white men have AGA, with the incidence increasing to 50% by age 50. White men are four times more likely than black men to develop premature hair loss.[2]

Alopecia areata (autoimmune hair loss) affects men and women of all races equally and occurs in 2% of the U.S. population. Most cases (60%) are in children and young adults.[3]

Telogen effluvium is a common condition internationally, but its exact prevalence has not been determined. Telogen effluvium has no racial bias and can occur at any age. Episodes are common in the first months of life. An episode can occur in either gender, but because postpartum hormonal changes are a frequent cause, the condition is believed to affect women more often than men. The chronic form of this disease has been reported mainly in women.[4]

The hair follicle, which anchors the hair strand to the skin, contains cells that produce new hairs. Hair follicle activity is cyclic. In the growing phase (anagen), the follicle lengthens, the dermal papilla enlarges, and a new hair is formed. Anagen hair is deeply anchored in subcutaneous tissue and cannot be pulled out easily.[5] During the catagen phase—a transition phase between the growing and resting phases—cell proliferation ceases, the hair follicle shortens, and a bulbous enlargement forms at the base of the hair. The resting phase (telogen) has an unpigmented, club-shaped root that is embedded in a shortened follicle and can be easily removed. Typically, 100 to 150 hairs are lost from the scalp each day as telogen hairs are shed.

Hair follicles and their sebaceous glands produce enzymes (delta-5-3 beta-hydroxysteroid hydrogenase, 17 beta-hydroxysteroid hydrogenase, and 5-alpha-reductase type I) that convert weak androgens (such as dehydro-3-epiandrosterone and 4-androstenedione) to testosterone and dihydrotestosterone (DHT). Testosterone and DHT stimulate production of growth factors and proteases, affect vascularization of the follicle and the composition of basement membrane proteins, and alter the amounts of cofactors required for follicle metabolism. Another enzyme (aromatase) found in the lower portion of the outer root sheath converts androgens (4-androstenedione and testosterone) to estrogens. These enzymes are believed to maintain androgen balance in the follicle, thereby regulating the hair cycle. Testosterone and DHT apparently bind to receptor proteins in cell nuclei of bulbar dermal papillae. The complex then attaches to a DNA site that regulates the manufacture of messenger RNAs responsible for hair protein synthesis. In a scalp hair follicle, the complex downregulates synthesis, whereas the opposite occurs in a hair follicle on the face.[6]

Pathophysiology of Hair Loss (Androgenetic Alopecia)

In androgenetic alopecia, the hair follicle undergoes a stepwise miniaturization and change in growth dynamics. With each successive cycle, the anagen (growing) phase becomes shorter and the telogen (resting) phase becomes longer. Consequently over time, the anagen-to-telogen ratio decreases from 12:1 to 5:1. Because telogen hairs are more loosely anchored to follicles, their presence in increased numbers manifests eventually by increased shedding. Also, the catagen phase (the intermediate phase between anagen regrowth and telogen shedding) increases, reducing the number of hairs. As telogen hairs are shed, they are gradually replaced by vellus-like (short and fine) hairs[7] (mean diameter reduced from 0.08 mm to less than 0.06 mm) or by anagen hairs that are too short to reach the surface. Although miniaturization of the follicle may be an abrupt process, pharmacologic treatment may similarly trigger development of enlarged anagen follicles in a fast, one-hair-cycle response.[8]

The androgen DHT, which is converted from testosterone by 5-alpha-reductase, is believed to be a primary repressor of hair growth by the mechanism mentioned previously. This androgen also binds five times more readily than testosterone to androgen receptors. Although two forms of the 5-alpha-reductase are found in the scalps of bald men, the amount of DHT formed locally (in scalp hair) is small compared with what is available systemically (produced by the prostate gland). The relative contributions of local and systemic DHT to balding are still not known.

Increased 5-alpha-reductase–mediated conversion of testosterone to DHT in the balding areas of women with AGA also supports the contention that DHT is important to this process. Women with this disease rarely lose all their hair, not only because they have less 5-alpha-reductase but also because they have more aromatase that converts testosterone into estradiol.[9] In addition, women are more likely to have follicles with fewer localized androgen receptors and, therefore, are more likely to retain actively growing hair.[10]

Antimitotic drugs, such as chemotherapy drugs used to treat cancer, can cause narrowing of the hair shaft, which may fracture the hair or stop hair growth. This condition is referred to as anagen alopecia or anagen effluvium (when referring to the shedding of anagen hairs). Another disease also marked by loose anagen hairs is "loose anagen syndrome." This uncommon disorder may be transmitted by autosomal dominant inheritance and is predominantly found in fair-haired girls ages 2 to 9 years.[11] Current nonprescription drug therapies are not FDA-approved for the treatment of anagen alopecia; however, positive clinical results of the use of minoxidil in female patients with anagen alopecia following cancer chemotherapy have been reported.[5]

Certain diseases, hair care products, and hair-grooming methods associated with scarring or burns on the scalp may result in scarring alopecia. Traction alopecia is seen primarily in children who braid their hair tightly every day. Braiding traumatizes the hair follicles, causing hairs to loosen and break. Patients who use oily moisturizers to make hair more manageable and to stop the scalp from flaking may develop folliculitis and resultant hair loss. Hot combs used to straighten hair may cause scalp inflammation and resultant scarring alopecia.[12]

Chronic papulosquamous diseases of the scalp, such as psoriasis and seborrheic dermatitis, may also lead to scarring alopecia. Several topical agents are available to relieve the itching and flaking associated with these disorders. Nonprescription agents marketed for alopecia are not effective in treating alopecia secondary to psoriasis or seborrhea.

Untreated, or improperly treated, tinea capitis may lead to hair loss. This disease, most commonly caused by *Trichophyton tonsurans* (a fungus), must be treated with systemic antifungals to eradicate it from the hair. Sporadic, patchy hair loss is characteristic of tinea capitis.[13] Hair loss secondary to tinea capitis is most typically temporary, and hair regrowth occurs following eradication of the dermatophyte. A complete discussion of tinea capitis is found in Chapter 43.

Psychological stress may potentiate several types of hair loss, although the literature on this subject is conflicting. High stress levels may depress the immune system and lead to symptoms such as hair loss.

Clinical Presentation of Hair Loss

The scalp of a patient with AGA shows no signs of inflammation or scarring. Hair loss is gradual, and the number of hairs coming out during brushing or shampooing does not suddenly increase, in contrast to other alopecias. Typically, male androgenetic hair loss is insidious in onset and usually does not start until after puberty. Progression fluctuates considerably, with 3 to 6 months of accelerated loss followed by 6 to 18 months of no loss. Most men take 15 to 25 years to lose their hair. Male pattern hair loss and/or gradual hair thinning usually occurs at the top rear of the head (vertex), the frontal hairline, and the occipital regions. The loss begins with a recession of the frontal hairline and continues with thinning at the vertex until all that is left is a fringe of hair at the occipital and temporal margins.

In women with alopecia, hair loss is typically more diffuse. There is a characteristic retention of the frontal hairline. Later, diffuse thinning is seen over the entire crown. Hair density remains normal but hair length does not. The woman's scalp will show a high density of hair, but the hairs will be thinner than normal, short, and tapered (rather than blunt, as seen when hair is damaged by breakage). Hair loss in women, while classified as androgenetic, may have a more significant genetic component.[5,14]

Androgenetic alopecia in women is a cause for suspicion of hyperandrogenism—an excess of androgen, which commonly accompanies significant acne, hirsutism (hairiness in other parts of the body), menstrual irregularities, and infertility. Patients with multiple symptoms should be referred for medical evaluation.

It is conceivable that a patient with pattern hair loss may be using a hair regrowth treatment agent on the scalp while using an antihirsute agent to remove excess hair on the face. Androgen excess may indicate serious metabolic disturbances, such as cardiovascular disease, diabetes mellitus, polycystic ovarian syndrome, and endometrial cancer.[14,15]

Compared with AGA, autoimmune hair loss (alopecia areata) has three stages: sudden loss of hair in patches, enlargement of the patches, and regrowth. The cycle may take months, sometimes years, and can occur in any hair-bearing area. Axillary, pubic, and other body hairs are often not affected. However, the eyebrows and eyelashes can be lost and sometimes may be the only sites affected.[12] Up to 5% of patients lose all their scalp hair (alopecia totalis), and 1% of patients lose all their body and scalp hair (alopecia universalis). Hair loss may accompany or be preceded by nail pitting or other nail abnormalities, as well as by itching, tingling, burning, or other painful sensations in the patch of hair loss. Patients presenting with these characteristics or suspected to have alopecia areata should be referred for medical evaluation.

Telogen effluvium (also known as diffuse alopecia) is characterized by nonscarring, diffuse hair loss usually caused by metabolic or hormonal disturbances or medications. The acute form is defined by shedding that lasts less than 6 months; the chronic form lasts longer than 6 months. The metabolic or physiologic disturbance usually precedes shedding by 1 to 6 months, but identifying a specific causal event is often difficult, if not impossible. This point is especially important to note with medication use, because hair loss will often occur one to several months after the patient has begun a particular drug therapy. Health care providers should assess the start date of all medications as a part of the clinical workup of patients with this type of hair loss. Telogen effluvium is usually reversible.[16]

Primary care providers may assess hair loss using a variety of tests (e.g., daily hair loss count, hair–pull test, etc.).[6,12] All patients presenting with hair loss other than that considered to be androgenetic in nature should be referred to a primary care provider for complete medical evaluation.

Treatment of Hair Loss

Treatment Goals

The goal in self-treating hair loss is to restore the patient's previous appearance or to achieve an appearance considered acceptable to the patient. This objective can be accomplished through nonprescription means by recommending (1) cosmetic camouflage and/or (2) the use of topical minoxidil to stimulate hair growth, if applicable.

General Treatment Approach

Currently, only topical minoxidil 2% and 5% concentrations are approved for self-treatment of androgenetic alopecia. Treatment is specifically for loss of vertex but not frontal hair. If the patient's baldness is clearly androgenetic, treatment with topical minoxidil 2% for women and 5% for men can be recommended. Otherwise, patients should be referred to their primary care provider for diagnosis. Although 5% minoxidil is not FDA-approved for the treatment of women with androgenetic alopecia, practitioners should be aware that dermatologists may recommend this concentration despite the lack of scientific data showing any greater benefit in women than the 2% solution.[5] Primary care providers may consider treating male patients who have failed nonprescription minoxidil with finasteride 1 mg tablets daily. Finasteride is the only prescription product currently FDA-approved for the treatment of alopecia in male patients. Finasteride has been studied in female patients; however, the results have shown the drug to be no better than placebo in women.[16] In addition, at least one study has shown minoxidil in combination with finasteride to be superior than either agent alone, indicating that self-care coupled with supervised medical treatment may be beneficial.[17] The algorithm in Figure 46-1 outlines the self-treatment of hair loss and lists specific exclusions for self-treatment.

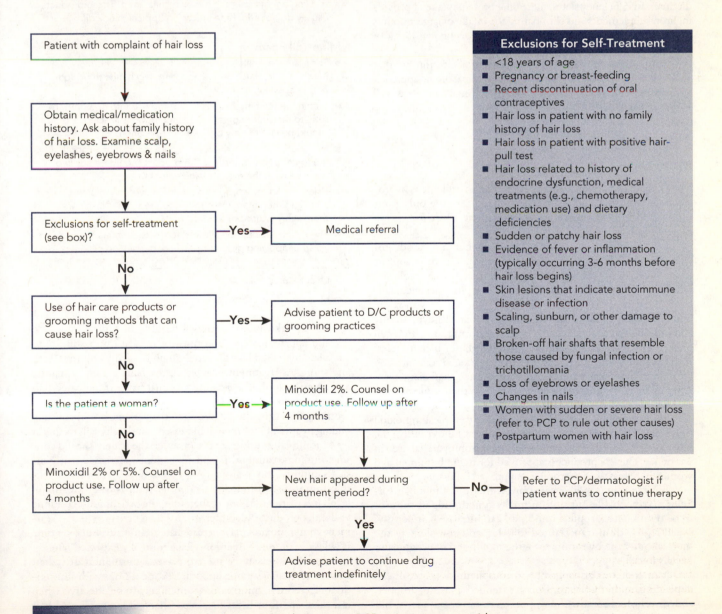

Exclusions for Self-Treatment

- <18 years of age
- Pregnancy or breast-feeding
- Recent discontinuation of oral contraceptives
- Hair loss in patient with no family history of hair loss
- Hair loss in patient with positive hair-pull test
- Hair loss related to history of endocrine dysfunction, medical treatments (e.g., chemotherapy, medication use) and dietary deficiencies
- Sudden or patchy hair loss
- Evidence of fever or inflammation (typically occurring 3-6 months before hair loss begins)
- Skin lesions that indicate autoimmune disease or infection
- Scaling, sunburn, or other damage to scalp
- Broken-off hair shafts that resemble those caused by fungal infection or trichotillomania
- Loss of eyebrows or eyelashes
- Changes in nails
- Women with sudden or severe hair loss (refer to PCP to rule out other causes)
- Postpartum women with hair loss

FIGURE 46-1 Self-care of hair loss. Key: D/C, discontinue; PCP, primary care provider.

Nonpharmacologic Therapy

Thinning hair can be camouflaged by using wigs (hair pieces) and hair weaves. Technological advances have made producing a custom wig that is a near-perfect match of the wearer's original hair color and style a standard practice, especially for individuals anticipating hair loss due to upcoming cancer chemotherapy. Hair loss that is dramatic and extensive can be emotionally distressing. These advances have tremendously improved the psychological impact of hair loss. Treatment of less severe hair loss can be approached by using hair sprays, gels, colorants, perms, and topical hair-building products in moderation; these products can create an illusion of fullness without decreasing hair loss.

Scalp massage, frequent shampooing, and electrical stimulation have been proposed as treatments for hair loss; however, these remedies are considered ineffective.[17,18]

Acute telogen effluvium usually resolves spontaneously, and treatment is limited to comforting and reassuring the patient. Chronic telogen effluvium is slower to resolve, but the patient still needs comfort and reassurance. When a primary care provider has determined that the patient's hair loss is caused by poor diet or iron deficiency, the patient may benefit from consulting a dietitian. In deficiency states, increasing protein intake or providing iron supplements and eliminating the intake of large amounts of vitamin A may be simple solutions to reversing hair loss seen in these situations.

Surgical transplantation of terminal hair follicles from another anatomic site is another alternative, nonpharmacologic approach to hair loss. This method may be useful in frontal hair loss as well as vertex hair loss.

Pharmacologic Therapy

Minoxidil

Minoxidil 2% and extra-strength topical minoxidil 5%, as hydroalcoholic solutions and solvent-free foams, are the only nonprescription agents currently approved by FDA for use in regrowing hair.

Minoxidil is a potassium channel opener and vasodilator (when used orally to control hypertension). The drug appears to act by increasing cutaneous blood flow directly to hair follicles, which increase in size after treatment,[19] and it promotes and maintains vascularization of hair follicles in alopecia.[19,20] Minoxidil, which has been shown to directly stimulate follicular hypertrophy and prolong the anagen phase,[19] may transform resting (telogen phase) hair follicles into active (anagen phase) hair follicles. Another study, which used a higher-than-marketed concentration of minoxidil, reported an increase in mean hair shaft diameter.[21] After up to 12 months of therapy, a subset of these same patients also revealed a reduction in the percentage of telogen hairs.

AGA in men and women is amenable to topical minoxidil treatment. Treatment is indicated for baldness at the crown of the head in men and for hair thinning at the frontoparietal area in women.[22] The 2% product is approved for use in both men and women, whereas the 5% product is approved for use in only men.

For men undergoing hair transplantation whose hair follicles may be viable but not optimally functioning in the area to be transplanted, topical minoxidil can increase hair density, speed regrowth in transplanted follicles, and complement the surgical outcome by minimizing the likelihood of progression of hair loss.[23]

Minoxidil can be applied by various methods (Table 46-1), depending on the applicator (spray, extended spray tip, dropper, and/or rub-on assembly).[24]

TABLE 46-1 Administration Guidelines for Minoxidil

Minoxidil Solution

- Apply minoxidil to clean, dry scalp and hair.
- Rub about 1 mL of the product into the affected area of the scalp twice daily (morning and night). Some products have a measuring cap indicating a 1 mL fill line.
- Wash and dry hands after applying the medication. If it gets into the eyes, mouth, or nose, rinse these areas thoroughly.
- Do not double the dose if you miss an application.
- Allow 2–4 hours for the drug to penetrate the scalp. Do not participate in any activity that might wash away or dilute the drug (e.g., bathing or swimming without a cap) for 2–4 hours after application.
- At night, apply the drug 2–4 hours before bedtime, because minoxidil can stain clothing and bed linen if not fully dry.
- Do not dry the scalp with a hair dryer after applying the drug. This action will reduce the drug's effectiveness.
- If applicable, apply hair grooming and styling products (e.g., sprays, mousses, gels) or coloring agents, permanents, or relaxing agents after the minoxidil has dried. These products usually do not affect the efficacy of topical minoxidil.

Minoxidil Foam

- The foam may melt on contact with warm skin. Therefore, wash hands in cold water before applying. Dry hands thoroughly before applying foam.
- Within the thinning hair area, part the hair into one or more rows to maximize contact of the foam with the scalp. The hair should be completely dry before application.
- Holding the can upside down, apply one-half of a capful of the foam to the fingertips. The product should be applied twice daily, in the morning and at night.
- Using the fingertips, spread the foam over the thinning scalp area, and then massage gently into the scalp. Wash hands thoroughly after application.
- The product should be allowed to dry completely before lying down or applying grooming, styling, or coloring products.

Source: Reference 24.

It may take approximately 4 months for topical minoxidil 2% and approximately 2 months for topical minoxidil 5% to stimulate increased hair growth, which is usually colorless, soft, and short. As treatment progresses, the hairs gradually mature and begin to look like existing terminal hairs. If increased hair density fails to appear by 12 months for men and 8 months for women after using the 2% product, the patient should consider ending treatment. For men, if increased hair density fails to appear by 4 months after using the 5% product, the patient should consider ending treatment. For many patients, increased hair density is minimal and treatment response is difficult to assess. Once the drug is discontinued, hair density returns to pretreatment levels in a matter of months; therefore, the patient must continue to use the product indefinitely to maintain new growth.[25] Treatment with minoxidil may increase hair loss initially, but over time it will slow or inhibit hair loss to the normally expected rate.[24]

In a 48-week study, men displayed a mean increase in hair density of 12.7% with minoxidil 2% and 18.6% with minoxidil 5%.[25] In men, minoxidil is more likely to be effective when less than one-fourth of the scalp surface has experienced hair loss or thinning. Although all the hair does not usually grow back, even with continued treatment, progressive loss of hair is usually slowed.

Of male patients younger than 50 years, about one-fourth experience moderate or better hair regrowth after using topical minoxidil.[19] One-third of the patients, however, attain only minimal hair regrowth. Minimal regrowth means that some new hairs are visible but not enough to cover thinning areas. Furthermore, in treated areas, the hair density (i.e., how closely the hairs grow) is less than that on the untreated part of the head where no significant hair loss has occurred. With moderate regrowth, hairs may cover some or all the thinning area and may grow more closely together. However, again, the hair density in the treated area will be less than that on the rest of the head. In one study, a minority of the patients had dense regrowth, which means that the thinning areas are almost completely covered and the hair density is equal to that on the untreated part of the head. The placebo vehicle also showed a modest response: About one-tenth of the patients had moderate or better regrowth, and about one-third had minimal regrowth.[25]

In women, topical minoxidil is more effective if less than about one-third of the scalp is thinning. Study data for women ages 18 to 45 years indicate that about one-fifth of the women experienced moderate regrowth after using topical minoxidil, whereas more than one-third experienced only minimal regrowth. In comparison, the placebo vehicle showed a 7% response rate for moderate regrowth and a 33% response rate for minimal regrowth.[19]

No differences in side effects or other problems were demonstrated in a limited number of older patients up to age 65 years. In short, those most responsive to topical minoxidil treatment are younger patients who have limited hair loss that has existed for a relatively short period of time.[19]

Topical minoxidil solution 2% has also been investigated in combination with oral finasteride 1 mg in male patients. The outcomes of this combination treatment indicate a higher percentage of responders than with either agent alone. It is inferred that efficacy may be enhanced by the two-drug regimen, which acts on multiple androgenetic alopecia etiologies.[26]

The most common side effect associated with minoxidil—local itching or irritation at the site of application—may be related to the hydroalcoholic/propylene glycol vehicle. Rare side effects include acne at the site of application, increased hair loss, inflammation (soreness) of the hair roots, reddened skin, swelling of the face, and allergic dermatitis.[22,24]

The most common side effect of long-term use is transient hypertrichosis (excessive hair growth), usually on the forehead and cheeks. Occasionally, patients may notice hypertrichosis on the chest, back, forearms, and ear rims, which could indicate that the product has been applied excessively.[27] A few patients will notice increased hair loss in the first few weeks of use. Most likely, this loss represents a displacement of telogen by new anagen hairs.

Minoxidil is absorbed through the skin in relatively low concentrations; documented systemic side effects are rare. In the unlikely event of an accidental ingestion, the patient should seek emergency medical attention. Symptoms may involve the following[24]:

- Low blood pressure (dizziness, confusion, fainting, and light-headedness)
- Blurred vision or other changes in vision
- Headache or chest pain
- Irregular heart rate
- Sudden unexplained weight gain
- Swollen hands or feet
- Flushing of the skin
- Numbness or tingling of the face, hands, or feet

Although hemodynamic changes have not been detected in most controlled clinical studies, patients with cardiovascular disorders may have an increased risk of cardiotoxicity.[28]

The use of topical minoxidil is not associated with any known drug interactions. However, the concurrent use of guanethidine could potentiate orthostatic hypotension, and the concurrent use of oral minoxidil could increase its systemic levels and enhance its effects. The application to the scalp of topical corticosteroids, petrolatum, or tretinoin (e.g., Retin-A) with minoxidil may increase absorption of minoxidil and the risk of side effects. Minoxidil should not be used for 24 hours before or after application of a permanent, hair color, or hair relaxant.[22,24]

Patients who are allergic to minoxidil or to any component of the preparation should avoid this medication, as should patients with scalp damage from psoriasis, severe sunburn, or abrasions, which may increase minoxidil absorption.

Topical minoxidil has a Pregnancy Category C rating, which means it is not known whether the drug can harm an unborn baby. Similarly, the effect on nursing babies is not known. Therefore, pregnant women and women who are breast-feeding their babies should be advised not to use the product without first consulting a primary care provider.

The use of the 5% product by women is not recommended, because the results with 2% and 5% are not measurably different, and because the risk of facial hair growth is greater with the 5% product. However, one study has shown that women prefer the 5% concentration product to the 2% product.[6]

The solution formulation is alcohol-based and will burn or irritate eyes, mucous membranes, or abraded skin. When spraying either formulation of the product, the patient should avoid inhaling it. If the product gets into the eyes, mouth, or nose, the patient should thoroughly rinse these areas. Patients should wash and dry their hands after using the product. These precautions also are intended to prevent the systemic entry of minoxidil by alternative routes. Products containing minoxidil should not be used on any other part of the body.[24]

Researchers have found little evidence of a potential effect of minoxidil on systemic endocrine functions.[29] Measurement of plasma testosterone as well as excretion of urinary hydroxysteroids and ketosteroids in hypertensive patients who have been treated with oral minoxidil has not revealed any effects. Moreover, although serum cortisol, testosterone, and thyroid indexes are apparently unchanged by topical minoxidil, modification of follicular testosterone metabolism does occur.[30] However, unstable cardiac patients should not use the product unless supervised by a primary care provider because of potential hemodynamic alterations seen with minoxidil.

Safety and efficacy of the product in children (younger than 18 years) or in older adults (older than 65 years) have not been established, so the use of minoxidil in these populations is contraindicated.

Product Selection Guidelines

The 2% formulation should normally be recommended for use by women; however, men are usually advised to use the 5% concentration. One study demonstrated a lower incidence of contact dermatitis with foam products, which do not contain

TABLE 46-2 Selected Hair Regrowth Products

Trade Name	Primary Ingredient
Equaline Hair Regrowth Treatment Men's Extra Strength (Albertson's)	Minoxidil 5%
Equaline Hair Regrowth Treatment Women's Regular Strength (Albertson's)	Minoxidil 2%
Leader Minoxidil Topical Solution (Leader Brands)	Minoxidil 5%
Minoxidil Topical Solution (Actavis)	Minoxidil 2%
Minoxidil Topical Solution 5% for Men (Actavis)	Minoxidil 5%
Rogaine Extra Strength Topical Solution for Men	Minoxidil 5%
Rogaine Men's Topical Solution (McNeil)	Minoxidil 2%
Rogaine Men's Topical Foam (McNeil)	Minoxidil 5%
Rogaine Women's Topical Solution (McNeil)	Minoxidil 2%

propylene glycol, compared with topical solutions.[5] Accordingly, this formulation *may* be more desirable in patients with a history of sensitive skin/dermatitis. Patient preference for method of application is a critical factor in product selection. Patients with impaired vision or physical dexterity may find the rub-on method of application preferable to using sprays or droppers. Table 46-2 lists examples of commercially available products.

Nonmonograph Products

In the past, FDA advisory panels have proposed removing from the market a number of ingredients that were known to be safe for external use but were purported to prevent hair loss or promote hair growth, without scientific data to support efficacy.[31] The false claims generally are no longer made, but many of these ingredients are still available today in nonprescription lotions and shampoos. In addition, oral and topical dietary supplements marketed to improve the structure and function of hair growth have become more popular. Ingredients that either are currently or have been known in the past to be included in shampoos, topical solutions, and dietary supplements for hair loss include amino acids, aminobenzoic acid, B vitamins, jojoba oil, lanolin, maidenhair fern (*Adiantum capillis-verneris*), polysorbates 20 and 660, royal jelly (white secretion of *Apis melliferis* worker bees), tetracaine hydrochloride, urea, and wheat germ oil.[12,17,31,32]

Assessment of Hair Loss: A Case-Based Approach

In addition to recommending treatment for hair loss, the practitioner should first identify any possible underlying medical cause. To assess alopecia areata or telogen effluvium, the practitioner can direct the patient to perform a gentle hair–pull test. The removal of 25% or more of the pulled hairs may indicate that the patient's hair loss is an active process (as in alopecia areata or telogen effluvium), and the patient should be referred to a dermatologist. However, the test may be falsely negative if the patient's hair has been recently combed, brushed, or shampooed.[12] If pathology-induced and active hair loss are ruled out, the practitioner should determine whether the balding fits the criteria for androgenetic alopecia.

Case 46-1 illustrates the assessment of patients with hair loss.

CASE 46-1

Relevant Evaluation Criteria	Scenario/Model Outcome
Information Gathering	
1. Gather essential information about the patient's symptoms, including:	
a. description of symptom(s) (i.e., nature, onset, duration, severity, associated symptoms)	Patient has had gradual hair loss, which recently has increased. There are no signs of inflammation or scarring on scalp.
b. description of any factors that seem to precipitate, exacerbate, and/or relieve the patient's symptom(s)	None
c. description of the patient's efforts to relieve the symptoms	None
2. Gather essential patient history information:	
a. patient's identity	Hector Fernandez
b. patient's age, sex, height, and weight	34-year-old male
c. patient's occupation	Insurance broker
d. patient's dietary habits	N/A
e. patient's sleep habits	N/A

Relevant Evaluation Criteria	Scenario/Model Outcome
f. concurrent medical conditions, prescription and nonprescription medications, and dietary supplements	Patient in good health; takes no medications
g. allergies	None
h. history of other adverse reactions to medications	None
i. other (describe) _____	Father and maternal uncles suffer from male pattern baldness. Hector prefers to use a topical treatment, because he is concerned about the side effects of systemic therapy.

Assessment and Triage

3. Differentiate the patient's signs/symptoms and correctly identify the patient's primary problem(s).	The patient has androgenetic alopecia, as evidenced by gradual hair loss and recent increase in hair loss. He has no signs of inflammation or scarring on scalp.
4. Identify exclusions for self-treatment (see Figure 46-1).	None
5. Formulate a comprehensive list of therapeutic alternatives for the primary problem to determine if triage to a medical practitioner is required, and share this information with the patient.	Options include: (1) Recommend self-care using OTC minoxidil topical treatment and/or camouflage measures. (2) Refer Hector to a PCP for treatment. (3) Recommend self-care until a PCP can be consulted. (4) Take no action.

Plan

6. Select an optimal therapeutic alternative to address the patient's problem, taking into account patient preferences.	Topical minoxidil solution
7. Describe the recommended therapeutic approach to the patient.	Apply approximately 1 mL of minoxidil 5% topical solution twice daily to a clean, dry scalp.
8. Explain to the patient the rationale for selecting the recommended therapeutic approach from the considered therapeutic alternatives.	The most effective nonsystemic therapy is topical minoxidil 5% solution.

Patient Education

9. When recommending self-care with nonprescription medications and/or nondrug therapy, convey accurate information to the patient, including:	
a. appropriate dose and frequency of administration	See Table 46-1.
b. maximum number of days the therapy should be employed	See the box Patient Education for Hair Loss.
c. product administration procedures	See Table 46-1.
d. expected time to onset of relief	See the box Patient Education for Hair Loss.
e. degree of relief that can be reasonably expected	Progressive hair loss will be slowed.
f. most common side effects	See the box Patient Education for Hair Loss.
g. side effects that warrant medical intervention should they occur	See the box Patient Education for Hair Loss.
h. patient options in the event that condition worsens or persists	See the box Patient Education for Hair Loss.
i. product storage requirements	See the box Patient Education for Hair Loss.
j. specific nondrug measures	Minimize exposure to agents that may trigger hair loss.
10. Solicit patient's follow-up questions.	How can I tell if I am responding to treatment?
11. Answer patient's questions.	Hair density will increase if the treated area involves early thinning. Look for fine, short hairs as a first response.

Key: N/A, not applicable; OTC, over-the-counter; PCP, primary care provider.

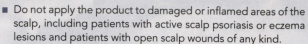

The goal in self-treating hair loss is to restore the patient's previous appearance or achieve an appearance the patient considers acceptable. This objective can be accomplished through nonprescription means by recommending (1) cosmetic camouflage and/or, if applicable, (2) the use of topical minoxidil to stimulate hair growth. To ensure optimal therapeutic outcomes, it is essential that patients carefully follow product packaging information and consider the following measures.

Nondrug Measures

- If desired, use wigs to cover severe hair loss until hair is regrown.
- For less severe hair loss, use hair sprays, gels, colorants, permanents, or hair-building products in moderation to create the illusion of full hair. These cosmetics will not increase the rate of hair loss.
- Avoid the use of oily hair products that can cause folliculitis.
- Avoid hairstyles that pull on the hair, such as tight braids.

Nonprescription Medications

- Note that use of minoxidil must be continuous and indefinite to maintain regrowth. It may take up to 4 months to see any results. If treatment is interrupted, regrowth will typically be lost within 4 months or less, and progression of hair loss will begin again.
- Minoxidil is not recommended in patients who are pregnant, breast-feeding, or planning to become pregnant while using this product. Consult a primary care provider before you use this product.

- See Table 46-1 for instructions on how to use this product.
- Do not apply the product more than twice daily. More frequent applications will not achieve better regrowth or a faster response, but may increase side effects.
- Do not apply the product to damaged or inflamed areas of the scalp, including patients with active scalp psoriasis or eczema lesions and patients with open scalp wounds of any kind.
- Note that local itching or irritation at the site of application may occur. More rarely, allergic contact dermatitis or transient hypertrichosis (unwanted facial hair growth) may occur. Keep product containers in a cool, dry place, and avoid refrigeration.
- Keep the product out of the reach of children. Ingestion of minoxidil is potentially hazardous and individuals should contact their poison control center immediately.
- Product is flammable. Keep away from fire or flame.
- Do not use on infants or children ages 18 years or younger.
- Do not use if you have heart disease except under the supervision of a primary care provider.
- If hair fails to appear despite consistent use of the product within the time specified on the product (generally 4–6 months), consider stopping the treatment and seeing your primary care provider for further evaluation.

Patient Counseling for Hair Loss

Patients should be advised that most treatment regimens for hair loss do not alter its progression, especially if the hair loss has gone on for a prolonged period of time. Some patients might instead be interested in hair transplants or surgical interventions. The practitioner should inform patients who want to use nonprescription minoxidil that the longer the hair thinning or loss has continued, the less likely it is that treatment will elicit a regrowth response. If the patient still wants to use minoxidil, the practitioner should review product instructions with the patient, making sure that the patient understands the possible adverse effects as well as the signs and symptoms that indicate the need for medical attention. In addition, the patient should be counseled that if hair regrowth is achieved, long-term continuation of minoxidil will be necessary to maintain hair regrowth. The box Patient Education for Hair Loss lists specific information to provide patients.

Evaluation of Patient Outcomes for Hair Loss

Patients should use minoxidil for the minimum recommended periods. If new hair growth does not occur after using minoxidil 2% or 5% for 4 months, the patient should consider ending treatment. If new hair does appear within the recommended periods, the practitioner should advise the patient to continue the drug treatment indefinitely.

Key Points for Hair Loss

- ➤ Minoxidil is suppressive, not curative, and is not effective for everyone.
- ➤ Offering cosmetic solutions may also be helpful.
- ➤ Patients, particularly women, are seeking treatment not only for hair loss but also for lost self-esteem resulting from the association of hair loss with illness and advanced age.
- ➤ Practitioners and primary care providers should dispense medication with a measure of emotional support and should make clear the limitations of the existing treatment.

REFERENCES

1. Sperling LC, Mezebish DS. Hair diseases. *Med Clin North Am.* 1998;82: 1155–69.
2. Sinclair R. Male pattern androgenetic alopecia. *BMJ.* 1998;317:865–9.
3. McDonagh A, Tazi-Ahnini R, Messenger AG. Alopecia areata: an update on etiology and pathogenesis. In: Forslind M, Lindberg M, eds. *Skin, Hair and Nails: Structure and Function.* New York: Marcel Dekker; 2005:359–76.
4. Camacho F. Alopecias due to telogen effluvium. In: Camacho F, Montagna W, eds. *Trichology: Diseases of the Pilosebaceous Follicle.* Madrid: Aula Medica Group; 1997:403–11.
5. Shapiro J. Hair loss in women. *N Eng J Med.* 2007:357;1620–30.
6. Forslind M. Formation and structure: an introduction to hair. In: Forslind M, Lindberg M, eds. *Skin, Hair and Nails: Structure and Function.* New York: Marcel Dekker; 2005:251–337.
7. Diseases of the skin appendages. In: James WD, Berger TG, Elston DM, eds. *Andrew's Diseases of the Skin—Clinical Dermatology.* 10th ed. Philadelphia: Elsevier; 2006:749–93.
8. Whiting DA. Possible mechanisms of miniaturization during androgenetic alopecia or pattern hair loss. *J Am Acad Dermatol.* 2001;45(3 suppl):S81–6.

9. Sawaya ME, Price VH. Different levels of 5 alpha-reductase type I and II, aromatase, and androgen receptor in hair follicles of women and men with androgenetic alopecia. *J Invest Dermatol.* 1997;109:296–300.

10. Randall VA, Hibberts NA, Thornton MJ, et al. The hair follicle: a paradoxical androgen target organ. *Horm Res.* 2000;54:243–50.

11. Hereditary and congenital alopecia and hypertrichosis. In: Sinclair RD, Banfield CC, Dawber RPR, eds. *Handbook of Diseases of the Hair and Scalp.* Malden, Mass: Blackwell Science; 1999:129–55.

12. Hair loss/hair dysplasia. In: Dawber R, Van Neste D, eds. *Hair and Scalp Disorders: Common Presenting Signs, Differential Diagnosis and Treatment.* 2nd ed. London: Martin Dunitz; 2004:51–154.

13. Kaufman K. Adrogens and alopecia. *Mol Cell Endocrinol.* 2002;198(1–2); 89–95.

14. Birch MP, Lalla SC, Messenger AG. Female pattern hair loss. *Clin Exp Dermatol.* 2002;27:383–8.

15. Guarrera M, Semino MT, Rebora A. Quantitating hair loss in women: a critical approach. *Dermatology.* 1997;194:12–6.

16. Orentreich D, Orentreich N. Androgenetic alopecia and its treatment, a historical view. In: Unger WP, ed. *Hair Transplantation.* 3rd ed. New York: Marcel Dekker; 1995:1–33.

17. Ross E. Shapiro J. Management of hair loss. *Dermatol Clin.* 2005;23; 227–43.

18. Price VH. Treatment of hair loss. *N Engl J Med.* 1999;341:964–73.

19. Otomo S. Hair growth effect of minoxidil. *Nippon Yakurigaku Zasshi.* 2002;119:167–74.

20. Lachgar S, Charveron M, Gall Y, et al. Minoxidil upregulates the expression of vascular endothelial growth factor in human hair dermal papilla cells. *Br J Dermatol.* 1998;138:407–11.

21. Kurata S, Uno H, Allenhoffmann BL. Effects of hypertrichotic agents on follicular and nonfollicular cells in vitro. *Skin Pharmacol.* 1996;9:3–8.

22. Minoxidil topical. *USP DI Volume I, Drug Information for the Health Care Professional.* Greenwood Village, Colo: Thomson Micromedex; 2007:2002–4.

23. Avram MR, Cole JP, Gandelman M, et al. The potential role of minoxidil in the hair transplantation setting. *Dermatol Surg.* 2002; 28:894–900.

24. McNeill PPC. Rogaine. Available at: http://www.rogaine.com. Last accessed October 5, 2008.

25. Price VH, Menefee E, Strauss PC. Changes in hair weight and hair count in men with androgenetic alopecia, after application of 5% and 2% topical minoxidil, placebo, or no treatment. *J Am Acad Dermatol.* 1999;41:717–21.

26. Khandpur S, Suman M, Reddy BS. Comparative efficacy of various treatment regimens for androgenetic alopecia in men. *J Dermatol.* 2002;29: 489–98.

27. Peluso AM, Misciali C, Vincenzi C, et al. Diffuse hypertrichosis during treatment with 5% topical minoxidil. *Br J Dermatol.* 1997;136:118–20.

28. Satoh H, Morikaw S, Fujiwara C, et al. A case of acute myocardial infarction associated with topical use of minoxidil (RiUP) for treatment of baldness. *Jpn Heart J.* 2000;41:519–23.

29. Nguyen KH, Marks JG Jr. Pseudoacromegaly induced by the long-term use of minoxidil. *J Am Acad Dermatol.* 2003;48:962–5.

30. Sato T, Tadokoro T, Sonoda T, et al. Minoxidil increases 17 beta-hydroxysteroid dehydrogenase and 5 alpha-reductase activity of cultured human dermal papilla cells from balding scalp. *J Dermatol Sci.* 1999;19:123–5.

31. Hanover L. Hair replacement. *FDA Consum.* 1997;31:7–10.

32. Maidenhair Fern and Royal Jelly monographs. In: Fetrow CW, Avila JR, eds. *Professional's Handbook of Complementary & Alternative Medicines.* Philadelphia: Lippincott Williams & Wilkins; 2004:530, 718.

Other Medical Disorders

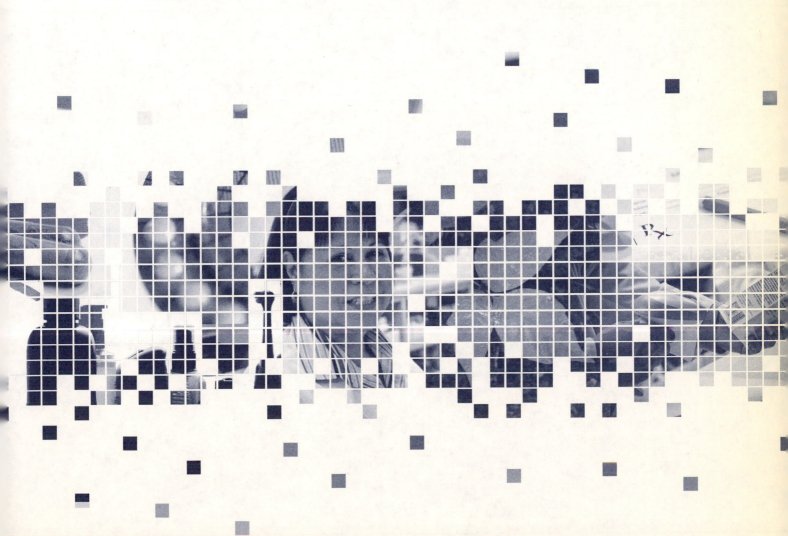

Diabetes Mellitus

Mitra Assemi and Candis M. Morello

As defined by the American Diabetes Association (ADA), diabetes mellitus (DM) is a group of metabolic diseases characterized by hyperglycemia resulting from defects in insulin secretion, insulin action, or both.[1] Chronic hyperglycemia results in long-term damage, dysfunction, and potential failure of various organs, including the eyes, nerves, heart, blood vessels, and kidneys. Although several types of diabetes are recognized, types 1 (5%–10% of patients) and 2 (90%–95% of patients) account for the majority of cases and are the focus of this chapter.[1] Other types (1%–5% of all cases) of diabetes include those associated with specific genetic conditions (e.g., maturity-onset diabetes of the young, or MODY; leprechaunism), medications (e.g., glucocorticoids), and illnesses. Gestational diabetes mellitus (GDM) develops in 4% of all pregnancies and can pose health risks for both mother and fetus. GDM first becomes apparent after 24 to 28 weeks of pregnancy but usually wanes after delivery. Women who develop GDM have a 20% to 50% chance of developing type 2 diabetes later in life.

More than 23.6 million people in the United States, or 7.8% of the population, have diabetes.[2] Of these, 5.7 million individuals do not have their diabetes diagnosed. Another 57 million Americans are currently estimated to have prediabetes. The number of individuals in whom diabetes is diagnosed is projected to more than double by 2050, because of both improved diagnostic criteria and the growing effect of a hypercaloric, sedentary lifestyle in the U.S. population.

Of all the individuals with diabetes, approximately 2 million have type 1 diabetes.[2] Although type 1 diabetes is most commonly diagnosed in childhood, it may present at any age in life. Risks of developing type 1 diabetes include genetic, autoimmune, and environmental factors that remain poorly defined.[1] Whites may have a higher genetic predisposition than other ethnic groups.

In contrast, the incidence of type 2 diabetes is reaching epidemic proportions in the United States. More than 21 million people currently have type 2 diabetes.[2] Its prevalence is higher among certain minority populations, including Hispanic Americans (1.7 times higher), African Americans (1.8 times higher), Asian Americans (2.0 times higher), and Native Americans/Alaska Natives (2.2 times higher, although prevalence rates vary across tribes). Excess body weight and a sedentary lifestyle are widely recognized risk factors, especially because type 2 diabetes is being diagnosed in a growing number of children and adolescents. Other risk factors include a family history of type 2 diabetes, prior history of GDM, and age older than 45 years.[1]

The tangible and intangible costs of diabetes care and treatment to both individuals and society are staggering. In 2007, the total annual combined direct and indirect costs were estimated to be $174 billion.[3] One of every 5 health care dollars is spent on care for an individual with diabetes, whereas 1 of every 10 health care dollars spent is attributed to diabetes-related costs. Because most health care expenditures are related to treatment of long-term diabetes complications, practitioners are focusing on prevention, early diagnosis, and aggressive metabolic control.

Regardless of type, self-care is integral to the effective management of diabetes. Practitioners can assist patients with diabetes by cultivating a relationship that will allow them to assess the patient's capability for self-care, identify gaps in the patient's knowledge of diabetes care, teach patients proper self-care strategies, and monitor self-care measures. The practitioner should be part of an interprofessional network of health care providers engaged in coordinating the patient's health care. Practitioners should also be a patient's resource for information on glucose monitors and other devices, self-monitoring of blood glucose (SMBG), medical nutrition therapy (MNT), physical activity, and drugs used in diabetes management and treatment.

Pathophysiology of Diabetes Mellitus

Working in conjunction with counterregulatory hormones (e.g., glucagon, epinephrine, norepinephrine, growth hormone, and cortisol), endogenous insulin maintains normal blood glucose (BG) concentrations between 60 and 100 mg/dL. Insulin and glucagon, the main hormones that control and balance glucose metabolism, are made and stored by the pancreatic beta and alpha cells, respectively. Beta cells release insulin into the portal vein in response to elevated plasma glucose, where the liver rapidly uses the hormone. Insulin has two main effects on fuel metabolism: (1) promotes storage (anabolic) and (2) prevents breakdown (anticatabolic). Insulin stimulates glucose uptake and storage as glycogen in muscle and liver cells. It converts excess glucose in the blood to fatty acids and triglycerides and promotes their storage in adipose tissue. Insulin also decreases hepatic glucose output, inhibits lipolysis (breakdown of fat) and production of ketone bodies, and enhances incorporation of amino acids into proteins. Although insulin's main effect is fuel storage, glucagon antagonizes the physiologic actions of insulin by increasing fuel breakdown and use. Glucagon secretion is triggered by low BG or high amino acid concentrations, resulting in increased liver glycogenolysis (breakdown of glycogen into glucose) and a subsequent rise in BG.

DM is a syndrome consisting of a heterogenous group of metabolic disorders characterized by chronic hyperglycemia and is associated with long-term consequences such as macrovascular and microvascular complications. Table 47-1 lists distinguishing features of type 1 and type 2 diabetes.

There are two categories of type 1 diabetes: immune-mediated and idiopathic diabetes.[4] The first and most common form of type 1 diabetes is caused by autoimmune destruction of insulin-secreting pancreatic islet cells, usually leading to an absolute insulin deficiency. Initially, postprandial (after meal) glucose concentrations rise, often undetected. Fasting hyperglycemia ensues once functional beta-cell mass falls below 80% to 90%. In most cases, the autoimmune process can be identified by the presence of autoantibodies. Type 1 diabetes is strongly associated with specific HLA tissue types, which can result in a protective or predisposing effect. Although genetics is a strong

causal component, only a small percentage of defective genes are expressed. If both parents have type 1 diabetes, only 20% of their children can be expected to develop the disease. The exact cause of idiopathic type 1 diabetes is unknown. To survive, patients with type 1 diabetes must receive daily and lifelong exogenous insulin to maintain their BG concentrations within normal ranges.

In type 2 diabetes, the primary metabolic defects include insulin resistance, beta-cell dysfunction, or both. Figure 47-1 provides an overview of the pathogenesis of this chronic condition. The degree of insulin resistance and/or beta-cell deficiency varies among people with type 2 DM. Initially, the pancreas compensates for insulin resistance by increasing insulin release. When this compensation is not adequate, hyperglycemia results. At diagnosis, beta-cell function may be as low as 50%.[5] Beta-cell function continues to decline with increased duration of diabetes. The liver and peripheral tissues (e.g., muscle and fat) are resistant to insulin effects. Increased hepatic glucose production occurs. Patients who are overweight are at increased risk of insulin resistance. In these patients, insulin resistance may improve with weight reduction.

TABLE 47-1 Differentiation of Type 1 and Type 2 Diabetes Mellitus

Characteristics	Type 1	Type 2
Demographics and Related Information		
Older terminology	Type I diabetes, insulin-dependent diabetes mellitus (IDDM), juvenile-onset diabetes mellitus	Type II diabetes, non–insulin-dependent diabetes mellitus (NIDDM), adult-onset diabetes mellitus
Family history of diabetes	Frequently negative	Commonly present
Age of onset	Usually <30 years, but can occur at any age	Usually >40 years, but can occur at any age
Symptoms		
Initial clinical presentation	Abrupt onset, moderate-to-severe symptoms of polyuria, polydipsia, fatigue, sudden weight loss, possible ketoacidosis	Usually gradual onset, possibly mild symptoms of polyuria, polydipsia, fatigue; often diagnosed when diabetic complications such as retinopathy, candidiasis, erectile dysfunction, and delayed wound healing are identified
Typical body habitus	Usually thin or not overweight	Usually overweight and/or obese (central, intra-abdominal obesity)
Risk of ketoacidosis	Constant, especially with insufficient insulin	Uncommon, except in the presence of unusual stress or moderate to severe sepsis
Macrovascular and microvascular complications	Infrequent until diabetes has been present for approximately 5 years	Frequent, can develop before diagnosis
Endogenous insulin production	Negligible to zero	May be increased, normal, or decreased
Etiology		
Primary cause	Autoimmune-mediated pancreatic beta-cell destruction, usually leading to absolute insulin deficiency	Insulin resistance, impaired insulin secretion, and/or increased hepatic glucose production
Treatment		
Medical nutrition therapy	Necessary in all patients	Necessary in all patients
Physical activity	Very important in all patients	Very important in all patients
Insulin replacement	Necessary for all patients	Necessary for many patients
Non-insulin BG-lowering agents	Pramlintide may be considered	Necessary for most patients
Glucose monitoring	Multiple SMBG required daily; quarterly A1C	Often beneficial; frequency of SMBG varies; quarterly A1C

Key: SMBG, self-monitoring of blood glucose; A1C, glycosylated hemoglobin.

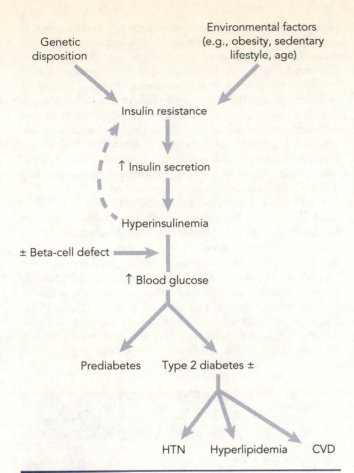

Defects in postreceptor binding may also cause insulin resistance. In some individuals with type 2 diabetes, a decreased number of insulin receptors and postreceptor defects may coexist, resulting in hyperglycemia.[6] Moreover, patients with insulin resistance are at risk of the "metabolic syndrome" (a cluster of symptoms or factors, including centralized obesity); increased blood pressure, triglycerides, and plasminogen activator inhibitor-1; and decreased high-density lipoprotein cholesterol (HDL-C). Patients with the metabolic syndrome have an increased rate of mortality and morbidity from cardiovascular disease.

Clinical Presentation of Diabetes Mellitus

Prediabetes precedes type 2 diabetes and is diagnosed by an impaired fasting glucose, characterized by a fasting plasma glucose concentration between 100 and 125 mg/dL, or an impaired glucose tolerance, characterized by a 2-hour plasma glucose concentration of 140 to 199 mg/dL after an oral glucose tolerance test.[1] Prediabetes is a risk factor for developing type 2 diabetes. Testing for prediabetes and type 2 diabetes routinely starts at age 45 and is repeated every 3 years.[7] Individuals with one or more risk factors for diabetes (adults younger than 45 and children who are either older than 10 years or have reached puberty) should also be tested. If initial tests are normal, repeat testing should occur every 3 years.

Table 47-2 summarizes the diagnostic criteria for DM. The metabolic changes are responsible for the onset of clinical symptoms. For individuals with new-onset DM, as plasma glucose concentrations rise to exceed the normal renal threshold of 180 mg/dL, glycosuria produces an osmotic diuresis and potential dehydration resulting in polyuria (frequent urination), especially at night (nocturia). Dehydration can progress to significant hypovolemia, electrolyte loss, and cellular dehydration, causing dry mouth and polydipsia (increased thirst). Because the lack of insulin prevents cells from using circulating plasma glucose, the nervous system signals polyphagia (hunger accompanied by increased appetite). Eating further promotes a further rise in plasma glucose concentration. Over time, lack of insulin stimulates protein and fat catabolism for energy, leading to weight loss, especially in patients with type 1 diabetes. The onset of clinical symptoms is usually more rapid and pronounced for patients with type 1 diabetes and often follows a stressful event. For patients with type 2 diabetes, symptoms of long-term diabetes complications may appear before elevated plasma glucose is detected. These symptoms may include visual changes; numbness or pain in the feet, legs, and hands; dry, itchy skin; slowed healing of cuts and scratches; gingivitis and/or dental caries; frequent infections (e.g., dermal, vaginal, bladder); and impotence.

TABLE 47-2 ADA Diagnostic Criteria for Diabetes Mellitus in Nonpregnant Patients[a]

Testing Condition	Plasma Glucose (mg/dL)	Presence of Symptoms	Comments
Casual	≥200	+	Symptoms include polyuria, polydipsia, polyphagia, and unexplained weight loss. Casual is defined as any time of day without regard to time since last meal.
Fasting	≥126	+/−	Fasting is defined as no caloric intake for at least 8 hours.
2-hour glucose during an OGTT	≥200	+/−	The test should be performed as described by World Health Organization, using a load of ~75 g anhydrous glucose dissolved in water for adults and 1.75 g/kg glucose dissolved in water for children.

Key: OGTT, oral glucose tolerance test.

[a] In the absence of unequivocal hyperglycemia, these criteria should be confirmed by repeat testing on a different day.

Source: Reference 1.

In patients with undiagnosed type 1 diabetes, as excess free fatty acids are mobilized to the liver, they are metabolized to acidic ketone bodies, which can eventually induce a metabolic acidosis. Left untreated, systemic ketoacidosis is a life-threatening situation that can lead to coma and death. In contrast, dehydration caused by hyperglycemia in patients with type 2 diabetes may place them at risk of developing hyperosmolar hyperglycemic state. Although the acute management of this syndrome is similar to that of ketoacidosis in patients with type 1 DM, diagnosis is often delayed because of nonspecific symptoms in elderly patients with type 2 DM.

Chronic hyperglycemia is associated with the development and progression of complications affecting major organs and physiologic systems. These long-term diabetes complications are responsible for significant rates of morbidity and mortality. Diabetes was the sixth leading cause of death listed on death certificates in the United States in 2002.[2] Complications of diabetes are categorized as microvascular and macrovascular. Studies in patients with type 1 and type 2 diabetes have clearly established a relation between amount of glycemic control and the risk of developing long-term microvascular and macrovascular complications.[5,8–10] For every 1% reduction of A1C (i.e., glycosylated hemoglobin), a marker for longer-term glycemic control, the overall risk of developing microvascular complications drops by as much as 40%. For this reason, glucose control forms the foundation of diabetes treatment and management.

Microvascular complications affect the eyes (retinopathy), nervous system (neuropathy), and kidneys (nephropathy). Among adults aged 20 to 74 years in the United States, diabetes is the leading cause of new-onset blindness.[2] Maintaining glucose at euglycemic concentrations can decrease and halt the progression of retinopathy and glaucoma.[5,8,9] Patients with type 1 diabetes, however, may experience a transient worsening of retinopathy after starting intensive glycemic control, resolving within 18 months of tight control.[8]

More than 60% of patients with diabetes have mild-to-moderate damage to their nervous system.[2] Severe neuropathy is a main contributor to lower-extremity amputations. Lowering BG to normal concentrations can improve symptoms of mild-to-moderate neuropathy.[5,8,9] Depending on the type of neuropathy, patients may be treated with medications that provide symptomatic relief (e.g., sensory pain, gastroparesis, incontinence, and sexual dysfunction).

Diabetes is the leading cause of end-stage renal disease in the United States.[2] Patients with impaired renal function (e.g., as indicated by microalbuminuria) are treated with medications to prevent or slow the progression of nephropathy, such as angiotensin-converting enzyme inhibitors or angiotensin receptor II blockers. Most people with diabetes also have hypertension, which further increases their risk of developing renal complications.[2,11] Studies have found that every 10 mm Hg reduction of systolic blood pressure results in a 12% reduction of risk for any complication related to diabetes.[2] Aggressive blood pressure control plays an important role in diabetes management.

Macrovascular complications include atherosclerosis, contributing to peripheral vascular disease (PVD), cardiovascular disease (CVD), and stroke. Symptoms of PVD include dry, callused skin, cold feet, decreased or absent foot pulses, leg pain, and difficulty walking (e.g., intermittent claudication). PVD coupled with neuropathy increases the risk of skin infections, gangrene, and subsequent amputation of extremities and limbs. Treatment includes reduction and elimination of risk factors (e.g., hyperglycemia, hypertension, hyperlipidemia, and smoking), proper foot self-care, and physical activity. Some patients may require antiplatelet therapy or vascular surgery.

Heart disease is the leading cause of diabetes-related deaths.[2] People with diabetes have two to four times the risk of heart attack and stroke, compared with people without diabetes. Additional risk factors for cardiovascular disease include obesity, hypertension (blood pressure greater than 130/80 mm Hg), hyperlipidemia, and smoking.[12–15] Therefore, in addition to controlling BG, weight, blood pressure, and lipids, smoking cessation also plays a crucial role in reducing cardiovascular risk in patients with diabetes. (See Table 47-3 for metabolic treatment goals.)

Rheologic changes also contribute to diabetes-related PVD and CVD. Platelets in patients with diabetes are hypersensitive to platelet aggregants.[16] People with type 2 diabetes and CVD overproduce thromboxane, a potent vasoconstrictor and platelet aggregant. Evidence to date from studies of types 1 and 2 diabetes supports the use of low-dose aspirin (81–325 mg daily) as a primary or secondary prevention strategy to reduce the incidence of cardiovascular events.[7] Unfortunately, less than half of all patients qualifying for aspirin therapy actually take it.[16]

Patients with diabetes may have abnormalities in immune function that increase their rates of morbidity and mortality

---

TABLE 47-3 ADA Treatment Goals for Nonpregnant Adults with Diabetes

Glycemic Control

Hemoglobin A1C	<7.0%[a,b]
Fasting plasma glucose	70–130 mg/dL (3.9–7.2 mmol/L)
Postprandial plasma glucose[c]	<180 mg/dL (<10.0 mmol/L)
Body mass index	<25.0 kg/m²
Blood pressure	<130/80 mm Hg

Lipids

Low-density lipoprotein cholesterol	<100 mg/dL (<2.6 mmol/L) (may be <70 mg/dL or 1.8 mmol/L in patients with overt cardiovascular disease)
Triglycerides	<150 mg/dL (<1.7 mmol/L)
High-density lipoprotein cholesterol	
For men	>40 mg/dL (>1.1 mmol/L)
For women	>50 mg/dL (>1.15 mmol/L)
Immunizations	Influenza vaccination annually Pneumococcal vaccination All other should be up to date (e.g., tetanus, hepatitis A and B, zoster)

Key: ADA, American Diabetes Association; A1C, glycosylated hemoglobin.

[a] Reference to a normal range for patients without diabetes of 4.0% to 6.0% using a Diabetes Control and Complications Trial–Based Assay.

[b] More stringent A1C goals (e.g., 6.0%) may be considered in individual patients.

[c] Postprandial plasma glucose measured 1–2 hours from the start of the meal, generally peak concentrations in patients with diabetes.

from infection.[17] These abnormalities contribute to slower rates of wound repair and increased risk of infection. In addition, diabetes increases the risk of complications, hospitalization, and death from influenza and pneumococcal disease.[17] Practitioners should ensure patients are up to date with their immunizations. People with diabetes should receive an annual influenza vaccination, as well as a pneumococcal vaccination. A one-time pneumococcal revaccination is recommended for patients older than 64 years who were previously immunized more than 5 years earlier when they were younger than 65 years. Patients should also be able to show current immunization status for other vaccinations, such as tetanus-diphtheria, hepatitis A, and hepatitis B.

Poorly controlled diabetes is a risk factor for the development of oral and dental complications, including gingivitis, periodontitis, dental caries, oral mucosal diseases, oral infections, salivary dysfunction, and taste disturbances.[18] Poor glycemic control and smoking increase the risk of periodontal disease. Maintaining glucose control and good dental hygiene, having regular checkups with a dentist, and smoking cessation can decrease the risk of developing oral and dental complications.

Patients can reduce their risk of developing or decreasing the progression of diabetes complications by instituting self-care and other preventive measures. Practitioners should educate patients about the role of self-care and other preventive measures and encourage their use (Table 47-4).

TABLE 47-4 Self-Care and Other Preventive Measures for Diabetes Complications

SMBG
- Determine frequency of BG testing (e.g., fasting, preprandial, postprandial, bedtime).
- Discuss low BG episodes and have patients test when symptoms arise and record the date, time, and BG value for evaluation.
- Educate patients on proper management of hypoglycemic episodes.

Medical Nutrition Therapy
- Tailor nutrition and physical activity based on individual characteristics such as glycemic control and comorbid conditions.
- Educate patients on ways to maintain a healthy weight.
- Refer patients to a dietitian if necessary.
- Instruct patients to perform SMBG before, during, and after physical activity.

Tobacco Use
- Recommend tobacco cessation (see Chapter 50).

Eye Care
- Recommend an annual dilated eye examination.
- Review any topical eye preparations for potential contraindication.
- Recommend medical attention immediately if vision changes or eye irritation occurs.

Dental Care
- Recommend professional teeth cleaning and oral health evaluation by a dentist twice each year.
- Recommend that teeth be brushed and flossed twice daily.
- Recommend a dental consult at the first sign of any gum abnormalities (e.g., bleeding).
- Have patients review dental care products with a dentist before use.

Skin Care
- Recommend daily bathing with mild soap, and dry skin thoroughly.
- Recommend that skin be inspected daily—head to toe—for signs of potential infection.
- Instruct patients to cleanse minor cuts and scratches promptly with soap and water.
- Instruct patients to avoid topical drying agents (e.g., alcohol) or salicylic acid–containing products.

Foot Care
- Perform annual foot examination. Patients identified at high risk of ulcers (e.g., neuropathy) should be seen regularly by a podiatrist.
- Have patients remove shoes at each visit with the health care provider for visual inspection.
- Teach patients to clean and inspect feet daily for any changes (e.g., corn, callus, open wound, fungal infection).
- Evaluate for any changes in foot appearance or tactile sensation.
- Instruct patients that nails should be trimmed carefully, preferably straight across and filed with an emery board to the contour of the toe.
- Instruct patients to avoid walking barefooted.
- Recommend use of soft cotton, synthetic blend, or wool socks to absorb moisture.
- Recommend patients wear properly fitting, comfortable shoes and use caution when "breaking in" new shoes.
- Recommend that patients inspect shoes for foreign objects before inserting feet.
- Recommend moisturizing lotion be used sparingly for dry feet. Allow feet to completely dry before wearing shoes to prevent excess moisture.

Medication Adherence: Information for Patients
- Discuss each medication's indication.
- Medications should be taken as prescribed. Patients should not discontinue medications without consulting provider.
- Take low-dose aspirin daily to prevent heart attack and stroke if indicated.
- Do not begin taking any nonprescription medications, herbal products, or supplements without first discussing them with a pharmacist or physician.
- Consult with your pharmacist about strategies to help keep track of medications and daily doses.
- Have an annual flu vaccination every fall.
- Confirm all immunizations are up to date.

Sick Day Management
- BG and urine ketones (especially with type 1 diabetes) need to be tested frequently during acute illness.
- Continue medications, including insulin, during an acute illness.
- Maintain ample hydration with noncaloric liquids.

Key: BG, blood glucose; SMBG, self-monitoring of blood glucose.

Treatment of Diabetes Mellitus

Patients with diabetes should receive medical care from an inter-professional team with expertise in diabetes.[7] Team members may include, but are not limited to, a physician, pharmacist, nurse educator or practitioner, physician assistant, dietitian, and mental health professional. These types of practitioners may also become certified diabetes educators specializing in the care of patients with diabetes. Effective diabetes management is patient centered, taking into account patient-specific factors such as the patient's health beliefs, attitudes, preferences, practices, health literacy, daily routines, and socioeconomic situation that may affect his or her self-care abilities. Collaborative diabetes management therefore includes patients, their families, and caregivers as central members of the team.

Treatment Goals

Glycemic control is the cornerstone of diabetes management.[7] It includes preventing hypoglycemic and hyperglycemic reactions. In conjunction with maintaining BG concentrations to as close to normal as possible, managing comorbid conditions such as overweight or obesity, hypertension, and hyperlipidemia are also part of the treatment to prevent the development and progression of long-term complications. Treatment goals should be individualized, taking into account patient-specific factors such as age (e.g., children, adolescents, and the elderly), pregnancy status, and comorbid conditions. Table 47-3 summarizes the recommendations for nonpregnant adults with diabetes.

General Treatment Approach

A diabetes care plan should include the following eight steps:

1. Assessment of the patient's knowledge, understanding, current care, and any factors (e.g., cultural, health literacy, and socioeconomic) that may affect their care
2. Meal planning and healthy eating instruction
3. Physical activity recommendations
4. Self-monitoring of BG and, when appropriate, ketone concentrations
5. Drug therapy
6. Patient self-management education
7. Assessment of adherence to SMBG, MNT, and other non-drug and drug therapy
8. Follow-up care to alter or adjust the plan as needed to achieve metabolic goals

DM treatment focuses on maintaining glycemic control and preventing or delaying the progression of long-term diabetes-related complications. Patient education about the disease itself and appropriate self-care are the cornerstones of effective management. Adherence to MNT, encompassing a meal and physical activity plan, is critical to glycemic control and in achieving and maintaining a healthy weight. Patients with diabetes should also avoid unhealthy habits, such as smoking, which can affect their risk of developing diabetic complications and other comorbid conditions. Finally, most patients should use SMBG to assess the effects of diet, physical activity, and medications on their BG. Not only does performing SMBG serve a clinical purpose, but it also gives the patient a sense of understanding and control over this chronic condition.

Pharmacologic treatment options for patients with type 1 diabetes include insulin therapy delivered by self-injection or an insulin pump. Select patients may also benefit from an amylin receptor agonist. Because they are unable to produce insulin, patients with type 1 diabetes must inject themselves with insulin each day. Insulin therapy should be tailored to balance the effects of diet and physical activity. To achieve balance, patients must routinely perform SMBG. Hypoglycemia and hyperglycemia are largely preventable once this balance is achieved. The algorithm in Figure 47-2 outlines a general treatment approach for type 1 diabetes.

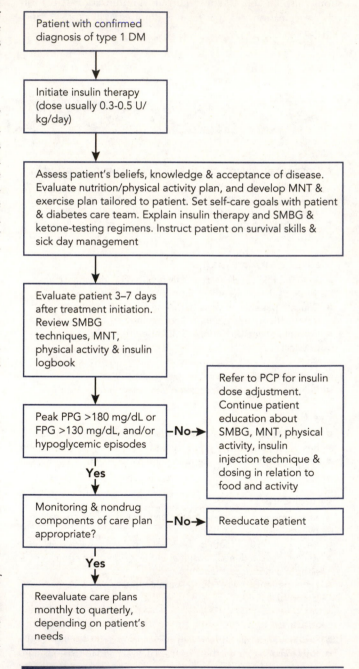

FIGURE 47-2 General treatment of type 1 diabetes mellitus. Key: DM, diabetes mellitus; FPG, fasting plasma glucose; MNT, medical nutrition therapy; PCP, primary care provider; PPG, postprandial plasma glucose; SMBG, self-monitoring of blood glucose.

Patients with prediabetes may be able to normalize their BG concentrations with diet, physical activity, and weight loss alone. Some may benefit from the addition of pharmacotherapy.[7] Patients with type 2 diabetes, however, often require MNT and physical activity combined with pharmacologic intervention. Figure 47–3 shows a general treatment algorithm for type 2 diabetes.

Nonpharmacologic Therapy

Medical Nutrition Therapy

Coupled with regular physical activity, MNT is an essential nonpharmacologic component of diabetes care. Rather than focusing on the need to "diet" or "lose weight," the term "nutrition" is used to emphasize the importance of eating for a healthy lifestyle and achieving and maintaining metabolic goals.

The concepts of MNT are similar for patients with types 1 and 2 diabetes, but treatment goals differ. For patients with type 1 diabetes, the goals are to integrate insulin regimens with usual habits of eating and physical activity, and to ensure normal growth and development during childhood and adolescence. Because obesity and a sedentary lifestyle are key issues in type 2 diabetes, the main objectives are healthy eating habits (including caloric and fat restriction), moderate weight loss, and increased physical activity to achieve optimal metabolic goals.

Dietitians who specialize in diabetes care can help patients learn about and incorporate nutritional guidelines into their daily lives. Practitioners can support and reinforce all phases of MNT by encouraging patients to follow their meal plan and to avoid fad diets, skipping meals, or prolonged fasting. Patients should be educated in reading food labels and interpreting nutritional values. Current ADA guidelines for meal planning entail an individualized approach and should involve the patient in the decision-making process, taking into account personal and cultural preferences.[19,20] Clinical studies have reported significant benefits of MNT, including 1% to 2% reductions in A1C, 15 to 25 mg/dL reductions in low-density lipoprotein cholesterol (LDL-C), and improved blood pressure.[19]

MACRONUTRIENTS

In general, the optimal mix of macronutrients (i.e., carbohydrate, protein, and fat) is individualized. Dietary carbohydrates are the main contributor to postprandial BG excursions. Although low-carbohydrate diets may seem a probable solution to controlling BG concentrations, foods containing carbohydrates also provide necessary amounts of vitamins, minerals, fiber, and energy.[19] Carbohydrates include starches (e.g., cereals, grains, starchy vegetables, legumes), sugars (e.g., glucose, fructose, sucrose, lactose), and fiber. A meal plan high in fresh fruits and vegetables and moderate in starches is recommended. High-fiber starches (e.g., legumes, whole-grain breads, and fiber-rich cereals with a goal of 14 grams fiber per 1000 kcal per day, or 20–30 grams fiber per day), are preferred over low-fiber starches (e.g., mashed potatoes, pasta, rice). A high-fiber diet can reduce hyperglycemia and cholesterol. Some beverages such as regular sodas, juices (more than 4 ounces), and sports drinks contain excessive or "hidden" carbohydrates. These beverages should be replaced with "low-" or non–carbohydrate-containing alternatives such as water, diet sodas, or sugar-free flavored water drinks. Consumers should read "sugar-free" product labels carefully because mislabeling can occur. To be considered sugar free, the product must contain less than 0.5 grams of sugar per labeled serving. Non-nutritive sweetening agents, as described below, are considered sugar free.

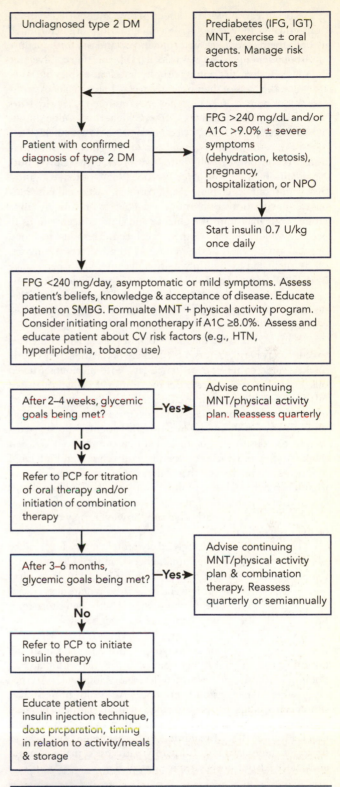

FIGURE 47-3 General treatment of type 2 diabetes mellitus. Key: A1C, glycosylated hemoglobin; CV, cardiovascular; DM, diabetes mellitus; FPG, fasting plasma glucose; HTN, hypertension; IFG, impaired fasting glucose; IGT, impaired glucose tolerance; MNT, medical nutrition therapy; NPO, nothing by mouth; PCP, primary care provider; SMBG, self-monitoring of blood glucose.

Not all carbohydrates affect plasma glucose concentrations equally. Elevated glucose concentrations are determined by both the quality (e.g., glycemic index) and the total quantity of carbohydrates (e.g., glycemic load [GL]) consumed. Glycemic index is a system that ranks carbohydrates on a scale of 0% to 100%, on the basis of their potential to raise plasma glucose concentrations immediately after they are consumed. Carbohydrates with a high glycemic index (70% or higher; e.g., doughnuts, most crackers, corn chips, dried fruits) break down quickly after ingestion, resulting in high and prolonged glucose concentrations. In contrast, carbohydrates that break down slowly during digestion have a low glycemic index (55% or less; e.g., most fresh fruits and vegetables, beans, oatmeal, pasta) and raise glucose concentrations only modestly. Diets with low glycemic index foods may improve glucose and lipid concentrations in people with diabetes. GL is the total glycemic response to a food or meal, on the basis of the grams of carbohydrates it contains. GL is calculated by multiplying the glycemic index percentage by the total grams of carbohydrate per serving. Typical diets contain approximately 100 GL units per day. The ADA states that the use of glycemic index or GL may be beneficial for glycemic control.[7]

With regard to fat, the main goal for people with diabetes is to reduce CVD risk factors. Less than 7% of the total daily caloric intake should come from saturated fats, with monounsaturated oils (e.g., olive oil) favored. Because trans fats or hydrogenated oils found in vegetable shortening cakes, hard margarines, pies, or snack foods increase LDL-C and decrease HDL-C, consumption of trans fats should be minimized. Patients who are overweight or consume high amounts of fat should decrease their intake of dietary fat. Recommend a daily cholesterol intake of less than 200 mg/day and that patients consume 2 or more servings of fish per week—avoiding commercially fried fish filets.[19] Consuming "light" or "fat-free" foods in which the fat has been replaced with a carbohydrate, however, may contribute to hyperglycemia.

The recommended average daily protein intake (e.g., intake of meat, poultry, fish, eggs, milk, cheese, and soy) for most patients is 15% to 20% of total daily calories.[19] The long-term consequences of high-protein and low-carbohydrate diets are not well established in patients with diabetes, although short-term (up to 1 year) use may be beneficial for weight loss.[7]

Lifestyle changes, moderate daily physical activity, and portion-size control for carbohydrates, protein, and fats are the critical factors in controlling obesity in patients with diabetes. Sodium intake should be limited (less than 2300 mg/day), especially when hypertension is present.[13] All health professionals should encourage patients to keep a meal plan and physical activity log to track the effects of food, physical activity, and medication on BG.[19] In addition, patients should learn how to interpret these data and to identify patterns to make a cause-and-affect relation for glycemic control.[21]

Use of Sweeteners

Both nutritive (caloric) and non-nutritive (noncaloric) sweetening agents are available and are good alternatives to using sugar. The calories from nutritive sweeteners such as fructose (4 kcal/g; e.g., honey, fruits, vegetables) and sugar alcohols (2 kcal/g; e.g., lactitol, maltitol, mannitol, sorbitol, xylitol) are generally counted in the carbohydrate total for meals and snacks.[19] Consuming large amounts of sugar alcohols may cause diarrhea, resulting from the laxative effects of polyols.

Currently the Food and Drug Administration (FDA) has approved five non-nutritive sweeteners, including saccharin (Sweet'n Low), sucralose (Splenda), acesulfame potassium (Sweet One, Sunett), aspartame (Equal, NutraSweet), and neotame.[22] Although neotame was approved for use in beverages and foods, no commercially available products are currently available in the United States. All non-nutritive sweeteners have undergone rigorous testing and are considered safe for consumption in moderate amounts, including by patients with diabetes and patients who are pregnant. They are heat stable (except aspartame) and may be used in food preparation in a manner similar to sugar. Aspartame contains phenylalanine in a high enough concentration that it should be avoided in patients with phenylketonuria. Stevia is a natural sweetening substance that is available as a dietary supplement.

Use of Alcohol

Although alcohol consumption precautions for patients with diabetes are similar to those for the general population, some notable exceptions exist. Patients with diabetes should be educated that alcohol (1) is considered a fat (7 cal/g) in the meal plan, (2) increases insulin response, and (3) impairs judgment and coordination. Acute alcohol consumption can cause and prolong hypoglycemia, especially if consumed on an empty stomach. Some epidemiologic evidence suggests that adults with diabetes who chronically consume mild-to-moderate amounts of alcohol (5–15 g/day) have a reduced risk of coronary heart disease. Controlled trials are necessary to validate this observation.[23–25]

Adult patients choosing to drink alcohol should be advised as follows[19]:

- Limit daily intake to no more than two alcoholic beverages for men and one for women.
- One drink is considered 12 ounces of beer, 5 ounces of wine, or 1.5 ounces of distilled spirits (hard alcohol). Each contains 15 grams of alcohol.
- Calories from alcoholic beverages and sugar-containing mixes must be included as an addition to the regular meal plan. No food should be omitted.
- To reduce hypoglycemia risk, consume alcohol with food and space drinks.
- Refrain from drinking if you are pregnant, overweight (adds calories), or have other medical problems such as pancreatitis, advanced neuropathy, hypertriglyceridemia, or alcohol abuse.

Use of Caffeine

Compared with placebo, acute caffeine doses of 375 mg/day (e.g., equivalent to more than seven caffeinated carbonated beverages) were shown to impair postprandial glucose metabolism in people with diabetes.[26] Thus, moderation is advised. Although ADA does not provide specific guidelines, a conservative recommendation is for patients to consume no more than one to two caffeinated beverages per day.

Use of Tobacco Products

Tobacco use is associated with an increased risk of mortality, macrovascular complications, and early microvascular complications, and it may predispose the user to developing type 2 diabetes.[7] Practitioners should encourage cessation of all tobacco products (see Chapter 50).

Physical Activity

Patients with diabetes benefit from an active lifestyle. The term *physical activity* is used because of the negative connotation of *exercise*. Regular physical activity can improve glycemic control (increases insulin sensitivity), facilitate weight loss (reduces body fat and increases muscle mass), reduce cardiovascular risk factors (reduces LDL-C and triglycerides; increases HDL-C with weight loss; improves blood pressure), and improve self-esteem.[27] Regular physical activity can even prevent the onset of type 2 diabetes.[28]

Before increasing physical activity, patients should undergo a thorough medical evaluation, including diagnostic studies to screen for any underlying diabetes-related complications that may limit certain activities.[29] The patient's lifestyle, preferences, metabolic goals, complications, and limitations should be accounted for to create an individualized fitness program. In general, patients should engage in 30 minutes or more of moderate physical activity on most days of the week.[29] Specific recommendations are to perform moderate-intensity aerobic physical activity at least 150 minutes per week, coupled with three times per week of resistance training, provided no contraindications exist.[7] Patients of advanced age should start slowly (5–10 minutes/day) and increase the amount of time gradually as tolerated. Patients are encouraged to use the large muscle groups and participate in aerobic activities (e.g., walking, swimming, and biking). Some modifications of physical activity are needed for patients with certain diabetes-related complications. For example, patients with moderate or worsening retinopathy should avoid activities that elevate blood pressure or are strenuous (e.g., heavy competitive sports and power weightlifting). Patients who have neuropathy with loss of protective sensation should avoid repetitive sports such as prolonged walking or jogging, although low-impact alternatives may be recommended by their physician with close follow-up.[29]

Effects of physical activity on BG vary in type 1 diabetes. Hyperglycemia results if insulin is inadequate when the patient begins the activity. More often, hypoglycemia may occur if the patient's BG concentration is normal or low just before physical activity. In general, only patients who use insulin need to consume extra carbohydrates or adjust insulin to account for the potential hypoglycemic effects of physical activity. Patients with type 1 diabetes may be at risk of hypoglycemia up to 8 to 15 hours after prolonged physical activity. Preventive measures should be taken to avoid this complication. Occasionally, patients with type 2 diabetes taking insulin secretagogues may experience hypoglycemia with physical activity. The degree of hypoglycemia, however, is not as significant as in insulin users. Table 47-5 provides guidelines for the conscientious patient performing physical activity. Patients should be reminded to include their physical activity in their daily log.

Monitoring of Glycemic Control

Results of the Diabetes Control and Complications Trial and the United Kingdom Prospective Diabetes Study showed the benefits of attaining close to normal glucose concentrations in patients with types 1 and 2 diabetes, respectively.[5,8] Regular monitoring of glycemic control is essential to achieving these goals. With knowledge of their glycemic status, patients are better able to self-manage their diabetes. Glycemic testing methods can be divided into two main categories; day-to-day glycemic measures (e.g., BG, blood ketones, urine ketones) and chronic glycemic control measures (e.g., A1C and glycated serum proteins). Home testing products for urine protein are also available.

TABLE 47-5 Patient Education for Patients with Diabetes Who Conscientiously Perform Physical Activity

- Wear properly fitted shoes and a diabetes identification bracelet or shoe tag.
- Perform SMBG before and after physical activity. BG testing during physical activity may be necessary for prolonged physical activity.
- Perform a 5- to 10-minute, low-intensity, aerobic (e.g., walking or bicycling) warm-up (to prepare the muscles and heart) and cool-down (to bring heart rate down) period.
- Adjust insulin or carbohydrate intake if needed. For insulin users who engage in moderate physical activity (e.g., 30–45 minutes of bicycling or jogging), reduce the preceding dose of regular or rapid-acting insulin by 30% to 50%.
- Before physical activity, if glucose concentration is normal or low (e.g., <100 mg/dL), patient should consume a 10- to 15-gram carbohydrate snack (e.g., 1 small apple, 6-ounce cup of yogurt, or four to six whole-grain crackers) and add an additional snack if needed after the activity.
- To avoid increased absorption of regular or rapid-acting insulin (and possible hypoglycemia) from physical activity, patients should inject insulin into the abdomen or do physical activities 30 minutes to 1 hour after insulin administration.
- Avoid physical activity if glucose concentration is greater than 250 mg/dL in the presence of ketosis (particularly in patients with type 1 diabetes). Use caution if BG concentrations are greater than 300 mg/dL without ketosis.
- Late-onset hypoglycemia can occur 8–15 hours after the physical activity, especially in patients with type 1 diabetes. If a patient performs physical activities during the day, recommend an increase in carbohydrate intake and perform SMBG during the night to detect nocturnal hypoglycemia. Individuals using insulin are more susceptible to hypoglycemia than are those taking insulin secretagogues.

Key: BG, blood glucose; SMBG, self-monitoring of blood glucose.
Source: References 27 and 29.

Self-Monitoring of Blood Glucose

Over the past decade SMBG has become the standard for day-to-day assessment of glycemic control. SMBG provides patients with immediate feedback. Patients can recognize glucose patterns to track whether daily goals are being met, to prevent or detect hypoglycemia, and to evaluate glycemic response to foods, physical activity, or medication changes. Practitioners use SMBG data to help patients make changes to their diabetes care plan.

Few patients with diabetes are not candidates for SMBG. The following patients should be strongly encouraged to self-test their BG[30]:

- All patients with type 1 diabetes
- All patients who use insulin
- Patients who use sulfonylureas or nonsulfonylurea insulin secretagogues to monitor for and detect hypoglycemia and to prevent asymptomatic hypoglycemia
- All patients having difficulty recognizing symptoms of hypoglycemia
- Pregnant patients with type 1, type 2, or GDM

The ADA also suggests that SMBG "may be desirable in all patients not achieving glycemic goals."[30] Testing frequency and timing depend on patients' individual needs, yet they should be sufficient to help patients reach target glycemic goals. More frequent monitoring may be necessary for patients prone to hypoglycemia and during illness, or for dose changes in insulin or other diabetes medication, physical activity, diet changes, or travel.[31] SMBG improves glucose control only with proper use and application.[8] Thus, the patient must be trained in SMBG technique and given specific guidelines for therapy alterations.[30,32]

Several factors play a role in SMBG product selection, including costs of necessary supplies not covered by the medical plan and individual patient special considerations (e.g., manual dexterity, visual acuity). Although SMBG offers many benefits, some drawbacks include expense (both out of pocket and time), possible invasive finger or skin punctures, motivation, and health literacy (e.g., cognition) required to perform SMBG and learn to interpret test results.

BG MONITORING WITH GLUCOSE MONITORS

A glucose monitor used in conjunction with reagent strips gives the specific BG concentration. Two types of monitors measure BG. Both are based on (oxidation) enzymatic activity. One type uses a photometric or reflectance measurement that is based on a dye–related reaction. The patient places a drop of blood on a reagent strip either before or after inserting the strip into a monitor, where it is read photometrically or colorimetrically. The other type of monitor measures BG with a biosensor that records an electronic charge produced by a chemical reaction. Reflectance monitors must be regularly cleaned, whereas monitors that use biosensor technology do not generally require cleaning.

All monitors are calibrated and will generally analyze the BG concentration according to programmed data. All monitors provide a digital display of the BG concentration, although the display size may vary. Most have memories for later recall of recent BG concentrations and can print retained data, once the monitor is downloaded. Patients who are blind or visually impaired may benefit from monitors with audio features (e.g., Prodigy Voice).

Many factors are used to determine the best monitor for an individual patient such as monitor size, size of display, blood sample size, capabilities for alternate site testing, timing devices, calibration, accuracy, ease of use, effect of temperature on accuracy, memory or data management and download features, battery types, need for cleaning, accessories required, audio capabilities, and price. Several monitors are available, and Table 47-6 lists

---

TABLE 47-6 Selected Blood Glucose Monitors[a]

Name (Mfr)	Sample Size (mcL)	Test Strip	Alternate Site	Test Time (seconds)	Touchable Strips
Accu-Chek Active (Roche Diagnostics)	1	Active	Yes	5	Yes (out-of-monitor dosing)
Accu-Chek Advantage (Roche Diagnostics)	4	Comfort Curve[b]	No	26	Yes
Accu-Chek Compact Plus (Roche Diagnostics)	1.5	Compact 17-test drum (1 installed)	Yes	5	Yes
Accu-Chek Aviva (Roche Diagnostics)	0.6	Aviva	Yes	5	Yes
Ascensia Breeze 2 (Bayer)	1	10-test disc Breeze 2	Yes	5	Yes
Ascensia Contour (Bayer)	0.6	Contour	Yes	5	Yes
FreeStyle Freedom Lite (Abbott Diabetes Care)	0.3	FreeStyle Lite	Yes	Ave 5	Yes
FreeStyle Lite (Abbott Diabetes Care)	0.3	FreeStyle Lite	Yes	Ave 5	
One Touch Basic (LifeScan)	9	One Touch Blue	No	45	No
One Touch Ultra (LifeScan)	1	Ultra	Yes	5	Yes
One Touch Ultra 2 (LifeScan)	1	Ultra	Yes	5	Yes
One Touch Ultra Mini (LifeScan)	1	Ultra	Yes	5	Yes
One Touch UltraSmart (Lifescan)	1	Ultra	Yes	5	Yes
Precision Xtra (Abbott Diabetes Care) [measures ketones also]	0.6	Precision Xtra (individually wrapped; end or top fill)	Yes	5 (10 for ketones)	Yes
Prestige IQ (Home Diagnostics)	4	Prestige Smart System	No	10–50	No (out-of-monitor dosing)
ReliOn Ultima (Wal-Mart)	0.6	ReliOn Ultima (individually wrapped)	No	20	Yes
Sidekick Testing System (Home Diagnostics)	1	Vial of 50 strips with monitor on vial lid	Yes	<10	Yes
TrueTrack Smart System (Home Diagnostics)	1	TrueTrack Smart System	Yes	10	Yes

Key: Ave, average; Mfr, manufacturer; s, seconds.

[a] List is not all-inclusive. A more exhaustive list may be found at ADA's *Diabetes Forecast,* available free online (www.diabetes.org/diabetes-forecast/resource-guide.jsp). Table contents may have changed since time of publication. All monitors are plasma referenced except One Touch Basic and SureStep, which are reported as whole blood.

products and features that may influence patient selection. FDA has set specific allowable variances for the monitors.

Even when BG monitors are used properly, calibrated frequently, and interpreted correctly, accuracy can vary by up to 20%. Most glucose monitors report plasma glucose concentrations, but a few report capillary (whole blood) glucose concentrations. Because plasma BG concentrations are typically 10% to 15% higher than whole blood, patients should know which results their monitors yield to determine their glycemic goals.[30]

Many BG monitors (Table 47-6) allow for blood sampling at alternate sites from the fleshy part of the palm, forearm, upper arm, thigh, and calf. Blood flow to the finger is faster than that to the forearm. Therefore, when glucose concentrations are rapidly fluctuating (e.g., after meals, during hypoglycemia, with increased physical activity), a fingerstick will reflect the change in BG before the alternate sites.[32,33] Patients should be educated that alternate site testing is recommended only for a fasting state, before meals, and for more than 2 hours after physical activity or meals.

Because drug therapy changes are made on the basis of results, accuracy is imperative. Tips for improving accuracy can be found in Table 47-7.

CONTINUOUS GLUCOSE MONITORING

An alternative method of monitoring glucose control is using a continuous glucose monitoring (CGM) system. A CGM device contains a sensor, inserted into the subcutaneous tissue, which records glucose concentrations every 5 minutes for up to 72 hours. Patients must calibrate the system daily by entering at least four SMBG readings taken at different times of the day with a standard glucose monitor. Data collected by the CGM device is downloaded into a computer and is viewed in graph and chart formats. Although not intended for day-to-day glucose monitoring, CGM offers the advantage of detecting glucose fluctuations, excursions, and trends throughout the day (e.g., unrecognized nocturnal or daytime hypoglycemia, 3- to 4-hour postprandial hyperglycemia), that go unnoticed using only A1C and SMBG values as guides for treatment. Results from CGM allows for better pattern management particularly for insulin users. Challenges with CGM include insurance coverage and the need for a motivated patient who will wear the device and obtain, record, and enter SMBG readings.

Finally, the glucose monitoring method recommended to the patient must be flexible and capable of being easily incorporated into the patient's lifestyle or daily routine. Providers can help individual patients select the best monitor for home use.

Ability to Reapply Blood to Strip	Provide Reading with Only Adequate Sample	Range (mg/dL)	Coding or Calibration	Battery	Memory (No. of BG Tests)
Yes	No	10–600	Insert chip	(1) Li 3V	200
Yes (up to 15 s)	No	10–600	Insert chip	(2) 2032 Li 3V	480
No	Yes	10–600	Automatic	(2) AAA	300
Yes (up to 5 s)	Yes	10–600	Insert chip	(2) 2032 Li 3V	500
No	No	20–600	Automatic	(1) Li 3V	420
No	Yes	10–600	Automatic	(2) Li 3V	480
Yes (up to 60 s)	Yes	20–500	Automatic	(1) 2032 Li 3V	400
Yes (up to 60 s)	Yes	20–500	Automatic	(1) CR2032 Li	400
No	No	0–600	Enter code	(2) AAA	75
No	Yes	20–600	Enter code	(1) 2032 Li 3V	150
No	Yes	20–600	Enter code	(2) 2032 Li 3V	500
No	Yes	20–600	Enter code	(1) 2032 Li 3V	50
No	Yes	20–600	Enter code	(2) AAA	3000 (and electronic logbook)
Yes (up to 30 s)	Yes	20–500	Insert calibrator strip	(1) CR2032 Li (installed)	450
No	Yes	20–600	Insert code strip	(1) AAA	365
Yes (up to 30 s)	Yes	20–500	Insert code strip	(2) AAA	450
No	Yes	20–600	Automatic	Not replaced	50 (no date or time)
No	Yes	20–600	Insert code chip	(1) CR2032 Li or (1) 3V Li	365

[b] Takes Advantage strips also (BG reading).

Source: Adapted with permission from Glucose Monitor Comparison Table prepared by Lisa Kroon, PharmD, CDE, University of California at San Francisco.

TABLE 47-7 Tips for Improving Accuracy of Fingerstick Technique

Using Test Strips

- Properly store test strips at room temperature in the original vial or container.
- Avoid exposing test strips to changes in temperature, humidity, and light.
- Check expiration date on test strips.
- Discard test strips from vials 90 days after opening
- Code monitor for the batch of test strips (if applicable).
- Use control solutions to verify test strips are working properly

Using Glucose Monitor

- Follow manufacturer's directions for calibrating monitor and using control solutions.
- Make sure monitor is clean.

Obtaining an Adequate Blood Sample

- Gather all necessary supplies (e.g., monitor, test strips, lancet, lancet device, tissue).
- Vigorously clean hands with warm soapy water to increase blood circulation.
- If alcohol must be used to clean hands, wait 1 minute to ensure alcohol has completely evaporated.
- Dry hands thoroughly.
- Hang hand below heart for 30–60 seconds to increase blood flow to fingers.
- Using the other hand, apply pressure on the finger from the base to the finger pad.

Lancing the Finger

- Use a lancet device with an adjustable puncture depth and adjust as needed to ensure adequate blood drop.
- Point fingers to the ground and lance the side of the fingertip.
- Avoid lancing finger pads since more nerves in these areas may cause pain.
- If lancing the index finger or thumb causes pain, avoid these areas as well.

Applying the Drop of Blood

- Ensure adequate size of blood drop is applied to test strip.
- If necessary, apply light pressure on the finger from the base to the finger pad to increase size of blood drop.
- Quickly place drop of blood on test strip. Method varies with monitor type. Refer to monitor instructions for proper technique.

Source: Reference 34.

Proper education in the methods for self-monitoring, the differences between individual monitors, the importance of multiple daily tests, and the interpretation and application of test results will encourage patients to perform SMBG consistently.[32] Return demonstration by the patient is necessary to ensure patient understanding and to correct any errors as they are observed. Patients should be encouraged to maintain accurate records of SMBG and to return with their logbook, which should also contain records of medication use (e.g., name, dose, time taken), diet changes, activities, and body weight. Despite the memory and downloading capability of most monitors, these features do not replace the importance of a patient-maintained logbook. This patient documentation is invaluable for the patient and clinician to identify BG patterns and assess the outcome of behavior and lifestyle modifications and to adjust treatment as necessary. In addition, computerized data-management systems accompanying monitors can be used at home or in the clinician's workplace. The programs include software for downloading monitor information, modules for personal digital assistants (PDAs), electronic logbooks, and Web-based programs to help patients track SMBG trends.

BG MONITORING WITH REAGENT STRIPS

Reagent strips (e.g., Chemstrip bG, Glucostix, Select GT Strips) are used infrequently to test BG. Unlike glucose monitor readings, which provide a specific glucose concentration at the time of the test, reagent strips provide a visual glucose concentration *range*. For these reasons, reagent strips are not recommended.

LANCETS AND BLOOD SAMPLING EQUIPMENT

Most BG testing requires the use of lancets, lancet devices, and tissue. Several lancing devices are available and are often provided with BG monitors. These devices allow for a fingerstick with less associated pain, because most have an autoretractable needle, and the amount of skin penetration can be adjusted in some products. Lancing devices should not be shared because they can harbor bloodborne pathogens and promote infection. Obtaining an adequate blood sample is essential for test accuracy. Clinicians should instruct patients on proper techniques for improving accuracy (Table 47-7). Patients should consult with their local jurisdiction about sharps disposal or call the Coalition for Safe Community Needle Disposal at 800-643-1643 for instructions for proper needle disposal.

Urine Testing

GLUCOSE

Urine glucose testing kits (e.g., Clinistix Reagent Strips, DiaScreen 1K) remain available. These tests are not recommended, because they do not provide accurate BG assessments.

KETONES

The development of self-blood ketone monitoring has revolutionized the process of detecting or predicting ketoacidosis. When the body does not have sufficient insulin, BG concentrations rise and the body's cells become energy deprived. During these times of low carbohydrate availability, the liver breaks down fat to produce ketone bodies (acetoacetate, 3-beta-hydroxybutyrate, and acetone). A sufficient blood concentration of ketones can result in a diabetic ketoacidosis, a potentially fatal condition. Because ketones in the blood overflow into the urine, urinary ketone concentrations can be tested to detect whether metabolic changes leading to ketoacidosis are occurring. The basis for the urinary ketone testing is that sodium nitroprusside alkali turns lavender in the presence of acetone or acetoacetic acid. These tests require comparing the color change to a reference chart. Several urine ketone testing products are available (e.g., Ketostix Reagent Strips, KetoCare Ketone Test Strips, DiaScreen 1K).

Certain BG monitors, such as Precision Xtra, are capable of using test strips designed to detect 3-beta-hydroxybutyrate concentrations in the blood. Unlike urine ketone tests, blood ketone tests provide a real-time picture. Another advantage of blood ketone testing over urine ketone and tablet testing is the lack of false positives in the presence of vitamin C or during exposure to ambient air.

Patients with type 1 diabetes should test for ketones when the plasma glucose is 240 mg/dL or greater. All patients with diabetes should check for ketones during times of stress or illness, during pregnancy, when the glucose concentration is greater than 300 mg/dL, or whenever ketoacidosis is suspected. In addition, patients should be counseled on the proper methods of testing for ketones in the urine and blood. Pregnant patients with diabetes (i.e., type 1, type 2, or GDM) are commonly instructed to test for ketones each morning and sometimes more often, to assess their metabolic status. The presence of ketones on two or more consecutive urine tests should be reported to the primary care provider.

MICROALBUMIN AND PROTEIN

Detection of microalbuminuria (trace protein in the urine) is an early sign of kidney damage. ADA recommends annual screening, although more frequent screening may be necessary in high-risk patients. Several nonprescription test products are available (e.g., Appraise Microalbumin Diabetes Monitoring System, KidneyScreen At Home), but the urine specimen is mailed to a laboratory for analysis and reporting. Large protein particles in the urine can be determined by using an array of products (e.g., Albustix, Chemstrip).

Self-Monitoring of Glycosylated Hemoglobin

Compared with SMBG, A1C and glycated protein testing provides useful information about a patient's glycemic control over a longer time period. Traditionally, these tests were performed in a laboratory setting from venipuncture samples. New technology allows for home or clinic testing with smaller blood samples.

Plasma glucose binds to red blood cells. A1C is formed at a rate directly proportional to the BG concentration over the previous 120 days (lifespan of the average erythrocyte).[30] Because A1C concentrations correlate with the weighted mean plasma glucose values over the preceding 2 to 3 months, it may be used to asses overall glycemic control in patients with diabetes. Patients may find it easier to understand their glycemic control using an estimated average glucose (eAG). A linear relation exists between A1C and average BG concentrations. The eAG is calculated by using the formula $eAG = 28.7 \times A1C - 46.7$. For example, an A1C of 7% and 10% are equivalent to eAGs of 154 mg/dL and 240 mg/dL, respectively. Practitioners can refer patients to a useful online eAG calculator (professional.diabetes.org/glucosecalculator.aspx).

In general, ADA recommends testing the A1C twice yearly in patients who are stable and meeting glycemic goals and every 3 months for patients not at goal or whose therapy has changed.[30] The exact testing frequency should be on the basis of clinical judgment. Normal nondiabetic A1C range is 4% to 6%. The goal for most people with diabetes is less than 7%. Several nonprescription A1C kits are available (e.g., AccuBase A1c Test Kit, A1c At Home, BIOSAFE Hemoglobin A1c Test Kit). Once a drop of blood is placed on a test strip, an individual mails the sample to a laboratory for analysis. Results are usually mailed or faxed back to the patient. Patients should discuss the use and results of these home monitoring kits with their health care providers.

Identification Tags

All persons with diabetes should wear a visible identification bracelet, necklace, or tag that indicates the person has diabetes and takes medication. Patients can find information for Medic-Alert, a reputable nationwide service available since 1956, at www.medicalert.org. Patients should also carry an identification card (e.g., in a wallet) that includes their name, address, and telephone number; the amount and type of medication used; and the name and telephone number of the patient's primary care provider. This information may be lifesaving if hypoglycemia or ketoacidosis occurs, requiring emergency services or hospitalization. Because a hypoglycemic reaction may be confused with drunkenness, patients with hypoglycemia have been known to be jailed rather than given medical care.

Travel Supplies and Preparations

Patients with diabetes planning travel should pack enough diabetes supplies for the entire trip, plus at least 1 extra week's worth (or double of what they anticipate needing). Patients should be advised to carry their supplies with them, not in checked luggage. The following is a travel checklist:

- A written note from patient's provider indicating the need for diabetes supplies (especially syringes and needles)
- Extra vials of U-100 insulin (only U-40 is available in some countries) or pen(s)
- Extra supply of syringes and needles because access may be limited; patients should refrain from prefilling syringes for a trip because of potential for leakage
- Extra supply of all oral medications in their original prescription bottles
- Extra SMBG supplies (e.g., glucose monitor, test strips, control solutions, lancets and devices, batteries if needed)
- Written prescriptions for medications, including insulin and diabetes supplies (e.g., syringes, test strips), in case of an emergency
- A summary of the patient's current medication regimen and emergency contact information
- Identification cards and a diabetes identification bracelet or tag
- Snacks and glucose tablets (and glucagon kit for insulin users) to be prepared for schedule changes or to prevent hypoglycemia (refer to hypoglycemia section)
- If traveling abroad, the names of English-speaking primary care providers in each city and some cards with several key phrases (e.g., "I have diabetes"; "Please get me a doctor") to access care in the language of the country being visited

Travelers should monitor their caloric intake carefully and allow time for physical activity. If notified in advance, most airlines offer special-order meals for people with diabetes. Advise the patient to wear comfortable well-fitting shoes if the patient intends to walk more than usual during the trip. Patients should anticipate changes in activity level because of extra walking and potentially erratic meals. Insulin users should be educated that time zone changes of 2 or more hours usually require insulin dose adjustments. They can work with their practitioners on specific adjustments to their basal and/or mealtime insulin doses. More frequent SMBG may be necessary.

Pharmacologic Therapy

Six classes of prescription oral agents are currently available to treat type 2 diabetes: sulfonylureas (i.e., glipizide and glyburide); nonsulfonylurea secretagogues or glinides (i.e., repaglinide and nateglinide); alpha-glucosidase inhibitors (i.e., acarbose); biguanides (e.g., metformin); thiazolidinediones (i.e., pioglitazone and rosiglitazone); and dipeptidyl peptidase-4 inhibitors (e.g., sitagliptin). In addition, two classes of prescription injectable agents (glucagon–like peptide-1) receptor agonists (i.e., exenatide) and amylin receptor agonists (i.e., pramlintide) are also available to treat type 2 diabetes. Oral and injectable agents, including insulin, are often used in combination.

Insulin

Insulin is the primary medication used to treat type 1 diabetes and GDM. Insulin is also commonly used in the treatment of type 2 diabetes. Although primary care providers prescribe insulin therapy, other practitioners, especially pharmacists, are often consulted by both primary care providers and patients about insulin and issues related to its use. Thus, practitioners should be knowledgeable about insulin products and their use.

Insulin stimulates glucose uptake and storage as glycogen in muscles and the liver and fatty acid and triglyceride synthesis. Insulin decreases hepatic glucose output, lipolysis, and ketone production. It also enhances amino acid incorporation into proteins.

The insulin molecule is composed of two amino acid chains, with the acidic A chain joined by a disulfide linkage to the basic B chain. Insulin analogues were developed with minor, but important, differences in the amino acids of human insulin that affect the insulin's absorption. All insulins except glargine have a neutral pH.

Available insulins can be divided into four groups according to their pharmacodynamics or time–action profile: onset (e.g., rapid, short, intermediate, or long acting), peak, and duration of action after subcutaneous (SQ) injection. Lispro (Humalog), aspart (NovoLog), and glulisine (Apidra) are rapid-acting insulin analogues. They differ from regular human insulin, a short-acting insulin, by substitution of amino acid residues in the insulin molecule that results in faster SQ absorption. Rapid- and short-acting insulins are dosed according to carbohydrate content and are used to provide mealtime insulin coverage and to correct for high BG. Their effects on BG are generally measured by testing postprandial plasma glucose concentrations.

To sustain its action, regular human insulin can be bound to zinc alone or in combination with protein molecules. Protamine and excess zinc slow insulin dissolution and absorption from the injection site. Neutral protamine Hagedorn (NPH) is an intermediate-acting insulin. NPH is an isophane insulin suspension, consisting of a complex mixture of human regular insulin, protamine, and some zinc, in which the ratio of insulin to protamine is equal. NPH insulin is typically dosed twice daily to supply basal insulin requirements.

Insulin glargine (Lantus) and detemir (Levemir) are long-acting insulin analogues. Glargine is an insulin analogue whose amino acid sequence causes a shift in the isoelectric point, making it more soluble at an acidic pH.[35] On injection, glargine, which has a pH of 4, forms a microprecipitate in the SQ tissue resulting from the pH change, which is then slowly absorbed. Insulin glargine and detemir do not have a pronounced peak effect and are used as a basal insulin.[36] Insulin glargine and detemir are usually dosed once daily. Some patients, particularly those with type 1 diabetes, may require twice daily injections for better basal insulin coverage. The effects of the intermediate- and long-acting insulins on BG are primarily measured by testing fasting plasma glucose concentrations.

Information about the pharmacodynamic profiles of insulins is contained in Table 47-8.[35,37,38] Many factors, such as insulin type, site of injection, injection technique, and individual patient response, can affect exogenous insulin's pharmacodynamic effects on BG concentrations.[31] Thus, the values listed in Table 47-8 have some degree of variability.

Human insulin is available without a prescription, whereas insulin analogues require a prescription. In the United States, insulin is commercially available in concentrations of 100 units/mL (designated as U-100). Regular U-500 insulin (Humulin R;

TABLE 47-8 Selected Insulin Pharmacodynamics

Insulin Type[a]	Onset of Action	Peak Action (hours)	Duration (hours)
Rapid-Acting			
Lispro	5–15 minutes	0.5–1.5	3–4
Aspart	5–15 minutes	0.5–1.5	3–4
Glulisine	5–15 minutes	0.5–1.75	1–3
Short-Acting			
Regular	0.5–1 hour	2–3	3–6
Intermediate-Acting			
NPH[b]	2–4 hours	4–10	10–16
Long-Acting			
Glargine	1.5 hours	No pronounced peak	20–24
Detemir	1–2 hours	4–16 hours; minimal peak at higher doses	6–24[c]

Key: NPH, neutral protamine Hagedorn.

[a] Human insulin and insulin analogues are produced through recombinant DNA technology.

[b] These insulins are isophane suspensions.

[c] When dosed at 0.4 units/kg, detemir has a dose-dependent duration of action.

Source: References 36 and 37.

Lilly) is available by prescription only for use in severely insulin-resistant patients requiring greater than 100 to 200 units per injection.

Insulin is also available as fixed-dose mixtures. Mixtures of NPH and regular human insulin are available without a prescription in ratios of 70% NPH to 30% regular and 50% NPH to 50% regular. Mixtures of the rapid-acting insulin analogues are available with a prescription only in ratios of 75% lispro protamine to 25% lispro, 50% lispro protamine to 50% lispro, 70% aspart protamine to 30% aspart, and 50% aspart protamine to 50% aspart. These formulations provide the rapid onset of lispro or aspart with the longer duration of action of a lispro or aspart protamine suspension, both of which are similar in action to human NPH. Table 47-9 summarizes the insulin formulations currently available in the United States. Inhaled insulin was removed from the marketplace in 2007. Other new formulations are currently undergoing clinical trials. Patients who switch from one source, type, or formulation (e.g., mixture) of insulin to another require close medical supervision.

The goal of insulin therapy in patients with type 1 diabetes is to mimic physiologic pancreatic insulin secretion to maintain normal plasma glucose concentrations. Physiologic insulin therapy provides basal and prandial (mealtime) needs. Patients with newly diagnosed diabetes are usually started on 0.5 to 0.1 units/kg of insulin daily.[40] Doses are adjusted according to BG response, glycemic goals, and other patient-specific variables (e.g., BG concentrations, growth, diet, activity, ketosis).

One half of the total daily dose is usually given as an intermediate or long-acting formulation to supply the basal metabolic needs. Depending on the insulin type and formulation

TABLE 47-9 Selected Insulin Preparations Available in the United States (U-100 Concentration)

Insulin Type[a] (Source)	Trade Name[a]	Manufacturer	How Supplied	Appearance
Rapid-Acting[b]				
Lispro	Humalog	Lilly	Vials and pens	Clear
Aspart (human analogue)	NovoLog	Novo Nordisk	Vials and pens	Clear
Glulisine (human analogue)	Apidra	sanofi-aventis	Vials and pens	Clear
Short-Acting				
Regular (human)	Humulin R	Lilly	Vials	Clear
Regular (human)	Novolin R	Novo Nordisk	Vials and pens	Clear
Intermediate-Acting				
NPH[c] (human)	Humulin N	Lilly	Vials and pens	Cloudy
NPH[c] (human)	Novolin N	Novo Nordisk	Vials and pens	Cloudy
Long-Acting				
Glargine (human analogue)[b]	Lantus	sanofi-aventis	Vials and pens	Clear
Detemir (human analogue)	Levemir	Novo Nordisk	Vials and pens	Clear
Mixtures				
75% NPL, 25% lispro (human analogues)[b]	Humalog Mix 75/25	Lilly	Vials and pens	Cloudy
50% NPL, 50% lispro (human analogues)[b]	Humalog Mix 50/50	Lilly	Pens	Cloudy
70% protamine crystalline aspart, 30% aspart (human analogues)[b]	NovoLog Mix 70/30	Novo Nordisk	Vials and pens	Cloudy
50% protamine crystalline aspart, 50% aspart (human analogues)[b]	NovoLog Mix 50/50	Novo Nordisk	Pens	Cloudy
70% NPH, 30% regular (human)	Humulin 70/30	Lilly	Vials	Cloudy
70% NPH, 30% regular (human)	Novolin 70/30	Novo Nordisk	Vials and pens	Cloudy
50% NPH, 50% regular (human)	Humulin 50/50	Lilly	Vials	Cloudy

Key: NPH, neutral protamine Hagedorn; NPL, neutral protamine lispro.

[a] Human insulin is produced through recombinant DNA technology.

[b] These insulins are available by prescription only.

[c] These insulins are isophane suspensions.

Source: References 37 and 39.

used, this dose may be administered all at once daily or divided to be administered twice daily (e.g., NPH or detemir).

The other half of the estimated total daily insulin dose is given as a rapid- or short-acting formulation to supply the patient's prandial needs. As a general rule in patients with newly diagnosed type 1 diabetes, 1 unit of rapid-acting insulin covers approximately 15 grams of carbohydrate. As part of MNT education, patients can be taught to estimate the total carbohydrates per meal to determine a prandial insulin dose. For patients who eat three meals a day, rapid- or short-acting insulin is dosed three times a day to be administered 0 to 30 minutes before meals, depending on the type used.

Insulin formulations are selected on the basis of patient-specific factors, such as diet, physical activity, ease of use (e.g., vials compared with delivery devices) and insurance status (e.g., formulary options available, affordability for uninsured patients). Dosing regimens are also tailored to patients' lifestyle and routine (e.g., number of daily meals and snacks, sleep, and work schedules). Insulin doses are adjusted on the basis of patient response to therapy as evidenced by trends in A1C and fasting, preprandial, and postprandial plasma glucose concentrations and incidence of hypoglycemia and hyperglycemia. Euglycemia can be achieved through intensive insulin therapy with multiple daily injections or an insulin infusion pump. Figure 47-4 depicts the glucose surges from three daily meals and the resultant insulin release from a healthy pancreas in response to prandial glucose. Patients can learn to manage and adjust their daily basal and prandial insulin requirements on the basis of BG concentrations, diet, and activity levels.

Insulin therapy in patients with type 2 diabetes is mainly determined by amount of glycemic control and duration of disease. Patients with type 2 diabetes whose BG is not controlled with non-insulin BG-lowering agents may require insulin therapy to achieve glycemic goals. In some cases, patients with newly diagnosed type 2 diabetes with severe hyperglycemia may require insulin therapy alone or in combination with other medications to reduce A1C values and BG concentrations. Once BG concentrations stabilize, these patients are usually transitioned to oral antidiabetic medications (e.g., metformin) for management.

Insulin formulation and dosing considerations in patients with type 2 diabetes are based on patient-specific factors, such as overall glycemic control and insulin sensitivity. Total daily dosage of insulin in patients with type 2 diabetes can vary, but typically range from 0.5 to 1.2 units/kg daily. Typically, patients with type 2 diabetes starting insulin therapy are started on once- or twice-daily dosing of an intermediate- or long-acting insulin. Patients with type 2 diabetes may require mealtime insulin therapy with a rapid- or short-acting formulation to minimize postprandial glucose excursions. As with type 1 diabetes, total daily insulin dose requirements are generally split between appropriate formulations to provide 50% as basal insulin and 50% as mealtime insulin. Dose is adjusted on the basis of patient response to therapy as evidenced by A1C trends, fasting and postprandial plasma glucose trends, and hypoglycemic episodes.

The most common side effect of insulin therapy is hypoglycemia. Many other factors (e.g., a decrease or inconsistency in mealtime carbohydrate content, physical activity, alcohol intake, and medications) can contribute to hypoglycemic episodes. For this reason, practitioners should carefully assess the relation between insulin dose and timing and patient BG trends, including hypoglycemic or hyperglycemic episodes, when adjusting insulin therapy. Patients with comorbid conditions, such as gastroparesis or reduced renal function, may be at increased risk of hypoglycemia. Insulin doses should be adjusted accordingly.

Weight gain is another common side effect. It is usually caused by increased efficiency of glucose and fat storage resulting from insulin therapy. Hypoglycemic episodes, which stimulate appetite, also contribute to weight gain because patients consume additional calories to correct the low BG.

Some patients experience local reactions on insulin injection, including pain, redness, bruising, burning, stinging, or irritation. Using a new syringe or pen needle with each injection may help minimize or alleviate pain associated with injections. Reminding patients to inject insulin at room temperature minimizes pain associated with cold insulin injections. Glargine was associated with a higher incidence of minor pain or stinging at injection sites compared with currently marketed neutral pH insulin preparations.[37] Most patients, however, tolerate glargine well. Proper insulin injection technique minimizes redness, swelling, and bruising. Good hygiene and proper use and storage of syringes and other delivery devices minimize the risk of infection. Practitioners should stress the importance of rotating or alternating injection sites within an anatomic area to limit local irritation, tissue reactions, and lipodystrophy.

Sensitivity and hypersensitivity reactions with human and analogue insulins are rare. Allergic reactions attributed to insulin additives (e.g., metacresol, phenol, methylparaben) are also rare. Patients who have had systemic allergic reactions (e.g., hives, angioedema, or anaphylaxis) to any insulin should be skin tested with each new preparation before starting its use. Insulin resistance secondary to insulin-blocking antibodies with human or analogue insulins are exceedingly rare. Patients showing adherence to therapy yet requiring greater than 200 units of insulin daily may be evaluated for the presence of insulin antibodies.

HYPERGLYCEMIA

Hyperglycemia can occur if an insulin dose is missed or if the dose is insufficient to meet metabolic needs or carbohydrates that are consumed. Hyperglycemic symptoms—frequent urina-

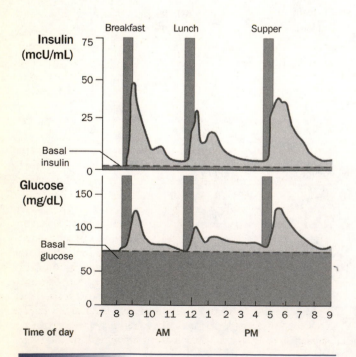

FIGURE 47-4 Relationship between insulin and glucose.

tion, dehydration, thirst, increased appetite—usually occur at BG concentrations greater than 180 mg/dL. If ketosis develops, the patient's breath may have a fruity odor. Untreated hyperglycemia requires immediate medical attention because it could progress to diabetic ketoacidosis (mainly in type 1 diabetes) or hyperosmolar hyperglycemic state (in type 2 diabetes), followed by coma and death. SMBG allows patients to detect consistent upswings in BG concentrations and adjust the insulin therapy accordingly or to contact the medical provider for reevaluation of pharmacologic and nonpharmacologic management of diabetes.

Morning hyperglycemia may result from an asymptomatic nocturnal hypoglycemia (Somogyi effect) in patients who are otherwise well controlled on intensive insulin regimens. In response to hypoglycemia, the body secretes epinephrine, which induces hepatic glucose production and results in morning hyperglycemia. For example, the Somogyi effect can occur if NPH causes nocturnal hypoglycemia because it peaks during the night when taken as a before-dinner injection. Another reaction that can present with a similar morning hyperglycemia is termed the "dawn phenomenon."[40] As part of the circadian rhythm, hormones such as growth hormone, cortisol, and epinephrine are released during the night. In response, the plasma glucose concentration rises in the early morning hours, and insulin is released from the functioning pancreas. In people with diabetes, the insulin release may not occur, resulting in morning hyperglycemia. Thus, a Somogyi effect is caused by too much insulin, whereas the dawn phenomenon is caused by too little insulin. Patients with morning hyperglycemia should monitor their plasma glucose concentration between 2 and 3 am to determine whether it is low (Somogyi effect) or normal or high (dawn phenomenon). They should record the results along with any changes in their diet and physical activities and be assisted in interpreting the results and adjusting therapy accordingly.

HYPOGLYCEMIA

Several factors can contribute to hypoglycemia, including insufficient caloric intake (e.g., skipping or delaying meals, vomiting), inaccurate insulin dose (e.g., too high, frequent adjustments, inadequate preparation, irregular timing), concomitant use of hypoglycemic drugs, drug interactions, very tight glycemic control, and physical activity. Although a BG concentration of less than 70 mg/dL indicates hypoglycemia, some patients experience symptoms at higher glucose concentrations.[41] Early warning symptoms may be both autonomic (e.g., trembling, shaking, sweating, palpitations, tachycardia) and neuroglycopenic (e.g., slow thinking, difficulty concentrating, slurred speech, uncoordinated, dizziness). Some patients may be hypoglycemic without experiencing any symptoms, a serious condition called hypoglycemic unawareness.

Mild-to-moderate hypoglycemic symptoms usually are rapidly relieved by ingestion of glucose. As a preventive measure, people with diabetes should always carry a source of fast-acting carbohydrate (Table 47-10). At the onset of hypoglycemic symptoms, patients should check their plasma glucose. If the result is low, patients should apply the "Rule of 15" and consume 15 grams of carbohydrates. If symptoms persist or BG concentrations are still below 70 mg/dL after 15 minutes, an additional 15 grams of carbohydrates should be consumed. BG concentrations of less than 50 mg/dL may require 20 to 30 grams of carbohydrates.[42] Foods high in fat (e.g., chocolate, potato chips, pizza) are poor choices for treating hypoglycemia, because fat delays carbohydrate absorption and adds unnecessary calories.[19]

TABLE 47-10 Selected Fast-Acting Carbohydrates for Treating Hypoglycemia (15 g)	
Source (Mfr)	**Quantity**
Milk (low-fat or nonfat)	8 oz (1 cup)
Fruit juice (e.g., apple, orange)	4 oz (1/2 cup)
Soft drink (nondiet)	4 oz (1/2 cup)
Sugar	1 tbsp or 3 cubes
Raisins	2 tbsp
Hard candies (e.g., Lifesavers, Brach's, Starbursts, Skittles, jelly beans)	5–6 pieces
Glucose tablets	
B-D Glucose Tablets (BD)	3 tablets (5 g per tablet; orange flavored)
DEX 4 (Iverness Medical)	4 tablets (4 g per tablet; grape, lemon, orange, or raspberry flavored)
Glucose gels	
GlucoBurst (PBM Products)	1 foil packet (15 g per packet; natural cherry flavor)
Glutose 15 (Paddock)	1 tube (15 g per tube; natural lemon flavored)
Glutose 45 (Paddock)	1/3 tube (45 g per reusable tube; natural lemon flavored)

Key: Mfr, manufacturer.

Protein-rich foods do not increase BG or prevent further hypoglycemic episodes and thus do not need to be added to carbohydrates for treatment of hypoglycemia. Patients who take alpha-glucosidase inhibitors (acarbose, miglitol) cannot rapidly digest table sugar (sucrose) or sugar from juices (fructose) or sodas. These patients should treat hypoglycemia with glucose (tablets or gel) or milk. Once hypoglycemia is treated, if mealtime is not within 1 hour, a small snack (e.g., crackers, piece of fruit, small sandwich) should be consumed to prevent further hypoglycemia. BG should be monitored frequently to prevent recurrent hypoglycemia.

Severe hypoglycemia may result in unconsciousness, coma, seizures, and inability to swallow and should be treated with glucagon.[43] All patients using insulin should have a glucagon emergency kit, particularly those with type 1 diabetes. Available by prescription, these kits contain a 1 mg ampule of glucagon, a syringe of diluent, and administration directions. Glucagon is indicated when an individual becomes unconscious because of hypoglycemia. For this reason, family members, other patient caregivers, and coworkers should be taught to mix and administer glucagon by SQ or intramuscular injection. Encourage them to practice the process of glucagon administration ahead of time so they will be prepared if an emergency arises. The usual dose is 1 mg for adults and children older than 10 years, 0.5 to 1 mg for children aged 5 to 10 years, and 0.25 to 0.5 mg for children younger than 5 years. Glucagon may cause vomiting, lasting up to 24 hours. Unconscious individuals should therefore be turned on their side before glucagon is administered, to prevent choking. Glucagon usually works within 5 to 10 minutes, but the effects are short lived. If no response is seen after

5 to 10 minutes, a second injection may be given. If this is ineffective, the caregiver should call 911 immediately. Once an individual is conscious and can swallow, the caregiver should give a carbohydrate liquid (e.g., juice, milk, nondiet soft drink) followed by a carbohydrate snack (small sandwich, crackers with peanut butter). For the next 24 hours, regular SMBG is necessary as well as adequate food intake to replenish hepatic glycogen stores. The primary care provider should be informed of the episode.

ADMINISTRATION GUIDELINES

Unless age (e.g., the very young) or physical or mental impairments preclude self-injection, a patient should be trained on (1) how to prepare his or her dose for SQ injection, (2) the location of acceptable self-injection sites, and (3) proper SQ injection technique. Advances from vials and syringes in the form of insulin-delivery devices, such as prefilled insulin pens, are now readily available. In addition to providing convenience, these devices can improve the accuracy of insulin administration or adherence in patients, particularly those with dexterity problems or visual or neurologic impairment. Table 47-11 describes the steps for preparing an insulin dose using a syringe and insulin vial or a prefilled insulin-delivery device.

Injection Sites, Routes, and Absorption Rates   Insulin injection site may influence insulin absorption. Acceptable SQ injection sites include the abdomen, upper arms (deltoid region), thighs (anterior and lateral aspects), and buttocks (Figure 47-5).[31]

Different anatomic sites differ in their rates of absorption. To decrease dose-to-dose absorption, patients should select then stick to one anatomic injection site. The abdomen is considered the preferred site for SQ injection of insulin by most experts because of the more predictable insulin absorption. Patients should avoid the area within 2 inches around the navel. Rotation of injection sites within an anatomic area helps prevent lipohypertrophy or lipoatrophy.

Proper SQ injection technique is depicted in Figure 47-6 and described step by step in Table 47-12.

Injection technique may need to be altered for certain patients (e.g., 45-degree injection angle for infants and extremely thin individuals with minimal SQ fat). Pinching the skin provides a firm injection surface and lifts the fat off the muscle to avoid intramuscular or intravenous injection. Properly injected insulin should leave only a needle puncture dot; bruising generally should not occur. If insulin leakage is observed, patients should be instructed to apply pressure to the injection site for 5 to 10 seconds (without rubbing). BG monitoring should be done more frequently on any day that insulin leakage or blood is observed. Patients who routinely experience insulin leakage after the injection should have their injection technique evaluated; a longer needle may be needed.

Injection pain can be reduced by injecting insulin at room temperature, keeping muscles relaxed before injection, ensuring air bubbles are not present in the syringe, penetrating the skin quickly, not changing direction of the needle during insertion or withdrawal, and using a new needle for each injection. Patients who routinely experience soreness, pain, bruising, welts,

---

TABLE 47-11   Guidelines for Preparing an Insulin Dose

Using a Vial and Syringe

- Wash hands with soap and warm water.
- Check the insulin label on the vial to verify the type of insulin to be injected.
- Visually inspect the insulin vial for signs of contamination or degradation (e.g., white clumps, color changes).
- For all cloudy insulins (Table 47-9), roll the vial gently back and forth between the hands to resuspend the insulin.
- Remove the cap and wipe the top of the vial off with an alcohol swab or cotton ball dipped in alcohol.
- Remove the protective coverings over the plunger and needle of the syringe.
- Taking care not to touch the needle, draw up air equal to the insulin dose to be administered into the syringe.
- Inject the air into the insulin vial.[a]
- With the syringe still inserted, invert the vial and withdraw the insulin dose.[b]
- Be sure to keep the hub of the needle below the surface of the insulin to prevent creating air bubbles within the syringe.
- If bubbles are present, gently tap the syringe to coax air to the top of the barrel where it can be injected back into the vial.
- Remove the syringe from the vial and self-inject dose, using proper injection technique (Table 47-12).

Using a Prefilled Insulin Pen Delivery Device

- Wash hands with soap and warm water.
- Check the insulin label on the device (e.g., pen) to verify the type of insulin to be injected.
- Remove the protective pen cap and visually inspect the insulin for signs of contamination or degradation.
- For all cloudy insulins (Table 47-9), invert and roll the device (e.g., pen) gently back and forth between the hands to resuspend the insulin.
- Wipe the rubber stopper with an alcohol swab.
- Attach a needle onto the device according to the manufacturer's directions.
- Remove the outer and inner needle cap.
- Follow any manufacturer's recommendations for priming the device (e.g., 2-unit air shot).
- Making sure pen dose selectors are first set to zero, dial the insulin dose to be injected.
- Use proper injection technique (Table 47-12).
- To deliver insulin when injecting, push down on the plunger button and hold for 5–10 seconds.
- Remove the needle from the device after injection to avoid allowing air into the insulin reservoir.

Key: NPH, neutral protamine Hagedorn.

[a] Patients mixing rapid- or short-acting insulin with NPH into the same syringe for injection should be instructed to inject air first into the NPH vial, then into the rapid- or short-acting vial.

[b] Patients mixing rapid- or short-acting insulin with NPH into the same syringe for injection should be instructed to withdraw the dose of the rapid- or short-acting insulin *before* the NPH.

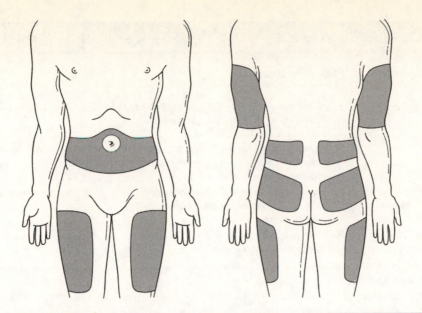

FIGURE 47-5 Body map of subcutaneous insulin injection sites.

or redness should have their injection technique evaluated by a practitioner.

SQ absorption rates can be highly variable within and across patients.[40] Patients should be educated about the influence of factors such as physical activity, massage, temperature, and smoking on insulin absorption. Performing physical activity or massaging the injection area can increase absorption rates. Heat from hot weather, a hot bath or shower, or sauna can increase peripheral blood flow, which can increase absorption rates. Cold has the opposite effect. Smoking, which can cause cutaneous vasoconstriction, may decrease insulin absorption rates, but this likely has little clinical significance.

The amount of insulin injected in a single dose may also affect insulin absorption rates. Patients failing to respond adequately to large doses of insulin (e.g., exceeding 50–60 units per dose) may split the dose to be injected over two sites within the same anatomic region.

Mixing Insulins Depending on the type of insulin, patients may mix two formulations together in a single syringe to limit the number of injections required. Table 47-13 summarizes the compatibility of various insulin mixtures. Glargine should not be mixed with any other form of insulin because of its low pH. Compatibility of detemir when mixed with other insulins has not been studied to date.

CONTAMINATION OF INSULIN

All insulins are produced at a near-neutral pH of 7.4 with the exception of glargine, which has a pH of 4. Lispro, aspart, glulisine, regular, glargine, and detemir insulins are clear aqueous fluids. If any of these products appear cloudy, flocculated, clumped, crystallized, or tinted, they may be contaminated and should not be dispensed or used. Other insulins (NPH and insulin mixtures containing an intermediate-acting insulin such as NPH, NPL, or protamine crystalline aspart) are cloudy suspensions. If any of these types of insulin suspensions rapidly settle out, precipitate, clump, flocculate, crystallize, or discolor, they may be altered and should not be dispensed or used.

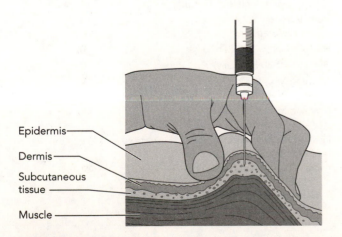

FIGURE 47-6 Correct method of subcutaneous insulin injection.

Epidermis
Dermis
Subcutaneous tissue
Muscle

TABLE 47-12 Insulin Subcutaneous Self-Injection Technique

- Prepare insulin dose for administration (see Table 47-11).
- Pinch the area to be injected.
- Insert the needle at a 90-degree angle to the skin in the center of the pinched area (a 45-degree angle for insertion may be used in small children and very thin adults).
- Release the pinch.
- Press down on the syringe or device plunger to inject insulin.
- Hold the syringe or device in the area for 5–10 seconds to ensure full delivery of insulin. This step is particularly important for insulin pen devices.
- Remove the syringe or device.

TABLE 47-13 Mixing Insulins

Mixture	Proportion	Pharmacodynamics	Stability
Lispro + NPH	Any	Slight decrease in absorption rate but not total bioavailability of lispro; postprandial BG response of lispro unaffected	Prepare mixture and inject immediately
Aspart + NPH	Any	Slight decrease in absorption rate but not total bioavailability of aspart; postprandial BG response of aspart unaffected	Prepare mixture and inject immediately
Glulisine + NPH	Any	No significant change in bioavailability or time to maximum concentration compared with glulisine alone	Prepare mixture and inject immediately
Regular + NPH	Any	No change in onset or duration of action of either insulin when administered in mixture	May be premixed into syringe, to be stored under refrigeration up to 7 days

Key: NPH, neutral protamine Hagedorn.
Source: References 36, 37, and 40.

STORAGE OF INSULIN

Insulin is a heat-labile protein, so all preparations must be stored carefully to maintain stability and maximum potency. Patients should inspect their insulin for visible changes in appearance before each injection. Color changes may be associated with protein denaturation and should be interpreted as evidence of potency loss.

Unopened insulin vials and cartridges may be stored in the refrigerator (36°F–46°F [2°C–8°C]) up until the expiration date listed on the product. Insulin should never be frozen. The refrigerator door is usually a good storage location to ensure that insulin does not become frozen. The stability of unopened and in-use insulin vials or cartridges stored at room temperature varies depending on the product. Once opened (in use), all insulin in vials may be stored away from heat sources and direct sunlight at room temperature (<77°F or 25°C for glulisine and <86°F or 30°C for all other insulins) for up to 28 to 30 days (in practice, ~1 month). In contrast, the stability of open insulin pens, refill cartridges, and other delivery devices varies depending on the product. Insulin pump cartridges, once opened, are generally stable for 48 hours. Table 47-14 summarizes the stability of open insulin at room temperature for select insulin products. Most pens and other delivery devices should not be refrigerated. Practitioners should contact individual manufacturers with specific questions about the stability of individual insulin products and devices under different storage or exposure conditions.

Patients who transport insulin regularly (e.g., to and from school or work, while running errands) should be reminded to insulate insulin from heat, direct sunlight, and excess agitation. Patients should never store insulin in the car. Insulin should be carried in an insulated pack by patients when traveling by bus, train, or air to ensure proper storage conditions.

PRODUCT SELECTION GUIDELINES

Practitioners should ensure that patients purchase the right type of supplies to facilitate insulin administration. Insulin available in vials must be administered with syringes. Spring-loaded plastic syringe holders are available from several manufacturers and can be used by patients who have needle phobia. Durable (reusable) and disposable insulin pens and other delivery devices provide added convenience and ease of use, especially in patients with impaired vision or dexterity. A resource guide with information on select insulin syringes, other delivery aids, and related products currently available in the United States is published annually in an issue of the ADA's *Diabetes Forecast* (available free online at www.diabetes.org/diabetes-forecast/resource-guide.jsp). Insulin pumps are an alternative delivery device available for use in select patients. Patients using syringes and disposable needles with other

TABLE 47-14 Stability of Selected Open (In-Use) Insulin Devices and Refill Cartridges at Room Temperature

Insulin Product (Mfr)	Stability at Room Temperature (<86°F [30°C]) (days)
Humalog Pen and KwikPen (Lilly)	28
Novolog FlexPen (Novo Nordisk)	28
Humulin N Pen (Lilly)	14
Novolin N Innolet (Novo Nordisk)	14
Humalog Mix 75/25 Pen and KwikPen (Lilly)	10
Humalog Mix 50/50 Pen (Lilly)	10
Humulin 70/30 Pen (Lilly)	10
Novolog Mix 70/30 FlexPen (Novo Nordisk)	14
Novolog Mix 50/50 FlexPen (Novo Nordisk)	14
Novolin 70/30 Innolet (Novo Nordisk)	10
Lantus SoloSTAR and Lantus cartridges for OptiClik (sanofi-aventis)[a]	28
Levemir FlexPen and Innolet (Novo Nordisk)	42

Key: Mfr, manufacturer.

[a] OptiClik device is distributed to physicians only and not available at pharmacies.

Source: References 31, 36, 44, and 45.

delivery devices should properly dispose of them according to local regulations. Practitioners should be familiar with the sharps disposal programs available to patients within their geographic area.

Insulin syringes are plastic, disposable syringes that come with very fine, well-lubricated needles. Recall that insulin is supplied as 100 units/mL (U-100) in the United States. Insulin syringes are designed for U-100 insulin and are marked in insulin units. Depending on the syringe, marker increments may differ and therefore should be pointed out to patients. Depending on the manufacturer, insulin syringes are available in 0.3, 0.5, and 1 mL capacities, which hold 30, 50, and 100 units, respectively. Patients should be reminded to purchase syringes closely matched to their individual insulin dose(s). For example, a patient taking 38 units of glargine once daily should use 0.5 mL syringe to draw up insulin to the 38-unit mark.

Today's needles have virtually no "dead space" or air space at the hub of the needle, thus reducing a potential source of dosing error. Several needle lengths, including 1/2, 3/8, and 5/16 inch, are available. The shortest needles are usually reserved for use in children or very thin adults. Needles come in a variety of gauges (e.g., 28–31). The higher the gauge, the finer is the needle, which lessens injection site pain. Silicone coating eases insertion, also reducing pain.

Manufacturers currently do not recommend reusing disposable syringes and pen needles. Studies have investigated the reuse of insulin syringes. ADA suggests that some patients may opt to reuse syringes or needles until the needle becomes dull, bent, or comes in contact with any surface other than the skin.[31] In practice, fine-gauge (e.g., 30 or 31) syringes and pen needles are more susceptible to bending and possibly breaking on reuse, which could result in injury or other adverse effects. Syringes and needles to be reused should not be cleaned with alcohol, which removes the silicone coating. Reused syringes and needles must be safely recapped and stored at room temperature away from children and pets. Certain patients, such as those with poor hygiene, an acute illness, open wounds, decreased immunity, or poor dexterity or vision should not reuse syringes or needles.

Sharps, such as needles and lancets, should be properly disposed of, ideally in a sharps container. Health care providers should be familiar with the sharps disposal requirements and local and mail-order service providers available within their community. A select list of related products and services is published in the *Diabetes Forecast* Resource Guide (www.diabetes.org/diabetes-forecast/resource-guide.jsp).

Several types of insulin injection aids and devices are available for patients who have an aversion to or difficulty with self-injection. Such products include syringe magnifiers, needle guides and vial stabilizers, syringe insertion aids, insulin pens, and jet injectors. Syringe magnifiers enlarge the marks on a syringe barrel, making them easier to see for visually impaired patients. Patients should be reminded that, depending on the manufacturer, magnifiers work only with specific syringe brands. Needle guides and vial stabilizers are available to help patients with limited dexterity safely insert syringes into vials and draw up accurate insulin doses. Insertion aids and jet injectors may be useful for patients with needle or self-injection phobias.

Insulin pens, most of which resemble writing pens, use single-use or disposable cartridges filled with 300 units of insulin. These devices may be ideal for children, adolescents, patients with visual or physical dexterity impairment, or really any patient who prefers them. Pen devices eliminate the step of withdrawing insulin from a vial. Individuals simply dial their dose using a dose knob or button. Patients feel the knob dialing and hear a click at each unit, which can help improve accuracy of insulin dosing. Depending on manufacturer, pens are available for most insulin types and mixtures. (For a comprehensive list of insulin pen and other delivery devices, see the ADA's *Diabetes Forecast* [www.diabetes.org/diabetes-forecast/resource-guide.jsp].) Pen needles should be selected on the basis of their compatibility with the device.

Intensive insulin therapy to achieve tight glycemic control in either type 1 or type 2 diabetes requires multiple daily injections. An alternative to multiple daily injections for certain patients is an insulin pump. Use of an insulin pump requires extensive patient training and education (e.g., adjusting insulin dosing based on BG and troubleshooting the device, catheter, and lines) to ensure optimal and safe insulin delivery and BG concentrations. For these reasons, not all patients are candidates for an insulin pump. People who are extremely motivated and responsible, have demonstrated appropriate health literacy about diabetes care and monitoring, and have proven consistent ability to adhere to SMBG, MNT, and insulin therapy recommendations can be considered for insulin pump therapy. Medicare currently covers insulin pumps and related supplies for patients with types 1 and 2 diabetes who meet its eligibility requirements.[46]

Insulin pumps are open-loop systems within a computerized, battery-driven portable device small enough to be worn on a belt loop, in a pocket, or attached to undergarments. The computer is programmed to deliver a continuous insulin infusion to meet basal requirements and can be programmed to deliver bolus doses for mealtime, snack, and physical activity requirements. Many patients, however, manually program for their bolus dosing. Rates can be programmed to fluctuate or can be manually adjusted, on the basis of SMBG results. Insulin is delivered from a reservoir by a computer-controlled plunger through tubing to an SQ-implanted catheter that must be changed regularly (usually every 2–3 days) by the patient to prevent irritation, lipodystrophy, and infection. The infusion line can be disconnected from the syringe when the patient is swimming, showering, or engaged in intimate activities, or if the infusion line becomes occluded.

Special Populations   Children and adolescents with diabetes differ from their adult counterparts in many ways. These differences include insulin sensitivity related to growth and puberty, neurologic vulnerability to hypoglycemia, and the ability to provide self-care.[7] Diabetes care and education for children and adolescents should therefore be provided by practitioners experienced in the unique physiologic, developmental, emotional, and psychosocial aspects and challenges faced by this population and their families.

Women with diabetes who become pregnant require special care to ensure the health and safety of themselves and the developing fetus. Diabetes can increase the risk of complications during pregnancy, including fetal malformations. Nearly two-thirds of pregnancies in women with diabetes are unplanned.[7] For this reason, women with diabetes who are of childbearing age should be screened and evaluated for their plans to conceive. Women with diabetes need to be educated about the importance of family planning and good glycemic control before conception and throughout pregnancy. Insulin is used for glycemic control during pregnancy, and dosing may need to be adjusted to ensure good glycemic control throughout pregnancy.

Older individuals with diabetes have higher rates of coexisting comorbid conditions, disability, and early death than do older individuals without diabetes.[7] Individuals who are physically, functionally, and cognitively intact with a normal life expectancy should have the same goals of therapy and self-care as their younger counterparts. Special considerations for self-care measures and medication therapy, including insulin, however, may be relevant for certain individuals. In older patients whose physical, functional, or cognitive abilities are impaired or diminished, or those who have significantly reduced life expectancies, less aggressive metabolic goals should be considered; abilities for self-care management should be assessed. Depending on their individual situations, such patients may be less likely to benefit from reducing the risk of microvascular and macrovascular complications and more likely to have serious adverse events from hypoglycemic episodes. Glycemic goals, however, must be tempered to avoid potential consequences of uncontrolled hyperglycemia, such as dehydration, poor wound healing, and hyperglycemic hyperosmolar coma.

Acute illness or conditions (e.g., cold, flu, food poisoning) can alter glycemic control in patients with diabetes. In such situations, patients should be instructed to monitor their BG more frequently than usual and be reminded of the symptoms and treatment of hypoglycemic episodes. Medication and insulin doses may need to be adjusted for changes in BG readings, food and liquid intakes, and physical activity experienced secondary to the illness until it has resolved.

Chronic conditions can also affect glycemic control in patients with diabetes. Patients with significantly decreased renal function may have decreased insulin clearance and should be closely monitored for hypoglycemic episodes. Patients undergoing hemodialysis may have fluctuating BG concentrations and should be closely monitored. Patients using or abusing alcohol and those with liver damage also should be instructed to perform SMBG regularly. Certain medications, such as beta-adrenergic blockers, corticosteroids, diuretics, niacin, hormonal contraceptives, protease inhibitors, and atypical antipsychotics, can alter BG concentrations. Beta-blockers can mask symptoms associated with hypoglycemia, such as tachycardia and tremor, so patients should be counseled about how to recognize hypoglycemia. Patients taking hypoglycemic agents or insulin in combination with medications known to raise or lower BG or medications that can alter their physiologic response to hypoglycemia should be instructed to perform SMBG regularly and to carefully monitor for other symptoms of hypoglycemia. Finally, for patients using insulin, their insulin doses can be adjusted based on BG concentrations, if they are taking medications or have comorbid conditions that affect their BG.

Complementary Therapies

People with diabetes are 1.6 times more likely to use some form of complimentary and alternative medicine, including herbal products or dietary supplements, than are people without diabetes.[47] Table 47-15 lists several common herbs and dietary supplements and their potential interactions with diabetes therapy and management. (For an in-depth discussion of American

---

TABLE 47-15 Selected Complementary Therapies That Potentially Affect Blood Glucose Control[a]

Agent	Possible Effect(s) on Blood Glucose
Botanical Medicines (Scientific Name)	
Aloe (*Aloe vera*)	May have hypoglycemic effects
Barley (*Hordeum vulgare; Hordeum distychum*)	May slow gastric emptying
Bitter melon (*Momordica charantia*)	May have hypoglycemic effects
Cinnamon (*Cinnamomum aromaticum*)	Has hypoglycemic effects
Fenugreek (*Trigonella foenum-graecum*)	May have hypoglycemic effects
Garlic (*Allium sativum*)	May have hypoglycemic effects
Ginseng (American/Panax/Siberian) (*Panax quinquefolius/ Panax ginseng/Eleutherococcus senticosus*)	May have hypoglycemic effects
Gotu kola (*Centella asiatica*)	May have hyperglycemic effects
Guar gum (*Cyamopsis tetragonoloba*)	May inhibit gastric glucose absorption to lower blood glucose
Guarana (*Paullinia cupana*)	May have hyperglycemic effects
Gymnema (*Gymnema sylvestre*)	May stimulate insulin production and enhance insulin sensitivity
Milk thistle (*Silibum marianum*)	May reduce insulin resistance secondary to hepatic damage
Nopal, or prickly pear cactus (*Pountia streptacantha*)	May have hypoglycemic effects
Oat bran (*Avena sativa*)	Reduces postprandial blood glucose and insulin concentrations
Stevia (*Stevia rebaudiana*)	May lower postprandial blood glucose
Nonbotanical Dietary Supplements	
Alpha-lipoic acid	May have hypoglycemic effects; may reduce neuropathic pain
Chromium	Deficiency associated with impaired glucose tolerance; if present, may have hypoglycemic effects
L-carnitine	May enhance insulin sensitivity
Vanadium	May enhance insulin sensitivity

[a] *Note:* This table does not include all case reports or possible interactions.

Source: References 48–50.

ginseng, cinnamon, and alpha-lipoic acid, see Chapter 54.) To date, no herbal product or dietary supplement has been proven to be a safe and effective alternative to MNT and pharmacologic therapy of diabetes. Patients choosing to use herbal and dietary supplements should have their BG monitored regularly.

Assessment of Diabetes Mellitus: A Case-Based Approach

If a patient describes classic symptoms of diabetes, the practitioner should ask whether a primary care provider has made this diagnosis. If not, screening for diabetes is appropriate.[1] ADA recommends that a laboratory-based glucose test should be considered in all individuals aged 45 years or older. If normal, patients should be retested every 3 years.[1] Patients with risk factors for diabetes should be considered for testing more frequently and at an earlier age (see Pathophysiology). Screening can start with the diabetes risk calculator developed by ADA (www.diabetes.org/risk-test.jsp). Table 47-16 lists the questions patients are asked to determine their risk of prediabetes or type 2 diabetes. Individuals with a high risk of prediabetes or diabetes can then be tested for capillary BG (fingerstick). Test results should be compared with the diagnostic criteria in Table 47-2. High-risk patients, identified during screening, should be referred to a primary care provider for follow-up.

When working with a patient with newly diagnosed diabetes, the practitioner should determine all medications and supplements the patient takes, any known drug allergies, any concurrent diseases or infections, and relevant social history (e.g., tobacco use, alcohol use, payer status). Practitioners should sensitively assess the patient's beliefs, attitudes, and knowledge toward the disease and the effect of diabetes care on the patient's lifestyle. These assessments allow for development of a culturally sensitive diabetes education and care plan centered on the patient's expectations and needs. Practitioners should be prepared to negotiate treatment and adherence strategies, provide information, and answer the patient's questions about diabetes and related conditions. Case 47-1 illustrates assessment of patients with type 1 diabetes mellitus.

TABLE 47-16 Diabetes Risk Calculator[a]

Questions	Response Options
1. Are you:	Male? Female?
2. How old are you?	Enter the number of years of age
3. Have you ever developed diabetes during pregnancy?	Yes No Does not apply to me
4. Does your mother, father, sister(s), or brother(s) have diabetes?	Yes or No
5. What race or ethnicity best describes you?	White/Caucasian Black/African American Native American Hispanic Asian Other
6. Have you ever been told by a doctor or other health professional that you had hypertension, also called high blood pressure?	Yes No
7. How much do you weigh?	Enter the number of pounds
8. How tall are you?	Enter the number of feet and inches, respectively
9. Compared with most men or women your age, would you say that you are:	More active Less active About the same

[a] On the basis of the responses to the questions listed above, the calculator places the individual into one of three risk categories: low risk, prediabetes, or type 2 diabetes.

Source: Diabetes Risk Calculator. Available at: http://www.diabetes.org/risk-test.jsp.) Copyright © 2008 American Diabetes Association from http://www.diabetes.org. Reprinted with permission from The American Diabetes Association.

CASE 47-1

Relevant Evaluation Criteria	Scenario/Model Outcome
Information Gathering	
1. Gather essential information about the patient's symptoms, including:	
a. description of symptom(s) (i.e., nature, onset, duration, severity, associated symptoms)	Patient wants to purchase Monistat. Her PCP instructed her to pick up an OTC product. Two days ago she started to have mild symptoms of itching and burning. She denies presence of fever or back pain.
b. description of any factors that seem to precipitate, exacerbate, and/or relieve the patient's symptom(s)	Her last A1C was 8% and her predinner BG concentrations have been high (averaging about 200 mg/dL). She reports occassionally skipping her lunchtime insulin dose because of being in class or on the go. Other readings are generally close to target.
c. description of the patent's efforts to relieve the symptoms	She started noticing vaginal yeast infection symptoms 2 days ago and contacted her PCP at Student Health yesterday. Per his instructions, she is stopping by the pharmacy to pick up an OTC product.

CASE 47-1 (continued)

Relevant Evaluation Criteria	Scenario/Model Outcome
2. Gather essential patient history information:	Last vaginal yeast infection was more than 2 years ago.
a. patient's identity	Brittany Smith
b. age, sex, height, and weight	18-year-old female, 5 ft 4 in, 120 lb, BMI 20.6
c. patient's occupation	College student, plays on softball team. She has a game or practice during the season every day except Sunday.
d. patient's dietary habits	Eats a 2400-calorie diet consisting of three meals and three snacks per day
e. patient's sleep habits	Sleeps well; no nightmares, night sweats, or other symptoms of Somogyi effect
f. concurrent conditions, prescriptions, and nonprescription medications and dietary supplements	For her prandial insulin needs, she takes insulin aspart (via vial and syringe) 6 units at breakfast and lunch, and 8 units at dinner. For her basal insulin, she takes 30 units of insulin glargine via vial and syringe daily at bedtime.
g. allergies	No known allergies
h. history of other adverse reactions to medications	No previous reactions
i. other (describe) _____	

Assessment and Triage

3. Differentiate patient's signs and symptoms and correctly identify the patient's primary problem(s).	PCP diagnosed patient with *Candida* vulvovaginitis and recommend Monistat for her. High BG concentrations at the dinner reading. She is concerned about her ability to administer insulin injections with busy, unpredictable schedule.
4. Identify exclusions for self-treatment.	None
5. Formulate a comprehensive list of therapeutic alternatives to address the primary problem to determine if triage to a medical practitioner is required and share this information with the patient.	Options include: (1) Recommend nonpharmacologic and/or nonprescription therapy for the *Candida* vaginal infection. (2) Given the patient's busy lifestyle, suggest changing to pen device for bolus insulin doses to improve convenience and adherence of dosing and administration, and offer strategies to improve adherence. (3) Take no action.

Plan

6. Select an optimal therapeutic alternative to address the patient's problem, taking into account patient preferences.	Advise the patient to eat low-fat, sugar-free yogurt daily and use the same Monistat product that worked previously. Remind the patient of the carbohydrate content of yogurt and the need to adjust her daily carbohydrate intake appropriately. Advise her to discontinue midmorning snack and subsequently monitor her BG between 10 am and 12 pm every day for 7 days.
7. Describe the recommended therapeutic approach to the patient.	You should eat 8 ounces of low-fat, sugar-free yogurt daily and use the same Monistat product you used before (see Chapter 8). I recommend substituting the yogurt for another carbohydrate source during a regularly scheduled meal or snack. I suggest discussing switching to a pen device for your short-acting insulin doses (such as the Novolog FlexPen) with your PCP in order to help you maintain your insulin dosing schedule. If your blood glucose concentration stays elevated or drops too low, see your PCP. Make sure you carry glucose tablets with you in case hypoglycemia occurs.
8. Explain to the patient the rationale for selecting the recommended therapeutic approach from the considered therapeutic alternatives.	You should use the same Monistat product because it worked before and you are familiar with its use. Monitor your BG concentrations closely while taking Monistat and substituting a yogurt for your midmorning snack to make sure hyper- or hypoglycemia does not occur. Skipping your lunchtime insulin dose is probably the cause of your predinner hyperglycemia. The insulin pen can be carried in your lunch or backpack to help remind you to take your lunchtime dose. You could also consider setting the alarm on your watch, PDA, or cell phone to help remind you of your next insulin dose when you are busy with classes, exams, and practice.

CASE 47-1 (continued)

Relevant Evaluation Criteria	Scenario/Model Outcome
Patient Education	
9. When recommending self-care with non-prescription medications and/or nondrug therapy, convey accurate information to the patient:	
a. appropriate dose and frequency of administration	One 8-ounce serving of low-fat, sugar-free yogurt daily in place of another carbohydrate serving.
	See Chapter 8 for information on Monistat.
	Monitor BG between 10 am and 12 noon daily for 7 days.
b. maximum number of days the therapy should be employed	See Chapter 8.
c. product administration procedures	See Chapter 8.
d. expected time to onset of relief	The itching and burning symptoms should improve within 2 days of starting treatment with Monistat.
	The BG values should normalize by the following day.
e. degree of relief that can be reasonably expected	All symptoms of the yeast infection should resolve.
	BG values should fall in the target goal range.
f. most common side effects	See Chapter 8 for side effects of Monistat.
	Because the insulin dosing is not being changed and a snack is being dropped, it is important to monitor for signs and symptoms of low blood sugar or hypoglycemia. If signs or symptoms occur, remember to check your BG and use glucose tablets as directed. Be sure to follow-up with a snack.
g. side effects that warrant medical intervention should they occur	See Chapter 8.
	If hyperglycemia does not resolve or if hypoglycemia occurs, contact your PCP.
h. patient options in the event that condition worsens or persists	See Chapter 8.
i. product storage requirements	See Chapter 8.
j. specific nondrug measures	See Chapter 8.
10. Solicit follow-up questions from patient.	I usually drink some juice or a soda when I feel low, but the tablets seem more convenient. I would like to buy some. How should I use them?
11. Answer patient's questions.	The usual dose is to dissolve 3 tablets (15 grams) in the mouth. Wait 15 minutes and then check your BG. If your BG is still low or if hypoglycemic symptoms are still present, take an additional 3 tablets. If these measures do not correct the hypoglycemia, seek medical attention. If the hypoglycemia is corrected, eat a small meal or snack (e.g., fruit and cheese, peanut butter and crackers) to prevent a recurrence of hypoglycemia.

Key: A1C, glycosylated hemoglobin; BG, blood glucose; BMI, body mass index; OTC, over-the-counter; PCP, primary care provider; PDA, personal digital assistant.

For overweight patients with type 2 diabetes, practitioners should also discuss weight loss (see Chapter 27). Education should focus on the link between overweight or obesity and type 2 diabetes and the importance of weight loss in helping control the disease. The overall health benefits of weight reduction should also be discussed. Learning that weight loss and consistent physical activity may obviate the need for medications may motivate an individual to lose weight. Case 47-2 illustrates assessment of patients with type 2 diabetes mellitus.

Patient Counseling for Diabetes Mellitus

Adhering to healthy eating, regular physical activity, and medication regimens are often challenges for individuals with diabetes. Practitioners can assist patients to overcome barriers to adhering to their diabetes therapies and can provide encouragement and counseling on meal planning and physical activity. Each patient encounter is an opportunity for the practitioner to evaluate and

CASE 47-2

Relevant Evaluation Criteria	Scenario/Model Outcome
Information Gathering	
1. Gather essential information about the patient's symptoms, including:	
a. description of symptom(s) (i.e., nature, onset, duration, severity, associated symptoms)	Patient comes to pharmacy with a new prescription for Actos (pioglitazone) and to pick up test strips for his BG monitor. BG values at PCP's office were greater than 200 mg/dL. Today's A1C was 8.5%. The PCP told him that he has to "start taking better care of himself," monitor his BG more regularly, and take his medications as prescribed. The patient also has an appointment with a registered dietitian who is a certified diabetes educator for meal planning and weight loss. He asks if the new pill will help control his diabetes so he does not have to bother with changing his diet or regularly checking his BG because money is tight for groceries and strips.
b. description of any factors that seem to precipitate, exacerbate, and/or relieve the patient's symptom(s)	N/A
c. description of the patent's efforts to relieve the symptoms	Patient checks his fasting BG in the mornings every few days. He has been fairly adherent with his prescription medications. His wife also makes him "special drinks" containing nopales and aloe vera.
2. Gather essential patient history information:	
a. patient's identity	Victor Sanchez
b. age, sex, height, and weight	48-year-old male, 5 ft 5 in, 170 lb, BMI 28.3
c. patient's occupation	Farm laborer who works seasonally. Married with 4 children, 2 of whom still live at home.
d. patient's dietary habits	Primarily tortillas, potatoes, and beans when he is out of work. Other times he has more access to chicken and fresh fruits and vegetables. Currently, he is unfamiliar with ADA dietary guidelines.
e. patient's sleep habits	Sleeps "like a baby"
f. concurrent conditions, prescriptions, and nonprescription medications and dietary supplements	Glipizide XL 10 mg before breakfast and metformin 1000 mg mornings and evenings for type 2 diabetes; enalapril 20 mg daily for hypertension for past 2 years and diabetic nephropathy for 1 year, atorvastatin 20 mg daily for dyslipidemia for past 2 years. His wife also makes him special drinks containing nopales and aloe vera.
g. allergies	Penicillin (rash)
h. history of other adverse reactions to medications	None
i. other (describe) _____	Type 2 diabetes diagnosed in Mexico 11 years ago. Resting BP taken at pharmacy is 126/80 mm Hg. Victor says his cholesterol has been elevated.
	Victor is concerned about his health, because he is the primary income earner for his family. He does not have insurance coverage for diabetes supplies and medications. He currently obtains all of his prescription medications through various patient assistance programs available through your pharmacy. He "tries to remember to" take his medications as prescribed, and his wife helps him by reminding him at breakfast and dinner. His daughter translates the instructions on his prescription bottles from English into Spanish for him and his wife, which they are both able to read. He currently does not formally do physical activity daily. He ran out of BG test strips 2 days ago but was unable to make it to the pharmacy to pick up more.
Assessment and Triage	
3. Differentiate the patients signs and symptoms and correctly identify the patient's primary problem(s).	Victor's immediate self-care need is to obtain BG test strips for his monitor.
	Victor also can benefit from education and support on the basics of diabetes, hypertension, and hyperlipidemia and self-care, including SMBG, diet, physical activity, and medication adherence. According to his known medical diagnoses and comments, it would appear he has metabolic syndrome.
4. Identify any exclusions for self-care.	None

Relevant Evaluation Criteria	**Scenario/Model Outcome**
5. Formulate a comprehensive list of therapeutic alternatives to address the primary problem to determine if triage to a medical practitioner is required and share this information with the patient.	Options include: (1) Remind Victor of the need for regular SMBG. Assess his beliefs and expectations about and commitment to monitoring. Negotiate a monitoring schedule that addresses his economic concerns and limitations, such as SMBG schedule only 3 days a week to help him save money on test strips. (2) Work with Victor to identify resources for groceries and meals available within his community (e.g., charitable organizations) to access during periods when he is out of work. Suggest he bring his wife, who prepares all the meals, with him to his upcoming appointment with the dietician. (3) Discuss the safety and efficacy of nopales and aloe vera with Victor to ensure he is educated about their safety and effectiveness in diabetes. (4) Counsel Victor on his new prescription for Actos, and explain how this agent fits in with his glipizide and metformin. Explain the slow onset of action for pioglitazone (e.g., noticeable effects on his BG). Review the dose and directions for pioglitazone; discuss and negotiate adherence strategies (e.g., take at breakfast with his other morning medication doses). Educate him about the signs and symptoms of hypoglycemia and the side effects of pioglitazone. Explain the importance of follow-up with his physician and laboratory testing to monitor for efficacy and potential side effects related to his medications. (5) Explore Victor's attitudes and expectations for drug therapy, and then discuss and negotiate strategies to help him adhere to therapy, such as Spanish labeling on prescription bottles and the use of a mediset to track daily medication doses. (6) Ask Victor whether his PCP has recommended aspirin therapy for him. Screen him for aspirin allergy or contraindications. Discuss the risks and benefits of aspirin therapy as primary cardioprotection, and recommend that he follow up with his PCP. (7) Ask Victor whether his immunizations (e.g., influenza, pneumococcal, tetanus) are up-to-date and make recommendations for immunizations as appropriate. (8) Ask Victor whether he uses tobacco or alcohol-related products and counsel him as appropriate. (9) Take no action.
Plan	
6. Select an optimal therapeutic alternative to address the patient's problem, taking into account patient preferences.	Provide him with strips and a list of community resources for groceries and meals. Counsel Victor on his new and existing prescription medications and any non-prescription medications he may use. Discuss dosing, adherence strategies, and monitoring for hypoglycemia and medication side effects. (After reviewing dietary supplements, practitioner concluded the patient may continue to drink nopales shakes but should eliminate aloe vera from them.) Discuss the need for aspirin therapy with the patient.
7. Describe the recommended therapeutic approach to the patient.	I recommend monitoring your BG, that is, blood glucose, three times a week. Your monitoring schedule could be as follows: Mondays, test your FBG, that is, fasting blood glucose, and test 2 hours after breakfast; Wednesdays, FBG and before and after lunch; and Fridays, FBG and before and after dinner. This schedule will help you save some money on test strips while providing your PCP, that is, primary care provider, with the information he or she needs to evaluate your diabetes and medications. You should also check your BG anytime you think you may have low BG. Each time you check your BG, record the date, time, and value from your monitor into a logbook to share with your PCP at your regular visits. Take your new medication, Actos, also called pioglitazone, once daily in the morning with your other morning medications. Report any unusual symptoms, such as swelling of your feet or legs, difficulty breathing, or unusual tiredness to your doctor or pharmacist if they occur. Take your wife with you to your appointment with the registered dietitian to discuss healthy meal planning tailored to your food preferences and budget. Follow-up with resources in your community for groceries and meals as needed during the year to help you maintain a healthy, well-balanced diet. (Patient says his wife is interested in knowing what foods he should and should not eat.)

Relevant Evaluation Criteria	Scenario/Model Outcome
8. Explain to the patient the rationale for selecting the recommended therapeutic approach from the considered therapeutic alternatives.	The BG monitor will show you the effects of different foods, physical activity, and medications on your BG. Your providers and you can use this information to plan your meals and activities and to adjust your medications as needed.
Patient Education	
9. When recommending self-care with non-prescription and prescription medications or nondrug therapy, convey accurate information to the patient.	Discuss the benefits and risk of aspirin therapy with the patient, counsel him on appropriate generic options available and on dosing, and recommend that he follow up and discuss his need for aspirin therapy with his PCP at his next visit.
10. Solicit follow-up questions from patient.	Can you help me interpret my BG readings?
11. Answer patient's questions.	Yes. If you carry the monitor with you, monitor your BG concentrations as we discussed, and record your meals and physical activity. We can set an appointment to review and interpret the readings.

Key: ADA, American Diabetes Association; A1C, glycosylated hemoglobin; BG, blood glucose; BMI, body mass index; BP, blood pressure; N/A, not applicable; PCP, primary care provider; SMBG, self-monitoring of blood glucose.

educate patients. A good way to start a conversation and help identify patient knowledge and commitment to self-care is asking simple questions such as the following: "What are your glucose concentrations running these days?" "What was your last A1C value?" If insulin was prescribed, the practitioner should explain the various diabetes care products and teach the patient how to use the selected products. Patients should be encouraged

to return for reevaluation of injection technique, self-monitoring of their BG, and adherence to a prescribed self-care routine. Moreover, practitioners should be familiar with new medications and devices, and should keep abreast of current practice guidelines for the care of people with diabetes. The box Patient Education for Diabetes Mellitus lists specific information to provide patients.

P A T I E N T   E D U C A T I O N   F O R
Diabetes Mellitus

The primary objective of diabetes self-care is to achieve and maintain metabolic control. Secondary benefits of meeting metabolic goals are to (1) prevent or reverse diabetes complications, (2) maintain normal daily activities with maximum lifestyle flexibility, (3) avoid weight gain by following a proper nutrition and physical activity plan, (4) avoid infection, and (5) achieve a sense of well-being. For most patients, carefully following product instructions (including instructions on the proper use of insulin) and the self-care measures listed here will help ensure optimal therapeutic outcomes.

Nondrug Measures

- Recognize that having diabetes requires lifestyle and behavioral changes.
- Consult with your primary care provider, dietitian, nurse, or pharmacist to develop a nutrition plan and physical activity program that suits your lifestyle.
- Learn how to read food labels.
- Involve your entire family in your healthy lifestyle changes.
- Knowledge is power. Know your glucose and other diabetes-related goals (see Table 47-3). Learn about your disease and the ways you can take control of your diabetes.
- Check your BG (blood glucose) regularly and know what makes your glucose concentrations go up and down (e.g., foods, activity, medications, stress).

- Use a logbook to document BG results, diet, physical activity, insulin, or other medication administration changes and bring it with you to every health care visit.
- To avoid being overwhelmed, set realistic, achievable goals. Make one or two specific changes at a time and recognize your accomplishments.
- If you have a diabetes complication, consult a diabetes specialist. Practice the preventive measures listed in Table 47-4.
- When performing physical activities conscientiously, follow the guidelines in Table 47-5.
- Monitor your BG several times each day (e.g., before meals, 2 hours after meals, at bedtime). If a BG reading is greater than 240 mg/dL, check urine ketones. If your values indicate a problem, see your primary care provider for adjustments to your therapy.
- If you use tobacco products, it is strongly advised to quit. A tobacco cessation program, which includes counseling and smoking cessation medications, is highly recommended (see Chapter 50).
- See your primary care provider if you have cuts or bruises that are not healing.

PATIENT EDUCATION FOR
Diabetes Mellitus *(continued)*

Nonprescription and Prescription Medications

- Follow your prescribed medication regimen, including insulin, carefully.
- Inject your insulin at the proper sites, and rotate your injection sites (see Figure 47-5).
- Follow the guidelines in Tables 47-11 and 47-12 for preparing and injecting insulin doses.
- Know the signs and symptoms related to low or high BG concentrations and appropriate monitoring and management strategies.
- Discuss taking a low dose of aspirin daily to prevent heart attack and stroke with your primary care provider.
- Take your medications as directed by your provider. Do not stop taking any of your medications unless you first discuss it with your provider.
- Do not start taking any nonprescription medications or complimentary therapies without first discussing them with your pharmacist or primary care provider. Consult your pharmacist for safe over-the-counter medication options to treat self-limiting conditions such as allergies, cough, or upset stomach.

- Read the labels of nonprescription medications to identify sugar and alcohol content. Avoid medications that contain sugar or alcohol.
- Certain cold medications, such as pseudoephedrine, may raise BG concentrations and blood pressure levels. Talk to your provider or pharmacist before selecting any allergy, cough, or cold preparations.
- Talk to your pharmacist about strategies to help you remember to take your medications.

⚠ If you use insulin and experience symptoms of hypoglycemia (e.g., sweating, hunger, rapid heart beat, confusion), hyperglycemia (e.g., frequent urination, dehydration, thirst, increased appetite), or ketoacidosis (e.g., BG greater than 240 mg/dL + urine ketones and flulike symptoms, confusion, stupor), contact your primary care provider.

Evaluation of Patient Outcomes for Diabetes Mellitus

ADA recommends specific therapeutic goals for people with diabetes (Table 47-3). If the patient is not achieving these outcomes, adherence to the care plan should be assessed. Nonadherent patients should be reevaluated and, if necessary, reeducated about the need for and benefits of the care plan. If nonadherence is not the problem, medical referral is appropriate. In addition, weight management should be closely monitored in patients with type 2 diabetes.

Key Points for Diabetes Mellitus

➤ Early detection, extensive patient education, and early, aggressive glycemic control through MNT, physical activity, and pharmacologic therapy can prevent the development

and progression of long-term complications, morbidity, and mortality associated with diabetes.

➤ Familiarity with the most current standards for diabetes screening and management is imperative to reducing and eliminating health disparities associated with diabetes risk, outcomes, morbidity, and mortality and to improving care for all patients with diabetes (Table 47-17).

➤ Patients should be educated about diabetes, the role of BG control in the prevention of long-term complications, self-care strategies (including SMBG and MNT), and pharmacologic therapy.

➤ Practitioners should be familiar with and assist patients selecting BG monitors and related supplies.

➤ Patients using insulin therapy should be educated about insulin and related supplies, proper injection site and technique, insulin storage, potential adverse events, and their management.

TABLE 47-17 Professional Online Resources for Diabetes Care and Management

Organization	Web Address	Comments
American Diabetes Association (ADA)	www.diabetes.org	Information for both practitioners and patients about diabetes and its management; free access to a variety of information and tools, including ADA guidelines to diabetes care and management (published annually in a supplement to *Diabetes Care*), recent research news and patient education materials (e.g., *Diabetes Forecast*); restricted access to a variety of resources, including scientific journals for members
American Association of Clinical Endocrinologists (AACE)	www.aace.com	Free access to guidelines and practice standards; continuing medication education and other resources available for members
American Association of Diabetes Educators (AADE)	www.diabeteseducator.org	Information for both practitioners and patients

(Continued)

TABLE 47-17   Professional Online Resources for Diabetes Care and Management *(continued)*

Organization	Web Address	Comments
National Institute of Diabetes and Digestive and Kidney Disorders (NIDDK), National Institutes of Health (NIH)	www.niddk.nih.gov	Statistics, health information, and research opportunities for practitioners
Centers for Disease Control and Prevention (CDC) Diabetes Public Resource	www.cdc.gov/diabetes	Statistics, recommendations for the Task Force on Community Preventative Services for diabetes, and other resources for practitioners and patients
National Diabetes Education Program (NDEP)	www.ndep.nih.gov	Collaboration of the NIH and CDC providing information for practitioners and patients; patient education materials available that are designed for specific ethnic populations and in a variety of languages
Insulin Pumpers	www.insulin-pumpers.org	Support and information for children and adults with diabetes and insulin pump delivery devices

➤ Practitioners and patients should negotiate adherence strategies tailored to patient-specific factors such as, but not limited to, food and activity preferences, sleep, mealtime, and work schedules, insurance status, and income.

➤ Patients with diabetes should be educated about the safety and efficacy of nonprescription medications for self-care of limited acute conditions and complimentary and alternative medicines.

REFERENCES

1. American Diabetes Association. Diagnosis and classification of diabetes mellitus. *Diabetes Care*. 2008;31(suppl 1):S55–S60.

2. Centers for Disease Control and Prevention. National diabetes facts sheet: general information and national estimates on diabetes in the United States, 2007. Atlanta, Ga: US Department of Health and Human Services, Centers for Disease Control and Prevention; 2008.

3. American Diabetes Association. Economic costs of diabetes in the U.S. in 2007. *Diabetes Care*. 2008;31:1–20.

4. American Diabetes Association. Report of the expert committee on the diagnosis and classification of diabetes mellitus. *Diabetes Care*. 2003; 26(suppl 1):S5–S20.

5. UK Prospective Diabetes Study (UKPDS) Group. Intensive glycemic control with sulphonlyureas or insulin compared with conventional treatment and risk of complications in patients with type 2 diabetes (UKPDS 33). *Lancet*. 1998;352:837–53.

6. Nathan DM. Initial management of glycemia in type 2 diabetes mellitus. *N Engl J Med*. 2002;347:1342–9.

7. American Diabetes Association. Standards of medical care in diabetes-2008 [position statement]. *Diabetes Care*. 2008;31(suppl 1):S12–S54.

8. The Diabetes Control and Complications Trial Research Group. The effect of intensive treatment of diabetes on the development and progression of long-term complications in insulin-dependent diabetes mellitus. *N Engl J Med*. 1993;329:977–86.

9. The Writing Team for the Diabetes Control and Complications Trial/Epidemiology of Diabetes Interventions and Complications Research Group. Sustained effect of intensive treatment of type 1 diabetes mellitus on development and progression of diabetic nephropathy. *JAMA*. 2003;290:2159–67.

10. Stratton IM, Adler AI, Neil HAW, et al. Association of glycaemia with macrovascular and microvascular complications of type 2 diabetes (UKPDS 35): prospective observational study. *BMJ*. 2000;321:405–11.

11. Adler AI, Stratton IM, Neil HAW, et al. Association of systolic blood pressure with macrovascular and microvascular complications in type 2 diabetes (UKPDS 36): a prospective observational study. *BMJ*. 2000; 321:412–9.

12. Chobanian AV, Bakris GL, Black HR, et al. The seventh report of the Joint National Committee on Prevention, Detection, Evaluation and Treatment Of High Blood Pressure: the JNC 7 Report. *JAMA*. 2003; 289:2560–72.

13. American Diabetes Association. Hypertension management in adults with diabetes. *Diabetes Care*. 2004;27(suppl 1):S65–7.

14. American Diabetes Association. Dyslipidemia management in adults with diabetes. *Diabetes Care*. 2004;27(suppl 1):S68–71.

15. Grundy SM, Cleeman JI, Merz CN, et al. The implications of recent clinical trials for the National Cholesterol Education Program Adult Treatment Panel III guidelines. *Circulation*. 2004;110:227–39.

16. American Diabetes Association. Aspirin therapy in diabetes. *Diabetes Care*. 2004;27(suppl 1):S72–3.

17. American Diabetes Association. Influenza and pneumococcal immunization in diabetes. *Diabetes Care*. 2004;27(suppl 1):S111–3.

18. Ship JA. Diabetes and oral health. *J Am Dent Assoc*. 2003;134(suppl): 4S–10S.

19. American Diabetes Association. Nutrition Recommendations and Interventions for Diabetes [position statement]. *Diabetes Care*. 2008;31(suppl 1); S61–S78.

20. Funnell MM, Anderson RM, Austin A, et al. AADE Position Statement: Individualization of diabetes self-management education. *Diabetes Educ*. 2007;33:45–9.

21. Hinnen DA, Childs BP, Guthrie DW, et al. Combating clinical inertia with pattern management. In: Mensing C, ed. *The Art and Science of Diabetes Self-Management Education*. 1st ed. Chicago: American Association of Diabetes Educators; 2006.

22. American Dietetic Association. Position of the American Dietetic Association: use of nutritive and nonnutritive sweeteners. *J Am Diet Assoc*. 2004;104:255–75.

23. Valmadrid CT, Klein R, Moss SE, et al. Alcohol intake and the risk of coronary heart disease mortality in persons with older-onset diabetes mellitus. *JAMA*. 1999;282:239–46.

24. Solomon CG, Hu FB, Stampfer MJ, et al. Moderate alcohol consumption and risk of coronary heart disease among women with type 2 diabetes mellitus. *Circulation*. 2000;102:494–9.

25. Ajani UA, Gaziano M, Lotufo PA, et al. Alcohol consumption and risk of coronary heart disease by diabetes status. *Circulation*. 2000;102:500–5.

26. Lane JD, Barkauskas CE, Surwit RS, et al. Caffeine impairs glucose metabolism in type 2 diabetes. *Diabetes Care*. 2004;27;2047–8.

27. Mullooly CA. Physical activity. In: Mensing C, ed. *The Art and Science of Diabetes Self-Management Education*. 1st ed. Chicago: American Association of Diabetes Educators; 2006.

28. The Diabetes Prevention Program Research Group. Reduction in the incidence of type 2 diabetes with lifestyle intervention or metformin. *N Engl J Med*. 2002;346:393–403.

29. American Diabetes Association. Physical activity/exercise and diabetes [position statement]. *Diabetes Care*. 2004;27(suppl 1):S58–S62.

30. American Diabetes Association. Tests of glycemia in diabetes [position statement]. *Diabetes Care*. 2004;27(suppl 1):S91–3.

31. American Diabetes Association. Insulin administration [position statement]. *Diabetes Care*. 2004;27(suppl 1):S106–9

32. Austin MM, Haas L, Johnson T, et al. American Association of Diabetes Educators Position Statement. Self-monitoring of blood glucose: benefits and utilization. *Diabetes Educ*. 2006;32:836–47.

33. McGarraugh G, Price D, Schwartz S, et al. Physiological influences on off-finger glucose testing. *Diabetes Technol Ther*. 2001;3:367–76.

34. Kuklarni K. Monitoring. In: Mensing C, ed. *The Art and Science of Diabetes Self-Management Education*. 1st ed. Chicago: American Association of Diabetes Educators; 2006.

35. DeWitt DE, Hirsch IB. Outpatient insulin therapy in type 1 and type 2 diabetes mellitus. *JAMA*. 2003;289:2254–64.

36. Goldman-Levine JD, Lee KW. Insulin detemir—a new basal insulin analog. *Ann Pharmacother*. 2005;39:502–7.

37. Insulin monograph and product tables. Facts and Comparisons 4.0 [online database]. St Louis: Wolters Kluwer Health; 2008. Last accessed February 27, 2008.

38. Apidra [prescribing information]. sanofi-aventis Pharmaceutics. Available at: http://products.sanofi-aventis.us/apidra/apidra.html. Last accessed October 22, 2008.

39. American Diabetes Association. Resource guide 2008. Insulins. *Diabetes Forecast*. 2008;58:RG11–4.

40. Kroon LA, Assemi M, Carlisle BA. Diabetes mellitus. In: Koda-Kimble MA, Young LY, Kradjan WA, et al., eds. *Applied Therapeutics*. 9th ed. Baltimore: Lippincott Williams & Wilkins; 2009.

41. Cryer PE, Davis SN, Shamoon H. Hypoglycemia in diabetes. *Diabetes Care*. 2003;26:1902–12.

42. Gonder-Frederick LA, Zrebiec J. Hypoglycemia. In: Franz MJ, ed. *A CORE Curriculum for Diabetes Education, Diabetes Management Therapies*. 5th ed. Chicago: American Association of Diabetes Educators; 2003.

43. Pearson T. Glucagon as a treatment of severe hypoglycemia: safe and efficacious but underutilized. *Diabetes Educ*. 2008;34:128–34.

44. Grajower MM, Fraser CG, Holcombe JH, et al. How long should insulin be used once a vial is started? *Diabetes Care*. 2003;26:2665–9.

45. Holcombe JH, Daugherty ML, De Felippis MR. How long should insulin be used once a vial is started? Response to Molitch. *Diabetes Care*. 2004;27:1241–2.

46. American Diabetes Association. Resource guide 2008. Insulin delivery. *Diabetes Forecast*. 2008;58:RG17–29.

47. Egede LE, Ye X, Zheng D, et al. The prevalence and pattern of complimentary and alternative medicine use in individuals with diabetes. *Diabetes Care*. 2002;25:324–9.

48. Yeh GY, Eisenberg DM, Kaptchuk TJ, et al. Systematic review of herbs and dietary supplements for glycemic control in diabetes. *Diabetes Care*. 2003;26:1277–94.

49. Rotblatt M, Ziment I, eds. *Evidence-Based Herbal Medicine*. Philadelphia: Hanley and Belfus; 2002.

50. McCarty MF. Nutraceutical resources for diabetes prevention—an update. *Med Hypothesis*. 2005;64:151–8.

Insomnia

Cynthia K. Kirkwood and Sarah T. Melton

Insomnia is one of the most common patient complaints, ranking third behind headache and the common cold. Insomnia is a symptom with diverse etiologies and patient complaints, and it can progress to a disorder.[1,2] Insomnia occurs when a person has trouble falling or staying asleep, wakes up too early and cannot return to sleep, or does not feel refreshed after sleeping. Patients with other sleep disorders, such as sleep apnea, narcolepsy, and restless legs syndrome, also seek nonprescription sleep aids. Because of potentially significant clinical effects, patients with these disorders should, preferably, see a sleep specialist.

Although the average adult requires 8 or more hours of sleep nightly, the typical American gets 6.9 hours.[3] According to the 2005 National Sleep Foundation survey, about three-fourths of all adult Americans reported one or more symptoms of insomnia during the past year.[3] About 33% of the U.S. population experienced insomnia nightly. About 11% of adult Americans report using alcohol; 9%, a nonprescription sleep aid; and 7%, a prescription hypnotic medication to manage their insomnia.[3] Patients reporting medical conditions were the most likely to report sleep problems and to take sleep products. The following medical conditions were associated with complaints of sleep problems: hypertension (29%), arthritis (28%), heartburn or gastroesophageal reflux disease (19%), depression (18%), diabetes (11%), and heart disease (10%).[3]

Insomnia has a significant economic impact, accounting for $14 billion annually in direct medical costs.[2] The estimated direct drug cost of insomnia for prescription medications was $809.92 million, and the cost for nonprescription medications was $325.8 million. Estimated costs for the use of alcohol or melatonin to enhance sleep were $780.39 million and $50 million, respectively.[4] Insomnia is associated with increased health care use, impaired quality of life, and an increased rate of traffic accidents, depression, alcohol abuse, and mortality.[2]

The prevalence of sleep complaints and hypnotic use is high among persons of advanced age, and more than half of this population reports at least one sleep complaint.[5] In adults older than 65, 3% to 21% of men and 7% to 29% of women use hypnotics compared with only 2% to 4% of the younger population.[5] As many as 24% of those who reported sleep difficulties used nonprescription sleep aids; 5% of those who used nonprescription medications reported use every night or a few nights a week.[6] This group also has an increased incidence of sleep apnea and restless legs syndrome. Significant morbidity is associated with obstructive sleep apnea, which has been linked to 38,000 cardiovascular deaths annually.[7] For these reasons, complaints of insomnia in patients of advanced age should be carefully evaluated.

Despite these data, only a small percentage of patients with a sleep disorder actually verbalize their complaints to a health care provider.[1,2] The combination of frequent misuse of hypnotics and availability of nonprescription agents makes insomnia a disorder of significant concern.

Pathophysiology of Insomnia

Physiologically, sleep can be categorized into different stages by using the sleeping electroencephalogram (EEG) in conjunction with electro-oculography and electromyography. Stage 1 sleep is a transitional stage, occurring as the patient falls asleep; the EEG resembles the waking state more than sleep. Stage 2 sleep, which comprises about 50% of sleep time, is light sleep. Stages 3 and 4, collectively known as deep sleep or delta sleep, are characterized by the patterns of delta waves, or slow-frequency waves, on the EEG. Rapid eye movement (REM) sleep is neither light nor deep, and the EEG manifests an increase in high-frequency waves. REM sleep is characterized by physiologic activity compared with other sleep stages; skeletal muscle movement is inhibited. The eyes move rapidly from side to side, while blood pressure, heart rate, temperature, respiration, and metabolism are increased.[8,9]

Upon falling asleep, an individual progresses through the four stages of sleep, reaching the first REM period in about 70 to 90 minutes. The time from falling asleep to the first REM period is referred to as REM latency. The first REM period is of short duration—usually 5 to 7 minutes. The sleep cycle then repeats about every 70 to 120 minutes, with each progressive REM period becoming longer and the time spent in deep sleep becoming shorter. The relative importance of medication effects in the different stages of sleep is unclear. However, prolonged suppression of REM sleep can result in psychological and behavioral changes.[8,9]

Sleep physiology changes with increasing age. Among the elderly, the total duration of sleep is shorter, the number of nocturnal awakenings increases, and less time is spent in stage 4 and REM sleep. Sleep latency usually remains normal with increasing age. Despite these changes, it cannot be assumed that this population requires less sleep.[10]

Insomnia can be classified as transient, short term, or chronic according to the duration of sleep disturbance. Transient insomnia is often self-limiting, lasting less than 1 week. Short-term insomnia usually lasts from 1 to 3 weeks.[8,9] Chronic, or long-term, insomnia lasts from more than 3 weeks to years and is often the result of medical problems, psychiatric disorders, or substance abuse.[1,2]

Insomnia can also be classified on the basis of an identifiable cause. Primary insomnia is the term used to describe patients who have sleep difficulty that lasts at least 1 month, affects psychosocial functioning, and is not caused by another sleep disorder, general medical disorder, psychiatric disorder, or medication.[11] All underlying causes of insomnia must be identified and managed to relieve the sleep disturbance.[8,9]

Difficulty falling asleep is often associated with acute life stresses or medical illness, anxiety, and poor sleep habits. The severity of stressful situations can affect the length of insomnia. Travel, hospitalization, or anticipation of an important or stressful event can cause transient insomnia. However, if more severe stressors are present (e.g., the death of a loved one, recovery from surgery, the loss of a job, or divorce), transient insomnia can become short-term insomnia. Unless managed appropriately, short-term insomnia can progress to chronic insomnia.

Shift workers often complain of sleep disturbances and/or excessive sleepiness. Sleep problems occur more frequently in individuals who must rotate shifts. Some nighttime workers adjust to their change in sleep schedule, whereas others never do. Among night-shift workers with complaints of excessive sleepiness, the worst period of the day is between 3 and 5 am.[7]

Sleep apnea is a common, undiagnosed cause of chronic insomnia. Patients with this disorder complain of daytime fatigue and sedation. Sleep apnea affects the quality of sleep of both the patient and family members because of the patient's gasping and snoring during sleep. Sleep apnea appears to be more common in men; the stereotypical patient is middle-aged, overweight, and hypertensive. Sleep apnea can be caused by an obstruction in the airway or central nervous system (CNS) mechanisms.[7]

Some individuals are extremely sensitive to the stimulant effects of caffeine and nicotine (see Chapter 50). Drinking caffeinated beverages in the late afternoon or evening hours can cause insomnia. Alcohol, if taken in excess, especially in the evening or on a chronic basis, can disturb sleep. Late-night exercise and late-evening meals as well as environmental distractions (e.g., noise, lighting, uncomfortable temperatures, or new surroundings) can also interfere with sleep.[12]

Several general medical disorders, in addition to psychiatric disorders, are associated with chronic insomnia (Table 48-1). Chronic insomnia can also be secondary to use of medications or other substances, sleep-wake schedule disorders, or primary sleep disorders.[13] Early morning awakening is often associated with depression. Nonprescription hypnotics are generally not helpful in patients with chronic insomnia; medical referral is indicated.

Finally, medications—prescription and nonprescription—can produce either insomnia or withdrawal insomnia (Table 48-2). Antidepressants, antihypertensives, and sympathomimetic amines are the medication classes commonly associated with insomnia as an adverse effect. Alcohol can cause insomnia after acute use and as a withdrawal effect after chronic use.

Clinical Presentation of Insomnia

Patients with insomnia can have any number of complaints, such as difficulty falling asleep, frequent awakening, early morning awakening and inability to fall back to sleep, disturbed qual-

TABLE 48-1 Medical Disorders Associated with Insomnia

General Medical Disorders
Arthritis
Cancer
Chronic pain syndromes
Congestive heart failure
Gastroesophageal reflux disease
Headaches
Nocturnal angina
Peptic ulcer
Postoperative pain

Respiratory Disorders
Asthma
Bronchitis
Chronic obstructive pulmonary disease

Other Medical Conditions
Arrhythmias
Benign prostatic hyperplasia
Constipation
Diabetes mellitus
Epilepsy
Hyperthyroidism
Irritable bowel syndrome
Menopause
Nocturia
Parkinson's disease
Pregnancy
Renal insufficiency

Psychiatric Disorders
Anxiety disorders
Bipolar disorder
Dementia/Alzheimer's disease
Depression
Personality disorders
Psychosis
Substance abuse

Sleep Disorders
Delayed sleep phase syndrome
Drug-related insomnia
Psychophysiologic insomnia
Restless legs syndrome
Shift-work sleep disorder
Sleep apnea

Source: References 1, 2, 7, 8, 12, and 13.

ity of sleep with unusual or troublesome dreams, or just poor sleep in general. Their actual duration of sleep as determined by sleep laboratory studies may or may not differ from that of individuals who report normal sleep. However, these patients usually report that it takes them more than 30 minutes to fall asleep and/or that their duration of sleep is less than 6 to 7 hours nightly. Patients who complain of insomnia characterized by frequent

TABLE 48-2 Drugs That Can Exacerbate Insomnia

Drugs That Can Cause Insomnia

Alcohol
Anabolic steroids
Antidepressants
Anticonvulsants
Antihypertensives
Antineoplastics
Amphetamines
Appetite suppressants (phentermine)
Beta-adrenergic agonists (albuterol)
Beta-blockers (especially propranolol)
Bupropion
Caffeine
Clonidine
Corticosteroids
Decongestants (e.g., pseudoephedrine, phenylephrine)
Desipramine
Diuretics (at bedtime)
Methyldopa
Hypnotic use (chronic)
Levodopa (in carbidopa and entacapone combination products)
Monoamine oxidase inhibitors (tranylcypromine)
Nicotine
Oral contraceptives
Quinidine
Selective serotonin reuptake inhibitors
Serotonin-norepinephrine reuptake inhibitors (venlafaxine, duloxetine)
Sympathomimetic amines
Theophylline
Thyroid preparations

Drugs That Can Produce Withdrawal Insomnia

Alcohol
Amphetamines
Antihistamines (first-generation)
Barbiturates
Benzodiazepines
Chloral hydrate
Monoamine oxidase inhibitors
Opiates, opioids
Tricyclic antidepressants
Illicit drugs (cocaine, marijuana, phencyclidine)

Source: References 1, 2, 7, 8, 12, and 13.

nighttime awakenings or early morning awakenings with difficulty going back to sleep, or those with a duration of insomnia of 4 weeks or longer should be referred to their health care provider for further investigation.

Sleep-deprived individuals are highly symptomatic, and their quality of life is negatively affected. Some impairment in daytime functioning is necessary for a diagnosis of insomnia, and a majority of untreated patients with insomnia report symptoms of fatigue, drowsiness, anxiety, irritability, depression, decreased concentration, and memory impairment. If left untreated, insomnia is associated with an increase in accidents as well as a rise in morbidity and mortality rates from general medical and psychiatric disorders (i.e., depression, anxiety, and substance abuse).[1]

Treatment of Insomnia

Treatment Goals

Treatment goals are to improve the patient's presenting symptoms (e.g., difficulty falling or staying asleep, or nonrestorative sleep), quality of life, and functioning.

General Treatment Approach

For patients with transient or short-term insomnia, but no underlying medical or psychiatric conditions that cause insomnia, reestablishing the normal sleep cycle with good sleep hygiene practices, with or without a nonprescription sleep aid, should help normalize sleep patterns (Figure 48-1). If diphenhydramine is recommended, it should be taken at bedtime only as needed. Patients who complain of continuing insomnia after 14 days of treatment with diphenhydramine combined with good sleep hygiene and those who experience side effects from this medication should be referred for a more thorough evaluation of the sleep disturbance and its etiology.[14] The algorithm in Figure 48-1 outlines the assessment and self-treatment of transient and short-term insomnia, and lists exclusions for self-treatment.

Nonpharmacologic Therapy

The sleep hygiene measures in Table 48-3 are recommended for all patients with insomnia.[9,15] In many patients with sleep disturbances, these measures should be tried before initiating pharmacotherapy. Patients should be encouraged to try one or two measures at a time.

Pharmacologic Therapy

When the Food and Drug Administration (FDA) issued its final monograph on nonprescription sleep aids in 1989, the antihistamine diphenhydramine (HCl and citrate salts) was the only Category I sleep aid listed.[16] Although the safety and efficacy of another antihistamine, doxylamine, have not been fully established, FDA has allowed it to remain on the market.[17] Minimal studies supporting the efficacy of doxylamine as a hypnotic are available.[1,17] Products containing pyrilamine maleate, potassium or sodium bromide, and scopolamine hydrobromide were removed from the U.S. market[7]; however, clinicians, particularly in the southwestern United States, may see these products imported from other countries.

Antihistamines

Both diphenhydramine and doxylamine are members of the ethanolamine group of antihistamines. Ethanolamines are thought to affect sleep through their affinity for blocking histamine$_1$ and muscarinic receptors.[16]

Selected clinical and pharmacokinetic properties of diphenhydramine and doxylamine are summarized in Table 48-4.[14,16,17] Both drugs are well absorbed from the gastrointestinal tract and have short-to-intermediate half-lives. Diphenhydramine is

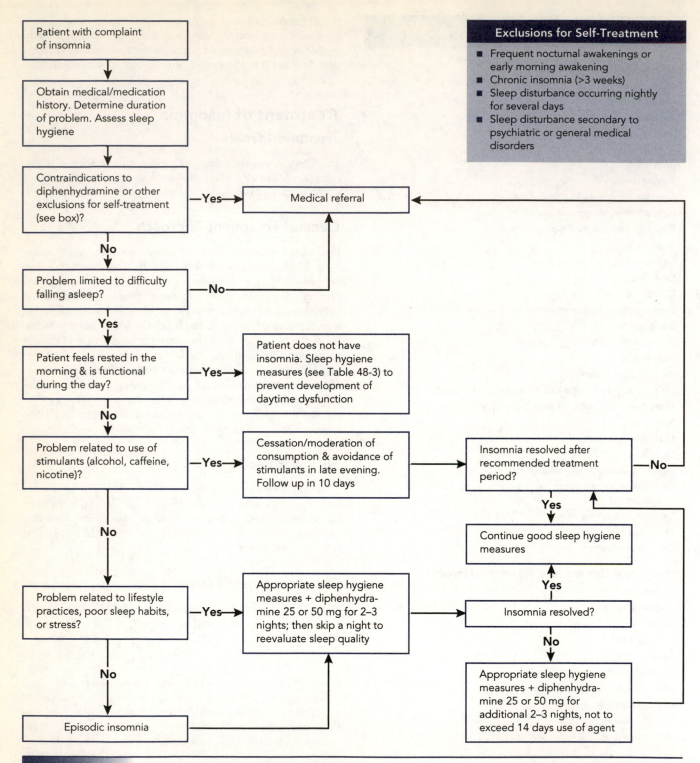

Exclusions for Self-Treatment

- Frequent nocturnal awakenings or early morning awakening
- Chronic insomnia (>3 weeks)
- Sleep disturbance occurring nightly for several days
- Sleep disturbance secondary to psychiatric or general medical disorders

FIGURE 48-1 Self-care of transient and short-term insomnia.

metabolized in the liver through two successive N–demethylations, and its apparent half-life can be prolonged in patients with hepatic cirrhosis.[14] Some but not all studies have shown a positive relationship between diphenhydramine plasma concentrations and drowsiness and cognitive impairment. Significant drowsiness lasted from 3 to 6 hours after a single dose of diphen-

hydramine 50 mg.[18] However, next-morning hangover was reported after multiple nightly dosing for insomnia.

The primary indication for diphenhydramine in insomnia is the symptomatic management of transient and short-term sleep difficulty, particularly in individuals who complain of occasional problems falling asleep. The evidence for the efficacy

---

TABLE 48-3 Principles of Good Sleep Hygiene

TABLE 48-3 Principles of Good Sleep Hygiene

- Use bed for sleeping or intimacy only.
- Establish a regular sleep pattern: Go to bed and arise at about the same time daily, even on the weekends.
- Make the bedroom comfortable for sleeping. Avoid temperature extremes, noise, and light.
- Engage in relaxing activities before bedtime.
- Exercise regularly but not within 2–4 hours of bedtime.
- If hungry, eat a light snack, but avoid eating meals within 2 hours before bedtime.
- Avoid daytime napping.
- Avoid using caffeine, alcohol, or nicotine for at least 4–6 hours before bedtime.
- If unable to fall asleep, do not continue to try to sleep; rather, perform a relaxing activity until you feel tired.
- Do not watch the clock at night.

Source: References 9 and 15.

of diphenhydramine in patients with chronic insomnia is poor, and tolerance to the hypnotic effect was reported to develop with repeated use.[1,13]

Although the usual optimal diphenhydramine dose is 50 mg nightly, some individuals benefit from a 25 mg dose. Intermittent use for 3 days with an "off" night to assess sleep quality without medication is suggested to reduce tolerance to the hypnotic effect. Diphenhydramine should be used for no more than 14 consecutive nights.[14]

Additive sedation or anticholinergic effects occur when diphenhydramine is used in combination with other medications that have these properties.[16] Diphenhydramine, an inhibitor of the hepatic enzyme CYP2D6, causes more than a twofold decrease in the clearance of venlafaxine and metoprolol.[14,19,20] In patients on multiple medications, particularly patients of advanced age, diphenhydramine may reduce the clearance of drugs metabolized by CYP2D6 (e.g., codeine or propranolol); these potential interactions should be carefully monitored.

TABLE 48-4 Selected Pharmacokinetic and Clinical Properties of Nonprescription Hypnotics

	Diphenhydramine	Doxylamine
Time to maximum plasma concentration (t_{max})	1–4 hours	2–3 hours
Maximum sedation	1–3 hours	NA
Protein binding	80%–85%	NA
Elimination half-life	2.4–9.3 hours	10 hours
Duration of sedation	3–6 hours	3–6 hours
Bioavailability	40%–60%	NA

Key: NA, not available.
Source: References 14, 16, and 17.

Anticholinergic toxicity can result from excessive antihistamine dosages. Other factors, including drug interactions, intentional overdosage, or individual sensitivity, can lead to toxicity.[21,22] CNS anticholinergic toxicity is one of the primary presenting features of antihistamine excess. Patients exhibiting excessive anticholinergic effects can be anxious, excited, delirious, hallucinating, or stuporous; in more severe cases, coma or seizures may occur. Other physical signs of anticholinergic toxicity include dilated pupils, flushed skin, hot and dry mucous membranes, and elevated body temperature. Tachycardia and moderate QTc prolongation on the electrocardiogram are common. In severe cases, rhabdomyolysis, dysrhythmias, cardiovascular collapse, and death can occur.[14,22]

In the case of diphenhydramine overdose, patients should be referred for emergency treatment, which includes gastric lavage and activated charcoal via gastric tube, and further symptomatic treatment. Syrup of ipecac should not be recommended.

Sedation, the intended effect when diphenhydramine is used as a hypnotic, may be associated with next-morning hangover in susceptible individuals.[14] Other primary side effects of diphenhydramine and doxylamine are anticholinergic.[14,17] Dry mouth and throat, constipation, blurred vision, urinary retention, and tinnitus commonly occur. Patients of advanced age, patients with comorbid general medical disorders, and patients taking multiple medications are particularly susceptible to developing adverse effects.

Diphenhydramine is contraindicated in several situations. Male patients of advanced age with prostatic hyperplasia and difficulty urinating should not use diphenhydramine because of increased urinary retention. Because anticholinergics can increase intraocular pressure, angle closure glaucoma is another contraindication. Patients with cardiovascular disease (e.g., angina or rhythm disturbance) may be particularly susceptible to the anticholinergic adverse effects of ethanolamine sleep aids and should not use these agents.[16] Anticholinergics tend to decrease cognition and increase confusion in patients with dementia; diphenhydramine is contraindicated in these patients as well.

Patients should be cautioned to avoid performing tasks that require their full attention or coordination (e.g., driving, cooking, or operating equipment) until their response to diphenhydramine is known. They should be warned of the additive CNS depressant effects of alcohol and encouraged not to drink alcoholic beverages while taking diphenhydramine. Some patients can develop excitation from diphenhydramine and other highly anticholinergic antihistamines.[16] This paradoxical effect occurs more often in children, patients of advanced age, and patients with organic mental disorders. Symptoms include nervousness, restlessness, agitation, tremors, insomnia, delirium, and, in rare cases, seizures.

Combination products containing diphenhydramine and acetaminophen (e.g., Excedrin PM), ibuprofen (e.g., Advil PM), or aspirin (e.g., Bayer PM) are available,[16] although no published studies establish whether these products are of additive benefit in inducing sleep in patients who complain of insomnia caused by pain.

Several case reports exist in the literature of diphenhydramine abuse in patients taking antipsychotic medications.[23] Animals studies indicate that selected antagonists of the histamine[1] receptors enhance dopamine release in the mesolimbic areas similar to that produced by cocaine.[24] Clinicians should carefully assess for abuse in individuals making repeated requests for diphenhydramine refills, especially in patients under treatment for psychosis.[23]

Ethanol

About 30% of patients with persistent insomnia report using alcohol to help fall asleep in the past year, with 67% reporting it was effective.[25] Ethanol initially improves sleep in nonalcoholics at both low and high doses, with disturbance in the second half of the night at high doses. However, tolerance quickly develops after the initial beneficial effects, often leading to the use of higher doses.[25] Individuals with heavy or continuous alcohol use usually experience restless sleep, often awaken within 2 to 4 hours, and have reduced total sleep duration.[25] Chronic alcohol drinkers usually have a marked disorganization of the sleep cycle. A worsening of sleep (or rebound insomnia) can occur when alcohol use ceases.

Alcohol is present in some nonprescription combination cold products (e.g., NyQuil Liquid contains 10% alcohol by volume). Products of this type are marketed to induce sleep. Data are limited, however, regarding the efficacy and safety of these products as hypnotics. The multiple ingredients in these products increase the risk of side effects and interactions with other drugs.

Pharmacotherapeutic Comparisons

Most published clinical trials indicate that diphenhydramine is effective in decreasing time to fall asleep (sleep latency) and in improving the reported quality of sleep for individuals with occasional sleep difficulty.[14] Compared with placebo, diphenhydramine improved sleep efficiency for 2 weeks in patients with mild insomnia.[26] Patients who have never been treated with hypnotics tend to respond better to diphenhydramine than those who have been previously treated.[27] In general, diphenhydramine is not as efficacious as benzodiazepine hypnotics, and it should not be recommended in individuals with a chronic sleep disturbance.[1,2]

Product Selection Guidelines

Because no published efficacy and safety studies document the value of doxylamine as a hypnotic, only diphenhydramine should be recommended to patients for such use at the present time. Nonprescription diphenhydramine is available as capsules, gelcaps, tablets, chewable tablets, solutions, and elixirs (Table 48-5), allowing various forms for different patient preferences.[14]

SPECIAL POPULATIONS

The safety of antihistamines during pregnancy has not been clearly established.[16] Therefore, the benefit–risk ratio of using these drugs to manage insomnia during pregnancy should be carefully evaluated. Doxylamine was formerly marketed as a prescription combination product for treating morning sickness during pregnancy. However, the manufacturer voluntarily removed this combination from the market in 1976 after allegations of teratogenicity. Although it is not possible to prove conclusively that doxylamine is not teratogenic, epidemiologic studies indicate that the possibility of such a relationship is remote.[16,17] Diphenhydramine is classified as Pregnancy Category B on the basis of safety studies conducted in animals. Most epidemiologic studies have not demonstrated increased risk of teratogenicity with the use of diphenhydramine during the first trimester, but one trial reported cleft palate alone and with other fetal abnormalities.[14] Nevertheless, rather than recommending a nonprescription product, pregnant women should be referred for further medical evaluation.

An increased risk of CNS side effects can occur with sedating antihistamine use in neonates. The intermittent use of low doses of diphenhydramine after the last daytime feeding would lessen potential drug effects in the newborn.[28] Use of large doses for sustained periods of time may inhibit lactation and affect breast-fed infants (e.g., drowsiness).[28] Continued use of sedating antihistamines for insomnia are not recommended for use in nursing mothers.[14,16,17]

Children and adolescents may present with insomnia because of a circadian rhythm disorder. Teenagers should be questioned about their use of nonprescription remedies and intake of caffeine or alcohol, which may interfere with sleep. Behavioral interventions and good sleep hygiene are first-line treatment for insomnia in children and adolescents. Diphenhydramine and doxylamine are not indicated to treat insomnia in children younger than 12 years. Diphenhydramine is known to cause paradoxical excitation in younger children and is not recommended to induce sleep in infants.[14] Anticholinergic toxicity is particularly common in children, in whom the symptoms are usually more severe. Diphenhydramine toxicity was reported in children using the topical application over large areas of their bodies, and in those using both the topical and oral preparations.[14] In December 2002, FDA issued a ruling that required a warning statement on all diphenhydramine-containing products (by December 6, 2004) that the product is not to be used in conjunction with any other preparations that contain diphenhydramine.[14]

TABLE 48-5   Selected Sleep Aid Products

Trade Name	Primary Ingredients
Single-Entity Antihistamine Products	
Compoz Nighttime Sleep Aid Tablets/Gelcaps	Diphenhydramine HCl 50 mg
Sominex Nighttime Sleep Aid Tablets	Diphenhydramine HCl 25 mg
Antihistamine/Analgesic Combination Products	
Advil PM Caplets	Diphenhydramine citrate 38 mg; ibuprofen 200 mg
Bayer PM Extra Strength Caplets	Diphenhydramine citrate 38.3 mg; aspirin 500 mg
Excedrin PM Geltabs/Caplets/Tablets	Diphenhydramine citrate 38 mg; acetaminophen 500 mg
Tylenol PM Extra Strength Geltabs/Gelcaps/Caplets	Diphenhydramine HCl 25 mg; acetaminophen 500 mg

Treatment of insomnia in the geriatric population ideally consists of behavioral therapy and pharmacotherapy with approved agents. The Beers criteria recommend avoiding the use of anticholinergics in older patients,[29] and diphenhydramine has caused cognitive impairment and falls in patients of advanced age.[1,2,29,30] Therefore, nonprescription antihistamines should not be recommended to treat insomnia in this age group, and the patients should be referred to their medical provider for further evaluation.

Complementary Therapies

Complementary therapies such as melatonin, 5-hydroxytryptophan (5-HTP), valerian, and kava are commonly used for insomnia. In a representative sample of the U.S. population, 5.2% used melatonin and 5.9% used valerian.[31] The decision to use the herbal compounds was made in consultation with a health care provider less than 50% of the time.[31] Despite widespread use, there are few scientific data supporting a beneficial effect of complementary therapies in the treatment of insomnia.[1,2]

A comprehensive report on the safety and effectiveness of melatonin found that, although there is some evidence for the benefits of melatonin supplements, for most sleep disorders the evidence suggests limited or no benefits.[32] Melatonin may be effective in short-term treatment of delayed sleep phase syndrome.[32] No evidence suggests that melatonin is effective in alleviating the sleep disturbance aspect of jet lag and shift-work disorders. The optimal dose and time of administration of melatonin for the treatment of insomnia have not been determined. The usual dose is 0.3 to 5 mg at bedtime.[33] Potential drug interactions, side effects, and toxicity, particularly with long-term use, are largely unknown.

L-tryptophan was recalled by FDA in 1990 because of safety concerns linking the supplement to eosinophilia-myalgia syndrome (EMS) and death.[34] L-tryptophan in the United States is limited for use, under medical supervision, in special dietary products such as infant formulas, enteral products, and approved parenteral drug products. In light of its questionable efficacy, concerns regarding contaminants, and known adverse effects, L-tryptophan should not be recommended as a sleep aid. Since the withdrawal of L-tryptophan from the market, 5-HTP, the immediate precursor of serotonin, is being used to treat insomnia. There is concern that 5-HTP, like L-tryptophan, can cause EMS[35] (see Chapter 54). The efficacy of 5-HTP in insomnia is not proven, and it should not be recommended as a sleep aid.

Valerian (*Valeriana officinalis*) is a perennial plant native to Europe and Asia. Preparations of valerian marketed as dietary supplements are made from its roots and stems.[33] Dried roots are prepared as tinctures or teas, and dried plant materials are compounded into tablets and capsules. Limited evidence shows no benefit in insomnia compared with placebo.[36] The optimum dose of valerian is unknown, although clinical trials have used 400 to 900 mg of the valerian root extract. Continuous nightly use for several days or weeks is required for effect, so valerian is not useful for acute insomnia. Patients using large doses of valerian over several years can experience severe benzodiazepine-like withdrawal symptoms and cardiac complications.[36] Therefore, valerian should be slowly tapered after extended use.

Kava (*Piper methysticum*) is a plant native to the islands of the South Pacific. Kava-containing supplements are advertised to promote relaxation (e.g., to reduce anxiety, stress, and tension), and for sleeplessness and menopausal symptoms.[33] There is little evidence to support the use of kava in insomnia, especially given the recent concern about the potential for hepatotoxicity and drug interactions with this herb.[37] Therefore, kava should not be recommended as a sleep aid.

Chamomile, ginseng, lavender, hops, lemon balm, and passionflower are being used to treat insomnia.[38] Inadequate evidence is available regarding their efficacy and safety in insomnia.

The American Academy of Sleep Medicine recommends dietary supplements not be used for the purpose of treating insomnia or any other sleep problem, unless approved by a medical provider, because of the risk of dangerous side effects and adverse drug interactions.[39] Chapter 54 provides an in-depth discussion of dietary supplements used to treat insomnia.

Complementary and alternative therapies such as acupuncture, tai chi, and light therapy may be useful in the treatment of insomnia.[1,2] However, these treatments have not been adequately evaluated. Chapter 55 provides an in-depth discussion of alternative therapies.

Assessment of Insomnia: A Case-Based Approach

In assessing whether to recommend a nonprescription sleep product, the practitioner should determine if use of such products is appropriate, what nondrug interventions should be recommended, and whether medical referral is indicated. Identifying acute precipitators of insomnia, poor sleep hygiene practices, or underlying medical disorders can assist the practitioner in making a recommendation.

Cases 48-1 and 48-2 illustrate the assessment of patients with insomnia.

CASE 48-1

Relevant Evaluation Criteria	Scenario/Model Outcome
Information Gathering	
1. Gather essential information about the patient's symptoms, including:	
a. description of symptom(s) (i.e., nature, onset, duration, severity, associated symptoms)	Patient complains of difficulty sleeping for the past 2 weeks. He feels drowsy and irritable during the day and falls asleep at his desk in the afternoon.

Relevant Evaluation Criteria	Scenario/Model Outcome
b. description of any factors that seem to precipitate, exacerbate, and/or relieve the patient's symptom(s)	Symptoms appeared about the same time patient started a new job. Previously, he typically slept well.
c. description of the patient's efforts to relieve the symptoms	He tries to stay up until he is sleepy at night. He usually lies in bed and becomes anxious when he cannot sleep. He notes that it is especially frustrating to watch the alarm clock, knowing that he will have to get up in just a few hours to go to work. Sometimes he will get up and watch a ball game on television. He is concerned about being drowsy during the daytime, because the drowsiness interferes with his work.
2. Gather essential patient history information:	
a. patient's identity	John Carroll
b. age, sex, height, and weight	28-year-old male, 6 ft 1 in, 200 lb
c. patient's occupation	Computer programmer
d. patient's dietary habits	Patient is conscientious about eating a healthy diet, low in fat and sodium. He drinks 2 cups of coffee in the morning and 2–3 Red Bull Energy Drinks during the afternoon.
e. patient's sleep habits	Stays up late working, especially when a project is due; sleeps late on the weekends often into the early afternoon. He has been napping 30 minutes at his desk in the afternoon and will often fall asleep for an hour after he arrives home from work.
f. concurrent medical conditions, prescription and nonprescription medications, and dietary supplements	Seasonal allergies; Flonase 1 spray per nostril daily, Chlor-Trimeton Allergy 12-hour (chlorpheniramine 12 mg extended-release) twice a day as needed in the spring and fall
g. allergies	Penicillin (anaphylaxis)
h. history of other adverse reactions to medications	None
i. other (describe) _____	Drinks 3–4 beers nightly to help him go to sleep

Assessment and Triage

3. Differentiate patient's signs and symptoms and correctly identify the patient's primary problem(s).	Poor sleep, likely secondary to stress of new job and poor sleep hygiene. Possible use of alcohol on daily basis and excessive caffeine are disrupting sleep.
4. Identify exclusions for self-treatment (see Figure 48-1).	None
5. Formulate a comprehensive list of therapeutic alternatives for the primary problem to determine if triage to a medical practitioner is required, and share this information with the patient.	Options include: (1) Refer John to his PCP. (2) Recommend diphenhydramine until John can make an appointment with his PCP. (3) Recommend diphenhydramine and good sleep hygiene, including limiting daily alcohol and caffeine use and obtaining regular physical activity. (4) Take no action.

Plan

6. Select an optimal therapeutic alternative to address the patient's problem, taking into account patient preferences.	Diphenhydramine 50 mg capsules and good sleep hygiene measures, as well as limited alcohol and caffeine consumption. He is not interested in trying a dietary supplement, such as an herb.
7. Describe the recommended therapeutic approach to the patient.	Take 1 diphenhydramine 50 mg capsule one-half to 1 hour before anticipated bedtime every night for 3 nights. Skip 1 night and evaluate ability to sleep. If not improved, continue diphenhydramine for 3 more nights and reevaluate ability to sleep without it. If symptoms persist for 10 days, seek medical evaluation. Follow measures for positive sleep hygiene (see Table 48-3). Limit alcohol consumption to two cans of beer or less, consumed no later than 2 hours before bedtime. Limit overall intake of caffeine, and at a minimum, avoid caffeine 6 hours before bedtime. A consistent sleep pattern will help to resolve your insomnia.

CASE 48-1 (continued)

Relevant Evaluation Criteria	Scenario/Model Outcome
8. Explain to the patient the rationale for selecting the recommended therapeutic approach from the considered therapeutic alternatives.	Seeing your primary care provider may not be necessary if you take the diphenhydramine and follow good sleep hygiene measures. Poor sleep practices are a common cause of insomnia. If these practices are continued, they can create a chronic sleep disturbance. A hypnotic such as diphenhydramine can facilitate falling asleep, but it must be combined with measures of good sleep hygiene. Alcohol in more than modest quantities can disrupt sleep and make insomnia worse. Therefore, alcohol consumption should be limited and avoided before bedtime. Caffeine is a stimulant that promotes wakefulness. So, caffeine intake should be limited and not consumed within 6 hours of bedtime. Stop drinking Red Bull Energy Drinks, because each 8.3-ounce can contains 80 mg of caffeine, which may also be contributing to your insomnia. All dietary (e.g., sodas, energy drinks) and hidden sources (e.g., chocolate) should be identified.

Patient Education

9. When recommending self-care with nonprescription medications and/or nondrug therapy, convey accurate information to the patient:

a. appropriate dose and frequency of administration	Take diphenhydramine 50 mg nightly for 3 nights, then reevaluate sleep for 1 night without the medication. Do not exceed this nightly dose. Always use sleep aids in combination with positive sleep hygiene measures. Never take hypnotics nightly for longer than 14 days without seeking medical evaluation. Alcoholic beverages should not be taken with diphenhydramine because of increased chances of sedation and negative effects of alcohol on sleep patterns.
b. maximum number of days the therapy should be employed	14 days of continuous nightly use
c. product administration procedures	Take one-half to 1 tablet before bedtime with a full glass of water.
d. expected time to onset of relief	Onset of sedation should occur within 1–2 hours.
e. degree of relief that can be reasonably expected	When combined with sleep hygiene measures, sleep should improve within 1–3 nights.
f. most common side effects	Sedation, next-morning hangover and anticholinergic effects (e.g., dry mouth and throat, urinary retention, blurry vision, constipation)
g. side effects that warrant medical intervention should they occur	Hives, severe itching, shortness of breath
h. patient options in the event that condition worsens or persists	If insomnia persists beyond 10 days, see your primary care provider.
i. product storage requirements	Keep in a tightly closed container. Keep out of the reach of children and pets.
j. specific nondrug measures	See Table 48-3 for sleep hygiene measures. Limit alcohol and caffeine intake.
10. Solicit follow-up questions from patient.	(1) May I repeat the dose if I do not fall asleep within 2 hours? (2) May I take diphenhydramine with my allergy medications?
11. Answer patient's questions.	(1) No. Repeating the dose increases the risk of side effects and likely will not improve sleep. (2) Yes. You can take diphenhydramine with Flonase. Do not take diphenhydramine with the Chlor-Trimeton though, because this allergy medicine contains chlorpheniramine. You should not combine diphenhydramine as a sleep aid and products that contain chlorpheniramine; this combination can result in increased side effects (e.g., sedation, drowsiness, blurred vision, constipation) or toxicity.

Key: PCP, primary care provider.

Relevant Evaluation Criteria	Scenario/Model Outcome
Information Gathering	
1. Gather essential information about the patient's symptoms, including:	
a. description of symptom(s) (i.e., nature, onset, duration, severity, associated symptoms)	Patient complains of difficulty sleeping for the past 3 months. She awakens around 3:00 am, often with shortness of breath, and is not able to go back to sleep. She also complains of severe fatigue and excessive daytime sleepiness.
b. description of any factors that seem to precipitate, exacerbate, and/or relieve the patient's symptom(s)	Sleep has been much worse since she had a respiratory infection that progressed to pneumonia. She has been using her albuterol inhaler every 2 hours during the day, and her insomnia has worsened progressively.
c. description of the patient's efforts to relieve the symptoms	She has tried to increase her exercise by walking in the evenings, but she lacks the energy to do this activity and often becomes short of breath.
2. Gather essential patient history information:	
a. patient's identity	Meredith Thompson
b. age, sex, height, and weight	48-year-old female, 5 ft 6 in, 135 lb
c. patient's occupation	Homemaker
d. patient's dietary habits	Vegetarian
e. patient's sleep habits	She usually goes to sleep around 11 am but finds that she awakes by 2:30 or 3 am. She has trouble going back to sleep and often has to use her albuterol inhaler. She estimates that she has gotten only 3 or 4 full nights of sleep the past month.
f. concurrent medical conditions, prescription and nonprescription medications, and dietary supplements	Spiriva (tiotropium) and albuterol inhalers for COPD for past 2 years; lisinopril for hypertension for the past 3 years.
g. allergies	NKA
h. history of other adverse reactions to medications	None
i. other (describe) _____	Smokes 1 pack of cigarettes per day
Assessment and Triage	
3. Differentiate patient's signs and symptoms and correctly identify the patient's primary problem(s).	Chronic poor sleep, most likely secondary to poor control of COPD and excessive use of albuterol
4. Identify exclusions for self-treatment (see Figure 48-1).	The symptoms that the patient complains of suggest an underlying cause (i.e., COPD and respiratory symptoms) for the insomnia that requires medical referral for evaluation.
5. Formulate a comprehensive list of therapeutic alternatives for the primary problem to determine if triage to a medical practitioner is required, and share this information with the patient.	Options include: (1) Refer Meredith to her PCP for management of COPD and counsel her on appropriate inhaler technique. Initiate the "5 A's" of tobacco cessation (see Chapter 50). (2) Refer Meredith to her PCP for management of COPD and counsel on appropriate inhaler technique. Initiate the 5 A's of tobacco cessation. Recommend good sleep hygiene measures (see Table 48-3). (3) Initiate the 5 A's of tobacco cessation. Recommend good sleep hygiene measures and a nonprescription sleep aid. (4) Take no action.
Plan	
6. Select an optimal therapeutic alternative to address the patient's problem, taking into account patient preferences.	Refer Meredith to her PCP. The underlying disorder(s) causing her insomnia needs to be addressed. Use of proper inhaler technique should be assessed. Recommend measures for sleep hygiene. Assist with quitting smoking if patient is ready to quit.
7. Describe the recommended therapeutic approach to the patient.	See your primary care provider as soon as possible for evaluation of your sleep disturbance. Follow measures of good sleep hygiene (see Table 48-3).

C A S E   4 8 - 2   *(continued)*

Relevant Evaluation Criteria	Scenario/Model Outcome
8. Explain to the patient the rationale for selecting the recommended therapeutic approach from the considered therapeutic alternatives.	You have described symptoms that indicate a medical disorder is possibly causing your sleep disturbance. The symptoms will need to be addressed if your sleep is to improve. Nonprescription hypnotics are unlikely to help you.
Patient Education	
9. When recommending self-care with nonprescription medications and/or nondrug therapy, convey accurate information to the patient.	Criterion does not apply in this case.
10. Solicit follow-up questions from patient.	Would herbals help my sleep instead?
11. Answer patient's questions.	No. Multiple factors may be contributing to your insomnia. It is very important that all of these be thoroughly addressed if your sleep problems as well as other symptoms are to improve. Dietary supplements, such as herbs, should be used only under the supervision of your medical provider because of the risk of side effects and drug interactions. Dietary supplements are not effective in treating medical causes of insomnia.

Key: COPD, chronic obstructive pulmonary disease; NKA, no known allergies; PCP, primary care provider.

Patient Counseling for Insomnia

Patients with sleep disorders should be encouraged to practice good sleep hygiene measures. For some patients, these measures alone will resolve insomnia. If use of a nonprescription sleep aid is appropriate, the dosage guidelines and recommended duration of therapy should be reviewed with the patient. Potential adverse effects, drug interactions, and any precautions or warnings should be carefully explained. In addition, patient education should include the signs and symptoms that indicate the need for further visits to the practitioner. Taking multiple products (i.e., prescription, nonprescription, dietary supplements) concomitantly to treat insomnia should be discouraged; this approach increases the risk of adverse effects. The box Patient Education for Insomnia lists specific information to provide patients.

PATIENT EDUCATION FOR Insomnia

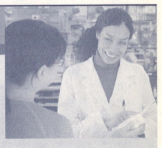

The objectives of self-treatment are to (1) improve the duration and quality of sleep, (2) reduce fatigue and drowsiness during the day, (3) improve daytime functioning, and (4) minimize side effects of treatment. It is important to carefully follow product instructions. The self-care measures listed here will help ensure the best treatment outcomes.

Disease Information

- Insomnia is difficulty getting enough sleep or trouble sleeping without interruption. Insomnia may be described as difficulty falling asleep, waking up too early, or waking up periodically during the night. Insomnia of any kind can cause fatigue and drowsiness during the day. It is classified as *chronic* when it happens almost every night for at least 1 month. Insomnia can be related to a medical or psychiatric condition, caused by mental stress or excitement, or caused by certain daytime and bedtime habits.

Nondrug Measures

- See Table 48-3 for nondrug measures to prevent insomnia.
- Using principles of good sleep hygiene can help improve bad sleep habits and enhance quality sleep.

- If insomnia worsens or continues beyond 2 weeks, seek medical attention.

Nonprescription Medications

- Do not drive or operate machinery after taking sleep aids, including melatonin and valerian.

Diphenhydramine

- Establish a regular bedtime and take diphenhydramine 30–60 minutes before you want to go to sleep. Do not take more than 50 mg of diphenhydramine each night.
- After 2–3 nights of improved sleep, skip taking the medication for 1 night to see if the insomnia is relieved.
- Do not take the medication for longer than 14 days. Longer use will cause tolerance to the medication's sleep-inducing effects but not necessarily to its side effects.
- Note that diphenhydramine can cause morning grogginess or excessive sedation, dry mouth, blurred vision, constipation, and difficulty urinating (particularly in older men).

PATIENT EDUCATION FOR
Insomnia *(continued)*

- Do not take diphenhydramine with alcohol; alcohol can increase the effects of the medication on the central nervous system. Alcohol also disrupts the sleep cycle.
- Do not take diphenhydramine with prescription sleep aids in an attempt to improve sleep further.
- Consult your health care provider before taking diphenhydramine with other medications.

Melatonin

- If melatonin is being used, take it approximately 1 hour before the established bedtime. Somnolence may occur within 30–45 minutes after taking it.
- Do not take more than 5 mg of melatonin each night.
- After taking melatonin, bedroom lights should be turned off.
- Sleep usually occurs within 30–45 minutes after taking the dose.

- Pregnant women should avoid melatonin because of potential hormonal effects on the fetus.

Valerian

- If valerian is being used, take it one-half to 2 hours before retiring to bed.
- It takes 2–4 weeks for optimal effects on sleep to occur.
- If you take valerian for several weeks or months, discontinue it slowly over several weeks to avoid withdrawal effects.
- Pregnant women should avoid valerian because of the potential to induce uterine contractions.

Evaluation of Patient Outcomes for Insomnia

Successful outcomes include decreased time to fall asleep, improved sleep quality, and decreased daytime fatigue and drowsiness. The patient should be advised to seek medical evaluation if sleep has not improved within 10 days.

Key Points for Insomnia

➤ Advise patients that diphenhydramine is the only antihistamine recommended as a sleep aid for occasional insomnia.

➤ Refer patients with chronic insomnia or sleep disturbance caused by an underlying disorder for medical evaluation.

➤ Counsel patients on the side effects of diphenhydramine and other sleep aids, particularly drowsiness and the additive CNS effects of alcohol and other sedating drugs.

➤ Counsel patients that nonprescription sleep aids can cause next-day hangover.

➤ Advise patients with self-treatable symptoms that if symptoms worsen or do not improve after 10 days, they should contact their primary care provider.

➤ Counsel patients with insomnia on nondrug measures such as good sleep hygiene (see Table 48-3).

➤ Refer children younger than 12 years, pregnant patients, and adults older than 65 with insomnia to their primary care provider.

➤ Advise patients of the different dosage forms of sleep aids so they can select a product that is best suited for them.

➤ Advise patients to discuss the potential risks and benefits of complementary and alternative therapies with their medical provider before selecting an agent.

➤ Advise patients not to take other oral medications that contain diphenhydramine with a nonprescription sleep aid that also contains diphenhydramine, or to apply products that contain diphenhydramine topically.

REFERENCES

1. NIH State-of-the-Science Conference Statement on Manifestations and Management of Chronic Insomnia in Adults. *NIH Consensus SCI State-ments.* 2005 Jun 13–15;22(2)1–30. Available at: http://www.consensus.nih.gov. Last accessed: September 24, 2008.
2. Buscemi N, Vandermeer B, Friesen C, et al. *Manifestations and Management of Chronic Insomnia in Adults. Evident Report/Technology Assessment No. 125.* Rockville, Md: Agency for Healthcare Research and Quality; June 2005. AHRQ Publication No. 05-E021-2.
3. National Sleep Foundation. 2005 Sleep in America Poll. Available at: http://www.sleepfoundation.org/site/c.huIXKjM0IxF/b.2419039/k.14E4/2005_Sleep_in_America_Poll.htm. Last accessed: September 24, 2008.
4. Martin SA, Aikens JE, Chervin RD. Toward cost-effectiveness analysis in the diagnosis and treatment of insomnia. *Sleep Med Rev.* 2004;8:63–72.
5. Tariq SH, Pulisetty S. Pharmacotherapy for insomnia. *Clin Geriatr Med.* 2008;24:93–105.
6. National Sleep Foundation. 2002 Sleep in America Poll. Available at: http://www.sleepfoundation.org/site/c.huIXKjM0IxF/b.2417355/k.143E/2002_Sleep_in_America_Poll.htm. Last accessed September 24, 2008.
7. Moore CA, Williams RL, Hirshkowitz M. Sleep disorders. In: Sadock BJ, Sadock VA, ed. *Comprehensive Textbook of Psychiatry.* 7th ed. Philadelphia: Lippincott Williams & Wilkins; 2000:1677–700.
8. Dopp JM, Phillips BG. Sleep disorders. In: DiPiro JT, Talbert RL, Yee GC, et al., eds. *Pharmacotherapy: A Pathophysiologic Approach.* 7th ed. New York: McGraw Hill, Inc; 2008:1191–1201.
9. Morin AK, Jarvis CI, Lunch AM. Therapeutic options for sleep maintenance and sleep-onset insomnia. *Pharmacotherapy.* 2007;27:89–110.
10. Espiritu JR. Aging-related sleep changes. *Clin Geriatr Med.* 2008;24:1–14.
11. Estivill E, Bov A, Garcia-Borreguero D, et al. Consensus on drug treatment, definition and diagnosis for insomnia. *Clin Drug Invest.* 2003;23:351–85.
12. Epstein DR, Bootzin RR. Insomnia. *Nurs Clin North Am.* 2002;37:611–31.
13. Sateia MJ, Pigeon WR. Identification and management of insomnia. *Med Clin North Am.* 2004;88:567–96.
14. STAT!Ref Online Electronic Medical Library [subscription database online]. Diphenhydramine. In: McEvoy GK, ed. *AHFS Drug Information 2008.* Bethesda, Md: American Society of Health-System Pharmacists. Posted April 21, 2008.
15. Stepanski EJ, Wyatt JK. Use of sleep hygiene in the treatment of insomnia. *Sleep Med Rev.* 2003;7:215–25.
16. STAT!Ref Online Electronic Medical Library [subscription database online]. Antihistamine drugs. In: McEvoy GK, ed. *AHFS Drug Information 2008.* Bethesda, Md: American Society of Health-System Pharmacists. Posted April 21, 2008.
17. STAT!Ref Online Electronic Medical Library [database online]. Doxylamine. In: McEvoy GK, ed. *AHFS Drug Information 2008.* Bethesda, Md: American Society of Health-System Pharmacists. Posted April 21, 2008.
18. Glass JR, Sproule BA, Herrmann N, et al. Acute pharmacological effects of temazepam, diphenhydramine, and valerian in healthy elderly subjects.

J Clin Psychopharmacol. 2003;23:260–8.

19. Lessard E, Yessine MA, Hamelin BA, et al. Diphenhydramine alters the disposition of venlafaxine through inhibition of CYP2D6 activity in humans. *J Clin Psychopharmacol.* 2001;21:175–84.

20. Hamelin BA, Bouayad A, Methot J, et al. Significant interaction between the nonprescription antihistamine diphenhydramine and the CYP2D6 substrate metoprolol in healthy men with high or low CYP2D6 activity. *Clin Pharmacol Ther.* 2000;67:466–77.

21. Baker AM, Johnson DG, Levisky JA, et al. Fatal diphenhydramine intoxication in infants. *J Forensic Sci.* 2003;48:425–8.

22. Bockholdt B, Klug E, Schneider V. Suicide through doxylamine poisoning. *Forensic Sci Int.* 2001;119:138–40.

23. Thomas A, Nallur DG, Jones N, et al. Diphenhydramine abuse and detoxification: a brief review and report. *J Psychopharmacol.* 2008 Feb 28 [Epub ahead of print].

24. Tanda G, Kopajtic TA, Katz JL. Cocaine-like neurochemical effects of antihistaminic medications. *J Neurochem.* 2008;106:147–57.

25. Roehrs T, Roth T. Sleep, sleepiness, sleep disorders and alcohol use and abuse. *Sleep Med Rev.* 2001;5:287–97.

26. Morin CM, Koetter U, Bastien C, et al. Valerian-hops combination and diphenhydramine for treating insomnia. *Sleep.* 2005;28:1465–71.

27. Kudo Y, Kurihara M. Clinical evaluation of diphenhydramine hydrochloride for the treatment of insomnia in psychiatric patients: a double-blind study. *J Clin Pharmacol.* 1990;30:1041–8.

28. National Institutes of Health, US National Library of Medicine. Diphenhydramine. LactMed. Available at: http://toxnet.nlm.nih.gov. Last accessed September 24, 2008.

29. Fick DM, Cooper JW, Wade WE, et al. Updating the Beers criteria for potentially inappropriate medication use in older adults. *Arch Intern Med.* 2003;163:2716–24.

30. Basu R, Dodge H, Stoehr GP, et al. Sedative-hypnotic use of diphenhydramine in a rural, older adult, community-based cohort: effects on cognition. *Am J Geriatr Psychiatry.* 2003;11:205–13.

31. Bliwise DL, Ansari FP. Insomnia associated with valerian and melatonin usage in the 2002 National Health Interview Survey. *Sleep.* 2007; 30:881–4.

32. Buscemi N, Vandermeer B, Pandya R, et al. *Melatonin for Treatment of Sleep Disorders. Summary. Evidence Report/Technology Assessment No. 108.* Rockville, Md: Agency for Healthcare Research and Quality; November 2004. AHRQ Publication No. 05-E002-1.

33. National Center for Complementary and Alternative Medicine. Available at: http://nccam.nih.gov. Last accessed September 24, 2008.

34. US Food and Drug Administration Office of Health Affairs. "Dear Colleague" Letter Regarding Research on Eosinophilia-Myalgia Syndrome and Current Regulatory Status of L-tryptophan. September 3, 1992. Available at: http://www.cfsan.fda.gov/~dms/ds-ltr3.html. Last accessed September 24, 2008.

35. US Food and Drug Administration Center for Food Safety and Applied Nutrition Information Paper on L-Tryptophan and 5-hydroxy-L-Tryptophan. February 2001. Available at: http://www.cfsan.fda.gov/~dms/ds-tryp1.html. Last accessed May 6, 2008.

36. Taibi DM, Landis CA, Petry H, et al. A systematic review of valerian as a sleep aid: safe but not effective. *Sleep Med Rev.* 2007;11:209–30.

37. US Food and Drug Administration Center for Food Safety and Applied Nutrition Consumer Advisory on Kava-Containing Dietary Supplements May Be Associated with Severe Liver Injury, March 25, 2002. Available at: http://www.cfsan.fda.gov/~dms/addskava.html. Last accessed September 24, 2008.

38. Gyllenhaal C, Merritt SL, Peterson SD, et al. Efficacy and safety of herbal stimulants and sedatives in sleep disorders. *Sleep Med Rev.* 2000; 4:229–51.

39. American Academy of Sleep Medicine (AASM). AASM Position Statement: Treating Insomnia with Herbal Supplements. Available at: http://www.aasmnet.org/Articles.aspx?id=254. Last accessed September 24, 2008.

Drowsiness and Fatigue

Michael Z. Wincor

Drowsiness and fatigue, typically the results of acute or chronic sleep deprivation, can increase the risk of work-related or driving-related accidents, as well as adversely impact productivity, mood, and overall health. Epidemiologic evidence indicates an increased incidence of sleep-related crashes in drivers who report an average of less than 7 hours of sleep per night.[1] The negative impact of sleep deprivation on driving performance is equivalent to driving legally drunk.[2] The combination of ethanol ingestion and sleepiness is particularly hazardous. A study of medical interns demonstrated a significant increase in both automobile accidents and near misses after they worked extended shifts in the hospital.[3] Caffeine is the most frequently used central nervous system (CNS) stimulant in the world; it has been used for centuries to relieve sleepiness and fatigue. This chapter covers caffeine's beneficial and harmful effects.

The primary sources of daily caffeine intake in the diet are coffee (50–130 mg per 5 ounces), tea (25–50 mg per 5 ounces), and soft drinks (30–60 mg per 12 ounces). Table 49-1 lists the caffeine content of common beverages. The per-capita consumption of caffeine from all sources is estimated to be 1.73 mg/kg/day, with a moderate intake generally defined as less than 300 mg/day; for children younger than 9 years, the average daily intake is 0.82 to 0.85 mg/kg/day, with the majority of intake from tea or soft drinks.[4] Caffeine is an ingredient in many nonprescription, prescription, and dietary supplements. It is the sum total of our daily intake of caffeine from all sources that may lead to adverse effects, withdrawal reactions, or rarely, drug interactions.

Pathophysiology of Drowsiness and Fatigue

Although specific disorders such as narcolepsy, sleep apnea, and sleep-related movement disorders must be considered, daytime drowsiness and fatigue are most often caused by inadequate sleep—involving insufficient duration of and/or fragmented sleep. The degree of sleepiness is determined by two factors that appear to regulate sleep and wakefulness: (1) a homeostatic process involving an increase in sleepiness as time since the most recent period of sleep increases and (2) a circadian process by which the master biological clock (in the suprachiasmatic nucleus) varies alertness over the course of the 24-hour day.[5] Other

possible contributing factors include the use of central nervous system (CNS) depressants (e.g., benzodiazepines, other anxiolytics and hypnotics, first-generation histamine H_1-receptor antagonists, antipsychotics, antidepressants, mood stabilizers, alcohol, anticonvulsants, and opioids), dopamine agonists, and some antihypertensive agents. Increased susceptibility to the sedating effects of these agents can be particularly troublesome in the elderly. Consumption of excessive amounts of caffeine in medications or dietary sources, particularly in the late afternoon and evening, can paradoxically cause daytime drowsiness by impairing sleep.

Clinical Presentation of Drowsiness and Fatigue

The subjective experience of sleepiness includes yawning, eye rubbing, nodding, and decreased ability to focus and concentrate. Subjective measures of sleepiness include the Stanford Sleepiness Scale and the Epworth Sleepiness Scale. Objectively, sleepiness has most frequently been measured with the Multiple Sleep Latency Test. This test measures the tendency to fall asleep by first recording an individual's sleep cycle for 1 night using a polysomnogram; the following day the individual participates in a series of "nap" sessions that are conducted in a dark quiet room and scheduled 2 hours apart. The assumption is that the sleepier the individual is, the more quickly he or she will fall asleep.

Treatment of Drowsiness and Fatigue

Treatment Goals

The goal in treating daytime drowsiness and fatigue is to identify and eliminate the underlying cause to improve mental alertness and productivity. The algorithm in Figure 49-1 outlines the approach to self-treatment.

General Treatment Approach

Many consumers use dietary sources of caffeine, such as coffee, tea, or carbonated soft drinks, to self-treat occasional symptoms of fatigue and drowsiness. If dietary sources are not available or

Editor's Note: This chapter is based on the 15th edition chapter with the same title, written by Robert J. Anderson and Diane Nykamp.

TABLE 49-1 Caffeine Content in Common Beverages

Coffees, Teas, and Soft Drinks	Caffeine Content (mg)
Coffee (8 oz)	110
Coffee, decaf (8 oz)	5
Starbucks Coffee, grande (16 oz)	550
Starbucks Coffee, tall (12 oz)	375
Espresso (1 oz)	90
Instant Coffee (8 oz)	75
Brewed Tea, US Brands	40
Snapple Iced Tea	21
Mountain Dew (12 oz)	55.5
Diet Coke (12 oz)	46.5
Coca-Cola (12 oz)	34.5
Dr. Pepper (12 oz)	42

Note: The listed caffeine content for the brewed coffees and teas may vary according to brewing methods.

are inconvenient to use, nonprescription caffeine-containing products may be used. Caffeine as a supplement, or in dietary form, is not a substitute for adequate sleep. Before recommending any caffeine-containing nonprescription product, the clinician should rule out any drug-induced cause of daytime drowsiness and fatigue. In addition, if drowsiness and fatigue are chronic symptoms, especially with adequate sleep, a referral to a physician or specialist may be indicated, given that medical conditions such as hypothyroidism (especially in women), anemia, and sleep apnea often present with similar symptoms.

Nonpharmacologic Therapy

Good sleep hygiene principles should be emphasized (see Chapter 48, Table 48-3).

Pharmacologic Therapy (Caffeine)

Caffeine, like theophylline, is a xanthine derivative that acts as a nonselective competitive antagonist of A1 and A2A receptors of adenosine.[6] An increase in the concentration of adenosine in the brain, especially during prolonged wakefulness, is theorized to be the cause of early morning grogginess. By reversing the effects of adenosine, caffeine exerts its pharmacologic effect by increasing arousal, decreasing fatigue, and elevating mood. Secondary effects on other neurotransmitters may also increase alertness.

Caffeine is rapidly and completely absorbed, reaching a peak concentration within 30 minutes.[7] It is water-soluble with a rapid and wide distribution to nearly every tissue in the body and an almost immediate effect on alertness. The elimination half-life is generally 3 to 5 hours; however, the metabolism of caffeine may be influenced by prior ingestion of caffeine, gender, smoking status, and other drugs.

As a xanthine derivative, caffeine possesses weak bronchodilation action. Caffeine also stimulates the sympathetic nervous system, resulting in the release of norepinephrine, epinephrine, and renin. In cardiac tissue, caffeine has a positive inotropic effect on the myocardium and a positive chronotropic effect on the sinoatrial node, resulting in a transient increase in heart rate, force of contraction, and cardiac output. Caffeine can cause modest increases in blood pressure, may increase the secretion of hydrochloric acid and pepsin, and can relax the lower esophageal sphincter, which could aggravate symptoms of peptic ulcer disease, gastric reflux, or esophagitis. High intake and prolonged use of caffeine may increase the risk of calcium oxalate stone formation in patients with a history of kidney stones.[8]

Caffeine is the only nonprescription stimulant approved by the Food and Drug Administration (FDA), and is commonly available in doses of 100 and 200 mg. Table 49-2 lists selected trade-name caffeine-only products. The labeled dose of most nonprescription supplements is 100 to 200 mg every 3 to 4 hours as needed, to a maximum daily dose of 600 mg. Used as a CNS stimulant, caffeine is marketed to help fatigued patients to stay awake and to restore mental alertness. Many consumers take caffeine to reduce fatigue or increase their alertness. Examples may include shift workers with irregular work patterns, overnight truck drivers, soldiers on active duty, medical residents on call at the hospital, or students studying late for an examination.

The effects of caffeine on daytime performance in alert individuals are unclear, and may depend on the type of task and prior state of alertness. When taken before sleep, caffeine delays sleep onset, reduces deep sleep, and increases nocturnal awakenings.[9] After 36 hours of sleep deprivation, caffeine, in sustained-release doses of 600 mg, improved psychomotor performance.[10] The dose-related response is such that "high users" of caffeine exhibit a better response; however, this benefit is offset by an increase in the incidence of side effects. For example, in one study, a 70 mg dose of caffeine improved hand steadiness and reduced fatigue, but a 250 mg dose decreased hand steadiness and increased jitteriness.[11]

The effect of low doses of caffeine (12.5–100 mg) versus placebo on cognitive performance and mood was measured in consumers with low, moderate, and habitual caffeine intake.[12] All doses of caffeine affected cognitive performance favorably; tolerance was not found to have an effect on performance or mood in the regular users of caffeine.

The positive effect of caffeine on performance appears to be maintained throughout the day. A randomized crossover study compared the effects of 1 or 2 cups of tea (37.5 mg/cup) or coffee (75 mg/cup) versus water administered four times during the day.[13] At all doses, and regardless of source, caffeine improved cognitive and psychomotor performance throughout the day and evening. As expected, the higher doses significantly and negatively impacted the ability to sleep. Lower doses of caffeine found in tea provided benefits similar to those of coffee but without disrupting sleep patterns.

The issue of whether caffeine can improve alertness and performance sufficiently to minimize traffic accidents was addressed in a double-blind study comparing the effects of 200 mg of caffeine with placebo on driving performance and sleepiness, as measured in a driving simulator during early morning hours.[14] After "restricted sleep," caffeine reduced early morning sleepiness for approximately 2 hours; after "no sleep," caffeine delayed sleep by only 30 minutes. Therefore, it is important to counsel patients that caffeine cannot compensate for inadequate sleep.

A common antidote for excessive alcohol ingestion is an increased intake of strong black coffee. In a randomized, double-blind study, the effect of caffeine (200 and 400 mg) versus placebo on driving performance was measured in a driving simulator in alcohol-impaired adults.[15] Both doses of caffeine were effective in counteracting "brake latency" but did not counteract other driving impairments caused by the alcohol.

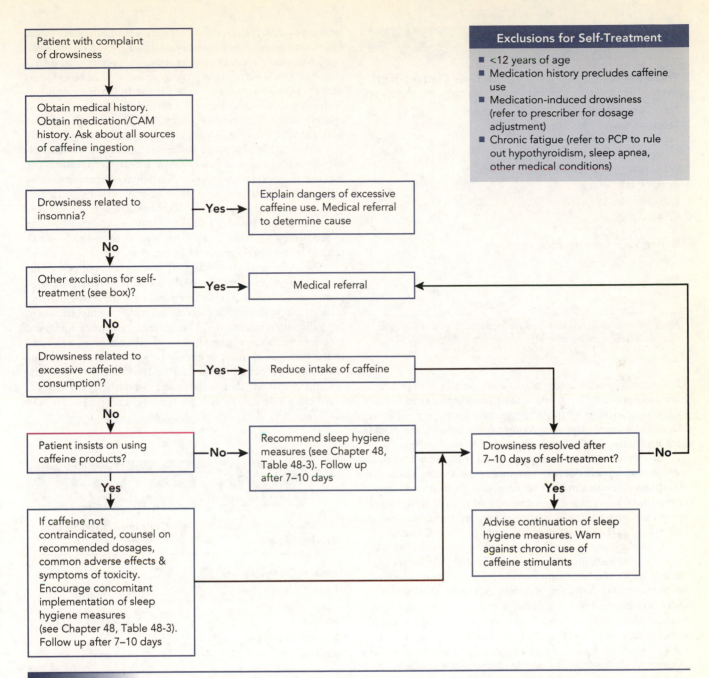

FIGURE 49-1 Self-care of drowsiness and fatigue. Key: CAM, complementary and alternative medicine; PCP, primary care provider.

Caffeine in doses varying from 4 to 10 mg/kg has improved athletic performance in endurance events such as cycling,[16] tennis,[17] swimming,[18] and rowing,[19] and may impact outcomes in competitions.

Caffeine taken in higher doses (5–8 mg/kg) can cause both cardiovascular and CNS side effects that may be manifested as increases in heart rate and blood pressure, as well as headache, symptoms of anxiety and insomnia, and an increase in hand tremor. Excessive dietary intake of caffeine has been reported to produce frequent headaches in children and adolescents.[20]

Patients who are more likely to experience adverse effects include (1) those "naive" to caffeine use,[21] (2) patients of advanced age,[22] (3) females, especially those who are caffeine-naive and nonsmokers,[23] and (4) people prone to anxiety or panic attacks.[24]

Clinicians should counsel these patients to temper their use of caffeine-containing nonprescription products in combination with dietary sources or drugs that also contain caffeine (Tables 49-1 and 49-2). The overuse of caffeine should be a part of the medication and dietary history in patients with persistent headache.

Rapid tolerance to the effects on respiratory and cardiovascular systems is common with caffeine, even in low-to-moderate doses,[25] possibly because of an upregulation of the adenosine receptors.[26] Habitual caffeine drinkers who routinely consume as little as 1 to 2 cups of coffee (or 80–160 mg caffeine per day) and abruptly discontinue caffeine may experience mild signs and symptoms of withdrawal. Common symptoms include a throbbing headache, fatigue, or anxiety that may start within

TABLE 49-2 Selected Caffeine-Containing Products

Trade Name	Caffeine Content (mg)
Nonprescription Caffeine-Only Products	
Maximum Strength NoDoz	200
Vivarin	200
Nonprescription Combination Products	
Anacin Caplets/Tab	32
Excedrin Extra Strength Gel Tabs/Tabs	65
Excedrin Migraine	65
Prescription Combination Products	
Cafergot	100
Fioricet	40
Fiorinal	40

Note: Information is not all-inclusive. Products may have changed formulations or caffeine content since time of publication.

12 hours after cessation. Symptoms usually peak in 24 to 48 hours but may persist up to 7 days.[27] The etiology of rebound or migraine headaches is often caffeine withdrawal, especially in adults or children with prolonged high-dose ingestion, and should be noted in the medication history.

In a preliminary study of prepubertal children, withdrawal and physical dependence–like symptoms were reported to occur if caffeine was consumed at 150 mg/day (or four times their normal intake) over a 2-week period of time.[28] Withdrawal symptoms in neonates have been reported after excessive (>800 mg/day) chronic maternal ingestion of caffeine.[29]

Caffeine is metabolized in the liver by the P450 CYP1A2 isoenzyme[30]; the primary demethylated metabolite is paraxanthine, which predominantly exerts a sympathomimetic effect. An exaggerated pharmacologic effect can occur when nonprescription caffeine is combined with other sources commonly found in the diet, or with prescription or nonprescription medications that contain caffeine (Table 49-2). Caffeine may increase the absorption of aspirin, which explains the rationale for its use in many headache formulations. Medications for headache and pain often contain 30 to 100 mg of caffeine per dose.

The CYP1A2 isoenzyme can be induced or inhibited by other drugs. The routine use of high doses of caffeine (>400 mg/day) could theoretically saturate the binding sites and increase the risk of interactions with drugs that share this metabolic pathway (e.g., the atypical antipsychotic clozapine). Cigarette smoking is a strong inducer of the CYP1A2 isoenzyme and has been shown to increase the clearance of caffeine by 56%. When quitting smoking, individuals should be counseled to reduce their caffeine intake by half (see Chapter 50). Conversely, hormonal contraceptives, ciprofloxacin, and fluvoxamine can inhibit the CYP1A2 isoenzyme. Although the clinical significance of these potential interactions is unknown, at-risk patients should be cautioned to moderate their use of caffeine, and the clinician should monitor for signs of such interactions.

Patients with existing coronary heart disease, uncontrolled hypertension, or preexisting arrhythmias should be counseled to avoid nonprescription caffeine-containing preparations and to moderate their intake of dietary caffeine. Several studies investigating the cardiovascular effects of caffeine intake in both healthy males[31] and females[32] have concluded that there was no increased risk for coronary artery disease, hypertension, myocardial infarction,[33] or cardiac arrythmias.[34] A small increase in blood pressure has been demonstrated in healthy individuals and patients with hypertension after the consumption of caffeine.[35] Lane and others[36] found that a relatively high dose of 500 mg of caffeine in healthy, nonsmoking, habitual coffee drinkers significantly raised systolic blood pressure by 4 mm Hg, diastolic blood pressure by 3 mm Hg, and heart rate by 2 beats per minute. The increase in blood pressure is not clinically significant in healthy individuals without hypertension, who may adapt to the cardiovascular effects possibly from tolerance. An average caffeine intake of 2 cups per day (<200 mg/day) in a large physician group during a period of 33 years was not found to be a risk factor for the development of hypertension.[37]

Patients should be cautioned about excessive consumption of caffeine in energy sports drinks and/or weight-loss supplements. Caffeine has replaced ephedra and ma huang in many weight-loss products. Natural caffeine, other methylxanthines, and caffeine-containing herbs like guarana, green tea, mate, and cola nut, are common ingredients in products that are marketed to the young consumer for energy or weight loss, but the caffeine content is often not listed on the label. Table 49-3 lists the amount of caffeine that is contained in both selected weight-loss dietary supplements and sports energy drinks. The amount of caffeine found in most products is usually equivalent to or

TABLE 49-3 Caffeine Content in Selected Dietary Supplements and Sports Energy Drinks

Trade Name	Caffeine Content (mg) per Serving
Dietary Supplements	
Dexatrim Max	50
Hydroxycut	200[a]
Metabolift	176[b]
Xenadrine NRG	300[c]
Xtreme Lean	Unknown[d]
Sports Energy Drinks[e]	
Cocaine	280
Full Throttle	150
Red Bull	80
SoBe Adrenalin Rush[f]	79
SoBe No Fear[g]	174

[a] As determined by guarana extract content plus unlisted amount of caffeine anhydrous.

[b] Total amount of methylxanthines from natural sources.

[c] As determined by guarana extract content.

[d] Contains bitter orange, methylxanthines, synephrine, and yerba mate.

[e] Caffeine content based on serving size sold.

[f] Also contains 50 mg Panax ginseng.

[g] Also contains 100 mg guarana and 100 mg *Panax ginseng*.

Note: Information is not all-inclusive. Products may have changed formulations or caffeine content since time of publication.

greater than 1 cup of coffee, or more than twice the level of caffeine contained in a can of carbonated cola. Guarana contains an even more concentrated dose of caffeine (200 mg), which can more easily lead to adverse effects when consumed in high doses or combined with other sources of caffeine commonly found in the diet or in nonprescription or prescription medications.

Product Selection Guidelines

SPECIAL POPULATIONS

Table 49-4 lists the safe amount of daily caffeine intake for special populations.

Caffeine is classified as FDA Pregnancy Category B and freely crosses the placenta. A review of the literature has concluded that moderate caffeine consumption (<300 mg/day) has little or no effect on the ability to conceive among non-smoking women.[38] Similarly, there appears to be no association between caffeine consumption (up to 300 mg/day) and the risk of miscarriage,[39] although higher consumption has been associated with an increased risk.[40,41]

No association has been found between moderate caffeine consumption and birth weight, gestational age, or fetal growth.[42] High caffeine consumption (>300 mg/day) during pregnancy has been associated with a higher risk of fetal growth retardation,[43] especially during the third trimester.[44] It would be prudent to limit total daily caffeine intake to less than 300 mg during pregnancy. A nonprescription caffeine-containing product should not be recommended during pregnancy, because combined with dietary sources it would likely increase the total daily intake to more than the maximum 300 mg.

The American Academy of Pediatrics considers usual amounts of caffeine in the diet to be compatible with breast-feeding.[45] The quantity of caffeine in breast milk after maternal ingestion of coffee has been estimated as 1.5 to 3.0 mg/cup consumed.[46] The range of caffeine concentration in breast milk is thought to be related to the mother's ability to metabolize caffeine.[8] Peak caffeine concentration in breast milk occurs 1 hour after maternal consumption. Neonates eliminate caffeine very slowly.[47] Infants unable to metabolize caffeine or those who receive large quantities of caffeine through breast milk may have symptoms of nervousness, increased heart rate, sleeplessness, poor feeding, and irritability. Women who breast-feed should be advised to consume caffeine in small-to-moderate amounts, preferably after breast-feeding to minimize effects of caffeine on the neonate.

Children are more susceptible to the cardiovascular and CNS side effects of caffeine because of their lower body weight. Soft drink consumption in adolescents has more than tripled in the past three decades.[48] In a recent study[49] in adolescents, a dose of more than 100 mg of caffeine per day (approximately three to four cans of soda) significantly increased systolic pressure.

Castellanos and others[50] completed a literature review on the behavioral effects of caffeine in children, concluding that the effects are modest at best. On the basis of available evidence to date, the maximum recommended daily intake of caffeine in children is less than 2.5 mg/kg/day.[51] Nonprescription caffeine products are not indicated in children younger than 12 years.

The elimination half-life of caffeine is prolonged in patients of advanced age,[22] increasing their susceptibility to an exaggerated pharmacologic effect and interference with sleep. It is not recommended that these patients consume caffeine in the diet or as an ingredient in a medication after dinner.

Concerns have been expressed that chronic high doses of caffeine may reduce bone mineral density (BMD) in women and increase the risk of osteoporosis and fractures. The results of studies discount the presence of a link between caffeine use and osteoporosis.[52,53] The effect of caffeine on calcium absorption is minimal, with no adverse effect on urinary calcium excretion.[54]

Tea may be protective against osteoporosis. In addition to caffeine, tea contains fluoride and many beneficial nutrients such as flavonoids. Hegarty and others,[55] studying elderly females in the United Kingdom, found that those who consumed tea had higher BMD measurements than those who did not. A Taiwanese study of men and women over the age of 30 years determined that habitual tea drinkers had an increased BMD.[56]

Complementary Therapies

The Chinese herb, ginseng, is frequently used as an adaptogen or tonic to boost "physical and mental energy and a sense of well being." A review of randomized controlled trials reveals weak and contradictory scientific evidence to support claims of enhanced mental and physical performance; this conclusion should be considered, given that various types of ginseng exist. (See Chapter 54 for detailed information on ginseng.) Other caffeine-containing dietary supplements that patients may be using as performance enhancers include cola nut, guarana, and mate; in such instances, clinicians should counsel these individuals regarding the risks of additive side effects and possible toxicity. Ingredients purported to counteract fatigue and often found in sports energy drinks include taurine and guarana; however, the amounts of these ingredients are unlikely to produce either therapeutic or adverse effects.

Assessment of Drowsiness and Fatigue: A Case-Based Approach

When assessing a patient with a complaint of daytime drowsiness, the clinician should determine the etiology of the patient's fatigue. Evaluating the patient's medical or psychiatric problems, current medication use, dietary caffeine consumption, sleep patterns, and lifestyle will help in determining the underlying cause. Given the paucity of data supporting the efficacy of caffeine, the side effects associated with recommended doses, and the effects of excessive doses of caffeine, clinicians should recommend improved sleep hygiene and lifestyle modifications or medical referral before recommending the use of a caffeine-containing product.

Case 49-1 provides an example of the assessment of patients with drowsiness and fatigue.

TABLE 49-4 Guidelines on Safe Total Daily Intake of Caffeine in Special Populations

Pregnancy	<300 mg
Breast-feeding	200–300 mg
Advanced age	<300 mg
Heart disease	<200 mg

Relevant Evaluation Criteria	Scenario/Model Outcome
Information Gathering	
1. Gather essential information about the patient's symptoms, including:	
a. description of symptom(s) (i.e., nature, onset, duration, severity, associated symptoms)	Patient picks up a 12-pack of Coca-Cola and is also requesting an OTC stimulant to help her stay awake later into the night to complete a major paper for one of her college classes. She says that she becomes drowsy after working late into the night. She reports that when she does sleep, she sleeps soundly. She denies loud snoring or any symptoms associated with sleep apnea or narcolepsy.
b. description of any factors that seem to precipitate, exacerbate, and/or relieve the patient's symptom(s)	On questioning, patient reports that her courses during the current semester have been extremely demanding and that she has been worried about her academic performance.
c. description of the patient's efforts to relieve the symptoms	Consuming 8–10 caffeinated sodas in a day (during afternoon and evening) helps to keep her awake to some extent, but this consumption causes several arousals from sleep for urination.
2. Gather essential patient history information:	
a. patient's identity	Agnes Heard
b. patient's age, sex, height, and weight	20-year-old female, 5 ft 4 in, 110 lb
c. patient's occupation	College student
d. patient's dietary habits	Healthy low-fat diet with occasional junk food, 2–3 cups of coffee in the morning, and 8–10 caffeinated sodas throughout the afternoon and evening
e. patient's sleep habits	Stays up late every night; sleeps late on Saturdays and Sundays
f. concurrent medical conditions, prescription and nonprescription medications, and dietary supplements	Seasonale 1 pink tablet daily for 84 consecutive days, followed by 1 white tablet for 7 days; recent physical examination indicated no medical problems
g. allergies	NKA
h. history of other adverse reactions to medications	None
i. other (describe) _____	N/A
Assessment and Triage	
3. Differentiate the patient's signs/symptoms and correctly identify the patient's primary problem(s).	Drowsiness while working on school assignments late into the night
4. Identify exclusions for self-treatment (see Figure 49-1).	None
5. Formulate a comprehensive list of therapeutic alternatives for the primary problem to determine if triage to a medical practitioner is required, and share this information with the patient.	Options include: (1) Refer Agnes to her PCP. (2) Recommend an OTC stimulant until Agnes can make an appointment to see her PCP. (3) Recommend good sleep hygiene and an OTC stimulant to prevent drowsiness while she completes her major paper. (4) Take no action.
Plan	
6. Select an optimal therapeutic alternative to address the patient's problem, taking into account patient preferences.	The patient prefers an OTC stimulant that, if used short term, should be able to increase her alertness. NoDoz or Vivarin 200 mg every 3–4 hours can be recommended (see Table 49-2). Sleep hygiene education (see Chapter 48, Table 48-3) should be offered, because the patient is apparently not allowing herself to satisfy her sleep need and is consuming caffeine late into the evening. Referral to her PCP is not necessary at this time, given that she recently had a physical without significant findings and her complaint appears to be directly related to her current school situation.
7. Describe the recommended therapeutic approach to the patient.	A caffeine dose of 200 mg every 3–4 hours should increase your alertness without producing significant adverse effects of the irritability or nervousness seen with higher doses.

CASE 49-1 (continued)

Relevant Evaluation Criteria	Scenario/Model Outcome
8. Explain to the patient the rationale for selecting the recommended therapeutic approach from the considered therapeutic alternatives.	Because this problem of drowsiness is tightly associated with self-induced sleep deprivation to complete a major assignment and the findings of a recent physical examination were unremarkable, there is no need to see your primary care provider. Caffeine tablets should be able to produce a modest increase in alertness if used as instructed and for a short period of time. A potential increase in side effects and toxicity exists if coffee and soda consumption continues in combination with the OTC stimulant.

Patient Education

9. When recommending self-care with non-prescription medications and/or nondrug therapy, convey accurate information to the patient:	
a. appropriate dose and frequency of administration	NoDoz or Vivarin 200 mg every 3–4 hours to a maximum of 600 mg
b. maximum number of days the therapy should be employed	Take for only 2–3 days; intermittent use should decrease the likelihood of tolerance and the consequences of chronic sleep deprivation.
c. product administration procedures	See 9a. and b.
d. expected time to onset of relief	Increased alertness should be noticed within 30 minutes; however, caffeine is not a substitute for sleep, and it is likely to be less effective as you become increasingly sleep deprived.
e. degree of relief that can be reasonably expected	Modest decrease in drowsiness and increase in alertness
f. most common side effects	Insomnia, nervousness, stomach upset, increased pulse rate
g. side effects that warrant medical intervention should they occur	Chest pain, palpitations, or irregular heart beat; combination of caffeine and oral contraceptive may increase the risk of adverse effects (e.g., increased heart rate, anxiety, hand tremor) attributable to decreased caffeine metabolism. If used in high doses chronically and abruptly discontinued, a caffeine withdrawal syndrome may be experienced.
h. patient options in the event that condition worsens or persists	Stop caffeine and see health care provider.
i. product storage requirements	Keep in original container, away from children and pets.
j. specific nondrug measures	You should practice the principles of good sleep hygiene.
10. Solicit follow-up questions from patient.	Can I double the dose of any of these products to see results more quickly?
11. Answer patient's questions.	No. Doubling the dose of any of these products will only increase your risk of suffering unwanted adverse effects.

Key: N/A, not available; NKA, no known allergies; OTC, over-the-counter; PCP, primary care provider.

Patient Counseling for Fatigue and Drowsiness

Counseling on the treatment of drowsiness and fatigue should focus on practicing good sleep hygiene and eliminating factors that may interfere with normal sleep. If a caffeine product is indicated, the clinician should review dosage guidelines with the patient, and emphasize the adverse effects and drug interactions that can occur with its use. The patient should be counseled on symptoms of excessive caffeine ingestion such as irritability, tremor, rapid pulse, dizziness, or heart palpitations, especially in elderly patients with cardiac disease. Regular users of caffeine should also be counseled on withdrawal symptoms such as headache and anxiety, which can occur if caffeine from any source is stopped abruptly. The box Patient Education for Fatigue and Drowsiness lists information to provide patients.

Evaluation of Patient Outcomes for Fatigue and Drowsiness

Successful outcomes include daytime alertness, increased productivity, and peak performance with respect to psychomotor tasks and cognitive function, including attention and concentration. An individual should be advised to seek medical evaluation if, after 7 to 10 days, drowsiness and fatigue persist despite the limited use of caffeine-containing products and the establishment of good sleep hygiene.

PATIENT EDUCATION FOR
Drowsiness And Fatigue

The objective of self-treatment is to maintain wakefulness. For most patients, improved sleep hygiene will help ensure optimal therapeutic outcomes. If the patient insists on taking a caffeine-containing product, carefully following product instructions and the self-care measures listed here will help ensure optimal therapeutic outcomes for most patients.

Nondrug Measures

- Practice good principles of sleep hygiene. (See Chapter 48, Table 48-3.)
- If drowsiness or fatigue persists or recurs, consult your primary care provider.

Nonprescription Medications

- Do not exceed the recommended dose of 200 mg every 3–4 hours to a maximum daily dose of 600 mg. Note that higher doses of caffeine may cause side effects and that chronic use may result in tolerance as well as withdrawal symptoms upon abrupt discontinuation.
- Do not use caffeine tablets in combination with coffee or other caffeinated products, including dietary supplements.
- Do not use if pregnant or breast-feeding.

- Do not use in children younger than 12 years.
- If you are taking clozapine, hormonal contraceptives, or ciprofloxacin, consult your primary care provider before using caffeine-containing products.
- If you have symptomatic gastroesophageal reflux disease or a history of kidney stones, avoid caffeine supplements and minimize dietary intake of caffeine.
- If you have a history of peptic ulcer disease, psychiatric disorders, symptomatic heart disease, or uncontrolled hypertension, consult your primary care provider before using caffeine products.

⚠ Seek medical attention immediately if symptoms of caffeine toxicity occur:
—Increases in heart rate and blood pressure
—Headache
—Symptoms of anxiety and insomnia
—Increase in hand tremor

Key Points for Fatigue and Drowsiness

➤ Chronic excessive sleepiness is a warning—it is generally the result of sleep deprivation (quantity and/or quality), and it is dangerous and potentially life threatening to continue without sleep.

➤ Caffeine is a nonselective adenosine receptor blocker, which is widely available and is most effective when used intermittently at doses of 200 mg or more.

➤ Caffeine in any form appears to be safe and effective in low-to-moderate doses in the diet, and for occasional use as a nonprescription supplement while completing tasks of short duration when enhanced alertness is desired.

➤ Pregnant or breast-feeding patients, children younger than 12 years, patients with heart disease, or patients with anxiety or psychiatric disorders should avoid caffeine.

➤ Clinicians should be aware of the various prescription and nonprescription medications, and diet supplements that contain caffeine, as well as the patient's dietary consumption of caffeine.

➤ Side effects of caffeine are more likely to occur in occasional users and patients of advanced age.

➤ In patients taking higher daily doses of caffeine, drug interactions can occur with medications that share a similar metabolic pathway with caffeine.

➤ There are insufficient data for clinicians to recommend the use of ginseng or other herbal supplements to increase energy or decrease fatigue.

REFERENCES

1. Stutts JC, Wilkins JW, Osberg JS, et al. Driver risk factors for sleep-related crashes. *Accid Anal Prev.* 2003;35:321–31.
2. Williamson AM, Feyer AM. Moderate sleep deprivation produces impairments in cognitive and motor performance equivalent to legally prescribed levels of alcohol intoxication. *Occup Environ Med.* 2000;57:649–55.
3. Barger LK, Cade BE, Najib TA, et al. Extended work shifts and the risk of motor vehicle crashes among interns. *N Engl J Med.* 2005;352:125–34.
4. International Food Information Council Foundation. Caffeine & Health: Clarifying the Controversies. Available at: http://www.ific.org/publications/reviews/upload/Caffeine_v8-2.pdf. Last accessed October 9, 2008.
5. Silver R, LeSauter J. Circadian and homeostatic factors in arousal. *Ann NY Acad Sci.* 2008;1129:263–74.
6. Daly JW. Mechanism of action of caffeine. In: Garattini S, ed. *Caffeine, Coffee and Health.* New York: Raven Press; 1993:97–150.
7. Mumford GK, Benowitz NL, Evans SM, et al. Absorption rate of methylxanthines following capsules, cola and chocolate. *Eur J Clin Pharmacol.* 1996;51:319–25.
8. Massey LK, Sutton RA. Acute effects on urine composition and calcium kidney stone risk in calcium stone formers. *J Urol.* 2004; 172:555–8.
9. Bonnet MH, Arand DL. Caffeine use as a model of acute and chronic insomnia. *Sleep.* 1992;15:526–36.
10. Patat A, Rosenzweig P, Enslen M, et al. Effects of a new slow release formulation of caffeine on EEG, psychomotor and cognitive functions in sleep-deprived subjects. *Hum Psychopharmacol.* 2000;15:153–70.
11. Richardson NJ, Rogers PJ, Elliman NA, et al. Mood and performance effects of caffeine in relation to acute and chronic caffeine deprivation. *Pharmacol Biochem Behav.* 1995;52:313–20.
12. Smit HJ, Rogers PJ. Effects of low doses of caffeine on cognitive performance, mood and thirst in low and higher caffeine consumers. *Psychopharmacologia.* 2000;152:167–73.
13. Hindmarch I, Rigney U, Stanley N, et al. A naturalistic investigation of the effects of day-long consumption of tea, coffee and water on alertness, sleep onset and sleep quality. *Psychopharmacologia.* 2000;149:203–16.
14. Reyner LA, Horne JA. Early morning driver sleepiness: effectiveness of 200 mg caffeine. *Psychophysiology.* 2000;37:251–6.
15. Liguori A, Robinson JH. Caffeine antagonism of alcohol-induced driving impairment. *Drug Alcohol Depend.* 2001;63:123–9.
16. Bell DG, Jacobs I, Zamecnik J. Effects of caffeine, ephedrine and their combination on time to exhaustion during high intensity exercise. *Eur J Appl Physiol.* 1998;77:427–33.
17. Ferrauti A, Weber K, Struder, HK. Metabolic and ergogenic effects of carbohydrate and caffeine beverages in tennis. *J Sports Med Phys Fit.* 1997; 37:258–66.

18. MacIntosh, BR, Wright BM. Caffeine ingestion and performance of a 1,500-metre swim. *Can J Appl Physiol*. 1995;20:168–77.

19. Bruce CR, Anderson ME, Fraser SF, et al. Enhancement of 2000-m rowing performance after caffeine ingestion. *Med Sci Sports Exerc*. 2000;32:1958–63.

20. Hering-Hanit R, Gadoth N. Caffeine-induced headache in children and adolescents. *Cephalalgia*. 2003;23:332–5.

21. Benowitz NL. Clinical pharmacology of caffeine. *Annu Rev Med*. 1990;41:277–88.

22. Massey LK. Caffeine and the elderly. *Drugs Aging*. 1998;13:43–50.

23. Carrillo JA, Benitez J. CYP 1A2 activity, gender and smoking as variables influencing the toxicity of caffeine. *Br J Clin Pharmacol*. 1996;41:605–8.

24. Charney DS, Heninger GR, Jatlow PI. Increased anxiogenic effects of caffeine in panic disorders. *Arch Gen Psych*. 1985;42:233–43.

25. Daly JW, Fredholm BB. Caffeine: an atypical drug of dependence. *Drug Alcohol Depend*. 1998;51:199–206.

26. Varani K, Portaluppi F, Merighi S, et al. Caffeine alters A2A adenosine receptors and their function in human platelets. *Circulation*. 1999;9:2499–502.

27. Schuh KJ, Griffiths RR. Caffeine reinforcement: the role of withdrawal. *Psychopharmacology*. 1977;132:320.

28. Bernstein GA, Carroll ME, Dean NW, et al. Caffeine withdrawal in normal school-age children. *J Am Acad Child Adoles Psychiatr*. 1998;37:858–65.

29. McGowan JD, Altman RE, Kanto WPJ. Neonatal withdrawal symptoms after chronic maternal ingestion of caffeine. *South Med J*. 1988;81:1092–4.

30. Tantcheva-Poor I, Zaigler M, Rietbrock S, et al. Estimation of cytochrome P-450 CYP 1A2 activity in 863 healthy Caucasians using a saliva-based caffeine test. *Pharmacogenetics*. 1999;9:131–44.

31. Grobbee DE, Rimm EB, Giovannucci E, et al. Coffee, caffeine, and cardiovascular disease in men. *N Engl J Med*. 1990;323:1026–32.

32. Willett WC, Stampler MJ, Manson JE, et al. Coffee consumption and coronary heart disease in women: a ten year follow-up. *JAMA*. 1996;275:458–62.

33. Myers MG, Basinski A. Coffee and coronary heart disease. *Arch Int Med*. 1992;152:1767–72.

34. Myers MG. Caffeine and cardiac arrhythmias. *Ann Int Med*. 1991;114:147–50.

35. Jee SH, He J, Whelton PK, et al. The effect of coffee on blood pressure: a meta-analysis of controlled clinical trials. *Can J Cardiol*. 1997;13 (suppl B):36B.

36. Lane JD, Peiper CF, Phillips-Bute BG, et al. Caffeine affects cardiovascular and neuroendocrine activation at work and home. *Psychosom Med*. 2002;64:595–603.

37. Klag MJ, Wang NY, Meoni LA. Coffee intake and risk of hypertension: the Johns Hopkins precursors study. *Arch Int Med*. 2002;162:657–62.

38. Leviton A, Cawan L. A review of the literature relating caffeine consumption by women to their risk of reproductive hazards. *Food Chem Toxicol*. 2002;40:1271–310.

39. Klebanoff MA, Levine RJ, DerSimonian R, et al. Maternal serum paraxanthine, a caffeine metabolite, and the risk of spontaneous abortion. *N Engl J Med*. 1999;341:1639–44.

40. Rasch V. Cigarette, alcohol and caffeine consumption: risk factors for spontaneous abortion. *Acta Obstet Gyn Scand*. 2003;82:182–8.

41. Gianelli M, Doyle P, Roman E, et al. The effect of caffeine consumption and nausea on the risk of miscarriage. *Paediatr Perinat Epidemiol*. 2003;17:316–23.

42. Clausson B, Granath F, Ekbom A, et al. Effects of caffeine exposure during pregnancy on birth weight and gestational age. *Am J Epidemiol*. 2002;155:429–36.

43. Bracken MB, Triche EW, Belanger K, et al. Association of maternal caffeine consumption with decrements in fetal growth. *Am J Epidemiol*. 2003;157:456–66.

44. Vik T, Bakketeig LS, Trygg KU, et al. High caffeine consumption in the third trimester of pregnancy: gender-specific effects on fetal growth. *Paediatr Perinat Epidemiol*. 2003;17:324–31.

45. Committee on Drugs, American Academy of Pediatrics. The transfer of drugs and other chemicals into human milk. *Pediatrics*. 1994;93:137–50.

46. Tyrala EE, Dodson WE. Caffeine secretion into breast milk. *Arch Dis Child*. 1979;54:787–800.

47. Ryu JE. Caffeine in human milk and in serum of breast fed infants. *Dev Pharmacol Ther*. 1985;8:329–37.

48. St-Onge M-P, Keller KL, Heymsfield SB. Changes in childhood food consumption patterns: a cause for concern in light of increasing body weights. *Am J Clin Nutr*. 2003;78:1068–73.

49. Savoca MR, Evans CD, Wilson ME, et al. The association of caffeinated beverages with blood pressure in adolescents. *Arch Ped Adoles Med*. 2004;158:473–7.

50. Castellanos FX, Rapoport JL. Effects of caffeine on development and behavior in infancy and childhood: a review of the published literature. *Food Chem Toxicol*. 2002;40:1235–42.

51. Nawrot P, Jordan S, Eastwood J, et al. Effects of caffeine on human health. *Food Addit Contam*. 2003;20:1–30.

52. Conlisk AJ, Galuska DA. Is caffeine associated with bone mineral density in young adult women? *Prevent Med*. 2000;31:562–8.

53. Lloyd T, Hohnson-Rollings N, Eggli DF, et al. Bone status among postmenopausal women with different habitual caffeine intakes: a longitudinal investigation. *J Am Coll Nutr*. 2000;19:256–61.

54. Heaney RP, Rafferty K. Carbonated beverages and urinary calcium excretion. *Am J Clin Nutr*. 2001;74:343–7.

55. Hegarty VM, May HM, Khaw KT. Tea drinking and bone mineral density in older women. *Am J Clin Nutr*. 2000;71:1003–7.

56. Wu-Hsing C, Yi-Ching Y, Wei-Jen Y, et al. Epidemiological evidence of increased bone mineral density in habitual tea drinkers. *Arch Int Med*. 2002;162:1001–6.

Smoking Cessation

Lisa A. Kroon, Karen Suchanek Hudmon, and Robin L. Corelli

In 1982, the U.S. Surgeon General C. Everett Koop stated that cigarette smoking was the "chief, single, avoidable cause of death in our society and the most important public health issue of our time."[1] This statement remains true today, more than 25 years later. In the United States, cigarette smoking is the leading known cause of preventable death,[2] responsible for approximately 438,000 deaths each year.[3] In addition to lives lost, the economic effect of smoking is enormous—each pack of cigarettes smoked costs society $7.18 for associated medical care ($3.45) and lost productivity ($3.73), totaling $157 billion in annual health-related economic losses.[3]

Despite the well-established and well-publicized negative effects of smoking, an estimated 20.8% of adult Americans (23.9% of males and 18.0% of females, in 2006) smoke either every day (80.1%) or some days (19.9%).[4] The prevalence of smoking varies by sociodemographic factors, including sex, race-ethnicity, education level, age, and socioeconomic status.[4] In 2006, the prevalence of smoking in the United States was highest among American Indian/Alaska Natives (32.4%) and next highest among non-Hispanic blacks (23.0%), followed by non-Hispanic whites (21.9%), Hispanics (15.2%), and non-Hispanic Asians (10.4%).[4] Smoking also is more common among persons of lower educational levels and those living below the federal poverty level.[4] The median prevalence of smoking varies by state, with Utah exhibiting the lowest prevalence at 9.8% and Kentucky exhibiting the highest at 28.6%.[5] An estimated 70% of smokers want to quit,[6] and in 2006 approximately 44.2% had stopped smoking at least 1 day during the past year because they were trying to quit.[4] This suggests that many patients will be receptive to cessation advice, and clinicians can have an important role in helping patients to achieve long-term abstinence.

Pathophysiology of Tobacco Use and Dependence

In 1988, the U.S. Surgeon General released a landmark report, concluding that tobacco products are effective nicotine delivery systems capable of inducing and sustaining chemical dependence. The primary criteria used to categorize nicotine as an addictive substance included its (1) psychoactive effects, (2) use in a highly controlled or compulsive manner, and (3) reinforcement of behavioral patterns of tobacco use. The underlying pharmacologic and behavioral processes associated with tobacco dependence are considered to be similar to those that determine addiction to drugs such as heroin and cocaine.[7]

As with other addictive substances (e.g., opiates, cocaine, amphetamines), nicotine stimulates the mesolimbic dopaminergic system in the midbrain, inducing pleasant or rewarding effects that promote continued use of the drug.[8] Nicotine binds to the $alpha_4beta_2$ nicotinic receptor in the ventral tegmental area of the brain, triggering the release of dopamine in the nucleus accumbens. Psychosocial, behavioral, and environmental factors also play an important role in establishing and maintaining dependence.[9] For example, smoking commonly is associated with specific activities such as driving, talking on the telephone, drinking coffee or alcohol, being around others who smoke, and eating. Over time, the habitual use of cigarettes under these circumstances can lead to the development of smoking routines that can be difficult to break. Indeed, specific environmental situations can become powerful conditioned stimuli associated with smoking and are capable of triggering "automatic" smoking patterns.[9] Comorbidities, particularly mental illness, also contribute to tobacco use—an estimated 44.3% of all cigarettes smoked in the United States are smoked by persons with mental illness.[10]

It is well established that tobacco is a detrimental substance,[11] and its use dramatically increases one's odds of dependence, disease, disability, and death. Cigarettes are carefully engineered and heavily marketed products—the tobacco industry spends nearly $19 to market its products for every $1 that the states spend on tobacco control.[12] Cigarettes are the *only* marketed consumable product that, when used as intended, will kill half or more of its users.[13]

Cigarette smoke, which is classified by the Environmental Protection Agency as a Class A carcinogen (i.e., a carcinogen with no safe level of exposure for humans), is a complex mixture of an estimated 4800 compounds found in gaseous and particulate phases. Approximately 500 compounds are present in the vapor phase, including nitrogen, carbon monoxide, ammonia, hydrogen cyanide, and benzene. The remaining constituents of tobacco smoke, including nicotine, are found in the particulate phase. The particulate fraction, excluding the nicotine and water components, is collectively referred to as tar. Numerous carcinogens, including polycyclic aromatic hydrocarbons and nitrosamines, have been identified in the tar fraction of tobacco smoke.[14]

Nicotine, the addictive component of tobacco, is distilled from burning tobacco and carried in tar droplets to the small airways of the lung, where it is absorbed rapidly into the arterial circulation and distributed throughout the body. Nicotine readily penetrates the central nervous system and is estimated to reach the brain within seconds after inhalation.[9] Nicotine binds to receptors in the brain and other organs, inducing a variety of predominantly stimulatory effects on the cardiovascular, endocrine, nervous, and metabolic systems.[8,9] Pharmacodynamic effects associated with nicotine administration include arousal and increases in the heart rate and blood pressure. In the brain, smoking leads to nicotinic cholinergic receptor activation and the release of numerous neurotransmitters, which induce a range of effects such as pleasure (dopamine), arousal (acetylcholine, norepinephrine), cognitive enhancement (acetylcholine), appetite suppression (dopamine, norepinephrine, serotonin), learning and memory enhancement (glutamate), mood modulation (serotonin), and reduction of anxiety and tension (beta-endorphin and gamma-aminobutyric acid).[9]

Clinical Presentation of Tobacco Use and Dependence

Most chronic tobacco users develop tolerance to the effects of nicotine, and abrupt cessation precipitates symptoms of nicotine withdrawal. The symptoms, and their severity, vary from person to person but generally include irritability, frustration, anger, anxiety, depression, difficulty concentrating, impatience, insomnia, and restlessness. Other symptoms that patients might report include cravings, hunger, impaired performance, constipation, cough, dizziness, and increased dreaming. Typically, the physiologic nicotine withdrawal symptoms peak within a few days after quitting and gradually dissipate over 2 to 4 weeks.[15]

According to a report issued by the U.S. Surgeon General in 2004, smoking adversely affects nearly every organ system in the body and plays a causal role in the development of numerous diseases (Table 50-1).[11] Furthermore, the report concluded that smoking cigarettes with lower machine-measured yields of tar and nicotine (e.g., "light" cigarettes) provided no clear benefit to health.[11] Involuntary exposure to secondhand smoke, which includes the smoke emanating from burning tobacco and that exhaled by the smoker, is associated with adverse health effects in nonsmoking adults and children, including cardiovascular disease, respiratory disease, and lung cancer.[16] There is no safe level of exposure to secondhand smoke.[16]

Many clinically significant interactions between tobacco smoke and medications have been identified. Tobacco smoke interacts with medications through pharmacokinetic or pharmacodynamic mechanisms that may lead to reduced therapeutic efficacy or, less commonly, increased toxicity.[17] Most of the pharmacokinetic interactions are the result of induction of hepatic cytochrome P450 (CYP) enzymes (primarily the CYP1A2 isozyme) by polycyclic aromatic hydrocarbons present in tobacco smoke.[17] Induction of the CYP1A2 enzyme can increase the hepatic metabolism of certain drugs (Table 50-2), potentially resulting in a reduced therapeutic response or need for higher dosages in smokers; conversely, the dosages of some drugs might need to be reduced in patients who quit smoking.[17] Similarly, the clearance of caffeine is significantly increased (by 56%) in smokers. Following cessation, smokers who drink caffeinated beverages should be advised to decrease their usual caffeine intake to avoid higher levels of caffeine, which may induce symptoms similar to nicotine withdrawal.

A significant pharmacodynamic drug interaction occurs with tobacco smoke and hormonal contraceptives (pills, patch, and ring). Data indicate that cigarette smoking substantially increases the risk of serious adverse cardiovascular events (stroke,

---

TABLE 50-1 Health Consequences of Smoking

Cancer

Acute myeloid leukemia
Bladder
Cervical
Esophageal
Gastric
Kidney
Laryngeal
Lung
Oral cavity and pharyngeal
Pancreatic

Cardiovascular Diseases

Abdominal aortic aneurysm
Coronary heart disease (angina pectoris, ischemic heart disease, myocardial infarction)
Cerebrovascular disease (transient ischemic attacks, stroke)
Peripheral arterial disease

Pulmonary Diseases

Acute respiratory illnesses
    Upper respiratory tract (rhinitis, sinusitis, laryngitis, pharyngitis)
    Lower respiratory tract (bronchitis, pneumonia)
Chronic respiratory illnesses
    Chronic obstructive pulmonary disease
    Respiratory symptoms
    Poor asthma control
    Reduced lung function

Reproductive Effects

Reduced fertility in women
Pregnancy and pregnancy outcomes
    Preterm, premature rupture of membranes
    Placenta previa
    Placental abruption
    Preterm delivery
    Low infant birth weight
Infant mortality
    Sudden infant death syndrome (SIDS)

Other Effects

Cataract
Osteoporosis (reduced bone density in postmenopausal women, increased risk of hip fracture)
Periodontitis
Peptic ulcer disease (in patients infected with *Helicobacter pylori*)
Surgical outcomes
    Poor wound healing
    Respiratory complications

Source: Reference 11.

---

myocardial infarction, and thromboembolism) in women using oral contraceptives.[18–24] This risk is markedly increased in women who are aged 35 years or older and smoke 15 or more cigarettes per day.[22] Accordingly, most experts consider use of hormonal contraceptives to be a contraindication in this population, and an alternative form of contraception should be used.[19,23,25] Additional interactions, with corresponding underlying mechanisms for the interactions, are depicted in Table 50-2.[17,26] During the course of routine patient care, it is important to assess for potential drug–smoking interactions, and make appropriate adjustments to the

TABLE 50-2 Drug Interactions with Tobacco Smoke	
Drug/Class	**Mechanism of Interaction and Effects**
Benzodiazepines (diazepam, chlordiazepoxide)	Pharmacodynamic: decreased sedation and drowsiness, possibly caused by nicotine stimulation of the central nervous system
Bendamustine	May reduce serum concentrations; use with caution in patients who smoke
Beta-blockers	Pharmacodynamic: decreased control of hypertension and heart rate, possibly caused by nicotine-mediated sympathetic activation
Caffeine	Increased metabolism (induction of CYP1A2); clearance increased 56%; possible increased caffeine levels after smoking cessation
Chlorpromazine	Decreased AUC (36%) and serum concentrations (24%); decreased sedation and hypotension possible in smokers; patients who smoke may need increased dosages
Clozapine	Increased metabolism (induction of CYP1A2); decreased plasma concentrations (18%); closely monitor drug levels upon cessation and reduce dose as required to avoid toxicity
Corticosteriods, inhaled	Smokers with asthma may have reduced response to inhaled corticosteroids
Erlotinib	Increased clearance (24%) and reduced trough serum concentrations (2-fold)
Flecainide	Increased clearance (61%); decreased trough serum concentrations (25%); smokers may need increased dosages
Fluvoxamine	Increased metabolism (induction of CYP1A2); increased clearance (24%); decreased AUC (31%); decreased plasma concentrations (32%); dosage modifications not routinely recommended but smokers may need increased dosages
Haloperidol	Increased clearance (44%); decreased serum concentrations (70%)
Heparin	Mechanism unknown but increased clearance and decreased half-life observed; smokers may need increased dosages
Insulin, subcutaneous	Possible decreased insulin absorption secondary to peripheral vasoconstriction; possible release of endogenous substances that antagonize insulin's effects; interactions likely not clinically significant; smokers may need increased dosages
Irinotecan	Increased clearance (18%) and decreased serum concentrations of active metabolite (~40% by glucuronidation); decreased systemic exposure resulting in lower hematologic toxicity and may reduce efficacy; smokers may need increased dosages
Mexiletine	Increased clearance (25%; by oxidation and glucuronidation); decreased half-life (36%)
Olanzapine	Increased metabolism (induction of CYP1A2); increased clearance (98%); decreased serum concentrations (12%); dosage modifications not routinely recommended, but smokers may need increased dosages
Opioids (propoxyphene, pentazocine)	Pharmacodynamic: unknown mechanism, decreased analgesic effect; smokers may need increased dosages for pain relief
Hormonal contraceptives	Pharmacodynamic: increased risk of cardiovascular adverse effects (e.g., stroke, myocardial infarction, and thromboembolism) in women who smoke and use hormonal contraceptives; substantially increased risk in women aged at least 35 years who smoke at least 15 cigarettes per day
Propranolol	Increased clearance (77%; by side-chain oxidation and glucuronidation)
Ropinirole	Decreased maximum serum concentration (38%) and area under the curve (30%) in study of patients with restless legs syndrome; smokers need increased dosages
Tacrine	Increased metabolism (induction of CYP1A2); decreased half-life (50%); serum concentrations 3-fold lower; smokers may need increased dosages
Theophylline	Increased metabolism (induction of CYP1A2); increased clearance (58%–100%); decreased half-life (63%); levels should be monitored if smoking is started, discontinued, or changed; increased clearance with passive smoking (secondhand smoke); considerably increased maintenance doses in smokers
Tizanidine	Decreased area under the curve (30%–40%) and reduced half-life (10%) was observed in male smokers

Source: References 17 and 26. Adapted with permission from reference 26. Copyright © 1999–2009 The Regents of the University of California, University of Southern California, and Western University of Health Sciences. All rights reserved.

medication regimen. For patients who are quitting, dosage adjustments might be necessary for some medications.

Benefits of Smoking Cessation

The 1990 Surgeon General's Report on the health benefits of smoking cessation outlined the numerous and substantial health benefits incurred when patients quit smoking.[27] Some health benefits are incurred shortly (e.g., within 2 weeks to 3 months) after quitting, and others are incurred over time (Figure 50–1). On average, cigarette smokers die approximately 10 years earlier than nonsmokers, and, of those who continue smoking, at least half will eventually die of a tobacco-related disease. Quitting at ages 30, 40, 50, and 60 years results in a gain of 10, 9, 6, and 3 years of life, respectively.[13] Thus, although it is important to educate tobacco users that it is never too late to quit and incur many of the associated health benefits, there are significant benefits to quitting earlier in life.

TIME ELAPSED

20 minutes after quitting: Blood pressure drops to a level close to that before the last cigarette. Temperature of hands and feet increases to normal.

8 hours after quitting: Blood levels of carbon monoxide drop to normal.

24 hours after quitting: Chance of having a heart attack decreases.

2 weeks to 3 months after quitting: Circulation improves, and lung function improves by up to 30%.

1 to 9 months after quitting: Coughing, sinus congestion, fatigue, and shortness of breath decrease, and cilia regain normal function in the lungs, increasing the ability to handle mucus, clear the lungs, and reduce infection.

1 year after quitting: Excessive risk of coronary heart disease is half that of a smoker's.

5 years after quitting: Risk of stroke is reduced to that of a nonsmoker 5 to 15 years after quitting.

10 years after quitting: Lung cancer death rate is about half that of continuing smokers. Risk of cancer of the mouth, throat, esophagus, bladder, kidney, and pancreas also are lower than that of continuing smokers.

15 years after quitting: Risk of coronary heart disease is similar to that of a nonsmoker.

FIGURE 50-1 Health benefits of smoking cessation. (*Source:* Reference 27.)

Smoking Cessation Treatment

Treatment Goals

Tobacco dependence is a chronic disease characterized by multiple failed attempts to quit before long-term cessation is achieved.[28] Because tobacco use is a complex, addictive behavior, helping a patient to quit and prevent relapse is best achieved by combining appropriate pharmacotherapy with counseling. For any patient who uses tobacco, the primary goal is complete, long-term abstinence from all nicotine-containing products.

General Treatment Approach

Most smokers use no cessation treatments for their quit attempts,[29] and approximately 95% of all quit attempts end in relapse.[28] Yet decades of research clearly show that patients who receive assistance have increased odds of quitting.[28] In 2008, the U.S. Public Health Service published an updated clinical practice guideline for treating tobacco use and dependence,[28] which presents evidence-based recommendations and effective strategies for clinician-facilitated tobacco cessation counseling. Although even brief advice from a clinician is associated with increased odds of quitting,[28,30] more intensive counseling (longer and more frequent counseling sessions, or greater overall contact time) and use of pharmacotherapy (excluding patients who should not self-treat, as listed in Figure 50-2) result in increased quit rates.[28] Two particularly effective types of counseling are practical counseling (problem solving and skills training) and social support delivered as part of treatment.[28]

In a meta-analysis of 29 studies,[28] it was determined that patients who receive a tobacco cessation intervention from a non-physician clinician or a physician clinician are 1.7 and 2.2 times as likely to quit (at ≥5 months after cessation), respectively, than are patients who do not receive an intervention from a clinician.

Self-help materials are only slightly better than no clinician intervention. Although the length of an intervention increases effectiveness, even minimal interventions (<3 minutes) increase cessation rates.[28] In a meta-analysis of 46 studies, 4 or more sessions was found to approximately double cessation rates.[28]

Although the use of pharmacotherapy approximately doubles a patient's chances of quitting, the addition of counseling further increases cessation rates (1.4 times as likely to quit).[28] Similarly, adding pharmacotherapy to counseling increases cessation rates. Therefore, cessation interventions should consist of pharmacotherapy (one or a combination of medications) and counseling, when medications are not contraindicated (see Special Populations).[28] Figure 50-2 outlines a self-treatment approach for smoking cessation.

Nonpharmacologic Therapy

Helping Patients Quit: The 5 A's Approach (Comprehensive Counseling)

Five key components of comprehensive counseling for tobacco cessation are (1) asking patients whether they use tobacco, (2) advising tobacco users to quit, (3) assessing patients' readiness to quit, (4) assisting patients with quitting, and (5) arranging follow-up care. These steps are referred to as the "5 A's."[28]

ASK ABOUT TOBACCO USE

A key first step is asking about tobacco use. Because tobacco use is the primary known preventable cause of mortality in the United States, and because tobacco smoke interacts with multiple medications, screening for tobacco use is crucial and should be a routine component of care. The following question can be used to identify all types of tobacco use, even for infrequent users: "Do you ever smoke or use any type of tobacco?" Tobacco use status should be considered a vital sign and collected routinely along with blood pressure, pulse, weight, temperature, and respiratory rate.[28] At a minimum, tobacco use status (current, former, never a user) and level of use (e.g., number of cigarettes smoked per day) should be documented in the medical record and reassessed periodically. Clinicians should also consider asking about exposure to secondhand smoke.

ADVISE TO QUIT

All tobacco users should be advised to quit. The advice should be clear, strong, and personalized, yet delivered with sensitivity and a tone of voice that communicates concern for the patient and a willingness to assist the patient with quitting when he or she is ready. When possible, clinicians should individualize the messages by linking their advice to the patient's health status, current medication regimen, personal reasons for wanting to quit, or the effect of tobacco on others. For example, "Ms. Bettis, I see that you now are on two different inhalers for your emphysema. Quitting smoking is the single most important treatment for your emphysema. I strongly encourage you to quit, and I would like to help you."

ASSESS READINESS TO QUIT

Because many patients will not be ready to quit in the near future, it is important for clinicians to gauge patients' readiness to quit before recommending a treatment regimen. Patients should be categorized as (1) not ready to quit in the next month; (2) ready to quit in the next month; (3) a recent quitter, having quit in the past 6 months; or (4) a former user, having quit more than 6 months ago.[28] This classification defines the clinician's next course of action, which is to provide counseling that is tailored to the patient's readiness to quit. The following is an example for a current smoker: "Mr. Crosby, have you given any thought to quitting? Is this something that you might consider doing in the next month?" Counseling a patient who is ready to quit in the next month should be different from counseling a patient who is not considering quitting in the near future.

ASSIST WITH QUITTING

Important elements of the "assist" component of treatment include helping patients to make the decision and commitment to quit and setting an actual quit date. Clinicians should be empathetic to the fact that quitting is a difficult process. As such, the goal is to help maximize patients' chances of success by designing an individualized treatment plan.

Except in the presence of special circumstances, or with specific populations for which there is inadequate evidence of effectiveness (pregnant women, smokeless tobacco users, light smokers, and adolescents), all patients attempting to quit should be encouraged to use pharmacotherapy (described later) combined with counseling, because this combination will yield higher quit rates than either approach alone.[28] Counseling inter-

ventions, which focus on promoting behavior change and enhancing adherence with medication regimens, include individualized counseling (e.g., in person or by telephone), a group cessation program, an Internet-based program, or a combination of these approaches.

ARRANGE FOLLOW-UP COUNSELING

Because a patient's ability to quit increases substantially when multiple counseling interactions are provided, arranging follow-up counseling is an important, yet typically neglected, element of treatment for tobacco dependence. Follow-up contact should occur soon after the quit date, preferably during the first week. This does not have to be done in person and could be performed by telephone or e-mail. A second follow-up contact is recommended within the first month after quitting.[28] Periodically, additional follow-up contacts should occur, to monitor patient progress (including adherence with pharmacotherapy) and to provide ongoing support. Quit rates at 5 or more months after cessation are associated with the total number of contacts: 12.4% for 0 to 1 contact, 16.3% for 2 to 3 contacts, 20.9% for 4 to 8 contacts, and 24.7% for more than 8 contacts.[28]

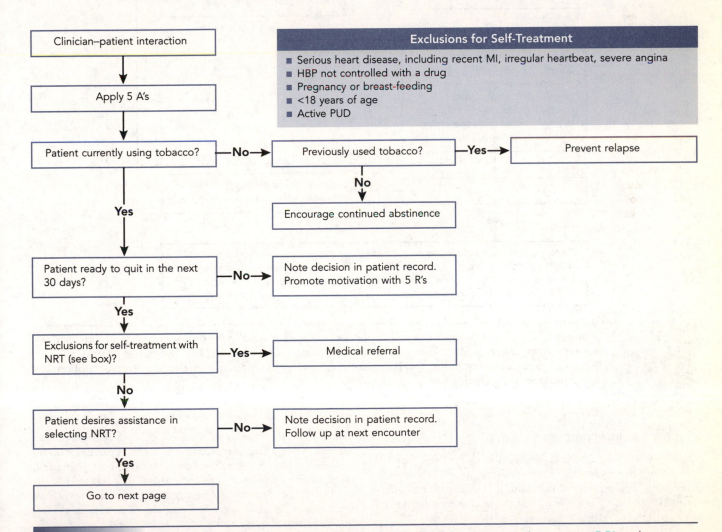

FIGURE 50-2 Self-care of tobacco use and dependence. Key: 5 A's, ask, advise, assess, assist, arrange; 5 R's, relevance, risks, rewards, roadblocks, repetition; HBP, high blood pressure; MI, myocardial infarction; NRT, nicotine replacement therapy; OTC, over-the-counter; PUD, peptic ulcer disease; Rx, prescription; TMJ, temporomandibular joint. *(continued on next page)*

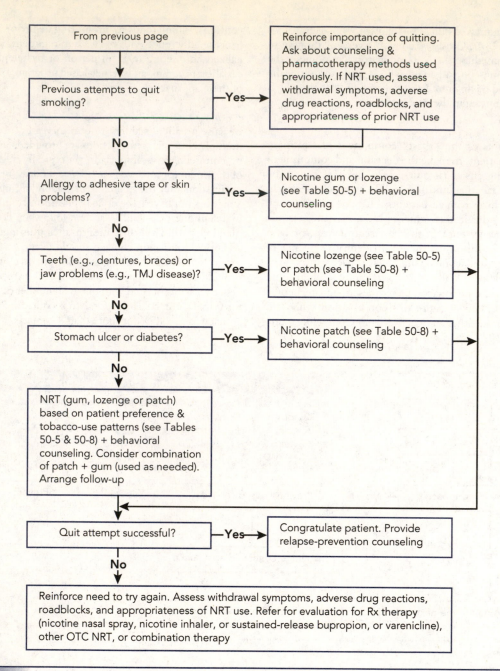

FIGURE 50-2 *(Continued)* Self-care of tobacco use and dependence. Key: 5 A's, ask, advise, assess, assist, arrange; 5 R's, relevance, risks, rewards, roadblocks, repetition; HBP, high blood pressure; MI, myocardial infarction; NRT, nicotine replacement therapy; OTC, over-the-counter; PUD, peptic ulcer disease; Rx, prescription; TMJ, temporomandibular joint.

Counseling Interventions for Quitting

When counseling a patient, the goal is to facilitate forward progress in the process of change, assisting patients to develop "readiness" for permanent cessation. It is important that clinicians view quitting as a process that might take months or even years to achieve, rather than a "now or never" event.

Counseling Patients Who Are Not Ready to Quit

When counseling patients who are not ready to quit, an important first step is to motivate the patient to start thinking about

quitting and to consider making the difficult decision to quit sometime in the foreseeable future. Sometimes patients who are not ready truly do not understand the need to quit. In general, most smokers will recognize the need to quit but are not yet ready to make the commitment to quit. Many patients will have tried to quit multiple times and relapsed; thus, they might feel too discouraged to try again.

Strategies for working with patients who are not ready to quit include increasing patient awareness of the available treatment options, having patients identify their reasons for smoking and for wanting to quit, and identifying barriers to quitting. Clinicians also can engage patients in thinking about quitting by raising awareness of specific drug interactions between medications and tobacco smoke (Table 50-2) and how tobacco use can induce or exacerbate medical conditions (e.g., chronic obstructive pulmonary disease and coronary heart disease). Although it may be useful to provide patients with information about the medications available for quitting, it is not appropriate to recommend a treatment regimen until a patient is ready to quit in the near future (e.g., within the next month). A treatment goal at this stage should be to promote motivation to quit. Encourage patients to seriously consider quitting by asking the following series of three questions:

1. *Do you ever plan to quit?*
   Most patients will respond "yes," in which case the clinician should continue with question 2. If they respond "no," the clinician should strongly advise the patient to quit and offer to assist, should the patient change his mind.

2. *How would it benefit you to quit later, as opposed to now?*
   Most patients will agree that there is never an ideal time to quit, and procrastinating a quit date has more negative effects than positive.

3. *What is the worst thing that would happen if you were to quit now?*
   This question probes patients' perceptions of quitting, which reveals some of the barriers to quitting that can then be addressed by the clinician.

Motivation also can be enhanced by applying the "5 R's."[28]

RELEVANCE

Encourage patients to think about why quitting is important to them. Because information has a greater effect if it takes on a personal meaning, counseling should be framed to relate to the patient's risk of disease or exacerbation of disease, other health concerns, family or social situation (e.g., having children with asthma), age, and other patient factors such as prior experience with quitting.

RISKS

Ask patients to identify negative health consequences of smoking, such as acute risks (e.g., shortness of breath, asthma exacerbations, pregnancy complications, infertility), long-term risks (e.g., cancer, cardiac and pulmonary disease), and environmental risks (e.g., effects of secondhand smoke on others, including children and pets, role modeling unhealthy behaviors around children and adolescents).

REWARDS

Ask patients to identify specific benefits of quitting, such as improved health, enhanced physical performance, acuity of taste and smell, reduced expenditures for tobacco, less time wasted or work missed, reduced health risks to others (fetus, children, housemates), and reduced aging of the skin.

ROADBLOCKS

Help patients identify significant barriers to quitting, and assist in developing coping skills to address or circumvent each barrier. Common barriers include nicotine withdrawal symptoms, fear of failure, a need for social support while quitting, depression, concern about weight gain, and a sense of deprivation or loss.

REPETITION

Continue to work with patients who are either not motivated to quit or have been unsuccessful in quitting. Discussing circumstances in which smoking occurred will help identify triggers for relapse and should be viewed as part of the learning process. Repeat interventions whenever possible.

Counseling Patients Who Are Ready to Quit

The goal for patients who are ready to quit in the next month is to achieve cessation by providing an individualized treatment plan, addressing the key issues listed in Table 50-3. The first step is to discuss the patient's tobacco use history, inquiring about levels of smoking, number of years smoked, methods used previously for quitting, and reasons for previous failed quit attempts. Clinicians should understand fully the patient's preferences for the different pharmacotherapies for quitting and work with patients in selecting the quitting methods (e.g., medications, behavioral counseling programs). Although it is important to recognize that pharmacotherapy might not be desirable or affordable for all patients, clinicians should educate patients that medications, when taken correctly, can substantially increase the likelihood of quitting.

In general, patients should be encouraged to select a quit date that is more than 2 days but less than 2 weeks away. This time frame provides patients with ample time to prepare themselves and their environment before the actual quit date. This includes removing all tobacco products and ashtrays from the home, car, and workplace. Patients should be advised to discuss their desire to quit with their family, friends, and coworkers and request their support and assistance. It is helpful to have patients think about when and why they smoke; this information is useful for anticipating situations that might trigger a desire to smoke and contribute to relapse. Additional counseling strategies to address with patients during a quit attempt are listed in Table 50-4. Patients should be counseled on proper medication use (including administration), side effects, and adherence, and it is crucial to emphasize the importance of receiving behavioral counseling throughout the quit attempt.

Counseling Patients Who Recently Quit

Patients who recently quit will face frequent, difficult challenges in countering withdrawal symptoms and cravings or temptations to use tobacco. It is important to help them identify situations that might trigger relapse and suggest appropriate coping strategies. Because smoking is a habitual behavior, patients should be advised to alter their daily routines. This helps to disassociate the behaviors from the tobacco.

Often, patients expect that they can change their behavior over a short period of time (weeks to months), yet experts believe patients must remain vigilant for at least 6 months before a new behavior is adopted or an old behavior is extinguished.[31] If a patient indicates he or she has quit smoking, it is important to ask *for how long* he or she has been abstinent. Many persons who quit using tobacco will experience cravings years and even decades after quitting. Thus, *relapse prevention* counseling should be part of every follow-up contact with patients who have recently quit smoking. Patients who slip and smoke a cigarette (or use any form of tobacco) or experience a full relapse back to habitual smoking should be encouraged to think through the scenario in which smoking first recurred and identify the trigger for relapse. Identifying triggers will provide valuable information for future quit attempts.

Counseling Patients Who Are Former Smokers

Although patients who have been smoke-free for 6 or more months can be considered former smokers, many remain

TABLE 50-3   Key Topics for Individualized Smoking Cessation Plans

Topic	Description
Assess tobacco use history	■ Current use: —Type(s) and amount of tobacco used ■ Past use: — Duration of smoking — Recent changes in levels of use ■ Past quit attempts: — Number of attempts, date of most recent attempt, duration of abstinence — Previous methods: What did or did not work? Why or why not? — Prior experience with cessation pharmacotherapy: agent used, adequacy of dose, adherence, duration of treatment — Reasons for relapse ■ Reasons or motivation for wanting to quit (or stay quit) ■ Confidence in ability to quit (or stay quit) ■ Triggers for smoking ■ Routines and situations associated with smoking ■ Stress-related smoking ■ Social support for quitting ■ Concerns about weight gain ■ Concerns about withdrawal symptoms
Facilitate the quitting process	■ Discuss methods for quitting: pros and cons of the different methods ■ Set a quit date: more than 2 days but less than 2 weeks away ■ Discuss coping strategies ■ Discuss withdrawal symptoms ■ Discuss concept of slip (occasional smoking) versus full relapse ■ Provide medication counseling: adherence and proper use ■ Offer to assist throughout the quit attempt

Arrange and provide follow-up counseling	■ Monitor the patient's progress throughout the quit attempt
	■ Evaluate the current quit attempt
	— Status of attempt
	— Slips (occasional smoking) and relapses
	— Medication use:
	  ● Adherence with regimen
	  ● Plans for discontinuation
	— Address temptations and triggers; discuss relapse prevention strategies
	— Provide encouragement throughout the quit attempt
	■ Follow-up contacts: First follow-up contact should occur during first week after quitting, a second follow-up contact within the first month, and additional contacts scheduled as needed. Can occur face to face, by telephone, or by e-mail

Source: Adapted with permission from reference 26. Copyright © 1999–2009 The Regents of the University of California, University of Southern California, and Western University of Health Sciences. All rights reserved.

vulnerable to relapse. The strategies to be applied for former tobacco users are similar, but typically less intensive, than those to be applied for recent quitters. The goal for these patients is to remain tobacco-free for life. Clinicians should evaluate their patient's quit attempt and coping strategies—has the patient had any strong temptations to use tobacco, or any occasional use of tobacco products (even a puff)? Also, it is important to ensure that patients are appropriately terminating or tapering pharmacotherapy products. Patients who have been smoke-free should be congratulated for their enormous success.

Helping Patients Quit: The Ask-Advise-Refer Approach (Brief Intervention)

Clinicians should familiarize themselves with local resources for smoking cessation, including group programs and telephone quit lines. When time or expertise limit the ability to provide comprehensive cessation counseling, clinicians are encouraged to apply an abbreviated 5 A's model, whereby they *Ask* about tobacco use, *Advise* tobacco users to quit, and *Refer* patients to other resources for additional assistance. Telephone-based counseling is available throughout the United States; these services provide low-cost interventions that can reach patients who might otherwise have limited access to medical treatment because of geographic location or lack of financial resources. In clinical trials, telephone counseling services for which at least some of the contacts are initiated by the quit line counselor were shown to be effective in promoting abstinence.[28] Combining medication with quit line counseling significantly improves abstinence rates compared with medication alone.[28] The national telephone number for the toll-free tobacco quit line is 1–800-QUIT NOW.

Pharmacologic Therapy

Although there are select situations in which pharmacotherapy should be used with caution or only while under the supervision of a primary care provider (see Special Populations), most quitters should be advised to incorporate pharmacotherapy as a component of their treatment plan. Currently, seven first-line agents are FDA-approved for smoking cessation,[28] including five formulations of nicotine replacement therapy (NRT), sustained-release bupropion, and varenicline. Three of the NRT formulations (gum, lozenge, and transdermal patch) are available without a prescription, whereas the nicotine inhaler, nicotine nasal spray, bupropion, and varenicline require a prescription. Although nortriptyline and clonidine are considered as second-line agents and significantly increase long-term cessation rates compared with placebo, these medications are associated with an increased incidence of adverse effects, require a prescription, and currently do not have an FDA-approved indication for smoking cessation.

Nicotine Replacement Therapy

NRT is the most commonly used pharmacotherapy for smoking cessation.[29] Similar to nicotine present in tobacco, NRT stimulates the release of dopamine in the central nervous system.[9] The rationale underlying the use of NRT for smoking cessation is twofold. First, NRT provides smokers with a nontobacco source of nicotine that reduces the physiologic symptoms of nicotine withdrawal that typically occur after abstinence from tobacco. Second, by attenuating the symptoms of withdrawal, NRT assists quitters by allowing them to focus on the behavioral and psychological aspects of smoking cessation. A key advantage of NRT is that patients are not exposed to the

TABLE 50-4 Cognitive and Behavioral Strategies for Smoking Cessation

Cognitive strategies focus on *retraining the way a patient thinks*. Often, patients mentally deliberate on the fact that they are thinking about a cigarette, and this leads to relapse. Patients must recognize that thinking about a cigarette does not mean they need to have one.

Review commitment to quit, focus on the downside of tobacco	Remind oneself that cravings and temptations are temporary and will pass. Announce, either silently or aloud, "I want to be a nonsmoker, and the temptation will pass."
Distractive thinking	Practice deliberate, immediate refocusing of thinking when cued by thoughts about tobacco use.
Positive self-talks, "pep-talks"	Say "I can do this," and remember previous difficult situations in which tobacco use was avoided with success.
Relaxation through imagery	Mentally focus on a scene, place, or situation that is peaceful, relaxing, and positive.
Mental rehearsal, visualization	Prepare for situations that might arise by envisioning how best to handle them. For example, envision what would happen if offered a cigarette by a friend, mentally craft and rehearse a response, and perhaps even practice it by saying it aloud.

Behavioral strategies involve *specific actions to reduce risk for relapse*. For maximal effectiveness, these should be considered before quitting, after determining patient-specific triggers for smoking. Below are some behavioral strategies for responding to several common cues or triggers for relapse.

Stress	Anticipate upcoming challenges at work, at school, or in personal life. Develop a substitute plan for smoking during times of stress (e.g., deep breathing, take a break or leave the situation, call supportive friend or family member, self-massage, use nicotine replacement therapy).
Alcohol	Drinking alcohol can lead to relapse. Consider limiting or abstaining from alcohol during the early stages of quitting.
Other smokers	Quitting is more difficult when other smokers are around. This is especially difficult if there is another smoker in the household. Limit prolonged contact with individuals who are smoking during the early stages of quitting. Ask coworkers, friends, and housemates not to smoke in your presence.
Oral gratification needs	Have nontobacco oral substitutes (e.g., gum, sugarless candy, straws, toothpicks, lip balm, toothbrush, nicotine replacement therapy, bottled water) readily available.
Automatic smoking routines	Anticipate routines that are associated with tobacco use and develop an alternative plan. Examples: ■ *Smoking with morning coffee:* change morning routine, drink tea instead of coffee, take shower before drinking coffee, take a brisk walk shortly after awakening. ■ *Smoking while driving:* remove all tobacco from car, have car interior detailed, listen to a book on tape or talk radio, use oral substitute. ■ *Smoking while on the phone:* stand while talking, limit call duration, change phone location, keep hands occupied by doodling or sketching. ■ *Smoking after meals:* get up and immediately do dishes or take a brisk walk after eating, call supportive friend.
Postcessation weight gain	Most tobacco users gain weight after quitting. Most quitters will gain less than 10 pounds, but there is a broad range of weight gain reported, with up to 10% of quitters gaining as much as 30 pounds.[28] In general, attempting to modify multiple behaviors at one time is not recommended. If weight gain is a barrier to quitting, engage in regular physical activity and adhere to a healthy diet (as opposed to strict dieting). Carefully plan and prepare meals; increase fruit, vegetable, and water intake to create a feeling of fullness; and chew sugarless gum or eat sugarless candy. Consider use of pharmacotherapy that was shown to delay weight gain (e.g., the 4 mg nicotine gum or lozenge or bupropion).
Cravings for tobacco	Cravings for tobacco are temporary and usually pass within 5 to 10 minutes. Handle cravings through distractive thinking, taking a break, changing activities or tasks, taking deep breaths, or performing self-massage.

Source: Reprinted with permission from reference 26. Copyright © 1999–2009. The Regents of the University of California, University of Southern California, and Western University of Health Sciences. All rights reserved.

carcinogens and other toxic constituents present in tobacco and tobacco smoke. Furthermore, NRT formulations provide lower, slower, and less variable plasma nicotine concentrations than do cigarettes,[32] thereby eliminating the near-immediate reinforcing effects of nicotine obtained through smoking.

Nicotine is well absorbed (Figure 50-3) from many sites, including the lung, skin, and nasal and buccal (oral) mucosa. Nicotine absorption is pH dependent, and lower systemic concentrations are achieved under acidic conditions. Nicotine also is well absorbed from the gastrointestinal tract (small intestine) but undergoes extensive first-pass hepatic metabolism, resulting in negligible systemic levels of nicotine.[32]

The main difference between the various NRT formulations is the site and rate of nicotine absorption (Figure 50-3). All of the NRT formulations deliver nicotine less rapidly and achieve lower serum nicotine levels than do cigarettes. Peak serum

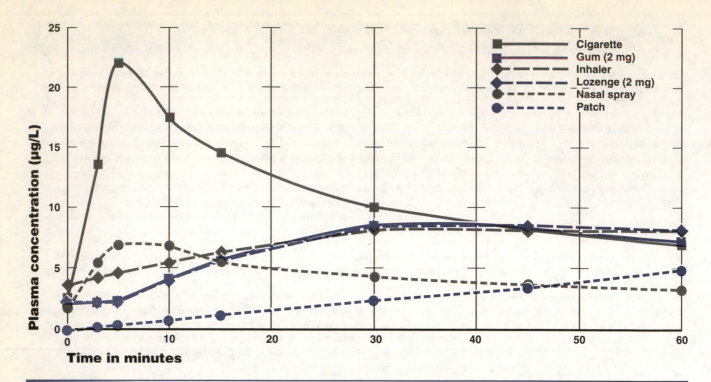

concentrations are achieved most rapidly with the nasal spray (11–18 minutes) followed by the gum, lozenge, and inhaler (30–60 minutes), and then the transdermal patch (3–12 hours). In contrast, significantly higher peak nicotine levels are attained within 10 minutes of smoking a cigarette.[32]

Patients should be instructed not to smoke cigarettes or use other forms of tobacco (e.g., snuff, chewing tobacco, cigars, pipes) while using NRT. Use of tobacco in combination with NRT may result in serum nicotine concentrations that are higher than those achieved from tobacco products alone, increasing the likelihood of nicotine-related adverse effects, including nausea, vomiting, hypersalivation, perspiration, abdominal pain, dizziness, weakness, and palpitations.

NICOTINE POLACRILEX GUM

Nicotine polacrilex gum is a resin complex of nicotine and polacrilin in a sugar-free (~1–2 cal/piece) chewing gum base. The product is available as 2 and 4 mg strengths, in regular (tobacco-like), cinnamon, fruit, mint (various), and orange flavors (Table 50-5). All gum formulations contain buffering agents (sodium carbonate and sodium bicarbonate) to increase salivary pH, thereby enhancing absorption of nicotine across the buccal mucosa. When the 2 and 4 mg strength gums are used properly, approximately 1 mg and 2 mg of nicotine is absorbed from each dose, respectively.[32] Peak serum concentrations of nicotine are achieved approximately 30 minutes after chewing a single piece of gum and then slowly decline over 2 to 3 hours.[32]

Individuals who smoke fewer than 25 cigarettes per day should start therapy with the 2 mg strength, and heavier smokers (≥25 cigarettes/day) should start with the 4 mg strength. Table 50-5 provides the manufacturer's recommended dosing schedule. During the initial 6 weeks of therapy, patients should use one piece of gum every 1 to 2 hours while awake. In general, this amounts to at least nine pieces of gum daily. Table 50-6

TABLE 50-5 Dosages for Nonprescription Nicotine Polacrilex Gum and Lozenge

	Gum	Lozenge
Product strength	Nicorette: 2 mg, 4 mg; regular, cinnamon, fruit, mint (various), orange Generic: 2 mg, 4 mg; regular, fruit, mint, orange	Commit: 2 mg, 4 mg; cappuccino, cherry, mint, original (light-mint)
Dose	≥25 cigarettes/day: 4 mg <25 cigarettes/day: 2 mg Weeks 1–6: 1 piece every 1–2 hours Weeks 7–9: 1 piece every 2–4 hours Weeks 10–12: 1 piece every 4–8 hours	First cigarette ≤30 minutes after waking: 4 mg First cigarette >30 minutes after waking: 2 mg Weeks 1–6: 1 lozenge every 12 hours Weeks 7–9: 1 lozenge every 2–4 hours Weeks 10–12: 1 lozenge every 4–8 hours

TABLE 50-6 Usage Guidelines for Nicotine Polacrilex Gum

- Do not smoke cigarettes or use other forms of tobacco (e.g., snuff, chewing tobacco, cigars, pipes) while on nicotine gum therapy.
- Note that nicotine gum is a nicotine delivery system, not a chewing gum.
- Proper administration technique is necessary when using this product. Nicotine from the gum is released using the "chew and park" method:
  — Chew each piece of gum *slowly* several times.
  — Stop chewing at first sign of peppery, minty, fruity, or citrus taste or after experiencing a slight tingling sensation in the mouth. This usually occurs after about 15 chews, but varies.
  — "Park" the gum between the cheek and gum to allow absorption of nicotine across the lining of the mouth.
  — When the taste or tingling dissipates (generally after 1–2 minutes), slowly resume chewing.
  — When the taste or tingle returns, stop chewing and park the gum in a different place in the mouth. Parking the gum in different areas of the mouth will decrease the incidence of mouth irritation.
  — The chew and park steps should be repeated until most of the nicotine is gone, which is when the taste or tingle does not return after continued chewing. On average, each piece of gum lasts 30 minutes.
- To minimize withdrawal symptoms, use the nicotine gum on a scheduled basis rather than as needed.
- Follow the dosage regimen carefully; reduce the dosage at the recommended intervals, and stop using the product after 12 weeks of treatment.
- Do not chew more than 24 pieces per day.
- Acidic beverages such as coffee, juices, wine, or soft drinks may transiently reduce the salivary pH, resulting in decreased absorption of nicotine across the buccal mucosa. Do not eat or drink anything (except water) 15 minutes before or while using the nicotine gum.
- Note that chewing the gum too quickly will result in an unpleasant taste caused by too much nicotine in the saliva and, if the nicotine is swallowed, may cause effects similar to those produced by excess smoking (e.g., nausea, throat irritation, lightheadedness, hiccups).
- Carry or have at least one full sleeve of nicotine polacrilex gum (12 pieces per sleeve) readily available at all times. Keep the nicotine gum in the same place you previously kept your cigarettes (e.g., shirt pocket, purse, or desk).
- Keep this product, including used pieces, out of the reach of children and pets.

provides specific instructions for proper use of the nicotine gum. The "chew and park" method described in this table allows for the slow, consistent release of nicotine from the polacrilin resin. Patients can use additional pieces of gum (up to the maximum of 24 pieces per day) if cravings occur between the scheduled doses. In general, individuals who smoke heavily will need more pieces to alleviate their cravings.

It is important to emphasize that patients often do not use enough of the gum to derive its full benefit. Commonly, patients chew too few pieces per day or shorten the duration of treatment. For this reason, it is preferable to recommend a fixed schedule of administration, tapering over 1 to 3 months rather than using the gum "as needed" to control cravings.[28]

The most common side effects associated with use of the nicotine gum include unpleasant taste, mouth irritation, jaw muscle soreness or fatigue, hypersalivation, hiccups, and dyspepsia. Many of these side effects can be minimized or prevented by using proper chewing technique.[28] The nicotine polacrilin resin is more viscous than ordinary chewing gum and more likely to adhere to fillings, bridges, dentures, crowns, and braces. If excessive sticking or damage to dental work occurs, the patient should stop using the nicotine gum and consult a dentist. Patients should be warned that chewing the gum too rapidly may result in excessive release of nicotine, leading to lightheadedness, nausea, vomiting, irritation of the throat and mouth, hiccups, and indigestion.

Patients with active temporomandibular joint disease should not use the nicotine gum because the highly viscous consistency of the formulation and the need for frequent chewing may exacerbate this condition. In addition, the manufacturer recommends that patients with stomach ulcers or diabetes contact their medical provider before use because these conditions are more serious and might require further monitoring.

NICOTINE POLACRILEX LOZENGE

The nicotine polacrilex lozenge is a resin complex of nicotine and polacrilin in a sugar-free (4 cal/lozenge), mint- or cherry-flavored lozenge (Table 50-5). The lozenges are available as 2 and 4 mg dime-sized tablets intended for use similar to other medicinal lozenges or troches (i.e., sucked and rotated within the mouth until it dissolves). The pharmacokinetics of the nicotine lozenge and gum formulations are comparable, but a nicotine lozenge delivers approximately 25% more nicotine than does an equivalent dose of nicotine gum because of complete dissolution of the dosage form.[33] Like nicotine gum, the lozenge also contains buffering agents (sodium carbonate and potassium bicarbonate) to increase salivary pH, enhancing the buccal absorption of nicotine.

Unlike other forms of NRT, which are dosed based on the number of cigarettes smoked per day, the recommended dosage of the nicotine lozenge is based on the "time to first cigarette" of the day. Some studies suggest that the best indicator of nicotine dependence is having a strong desire or need to smoke soon after waking.[33] Thus, patients who smoke their first cigarette of the day within 30 minutes of waking are likely to be more highly dependent on nicotine and require higher dosages than those who delay smoking for more than 30 minutes after waking (Table 50-5).

During the initial 6 weeks of therapy, patients should use 1 lozenge every 1 to 2 hours while awake. In general, this amounts to at least 9 lozenges daily. Table 50-7 provides further instructions for proper use of the nicotine lozenge. Patients can use additional lozenges (up to 5 lozenges in 6 hours or a maximum of 20 lozenges per day) if cravings occur between the scheduled doses. The manufacturer recommends that patients with stomach ulcers or diabetes contact their medical provider before use because these conditions, which are more serious, may require further monitoring.

Side effects associated with the nicotine lozenge include mouth irritation, nausea, hiccups, cough, heartburn, headache, flatulence, and insomnia. Patients who use more than one lozenge at a time, continuously use one lozenge after another, or chew or swallow the lozenge are more likely to experience heartburn or indigestion.

TABLE 50-7 Usage Guidelines for Nicotine Polacrilex Lozenge

- Do not smoke cigarettes or use other forms of tobacco (e.g., snuff, chewing tobacco, cigars, pipes) while using the nicotine lozenge.
- Proper administration technique is necessary when using the nicotine lozenge:
  — Place the lozenge in the mouth and allow it to dissolve slowly (20–30 minutes). As the nicotine is released from the lozenge, you may experience a warm, tingling sensation.
  — To reduce the risk of side effects (nausea, hiccups, heartburn), the lozenge should *not* be chewed or swallowed.
  — Occasionally rotate the lozenge to different areas of the mouth to decrease mouth irritation.
- To minimize withdrawal symptoms, use the nicotine lozenge on a scheduled, rather than an as-needed basis.
- Follow the dosage regimen carefully; reduce the dosage at the recommended intervals, and stop using the product after 12 weeks of treatment.
- Do not use more than 5 lozenges in 6 hours or more than 20 lozenges per day.
- Acidic beverages such as coffee, juices, wine, or soft drinks may transiently reduce the salivary pH, resulting in decreased absorption of nicotine across the buccal mucosa. Do not eat or drink anything (except water) 15 minutes before or while using the nicotine lozenge.
- Patients who use more than 1 lozenge at a time, continuously use 1 lozenge after another, or chew or swallow the lozenge are more likely to experience heartburn or indigestion.
- Carry or have at least one full sleeve of nicotine polacrilex lozenges (12 pieces per sleeve) or a pop-pak (cylinder-shaped tube) readily available at all times. Keep the nicotine lozenge in the same place you previously kept your cigarettes (e.g., shirt pocket, purse, or desk).
- Keep this product out of the reach of children and pets.

NICOTINE TRANSDERMAL SYSTEMS (NICOTINE PATCH)

Nicotine transdermal systems deliver continuous, low levels of nicotine across the skin over 24 hours. The patch consists of a waterproof surface layer, a nicotine reservoir, an adhesive layer, and a disposable protective liner. Currently, there are two marketed products (Table 50-8).

TABLE 50-8 Dosages for Nonprescription Transdermal Systems (Nicotine Patch)

	NicoDerm CQ Patch (Regular and Clear)	Generic Patch (Formerly Habitrol)
Product strength	7, 14, 21 mg (24 hour)	7, 14, 21 mg (24 hour)
Dose	*>10 cigarettes/day:* 21 mg/day × 6 weeks; 14 mg/day × 2 weeks; 7 mg/day × 2 weeks	*>10 cigarettes/day:* 21 mg/day × 4 weeks; 14 mg/day × 2 weeks; 7 mg/day × 2 weeks
	≤10 cigarettes/day: 14 mg/day × 6 weeks; 7 mg/day × 2 weeks	*≤10 cigarettes/day:* 14 mg/day × 6 weeks; 7 mg/day × 2 weeks

---

The dosing schedules for the nicotine patches vary slightly (Table 50-8). Before recommending a specific product and a dosing schedule, it is important to know how many cigarettes the patient smokes per day. In general, heavier smokers (e.g., ≥10 cigarettes per day) will require higher-strength formulations for a longer duration of therapy. Patients experiencing side effects such as dizziness, perspiration, nausea, vomiting, diarrhea, or headache should consider a lower strength patch. Additional instructions for proper use of the nicotine patch are listed in Table 50-9.

The most common side effects associated with the nicotine patch are local skin reactions (erythema, burning, and pruritus) at the application site, which are generally caused by skin occlusion or sensitivity to the patch adhesives. Other less common side effects include vivid or abnormal dreams, insomnia, and headache. Sleep disturbances might be caused by nocturnal nicotine absorption. If this side effect becomes troublesome,

---

TABLE 50-9 Usage Guidelines for Nicotine Transdermal Systems (Nicotine Patch)

- Do not smoke cigarettes or use other forms of tobacco (e.g., snuff, chewing tobacco, cigars, pipes) while using the nicotine patch.
- Apply the patch to a clean, dry, hairless area of the skin on the upper body or the upper outer part of the arm at approximately the same time each day.
- The patch should be applied to a different area of skin each day. To minimize the potential for local skin reactions, the same area should not be used again for at least 1 week.
- During application, apply firm pressure to the patch with the palm of the hand for 10 seconds. Be sure that the patch adheres well to the skin, especially around the edges; this is necessary for a good seal.
- Wash your hands after applying or removing the patch.
- The patch should not be left on the skin for more than 24 hours, because prolonged use may lead to skin irritation.
- Any adhesive remaining on the skin after the patch removal can be removed with rubbing alcohol.
- Water will not reduce the effectiveness of the nicotine patch if it is applied correctly. You may bathe, swim, shower, or exercise while wearing the patch.
- Do not cut patches in half or into smaller pieces to adjust or reduce the nicotine dosage. Nicotine in the patch may evaporate from the cut edges and the patch may be less effective.
- Local skin reactions (itching, burning, and redness) are common with the nicotine patch. These reactions are generally caused by adhesives; they can be minimized by rotating patch application sites and, if they occur, treated with nonprescription hydrocortisone cream.
- Remove the nicotine patch before having a magnetic resonance imaging (MRI) procedure. Burns from nicotine patches worn during MRIs were reported and are likely caused by the metallic component in the backing of some patches.
- Individuals experiencing troublesome dreams or other sleep disruptions should remove the patch before bedtime.
- Discard the removed nicotine patch by folding it onto itself, completely covering the adhesive area.
- Keep new and used patches out of the reach of children and pets.

patients should be instructed to remove the patch at bedtime and apply a new patch as soon as possible after waking the following morning.[28]

Prescription Medications for Smoking Cessation

NICOTINE INHALER

The nicotine inhaler consists of a plastic mouthpiece and a nicotine-containing cartridge that delivers 4 mg of nicotine as an inhaled vapor, of which 2 mg is absorbed across the oropharyngeal mucosa. The inhaler reduces nicotine withdrawal symptoms and may give some degree of comfort by providing a hand-to-mouth ritual that emulates smoking. Side effects of the inhaler include mild mouth and throat irritation, cough, and rhinitis.

NICOTINE NASAL SPRAY

The nicotine nasal spray is an aqueous solution of nicotine for administration to the nasal mucosa. Each actuation delivers a 0.5 mg bolus of nicotine that is absorbed across the nasal mucosa. Because of its rapid onset of action (relative to other NRT formulations), the spray is a potential option for patients who prefer a medication to manage withdrawal symptoms rapidly. Initially, most patients will experience nose and throat irritation (peppery sensation), watery eyes, sneezing, or coughing when using this product. This product is to be administered without sniffing (i.e., not administered like standard allergy nasal sprays). With regular use, tolerance generally develops, and, after the first week, most patients have minimal difficulty tolerating the spray.

SUSTAINED-RELEASE BUPROPION

Sustained-release bupropion was the first non-nicotine pharmaceutical aid approved for smoking cessation. This agent is a prescription antidepressant medication that is believed to promote smoking cessation by blocking the reuptake of dopamine and norepinephrine in the brain, thereby decreasing the cravings for cigarettes and symptoms of nicotine withdrawal.[28]

Therapy is started with a dose of 150 mg orally every morning for 3 days, followed by 150 mg twice daily for 7 to 12 weeks. Because steady-state blood levels are reached after approximately 7 days of therapy, patients set their quit date for 1 to 2 weeks after starting therapy. Insomnia and dry mouth are the most common side effects reported with bupropion. Because seizures have been reported in approximately 0.1% of patients, bupropion is contraindicated in patients who (1) have a seizure disorder, (2) have a current or prior diagnosis of anorexia or bulimia nervosa, (3) are undergoing abrupt discontinuation of alcohol or sedatives (including benzodiazepines), (4) are currently using or have used a monoamine oxidase inhibitor within the past 14 days, or (5) are currently being treated with any other medications that contain bupropion. Other factors that might increase the odds of seizure and are classified as warnings for this medication include a history of head trauma or prior seizure, central nervous system tumor, the presence of severe hepatic cirrhosis, and concomitant use of medications that lower the seizure threshold. Bupropion can be used safely in combination with NRT and may be beneficial for use in patients with underlying depression or concern about weight gain (see Patient Preferences).

VARENICLINE

Varenicline is a partial agonist and is highly selective for the $alpha_4 beta_2$ nicotinic acetylcholine receptor. The efficacy of varenicline in smoking cessation is believed to be the result of sustained, low-level agonist activity at the receptor site combined with competitive inhibition of nicotine binding. The partial agonist activity induces modest receptor stimulation, leading to increased dopamine levels that attenuate the symptoms of nicotine withdrawal. In addition, by competitively blocking the binding of nicotine to nicotinic acetylcholine receptors in the central nervous system, varenicline inhibits the surges of dopamine release that occur immediately after inhalation of tobacco smoke. The latter mechanism may be effective in preventing relapse by reducing the pleasure associated with smoking.[34]

Similar to sustained-release bupropion, treatment with varenicline should be started 1 week before the patient stops smoking. This regimen allows for gradual escalation of the dose to minimize treatment-related nausea and insomnia. Therapy is started at 0.5 mg daily days 1 to 3, 0.5 mg twice daily days 4 to 7, and 1 mg twice daily weeks 2 to 12. Nausea, insomnia, abnormal dreams, and headache are the most common side effects reported with varenicline. Postmarketing case reports of neuropsychiatric symptoms (behavior changes, agitation, depressed mood, suicidal ideation or behavior) and worsening of preexisting psychiatric illness among patients being treated with varenicline were described.[35] These reports are rare in comparison to the total number of patients receiving varenicline treatment, but nonetheless they warrant ongoing surveillance.

Pharmacotherapeutic Comparison

Currently, few trials directly compare the various agents for smoking cessation. In general, regimens with the first-line agents (Table 50-10) more than double the long-term quit rates compared with placebo.[28]

Product Selection Guidelines

All first-line, FDA-approved cessation medications approximately double quit rates. The choice of therapy is therefore based largely on contraindications or precautions, patient preference, and tolerability of the available dosage forms.

SPECIAL POPULATIONS

NRT should be used with caution in patients with serious underlying cardiovascular disease, including those who have had a recent myocardial infarction (i.e., within the preceding 2 weeks), those with serious arrhythmias, and those with serious or worsening angina pectoris.[28] Nicotine may increase the myocardial workload by increasing the heart rate and blood pressure and may constrict coronary arteries, leading to cardiac ischemia.[36,37] Although most experts believe the risks of NRT in patients with cardiovascular disease are small relative to the risks of continued smoking,[37,38] patients with serious underlying cardiovascular disease are advised to use NRT only while under the supervision of a medical provider.

Prescription forms of nicotine are classified by the FDA as Pregnancy Category D, meaning there is evidence of risk to the human fetus.[39] Although NRT may pose a risk to the developing fetus, some experts have argued that NRT use during pregnancy is safer than continued smoking.[37,38] However, because data showing effectiveness of NRT in pregnancy are inconclusive and because nicotine has the potential to cause fetal harm, the 2008 Clinical Practice Guideline states that pregnant women should be encouraged to quit without medication. Instead, clinicians are advised to offer interventions of person-to-person behavioral counseling for their pregnant patients who smoke.[28]

TABLE 50-10 Methods for Smoking Cessation: Estimates of Treatment Efficacy for First-Line Agents Compared with Placebo at 6 Months after Quitting

Pharmacotherapy	Estimated Odds Ratio[a] (95% CI)	Estimated Abstinence Rate[b] (95% CI)
Placebo	1.0	13.8
Monotherapy (First-Line Agents)		
Sustained-release bupropion	2.0 (1.8–2.2)	24.2 (22.2–26.4)
Nicotine gum (6–14 weeks)	1.5 (1.2–1.7)	19.0 (16.5–21.9)
Nicotine inhaler	2.1 (1.5–2.9)	24.8 (19.1–31.6)
Nicotine lozenge (2 mg)	2.0 (1.4–2.8)	24.2[c]
Nicotine patch (6–14 weeks)	1.9 (1.7–2.2)	23.4 (21.3–25.8)
Nicotine nasal spray	2.3 (1.7–3.0)	26.7 (21.5–32.7)
Varenicline (2 mg/day)	3.1 (2.5–3.8)	33.2 (28.9–37.8)
Combination Therapy (First-Line Agents)		
Nicotine patch (>14 weeks) + ad lib NRT (gum or nasal spray)	3.6 (2.5–5.2)	36.5 (28.6–45.3)
Nicotine patch + bupropion SR	2.5 (1.9–3.4)	28.9 (23.5–35.1)
Nicotine patch + nicotine inhaler	2.2 (1.3–3.6)	25.8 (17.4–36.5)

Key: CI, confidence interval; NRT, nicotine replacement therapy.

[a] Estimated relative to placebo.

[b] Abstinence percentages for specified treatment.

[c] One qualifying randomized trial; 95% CI not reported in the 2008 Clinical Practice Guideline.

Source: Data from reference 28. Reprinted with permission from reference 26. Copyright © 1999–2009 *Rx for Change: Clinician-Assisted Tobacco Cessation.* San Francisco, Calif: University of California San Francisco, University of Southern California, and Western University of Health Sciences.

The efficacy of NRT, bupropion SR, and varenicline has not been established in pediatric or adolescent smokers, and none of the NRT products are currently indicated for use in this population.[28] Accordingly, counseling is the recommended treatment method for smokers younger than 18 years.

People older than 65 years can benefit greatly from quitting smoking. Pharmacologic therapy and counseling are recommended. If mobility is an issue, referral to a quit line may be useful.[28]

The manufacturers of nicotine gum, lozenge, and patch recommend that patients taking a prescription medicine for depression or asthma speak with their doctor or pharmacist before using nonprescription NRT. Fluvoxamine and theophylline (both now used infrequently) and inhaled corticosteroids have known clinically significant interactions with tobacco smoke (Table 50-2).

Light smokers include those who smoke fewer than 10 cigarettes per day and those who do not smoke every day. Counseling is the recommended treatment method for this population.[28] However, the nicotine patch is approved for use in light smokers, and the nicotine lozenge was shown to be effective in individuals smoking ≤15 cigarettes daily.[40] Use of smokeless tobacco (e.g., snuff, moist snuff, chewing tobacco), cigars, and pipes can produce nicotine addiction and has serious health consequences. Behavioral counseling is the recommended treatment method for these tobacco users.[28]

Some patients may need to use their smoking cessation medication longer than the usual recommended treatment duration. Although the general goal is complete, long-term abstinence from all nicotine-containing products, some smokers may benefit from long-term medication use.[28] If continued use helps prevent relapse, this is considered preferable to that patient returning to smoking, which has detrimental health consequences.[28]

PATIENT FACTORS

When recommending a nonprescription agent for smoking cessation, it is essential to determine the patient's smoking patterns, lifestyle habits, and coexisting medical conditions. In general, higher levels of smoking will require higher dosages of NRT and longer treatment durations. Patients who smoke continuously throughout the day might have better success with the nicotine patches, because these provide a sustained, steady release of nicotine. Conversely, patients who smoke intermittently throughout the day or who smoke intensely for short periods of time followed by long periods of abstinence might prefer a relatively short-acting formulation such as nicotine gum or lozenge to more closely mimic their tobacco use patterns. For some quitters, frequent gum chewing may not be feasible or socially acceptable. The nicotine patch, which can be concealed under clothing, might be a reasonable choice for these individuals. Others may find nicotine lozenges, which can be used more discreetly, to be an acceptable alternative. Patients with underlying dermatologic conditions (e.g., psoriasis, eczema, atopic dermatitis) or allergy to adhesive tape are more likely to experience skin irritation and should not use the nicotine patch. The nicotine lozenge or patch is more appropriate than the nicotine gum for patients with temporomandibular joint disease or dentures. Finally, patients with serious cardiovascular disease, women who are pregnant or nursing, light smokers, and adolescents should be referred for further evaluation by their primary provider before starting treatment with NRT.

PATIENT PREFERENCES

When assisting patients with quitting, it is particularly important to understand the patient's perceptions and expectations about pharmacotherapy, including the ability to comply with the regimen, previous experience with cessation medications, and concern about weight gain. Because NRT formulations require frequent dosing or nontraditional routes of administration, patient education about proper use of these products is essential. Patients who have difficulty taking multiple doses of medications throughout the day or those who want a simplified regimen might achieve greater success with the nicotine patch. In contrast, the gum or lozenge may be preferable for patients desiring the ability to titrate nicotine levels to manage withdrawal symptoms. Some quitters may find they need an oral substitute for tobacco; the oral gratification afforded by the nicotine gum, lozenge, or inhaler might be beneficial in these patients. Other quitters may prefer the idea of using a combination of medications, such as the nicotine patch plus gum or lozenge, on an as-needed basis (see discussion below).

All smokers making a repeat quit attempt should be queried about their prior use of pharmacotherapy and their perceptions of the treatment options. For patients reporting a favorable past experience with a given product, retreatment with the same agent may be appropriate, with consideration given to increasing the dose, frequency, or duration of therapy. For patients reporting a negative experience with a particular medication (e.g., poor adherence, side effects, palatability issues, or cost) a different regimen should be considered. For example, if a patient had short-term success with the patch but discontinued therapy because of intolerable nightmares, he or she may attempt to quit again by using the patch, but it should be removed at bedtime. A patient who is unable to tolerate nicotine gum because of jaw muscle ache could be advised to switch to the nicotine lozenge or patch. For patients expressing concern about postcessation weight gain, the 4 mg nicotine gum, 4 mg lozenge, or bupropion SR might be particularly helpful, because these products were shown to delay weight gain after quitting.[28] For patients in which the out-of-pocket expense might be a barrier to pharmacologic treatment, use of the generic formulations may be preferable.

Combination therapy should be considered as a first-line treatment and might be particularly appropriate in patients who have experienced numerous failed attempts using monotherapy. Combination therapy generally involves the use of a long-acting medication (nicotine patch or sustained-release bupropion) in combination with a short-acting nicotine formulation (nicotine gum, lozenge, inhaler, or nasal spray). The long-acting nicotine formulation, which delivers relatively constant concentrations of drug, is used to prevent the onset of severe withdrawal symptoms, whereas the short-acting nicotine formulation, which delivers nicotine more rapidly, is used "as needed" to control withdrawal symptoms that may occur during potential relapse situations (e.g., after meals, or when stressed or around other smokers). Research suggests that combination therapy may be somewhat more efficacious than monotherapy.[28] A disadvantage of combination therapy is the possibility of more side effects (e.g., nicotine toxicity) and increased cost. Although the current FDA labeling of nonprescription NRT specifically warns against the concomitant use of nicotine-containing products (including other forms of NRT), evidence from controlled trials supports combination therapy with the nicotine patch and nicotine gum.[28] Although use of lozenge plus patch would be expected to be similarly effective, this combination has not been adequately studied. For other combination therapy, patients should be referred to their primary provider to determine appropriate options.

Complementary Therapies

Although a variety of herbal and homeopathic products are available to aid cessation, data are lacking to support their safety and efficacy. Many herbal preparations for cessation contain lobeline (*Lobelia inflata*), an herbal alkaloid with partial nicotinic agonist properties. A meta-analysis found no evidence to support the role of lobeline as an aid for smoking cessation.[41] Controlled trials to test the effects of hypnosis and acupuncture similarly were not found to be effective treatments for smoking cessation.[28,42] Patients should be cautioned that "herbal" cigarettes are not safe alternatives; similar to cigarettes, these products also result in the inhalation of tar, carbon monoxide, and other harmful byproducts of combustion.

Assessment of Smoking Cessation: A Case-Based Approach

To help the patient succeed at smoking cessation, the clinician must help patients evaluate how they smoke, identify medications and quitting methods they have or have not tried in the past, and determine appropriate cessation therapies. Analysis of the patient's smoking patterns and the reasons for smoking helps the clinician work with the patient to develop an appropriate treatment plan. Cases 50-1 and 50-2 illustrate the assessment of patients who want to quit.

Patient Counseling for Smoking Cessation

Smoking is the leading known cause of preventable morbidity and mortality in the United States. Substantial benefits of quitting can be realized at any age. Although approximately 70% of adult smokers would like to quit,[6] few are able to do so on their own. Research has shown that tobacco cessation rates can be substantially improved with treatment that includes counseling and pharmacotherapy.[28] (See Nonpharmacologic Therapy for a detailed discussion of counseling.) Health care providers are in an ideal position to identify tobacco users and provide assistance throughout the quit attempt.

Evaluation of Patient Outcomes for Smoking Cessation

Follow-up contact is an essential component of treatment for tobacco use and dependence.[28] At each follow-up contact, the clinician should assess an individual's tobacco use status and, if appropriate, assess and monitor pharmacotherapy use. If the patient has remained abstinent, congratulate the success and provide encouragement to remain tobacco-free. If the patient has used tobacco, review the specific circumstances, and reassess the commitment to abstinence. Encourage the patient to learn from his or her mistakes, and identify strategies to prevent future lapses. Determine whether the patient is experiencing nicotine withdrawal symptoms or adverse effects from the pharmacotherapy. Finally, offer ongoing support; if a clinician is unable to provide the level of ongoing support a patient needs or desires, refer the patient to a specialist for more intensive treatment.

Relevant Evaluation Criteria	Scenario/Model Outcome
Information Gathering	
1. Gather essential information about the patient's symptoms, including:	
a. description of symptom(s) (i.e., nature, onset, duration, severity, associated symptoms)	Patient would like information about the various OTC medications for smoking cessation. He has a 3-year-old son, and he is ready to quit smoking now to prevent his child from further exposure to secondhand smoke. He has smoked 1.5 packs per day (or 30 cigarettes) for 12 years and smokes his first cigarette immediately after waking. He has not received cessation counseling from a clinician. His friends have used the nicotine patch with success, so he would like to try it. He is in a rush to pick up his child from preschool.
b. description of any factors that seem to precipitate, exacerbate, and/or relieve the patient's symptom(s)	He mostly smokes while driving and at home in the morning and in the evenings after dinner.
c. description of the patient's efforts to relieve the symptoms	He has never tried to quit smoking before.
2. Gather essential patient history information:	
a. patient's identity	Tim Burns
b. patient's age, sex, height, and weight	32-year-old male, 6 ft, 190 lb, BMI 25.8
c. patient's occupation	Insurance salesman
d. patient's dietary habits	Reasonably healthy
e. patient's sleep habits	Sleeps 6–7 hours during work week
f. concurrent medical conditions, prescription and nonprescription medications, and dietary supplements	Exercise-induced asthma; uses albuterol inhaler as needed
g. allergies	NKA
h. history of other adverse reactions to medications	None
i. other (describe) _____	Married with 3-year-old son
Assessment and Triage	
3. Differentiate the patient's signs/symptoms, and correctly identify the patient's primary problem(s).	Patient is a younger smoker who would like to quit to protect his child from secondhand smoke and to improve his own health.
4. Identify exclusions for self-treatment (see Figure 50-2).	None
5. Formulate a comprehensive list of therapeutic alternatives for the primary problem to determine if triage to a medical practitioner is required, and share this information with the patient.	Recommend pharmacotherapy and counseling. Refer Tim to telephone counseling (1-800-QUIT-NOW) because he is in a hurry. Recommend he set a quit date in 1–2 weeks. Take no action. Pharmacotherapy options include: (1) Recommend nicotine patch. (2) Recommend nicotine gum. (3) Recommend nicotine lozenge. (4) Refer to PCP for prescription pharmacotherapy (nicotine inhaler, nicotine nasal spray, bupropion SR, varenicline).
Plan	
6. Select an optimal therapeutic alternative to address the patient's problem, taking into account patient preferences.	Tim expressed interest in using the nicotine patch. Select a patch type and dose (Table 50-8) based on his smoking of 30 cigarettes daily.
7. Describe the recommended therapeutic approach to the patient.	Behavioral counseling: refer patient to quit line. See Tables 50-3 and 50-4.

CASE 50-1 *(continued)*

Relevant Evaluation Criteria	Scenario/Model Outcome
	Medication counseling: see Tables 50-8 and 50-9 for specific medication dosing and counseling points.
	Pharmacotherapy is recommended because Tim has no contraindications or precautions for self-care use.
8. Explain to the patient the rationale for selecting the recommended therapeutic approach from the considered therapeutic alternatives.	You do not have any medical conditions for which nicotine replacement medications should be used with caution (e.g., recent heart attack, serious arrhythmias, or angina). The nicotine patch will provide a low, constant level of nicotine in your body to help reduce nicotine withdrawal symptoms.
	Receiving counseling, in addition to taking the nicotine patch as directed, will increase your chances of success with quitting.

Patient Education

9. When recommending self-care with non-prescription medications and/or nondrug therapy, convey accurate information to the patient:	
a. appropriate dose and frequency of administration	The 21 mg nicotine patch used once daily for 24 hours should be started. See Table 50-8 for tapering schedule.
b. maximum number of days the therapy should be employed	See Table 50-8.
c. product administration procedures	See Table 50-9.
d. expected time to onset of relief	The level of nicotine in your body will gradually rise over the next 12 hours and will remain steady with continued use of the patch. The blood nicotine levels are lower than those from smoking but should be sufficient to help control your nicotine withdrawal.
e. degree of relief that can be reasonably expected	Most patients find that nicotine withdrawal symptoms peak a few days after the last cigarette; withdrawal symptoms then gradually diminish over the next 2–4 weeks.
f. most common side effects	The most common side effects include skin reactions (redness, burning, itching) at the application site, sleep disturbances (vivid dreams, insomnia), and headaches.
g. side effects that warrant medical intervention should they occur	You should contact your PCP if you experience severe skin irritation (rash or redness of the skin that does not go away after 4 days, or if the skin swells); irregular heartbeats or palpitations; symptoms of nicotine overdose (nausea, vomiting, dizziness, weakness, or rapid heartbeat).
h. patient options in the event that condition worsens or persists	If you experience withdrawal symptoms or severe cigarette cravings, you should contact your PCP because you might need a higher dosage of nicotine. If you have side effects related to nicotine excess (see above), you should use the next lower patch dose.
i. product storage requirements	Store at room temperature. Keep unused patch in closed, protective pouch. See Table 50-9 for proper disposal.
j. specific nondrug measures	See Table 50-4. The quit line counselor will talk with you about problem-solving and coping skills. It is important to have your wife be a support for you when you quit. The counselor will arrange follow-up contacts after your quit date.
10. Solicit follow-up questions from patient.	(1) Can I cut the patch in half when I decrease the dose? (2) If I am trying to break the nicotine addiction, why would I take nicotine?
11. Answer patient's questions.	(1) The patch should not be cut in half, because nicotine can evaporate rapidly from the cut edges, resulting in erratic or reduced delivery of nicotine from the patch. (2) The addiction to nicotine is strong, and abruptly stopping smoking generally causes withdrawal symptoms. The nicotine patch just replaces a portion of the amount of nicotine you received when smoking and will make you more comfortable while quitting to help reduce your withdrawal symptoms while you work on changing your behaviors and routines.

Key: BMI, body mass index; NKA, no known allergies; OTC, over-the-counter; PCP, primary care provider.

CASE 50-2

Relevant Evaluation Criteria	Scenario/Model Outcome
Information Gathering	
1. Gather essential information about the patient's symptoms, including:	
a. description of symptom(s) (i.e., nature, onset, duration, severity, associated symptoms)	Patient quit smoking 5 days ago and is using the 21 mg nicotine patch. She complains of trouble sleeping and is experiencing disturbing dreams since starting the patch. She had been smoking approximately 1 pack per day (~20 cigarettes daily) for 20 years before quitting.
b. description of any factors that seem to precipitate, exacerbate, and/or relieve the patient's symptom(s)	Before quitting, patient states she had to have a cigarette right when she woke up in the morning because she had such intense cravings.
c. description of the patient's efforts to relieve the symptoms	Patient used 21 mg nicotine patch for 5 days. She has not previously tried pharmacotherapy for quitting. She purchased the patch on her own and has not received any counseling from a clinician. She states she feels the nicotine withdrawal symptoms are minimal and thinks the patch is working well.
2. Gather essential patient history information:	
a. patient's identity	Carol Manning
b. patient's age, sex, height, and weight	49-year-old female, 5 ft 5 in, 160 lb
c. patient's occupation	Executive assistant in marketing firm
d. patient's dietary habits	Tries to eat healthy at home; lunch is usually fast food or deli sandwich
e. patient's sleep habits	Sleeps 7–8 hours a night. Since using the patch, she has experienced trouble sleeping and disturbing dreams.
f. concurrent medical conditions, prescription and nonprescription medications, and dietary supplements	Dyslipidemia; simvastatin 40 mg by mouth daily; ibuprofen 400 mg as needed for headache
g. allergies	NKA
h. history of other adverse reactions to medications	None
i. other (describe) _____	Divorced. Some close friends and coworkers also smoke. No major dental work.
Assessment and Triage	
3. Differentiate the patient's signs/symptoms and correctly identify the patient's primary problem(s).	Patient is recent quitter experiencing intolerable side effects from the nicotine patch (i.e., sleep disturbances).
4. Identify exclusions for self-treatment (see Figure 50-2).	None
5. Formulate a comprehensive list of therapeutic alternatives for the primary problem to determine if triage to a medical practitioner is required, and share this information with the patient.	Recommend continued pharmacotherapy and counseling. Take no action. Pharmacotherapy options include: (1) Recommend removing nicotine patch at night and adding gum as needed (particularly in the morning on waking). (2) Recommend alternative NRT, such as gum or lozenge. (3) Refer to PCP for prescription pharmacotherapy (nicotine inhaler, nicotine nasal spray, bupropion SR, varenicline).
Plan	
6. Select an optimal therapeutic alternative to address the patient's problem, taking into account patient preferences.	Because Carol has expressed that she feels the patch is working well to manage her withdrawal symptoms, continue the nicotine patch, but advise her to take the patch off before bedtime. This should help reduce the sleep disturbances and disturbing dreams. She can use combination therapy with nicotine gum as needed. A 2 mg gum dose is reasonable to be used on an as-needed basis.
7. Describe the recommended therapeutic approach to the patient.	Counseling: See Tables 50-3 and 50-4. It will be important to enlist the support of your coworkers and friends. Pharmacologic therapy is recommended, because you have no contraindications or precautions for self-care use of the nicotine patch and as-needed 2 mg gum.

CASE 50-2 (continued)

Relevant Evaluation Criteria	Scenario/Model Outcome
8. Explain to the patient the rationale for selecting the recommended therapeutic approach from the considered therapeutic alternatives.	You do not have any medical conditions in which nicotine medications should be used with caution (e.g., recent heart attack, serious arrhythmias, or angina). The nicotine patch will provide a low, constant level of nicotine to help reduce nicotine withdrawal symptoms. By taking it off at night, you should no longer experience sleep disturbances. The nicotine gum should be used only when you experience situations in which you are craving a cigarette, such as when you wake up. Receiving counseling, in addition to taking your medications as directed, will increase your chances of quitting.

Patient Education

9. When recommending self-care with non-prescription medications and/or nondrug therapy, convey accurate information to the patient:	
a. appropriate dose and frequency of administration	Use the 2 mg nicotine gum if you experience situations in which you are craving a cigarette, such as when you wake up. See Tables 50-5 and 50-8.
b. maximum number of days the therapy should be used	See Table 50-8.
c. product administration procedures	See Tables 50-6 and 50-9.
d. expected time to onset of relief	With the patch, the level of nicotine in your body will gradually rise over the next 12 hours and will remain steady with continued use of the patch. The blood nicotine levels are lower than those from smoking but should be sufficient to help control your nicotine withdrawal. With the gum, nicotine levels will peak 30–60 minutes after you start using the gum.
e. degree of relief that can be reasonably expected	Most patients find that nicotine withdrawal symptoms peak in the first few days after the last cigarette; withdrawal symptoms then gradually diminish over the next 2–4 weeks. Over time, you may find you need to use the gum less often. But be sure to stick with the recommended daily dosing schedule and duration. This will help you to be more comfortable while you are quitting.
f. most common side effects	See Case 50-1 for nicotine patch. The most common side effects of the nicotine gum are unpleasant taste, mouth irritation, jaw muscle soreness or fatigue, hypersalivation, hiccups, and dyspepsia.
g. side effects that warrant medical intervention should they occur	See Case 50-1 for nicotine patch. If you experience symptoms of nicotine excess (e.g., nausea, vomiting, dizziness, weakness, or rapid heartbeat), contact your PCP for evaluation of your medication regimen.
h. patient options in the event that condition worsens or persists	If you experience withdrawal symptoms or severe cigarette cravings, you should contact your PCP because you might need a higher dosage of nicotine. If you have side effects related to nicotine excess (see above), you should also contact your PCP.
i. product storage requirements	See Case 50-1 for nicotine patch. For the gum, store at room temperature. See Table 50-6 for proper disposal.
j. specific nondrug measures	Some coping strategies are listed in Table 50-4. In addition to the counseling I can provide, other counseling programs are available, including the telephone quit line (1-800-QUIT NOW), group classes, and Web-based programs. We can discuss which options you feel might be useful to you.
10. Solicit follow-up questions from patient.	How often may I use the gum?
11. Answer patient's questions.	You should use the gum only when you feel a strong craving to smoke, such as when you wake up in the morning. The patch will provide a consistent low level of nicotine to help reduce withdrawal symptoms. You should use the nicotine gum only when you feel a need, or urge, to smoke. Even though the box says you can use up to 24 pieces a day, you should not need this much when using the gum with the patch.

Key: NKA, no known allergies; NRT, nicotine replacement therapy; PCP, primary care provider.

PATIENT EDUCATION FOR
Smoking Cessation

Tobacco dependence is a chronic disease optimally treated with a combination of counseling and medications. The primary goal of smoking cessation treatment is to attain complete, long-term abstinence from all nicotine-containing products. For most people, carefully following product instructions and the self-care measures listed here will help ensure optimal treatment outcomes.

Nondrug Methods

- Receiving counseling from a clinician will increase success of smoking cessation. A clinician can help develop a tailored smoking cessation treatment plan.
- Telephone quit lines (1-800-QUIT-NOW) are also available to provide comprehensive counseling services at no cost.

Nonprescription Medications

Nicotine Replacement Therapy

- NRT helps relieve and prevent symptoms of nicotine withdrawal by partially replacing the high levels of nicotine your body is used to obtaining from cigarettes. Use of NRT helps you focus on changing your smoking routines and practice new coping skills while decreasing your withdrawal symptoms.
- NRT does not contain any of the harmful tars and other toxins present in tobacco smoke.
- Symptoms of nicotine withdrawal are common and should subside over 2–4 weeks.
- Recommended daily dosages for NRT are shown in Tables 50-5 and 50-8.
- See Table 50-6 for guidelines for the use of nicotine gum, Table 50-7 for the nicotine lozenge, and Table 50-9 for the nicotine patch.
- Follow the dosage regimen of the selected product carefully. Failure to do so will increase the chance of having withdrawal symptoms. Discontinuing therapy early might lead to relapse.

- Discontinue use of any form of NRT if you relapse back to smoking.
- Symptoms of nicotine excess include nausea, vomiting, dizziness, diarrhea, weakness, and rapid heartbeat.
- Do not eat or drink (except water) 15 minutes before or while using the nicotine gum or lozenge.
- Store NRT products at room temperature and protect from light.
- Keep new and used products out of the reach of children or pets.
- For all forms of NRT, consult your primary care provider before use if you have had a recent (in the past 2 weeks) heart attack, experience frequent pain caused by severe angina, have irregular heartbeats, are pregnant or breastfeeding, are younger than 18 years, or smoke fewer than 10 cigarettes a day.
- You may consider use of the gum with the patch (gum used only as needed). For other possible medication combinations, speak to your primary care provider first. For all forms of NRT, stop use and seek medical attention if irregular heartbeat or palpitations occur or if you have symptoms of nicotine overdose, such as nausea, vomiting, dizziness, diarrhea, and weakness.
- *Nicotine gum:* stop use if mouth, teeth, or jaw problems develop.
- *Nicotine lozenge:* stop use if mouth problems, persistent indigestion, or severe sore throat develop.
- *Nicotine patch:* stop use if the skin swells, a rash develops, or skin redness caused by the patch does not subside with use of nonprescription hydrocortisone cream or does not go away after 4 days.

Key Points for Smoking Cessation

➤ Clinicians should apply the 5 A's approach in providing smoking cessation counseling: ask, advise, assess, assist, and arrange.

➤ For a patient who is not ready to quit, provide brief counseling by addressing the 5 R's: relevance, risks, rewards, roadblocks, and repetition.

➤ For a patient who is ready to quit, offer counseling and pharmacotherapy. If time is limited, refer patient to the toll-free quit line (1-800-QUIT-NOW).

➤ Numerous effective medications are available for tobacco dependence, and clinicians should encourage their use by all patients attempting to quit smoking—except when medically contraindicated or with specific populations for which there is insufficient evidence of effectiveness (i.e., pregnant women, smokeless tobacco users, light smokers, and adolescents). If a patient has exclusions to self-treatment with NRT, refer to a primary care provider for further assessment.

➤ It is never too late to quit, but quitting earlier in life is clearly advantageous. Quitting smoking at any age has immediate as well as long-term benefits by reducing the risk for smoking-related diseases and improving health in general.

REFERENCES

1. US Department of Health and Human Services. *The Health Consequences of Smoking. A Report of the Surgeon General.* Rockville, Md: Public Health Service, Office on Smoking and Health; 1982. DHHS Publication No. (PHS) 82-50179.
2. Mokdad AH, Marks JS, Stroup DF, et al. Actual causes of death in the United States, 2000. *JAMA.* 2004;291:1238–45.
3. Centers for Disease Control and Prevention. Annual smoking-attributable mortality, years of potential life lost, and economic costs—United States, 1997–2001. *MMWR Morb Mortal Wkly Rep.* 2005;54:625–8.
4. Cigarette smoking among adults—United States, 2006. *MMWR Morb Mortal Wkly Rep.* 2007;56:1157–61.
5. Centers for Disease Control and Prevention. State-specific prevalence of cigarette smoking among adults and quitting among persons aged 18–35 years—United States, 2006. *MMWR Morb Mortal Wkly Rep.* 2007;56:993–6.
6. Cigarette smoking among adults—United States, 2000. *MMWR Morb Mortal Wkly Rep.* 2000;51:642–5.
7. US Department of Health and Human Services. The Health Consequences of Smoking: Nicotine Addiction. A Report of the Surgeon General. Washington, DC: US Government Printing Office; 1988. DHHS Publication No. (PHS) 88-8406.
8. Benowitz NL. Neurobiology of nicotine addiction: implications for smoking cessation treatment. *Am J Med.* 2008;121(4 suppl 1):S3–S10.
9. Benowitz NL. Clinical pharmacology of nicotine: implications for understanding, preventing, and treating tobacco addiction. *Clin Pharmacol Ther.* 2008;83:531–41.

10. Lasser K, Boyd JW, Woolhandler S, et al. Smoking and mental illness: a population-based prevalence study. *JAMA*. 2000;284:2606–10.

11. US Department of Health and Human Services. *The Health Consequences of Smoking: A Report of the Surgeon General*. Bethesda, Md: US Department of Health and Human Services, Centers for Disease Control and Prevention, National Center for Chronic Disease Prevention and Health Promotion, Office on Smoking and Health; 2004.

12. Federal Trade Commission. Cigarette Report for 2003. Issued 2005. Available at: http://www.ftc.gov/reports/cigarette05/050809cigrpt.pdf. Last accessed October 17, 2008.

13. Doll R, Peto R, Boreham J, et al. Mortality in relation to smoking: 50 years' observations on male British doctors. *BMJ*. 2004;328:1519.

14. National Cancer Institute. *Risks Associated with Low Machine-Measured Yields of Tar and Nicotine*. Smoking and Tobacco Control Monograph No. 13. Bethesda, Md: US Department of Health and Human Services, National Institutes of Health, National Cancer Institute; October 2001. NIH Publication No. 02-5074.

15. Hughes JR. Effects of abstinence from tobacco: valid symptoms and time course. *Nicotine Tob Res*. 2007;9:315–27.

16. US Department of Health and Human Services. *The Health Consequences of Involuntary Exposure to Tobacco Smoke: A Report of the Surgeon General*. Bethesda, Md: US Department of Health and Human Services, Centers for Disease Control and Prevention, Coordinating Care for Health Promotion, National Center for Chronic Disease Prevention and Health Promotion, Office on Smoking and Health; 2006.

17. Zevin S, Benowitz NL. Drug interactions with tobacco smoking. An update. *Clin Pharmacokinet*. 1999;36:425–38.

18. Seibert C, Barbouche E, Fagan J, et al. Prescribing oral contraceptives for women older than 35 years of age. *Ann Intern Med*. 2003;138:54–64.

19. World Health Organization. Low dose combined oral contraceptives. In: *Medical Eligibility Criteria for Contraceptive Use*. 3rd ed. Geneva: World Health Organization; 2004.

20. Burkman R, Schlesselman JJ, Zieman M. Safety concerns and health benefits associated with oral contraception. *Am J Obstet Gynecol*. 2004; 190(4 suppl):S5–S22.

21. Rosenberg L, Palmer JR, Rao RS, et al. Low-dose oral contraceptive use and the risk of myocardial infarction. *Arch Intern Med*. 2001;161: 1065–70.

22. Schwingl PJ, Ory HW, Visness CM. Estimates of the risk of cardiovascular death attributable to low-dose oral contraceptives in the United States. *Am J Obstet Gynecol*. 1999;180(1 pt 1):241–9.

23. Schiff I, Bell WR, Davis V, et al. Oral contraceptives and smoking, current considerations: recommendations of a consensus panel. *Am J Obstet Gynecol*. 1999;180(6 pt 2):S383–4.

24. Tanis BC. Oral contraceptives and the risk of myocardial infarction. *Eur Heart J*. 2003;24:377–80.

25. ACOG practice bulletin. No. 73: use of hormonal contraception in women with coexisting medical conditions. *Obstet Gynecol*. 2006;107:1453–72.

26. *Rx for Change: Clinician-Assisted Tobacco Cessation*. San Francisco, Calif: University of California San Francisco, University of Southern California, and Western University of Health Sciences; 1999–2009.

27. US Department of Health and Human Services. *The Health Benefits of Smoking Cessation. A Report of the Surgeon General*. Bethesda, Md: US Department of Health and Human Services, Public Health Service, Centers for Disease Control and Prevention and Health Promotion, Office on Smoking and Health; 1990. DHHS Publication No. (CDC) 90-8416.

28. Fiore MC, Jaen CR, Baker TB, et al. *Treating Tobacco Use and Dependence: 2008 Update. Clinical Practice Guideline*. Rockville, Md: US Department of Health and Human Services, Public Health Service; May 2008.

29. Shiffman S, Brockwell SE, Pillitteri JL, et al. Use of smoking-cessation treatments in the United States. *Am J Prev Med*. 2008;34:102–11.

30. Stead LF, Bergson G, Lancaster T. Physician advice for smoking cessation. *Cochrane Database Syst Rev*. 2008;2:CD000165.

31. Prochaska JO, DiClemente CC. The transtheoretical approach: crossing traditional boundaries of therapy. Homewood, Ill: Dow Jones-Irwin; 1984.

32. Hukkanen J, Jacob P 3rd, Benowitz NL. Metabolism and disposition kinetics of nicotine. *Pharmacol Rev*. 2005;57:79–115.

33. Shiffman S, Dresler CM, Hajek P, et al. Efficacy of a nicotine lozenge for smoking cessation. *Arch Intern Med*. 2002;162:1267–76.

34. Foulds J. The neurobiological basis for partial agonist treatment of nicotine dependence: varenicline. *Int J Clin Pract*. 2006;60:571–6.

35. US Food and Drug Administration, Center for Drug Evaluation and Research. Information for Healthcare Professionals Varenicline (marketed as Chantix). Available at: http://www.fda.gov/cder/drug/info sheets/HCP/ vareniclineHCP.htm. Last accessed October 17, 2008.

36. Benowitz NL, Gourlay SG. Cardiovascular toxicity of nicotine: implications for nicotine replacement therapy. *J Am Coll Cardiol*. 1997;29:1422–31.

37. Benowitz NL. Cigarette smoking and cardiovascular disease: pathophysiology and implications for treatment. *Prog Cardiovasc Dis*. 2003;46:91–111.

38. Joseph AM, Fu SS. Safety issues in pharmacotherapy for smoking in patients with cardiovascular disease. *Prog Cardiovasc Dis*. 2003;45:429–41.

39. Dempsey DA, Benowitz NL. Risks and benefits of nicotine to aid smoking cessation in pregnancy. *Drug Saf*. 2001;24:277–322.

40. Shiffman S. Nicotine lozenge efficacy in light smokers. *Drug Alcohol Depend*. 2005;77:311–4.

41. Stead LF, Hughes JR. Lobeline for smoking cessation. *Cochrane Database Syst Rev*. 2000;2:CD000124.

42. White AR, Rampes H, Campbell JL. Acupuncture and related interventions for smoking cessation. *Cochrane Database Syst Rev*. 2006;1: CD000009.

Home Medical Equipment

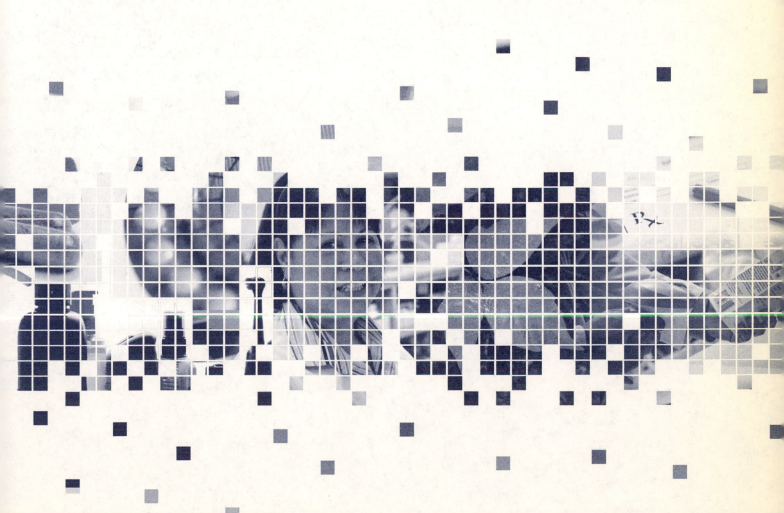

Home Testing and Monitoring Devices

Geneva Clark Briggs and Holly Hurley

In 1977, Warner-Lambert introduced the first home pregnancy test kit—an event that had a dramatic effect on the home diagnostics market. Annual sales of home pregnancy tests and ovulation prediction kits alone were almost $262 million in 2006.[1] The market continues to grow, with an expanded array of products and more user-friendly versions of established ones. Several forces are driving the growth in home diagnostics. First is the increased public interest in health and preventive medicine: Testing and monitoring kits now allow patients to test themselves conveniently at home, which encourages active participation in their own health care. Second is a reduction in health care costs: Home tests help patients avoid unnecessary visits to health care providers or allows them to seek earlier treatment of a medical condition. Third is the reduced access and availability of health care resources (i.e., extensive wait times for physician appointments and lengthy office waits). Fourth is the increased number of available tests. Finally, important advances in technology, such as monoclonal antibodies, have led to simplified tests that can be accurately and easily performed at home.

Home testing and monitoring kits are designed to detect presence or absence of a medical or physiologic condition and to monitor disease therapy. The Food and Drug Administration (FDA) requires home tests to perform as well as the professional-use equivalent. However, these products must be used properly to achieve accurate results.[2]

This chapter discusses home test kits that aid in detecting the following conditions: pregnancy, female fertility, male infertility, menopause, colorectal cancer (fecal occult blood tests), high cholesterol levels, urinary tract infections (UTIs), human immunodeficiency virus (HIV), and hepatitis C, as well as drug abuse. This chapter also covers proper selection and use of blood pressure monitors. In addition, a table of miscellaneous tests is included. (See Chapter 8, Chapter 13, and Chapter 47 for products used in self-monitoring of vaginal fungal infections, asthma, and diabetes mellitus, respectively.)

SELECTION CRITERIA

With the variety of diagnostic and monitoring products available, deciding which test to recommend to a given patient is quite challenging. The major product variables to consider include the test complexity, ease of reading results, presence of a control, and cost. Table 51-1 addresses these variables as well as the major patient assessment variables, which comprise three general areas:

1. Appropriateness of testing
2. Ability to accurately conduct the test and interpret the results
3. Potential interference with test results

PREGNANCY DETECTION TESTS

In 2005, the birth rate in the United States was 14.0 live births per 1000 population.[3] The female fertility rate in women ages 15 to 44 years increased in 2005 to 66.7 births per 1000 women.[3] In the United States, two-thirds (67%) of women ages 18 to 44 years who became pregnant found out by using a home pregnancy test.[4] Early detection of pregnancy is desirable for many reasons, including allowing the woman to make decisions regarding prenatal care and lifestyle changes to avoid potential harm to the fetus.

Physiology of the Female Reproductive Cycle

The female reproductive cycle is approximately 28 days long and is hormonally controlled. At the beginning of the cycle (day 1 through approximately day 12), low levels of circulating estrogen and progesterone cause the hypothalamus to secrete gonadotropin-releasing hormone (GnRH). GnRH stimulates release of follicle-stimulating hormone (FSH) and low levels of luteinizing hormone (LH) from the anterior pituitary gland. This combination of hormones promotes development of several follicles within an ovary during each cycle. One follicle is self-selected and continues to mature while the others regress. At midcycle (approximately day 14 or 15), circulating and urinary LH levels significantly increase and cause final maturation of the follicle. Ovulation (rupturing of the follicle and release of the ovum) occurs approximately 20 to 48 hours after the LH surge. Cells in the ruptured follicle then luteinize and form the corpus luteum, which begins to secrete progesterone and estrogen. For approximately 7 to 8 days after ovulation, the corpus luteum continues to develop and secrete estrogen and progesterone, which inhibits further secretion of FSH and LH.

Editor's Note: This chapter is based on the 15th edition chapter with the same title, written by Wendy Munroe Rosenthal and Geneva Clark Briggs.

TABLE 51-1 Selection and Use of Home Tests/Devices

- Not all available tests are FDA-approved for home use. The status of a particular test can be checked at www.accessdata.fda.gov/scripts/cdrh/cfdocs/cfIVD/Search.cfm.
- Always check the expiration date before purchase to ensure reagents are not outdated. For example, a test that has an expiration date of 07/08 expires at the end of July 2008.
- Follow the manufacturer's instructions for storing the tests to ensure reagents remain stable.
- When selecting a test, consider simplicity of use. Single-step tests are usually desirable because each step is a potential source of error.
- When considering cost, determine the cost per test unit and whether kits with multiple tests are needed. Generic or store-brand kits may cost significantly less.
- When possible, select a test that includes a control to ensure the test is functioning correctly.
- Read all instructions carefully and completely before attempting to perform a test.
- Note the time of day the test is to be conducted, the length of time required, and any necessary supplies or equipment; then schedule the best time and place to conduct the test.
- Follow instructions exactly as described and in sequence. If you have questions about the testing procedure or interpretation of the results, consult a health care provider or, if provided, call the test manufacturer's toll-free number for customer assistance.
- Use an accurate timing device that measures seconds to ensure that you wait the specified length of time between steps. In addition, waiting longer than the specified time to read test results could affect test reliability.
- If the selected test requires observation of a color change and you have color-defective vision or other visual impairment, ask someone without vision problems to observe the color change and/or read the test results. Also, read the test in good lighting.
- If you have physical limitations that could interfere with performing the test, ask someone to help you perform the test.
- If the test requires a fingerstick and you have a medical condition or take medications that may cause excessive bleeding, consult your health care provider before performing the test.

Once ovulation occurs, the ovum remains viable for fertilization for only 12 to 24 hours. Sperm may live up to 72 hours; therefore, optimal days for fertilization to occur include the 2 days before ovulation, the day of ovulation, and the day after ovulation. For the greatest chance of achieving pregnancy, intercourse should take place within 24 hours after the LH surge.

If fertilization occurs, trophoblastic cells produce human chorionic gonadotropic (hCG) hormone. This hormone causes the corpus luteum to continue to produce progesterone and estrogen, forestalling the onset of menses while the placenta develops and becomes functional. As early as day 7 after conception, the placenta produces hCG, some of which is excreted in the urine. The concentration of hCG continues to increase during early pregnancy, reaching maximum levels of hCG 6 weeks after conception. hCG levels decline over the following 4 to 6 weeks and then stabilize for the remainder of the pregnancy.

If fertilization does not occur during a cycle, the corpus luteum degenerates, circulating levels of progesterone and estrogen diminish, and menstruation occurs (days 1–5). Resulting low levels of progesterone and estrogen cause release of GnRH from the hypothalamus, and the hormonal cycle begins again.

Usage Considerations

The hormone produced by the trophoblast of the fertilized ovum, hCG, is detectable in the urine within 1 to 2 weeks after fertilization. It is composed of multiple forms including intact hCG, hyperglycosolated hCG (hCG-H), and free alpha and beta subunits. The primary form detected in early pregnancy is hCG-H.[5] However, most pregnancy tests have a decreased sensitivity for hCG-H.[6]

Numerous pregnancy tests with different reaction times and hCG sensitivity are available for home use. Table 51-2 lists some available products that have been tested for accuracy.[4,7–9] Overall, First Response Early Result may be the best test for detecting pregnancy before the fourth week of gestation, when hCG levels are low. After that point, most of the tests are equivalent.

Mechanism of Action

Home pregnancy tests are designed to detect the presence of hCG in urine. The tests use monoclonal or polyclonal antibodies in an enzyme immunoassay. The antibodies are bound to a solid surface such as a stick, bead, or filter. If urinary hCG is present, it will form a complex with the antibodies. Another antibody, one linked to an enzyme that will react with a chromogen to produce a distinctive color, is added. The hCG is "sandwiched" between the antibody linked to the enzyme and the antibodies bound to the solid surface. Washing or filtering within the testing device removes unbound substances; a chromogen then reacts with the enzyme causing a color change.

TABLE 51-2 Selected Pregnancy Tests

Trade Name	hCG Sensitivity	Product Features
First Response Early Result	<6.3 mIU/mL	Test stick; best combination of sensitivity and reliability; can test up to 4 days before missed period
Clearblue Easy +/– Results	25 mIU/mL	Test stick; can test up to 4 days before missed period; Clearblue Easy digital display test also available
Store brands	100 mIU/mL	Test sticks; some CVS samples failed to work[7]
E.P.T.	100 mIU/mL	Test sticks; some samples failed to work; E.P.T. Certainty has digital display
Accu-Clear	>100 mIU/mL	Test sticks or cassettes; 1% of samples failed to work[7]
Fact Plus	>100 mIU/mL	Test sticks or cassettes; can test up to 4 days before missed period with test sticks

Source: References 4 and 7–9.

Accuracy Rate

A pregnancy cannot be detected before implantation. Because of natural variability in the timing of ovulation, implantation does not necessarily occur before the expected onset of the next menses. One study found the highest possible screening sensitivity for an hCG-based pregnancy test conducted on the first day of a missed period is 90%, because 10% of women may not have an implanted embryo at that point. The authors estimate that the highest possible screening sensitivity of a home pregnancy test by 1 week after the first day of the missed period is 97%.[10] A test sensitivity for hCG of 12.4 mIU/mL is needed to detect 95% of pregnancies on the expected day of a missed period.[11] Although most pregnancy tests are advertised as 99% accurate, studies of consumer use of home pregnancy tests have found the actual accuracy rate to be 50% to 75%, because the directions were not followed carefully.[12]

Exclusions for Self-Testing

A false-positive result may occur if the woman has had a miscarriage or given birth within the previous 8 weeks, because hCG may still be present in the body. Medications such as Pergonal (menotropins for injection) and Profasi (chorionic gonadotropin for injection) can produce false-positive results. Unreliable results may occur in patients with ovarian cysts or an ectopic pregnancy. Oral contraceptive use does not affect test results.

Interferences

Because hCG levels are very low in early pregnancy and may be below the sensitivity of a particular test, false-negative results may occur with home pregnancy tests if they are performed on or before the first day of a missed period. Erroneous results may also result from refrigerated urine not allowed to warm to room temperature before testing, waxed cups used for collecting urine, or soap residue in household containers used for collecting urine.

Usage Guidelines

See the box Patient Education for Pregnancy Tests.

Product Selection Guidelines

Product labeling for most tests states that women may use the test as early as the first day of a missed menstrual period. Some tests that can detect hCG levels at 25 mIU/mL or less can be used 3 days before the missed period. The earlier a pregnancy test is used, the greater is the likelihood of a false-negative result. Most pregnancy tests are one-step procedures. Some tests have clear test sticks that allow the woman to see the reaction occurring as a check that sufficient urine was absorbed by the stick. Other tests include two devices, which can be helpful if a negative test is obtained first. The newest tests are digital and display the results as "pregnant" or "not pregnant" instead of colored lines, which eliminates the need to interpret the results. The time to obtain test results varies from 1 to 5 minutes. Generic (store-brand) kits are available and are usually less expensive than the brand-name kits.

In a recent study of seven nonprescription pregnancy tests, it was found that First Response Early Result was the most sensitive and reliable test. It detected hCG at concentrations as low as 6.5 mIU/mL. In addition, this product was expected to detect more than 95% of pregnancies on the first day of a missed period.[7]

Assessment of Pregnancy Test Use: A Case-Based Approach

The practitioner should first determine if a pregnancy test is appropriate for the patient by asking questions about her menstrual cycle and the number of days since unprotected intercourse. If product use is appropriate, the practitioner should ask about previous use of pregnancy tests and any difficulties the patient had with the tests. The practitioner must ask questions about medical disorders and medication use to determine whether inaccurate test results are possible or special measures may be required to protect the unborn child.

Case 51-1 illustrates assessment of a patient who wishes to use a pregnancy test.

CASE 51-1

Relevant Evaluation Criteria	Scenario/Model Outcome
Information Gathering	
1. Gather essential information about the patient's symptoms, including:	
a. description of symptom(s) (i.e., nature, onset, duration, severity, associated symptoms)	Patient thinks she may be pregnant, because she had unprotected sexual intercourse with her boyfriend a few weeks ago.
b. medical history, including family history	(1) Date of last menstrual period: 06/14/08 (2) Date of expected menstrual period: 07/14/08 (3) Menstrual cycle: 30-day, regular cycle with no unusual symptoms or complications
2. Gather essential patient history information:	
a. patient's identity	Alexandria Smith
b. patient's age, sex, height, and weight	16-year-old female, 5 ft 5 in, 130 lb
c. patient's occupation	Full-time student

C A S E   5 1 - 1   *(continued)*

Relevant Evaluation Criteria	Scenario/Model Outcome
d. concurrent medical conditions, prescription and nonprescription medications, and dietary supplements	No current medical conditions; Centrum Multi-Vitamin (500 mcg of folic acid) 1 tablet every day
e. prior use of diagnostic/monitoring test	Alexandria has used the Fact Plus home pregnancy test in the past few days. She says the test was negative. Her period is due in 2 days.
f. Potential problems with performing/interpreting test	Alexandria's first test showed a very faint pink line, but she determined it was negative after waiting 5 minutes.

Assessment and Triage

3. Determine if self-testing is appropriate.	Self-testing is not appropriate at this time. Because of hCG sensitivity, the patient should test at a later date as directed in the test instructions.
4. Identify exclusions for self-testing.	None
5. Formulate a comprehensive list of therapeutic alternatives for the primary problem to determine if triage to a medical practitioner is required, and share this information with the patient.	Options include: (1) Recommend retesting the first day after a missed period. (2) Recommend a test with a low hCG sensitivity and also a digital testing device. Educate the patient to follow all manufacturers' instructions when performing the self-test. Advise the patient to retest in 1 week if the test is negative and she has not started her period. (3) Take no action.

Plan

6. Select an optimal therapeutic alternative to address the patient's problem, taking into account patient preferences.	The patient prefers testing with a digital device for easier-to-read results.

Patient Education

7. Describe the testing procedure to the patient including,	
a. specific instructions	When you do perform the test, follow the instructions carefully (see the box Patient Education for Pregnancy Tests).
b. how to avoid incorrect results	See the box Patient Education for Pregnancy Tests.
8. Solicit follow-up questions from patient.	If the test comes back positive, does this mean I am definitely pregnant?
9. Answer patient's questions.	Most likely. Your medication and medical history indicates that you would not have a false-positive test result. The test determines hCG levels in your urine. If the test comes back positive, you should see a health care provider immediately for follow-up. You should also start taking a prenatal vitamin with a higher daily dosage of folic acid (800 mcg).

Patient Counseling for Pregnancy Tests

When counseling a patient on the use of pregnancy tests, the practitioner should emphasize the importance of following package instructions carefully, especially the instruction for when to begin testing. Pregnancy tests are very sensitive; therefore, the patient should be advised of medical and environmental factors that can cause inaccurate test results. The box Patient Education for Pregnancy Tests lists specific information to provide patients.

P A T I E N T   E D U C A T I O N   F O R
Pregnancy Tests

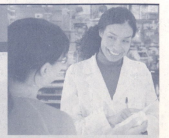

The obvious objective of self-testing is to determine whether a patient is pregnant. For most patients, carefully following package instructions and the self-care measures listed here will help ensure accurate test results.

Avoidance of Incorrect Results

- The most accurate results will be obtained by waiting at least 1 week after the date of

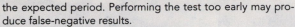

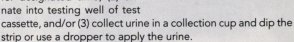

the expected period. Performing the test too early may produce false-negative results.

- Be sure to use the urine collection device provided in the kit. Wax particles in waxed cups can clog the test matrix, causing false results. Soap residue in household containers can also interfere with test results.
- Try to test the urine sample immediately after collection.
- If the sample must be tested later, store it in the refrigerator, but allow the sample to warm to room temperature for 20–30 minutes before testing. Chilled urine may produce false-negative results. Be careful not to redisperse any sediment present in the sample. Do not shake the sample.

Usage Guidelines

- Unless package instructions specify otherwise, use the first morning urine, because the levels of hCG, if present, will be concentrated at that time.
- If testing occurs at other times of the day, restrict fluid intake for 4–6 hours before urine collection.
- Remove test stick or cassette from packaging just before use. For test sticks, remove cap, if present, from absorbent tip.

- Apply urine to testing device using whichever of the following methods is specified in package instructions: (1) hold test stick in the urine stream for designated time, (2) urinate into testing well of test cassette, and/or (3) collect urine in a collection cup and dip the strip or use a dropper to apply the urine.
- After the urine is applied, lay the testing device on a flat surface. Wait the recommended time (1–5 minutes) before reading results. Waiting the maximum allowed time may improve the sensitivity of the test.
- After reading the results, discard the testing device. If the test result is negative, test again in 1 week if menstruation has not started.

 If the second test is negative and menstruation has not begun, consult a health care provider.

Source: References 4 and 9.

Evaluation of Patient Outcomes with Pregnancy Tests

If the pregnancy test result is positive, the woman should assume she is pregnant and contact her primary care provider or an obstetrician as soon as possible. Also, if the patient is taking a medication with teratogenic potential (e.g., Accutane or methotrexate) or any medications for chronic conditions, she should be advised to discuss with her health care practitioners any possible effects the drugs may have on a fetus. If the test result is negative, the woman should review the procedure and make sure she performed the test correctly. She should test again in 1 week if menstrual flow has not begun. If the results of the second test are negative and menses still has not begun, the woman should seek the advice of a health care provider.

FEMALE FERTILITY TESTS

Women who have difficulty becoming pregnant use various methods of predicting ovulation so they can time sexual intercourse to coincide with optimal fertility. This section discusses women's use of basal thermometers and ovulation prediction test kits and devices. These tests and devices are also useful for women who want to be more aware of their time of ovulation. However, they are not a reliable means of birth control.

It may take several months for fertile women to become pregnant. In contrast, infertility is defined as the medical inability to conceive after 1 year of unsuccessful attempts. In a National Survey of Family Growth conducted in 2002, it was shown that infertility is estimated to occur in 7.4 percent of married women ages 15 to 44 years.[13]

Available nonprescription products for ovulation prediction (Table 51-3) include ovulation detecting devices, basal thermometers, and urine tests.[4,8,16–19] Each detection method has a different mechanism of action and method of use. Women should pick a method that best suits their lifestyle or philosophy of self-care.

Saliva microscopy and home saliva monitors are also available. These two products are not discussed here, because the results obtained with these devices are not reliable or the data on accuracy are conflicting.[14]

Basal Thermometry

For many years, women have measured basal body temperature (BBT) to predict the time of ovulation. Resting BBT is usually below normal during the first part of the female reproductive cycle. Approximately 24 to 48 hours after ovulation, it rises to a level closer to normal (i.e., 98.6°F [37°C]).[17]

Usage Considerations

Mechanism of Action

When using basal thermometry, women take their temperature (orally, rectally, or vaginally) with a basal thermometer each morning before arising. These temperature measurements are then plotted graphically. A rise in temperature signals that ovulation has occurred. When the increase occurs, women who want to become pregnant should have intercourse as soon as possible to maximize their chances of conception.

Accuracy Rate

The only equipment necessary for monitoring BBT is a basal thermometer, which has smaller gradations than a regular

TABLE 51-3 Selected Ovulation Prediction Tests and Devices

Trade Name	Reaction Time	Product Features
Clearblue Easy Ovulation Test Pack	3 minutes	7-day kit. Urine test sticks; predicts ovulation within 24–36 hours; most sensitive product in *Consumer Reports* test[15]; easy to read
Clearblue Easy Digital Ovulation Test	3 minutes	7-day kit. Urine test sticks; clear and easy to read with no lines to interpret; digital smiley face technology
Clearblue Easy Fertility Monitor	5 minutes	Reusable monitor. Urine test sticks; predicts 1- to 5-day window of peak fertility; stores daily fertility information; easy to read; tests for LH and E3G, an estrogen metabolite
Answer 1-Step Ovulation	5 minutes	7-day kit. Urine test sticks; predicts ovulation within 24–36 hours
Accu-Clear Early Ovulation Predictor Test	3 minutes	5-day kit. Urine test sticks; predicts ovulation within 24–48 hours
First Response 1-Step Ovulation Predictor Test	5 minutes	7-day kit. Urine test sticks; predicts ovulation within 24–36 hours
BD Basal Thermometer	1 minute	Digital thermometer. Auto memory for last reading; continuous beep to indicate it is working; signals when done; large lighted display
OV-Watch	Measures chloride ions every 30 minutes up to 12 readings	Lightweight watch that is worn during sleep; detects up to 4 days prior to ovulation; easy to use and read

Key: LH, luteinizing hormone; E3G, estrone-3-glucuronide.
Source: References 4, 8, and 16–19.

thermometer. Although basal thermometry is a relatively simple method of ovulation prediction, interpreting temperature data can be confusing. The temperature increase that follows ovulation is small ($0.4°F–1.0°F$ [$0.2°C–0.6°C$]). Women who have trouble reading a thermometer may miss the rise altogether; in this case, a digital model should be used.

Interferences

Several factors, such as emotions, movements, and infections, can influence the basal temperature. Eating, drinking, talking, and smoking should be postponed until after each measurement is obtained.

Usage Guidelines

See the box Patient Education for Ovulation Prediction Tests and Devices.

Product Selection Guidelines

The BD basal digital thermometer includes an FDA-approved fertility software program (Taking Charge of Your Fertility). Digital thermometers that track multiple temperature readings for the user are available, although they are more expensive than digital thermometers that lack this feature.

Urinary Hormone Tests

Ovulation prediction tests that use urine samples to estimate the time of ovulation are marketed to women who are having difficulty conceiving and need to pinpoint ovulation.

Usage Considerations

Mechanism of Action

Urine-based ovulation prediction tests use monoclonal antibodies specific to LH to detect the surge in LH. An enzyme-linked immunosorbent assay (ELISA) elicits a color change indicating the amount of LH in the urine.[20] The LH surge is revealed by a difference in color or color intensity from that noted on the previous day of testing. The intensity of color on the test stick is directly proportional to the amount of LH in the urine sample. Generally, early morning collection of urine is recommended, because the LH surge usually begins early in the day, and the urine concentration is relatively consistent at this time. Some products do not specify a time of day, requiring only that a consistent time of day be used.

Testing should begin 2 to 4 days before the estimated day of ovulation. The kit contains directions to determine when to begin testing according to the average length of the past three menstrual cycles. If the cycle varies by more than 3 to 4 days each month, the woman should use the shortest menstrual cycle to determine the starting date.

The Clearblue Easy Fertility Monitor increases the specificity of ovulation prediction by measuring both LH and estrone-3-glucuronide (E3G), a component of estrogen. E3G levels rise and fall in a pattern similar to that of LH. This product uses test sticks that the woman places in her urine stream and then inserts into a small, palm-size monitor with a light-emitting diode screen. The patient must establish a baseline with data about fluctuations in her hormone levels to accurately predict ovulation. For the first month, she tests for 20 consecutive days, starting on approximately the sixth day after the beginning of menstruation.[21] Using these data, the monitor calculates the time window during which the woman is most likely to conceive. After establishing her baseline, she tests for

10 to 20 days each month, depending on her cycle length. Each day's results are displayed as low, high, or peak fertility.[8] A low result indicates a small chance of conception; accordingly, a high result indicates increased chance of conception. This reading is typically displayed for 1 to 5 days leading up to peak fertility for each cycle. A "peak" reading indicates the highest chance of conception and is usually observed 2 days before ovulation.

Exclusions for Self-Testing

Medications used to promote ovulation (e.g., menotropins) artificially elevate LH and may cause false-positive results in ovulation prediction tests that measure only LH. The true LH surge can be detected in patients receiving clomiphene as long as testing does not begin until the second day after drug therapy ends. Medical conditions associated with high levels of LH, such as menopause and polycystic ovarian syndrome (PCOS), may also cause false-positive results for ovulation. Pregnancy can give a false-positive result for ovulation. If the patient has recently discontinued using oral contraceptives, the start of ovulation may be delayed for one to two cycles. Therefore, it would not be appropriate to use a home ovulation prediction test until fertilization has been attempted unsuccessfully for 1 to 2 months after discontinuation of the oral contraceptives.

PCOS, medications that affect the cycle (e.g., oral contraceptives, certain fertility treatments, and estrogen-containing medications), impaired liver or kidney function (which alters levels of E3G), breast-feeding, tetracycline (not oxytetracycline or minocycline), and perimenopause may produce false-positive results with the Clearblue Easy Fertility Monitor. Women who have recently been pregnant, stopped breast-feeding, or stopped using hormonal contraception should consider waiting until they have at least two consecutive natural menstrual cycles (lasting 21–42 days) before using the Clearblue Easy Fertility Monitor.[8]

Usage Guidelines

See the box Patient Education for Ovulation Prediction Tests and Devices.

Product Selection Guidelines

The available ovulation prediction tests vary in the length of time needed to complete the test, method of applying urine to the test stick, and number of individual tests provided. Patients with longer cycles may benefit from purchasing kits that contain more testing sticks.

The Clearblue Easy Fertility Monitor does have some possible advantages over the standard ovulation prediction kits. The traditional kits identify the 24- to 48-hour window around ovulation, whereas the Clearblue Easy Fertility Monitor identifies a larger window of several days. This monitor does not require patients to interpret color changes. It is effective for women with monthly cycle lengths of 21 to 42 days, because the monitor calculates the fertility period on the basis of each woman's hormone levels.[8] In addition, it measures both LH and E3G, increasing the specificity of ovulation prediction. However, it has not been proven whether these possible advantages increase a woman's chance of accurately identifying ovulation and, ultimately, conceiving.

In a test of 11 ovulation prediction kits, *Consumer Reports* found that the ClearBlue Easy Ovulation Test Pack was the most sensitive and easiest to read.[15] The test also found that the Clearblue Easy Fertility Monitor was the second most sensitive test. The initial cost of the Clearblue Easy Fertility Monitor is higher than that of the traditional ovulation prediction kits that detect only LH, but it is reusable for an indefinite period, with only the additional expense of more test sticks. *Consumer Reports* estimated that a user would need to test for ovulation for 8 months or longer to make this monitor's price competitive.[15]

Wristwatch Ovulation Prediction Device

A new lightweight wristwatch, OV-Watch, has been developed that uses a specialized biosensor to detect and measure the fluctuation of chloride ions to predict ovulation.

Usage Considerations

Mechanism of Action

Studies have shown that during a woman's menstrual cycle, numerous electrolytes detected in a woman's perspiration are known to fluctuate. One of the electrolytes, chloride, peaks at various times throughout the monthly cycle.[18] This concept has allowed the development of a watch device to detect chloride ions transdermally. Approximately, 6 days before ovulation there is a chloride ion surge that appears days before the surge in estrogen and LH. The watch has a specialized biosensor that detects the chloride ion surge. This surge directly relates to ovulation; therefore, the watch has been shown to detect the fertile window earlier than other tests or devices. When using the watch, a woman should begin wearing the device on the first, second, or third day of her menstrual cycle. The watch is usually worn at least 6 hours during sleep; data are recorded every 30 minutes for a maximum of twelve daily readings.

Accuracy Rate

A clinical trial was conducted in 105 women to compare the watch device with the standard urine LH device and the basal body thermometer in predicting fertile days and ovulation. The results concluded that the watch was equivalent to the other products in determining the actual day of ovulation within 2 to 3 days. However, the watch detected more of the fertile days than the other products. Finally, the study suggested that approximately two-thirds of patients who used the watch were more likely to become pregnant within 6 months.[19]

Interferences

Several factors, such as excessive moisture, hormonal contraceptives, menopause, liver and kidney disease, breast-feeding, and PCOS can affect the accuracy of the watch.

Usage Guidelines

See the box Patient Education for Ovulation Prediction Tests and Devices.

Product Selection Guidelines

The OV-Watch uses advanced technology to help predict a woman's fertile window. In addition, the more fertile days a woman can identify, the better are her chances of becoming pregnant.

Assessment of Female Fertility Test Use

The practitioner should ask a patient privately about her reasons for using an ovulation prediction test. If the reason is difficulty in conceiving, the practitioner should find out whether the patient has consulted a health care provider about a possible fertility problem and whether she has previously used ovulation prediction tests or devices. Questions about other possible pathology and medication use are appropriate for determining possible interferences with test results or temperature measurements.

Patient Counseling for Female Fertility Tests

To use ELISA–based ovulation prediction products effectively, a woman must know approximately when ovulation occurs or be willing to track three menstrual cycles to determine when it occurs. The practitioner should explain the hormonal fluctuations during the cycle and how they relate to the use of ovulation prediction tests and devices. The practitioner should also explain the reason for the number of tests or measurements that must be performed with each type of product. The practitioner should emphasize that the woman must consistently use the products for at least 3 months. The box Patient Education for Ovulation Prediction Tests and Devices lists specific information to provide patients.

PATIENT EDUCATION FOR
Ovulation Prediction Tests and Devices

The objective of self-testing is to more accurately determine the time of ovulation to increase the chances of conception. For most patients, carefully following product instructions and the self-care measures listed here will help increase the chances of achieving this goal.

Basal Thermometers
Avoidance of Incorrect Results
- Do not move while taking temperature measurements.
- Emotions can affect temperature measurements.
- If an infection is suspected, discontinue the measurements until the disorder is resolved. Begin taking temperatures again on the first day of menstruation of the cycle after resolution of the disorder.
- Do not eat, drink, talk, or smoke within 30 minutes before taking temperature measurements.

Usage Guidelines
- Read the instructions thoroughly before using the thermometer, and follow instructions carefully.
- Choose one method of taking temperatures (orally, vaginally, or rectally), and use that method consistently.
- Take temperature readings at approximately the same time each morning. Take temperatures just before rising each morning after at least 5 hours of sleep. If using a regular basal thermometer, plot the temperatures on a graph. A rise in temperature indicates that ovulation has occurred.

Ovulation Prediction Tests
Avoidance of Incorrect Results
- Fertility medications, PCOS, menopause, and pregnancy can cause false-positive results for ovulation.
- Oral contraceptives, hormone replacement therapy, impaired liver or kidney function, breast-feeding, tetracycline (but not oxytetracycline or minocycline), and perimenopause can cause false-positive results with the Clearblue Easy Fertility Monitor.
- Recent pregnancy or discontinuation of oral contraceptives or breast-feeding will delay ovulation for one or two cycles. Start testing after two natural menstrual cycles have occurred.

Usage Guidelines (Except Clearblue Easy Fertility Monitor)
- Start using the test 2–3 days before ovulation is expected.
- Follow the manufacturer's specific directions regarding the timing of urine collection. If the first morning urine is not tested, restrict fluid intake for at least 4 hours before testing and avoid urinating until ready to test the urine, so the urine will not be diluted.
- Test the urine sample immediately after collection.
- If immediate testing is not feasible, refrigerate urine for the length of time specified in the directions for each product. Allow refrigerated sample to stand at room temperature for 20–30 minutes before beginning the test.
- Do not redisperse any sediment that may be present in the sample.
- If using a kit designed to be passed through the urine stream, either hold a test stick in the urine stream for the specified time, or collect urine in a collection cup and dip the stick in the urine.
- If using a kit not designed to be passed through the urine stream, collect urine in a collection cup, then place the urine in the testing well using the dropper provided.
- After the urine is placed on the testing device, read the results in 3–5 minutes, depending on the manufacturer's instructions.
- Watch for the test's first significant increase in color intensity, which indicates that the surge of LH has occurred and ovulation will occur within a day or two.

PATIENT EDUCATION FOR
Ovulation Prediction
Tests and Devices *(continued)*

- Once the LH surge is detected, discontinue testing. Remaining tests can be used later, if necessary.
- If the LH surge is not detected, carefully review the testing instructions to ensure they were performed properly.
- If the testing procedure was accurate, ovulation may not have occurred or testing may have occurred too late in the cycle. Consider testing for a longer period and earlier in the next cycle to increase the chances of detecting the LH surge.

Usage Guidelines for Clearblue Easy Fertility Monitor Test

- For the first month, begin testing on the sixth day after beginning menstruation and test for 20 days.
- For subsequent months, test the number of days indicated by the monitor.
- Remove test stick or cassette from packaging just before use.
- Hold the test stick in the urine stream; insert stick in monitor.
- Discard test stick after use.

OV-Watch Fertility Predictor Device
Avoidance of Incorrect Results

- Fertility medications, hormonal contraceptives, menopause, impaired liver and kidney function, breast-feeding, and PCOS may interfere with results.
- Do not expose the watch to water or excessive moisture. Wait 1 hour after exercising or showering before wearing the watch.

Usage Guidelines

- Before using the watch, read the manufacturer's instructions thoroughly to attach the sensor and program the device.
- Use the watch on the first, second, or third day of the menstrual period.

Key: LH, luteinizing hormone; PCOS, polycystic ovarian syndrome.
Source: References 16–18, 20, and 21.

Evaluation of Patient Outcomes with Female Fertility Testing

Ovulation prediction products should not be used for more than 3 months. If conception does not occur within this period, the woman should see a primary care provider.

MALE FERTILITY TESTS

Sperm concentration is one of the many factors used to determine male fertility. Because many additional factors play a role in male infertility, a positive test for sperm count is not a guarantee of fertility. Sperm production is influenced by physical, emotional, and psychological factors. Factors such as concentration of hormones, stress, high fever, exercise, travel, surgery, medication, and changes in diet may result in a decreased sperm concentration.

Usage Considerations

The male fertility test measures sperm concentration as either above or below the cutoff of 20 million sperm cells per milliliter, which is the World Health Organization criterion for determining low sperm count. Two test results of fewer than 20 million cells per milliliter obtained at least 3 days, but not more than 7 days, apart may indicate male infertility.[22]

Mechanism of Action

The test works by staining cells in the sperm sample to produce a color. The intensity of the color is compared with a color reference on the test cassette. The color comparison identifies whether the sperm concentration in the test sample is above 20 million cells per milliliter (positive test) or below this level (negative test). The test kit contains all the necessary supplies for two tests: test cassette, testing solution, plastic droppers, two liquefaction cups, and two nonspermicidal condoms.

Accuracy Rate

Testing performed by the manufacturer found the overall accuracy of the test was 78%.[22]

Interferences

Only the condoms provided in the kit should be used for semen collection. Spermicidal condoms may interfere with the test.

Usage Guidelines

See the box Patient Education for Male Fertility Tests.

Product Selection Guidelines

FertilMARQ and BabyStart are the same male infertility test marketed under different names. Because this test requires the user to make a color comparison, patients with visual difficulties should seek assistance in interpreting the test results.

Assessment of Male Fertility Test Use

The practitioner should ask a patient privately whether he has consulted a primary care provider about a possible fertility problem, and whether the patient has used male fertility tests previously. Questions about possible pathology, medication use, stress, and physical activity are appropriate for determining possible interference with test results.

Patient Counseling for Male Fertility Tests

Because physical, psychological, and emotional factors can affect sperm concentration, the practitioner should explain the need for two tests to confirm a sperm count above or below 20 million cells per milliliter. The box Patient Education for Male Fertility Tests lists specific information to provide patients.

PATIENT EDUCATION FOR
Male Fertility Tests

The objective of self-testing is to screen for low sperm levels in semen. For most patients, carefully following product instructions and the self-care measures listed here will help ensure accurate test results.

Avoidance of Incorrect Results

- Use only the condoms provided in the kit for semen collection.
- Wait 3 days after the last ejaculation before collecting a semen sample for testing.
- Use only thinned (liquefied) semen for testing. Some patients have high-viscosity semen, which will not properly liquefy. These patients cannot get accurate results with this test, but these patients cannot be identified until they attempt the test and discover the semen sample will not liquefy sufficiently to pass through the test cassette.
- Test within 12 hours of sample collection.
- If the sample or solutions take more than 5 minutes to drain through the test wells, the test is invalid.

Usage Guidelines

- Semen sample can be collected in one of three ways:
  —By masturbation, directing semen into the liquefaction cup
  —By masturbation, using the supplied condom
  —During intercourse, using one of the supplied condoms
- Because freshly ejaculated semen is gel-like, the sample must be allowed to thin to a liquid consistency for testing. The liquefaction cups speed this process from 1 hour to 15 minutes.
- After collection, squeeze all the semen collected into a liquefaction cup and place cap on cup. Small flakes at the bottom of the liquefaction cup are normal.
- Swirl the cup gently at least 10 times.

- Allow the semen sample to liquefy for 15 minutes.
- The semen sample may be stored in the cup for up to 12 hours before testing.
- Swirl the cup again before beginning the test.
- The test cassette contains four wells labeled A, B, C, and D. Reference wells A and C are blue. Test wells B and D are white, and the liquefied semen sample is placed in these wells. The cassette contains enough wells to test two separate semen samples.
- The color of test well B or D is compared with the adjacent blue reference well.
- Fill dropper with semen and add one drop to test well B. Let the drop soak in for at least 1 minute.
- Add two drops of blue solution to test well B. Let the drops soak in for at least 1 minute.
- Add two drops of clear solution to test well B. Let the drops soak in at least 1 minute. Read results within 5 minutes.
- Compare the color in the test well with the color in the adjacent reference well A. Obtaining a blue color as dark as or darker than the reference color is a positive result (sperm ≥ 20 million/mL). A blue color lighter than the reference color is negative (sperm ≤ 20 million/mL).
- Two separate semen samples should be tested before a complete interpretation of the results can be made. Collect and test the second sample at least 3 days, but not more than 7 days, after the first test was performed.
- When performing the second test, use test well D and reference well C.
- If two negative tests are obtained, see a health care provider for evaluation and further testing.

Source: Reference 22.

Evaluation of Patient Outcomes with Male Fertility Tests

With the male fertility test, the patient should contact his primary care provider or a fertility specialist if two negative tests are obtained. If one positive and one negative test are obtained, the test should be repeated in 10 weeks with a new test kit.

FSH URINE TESTS FOR MENOPAUSE

Menopause is defined as the cessation of a woman's menses for at least 12 consecutive months. The average age for onset of menopause is 51 years; however, it can occur earlier or later in life.[23] Menopause results from the decline and eventual cessation of estrogen production. As estrogen levels decline, FSH levels increase. To most patients, menopause refers to a series of changes beginning with early menopause (perimenopause) and ending with the cessation of menstrual periods for a full 12 months (menopause). Symptoms of perimenopause and menopause may include irregular menstrual cycles, hot flashes, vaginal dryness, mood swings, insomnia, and fatigue. Many women find that symptoms of menopause interfere with their daily lives.

Usage Considerations

At this time several home tests are being marketed for menopause. The urine-based tests for FSH are FDA-approved; the saliva tests are not.

TABLE 51-4 FSH Urine Tests for Menopause

Trade Name	Availability	Product Features
Estroven Menopause Monitor	www.testsymptomsathome.com; selected retail stores	2 test cassettes, 2 droppers, 2 urine collection dishes
CARE Menopause Test	www.home-drugtest.com; selected retail stores	2 test cassettes, 2 droppers, 2 urine collection dishes
RU25 Plus Home Menopause Test Kit	www.home-menopause-test.com; www.hormonecheck.com	2 test sticks

Source: References 24–26.

Mechanism of Action

Tests for menopause use monoclonal antibodies specific to FSH to detect the hormone in urine. An ELISA elicits a color change that indicates the amount of FSH in the urine. A positive test indicates the presence of FSH at a concentration greater than 25 IU/L, which may indicate a woman is menopausal.[24-26] Because FSH levels change during the menstrual cycle, the test should be done twice to confirm the results. The two tests should be performed 1 to 2 weeks apart.

Interferences

Dilute urine can produce incorrect results. The patient should test the first morning urine, avoid drinking large amounts of fluids the night before testing, and not consume any fluids after midnight. Oral contraceptives, hormone replacement therapy, and estrogen supplements may affect the test and produce inaccurate results because of their estrogen content and effects on FSH levels.[24-26]

Usage Guidelines

See the box Patient Education for Menopause Tests. Table 51-4 lists selected menopause tests.

Product Selection Guidelines

Urine-based tests consist of either sticks placed in the urine stream or cassettes to which collected urine is applied. Patient preference should dictate which product is selected. Most test kits come with two testing devices for the recommended repeat test.

Saliva tests, which are mailed to a laboratory for analysis, measure numerous hormone levels; however, they are not FDA-approved.

Assessment of FSH Test for Menopause Use

The practitioner should find out whether the patient is experiencing classic symptoms of perimenopause and has consulted her primary care provider about them. Questions about use of estrogenic medications are appropriate for determining possible interference with test results.

Patient Counseling for FSH Tests for Menopause

The practitioner should emphasize that the FSH test is not a definitive diagnostic test for menopause. The diagnosis would need to be confirmed by the woman's primary care provider. The box Patient Education for Menopause Testing lists specific information to provide patients.

PATIENT EDUCATION FOR Menopause Tests

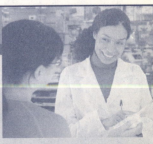

The objective of self-testing is to screen for high levels of follicle-stimulating hormone in the urine. For most patients, carefully following product instructions and the self-care measures listed here will help ensure accurate test results.

Avoidance of Incorrect Results
- Use first morning urine.
- Do not drink large amounts of fluids the night before performing the test.
- Do not drink fluids after midnight before testing in the morning.

Usage Guidelines
Test Cassettes
- Remove test cassette from foil and place on flat, hard surface.
- Catch midstream urine in the collection cup.

- Urine can be stored in the refrigerator for up to 24 hours before testing. Bring sample to room temperature before testing.
- Fill plastic dropper with urine. Hold the dropper vertical to the test cassette, and gently squeeze 4 full drops of urine into the round urine well on right side of cassette.
- Wait 15 minutes. Do not move cassette during this time.
- Read results in test window. Do not move the test cassette until results are checked.
- Repeat test in 7 days with a new test cassette. Each test cassette should be used only once.

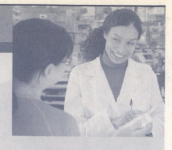
Evaluation of Patient Outcomes with FSH Tests for Menopause

Although FSH is elevated during menopause, FSH levels may be normal during the perimenopause period, which is when women often are most symptomatic. Therefore, a negative test (FSH < 25 IU/mL) does not indicate necessarily that the menopausal process has not begun. If a woman gets a negative result and is experiencing classic menopausal symptoms or obtains a positive result for elevated FSH, she should consult a health care provider for symptom management and osteoporosis prevention.

FECAL OCCULT BLOOD TESTS

Colorectal cancer is the second leading cause of cancer death in the United States. In 2008, the American Cancer Society estimated that 148,000 cases of colorectal cancer would be diagnosed and approximately 49,960 people would die from the disease.[27] This disorder may be hard to detect. One early and common symptom of colorectal cancer is rectal bleeding. Checking for hidden (occult) blood in the stool is an easy way to screen for a potential colon problem. Fecal occult blood tests (FOBTs) can be used as an adjunct to more invasive tests to detect colorectal cancer and other causes of gastrointestinal (GI) bleeding.

Colorectal cancer occurs most commonly in patients with a family history of colorectal cancer, intestinal polyps, or ulcerative colitis. The incidence of colorectal cancer increases with advancing age and is known to be directly related to consumption of high amounts of red and processed meat.[28]

Usage Considerations

Several nonprescription FOBTs are available. They fall into three categories: toilet tests (EZ-Detect Stool Blood Test), stool wipes (LifeGuard), and manual stool application devices (Colon-Test-Sensitive). They are all noninvasive and easy to use in the privacy of the home.

Accuracy Rate

One study found that a 3-day FOBT identified only 24% of colon lesions. When a 3-day FOBT was combined with sigmoidoscopy, many more cancers were identified (75.8%).[29]

Mechanism of Action

The in-home tests detect blood in feces with a colorimetric assay for hemoglobin. The heme portion of hemoglobin acts as an oxidizing agent; it catalyzes oxidation of the test reagent, tetramethylbenzidine, which produces a blue-green color. The appearance of this color indicates a positive test.[30–32]

Blood may be present on the surface or contained within the stool matrix. In general, matrix blood originates in the upper GI tract, whereas surface blood comes from the lower tract. The kits are more likely to detect blood from lower GI abnormalities. With the toilet and wipe tests, the reagent is sandwiched between two layers of biodegradable paper. The toilet tests are placed in the toilet bowl after a bowel movement. This type of kit is based on the premise that a significant amount of fecal blood will remain on the surface of the toilet bowl water after a bowel movement. In a wipe test, a stool sample is collected by using the test wipe to clean the anus after a bowel movement. With the stool application device tests, stool is applied to two wells with a wooden stick.

Exclusions for Self-Testing

Women who are menstruating should delay testing until menses has ceased. Menstrual blood present in the toilet bowl water or contaminating the stool sample can produce a positive result.

Interferences

Blood in the stool can signify a number of conditions in addition to cancer of the colon and rectum, including ulcers, Crohn's disease, colitis, anal fissures, diverticulitis, and hemorrhoids. Any of these conditions can give a positive result for an FOBT.

Aspirin, nonsteroidal anti-inflammatory drugs (NSAIDs), and steroids may cause sufficient gastric bleeding to produce positive results. These medications should be avoided for at least 2 to 3 days before testing as well as during the test period. A recent study, however, found that usual doses of aspirin and NSAIDs did not increase the risk of a false-positive FOBT.[33] The authors concluded there is little concern for a false-positive FOBT in patients who cannot safely discontinue aspirin or NSAIDS for specimen collection. Rectally administered medications should also be avoided. However, patients should always consult a health care provider before discontinuing any prescribed medications.

Vitamin C ingestion in excess of 250 mg/day may interfere with the peroxidase action of hemoglobin, causing false-negative results in the ColonTest-Sensitive, and LifeGuard tests.[31,32] The FOBTs are not specific for human blood and may produce false-positive results if red meat is consumed. Toilet bowl cleaners may also produce false-positive results. The box Patient Education for Fecal Occult Blood Tests lists measures for avoiding inaccurate test results.

Usage Guidelines

See the box Patient Education for Fecal Occult Blood Tests.

Product Selection Guidelines

Patients who want to avoid restricting their diet or stopping vitamin C may prefer the EZ-Detect product, which does not require a diet or medication change. Some patients may prefer the wipe or toilet tests to the stool collection type. All tests are similar in cost. All products, except ColonTest-Sensitive, have a card for recording results to give to the primary care provider.

Assessment of Fecal Occult Blood Test Use

Assessing the degree of risk a patient has for colorectal cancer is a major consideration in determining whether to recommend an FOBT. Patients with a personal or family history of colorectal cancer have a higher risk of developing the disease and would most likely benefit from testing. Patients with a family history should start testing annually at age 40 years; everyone should be tested yearly starting at age 50.[34] Determining the potential for false test results is another important consideration. False-negative tests could delay necessary treatment, whereas false-positive tests could cause unwarranted anxiety.

Patient Counseling for Fecal Occult Blood Tests

When counseling a patient on the use of FOBTs, the practitioner should emphasize the importance of following package instructions carefully. The box Patient Education for Fecal Occult Blood Tests lists specific information to provide patients.

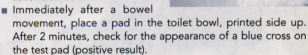

PATIENT EDUCATION FOR
Fecal Occult Blood Tests

The objective of self-testing is to screen for blood in the stool. For most patients, carefully following product instructions and the self-care measures listed here will help ensure accurate test results.

Avoidance of Incorrect Results
- Do not perform test during times of known bleeding, such as hemorrhoidal or menstrual bleeding.
- Increase dietary fiber intake for several days before testing. Roughage increases the accuracy of the test by stimulating bleeding from lesions that might not otherwise bleed.
- Because bleeding from cancerous lesions may be intermittent, perform the test on three consecutive bowel movements to increase the chance of detecting a possible lesion.
- Complete all three stool tests even if the first two produce negative results.
- Do not take nonprescription medications such as aspirin and NSAIDs for 2 to 3 days before testing and during testing.
- Some medications can cause bleeding and may need to be stopped before testing. Consult a health care provider about which medications to stop before performing the test.
- Chemicals in the toilet can interfere with the test. Following the instructions carefully can prevent this problem.

Usage Guidelines
- Do not eat red meat 2 to 3 days before testing and during the test period because undigested meat may produce a false-positive result.
- Do not take more than 250 mg/day of vitamin C for 2 to 3 days before and during the test period.

EZ-Detect
- Remove toilet tank cleansers or deodorizers and flush toilet twice before testing.
- Before testing, use one test pad to perform a water quality check. If any trace of blue appears in the cross-shaped area when the

pad is placed in the toilet water, use another toilet to complete the testing. Perform a water quality check on the second toilet as well.
- Immediately after a bowel movement, place a pad in the toilet bowl, printed side up. After 2 minutes, check for the appearance of a blue cross on the test pad (positive result).
- If color changes differ from the blue cross, discard the pad and repeat the test after the next bowel movement.
- Repeat the test on the next two bowel movements.
- If results are negative for all three tests, use remaining pad to perform a quality check of the test pads. Flush the toilet and empty the contents of the positive control chemical package into the bowl as it refills. Float the remaining test pad in the water, printed side up. After 2 minutes, check for a blue cross, which indicates the test pads are working properly. If the blue cross does not appear, call the assistance line provided with the product.

 Notify a health care provider if any of the three tests is positive.

LifeGuard
- Wipe with test pad after bowel movement.
- Peel and flush biodegradable tissue liner. Fold test in half to seal sample.
- Add 4 drops of developer to test pad. Observe for blue color change that indicates a positive result. Developer can be added to pad up to 14 days after the test.
- Add one drop of developer between the positive and negative lines on the control side of pad. The controls should not be developed until after the stool sample is developed. If the

Evaluation of Patient Outcomes with Fecal Occult Blood Tests

A patient evaluating the results of an FOBT must remember that the test is a screening method and is not specific to a particular disease. A positive test result may indicate any medical condition that causes a loss of blood through the GI system. The primary value of FOBT is to alert patients and health care providers that a thorough workup may be needed. The kits are not intended to replace other diagnostic procedures. Patients should be advised to contact their primary care provider if a positive test result is obtained.

CHOLESTEROL TESTS

Elevated cholesterol levels result from excessive production of cholesterol by the liver, deficient removal of the cholesterol from the bloodstream, and excessive intake of cholesterol-rich foods. Elevated low-density lipoprotein cholesterol (LDL-C) is the major cause of atherosclerotic heart disease, which can result in heart attack and stroke.[35] Although lowering LDL-C is the main target of therapy, other important goals include raising levels of high-density lipoprotein cholesterol (HDL-C), which removes deposits from the blood vessels, and lowering triglycerides, which contribute to development of heart disease.

Sixteen percent of American adults have high cholesterol.[36] Twenty-seven percent of women and 19.9% of men ages 55 to 64 years have high cholesterol.[36] Because of these statistics, the National Cholesterol Education Program recommends that all adults have a lipid profile measured at least every 5 years, starting at age 20.[35] A home cholesterol test is one means of achieving this first critical step to minimize the risk for cardiovascular heart disease. However, this test should not replace a complete lipid panel conducted by a primary care provider.

Because elevated cholesterol is a chronic condition that requires lifestyle modification and, frequently, medication for treatment, adhering to a treatment plan can be difficult for patients. Home cholesterol tests can help monitor the efficacy of and adherence to diet, exercise, and medication plans.

Usage Considerations

Some nonprescription cholesterol tests (Table 51-5) measure only total cholesterol, whereas others also measure LDL-C, HDL-C, and triglycerides. Individuals with diabetes might want to consider the CardioChek, which measures glucose and ketone levels in addition to cholesterol and triglyceride levels. The CholesTrack and Home Access kits allow patients to measure their total blood cholesterol levels at home, whereas patients who use the Personal Cholesterol Monitor store their total cholesterol level results on a smart card to share with their primary care provider or other practitioner. BIOSAFE offers a self-collected, laboratory-performed test for a complete lipid profile.

Mechanism of Action

With the total cholesterol test cassettes, cholesterol present in a blood sample is converted into hydrogen peroxide through a chemical reaction involving cholesterol esterase and cholesterol oxidase.[37,38] The peroxide then reacts with horseradish peroxidase and a dye to produce the color that rises along the cholesterol test's measurement scale. The test cassette has two separate indicator spots that change color to show that the test is functioning properly. One of the indicator spots also indicates completion of the test, signaling it is time to read the scale.

The CardioChek and the Personal Cholesterol Monitor are reflectance photometers that read the color intensity of the chemical test reaction.[39,40] Similar to a glucose meter, the results of the test are displayed on a screen. BIOSAFE's lipid profile is performed by a CLIA (Clinical Laboratory Improvement Act)–certified laboratory.[41]

Exclusions for Self-Testing

Excessive bleeding from a fingerstick can occur in patients who have coagulation disorders or use anticoagulants. These patients should not self-test for cholesterol levels.

Accuracy Rate

The accuracy rate of home cholesterol tests is debated. Except for BIOSAFE, which is mailed to a laboratory, all products are

TABLE 51-5 Selected Cholesterol Tests	
Trade Name	**Product Features**
CholesTrak AccuMeter Home Cholesterol Test Home Access Instant Cholesterol Test	Measures total cholesterol; not reusable; includes test cassette, lancet, and chart for interpreting test results from a drop of blood; chart is specific for test cassette and should not be reused
Personal Cholesterol Monitor	Measures total cholesterol; stores results on smart card; reusable; all materials needed to conduct test packaged together in 6-unit quantities
CardioChek	Measures total cholesterol, HDL-C, and triglycerides; can also measure glucose and ketones; stores results; reusable; separate testing strip and corresponding color-coded memory chip required for each type of test; cholesterol strips available in vials of 6, 25, 50, and 100; HDL-C and triglyceride strips available in vials of 6 and 25; each vial contains a memory chip
BIOSAFE Total Cholesterol Panel	Lipid profile (total cholesterol, triglycerides, HDL-C, LDL-C) results are obtained after mailing sample to laboratory; not reusable; contains lancet and sample collection card

Source: References 37–41.

FDA-approved for home use, are CLIA-waived devices, and are rated substantially equivalent to a laboratory-based cholesterol test. A published study of the CholesTrak device found that untrained consumers obtained results that correlated well with a laboratory-based cholesterol reference method.[42] *Consumer Reports* tested the CholesTrak, Accustat (previously named First Check), Home Access, CardioChek, and BIOSAFE Total Cholesterol Panel kits. The first three, which are essentially the same device, gave results that varied no more than 15% from laboratory values. The CardioChek and BIOSAFE Total Cholesterol Panel yielded results that were "often wide of the mark."[43] The report gave no more specifics.

Interferences

Good fingerstick technique is necessary to avoid erroneous results with cholesterol tests. Two or three hanging drops of blood are needed, but excessive squeezing and milking of the finger will negatively affect the quality of the blood sample. If sufficient blood cannot be obtained from the first fingerstick, the patient should use a different finger. A low cholesterol value may result if the blood sample is too small or if it takes longer than 5 minutes to collect the necessary amount of blood.

The patient should avoid doses of 500 mg or more of vitamin C before the test to avoid obtaining an artificially low result. Vitamin C slows the development of the color reaction by slowing the rate of peroxide production by oxidases.

Usage Guidelines

See the box Patient Education for Cholesterol Tests.

Product Selection Guidelines

Although significantly more expensive than individual total cholesterol test cassette kits, the CardioChek and the Personal Cholesterol Monitor are reusable with the purchase of additional testing materials and will store test results. The CardioChek has the ability to test for HDL-C and triglycerides, whereas the other home tests measure only total cholesterol. BIOSAFE provides a lipid profile, but results are not immediately available.

Assessment of Cholesterol Test Use: A Case-Based Approach

Before recommending a cholesterol test, the practitioner should first determine whether the patient has been diagnosed with heart disease or has some reason to be concerned about hypercholesterolemia. Conscientious monitoring of cholesterol is imperative for patients with heart disease, because elevated cholesterol levels have a significant impact on cardiovascular health. The practitioner should also ask about lifestyle and other factors that can affect test results.

Case 51-2 is an example of a cholesterol test assessment.

C A S E   5 1 - 2

Relevant Evaluation Criteria	**Scenario/Model Outcome**
Information Gathering	
1. Gather essential information about the patient's symptoms, including:	
a. description of symptom(s) (i.e., nature, onset, duration, severity, associated symptoms)	Patient recently lost 20 pounds and is interested in knowing his cholesterol level.
b. medical history, including family history	He has heart disease and is treated with a lipid-lowering agent. His primary care provider checks his cholesterol level annually.

CASE 51-2 (continued)

Relevant Evaluation Criteria	Scenario/Model Outcome
2. Gather essential patient history information:	
a. patient's identity	Joseph Williams
b. patient's age, sex, height, and weight	68-year-old male, 5 ft 8 in, 270 lb
c. patient's dietary habits	Patient states compliance with low-fat diet and has seen a dietitian.
d. concurrent medical conditions, prescription and nonprescription medications, and dietary supplements	Hypertension, lipid disorder; simvastatin 40 mg, enalapril 40 mg, enteric-coated aspirin 81 mg daily (adherence verified by refill records)
e. prior use of diagnostic/monitoring test	Joseph has never used a home monitoring test.
f. potential problems with performing/interpreting test	He does not have any visual or physical impairments.
	Use of daily aspirin should not cause a bleeding issue.

Assessment and Triage	
3. Determine if self-testing is appropriate.	Self-testing is appropriate.
4. Identify exclusions for self-testing.	None
5. Formulate a comprehensive list of therapeutic alternatives for the primary problem to determine if triage to a medical practitioner is required, and share this information with the patient.	Options include: (1) Suggest an appropriate at home cholesterol test (single- or multiple-use). (2) Refer for cholesterol testing. (3) Take no action.

Plan	
6. Select an optimal therapeutic alternative to address the patient's problem, taking into account patient preferences.	The patient prefers to try an at-home test given that his next appointment is not for 4 months. He is interested in testing only once, so a single-use test is suggested.

Patient Education	
7. Describe the testing procedure to the patient including,	
a. specific instructions	When you perform the test, follow the instructions carefully (see the box Patient Education for Cholesterol Tests).
b. how to avoid incorrect results	See the box Patient Education for Cholesterol Tests.
8. Solicit follow-up questions from patient.	If my cholesterol has not gone down, does this mean my weight loss has not helped?
9. Answer patient's questions.	No. Because of the variation in the home test, your true cholesterol level may be lower or higher than the reading you get with the home test. In addition, although the different lipids that make up the cholesterol level may have improved, you are measuring only total cholesterol.

Patient Counseling for Cholesterol Tests

When counseling a patient about cholesterol tests, the practitioner should emphasize the importance of properly collecting blood samples and advise the patient to seek assistance with the finger-stick, if needed. To further ensure accurate test results, the practitioner should advise the patient of medical and lifestyle factors that can cause inaccurate test results. The box Patient Education for Cholesterol Tests lists specific information to provide patients.

PATIENT EDUCATION FOR
Cholesterol Tests

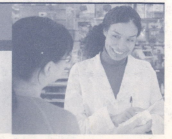

One objective of self-testing is to screen for high total cholesterol levels, allowing patients with elevated levels to start making lifestyle changes that can prevent heart attack and stroke. In addition, the patient should see a primary care provider for a full lipid profile and medical evaluation. Another objective is to monitor the effects of diet, exercise, or medication in patients with diag-

PATIENT EDUCATION FOR
Cholesterol Tests *(continued)*

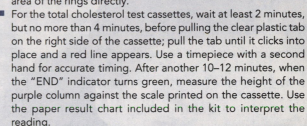

nosed hypercholesterolemia. For most patients, carefully following package instructions and the self-care measures listed here will help ensure achievement of accurate test results, which, in turn, can help patients achieve their medical goals with the assistance of a health care professional.

Avoidance of Incorrect Results

- If two or three hanging drops of blood cannot be obtained, or if it takes longer than 5 minutes to collect this amount of blood, do not perform the test.
- Do not excessively squeeze or milk the finger.
- If taking vitamin C in doses of 500 mg or more, do not take the dose within 4 hours of testing.

Usage Guidelines

- Because of the risk of excessive bleeding from the fingerstick, do not use cholesterol tests if you have hemophilia or take anticoagulants. Have a primary care provider perform the test.
- Before starting the test, wash your hands thoroughly with soap and warm water; then dry them.
- To stabilize the cholesterol level, sit and relax for 5 minutes before performing the test.
- For the CardioChek test, insert the memory chip corresponding to the desired test into the meter and turn on the meter.
- Lance the outside of one fingertip and wipe away the first sign of blood with the gauze pad. Then apply blood to the testing device as quickly as possible. For the total cholesterol test cassettes, fill the well of the test cassette. For the CardioChek test and Personal Cholesterol Monitor, apply enough blood to

cover the testing area of a strip. For the BIOSAFE test, place enough blood to fill each of the three rings on the test paper. Do not touch the area of the rings directly.

- For the total cholesterol test cassettes, wait at least 2 minutes, but no more than 4 minutes, before pulling the clear plastic tab on the right side of the cassette; pull the tab until it clicks into place and a red line appears. Use a timepiece with a second hand for accurate timing. After another 10–12 minutes, when the "END" indicator turns green, measure the height of the purple column against the scale printed on the cassette. Use the paper result chart included in the kit to interpret the reading.
- For the CardioChek or Personal Cholesterol Monitor test, insert the test strip into the meter either before or after the blood sample has been applied. The meter displays the test results in approximately 1–3 minutes, respectively.
- For the BIOSAFE test, allow blood to dry on the test paper. Provide your name and address on the test paper, and place it into the plastic container provided. Mail to BIOSAFE. Results will be mailed back in approximately 1 week.
- Dispose of the lancet in a puncture-resistant container.

 If the total cholesterol reading is 200 mg/dL or greater, HDL-C is 40 mg/dL or less, or triglycerides are 150 mg/dL or greater, see a primary care provider for evaluation and further testing.

Source: References 37–41.

Evaluation of Patient Outcomes with Cholesterol Tests

Any patient who obtains a result of a total cholesterol of 200 mg/dL or greater, an HDL-C of 40 mg/dL or less, or triglycerides of 150 mg/dL or greater should see a primary care provider for a repeat measurement, full lipid profile, and appropriate medical workup. Patients should not adjust their cholesterol-lowering medications on the basis of a home test without consulting their primary care provider.

URINARY TRACT INFECTION TESTS

Urinary tract infections (UTIs) are the cause for 4 million visits to primary care providers every year.[44] Women have a shorter urethra than men and are therefore more likely to contract UTIs because of retrograde migration of bacteria from the skin. Compared with women, men older than 50 years have a greater likelihood of contracting UTIs because of prostate problems. Conditions that increase risk of UTIs include pregnancy, diabetes, urinary stones, urinary obstructions such as those caused by an enlarged prostate, presence of urinary catheters, and a history of UTIs.[45]

The gram-negative bacterium *Escherichia coli* is responsible for 80% of UTIs.[45] Both gram-positive and gram-negative bacteria account for the other 20% of causative organisms. Symptoms of a UTI include pain on urination, sensation of an urgent need to urinate, frequent urination, blood in the urine, and lower abdominal pain or discomfort.

Two primary uses for UTI tests are (1) early detection of such infections in patients with a history of recurrent UTIs or risk factors associated with UTIs and (2) confirmation that an infection has been cured by antibiotic therapy.

Usage Considerations

Two types of UTI tests are available. The mechanism of action is the primary difference between the two.

Mechanism of Action

One type of UTI test (UTI Bladder Infection Test) detects nitrites in the urine on the basis of the principle that gram-negative bacteria reduce nitrate in the urine to nitrite.[46] In the strip, arsanilic acid reacts with urinary nitrite to form a diazonium compound, which in turn reacts with another chemical on the strip to produce a pink color. A positive test requires a bacterial concentration of 10^5 per milliliter of urine.

The other type of test (AZO Strips) detects both nitrite and leukocyte esterase (LE), an enzyme unique to leukocytes (white blood cells).[47] White blood cells may be found in the urine when a UTI is present.

Accuracy Rate

In general, nitrite-based tests have low sensitivity (45%–60%) and high specificity (85%–98%).[48] Higher levels of accuracy are achieved in elderly, pregnant, and urology patients. Combining nitrite- and LE-based tests increases overall sensitivity and specificity, and decreases the risk of false-negative results.

Interferences

A strict vegetarian diet that provides insufficient urinary nitrates can cause false-negative nitrite results with a UTI test. Tetracycline may produce a false-negative reading for nitrites. False-negative results can also be caused by doses of vitamin C in excess of 250 mg, because ascorbic acid blocks the nitrite test reaction. The patient should allow 10 hours between the last dose of vitamin C and the test procedure. Doses of vitamin C in excess of 500 mg within 24 hours of testing may result in a false-negative result for the LE test, by blocking the development of the color reaction.[46] Dyes or medications such as phenazopyridine, commonly used by patients with UTIs, may cause a false-positive result by changing the sensor pad to pink.

Usage Guidelines

See the box Patient Education for Urinary Tract Infection Tests.

Product Selection Guidelines

The nitrite strips detect only infections caused by gram-negative bacteria. The combination of nitrite and LE tests gives AZO Strips enhanced specificity and sensitivity. The UTI Bladder Infection Test is a test stick similar to those used in pregnancy tests; test sticks may be easier to hold in the urine stream than the AZO test strips.

Assessment of Urinary Tract Infection Tests

Before recommending a UTI test, the practitioner should first determine the patient's reason for using the test. If the patient is testing for a suspected UTI, the practitioner should evaluate the patient's symptoms and risk factors for UTIs. If symptoms of a UTI are present, the patient should be referred to his or her primary care provider immediately for evaluation and treatment. If the patient is testing to find out whether a treated UTI has been cured, the practitioner should assess patient adherence to the therapy. The patient's diet and medication use are important factors to evaluate for possible interference with test results.

Patient Counseling for Urinary Tract Infection Tests

Counseling on the use of UTI tests should emphasize the importance of collecting a clean sample of midstream urine if the sensor pad is to be immersed in a cup of urine. The practitioner should advise a patient with visual difficulties to seek assistance in interpreting test results. To further ensure accurate test results, the practitioner should advise the patient of medical and dietary factors that can cause inaccurate test results. The box Patient Education for Urinary Tract Infection Tests lists specific information to provide patients.

PATIENT EDUCATION FOR
Urinary Tract Infection Tests

The objective of self-testing is to detect UTIs in the early stages or to confirm that an infection was successfully treated. For most patients, carefully following the package instructions and the self-care measures listed here will help ensure achievement of accurate test results and allow prompt treatment of a detected UTI.

Avoidance of Incorrect Results

- Persons on a strict vegetarian diet or tetracycline may not obtain accurate results.
- Certain dyes or medications, such as phenazopyridine, may cause a false-positive result by changing the sensor pad to pink.
- If using the UTI Bladder Infection Test, do not take 250 mg or more of vitamin C within 10 hours of testing.
- If using AZO Test Strips, do not take 500 mg or more of vitamin C within 24 hours of testing.
- Women should not use AZO Test Strips during menses, because blood will cause a false-positive result.

Usage Guidelines

- Clean the genital area thoroughly before collecting a urine sample.
- Test the first urine of the morning or, for later testing, use urine held in the bladder for at least 4 hours.

- To improve sensitivity, test on 3 consecutive days if the test on the previous day was negative. However, a primary care provider should be contacted immediately for evaluation and treatment of any positive test.
- Depending on the test purchased, pass the test strip or stick through the urine stream.
- Do not touch the sensor pad with your fingers, because skin oils can interfere with the test reaction. If urine is collected in a cup, immerse the sensor pad into the cup for 1 second.
- Make sure urine completely covers the pad.
- Wait the indicated time (30–60 seconds); then compare the color on the sensor pad with the color chart provided. For the UTI Bladder Infection Test, a pink color on the pad indicates a positive result. For the AZO Test, a dark tan to purple color on the leukocyte pad indicates a positive result.
- Wait no longer than 3 minutes to read the test strip, and ignore any color changes that occur after that time.
- If the test is negative but symptoms persist, see a primary care provider immediately for evaluation and treatment.

Source: References 46 and 47.

Evaluation of Patient Outcomes with Urinary Tract Infection Tests

Because tests will detect only about 90% of infections, the patient should contact a primary care provider if a negative result is obtained, but UTI symptoms persist.[46,47] If a positive result is obtained, the patient should contact a primary care provider immediately for evaluation and treatment.

HUMAN IMMUNODEFICIENCY VIRUS-1 TESTS

An estimated 984,000 persons in the United States are living with human immunodeficiency virus (HIV), including 24% to 27% who do not know they are infected.[49] Home HIV-1 tests allow a person to test for HIV type 1 (HIV-1) in privacy.

Acquired immunodeficiency syndrome (AIDS) is an incurable disease caused by HIV-1 virus. The disease destroys the body's immune system. AIDS can be contracted by contact with infected body fluids such as blood or semen. People at risk for contracting the virus include those who (1) share needles or syringes for the purpose of injecting drugs, including steroids; (2) have sexual intercourse with a person infected with HIV-1, with someone who injects drugs, or with multiple partners; (3) had a blood transfusion anytime between 1978 and May 1985; and (4) were born to a mother infected with HIV.

Usage Considerations

Two test kits that use blood samples for HIV-1 detection currently are available: Home Access HIV-1 Test System and Home Access Express HIV-1 Test System. Saliva-based kits are available but are not approved for home use.

Mechanism of Action

The HIV-1 tests detect antibodies to the virus. Because 3 weeks to 6 months may be required to develop sufficient antibodies for detection, the time since possible exposure to the virus must be considered in determining when to perform the test.

After collection, the home HIV-1 test samples are mailed to a certified laboratory for processing. Positive samples are rescreened twice. Repeated positive samples are confirmed with an immunofluorescent assay.[50]

Interferences

No factors are known to interfere with home HIV-1 tests.

Usage Guidelines

See the box Patient Education for HIV-1 Tests.

Product Selection Guidelines

The two available HIV-1 tests differ in price and turnaround time to obtain results. The first test, Home Access, takes approximately 7 business days to obtain the results. The second, Home Access Express, takes approximately 3 business days. The Home Access sample is sent to the testing laboratory by regular mail, whereas the Home Access Express sample is shipped through Federal Express. Consequently, the Home Access Express version costs more.

Assessment of HIV-1 Test Use

Before recommending an HIV-1 test, the practitioner should first determine how much time has elapsed since the patient was possibly exposed to the HIV-1 virus. The patient may not know all the risk factors for HIV-1 infection; therefore, the practitioner should tactfully find out whether the patient has engaged in any activities that increase risk for contracting HIV-1. The patient should be asked about medical disorders that might rule out use of a fingerstick-based test, such as anticoagulation or bleeding disorder, or physical limitations that might interfere with performing the test.

Patient Counseling for HIV-1 Tests

Counseling on the use of HIV-1 tests should emphasize the importance of applying enough blood on the specimen card to ensure an accurate reading. The practitioner should also advise the patient of the fragility of blood samples and not to delay mailing the specimen card. The box Patient Education for HIV-1 Tests lists specific information to provide patients.

PATIENT EDUCATION FOR
H I V - 1   T e s t s

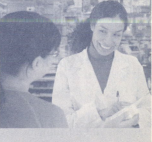

The objective of self-testing is to determine whether an HIV-1 infection is present. For most patients, carefully following package instructions and the self-care measures listed here will help ensure the achievement of accurate test results. Furthermore, self-testing will allow prompt treatment of a detected infection.

Precautions
- Do not share the test lancet with other individuals. Do not allow the blood being tested to contact other individuals.
- The lancet is a biohazard; dispose of it in a puncture-resistant container.

Usage Guidelines
- Call the product manufacturer's toll-free number to register and receive pretest counseling. The manufacturer's customer representative will ask for the confidential code included in the kit.
- Using alcohol, clean the fingertip chosen for puncture. Allow alcohol to dry.
- Prick the cleaned fingertip using the lancet provided, and place a few drops of blood on the blood specimen card. Fill the circle

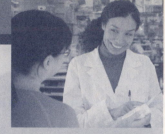

PATIENT EDUCATION FOR
H I V - 1   T e s t s   *(continued)*

- on the card completely to ensure a readable test. Examine the back of the card to ensure the blood soaked through. If it did not, place more blood on the front of the card. If a second fingerstick is needed, use the second lancet provided in the kit.
- Allow the card to air-dry for 30 minutes, place sample in specimen return pouch, and seal it in the prepaid and addressed shipping package. Be sure that the processing laboratory receives the specimen within 10 days of sampling.
- Call the manufacturer's toll-free number in 3–7 business days to obtain the results, depending on which test kit was used.

- Note that counseling is available 24 hours/day, for both negative and positive results, and is included in the cost of the testing unit.

 If the test is positive, see a primary care provider immediately for evaluation and treatment. Avoid activities that can result in transfer of blood or other body fluids to other individuals.

Source: Reference 50.

Evaluation of Patient Outcomes with HIV-1 Tests

A patient with a positive result should see a primary care provider to be retested for confirmation of HIV-1 infection. Infected patients should be counseled on precautions to avoid infection of others. Patients with negative results should confirm that sufficient time has passed since the potential exposure before they test themselves.

HEPATITIS C TESTS

Hepatitis C is one of six identified hepatitis viruses and is considered the most common cause of chronic viral hepatitis in the United States. An estimated 4.1 million Americans have been infected with hepatitis C. This infection accounts for approximately one-third of all deaths caused by chronic liver disease each year and is a major reason for liver transplantation.[51]

Risk factors for hepatitis C are as follows[51]:

- Injection use of drugs
- Receipt of clotting factor concentrate produced before 1987
- Long-term hemodialysis
- Transfusion or organ transplant before 1992
- Sexual intercourse with multiple partners
- Birth by a mother infected with hepatitis C

The Centers for Disease Control and Prevention estimate that transmission through shared needles accounts for 60% of all new cases of hepatitis C. Anyone who has or may have occupational exposure to blood, including health care workers and military personnel, is also at increased risk for developing hepatitis C.[51]

Hepatitis C induces liver damage by causing hepatic cell necrosis and inflammation, which over time may progress to fibrosis, cirrhosis, and hepatocellular carcinoma. Of people infected with hepatitis C, 85% are likely to progress to the chronic disease state.[52] Clinically, hepatitis C may go undetected for many years; liver disease may be advanced by the time symptoms arise.

Usage Considerations

One test kit currently is available for hepatitis C detection, Hepatitis C Check. After collection, the test blood sample is mailed to a certified laboratory for processing.

Mechanism of Action

The kit tests for presence of antibodies to the hepatitis C virus, not the virus itself. The Hepatitis C Check uses an ELISA to test for antibodies and then confirms the results with a recombinant immunoblot assay.[52] Because 6 months may be required to develop sufficient antibodies for detection, the time since possible exposure to the virus must be considered in determining when to perform the test.

Interferences

Providing an inadequate blood sample (i.e., incompletely filling the circle on the blood sample card) may cause inaccurate results.

Usage Guidelines

See the box Patient Education for Hepatitis C Tests.

Product Selection Guidelines

Home Access Hepatitis C Check is a single-use test kit containing two lancets, a blood sample card, gauze pad, an adhesive bandage, and a postage-paid envelope. Each kit also includes a unique personal identification number, which the purchaser uses to register the kit and access test results.

Assessment of Hepatitis C Test Use

A patient who recently has been infected may receive a false-negative result, because antibodies to the virus have not had sufficient time to form. Clinical studies on file with the manufacturer report no false-positive results.[52] The patient may not know all the risk factors for hepatitis C; therefore, the practitioner should tactfully find out whether the patient has engaged in any activities that can cause the disease. The patient should be asked about medical disorders that might rule out use of a fingerstick-

PATIENT EDUCATION FOR
Hepatitis C Tests

The objective of self-testing is to determine whether a hepatitis C infection is present. Self-testing will also allow prompt treatment of a detected infection. For most patients, carefully following package instructions and the self-care measures listed here will help ensure achievement of accurate test results.

Precautions

- Do not share the test lancet with other individuals.
- Do not allow the blood being tested to contact other individuals.
- The lancet is considered a biohazard; dispose of it in a puncture-resistant container.

Usage Guidelines

- Register the PIN (personal identification number) with the manufacturer by calling the enclosed toll-free telephone number and following the automated directions.
- Remain seated during the testing process to prevent falling if dizziness occurs.
- Before starting the test, wash your hands thoroughly with soap and warm water, and dry them.

- Date the blood sample card.
- Lance the side of one of the middle fingers.
- Apply a sufficient number of blood drops until both the front and back of the circular area on the testing card are saturated.
- Allow the sample to dry at least 30 minutes before sealing it in the pouch and mailing.
- After 4–10 business days, call the toll-free number provided, using the PIN number to access the test results. Test results are available for up to 1 year.
- Note that counseling is available 24 hours a day, for both negative and positive results, and is included in the cost of the testing unit.

 If the test is positive, see a primary care provider immediately for evaluation and treatment. Avoid activities that can result in transfer of blood or other body fluids to other individuals.

Source: Reference 52.

---

based test, such as anticoagulation or bleeding disorder, or physical limitations that could interfere with performing the test.

Patient Counseling for Hepatitis C Tests

The practitioner should advise the patient of the fragility of blood samples and not to delay mailing the specimen card. The box Patient Education for Hepatitis C Tests lists specific information to provide patients.

Evaluation of Patient Outcomes with Hepatitis C Tests

Patients who test positive should be referred to a primary care provider given that treatment options are available only by prescription. Infected patients should be counseled on precautions to avoid infection of others. These patients should also be advised to avoid alcohol and other drugs that may advance the progression of liver disease. They should also be tested for and vaccinated against other forms of hepatitis, such as the hepatitis A and hepatitis B viruses.

DRUG ABUSE TESTS

An estimated 8.1% of Americans abuse drugs, whether legal or illegal.[36] Drug abuse, in turn, leads to higher accident and absentee rates at work. Drug abuse is a problem in the United States regardless of socioeconomic status, gender, or race.

The symptoms of drug use are varied but may include withdrawal from activities, fatigue, red eyes, drowsiness, slurred speech, and chronic cough. The National Institute of Drug Abuse (www.nida.nih.gov) is a good resource for specific symptoms for the various drugs of abuse. Drug abuse tests may allow parents and caregivers to detect such use early enough to affect the course of addiction.

Usage Considerations

Numerous products for detecting use of drugs are available in retail stores and pharmacies, by telephone, and through the Internet. A number of the tests currently available are not FDA-approved for home use. FDA has proposed a policy (which it currently follows) that allows the marketing of non–FDA-approved home test kits if the specimen is mailed to a certified laboratory. Table 51-6 lists some example tests and the substances each test identifies.

Home drug tests are marketed primarily to parents as an aid for determining drug use in their children. These tests are a means of obtaining results anonymously when drug use is suspected. Home drug testing, however, is not a substitute for open communication between parents and children regarding drug use.

Samples of urine or hair are collected at home. The hair tests and some of the urine tests are mailed to a clinical laboratory, with results obtained by telephone or over the Internet. Some of the urine tests have the user conduct a preliminary screening test in the home and then mail positive samples to a laboratory for confirmation. Other urine tests are performed only at home. Saliva tests are available, but they are expensive and are currently marketed only to drug testing programs and employers.

TABLE 51-6 Selected Home Drug Abuse Tests

Product	Time to Result	Body Site	Testing Location	Substances Detected
At Home Drug Test	10 minutes for initial screen; 5–7 days for laboratory confirmation	Urine	Home; send away for confirmation	Depends on kit purchased; one kit tests for methamphetamines, amphetamines, marijuana, cocaine, and opiates; other kits test for a single substance
Dr. Brown's Home Drug Testing System	5–7 days	Urine	Send away	Marijuana, cocaine, amphetamine, phencyclidine, codeine, morphine, heroin
Quick Screen Pro Multi-Drug Screening	3–15 minutes for initial screen; 5–7 days	Urine	Home; send away for confirmation	Amphetamine, cocaine, marijuana, opiates, phencyclidine
PDT-90 Personal Drug Testing Service	5–7 days	Hair	Send away	Marijuana, cocaine, opiates, methamphetamine, amphetamine, phencyclidine, barbiturates, benzodiazepines

Source: References 53–56

Some of the test kits include telephone counseling to (1) help parents recognize the signs of drug use, (2) assist in creating a family drug policy, and (3) emphasize that parents should use the test to develop trust and open communication within their families, rather than to intimidate with the threat of random testing. Some telephone counseling programs provide referrals to rehabilitation and counseling services in the family's community.

Mechanism of Action

For the home urine tests, an immunochromatographic assay similar to the home pregnancy and ovulation tests is used for initial screening of a sample. Available testing devices include (1) a test cassette to which urine is applied and (2) a test device that is placed in the urine sample. In each test, a positive result for a particular drug is absence of a line next to the drug name in the testing area. For a negative test, a line appears by the drug name and in the control area.

Urine samples sent to clinical laboratories for testing are checked for evidence of adulteration before processing for the presence of drugs.[53–56] Substances such as water or household chemicals can be added to urine samples in an attempt to mask drug use. The laboratories use an enzyme-multiplied immunoassay technique to detect drugs in the urine samples. Gas chromatography–mass spectrometry is then used to identify the specific drug.

Home urine tests detect drug use that occurred from several hours before testing to within 2 to 3 days of testing. The amount of drug found in the urine is affected by the time since consumption, the amount taken, and the amount of water consumed before sampling. Test results are reported as only positive or negative for a drug. Quantity or route of ingestion is not determined.

Hair testing detects trace amounts of ingested drugs that become trapped in the core of the hair shaft as it grows at an average rate of one-half inch per month. Drug use over a 90-day period can be determined from a hair sample of 1 and one-half inches.[56] The presence of drugs is determined by radioimmunoassay techniques, and then gas chromatography–mass spectrometry analysis identifies the specific substance. Hair tests report positive or negative results for a drug. Positive results are reported as a number indicating low, medium, or high levels of use for all drugs except marijuana.

Usage Guidelines

See the box Patient Education for Drug Abuse Tests.

Interferences

Ingestion of decongestants, dextromethorphan, antidiarrheals, or cough medicines containing codeine may cause false-positive results for home drug abuse tests. These items contain substances structurally related to certain drugs of abuse. Consumption of large quantities of poppy seeds or poppy seed paste may or may not cause a false-positive result for opiates, depending on the test's sensitivity. Sensitivity standards for opiates were raised in the year 2000 from 300 to 2000 ng/mL to eliminate the possibility of false-positive results. Only the QuickScreen Pro lists the higher sensitivity standard in its package labeling.[55]

Product Selection Guidelines

The criteria for selecting one drug abuse test over another include the drugs that are suspected of being used, type of suspected use (i.e., casual versus chronic), length of time since last use, and possibility of the suspected drug user tampering with the sample. The list of drugs that may be identified with each kit varies. These tests can test for a single drug (e.g., At Home Marijuana Test [Pharmatech]) or up to 12 drugs (First Check 12 [First Check Diagnostics]).

In general, urine tests are better for detecting low-level, casual drug use. Hair testing detects longer-term use. It takes at least 5 to 7 days for hair to grow far enough from the scalp for testing purposes.

Urine samples are subject to tampering by adding chemicals, diluting with water, or substituting someone else's sample. Some of the test kits include a temperature strip on the urine collection cup to ensure the sample is at body temperature. Hair samples, if taken directly from the person being tested, are not subject to tampering. Parents should weigh the possibility of tampering when deciding which type of test to choose.

Information on FDA approval of a drug abuse test for home use is available at www.accessdata.fda.gov/scripts/cdrh/cfdocs/cfIVD/Search.cfm. Additional information on urine testing can be found at www.fda.gov/cdrh/oivd/homeuse-drug-2step.html.

The objective of self-testing is to detect and identify abuse of drugs. Self-testing will also allow prompt intervention to rehabilitate a confirmed drug user. For most patients, carefully following package instructions and the measures listed here will help ensure achievement of accurate test results.

Avoidance of Incorrect Results

- Drug tests on urine samples report only a positive or negative outcome. Neither the quantity of drug taken nor the method in which it was taken is determined.
- Drug tests on hair samples can report low, medium, or high level of drug use, but the use could have occurred as long as 90 days before testing.
- Cough medicines that contain codeine or dextromethorphan, decongestants, antidiarrheals, and possibly poppy seeds may cause false-positive test results.

Usage Guidelines for Urine Drug Abuse Tests

- Collect urine using the collection device included with the test. Do not take urine from the toilet.
- Check the temperature of the urine sample immediately after collection using the temperature strip, if included. If the sample is not between 90°F (32°C) and 100°F (38°C), adulteration may have occurred.
- Immerse the test card in the urine sample for 10 seconds or until visible migration across the test panels has occurred.

Place device on flat surface or leave immersed in sample. Do not allow urine to exceed the "max line."

- Read the results when the "results ready" indicator changes to a pinkish red.
- Do not read results after 15 minutes or when the "results expired" indicator changes color.
- If no line appears in the control region, the test is invalid and should be repeated with a new card.

Usage Guidelines for Hair Drug Abuse Tests

- Collect a hair sample that is one-half inch wide and one strand deep from the crown of the head, as close to the scalp as possible.
- Align the cut ends of the hair sample, and place the sample in the collection package as directed. Do not collect hair from a hairbrush, comb, or clothing; there is no guarantee the hair is actually from the person to be tested.
- Results are available approximately 5 days after receipt by the laboratory. To access results, call the toll-free number and provide the code number accompanying the kit.
- If the test is positive, seek the services of a drug rehabilitation organization.

Source: References 53–56.

Assessment of Drug Abuse Test Use

To determine which type of drug abuse test to recommend, the practitioner should ask about the length of suspected drug use and the types of drugs that are suspected. The practitioner should also ask whether the suspected user is likely to tamper with urine samples. The practitioner should determine if the suspected user takes legal prescription or nonprescription medications, which may interfere with the test.

Patient Counseling for Drug Abuse Tests

When parents or caregivers ask for assistance in selecting a drug abuse test, the practitioner should be prepared to offer information about family counseling agencies as well as clinical advice. The practitioner should emphasize the limitations of the tests when confirming drug use and, in the case of urine tests, when identifying anything more than the type of drug that is being abused. The box Patient Education for Drug Abuse Tests lists specific information to provide patients.

Evaluation of Patient Outcomes with Drug Abuse Tests

If a positive result is obtained with a drug abuse test, parents or caregivers need to consider potential problems with the test itself before concluding that drug use is confirmed. In addition, they must not assume that a negative result is accurate. Parents should also consider the testing window when evaluating results.

BLOOD PRESSURE MONITORS

Hypertension, defined as either a systolic blood pressure greater than 140 mm Hg or a diastolic blood pressure greater than 90 mm Hg, is often an asymptomatic disease.[57] Table 51-7 lists the classification of blood pressures from the seventh report of the Joint National Committee on Prevention, Detection, Evaluation and Treatment of High Blood Pressure (JNC 7).

Twenty-seven percent of Americans 20 years of age and older have hypertension.[36] Thirty percent of people with hypertension are unaware of their condition; almost 40% are not receiving treatment; and 66% have not achieved national goals for blood pressure control.[57] The reasons for the lack of adequate control are multiple, but a significant factor is lack of patient motivation to take steps to control blood pressure, especially if the patient is asymptomatic, which leads to nonadherence with treatment strategies.

The consequences of untreated hypertension are well documented. Long-standing elevations in blood pressure can lead to damage of the heart, kidney, lungs, eyes, and blood vessels, and to an increase in morbidity and mortality.

Treatment of high blood pressure often involves significant lifestyle changes (diet and exercise) and the institution of drug

TABLE 51-7 Classification of Blood Pressure

Category	Systolic BP (mm Hg)		Diastolic BP (mm Hg)
Normal	<120	and	<80
Prehypertension	120–139	or	80–89
Hypertension, stage 1	140–159	or	90–99
Hypertension, stage 2	≥160	or	≥100

Key: BP, blood pressure.
Source: Reference 57.

therapies. These measures inevitably produce side effects, so the patient who was without symptoms of disease may become symptomatic. Patient education and empowerment play a large role in improving patient adherence with antihypertensive efforts. Adherence, in turn, helps reduce morbidity and mortality, maintains or improves the patient's quality of life, and improves the patient's use of health care resources.

Teaching patients to take their own blood pressure at home is an excellent means of achieving these goals, because home blood pressure monitoring gives patients a sense of control over their health, allows them to measure their progress toward a goal blood pressure, and provides useful data on blood pressure values away from the primary care provider's office. Three general advantages of measuring blood pressure outside the clinician's office are the ability to (1) distinguish sustained hypertension from "white-coat hypertension," (2) assess response to antihypertensive medication, and (3) improve patient adherence to treatment.

Usage Considerations

Of the three categories of blood pressure monitors—mercury column, aneroid, and digital—aneroid and digital monitors are the most popular choices for home use. Monitors that measure pressure at the wrist and fingers have become popular, but it is important to realize that the systolic and diastolic pressures vary substantially in different parts of the arterial tree. Finger monitors have so far been found to be inaccurate and are not recommended.[58] Wrist monitors are typically smaller than the arm devices and can be used in obese people, because the wrist diameter is little affected by obesity.[58]

Mechanism of Action

Blood pressure readings include two types of pressures: systolic, which indicates pressure at the time of contraction of the heart cavities, and diastolic, which indicates pressure at the time of dilation of the heart cavities. Blood pressure is measured indirectly by two methods: auscultatory (measurement of sound) and oscillometric (measurement of vibration). Mercury and aneroid meters involve auscultation with the use of a stethoscope to detect Korotkoff's sounds, which are produced by the motion of the arterial wall in response to changes in arterial pressure. Oscillometric sensors, which are often used with digital meters, measure blood pressure by detecting blood surges underneath the cuff as it is deflated. The detection device, which is usually indicated on the cuff with a tab or other marking, is placed directly over the brachial artery. The brachial artery can be found by palpating 1 to 2 inches

above and just to the inside of the antecubital space. As cuff pressure increases during the measurement procedure, the brachial artery is compressed and blood flow is obstructed. As cuff pressure is gradually released, blood flow is reestablished and Korotkoff's sounds can be heard in different phases. Phase I, which corresponds to systolic pressure, can be identified when at least two consecutive "beats" are heard as cuff pressure is decreased. The nature of the sounds changes over the next three phases. Diastolic pressure is identified as phase V, the disappearance of sound.

Interferences

Stress, tobacco smoking, and ingestion of caffeine-containing beverages can increase blood pressure. Some medications such as pseudoephedrine may also increase blood pressure. Conversely, eating or taking a hot bath can lower blood pressure.

Usage Guidelines

The actual measurement of blood pressure is a relatively simple procedure; however, many people consistently do it incorrectly. Blood pressure is naturally variable. Therefore, proper technique is essential to reduce measurement variability and improve the quality of results. The normal range for blood pressure is established with patients sitting in the resting state; any variation from this setting can produce inaccurate results.

Using the appropriate size cuff is essential to accurately measure a patient's blood pressure (Table 51-8). If the cuff is too small, blood pressure readings can be overestimated significantly by as much as 20 to 30 mm Hg. Several monitors are supplied with a large cuff; many others allow for purchase of a large cuff separately. For patients with arms too large for the largest size cuff, a wrist monitor may be a useful alternative. To obtain accurate readings with wrist cuffs, the patient must hold the wrist at heart level during the reading. Because these devices are also highly sensitive to changes in the wrist level, it is best to support the arm on a table with a pillow that will raise the wrist to the appropriate level. For the person who is doing the actual monitoring, following the steps outlined in the box Patient Education for Self-Monitoring of Blood Pressure will help improve the accuracy of blood pressure readings, regardless of whether they are taken in the primary care provider's office, the pharmacy, or the home by the patient.

TABLE 51-8 Arm Circumferences to Determine Appropriate Cuff Size

Arm Circumference (Adult)[a]	Cuff Size
22–26 cm	Small adult cuff
27–34 cm	Regular adult cuff
35–44 cm	Large adult cuff
≥45 cm	Thigh cuff[b]

[a] Determine arm circumference by measuring around the midpoint of the upper arm. Remeasure the patient's arm periodically, especially if he or she has recently gained or lost significant weight.

[b] Consider a wrist monitor for patients whose arm circumference is >45 cm.

Source: Reference 58.

Product Selection Guidelines

Of the three types of blood pressure measuring devices, no single one is best for every patient. The choice of device is individualized according to characteristics such as the patient's ability and willingness to learn, physical disabilities, patient preference, and the cost of the device. Mercury column devices are expensive and, as discussed in the next section, have other disadvantages for home use. In general, aneroid devices are the least expensive. Depending on the features, a digital device can cost as much as a mercury column device. A discussion of the pros and cons of all three types of devices follows.

Mercury Column Devices

The mercury column blood pressure monitor is still the reference standard in blood pressure measurement. This monitor typically comes with a cuff and an inflation bulb. The tubing from the cuff is attached to a column of mercury encased in a glass gauge.

Although mercury monitors are the most accurate and reliable of the devices, their routine use for home measurement is discouraged, because they are cumbersome and pose the risk of mercury toxicity should the glass tubing break. They also require good eyesight and hearing for effective use. If the mercury does not rest at zero when the cuff is lying flat and completely deflated, the device needs recalibration.

Aneroid Devices

Next to mercury column monitors, aneroid devices are the most accurate and reliable. They are light, portable, and very affordable, and they pose no risk from mercury toxicity. They include several features that make patient instruction much easier. First, many devices now come with a stethoscope attached to the cuff, which frees the patient from having to hold the bell of the stethoscope in place. Second, a D-ring on the cuff allows a single user to place the cuff on the arm easily. Third, a few manufacturers offer a gauge attached to the inflation bulb, making it easier to manipulate the equipment because there are fewer pieces to control. Such monitors are considered the option of choice for home use, but they do require careful patient instruction and follow-up. Good eyesight and hearing are necessary for accurate readings with standard models. For patients with reduced visual capacity, however, devices with large-type print on the face of the gauge are available.

At the bottom of the face of each aneroid device is a small box. When the cuff is completely deflated and lying on the table, the needle of the gauge should rest in the box. If the needle is outside the box, the gauge needs recalibration. Many manufacturers sell recalibration tools to allow health care professionals to adjust the devices.

Digital Devices

With advancing technology, digital devices have become more accurate, reliable, and easy to use, and as a result have skyrocketed in popularity. Such devices include semiautomatic (manually inflating), fully automatic (autoinflating), wrist, and finger blood pressure monitors. Features such as printouts, pulse monitor, digital clock, automated inflation and deflation, memory, large display, and D-ring for the cuff differentiate many of the devices. These features significantly affect the price.

A major drawback to the digital monitors is the user's inability to determine whether the device is out of calibration.

As a result, many clinicians recommend the aneroid devices over the easier-to-use digital products. The JNC 7 report notes that home measurement devices should be checked regularly for accuracy[57]; therefore, patients should be advised to have their monitors checked at least yearly.

If recommending a digital device, the practitioner should check the manufacturer's specifications to ensure the monitor at least meets the accuracy standards set by the American National Standards Institute (ANSI). The ANSI standards for digital sphygmomanometers state that blood pressure readings between 20 and 250 mm Hg must not differ by more than 3 mm Hg or 2%, whichever is greater.[59]

Assessment of Blood Pressure Self-Monitoring

The practitioner should first determine why a patient wants to use a blood pressure monitor. If the use is warranted, the practitioner should determine whether the patient has physical impairments that can interfere with proper use of the monitor. The practitioner should also evaluate the patient's ability to comprehend and follow instructions.

Patient Counseling for Blood Pressure Self-Monitoring

The practitioner should emphasize the importance of tracking blood pressure values to monitor control of hypertension. Regular self-monitoring of blood pressure will illustrate positive effects of proper diet, exercise, and medication use in controlling the disorder. Such reinforcement can improve patient adherence with prescribed therapies. The patient should be shown the proper technique for blood pressure monitoring and encouraged to return for a follow-up evaluation of the patient's technique. Because of white coat hypertension, patients measuring blood pressure at home usually obtain lower results than those taken at the doctor's office. In the home setting, a blood pressure greater than 135/85 mm Hg should be considered elevated.[57] The box Patient Education for Self-Monitoring of Blood Pressure lists specific information to provide patients.

Evaluation of Patient Outcomes for Self-Monitoring of Blood Pressure

Patients measuring blood pressure for diagnostic and monitoring purposes should be instructed on how to track values and discuss the values with a primary care provider. Patients monitoring their blood pressure should be cautioned not to adjust their medications unless instructed otherwise. Patients should be instructed to immediately contact their primary care provider if they are obtaining very high values and having any symptoms of high blood pressure such as headache or blurred vision. The practitioner can play a major role in aiding hypertensive patients by (1) motivating them to perform home monitoring of blood pressure, (2) guiding them in product selection, (3) training them to use devices appropriately, and (4) facilitating communication between the patient, the patient's family, and the patient's primary care provider regarding any antihypertensive therapy.

PATIENT EDUCATION FOR
Self-Monitoring of Blood Pressure

The objective of self-testing is to identify elevated blood pressure or monitor the efficacy of diet, exercise, or medication in managing hypertension. For most patients, carefully following product instructions and the self-care measures listed here will help ensure accurate blood pressure readings.

Precautions/Avoidance of Incorrect Results
- Keep a log of blood pressure readings and any circumstances that might have affected the reading (e.g., nervous, late for work).
- If home readings are being performed for diagnostic purposes, take readings at different times throughout the day and under different circumstances.
- If readings are being done to determine adequacy of antihypertensive therapy, take the reading at the same time of day, preferably in the early morning soon after arising from bed.
- Allow plenty of time to relax before taking a blood pressure reading. Feelings of stress or pressure can elevate the blood pressure.
- Do not use tobacco products or drink caffeine-containing beverages for at least 30 minutes before taking a measurement. These activities can increase blood pressure.
- Wait 10–15 minutes after a bath and 30 minutes after eating to take a measurement. These activities can lower blood pressure.
- Some medications may increase blood pressure. Be alert for possible changes in readings when starting or stopping medications.

Usage Guidelines
- Make sure the room is at a comfortable temperature.
- Sit in a comfortable chair, with the back supported and the feet straight ahead and flat on the floor.
- If using an arm cuff, place the arm to be measured on a table, making sure the upper arm is at heart level. Remove restrictive clothing from the arm.
- If using a wrist cuff, place pillow(s) under the arm to be measured to bring the wrist up to heart level.
- Place the cuff on the arm to be measured. The cuff should be snug but not tight enough to restrict blood flow. Use the guidelines in Table 51-8 for selecting cuff size.
- Rest for at least 5 minutes in this position.
- Measure the blood pressure as directed by the product instructions. If using a stethoscope, listen for the Korotkoff's sounds as defined:
  —Phase 1: Sound begins as a soft tapping. Record the systolic pressure at the point when two taps are heard in sequence.
  —Phase 2: Tapping sound gets louder and is accompanied by a swishing sound or murmur.
  —Phase 3: Tapping sounds persist, but the swishing or murmur sound stops.
  —Phase 4: Muffling or softening of tapping sounds.
  —Phase 5: Sound stops. Record the diastolic pressure at the point when sound stops.
- Take two to three measurements separated by at least 2 minutes using the same arm.
- Record the results, arm used, time and date of measurement, and name and time of last dose of any medications, including antihypertensive medications.
- Do not adjust blood pressure medications on the basis of home measurements unless specifically instructed to do so by a health care provider.

 See a primary care provider immediately for evaluation and treatment if blood pressure values are high, and you are having symptoms such as headache or blurred vision.

Source: References 57 and 58.

MISCELLANEOUS HOME TESTS

As the market for home test products and shopping over the Internet have exploded, new tests are becoming available with increasing frequency. Selected miscellaneous home tests are detailed in Table 51-9. Instructions for use are generally available from the manufacturer's Web site or an Internet site that sells the product. Following the general guidelines given in this chapter will also help patients obtain accurate results.

KEY POINTS FOR HOME TESTING AND MONITORING DEVICES

➤ To advise patients properly on selecting and using home testing or monitoring products, the practitioner must be familiar with the procedures for each available product.
➤ Manufacturers continually introduce new products and modify current ones to provide more user-friendly versions. To keep up to date, the practitioner should request product information from manufacturers by calling their toll-free numbers, visiting their Web sites, or contacting their sales representatives.
➤ FDA's Web site should also be checked frequently for problem reports, updates, and news on home tests.
➤ Patients who are using home tests or devices should be encouraged to follow instructions carefully and to contact either the pharmacist or the manufacturer's toll-free number for assistance, if needed.
➤ The practitioner should stress that the patient is self-testing, not self-diagnosing. Positive test results should be reported to a primary care provider immediately for definitive diagnosis and management. Negative test results should be questioned when the patient is experiencing symptoms of a suspected condition.
➤ If there is any question about the results, the patient should seek the advice of a health care provider.

TABLE 51-9 Selected Miscellaneous Home Tests

Test	Purpose	Testing Medium	Important Points	Additional Information
Alcohol screening tests	Prevent inappropriate alcohol consumption	Breath (SAFE-Slim, BreathScan) Saliva (ALCO-Screen)	Put nothing in mouth for 15 minutes before or during the test; follow timing directions carefully and use a timing device.	Semiquantitative BAC; saliva test strips can be used to detect alcohol in drinks.
Visiderm	Monitor moles for changes over time	Skin	Use a transparent overlay to trace outline of individual moles; record color and other details; do subsequent examinations of each mole on same overlay.	Test includes transparent overlays, pen, color chart, instructions, and storage box.
Biosafe Anemia Meter	Measure hemoglobin to monitor for anemia	Blood	Blood is placed in well of testing device and plunger is depressed; read results in 20 minutes.	Test gives numerical result; kit includes test cassette, lancet, user manual; view window indicates if sufficient blood has been applied.
Breast Self-Examination Aid	Aid to make breast self-examination easier and more comfortable		Examine breasts monthly; self-examination does not take place of mammogram and professional examination.	Two-layer polyurethane breast shield or glove containing a small amount of silicone lubricant to reduce friction; some kits come with instructional video (Aware, Sensatouch).
TobacAlert (tobacalert.com)	Detect tobacco use or exposure	Urine	Test detects cotine, a metabolite of nicotine; detects use or exposure in previous 48–72 hours; dip strip in urine sample and read results in specified time (10–15 minutes).	Use of nicotine patch or gum can affect results.
Early Alert Alzheimer's Home Screening Test	Screen for early stage of Alzheimer's disease		Release 1 strip, sniff, and identify odor based on four suggested answers; do not use if nasal congestion or long-lasting loss of smell from other causes exists.	Loss of smell is among first signs of Alzheimer's disease; kit contains 12 microencapsulated, one-time-use-only odor strips; if ≥4 answers are incorrect, see a PCP for evaluation.
My Allergy Test (immunetech.com)	Detects allergy to 10 most common allergens: dust mites, cat hair, mold (*Alternaria*), ragweed, mountain cedar (juniper), Timothy grass, Bermuda grass, egg white, milk, wheat	Blood (4–5 drops)	If negative result but positive symptoms, see PCP.	Test measures IgE antibodies; tests for only 10 allergens; results are available by e-mail in 10 days or by regular mail. Version that analyzes house dust for common allergens is also available.
Proview Eye Pressure Monitor Kit (Bausch.com)	Monitor IOP in patients with glaucoma	Eye	Press device on partially closed eyelid until you see the appearance of a pressure phosphene, usually described as a dark circle with a ring of light around the outside. Test does not replace in-office IOP measurement.	Kit includes eye pressure monitor, log book, instructions, educational brochure, magnifier, and case; makes contact with the eyelid only; no anesthetic required; can be used to increase patient involvement and track effect of medications.

(Continued)

TABLE 51-9 Selected Miscellaneous Home Tests (continued)

Test	Purpose	Testing Medium	Important Points	Additional Information
IDENTIGENE DNA Paternity Test Collection Kits	Check paternity of a child	Cheek cells	Collect cheek cell samples from each participant: alleged father, child, and biological mother. Swabs are mailed to laboratory.	Additional ~$120 laboratory fee plus cost of kit ($30); not available in all states; results available 3–5 days after sample is received by laboratory. Results are not valid for legal purposes (requires verified collection procedure and additional costs).
Fertell Couples Fertility Test	Screens for both male (concentration of motile sperm) and female infertility (FSH)	Sperm, urine	Ovarian reserve is measured using day-3 menstrual cycle FSH levels; sperm are "counted" as they move through a container that mimics a female's cervical fluid.	FDA-cleared test with a 95% accuracy rate; male portion of the test takes approximately 80 minutes; female portion takes approximately 30 minutes. Consult PCP if results indicate possible infertility or fertile results are obtained with continued difficulty conceiving.
EarCheck Middle Ear Monitor	Detects middle ear fluid (otitis media with effusion)	Ear	Device emits sound waves into the ear canal. Some of the sound reflects off the eardrum and travels back to the built-in microphone. The sound is analyzed to determine if middle ear fluid is present.	Device is not validated in patients over 19 years, and cannot be used in those < 6 months of age, or those with ear tubes, known perforation or rupture of the eardrum, or visible drainage of pus or blood in the outer ear canal. If positive result or negative result + symptoms is obtained, see PCP.

Key: BAC, blood alcohol concentration; FDA, Food and Drug Administration; Ig, immunoglobulin; IOP, intraocular pressure; PCP, primary care provider.

REFERENCES

1. Levy S. Health begins at home. *Drug Top*. July 24, 2006.
2. US Food and Drug Administration. *FDA Review of Home-Use Devices*. Rockville, Md: Center for Devices and Radiological Health; 2003.
3. Martin, J, Hamilton B, Sutton P, et al. *Births: Final Data for 2005 National Vital Statistics Reports*. Hyattsville, Md: National Center for Health Statistics; 2007.
4. First Response Resource Center. Available at: http://www.firstresponse.com. Last accessed September 26, 2008.
5. Davies S, Byrn F, Cole LA. Human chorionic gonadotropin testing for early pregnancy viability and complications. *Clin Lab Med*. 2003; 23: 257–64.
6. Butler SA, Khanlian SA, Cole LA. Detection of early pregnancy forms of human chorionic gonadotropin by home pregnancy test devices. *Clin Chem*. 2001;47:2131–6.
7. Cole L, Sutton-Riley J, Khanlian S, et al. Sensitivity of over-the-counter pregnancy tests: comparison of utility and marketing messages. *JAPhA*. 2005;45:608–15.
8. Clearblue Easy Product Information. Waltham, Mass: Inverness Medical; 2005.
9. Fact Plus Product Information. Waltham, Mass: Inverness Medical; 2006.
10. Wilcox AJ, Baird DD, Dunson D, et al. Natural limits of pregnancy testing in relation to the expected menstrual period. *JAMA*. 2001;286:1759–61.
11. Cole L, Khanlian S, Sutton J, et al. Accuracy of home pregnancy tests at the time of a missed menses. *Am J Obstet Gynecol*. 2004;190:100–5.
12. Bastian L, Nanda K, Hasselblad V, et al. Diagnostic efficiency of home pregnancy test kits: a meta-analysis. *Arch Fam Med*. 1998;7:465–9.
13. Chandra A, Martinez GM, Mosher WD, et al. Fertility, family planning, and reproductive health of U.S. women: data from the 2002 National Survey of Family Growth. National Center for Health Statistics. *Vital Health Stat* 2005;23(25):22.
14. Scolaro KL, Lloyd KB, Helms KL. Devices for home evaluation of women's health concerns. *Am J Health Syst Pharm*. 2008;65:299–314.
15. When the test really counts. Part two: the fertility window. *Consum Rep*. February 2003:48–50.
16. Accu-Clear product information. Waltham, Mass: Inverness Medical; 2006.
17. BD Basal Digital Thermometer product information. Franklin Lakes, NJ: BD; 2007.
18. Lennard J, Lind J, Honeywell M. Advanced Technology for Fertility Prediction. *US Pharm*. 2006;12:49–54.
19. Haney A. Results of US Pivotal Clinical Trial of Fertilite (OV–Watch). Data on file, Atlanta, Ga: HealthWatchSystems; 2007.
20. Eichner S, Timpe E. Urinary-based ovulation and pregnancy: point-of-care testing. *Ann Pharmacother*. 2004;38:325–31.
21. Pray J, Pray WS. Ovulation and fertility home diagnostic kits. *US Pharm*. 2003;28;59:3083–92.
22. FertilMARQ product information. Wilmington, Mass: Embryotech Laboratories; 2007.
23. American College of Obstetricians and Gynecologists. The menopause years. Available at: http://www.acog.com. Last accessed September 26, 2008.

24. Estroven product information. Bloomfield, Conn: Amerifit Nutrition; 2008.

25. RU25 Plus Home Menopause Test Information. Lockport, Ill: Hormone Check; 2005.

26. CARE FSH Product Information. Waterbury, Conn: Care Products; 2003–2004.

27. American Cancer Society. Cancer Facts and Figures 2008. Available at: http://www.cancer.org. Last accessed September 26, 2008.

28. Chao A, Thun M, Connell C, et al. Meat consumption and risk of colorectal cancer. *JAMA*. 2005;293:172–82.

29. Lieberman DA, Harford WV, Ahnen DJ, et al. One-time screening for colorectal cancer with combined fecal occult blood testing and examination of the distal colon. *N Engl J Med*. 2001;345:555–60.

30. EZ-Detect product information. Newport Beach, Calif: Biomerica; 2000–2001.

31. ColonTest-Sensitive product information. Las Vegas, NV: Diagnostica.

32. LifeGuard product information. Durham, NC: MedTek.

33. Kahi CJ, Imperiale TF. Do aspirin and nonsteroidal anti-inflammatory drugs cause false-positive fecal occult blood test results? A prospective study in a cohort of veterans. *Am J Med*. 2004;117:837–41.

34. American Cancer Society. Colon and Rectal Cancer. Available at: http://www.cancer.org Last accessed September 26, 2008.

35. National Institutes of Health. Executive summary. In: *Third Report of the National Cholesterol Education Program (NCEP) Expert Panel on Detection, Evaluation, and Treatment of High Blood Cholesterol in Adults (Adult Treatment Panel III)*. Bethesda, Md: National Institutes of Health; May 2001. NIH Publication No. 01-3670.

36. *Health, United States, 2007*. Hyattsville, Md: National Center for Health Statistics; 2007.

37. CholesTrak product information. Vista, Calif: Accutech; 2004.

38. Home Access Instant Cholesterol Test product information. Hoffman Estates, Ill: Home Access Health.

39. Cardiochek product information. Indianapolis, Ind: Polymer Technology Systems.

40. Personal Cholesterol Monitor product information. Post Falls, Idaho: Lifestream Technologies; 2000.

41. BIOSAFE Total Cholesterol Panel product information. Lincolnshire, Ill: BIOSAFE.

42. McNamara JR, Warnick GR, Leary ET, et al. Multicenter evaluation of a patient-administered test for blood cholesterol measurement. *Prev Med*. 1996;25:583–92.

43. Do home cholesterol tests work? *Consum Rep*. August 2003:9.

44. Centers for Disease Control and Prevention. Urinary tract infections. Available at: http://www.cdc.gov. Last accessed September 26, 2008.

45. Stamm WE. Urinary Tract infections and pyelonephritis. In: Kasper DL, Braunwald E, Fauci AS, et al., eds. *Harrison's Principles Of Internal Medicine*. 16th ed. New York: McGraw-Hill, Inc; 2005.

46. UTI Bladder Infection Test product information. Redmond, Wash: Consumers Choice Systems; 2005.

47. AZO test strips product information. Woburn, Mass: PolyMedica Health; 2005.

48. Division of HIV/AIDS Prevention, National Center for HIV, STD and TB Prevention, Centers for Disease Control & Prevention. Basic Statistics. Available at: http://www.cdc.gov/hiv/stats.htm. Last accessed September 26, 2008.

49. Home Access Express HIV-1 test system product information. Hoffman Estates, Ill: Home Access Health.

50. Centers for Disease Control and Prevention. Viral Hepatitis C. Available at: http://www.cdc.gov/hepatitis/index.htm. Last accessed September 26, 2008.

51. Home Access Hepatitis C Check product information. Hoffman Estates, Ill: Home Access Health.

52. At Home Drug Test product information. San Diego, Calif: Pharmatech.

53. Dr. Brown's Home Drug Testing System product information. Elan. Available at: http://www.drbrowns.com/pages/discussion.html. Last accessed October 8, 2008.

54. Quick Screen Pro product information. Vista, Calif: Craig Medical Distribution.

55. PDT-90 Personal Drug Testing Service product information. Cambridge, Mass: Psychemedics.

56. US Department of Health and Human Services. National Institutes of Health, National Heart, Lung, and Blood Institute, National High Blood Pressure Education Program. *The Seventh Report of the Joint National Committee on the Detection, Evaluation, and Treatment of High Blood Pressure (JNC-VII)*. Bethesda, Md: US Department of Health and Human Services; 2004. NIH Publication No. 04-5230. Available at: http://www.nhlbi.nih.gov/ guidelines/hypertension/jnc7full.pdf. Last accessed September 26, 2008.

57. American Heart Association. AHA scientific statement. Recommendations for blood pressure measurement in humans and experimental animals, part 1: blood pressure measurement in humans: a statement for professionals from the Subcommittee of Professional and Public Education of the American Heart Association Council on High Blood Pressure Research. *Circulation*. 2005;111:697–716.

58. Association for the Advancement of Medical Instrumentation. Electronic or automated sphygmomanometers. Arlington, Va: American National Standards Institute; 1992:1–40.

Adult Urinary Incontinence and Supplies

Christine K. O'Neil

Urinary incontinence (UI) is defined as the complaint of any involuntary leakage of urine.[1] Although often mistakenly thought of as a problem of aging, UI affects persons of all ages, socioeconomic backgrounds, and ethnicities. UI is twice as common in women, but men also suffer from the symptoms.[2] An estimated 17 million people in the United States are affected by UI, whereas another 34 million may suffer from overactive bladder (OAB).[3]

UI is an underdiagnosed and underreported condition with major psychosocial and economic effects on society. Feelings of embarrassment, denial, and misinformation prevent many people from seeking help, which may lead to anxiety, depression, and, possibly, social isolation. Severe UI usually results in a loss of self-esteem and the ability to maintain an independent lifestyle. In addition, it is generally recognized as a major cause of institutionalization of older people.

Direct costs associated with UI include the expenses for diagnosis, specific treatment, routine care, rehabilitation, and hospital and nursing home admissions. The direct costs of treating UI and OAB in men and women of all ages were estimated at 19.5 billion and 12.6 billion, respectively, in 2000.[3]

Several studies have determined the prevalence of UI in nursing homes and the community.[4,5] The reported prevalence rates are approximately 50% for people in nursing homes, and range between 2% and 55% for adults living in the community, depending on the definition of UI, population characteristics, and methodologic approach.[6] Among adults 30 to 60 years of age, the prevalence of UI ranges from 12% to 42% for women and from 3% to 5% for men. For older people (>60 years of age), prevalence rates from 17% to 55% have been reported for women and from 11% to 34% for men.

Despite the high prevalence of UI, less than half of community-dwelling persons with UI consult with their health care professional.[7] Many accept the symptoms as a natural part of aging and use self-care strategies with little or no health professional guidance. Although they are reluctant to talk about UI, Americans spend $1.1 billion annually on disposable incontinence products (e.g., pads, shields, guards, undergarments, and briefs).[8]

Pathophysiology of Urinary Incontinence

Urination is a complex process, involving a coordinated effort by the bladder, urethra, muscular components of the lower urinary tract, brain, and spinal cord.[9,10] Urine produced by the kidneys is propelled through the ureters to the bladder. The detrusor muscle, the smooth muscle layer of the bladder, gives tone to the bladder, relaxing as the bladder fills with urine and contracting during urination. The bladder neck, which joins the bladder and the urethra, is surrounded by smooth muscle, referred to as the internal sphincter, which either constricts to hold urine in the bladder or relaxes, permitting urine flow through the urethra. Voluntary control of micturition is maintained by contraction of the external sphincter, a striated muscle located at mid-urethral length. When relaxed, the urethra, surrounded by both smooth and striated muscle, allows urine to leave the body.

The bladder and the internal sphincter are innervated by the autonomic nervous system, and the external sphincter is innervated by the somatic or voluntary nervous system. Parasympathetic and sympathetic nerves innervate the smooth muscle of the bladder and urethra. Both alpha-adrenergic and beta-adrenergic receptors are present in the urinary structures. The alpha-receptors are located in the base of the bladder and the proximal urethra, and the beta-receptors are found primarily in the body of the bladder detrusor. Stimulation of the alpha-receptors causes contraction of the smooth muscles in the bladder neck and urethra, thus closing the bladder outlet. Stimulation of the beta-receptors results in smooth muscle relaxation and allows the bladder to fill. Thus, sympathetic stimulation causes the bladder to retain urine. Parasympathetic cholinergic receptors are located throughout the bladder. Stimulation of these receptors causes the detrusor to contract, emptying the bladder. The sacral center, lying between vertebrae S2 and S4, acts as the relay center for information to and from the bladder, pelvic floor, and brain.

The capacity of the bladder is approximately 400 to 500 mL. When the bladder fills, stretch receptors in the detrusor wall transmit signals to the brain through the spinal cord, initiating the urge to urinate when the bladder is approximately half full. Under normal circumstances, adults can delay voiding for 30 to 60 minutes as a result of the short sacral reflex, which diminishes the urge to urinate by increasing contraction of the external sphincter and relaxing the detrusor muscle of the bladder. Bladder emptying is initiated voluntarily, causing relaxation of the external sphincter and contraction of the detrusor. Normal urination results in complete emptying of the bladder, with little or no residual urine (50 mL or less). Any disruption in the integration of musculoskeletal and neurologic function can lead to loss of control of normal bladder function and UI.[11]

Clinical Presentation of Urinary Incontinence

UI is a symptom that can be caused by anatomic, physiologic, and pathologic factors affecting the urinary tract, as well as external factors.[2,12–14] In many cases, multiple and interacting factors contribute to UI. The risk of UI is strongly associated with aging. Additional risk factors for UI, some at least partially reversible, have been identified (Table 52-1).[2,12–14] Identification of the cause(s) of UI is essential for the assessment and successful management of UI.

Age-related changes in the bladder and urinary tract may contribute to an older person's vulnerability to UI. With age, the kidney's ability to concentrate urine diminishes, resulting in larger urine volumes. In addition, age-related hypotrophic changes in bladder tissue lead to frequent urination and nocturia, whereas decreased muscle tone of the bladder, as well as the bladder sphincters and pelvic muscles, contributes to the potential for reduced urine control. This loss of control, combined with diminished mobility and reaction time, predisposes older people to UI.[15]

In women, the loss of estrogen causes a decrease in bladder outlet and urethral resistance, as well as a decline in pelvic musculature—all of which increase the likelihood of UI. In addition, estrogen loss results in atrophic changes in the vaginal and urethral mucosa, disrupting the vaginal flora and leading to atrophic vaginitis and chronic urethritis. These conditions, in turn, may cause urinary frequency and urgency, dysuria, urinary tract infections, and UI. The woman's short urethra exerts less resistance to intravesicular pressure than the longer male urethra. Consequently, obesity, chronic cough, and jarring exercise, which all increase intra–abdominal pressure, result in extra load on the bladder. As such, these factors can overwhelm the relatively low resistance offered by the short female urethra. Childbirth, gynecologic procedures, and muscle atrophy from aging also weaken the woman's pelvic floor muscles, thereby decreasing support for the bladder. Without adequate support, positioning of the bladder becomes distorted (known as cystocele or anterior wall prolapse) and can result in urethral kinking, with subsequent poor bladder emptying. These conditions may result in chronic obstruction of the bladder, again leading to UI from urine volume overload.

Men often develop prostatic enlargement beginning in their middle to late 40s, which results in urethral obstruction, leading to decreased urinary flow rates, increased residual volumes, detrusor instability, and possibly overflow incontinence. Paradoxically, prostatectomy to relieve bothersome symptoms related to benign prostatic hyperplasia (BPH) can result in stress incontinence caused by incidental injury to the internal sphincter.

UI can be described broadly as transient or chronic. Transient UI is usually of sudden onset and secondary to acute illness (e.g., urinary tract infections) or to any disease that causes acute confusion (e.g., respiratory disease, myocardial infarction, or septicemia) or immobility, preventing the person from reaching a toilet independently or in time. Many other conditions and medications can cause or contribute to transient UI (Table 52-2).[2,16] Managing these conditions may resolve UI in some patients, but only reduce the severity of symptoms in others. Chronic UI is often related to neurologic or other chronic conditions, such as intrinsic sphincter deficiency, BPH, or cystocele.[17] UI can be classified as OAB, stress incontinence, mixed incontinence (OAB plus stress incontinence), overflow incontinence, or functional incontinence, depending on the underlying etiologies.

TABLE 52-1 Risk Factors for Urinary Incontinence

BPH/TURP/prostatectomy

Caucasian race

Childhood nocturnal enuresis

Diabetes

Environmental barriers

Estrogen depletion

Fecal impaction

High fluid intake (leading to polyuria and bladder capacity overload)

High-impact physical activities

Immobility/chronic degenerative disease

Impaired cognition: acute or chronic

Low fluid intake (leading to concentrated urine and bladder irritation that worsens symptoms)

Medications (Table 52-2)

Metabolic disorders (hyperglycemia, hypercalcemia)

Neurologic disorders (spinal cord injury, neuropathy)

Obesity (moderate-to-morbid)

Pelvic floor muscle weakness

Pregnancy/vaginal delivery/episiotomy

Smoking

Stroke

Key: BPH, benign prostatic hyperplasia; TURP, transurethral resection of the prostate.
Source: Adapted from references 2 and 12–14.

TABLE 52-2 Reversible Conditions That Cause or Contribute to Urinary Incontinence

Conditions Affecting the Lower Urinary Tract
Urinary tract infections, atrophic vaginitis/urethritis, stool impaction

Drug Side Effects
Polyuria, frequency, urgency: caffeine, diuretics, alcohol, acetylcholinesterase inhibitors

Urinary retention: anticholinergics, antidepressants, hypnotics/sedatives, antipsychotics, narcotics, muscle relaxants, antihypertensives (calcium channel blockers), beta-adrenergic agonists, alpha-adrenergic agonists

Urethral relaxation: alpha-adrenergic blockers

Cough: ACE inhibitors

Increased Urine Production
Metabolic disorders (hyperglycemia, hypercalcemia), excessive fluid intake, volume overload, venous insufficiency with edema leading to nocturia

Inability or Willingness to Reach a Toilet
Dementia, delirium, chronic illness/injury that interferes with mobility, psychological conditions

Key: ACE, angiotensin-converting enzyme.
Source: References 2 and 16.

Recognition of signs and symptoms of UI is an essential first step in providing treatment advice. Patients often delay discussion or do not seek medical evaluation for UI with their primary care provider. Therefore, it is important for practitioners to inquire about potential UI symptoms when such conditions are suspected on the basis of clinical evidence or patient inquiries. Open-ended questions such as "What problems are you having, if any, with your bladder?" and "How often do you experience urine leakage?" can be used to begin this dialogue. An awareness of signs such as the odor of urine or appearance of wetness is also necessary to identify potential patients suffering from UI. Table 52-3 lists observed and reported symptoms commonly associated with particular types of UI.

Overactive bladder occurs in both men and women, and its incidence increases with age. This condition is characterized by sudden and profound urinary urgency (strong desire to void), frequency (urinating more than eight times daily), nocturia (two or more awakenings at night to pass urine), or enuresis; OAB is often, but not always, accompanied by urge incontinence (involuntary urine leakage with urgency).[2,10,11,15] OAB is usually, but not always, attributable to uninhibited contractions of the detrusor muscle, referred to as detrusor instability. Other terms describing detrusor instability are detrusor hyperreflexia, detrusor hyperactivity with impaired bladder contractility, and bladder instability.

Neurogenic causes of detrusor instability include dementia, stroke, Parkinson's disease, suprasacral spinal cord injury, multiple sclerosis, and medullary lesions. Detrusor instability of neurologic origin is referred to as hyperreflexia. Nonneurogenic causes of detrusor instability include bladder irritation caused by infection or interstitial cystitis (bladder pain syndrome), obstruction (e.g., BPH or cystocele), bladder stones, and tumors. Excessive beverage intake and some therapeutic agents (e.g., diuretics and alcohol) can exacerbate symptoms of urge incontinence as a result of increased filling of the bladder. Bethanechol can also lead to urge incontinence through cholinergically mediated contraction of bladder smooth muscle.

Stress incontinence is the most frequently encountered type of UI in women, except in the very old (>75 years) in whom OAB is most common. Symptoms of stress incontinence may occur in some men after transurethral resection of the prostate and radical prostatectomy.[11] Stress incontinence is characterized by involuntary leakage of urine with sudden increases in abdominal pressure associated with sneezing, laughing, coughing, exercising, and lifting. Symptoms are exacerbated with pregnancy and obesity, which also increase intraabdominal pressure. This involuntary leakage is believed to be caused by hypermobility of the bladder neck or weakness of the urethral sphincter and pelvic floor muscles. Hypermobility refers to displacement of the bladder neck and urethra during physical exertion; it occurs when the supporting pelvic muscles have been weakened as a result of vaginal childbirth and aging. The weakening of the urethral sphincter can be secondary to vaginal or urologic surgery, trauma, aging, or inadequate estrogen, or it may be neurologic in etiology.[18] Drug-related causes of stress incontinence include alphaadrenergic antagonists such as prazosin, terazosin, doxazosin, tamsulosin, and alfuzosin, which cause urethral relaxation (Table 52-2).

Mixed incontinence, most common in women, consists of the combination of OAB and stress incontinence.[2] Although the term *mixed UI* is generally applied to women, men with outlet obstruction resulting from BPH may exhibit mixed symptoms of OAB and overflow incontinence. Men may also exhibit mixed symptoms as a result of stress UI attributable to radical prostatectomy or transurethral resection of the prostate combined with OAB.

Overflow incontinence, an involuntary urine loss associated with overdistention of the bladder, is observed in 7% to 11% of incontinent older patients.[2] Symptoms include dribbling, reduced force and caliber of urinary stream, urgency, and a sensation of incomplete voiding. The two main causes are outlet obstruction and/or an underactive bladder (detrusor) muscle. Outlet obstruction can be caused by BPH, urogenital tumors, pelvic organ prolapse, or previous anti-incontinence surgery. Dysfunctional bladder contractility can result from diabetic or alcoholic neuropathy, lower spinal cord injury, radical pelvic surgery, or medications with anticholinergic properties, such as antihistamines, antipsychotics, narcotics, tricyclic antidepressants, muscle relaxants, and medications used to treat urge incontinence. These medications can cause overflow incontinence by blocking cholinergically mediated bladder contractions, thereby inhibiting normal bladder function.

Functional incontinence is described as urine loss caused by factors such as physical or cognitive impairment, which interfere with a person's ability to reach toilet facilities in time or to perform toileting tasks.[2,10] Causes of this type of UI are many and include stroke, diminished mobility, impaired cognitive function or perception, environmental barriers, use of sedative and hypotensive agents, poorly controlled severe pain, and psychological unwillingness to release urine in the proper place. Because many functionally impaired people may

TABLE 52-3	Common Signs/Symptoms of Urinary Incontinence, by Type

Classification of UI	Signs/Symptoms
Urge	Urgency
	Frequency
	Large amount of urine loss
	Nocturia or nocturnal incontinence (enuresis)
	Inability to reach toilet following urge to void
Stress	Urine leakage during physical activity, lifting coughing, sneezing
	Small-to-moderate urine loss depending on level of activity
	Able to reach toilet in time to complete void
	Occasional urgency
	In severe forms, urine loss on ambulating
	Rare nocturia and enuresis
Overflow	Sensation of bladder or abdominal fullness
	Sensation of incomplete bladder emptying
	Sensation of perineal bulge (cystocele/anterior wall prolapse)
	Hesitancy
	Straining to void
	Decreased or incomplete urine stream; dribbling
	Frequency common
	Urgency common
Mixed	Presence of both stress and urge symptoms

have other types of UI, functional incontinence should be a diagnosis of exclusion.

The consequences of UI are considerable. Many people are embarrassed by such a condition and refrain from discussing their urinary problems with their primary health care providers. Some people with UI believe it is a normal consequence of aging, rather than a symptom of underlying disease or anatomic change. Social isolation occurs because the incontinent patient avoids social interaction to prevent the embarrassment and rejection that often accompany UI. In turn, social isolation leads to depression. Intimate contact and sexual activity with the patient's partner can also decrease. Attempts to limit episodes of involuntary urine loss by restricting fluid intake can cause dehydration and hypotension, whereas skin irritation and ulceration caused by long exposure to urine results in "diaper rash" and possibly pressure ulcers.[2]

The caregivers of incontinent older patients are under stress because of the tedious and time-consuming care needed to deal with the problems at home. Often, the loss of urine control leads to a drastic reduction in quality of life, nursing home placement, or elder abuse.[2,19] Falls and fractures can result from UI and with urgency symptoms in the absence of incontinence.

Treatment of Adult Urinary Incontinence

Treatment Goals

The goals of treatment of UI are to cure incontinence or to reduce the severity of symptoms, avoid complications, and improve the patient's quality of life. When incontinence aids are used as part of self-management in UI, additional goals are to control or treat skin breakdown (diaper rash), control the odor of leaked urine, and contain urine in the undergarment.

General Treatment Approach

After medical evaluation, treatment is individualized for the type of UI. The four major categories of intervention are behavioral, devices, pharmacologic, and surgical. Nonsurgical treatments for UI in women have been systematically reviewed in a recent publication.[20] Figure 52-1 outlines the self-management of adult UI.

Nonpharmacologic Therapy

Behavioral techniques decrease the frequency of UI in most patients, have no reported side effects, and do not limit future therapies.[2] To be most successful, these techniques generally require patient and/or caregiver involvement and continued practice. Three types of behavioral techniques, listed in order of increasing need for patient involvement, are toileting assistance, bladder training, and pelvic floor muscle training. Behavioral techniques are now the accepted first-line therapy in treating all forms of UI except overflow incontinence.[10] A behavioral modification program involving pelvic floor muscle training and behavioral techniques was found to prevent the development of UI in continent older women.[21] Practitioners should educate patients about the role of behavioral therapy in the prevention and management of UI.

Toileting assistance includes routine/scheduled toileting performed at fixed, regular intervals (every 2–4 hours); habit training, which is toileting scheduled to match voiding patterns in those who have natural voiding patterns; and prompted voiding. In prompted voiding, patients are trained to void only if the need is voiced on direct questioning. They are checked for wetness and praised for maintaining continence and trying to toilet.

Bladder training consists of education, scheduled voiding with systematic delay, and positive reinforcement. Patients are taught to delay voiding when the urge occurs and to use tactics to increase urine volume and the interval between voids. Bladder training is recommended for urge or mixed incontinence, but is often difficult to achieve in cognitively impaired or frail older people.

Pelvic floor muscle training aims to improve urethral closure pressure by activating the striated muscles of the urethra and the underlying pelvic floor muscles. Two components of training have been established. Early improvement (reduction of urine leakage within 1 week of beginning pelvic floor muscle exercises) may be achieved by some women who learn "the knack maneuver" or volitional precontraction. *The knack,* is a term to describe learning to contract pelvic floor muscles in anticipation of and during increases in intra-abdominal pressure (such as a cough). This maneuver alone has demonstrated the capacity to reduce stress incontinence.[22] In addition, pelvic floor muscle training, also known as Kegel exercises or pelvic floor exercises, is designed to strengthen the voluntary periurethral and perivaginal muscles, giving the patient more control of micturition and reducing UI.[2] These exercises have been used successfully for stress and OAB; they are performed by squeezing the pelvic muscles as if to stop the flow of urine. These contractions should be held for about 10 seconds and then released for 10 seconds; three to four sets of 10 contractions per day are generally recommended.[2,23] It is important to advise patients that the response to pelvic muscle exercises is delayed. The exercises may be augmented by the use of vaginal weights or biofeedback techniques. Biofeedback can facilitate learning of pelvic muscle exercises. Direct electrical stimulation of the pelvic floor muscles with vaginal or anal probes or surface electrodes has been used with limited success in stress, urge, and mixed UI.

A relatively new option available only through a primary care provider's office is the NeoControl Pelvic Floor Therapy System.[24] This is a pulsating magnetic chair that uses directed magnetic fields to induce pelvic muscle contractions. Patients generally require treatments twice a week for about 20 to 30 minutes for a total of 8 weeks or more. This option is approved by the Food and Drug Administration (FDA) for the treatment of stress, OAB, and mixed UI.

Application of mechanical pressure to support the urethra is evident in the age-old advice to cross the legs before coughing or sneezing to prevent urine leakage in women with stress incontinence.[25] Similarly, various devices have been used for UI, including elevating devices to support the bladder neck (pessary, tampon, or prosthesis); urethral occlusive devices (urethral plug, expandable urethral devices, or urethral shields); external collection systems (condom catheters, or female urinals); penile compression devices; and catheterization (intermittent, indwelling, or suprapubic).[2] A recent review of mechanical devices found inconsistent results, insufficient evidence to compare one device with another, and no evidence to compare mechanical devices with other forms of treatment.[16]

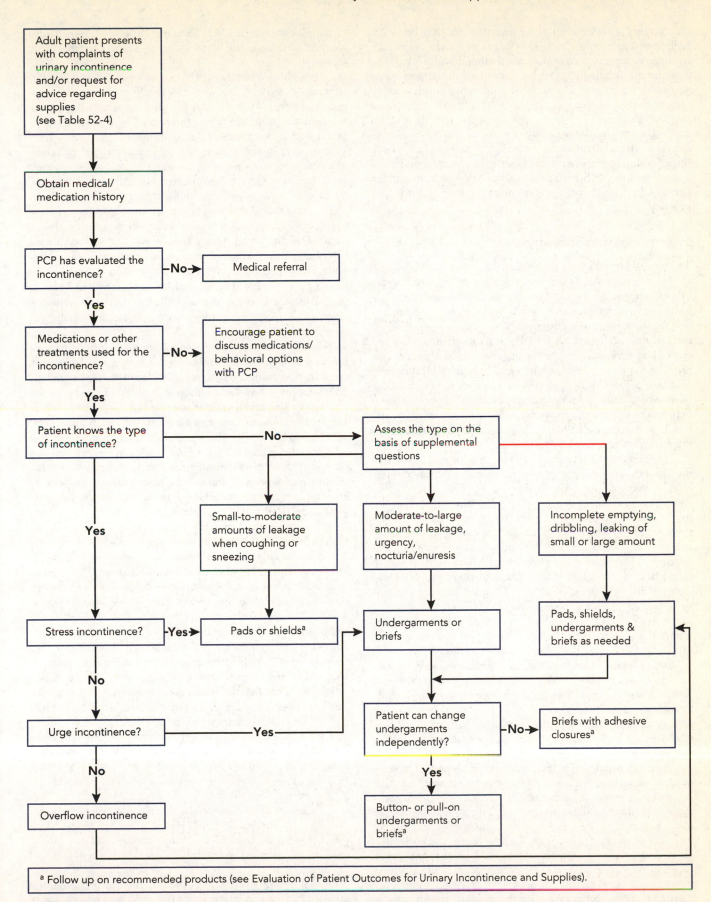

FIGURE 52-1 Self-care of adult urinary incontinence. Key: PCP, primary care provider.

Surgery is uncommon in the treatment of OAB; however, both stress and overflow incontinence can be treated successfully by surgery. Surgery is an option when other nonpharmacologic and pharmacologic therapies have failed, or the patient wants definitive treatment. The aims of continence surgery are to elevate the bladder neck, support the urethra, and increase urethral resistance.[2,26] Some surgical options include urethral bulking agents (collagen), sling operation, tension-free vaginal tape, artificial sphincter insertion, needle bladder-neck suspension, retropubic suspension, urinary diversion, and bladder denervation. It should be noted that surgical treatment for stress incontinence can instigate or exacerbate symptoms of urgency.

Pharmacologic Therapy

The type of UI influences the choice of treatments. For that reason, an overview of the pharmacologic measures for specific types of UI is presented here. Most medications used to treat these disorders are prescription products, but in some cases nonprescription medications may be suggested. Nonprescription medications for UI are considered an off-label indication, however, and should be used only after a thorough evaluation by a primary care provider has determined the cause and/or type of UI. Inappropriate use of systemic nonprescription products and incorrect use of absorbent undergarments and pads before a proper evaluation may result in unnecessary expense, inappropriate treatment, and possibly unnecessary changes in the patient's lifestyle and psychological well-being.

Detrusor instability may be treated with anticholinergic medications, which facilitate urine storage by decreasing uninhibited detrusor contractions. Most often, a prescription medication such as darifenacin, oxybutynin chloride, solifenacin, tolterodine, or trospium is used first. Other prescription medications with less evidence of clinical efficacy and concerns about risk of side effects include propantheline, imipramine, and nifedipine. Flavoxate is not effective according to the results of four placebo-controlled trials.[26] Diphenhydramine and dicyclomine are used occasionally (see Chapter 12). Practitioners should counsel patients about the potential side effects that occur more frequently with diphenhydramine than with the other prescription products. Sedation, dry mouth (a problem for denture use, and patients with gastroesophageal reflux disease, dysphagia, or stroke), dizziness, constipation, and confusion can be significant problems in older patients. Contraindications to the use of diphenhydramine (and other anticholinergic medications) include many conditions (e.g., narrow-angle glaucoma, peptic ulcer, urinary tract obstruction, gastroesophageal reflux disease, and uncontrolled hyperthyroidism) that occur more often in older patients than in other patients.

Stress incontinence is often treated with agents that increase outflow resistance through alpha-receptor stimulation that enhances contraction of the bladder-neck muscles.[2] A commonly recommended nonprescription drug is pseudoephedrine (see Chapter 12). The dose of pseudoephedrine is 15 to 30 mg three times daily, starting with the lowest dose, especially in older people. Use of nonprescription medications for UI is an off-label indication and must be approved by a primary care provider. Caution should be used, however, when initiating such therapy in patients with hypertension and/or cardiac arrhythmias. The practitioner should advise patients to monitor their blood pressure and pulse, and to report any new occurrences of heart palpitations or fainting. Common adverse effects of pseudoephedrine include insomnia, headache, tachycardia, elevated blood pressure, dizziness, nervousness, agitation, and tremor.

In women, estrogen therapy may be used, and benefits are usually seen in 4 to 6 weeks. A Cochrane review of estrogen, compared with placebo, for UI indicated that estrogen use resulted in higher rates of cure and symptom improvement, with more positive effects on urge UI than stress UI.[27] Practitioners should counsel female patients about the common side effects of oral estrogen therapy, such as weight gain, fluid retention, increased blood pressure, and vaginal spotting. In light of recent concerns about the complications (heart attack, stroke, and breast cancer) associated with postmenopausal estrogen/progestin therapy, these products should be used in the lowest dosage for the shortest period of time (3–5 years). Topical vaginal estrogen therapy is useful for underlying vaginitis and urethritis, and may exert a greater benefit than oral estrogen; several randomized controlled trials of vaginal estrogen have shown a decrease in urgency and incontinence.[28] Therapy with estrogen vaginal cream is usually initiated with daily application and tapered to several times weekly applications. Other vaginal estrogen options include the vaginal ring and vaginal tablets. Estrogen can be used in combination with alpha-adrenergic agonists; however, the combination is only slightly more effective and can be associated with more adverse effects and increased therapy cost. The antidepressant imipramine, which also acts as an adrenergic agonist, has been suggested when alpha-adrenergic agents and estrogens have failed. Duloxetine, a selective serotonin and norepinephrine reuptake inhibitor currently approved for the treatment of depression and diabetic neuropathy, is moderately effective in managing stress UI.[29] If medical treatment fails, surgical correction may be possible.

The treatment of overflow incontinence is directed by the underlying cause. In BPH, alpha-adrenergic antagonists (terazosin, doxazosin, tamsulosin, alfuzosin, or prazosin) or 5-alpha-reductase inhibitors (finasteride or dutasteride) can be used to reduce the degree of outlet obstruction. Alpha-adrenergic antagonists have a much faster onset of effect (several days) than do 5-alpha-reductase inhibitors. Because of a relatively high rate of orthostatic hypotension, prazosin is not recommended for therapy of UI. Prescription agents such as bethanechol chloride may be initiated if the bladder has insufficient contractile strength such as after general anesthesia. Its efficacy is not well established in long-standing hypotonic bladder, however, and it is associated with potentially serious adverse effects. In neurogenic bladder, bethanechol appears to be most effective when starting therapy as soon as possible after the occurrence of incontinence following the neurologic event. Surgery for BPH is often necessary. Catheterization, usually intermittent, is combined with frequent attempts to toilet as a last resort when medical and surgical corrections have failed.

Treatment of functional and iatrogenic incontinence requires evaluating the patient's entire medical status, medication history, and environment. UI resulting from medications can be resolved by initiating alternative treatments. Underlying dysfunctions such as pain related to rheumatoid arthritis and decreased mobility can be remedied by medical and environmental changes that make using the toilet possible or easier within the limitations of the patient's functional status. Often an assessment by physical or occupational therapists can be useful in enhancing physical function.

Use of Urinary Incontinence Supplies

Absorbent undergarments and pads are used to protect clothing, bedding, and furniture while allowing the patient to have independence and mobility. Although absorbent products are beneficial, they should be used only after a thorough and complete physical examination. Prematurely initiating the use of absorbent protective products relieves the discomfort and obscures the cause of UI. Because correction of the cause may be possible, the premature acceptance of UI may have significant financial, social, and psychological consequences.

Product Selection Guidelines

The type of absorbent product selected depends on several factors[2]:

- Type and severity of UI
- Functional status
- Gender
- Availability of caregivers
- Patient preference
- Cost
- Convenience

The clinician needs to discuss these factors with patients and their caregivers when helping them select absorbent garments and pads, which are available as reusable or disposable products (Table 52-4). This discussion is particularly important for low-income patients who often do not have the economic flexibility to purchase absorbent products; they may be forced to resort to toilet paper or tissue products, an ineffective substitute. Many people attempt to extend the life of disposable products by layering flushable tissue over the pad. The tissue is also easier to dispose of in public places. However, its reduced wicking capacity can expose the skin to more moisture and thus potential for breakdown. Some patients may be inclined to use low-cost menstrual pads that may be effective in some cases; however, these products contain materials that are specific to absorbing blood, not urine. Given the wide variety of available products, a resource guide published by the National Association for Continence may be invaluable in helping patients with selection of a product.[30]

The disposable product market has been a multimillion-dollar industry since the 1990s. These products work in the same manner as children's disposable diapers. They are designed to absorb urine; provide a moisture barrier to protect clothes, bedding, and furniture; and minimize skin contact with urine. For maximum absorbency, products containing an absorptive gel of super absorbent polymers may be preferable. Urine is jelled in the matrix of the absorbent layer, minimizing its contact with skin. Reusable incontinence undergarments may offer a more affordable option.[31] These resemble underpants with a waterproof crotch and are designed to hold a reusable panty liner. The newest option is reusable incontinence undergarments that resemble standard underwear but have the absorbency of disposable briefs. These undergarments have a unique crotch design made of several layers of wicking fabric that quickly pulls moisture away from the skin. They are available for men and women in a variety of leakage control levels. Reusable incontinence underwear is constructed of waterproof outer fabrics ranging from lace to nylon floral prints, making them an attractive and affordable option for patients

with an active lifestyle. A recent comparative evaluation of the performance and cost-effectiveness of four key absorbent product designs demonstrated significant and substantial differences between products and considerable individual variability in preference. Cost-effective management with absorbent products may best be achieved by allowing users to choose combinations of designs for different circumstances.[32]

The capacity of each disposable product corresponds to the needs of the patient:

- *Guards/shields:* 2 to 12 ounces (60–360 mL), light-to-heavy capacity.
- *Undergarments:* 12 to 18 ounces (360–540 mL), moderate-to-heavy capacity.
- *Briefs:* 28 to 36 ounces (840–1100 mL), moderate-to-heavy capacity.

Patients with small amounts of leakage (e.g., dribbling), as occurs in stress or overflow incontinence and after urologic surgical procedures, may require only a pad or shield.[33,34] A recent systematic review of absorbent products suggested that disposable insert pads are best for leak-through prevention, and are the most acceptable and preferred design for women with light UI.[35] In a similar study, guards were a preferred product for light UI in men.[36] If larger amounts of urine are lost with UI, as often occurs with detrusor instability, products with a larger capacity would be more appropriate. Many products designed for overnight (heavy) use tend to have the largest capacities.[30]

Another important issue is the functional capacity of the patient. If the patient needs assistance with absorbent garments, the caregiver may find that briefs or diapers with "roll-on" bed application and adhesive closures are useful. Securing the product may be an important issue. Close-fitting underwear is recommended. Some garments or shields have adhesive strips or belts to hold them in place. The use of belts may require assistance from a caregiver. Of course, comfort and leg security from urine leakage are important. Many product lines offer elastic legs or contoured shapes. Caregivers and patients should consider products designed for the differences between male and female anatomy when selecting large-capacity products.[33,34]

Protective underpads are often used in conjunction with briefs and undergarments for extended duration activities, such as sleeping and sitting. Both bed and chair pads are available, and the practitioner should inquire about the need for additional protection. The underpad should have a known capacity, a waterproof duration of several hours, and an ability to remain intact when wet. Bed pads are available in sizes from 16 by 24 inches to 30 by 36 inches. For chairs, a 16- by 18-inch pad should be used.[34]

Complications from Absorbent Products

Because the use of absorbent products increases the risk of skin irritation and maceration, these products should be checked every 2 hours. With continual urine loss, it is recommended that the absorbent material be changed every 2 to 4 hours. The use of skin protectants (barrier creams and ointments), as in diaper rash, is appropriate. If a rash occurs, the same treatment as that described for infants (see Chapter 36) is indicated.

TABLE 52-4 Selected Adult Incontinence Products

Trade Name	Product Features[a]
Assurance Slip-On Protective Undergarment[b]	For moderate/heavy leakage; one-size, one-piece design; no buttons or tapes
Attends Briefs	For heavy leakage; sizes Y, S, M, L; refastenable tapes
Attends Briefs with Waistband	For heavy leakage; sizes M, L
Attends Guards Super Absorbency	For light/moderate leakage; curved fit
Attends Pads	For light leakage; medium-, extra-, superabsorbency
Attends Undergarments Super Absorbency	For moderate leakage; reusable elastic belts
Conveen Drip Collector	For dribbling/light leakage; 3- and 4-ounce capacity; adheres to underwear; designed for men
Depend Underwear Extra & Super Plus Absorbency	For heavy leakage; sizes S/M, L; feels and wears like underwear
Depend Refastenable Underwear Extra & Super Plus Absorbency	For heavy leakage; sizes S/M, L/XL; feels and wears like underwear; four refastenable tabs
Depend Fitted Briefs Regular & Overnight Absorbency	For heavy leakage; sizes M, L; six refastenable tapes plus elastic leg and waist; wetness indicator; overnight absorbency absorbs 30% more urine than regular absorbency
Depend Guards for Men	For light/moderate leakage; one size; anatomic design with elasticized pouch and cup-like fit
Depend Undergarments Easy Fit Elastic Leg/Adjustable Straps Regular & Extra Absorbency	For moderate leakage; soft, cloth-like outer cover; one size; reusable hook and loop strap tabs; fits hip sizes up to 65 inches
Depend Undergarments Elastic Leg/Button Straps Regular & Extra Absorbency	For moderate leakage; soft, cloth-like outer cover; one size; reusable button strap tabs; fits hip sizes up to 65 inches
Depend Undergarments Elastic Leg Extra Absorbency	For moderate leakage; soft, cloth-like outer cover; one size; reusable button strap tabs
Poise Pantiliners	Very light absorbency; 6½ inches long
Poise Extra Coverage Pantiliners	Very light absorbency; 7½ inches long
Poise Thin Pads Light Absorbency	For light leakage; 8½ inches long; elasticized sides
Poise Pads Regular Absorbency	For light leakage; 8½ inches long; elasticized sides
Poise Pads Extra Absorbency	For light leakage; 9½ inches long; elasticized sides, one end wider
Poise Pads Extra Plus Absorbency	For light/moderate leakage; 11 inches long; elasticized sides, one end wider
Poise Pads with Side Shields Ultra Absorbency	For light/moderate leakage; 11 inches long
Poise Pads with Side Shields Ultra Plus Absorbency	For moderate leakage; 13 inches long; pad-like comfort with guard-like absorbency; one end wider
Prevail Underwear	For heavy leakage; sizes S, M, L; for men and women; look and feel like underwear; pull-on
Serenity/TENA Dry Active Liners	For extra light leakage
Serenity/TENA Thin Pads Light	For light leakage
Serenity/TENA Pads Slender	For light leakage
Serenity/TENA Pads Extra	For moderate leakage
Serenity/TENA Pads Extra Plus	For moderate leakage
Serenity/TENA Pads Ultra	For heavy leakage
Serenity/TENA Pads Ultra Plus Night and Day	For heavy leakage; longest pad
Serenity/TENA Guards Super Absorbency	For moderate/heavy leakage
Serenity Guards Super Plus Absorbency	For heavy leakage
TENA Briefs	For heavy leakage; sizes Y, S, M, L; refastenable tabs

Key: Y, youth; S, small; M, medium; L, large.

[a] Products change often; refer to Web sites for current product availability (i.e., www.depend.com, www.poise.com, www.serenity.com).

[b] Manufacturer markets other products similar to the Depend line but offers a lower price point.

Urine odor is an embarrassing problem. Nonprescription products containing chlorophyll (e.g., Derifil, Pals, or Nullo) can be recommended to help decrease urine odor. However, frequent checks and changes are preferable to efforts to mask the odor.

The healing of skin wounds may be delayed in the patient with skin wetted by urine. Any skin breakdown needs to be reported to the primary care provider. This serious complica-tion should not be treated with nonprescription products with-out medical supervision.

UI products not available from the pharmacy or specialty supply store may be obtained by contacting the National Association for Continence, PO Box 1019, Charleston, SC 29402-1019; 1-843-377-0900, 1-800-BLADDER; fax: 1-843-377-0905; or www.nafc.org.

TABLE 52-5 Botanical Medicines Used to Treat Incontinence Related to BPH			
Herb (Scientific Name) [Trade Name]	**Dosage**	**Side Effects and Risks**	**Effectiveness for Incontinence Comments**
Pygeum (*Prunus africana*)	100–200 mg in divided doses	Mild diarrhea, indigestion; no known contraindications; no reported drug interactions	3-month symptomatic improvement in BPH[a]
Saw palmetto (*Serenoa repens* [LSESR], *Sabal serrulata*)	160 mg 2 times/day	Headache, hypertension, abdominal pain, constipation, diarrhea, nausea, decreased libido, dysuria, impotence, urine retention, and back pain	Use supported by in vitro, animal, and human clinical studies[b]; use only in diagnosed BPH: PSA and size of prostate not affected

Key: BPH, benign prostatic hyperplasia; LSESR, lipidosterolic extract of *Serenoa repens*; PSA, prostate-specific antigen.

[a] Trials included 12 double-blind, placebo-controlled trials; 34 open-label trials; and no comparative trials.

[b] Studies showed that saw palmetto was more effective than placebo and as effective as finasteride, and that time to maximum effect is delayed for several months. More comparative studies with alpha-blockers are needed; some contradictory information exists regarding the efficacy of saw palmetto in moderate-to-severe BPH.

Source: References 39–46.

Complementary Therapies

Nutritional deficiencies of protein, calcium, vitamin C, zinc, magnesium, and vitamin B_{12} have been proposed as possibly contributing to the development of UI.[37] Of these, the relationship between vitamin B_{12} deficiency and UI has been established.[38] A B_{12} deficiency may lead to diminished neurosensory input regarding bladder fullness or to inappropriate neurologic stimulation of the bladder, causing detrusor instability. Many factors such as spicy and acidic foods (caffeine, alcohol, and tobacco), dyes (Food Drug and Cosmetic Yellow Dye No. 5), food preservatives, and sugar substitutes (i.e., aspartame) may cause urinary frequency and urgency with the potential for UI.

Several herbal treatments have been suggested for UI (Table 52-5[39–46]), among them phytoestrogens (soybean and flaxseed), saw palmetto and pygeum or African plum, St. John's wort, and bearberry (uva-ursi) teas.[37] With the exception of the use of saw palmetto and pygeum for overflow incontinence related to BPH, evidence is lacking for their effectiveness. An in-depth discussion of saw palmetto and pygeum is presented in Chapter 54.

Assessment of Adult Urinary Incontinence and Supplies: A Case-Based Approach

Because of the public's general lack of sufficient medical knowledge about the different types of UI, some patients (or their caregivers) may attempt self-diagnosis and treatment without consulting their primary care providers. Self-diagnosis obviously could lead to inappropriate assessment and treatment. Therefore, it is imperative that practitioners inquire about a proper medical evaluation before recommending nonprescription products, including absorbent products. A primary care provider must recommend use of nonprescription medications for off-label indications.

Armed with the patient's history and proper diagnosis, the practitioner can answer questions appropriately and help in the selection and proper use of devices and medications for treating this disorder.

Case 52-1 illustrates the assessment of adult patients with UI.

CASE 52-1

Relevant Evaluation Criteria	Scenario/Model Outcome
Information Gathering	
1. Gather essential information about the patient's symptoms, including:	
a. description of symptom(s) (i.e., nature, onset, duration, severity, associated symptoms)	Patient complains of episodes of a weak bladder. The first incident occurred after the birth of her third child. As a result, she refrains from many activities that she once enjoyed, particularly sports and dancing. She has gained 30 pounds since the start of the symptoms owing to inactivity.
b. description of any factors that seem to precipitate, exacerbate, and/or relieve the patient's symptom(s)	The "leakage" occurs when she lifts her children, coughs, sneezes, or laughs. No leakage occurs at any other times.
c. description of the patent's efforts to relieve the symptoms	I have been using panty liners, but they don't seem to protect my clothes.

CASE 52-1 (continued)

Relevant Evaluation Criteria	Scenario/Model Outcome
2. Gather essential patient history information:	
a. patient's identity	Ms. Smith
b. age, sex, height, and weight	45-year-old female, 5 ft 4 in, 170 lb
c. patient's occupation	Accountant
d. patient's dietary habits	Balanced diet, 4–5 cups coffee/tea per day; social alcohol use
e. patient's sleep habits	No nighttime awakenings
f. concurrent medications and medical conditions	Occasional use of ibuprofen for migraine headaches
g. allergies	NKA
h. history of other adverse reactions to medications	None
i. other (describe) _____	Lives with husband and three children

Assessment and Triage

3. Differentiate patient's signs/symptoms and correctly identify the patient's primary problem(s) (see Table 52-3).	Characteristics of Ms. Smith's urine leakage are consistent with stress incontinence.
4. Identify exclusions for self-treatment (see Figure 52-1).	None. However, Ms. Smith should be encouraged to seek a diagnosis for her UI before relying on incontinence products.
5. Formulate a comprehensive list of therapeutic alternatives for the primary problem to determine if triage to a medical practitioner is required, and share this information with the patient.	Options include:
	(1) Refer Ms. Smith to her PCP/gynecologist for evaluation of stress incontinence.
	(2) Recommend a pad or shield for light urine leakage. Reusable incontinence underwear might also be an option for her active lifestyle.
	(3) Advise Ms. Smith that weight loss may help.
	(4) Suggest pelvic floor–strengthening exercises.
	(5) Suggest avoidance of frequent use of caffeine.
	(6) Take no action.

Plan

6. Select an optimal therapeutic alternative to address the patient's problem, taking into account patient preferences.	See Figure 52-1. Ms. Smith should be referred for medical evaluation of stress incontinence. She should be encouraged to learn pelvic floor muscle exercises and to use pads, shields, or reusable incontinence underwear, as needed, for light urine leakage, because these products would offer more protection than panty liners.
7. Describe the recommended therapeutic approach to the patient.	Once you have seen your primary care provider, a pad or shield may be appropriate for persistent symptoms.
8. Explain to the patient the rationale for selecting the recommended therapeutic approach from the considered therapeutic alternatives.	Medical evaluation is necessary to determine the type of incontinence and the need for prescription medication.

Patient Education

9. When recommending self-care with nonprescription medications, convey accurate information to the patient:	
a. appropriate dose and frequency of administration	Refer to the box Patient Education for Adult Urinary Incontinence and Supplies.
b. maximum number of days the therapy should be employed	Refer to the box Patient Education for Adult Urinary Incontinence and Supplies.
c. product administration procedures	Refer to the box Patient Education for Adult Urinary Incontinence and Supplies.
d. expected time to onset of relief	N/A
e. degree of relief that can be reasonably expected	Refer to the box Patient Education for Adult Urinary Incontinence and Supplies.
f. most common side effects	Skin irritation, rash, maceration, and breakdown

CASE 52-1 (continued)

Relevant Evaluation Criteria	Scenario/Model Outcome
g. side effects that warrant medical intervention should they occur	You should check for skin irritation every 2 hours. Refer to the box Patient Education for Adult Urinary Incontinence and Supplies.
h. patient options in the event that condition worsens or persists	If urine loss is continual, change absorbent undergarments every 2–4 hours. See your primary care provider for further follow-up.
i. product storage requirements	N/A
j. specific nondrug measures	Refer to the box Patient Education for Adult Urinary Incontinence and Supplies for behavioral measures to reduce and improve incontinence symptoms. Pelvic floor exercises may be beneficial in stress incontinence.
10. Solicit follow-up questions from patients.	What if the incontinence product does not provide enough protection?
11. Answer patient's questions.	You may select another absorbent product according to the amount of urine leakage (see Table 52-4).

Key: N/A, not applicable; NKA, no known allergies; PCP, primary care provider.

Patient Counseling for Adult Urinary Incontinence and Supplies

The clinician's role in self-treatment of UI includes educating patients about UI; recommending medical evaluation, as appropriate, on the basis of an initial evaluation of signs and symptoms; assisting patients and caregivers in selecting products to reduce the risk of leakage of urine to outer garments; and avoiding aggravating factors. Patients should be provided with information to help them understand UI. The box Patient Education for Adult Urinary Incontinence and Supplies lists specific information to provide patients regarding the use of incontinence supplies. An excellent resource for patient education is the Simon Foundation for Continence, PO Box 815, Wilmette, IL 60091; 1-800-23Simon; or www.simon foundation.org.

PATIENT EDUCATION FOR
Adult Urinary Incontinence and Supplies

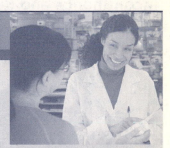

The objectives of self-treatment are to (1) reduce or eliminate symptoms of urinary incontinence (UI), (2) control or treat skin irritation caused by contact with urine, (3) control the odor of urine leaked from the bladder, (4) control leakage of urine to outer garments, and (5) prevent other complications such as falls and social isolation. For most patients, carefully following product instructions and the self-care measures listed here will help to ensure optimal therapeutic outcomes.

■ Consult a primary care provider for a thorough examination before resorting to permanent use of absorbent undergarments or shields. Many cases of UI are reversible with treatment.

■ These products are designed to absorb urine; to provide a moisture barrier to protect clothes, bedding, and furniture; and to minimize skin contact with urine.

■ Base selection of absorbent products on the amount of leaked urine:
—Guards/shields: 2–12 ounces (60–360 mL), light-to-heavy capacity
—Undergarments: 12–18 ounces (360–540 mL), moderate-to-heavy capacity
—Briefs: 28–36 ounces (840–1000 mL), moderate-to-heavy capacity

■ Choose briefs or diapers with roll-on bed application and adhesive closures for patients who are unable to change themselves.

■ If additional protection is needed during sleeping and sitting, select absorbent bed or chair pads to use with absorbent undergarments.

■ Check skin for irritation or maceration every 2 hours, even when absorbent garments are used.

■ If urine loss is continual, change absorbent undergarments every 2–4 hours, and consult your primary care provider if UI symptoms worsen.

■ If desired, use skin protectants labeled for diaper rash to protect the patient's skin.

■ If desired, use products containing chlorophyll, such as Derifil, Pals, and Nullo, to help decrease odor. However, continue frequent skin checks and frequent changes of absorbent undergarments.

■ If pressure ulcers (open sores) occur in an immobile patient, consult a primary care provider. Do not attempt to treat the ulcers with nonprescription products.

■ Identify and eliminate foods, liquids, or other substances that can irritate the bladder (e.g., coffee, tea, soda, alcohol, chocolate, acidic juices, tomato-based sauces, spicy food, artificial sweeteners, and nicotine).

■ Avoid excessive intake of liquid. Drink enough to produce about a cup of urine every 3–4 waking hours on average.

■ Avoid products that irritate the urethra and bladder. Use cotton underwear, avoid scented powders or bath products, and use white toilet paper.

■ Follow instructions for behavioral therapy and medications for incontinence if prescribed by your primary care provider.

Evaluation of Patient Outcomes for Adult Urinary Incontinence and Supplies

At follow-up, the clinician should find out whether the recommended incontinence product is comfortable and easy to use, and whether leakage from the undergarment or odor is a problem. If leakage is occurring, the absorbency and/or type of product should be reassessed. Patients who have problems with odor may need to use deodorizers. The patient or caregiver should also be asked whether the skin, especially in the perivaginal and perianal areas, is being checked for breakdown. Redness or skin fissures call for the use of skin protectants. Questioning about occurrence of urinary tract or vaginal infections is also appropriate. Such infections may indicate a need to change undergarments more often or to use another type of incontinence product. These measures will prevent prolonged skin contact with urine. In addition, the practitioner should monitor the effectiveness of other prescription medication and behavioral therapies for UI. The patient should be asked about side effects associated with the specific medication he or she may be prescribed.

Practitioners should also evaluate whether the use of incontinence products and other treatments has allowed the patient to resume his or her normal lifestyle and social interactions. If these objectives are not being met after an adequate duration of any pharmacotherapy, the medication dose and type of should be reviewed. Alternative absorbent products should also be considered. The patient should be encouraged to seek further advice from his or her primary care provider on treatment options.

Key Points for Adult Urinary Incontinence and Supplies

➤ UI is a common treatable condition that is often cured or improved with therapy.

➤ Because the cause of UI may be multifactorial, the patient should receive a comprehensive medical evaluation before planning therapy.

➤ A variety of treatment options are available, including drug therapy, behavioral therapies, devices, incontinence aids, and surgery.

➤ Incontinence aids are designed to absorb urine; to provide a moisture barrier to protect clothes, bedding, and furniture; and to minimize skin contact with urine.

➤ The selection of absorbent products is based on the amount of urine leakage.

➤ Practitioners can play an important role in educating patients about UI, performing assessment and triage to medical evaluation, counseling on the selection and appropriate use of prescription and nonprescription incontinence products and the avoidance of aggravating factors, and monitoring patient response.

REFERENCES

1. Sand PK, Dmochowski R. Analysis of the standardisation of terminology of lower urinary tract dysfunction: report from the standardisation sub-committee of the international continence society. *Neurourol Urodynam.* 2002;21:167–78.

2. Fantl AJ, Newman DK, Lolling L, et al. *Urinary Incontinence in Adults: Acute and Chronic Management, Clinical Practice Guideline.* Rockville, Md: US Department of Health and Human Services, Public Health Service, Agency for Health Care Policy and Research; 1996. Publication No. 96–0682.

3. Hu T-W, Wagner TH, Bentkover JD, et al. Costs of urinary incontinence in the United States: a comparative study. *Urology.* 2004;63:461–5.

4. Brandeis GH, Baumann MM, Hossain M, et al. The prevalence of potentially remediable urinary incontinence in frail older people: a study using the Minimum Data Set. *J Am Geriatr Soc.* 1997;45:179–84.

5. Roberts RO, Jacobsen SJ, Rhodes T, et al. Urinary incontinence in a community-based cohort: prevalence and health care-seeking. *J Am Geriatr Soc.* 1998;46:467–72.

6. Thom D. Variation in estimates of urinary incontinence prevalence in the community: effects of differences in definition, population characteristics, and study type. *J Am Geriatr Soc.* 1998;46:473–80.

7. Burgio KL, Ives DG, Locher JL, et al. Treatment seeking for urinary incontinence in adults. *J Am Geriatr Soc.* 1994;42:208–12.

8. Lee SY, Phanumus D, Fields SD. Urinary incontinence: a primary care guide to managing acute and chronic symptoms in older adults. *Geriatrics.* 2000;55:65–72.

9. de Groat WC, Yoshimura N. Pharmacology of the lower urinary tract. *Annu Rev Pharmacol Toxicol.* 2001;41:691–721.

10. Busby-Whitehead J, Johnson TM. Urinary incontinence. *Clin Geriatr Med.* 1998;14:285–96.

11. Couture JA, Valiquette L. Urinary incontinence. *Ann Pharmacother.* 2000; 34:646–55.

12. Holroyd-Leduc JM, Strauss SE. Management of urinary incontinence in women. *JAMA.* 2004;291:986–95.

13. Grodstein F, Fretts R, Lifford K, et al. Association of age, race, and obstetric history with urinary symptoms among women in the Nurses' Health Study. *Am J Obstet Gynecol.* 2003;189:428–34.

14. Sampselle CM, Harlow SD, Skurnick J, et al. Urinary incontinence predictors and life impact in ethnically diverse perimenopausal women. *Obstet Gynecol.* 2002;100:1230–8.

15. Staskin DR. Overactive bladder in the elderly: a guide to pharmacological management. *Drugs Aging.* 2005;22:1013–28.

16. Shaikh S, Ong EK, Glavind K, et al. Mechanical devices for urinary incontinence in women. *Cochrane Database Syst Rev.* 2006;3:CD001756.

17. DeLancey JO, Miller JM, Kearney R, et al. Vaginal birth and de novo stress incontinence: relative contributions of urethral dysfunction and mobility. *Obstet Gynecol.* 2007;110(2 pt 1):354–62.

18. Culligan PJ, Heit M. Urinary incontinence in women: evaluation and management. *Am Fam Physician.* 2000;62:2433–44.

19. Jackson S. The patient with an overactive bladder: symptoms and quality of life issues. *Urology.* 1997;50(suppl 6A):18–22.

20. Shamilyan TA, Kane, RL, Wyman J, et al. Systematic review: randomized, controlled trials of nonsurgical treatments for urinary incontinence in women. *Ann Intern Med.* 2008;148:459–73.

21. Diokno AC, Samselle CM, Herzog AR, et al. Prevention of urinary incontinence by behavioral modification program: a randomized, controlled trial among older women in the community. *J Urol.* 2004;171:1165–71.

22. Miller J, Sampselle C, Ashton-Miller J, et al. Clarification and confirmation of the Knack maneuver: the effect of volitional pelvic floor muscle contraction to preempt urine expected stress incontinence. *Int Urogynecol J.* 2008;19:773–82.

23. Culligan PJ, Neit M. Information from your family doctor: exercising your pelvic muscles. *Am Fam Physician.* 2000;62:2447.

24. NeoControl® Pelvic Floor Therapy System. Available at: http://www.neocontrol.com. Last accessed September 25, 2008.

25. Norton PA, Baker JE. Postural changes reduce leakage in women with stress urinary incontinence. *Obstet Gynecol.* 1994;84:770–4.

26. Smith PP, McCrery RJ, Appell RA. Current trends in the evaluation and management of female urinary incontinence. *CMAJ.* 2006;175:1233–40.

27. Moehrer B, Hextall A, Jackson S. Oestrogens for urinary incontinence in women. *Cochrane Database Syst Rev.* 2003;2:CD001405.

28. The North American Menopause Society. The role of local vaginal estrogen for treatment of vaginal atrophy: 2007 position statement of the North American Menopause Society. *Menopause.* 2007;14:357–69.

29. McCormick PL, Keating GM. Duloxetine: in stress urinary incontinence. *Drugs.* 2004;64:2567–73.

30. National Association for Continence. Resource Guide® Products and Services for Incontinence. Available at: http://www.nafc.org/online-store/consumer-publications-and-products/nafc-educational-booklets/

resource-guide-products-and-services-for-incontinence. Last accessed September 25, 2008.

31. Gallo M, Staskin DR. Patient satisfaction with a reusable undergarments for urinary incontinence. *J Wound Ostomy Continence Nurs*. 1997;24:226–36.

32. Fader M, Cottenden A, Getliffe K, et al. Absorbent products for urinary/faecal incontinence: a comparative evaluation of key product designs. *Health Technol Assess*. 2008; 12(29):1–208.

33. Newman DK. Bladder dysfunction in women. Products and devices play important role. *Adv Nurse Pract*. 2006;14:55–6, 58, 60–2.

34. Brink CA. Absorbent pads, garment, and management strategies. *J Am Geriatr Soc*. 1990;38:368–73.

35. Fader M, Cottenden AM, Getliffe K. Absorbent products for light urinary incontinence in women. *Cochrane Database Syst Rev*. 2007;2: CD001406.

36. Fader M, Macaulay M, Pettersson L, et al. A multi-centre evaluation of absorbent products for men with light urinary incontinence. *Neurourol Urodyn*. 2006;25:689–95.

37. Bottomley JM. Complementary nutrition in treating urinary incontinence. *Top Geriatr Rehab*. 2000;16:61–77.

38. Rana S, D'Amico F, Merenstein JH. Relationship of vitamin B12 deficiency with incontinence in older people. *J Am Geriatr Soc*. 1998;46:931–2.

39. Wilt TJ, Ishani A, Stark, G, et al. Saw palmetto extracts for treatment of benign prostatic hyperplasia: a systematic review. *JAMA*. 1998;280:1604–9.

40. Boyle R, Robertson C, Lowe F, et al. Updated meta-analysis of clinical trials of *Serenoa repens* extract in the treatment of symptomatic benign prostatic hyperplasia. *BJU Int*. 2004;93:751–6.

41. McQueen CE, Bryant PJ. Pygeum. *Am J Health Syst Pharm*. 2001;58:120–3.

42. Andro M-C, Riffaud J-P. *Pygeum africanum* extract for the treatment of patients with benign prostatic hyperplasia: a review of 25 years of published experience. *Curr Ther Res*. 1995;56:796–817.

43. Gordon AE, Shaughnessy AF. Saw palmetto for prostate disorders. *Am Fam Physician*. 2003;67:1281–3.

44. Dvorkin L, Song KY. Herbs for benign prostatic hyperplasia. *Ann Pharmacother*. 2002;36:1443–52.

45. Wilt TJ, Ishani A, Rutks I, et al. Phytotherapy for benign prostatic hyperplasia. *Public Health Nutr*. 2000;3(4A):459–72.

46. Bent S, Kane C, Shinohara K, et al. Saw palmetto for benign prostatic hyperplasia. *N Engl J Med*. 2006;354:557–66.

Complementary and Alternative Medicine

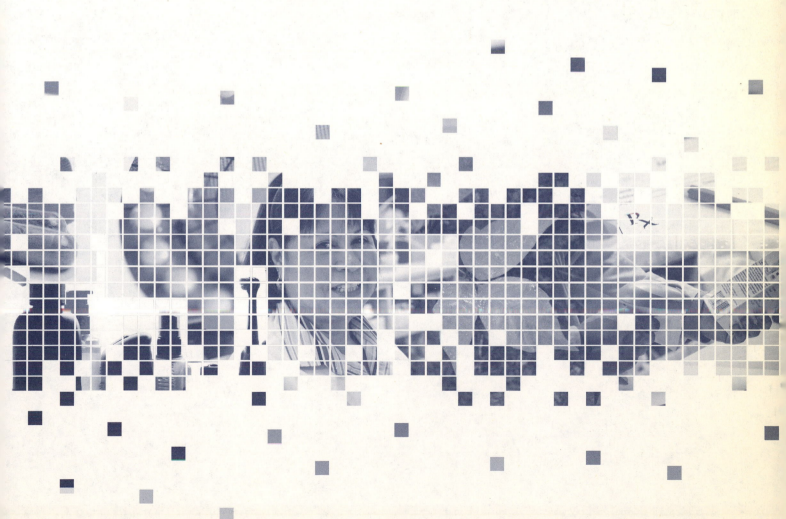

Introduction to Dietary Supplements

Candy Tsourounis and Cathi Dennehy

Since 1994, the use of complementary and alternative medicine (CAM) in the United States has increased substantially.[1] The National Institutes of Health categorizes CAM as (1) whole medical systems such as traditional Chinese medicine and Ayurveda; (2) mind–body medicine such as meditation and prayer; (3) biologically based practices such as herbs, vitamins, and foods; (4) manipulative and body-based practices such as massage, chiropractic, and osteopathic care; and (5) energy medicine such as therapeutic touch, qi gong, and magnetic fields.[2] The most commonly used form of CAM includes the use of herbs, vitamins, and other related dietary supplements.[1]

Many terms have been used to describe these types of products, including nutraceuticals, natural products, dietary supplements, herbs, botanicals, and phytochemicals. The Food and Drug Administration (FDA) defines dietary supplements (DS) as vitamins, minerals, herbs or other botanicals, amino acids; or dietary substances used to supplement the diet by increasing dietary intake or concentrates, metabolites, constituents, extracts; or any combination of these stated ingredients.[3] For the purposes of this chapter, herbs, vitamins, and similar products will be referred to as DS. This designation is also used by FDA as it relates to the intended use, namely to supplement the diet. Indeed, DS today are not only used to supplement the diet, but also to treat various symptoms and medical conditions by consumers.

Use of Dietary Supplements

Prevalence and Patterns of Use

Recent trends indicate that DS use has increased more than use of other CAM modalities.[1] Sales of DS have also increased from $8.8 billion in 1994 to $18.8 in 2003.[1] According to one national survey, nearly one in five U.S. adults reports using an herb to treat a health condition or for health promotion.[4] Other popular reasons for DS use include the treatment of a head or chest cold, musculoskeletal conditions, and stomach or intestinal illnesses.[4]

Top Selling Dietary Supplements

Dietary supplements are just one category of CAM-based therapies and should be assessed separately when considering use of CAM and sales of CAM-based products. Although DS sales as a whole may be on the rise, use of a particular group of DS may actually be on the decline. For example, among all DS, multi-

vitamins are the top selling supplements, primarily because they are used across all life stages. Glucosamine with or without chondroitin is the top selling non-vitamin, non-mineral DS and exceeded sales of any individual herb in 2006.[5] Surprisingly, single-ingredient herbal preparations have been declining in sales since 2006.[5] Garlic, saw palmetto, echinacea, *Ginkgo biloba*, St. John's wort, black cohosh, evening primrose, red clover, and dong quai root have experienced a loss of sales growth in the United States between 6% to 20% in 2006 compared with 2005.[5] Reasons for the decline may be due to negative studies published in the literature and discussed in the popular media, problems with DS purity, or the increased marketing of proprietary blends that include more than one ingredient.

The 2002 National Health Interview Survey (NHIS), a survey of more than 30,000 Americans, is the most current and comprehensive data available on the use of non-vitamin, non-mineral DS. Approximately one in five persons used a non-vitamin, non-mineral supplement, with the most prevalent being echinacea (38.4%), ginseng (23%), ginkgo (20.1%), garlic (18.6%), and glucosamine (13.7%).[6] From this example, it is clear that reported DS use does not always correspond to trends in sales.

Attitudes and Predictors of Use

Many studies have measured predictors for DS use in diverse populations including older adults, women, and adolescents.[1,4,6–8] For most American adults, common predictors for DS use include being female, being well educated, living in the West, being uninsured, and having higher socioeconomic status and chronic medical conditions.[4,7,8] Among older adults, DS use has doubled since 1998.[9] Older adults are more likely to use non-vitamin, non-mineral DS if they live in California, have greater difficulties with muscle strength, and read health or fitness magazines.[10] The most common reasons stated among older adults for taking a DS were to improve general wellness, manage arthritis, prevent or manage colds, or improve memory.[7] Individuals who cited "general wellness" as their rationale for use were 16 times more likely to consume DS. Other factors that appeared to be highly predictive of DS use include having an attitude that the DS will work and having a history of receiving health care from CAM practitioners. Consistent with other studies, consumers who indicated that they do not use prescription or nonprescription medications were unlikely to take DS.[7] These findings suggest that the preservation of health, regardless of an individual's assessment of his or her own health status, medical history, or concomitant medications, was the most important predictor of use.[7] Television was the most commonly reported source of DS information (73%), followed by magazines and radio (both 30%), newspapers (13%), friends (8%), and store displays (5%).[7] Consistent across all surveys, users of DS tend not to report using DS to their health care providers. For example, in 1993, nondisclosure of DS use was estimated at 70% compared with 1998 when 40% of consumers did not disclose DS use to their providers.[11] The 2002 NHIS again reported nondisclosure of DS use at 69%.[6] Consumers were more likely to disclose use of the DS if they were seeking care for a different problem. Interestingly, only 30% of consumers report using DS when asked as part of a periodic health review, and 61% disclosed use in a direct provider interview but only if asked specifically regarding use.[11] Reasons for nondisclosure are varied but have included an impression of disinterest by the provider, anticipation of a negative response, and a perception that their physician is unable or unwilling to contribute helpful information.[12] Other reasons include the perception that CAM therapies are irrelevant to medical care and that the coordination of care is a personal choice.

Legislation and Regulatory Issues

Dietary Supplement Health and Education Act

In 1994, the Dietary Supplement Health and Education Act (DSHEA) was approved by Congress and signed into law.[3] This act allowed DS to be regulated by FDA under the purview of the Center for Food Safety and Applied Nutrition (CFSAN). As a result, DS were excluded from the strict purity and potency standards that are applied to prescription and nonprescription medicines through the Center for Drug Evaluation Research. In this way, DS simply had to meet the standards that applied to food preparation. Any additional standards regarding purity and potency were the sole responsibility of the manufacturer. Many DS were identified to have significant variability in content, purity, potency, consistency, and actual identity. As a result, reports of contamination, herb misidentification, and sub- and supratherapeutic effects have been reported in the literature.[13] The lack of strict standards and limited oversight of the manufacturing process created a "buyer beware" market, placing the consumer at risk and often alienating many allopathic or conventional health care practitioners to the use of CAM therapies.

Another major difference between DS and prescription or nonprescription medicines is the level of evidence required to demonstrate safety and efficacy. For prescription and nonprescription drugs, clinical trials are required to demonstrate evidence of the drug's safety and efficacy prior to marketing. For DS, clinical trials are not required to prove safety and efficacy prior to marketing, although the manufacturer is prohibited from marketing unsafe or ineffective products. In this way, the burden of proof is shifted to FDA, which has to prove that the DS is not safe to restrict its use or remove it from the market.

Ingredients that were sold in the United States prior to October 15, 1994, are not required to be reviewed for safety by FDA before being marketed, because they are assumed to be safe on the basis of a history of use in humans. For any new DS ingredient that was not on the market prior to October 15, 1994, a manufacturer must notify FDA of the intent to market the product 75 days in advance and also provide FDA with evidence that the DS is safe in humans when used as directed.[3] Unfortunately, there is no comprehensive list that indicates which DS ingredients were sold prior to October 15, 1994, so the decision as to whether a product contains a new ingredient is left up to the manufacturer. Finally, no explicit criterion details what a manufacturer must submit to FDA to conclude that the product poses no significant or unreasonable risk of illness or injury when used as directed.

Good Manufacturing Practice

When DSHEA was enacted, it required the establishment of Good Manufacturing Practice (GMP) standards for the DS industry. In 2007, FDA issued a final rule on proposed changes to GMP standards for DS.[14] The proposed changes came after significant pressure from stakeholders and consumers to improve product quality. Among the various changes, DS must be manufactured in a quality manner without adulterants or impurities and must be labeled accurately. These changes will help to better regulate manufacturing practices, especially as they relate to setting limits on the presence of bacteria, pesticides, and heavy metals. To allow manufacturers time to comply, a long phase-in period has been developed. Larger supplement manufacturers are required to comply by June 2008 and smaller manufacturers by 2009 or later. In response, manufacturers have expressed concern regarding the cost of these changes, which could increase the purchase price for DS products.

Labeling

The Federal Trade Commission (FTC) and FDA work together in the enforcement of DS regulations.[15] FDA has primary responsibility for regulating claims found on packaging, package labeling, inserts, and other promotional materials that are distributed at the point of sale. FTC has primary responsibility for advertising claims made through print and broadcast advertisements, infomercials, catalogs, and other direct marketing materials.[15] FTC requires DS claims of safety and efficacy to be supported by "competent and reliable scientific evidence." This evidence is defined as "tests, analyses, research, studies or other evidence based on the expertise of professionals in the relevant area that have been conducted and evaluated in an objective manner by qualified individuals, using procedures generally accepted to yield accurate and reliable results." Complaints against DS advertising may be filed with FTC online (www.ftccomplaintassistant.gov).

All DS marketed in the United States are required to meet supplement labeling requirements.[16] The labels must list (1) the name of the product as well as the word *supplement;* (2) the net quantity of contents; (3) the manufacturer's, packer's, or distributor's name and place of business; and (4) directions for use. In addition, each label must also contain a supplement facts panel that describes the serving size, the list of dietary ingredients, amount per serving size, and the percent daily value if one is established (see Chapter 4, Figure 4–5, and vm.cfsan.fda.gov/~acrobat/fdsuppla.pdf). Plant-based DS should indicate the scientific name of the plant containing the Latin binomial, as well as the specific plant part used. Manufacturers may market a combination of DS ingredients as a proprietary blend. Although the individual ingredients in the proprietary blend are listed, the actual quantity of each ingredient is not disclosed. Under DSHEA, the total weight of the blend and the components of the blend, in order of predominance by weight, are required. Fillers, artificial colors, sweeteners, flavors, or binders should also be listed in descending order of predominance. Consistent with the trend in formulating proprietary blends, many multivitamin products are being combined with DS.[9]

When a DS does not follow the labeling requirements, the product is considered misbranded. DS manufacturers are not allowed to make claims that their product will diagnose, cure, mitigate, treat, or prevent disease. These claims would require the product to adhere to the regulations related to a drug and would be subject to all the regulatory processes necessary to demonstrate safety and efficacy. Other examples of misbranding include DS that do not conform to labeling requirements; fail to contain the name or place of business of the manufacturer, packer, or distributor; or fail to include accurate statements regarding the quantity of the contents.

All DS products fall under one of three types of product claims: (1) health claim, (2) nutrient content claim, or (3) structure-function claim.[17] Both health claims and nutrient content claims require FDA approval, whereas structure-function claims do not. A manufacturer must notify FDA of the exact wording of any structure-function claim within 30 days after the product is marketed. Product labels that contain these claims must also carry the disclaimer: "This statement has not been evaluated by the FDA. This product is not intended to diagnose, treat, cure or prevent disease."

Health claims describe the relationship between a food, food component, or DS ingredient, and the resulting reduction in risk of a disease or health-related condition. Claiming that a diet low in saturated fat and cholesterol that includes 25 grams of soy protein daily may reduce the risk of heart disease is an example of an approved health claim. Nutrient content claims describe the relative amount of a nutrient or dietary substance in a product. For example, "very low sodium" means the product is required to have 35 mg or less per reference amount. Lastly, a structure-function claim describes how a product may maintain the normal healthy structure or function of the body without discussing a specific disease state. Accordingly, a supplement manufacturer may claim that the product "supports healthy cholesterol levels" but is prohibited from indicating that the supplement may "reduce high cholesterol levels."

Dietary Supplement and Nonprescription Drug Consumer Protection Act

One of the most important changes to the supplement industry involves the Dietary Supplement and Non-Prescription Drug Consumer Protection Act (Public Law 109-462), which was signed into law on December 22, 2006.[18] This law requires manufacturers, packers, or distributors of DS to submit to FDA serious adverse event reports that are based on specific information received from the public. Serious adverse events are defined as death, a life-threatening situation, an inpatient hospitalization, a persistent or significant disability or incapacity, a congenital anomaly or birth defect, or an adverse event that, on the basis of reasonable medical judgment, requires medical or surgical intervention to prevent such serious outcomes. Increased reporting of adverse events may better characterize the frequency and type of serious adverse events associated with DS. More importantly, FDA may be alerted to trends in serious adverse events so that appropriate corrective action may be taken. Consumers and health care providers are also encouraged to report DS-related adverse events through FDA's MedWatch program (www.fda.gov/medwatch).[19]

Production Issues

Plant Species and Parts

When the average consumer enters a pharmacy and is searching for an echinacea product, they may encounter products that contain *Echinacea pallida*, *Echinacea purpurea*, and *Echinacea angustifolia* as single-ingredient products; products that contain a mixture of two or all of these species; and products that contain echinacea as one of many listed supplement ingredients. In the case of echinacea, single-ingredient products involving the above-ground parts of *E. purpurea*, formulated as an alcohol extract of the fresh pressed juice, have been the most widely studied; according to a recent meta-analysis the above-ground parts of *E. purpurea* demonstrate some evidence of efficacy in reducing cold incidence and duration with natural virus exposure, when administered at the first sign of symptoms in adults.[20] The other two species of echinacea have been less well studied and have not demonstrated consistent benefits in clinical trials.[20,21] A pharmacist should explain that herbal products typically carry two names, the common name and the Latin binomial name (i.e., genus and species). An example would be a product such as St. John's wort (common name), which is also known as *Hypericum perforatum* (Latin genus and species name).[14] Some product labels may list only the Latin name, which can be confusing to a consumer who is unfamiliar with this terminology.

Common Product Formulations

The content of any DS is based on the raw starting material and how the material is subsequently processed or formulated. Plant-based DS such as echinacea and ginseng have greater variability in product composition than single-ingredient DS such as creatine and melatonin. This variability is due to the chemical composition of botanical DS, which is influenced by the plant's growing conditions, the plant species, and the specific plant part used.

Knowing which plant species is preferred or which part of the plant to use can be based on historical precedent when clinical trial data are lacking. In developing countries, plant-based medicine is common, and information regarding preferred plant species, preferred plant part, and proper use is handed down from generation to generation, setting a historical precedent for use. The World Health Organization estimates that approximately 25% of modern medications are plant-derived.[22] In developing countries, such as Africa, the use of plants as medicines is as high as 80%.[22] Use of herbs based on historical precedent is also seen in the practice of midwifery.[23,24] Few clinical trials exist on the use of DS in pregnant women, lactating women, and children. The decision to use DS on the basis of historical precedent is something individual practitioners must discuss with their patients.[23,24]

Method of Preparation

The method in which a DS is manufactured will ultimately affect its final chemical composition and potential efficacy. Some formulations may be well studied, whereas others may not have been studied at all. The most common herbal formulations that a consumer will encounter are either made directly from the fresh plant (e.g., expressed juice, tincture, or tea) or the dried plant (e.g. fluid extract/tincture; evaporated extract [capsules, tablets]; or tea).[25] Most of the common non–plant-based DS such as vitamins, minerals, glucosamine, creatine, coenzyme Q10, melatonin, and S-adenosyl-methionine are manufactured as tablets or capsules; they represent compounds that are structurally similar to or identical to compounds naturally found in the human body.

Freshly pressed juice formulations are prepared by pressing the herb and collecting the liquid that is removed.[25] This type of preparation often takes a large amount of the herb to create a substantial portion of juice. In the case of *E. purpurea,* the most well-studied formulation is an alcohol extract of the expressed freshly pressed juice.[20] One potential advantage of the alcohol extract is that the presence of alcohol increases the product's shelf life.[26]

Tea formulations are prepared from steeping or boiling the fresh or dried leaf portions of one or more plant species in hot water.[26] This process releases the "water-soluble" constituents into the tea. The potency is determined by the steeping time or the time spent boiling and evaporating the mixture, as well as the amount of herb used. The term *decoction* may also be used when referring to the simmering of the bark root or berries of a plant for the purposes of making a tea.[26] Common single-herb tea formulations include chamomile, ginger, peppermint, green tea, and black tea. Multi-ingredient blends that are customized to a specific person's ailment are commonly used in traditional Chinese medicine and may also be administered as teas.

Extracts are intended to concentrate the effects of an herb and can be prepared by soaking fresh or dried plant parts in alcohol, water, alcohol/water mixtures, or oil.[25] The extraction liquid is then reserved and the plant material discarded. Tinctures are fluid extracts in which alcohol is typically used as the extraction medium.[25] The chemicals that seep into the extraction liquid are specific to the solution used. If the extracted liquid is evaporated and dried, it can be formulated into pills or capsules.[25] Extracts and tinctures may list the extraction ratio on the package label. For example, a 5:1 ratio would indicate that 5 parts of herb were used to prepare 1 part of the extract.[26] *Ginkgo biloba* is prepared as a dried extract in tablet form. Ginkgo is typically standardized to a 50:1 extract ratio, meaning that 50 parts of the ginkgo leaf were used to prepare 1 part of the extract.[26] Garlic is available in multiple formulations, the most popular being a dried powdered extract in tablet or capsule form and an aged garlic extract.[26] The chemical composition of the powdered extract will differ from that of the aged extract because of the differences in method of preparation. This variance in composition, in turn, will influence the pharmacology and efficacy of each product.

Standardization

The process of standardization is primarily reserved for plant-based DS, because herbs contain many active and inactive constituents. For specific DS, standardization involves identifying specific chemicals or "markers" that are thought to possess therapeutic activity, isolating them, and then formulating them into a final and consistent product. Standardization can occur, however, only if the chemical markers that contribute to the pharmacologic effect have been identified. For example, a *Ginkgo biloba* product may indicate that it is standardized to contain 6% terpene lactones and 24% flavonoid glycosides, whereas a chasteberry product may not list any standardized markers at all. Sometimes, the identified active chemical markers change over time as new pharmacologic research is performed. Such a change occurred with St. John's wort in which the active antidepressant marker was initially thought to be hypericin but is now thought to be hyperforin. Bottles of St. John's wort may list one or both of these standardizations on the package label. Interestingly, no legal or regulatory definition is accepted as it relates to standardization of DS. Claiming that a product is standardized does not necessarily mean a uniform manufacturing process was used.

Common Quality Control Issues

Adulteration

According to DSHEA, adulteration of a dietary supplement occurs when it (1) presents a significant or unreasonable risk of illness or injury when used in accordance with the suggested labeling, (2) is a new entity and lacks adequate evidence to ensure its safety of use, (3) has been declared an imminent hazard by the Secretary of the Department of Health and Human Services, or (4) contains a dietary ingredient that is present in sufficient quantity to render the product poisonous or deleterious to human health, as described for adulterated foods in the Food, Drug, and Cosmetic Act.[3] Adulteration of DS has occurred both intentionally and unintentionally. Examples of unintentional adulterants include heavy metals introduced at the time of cultivation or during the manufacturing process.[27] Intentional adulteration can occur when a manufacturer substitutes a different DS for an ingredient that is in short supply or is too expensive. It can also occur when a prescription drug is added to the product to enhance the pharmacologic effect. Examples of intentional adulteration with prescription drugs have occurred with Chinese patent medicines.[27] The new GMP standards for DS may help to address this issue.

Quality Assurance Programs

Several organizations have developed programs to assess analytical reference standards and to certify DS composition. These programs indicate when the DS product contents match the label contents; unfortunately assurances cannot be made regarding DS safety or efficacy. These programs also do not address product quality between different batches or lots, because they test only a single batch at any one time.

United States Pharmacopoeia Dietary Supplement Verification Program

In 2002, the U.S. Pharmacopoeia (USP) initiated a voluntary Dietary Supplement Verification Program.[28] The purpose of the program is to provide consumers with a method for identifying DS that have passed rigorous standards for purity, accuracy of ingredient labeling, and GMP. Products earning USP certification carry a distinctive seal of approval on the product label. These products are certified to contain the listed ingredients in the indicated amounts, to be bioavailable, to be free of contaminants, and to have been manufactured under appropriate conditions. As of 2008, nine DS manufacturers are regular program participants. USP will periodically conduct audits of certified products to ensure continuing adherence to quality standards. Approved products can be found at the USP Web site (www.usp.org/USPVerified/dietarySupplements/supplements.html).

ConsumerLab.com

ConsumerLab.com, LLC, is an independent company that tests products relating to health, wellness, and nutrition such as dietary supplements.[29] Products are tested on the basis of identity, purity,

TABLE 53-1	Characteristics of Supplements Making Fraudulent or Misleading Claims

- List specific disease states or allude to the product's use for a disease normally treated with prescription drug therapy
- State efficacy similar to, or can be used as an alternative to, a prescription or nonprescription drug
- List a wide variety of unrelated clinical conditions for use
- State only benefits and no harms
- Neglect to provide expiration date, lot number, and contact information for the manufacturer on the package label
- Use pseudo-medical terminology such as "detoxify," "purify," or "improves body chemistry"
- Use terms such as "miraculous discovery," "revolutionary therapy," or "breakthrough treatment," which suggest that the product has superior efficacy to standard medical care
- Suggest that the product is more expensive because it works so well

and consistency to the labeled ingredients. The test results are posted on the Web site (www.consumerlab.com/aboutcl.asp) with new results available every 4 to 6 weeks. Manufacturers whose products pass the review are allowed to license the CL seal of approval for that product. The site provides free access to some names of a few products in each category that have passed testing, whereas names of products that fail testing are available to only subscribers. Currently a yearly subscription costs $29. The company is not affiliated with manufacturers of any DS, health, or nutrition products.

National Sanitation Foundation International

National Sanitation Foundation (NSF) International (www.nsf.org) is an independent, nonprofit organization that provides certifications of DS, as well as of food and water quality.[30] The organization verifies that the product contains the labeled ingredients and that contaminants and unlisted ingredients are not present. A DS product that meets certification standards is allowed to carry the NSF Certification seal of approval on the label.

Hazards from Dietary Supplements

False Advertising/Quackery

Manufacturers who make DS health claims sometimes ignore the regulations established by FDA and FTC, and market products using false or misleading claims. FTC requires all advertising to be truthful, not misleading, and based on sound scientific evidence. The weight-loss DS market is one example in which false or misleading health claims are commonly identified.[31] Historically, this type of practice might be considered "quackery," which implies that the person promoting use of the product knows it to be ineffective and is still promoting its use. In the case of some DS, some manufacturers may believe that their products are effective for a wide variety of ailments with or without strong clinical support. One Web site known as "Quackwatch" (www.quackwatch.com) was created to help consumers spot fraudulent claims.[32] A portion of the Web site deals with claims specific to CAM therapies and DS. Consumers and practitioners should be wary of information found on Internet Web sites that market DS products. These Web sites have been shown to be unreliable and often list disease claims, fail to cite the standard federal disclaimer, and are less likely to provide referenced information compared with non-retail Internet Web sites.[33] One of the best ways for a consumer to identify fraudu-

lent claims is to be wary of products that contain any of the characteristics listed in Table 53-1. In addition, they should consult a reliable drug information resource, as well as their health care provider, to confirm whether the health claims have some basis in science. Consumers and practitioners can also check the FDA Office of Dietary Supplements Web site for new press releases regarding products that have been identified as containing adulterants, such as prescription drugs, or manufacturers that have been issued warnings or recalls for making false or inaccurate claims.[34] FDA has also created supplement categories that should be viewed with scrutiny on the basis of a history of prior violations or problems. These supplement categories are listed in Table 53-2.[35] A consumer or practitioner who wishes to file a complaint related to false advertising should contact FTC.[15]

Hazards Introduced by the Consumer

Exceeding the recommended dietary allowance for a vitamin or mineral supplement or taking more of a supplement than is directed on the label can occur intentionally or accidentally. Accidental over-supplementation is more likely to occur when a consumer is taking more than one multi-ingredient product containing similar ingredients. Regardless of how it occurs, over-supplementation should be discouraged, given that it is more likely to result in an adverse event. Some DS have very

TABLE 53-2	Categories of Supplements That FDA Considers "Clearly Problematic"

- Treatments for life-threatening diseases: (e.g., HIV or cancer)
- Weight-loss products
- Autism treatments
- Treatments for behavioral disorders (e.g., hyperactivity or attention deficit disorder)
- Treatments for mental retardation and Down syndrome
- Colloidal minerals
- Colloidal silver products
- Supplements for smokers
- Supplements for drinkers

Key: HIV, human immunodeficiency virus.
Source: Adapted from reference 4.

serious consequences if overused. For example, the overuse of colloidal silver has led to irreversible blue-gray skin discoloration.[36] Other adverse effects such as zinc supplementation causing copper deficiency and subsequent anemia, leukopenia, and neutropenia may be serious but reversible, and may occur only when large amounts of the product are ingested.[37] As mentioned previously, adverse events should be reported by consumers and health care professionals to MedWatch.[19] In most cases, individual case reports and post-marketing surveillance provide the best means of identifying adverse events and drug interactions. Consumers should be advised to monitor for acute adverse events for up to 2 weeks after initiating a new DS and to continue monitoring for chronic adverse events while using the product.

Product Hazards: Adverse Effects and Drug Interactions

The fact that herbal DS are derived from a natural source does not guarantee safety. Some plants such as poison oak or ivy were never meant to be ingested. Adverse effects are often linked to the basic pharmacology of the supplement, as was noted when products containing ephedra were removed from the market owing to their association with stroke and myocardial infarction.[38] Other DS may be harmful because they contain chemical entities that are toxic when ingested. Pyrrolizidine alkaloids present in comfrey, borage, and life root have been associated with case reports of hepatotoxicity.[39] In cases in which a supplement is suspected of causing an adverse event, product testing is essential to rule out possible plant misidentification; adulteration with prescription or nonprescription drugs; or contamination with heavy metals, microbial contaminants, and pesticides that can occur during production.[40]

Interactions between DS and conventional medications may have either a pharmacodynamic or pharmacokinetic basis. Pharmacodynamic interactions are possible when a supplement's pharmacology is similar to or opposite that of a medication the consumer is taking. For example, St. John's wort and L-tryptophan have both been linked to case reports of serotonin syndrome in persons taking these products with prescription psychotropic medications.[41-43] Because both of these DS increase the levels of circulating serotonin, the resulting effects may be additive with the psychotropic drug. Similar types of additive effects have occurred or could theoretically occur in persons combining central nervous system depressants with DS that have sedative properties, such as kava or valerian, or in persons combining drugs that have antiplatelet or anticoagulant activity with DS that have antiplatelet properties, such as fish oil, flaxseed oil, garlic, ginseng, ginkgo, and ginger.[44] Case reports of a DS opposing the effect of a medication or adversely influencing an existing disease state have been reported infrequently in the literature. Theoretical concerns are cited as a reason to avoid DS that enhance immune system activity such as echinacea in persons with autoimmune disorders or in whom immunosuppressants are required.[45] Finally, some DS may have pharmacokinetic interactions that affect the bioavailability of other medications. St. John's wort induces multiple cytochrome P450 isoenzymes, as well as the p-glycoprotein drug transporter system.[44] It has been reported to induce the metabolism of several drugs including oral contraceptives, indinavir, and cyclosporine.

Communication Issues
Counseling on Dietary Supplements

The primary consideration in counseling consumers regarding DS is to recognize the importance of respecting the person's beliefs and values so that a trusting, nonjudgmental relationship can develop. The person must feel comfortable sharing with the clinician any use of DS. Clinicians must also be able to provide evidence-based recommendations regarding DS when information is available. When such evidence is not available, the risk of adverse effects versus the potential for positive effects must be weighed and the process of decision making clearly explained to consumers. Clinicians should discourage the use of unsafe products and practices. However, health care professionals do not control access to DS, and consumers may choose to use any available DS. In many instances, practitioners may be in the position of educating consumers on DS whose use they have discouraged. These are the situations in which complete counseling on expectations and adverse events is essential. For example, educating a consumer on the early signs of a serious adverse effect will enable the consumer to recognize a problem and discontinue the DS early enough to minimize harm. Consumers should always be advised to seek medical care for serious conditions and should be counseled to tell all health care providers about their use of DS.

Consumers should be instructed to read labels carefully and to ask questions. Pharmacists should be aware of the potential for confusion, as it relates to DS labels and claims, and counsel consumers in such a way to help them avoid confusion. *Thymus* is an example of a term that might be dangerous if misunderstood. On a supplement label, "*Thymus extract*" may refer to an extract of the herbs thyme, Spanish thyme, or wild thyme, products with relatively few adverse events when used in small doses, whereas "thymus extract" may refer to a preparation made from animal thymus gland, a product with considerable quality and safety concerns.

In addition to these broad counseling issues, the following points should be emphasized. First, clinicians should emphasize that most self-care with DS should be for a limited period of time. If a problem persists, the consumer should seek medical care. Second, consumers should not take DS for a condition that also is being treated with a prescription medication without informing their provider. Third, consumers should be informed that FDA does not control the quality of DS as it does with prescription medications. The following points should be used in counseling consumers who wish to use a DS:

- Purchase products that have either a seal of quality on the label, acquired through a program such as United States Pharmacopeia's DSVP or NSF International, or products that meet their content claim as assessed by ConsumerLab.com.
- Purchase from large, reputable companies. These companies have the resources to meet strict manufacturing standards, have a reputation to uphold, and are more likely to follow quality assurance procedures. Companies that also manufacture regulated prescription or nonprescription medications (e.g., Bristol-Meyers-Squibb, American Home Products, drugstore chain store brands) are more likely to have GMPs in place and are more likely to follow these procedures when producing DS.

■ Once a quality DS has been selected, consumers should continue to use the same brand and formulation. Although this approach does not guarantee a lack of potential quality issues, as variability between production lots can occur, it does increase the likelihood of a consistent product and dose. Clinicians working with consumers who have not had positive results might consider a trial of a different brand, if appropriate for the specific symptom, before determining that the supplement is ineffective for that consumer.

Additional recommendations for counseling can be found in Table 53-3.

Considerations for Special Groups

The following sections provide a brief overview of issues regarding the use of DS by different groups of consumers. The lack of data on safety and efficacy in these groups, as well as the current regulatory issues, underscores the need for comprehensive assessment of the consumer's health status and knowledgeable counseling.

Older Adults

Although many older adults are healthy and living independently, other individuals may have a significant burden of disease. Many may have age- and disease–related physiologic declines such as in renal function. Older individuals may be chronically taking multiple prescription and nonprescription medications, making a thorough medication and DS history essential. The potential for drug–food and drug–DS interactions, age-related functional declines, and concomitant diseases should be considered in counseling older adults about DS.

Children

Use of DS by children presents unique challenges. Under the age of 2 years, the child's renal function is less developed than that of an adult. The central nervous system of a child may be uniquely sensitive to many drugs and chemicals. Very little research is available regarding the safe and effective use of DS in children, making evidence-based recommendations difficult. In addition, from a practical perspective, an appropriate dose of a DS product for a child cannot be determined if the content of the product is in question. Finally, DS should have childproof safety closures, given that accidental ingestions may occur in young children.[46]

Pregnant Consumers

The use of DS by a woman who is either planning to become pregnant or who is pregnant presents several dilemmas. Throughout the world, herbal DS have been used to maintain health during pregnancy, prevent miscarriages, and induce labor. In the United States, concern has focused on minimizing fetal exposures to prescription and nonprescription medications, as well as DS. Although many herbs have been used in pregnancy, little data exist on their safety on the developing embryo and fetus. As part of standard preconception care, a woman should be asked about her use of DS, especially if it might affect her nutritional status at the time of conception or her ability to become pregnant. Many Web sites and personnel of health food

---

TABLE 53-3 General Recommendations for Advising Consumers

Appropriate Use
- Read all labels carefully; never take more than the recommended amount.
- Never share DS with others.
- Do not select a product that lacks dosing recommendations on the label.
- Avoid products that do not carry a lot number or expiration date.
- Discard products 1 year from the date of purchase if no other expiration date is present.
- Select products that list the manufacturer's name, address, and telephone number.
- Store products in a dry environment out of direct sunlight and humidity, and away from young children and pets.

Special Groups
- Always seek the advice of a pediatrician before using a DS in children.
- Avoid DS if you are pregnant or nursing, or trying to become pregnant.
- Speak to your health care professional if you are trying to treat a life-threatening condition, such as cancer or HIV.

Adverse Effects
- The term *natural* does not mean safe; be diligent and report any unusual experiences to your doctor and pharmacist.
- Ask your provider before using a DS if you are allergic to plants, weeds, and/or pollen.

Interactions
- If you are taking a prescription medicine, do not take a DS for the same condition.
- When possible, avoid taking multi-ingredient preparations; select single-ingredient products that list the strength per dose.
- Do not take these products with alcohol until you know it is safe to do so, or you are familiar with the effects.
- Check with your health care provider if you are taking "blood thinning" drugs; some DS may interact with the drugs.
- Always inform your health care provider of the products you are taking; keep a list if necessary or bring them with you to your appointment.

Expectations
- Never use these products in place of proper rest and nutrition; eat a balanced diet.
- Do not expect a cure or unrealistic results; these agents are not "cure-alls."
- If it sounds too good to be true, it probably is; use discretion when evaluating claims.
- Keep a diary to track DS effectiveness and side effects.

Key: DS, dietary supplements; HIV, human immunodeficiency virus.

stores willingly offer advice, based on limited evidence, regarding the use of herbs during pregnancy and lactation.[47] The most important issue in use of DS during pregnancy and lactation is simply not knowing the exact content in any given batch or product brand. At the present time, clinicians should advise women to limit their use of DS to those that have reasonable proof of safety and efficacy during pregnancy and lactation.

Renal Disease

Many Americans have chronic renal insufficiency (CRI) or failure attributable to systemic diseases such as diabetes mellitus. CRI presents many challenges to the safe use of many prescription and nonprescription medications. Most commonly, the individual may be unable to eliminate the drug appropriately, potentially resulting in supratherapeutic concentrations. This effect is also true for hepatically metabolized drugs with active, renally eliminated metabolites. When CRI is severe enough to require dialysis, the absorption, distribution, and hepatic metabolism of drugs may also be altered. Although evidence is limited, these concerns are also potentially applicable to DS. In addition, many herbs possess antiplatelet properties that might increase the risk of bleeding in adults with CRI.[44]

Surgery

A detailed preoperative history that includes questions related to DS use should be obtained from all patients undergoing surgery. Supplements that are known to affect sedation or platelet function, or that may possibly affect the metabolism of anesthetic agents should be discontinued 2 weeks prior to the procedure. Other DS that the consumer is taking should also be reviewed by the health care provider to avoid any potential harm to the consumer.

Reliable Information Resources

Cochrane Database

The Cochrane Database is accessible through Medline and offers evidence-based analyses of DS. These reports provide detailed information on trials that were included and excluded from the analysis, and on the methodology used.[48] One advantage of the Cochrane Database is that statements that support or oppose the use of a specific DS are very clearly expressed. A disadvantage is that many practitioners may have difficulty understanding the style and arrangement of the information that support the reasoning for the analyses.

ConsumerLab.com

This site provides access to a Natural Products Encyclopedia. The information in this encyclopedia is evidence-based and well referenced. It is a useful resource for both consumers and health care providers.[29]

Natural Medicines Comprehensive Database

The Natural Medicines Comprehensive Database (NMCD) is produced by Therapeutics Faculty, Inc., which also publishes *The Pharmacist's Letter* and *The Prescriber's Letter*. The database is a comprehensive resource in that both herbal and nonherbal DS

are reviewed. Many combination products are also listed, with lists of ingredients and links to the individual monographs for those ingredients. Each monograph has an accompanying consumer handout in the electronic version. The electronic database includes a drug–supplement interaction checker. Print- and personal digital assistant–based versions are also available, as well as a consumer information version. One potential disadvantage is that occasional monographs cite references from resources other than the primarily literature, particularly as it pertains to side effects.[49]

Natural Standard

Natural Standard is an electronic database, produced by an international research collaboration of health professionals from many disciplines, including those trained in Western- and Asian-based forms of care. Professional level monographs are highly detailed and descriptive of all available evidence. Recommendations are graded to reflect the type and quality of the clinical evidence on which they are based. Currently, the number of products included in Natural Standard is fewer than some other resources, primarily because of the length of time required to prepare such detailed reviews. In addition to reviews of DS, the database also includes monographs on other CAM modalities and a dictionary of terms. Natural Standard also publishes the *Natural Standard Herb and Supplement Handbook,* which provides evidence on 98 key DS.[50]

National Center for Complementary and Alternative Medicine

The National Center for Complementary and Alternative Medicine (NCCAM) is part of the National Institutes of Health and one of the federal government's leading agencies in promoting evidence-based research on CAM therapies. The Web site is useful and provides information on clinical trials, opportunities for research and funding, training opportunities for CAM practitioners, and health information on a variety of CAM modalities. DS monographs are in the health information section and provide concise evidence-based summaries of what the product is used for, how it is used, what the science says, and what the side effects and cautions are. Sources for more information are also provided.[51]

Key Points for Dietary Supplements

➤ DS use is common among consumers, making it essential for all practitioners to be knowledgeable about the most frequently used products. This education should include information about evidenced-based resources and where to report adverse effects, drug interactions, or suspected fraudulent health claims.

➤ Regulation under DSHEA has created a marketplace in which product safety, efficacy, and quality can be uncertain.

➤ Practitioners are in a unique position to counsel consumers on DS and should have an open, nonjudgmental, evidence-based approach.

➤ Obtaining a DS history should be included as part of the overall medication history.

➤ Counseling recommendations should include consideration of overall scientific support, specific patient groups, potential for adverse effects, and potential for interactions with other medications or medical illnesses.

REFERENCES

1. Bardia A, Nisly NL, Zimmerman B, et al. Use of herbs among adults based on evidence-based indications: findings from the National Health Interview survey. *Mayo Clin Proc* 2007;82:561–6.
2. CAMBASICS. What is CAM? October 24, 2007. Available at: http://nccam.nih.gov/health/whatiscam. Last accessed September 26, 2008.
3. US Food and Drug Administration. Dietary Supplement Health and Education Act of 1994. Pub L No. 103-417.103rd Congress. Available at: http://www.fda.gov/opacom/laws/dshea.html. Last accessed September 26, 2008.
4. Gardiner P, Graham R, Legedza AT, et al. Factors associated with herbal therapy use by adults in the United States. *Altern Ther Health Med.* 2007;13:22–9.
5. Top 100 Selling US Supplements Sales & Growth 1999–2006: Chart 14. *Nutrition Business Journal.* Boulder, Colo: Penton Media; 2008.
6. Kennedy J. Herb and Supplement Use in the US Adult Population. *Clin Therapeut* 2005;27:1847–58.
7. Marinac JS, Buchinger CL, Godfrey LA, et al. Herbal products and dietary supplements: a survey of use, attitudes and knowledge among older adults. *J Am Osteopath Assoc.* 2007;107:13–23.
8. Gardiner P, Graham RE, Legedza ATR, et al. Factors associated with dietary supplement use among prescription medication users. *Arch Intern Med.* 2006;166:1968–74.
9. Kelly JP, Kaufman DW, Kelley K, et al. Recent trends in use of herbal and other natural products. *Arch Intern Med.* 2005;165:281–6.
10. Nahin RL, Fitzpatrick AL, Williamson JD, et al. Use of herbal medicine and other dietary supplements in community-dwelling older people: baseline data from the Ginkgo Evaluation of Memory Study. *J Am Geriatr Soc.* 2006;54:1725–35.
11. Eisenberg DM, Davis RB, Ettner SL, et al. Trends in alternative medicine use in the United States, 1990–1997: results of a follow-up national survey. *JAMA.* 1998;280:1569–75.
12. Adler SR, Fosket JR. Disclosing complementary and alternative medicine use in the medical encounter: a qualitative study in women with breast cancer. *J Fam Pract.* 1999;48:453–8.
13. Larimore WL, O'Mathuna DP. Quality assessment programs for dietary supplements. *Ann Pharmacother.* 2003;37:893–8.
14. US Food and Drug Administration. Current good manufacturing practice in manufacturing, packaging, labeling, or holding operations for dietary supplements. Final rule. *Fed Regist.* 2007;72:34958. Available at: http://www.cfsan.fda.gov/~lrd/fr07625a.html. Last accessed September 26, 2008.
15. Federal Trade Commission. Dietary Supplements: An Advertising Guide for Industry. Available at: http://www.ftc.gov/bcp/conline/pubs/buspubs/dietsupp.shtm. Last accessed September 26, 2008.
16. National Institutes of Health, Office of Dietary Supplements. Dietary supplements: background information. Available at: http://dietary-supplements.info.nih.gov/factsheets/dietarysupplements.asp. Last accessed September 26, 2008.
17. US Food and Drug Administration. Claims That Can Be Made for Conventional Foods and Dietary Supplements. Center for Food Safety and Applied Nutrition, Office of Nutritional Products, Labeling and Dietary Supplements, September 2003. Available at: http://www.cfsan.fda.gov/~dms/hclaims.html. Last accessed September 26, 2008.
18. US Food and Drug Administration. Dietary Supplement and Non-Prescription Drug Consumer Protection Act. Pub L No. 109-462. 109th Congress. December 22, 2006. Available at: http://www.fda.gov/cder/regulatory/public_law_109462.pdf. Last accessed September 26, 2008.
19. US Food and Drug Administration. MedWatch. Available at: http://www.fda.gov/medwatch. Last accessed September 26, 2008.
20. Linde K, Barrett B, Wolkart K, et al. Echinacea for preventing and treating the common cold. *Cochrane Database System Rev.* 2006;1:CD000530.
21. Blumenthal M, Goldberg A, Brinckmann J, eds. *Herbal Medicine: Expanded Commission E Monographs.* 1st ed. Newton, Mass: Integrative Medicine Communications; 2000.
22. World Health Organization. Traditional Medicine Fact Sheet. Available at: http://www.who.int/mediacentre/factsheets/fs134/en. Last accessed September 26, 2008.
23. McFarlin BL, Gibson MH, O'Rear J, Harman P. A national survey of herbal preparation use by nurse-midwives for labor stimulation. *J Nurse Midwifery.* 1999;44:205–16.
24. Allaire AD, Moos MK, Wells SR. Complementary and alternative medicine in pregnancy: a survey of North Carolina Certified Nurse-Midwives. *Obstet Gynecol.* 2000;95:19–23.
25. Schulz V, Hansel R, Blumenthal M, eds. *Rationale Phytotherapy: A Reference Guide for Physician's and Pharmacists.* 2nd ed. Berlin Heidelberg: Springer-Verlag; 2004.
26. Rotblatt M, Ziment I, eds. *Evidence-Based Herbal Medicine.* Philadelphia: Hanley and Belfus; 2002.
27. Cole MR, Fetrow CW. Adulteration of dietary supplements. *Am J Health Syst Pharm.* 2003;60:1576–80.
28. USP's Dietary Supplement Verification Program Overview. Available at: htpp://www.usp.org/USPVerified. Last accessed September 26, 2008.
29. Consumer.Lab.com. 2008. Available at: http://www.consumerlab.com/aboutcl.asp. Last accessed September 26, 2008.
30. NSF International. NSF Consumer Information: The Importance of Dietary Supplement Certification. Available at: http://www.nsf.org/consumer. Last accessed September 26, 2008.
31. FTC cracks down on false dietary supplement ads. *Am J Health Syst Pharm.* 2001;58:1382, 1384.
32. Quackwatch: Your Guide to Quackery, Health Fraud and Intelligent Decisions. [Operated by Barrett Stephen, MD.] Available at: http://www.quackwatch.org. Last accessed September 26, 2008.
33. Morris CA, Avorn J. Internet marketing of herbal products. *JAMA* 2003;290:1505–9.
34. FDA Office of Dietary Supplements. Available at: http://www.cfsan.fda.gov. Last accessed September 26, 2008.
35. FDA Office of Dietary Supplements: Dietary Supplement Enforcement Report. Available at: http//:www.fda.gov/oc/nutritioninitiative/report.html. Last accessed September 26, 2008.
36. McKenna JK, Hull CM, Zone JJ. Argyria associated with colloidal silver supplementation. *Int J Dermatol.* 2003;42:549.
37. Salzman MB, Smith EM, Koo C. Excessive zinc supplementation. *J Ped Hem Onc.* 2002;24:582–4.
38. Siegner AW Jr. The Food and Drug Administration's actions on ephedra and androstenedione: understanding their potential impacts on the protections of the Dietary Supplement Health and Education Act. *Food Drug Law J.* 2004;59:617–28.
39. Chitturi S, Farrell G. Hepatotoxic slimming aids and other herbal hepatotoxins. *J Gatroenterol Hepatol.* 2008;23:366–73.
40. Van Breemen RB, Fong HHS, Farnsworth NR. Ensuring the safety of botanical dietary supplements. *Am J Clin Nutr.* 2008;87(suppl):509S–13S.
41. Schulz V. Safety of St. John's wort extract compared to synthetic antidepressants. *Phytomed.* 2006;13:199–204.
42. Hammerness P. St. John's wort: A systematic review of adverse effects and drug interactions for the consultation psychiatrist. *Psychosomatics.* 2003;44:271–82.
43. Turner EH, Loftis JM, Blackwell AD. Serotonin a la carte: supplementation with the serotonin precursor 5-hydroxytrytophan. *Pharmacol Therap.* 2006;109:325–38.
44. Haller CA. Clinical approach to adverse events and interactions related to herbal and dietary supplements. *Clin Toxicol.* 2006;44:605–10.
45. Basch EM, Ulbright CE, eds. *Natural Standard Herb and Supplement Handbook: The Clinical Bottom Line.* 1st ed. St Louis: Elsevier Mosby; 2005.
46. Palmer ME, Haller C, McKinney PE, et al. Adverse events associated with dietary supplements: an observational study. *Lancet.* 2003;361:101–6.
47. Buckner KD, Chavez ML, Raney EC, et al. Health food stores' recommendations for nausea and migraines during pregnancy. *Ann Pharmacother.* 2005;39:274–9.
48. The Cochrane Database of Systematic Reviews [electronic resource]. Chichester, West Sussex, UK: Wiley; 2004.
49. Jellin JM, et al., eds. *Natural Medicines Comprehensive Database.* Stockton, Calif: Therapeutic Research Faculty; 2008. Available at: http://www.naturaldatabase.com. Last accessed September 26, 2008.
50. Basch E, Ulbricht C, eds. *Natural Standard.* Cambridge, Mass; Natural Standard. Available at: http://www.naturalstandard.com. Last accessed September 26, 2008.
51. National Center for Complementary and Alternative Medicine. Available at: http://nccam.nih.gov. Last accessed September 26, 2008.

Natural Products

Cydney E. McQueen and Katherine Kelly Orr

In a 2002 national survey, almost one in every five adults in the United States reported use of a natural product at least once during the previous 12 months.[1] Echinacea (40.3%), ginseng (24.1%), ginkgo (21.1%), and garlic (19.9%) were the most commonly used products.[1] This chapter focuses on natural products by an organ system approach. Natural products discussed in this chapter are included because they (1) have evidence to support their use, (2) are widely promoted alone or in combination products with or without evidence supporting their use, or (3) present known or theoretical safety concerns. Some of the information on individual natural products is adapted from an earlier version of this chapter.[2]

In addition to the information discussed in this chapter, decisions regarding a patient's use of a supplement should consider other factors that affect supplement choice. Chapter 53 addresses issues such as product quality concerns, research concerns, regulations, and tips on counseling patients.

CARDIOVASCULAR SYSTEM

Coenzyme Q10

Coenzyme Q10 (CoQ10) is found in every cell of the human body, primarily in the mitochondria. Originally extracted from bovine heart tissue, it is now manufactured using a beet and sugarcane fermentation process.[3] The chemically reduced form is called ubiquinone; this name is occasionally used in supplement labeling and reference books.

Therapeutic Uses

Consumers use CoQ10 as a treatment for several cardiovascular conditions and as a general antioxidant. It has also been investigated for use in Parkinson's disease and migraine prevention.

Physiologic Activity

CoQ10 exists in greatest concentrations in the mitochondria of the heart, liver, pancreas, and kidneys.[4] It is a cofactor in many functions associated with energy production and is the rate-limiting cofactor in mitochondrial adenosine triphosphate (ATP) formation. A powerful antioxidant itself, it is also involved with regeneration of other antioxidants such as vitamin E. CoQ10 stabilizes membranes and may have vasodilatory and inotropic effects.[5,6] One dosage form of CoQ10 has Food and Drug Administration (FDA) orphan drug status for the treatment of Huntington's disease.[7]

Dosage and Product Considerations

For heart failure, cardiomyopathy, or hypertension, the dosage is 100 to 200 mg daily.[8] Doses greater than 100 mg should be given in divided doses. CoQ10 products that meet USP guidelines are available.

Safety Considerations

Adverse effects include nausea, gastrointestinal (GI) distress, anorexia, headache, irritability, and dizziness in less than 1% of patients.[8] Mild increases in liver enzymes have been rarely reported. CoQ10 should be avoided in pregnancy and lactation because of the lack of information about effects.

The CoQ10 structure is similar to that of menaquinone, a synthetic vitamin K, which theoretically may have some vitamin K–like procoagulant effects.[9] There are case reports of decreases in warfarin effectiveness attributed to concomitant CoQ10 use, although one placebo-controlled crossover study noted no differences in international normalized ratio (INR) values in patients stable on warfarin dosages.[10,11] Patients on warfarin therapy should discuss CoQ10 with their primary care provider prior to use. If the decision is made to use CoQ10, the patient's INR should be monitored more frequently until effects are determined.

Hydroxymethyl glutaryl coenzyme A reductase inhibitors, or "statins," lower serum concentrations of CoQ10, but possibly not within muscle tissue.[12,13] This lowering is believed to be a class effect, but may be dose-related or differ in extent among drugs.[14]

CoQ10 may increase the effectiveness or decrease the toxicities of some chemotherapy agents, but may or may not have the same effect on radiation therapy.[15,16] Animal studies have shown decreases in effectiveness of radiation therapy with large doses,

Editor's Note: This chapter is based on the 15th edition chapters "Botanical Natural Medicines," written by Anne Lamont Hume and Kathryn Michele Strong, and "Nonbotanical Natural Medicines," written by Cydney E. McQueen.

but not with doses that would be equivalent to approximately 700 mg in a human being.[15] Information on interactions changes rapidly, so patients interested in using CoQ10 should discuss its use with their oncologist.

Summary of Clinical Evidence

Evidence for use of CoQ10 in congestive heart failure (CHF) is contradictory. Several early clinical trials demonstrated promise.[17,18] More recent studies, including some of higher quality and design, have demonstrated both positive and negative results in outcomes such as overall symptoms, ejection fraction, or oxygen consumption.[19–21] A trial in patients on a heart transplant waiting list found significant improvements in multiple symptoms, especially the 6-minute walk test, and New York Heart Association functional class, but no difference in echocardiography measurements.[20] Despite unanswered questions regarding extent of efficacy, CoQ10 is sometimes used as an adjunctive therapy. This use is acceptable because of the favorable side effect profile.

Small preliminary trials have investigated CoQ10 for cardiomyopathy and ischemic heart disease. Some benefit was noted in high-density lipoprotein (HDL) and other lipoprotein concentrations in patients with ischemic heart disease, but overall risk reduction for death or secondary cardiac events was minimal.[22,23] Additional trials suggest lipid improvements and decreased insulin resistance in patients with coronary artery disease; however, the clinical significance of these changes on long-term outcomes is unknown.[24,25] A 1-year trial examining 120 mg/day CoQ10 compared with B vitamins in 144 post–myocardial infarction patients reported a significantly lower rate of cardiac events (24.6% in the CoQ10 group vs. 45% in the B vitamin group).[26] CoQ10 has been demonstrated to have blood pressure–lowering effects in patients with essential hypertension. The clinical evidence is sufficient to consider it an optional adjunctive therapy in patients needing additional decreases of 8 to 20 mm Hg.[27]

Although statins are known to reduce endogenous CoQ10 concentrations, the clinical significance of this is not well characterized. The effectiveness of supplementing patients with CoQ10 to reduce statin side effects such as fatigue or myalgia has never been studied.[8] Fortunately the mild adverse event profile does allow consideration of use for individual patients.

Four trials have evaluated use in Parkinson's disease using doses of 300 mg daily up to 2400 mg daily. Despite methodologic limitations of the trials, all showed some evidence of symptom improvement. Although the most appropriate dosage has yet to be determined, CoQ10 could be considered an adjunctive therapy for some patients.[28,29]

CoQ10 has also been investigated for Huntington's disease, breast cancer, and migraine headaches. Although some evidence looks promising, no conclusions regarding efficacy are possible.[30–32]

Garlic

Garlic supplements are derived from dried or fresh bulbs of the same plant used in cooking, *Allium sativum.*

Therapeutic Uses

Garlic has been used to treat hyperlipidemia, hypertension, and type 2 diabetes mellitus, as well as prevention of various cancers.[33,34]

Physiologic Activity

Garlic bulbs contain an odorless sulfur-containing amino acid derivative alliin (S-allyl-l-cysteine sulfoxide). When the bulb is crushed, the enzyme allinase is released. This enzyme converts alliin to the pungent allicin, the main component of garlic's volatile oil. Allicin is used as the primary marker for product quality but may not be the primary active compound; other organosulfur-containing substances may also exert pharmacologic effects. In animal and in vitro models, garlic possesses hypotensive, hypolipidemic, antiplatelet, and anti-infective properties. Ajoene, a component of the volatile oil, has been shown to have antiplatelet effects and antibacterial activity.[8] Garlic's antioxidant effects may be of importance, in that some researchers believe that prevention of lipid oxidation may be as important to cardiovascular health as garlic's hypolipidemic activity.[34]

Dosage and Product Considerations

Most research on garlic's various uses has been conducted with the use of tablets or capsules of powdered, dehydrated garlic standardized to an allicin content of 1% to 1.6%, providing 3 to 5 mg of allicin per day.[8,34] These doses should be considered recommended until more information is available regarding optimum doses for specific indications.

Garlic supplements vary in their chemical composition, which may contribute to the contradictory results of many studies. As with many supplements, garlic products sometimes do not meet labeled standards, despite claims of high quality.[35] An enteric coating will help prevent destruction of alliin by gastric acid and may also help to decrease breath odor.[34] Although the idea of "odorless" products sound appealing, these or aged products are less likely to contain appropriate amounts of allicin.[34]

Safety Considerations

Although generally well tolerated, garlic may cause gastrointestinal (GI) side effects including nausea, vomiting, and heartburn, more commonly with higher dosages. Bad breath and body odor may also occur. Allergic reactions have been reported with the use of oral garlic on rare occasions.[34]

Garlic supplements should be stopped at least 7 to 10 days before any surgical procedure because of antithrombotic effects.[36] As a general warning, patients taking warfarin or other platelet-active drugs or supplements such as ginkgo should use garlic supplements with caution because of potential bleeding risk.[36,37] Garlic used in dietary amounts does not affect platelet function.[38]

Garlic's effect on drugs metabolized through cytochrome (CYP) P450 isoenzymes is unclear. Garlic has been reported to decrease concentrations of saquinavir by approximately 50%; however, the mechanism may involve induction of p-glycoprotein and therefore decreased absorption, rather than increased clearance.[37,39] This idea is supported by two studies that failed to find any interactions between garlic and docetaxel and other 3A4 and 2D6 substrates.[40,41] Until more evidence is available, concomitant use of garlic and drugs with a high potential for harm from reduced levels, such as human immunodeficiency virus (HIV) medications, should generally be avoided.

Summary of Clinical Evidence

A substantial body of evidence, with sometimes contradictory findings, does support that garlic supplements slightly reduce total and low-density lipoprotein (LDL) cholesterol concentrations.[34,42,43] Effects are modest, with the most rigorous studies showing the smallest benefit, reductions of about 5% in total cholesterol, with a possible reduction of benefit over time.[8]

Although garlic is often used for decreasing blood pressure and type 2 diabetes, the limited clinical evidence that exists is not enough to recommend use.[8,44,45]

Epidemiologic studies suggest that high dietary intake of raw and/or cooked garlic is related to lower rates of stomach and colorectal cancer.[46] The available evidence is based primarily on epidemiologic and animal studies, not on clinical trials with supplements, so product claims of cancer prevention are premature.[47]

Fish Oil

Fish oil is used as a source of omega-3 fatty acids, primarily docosahexaenoic acid (DHA) and eicosapentaenoic acid (EPA).

Therapeutic Uses

Fish oil is used to lower triglyceride levels, for hypertension, and for a variety of inflammatory conditions such as rheumatoid arthritis. Consumers who do not eat fish sometimes take fish oil to help ensure an adequate intake of omega-3 fatty acids.

Physiologic Activity

The intake of exogenous EPA and DHA influences production of prostaglandins, thromboxanes, and leukotrienes. Fish oil affects concentrations of many cytokines involved in the body's inflammatory response. There is some competitive inhibition of arachidonic acid, which decreases production of cytokines such as thromboxane A_2 and leukotriene B_4, while effects at another part of the production cascade increase thromboxane A_3 and prostaglandin E_3.[8,48] In general, actions can be summarized as increasing the anti-inflammatory cytokines and decreasing pro-inflammatory cytokines. These effects help to explain clinical effects on symptoms of inflammatory conditions such as rheumatoid arthritis and psoriasis. As for effects on lipids, omega-3 fatty acids may decrease the intestinal absorption of cholesterol.[8] In addition, fish oil inhibits enzymes involved in synthesis, excretion, and degradation of very-low-density lipoproteins, thereby decreasing other lipoproteins. Although studies in patients with hypercholesterolemia have noted decreases in total cholesterol and LDL, and increases in HDL, these are small changes (5–10%) compared with the decreases in triglyceride concentrations, which can be 20% to 40% with dosages of 2 to 4 grams per day.[49]

Dosage and Product Considerations

General use to balance omega-6 fatty acid intake is 1 to 2 grams daily. For treatment of hyperlipidemia, 2 to 4 grams per day is given in divided doses. For rheumatoid arthritis, generally 4 grams per day is administered; however, doses of up to 40 grams per day have been used in clinical trials. In psoriasis, generally 3 to 4 grams per day is given, although 18 grams per day have been used in clinical trials.

The most common side effect is "fish burp," which can generally be lessened by using enteric-coated products and taking with meals. With increased information and media coverage of mercury and other toxins in fish, there has been concern about mercury concentrations in fish oil supplements. Fortunately, mercury collects in the flesh to a far greater extent than in the skin, from which fish oil is produced. Supplements tested for mercury have had no or barely detectable concentrations of mercury present.[50] Products can have more significant levels of dioxins and pesticides, so, as with all supplements, taking a high-quality product, such as those meeting USP standards, is important.[8,51] A prescription fish oil product, Lovaza, is available and is more suitable for patients with significantly elevated triglycerides.

Safety Considerations

Primary side effects of fish oil are belching, fishy halitosis, and GI distress.[8] At dosages greater than 4 grams per day, increased bleeding risk may be present.[8] Patients taking anticoagulants and antiplatelet agents should probably restrict use to 3 grams daily or less and monitor closely.

Summary of Clinical Evidence

Studies have demonstrated that fish oil supplements are effective in decreasing triglycerides by 20% to 40%, with little to no effect on total cholesterol and LDL concentrations.[8] A 2006 meta-analysis of trials that examined effects on cardiovascular outcomes concluded that supplements reduced rates of cardiac death, all-cause mortality, and heart attack.[52]

Multiple small studies have demonstrated contradictory results for lowering blood pressure.[8] At this time, any small decrease in blood pressure can be considered a beneficial side effect of taking fish oil, not a primary reason for using a supplement. Fish oil has been investigated for rheumatoid arthritis in about 15 clinical trials. Benefits noted are reductions in pain and swelling, increased range of motion, and ability to reduce doses of prescription anti-inflammatory drugs.[8,53,54]

Horse Chestnut Seed Extract

The seeds, leaf, flower, and branch bark of horse chestnut trees (*Aesculus hippocastanum* or *Hippocastani semen*) are all used medicinally; however, the seed extract is most commonly seen in dietary supplements.

Therapeutic Uses

Horse chestnut seed extract (HCSE) has been used to treat chronic venous insufficiency (CVI), including varicose veins and hemorrhoids.[55]

Physiologic Activity

Horse chestnut seeds contain flavonoids, such as quercetin and kaempferol, and triterpenoid saponins, the primary component of which is aescin (also known as escin). Aescin has anti-inflammatory effects and reduces venous capillary permeability by both stabilizing membranes of cholesterol-containing lysomes and by decreasing the release of enzymes that degrade capillary cell membranes.[8] It may also have some weak diuretic activity. Horse chestnut seeds also naturally contain aesculin, a hydroxycoumarin that may increase bleeding time via antithrombin activity.[8,55]

Dosage and Product Considerations

HCSE is dosed by the aescin component, 50 to 75 mg twice daily.[8] Total extract dose may vary depending on the standardization of the extract; 16% to 20% aescin is common. HCSE products should not contain aesculin.[55]

Safety Considerations

HCSE can occasionally cause pruritus, nausea, and vomiting.[8,55] Some patients may notice a reddish discoloration of urine. Hypoglycemia has been reported, but the association with HCSE is not certain. Hypersensitivity is more likely in those with latex allergy. HCSE is contraindicated in pregnancy secondary to increased risk of bleeding should the product contain aesculin.[8] These products may also interact with anticoagulants or antiplatelet agents. There are rare reports of hepatotoxicity, nephropathy, spasms, severe bleeding, and shock with parenteral preparations.[8]

Summary of Clinical Evidence

Multiple clinical trials for CVI, as well as a meta-analysis, have demonstrated a modest reduction of leg volume and decreased pain.[8,55,56] Because CVI treatment options are limited to leg compression stockings, limb elevation, and diuretics, patients may attempt therapy with HCSE.

Policosanol

Policosanol is usually made from sugarcane and is a mixture of long-chained alcohols, primarily octacosanol, tiracontanol, and hexacosanol.[57,58]

Therapeutic Uses

Policosanol is used for treatment of hypercholesterolemia and intermittent claudication (IC).

Physiologic Activity

A high percentage of the active long-chain alcohols in policosanol are oxidized to fatty acids, which may also have beneficial activity.[57,58] Policosanol decreases cholesterol through decreased hepatic synthesis. It does not inhibit HMG-CoA (3-hydroxy-3-methylglutaryl coenzyme A) reductase directly, but may affect the enzyme levels, either by increasing its degradation or decreasing its synthesis.[57] Policosanol activates the enzyme AMP-kinase, which suppresses HMG-CoA reductase function.[58] Although most policosanol products are produced from sugarcane, others are made from wheat germ, rice, or beeswax. These products can have different percentages of constituents. Although some clinicians argue that non-sugarcane products are ineffective owing to lower amounts of octacosanol, at least one study noted that octacosanol had a much smaller effect on cholesterol synthesis than triacontanol.[58] Because 10 of 11 studies demonstrating benefit used products with higher octacosanol content, perhaps it serves as a marker compound for another, more active, component.

Dosage and Product Considerations

For hyperlipidemia, the dosage is 10 to 20 mg per day.[57,58] Because trials that have found benefit have used sugarcane-derived products, it is prudent to recommend these over wheat germ- or beeswax-derived products. For IC, the dosage is 10 mg twice daily.[8]

Safety Considerations

Policosanol is well tolerated; safety tests have used up to 1000 mg with no adverse effects.[58] The most common side effects reported are weight loss, polyuria, and headache.[8,58] Although animal studies have not found evidence of harm, policosanol should not be used in pregnancy or lactation.

No direct drug interactions are known. Most information sources include cautions against possible additive effects when used with antiplatelet or anticoagulant agents.[8] A recent study found no effect on any coagulation factors; however, it used a rice-derived policosanol, and it is not clear that results can be extrapolated to all other policosanol products.[59]

Summary of Clinical Evidence

Early studies of policosanol for hyperlipidemia were positive, with reductions of 20% to 29%.[8] Since 2004, additional studies have been contradictory, often finding no clinical benefit.[8] Some negative studies used non-sugarcane–derived products, which some scientists believe are not effective (see Physiologic Activity), but others used the same products as earlier studies.[60,61] All studies have had design flaws that limit their ability to make a true determination of effects. Until reliable information is available about policosanol, it cannot be recommended for lipid lowering. Because of the favorable safety profile, patients who are maintaining their cholesterol concentrations with diet and lifestyle changes do not need to be discouraged from using policosanol adjunctively.

Four trials examining policosanol's effects in IC, including a comparison with lovastatin, found improvement in symptoms of pain and swelling, and increases in walking distance of up to 33%.[8,62] These were short-term studies, so longer trials are needed to investigate safety.

Red Rice Yeast

Monascus purpureus is a yeast that grows on fermented rice. It has been used in traditional Chinese medicine for treatment of cardiovascular conditions.

Therapeutic Uses

Red yeast rice is used to lower cholesterol concentrations.

Physiologic Activity

Red yeast rice contains multiple components. Of primary importance is monacolin K, which is an analogue of lovastatin and functions as a statin.[8] The monacolin K component is fairly small, however, and cannot be responsible for the extent of cholesterol-lowering effects reported in clinical trials. Other mechanisms may be contributing to effects.

Dosage and Product Considerations

For hyperlipidemia, the dosage is 1.2 to 2.4 grams per day in two doses.[8] In the United States, certain red yeast rice products have been declared illegal, because they contained an "unauthorized drug."[63] Red yeast rice is still widely available, but manufacturers are generally not making claims about cholesterol-lowering activity or mevacolin K content. As a result, many manufacturers no longer take care to ensure that their products contain a standardized amount of mevacolin K, making the choice of a high-quality and effective product difficult. An additional reason for choosing a high-quality product is that improperly fermented red yeast rice can contain citrinin, a nephrotoxic compound.[8]

Safety Considerations

Reported effects include GI symptoms including stomachache, bloating, flatulence, heartburn, allergic reactions, and headache.[8] Increases in liver function enzymes and rhabdomyolysis have been reported.[8] In general, just as patients who take statin drugs, patients on red yeast rice should have their liver function monitored. Patients who do not tolerate statins should not take red yeast rice. Patients who have heavy daily alcohol intake, defined as greater than two alcoholic drinks, should not use this supplement because of potential increased risk of hepatic effects.

Red yeast rice should not be taken by pregnant women; it should be considered Pregnancy Category X, like statins.[64]

Summary of Clinical Evidence

Studies have demonstrated that red yeast rice can lower lipid concentrations.[8] One meta-analysis reported total cholesterol of 13% to 26%, LDL cholesterol of 21% to 33%, and triglycerides of 13% to 34%.[65] Generally, HDL cholesterol concentrations have not been significantly changed.[65]

Royal Jelly

Therapeutic Uses

Royal jelly is used for reducing elevated cholesterol concentrations as well as treating dermatitis, premenstrual syndrome, and asthma.

Physiologic Activity

Royal jelly is produced by worker honeybees to feed to developing queen bees. Largely water, it contains proteins, sugars, lipids, amino acids, and other components.[66] Although animal studies have demonstrated lipid-lowering activities, the mechanism is not well defined. Overall GI absorbtion/resorption of cholesterol may be decreased along with increased excretion via bile.[66] In addition, royal jelly may have some antioxidant and estrogenic activity, and its effects on premenstrual symptoms are being investigated.[8,66]

Dosage and Product Considerations

The appropriate dosage of royal jelly for lowering lipid concentrations has not been determined with trials using 20 mg to 6 g/day.[8,66]

Safety Considerations

The most common adverse events are allergic, ranging from mild rash to death from anaphylactic reactions.[67] In addition, a case of hemorrhagic colitis that resolved upon discontinuation of royal jelly has been reported.[68]

Although sometimes recommended for asthma, patients with asthma or atopy should avoid using royal jelly. There have been multiple reports of asthmatic attacks triggered by royal jelly use.[67] Use with warfarin is not recommended owing to one report of an interaction resulting in a dangerous increase in INR.[69]

Summary of Clinical Evidence

One meta-analysis of European studies of royal jelly found modest decreases in serum lipid concentrations.[66] However, only five of those trials used oral or sublingual products, whereas the remainder used injectable formulations. A recent small study of 15 individuals noted decreases in total cholesterol and LDL cholesterol concentrations of about 11 mg/dL after 4 weeks.[70]

No published studies of royal jelly's use in dermatitis, premenstrual syndrome, and asthma are available.

NERVOUS SYSTEM DISORDERS

Butterbur

Petasites hybridus (L.) Gaertner, Meyer & Scherb, also referred to as butterbur, is native to marshy areas in northern Asia, Europe, and parts of North America. It is a member of the Asteraceae family (formerly Compositae).

Therapeutic Uses

Butterbur is used to prevent migraines as well as treat allergic rhinitis and asthma.[8]

Physiologic Activity

The sesquiterpenes petasin and isopetasin are isolated from the plant's rhizomes, roots, and leaves.[71] Extracts also contain volatile oils, tannins, flavonoids, and pyrrolizidine alkaloids. Petasin may reduce spasms in smooth muscle and vascular walls, and inhibit leukotriene synthesis. Isopetasin decreases prostaglandin synthesis, thereby reducing inflammation. Both compounds have an affinity for cerebral blood vessels.

Dosing and Product Considerations

For migraine prevention, studies use standardized extracts containing a minimum of petasin 7.5 mg and isopetasin 7.5 mg per 50 mg tablet of the crude drug. Dosages of standardized crude drug ranging from 50 to 100 mg twice daily are administered for 4 to 6 months, then tapered until migraine incidence increases.[8] Standardized petasin (Ze 339) 8 to 16 mg has been administered three to four times daily for allergic rhinitis.[72,73] Upon selection, butterbur products should be certified and labeled as being free of unsaturated pyrrolizidine alkaloids (UPAs) as discussed in subsequent text.

Safety Considerations

Pyrrolizidine alkaloids are minor, highly toxic compounds in butterbur extract. Presence of a UPA nucleus can cause serious damage to the liver and carcinogenesis. Germany and Switzerland license butterbur products only after they are certified to provide a daily dosage of less than 1 mcg of UPAs in a daily dose.[74] Patients should also avoid the use of butterbur if they are allergic to plants in the Asteraceae family. Use of butterbur should be avoided in pregnancy and lactation due to potential liver toxicity.

Summary of Clinical Evidence

Studies have shown the ability of butterbur to reduce migraine frequency, decrease associated symptoms, and reduce duration and intensity of migraine pain.[71,75] Results may be dose-related, with higher dosages of 75 mg twice daily having a greater effect. An open-labeled study including children and adolescents aged 6 to 17 years old provided similar results.[76] Studies also suggest that short-term usage for less than 14 days of butterbur extract may be as effective as cetirizine and fexofenadine for symptoms associated with seasonal allergic rhinitis.[72,73] Preliminary evidence for symptoms related to perennial allergic rhinitis finds butterbur comparable to fexofenadine.[77]

Feverfew

Feverfew (*Tanacetum parthenium* [L.] Schultz-Bip.) is a member of the family Asteraceae. The plant is native to the Balkans.

Therapeutic Uses

Feverfew has been used to prevent migraines as well as to treat dysmenorrhea, arthritis, and psoriasis.[8]

Physiologic Activity

The active components of feverfew for preventing headaches are unknown. The sesquiterpene lactone, parthenolide, is the most abundant and best studied component. However, a study using an alcoholic extract of feverfew standardized to parthenolide content was found to be ineffective in prevention of migraines.[78] Chrysanthenyl acetate, an essential oil of feverfew, may inhibit prostaglandin synthetase and possess analgesic properties. Feverfew may have pharmacologic effects on prostaglandin synthesis, platelet aggregation, serotonin release, macrophage function, and vascular smooth muscle contraction. Extracts may also inhibit pain transmission.

Dosage and Product Considerations

Clinical studies have used feverfew leaf in dosages of 50 to 100 mg in divided doses daily or 6.25 mg standardized extract of 0.2 to 0.35 parthenolide two or three times daily.[8] Standardization of a feverfew product to its parthenolide content does not appear necessary. Feverfew must be taken continuously to be effective for migraine prophylaxis and is not effective for treatment of acute migraine attacks.

Safety Considerations

GI adverse effects may result from ingestion of feverfew. Oral ulcers can occur from chewing fresh leaves. The postfeverfew syndrome has been reported after abrupt withdrawal from chronic use and may result in anxiety, headaches, insomnia, and muscle stiffness. Patients should avoid use of feverfew if they are allergic to plants in the Asteraceae family. Feverfew should be avoided in pregnancy and lactation. Feverfew may possess antiplatelet effects, and patients taking warfarin and other platelet-active drugs or herbs should use feverfew with caution.[37]

Summary of Clinical Evidence

After an analysis of the clinical evidence supporting the use of feverfew for migraine prevention, the 2000 U.S. Headache Consortium ranked it as a second-line therapy for the prevention of migraines.[79] However, a Cochrane systematic review of feverfew in preventing migraine found insufficient evidence from randomized, double-blind trials to suggest an effect.[80] Overall, research demonstrates mixed results, although dried leaf capsules may have some benefit in migraine prophylaxis.

Huperzine

Huperzine A is derived from the Chinese club moss (*Huperzia serrata* [Thumb.] Trev.) and is a member of the Lycopodiaceae family. It is approved as a treatment for Alzheimer's disease (AD) in China.

Therapeutic Uses

Huperzine A has been used to treat dementia, increase memory, and enhance learning. Huperzine A is considered a protective agent against organophosphate chemical-warfare agents and a treatment for myasthenia gravis.

Physiologic Activity

Huperzine A is an unsaturated sesquiterpene compound of which only the levorotatory isomer is pharmacologically active. It is a potent peripherally and centrally acting reversible acetylcholinesterase inhibitor, which crosses the blood–brain barrier.[81]

Dosage and Product Considerations

The dosages used to treat AD range from 50 to 200 mcg of huperzine A twice daily.[8,81] Lead has been detected in some huperzine products. In an effort to develop more selective acetylcholinesterase inhibitors, chemical hybrids of huperzine A and tacrine or huperzine A and donepezil are being investigated. The huperzine A and tacrine hybrid is also referred to as huprine X.[82]

Safety Considerations

Adverse effects are primarily cholinergic and include sweating, blurred vision, nausea, vomiting, diarrhea, dizziness, bradycardia, and loss of appetite. Theoretically, huperzine should be avoided in patients with bradycardia, peptic ulcer disease, and increased gastric acid secretion. Concurrent use of anticholinergic drugs such as benztropine may decrease the effectiveness of huperzine A. Additive cholinergic effects may occur if taken with other acetylcholinesterase inhibitors such as donepezil or cholinergic agents such as bethanechol. In addition, huperzine A can have additive effects in the presence of other medications that may cause bradycardia, including beta-blockers. Huperzine should be avoided in pregnancy and lactation because of the lack of information about effects.

Summary of Clinical Evidence

A recent Cochrane review of six clinical trials concluded that huperzine A may have some efficacy in common neuronal problems associated with AD, including cognitive function, global clinical status, behavioral disturbance, and functional performance. However, only one study was of good quality and size. At this time huperzine A should not be recommended for use in AD until further evidence is available to support its efficacy.[83]

Ginkgo

Ginkgo biloba L. is a tree and the only living member of the family Ginkgoaceae.

Therapeutic Uses

Ginkgo has been used for many conditions including AD, vascular dementias, IC, tinnitus, and acute mountain sickness.[84,85]

Physiologic Activity

The extract or tincture from leaves is used primarily for medicinal purposes. The standardized *Ginkgo biloba* L. concentrated (50:1) leaf extract contains diterpene lactones such as ginkgolides (A, B, C, and M) and the sesquiterpene bilobalide. These constituents may be responsible for neuroprotective properties reported with the leaf extract. Ginkgolide B is also a potent platelet-activating factor (PAF) antagonist. The extract also contains bioflavonoids and flavone glycosides such as quercetin, 3-methyl quercetin, and kaempferol. The flavonoid fractions have been shown to possess antioxidant and free radical scavenger effects.[85]

Dosage and Product Considerations

Recommended dosages for dementias and IC range between 120 and 240 mg daily of ginkgo leaf extract in two to three divided doses. *Ginkgo biloba* L. is available as capsules or tablets containing 40, 60, or 120 mg of a concentrated (50:1) leaf extract.[85] Ginkgo preparations should contain 24% ginkgo flavone glycosides and 6% terpenoids. Products should be free of ginkgolic acid.[85] Egb 761 is the standardized *Ginkgo biloba* L. extract used in many clinical trials. Commercially available ginkgo supplements may contain subtherapeutic amounts of ginkgolides and bilobalide.

Safety Considerations

Mild GI adverse effects, headache, dizziness, and allergic skin reactions have been reported with ginkgo. Ginkcolic acids, similar to poison ivy allergens, may increase the risk of allergic reactions. Seizures and bleeding associated with ginkgo have also been described in case reports.[67,86] Gingko should be avoided in pregnancy and lactation because of the lack of information about effects.

An in vitro study indicated that ginkgolides in standardized ginkgo products have minimal effect on PAF.[88] A small randomized clinical trial supported these results; patients taking high-dose EGb 761 and 325 mg of aspirin for treatment of peripheral arterial disease demonstrated no effect on bleeding indices compared with aspirin alone.[89] Standardized gingko is unlikely to cause bleeding. As a general warning, patients taking warfarin and other platelet-active drugs and natural products such as garlic should use ginkgo with caution because of the potential risk for bleeding.[37,90] Use of ginkgo should also be stopped at least 7 to 10 days before any surgical procedure.[36]

A study involving 12 healthy volunteers failed to find an interaction between ginkgo and substrates for either CYP3A4 or CYP2D6.[91] On the basis of a single case report involving an 80-year-old woman with AD, a drug interaction may exist between trazodone and ginkgo.[92] Ginkgo has generally been associated with a reduction of blood pressure, although a paradoxical loss of antihypertensive efficacy has also been documented between ginkgo and a thiazide diuretic (Table 54-1).[85]

Summary of Clinical Evidence

Ginkgo has been used to treat both vascular and nonvascular conditions. In a recent Cochrane review, ginkgo performed better than placebo regarding clinical global improvement in trials of patients with dementia or cognitive impairment at dosages higher than 200 mg.[8] Underlying severity of dementia may influence clinical response to ginkgo with greater improvement in patients with mild cognitive impairment. Selected measures of cognition demonstrated improvement with any dosage at 12 weeks, but not 24 weeks. Various scales assessing activities of daily living resulted in improvement with dosages less than 200 mg at 12 and 24 weeks. Older studies included in the analysis that demonstrated benefit have been criticized on the basis of methodologic and statistical issues. Placebo-controlled trials using either ginkgo or cholinesterase inhibitors, such as donepezil, have suggested benefits in patients with dementia.[93,94] Methodology has been criticized, and rigorous clinical trials directly comparing ginkgo and cholinesterase inhibitors in mild-to-moderate AD are needed to determine the relative value of these therapies. A clinical trial of 230 older adults with normal cognitive function failed to demonstrate a benefit from ginkgo (Ginkoba) 40 mg three times daily on enhancing memory.[95] Overall, the benefit from ginkgo has been inconsistent. Research into the potential benefits of ginkgo for other uses is limited. A meta-analysis of eight randomized, double-blind, placebo-controlled trials of IC indicated that ginkgo has a modest benefit and is more effective than placebo.[96] EGb 761 has demonstrated similar results in a systematic review of nine randomized, controlled studies.[97] Direct comparisons with other interventions are not available.

A study (n = 978) evaluating tinnitus, without other symptoms of cerebral insufficiency, did not demonstrate any benefit from 50 mg of *Ginkgo biloba* L. extract (LI 1370) three times daily compared with placebo.[98] A meta-analysis of six randomized trials also failed to identify a benefit from ginkgo in patients with tinnitus.[99]

Prevention of acute mountain sickness has been studied (n = 614) by comparing ginkgo, acetazolamide, and ginkgo and acetazolamide with placebo. Ginkgo was similar to placebo and inferior to acetazolamide in decreasing incidence and severity of acute mountain sickness.[100] A smaller placebo-controlled trial further confirms these findings.[101]

Kava

Kava is derived from the rhizome and roots of *Piper methysticum* G. Forster. A member of the black pepper family (Piperaceae), kava is widely used by Pacific Islanders as a social and ceremonial tranquilizing beverage.

TABLE 54-1 Selected Herb–Drug Interactions

Herb	Interaction/Results	Theoretical Interactions/Results
Alpha-lipoic acid		SMBG recommended in patients taking antihyperglycemic medications
		Potential chelating activity with minerals and antacids
		Possible interference with conversion of thyroxine to triiodothyronine
Andrographis		Possible additive effects if taken with other platelet-active drugs or herbs
		Possible interaction with immunosuppressant drugs related to herb's immunostimulating properties
African plum (pygeum)		Potential risk for increased side effects if used in combination with finasteride.
Black cohosh		Possible additive estrogenic activity with HRT or OCP
		May increase toxicity of doxorubicin and docetaxel
		May decrease effectiveness of cisplatin
		Possible potentiation of antihypertensive agents
		Avoid with other hepatotoxic drugs
Butterbur	Substrate of CYP3A4; avoid with known inducers	Possible interaction with anticholinergics or antimigraine medications
Chamomile		Clinical significance of preliminary evidence suggesting decreased CYP1A2 and 3A4 activity is unknown
Chastetree berry		Minimal evidence for possible interference with hormonal contraceptives
		Possible interaction with antipsychotics, dopamine agonists, and metoclopramide due to dopaminergic activity
Chondroitin		Possible increased risk of bleeding if taken with antiplatelet agents or warfarin
Coenzyme Q10		Possible vitamin K–like procoagulant effects if taken with warfarin; monitor INR
Cranberry		Possible increased INR and risk of bleeding in people on warfarin
		Possible CYP2C9 inhibition
		May alter excretion of weakly alkaline drugs or neutralize effects of antacids
Devil's claw		Possible increased risk of bleeding in patients taking warfarin.
DHEA	Triazolam: increased blood levels	Interference with hormonal or antihormonal therapies such as aromatase inhibitors
		May increase risk of blood clots with OCPs
		Possible increased levels of 3A4 substrates
Echinacea		Possible interaction with immunomodulating therapies
		Clinical support lacking for in vitro analysis suggesting CYP3A4 inhibition
Eleutherococcus (Siberian ginseng)	Digoxin: possible false elevation in plasma levels (assay dependent)	SMBG recommended in patients taking antihyperglycemic medications
	Caffeine: increased CNS stimulation	Possible inhibition of CYP1A2, 2C9, 3A4, and 2D6 (although 3A4 and 2D6 not affected at normal doses)
	Hexobarbital: inhibited metabolism	Variable activity on blood pressure; avoid if taking antihypertensives
Evening primrose oil		Possible additive effects if taken with other platelet-active drugs or herbs
		Seizure possible if taken with phenothiazines
		Potential additive effects to antihypertensives
Feverfew		Possible additive effects if taken with other platelet-active drugs or herbs
Garlic	Warfarin: increased INR in case reports	Contradictory evidence regarding induction of drugs metabolized through CYP3A4 and 2D6
	Saquinavir: 50% decrease in levels	
	OCPs: decreased effectiveness	
Ginger	Platelet-active drugs: possible additive effect at high doses (>4 g/day)	Avoid with antihyperglycemic drugs due to additive effects

TABLE 54-1 Selected Herb–Drug Interactions (continued)

Herb	Interaction/Results	Theoretical Interactions/Results
Ginkgo	Platelet-active drugs: possible additive effect Trazodone: case report of coma in patient taking low-dose trazodone	Ingestion associated with seizures; avoid in patients with a history of seizures or on drugs that may lower seizure threshold Potential additive effects with antihypertensives although paradoxical hypertension has been reported with HCTZ
Ginseng	Glucose-lowering medications: possible lowered BG levels in type 2 DM; SMBG levels required Phenelzine: possible headache, tremor, and mania in case report; cause of effect (herb or other factors) unclear	Unpredictable effect on concurrent anticoagulant and antiplatelet therapy Possible interference with antipsychotics and immunosuppressants Inhibition of CYP2D6 (not clinically significant)
Glucosamine		SMBG recommended for first few days of use in patients taking antihyperglycemic medications
Green tea	Decongestants: additive stimulant effects	Possible antagonism of warfarin's effect Possible antagonism of concurrent sedatives related to caffeine content
Fish oil		Possible additive effects if taken with anticoagulant and antiplatelet therapy at doses >4 g
Horse chestnut	Platelet-active drugs: possible additive effects if taken with other platelet-active drugs or herbs	Limited available evidence supports concern HCSE may lower blood glucose
5-HTP	SSRIs, tramadol, DM: increased risk of serotonergic side effects Carbidopa: decreased peripheral metabolism	
Huperzine A		Possible decreased effectiveness if taken with anticholinergic drug such as benztropine Possible additive cholinergic effects if taken with other acetylcholinesterase inhibitors (donepezil) or cholinergic agents (bethanechol) Additive effects if taken with drugs causing bradycardia
Kava	Levodopa: reduced efficacy of levodopa Concern over kava's hepatotoxicity contraindicates use with other drugs and supplements that damage liver	Possible increased sedative effect with alcohol and other CNS depressants Possible additive effects with other platelet-active drugs or herbs Preliminary evidence suggests kava may inhibit CYP2C9, 2C19, 2D6, and 3A4 (significance unknown)
Melatonin	Nifedipine: reduced delivery via the GITS Fluvoxamine, MAOIs, and tricyclic antidepressants: increase melatonin BZDPs and sodium valproate: decrease nighttime levels	Caffeine or OCP usage has various effects on melatonin levels Verapamil may decrease melatonin Possible interaction with immunosuppressant drugs related to immunostimulating properties
Melissa		Concomitant use of oral lemon balm and sedating supplements and drugs contraindicated
Milk thistle		Effect on activity of CYP3A4 and 2C9 in vitro unclear
Peppermint	Decreased absorption of iron salts Premature dissolution of enteric-coated peppermint oil by drugs that increase gastric pH	Significance of decreased activity of CYP3A4 in vitro and in vivo studies unknown
Phytoestrogens (red clover, others)		Possible increased risk of bleeding in patients taking warfarin with red clover–based products
Policosanol		Possible additive effects when used with antiplatelet or anticoagulant agents
Probiotics	Separate doses of antibiotics and antifungals by 2 or more hours	
Red yeast rice	Additive HMG-CoA reductase activity when used with statins	
Royal jelly	Warfarin: case report of significantly increased INR	Possible loss of glucose control with antihyperglycemic agents

(Continued)

TABLE 54-1 Selected Herb–Drug Interactions (continued)

Herb	Interaction/Results	Theoretical Interactions/Results
SAMe		Possible increased risk of serotonin syndrome if taken with antidepressants and 5-HT1 agonists Significance on glucocorticoid increases unknown
Saw palmetto		Potential interaction with hormonal or antihormonal therapies Possible additive effects when used with antiplatelet or anti-coagulant agents (one case report)
St. John's wort	3A4 substrates: decreased drug levels and effects (examples: alprazolam, amitriptyline, digoxin, imatinib, irinotecan, nifedipine, simvastatin, tacrolimus, theophylline, warfarin) Antidepressants: increased risk of serotonin syndromes with nefazodone, sertraline, and paroxetine Cyclosporine: decreased blood levels of immunosuppressant, including case reports of transplant graft rejection OCPs: decreased effectiveness Protease inhibitors and nonnucleoside reverse transcriptase inhibitors: decreased serum levels	Possible increased risk of serotonin syndrome if taken with 5-HT1 agonists, DM, meperidine, pentazocine, and tramadol; interaction possibly similar to conventional antidepressants and MAOIs with increased potential for hypertension, hyperthermia, agitation, and coma Possible decreased levels and effect of amiodarone Monitoring for fexofenadine toxicity recommended if taken concomitantly Morphine: increased narcotic-induced sleep time in animal studies Use with other photosensitizing agents contraindicated
Valerian		Possible increased sedative effect if taken with alcohol or other CNS depressants (BZDPs, opioids, kava) May inhibit CYP3A4 (not clinically significant)

Key: BG, blood glucose; BZDP, benzodiazepine; CNS, central nervous system; CYP, cytochrome P450; DM, dextromethorphan; GITS, gastrointestinal therapeutic system; HCSE, horse chestnut seed extract; HCTZ, hydrochlorothiazide; HRT, hormone replacement therapy; 5-HT1, 5-hydroxytryptamine1; 5-HTP, 5-hydroxytriptophan; INR, international normalized ratio; MAOI, monoamine oxidase inhibitor; OCP, oral contraceptive pills; SMBG, self-monitoring of blood glucose.

Therapeutic Uses

Kava is used to treat mild anxiety and sleep disturbances.

Physiologic Activity

The pharmacologically active constituents of kava are the fat-soluble lactones, also referred to as kavalactones and kavapyrones. The mechanism of action includes interacting with dopaminergic transmission, inhibiting central monoamine oxidase-B (MAO-B), and modulating gamma–aminobutyric acid–B (GABA-B) receptors.[102] Kava may also inhibit uptake of noradrenaline and have antithrombotic activity.

Dosage and Product Considerations

The usual dosage of kava preparations is equivalent to 60 to 120 mg of kavapyrones. In trials using extracts standardized to 70% kavalactones, the recommended dosage is 100 mg two to three times a day. WS 1490 is a standardized kava extract used in many clinical trials. Kava-containing products have limited availability because of ongoing concerns about the risk of liver disease (see Safety Considerations).

Safety Considerations

Dizziness and drowsiness are most commonly reported. Mouth ulceration and numbness may occur if the raw plant is chewed.

The use of kava is discouraged when operating machinery or motor vehicles. Acute overdoses with kava may result in impaired mental status and ataxia similar to alcohol intoxication.[103] Kava dermopathy syndrome (a dry, scaly rash primarily on the palms, soles, forearms, shins, and back) can occur in patients chronically using high-dose kava teas, tablets, or the native plant.[104] Thrombocytopenia, leukopenia, and hearing impairment have also been reported with kava.[104] Kava should not be used in pregnancy and lactation.

In 2002, the Center for Food Safety and Nutrition issued a warning advising consumers and professionals of the risk of severe liver injury associated with kava-containing supplements. Germany, Switzerland, Canada, Australia, and France have restricted the sale of kava products in response to case reports of liver failure associated with kava use.[105] As of 2004, at least 78 cases of hepatotoxicity have been associated with kava ingestion. Of these, four are probably linked to kava and another 23 are potentially linked.[105]

Kava potentially can interact with anticoagulants and other drugs that increase the risk of bleeding.[37] Concomitant use of kava with alcohol and other central nervous system (CNS) depressants such as benzodiazepines (BZDP), anticonvulsants, opioids, and valerian could increase the risk of sedation. Preliminary evidence suggests kava may inhibit CYP2C9, 2C19, 2D6, and 3A4; therefore, it should be avoided if an individual is taking drugs metabolized through these pathways.[106] Kava should not be taken with other hepatotoxic medications, natural products, or alcohol. Kava may interfere with dopamine transmission, resulting in an interaction with levodopa or worsening of symptoms of parkinsonism.[107]

Summary of Clinical Evidence

Small studies support kava extracts to be superior to placebo for short-term treatment of anxiety. A Cochrane systematic review found a significant difference in the Hamilton Anxiety (HAM-A) scale compared with placebo.[108] Another meta-analysis of kava extract WS 1490 reported an efficacy success rate based on an odds ratio of 3.3 (95% confidence interval: 2.09–5.22) compared to placebo; however, overall HAM-A scores were not significant. Women and younger patients showed the most improvement.[109] Similar efficacy to BZDPs and buspirone has also been reported.[8] Despite its efficacy, current safety issues require that kava not be used until its full potential for hepatotoxicity is completely understood.

Melatonin

Therapeutic Uses

Melatonin, or N-acetyl-5-methoxytryptamine, synthesized from tryptophan via a serotonin pathway, is a hormone produced by the pineal gland. Melatonin has FDA orphan drug status for treatment of sleep disorders in blind patients.[110] As a dietary supplement, melatonin is primarily used for treatment of insomnia and prevention of "jet lag" in air travelers.

Physiologic Activity

Melatonin regulates sleep and circadian rhythms. Release of melatonin is induced by darkness and suppressed by light; exogenous administration of melatonin increases endogenous concentrations and stimulates sleep regulation mechanisms. When taken for insomnia near bedtime, melatonin does not generally cause a feeling of drowsiness; rather, it may make a patient's attempt to sleep more successful. Melatonin's effects for prevention and treatment of jet lag may be a result of more rapid adjustment of circadian rhythm after changing time zones. Melatonin has regulatory effects on sexual development and ovulation, with high dosages studied as a contraceptive; has effects on the immune system; and is also a potent antioxidant.[111,112]

Dosage and Product Considerations

For insomnia, 0.3 to 5 mg can be taken 30 minutes prior to bedtime. For jet lag, 2 to 5 mg in the evening, between 1700 and 2200, of the day of arrival at the destination and at bedtime for the following 2 to 5 days is recommended.[8] The dosage for occasional insomnia remains unclear. As little as 0.3 mg will produce supraphysiologic concentrations and may be more effective than higher dosages.[113] The dosage should be limited to not more than 5 mg on an occasional basis to reduce the risk of adverse effects.

Most melatonin products are produced synthetically, although some produced with bovine pineal gland extracts are available. These products carry an added risk of bacterial contamination and, theoretically, a risk of bovine spongiform encephalitis (mad cow disease); use should be discouraged.

Safety Considerations

Rare reported side effects include nausea and vomiting, headache, tachycardia, irritability, dysthymia and worsening of depressive symptoms, and a morning "hangover" effect.[111] Long-term administration is not recommended unless under the direct supervision of a primary care provider.

The use of melatonin in children and adolescents remains controversial because of hormonal effects. Usage should be discussed first with a primary care provider. Pregnant and lactating women should not use melatonin because of possible hormonal effects on the fetus.

Several interactions with melatonin are known. Fluvoxamine, monoamine oxidase inhibitors (MAOIs), and tricyclic antidepressants may increase endogenous melatonin concentrations, whereas BZDPs and sodium valproate decrease nighttime concentrations.[114,115] Oral contraceptives and caffeine have variable effects on melatonin concentrations in women, depending on the phase of the reproductive cycle.[116] Verapamil may also decrease concentrations by increasing melatonin excretion.[114] The clinical significance of these interactions is not known. However, melatonin's effect on nifedipine delivered via the GI therapeutic system (GITS) is clinically significant.[117] The drug's effectiveness is reduced, but whether melatonin affects nifedipine or the delivery system is unknown.

Because melatonin may have stimulatory effects on the immune system, concomitant use with immunosuppressant therapy is not recommended. Like coenzyme Q10, melatonin may help to reduce toxicities of some cancer chemotherapy agents such as doxorubicin and cisplatin.[118] As information on effects on chemotherapy changes rapidly, patients receiving cancer treatment should be advised to discuss melatonin use with their oncologists.

Summary of Clinical Evidence

Evidence with melatonin for the treatment of insomnia is not definitive. Increases in rapid eye movement sleep, slightly faster sleep onset, increased duration of sleep, decreased daytime somnolence, and more "normal" patterns of time in sleep stages have been demonstrated in healthy people with insomnia and in women with asthma.[111,119,120] A recent meta-analysis of 17 studies, conducted primarily in healthy, normal patients and people with insomnia, supports the claim that melatonin has small but clinically significant benefits.[113] More benefits may occur in patients whose natural sleep patterns are disrupted for physical reasons, such as ill health, although one study in patients with AD found no difference from placebo.[121] Melatonin has been investigated in children with developmental disabilities and several trials have also found benefit for healthy children 6 to 12 years old with chronic sleep-onset insomnia.[122,123] Sleep patterns improve in children with attention deficit hyperactivity disorder (ADHD) with no detectable effects on ADHD symptoms.[124]

Clinical evidence for jet lag is slightly more consistent than for insomnia. A systematic review concluded that melatonin can decrease jet lag in people crossing five or more time zones and has greater benefit for eastward travel than westward.[125]

Although insomnia resulting from the circadian rhythm disruption caused by shift work may seem similar to insomnia associated with jet lag, melatonin is not effective for this use.[126]

Melatonin's use in children with insomnia has been sufficiently studied in only individuals with neurologic disorders or blindness.[113] Children should take melatonin only upon the recommendation of a primary care provider (see Adverse Effects/Precautions/Contraindications).

St. John's Wort

Hypericum perforatum L. is a perennial with more than 400 species that grows wild throughout Europe, Asia, North America, and South America. The yellow flowers and the leaves contain the highest levels of medicinally useful compounds. St. John's wort (SJW) is classified in the Clusiaceae family but may also be listed under the Hypericaceae family.

Therapeutic Uses

SJW is used to treat depression, pain, anxiety, obsessive-compulsive disorder, and premenstrual syndrome.[8]

Physiologic Activity

Antidepressant activity has been attributed to hypericin, although current evidence suggests hyperforin is responsible.[127] Other potential biologically active constituents include flavonoids, tannins, volatile oils, and phenols. SJW may modulate serotonin, dopamine, and norepinephrine. In vitro analysis suggests SJW may also have an affinity for sigma receptors and acts as a receptor antagonist at adenosine, BZDP, GABA, and inositol triphosphate receptors.[127,128]

Dosage and Product Considerations

The recommended dosage for adults with mild-to-moderate depression is 900 to 1800 mg per day standardized extract of 0.3% hypercin or 5% hyperforin.[8] It should be taken in three divided doses with meals. LI 160, ZE 117, WS 5570, STW3, and STW3-VI are extracts commonly used in clinical studies. The content of hypercin and hyperforin varies in commercial preparations, and products may not be interchangeable.[129] As with prescription antidepressants, the therapeutic effects of SJW are not evident for several weeks. Depression should never be self-diagnosed or self-treated. Patients should be counseled to seek appropriate medical care for this potentially life-threatening condition before using SJW.

Safety Considerations

An analysis of randomized trials found rates of adverse effects in patients taking SJW similar to those for placebo. In addition, rates for SJW were much lower, compared with older antidepressants, and slightly lower than with selective serotonin receptor inhibitors (SSRIs).[130] The most frequently reported adverse effects included paresthesias, headache, nausea, dry mouth, agitation, and skin reactions. SJW should be avoided in patients with bipolar disorder and schizophrenia. Photosensitivity reactions have been reported; however, there is also evidence to support a lack of effect.[131] Until the significance of potential photosensitivity with SJW is clearly established, patients should limit their exposure to sun and apply sunscreen. Similar to SSRIs, SJW may cause sexual dysfunction such as loss of libido. Abrupt discontinuation after chronic use of SJW may result in withdrawal symptoms similar to those of conventional antidepressants. SJW should be avoided in pregnancy and lactation because of the lack of information about effects.

Unlike drug interactions discussed in this chapter, interactions with SJW are well documented and clinically significant. SJW contains many compounds that influence activities of major human drug-metabolizing enzymes, resulting in multiple pharmacokinetic interactions. The specific enzymes, the degree of influence of hypericin versus hyperforin, and in vitro analysis versus clinical outcomes are still being studied. SJW is a potent inducer of CYP3A4, resulting in significantly lower concentrations of drugs metabolized through this pathway. Extent of CYP3A4 induction may correlate to hyperforin dose and vary among products.[132,133] SJW may also induce p-glycoprotein transport proteins that result in lower serum concentrations of drugs such as digoxin.[37,133] Additional evidence suggests induction of CYP1A2 and CYP2C9 although to a lesser extent than CYP3A4.[37] Many drug interactions are based on extrapolating across a drug class or metabolic pathway. SJW will also increase the risk of developing serotonin syndrome if taken concurrently with other serotonergic drugs or natural products.

Summary of Clinical Evidence

Many clinical trials evaluating SJW have been published. Comparisons have been made to placebo, light therapy, and traditional antidepressants. Efficacy evaluations also vary from study to study, with rankings of "less than" to "as effective" as traditional agents to treat mild, moderate, and severe depression. A Cochrane review evaluated hypericum extracts for major depression, including 18 clinical trials comparing it to placebo and 17 studies comparing it to standard antidepressants. Results demonstrate SJW has a significant benefit compared with placebo and similar efficacy in comparison with standard antidepressants for mild-to-moderate depression. The reported rate of side effects and trial discontinuation were also significantly lower with SJW than with older traditional antidepressants, indicating hypericum extract may be more tolerable. In addition, the results vary depending on the country of origin, with German-speaking countries showing more positive outcomes. Conclusions cannot be made regarding severe depression.[134] Recent large randomized clinical trials enrolling more than 300 participants have also shown benefit compared with placebo and antidepressants.[135,136] Evidence supports efficacy for mild-to-moderate depression with comparable efficacy to fluoxetine, sertraline, and citalopram. However, because SJW interacts with many drugs, it is not an appropriate choice for many patients.

Valerian

Native to Europe and Asia, valerian grows in most parts of the world. More than 200 plant species belong to the genus *Valeriana*. The most common plant used for medicinal purposes is *Valeriana officinalis* L. from the Valerianaceae family.

Therapeutic Uses

Valerian is used for alleviating insomnia and anxiety.

Physiologic Activity

The CNS activity of valerian may be a result of valepotriates and sesquiterpene constituents of the volatile oils.[137] Major sesquiterpenes are valerenic acid, valerenone, and kessyl glycol. Aqueous extracts lacking valepotriates and sesquiterpenes have similar effects, indicating other unidentified, active components may also be involved. Data suggest that sedation from valerian extracts results from interaction with $GABA_A$ receptors in the brain.[138] Valerian may also have barbiturate-like CNS depressant effects.

Dosage and Product Considerations

Most clinical trials using valerian for insomnia used valerian root extract in a dosage of 400 to 900 mg, administered 30 to 120 minutes before bedtime. Teas can be prepared from dried roots, although the teas often have an unpleasant taste and smell.[8]

Safety Considerations

Valerian products containing little or no valepotriates are generally well tolerated. Adverse effects include headache, excitability, and paradoxical insomnia. Cardiac disturbances and BZDP-like withdrawal symptoms have been reported during valerian withdrawal.[139] Residual daytime sedation has been reported with higher doses. *V. officinalis* preparations are considered safe despite the known in vitro cytotoxic activity of valepotriates. Pregnant women should not use valerian because of its potential to induce uterine contractions. Chronic administration of valerian has been linked to hepatotoxicity. Valerian can potentiate the effects of other CNS depressants such as alcohol, opiates, barbiturates, and BZDPs; they should not be taken concomitantly. Valerian has a possible effect on cytochrome P450, although clinical significance is not demonstrated.[140]

Summary of Clinical Evidence

Older studies demonstrated a decrease in sleep latency and an increase in sleep quality in patients taking 270 to 1200 mg of valerian per day for less than 6 weeks.[137] Recent placebo-controlled studies have not found significant benefit.[141,142] A study of older adults found *V. officinalis* to be inferior to temazepam or diphenhydramine.[143]

5-Hydroxytryptophan

Therapeutic Uses

5-Hydroxytryptophan (5-HTP) is used for depression, anxiety, and insomnia.

Physiologic Activity

5-HTP crosses the blood–brain barrier and is converted to serotonin, although much of it is broken down in the periphery.[8] Increased serotonin levels may result in serotonergic effects within the CNS.

Dosage and Product Considerations

5-HTP is marketed as a safer alternative to tryptophan, a supplement banned after more than 1500 cases of eosinophilia myalgia syndrome (EMS) that included 38 deaths were reported in 1989. The cases were linked to product contamination with peakX (4,5-tryptophan-dione).[8] However, 5-HTP may not actually be safer, because peakX has also been found in samples of 5-HTP including products tested after being associated with cases of an EMS-like illness.[144,145] In addition, EMS has occurred with use of tryptophan and 5-HTP products in which no peakX was found.

Patients should be encouraged to avoid 5-HTP because of safety concerns. Additional counseling points should mention that depression and serious anxiety and panic disorders are not self-treatable conditions. Patients should discuss symptoms with their primary care provider. If 5HTP is started for any condition, patients should be monitored closely and dosages should not exceed 150 to 300 mg/day.

Safety Considerations

Adverse effects include nausea, vomiting, diarrhea, anorexia, belching, and flatulence.[8,146] Pregnant or lactating women should avoid 5-HTP owing to the lack of information on its safety. 5-HTP should not be used with serotonergic agents, such as SSRIs, $5HT_1$-agonists, tramadol, and dextromethorphan, because of the potential increased risk of serotonin syndrome.[8] Carbidopa may increase 5-HTP side effects by decreasing peripheral metabolism.[147]

Summary of Clinical Evidence

Clinical evidence for depression is preliminary, in that studies have been small, thereby limiting their usefulness in decision making.[146]

Use of 5-HTP has not been well studied in anxiety and insomnia. One study examining treatment of night terrors in children noted substantial benefit, but more evidence is needed.[148]

DIGESTIVE SYSTEM

Chamomile

Two common forms of chamomile are Roman or common chamomile (*Chamaemelum nobile* L. All., *Anthemis nobilis* L.) and German or Hungarian chamomile (*Matricaria recutita* L., *Chamomilla recutita* L.) Rauchert. Both herbs are from the family Asteraceae. Indigenous natives and Spanish-speaking people of the Americas have used dog fennel, a member of the genus *Anthemis,* as "chamomile."

Therapeutic Uses

German chamomile has been used for motion sickness, as well as many GI, inflammatory, and dermatologic diseases, including those in children. Chamomile has been used to decrease mucositis after some types of chemotherapy. It has also been used for anxiety, insomnia, and GI spasms, especially as an herbal tea. Topically, chamomile has been used for hemorrhoids and inflammation of skin and mucous membranes.

Physiologic Activity

Chamomile contains 0.3% to 2.0% of a volatile oil. The oil contains alpha-bisabolol and sesquiterpene alpha-bisabolol, which have anti-inflammatory and antibacterial activity. Important flavonoids have been identified in German chamomile, including apigenin, luteolin, and quercetin. Apigenin may affect central neurotransmitter systems, including serving as a BZDP-receptor–binding ligand.[149]

Dosage and Product Considerations

German chamomile may be prepared as a 3 gram infusion in 150 mL of hot water, three to four times per day. The dosage for oral irritations is rinsing three times daily with 10 to 15 drops Kamillosan Liquidum in 100 mL warm water. Topically, 2% ethanolic extract in cream base may be applied as needed.[8] Chamomile products containing dog fennel may have a higher rate of allergic reactions attributable to anthecotulid and should be avoided.

Safety Considerations

Chamomile generally is safe. Allergic reactions have been reported with a frequency less than 2%, although they may be more common than previously thought.[150] Patients with an allergy to ragweed and related plants in the family Asteraceae should avoid chamomile. Pregnant women should avoid chamomile owing to potential for uterine contractions.[8] Patients taking warfarin and platelet-active drugs or herbs should use chamomile with caution.[151] In addition, patients taking sedatives might experience additive effects if chamomile is also used. Little evidence supports these potential interactions. Preliminary in vitro and animal studies suggest that chamomile extracts and tea infusions may decrease activity of CYP1A2, 2E1, and 3A4.[37,152,153] However, significant interactions have not been reported.

Summary of Clinical Evidence

Evidence of chamomile's effectiveness from clinical trials is limited. Benefit has been demonstrated for management of oral mucositis in patients receiving radiation and various forms of chemotherapy.[154] However, a randomized double-blind, placebo-controlled trial found no difference for prevention of oral mucositis in patients receiving 5-fluorouracil.[155] Chamomile should not be recommended as an initial treatment option. In atopic eczema, a partially double-blind placebo-controlled trial demonstrated topical chamomile to be more effective than placebo and 0.5% hydrocortisone cream.[156]

Ginger

Ginger (*Zingiber officinale* Roscoe) is a perennial from the Zingiberaceae family whose rhizomes and roots are used medicinally.

Therapeutic Uses

The primary use of ginger has been as an antiemetic agent to relieve nausea and vomiting associated with pregnancy, motion sickness, chemotherapy, and surgery.[8] Ginger has also been used for indigestion, colic, and arthritis.

Physiologic Activity

Ginger rhizomes possess volatile oil containing sesquiterpene hydrocarbons, including zingiberene and alpha-curcumene. Lesser amounts of farnesene, beta-sesquiphellandrene, and beta-bisabolene are present. An oleoresin is also present with non-volatile pungent components, including gingerol, shogaols, and zingerone. Galanolactone, a diterpenoid isolated from ginger, and 6-shagoal has been shown to have anti-5-hydroxytriptamine activity in the GI tract, although not the CNS, and may also contribute to the antiemetic activity of ginger preparations. Ginger does not affect GI motility or increase gastric emptying. The 6-shogaol and 6-gingerol components inhibit cyclooxygenase and lipoxygenase pathways, resulting in anti-inflammatory actions, as well as potential inhibition of platelet thromboxane.[8]

Dosage and Product Considerations

For nausea and vomiting in pregnancy, dried ginger 250 mg four times daily has been used. For motion sickness, a typical dose is two 500 mg capsules of dried powdered ginger root taken 30 minutes before travel, followed by one or two more 500 mg capsules as needed every 4 hours. Daily dosages greater than 4 grams should be avoided.[8]

Safety Considerations

Heartburn and dermatitis have been reported with ginger. Belching was also identified in a clinical trial comparing ginger with pyridoxine.[157] During pregnancy, studies have found no significant adverse effects in pregnancy outcomes between ginger and placebo or pyridoxine.[158] A cohort study evaluating pregnancy outcomes through the Canadian Motherisk Helpline reported that exposure to ginger between the fourth and 14th week of pregnancy did not increase risk of major malformations.[159] Of note, 49% of women used ginger capsules with the remainder using ginger teas, cookies, candies, and other products.[159] Ginger may increase the risk of hypoglycemia and alter platelet function at dosages greater than 1 gram per day.[8] Ginger should be used with caution by an individual also taking warfarin and platelet-active drugs or herbs.[37,160,161]

Summary of Clinical Evidence

Mixed results have been found for the management of postoperative nausea and vomiting (PONV). A recent meta-analysis evaluated a fixed dose of ginger in the management of PONV.[162] Pooled data from five placebo-controlled trials were included, providing evidence that at least 1 gram of ginger was effective in the management of nausea and vomiting. However, the study with overall strongest design has failed to find a difference between ginger and placebo.[163]

A systematic review of pregnancy-induced nausea and vomiting evaluated six randomized controlled clinical trials and one observational study.[158] Five of the six studies were of high quality. Ginger was more effective than placebo and similar to pyridoxine in early pregnancy.[158] Of note, the effectiveness of ginger for the more severe form of nausea and vomiting in pregnancy, hyperemesis gravidarum, is unknown and ginger should not be recommended as a therapy for this condition.

Evidence is inconsistent for the role in ginger in prevention of motion sickness. The largest trial with 1489 volunteers, found that ginger extract Zintona provided benefit similar to that of available nonprescription medications in preventing sea sickness.[164] However, the survey had subjective outcomes and was not validated. Baseline assessments and compliance were also omitted. Further evidence is needed to better define the role of ginger in preventing motion sickness.

Milk Thistle

Milk thistle (*Silybum marianum* (L.) Gaertn.) is a member of the aster family Asteraceae.

Therapeutic Uses

Milk thistle has been used to treat liver disease, including hepatitis and cirrhosis. In Europe, it is administered to treat poisoning by the mushroom *Amanita phalloides* (death cap). Milk thistle has been used as a protective agent after the liver was exposed to alcohol, acetaminophen, and carbon tetrachloride.

Physiologic Activity

The seeds and, to a lesser extent, the leaves and stems contain several compounds collectively referred to as silymarin. Silymarin is composed primarily of silybin, along with isosilybin, dehydrosilybin, silydianin, and silychristin. These biologically active compounds may have antioxidant, antifibrotic, anti-inflammatory activity, as well as other beneficial effects such as regulation of cell permeability and inhibition of mitochondrial injury. The antioxidant properties of silymarin may be the primary beneficial effect.

Dosage and Product Considerations

The average dosage is 150 mg silymarin three times per day for cirrhosis and 240 mg silybin (silibinin) twice daily for hepatitis. Milk thistle preparations contain varying amounts of a concentrated seed extract, standardized to flavonolignans 70% to 80% calculated as silymarin, approximately 70% is silybin. Multiple variations of silymarin and silybin have been used in clinical studies, it is unknown if similar products are available in the United States, even with identical standardization.[8] Liver disease resulting from alcohol, acetaminophen, and other drugs or chemicals is potentially fatal, and patients should be cautioned against self-treatment.

Safety Considerations

Nausea, abdominal fullness, and diarrhea have been reported. Allergic reactions have been reported with milk thistle. Patients with allergy to ragweed and other members of the Asteraceae family should be cautioned not to use milk thistle although documented cases of cross-sensitivity are rare. Milk thistle should be avoided in pregnancy and lactation owing to unkown effects.[8] Potential inhibitory effects of milk thistle on major CYP isoenzymes 2C9 and 3A4 has been studied in vitro, and patients should be cautioned about concomitant use with medications metabolized by these enzymes.[165]

Summary of Clinical Evidence

A systematic review conducted by the Agency for Healthcare Research and Quality identified 16 prospective studies of milk thistle in varying types of liver disease. Milk thistle improved aminotransferase concentrations and other measures of liver function in four of six studies of alcoholic liver disease. The effect of milk thistle on survival is unknown.[166] A recent Cochrane systematic review of 18 randomized controlled studies investigated the effect of milk thistle on liver disease caused by alcohol or hepatitis B or C viral infection. Reduction in mortality or complications of liver disease, or changes in liver histology were not found. With inclusion of all trials, liver-related mortality was significantly reduced, but not in the five high-quality trials.[167]

Peppermint

Peppermint (*Mentha piperita* L.) is a member of the mint family Lamiaceae. It has been cultivated for its fragrant volatile oil, which is extracted primarily from its leaves.

Therapeutic Uses

Both peppermint leaf and oil have been used for many purposes including treatment of irritable bowel syndrome (IBS), non-ulcerative dyspepsia, colonic spasm, and tension headache.

Physiologic Activity

The biological activity of peppermint may be a result of its 0.5% to 4% essential oil. The oil or leaf preparations should be standardized to contain not less than 44% menthol. Menthol stereoisomers are also present, including 3% d-neomenthol, as well as other monoterpenes such as menthone, menthofuran, eucalyptol, and limonene. The mechanism of action of peppermint involves direct relaxation of GI smooth muscle.

Dosage and Product Considerations

The usual dosage of peppermint oil enteric-coated capsules for IBS is 0.2 to 0.6 mL (187–374 mg) three times daily. Enteric-coated preparations allow for release in the small intestine and reduce risk of heartburn. Clinical trials have studied 10 to 30 mL of peppermint oil solution as an antispasmatic. Pure peppermint oil should be diluted prior to topical usage.[8]

Safety Considerations

Heartburn reported in some patients may be attributed to relaxation of the lower esophageal sphincter. Patients who have severe preexisting GI disease should avoid use of peppermint oil. Peppermint leaf tea should be used with caution in infants and small children because of possible laryngeal and bronchial spasms from volatilized menthol. The oil may also irritate mucous membranes. In vitro studies suggest that peppermint tea and peppermint oil may decrease activity of some CYP isoenzymes, including CYP3A4.[168] The evidence should be considered preliminary given that significant interactions have not been reported. Antacids or other medications increasing stomach pH may affect dissolution of enteric-coated capsules.[8] The ingestion of peppermint may decrease absorption of iron.[37]

Summary of Clinical Evidence

A systematic review evaluating peppermint oil in the treatment of IBS concluded that peppermint oil had significant efficacy compared with placebo and was comparable to selected smooth muscle relaxants.[169] In a study of 42 children with IBS, 75% experienced a reduction in severity of their abdominal pain with the use of pH-dependent, enteric-coated peppermint oil capsules.[170] A recent double-blind randomized controlled trial was conducted and included 57 patients with IBS. At the end of 4 weeks, 75% of patients reported a significant improvement in symptoms compared with 38% taking placebo.[171]

Reduction of colonic spasm during procedures has been investigated with patients receiving barium enemas. Studies demonstrate the incidence of spasms was significantly decreased compared with placebo and was similar to scopolamine butylbromide.[172,173] Compared with intramuscular hyoscyamine, peppermint has also been shown to significantly increase the opening ratio of the pyloric ring during upper endoscopy with fewer side effects.[174]

ENDOCRINE SYSTEM

Alpha-Lipoic Acid

Therapeutic Uses

Alpha-lipoic acid, also known as thioctic acid, is a lipophilic and hydrophilic endogenous substance promoted as a supplement for diabetic patients. In Europe, intravenous alpha-lipoic acid is an approved treatment for diabetic peripheral neuropathy.[8]

Physiologic Activity

Alpha-lipoic acid is a cofactor for several enzymes involved in glucose metabolism. Concentrations are reduced in diabetic animals with decreased glucose uptake in muscle tissue. Theoretically, supplementation would increase the activity of enzymes responsible for glucose uptake. Human studies have shown improvement in measurements of glucose metabolism, and animal studies have noted improvements in nerve blood flow and distal conduction.[175,176] Alpha-lipoic acid is a chelating agent and antioxidant.[8,177]

Dosage and Product Considerations

Because bioavailability is approximately 30%, an 1800 mg daily oral dose, given as 600 mg three times daily, should be comparable to an intravenous dose of 600 mg, the dose used in most European trials for diabetic neuropathy.[178] For burning mouth syndrome, 600 to 800 mg is administered daily in three or four doses.[8] Alpha-lipoic acid should be taken on an empty stomach, because food decreases its absorption, and separated by 2 to 3 hours from antacids or other mineral-containing supplements because of its chelating activity.[179]

Safety Considerations

Occasional adverse effects include headache, nausea, and allergic rash.[179,180] Additive glucose-lowering effects and hypoglycemia may occur when used with antidiabetic medications. Diabetic patients who wish to add alpha-lipoic acid to their current treatment should discuss its use with their primary care provider. Patients should frequently monitor glucose concentrations, especially during the first few weeks of therapy. Dosages of other medications may need to be adjusted by a primary care provider.

One animal study found that alpha-lipoic acid given with thyroxine inhibits the conversion of thyroxine to triiodothyronine. The supplement may displace thyroxine from the serum-binding protein.[181] Until more information is known, patients with thyroid conditions should avoid alpha-lipoic acid.

Summary of Clinical Evidence

The efficacy of alpha-lipoic acid for symptoms of diabetic neuropathy is contradictory. A large placebo-controlled trial found improvement in Total Symptom Scores and Neuropathy Impairment Scores by 5 weeks, whereas a 7-month-long trial did not.[182,183] A 2-year study of 600 and 1200 mg doses demonstrated improvements in nerve conduction but not neuropathic symptoms.[184] Two placebo-controlled trials noted improvements in symptoms such as pain, numbness, paresthesia, and burning sensation.[185,186] Overall, evidence is preliminary.

Two studies have noted reductions in glucose concentrations, and improvement in insulin sensitivity and glucose disposal rates.[187,188] However, reductions in serum glucose and glycosylated hemoglobin concentrations in several studies have not been significant.[8]

Of the trials for burning mouth syndrome, all have found a reduction in symptoms with alpha-lipoic acid.[8] Although trials have been small, alpha-lipoic acid may be an appropriate adjunctive treatment option.

American ginseng (*Panax quinquefolius*)

Therapeutic Uses

American ginseng, *Panax quinquefolius,* is closely related to Asian ginseng, *Panax ginseng*. It is most frequently recommended to reduce postprandial glucose elevations and to reduce the severity of cold and upper respiratory infection symptoms. In traditional Chinese medicine, American ginseng, like *Panax ginseng,* is considered an adaptogen, a substance that aids the body in returning to normal function and to adapt to stress.

Physiologic Activity

Similar to other ginseng species, American ginseng contains many components with pharmacologic activity. The ginsenosides, triterpene saponins, are best known for effects on blood pressure and stimulation of immune cell function, such as increased monocyte activity or release of tumor necrosis factor (TNF) and interleukins.[8] The non-saponin components, however, are probably more responsible for hypoglycemic effects.[8] These components, although present in other species, are more plentiful in American ginseng.[189] The ginsenosides often occur in pairs that have opposing pharmacologic actions. Some ginsenoside components in American ginseng may have estrogenic activity; however, concentrations depend on processing and extraction methods, so this activity may vary between different products.[190]

Dosage and Product Considerations

Trials demonstrating positive results in reducing postprandial glucose concentrations have used 1 to 3 grams 30 minutes before meals in patients with diabetes. Unfortunately, not enough information is available to provide recommendations on the most appropriate product.[8]

For reduction of the incidence and severity of colds and other upper respiratory infections, clinical evidence supports use of only a specific extract of polysaccharides from American ginseng. This is available under the brand name COLD-fX and is dosed at 200 mg of extract given twice daily.[8]

Safety Considerations

American ginseng is better tolerated than other ginseng species. Adverse effects include increased and decreased blood pressure, increased and decreased blood glucose concentrations, and mild

GI disturbances.[8] Two studies have found no effects on blood pressure.[191,192] Differences in ginsenoside or other component concentrations may help to explain differences in adverse effects, as well as opposing clinical effects, between American ginseng and other *Panax* species.

Use in patients with schizophrenia has been associated with insomnia and agitative states.[193] Although these effects occurred with high dosages, use of American ginseng should be avoided in these patients. Use with psychotropic agents is also contraindicated.[37]

American ginseng may decrease warfarin's effect, and because of the variability in batches and products, concomitant use should be avoided entirely.[194]

Summary of Clinical Evidence

The reductions in postprandial hyperglycemia in clinical trials have been clinically significant; however, all trials used glycemic loads smaller than a typical meal.[8,195] The long-term effects and utility for management of glucose concentrations are unknown.

For treatment of colds or other upper respiratory infections, three trials, two large and of high quality, found that a specific extract is effective in reducing the number, duration, and severity of colds and upper respiratory infections.[196–198] These results, however, cannot be extrapolated to any other American ginseng preparations.

Cinnamon
Therapeutic Uses

Cinnamon has become popular to help lower blood glucose concentrations. The type of cinnamon being used is the same as the baking spice, *Cinnamomum cassia,* also known as bastard cinnamon. Although true cinnamon, *Cinnamomum verum* or *Cinnamomum zeylanicum,* may have similar effects, it has not been used in trials.[199]

Physiologic Activity

One chemical constituent in cinnamon, a type of procyanidin type-A polymer, may be responsible for hypoglycemic effects. Insulin sensitivity is increased via autophosphorylation of insulin receptors.[200] Cinnamon also has other components, especially in the oil, that have antifungal and antimicrobial activities.[8]

Dosage and Product Considerations

On the basis of dosages used in studies, 1 to 6 grams of ground cinnamon is given in divided doses.[8] Cinnamon is available in capsules, but patients may also take ground cinnamon in food (such as on oatmeal or apple sauce). A 1 gram dose is approximately one-half teaspoonful.[199]

Safety Considerations

No adverse events have been reported in clinical trials, although safety for more than 4 months has not been assessed. Patients should be counseled not to confuse cinnamon supplements with cinnamon oil, because there are reports of hypersensitivity reactions to cinnamon oil, as well as poisoning in a child from ingestion.[199]

Summary of Clinical Evidence

Clinical trials have had contradictory results in the management of diabetes, some of which may be associated with differences in dosage. Recent negative trials have used 1 to 1.5 grams per day, whereas trials with positive results have used 3 to 6 grams per day.[8,201–204] A pilot study of a cinnamon extract in patients with polycystic ovary syndrome that measured insulin resistance did note significant reductions.[205] At this time, cinnamon cannot be generally recommended but could be considered as an adjunctive therapy.

Dehydroepiandrosterone
Therapeutic Uses

Dehydroepiandrosterone (DHEA) is a steroid hormone secreted by the adrenal cortex. Concentrations normally decline with advancing age. DHEA is marketed primarily to treat sexual dysfunction or improve sexual performance, to combat symptoms of aging, and to enhance athletic performance or increase muscle mass.

Physiologic Activity

DHEA circulates in its sulfate storage form, dehydroepiandrosterone sulfate, and does not bind directly to estrogen or androgen receptors, but is a precursor for male and female sex hormones. Generally, in women, DHEA increases testosterone concentrations more than estrogen concentrations, whereas, in men, estrogen increases, but not testosterone.[206] The extent to which androgen and estrogen transformation occurs depends partly on a patient's baseline hormone concentrations.

Dosage and Product Considerations

For most uses, 25 mg once daily is administered. Because of greater risk of adverse effects with dosages of 50 mg and higher, patients should use these dosages only under supervision and monitoring by a primary care provider.[8,207,208] If hormone-associated effects appear (see Safety Considerations), the patient should discontinue the supplement.

Although most DHEA products are synthetically manufactured, some are extracted from animals, and therefore carry risks of contamination. Patients should be counseled to avoid these. Wild yam products are often falsely promoted as DHEA precursors. This is based on the fact that wild yam contains diosgenin, which was once used by pharmaceutical manufacturers in the production of estrogens and androgens. However, the chemical reactions necessary for transformation do not occur in the human body. Further complicating patient education is the fact that some wild yam plants do contain very small amounts of naturally occurring DHEA.

Safety Considerations

Adverse effects are sex hormone–related. Women may experience hirsutism, voice deepening, increased acne, and menstrual changes, whereas men have reported gynecomastia and testicular changes. Other side effects include increased HDL cholesterol concentrations and liver function enzymes, headache, congestion, and insomnia. At least four case reports of severe mania requiring hospitalization exist.[8,207,208] DHEA should be avoided in bipolar disorder and is contraindicated in pregnancy or lactation. DHEA should not be taken in conjunction with any other hormonal or hormone-blocking medications, or in patients with a history of breast, prostate, cervix, or endometrial cancer. One study noted increased levels of 5-alpha-androstane-3-alpha-17-beta-diol glucuronide (ADG) with DHEA supplementation in healthy young men. Because ADG may function as a prostate growth factor, high dosages and long-term use may have negative effects on prostate health.[209]

Women using DHEA must be counseled that voice changes caused by increased testosterone levels are generally irreversible.

Summary of Clinical Evidence

For documented DHEA deficiencies, some clinicians recommend DHEA supplementation. An example is in women with adrenal failure. One study found that when DHEA 50 mg per day was added to the standard hydrocortisone treatment regimen, patients showed significant improvement in general well-being, sexual function, and lipid profiles.[206] Another study using 25 mg per day, however, did not observe any benefits.[210] The efficacy of DHEA in women with adrenal failure remains unclear.

Despite marketing claims, in healthy pre- or postmenopausal women, DHEA does not improve sexual arousal or function.[211,212] However, one trial in postmenopausal women older than 70 years did note improvement of libido and sexual dysfunction, although these effects were measured on a nonvalidated questionnaire.[213] That trial and another in men of advanced age also found improved skin health, such as epidermal thickness and sebum production.[214] Two additional trials in postmenopausal women noted improvements in scores on the Kupperman index, a validated measurement of postmenopausal vasomotor and psychological symptoms.[215,216]

Clinical evidence in men with erectile dysfunction (ED) is preliminary. Significant improvement has been noted in men with ED from hypertension or unknown causes, but not for diabetes-related or neurologically induced dysfunction.[214,217] Even in these men, prescription drugs should be first-line therapy unless contraindicated.

Despite early small studies finding some benefit in healthy older men and women, all later trials have found no benefits on muscle mass or strength.[218,219] Studies using up to 100 mg daily in young healthy men have shown no increases in strength or lean body mass or improvements in athletic performance.[220,221] Two studies in older men and women have found increases in bone mineral density; more research is needed on these effects before recommendations can be made.[222,223]

Studies in healthy older men and women do not show any benefit in general well-being, memory, or cognition.[224,225]

IMMUNE STIMULANTS

Andrographis ("Indian Echinacea")

Andrographis paniculata (Burm f.) Nees from the family Acanthaceae is an annual shrub that grows in Asia and is cultivated in northern India.

Therapeutic Uses

Andrographis is typically used as an immune stimulant to prevent and treat common viral respiratory infections including the common cold and influenza.

Physiologic Activity

Andrographolide and deoxyandrographolide found in the leaf and rhizome are the active components.[226] Andrographis may have both antiviral and immunostimulating properties. Administration may increase antibody activity and phagocytosis by macrophages, as well as inhibit PAF-induced platelet aggregation.[226,227]

Dosage and Product Considerations

The recommended dosage for common cold treatment is 1.2 to 6 grams per day of the andrographis dried leaves, standardized to 5% andrographolides, for up to 7 days.[8] Commercial products are standardized to contain between 4% and 6% andrographolide. Andrographis is often evaluated in clinical trials with a single ingredient product containing only andrographis. However, andrographis is commonly available in multi-ingredient cold formulas containing other immune stimulants.

Safety Considerations

Safety data for use of andrographis is limited to 3 months. Patients may experience headache, fatigue, rash, diarrhea, and vomiting with high doses. Animal studies have suggested andrographis may decrease male and female fertility, and have possible abortifacient effects and therefore should not be used in pregnancy. Because of its proposed effect on PAF, patients taking warfarin and other platelet-active drugs or herbs should use this with caution. Andrographis should not be taken with immunosuppressive agents although no reports of this interaction have been documented.

Summary of Clinical Evidence

Clinical studies of andrographis often use visual analogue scales and rely on patients' subjective assessments to determine improvement in symptoms. In a systematic review of safety and efficacy including seven double-blind controlled trials, andrographis was superior to placebo in improving subjective symptoms of uncomplicated upper respiratory tract infections.[228] Preliminary evidence suggests it may also reduce the frequency of cold-like infections if taken chronically.[229] A phase I trial of patients with HIV infection taking high doses of andrographolide have experienced increases in CD4+ counts.[230]

Colostrum

Therapeutic Uses

Colostrum is the thin, white fluid produced by mammary glands immediately after birth prior to milk production. It provides passive immunity against many pathogens until the newborn is able to produce sufficient antibodies. In addition to treatment of diarrhea of various etiologies, colostrum is marketed for general well-being, improved athletic performance, and immune system stimulation.

Physiologic Activity

Colostrum is rich in antibodies, immunoglobulins A and E, and growth factors, which may be the components that provide immune-stimulating benefits. Hyperimmune bovine colostrum is collected from cows inoculated with pathogens to induce production of specific antibodies and immunoglobulins. There are several types of prescription hyperimmune colostrum products with FDA-approved orphan drug status for conditions such as acquired immunodeficiency syndrome (AIDS)-related diarrhea and *Cryptosporidium* infection in patients who are immunocompromised.[231] Human studies have found colostrum can increase serum concentrations of insulin-like growth factor; theories that this effect may allow better utilization of glucose have sparked research into athletic performance.[232]

Dietary supplement bovine colostrum is generally not collected from inoculated cows. The results of research with hyperimmune colostrum cannot be extrapolated to dietary supplement colostrum products (see Summary of Clinical Evidence).

Dosage and Product Considerations

Trials have used a wide range of doses and formulations. Dosages of 20 to 60 grams once daily of colostrum powder are common, although, because of the variety of available concentrations and dosage forms, following the manufacturer's listed dosing is recommended.[8]

A cow never exposed to a specific pathogen will not produce antibodies to that pathogen, so any benefit on immune function will be general in nature. Patients should be counseled to be wary of colostrum marketing claims regarding specific pathogens.

Colostrum products carry a small possibility of contamination from diseased cattle. Risk of contamination with bovine spongiform encephalitis is almost nil, because colostrum is collected from live cattle and therefore should not come in contact with nerve tissue.

Safety Considerations

Reported side effects include GI upset and increased liver function enzymes in patients with AIDS.[8,233] Individuals with milk allergies should avoid colostrum. Pregnant or lactating women should also avoid use.

Summary of Clinical Evidence

FDA-approved hyperimmune colostrums are effective for infectious diarrhea and AIDS-related diarrhea.[234] Use of these to improve athletic performance has been investigated, but the overall evidence does not demonstrate improvement in strength or endurance.[235,236]

In the United States, dietary supplement colostrum is promoted to strengthen the immune system and to improve athletic performance. To date, no clinical studies have investigated the effects of available dietary supplement colostrums.

Echinacea

Echinacea, or purple coneflower, was the most commonly used natural product according to a national survey.[1] Nine species of echinacea, a member of the Asteraceae family, are found in North America. *Echinacea* species typically used in clinical trials include *E. purpurea* (L.) Moench, *E. angustifolia* (DC.) Heller, and *E. pallida* (Nutt.) Britt. The roots, leaves, and flowers of echinacea are the medicinally active parts of the plant.

Therapeutic Uses

Echinacea has been used as an immune stimulant to prevent and treat colds and other respiratory infections.

Physiologic Activity

Echinacea has many different components that target the non-specific cellular immune system; these include alkylamides, caffeic acid derivatives (chicoric acid, chlorogenic acid, and cynarin), flavonoids, glycoproteins, isobutylamides, polyenes, and polysaccharides. Although echinacea's mechanism of action remains unclear, its effects on cellular immune system include increasing cytokine secretion, lymphocyte activity, and phagocytosis. Antiviral, antifungal, and anti-inflammatory activity has been observed.[237]

Dosage and Product Considerations

Echinacea preparations are not typically standardized to one active constituent. Echinacea is available in single- and multiple-ingredient formulations such as teas, tinctures, extracts, juices, capsules, and tablets. Each product has its own dosing regimen; however, all must be taken at first sign of a cold. Products labeled "echinacea" may be chemically different plants or plant parts. One echinacea product meets USP standards and carries the USP Verified Mark on the label.

Safety Considerations

Adverse effects may include mild GI discomfort, tingling sensation of the tongue, and headache. Patients with allergies to plants in the Asteraceae family, as well as those with a history of asthma, atopy, and allergic rhinitis should avoid echinacea. Patients with severe systemic illnesses including HIV/AIDS, multiple sclerosis, tuberculosis, and autoimmune disorders including rheumatoid arthritis should also avoid the use of echinacea. Evidence supporting this concern is limited to case reports.[238] Patients should avoid taking echinacea if they are on immunosuppressants, although no interactions have been documented. In vitro analyses have implicated echinacea as a potential inhibitor of CYP3A4 isoenzymes.[239] This interaction has not been reported in humans. Insufficient data are available to support safe use during pregnancy, although a recent systematic review found no differences in rates of major malformations.[240] Safety data on use during lactation are still lacking.

Summary of Clinical Evidence

A Cochrane review analyzed clinical trials utilizing echinacea for the treatment and prevention of the common cold.[241] Twenty-two comparisons from 16 trials of reasonable-to-good methodology were included; all but one study was double-blind. For treatment, results demonstrated from nine studies reported a significant effect on severity and duration compared with placebo, whereas six showed no benefit. A variety of echinacea-containing products were used, although *E. purpurea* demonstrated best results when administered at first appearance of symptoms. Three comparisons for prevention showed no benefit over placebo. Evidence did not support chronic use of echinacea to prevent or reduce frequency of respiratory infections.[241] Conversely, another recent meta-analysis of 14 randomized placebo-controlled studies evaluating echinacea found a significant reduction in duration of 1.4 days, and the odds of developing a cold was reduced by 58%.[242] Results of studies have been inconsistent, however, and larger prospective trials using quality products are needed.

Probiotics

Therapeutic Uses

In addition to use for antibiotic-induced diarrhea and other GI disorders (see Chapter 24), probiotics are also used for atopic dermatitis and allergies.

Physiologic Activity

Probiotics refers to several types of beneficial bacteria, including *Lactobacillus* sp., *Bifidobacteria* sp., or even one yeast, *Saccharomyces boulardii*. The exact mechanisms by which probiotics reduce symptoms of allergic reactions such as rhinitis or dermatitis are not very well understood. Probiotics decrease intestinal permeability, which may help to decrease exposure to allergens. The normalization of gut flora decreases inflammatory responses, but probiotics have some immunomodulating activity. Macrophage and lymphocyte activity are both affected, as are various cytokines, such as increased interferon-alpha and immunoglobulin, and decreased TNF.[243]

Dosage and Product Considerations

Various probiotic preparations are available, with one or multiple species. *Lactobacillus* and *Bifidobacteria* species are dosed at 1 to 10 billion colony-forming units per day, given in divided doses.[8] *Saccharomyces boulardii* is dosed at 250 to 500 mg two to four times daily.[8] For antibiotic–associated diarrhea, *Lactobacillus* and *Saccharomyces* products are recommended. For atopy and dermatitis, *Lactobacillus rhamnosus* GG is recommended.

Because the microorganisms should be live, the quality of probiotic products is essential. Some studies have found that products did not contain live cultures or adequate amounts.[244] Refrigerated products may be less likely to have suffered from degrading temperature extremes, but refrigeration is not a guarantee of quality.

Safety Considerations

Slight GI effects such as bloating and flatulence generally subside over time and can be minimized by titration when starting a supplement. Diarrhea has been reported in children.[245]

Because of reports of systemic infection, patients who are immunocompromised should avoid the use of probiotic preparations.[246] Although information is limited, no harmful effects have been observed in women in late-stage pregnancy or in breast-feeding infants during long-term use.[247] Doses of antimicrobial agents should be administered several hours apart from probiotics.

Summary of Clinical Evidence

Use of probiotics for antibiotic-associated diarrhea has strong support. Trials have noted reduced incidence and severity when used with antibiotic therapy.[248]

Clinical trials have examined use for atopic eczematous dermatitis in infants and children, and noted significant improvement in symptoms.[8] When probiotics were given to pregnant or breast-feeding women, reductions in dermatitis were observed in the infants as well.[249] Some reviews and studies have not noted similar results, which may mean that benefits may not be as extensive as previously thought.[250] A trial in infants with allergy to cow's milk found benefit in infants who were sensitized to immunoglobulin E, but not in infants who were not sensitized.[251]

Probiotics have also been tested for use in decreasing allergic rhinitis, with contradictory results.[252,253] However, because of the advantageous safety profile, it may be appropriate to attempt use of probiotics in individual patients.

PHYSICAL AND MENTAL PERFORMANCE ENHANCERS

Eleuthero

Eleutherococcus senticosus from the Araliaceae family is often referred to as Siberian ginseng. The plant is not a genus of *Panax*, as are Asian and American ginseng. *Eleutherococcus* is found in eastern Siberia, northeastern China, Korea, and Hokkaido Island.

Therapeutic Uses

Eleuthero's traditional use is as an adaptogen for improvement of athletic performance, chronic stress, and immune deficiency, although its effects are not as strong as the true ginsengs discussed in this chapter. Other uses for eleuthero include treatment of herpes simplex type II infections; normalization of blood pressure, including hypotension and hypertension; prevention of atherosclerosis; and normalization of blood glucose in diabetes mellitus.

Physiologic Activity

The active compounds of eleuthero, derived primarily from the root and leaf, are referred to as eleutherosides (subtypes A-M). Flavonoids, hydroxycinnamates, and other constituents such as sesamin, B-sitosterol, hedarasaponin B, and isofraxidin may also have biological activity. Animal studies and in vitro analysis suggest these compounds have antiplatelet, immunostimulant, and antioxidant properties.[254]

Dosage and Product Considerations

Siberian ginseng products are available in many forms with varying recommended dosages. Commercial products are often standardized to eleutheroside B and/or eleutheroside E content. Siberian ginseng extract standardized to contain eleutheroside E 0.3% in doses of 400 mg/day was used in the herpes simplex type II study.[255] In the past, eleuthero has been adulterated with other plants, such as silk vine (*Periploca graeca*) that contain cardiac glycosides, or with caffeine to enhance its stimulant effects.[256]

Safety Considerations

Both drowsiness and stimulant effects have been reported with eleuthero. Because of its variable effects on blood pressure, eleuthero should be avoided in patients with hypertension. Theoretically, patients with diabetes mellitus should be monitored for hypoglycemia. Eleuthero is recommended for only short-term use because of alleged estrogenic effects, although clinical evidence is lacking.[255] Use should be avoided in pregnancy and lactation. In patients taking digoxin, eleuthero may produce falsely elevated plasma digoxin concentrations, depending on the assay used.[256] Eleuthero does not affect activity of CYP2D6 and 3A4 at normal dosages.[257]

Summary of Clinical Evidence

Well-designed, randomized clinical trials documenting the safety and efficacy of eleuthero are lacking. In a small 6-month study, *Eleutherococcus* extract taken once daily demonstrated a beneficial effect on frequency, severity, and duration of herpes simplex type II infections.[255] Studies using standardized preparations of eleuthero are required to determine the actual benefit.

Ginseng (*Panax ginseng*)

The root and rhizome of Asian ginseng (*Panax ginseng* C.A. Meyer) is from the family Araliaceae and is exported primarily from Korea and China.

Therapeutic Uses

Asian ginseng, also classified as an adaptogen like American ginseng, has been used to treat mental and physical stress, anemia, diabetes mellitus, insomnia, impotence, and fever.

Physiologic Activity

The constituents most responsible for ginseng's adaptogen activity are triterpenoid saponins, including ginsenosides. At least 30 ginsenosides, also referred to as panaxosides, have been identified. Additional constituents include carbohydrates, B vitamins, and flavonoids.

Dosage and Product Considerations

Most studies of ginseng used dosages of extracts standardized to 4% triterpenoid glycosides between 100 and 400 mg per day. In some studies, powdered root has been used in doses of 1 to 9 grams.[8] Ginseng products may contain adulterants.

Safety Considerations

Adverse effects include insomnia, headache, blood pressure changes, anorexia, rash, mastalgia, and menstrual abnormalities. Large dosages may cause gastric upset and CNS stimulation. Use should be avoided in pregnancy and lactation because of the lack of information about effects. Ginseng should be used with caution in patients with cardiovascular disease or diabetes mellitus and in the presence of acute illness. Ginseng's effect on anticoagulant and antiplatelet therapy is not predictable. The use of ginseng with phenelzine or other MAOIs, corticosteroids, or large amounts of stimulants, including caffeine-containing beverages, should be avoided.[37,258]

The duration of treatment with ginseng should be limited to 3 months because of the possibility of hormone-like effects, although evidence for this effect is lacking. In the late 1970s a "ginseng-abuse syndrome" was described in long-term ginseng users. This report has since been discredited because the study was poorly controlled.

Summary of Clinical Evidence

Results have been inconsistent regarding Asian ginseng's ability to improve memory and cognitive function. Two small studies demonstrated that dosages of standardized extract G115 improved mental performance over placebo.[259,260] Previous studies do not support these findings.[261,262]

Small short-term studies have studied Asian ginseng's effect on fasting and postprandial glucose concentrations in people with type 2 diabetes mellitus with mixed results.[263,264] However, most studies with well-designed methodology had negative findings. A randomized, double-blind, placebo-controlled study conducted over 12 weeks demonstrated that Korean red ginseng use resulted in overall good glucose control, but failed to show a significant difference in glycosylated hemoglobin (A1C) concentrations.[265]

Green Tea

Leaves from the tea shrub *Camellia sinensis* (L.) Kuntze provide green tea. This plant belongs to the family Theaceae. Native to southeastern Asia, tea leaves are heated immediately after harvesting, then mechanically rolled and crushed before drying to produce green tea. From the same plant as green tea, black tea is produced by allowing the leaves to wilt before they are rolled and left in a humid environment for several hours. This process promotes enzymatic changes (fermentation) and a gradual change in color to reddish-brown. Oolong, another commonly available tea, is a partially fermented tea.

Therapeutic Uses

Green tea is considered a performance enhancer because of the stimulant effect from caffeine. Green tea has also been used to protect against development of many diseases, including cardiovascular disease, cancer, and liver disorders.

Physiologic Activity

In addition to caffeine, green tea contains polyphenolic compounds including flavonols (also known as catechins), flavonoids, and phenolic acids. The most prevalent flavonols include epicatechin, epicatechin-3-gallate, epigallocatechin, and epigallocatechin-3-gallate (EGCG).[266]

Dosage and Product Considerations

Dosages of green tea in epidemiologic studies vary between 1 and 10 cups daily. On average, the dosage commonly consumed in Asian countries is about 3 cups per day. Ingestion of 10 cups or more of green tea has shown benefit in reducing cholesterol concentrations. Green tea extract supplements standardized to polyphenol content retain effects similar to that of green tea while reducing exposure to caffeine.[267] Green, black, and Oolong teas are different products with varying amounts of caffeine.

Safety Considerations

Ingestion of large quantities of green tea can cause adverse GI symptoms as well as CNS and cardiac stimulation attributed to the caffeine content. Green tea (1 bag) has 20 mg of caffeine on average, with a range of 8 to 30 mg. In comparison, black tea (1 bag) has 40 mg of caffeine on average, with a range of

25 to 110 mg, and Oolong tea (1 bag) has 30 mg of caffeine on average, with a range of 12 to 55 mg.[268] Green tea should be avoided if other stimulating medications including theophylline are being ingested. Caution should be advised during pregnancy and lactation in regard to caffeine consumption. Conversely, green tea may oppose the action of sedating medications, including BZDPs. Green tea in large doses may antagonize the effects of warfarin, although brewing destroys most of its vitamin K content.[269]

Summary of Clinical Evidence

Epidemiologic evidence suggests that daily consumption of green tea may protect against cardiovascular disease as well as liver disorders.[270] Japanese men older than 40 years who consumed green tea daily had decreased serum concentrations of total cholesterol and triglyceride, and increased HDL cholesterol. However, another study of men and women who smoked cigarettes found no effect of green tea on lipids and lipoproteins.[271] A randomized controlled trial of theaflavin-enriched green tea extract demonstrated mild reductions in LDL cholesterol concentrations in patients on diets low in saturated fats.[272] Support for green tea is derived from epidemiologic studies; however, well-designed studies of a standardized product will further determine its role.[273]

Human and animal studies suggest that consumption of green tea may reduce the incidence of a variety of cancers including breast, bladder, esophageal, pancreatic, and head and neck cancers.[274,275] High levels of green tea consumption may reduce the risk of gastric cancer, although evidence suggests that low-to-moderate consumption of green tea did not reduce this risk.[276]

KIDNEY, URINARY TRACT, AND PROSTATE DISORDERS

African Plum

African plum is derived from the bark of *Prunus africana* (Hook f.) Kalkman (syn. *Pygeum africanum* Hook f.), a member of the Rosaceae family.

Therapeutic Uses

African plum tree bark has been used to treat benign prostatic hyperplasia (BPH).

Physiologic Activity

Pygeum bark contains phytosterols; pentacyclic triterpenes, including ursolic and oleanic acids; and ferulic acid esters, including

---

A WORD ABOUT Weight-Loss Products

Hoodia

One of the latest fads, hoodia (*Hoodia gordonii*), is a cactus from the Kalahari Desert. Despite claims by manufacturers, no human clinical trials have been published. There may have been one study (n = 9) conducted in Britain.[277] Limited animal studies suggest that hoodia may have an effect on the hypothalamus to increase satiety, the feeling of fullness, so human research is desirable.[8] South Africa has protected the endangered Hoodia species with special permits required to grow or harvest the plant. Very low production means that some, perhaps even the majority, of the hoodia products for sale do not actually contain hoodia.[277] Considering the lack of evidence and any information regarding adverse effects or drug interactions, hoodia should be avoided until far more information is available.

Chitosan

Another popular weight loss supplement, chitosan, is claimed to help by blocking intestinal absorption of fat.[8] That effect and weight change have been examined in several trials, with conflicting results.[278] Overall, it can be said that any possible benefit over placebo is so small that it does not outweigh even a small risk of adverse effects or the cost of the supplement. Fortunately, the adverse event profile is limited: slight GI effects and cross-reactivity with shellfish allergy. Patients should be encouraged to take a multivitamin to prevent deficiencies of fat-soluble vitamins, and to take any medications at least 2 hours from a dose of chitosan.[8]

Stimulants and "Fat-Burners"

After the FDA banned ephedra alkaloids from weight-loss supplements, manufacturers simply substituted other sources of ephedra alkaloids (heartleaf, country mallow—other banned substances) or other stimulants.[8] Guarana, as a source of caffeine, is most common, followed by bitter orange (*Citrus aurantium*) as a source of synephrine. Bitter orange may not be any safer than ephedra: Shortly after it began being widely used, case reports of cardiovascular events were published, along with two cases of ischemic colitis.[8,279] Although stimulants may provide an increased boost in weight loss, the safety issues far outweigh small benefits.

docosanol and tetracosanol. Phytosterols may compete with androgen precursors and inhibit prostaglandin synthesis in the prostate. Triterpenes may also have anti-inflammatory properties. Ferulic acid esters reduce prolactin concentrations as well as prostate cholesterol concentrations, a precursor to testosterone synthesis.[280] Minimal inhibition of 5-alpha-reductase is observed. Pygeum reduces excitability of the detrusor muscle, increases prostatic secretions, and possibly decreases proliferation of fibroblasts within the prostate.[281]

Dosage and Product Considerations

Products are standardized to contain 14% triterpenes and 0.5% n-docosanol; the average dosage is 50 to 100 mg twice daily.[280] Combination products with saw palmetto or pumpkin may provide additional benefit if all ingredients are in standardized dosing.[8]

In 1998, the demand for pygeum extract was so high that it caused the African plum tree to become a threatened species, with current international trade being monitored under the Convention on International Trade in Endangered Species of Wild Fauna and Flora.[281]

Safety Considerations

Most adverse effects involve GI complaints, including diarrhea, constipation, and gastric pain.[281] Men presenting with prostate symptoms should contact their primary care provider before starting pygeum to rule out prostate cancer. It is unclear whether pygeum affects prostate-specific antigen (PSA) levels. The risk of side effects with pygeum is increased if combined with finasteride.[8] Due to possibility of hormonal effects, pygeum should be avoided in pregnancy and lactation.

Summary of Clinical Evidence

Pygeum has demonstrated improvements in urinary flow, void volumes, residual volumes, nocturia, daytime frequency, and subjective symptom assessments of BPH. Larger studies including standardized dosing, active comparisons, and adequate duration to detect significant differences are needed to fully assess its efficacy.[282]

Cranberry

Cranberry (*Vaccinium macrocarpon* Ait.) is an evergreen bush native to North America belonging to the family Ericaceae.

Therapeutic Uses

Cranberry has been used to prevent and treat urinary tract infections (UTI).

Physiologic Activity

Cranberry contains proanthocyanidins. Epicatechin is the primary proanthocyanidin found in cranberry extracts. The exact mechanism is unknown, but evidence suggests that cranberry blocks bacteria, *Escherichia coli* in particular, from adhering to bladder, kidneys, and urethra. Fructose found in cranberry juice may also alter bacterial adhesion.[283]

Dosage and Product Considerations

The ideal dosage of cranberry has not been established given that many studies used unsweetened cranberry juices. Cranberry juice cocktail is approximately 30% pure cranberry juice and contains more sugar; it is unknown if this product will demonstrate the same effects. For prevention of UTI, the dosage of cranberry juice is 300 to 900 mL per day. Encapsulated cranberry formulations at a dosage of approximately 400 mg three times daily may be preferred to avoid the sugar content of juices.[8] Fresh or frozen cranberries may also be used, although the bitter taste makes this method unpopular.

Safety Considerations

Evidence suggests that regular use of cranberry concentrate tablets might increase risk of kidney stones.[284] Patients may experience diarrhea with large daily doses. Theoretically, cranberry juice may alter excretion of weakly alkaline drugs or neutralize effects of antacids. Case reports have emerged suggesting cranberry may cause bleeding in patients taking warfarin.[285] Cranberry may be a CYP2C9 inhibitor although only the warfarin interaction has been reported.

Summary of Clinical Evidence

Clinical trials suggest that daily consumption of cranberry juice may prevent UTI. A recent Cochrane database systematic review of 10 studies concluded preventive use of cranberry products over 12 months significantly reduces incidence of UTIs. Various cranberry formulations were included in the meta-analysis. Women with recurrent UTIs received more benefit than did elderly or catheterized patients. A high dropout rate in some trials suggests long-term cranberry use may not be well tolerated.[286] Cranberry does not prevent UTIs in patients with neurogenic bladder.[287] Evidence does not support its use in treating UTIs and patients should be referred to their health care provider.[288]

Saw Palmetto

Saw palmetto (*Serenoa repens* [Michx.] G. Nichols), a dwarf palm tree from the Arecaceae family, is native to the southeast coastal region of the United States.

Therapeutic Uses

Saw palmetto has been used to treat BPH.

Physiologic Activity

The lipophilic extracts from the ripened fruit contain saturated and unsaturated fatty acids and plant sterols. Although the active compounds responsible have not been identified, they are likely present in the lipophilic extract. Saw palmetto inhibits 5-alpha-reductase and cytosolic androgen receptor binding, and has local antiestrogenic and anti-inflammatory effects on the prostate.[289]

Dosage and Product Considerations

The usual dosage is 160 mg twice daily or 320 mg once daily. Saw palmetto products should contain 80% to 95% standardized fatty acids.[8]

Safety Considerations

In comparative clinical trials, saw palmetto has been shown to be better tolerated than finasteride and tamsulosin. GI complaints are most commonly reported. One report exists of a 54-year-old man taking saw palmetto who had intraoperative hemorrhage during surgery.[290] Saw palmetto should be used with caution in patients taking any drug or natural product that might prolong bleeding. Patients concomitantly taking androgenic medications should avoid use. Men with prostate symptoms should contact their provider before starting saw palmetto to rule out prostate cancer. Saw palmetto is occasionally used in multi-ingredient products intended for women; because of the inhibition of 5-alpha-reductase, it should be considered as a Pregnancy Category X and also should not be used in lactation.

Summary of Clinical Evidence

In a systematic review, saw palmetto provided mild-to-moderate improvement in urinary symptoms and flow measures in men with BPH.[291] Improvements were similar to those seen with finasteride, and saw palmetto was associated with fewer adverse effects. Typical study durations range from 4 to 48 weeks. However, a recent randomized double-blind trial including 225 men with moderate-to-severe BPH found saw palmetto did not improve symptoms or objective measures compared with placebo.[292] The baseline American Urological Association Symptom Index (AUASI) was 8 or greater; therefore, the results are not applicable to men with mild, symptomatic BPH (AUASI: 0–7). Long-term data on the efficacy and safety of saw palmetto are lacking. Saw palmetto does not alter prostate volume or PSA concentrations.

MUSCULOSKELETAL SYSTEM

Chondroitin Sulfate

Therapeutic Uses

Chondroitin sulfate (CS) is a glucosaminoglycan made from glucuronic acid and galactosamine present in animal cartilage. CS solution, in combination with hyaluronic acid, has FDA-approved labeling as an ophthalmic viscosurgical device for use in cataract surgery and corneal transplants. As a dietary supplement, CS is usually combined with other supplements in products for osteoarthritis and joint health, and has primarily been studied for knee and hip osteoarthritis.

Physiologic Activity

Similar to glucosamine, CS serves as building material for cartilage production, but it also inhibits leukocyte elastase, an enzyme involved in cartilage degradation.[293] CS may also stimulate chondrocytes to produce more cartilage components.[294] Some evidence suggests chondroitin has beneficial effects lasting beyond dates of use.[295]

Dosage and Product Considerations

For osteoarthritis, the recommended dosage is 1200 mg daily, either once or in divided doses.[8] Because many products include both glucosamine and chondroitin, patients should know that chondroitin, the ingredient with less evidence of efficacy, is also the more expensive ingredient. A patient concerned about cost could be advised to begin treatment with glucosamine sulfate (see glucosamine discussion regarding salt form) monotherapy. If after 4 to 5 months, benefit is seen but symptoms are still bothersome, a CS product may be added or a combination product used. If no additional benefit is apparent after 3 to 5 months, the CS should be discontinued. Patients should be counseled to take CS with food if nausea or GI upset occurs.

Because CS is an animal product, concern about contamination is always present. Often, CS is still produced from bovine trachea, so these carry an added risk of bacterial contamination. Because the trachea does not contain great amounts of neural tissue, the risk of contamination with bovine spongiform encephalitis (mad cow disease) is minimal. Of more concern is that several CS supplements have been shown to contain little actual chondroitin.[35]

Safety Considerations

Occasional adverse reactions include mild GI upset and nausea.[8] During clinical trials, allergic reactions, edema, diarrhea, constipation, nausea, heartburn, and hair loss were reported infrequently.[294-296] One report documented exacerbation of previously well-controlled asthma, which resolved completely on discontinuation of the glucosamine/chondroitin product.[297] Use in pregnancy or lactation should be avoided because of lack of information on effects.

Some animal studies have shown intravenous CS to have antithrombotic properties.[298] Although there are currently no reports of increased bleeding in humans, patients should monitor carefully for signs of bleeding, especially if also on anticoagulants or antiplatelet agents.

Summary of Clinical Evidence

Information on chondroitin's efficacy is limited, because few trials have examined chondroitin monotherapy. Meta-analyses have concluded that, despite the limited size and quality of some trials, CS therapy may provide moderate benefit in osteoarthritis, especially in combination with nonsteroidal anti-inflammatory drug (NSAID) therapy.[294,299] This finding is borne out by results of the most recent trial, which noted improvement in the joint space structure, although not in symptoms, despite use of a low dose, 800 mg/day.[300] In addition, a 1-year trial in which patients received 800 mg/day for months 1 to 3 and then months 6 to 9 noted statistically and clinically significant improvement in pain and function index scores during both active treatment and the 3 months of no treatment.[295]

Devil's Claw

Therapeutic Uses

Devil's claw, *Harpagophytum procumbens,* is an African desert plant often recommended for arthritis and back and joint pain. Both the dried ground root and standardized extracts are used.

Physiologic Activity

Devil's claw has anti-inflammatory, anticonvulsant, analgesic, and hypoglycemic activity.[301-303] Although the plant and its extracts have demonstrated anti-inflammatory effects in animal and human studies, much of the scientific data regarding the mechanism are conflicting.[8] Harpagoside is one of the iridoid glycosides present in devil's claw and is believed to be the primary active component; products are often standardized to harpagoside content. However, harpagoside is not responsible for all of the anti-inflammatory activity of devil's claw. For example, TNF release is inhibited by extracts, but not by the harpagoside alone.[304] Thromboxane release is inhibited, but none of the constituents affect cyclooxygenases (COX) ex vivo, although COX-2 inhibition is seen in vitro.[301] Effects in arthritis may be linked to inhibition of matrix metalloproteinases, enzymes that degrade cartilage.[305]

Dosage and Product Considerations

Dosage of devil's claw is determined by harpagoside content with 50 to 60 mg per day in divided doses recommended. Because standardization may differ, the total amount of extract needed to reach the desired harpagoside content may vary.

Safety Considerations

Adverse effects include diarrhea, headache, anorexia, and rash. A few trials have reported dropouts owing to diarrhea.[306] Reductions in blood pressure are mentioned in animal studies but have not been seen in trials.

Because of hypoglycemic and hypotensive effects noted in animal studies, devil's claw is not recommended in patients with diabetes or cardiac disease.[8] Usage in pregnancy and lactation is not recommended.

Although there is currently only one report of an interaction resulting in increased bleeding, devil's claw should not be used with warfarin.[8]

Summary of Clinical Evidence

For osteoarthritis, at least five trials have examined efficacy and demonstrated pain relief greater than placebo or equivalent to a prescription pain medication.[8] A recent systematic review concluded that the available evidence does support of use of devil's claw for osteoarthritis.[307]

Devil's claw has been compared with placebo, NSAIDS, a COX-2 inhibitor, and controls such as massage and acupuncture for the treatment of lower back pain. All but one study found greater benefit in pain relief and increased mobility in patients receiving devil's claw.[307] Overall, the clinical evidence does support use in patients with chronic back pain not associated with disk or nerve root conditions.

Glucosamine
Therapeutic Uses

Glucosamine is one of the more well-researched dietary supplements. A substance used by the body to make cartilage, it is primarily promoted for osteoarthritis.

Physiologic Activity

Exogenous administration of glucosamine, an endogenous mucopolysaccharide, increases the components available for cartilage synthesis. Because sulfur is essential for glycosaminoglycan bonds within cartilage, the sulfate salt form may also provide important activity.[308] In addition, glucosamine promotes its own use by stimulating production of cartilage and synovial fluid by chondrocytes and synoviocytes. It also inhibits matrix metalloproteinase and modulates activities of collagenase and cytokines involved in stress reactions.[309,310] A recent study demonstrated greater effectiveness of glucosamine in patients with high cartilage turnover rates, as indicated by increased levels of collagen type II.[311] More research is needed to determine if results of this assay could be used to predict a successful or unsuccessful response to glucosamine therapy.

Dosage and Product Considerations

For osteoarthritis, the appropriate dosage is 1500 mg daily of the sulfate salt form, given in one or divided doses.[8] The majority of trials demonstrating efficacy and safety have used glucosamine sulfate, primarily a crystalline form from Rotta Laboratories. One small trial and a large recent trial found no benefit over placebo for the hydrochloride form.[312,313] Although other evidence supports some efficacy with the hydrochloride form, the sulfate form should be recommended.[8] Any GI upset is usually alleviated by taking in divided doses with meals. Patients should be counseled that glucosamine will not provide pain relief as quickly as NSAIDs or acetaminophen might. Effects may not be experienced for 6 to 8 weeks, with full benefits not evident for several months.

Some topical preparations containing glucosamine (and other ingredients known to be topically effective for osteoarthritis) are currently marketed. Only one small trial with severe methodologic limitations has been conducted.[314] Although one study found that glucosamine is absorbed transdermally, additional confirmation and clinical trials are needed before topical glucosamine can be recommended.[315]

Safety Considerations

Nausea, stomach upset, constipation, and diarrhea are the most common adverse effects.[8] Drowsiness, headache, and skin reactions have been infrequently reported.

Glucosamine can be manufactured from shellfish chitin as well as produced synthetically. Some manufacturers have claimed that their products are allergen-free, because processing does remove much of the allergenic material. One study tested this claim using one particular product and found no reactions in 15 individuals with shellfish allergies.[316] Because source materials may not remain consistent, even for a particular manufacturer, patients with severe shellfish allergies should avoid glucosamine.

One report documented exacerbation of previously well-controlled asthma, which resolved completely on discontinuation of a glucosamine-chondroitin product.[297]

Because of glucosamine's glucose-based chemical structure, the potential risk of hyperglycemia has been concern; many reference texts still contain cautions regarding hyperglycemia. Two 3-year studies with glucosamine sulfate found no changes in glycemic indicators in any subjects, a recent study of a glucosamine hydrochloride and chondroitin combination noted no changes in A1C levels in patients with diabetes, and a study examining insulin resistance in patients without diabetes found no effects.[317–320] Patients with diabetes initiating glucosamine therapy should simply monitor glucose levels more closely for a few days to ensure stability of levels.

Although anecdotal reports of cholesterol elevations in patients taking glucosamine have been discussed, no published case reports exist and no indication of changes in lipid status has been observed in any long-term clinical trials or a short-term safety trial.[317,318,321] A check of lipid concentrations approximately 1 month after starting glucosamine is a sensible precaution. Pregnant or lactating women should avoid glucosamine because of the lack of information about its effects. There are no known interactions.

Summary of Clinical Evidence

Multiple clinical trials have compared glucosamine sulfate against placebo and/or standard treatments such as NSAID therapy for the treatment of osteoarthritis. The majority had positive results for symptoms, showing greater benefit than placebo and similar efficacy in symptom relief to NSAID treatment, although the studies were small and had methodologic limitations.[322,323] Two large (n = 202, 212) well-designed 3-year studies in patients with knee osteoarthritis demonstrated significant efficacy and safety.[317,318] Subjects had significant reduction of knee cartilage loss and some experienced increased cartilage growth compared with placebo patients. A recent large (n = 318), well-designed study also found benefit compared with placebo and acetaminophen.[324] Meta-analyses of randomized, controlled trials have concluded that glucosamine sulfate is safe and effective for the treatment of osteoarthritis, although the full extent of effectiveness is not known.[322,323]

Methyl-Sulfonyl-Methane

Therapeutic Uses

Methyl-sulfonyl-methane (MSM), also known as dimethylsulfone, is a naturally occurring compound found in foods such as vegetables and milk. MSM has become a popular ingredient in dietary supplements for use in arthritis and allergies despite little evidence. MSM is a major metabolite of dimethylsulfoxide (DMSO), an industrial solvent that workers with arthritis began using topically; MSM was developed as a therapy in an attempt to avoid the toxicity and unpleasant side effects of DMSO.[325]

Physiologic Activity

MSM is a source of sulfur, released on breakdown by intestinal bacteria. The sulfur is then incorporated into amino acids such as cysteine and methionine. The mechanism for activity in osteoarthritis is unclear, although sulfur is essential for bonding in cartilage, and animal studies have found lower levels of sulfur in arthritic cartilage.[326] One study did find a decrease in joint disease in a rheumatoid arthritis mice model.[327] Much of the touted evidence is for DMSO, rather than MSM. The two products have many different properties.[325]

Dosage and Product Considerations

Currently, there is not enough evidence or information about safety to recommend MSM for osteoarthritis. Patients should be counseled on treatment choices with greater evidence. Dosages used in clinical trials have varied widely.[8] If a patient chooses to use MSM, counseling should include cautions not to exceed a dose range of 1500 to 3000 mg daily in one or divided doses, as well as information about expected adverse effects (see Safety Considerations).

MSM can be destroyed by water or excessive heat in manufacture or storage. Proper storage away from excessive heat and moisture will preserve supplement quality.

Safety Considerations

The rarely reported adverse effects include headache, pruritus, nausea, and diarrhea.[328] One 90-day high-dose study in rats demonstrated no toxicities.[329] Use in pregnancy and lactation should be avoided because of lack of information about effects. No drug interactions are known.

Summary of Clinical Evidence

For osteoarthritis, one 12-week trial (n = 118) comparing MSM with glucosamine sulfate, placebo, and the combination of MSM and glucosamine sulfate found statistically significant improvement in pain and functioning in all groups but placebo. Improvement was greater in the combination group than with either MSM or glucosamine sulfate alone.[330] A smaller trial (n = 50) of MSM versus placebo also noted greater improvement in the MSM group.[331]

Only one uncontrolled study (n = 55) has evaluated MSM for seasonal allergic rhinitis.[328] Although significant reductions in allergy symptom questionnaire scores were noted, one trial is not enough evidence to be able to recommend its use.

S-Adenosyl-L-Methionine

Therapeutic Uses

S-adenosyl-L-methionine (SAMe) is an endogenous substance formed from L-methionine and ATP that is also sold as a dietary supplement. SAMe is used for osteoarthritis and depression.

Physiologic Activity

SAMe is produced primarily in the liver; liver disease and low B_{12} and folate levels may decrease SAMe concentrations.[332] SAMe donates methyl groups to endogenous substances, including neurotransmitters and catecholamines. It crosses the blood–brain barrier and increases brain neurotransmitter levels, including norepinephrine, dopamine, and serotonin.[333] For osteoarthritis, SAMe's mechanism of action is unknown. It may serve as a source of sulfur required for cartilage growth and repair, and to stimulate proteoglycan production. Some anti-inflammatory and analgesic effects may also exist.

Dosage and Product Considerations

For osteoarthritis, most trials have used doses of 400 to 800 mg per day in divided doses, whereas doses for depression are 1200 to 1600 mg daily (see Safety Considerations).[8]

Depression is not self-treatable. Because of the potential for serious psychological adverse effects, SAMe should not be used for self-treatment of depression.

Safety Considerations

The most common adverse effects include nausea, diarrhea, and heartburn.[331,333,334] Less frequently, dry mouth, vomiting, headache, dizziness, nervousness, insomnia, cognitive impairment, and a switch to manic state in patients with bipolar disorder have also been reported.[332,333,335,336] In addition, SAMe has been associated with development of hypomania or severe mania in subjects with no personal or family history of mania or bipolar disorder.[337–339] At least one report of mixed mania was associated with suicidal ideation within 2 weeks.[332]

Some adverse effects may be dose-related, because mania/hypomania has not been reported in any osteoarthritis trials using the lower dosages.[8] More research is needed to determine if this association is accurate. Until more is known, it is a reasonable precaution to encourage the avoidance of SAMe and use of treatments with greater evidence of efficacy and safety. Patients who choose to use SAMe should take the lowest dosage that provides relief of osteoarthritis symptoms.

In several trials, SAMe has been associated with significantly increased homocysteine concentrations.[332,339,340] At least two studies, however, have not found such changes and, although hyperhomocysteinemia may be a risk factor for cardiovascular disease, the clinical relevance is controversial.[341] Until more is known, patients with preexisting hyperhomocysteinemia should avoid this dietary supplement.

SAMe should not be used with other serotonergic agents, such as SSRIs or 5-hydroxytryptamine$_1$ (5-HT$_1$)-agonists for migraine, because of increased risk of serotonin syndrome. The concomitant use of SAMe and corticosteroids should be avoided until more is known about possible effects on glucocorticoid concentrations.

Long-term safety issues have yet to be determined. Although one study of intravenous SAMe in pregnant women noted no adverse outcomes, SAMe should not be used in pregnancy or lactation until more is known about possible fetal effects.[334]

Summary of Clinical Evidence

Many early trials with positive results were of short duration and poor design, and used injectable dosage forms.[341] Several literature reviews and a meta-analysis have concluded that, despite trial limitations, SAMe performed significantly better than placebo and similarly to NSAIDS in restoring functionality and decreasing pain, although with a slower onset of action.[342,343] Effects were similar in comparison with a COX2 inhibitor.[342]

Clinical trials for depression have been small and with many methodologic limitations. Two meta-analyses examining results with both intravenous and oral SAMe concluded that SAMe does have efficacy for depression.[344,345] One meta-analysis suggested clinical benefits may be comparable to those of tricyclic antidepressants. Symptom improvement occurs more rapidly with SAMe than with standard antidepressant treatment. Changes have been seen as early as 1 to 2 weeks, although those responses were observed in trials using intravenous doses or intravenous and oral dose combinations.[341] No comparisons with SSRIs have been conducted, although one trial found benefit when SAMe was added to either SSRI or venlafaxine therapy in patients who had not responded to their antidepressant therapy alone.[346]

A few small trials examining SAMe for depression associated with fibromyalgia noted an improvement in pain and other physical and psychological symptoms.[347–349] Although evidence is limited, few effective therapies for fibromyalgia exist and may lead clinicians to attempt SAMe therapy in patients who are refractory to treatment.

SKIN AND MUCOUS MEMBRANE CONDITIONS

Melissa (Lemon Balm)

Melissa is derived from the plant *Melissa officinalis* L. of the family Lamiaceae.

Therapeutic Uses

Melissa is used commonly as a topical cream for cold sores (herpes labialis) and orally for relaxation, AD, insomnia, or nervous stomach. It is inhaled as a part of aromatherapy.

Physiologic Activity

Melissa's effects may be a result of volatile oils extracted from the plant's leaves that are believed to have sedative, antioxidant, and antiviral effects. Preliminary research suggests orally administered lemon balm may have acetylcholine receptor activity.[350]

Dosage and Product Considerations

For herpetic lesions, studies have used a cream or ointment containing 1% of a 70:1 lyophilized aqueous extract, which is applied two to five times daily at first sign of symptoms until after all lesions heal.[8] Treatment of herpes with melissa does not alter the ability to transmit the infection to others.

Safety Considerations

Hypersensitivity reactions and skin irritation have been associated with topical application. Theoretically, concomitant use of herbs and medications with sedating properties should not be combined with oral ingestion of lemon balm. Use should be avoided in pregnancy and lactation because of the lack of information about effects.

Summary of Clinical Evidence

In the treatment of oral herpes, application of melissa cream produced significant benefits by reducing the intensity of discomfort as well as the number and size of lesions. Long-term follow-up suggested that chronic application also delays the time to the next herpes flare-up.[351,352] Orally administered lemon balm has been investigated for use for improving AD, cognitive function, and mood modulation.[350,353,354]

Tea Tree Oil

Tea tree oil is derived from leaves of the tree *Melaleuca alternifolia* (Maiden & Betche) Cheel from the family Myrtaceae. The tea tree is not related to the plant that is used to make black and green teas.

Therapeutic Uses

Tea tree oil has been used as an antiseptic and anti-infective agent.

Physiologic Activity

Tea tree leaves contain about 2% of volatile oil, with more than 100 monoterpenenoid, sesquiterpenoid, and alcohol compounds.

The primary constituent is terpinen–4–ol, which is active against pathogenic bacteria and fungi, likely through effects on membrane permeability

Dosage and Product Concerns

The oil is applied topically once or twice daily in solution concentrations of 0.4% to 100%, depending on the condition and area of treatment. For acne, a 5% concentration is applied daily for up to 3 months. For athlete's foot, tea tree oil cream 25% to 50% is applied twice daily for 4 weeks. For fungal toenail infections, tea tree oil 100% has been used twice daily for 6 months.[8]

Safety Considerations

Skin irritation may occur in sensitive patients. Although the oil can be safely used on oral mucosa, it should not be swallowed, because ingesting even small amounts may cause confusion, ataxia, and systemic contact dermatitis that resolve very slowly.[355] Prepubertal gynecomastia was reported in three boys using topical tea tree and lavender oils, but resolved upon discontinuation.[356]

Summary of Clinical Evidence

Studies have found that tea tree oil may be an effective treatment for athlete's foot and other fungal infections of the skin and nails.[357,358] However, for onychomycosis, tea tree oil was compared with clotrimazole 1% solution, not to available prescription medications. In the treatment of acne, daily application of a tea tree oil gel 5% for 3 months appeared to reduce the average number of lesions at a rate similar to that of benzoyl peroxide 5% but with less irritation.[359] Tea tree oil may be an option for those not tolerating current therapies for the treatment of athlete's foot, onychomycosis, or acne. Tea tree oil has also been investigated in fluconazole-resistant oral *Candida* infections occurring in patients with AIDS.[360]

WOMEN'S HEALTH

Black Cohosh

Black cohosh is made from the dried rhizome and roots of *Cimicifuga racemosa* (L.) Nutt., formerly *Actaea racemosa*. It is a member of the Ranunculaceae family.

Therapeutic Uses

Traditionally black cohosh has been used to treat the symptoms of premenstrual syndrome (PMS), dysmenorrhea, menopause, and rheumatoid arthritis.

Physiologic Activity

The primary active components of black cohosh rhizomes are triterpene glycosides, including acetein, cimicifugoside, and 27 deoxyacetin. Isoflavones such as formononetin may be present, but they may be absent from commercial products. Other constituents include isoferulic and salicylic acids, tannins, resin, starch, and sugars.[361] Although the issue is controversial, black cohosh probably does not exhibit estrogenic activity, and it has shown no effect on vaginal epithelium, endometrium, or hormone concentrations.[362,363]

Dosage and Product Considerations

Black cohosh, as a standardized extract, is usually administered as 40 mg daily in one or two doses.[8] The most commonly used commercial preparation is Remifemin. The preparation is standardized to 20 mg of the root per tablet, consisting of 1 mg of triterpene glycosides.[364]

Safety Considerations

Adverse effects are mild, with GI complaints, headache, rash, and weight gain occurring occasionally. Hepatitis, seizures, and cardiovascular disease have been reported in patients taking multiple herbal products including black cohosh.[365] Approximately 30 case reports of acute hepatitis associated with black cohosh have also been published. The Dietary Supplement Information Expert Committee has recommended a cautionary statement regarding potential hepatotoxicity be placed on products.[366] Clinical data on drug interactions with black cohosh are limited. Black cohosh may have additive effects with tamoxifen and may increase the toxicity of doxorubicin and docetaxel.[367] The use of black cohosh longer than 6 months is not recommended because of the lack of long-term safety studies.[368] Use should be avoided in pregnancy and lactation because of potential hormonal effects.

Summary of Clinical Evidence

Since publication of the Women's Health Initiative, interest in black cohosh as an alternative to estrogen replacement therapy (ERT) has increased.[369] Several clinical trials have evaluated black cohosh for menopausal symptoms with mixed results. The use of validated outcome measures has varied.

A 6-month study of 150 peri- and postmenopausal women showed that 40 mg daily provided the same symptom relief as 120 mg daily. Although symptoms were relieved in 70% of the subjects regardless of dose, the study was not placebo-controlled. No evidence of estrogenic effects from the product was detected.[370] A large study (n = 2016) of women evaluating Remifemin use on subjective symptoms of menopause also found a significant reduction in symptoms at the end of 12 weeks. However, this study too had no placebo for comparison.[371] A randomized placebo-controlled study enrolled women (n = 304) and demonstrated symptomatic relief of vasomotor symptoms, especially in women earlier in the peri- and postmenopausal period. The study used 40 mg daily of a standardized isopropanolic extract of black cohosh root.[372]

The Herbal Alternatives for Menopause Trial (HALT) evaluated three formulations of black cohosh: black cohosh alone, a multibotanical containing black cohosh, or the multibotanical combined with dietary soy. Hormone therapy and placebo served as comparison for the treatment of vasomotor symptoms. The randomized, double-blind study (n = 351) concluded at 1 year that black cohosh, in any formulation, was not effective.[373] Although an overall design was strong, the study was underpowered to detect small changes in symptom frequency, and quality of the multibotanical preparations has been questioned.

The safety and efficacy of black cohosh in women who have had breast cancer remains controversial.[362] A double-blind, randomized, placebo-controlled trial including women undergoing or completing breast cancer treatment (n = 132) evaluated crossover use of black cohosh or placebo for two 4-week periods. No significant differences between the treatments with regard to hot flashes or toxicity were found.[374] Women who were breast cancer survivors also failed to find a difference between black cohosh and placebo in reducing the number or intensity of hot flashes. Concentrations of follicle-stimulating hormone and luteinizing hormone were similar in the two groups.[375]

The North American Menopause Society recommends a trial of nonprescription products such as black cohosh for mild vasomotor symptoms. Their position statement acknowledges that the clinical trial data are insufficient but supports short-term use because of the overall safety profile.[376] The long-term effects of black cohosh on cardiovascular disease, osteoporosis, and breast cancer are unknown.

Chastetree Berry

Chastetree (*Vitex agnus-castus* L.), commonly referred to as vitex, is a member of the Verbenaceae family. The dried ripe fruits or berries and the leaves are the medicinally useful parts of the plant.

Therapeutic Uses

Chastetree berry has been used to treat symptoms of PMS, dysmenorrhea, mastalgia, and menopausal symptoms.

Physiologic Activity

The fruits contain essential oils, diterpines, glycosides, and various flavonoids including casticin, orientin, and quercetagetin. Effects on menstrual regulation are likely due to dopaminergic compounds responsible for suppressing prolactin release by binding to dopamine-2 receptors.[377] Progestin and estrogen-related compounds may also be present in the fruit.[8]

Dosage and Product Considerations

Clinical trials have used 20 to 40 mg of the extract daily. The standardization of chastetree berry has not been well established.[8]

Safety Considerations

GI complaints occur occasionally. Other symptoms include dry mouth, headache, rashes, itching, acne, menstrual disorders, and agitation. Use should be avoided in pregnancy because of potential effects on the uterus. Chastetree berry potentially may interact with dopaminergic antagonists and oral contraceptives, but these interactions have not been documented.[378]

Summary of Clinical Evidence

Clinical trials support efficacy of chastetree berry in improving mild-to-moderate symptoms associated with PMS. A double-blind study (n = 170) of women with PMS compared the effect of chastetree berry extract daily with placebo on mood, breast fullness, and other symptoms over three menstrual cycles. The results indicated that chastetree berry extract improved the main symptom scores and had a significantly greater overall

response rate than placebo. Symptoms improved in 24% of women taking placebo compared with 52% of women taking the botanical.[379] This study was well designed, with a placebo group, a large number of women with PMS using established diagnostic criteria, descriptive data on the study groups at baseline, and a method of scoring symptoms. Long-term effects are unknown.

Preliminary evidence suggests there may be benefit in premenstrual dysphoric disorder and cyclic mastalgia.[380,381]

Evening Primrose Oil

Evening primrose (*Oenothera biennis* L.) is a member of the primrose family Onagraceae and is used for its high content of essential fatty acids. The seed oils of black currant (*Ribes nigrum* L.) and borage (*Borago officinalis* L.) are also used for similar purposes.

Therapeutic Uses

Evening primrose oil (EPO) has been used for mastalgia, symptoms of PMS and menopause, preeclampsia, diabetic neuropathy, chronic fatigue syndrome, and atopic dermatitis.

Physiologic Activity

The oil from evening primrose seeds consists of at least 85% to 92% unsaturated fatty acids. Most of the polyunsaturated fatty acids are the essential *cis*-linoleic acid and the rare *cis*-gamma-linolenic acid (GLA) forms thought to be responsible for anti-inflammatory activity. The seed oil contains smaller amounts of palmitic, oleic, and stearic acids, as well as steroids, including campesterol and beta-sitosterol.

Dosage and Product Considerations

In clinical trials, daily dosages of EPO 2 to 4 grams have been used. Depending on the brand, the oil contains a minimum of 8% to 16% GLA.

Safety Considerations

Adverse effects of EPO include headache, nausea, diarrhea, and abdominal pain occurring occasionally. EPO products may possess antiplatelet effects, and patients taking warfarin and other platelet-active drugs or herbs should use this botanical with caution. Concurrent use with phenothiazines potentially may result in seizures.[365] Use of EPO for cervical ripening during labor may be associated with adverse pregnancy outcomes including prolonged rupture of membranes and vacuum extraction.[382]

Summary of Clinical Evidence

Despite its widespread use, study results with EPO for PMS have been contradictory and inconsistent. A well-designed study of 120 women with severe mastalgia failed to demonstrate a difference between EPO and its control oil on the number of days with breast pain.[383]

Although more evidence is needed, there have been promising outcomes with EPO in the treatment of atopic dermatitis and diabetic neuropathy.[384,385]

Phytoestrogens

Phytoestrogens are derived from many different plants.

Therapeutic Uses

Phytoestrogens, including soy and red clover products, have been used primarily for symptoms associated with menopause. Preliminary evidence suggests that phytoestrogens may have a role in preventing prostate cancer.

Physiologic Activity

Phytoestrogen supplements have been derived primarily from soy (*Glycine max* [L.] Merrill) and red clover (*Trifolium pratense* L.). Soy-based phytoestrogens may include isoflavones such as genistein, daidzein, and glycitein. Red clover–based products may include biochanin, genistein, daidzein, and formononetin. These compounds have multiple complex effects including estrogenic, antiestrogenic, antioxidant, and anticancer activity.

Dosage and Administration Guidelines

A recommended dosage of "phytoestrogen" has not been established. Products contain varying amounts and types of isoflavones. Products derived from soy and red clover sources may have different effects. The benefits from soy are primarily from dietary sources, not from supplements. Soy supplements meeting USP standards are available.

Safety Considerations

Phytoestrogen products derived from soy or red clover are well tolerated. GI complaints, headaches, and allergic reactions may occur. The long-term safety of phytoestrogens is not established, especially with respect to the risk of estrogen-dependent cancers and thromboembolic disease. The safety of phytoestrogen supplements in women with estrogen-receptor–positive breast cancer is unknown, and the supplements should be avoided.[386] Coumestans in red clover may increase the risk of bleeding, especially if warfarin and similar drugs are taken concomitantly, although evidence of an interaction is limited. Genistein may counteract the beneficial effect of tamoxifen in slowing breast cancer growth.[387] Daidzein may inhibit the activity of CYP1A2.[388]

Summary of Clinical Evidence

Publication of the Women's Health Initiative has suggested that the risks of ERT may outweigh its benefits in some women.[369] The purported benefits of phytoestrogens, especially soy-based products, are based on population-based observational studies of dietary patterns in different parts of the world. It is simplistic to think that the lifetime risk of any given disease is related solely to the presence or absence of one dietary component such as isoflavones. A second critical factor is the recognition that the phytoestrogen content in foods, especially of the biologically active isoflavones, will vary significantly even in soy foods, let alone supplements.

The most common use of phytoestrogens is for managing vasomotor symptoms. A recent Cochrane database systematic review found a lack of difference between phytoestrogen treatments and placebo in alleviating symptoms. Thirty trials met inclusion criteria; however, only a few high-quality trials using red clover (Promensil) were suitable for analysis. Those that did show benefit were of low quality or underpowered. In addition, for up to 2 years of use, there was no evidence of adverse effects on the endometrium.[389] Another systematic review that included soy foods and extracts, as well as red clover–based products, reported that hot flushes and other symptoms were not improved.[390] A 3-month study compared two red clover products with placebo in women (n = 252) experiencing at least 35 hot flashes per week. One product contained a higher content of biochanin A and genistein (Promensil), whereas the other had higher amounts of formononetin and daidzein (Rimostil). The two active products were similar to placebo in reduction of mean daily hot flash count.[391]

The effect of phytoestrogens on prevention and treatment of breast cancer is unknown. There is evidence they can both protect or support tumor growth. The potential effect likely will depend on the specific isoflavone, timing of exposure, genetic factors, and whether the cancer is estrogen-receptor–positive or –negative.[386,392] The ingestion of at least 25 g of soy protein daily as part of a diet low in saturated fat and cholesterol may reduce the risk of coronary heart disease. The effect of phytoestrogen dietary supplements on the risk of myocardial infarction is unclear.[393]

The effect of soy isoflavones on the risk of osteoporosis has yielded positive findings. A double-blind placebo-controlled study of 389 postmenopausal women with osteopenia was randomized to receive placebo or 54 mg of genistein in addition to calcium and vitamin D. After 2 years of treatment, there were significant changes in the anteroposterior lumbar spine, the femoral neck, and urinary markers. No changes in endometrial thickness were evident.[394]

ASSESSMENT OF NATURAL PRODUCT USE: A CASE-BASED APPROACH

The clinician should determine a patient's reasons for purchasing a natural medicine. The appropriateness of supplements for a child, a pregnant woman, or an older adult must be determined. If a medically diagnosed condition is being treated, the clinician should encourage the patient to involve the primary care provider in the use of the supplement, if its use is appropriate. Information about possible allergies to plant materials, current conventional medication use, and comorbidity will help identify possible contraindications to use of the natural product.

If self-treatment with a natural product is appropriate, the clinician should review the length of therapy and recommended dosages with the patient. The efficacy of different dosage forms should also be explained. Cases 54-1 and 54-2 provide examples of the assessment of patients who are considering use of a natural product.

CASE 54-1

Relevant Evaluation Criteria	Scenario/Model Outcome
Information Gathering	
1. Gather essential information about the patient's symptoms, including:	
a. description of symptom(s) (i.e., nature, onset, duration, severity, associated symptoms)	Patient reports that his cholesterol level has not decreased quite as much as needed, and that his PCP has given him a new prescription for an increased dosage of simvastatin. "I just need to come down 8 or 10 more points."
b. description of any factors that seem to precipitate, exacerbate, and/or relieve the patient's symptom(s)	None
c. description of the patient's efforts to relieve the symptoms	He follows a low-fat, low-cholesterol diet and exercises regularly. He also takes fish oil 3 g/day.
2. Gather essential patient history information:	
a. patient's identity	Robert John Nellsen
b. patient's age, sex, height, and weight	67-year-old male, 6 ft 1 in, 186 lb
c. patient's occupation	Retired building contractor
d. patient's dietary habits	Low-fat, low-cholesterol diet
e. patient's sleep habits	He usually gets 7.5–8 hours of sleep per night; has insomnia 4–5 times per year.
f. concurrent medical conditions, prescription and nonprescription medications, and dietary supplements	Stage 1 HTN, well controlled on hydrochlorothiazide 12.5 mg every day
	Mild knee and right shoulder osteoarthritis, treated with as-needed ibuprofen and/or APAP
	Centrum Silver 1 tablet every day
	Enteric-coated fish oil 1 gram 3 times/day
	Simvastatin 20 mg every day
g. allergies	NKDA; no known food or plant allergies
h. history of other adverse reactions to medications	Intolerant of erythromycin (severe nausea and vomiting, requiring change in antibiotic)
i. other (describe) _____	Patient comes to your pharmacy counter with two products, red yeast rice and garlic. He says that he does not want to increase his simvastatin dose, because when he was on a 40 mg dose several years ago, he felt quite fatigued much of the time. He wants to know which of the two natural medicines would be better for him to take to get his cholesterol down a little lower.
Assessment and Triage	
3. Differentiate the patient's signs/symptoms and correctly identify the patient's primary problem(s).	Hyperlipidemia, uncontrolled
	Osteoarthritis, mild and adequately treated with as-needed medications
	Hypertension, controlled
	Lack of education regarding dietary supplements
4. Identify exclusions for self-treatment.	None
5. Formulate a comprehensive list of therapeutic alternatives for the primary problem to determine if triage to a medical practitioner is required, and share this information with the patient.	Options include: (1) Continue the simvastatin and add garlic. (2) Stop simvastatin and begin red yeast rice. (3) Increase simvastatin dose and add coenzyme Q10 (CoQ10). (4) Take no action.
Plan	
6. Select an optimal therapeutic alternative to address the patient's problem, taking into account patient preferences.	Fill prescription for increased simvastatin dosage and add CoQ10.

CASE 54-1 (continued)

Relevant Evaluation Criteria	Scenario/Model Outcome
7. Describe the recommended therapeutic approach to the patient.	Simvastatin is known to decrease CoQ10 levels. This effect may be associated with side effects such as the fatigue he experienced with the 40 mg dose taken previously. Increasing the simvastatin will be the most effective way for him to decrease his cholesterol levels to the desired goal, and taking the CoQ10 may help him tolerate the medication better.
	Encourage continuance of low-fat diet and regular exercise for control of hyperlipidemia and HTN.
8. Explain to the patient the rationale for selecting the recommended therapeutic approach from the considered therapeutic alternatives.	The red yeast rice product contains a statin very similar to the simvastatin that he is currently taking, so it would not be appropriate to take these together. Also, the red yeast rice alone may not provide a large enough cholesterol-lowering effect to maintain his present levels, much less decrease them further.
	The evidence for garlic does support lipid-lowering effects, although the reductions are probably limited to about 5%.

Patient Education

9. When recommending self-care with nonprescription medications and/or nondrug therapy, convey accurate information to the patient:	
a. appropriate dose and frequency of administration	CoQ10 100 mg/day
b. maximum number of days the therapy should be employed	During time patient is on simvastatin
c. product administration procedures	You may take the CoQ10 with meals if any gastrointestinal upset occurs.
d. expected time to onset of relief	
e. degree of relief that can be reasonably expected	You should monitor for occurrence of excessive fatigue after increasing the simvastatin dosage.
f. most common side effects	
g. side effects that warrant medical intervention should they occur	
h. patient options in the event that condition worsens or persists	If he still experiences intolerable fatigue on the 40 mg dose of simvastatin, consider a recommendation to the physician to decrease the dosage back to 20 mg, and add garlic, a standardized product providing allicin about 4 mg/day.
i. product storage requirements	Keep product in an appropriate storage area away from excessive heat and moisture, and out of reach of children and pets.
j. specific nondrug measures	After choosing an appropriate, high-quality product, maintain therapy with that same product.
10. Solicit follow-up questions from patient.	Does it matter what brand I buy?
11. Answer patient's questions.	Some products may not contain the stated amount of coQ10. It is a good idea to buy a product that has a quality assurance seal of approval (such as "USP Verified") or that is listed on www.consumerlab.com as having passed tests to confirm appropriate amounts.

Key: APAP, acetaminophen; HTN, hypertension; NKDA, no known drug allergies; PCP, primary care provider.

CASE 54-2

Relevant Evaluation Criteria	Scenario/Model Outcome

Information Gathering

1. Gather essential information about the patient's symptoms, including:

   a. description of symptom(s) (i.e., nature, onset, duration, severity, associated symptoms)

   Patient is inquiring about a product to help her "boost immunity" and prevent a cold this winter. She has never taken a natural product before, although work colleagues have advised her to purchase one.

   b. description of any factors that seem to precipitate, exacerbate, and/or relieve the patient's symptom(s)

   Katie currently has no symptoms. She is in close contact daily with young children. In the past, development of a URI has exacerbated her asthma.

   c. description of the patient's efforts to relieve the symptoms

   Patient has not taken any steps in prevention of illness.

2. Gather essential patient history information:

   a. patient's identity

   Katie McCarthy

   b. patient's age, sex, height, and weight

   31-year-old female, 5 ft 4 in, 130 lb

   c. patient's occupation

   Preschool teacher

   d. patient's dietary habits

   Normal healthy diet with occasional snacking

   e. patient's sleep habits

   Approximately 5–6 hours of sleep per night

   f. concurrent medical conditions, prescription and nonprescription medications, and dietary supplements

   Asthma with identified triggers of ragweed, pollen, and URIs; no history of hospitalizations; Mircette 1 tablet daily, Flovent 44 mcg 2 puffs 2 times/day, Ventolin HFA 2 puffs every 4–6 hours as needed, multivitamin 1 tablet daily

   g. allergies

   NKDA or food allergies; seasonal allergies to ragweed and pollen

   h. history of other adverse reactions to medications

   None

   i. other (describe) _____

   Katie is holding a store-brand product with a 300 mg proprietary blend of the following ingredients: echinacea (above-ground parts), eleuthero (root), ginger (dried rhizome), goldenseal (root), and peppermint (leaf). The product also contains vitamins A 1667 IU, C 1000 mg, E 30 IU, B6 2.5 mg, and B12 12.5 mcg.

Assessment and Triage

3. Differentiate the patient's signs/symptoms and correctly identify the patient's primary problem.

   Patient has no symptoms at this time.

4. Identify exclusions for self-treatment.

   No exclusions for self treatment at this time

5. Formulate a comprehensive list of therapeutic alternatives for the primary problem to determine if triage to a medical practitioner is required, and share this information with the patient.

   Options include:
   (1) Refer Katie to her PCP to develop an updated asthma action plan for the winter.
   (2) Educate Katie on nonpharmacologic methods to prevent transmission of the cold virus, and offer a flu shot.
   (3) Assist in selecting natural product for cold prevention.
   (4) Take no action.

Plan

6. Select an optimal therapeutic alternative to address the patient's problem, taking into account patient preferences.

   Suggest nonpharmacologic measures to help prevent virus transmission and provision of a flu shot

7. Describe the recommended therapeutic approach to the patient.

   Practice good hygiene measures by washing hands frequently and/or using antibacterial lotions. Lifestyle modifications include a balanced diet, sufficient intake of fluids, and adequate sleep (at least 8 hours). Continue to adhere to inhaled corticosteroid therapy.

   If a cold does develop, relief of symptoms can be managed with OTC products. Monitor asthma symptoms and increased albuterol use closely, and seek PCP attention if they worsen.

CASE 54-2 *(continued)*

Relevant Evaluation Criteria	Scenario/Model Outcome
8. Explain to the patient the rationale for selecting the recommended therapeutic approach from the considered therapeutic alternatives.	Regarding the natural product you selected to help prevent a cold, evidence does not support chronic use of any herbal ingredients to prevent or reduce frequency of respiratory infections. Echinacea may be useful in reducing duration and severity of a cold; however, optimal standardization and dosing are yet to be identified. However, you should not use echinacea because of your ragweed sensitivity. Chronic use of high-dose vitamins is also a concern. The flu vaccine is recommended in all patients with asthma; not only will it prevent the flu, it will prevent a related asthma exacerbation commonly associated with flu.
Patient Education	
9. When recommending self-care with nonprescription medications and/or nondrug therapy, convey accurate information to the patient.	No OTC medications are warranted at this time. Nondrug measures were discussed in step 7.
10. Solicit follow-up questions from patient.	What would happen if I take the immune-boosting product anyway?
11. Answer patient's questions.	Because ragweed is identified as an asthma trigger, it is possible echinacea may precipitate an asthma exacerbation.

Key: NKDA, no known drug allergies; OTC, over-the-counter; PCP, primary care provider; URI, upper respiratory infection.

CONCLUSION

The use of natural products has continued to grow over the last 15 to 20 years, presenting many challenges and opportunities for clinicians, especially in the ambulatory care setting. The most important issue is to encourage a culture of respect for the patient's beliefs and values so that a trusting, nonjudgmental relationship can develop. Patients must feel comfortable sharing their use of natural products with the clinician, and the pharmacist must be well informed regarding the safety, efficacy, and clinical use of common natural products. In addition, clinicians should also be aware of the potential for interactions with prescription or nonprescription medications (Table 54-1).

KEY POINTS FOR NATURAL MEDICINES

➤ Use of natural medicines has increased significantly over the last 15 to 20 years.
➤ Clinical research has compared natural medicines with prescription drugs for prevention and treatment of common conditions.
➤ Some natural products, such as ginger and saw palmetto, have evidence of safety and efficacy, whereas others, including huperzine A, demonstrate promise.
➤ Natural medicines have also demonstrated significant adverse effects and drug interactions.
➤ Concerns remain regarding commercial availability of the studied product to the typical American consumer.

➤ Some natural products are available in formulations meeting USP standards and their labels include the USP Verified Mark.
➤ Patients and clinicians must communicate clearly to ensure safe use of these products.
➤ Patients must recognize that "natural" does not always mean "safe." Clinicians must take advantage of the fact that patients use natural products, because they want greater involvement in their own health care, and are increasingly interested in health promotion and disease prevention.
➤ Safe and effective use of natural products, especially in patients taking prescription and nonprescription drugs for chronic diseases, requires a partnership between patients and clinicians.

REFERENCES

1. Barnes PM, Powell-Griner E, McFann K, et al. Complementary and alternative medicine use among adults: United States, 2002. *Adv Data.* 2004;343:1–19.
2. Nemecz G, Combest WL. Herbal remedies. In: Allen LV, Berardi RR, DeSimone EM, et al., eds. *Handbook of Nonprescription Drugs.* 12th ed. Washington, DC: American Pharmaceutical Association; 2001:953–82.
3. Roffe L, Schmidt K, Ernst E. Efficacy of coenzyme Q10 for improved tolerability of cancer treatments: a systematic review. *J Clin Oncol.* 2004; 22:4418–24.
4. Overvad K, Diamant B, Holm L, et al. Coenzyme Q_{10} in health and disease. *Eur J Clin Nutr.* 1999;53:764–70.
5. Turunen M, Olsson J, Dallner G. Metabolism and function of coenzyme Q. *Biochim Biophys Acta.* 2004;1660(1–2):171–90.
6. Crane FL. Biochemical functions of coenzyme Q10. *J Am Coll Nutr.* 2001;20:591–8.
7. Food and Drug Administration. List of Orphan Designations and Approvals. Available at: http://www.fda.gov/orphan/designat/list.htm. Last accessed October 23, 2008.
8. McQueen CE, editor. *Sigler's Dietary Supplement Drug Cards.* 2nd ed. Lawrence, Kan: SFI Medical Publishing; 2009.

9. Landbo C, Almdal TP. Interaction between warfarin and coenzyme Q10 [abstract]. *Ugeskr Laeger.* 1998;160:3226–7.

10. Spigset O. Reduced effect of warfarin caused by ubidecarenone. *Lancet.* 1994;334:1372–3.

11. Engelsen J. Effect of coenzyme Q10 and *Ginkgo biloba* on warfarin dosage in stable, long-term warfarin treated outpatients. A randomized, double-blind, placebo-crossover trial. *Thromb Haemost.* 2002;87:1075–6.

12. Rundek T, Naini A, Sacco R, et al. Atorvastatin decreases the coenzyme Q10 level in the blood of patients at risk for cardiovascular disease and stroke. *Arch Neurol.* 2004;61:889–92.

13. Laaksonen R, Jokelainen K, Sahi T, et al. Decreases in serum ubiquinone concentrations do not result in reduced levels in muscle tissue during short-term simvastatin treatment in humans. *Clin Pharmacol Ther.* 1995; 57:62–6.

14. Bleske BE, Willis RA, Anthony M, et al. The effect of pravastatin and atorvastatin on coenzyme Q10. *Am Heart J.* 2001;142:e2.

15. Lund EL, Quistorff B, Span-Thomsen M, Kristjansen PE. Effect of radiation therapy on small-cell lung cancer is reduced by ubiquinone intake. *Folia Microbiol.* 1998;43:505–6.

16. Conklin KA. Dietary antioxidants during cancer chemotherapy: impact on chemotherapeutic effectiveness and development of side effects. *Nutr Cancer.* 2000;37:1–18.

17. Rengo F, Abete P, Landino P, et al. Role of metabolic therapy in cardiovascular disease. *Clin Investig.* 1993;71:S124–8.

18. Morisco C, Trimarco B, Condorelli M. Effect of coenzyme Q10 therapy in patients with congestive heart failure: a long-term multicenter randomized study. *Clin Investig.* 1993;71:S134–6.

19. Khatta M, Alexander B, Krichten C, et al. The effect of coenzyme Q10 in patients with congestive heart failure. *Ann Intern Med.* 2000;132:636–40.

20. Berman M, Erman A, Ben-Gal T, et al. Coenzyme Q10 in patients with end-stage heart failure awaiting cardiac transplantation: a randomized, placebo-controlled study. *Clin Cardiol.* 2004;27:295–9.

21. Belardinelli R, Mucaj A, Lacalaprice F, et al. Coenzyme Q10 and exercise training in chronic heart failure. *Eur Heart J* 2006;27:2675–81.

22. Langsjoen PH, Vadhanavikit S, Folkers K. Response of patients in classes III and IV of cardiomyopathy to therapy in a blind and crossover trial with coenzyme Q10. *Proc Natl Acad Sci USA.* 1994;15:S287–94.

23. Permanetter B, Rossy W, Klein G, et al. Ubiquinone (coenzyme Q10) in the long-term treatment of idiopathic dilated cardiomyopathy. *Eur Heart J.* 1992;13:1528–33.

24. Singh RB, Niaz MA, Rastogi SS, et al. Effect of hydrosoluble coenzyme Q10 on blood pressures and insulin resistance in hypertensive patients with coronary artery disease. *J Hum Hypertens.* 1999;13:203–8.

25. Singh RB, Niaz MA. Serum concentration of lipoprotein(a) decreases on treatment with hydrosoluble coenzyme Q10 in patients with coronary artery disease: discovery of a new role. *Int J Cardiol.* 1999;68:23–9.

26. Singh RB, Neki NS, Kartikey K, et al. Effect of coenzyme Q10 on risk of atherosclerosis in patients with recent myocardial infarction. *Mol Cell Biochem.* 2003;246(1-2):75–82.

27. Burke BE, Neuenschwander R, Olson RD, et al. Randomized, double-blind, placebo-controlled trial of coenzyme Q10 in isolated systolic hypertension. *South Med J.* 2001;94:1112–7.

28. The NINDS NET-PD Investigators. A randomized clinical trial of coenzyme Q10 and GPI-1485 in early Parkinson disease. *Neurol.* 2007; 68:20–28.

29. Storch A, Jost WH, Vieregge P, et al. Randomized, double-blind, placebo-controlled trial on symptomatic effects of coenzyme Q10 in Parkinson disease. *Arch Neurol.* 2007;64:E1-E7.

30. Huntington Study Group. A randomized, placebo-controlled trial of coenzyme Q10 and remacemide in Huntington's disease. *Neurology.* 2001;57:397–404.

31. Lockwood K, Moesgaard S, Yamamoto T, et al. Progress on therapy of breast cancer with vitamin Q10 and the regression of metastases. *Biochem Biophys Res Comm.* 1995;212:172–7.

32. Sándor PS, Di Clemente L, Coppola G, et al. Efficacy of coenzyme Q10 in migraine prophylaxis: a randomized controlled trial. *Neurology.* 2005;64:713–5.

33. Charlson M, McFerren M. Garlic: what we know and what we don't know. *Arch Int Med* 2007;167:325–6.

34. *Garlic Effects on Cardiovascular Risks and Disease, Protective Effects against Cancer, and Clinical Adverse Effects. Summary, Evidence Report/Technology Assessment: Number 20.* Rockville, Md: Agency for Healthcare Research and Quality; October 2000. AHRQ Publication No. 01-E022.

35. Cooperman T, Obermyer W, ed. ConsumerLab. Available at: http://www.consumerlab.com. Last accessed October 23, 2008.

36. Ciocon JO, Ciocon DG, Galindo DJ. Dietary supplements in primary care. Botanicals can affect surgical outcomes and follow-up. *Geriatrics.* 2004;59:20–4.

37. Boullata J. Natural health product interactions with medication. *Nutr Clin Pract.* 2005;20:33–51.

38. Scharbert G, Kalb ML, Duris M, et al. Garlic at dietary doses does not impair platelet function. *Anesth Analg.* 2007;105(5):1214–18.

39. Piscitelli SC, Burstein AH, Welden N, et al. The effect of garlic supplements on the pharmacokinetics of saquinavir. *Clin Infect Dis.* 2002; 34:234–8.

40. Markowitz JS, Devane CL, Chavin KD, et al. Effects of garlic (*Allium sativum* L.) supplementation on cytochrome P450 2D6 and 3A4 activity in healthy volunteers. *Clin Pharmacol Ther.* 2003;74:170–7.

41. Cox MC, Low J, Lee, et al. Influence of garlic (*Allium sativum*) on the pharmacokinetics of docetaxel. *Clin Canc Res.* 2006;12:4636–40.

42. Alder R, Lookinland S, Berry JA, et al. A systemic review of the effectiveness of garlic as an anti-hyperlipidemic agent. *J Am Acad Nurse Practitioners.* 2003;15:120–9.

43. Superko HR, Krauss RM. Garlic powder, effect on plasma lipids, postprandial lipemia, low density lipoprotein particle size, high density lipoprotein subclass distribution and lipoprotein (a). *J Am Coll Cardiol.* 2001;35:321–6.

44. McMahon FG, Vargas R. Can garlic lower blood pressure? A pilot study. *Pharmacotherapy.* 1993;13:406–7.

45. Dwahan V, Jain S. Effect of garlic supplementation on oxidized low density lipoproteins and lipid peroxidation in patients of essential hypertension. *Mol Cell Biochem.* 2004;266:109–15.

46. Fleischauer AT, Arab L. Garlic and cancer: a critical review of the epidemiologic literature. *J Nutr.* 2001;131:1032–40.

47. Thomson M, Ali M. Garlic [*Allium sativum*]: a review of its potential use as an anti-cancer agent. *Curr Cancer Drug Targets.* 2003;3:67–81.

48. Vanschoonbeek K, de Maat MPM, Heemskerk HWM. Fish oil consumption and reduction of arterial disease. *J Nutr.* 2003;133:657–60.

49. Kris-Etherton PM, Harris WS, Appel LJ; AHA Nutrition Committee. Omega-3 fatty acids and cardiovascular disease: new recommendations from the American Heart Association. *Arterioscler Thromb Vasc Biol.* 2003;23:151–2.

50. Foran SE, Flood JG, Lewandrowski KB. Measurement of mercury levels in concentrated over-the-counter fish oil preparations: is fish oil healthier than fish? *Arch Pathol Lab Med.* 2003;127:1603–5.

51. Melanson SF, Lewandrowski EL, Flood JG, et al. Measurement of organochlorines in commercial over-the-counter fish oil preparations: implications for dietary and therapeutic recommendations for omega-3 fatty acids and a review of the literature. *Arch Pathol Lab Med.* 2005; 129(1):74–7.

52. Wang C, Harris WS, Chung M, et al. n-3 fatty acids from fish or fish oil supplements, but not α-linolenic acid, benefit cardiovascular disease outcomes in primary- and secondary prevention studies: as systematic review. *Am J Clin Nutr.* 2006;84:5–17.

53. Simopoulos AP. Omega-3 fatty acids in inflammation and autoimmune diseases. *J Am Coll Nutr.* 2002;21(6):495–505.

54. Cleland LG, James MJ, Proudman SM. The role of fish oils in the treatment of rheumatoid arthritis. *Drugs.* 2003;63(9):845–53.

55. Pittler MH, Ernst E. Horse-chestnut seed extract for chronic venous insufficiency. *Cochrane Database Syst Rev.* 2004;1:CD003230.

56. Siebert U, Brach M, Sroczynski G, et al. Efficacy, routine effectiveness, and safety of horsechestnut see extract in the treatment of chronic venous insufficiency: a meta-analysis of randomized controlled trials and large observational studies. *Intl Angiology.* 2002;21:305–15.

57. Singh DK, Li L, Porter TD. Policosanol inhibits cholesterol synthesis in hepatoma cells by activation of AMP-kinase. *J Pharmacol Exp Ther.* 2006; 318:1020–6.

58. Gouni-Berthold I, Berthold HK. Policosanol: clinical pharmacology and therapeutic significance of a new lipid-lowering agent. *Am Heart J.* 2002;143:356–65.

59. Reiner A, Tedeschi-Reiner E. Rice policosanol does not have any effects on blood coagulation factors in hypercholesterolemic patients. *Coll Antropol.* 2007;31:1061–4.

60. Lin Y, Rudrum M, van der Wielen RPJ, et al. Wheat germ policosanol failed to lower plasma cholesterol in subjects with normal to mildly elevated cholesterol concentrations. *Metabolism.* 2004;53:1309–14.

61. Greyling A, DeWitt C, Oosthuizen W, Jerling JC. Effects of a policosanol supplement on serum lipid concentrations in hypercholesterolaemic and heterozygous familial hypercholesterolaemic subjects. *Brit J Nutr.* 2006;95:968–75.

62. Castano G, Mas R, Fernandez L, et al. Effects of policosanol and lovastatin in patients with intermittent claudication: a double-blind comparative pilot study. *Angiology.* 2003;54:25–38.

63. US Food and Drug Administration. FDA Warns Consumers to Avoid Red Yeast Rice Products Promoted on Internet as Treatments for High Cholesterol [news release]. August 9, 2007. Available at: http://www.fda.gov/bbs/topics/NEWS/2007/NEW01678.html. Last accessed October 23, 2008.

64. Kazmin A, Garcia-Bournissen F, Koren G. Risks of statin use during pregnancy: a systematic review. *J Obstet Gynaecol Can.* 2007;29:906–8.

65. Journoud M, Jones P. Red yeast rice: a new hypolipidemic drug. *Life Sci.* 2004;74:2675–83.

66. Vittek J. Effect of royal jelly on serum lipids in experimental animals and humans with atherosclerosis. *Experientia.* 1995;51(9–10):927–35.

67. Thien FCK, Leung R, Baldo BA, et al. Asthma and anaphylaxis induced by royal jelly. *Clin Exp Allergy* 1996;26:216–22.

68. Yonei Y, Shibagaki K, Tsukada N, et al. Case report: haemorrhagic colitis associated with royal jelly intake. *J Gastro Hepatol.* 1997;12:495–9.

69. Lee N, Joli D. Warfarin and royal jelly interaction. *Pharmacotherapy.* 2006;26:583–6.

70. Guo H, Saiga A, Sato M, et al. Royal jelly supplementation improves lipoprotein metabolism in humans. *J Nutr Sci Vitaminol.* 2007;54:345–8.

71. Grossmann W, Schmidramsl H. An extract of *Petasites hybridus* is effective in prophylaxis of migraine. *Int J Clin Pharm Ther.* 2000;38:430–5.

72. Schapowal A. Randomised controlled trial of butterbur and cetirizine for treating seasonal allergic rhinitis. *BMJ.* 2002;321:1–4.

73. Schapowal A. Treating intermittent allergic rhinitis: a prospective, randomized, placebo and antihistamine-controlled study of Butterbur extract Ze 339. *Phytother Res.* 2005;19:530–7.

74. Hasler A, Passafaro A, Meier B. Trace analysis of pyrrolizidine alkaloids b GC-NPD of extracts from the roots of *Petasites hybridus*. *Pharma Acta Helv.* 1998;72:367.

75. Lipton R, Gobel H, Einhaupl K, et al. *Petasites hybridus* root (butterbur) is an effective preventative treatment for migraine. *Neurology.* 2004; 63:2240–4.

76. Pothmann R, Danesch U. Migraine prevention in children and adolescents: results of an open study with a special butterbur root extract. *Headache.* 2005;45:196–203.

77. Lee D, Gray R, Robb F, et al. A placebo-controlled evaluation of butterbur and fexofenadine on objective and subjective outcomes in perennial allergic rhinitis. *Clin Exp Allergy.* 2004;34:646–9.

78. de Weerdt CJ. Herbal medicines in migraine prevention. Randomized double-blind placebo-controlled crossover trial of feverfew preparation. *Phytomedicine.* 1996;3: 225–30.

79. Ramadan NM, Silberstein SD, Freitag FG, et al. Evidence-Based Guidelines for Migraine Headache in the Primary Care Setting: Pharmacological Management for the Prevention of Migraine. Available at: http://www.aan.com/professionals/practice/pdfs/gl0090.pdf. Last accessed October 23, 2008.

80. Pittler M, Ernst E. Feverfew for preventing migraine. *Cochrane Database Syst Rev.* 2004;1:CD002286.

81. Pepping J. Huperzine A. *Am J Health Syst Pharm.* 2000;57:530–4.

82. Camps P, Cusack B, Mallender W, et al. Huprine X is a novel high-affinity inhibitor of acetylcholinesterase that is of interest for treatment of Alzheimer's disease. *Mol Pharm.* 2000;57:409–17.

83. Li J, Wu HM, Zhou RL, et. al. Huperzine A for Alzheimer's disease. *Cochrane Database Syst Rev.* 2008;2:CD005592.

84. Birks J, Grimley Evans J. Ginkgo biloba for cognitive impairment and dementia. *Cochrane Database Syst Rev.* 2007;2:CD003120.

85. Sierpina VS, Wollschlaeger B, Blumenthal M. Ginkgo biloba. *Am Fam Physician.* 2003;68:923–6.

86. Granger AS. *Ginkgo biloba* precipitating epileptic seizures. *Age Ageing.* 2001;30:523–5.

87. Bent S, Goldberg H, Padula A, et al. Spontaneous bleeding associated with ginkgo biloba: a case report and systematic review of the literature: a case report and systematic review of the literature. *J Gen Intern Med.* 2005;20:657–61.

88. Koch E. Inhibition of platelet activating factor (PAF)-induced aggregation of human thrombocytes by ginkgolides: considerations on possible bleeding complications after oral intake of *Ginkgo biloba* extracts. *Phytomedicine.* 2005;12:10–6.

89. Gardner CD, Zehnder JL, Rigby AJ, et al. Effect of *Ginkgo biloba* (EGb 761) and aspirin on platelet aggregation and platelet function analysis among older adults at risk of cardiovascular disease: a randomized clinical trial. *Blood Coag Fibrinolysis.* 2007;18:787–93.

90. Bone KM. Potential interaction of *Ginkgo biloba* leaf with antiplatelet or anticoagulant drugs: what is the evidence. *Mol Nutr Food Res.* 2008; 52(7):764–71.

91. Markowitz JS, Donovan JL, DeVane CL, et al. Multiple-dose administration of *Ginkgo biloba* did not affect cytochrome P-450 2D6 or 3A4 activity in normal volunteers. *J Clin Psychopharmacol.* 2003;23:576–81.

92. Galluzzi S, Zanetti O, Binetti G, et al. Coma in a patient with Alzheimer's disease taking low dose trazodone and *Ginkgo biloba*. *J Neurol Neurosurg Psychiatry.* 2000;68:679–80.

93. Wettstein A. Cholinesterase inhibitors and ginkgo extracts—are they comparable in the treatment of dementia? Comparison of published placebo-controlled efficacy studies of at least six months' duration. *Phytomedicine.* 2000;6:393–401.

94. Mazza M, Capuano A, Bria P, et al. Ginkgo biloba and donepezil: a comparison in the treatment of Alzheimer's dementia in a randomized placebo-controlled double-blind study. *Eur J Neurol.* 2006;13:981–5.

95. Solomon PR, Adams F, Silver A, et al. Ginkgo for memory enhancement: a randomized controlled trial. *JAMA.* 2002;288:835–40.

96. Pittler MH, Ernst E. *Ginkgo biloba* extract for the treatment of intermittent claudication: a meta-analysis of randomized trials. *Am J Med.* 2000; 108:276–81.

97. Horsch S, Walther C. Ginkgo biloba special extract EGb 761 in the treatment of peripheral arterial occlusive disease (PAOD)—a review based on randomized, controlled studies. *Intl J Clin Pharmacol Ther.* 2004;42:63–72.

98. Drew S, Davies E. Effectiveness of *Ginkgo biloba* in treating tinnitus: double-blind, placebo controlled trial. *BMJ.* 2001;322:73.

99. Rejali D, Sivakumar A, Balaji N. Ginkgo biloba does not benefit patients with tinnitus: a randomized placebo-controlled double-blind trial and meta-analysis of randomized trials. *Clin Otolaryngol.* 2004;29:226–31.

100. Gertsch JH, Basnyat B, Johnson W, et al. Randomised, double-blind, placebo controlled comparison of ginkgo biloba and acetazolamide for prevention of acute mountain sickness among Himalayan trekkers: the prevention of high altitude illness trial (PHAIT) *BMJ.* 2004;328:797.

101. Chow T, Browne V, Heileson HL, et al. Ginkgo biloba and acetazolamide prophylaxis for acute mountain sickness: a randomized, placebo-controlled trial. *Arch Intern Med.* 2005;165:296–301.

102. Cagnacci A, Arangino S, Renzi A, et al. Kava-kava administration reduces anxiety in perimenopausal women. *Maturitas.* 2003;44:103–9.

103. Perez J, Holmes JF. Altered mental status and ataxia secondary to acute Kava ingestion. *J Emerg Med.* 2005;28:49–51.

104. Clouatre D. Kava kava: examining new reports of toxicity. *Toxicol Lett.* 2004;150:85–96.

105. Centers for Disease Control and Prevention. Hepatic toxicity possibly associated with kava-containing products—United States, Germany, and Switzerland, 1999–2002. *MMWR Morb Mortal Wkly Rep.* 2002;51:1065–7.

106. Matthews JM, Etheridge AS, Valentine JL, et al. Pharmacokinetics and disposition of the kavalactone kawain: interaction with kava extract and kavalactones in vivo and in vitro. *Drug Metab Disp.* 2005;33:1555–63.

107. Meseguer E, Taboada R, Sanchez V, et al. Life threatening parkinsonism induced by kava-kava. *Mov Disord.* 2002;17:195–6.

108. Pittler MH, Ernst E. Kava extract for treating anxiety. *Cochrane Database Syst Rev.* 2003;1:CD003383.

109. Witte S, Loew D, Gaus W. Meta-analysis of the efficacy of the acetonic kava-kava extract WS1490 in patients with non-psychotic anxiety disorders. *Phytother Res.* 2005;19:183–8.

110. *Drug Facts and Comparisons.* St Louis: Wolters Kuwer Health; 2008: KU-14g.

111. Dennehy CE, Tsourounis C. Botanicals ("herbal medications") and nutritional supplements. In: Katzung BG, ed. *Basic and Clinical Pharmacology.* 10th ed. New York: Lange/McGraw Hill; 2007:1060–2.

112. Luboshitzky R, Lavie P. Melatonin and sex hormone interrelationships—a review. *J Ped Endocrinol.* 1999;12:355–62.

113. Brzezinski A, Vangel MG, Wurtman RJ, et al. Effect of exogenous melatonin on sleep: a meta-analysis. *Sleep Med.* 2005;9:41–50.

114. Claustrat B, Brun J, Chazot G. The basic physiology and pathophysiology of melatonin. *Sleep Med.* 2005;9:11–24.

115. Djeridane Y, Touitou Y. Chronic diazepam administration differentially affects melatonin synthesis in rat pineal and Harderian glands. *Psychopharmacol.* 2001;154:403–7.

116. Wright KP Jr, Myers BL, Plenzler SC, et al. Acute effects of bright light and caffeine on nighttime melatonin and temperature levels in women taking and not taking oral contraceptives. *Brain Res.* 2000;873:310–7.

117. Lusardi P, Piazza E, Fogari R. Cardiovascular effects of melatonin in hypertensive patients well controlled by nifedipine: a 24-hour study. *Br J Pharmacol.* 2000;49:423–7.

118. Lissoni P, Barni S, Mandala M, et al. Decreased toxicity and increased efficacy of cancer chemotherapy using the pineal hormone melatonin in metastatic solid tumour patients with poor clinical status. *Eur J Cancer.* 1999;35:1688–92.

119. Andrade C, Srihari BS, Reddy KP, et al. Melatonin in medically ill patients with insomnia: a double-blind, placebo-controlled study. *J Clin Psychiatry.* 2001;62:41–5.

120. Campos FL, da Silva-Júnior FP, de Bruin VMS, et al. Melatonin improves sleep in asthma. A randomized, double-blind, placebo-controlled study. *Am J Resp Crit Care Med.* 2004;170:947–51.

121. Singer C, Tractenberg RE, Kaye J, et al. A multicenter, placebo-controlled trial of melatonin for sleep disturbance in Alzheimer's disease. *Sleep.* 2003;26:893–901.

122. Smits MG, Nagtegaal EE, van der Heijden J, et al. Melatonin for chronic sleep onset insomnia in children: a randomized placebo-controlled trial. *J Child Neurol.* 2001;16:86–92.

123. Smits MG, van Stel HF, van der Heijden J, et al. Melatonin improves health status and sleep in children with idiopathic chronic sleep-onset insomnia: a randomized placeb-controlled trial. *J Am Acad Child Adolesc Psychiatry* 2003;42:1286–93.

124. van der Heijden J, Smits MG, van Someren EJW, et al. Effect of melatonin on sleep, behavior, and cognition in ADHD and chronic sleep-onset insomnia. *J Am Acad Child Adolesc Psychiatry* 2007;46:233–41.

125. Herxheimer A, Petrie K. Melatonin for the prevention and treatment of jet lag. *Cochrane Database Syst Rev.* 2002;2:CD001520.

126. Burstein AH. Melatonin for shift-work insomnia. *Pharm Diet Suppl Alert.* 2000;1:33–6.

127. Barnes J, Anderson L, Phillipson J. St. John's wort (*Hypericum perforatum L.*): a review of its chemistry, pharmacology and clinical properties. *J Pharm Pharmacol.* 2001;53:583–600.

128. *Hypericum perforatum. Altern Med Rev.* 2004;9:318–25.

129. Wurglics M, Westerhoff K, Kaunzinger A, et al. Batch-to-batch reproducibility of St. John's wort preparations. *Pharmacopsychiatry.* 2001;34:S152–6.

130. Knuppel L, Linde K. Adverse effects of St. John's wort: a systematic review. *J Clin Psychiatry.* 2004;65:1470–9.

131. Schempp CM, Müller K, Winghofer B, et al. Single-dose and steady-state administration of Hypericum perforatum extract (St John's Wort) does not influence skin sensitivity to UV radiation, visible light, and solar-simulated radiation. *Arch Dermatol.* 2001;137(4):512–3.

132. Mueller SC, Majcher-Peszynska J, Uehleke B, et al. The extent of induction of CYP3A by St. John's wort varies among products and is linked to hyperforin dose. *Eur J Clin Pharmacol.* 2006;62:29–36.

133. Madabushi R, Frank B, Drewelow B, et al. Hyperforin in St. John's wort drug interactions. *Eur J Clin Pharmacol.* 2006;62:225–33.

134. Linde K, Berner M, Kriston L. St. John's wort for major depression. *Cochrane Database Syst Rev.* 2008;4:CD000448.

135. Kasper S, Anghelescu IG, Szegedi A, et al. Superior efficacy of St John's wort extract WS 5570 compared to placebo in patients with major depression: a randomized, double-blind, placebo-controlled, multi-center trial [ISRCTN77277298]. *BMC Med.* 2006;4:14.

136. Gastpar M, Singer A, Zeller K. Comparative efficacy and safety of a once-daily dosage of hypericum extract STW3-VI and citalopram in patients with moderate depression: a double-blind, randomised, multi-centre, placebo-controlled study. *Pharmacopsychiatry.* 2006;39:66–75.

137. Pepping J. Valerian: *Valeriana officinalis. Am J Health Syst Pharm.* 2000; 57:328–35.

138. Wagner J, Hening W. Beyond benzodiazepines: alternative pharmacologic agents for the treatment of insomnia. *Neuropsychiatry.* 1998;32: 680–91.

139. Garges HP, Varia I, Doraiswamy PM. Cardiac complications and delirium associated with valerian root withdrawal. *JAMA.* 1998; 280:1566–7.

140. Donovan JL, DeVane CL, Chavin KD, et al. Multiple night-time doses of valerian (Valeriana officinalis) had minimal effects on CYP3A4 activity and no effect on CYP2D6 activity in healthy volunteers. *Drug Met Dispos.* 2004;32:1333–6.

141. Coxeter PD, Schluter PJ, Eastwood HL, et al. Valerian does not appear to reduce symptoms for patients with chronic insomnia in general practice using a series of randomised n-of-1 trials. *Complement Ther Med.* 2003; 11:215–22.

142. Diaper A, Hindmarch I. A double-blind, placebo-controlled investigation of the effects of two doses of a valerian preparation on the sleep, cognitive and psychomotor function of sleep-disturbed older adults. *Phytother Res.* 2004;18:831–6.

143. Glass J, Sproule B, Herrmann N, et al. Acute pharmacological effects of temazepam, diphenhydramine, and valerian in healthy elderly subjects. *J Clin Psychopharmacol.* 2003;23:260–8.

144. Klarskov K, Johnson KL, Benson LM, et al. Eosinophilia-myalgia syndrome case-associated contaminants in commercially available 5-hydroxytryptophan. *Adv Exp Med Biol.* 1999;467:461–8.

145. Michelson D, Page SW, Casey R, et al. An eosinophilia-myalgia syndrome related disorder associated with exposure to L-5-hydroxytryptophan. *J Rheumatol.* 1994;21:2261–5.

146. Shaw K, Turner J, Del Mar C. Tryptophan and 5-hydroxytryptophan for depression. *Cochrane Database Syst Rev.* 2002;1:CD003198.

147. Gijsman HJ, van Gerven JM, de Kam ML, et al. Placebo-controlled comparison of three dose-regimens of 5-hydroxytryptophan challenge test in healthy volunteers. *J Clin Psychopharmacol.* 2002;22:183–9.

148. Bruni O, Ferri R, Miano S, et al. L-5-hydroxytryptophan treatment of sleep terrors in children. *Eur J Ped.* 2004;163:402–7.

149. Viola H, Wasowski C, Levi de Stein M, et al. Apigenin, a component of Matricaria recutita flowers, is a central benzodiazepine receptors-ligand, with anxiolytic effects. *Planta Med.* 1995;61:213–6.

150. Reider N, Sepp N, Fritsch P, et al. Anaphylaxis to chamomile: clinical features and allergic cross-reactivity. *Clin Exp Allergy.* 2000;30:1436–43.

151. Segal R, Pilote L. Warfarin interaction with Matricaria chamomilla. *CMAJ.* 2006;174:1281–2

152. Budzinski JW, Foster BC, Vandenhoek S, et al. An in vitro evaluation of human cytochrome P450 3A4 inhibition by selected commercial herbal extracts and tinctures. *Phytomedicine.* 2000;7: 273–82.

153. Ganzera M, Schneider P, Stuppner H. Inhibitory effects of the essential oil of chamomile (*Matricaria recutita* L.) and its major constituents on human cytochrome P450 enzymes. *Life Sci.* 2006;78:856–61.

154. Carl W, Emrich LS. Management of oral mucositis during local radiation and systemic chemotherapy: a study of 98 patients. *J Prosthet Dent.* 199;66:361–9.

155. Fidler P, Loprinzi CL, O'Fallon JR, et. al. Prospective evaluation of a chamomile mouthwash for prevention of 5-FU-induced oral mucositis. *Cancer.* 1996;77:522–5.

156. Patzelt-Wenczler R, Ponce-Pöschl E. Proof of efficacy of Kamillosan(R) cream in atopic eczema. *Eur J Med Res.* 2000,5.171–5.

157. Smith C, Crowther C, Willson K, et al. A randomized controlled trial of ginger to treat nausea and vomiting in pregnancy. *Obstet Gynecol*. 2004; 103:639–45.

158. Borelli F, Capasso R, Aviello G, et al. Effectiveness and safety of ginger in the treatment of pregnancy-induced nausea and vomiting. *Obstet Gynecol*. 2005;105:849–56.

159. Portnoi G, Chng LA, Karimi-Tabesh L, et al. Prospective comparative study of the safety and effectiveness of ginger for the treatment of nausea and vomiting in pregnancy. *Am J Obstet Gynecol*. 2003;18:1374–7.

160. Lesho EP, Saullo, Udvari-Nagy S. A 76 year-old woman with erratic anticoagulation. *Cleveland Clin J Med*. 2004;71:651–6.

161. Shalansky S, Lynd L, Richardson K, et al. Risk of warfarin-related bleeding events and supratherapeutic international normalized ratios associated with complementary and alternative medicine: a longitudinal analysis. *Pharmacotherapy*. 2007;27:1237–47.

162. Chaiyakunapruk N, Kitikannakorn N, Nathisuwan S, et al. The efficacy of ginger for the prevention of postoperative nausea and vomiting: a meta-analysis. *Am J Obstet Gynecol*. 2006;194:95–9.

163. Arfeen Z, Owen H, Plummer JL, et al. A double-blind randomized controlled trial of ginger for the prevention of postoperative nausea and vomiting. *Anaesth Intens Care*. 1995;23:449–52.

164. Schmid R, Schick T, Steffen R, et al. Comparison of seven commonly used agents for prophylaxis of seasickness. *J Travel Med*. 1994;1:203–6.

165. Sridar C, Goosen TC, Kent UM, et al. Silybin inactivates cytochromes P450 3A4 and 2C9 and inhibits major hepatic glucuronosyltransferases. *Drug Metab Dispos*. 2004;32:587–94.

166. Milk thistle: effects on liver disease and cirrhosis and clinical adverse effects. Summary, Evidence Report/Technology Assessment: Number 21, September 2000. Agency for Healthcare Research and Quality, Rockville, Md. Available at: http://www.ahrq.gov/clinic/epcsums/milktsum.htm. Last accessed October 23, 2008.

167. Rambaldi A, Jacobs BP, Gluud C. Milk thistle for alcoholic and/or hepatitis B or C virus liver diseases. *Cochrane Database Syst Rev*. 2007;4: CD003620.

168. Dresser GK, Wacher V, Wong S, et al. Evaluation of peppermint oil and ascorbyl palmitate as inhibitors of cytochrome P450 3A4 activity in vitro and in vivo. *Clin Pharmacol Ther*. 2002;72:247–55.

169. Grigoleit HG, Grigoleit P. Peppermint oil in irritable bowel syndrome. *Phytomedicine*. 2005;12(8):601–6.

170. Kline RM, Kline JJ, DiPalma J, et al. Enteric-coated, pH dependent peppermint oil capsules for the treatment of irritable bowel syndrome in children. *J Pediatr*. 2001;138:125–8.

171. Cappello G, Spezzaferro M, Grossi L, et al. L Peppermint oil (Mintoil) in the treatment of irritable bowel syndrome: a prospective double blind placebo-controlled randomized trial. *Dig Liver Dis*. 2007;39(6):530–6.

172. Sparks MJ, O'Sullivan P, Herrington AA, et al. Does peppermint oil relieve spasm during barium enema? *Br J Radiol*. 1995;68:841–3.

173. Asao T, Kuwano H, Ide M, et al. Spasmolytic effect of peppermint oil in barium during double-contrast barium enema compared with Buscopan. *Clin Radiol*. 2003;58:301–5.

174. Hiki N, Kurosaka H, Tatsutomi Y, et. al. Peppermint oil reduces gastric spasm during upper endoscopy: a randomized, double-blind, double-dummy controlled trial. *Gastrointest Endosc*.2003;57:475–82.

175. Konrad T, Vicini P, Justerer K, et al. Alpha-lipoic acid treatment decreases serum lactate and pyruvate concentrations and improves glucose effectiveness in lean and obese patients with type 2 diabetes. *Diabetes Care*. 1999;22:280–7.

176. van Dam PS, van Asbeck BS, Van Oirschot JF, et al. Glutathione and alpha-lipoate in diabetic rats: nerve function, blood flow and oxidative state. *Eur J Clin Invest*. 2001;31:417–24.

177. Scott BC, Aruoma OI, Evans PJ, et al. Lipoid and dihydrolipoic acids as antioxidants: a critical evaluation. *Free Radical Res*. 1994;20:119–33.

178. Tiechert J, Kern J, Tritschler HJ, et al. Investigations on the pharmacokinetics of alpha-lipoic acid in healthy volunteers. *Intl J Clin Pharmacol Ther*. 1998;36:625–8.

179. Gleiter CH, Schug BS, Hermann R, et al. Influence of food intake on the bioavailability of thioctic acid enantiomers. *Eur J Clin Pharmacol*. 1996;50:513–4.

180. Ziegler D, Nowak H, Kempler P, et al. Treatment of symptomatic diabetic polyneuropathy with the antioxidant α-lipoic acid: a meta-analysis. *Diabetic Med*. 2004;21:114–21.

181. Segermann J, Hotze A, Ulrich H, et al. Effect of alpha-lipoic acid on the peripheral conversion of thyroxine to triiodothyronine and on serum lipid-, protein- and glucose levels. *Arzneimittelforschung*. 1991;41:1294–8.

182. Zeigler D, Ametov A, Barinov A, et al. Oral treatment with alpha-lipoic acid improves symptomatic diabetic polyneuropathy. *Diabetes Care*. 2006;29:2365–70.

183. Ziegler D, Hanefeld M, Ruhnau K-J, et al. Treatment of symptomatic diabetic polyneuropathy with the antioxidant alpha-lipoic acid: a 7-month multicenter randomized controlled trial (ALADIN III Study). *Diabetes Care*. 1999;22:1296–301.

184. Reljanovic M, Reichel G, Rett K, et al. Treatment of diabetic polyneuropathy with the antioxidant thioctic acid (α-lipoic acid): a two year multicenter randomized double-blind placebo-controlled trial (ALADIN II). *Free Radical Res*. 1999;31:171–9.

185. Ruhnau K-J, Meissner HP, Finn J-R, et al. Effects of 3-week oral treatment with the antioxidant thioctic acid (alpha-lipoic acid) in symptomatic diabetic polyneuropathy. *Diabetic Med*. 1999;16;1040–3.

186. Hahm JR, Kim, BJ, Kim KW. Clinical experience with thioctacid (thioctic acid) in the treatment of distal symmetric polyneuropathy in Korean diabetic patients. *J Diab & Its Complications*. 2004;18:79–85.

187. Evans JL, Heymann CJ, Goldfine ID and Gavin LA. Pharmacokinetics, tolerability and fructosamine-lowering effect of a novel, controlled-release formulation of alpha-lipoic acid. *Endocrine Pract*. 2002;8:29–34.

188. Kamenova P. Improvement of insulin sensitivity in patients with type 2 diabetes mellitus after oral administration of alpha-lipoic acid. *Intl J Endo Metab*. 2007;5:251–8.

189. Lim W, Mudge KW, Vermeylen F. Effects of population, age, and cultivation methods on ginsenoside content of wild American ginseng (*Panax quinquefolium*). *J Agric Food Chem*. 2005;53:8498–505.

190. King ML, Adler SR, Murphy LL. Extraction-dependent effects of American ginseng (*Panax quinquefolium*) on human breast cancer cell proliferation and estrogen receptor activity. *Integr Cancer Ther*. 2006;5:236–43.

191. Stavro PM, Woo M, Leiter LA, et al. Long-term intake of north American ginseng has no effect on 24-hour blood pressure and renal function. *Hypertension*. 2006;47:791–6.

192. Stavro PM, Woo M, Heim TF, et al. North American ginseng exerts a neutral effect on blood pressure in individuals with hypertension. *Hypertension*. 2005;46:406–11.

193. Brown R. Potential interactions of herbal medicines with antipsychotics, antidepressants and hypnotics. *Eur J Herbal Med*. 1997;3:25–8.

194. Yuan C-S, Wei G, Dey L, et al. American ginseng reduces warfarin's effect in healthy patients. *Ann Int Med*. 2004;141:23–7.

195. Dascalu A, Sievenpiper JL, Jenkins AL, et al. Five batches of Ontario-grown American ginseng root product comparable reductions of postprandial glycemia in healthy individuals. *Can J Physiol Pharmacol*. 2007; 85:856–64.

196. McElhaney JE, Gravenstein S, Cole SK. A placebo-controlled trial of a proprietary extract of North American ginseng (CVT-E002) to prevent acute respiratory illness in institutionalized older adults. *JAGS*. 2004: 52:13–9.

197. Predy GN, Goel V, Lovlin R, et al. Efficacy of an extract of North American ginseng containing poly-furanosyl-pyranosyl-saccharides for preventing upper respiratory tract infections: a randomized controlled trial. *CMAJ*. 2005;173:1043–8.

198. McElhaney JE, Goel V, Toane B. Efficacy of COLD-fX in the prevention of respiratory symptoms in community-dwelling adults: a randomized, double-blinded, placebo controlled trial. *Altern Complement Med*. 2006;12:153–7.

199. Chase CK, McQueen CE. The use of cinnamon in diabetes. *Am J Health System Pharm*. 2007;64:1033–35.

200. Imparl-Radosevich J, Deas S, Polansky MM, et al. Regulation of PTP-1 and insulin receptor kinase by fractions from cinnamon: implications for cinnamon regulation of insulin signalling. *Horm Res*. 1998;50:177–82.

201. Blevins SM, Leyva MJ, Brown J, et al. Effect of cinnamon on glucose and lipid levels in non-insulin-dependent type 2 diabetes. *Diabetes Care*. 2007;30:2236–7.

202. Altschuler JA, Casella SJ, MacKenzie SJ, et al. The effect of cinnamon on A1C among adolescents with type 1 diabetes. *Diabetes Care*. 2007; 30:813–6.

203. Khan A, Safdar M, Khan MMA, et al. Cinnamon improves glucose and lipids of people with type 2 diabetes. *Diabetes Care*. 2003;26:3215–8.

204. Baker WL, Gutierrez-Williams G, White CM, et al. Effect of cinnamon on glucose control and lipid parameters. *Diabetes Care*. 2008;31:41–3.

205. Wang JG, Anderson RA, Graham GM 3rd, et al. The effect of cinnamon extract on insulin resistance parameters in polycystic ovary syndrome: a pilot study. *Fertil Steri*. 2007;88:240–3.

206. Arlt W, Callies F, van Vlijmen JC, et al. Dehydroepiandrosterone replacement in women with adrenal insufficiency. *N Engl J Med*. 1999; 341:1013–20.

207. Dean CE. Prasterone (DHEA) and mania. *Ann Pharmacother*. 2000; 34:1419–22.

208. Kline MD, Jaggers ED. Mania onset while using dehydroepiandrosterone. *Am J Psychiatry*. 1999;156:971.

209. Acacio BD, Stanczyk FZ, Mullin P, et al. Pharmacokinetics of dehydroepiandrosterone and its metabolites after long-term daily oral administration to healthy young men. *Fertil Steril*. 2004; 81:595–604.

210. Løvås K, Gebre-Medhin G, Trovik TS, et al. Replacement of dehydroepiandrosterone in adrenal failure: no benefit for subjective health status and sexuality in a 9-month, randomized, parallel group clinical trial. *J Clin Endocrinol Metab*. 2003;88:1112–8.

211. Meston CM, Heiman JR. Acute dehydroepiandrosterone effects on sexual arousal in premenopausal women. *J Sex Marital Ther*. 2002;28:53–60.

212. Hackbert L, Heiman JR. Acute dehydroepiandrosterone (DHEA) effects on sexual arousal in postmenopausal women. *J Womens Health Gend Based Med*. 2002;11:155–62.

213. Bauleiu EE, Thomas G, Legrain S, et al. Dehydroepiandrosterone (DHEA), DHEA sulfate, and aging: contribution of the DHEAge study to a sociobiomedical issue. *Proc Nat Acad Sci U S A*. 2000;97:4279–84.

214. Reiter WJ, Pycha A, Schatzl, et al. Dehydroepiandrosterone in the treatment of erectile dysfunction: a prospective, double-blind, randomized, placebo-controlled study. *Urology*. 1999;53:590–4.

215. Stomati M, Rubino S, Spineti A, et al. Endocrine, neuroendocrine and behavioral effects of oral dehydroepiandrosterone sulfate supplementation in postmenopausal women. *Gynecol Endocrinol*. 1999;13:15–25.

216. Stomati M, Monteleone P, Casarosa E, et al. Six-month oral dehydroepiandrosterone supplementation in early and late postmenopause. *Gynecol Endocrinol*. 2000;14:342–63.

217. Reiter WJ, Schatzl G, Mark I, et al. Dehydroepiandrosterone in the treatment of erectile dysfunction in patients with different organic etiologies. *Urol Res*. 2001;29:278–81.

218. Morales AJ, Haubrich RH, Hwang JY, et al. The effect of six months treatment with a 100 mg daily dose of dehydroepiandrosterone (DHEA) on circulating sex steroids, body composition and muscle strength in age-advanced men and women. *Clin Endocrinol*. 1998;49:421–32.

219. Villareal DT, Holloszy JO. DHEA enhances effects of weight training on muscle mass and strength in elderly women and men. *Am J Physiol Endolcrinol Metab* 2006;291:E1003–8.

220. Wallace MB, Lim J, Cutler A, et al. Effects of dehydroepiandrosterone vs androstenedione supplementation in men. *Med Sci Sports Exerc*. 1999; 31:1788–92.

221. Brown GA, Vukovich MD, Sharp RL, et al. Effect of oral DHEA on serum testosterone and adaptations to resistance training in young men. *J Appl Physiol*. 1999;87:2274–83.

222. Villareal DT, Holloszy JO, Kohrt WM. Effects of DHEA on bone mineral density and body composition in elderly women and men. *Clin Endocrinol* 2000; 53:561–8.

223. Jankowski CM, Gozansky WS, Schwartz RS, et al. Effects of dehydroepiandrosterone replacement therapy on bone mineral density in older adults: a randomized, controlled trial. *J Clin Endocrinol Metab* 2006; 91(8):2986–93.

224. van Niekirk JK, Huppert FA, Herbert J. Salivary cortisol and DHEA: association with measures of cognition and well-being in normal older men, and effects of three months of DHEA supplementation. *Psychoneuroendocrinology*. 2001;26:591–612.

225. Hirshman E, Wells E, Wierman ME, et al. The effect of dehydroepiandrosterone (DHEA) on recognition memory decision processes and discrimination in postmenopausal women. *Psychonomic Bull Rev*. 2003;10:125–34.

226. Panossian A, Hovhannisyan A, Mamikonyan G, et al. Pharmacokinetic and oral bioavailability of andrographolide from *Andrographis paniculata* fixed combination Kan Jang in rats and humans. *Phytomedicine*. 2000;7:351–64.

227. Puri A, Saxena R, Saxena RP, et al. Immunostimulant agents from *Andrographis paniculata*. *J Nat Prod*. 1993;56:995–9.

228. Coon JT, Ernst E. Andrographis paniculata in the treatment of upper respiratory tract infections: a systematic review of safety and efficacy. *Planta Med*. 2004;70:293–8.

229. Caceres DD, Hancke JF, Burgos RA, Wikman GK. Prevention of common colds with *Andrographis paniculata* dried extract: a pilot, double-blind trial. *Phytomedicine*. 1997;4:101–4.

230. Calabrese C, Berman SH, Babish JG, et al. A phase I trial of andrographolide in HIV positive patients and normal volunteers. *Phytother Res*. 2000;14:333–8.

231. *Drug Facts and Comparisons*. St Louis: Wolters Kuwer Health; 2008: KU-7, 10.

232. Mero A, Kahkonen J, Nykanen T, et al. IGF-I, IgA, and IgG responses to bovine colostrum supplementation during training. *J Appl Physiol*. 2002;93:732–9.

233. Greenberg PD, Cello JP. Treatment of severe diarrhea caused by *Cryptosporidium parvum* with oral bovine immunoglobulin concentrate in patients with AIDS. *AIDS Hum Retrovirol*. 1996;13:348–54.

234. Ashraf H, Mahalanabis D, Mitra AK, et al. Hyperimmune bovine colostrum in the treatment of shigellosis in children: a double-blind, randomized, controlled trial. *Acta Paediatr*. 2001;90(12):1373–8.

235. Hofman Z, Smeets R, Verlaan G, et al. The effect of bovine colostrum supplementation on exercise performance in elite field hockey players. *Int J Sport Nutr Exerc Metab*. 2002;12:461–9.

236. Brinkworth GD, Buckley JD, Bourdon PC, et al. Oral bovine colostrum supplementation enhances buffer capacity but not rowing performance in elite female rowers. *Int J Sport Nutr Exerc Metab*. 2002;12:349–65.

237. Barnes J, Anderson LA, Gibbons S, Phillipson JD. Echinacea species (Echinacea angustifolia (DC.) Hell., Echinacea pallida (Nutt.) Nutt., Echinacea purpurea (L.) Moench): a review of their chemistry, pharmacology and clinical properties. *J Pharm Pharmacol*. 2005;57:929–54.

238. Lee A, Werth V. Activation of autoimmunity following use of immunostimulatory herbal supplements. *Arch Dermatol*. 2004;140:723–7.

239. Yale SH, Glurich I. Analysis of the inhibitory potential of *Ginkgo biloba, Echinacea purpurea,* and *Serenoa repens* on the metabolic activity of cytochrome P450 3A4, 2D6, and 2C9. *J Altern Complement Med*. 2005;11:433–9.

240. Perri D, Dugoua JJ, Mills E, Koren G. Safety and efficacy of echinacea (Echinacea angustafolia, e. purpurea and e. pallida) during pregnancy and lactation. *Can J Clin Pharmacol*. 2006;13:e262–7.

241. Linde K, Barrett B, Wölkart K, et al. Echinacea for preventing and treating the common cold. *Cochrane Database Syst Rev*. 2006;1:CD000530.

242. Shah SA, Sander S, White CM, et al. Evaluation of echinacea for the prevention and treatment of the common cold: a meta-analysis. *Lancet Infect Dis*. 2007;7:473–80.

243. Isolauri E, Sutas Y, Kankaanpaa P, et al. Probiotics: effects on immunity. *Am J Clin Nutr*. 2001;73:444S–50S.

244. Temmerman R, Scheirlinck I, Huys G, et al. Culture-independent analysis of probiotic products by denaturing gradient gel electorophoresis. *Applied Environ Microbiol*. 2003;69:220–6.

245. Mason P. *Dietary Supplements*. 3rd ed. London, UK: Pharmaceutical Press; 2007:251–62.

246. MacGregor G, Smith AJ, Thakker B, et al. Yoghurt biotherapy: contraindicated in immunosuppressed patients? *Postgrad Med*. 2002;78:366–7.

247. Rautava S, Kalliomäki M, Isolauri E. Probiotics during pregnancy and breastfeeding might confer immunomodulatory protection against atopic disease in the infant. *J Allergy Clin Immunol*. 2002;109:119–21.

248. McFarland LV. Meta-analysis of probiotics for the prevention of antibiotic associated diarrhea and the treatment of *Clostridium difficile* disease. *Am J Gastroenterol* 2006;101:812–22.

249. Kalliomäki M, Salminen S, Arvilommi H, et al. Probiotic in primary prevention of atopic disease: a randomized placebo-controlled trial. *Lancet*. 2001;357:1076–9.

250. Osborn DA. Sinn JK. Probiotics in infants for prevention of allergic disease and food hypersensitivity. *Cochrane Database Syst Rev*. 2007;4:CD006475.

251. Viljanen M, Savilahti E, Haahtela T, et al. Probiotics in the treatment of atopic eczema/dermatitis syndrome in infants: a double-blind placebo-controlled trial. *Allergy*. 2005;60:494–500.

252. Moreira A, Kekkonen R, Korpela R, et al. Allergy in marathon runners and effect of Lactobacillus GG supplementation on allergic inflammatory markers. *Respir Med*. 2007;101:1123–31.

253. Xiao JZ, Kondo S, Yanagisawa N, et al. Probiotics in the treatment of Japanese cedar pollinosis: a double-blind placebo-controlled trial. *Clin Exper Allergy*. 2006;36:1425–35.

254. Eleutherococcus senticosus. *Altern Med Rev*. 2006;11:151–5.

255. Williams M. Immunoprotection against herpes simplex type II infection by eleutherococcus root extract. *Int J Altern Complement Med*. 2001;13:9–12.

256. Dasgupta A, Wu S, Actor J, et al. Effect of Asian and Siberian ginseng on serum digoxin measurement by five digoxin immunoassays. *Am J Clin Path*. 2003;119:289–303.

257. Donovan JL, DeVane CL, Chavin KD, et al. Siberian ginseng (*Eleutherococcus senticosus*) effects on CYP2D6 and CYP3A4 activity in normal volunteers. *Drug Metab Dispos*. 2003;31:519–22.

258. Coon JT, Ernst E. *Panax ginseng:* a systematic review of adverse effects and drug interactions. *Drug Saf*. 2002;25:323–44.

259. Reay JL, Kennedy DO, Scholey AB. Single doses of *Panax ginseng* (G115) reduce blood glucose levels and improve cognitive performance during sustained mental activity. *J Psychopharmacol*. 2005;19:357–65.

260. Kennedy DO, Haskell CF, Wesnes KA, et al. Improved cognitive performance in human volunteers following administration of guarana (*Paullinia cupana*) extract: comparison and interaction with Panax ginseng. *Pharmacol Biochem Behav*. 2004;79:401–11.

261. Volger BK, Pittler MH, Ernst E. The efficacy of ginseng: a systematic review of randomized clinical trials. *Eur J Clin Pharmacol*. 1999;55:567–75.

262. Persson J, Bringlöv E, Nilsson LG, Nyberg L. The memory-enhancing effects of Ginseng and *Ginkgo biloba* in healthy volunteers. *Psychopharmacology* (Berl). 2004;172:430–4.

263. Sievenpiper JL, Arnason JT, Leiter LA, Vuksan V. Null and opposing effects of Asian ginseng (*Panax ginseng* C.A. Meyer) on acute glycemia: results of two acute dose escalation studies. *J Am Coll Nutr*.2003;22:524–32.

264. Sievenpiper JL, Sung MK, Di Buono M, et. al. Korean red ginseng rootlets decrease acute postprandial glycemia: results from sequential preparation- and dose-finding studies. *J Am Coll Nutr*. 2006;25:100–7.

265. Vuksan V, Sung MK, Sievenpiper JL, et al. Korean red ginseng (*Panax ginseng*) improves glucose and insulin regulation in well-controlled, type 2 diabetes: results of a randomized, double-blind, placebo-controlled study of efficacy and safety. *Nutr Metab Cardiovasc Dis*. 2008;18:46–56.

266. Mukhtar H, Ahmad N. Tea polyphenols: prevention of cancer and optimizing health. *Am J Clin Nutr*. 2000;71(suppl):1698–702.

267. Henning S, Niu Y, Lee N, et al. Bioavailability and antioxidant activity of tea flavanols after consumption of green tea, black tea, or green tea extract supplement. *Am J Clin Nutr*. 2004;80:1558–64.

268. The Stash Tea Company. Caffeine Information on Tea. Available at: http://www.stashtea.com/caffeine.htm. Last accessed October 23, 2008.

269. Heck A, DeWitt B, Lukes A. Potential interactions between alternative therapies and warfarin. *Am J Health Syst Pharm*. 2000;57:1221–30.

270. Imai K, Nakachi K. Cross sectional study of effects of drinking green tea on cardiovascular and liver disease. *BMJ*. 1995;310:693–6.

271. Princen HM, Duyvenvoorde W, Buytenhek R, et al. No effect of consumption of green and black tea on plasma lipid, on antioxidant levels and on LDL oxidation in smokers. *Arterioscler Thromb Vasc Biol*. 1998;18:833–41.

272. Maron D, Lu G, Cai N, et al. Cholesterol lowering effect of a theaflavin-enriched green tea extract: a randomized controlled trial. *Arch Intern Med*. 2003;163:1448–53.

273. Wolfram S. Effects of green tea and EGCG on cardiovascular and metabolic health. *J Am Coll Nutr*. 2007;26:373S-88S.

274. Bushman J. Green tea and cancer in humans: a review of the literature. *Nutr Cancer*. 1998;31:151–9.

275. Kurahashi N, Sasazuki S, Iwasaki M, et al; JPHC Study Group. Green tea consumption and prostate cancer risk in Japanese men: a prospective study. *Am J Epidemiol*. 2008;167:71–7.

276. Yoshitaka T, Yoshikazu N, Shoko K, et al. Green tea and the risk of gastric cancer in Japan. *N Engl J Med*. 2001;344:632–6.

277. Duenwald M. "An appetite killer for a killer appetite? Not yet." *The New York Times*. April 19, 2005.

278. Ni Mhurchu C, Dunshea-Mooij C, Bennett D, Rodgers A. Effect of chitosan on weight loss in overweight and obese individuals: a systematic review of randomized controlled trials. *Obesity Rev*. 2005;6:35–42.

279. Sultan S, Spector J, Mitchell RM. Ischemic colitis associated with use of a bitter orange-containing dietary weight-loss supplement. *Mayo Clinic Proceed*. 2006;81:1630–1.

280. *Pygeum africanum* (*Prunus africana*) (African plum tree). *Altern Med Rev*. 2002;7:71–4.

281. McQueen C, Bryant P, Pepping J. Alternative therapies: pygeum. *Am J Health Syst Pharm*. 2001;58:120–3.

282. Wilt T, Ishani A, Mac Donald R, et al. Pygeum africanum for benign prostatic hyperplasia. *Cochrane Database Syst Rev*. 2002;1:CD001044.

283. Howell AB. Bioactive compounds in cranberries and their role in prevention of urinary tract infections. *Mol Nutr Food Res*. 2007;51:732–7.

284. Terris MK, Issa MM, Tacker JR. Dietary supplementation with cranberry concentrate tablets may increase the risk of nephrolithiasis. *Urology*. 2001;57:26–9.

285. Pham DQ, Pham AQ. Interaction potential between cranberry juice and warfarin. *Am J Health Syst Pharm*. 2007;64:490–4.

286. Jepson R, Craig J. Cranberries for preventing urinary tract infections. *Cochrane Database Syst Rev*. 2008;1:CD001321.

287. Linsenmeyer T, Harrison B, Oakley A, et al. Evaluation of cranberry supplement for reduction of urinary tract infections in individuals with neurogenic bladders secondary to spinal cord injury. A prospective, double-blinded, placebo-controlled, crossover study. *J Spinal Cord Med*. 2004;27:29–34.

288. Jepson RG, Mihaljevic L, Craig J. Cranberries for treating urinary tract infections. *Cochrane Database Syst Rev*. 2000;2:CD001322.

289. Gerber GS, Zabaja GP, Bales GT, et al. Saw palmetto in men with lower urinary tract symptoms: effect on urodynamic parameters and voiding symptoms. *Urology*. 1998;51:1003–7.

290. Cheema P, El-Mefty O, Jazieh AR. Intraoperative haemorrhage associated with the use of extract of Saw Palmetto herb: a case report and review of literature. *J Intern Med*. 2001;250:167–9.

291. Wilt T, Ishani A, Mac Donald R. *Serenoa repens* for benign prostatic hyperplasia. *Cochrane Database Syst Rev*. 2002;2:CD001423.

292. Bent S, Kane C, Shinohara K, et al. Saw palmetto for benign prostatic hyperplasia. *N Eng J Med*. 2006;354:557–66.

293. Morreale P, Manopulo R, Galati M, et al. Comparison of the anti-inflammatory efficacy of chondroitin sulfate and diclofenac sodium in patients with knee osteoarthritis. *J Rheumatol*. 1996;23:1385–91.

294. Leeb BF, Schweitzer H, Montag K, et al. A meta-analysis of chondroitin sulfate in the treatment of osteoarthritis. *J Rheumatol*. 2000;27:205–11.

295. Uebelhart D, Malaise M, Marcolongo R, et al. Intermittent treatment of knee osteoarthritis with oral chondroitin sulfate: a one-year, randomized, double-blind, multicenter study versus placebo. *Osteoarthr Cart*. 2004;12:269–76.

296. Mazieres B, Combe B, Phan Van A, et al. Chondroitin sulfate in osteoarthritis of the knee: a prospective, double-blind, placebo-controlled multicenter clinical study. *J Rheumatol*. 2001;28:173–81.

297. Tallia AF, Cardone DA. Asthma exacerbation association with glucosamine-chondroitin. *J Am Board Fam Pract*. 2003;15:481–4.

298. Morrison LM, Rucker PG, Ershoff BH. Prolongation of thrombus-formation time in rabbits given chondroitin sulfate A. *J Atheroscler Res*. 1968;8:319–27.

299. McAlindon TE, LaValley MP, Gulin JP, et al. Glucosamine and chondroitin for treatment of osteoarthritis: a systematic quality assessment and meta-analysis. *JAMA*. 2000;283:1469–75.

300. Michel B, Stucki G, Frey D, et al. Chondroitins 4 and 6 sulfate in osteoarthritis of the knee. *Arth Rheumatism*. 2005;52:779–86.

301. Grant L, McBean DE, Fyfe L, Warnock AM. A review of the biological and potential therapeutic actions f *Harpagophytum procumbens*. *Phytother Res*. 2007;21:199–209.

302. Mahomed IM, Ojewole JAO. Anticonvulsant activity of *Harpagophytum procumbens* DC [Pedaliaceae] secondary root aqueous extract. *Brain Res Bull*. 2006;69:57–62.

303. Mahomed IM, Ojewole JAO. Analgesic, anti-inflammatory and anti-diabetic properties of *Harpagophytum procumbens* DC (Pedaliaceae) secondary root aqueous extract. *Phytother Res*. 2004;18:982–9.

304. Fiebich BL, Heinrich M, Hiller K-O, Kammerer N. Inhibition of TNF-α synthesis in LPS-stimulated primary human monocytes by *Harpagophytum procumbens* extract SteiHap 69. *Phytomedicine*. 2001;8:28–30.

305. Chrubasik JE, Neumann E, Müller-Ladner U, et al. Potential molecular basis of the chondroprotective effect of *Harpagophytum procumbens*. *Phytomedicine*. 2006;13:598–600.

306. Brien S, Lewith GT, McGregor G. Devil's claw (*Harpagophytum procumbens*) as a treatments for osteoarthritis: a review of efficacy and safety. *J Altern Complement Med*. 2006;12:981–93.

307. Gagnier JJ, Chrubasik S, Manheimer E. *Harpagophytum procumbens* for osteoarthritis and low back pain: a systematic review. *BMC Complement Altern Med*. 2004;4:13. Available at: http://www.biomedcentral.com/1472-6882/4/13. Last accessed October 23, 2008.

308. Hoffer LJ, Kaplan LN, Hamadeh MJ, et al. Sulfate could mediate the therapeutic effect of glucosamine sulfate. *Metab Clin Exp*. 2001;50:767–70.

309. Piperno M, Reboul P, Hellio Le Graverand MP, et al. Glucosamine sulfate modulates dysregulated activities of human osteoarthritic chondrocytes in vitro. *Osteoarth Cart*. 2000;8:207–12.

310. Lippiello L. Glucosamine and chondroitin sulfate: biological response modifiers of chondrocytes under simulated conditions of joint stress. *Osteoarth Cart*. 2003;11:335–42.

311. Christgau S, Henrotin Y, Tankó LB, et al. Osteoarthritic patients with high cartilage turnover show increased responsiveness to the cartilage turnover show increased responsiveness to the cartilage protecting effects of glucosamine sulphate. *Clin Exp Rheumatol*. 2004;22:36–42.

312. Houpt JB, McMillan R, Wein C, et al. Effect of glucosamine hydrochloride in the treatment of pain of osteoarthritis of the knee. *J Rheumatol*. 1999;26:2423–30.

313. Clegg DO, Reda DJ, Harris CL, *et al*. Glucosamine, chondroitin sulfate, and the two in combination for painful knee osteoarthritis. *N Engl J Med*. 2006;354:795–808.

314. Cohen M, Wolfe R, Mai T, et al. A randomized, double blind, placebo controlled trial of a topical cream containing glucosamine sulfate, chondroitin sulfate, and camphor for osteoarthritis of the knee. *J Rheumatol*. 2003;30:523–8.

315. Kanwischer M, Kim SY, Kim JS, et al. Evaluation of the physiochemical stability and skin permeation of glucosamine sulfate. *Drug Devel Indust Pharm*. 2005;31:91–7.

316. Villacis J, Rice TR, Bucci LR, et al. Do shrimp-allergic individuals tolerate shrimp-derived glucosamine? *Clin Exper Allergy*. 2006;36:1457–61.

317. Reginster JY, Deroisy R, Rovati LC, et al. Long-term effects of glucosamine sulphate on osteoarthritis progression: a randomized, placebo-controlled clinical trial. *Lancet*. 2001;357:251–6.

318. Pavelka K, Gatterová J, Olejarová M, et al. Glucosamine sulfate use and delay of progression of knee osteoarthritis. *Arch Intern Med*. 2002;162:2113–23.

319. Scroggie DA, Albright A, Harris MD. The effects of glucosamine-chondroitin supplementation on glycosylated hemoglobin levels in patients with type 2 diabetes mellitus. *Arch Intern Med*. 2003;163:1587–90.

320. Muniyappa R, Karne RJ, Hall G, et al. Oral glucosamine for 6 weeks at standard doses does not cause or worsen insulin resistance or endothelial dysfunction in lean or obese subjects. *Diabetes*. 2006;55:3142–50.

321. Albert SG, Oiknine RF, Parseghian S, et al. The effect of glucosamine on serum HDL cholesterol and apolipoprotein A1 levels in people with diabetes. *Diabetes Care*. 2007;30:2800–3.

322. Kayne SB, Wadeson K, MacAdam A. Is glucosamine an effective treatment for osteoarthritis? A meta-analysis. *Pharm J*. 2000;265:759–63.

323. Richy F, Bruyere O, Ethgen O, et al. Structural and symptomatic efficacy of glucosamine and chondroitin and knee osteoarthritis. A comprehensive meta-analysis. *Arch Int Med*. 2003;163:1514–22.

324. Herrero-Beaumont G, Ivorra JAR, Trabado MC, *et al*. Glucosamine sulfate in the treatment of knee osteoarthritis symptoms. *Arthritis Rheum*. 2007;56:555–67.

325. Ely A, Lockwood B. What is the evidence for the safety and efficacy of dimethyl sulfoxide and methylsulfonylmethane in pain relief? *Pharmaceutical J*. 2002;269:685–7.

326. Rizzo R, Grandolfo M, Godeas C, et al. Calcium, sulfur, and zinc distribution in normal and arthritic articular equine cartilage: a synchrotron radiation-induced X-ray emission (SRIXE) study. *J Exp Zoology*. 1995;273:82–6.

327. Moore RD, Morton JI. Diminished inflammatory joint disease in MRL/1pr mice ingesting dimethylsulfoxide (DMSO) or methylsulfonylmethane (MSM). *Fed Proc*. 1985;44:530, 692.

328. Barrager E, Veltmann JR Jr., Schauss AG, et al. A multi-centered, open-label trial on the safety and efficacy of methylsulfonylmethane in the treatment of seasonal allergic rhinitis. *J Altern Complement Med*. 2002;8:167–73.

329. Horvath K, Noker PE, Somfai-Relle S, et al. Toxicity of methylsulfonylmethane in rats. *Food Chem Toxicol*. 2002;40:1459–62.

330. Usha PR, Naidu MUR. Randomised, double-blind, parallel, placebo-controlled study of oral glucosamine, methylsulfonylmethane and their combination in osteoarthritis. *Clin Drug Invest*. 2004;24:353–63.

331. Kim SL, Axelrod LJ, Howard P, et al. Efficacy of methylsulfonylmethane (MSM) in osteoarthritis pain of the knee: a pilot clinical trial. *Osteoarthritis Cartilage*. 2006;14:286–94.

332. Gorën JL, Stoll AL, Damico KE, et al. Bioavailability and lack of toxicity of S-adenosyl-L-methionine (SAMe) in humans. *Pharmacotherapy*. 2004;24:1501–7.

333. Berger R, Nowak H. A new medical approach to the treatment of osteoarthritis: report of an open phase IV study with ademethionine (Gumbaral). *Am J Med*. 1987;83:84–4.

334. Fetrow CW, Avila JR. Efficacy of the dietary supplement S-adenosyl-L-methionine. *Ann Pharmacotherapy*. 2001;35:1414–25.

335. Brown RP, Gerbarg P, Bottiglieri T. S-adenosylmethionine (SAMe) for depression. *Psychiatric Ann*. 2002;1:29–44.

336. Lipinski JF, Cohen BM, Frankenberg F, et al. An open trial of S-adenosyl methionine for treatment of depression. *Am J Psychiatry*. 1984;141:448–50.

337. Carney MWP, Martin R, Bottiglieri T, et al. Switch mechanism in affective illness and S-adenosyl methionine. *Lancet*. 1983;1:820–1.

338. Carney MWP, Edeh J, Bottiglieri T, et al. Affective illness and S-adenosyl methionine: a preliminary report. *Clin Neuropharmacol*. 1986;9:379–85.

339. Kagan BL, Sultzer DL, Rosenlicht N, et al. Oral S-adenosylmethionine in depression: a randomized, double-blind, placebo-controlled trial. *Am J Psychiatry*. 1990;147:591–5.

340. Carrieri PB, Indaco A, Gentile S, et al. S-adenosylmethionine treatment of depression in patients with Parkinson's disease. A double-blind, crossover study versus placebo. *Curr Therapeut Res*. 1990;48:154–60.

341. Fetrow CW. S-Adenosyl-L-methionine (SAMe) and depression. *Pharm Dietary Suppl Alert*. 2000;1:1–8.

342. Najm WI, Reinsch S, Hoehler F, et al. S-adenosyl methionine (SAMe) versus celecoxib for the treatment of osteoarthritis symptoms: a double-blind cross-over trial. *BMC Musculoskelet Disord*. 2004;5:6. Available at: http://www.biomedcentral.com/1471-2474/5/6. Last accessed October 23, 2008.

343. Soeken KL, Lee W-L, Bausell RB, et al. Safety and efficacy of S-adenosyl methionine (SAMe) for osteoarthritis: a meta-analysis. *J Fam Pract*. 2002;51:425–30.

344. Bressa GM. S-adenosyl-l-methionine (SAMe) as antidepressant: meta-analysis of clinical studies. *Acta Neurol Scand Suppl*. 1994;154:7–14.

345. Williams A, Girard C, Jui D, *et al*. S-adenosylmethionine (SAMe) as treatment for depression: a systematic review. *Med Clin Exp* 2005;28:132–9.

346. Alpert JE, Papakostas G, Mischoulon D, et al. S-adenosyl-L-methionine (SAMe) as an adjunct for resistant major depressive disorder: an open trial following partial or nonresponse to selective serotonin reuptake inhibitors or venlafaxine. *J Clin Psychopharmacol*. 2004;24:661–4.

347. Tavoni A, Vitali C, Bombardieri S, et al. Evaluation of S-adenosylmethionine in primary fibromyalgia. *Am J Med*. 1987;83(suppl A):107–10.

348. Jacobsen S, Danneskiold-Samsøe B, Bach Andersen R. Oral S-adenosylmethionine in primary fibromyalgia. Double-blind clinical evaluation. *Scand J Rheum*. 1991;20:294–302.

349. Tavoni A, Jeracitano G, Cirigliano G. Evaluation of S-adenosylmethionine in secondary fibromyalgia: a double-blind study. *Clin Exp Rheum*. 1998;16:106–7.

350. Kennedy DO, Scholey A, Tildesley N, et al. Modulation of mood and cognitive performance following acute administration of *Melissa officinalis*. *Pharmcol Biochem Behav*. 2002;72:953–64.

351. Wolbling RH, Leonhardt K. Local therapy of herpes simplex with dried extract from *Melissa officinalis*. *Phytomedicine*. 1994;1:25–31.

352. Koytchev R, Alken RG, Dundarov S. Balm mint extract for topical treatment of recurring Herpes labialis. *Phytomedicine*. 1999;6:225–30.

353. Akhondzadeh S, Noroozian M, Mohammadi M, et al. *Melissa officinalis* extract in the treatment of patients with mild to moderate Alzheimer's disease: a double blind randomized, placebo controlled trial. *J Neurol Neurosurg Psychiatry*. 2003;74:863–6.

354. Kennedy DO, Wake G, Savelev S, et al. Modulation of mood and cognitive performance following acute administration of single doses of Melissa officinalis (Lemon balm) with human CNS nicotinic and muscarinic receptor-binding properties. *Neuropsychopharmacology*. 2003;28:1871–81.

355. Morris MC, Donoghue A, Markowitz JA, Osterhoudt KC. Ingestion of tea tree oil (Melaleuca oil) by a 4-year-old boy. *Pediatr Emerg Care*. 2003;19:169–71.

356. Henley DV, Lipson N, Korach KS, Bloch CA. Prepubertal gynecomastia linked to lavender and tea tree oils. *N Engl J Med*. 2007;356:479–85.

357. Satchell AC, Saurajen A, Bell C, Barnetson RS. Treatment of interdigital tinea pedis with 25% and 50% tea tree oil solution: a randomized, placebo-controlled, blinded study. *Australas J Dermatol*. 2002;43175–8.

358. Buck DS, Nidorf DM, Addino JG. Comparison of two topical preparations for the treatment of onychomycosis: *Melaleuca alternifolia* (tea tree) oil and clotrimazole. *J Fam Pract*. 1994;38:601–5.

359. Bassett IB, Pannowitz DL, Barnestson RSC. A comparative study of tea-tree oil versus benzoyl peroxide in the treatment of acne. *Med J Aust*. 1990;153:455–8.

360. Vazquez JA, Zawawi AA. Efficacy of alcohol-based and alcohol-free melaleuca oral solution for the treatment of fluconazole-refractory oropharyngeal candidiasis in patients with AIDS. *HIV Clin Trials*. 2002;3:379–85.

361. Li JX, Yu ZY. Cimicifugae rhizoma: from origins, bioactive constituents to clinical outcomes. *Curr Med Chem*. 2006;13:2927–51.

362. Lupu R, Mehmi I, Tsai MS, et al. Black cohosh, a menopausal remedy, does not have estrogenic activity and does not promote breast cancer cell growth. *Int J Oncol*. 2003;23:1407–12.

363. Reed SD, Newton KM, LaCroix AZ, et al. Vaginal, endometrial, and reproductive hormone findings: randomized, placebo-controlled trial of black cohosh, multibotanical herbs, and dietary soy for vasomotor symptoms: the Herbal Alternatives for Menopause (HALT) Study. *Menopause*. 2008;15:51–8.

364. Kligler B. Black Cohosh. *Am Fam Physician*. 2003;68:114–6.

365. Huntley A, Ernst E. A systematic review of the safety of black cohosh. *Menopause*. 2003;10:58–64.

366. Mahady GB, Dog TL, Barrett ML, et. al.United States Pharmacopeia review of the black cohosh case reports of hepatotoxicity. *Menopause*. 2008;15(4 pt 1):628–38.

367. Rockwell S, Liu Y, Higgins SA. Alteration of the effects of cancer therapy agents on breast cancer cells by the herbal medicine black cohosh. *Breast Cancer Res Treat*. 2005;90:233–9.

368. Huntley A. Drug-herb interactions with herbal medicines for menopause. *J Br Menopause Soc*. 2004;10:162–5.

369. Writing Group for the Women's Health Initiative Investigators. Risks and benefits of estrogen plus progestin in healthy postmenopausal women: principal results from the Women's Health Initiative. Randomized controlled trial. *JAMA*. 2002;288:321–33.

370. Liske E, Hanggi W, Henneicke-von Zepelin HH, et al. Physiological investigation of a unique extract of black cohosh (*Cimicifuga racemosa rhizoma*): a 6-month clinical study demonstrates no systemic estrogenic effect. *J Womens Health Gend Based Med*. 2002;11:163–74.

371. Vermes G, Bánhidy F, Acs N. The effects of remifemin on subjective symptoms of menopause. *Adv Ther*. 2005;22:148–54.

372. Osmers R, Friede M, Liske E, et al. Efficacy and safety of isopropanolic black cohosh extract for climacteric symptoms. *Obstet Gynecol*. 2005;105:1074–83.

373. Newton KM, Reed SD, LaCroix AZ, et al. Treatment of vasomotor symptoms of menopause with black cohosh, multibotanicals, soy, hormone therapy, or placebo: a randomized trial. *Ann Intern Med*. 2006;145:869–79.

374. Pockaj BA, Gallagher JG, Loprinzi CL, et. al. Phase III double-blind, randomized, placebo-controlled crossover trial of black cohosh in the management of hot flashes: NCCTG Trial N01CC1. *J Clin Oncol*. 2006;24:2836–41.

375. Jacobson JS, Troxel AB, Evans J, et al. Randomized trial of black cohosh for the treatment of hot flashes among women with a history of breast cancer. *J Clin Oncol*. 2001;19:2739–45.

376. North American Menopause Society. Treatment of menopause-associated vasomotor symptoms: position statement of the North American Menopause Society. *Menopause*. 2004;11:11–33.

377. Wuttke W, Jarry H, Christoffel V, et al. Chaste tree (*Vitex agnus-castus*)— pharmacology and clinical indications. *Phytomedicine*. 2003;10:348–57.

378. Daniele C, Thompson Coon J, Pittler MH, Ernst E. *Vitex agnus castus*: a systematic review of adverse events. *Drug Saf*. 2005;28:319–32.

379. Schellenberg R. Treatment for the premenstrual syndrome with *Agnus castus* fruit extract: prospective, randomized, placebo controlled study. *BMJ*. 2001;322:134–7.

380. Atmaca M, Kumru S, Tezcan E. Fluoxetine versus Vitex agnus castus extract in the treatment of premenstrual dysphoric disorder. *Hum Psychopharmacol*. 2003;18:191–5.

381. Halaska M, Beles P, Gorkow C, Sieder C. Treatment of cyclical mastalgia with a solution containing a *Vitex agnus castus* extract: results of a placebo-controlled double-blind study. *Breast*.1999;8:175–81.

382. Dove D, Johnson P. Oral evening primrose oil: its effect on length of pregnancy and selected intrapartum outcomes in low-risk nulliparous women. *J Nurse Midwifery*. 1999;44:320–4.

383. Blommers J, de Lange-De Klerk ES, Kuik DJ, et al. Evening primrose oil and fish oil for severe chronic mastalgia: a randomized double-blind, controlled trial. *Am J Obstet Gynecol*. 2002;187:1389–94.

384. Morse NL, Clough PM. A meta-analysis of randomized, placebo-controlled clinical trials of Efamol evening primrose oil in atopic eczema. Where do we go from here in light of more recent discoveries? *Curr Pharm Biotechnol*. 2006;7:503–24.

385. Keen H, Payan J, Allawi J, et. al. Treatment of diabetic neuropathy with gamma-linolenic acid. The gamma-Linolenic Acid Multicenter Trial Group. *Diab Care*. 1993;16:8–15.

386. Duffy C, Cyr M. Phytoestrogens: potential benefits and implications for breast cancer survivors. *J Womens Health*. 2003;12:617–31.

387. Ju YH, Doerge DR, Allred KF, et al. Dietary genistein negates the inhibitory effect of tamoxifen on growth of estrogen-dependent human breast cancer (MCF-7) cells implanted in athymic mice. *Cancer Res*. 2002;62:2474–7.

388. Peng WX, Li HD, Zhou HH. Effect of daidzein on CYP1A2 activity and pharmacokinetics of theophylline in healthy volunteers. *Eur J Clin Pharmacol*. 2003;59:237–41.

389. Lethaby AE, Brown J, Marjoribanks J, et al. Phytoestrogens for vasomotor menopausal symptoms. *Cochrane Database Syst Rev*. 2007;4: CD001395.

390. Krebs EE, Ensrud KE, MacDonald R, et al. Phytoestrogens for treatment of menopausal symptoms: a systematic review. *Obstet Gynecol*. 2004;104:824–36.

391. Tice JA, Ettinger B, Ensrud K, et al. Phytoestrogen supplements for the treatment of hot flashes: the Isoflavone Clover Extract (ICE) study. *JAMA*. 2003;290:207–14.

392. Duffy C, Perez K, Partridge A. Implications of phytoestrogen intake for breast cancer. *CA Cancer J Clin*. 2007;57:260–77.

393. Dewell A, Hollenbeck PL, Hollenbeck CB. Clinical review: a critical evaluation of the role of soy protein and isoflavone supplementation in the control of plasma cholesterol concentrations. *J Clin Endocrinol Metab*. 2006;91:772–80.

394. Marini H, Minutoli L, Polito F, et al. Effects of the phytoestrogen genistein on bone metabolism in osteopenic postmenopausal women: a randomized trial. *Ann Intern Med*. 2007;146:839–47.

Common Complementary and Alternative Medicine Health Systems

Catherine Ulbricht and Erica Rusie-Seamon

The term *complementary and alternative medicine* (CAM) is generally regarded as a broad group of healing philosophies, diagnostic approaches, and therapeutic interventions that do not conform to the conventional Western health system.[1] *Alternative therapies* have been defined as those used in place of conventional practices, whereas *complementary* or *integrative medicine* can be combined with mainstream approaches.[2,3] Other terms used to refer to CAM include *folkloric, holistic, irregular, nonconventional, non-Western, traditional, unconventional, unorthodox,* and *unproven medicine.* The most common CAM therapies and health systems include Ayurveda, homeopathy, naturopathy, traditional Chinese medicine (TCM)/acupuncture, chiropractic care, and massage. This chapter presents a brief overview of common complementary and alternative modalities other than dietary supplements, which are discussed in depth in Chapters 53 and 54.

Overview of Common CAM Health Systems

Major Domains

In the United States, the National Center for Complementary and Alternative Medicine (NCCAM) classifies CAM therapies into five categories or domains[4]:

1. *Alternative medical systems:* The theories and practices of alternative medical systems developed independently of conventional biomedical approaches (e.g., Ayurveda, homeopathy, and TCM). Some practices such as Ayurveda and TCM preceded the concepts of conventional Western medicine.
2. *Mind–body interventions:* This branch of CAM "focuses on the interactions among the brain, mind, body, and behavior, and on the powerful ways in which emotional, mental, social, spiritual, and behavioral factors can directly affect health." Examples include hypnosis, meditation, yoga, and prayer. *Tai chi* and *qi gong,* components of TCM, may also be considered mind–body interventions.
3. *Biologically based therapies:* This domain "includes, but is not limited to, botanicals, animal-derived extracts, vitamins, minerals, fatty acids, amino acids, proteins, prebiotics and probiotics, whole diets, and functional foods." A major subset includes dietary supplements (see Chapters 53 and 54).
4. *Manipulative and body-based methods:* These diverse practices "focus on the structures and systems of the body, including the bones and joints, the soft tissues, and the circulatory and lymphatic systems." Chiropractic is a major manipulative and body-based method, along with osteopathic manipulation, massage therapy, and reflexology.
5. *Energy therapies:* These therapies use both veritable and putative types of energy. Veritable energies are measurable forces such as light and magnetism that may be used to treat patients. Putative energy fields or "biofields" cannot be measured by using current technologies, but they are based on theories that a human being contains "vital energy" or "life force." Such energy fields include *qi* in TCM and *doshas* in Ayurvedic medicine. Techniques include acupuncture, *qi gong,* and reiki.

Healing systems do not refer to individual practices or remedies, but rather to complete sets of theories and practices. A system centers on a philosophy or lifestyle such as the power of nature or the presence of energy in the body. Some CAM therapies have become widely accepted and integrated into conventional medicine. Many conventional prescription drugs originally came from natural products, such as digoxin from the foxglove plant, paclitaxel from the bark of the yew tree, and yohimbine from yohimbe bark extract.[5]

Potential Benefits and Risks

CAM is often considered a form of preventive medicine and is widely used to maintain health and reduce disease risk.[2] For patients, the attraction of CAM includes the potential to treat diseases for which conventional therapies have failed, an increased sense of patient empowerment and participation, and the perception that CAM may represent safe and natural therapeutic approaches. In addition, some patients use CAM techniques such as meditation and prayer to cope with chronic or untreatable illnesses.[3]

The efficacy of CAM therapies, however, is unproven by conventional clinical testing.[5] Furthermore, natural products may cause adverse effects or may interact with conventional drugs, foods, or other supplements.[1,5] Therefore, CAM should not be used in place of more proven therapies; a qualified health care provider should be consulted about therapies and/or health conditions.

Research Issues

The safety and efficacy of many CAM approaches have not been fully evaluated, although research is increasing.[1] In 1992, the U.S. Congress established the Office of Alternative Medicine within the National Institutes of Health, with a budget of $2 million to rigorously evaluate CAM practices. In 1998, with the creation of NCCAM, Congress elevated the status of the Office of Alternative Medicine to a National Institutes of Health center. The NCCAM budget has progressively increased, from $50 million in fiscal year 1999 to more than $122 million in 2006, toward its mission to support CAM research and education.

When one attempts to learn about CAM health systems, evidence on its safety and efficacy may be difficult to obtain. This difficulty may be due, in part, to the fact that many CAM studies are reported in foreign languages and/or in journals that are not peer-reviewed. To obtain evidence-based information about CAM, the researcher should broaden literature searches to include languages other than English. Several databases should be searched in addition to PubMed or Medline. In addition, researchers may also use guides and/or validated scales such as the Jadad scale to rate the quality of available studies.

Another issue in evaluating CAM research is the lack of standardization. Many individual therapies involve a variety of techniques, making it difficult to compare study results. Some types of CAM such as Ayurveda do not require practitioners to be licensed or even formally trained, which may contribute to the variation within CAM therapies.

Experimental design is perhaps the most problematic issue in CAM research. Some critical elements of clinical research such as placebo control and blinding are often difficult in CAM research. For example, the participatory nature of meditation therapy precludes blinding of the subject to the active treatment.[6] Blinding is also a central problem with acupuncture, because this therapy clearly cannot be easily delivered by a practitioner blinded to the intervention. The Jadad score is sometimes modified for application to acupuncture studies because of the difficulty in blinding the acupuncturist.[7]

As for the challenge of placebo control in CAM therapies such as acupuncture, researchers have developed "sham" treatments to approximate subject blinding. For acupuncture, sham treatment typically involves placement of needles at "non-active" sites or at a proscribed distance (usually about 1 inch) from the active sites in the study, whereas depth and stimulation remain the same. Other sham acupuncture techniques involve treatment at actual acupuncture points but without needle penetration. Critics of this approach argue that even pressure at acupuncture points can elicit effects. Disagreement regarding the validity or best model of sham acupuncture continues in the medical community. Although some studies have demonstrated that sham procedures achieved blinding of subjects, methods used to create sham acupuncture vary widely. Sham acupuncture is often not regarded as a true placebo, given that the patient is subjected to physical stimulation, and experimental studies have shown this technique to also elicit effects.[8]

Working with CAM Practitioners

Ideally, conventional and CAM practitioners should work collaboratively to the benefit of the patient.[1] Pharmacists and other conventional health care providers are encouraged to have an objective attitude toward CAM practitioners, especially as some techniques are now provided in conventional medical centers. An example of an integrative approach is a clinic that includes both conventional and CAM practitioners such as chiropractors or acupuncturists. In addition, more conventional practitioners are becoming comfortable with CAM therapies such as therapeutic massage or acupuncture. Patients should feel comfortable discussing with their conventional health care practitioner any CAM therapies they are using or considering.

Homeopathy

Homeopathy is a distinct system of medicine with its own pharmacopoeia and principles of practice.[9] The term *homeopathy* comes from the two Greek words *homoios* (similar) and *pathos* (suffering or disease). Homeopathy was developed in the early 1800s by German physician Samuel Hahnemann, who also coined the term *allopathy* as a synonym for conventional medicine. Homeopathy is based on the principle of "like cures like" or the "law of similars." This principle states that if a substance produces the symptoms of an illness in large doses, that same substance can cure it in very minute doses. The more attenuated a homeopathic medicine is, the greater is its potency. The efficacy of homeopathic medicines is believed to depend not only on its dilution but also on the vigorous shaking, or *succussion*, which is performed with each dilution.

The homeopathic principle of like cures like is often compared with vaccination, which involves administration of antigenic material to induce immunity to infectious agents.[9] Vaccines typically contain attenuated or killed pathogens or their purified proteins and are used for prophylaxis. In contrast, homeopathic remedies are generally used to treat an existing illness rather than for prophylaxis. One exception is Oscillococcinum, a homeopathic preparation derived from wild duck heart and liver, used to prevent and treat influenza.[10]

Although homeopathic medicines are generally meant to be ingested, they are not classified as dietary supplements. Homeopathic products are regulated by the Food and Drug Administration (FDA) and are subject to the Food, Drug, and Cosmetic Act (FDCA), but the premarket approval process is distinct from the approval process for conventional drugs.[11] Homeopathic drugs are approved with the publication of a monograph by the Homeopathic Pharmacopoeia Convention of the United States in the *Homeopathic Pharmacopoeia of the United States* (HPUS). The criteria for inclusion in the HPUS are demonstrated safety and efficacy, which is subject to clinical verification using conventional clinical trials. Each homeopathic remedy must also be manufactured according to its approved methods of preparation published in the HPUS.[12]

As with conventional drugs, homeopathic remedies may be sold over the counter if they are intended to treat self-limiting conditions such as headaches and colds.[11] If claimed to treat a serious condition such as cancer, homeopathic remedies may be obtained only by prescription. Homeopathic medicines are commonly found in integrative pharmacies that stock alternative remedies along with standard drugs. Chain drugstores and health food markets may also carry homeopathic medicines even in pediatric and veterinary formulations.

According to the 2002 National Health Interview Survey of 31,044 American adults, 3.6% reported using homeopathy.[13] Homeopathic drug sales are estimated to represent 0.26% of the U.S. drug market. Sales of homeopathic medicines increase at a rate of approximately 8% per year and reached an estimated $450 million in 2003.

Technique

Medicines used in homeopathy are derived from many substances including botanical, mineral, and pharmaceutical and zoological sources. These substances are serially diluted and succussed (or triturated) to increase the strength or potency of the medication. This process is called attenuation or "potentization." After each attenuation step, the preparation is given a higher number, so a substance that was attenuated four times would be designated as 4X, 4C, or LM4, depending on the dilution factor. The decimal (1:10 dilutions) and centesimal (1:100 dilutions) scales of attenuation are used to make X and C potencies, respectively, as illustrated in Figure 55-1.[14,15] The letter M is also used in potency terminology and means 1000C, not the use of 1:1000 dilutions in the attenuation process. Although many homeopathic medicines such as aconite and arnica are highly toxic, they are often so dilute that they are well below toxic dosages.

Training

More than 30 schools in North America offer training in homeopathy, and the Council on Homeopathic Education (CHE) currently is developing professional standards for homeopathic education. The Certificate in Classical Homeopathy (CCH) examination process includes a written and an oral section, and is similar to the board examinations taken by conventional health care practitioners to achieve professional status. The organizations provide listings of certified homeopathic practitioners on their Web sites, which the clinician can use to identify qualified homeopaths throughout the United States.[16]

Certification from CCH is not recognized by any state as a license to practice homeopathy. Arizona, Connecticut, and Nevada require that homeopaths also be licensed allopathic or osteopathic physicians. Health freedom acts in California, Minnesota, and Rhode Island protect the rights of professionals without medical licenses to practice homeopathy and other modalities that the state deems harmless. All other states lack specific regulatory language for homeopathy; therefore, homeopathy falls under the statutes regulating the practice of medicine.

Theory/Evidence

Homeopathy originated in the late 1700s when Dr. Samuel Hahnemann developed malaria-like symptoms after taking a high dose of quinine, a treatment for malaria. Hahnemann began testing progressively higher dilutions of various substances in a series of human experiments he called "provings." From these so-called provings, Hahnemann concluded that the strength and efficacy of a substance increased with serial dilutions. Some homeopathic remedies are so dilute that they actually contain no molecules of the active ingredient. According to the principles of homeopathy, the diluent retains an "imprint" of the substance that stimulates the body's innate healing mechanisms. Each serial dilution must also be vigorously shaken (succussed), which is believed to activate or release the healing effects of the substance.[15,17]

Because homeopathic preparations contain little to no active ingredient, critics argue that any demonstrated efficacy is simply a placebo effect.[18] Proponents of homeopathy state that trials have demonstrated effectiveness in infants or animals, and that these subjects are unlikely to have preconceived expectations that may influence their perceptions. Overall the effectiveness of homeopathy has not been consistently demonstrated in randomized controlled trials.[19] Citing the lack of reliable research, NCCAM has stated that the effectiveness of homeopathy cannot be determined for any clinical condition.[4] Similarly both the American Medical Association and the American Academy of Pediatrics have neither accepted nor rejected homeopathy in the treatment of any medical condition.[20]

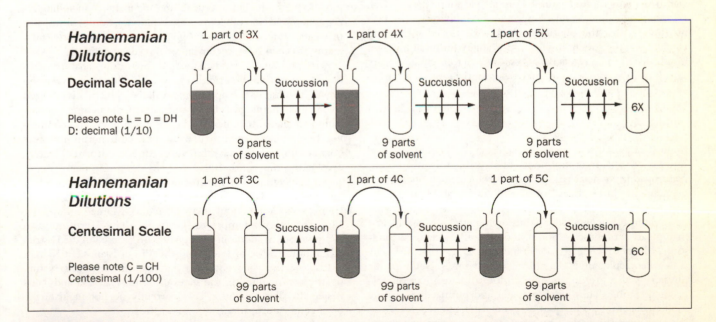

FIGURE 55-1 Method for making homeopathic X and C potencies. Decimal scale, designated by an *X* or *D*, involves dilutions of 1:10 for each attenuation (dilution with succussion) step taken to make the desired X potency. Centesimal scale, designated by *C*, involves dilutions of 1:100 for each attenuation step taken to make the desired C potency. (Reprinted with permission from *Introduction to Homeopathic Medicines for Pharmacists.* New Town Square, Pa: Boiron Institute; 2001:9.)

Safety

The risk of toxicity in homeopathy is generally considered to be low, owing to the extremely dilute nature of homeopathic remedies.[11] Allergic reactions are possible even if the allergens in the ingredients in the homeopathic treatment exist in low concentrations. Theoretically, drugs that alter the immune system such as corticosteroids or antibiotics may block the actions of homeopathic products, although limited evidence exists that this occurs.

Naturopathy

The term *naturopathy* was originated in the late 1890s by John Scheel, a New York City physician. However, Dr. Benedict Lust, who publicized this field of medicine and founded the American School of Naturopathy in 1905, is generally credited as the founder of naturopathy.[21]

Traditional naturopathy is a philosophy of life and an approach to living that incorporates a lifestyle as close to nature as possible. A system of naturopathic therapy employs natural forces such as light, heat, air, water, and massage; this therapy focuses on building health rather than on treating disease. Naturopathic physicians (NDs) may be considered primary care clinicians.

The practice of naturopathic medicine emerges from six underlying principles of healing that distinguish the profession from other medical approaches. These principles are based on the objective observation of the nature of health and disease, and are continually reexamined in light of scientific analysis. The first principle is that the body has the inherent ability to maintain and restore health. Second, the physician aims to identify and treat the cause rather than the symptoms of a disease. The third principle states that methods designed to treat only the symptoms may be harmful and should be avoided or minimized. Fourth, the physician treats the whole person, taking into account the physical, spiritual, mental, and social aspects of the individual. The fifth principle is that the physician plays a role in educating and encouraging the patient to take responsibility for his or her own health. Finally, the physician assesses risk factors and hereditary susceptibility to disease, and makes appropriate interventions to avoid further harm or risk to the patient.

Technique

In most cases of disease or wellness, nutritional counseling and support are major components of naturopathic treatments. Naturopathic physicians use dietetics, fasting, and nutritional supplementation in practice. Botanical medicine and homeopathy may be used in naturopathy.

Naturopathic medicine has its own methods of therapeutic manipulation of muscles, bones, and spine. Physicians use ultrasound, diathermy (electrically induced heat), exercise, massage, water, heat, cold, air, and gentle electrical pulses. Naturopathic physicians also provide natural childbirth care in an out-of-hospital setting. They offer prenatal and postnatal care using modern diagnostic techniques. As general practitioners, NDs may perform minor outpatient surgeries, such as repairing superficial wounds or removal of foreign bodies or cysts.[21]

Because naturopaths believe that mental attitudes and emotional states may influence or cause physical illnesses, counseling, nutritional balancing, stress management, hypnotherapy, biofeedback, and other therapies may be used to help patients heal on the psychological level.

Naturopaths may prescribe substances that are deemed appropriate by the Naturopathic Formulary Advisory Peer Committee. These substances are published in the *Naturopathic Physician Formulary,* which includes uncontrolled substances and drugs of natural origin. Listed substances vary among states depending on state law. In some states such as Utah, naturopaths may prescribe only medicines listed in the *Naturopathic Physician Formulary.*[22]

Training

In North America, seven schools are currently accredited by the Council on Naturopathic Medical Education (CNME).[23] The schools in the United States that offer training for the Doctor of Naturopathic Medicine (ND) degree are Bastyr University (Seattle, Wash), National College of Natural Medicine (Portland, Ore), National University of Health Sciences (Lombard, Ill), Southwest College of Naturopathic Medicine (Tempe, Ariz), and University of Bridgeport College of Naturopathic Medicine (Bridgeport, Conn). In Canada, the training is offered at the Boucher Institute of Naturopathic Medicine (New Westminster, British Columbia) and the Canadian College of Naturopathic Medicine (Toronto, Ontario).

Similar to allopathic medical schools, admission into a naturopathic training program requires 4 years of undergraduate study that includes premedical coursework. The ND degree requires 4 years of postgraduate training, which includes about 4500 hours of academic and clinical training. Academic training includes core subjects such as anatomy, biochemistry, microbiology, and pathology. Clinical training during the last 2 years encompasses various alternative modalities including herbal therapy and homeopathy, in addition to mainstream clinical training such as in cardiology and nutrition. Naturopathic Physicians Licensing Examinations (NPLEX) are taken at the end of both preclinical and clinical training. Naturopathic physicians are educated in modern methods of diagnostic testing and imaging, including X-ray, ultrasound, and other imaging techniques. Some naturopaths may participate in residency programs, including integrative programs that train NDs in conventional medical settings.

In addition to a standard medical curriculum, a naturopathic doctor must study holistic therapies with a strong emphasis on preventing disease and optimizing wellness. The ND is required to complete training in clinical nutrition, acupuncture, homeopathic medicine, botanical medicine, psychology, and counseling. Before they can practice, naturopathic physicians must pass board examinations set by the North American Board of Naturopathic Examiners (NABNE).[24]

The licensing of naturopathic doctors will vary depending on the state. NDs are licensed to practice in Alaska, Arizona, California, Connecticut, Hawaii, Idaho, Maine, Minnesota, Montana, New Hampshire, Oregon, Utah, Vermont, and Washington. In addition, naturopaths are licensed in the District of Columbia, Puerto Rico, and the Virgin Islands. In Kansas, practitioners may be registered as naturopathic physicians. Naturopathy is prohibited in the states of South Carolina and Tennessee. In all other states, laws currently do not regulate the practice of naturopathy.

Because of the increasing popularity of naturopathy, more physicians trained in conventional medicine or other CAM fields are incorporating naturopathic treatments into their practices. Practitioners who hold degrees in osteopathy, chiropractic, acupuncture, dentistry, and veterinary medicine may seek additional training in naturopathy; they use the terms *holistic, natural,* or *integrative* to promote their practices.

Theory/Evidence

The individual methods used in naturopathic medicine vary in their effectiveness. For instance, a proper diet may help prevent heart disease. This recommendation is supported by basic science and is recommended in conventional medicine as well as in naturopathy. Other forms of naturopathic treatment have not been conclusively shown to be effective. For example, acupuncture may help to reduce pain in some instances, but it is not widely recommended for use in place of standard analgesics for extreme pain or in surgery.[25,26] The efficacy of herbal remedies used in naturopathy may vary depending on the herb and the condition treated.[5]

Safety

The safety of naturopathic remedies varies depending on the treatment and the condition treated. Naturopathic methods are generally considered to be safer alternatives to some conventional drugs or treatments. However, herbal remedies are not free from adverse effects and interactions may occur with drugs, supplements, or foods.[1,5,27] The safety of other naturopathic modalities such as fasting or other dietary restrictions often depends on the state of the individual. Perhaps most importantly, naturopathic treatments should not be used in place of more proven therapies for serious medical conditions.

TCM/Acupuncture

Chinese medicine is a broad term encompassing many different modalities and traditions of healing.[5,28] They share a common root in Chinese philosophy including Taoism, Confucianism, and Buddhism, and may date back more than 5000 years. The term *traditional Chinese medicine* is a relatively recent development. In the 1940s and 1950s, the Chinese government undertook an effort to coalesce diverse forms of Chinese medicine into a unified system to be officially defined as TCM. The intent was to integrate traditional practitioners into an organized health system and to provide care for a large population by using familiar and inexpensive methods.

Although TCM is considered to be "complementary" or "alternative" in most of the Western world, in China the term for TCM literally means "central medicine." TCM and Western medicine are commonly used side by side in modern China. As a result, China is relatively advanced compared with Western countries in using integrative medicine. TCM features prominently in the treatment of major illnesses including cancer and heart disease. According to the World Health Organization, TCM is fully integrated into the Chinese health system and is practiced in 95% of Chinese hospitals.[29]

Technique

TCM emphasizes herbal medicine. Herbs are usually given as pills, extracts, capsules, tinctures, or powders; these may be used directly or combined with food or other treatments. More than 400 different kinds of herbs are used in TCM including 50 "fundamental" herbs. Dried herbs and powders in addition to conventional drugs are commonly sold in pharmacies.[30] Some Chinese herbs have received attention in Western medicine for treating serious disorders. For example, the mold *Monascus purpureus* found in red yeast rice is a natural source of lovastatin.[5] Beviramat, derived from the Chinese herb *Syzygium claviflorum*,

is in a new class of anti–human immunodeficiency virus (HIV) drugs called "maturation inhibitors" and is currently in phase IIb clinical trials.[31]

In addition to herbs, TCM also incorporates minerals, metals, and animal products into therapeutic preparations. However, the use of animal products has become more infrequent in recent years, in part because of restrictions on certain species (particularly endangered species).

Acupuncture is also considered a form of TCM, although it is regarded as more of a supportive treatment to herbal therapy.[5] Many different varieties of acupuncture exist both in Chinese and Western medicine. The most common forms of acupuncture in the United States combine the use of acupuncture with Chinese herbs. Classic acupuncture, also known as five-element acupuncture, uses a different needling technique and relies on acupuncture without the use of herbs. Japanese acupuncture uses smaller needles than the other varieties of acupuncture. Medical acupuncture refers to acupuncture practiced by a conventional medical doctor. Auricular acupuncture treats the entire body through acupuncture points in the ears only, and electroacupuncture uses electrical currents attached to acupuncture needles.

Cupping and moxibustion are commonly used to complement acupuncture, but these techniques may also be used independently in TCM.[5] They share the principle of using heat to stimulate circulation to break up congestion or stagnation of blood and *chi* (*qi*), which is the "life force" central to health and well-being in TCM. Cupping has some relation to the massage technique *tuina*, which uses rapid skin pinching at points on the back to break up congestion and stimulate circulation. Moxibustion involves the burning of dried moxa (mugwort), either on or near the skin and sometimes in conjunction with acupuncture needles on specific points. Cupping may also be used over acupuncture points or elsewhere.[32]

TCM practitioners may also use other modalities such as meditation and martial arts.[5] *Tai chi chuan* (or *tai chi*) is a meditative form of martial arts that incorporates the theories of *yin* and *yang* from both Taoism and Confucianism. *Tai chi* is practiced to improve balance, coordination, and relaxation, and overall well-being. TCM may also incorporate *feng shui*, which is the art of arranging furniture and objects to increase health and prosperity.

Training

Acupuncture and Oriental Medicine is a 3- or 4-year masters level program, offered by more than 45 accredited or candidate colleges in the United States. The Accreditation Commission of Acupuncture and Oriental Medicine (ACAOM) gives accreditation to professional acupuncture programs and is recognized by the Department of Education. The National Certification Commission for Acupuncture and Oriental Medicine (NCCAOM) offers three independent certification programs including Acupuncture, Chinese Herbology, and Oriental Bodywork Therapy.[33] Acupuncturists who pass national examinations administered by NCCAOM are entitled to identify themselves as board-certified in their discipline and as diplomates of the NCCAOM.

Licenses to practice acupuncture are granted by individual states. Although requirements vary, many states require acupuncturists to pass the NCCAOM examinations. This organization then verifies credentials and continuing education requirements of its diplomates. Each acupuncturist is required to obtain 30 continuing education credits every 2 years. In Oklahoma, only acupuncturists who hold Doctor of Medicine (MD), Doctor of

Osteopathy (DO), or Doctor of Chiropractic (DC) degrees may perform acupuncture. Alabama, Delaware, Mississippi, North Dakota, South Dakota, and Wyoming do not currently have any laws in place regarding the practice of acupuncture.

Theory/Evidence

Taoism, Confucianism, and Buddhism provided the basis for the development of Chinese medical theory.[5] Nature and the laws that govern the ongoing, harmonious flow of life energy through the natural world are used to understand the body and health. The person is viewed as an ecosystem that is embedded in, and related to, the larger ecosystem of nature and therefore subject to the same laws. The life force called *chi* (or *qi*), circulates through the body and enlivens it. Health is a function of a balanced, harmonious flow of chi, and illness results when there is a blockage or an imbalance in the flow of chi. *Yin* and *yang* are opposite and complementary qualities of life energy (*qi*). *Yin* is regarded as the feminine principle and *yang* the masculine principle. The human being has a system of pathways called "meridians," which may also be referred to as "channels," through which chi flows. Meridians correspond with specific organs or organ systems ("organ networks"). Health is an ongoing process of maintaining balance and harmony of the circulation of chi through all the organs and systems of the body. The body has five organ networks, each corresponding with a particular element.

Despite the growing popularity of TCM in the West, its effectiveness remains debatable. Scientific evidence supports the use of acupuncture for several indications including perioperative dental pain and several types of nausea and vomiting. Moxibustion, which is traditionally used to turn breech babies, has been used with some success, although systematic reviews and meta-analyses have yielded insufficient evidence to support its efficacy.[32] In addition, few well-designed trials of TCM herbal formulas have been conducted.[28] Several drugs derived from TCM such as lovastatin for hyperlipidemia[5] and Beviramat for HIV infection[31] have demonstrated efficacy in clinical trials.

Safety

Adverse events with acupuncture are rare, even with its adjunctive techniques of cupping and moxibustion.[31] Needles must be sterile to avoid disease transmission. Acupuncture should be avoided or used cautiously in individuals with heart disease, diabetes, seizures, infections, bleeding disorders, or neurologic disorders, or among individuals using concomitant use of antithrombotic drugs. Acupuncture should be avoided on areas that have received radiation therapy and during pregnancy. Frail older adults or otherwise medically complex patients should also use acupuncture with caution. Electroacupuncture should be avoided in patients with arrhythmia or seizure disorders, or in patients with pacemakers.

Cupping commonly leaves a temporary bruising of the skin. Moxibustion also may leave a temporary discoloration on the skin, which may be washed off or will disappear on its own. Historically, some traditional practitioners of moxibustion have intentionally employed more aggressive use of the technique to an extent that might leave minor scarring, but this aggressive form of practice is not regularly used in the West.

Chinese herbs have been associated with adverse effects. FDA collected more than 1500 reports of serious toxicity including death related to the use of ephedra (ma huang). Chinese herbs may interact with other herbs, foods, or drugs.[34] There

have been reports of manufactured or processed Chinese herbal products being tainted with toxins or heavy metals. In addition, prescription drugs such as corticosteroids have been included in the preparations but not include in the listed ingredients.

Chiropractic Care

Chiropractic is a discipline that focuses on the relationship between spinal structure and body function mediated by the nervous system.[35] It originated in 1895 with D. D. Palmer, a popular hands-on healer practicing in Davenport, Iowa. Palmer's formulation of *chiropractic* combined the Greek *cheir* (hand) and *praxis* (practice). Palmer's original philosophy described the approach as connecting "man the spiritual" to "man the physical" by eliminating interference to the flow of "Innate Intelligence" through each individual. This innate intelligence, an almost metaphysical phenomenon, flows through the nervous system. The clearer the nervous system is, the more the innate intelligence can express itself and fully enliven the person's body and organs.

Important distinctions exist between the profession of chiropractic, chiropractic care, and spinal manipulation. A chiropractor delivers chiropractic care that is a full range of treatment delivered in one or more therapeutic encounters. Treatment includes procedures and techniques of assessment, and a tailored mix of therapeutic interventions to improve a patient's health status. The term *spinal manipulation* or *adjustment* does not operationally define the profession or chiropractic care, although it is a well-known treatment procedure. Chiropractic care also includes other procedures such as exercise, dietary advice, ergonomic and lifestyle advice, supplements, all forms of physical therapy and rehabilitation intervention, and referral to other practitioners as necessary.

Techniques

Patients usually lie face down on a Cox table, which is similar to a massage table with an open space in which to place the face. Visits may last 15 minutes to 1 hour, depending on the technique used. Chiropractors may see clients up to three times a week at first, then less frequently over time.

Patients can be diagnosed by many different procedures including X-ray, computed tomography, magnetic resonance imaging, electrical current, or ultrasound therapy. Thermography may also be used, followed by treatment with ice packs and heat packs.

More than 100 chiropractic and spinal manipulative adjusting techniques may be employed. Spinal manipulative therapy uses many techniques to apply force to an area of the spine joint. Massage or mobilization of soft tissue is used in techniques such as myofascial trigger point therapy, cross-friction massage, active release therapy, muscle stripping, or Rolfing structural integration. Mechanical traction or the use of external resistance on the spine may also be used. The cracking sound has typically been associated with cavitation in the spinal zygapophyseal (the neural arch between the joint processes) joints. The cracking or popping of a joint has not been proven to be essential to a clinically effective manipulation.

Training

Chiropractic is now one of the largest and best established professions of CAM in the United States. There were 62,000 licensed chiropractors in 2000, and this number is expected to reach 100,000 by 2010. All 50 states have formal statutes that recognize and regulate the practice of chiropractic.[5]

A typical applicant to a chiropractic college has completed 4 years of undergraduate coursework.[36] The curriculum of a chiropractic college includes didactic coursework and clinical training totaling a minimum of 4200 hours. Clinical training with actual patients is typically for a minimum of 1 year. Specialty training is available through full-time residency programs, which may require an additional 2 to 3 years of clinical training. Before they are allowed to practice, doctors of chiropractic must pass national board examinations and become licensed. Chiropractors generally do not prescribe drugs, but those who are also licensed naturopaths may prescribe remedies according to naturopathic guidelines.

Theory/Evidence

Designing clinical trials to evaluate the efficacy of chiropractic is difficult, primarily because of the issues in developing an appropriate placebo. Despite a limited number of well-conducted studies, evidence is reasonable to support the use of chiropractic manipulative therapy in the treatment of episodic tension-type and cervicogenic headache. Insufficient evidence exists to support chiropractic manipulation in the treatment of migraine headache. Similarly, well-designed, double-blind randomized controlled trials of chiropractic manipulation for low back pain have yet to be published. The main methodologic issues are a potentially strong placebo effect and the high rate of spontaneous recovery. For low back pain, sufficient evidence from both blinded and non-blinded trials supports the use of spinal manipulation. Preliminary evidence supports the need for further research on the role of chiropractic for vision problems, shoulder pain, thoracic pain, and whiplash injuries. Chiropractic has been used to treat other conditions including asthma, carpal tunnel syndrome, and hypertension, although evidence is quite limited for these conditions.

Safety

The most common adverse reaction to spinal manipulation is mild transient localized discomfort in the area of treatment.[5] Less common side effects may include transient headache or fatigue. Any detrimental effects of manipulation, if they do occur, are what the patient might provoke upon an impulsive strain such as sneezing. Risk of a serious adverse event has been estimated to be approximately 5 in 1000 patients reporting symptoms exacerbated permanently or temporarily through spinal manipulative therapy. From 1947 to 1991, 50 well-documented cases of adverse events including 12 deaths were reported in the United States. As of 1993, there have been reports of 89 case reports in which chiropractic manipulation was implicated in the precipitation or aggravation of pain in previously asymptomatic or minimally symptomatic areas of the musculoskeletal system.

Reports of adverse neurologic events have been controversial.[5] In one survey of members of the Association of British Neurologists, 35 cases of neurologic complications were reported as being possibly associated with cervical spine manipulation over a 12-month period including seven cases of stroke in the brainstem region. From 1947 to 1977, 22 patients who suffered from stroke associated with therapeutic cervical manipulation were reported in the English literature. A survey of 177 California neurologists over a 2-year period suggested a possible 55 strokes, 16 myelopathies, and 30 radiculopathies within 24 hours after

receiving chiropractic manipulation; however, the methodology and accuracy of the survey have been questioned. From 1996 to 1997, 13 consultant neurologists observed a total of 16 patients with neurologic complications following cervical spine manipulation. The risk of stroke for individuals younger than 45 years is about 1.3 per 100,000 people who had one or more chiropractic visits in the previous week. Numerous case reports have been identified of vertebrobasilar ischemic strokes that occurred after chiropractic manipulation of the cervical spine. Furthermore, vertebral artery injury constitutes 65% of all complications in manipulative therapy. The vertebral arteries are susceptible to trauma in the transverse foraminae, at the atlantoaxial joint, and at the occipitoatlantal joint. The damage may be followed by thrombus formation, resulting in occlusion of the vessel and/or cerebral embolic events. In patients with vertebral artery dissection (predominantly at the C1–C7 level) that occurred from sports activity and chiropractic manipulation, headache and/or neck pain was the prominent feature in 88% of patients. Major risks may arise from forceful and vigorous movements or from manipulations that involve extreme positions of the head. The most dangerous manipulations are twisting movements (rotation + extension + traction). Manipulation strategies should avoid thrusts of this kind to minimize the risk of complications.

Patients with acute arthritis of any type, as well as conditions such as osteoporosis, should either avoid or use chiropractic adjustment cautiously. Caution is also warranted in patients with bleeding disorders, migraines, and tumors or metastasis to the spine. Patients with symptoms of vertebrobasilar vascular insufficiency, aneurysms, arteritis, or unstable spondylolisthesis should avoid chiropractic care. Patients receiving anticoagulant therapy should also be advised to avoid chiropractic care.

A final consideration with this health system is that traditionally chiropractors have discouraged the use of routine vaccinations.[37] Although this attitude may be less likely now with more recent graduates of chiropractic colleges who do educate consumers on both the risks and benefits of immunizations, Western health care providers including pharmacists should be aware of this aspect of chiropractic care.

Ayurveda

Ayurveda originated in India more than 5000 years ago and is probably the world's oldest system of natural medicine.[5,38] When translated, *Ayurveda* means "science of life"; the term stems from the spiritual teachings known as the Vedas. Ayurveda, which may be the original basis for Chinese medicine, is an integrated system of specific theories and techniques employing diet, herbs, exercise, meditation, yoga, and massage or bodywork. The goal of Ayurveda is to achieve optimal health on physical, psychological, and spiritual levels.

In India, Ayurveda involves the eight principal branches of medicine including pediatrics, gynecology, obstetrics, ophthalmology, geriatrics, otolaryngology, general medicine, and surgery. In Western countries, the practice of Ayurveda is less focused on its spiritual roots than on its use as a form of CAM. Ayurveda relies on the individual's willingness to participate in lifestyle and behavior changes.

Technique

Ayurveda teaches that vital energy (*prana*) is the basis of all life and healing.[5,38] As *prana* circulates throughout the human body, it is governed by the five elements of earth, air, fire, water, and ether. The five elements combine with one another into pairs called *doshas* that include *vata* (ether and air), *pitta* (fire and water), and *kapha* (earth and water). Health is a state of balance and harmony among the five elements, and illness occurs when there is an imbalance or lack of harmony among them.

The regulation of diet as a form of therapy is a central ideal in Ayurveda. An individual's mental and spiritual development as well as temperament can be influenced by the quality and quantity of food consumed. An important principle in Ayurveda is that "there is nothing in the world that is not a medicine or food." Foods and herbs are described in terms of their energetic qualities rather than the chemical properties. Sweet foods (called *madhura*) are said to provide nourishment and coolness, and aid in increasing body weight. Sour foods (called *amla*) are believed to provide warmth and to aid in weight gain. Salty foods (*lavana*) provide warmth, stimulate the senses, and aid weight gain. In contrast, bitter foods (*katu*) provide coolness and help weight loss. Pungent foods (*tikta*) also aid in weight loss but provide warmth and stimulation. Numerous herbs and spices including turmeric and cumin are used in Ayurveda.

Ayurveda holds that each 24-hour cycle is divided into 4-hour segments governed by the *doshas*. These time periods are believed to correspond with nature. Ayurvedic practitioners guide patients to plan their activities to be in harmony with these natural principles of timing.

A practitioner usually interviews the patient about his/her medical history. The practitioner then palpitates the wrist to determine subtle qualities of the pulse. Practitioners may also evaluate the appearance of the tongue, face, lips, nails, or eyes. Laboratory tests of blood, urine, and stools may be used to help with diagnosis. Most practitioners do not perform actual treatments or healing in the office, although some massage therapists will perform Ayurvedic massage. The initial consultation is usually the longest and lasts from 45 to 90 minutes. Follow-up consultations may be spaced by several weeks or months to monitor the individual's progress. Follow-up will usually be brief office visits involving a diagnostic review and an adjustment of the regimen.

Training

Ayurveda is practiced in Western medicine by health care professionals who are licensed in a variety of disciplines.[5,38] Allopathic and osteopathic physicians, naturopaths, acupuncturists, nurses, massage therapists, and chiropractors may all practice Ayurveda. In India, the standard length of training to practice Ayurveda is 5 years, whereas Ayurvedic training in the United States varies in its duration. Health counselors, educators, or consultants may also incorporate Ayurveda into their practices without specific Ayurvedic licensing. In Western countries, two major approaches to training and practice exist. The first is offered by diverse teachers and practitioners, many of whom are either from India or were trained there. The second consists of devotees of Maharishi Mahesh Yogi, the Indian spiritual teacher who introduced transcendental meditation (TM) to the West. In 1980, this group coined the term *Maharishi Ayur-Ved,* a practice that incorporates TM as part of an Ayurvedic approach.[39]

Theory/Evidence

The safety and efficacy of Ayurveda is difficult to systematically study because of its predominantly "person-specific" approach. Two individuals with the same symptom might be treated very differently in terms of herbal remedies, lifestyle changes, yoga postures, diet, or other factors. Nonetheless, several specific herbal formulations have been studied in Western-style clinical trials. Currently, there is inadequate evidence to recommend Ayurveda for any indication.

Safety

Many different Ayurvedic herbs exist, and they are frequently taken in combination with other herbs and/or minerals.[5,38] For example, a traditional Ayurvedic formula consists of valerian (*Valeriana wallichi*), rose petals (*Rosa centifolia*), muskroot (*Nardostachys jatamansi*), heart-leaved moonseed (*Tinospora cordifolia*), winter cherry (*Withania somnifera*), pepper (*Piper negrum*), ginger (*Zingibar officinalis*), aloeweed (*Convolvulus pluricalis*), and licorice root (*Glycyrrhiza glabra*). Safety and toxicity will vary greatly depending on the herb and its preparation. In general, Ayurvedic herbal medicines should be used cautiously, because their potencies may not be tested or standardized. Some herbs imported from India have been reported to contain high levels of toxic metals or Western drugs. It is important that consumers purchase Ayurvedic herbs that are from trustworthy sources. Ayurvedic herbs can interact with other herbs, foods, and drugs. For example, licorice may increase the risk of bleeding when used with anticoagulants or antiplatelet drugs.

Metal toxicity has been associated with Ayurvedic medicines in the past, and heavy metal contamination continues to be a concern in Ayurvedic medicines. In addition to herbs, Ayurvedic formulas known as *rasa shastra* may also contain metals such as arsenic, mercury, or zinc. Practitioners claim that these medicines are safe when properly prepared and administered. However, more than 80 cases of heavy metal poisoning worldwide have been linked to Ayurvedic medicine. According to the U.S. Centers for Disease Control and Prevention, 12 cases of lead poisoning were associated with Ayurvedic medicines from 2000 to 2003. Even herbal-only Ayurvedic formulas may contain heavy metals; a recent study[40] found that approximately 20% of herbal-only formulas contained detectable metals (compared with 40% of *rasa shastra* medicines). Therefore, consumers are advised to use Ayurvedic herbs cautiously. Products that have seals of quality approval from the U.S. Pharmacopeia have been tested and should not contain unacceptable levels of harmful metals. Product testing information is also available from consumer sites such as ConsumerLab.com.

Massage

Soft tissue manipulation has been practiced for thousands of years in diverse cultures. Chinese use of massage dates to 1600 BC, and Hippocrates made reference to the importance of physicians being experienced with "rubbing" as early as 400 BC.[5]

Massage spread throughout Europe during the Renaissance and was introduced in the United States in the 1850s. By the early 1930s, massage became a less prominent part of Western medicine. Interest in therapeutic massage resurged in the 1970s, particularly among athletes to promote well-being, relaxation, pain reduction, stress relief, healing of musculoskeletal injuries, sleep enhancement, and quality of life. According to a recent review, massage is currently the most common form of CAM therapy used in the United States.[41]

A common goal of massage therapy is to help the body heal itself. Touch is fundamental to massage therapy; it is used by therapists to locate painful or tense areas, to determine how much pressure to apply, and to establish a therapeutic relationship with clients. The term *toxic touch* refers to techniques with detrimental effects.

Technique

Many different therapeutic techniques can be classified as massage therapy. Most involve the application of fixed or moving pressure or manipulation of the clients' muscles/connective tissues. Practitioners may use their hands or other areas such as forearms, elbows, or feet. Lubricants may be added to aid the smoothness of massage strokes.

Training

Training requirements for massage therapy vary in the United States, but generally involve 500 to 1000 hours for certification by the National Certification Board for Therapeutic Massage and Bodywork.[42] More than 1000 massage training programs exist in the United States and accreditation is provided by the Commission on Massage Therapy Accreditation.[43] Upon fulfilling the necessary requirements, massage therapists receive the designation of Nationally Certified in Therapeutic Massage and Bodywork. Most states require massage therapists to be licensed before practicing.

Theory/Evidence

Research on massage therapy is limited, and published studies frequently use a variety of techniques and trial designs. Evidence-based conclusions about the effectiveness of massage cannot be drawn for any health condition, although its remains a popular CAM therapy for improving relaxation, mood, and overall well-being, particularly in palliative care.[44]

Safety

Few adverse effects have been reported with massage.[5] Fractures, discomfort, bruising, swelling of massaged tissues, and liver hematoma have been reported. Vigorous massage should be avoided in patients with bleeding disorders, peripheral vascular disease, or thrombocytopenia, or in those receiving antithrombotic therapy. According to preliminary data, blood pressure may increase in healthy patients following vigorous massage (e.g., trigger point therapy), although in patients with hypertension, massage may actually lower blood pressure. Areas that should not be massaged include those with osteoporotic and other fractures, open/healing skin wounds, skin infections, recent surgery, or blood clots. Massage and other touch-based therapies should be used cautiously in patients with a history of physical abuse. Women who are pregnant should consult their obstetrician before beginning massage therapy. Allergies or skin irritation can occur with the oils used in massage such as olive and mineral oil.

Massage has not been evaluated as a method to diagnose medical conditions. Massage should not be used as a substitute for more proven therapies for medical conditions or should not cause pain to the client.

Conclusion

Consumers increasingly seek care from complementary and alternative practitioners and health systems. Although some historical and scientific evidence support the effectiveness of some CAM approaches,[5] general statements are difficult to make on the safety and efficacy of CAM as a whole. Important components of clinical trials such as placebo controls and blinding are difficult to achieve; as a result, the available scientific evidence is limited. Because the use of CAM health systems continues to increase, both consumers and Western health care providers should be better informed about the potential risks and benefits of CAM techniques.

In this age of technology, more consumers are using Web sites for health information before consulting health care professionals. With knowledge so readily available, consumers have increased their responsibility for their health decisions and should be strongly encouraged to tell their health care providers whether they are also using any CAM approaches to their health. Similarly, all Western health care providers including pharmacists must be knowledgeable about CAM practitioners and health systems, as well as the evidence that supports or refutes their use.

Key Points for Common Complementary and Alternative Medicine Health Systems

➤ The term *complementary and alternative medicine* (CAM) is generally regarded as a broad group of healing philosophies, diagnostic approaches, and therapeutic interventions that do not conform to the conventional Western health system. The most common CAM therapies and health systems include Ayurveda, homeopathy, naturopathy, traditional Chinese medicine (TCM)/acupuncture, chiropractic care, and massage.

➤ The term *homeopathy* comes from the two Greek words *homoios* (similar) and *pathos* (suffering or disease). Homeopathy is based on the principle of "like cures like," which states that if a substance produces the symptoms of an illness in large doses, that same substance can cure it in very minute doses. Owing to the lack of reliable research, homeopathy cannot be determined for any clinical condition. The risk of toxicity is low because of the dilute nature of the remedies.

➤ A system of naturopathic therapy employs natural forces such as light, heat, air, water, and massage; this therapy focuses on building health rather than on treating disease. Naturopathy is based on six principles: (1) healing power of nature, (2) identifying and treating the cause, (3) doing no harm, (4) treating the whole person, (5) the physician as teacher, and (6) prevention. The licensing of naturopathic doctors will vary depending on state laws.

➤ TCM includes herbal medicine as well as various techniques such as acupuncture, moxibustion, and cupping. TCM is dependent on the life force (*qi*), which circulates through the body through meridians (channels) connecting all major organs. *Qi* consists of *yin* and *yang*, opposite and complementary qualities. Illness results when these are unbalanced. An acupuncturist inserts sterilized needles into channels of energy to try to restore balance to the patient's *qi*.

➤ Chiropractic is a discipline that focuses on the relationship between spinal structure and body function mediated by the nervous system. Various chiropractic and spinal manipulative techniques may be employed. The cracking sound has typically been associated with cavitation in the spinal zygapophyseal (the neural arch between the joint processes) joints. The most common adverse reaction is mild transient localized discomfort in the area of treatment. Cases of adverse events including death have been reported.

➤ Ayurveda originated in India and is an integrated system of specific theories and techniques employing diet, herbs, exercise, meditation, yoga, and massage or bodywork. Ayurveda teaches that vital energy (*prana*) is the basis of all life and healing. As *prana* circulates throughout the human body, it is governed by the five elements of earth, air, fire, water, and ether. The five elements combine with one another into pairs called *doshas* that include *vata* (ether and air), *pitta* (fire and water), and *kapha* (earth and water). Many Ayurvedic herbs exist and may interact with other drugs, herbs, and foods.

➤ Touch is fundamental to massage therapy. It is used by therapists to locate painful or tense areas, to determine how much pressure to apply, and to establish a therapeutic relationship with clients. A common goal of massage therapy is to help the body heal itself. Massage has not been evaluated as a method to diagnose medical conditions.

REFERENCES

1. Basch EM, Ulbricht CE, Cohen L, et al. Complementary, alternative, and integrative therapies in cancer care. In: DeVita VT Jr, Lawrence TS, Rosenberg S, et al., eds. *Cancer: Principles and Practice of Oncology*. 7th ed. New York: Lippincott Williams & Wilkins; 2004:2805.

2. Zollman C, Vickers A. ABC of complementary medicine: what is complementary medicine? *BMJ*. 1999;319:693.

3. Cassileth BR. "Complementary" or "alternative?" It makes a difference in cancer care. *Comp Ther Med*. 1999;44:22.

4. National Center for Complementary and Alternative Medicine. Major Domains of Complementary and Alternative medicine. Available at: http://nccam.nih.gov/health/backgrounds/wholemed.htm. Last accessed September 29, 2008.

5. Natural Standard: The Authority on Integrative Medicine. Available at: http://www.naturalstandard.com. Last accessed September 29, 2008.

6. Mehling WE, DiBlasi Z, Hecht F. Bias control in trials of bodywork: a review of methodological issues [review]. *J Altern Complement Med*. 2005;11:333–42.

7. Schnyer RN, Allen JJ. Bridging the gap in complementary and alternative medicine research: manualization as a means of promoting standardization and flexibility of treatment in clinical trials of acupuncture [review]. *J Altern Complement Med*. 2002;8:623–34.

8. Birch S. A review and analysis of placebo treatments, placebo effects, and placebo controls in trials of medical procedures when sham is not inert [review]. *J Altern Complement Med*. 2006;12:303–10.

9. Hjelvik M, Mørenskog E. The principles of homeopathy. *Tidsskr Nor Laegeforen*. 199730;117:2497–501.

10. Vickers AJ, Smith C. Homoeopathic Oscillococcinum for preventing and treating influenza and influenza-like syndromes. *Cochrane Database Syst Rev*. 2006;3:CD001957.

11. Borneman JP, Field RI. Regulation of homeopathic drug products. *Am J Health Syst Pharm*. 2006;63:86–91.

12. Homeopathic Pharmacopoeia of the United States. Southeastern, Pa: Homeopathic Pharmacopoeia Convention of the United States; 2004.

13. Barnes PM, Powell-Griner E, McFann K, et al. *Complementary and Alternative Medicine Use among Adults: United States, 2002*. Hyattsville, Md: National Center for Health Statistics; 2004:1–19. Advance Data from Vital and Health Statistics, No. 343.

14. Yasgur J. *Yasgur's Homeopathic Dictionary and Holistic Health Reference*. 4th ed. Greenville, Pa: Van Hoy Publishers; 1998.

15. O'Reilly WB, ed. *Organon of the Medical Art*. Hahnemann S, trans-ed. Redmond, Wash: Birdcage Books; 1996.

16. Council on Homeopathic Education Summit Meeting. Standards and Competencies for the Professional Practice of Homeopathy in North America. Available at: http://www.chedu.org/standards.html. Last accessed September 29, 2008.

17. Vithoulkas G. *The Science of Homeopathy*. New York: Grove Weidenfeld; 1980.

18. Ernst E, Pittler MH. Efficacy of homeopathic arnica: a systematic review of placebo-controlled clinical trials [review]. *Arch Surg*. 1998;133:1187–90.

19. Merrell WC, Shalts E. Homeopathy [review]. *Med Clin North Am*. 2002; 86:47–62.

20. Stehlin I. Homeopathy: real medicine or empty promises? *FDA Consum*. 1996;30(10). Available at: http://www.fda.gov/fdac/features/096_home. html. Last accessed September 29, 2008.

21. American Cancer Society (ACS). Naturopathic Medicine. Available at: http://www.cancer.org/docroot/ETO/content/ETO_5_3X_Naturopathic_Medicine.asp?sitearea=ETO. Last accessed September 29, 2008.

22. Utah Division of Administrative Rules. Rule R156-71: Naturopathic Physician Practice Act Rules. May 1, 2008. Available at: http://www.rules. utah.gov/publicat/code/r156/r156-71.htm. Last accessed September 29, 2008.

23. The Council on Naturopathic Medical Education. Available at: http://www.cnme.org. Last accessed September 29, 2008.

24. North American Board of Naturopathic Examiners. Available at: http://www.nabne.org. Last accessed September 29, 2008.

25. Wang SM, Kain ZN, White P. Acupuncture analgesia, I: the scientific basis [review]. *Anesth Analg*. 2008;106:602–10.

26. Wang SM, Kain ZN, White PF. Acupuncture analgesia [review], II: clinical considerations. *Anesth Analg*. 2008;106:611–21, table of contents.

27. Skalli S, Zaid A, Soulaymani R. Drug interactions with herbal medicines [review]. *Ther Drug Monit*. 2007;29:679–86.

28. Shea JL. Applying evidence-based medicine to traditional Chinese medicine: debate and strategy [review]. *J Altern Complement Med*. 2006;12: 255–63.

29. World Health Organization. Available at: http://www.who.int. Last accessed September 29, 2008.

30. Wong, Ming (1976). La Médecine chinoise par les plantes. Le Corps a Vivre series. Éditions Tchou.

31. Yu D, Morris-Natschke SL, Lee KH. New developments in natural products-based anti-AIDS research [review]. *Med Res Rev*. 2007;27:108–32.

32. Coyle ME, Smith CA, Peat B. Cephalic version by moxibustion for breech presentation [review]. *Cochrane Database Syst Rev*. 2005;2:CD003928.

33. National Certification Commission for Acupuncture and Oriental Medicine. Available at: http://www.nccaom.com. Last accessed September 29, 2008.

34. US Food and Drug Administration. Sales of Supplements Containing Ephedrine Alkaloids (Ephedra) Prohibited. Feb 2004. Available at: http://www.fda.gov/oc/initiatives/ephedra/february2004. Last accessed September 29, 2008.

35. Ernst E. Chiropractic: a critical evaluation [review]. *J Pain Symptom Manage*. 2008;35:544–62.

36. American Chiropractic Association. Available at: http://www.amerchiro.org. Last accessed September 29, 2008.

37. Busse JW, Wilson K, Campbell JB. Attitudes towards vaccination among chiropractic and naturopathic students. *Vaccine*. 2008 July 29.

38. Sharma H, Chandola HM, Singh G, et al. Utilization of Ayurveda in health care: an approach for prevention, health promotion, and treatment of disease, part 1:Ayurveda, the science of life [review]. *J Altern Complement Med*. 2007;13:1011–9.

39. A Transcendental Meditation (TM) Portal for Teachings of Maharishi Mahesh Yogi. Available at: http://www.alltm.org. Last accessed September 29, 2008.

40. Saper R, Phillips R, Sehgal A, et al. Lead, mercury, and arsenic in US- and Indian-manufactured Ayurvedic medicines sold via the Internet. *JAMA*. 2008;300:915–23.

41. Myklebust M, Iler J. Policy for therapeutic massage in an academic health center: a model for standard policy development. *J Altern Complement Med*. 2007;13:471–5.

42. The National Certification Board for Therapeutic Massage & Bodywork. Available at: http://www.ncbtmb.org. Last accessed September 29, 2008.

43. Commission on Massage Therapy Accreditation. Available at: http://www.comta.org. Last accessed September 29, 2008.

44. Gray RA. The use of massage therapy in palliative care [review]. *Complement Ther Nurs Midwifery*. 2000;6:77–82.

Index

Page numbers followed by *t* and *f* denote tables and figures, respectively.